Willard and Spackman's

Occupational Therapy

13TH EDITION

Willard and Spackman's
Occupational Therapy

13TH EDITION

Barbara A. Boyt Schell, PhD, OT/L, FAOTA

Professor Emerita
School of Occupational Therapy
Ivester College of Health Sciences
Brenau University
Gainesville, Georgia
Co-Owner
Schell Consulting
Athens, Georgia

Glen Gillen, EdD, OTR/L, FAOTA

Professor and Director, Programs in Occupational Therapy
Vice Chair, Department of Rehabilitation and Regenerative Medicine
Assistant Dean, Vagelos College of Physicians and Surgeons
Columbia University
New York, New York

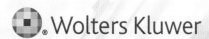

Wolters Kluwer

Philadelphia • Baltimore • New York • London
Buenos Aires • Hong Kong • Sydney • Tokyo

Acquisitions Editor: Michael Nobel
Editorial Coordinator: Tim Rinehart
Marketing Manager: Shauna Kelley
Project Manager: Laura S. Horowitz/York Content Development
Design Coordinator: Stephen Druding
Compositor: Absolute Service, Inc.
Composition Project Manager: Harold Medina

13th Edition

351 West Camden Street   Two Commerce Square
Baltimore, MD 21201   2001 Market Street
                                  Philadelphia, PA 19103

Printed in China

Not authorised for sale in United States, Canada, Australia, New Zealand, Puerto Rico, or U.S. Virgin Islands.

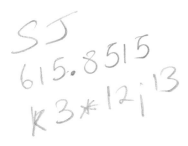

Library of Congress Cataloging-in-Publication Data

Names: Schell, Barbara A. Boyt, editor. | Gillen, Glen, editor.
Title: Willard & Spackman's occupational therapy / [edited by] Barbara A.
  Boyt Schell, Glen Gillen.
Other titles: Willard and Spackman's occupational therapy | Occupational
  therapy
Description: Thirteenth edition. | Philadelphia : Wolters Kluwer, [2019] |
  Includes bibliographical references and index.
Identifiers: LCCN 2018032182 | ISBN 9781975106584
Subjects: | MESH: Occupational Therapy | Rehabilitation, Vocational
Classification: LCC RM735 | NLM WB 555 | DDC 615.8/515—dc23 LC record available at https://lccn.loc.gov/2018032182

DISCLAIMER

When citing chapters from this book, please use the appropriate form. The APA format is as follows:

[Chapter author last name, I.] (2019). Chapter title. In B. A. B. Schell & G. Gillen (Eds.), *Willard & Spackman's occupational therapy* (13th ed., pp. x–x). Philadelphia, PA: Wolters Kluwer.

Johnson, K. R., & Dickie, V. (2019). What is occupation? In B. A. B. Schell & G. Gillen (Eds.), *Willard & Spackman's occupational therapy* (13th ed., pp. 2–10). Philadelphia, PA: Wolters Kluwer.

DEDICATION

Ellen S. Cohn, ScD, OTR, FAOTA

Clinical Professor, Entry-level OTD Program Director
Department of Occupational Therapy
Sargent College of Health & Rehabilitation Sciences
Boston University
Co-Editor *Willard & Spackman's Occupational Therapy*, 10th & 11th Edition
Consulting Editor *Willard & Spackman's Occupational Therapy*, 12th Edition

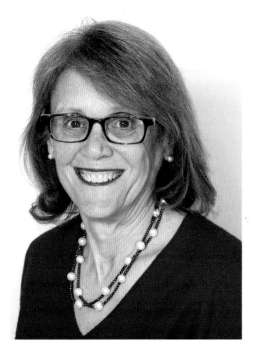

We are pleased to dedicate this edition to Dr. Ellen S. Cohn—a clinician, educator, and scholar whose intellectual integrity, standards of excellence, and enduring commitment to the profession is reflected in her many contributions to occupational therapy (OT) and the people served by the profession. Dr. Cohn has contributed 22 chapters to seven editions of *Willard & Spackman's Occupational Therapy* beginning in 7th edition (1988) through this 13th edition. As co-editor of the 10th and 11th editions, and consulting editor of the 12th edition, she collaborated on key efforts to reconstruct the text to guide both students and instructors toward more reflective, client-centered, and occupation-based practice. As a result, the text includes clear identification of the status of evidence regarding the methods of assessment and intervention, an element Dr. Cohn felt strongly about weaving into the fiber of the text. Similarly, Dr. Cohn was instrumental in bringing a more international perspective to the text by recruiting well-respected international OT scholars to contribute. In addition, she significantly expanded the role of first-person narratives including the addition of chapters related to caregiving and community-based practice. She facilitated the development of a section devoted to describing common health conditions seen in OT clients, including diagnostic information, implications for occupation, evaluation and intervention strategies, and a description of current evidence that supports practice decisions.

Dr. Cohn is an outstanding editor, starting with her impressive command of all things grammatical. More important is her grasp of complex ideas, which she elegantly makes accessible to readers, interweaving important theoretical and practice perspectives. She is a great listener and articulate advocate while also able to focus on the practical planning and processes required for bringing a textbook of this magnitude into being. And she does it all with a delightful sense of humor.

Because of her many contributions to the field, it was not surprising to us that she received the 2018 Eleanor Clarke Slagle Lectureship from the American Occupational Therapy Association in the same year that we chose to honor her with this dedication. We are grateful for her service to this text and the profession.

Barbara A. Boyt Schell
Lead Editor

Glen Gillen
Co-editor

Elizabeth B. Crepeau
Editor Emerita

ON THE COVER

Reconstruction aides, recruited to provide occupational therapy for soldiers injured in WWI, are lined up to march in a parade in 1918. They are shown in contrast to occupational therapists in 2018 working in a variety of settings, supporting clients in a range of occupations across the life span.

CONSULTING EDITORS

Lori T. Andersen, EdD, OTR/L, FAOTA
Retired, Associate Professor
Department of Occupational Therapy and Community
  Health
Florida Gulf Coast University
Fort Myers, FL

Catana E. Brown, PhD, OTR/L, FAOTA
Professor
Department of Occupational Therapy
Midwestern University
Glendale, AZ

Kristie Patten Koenig, PhD, OT/L, FAOTA
Associate Professor and Chair
Department of Occupational Therapy
New York University
New York, NY

CONTRIBUTORS

Diane E. Adamo, PhD, OTR, MS
Director of Research and Associate Professor
Department of Health Care Sciences
Wayne State University
Detroit, MI

Lori T. Andersen, EdD, OTR/L, FAOTA
Retired, Associate Professor
Department of Occupational Therapy and
    Community Health
Florida Gulf Coast University
Fort Myers, FL

Nancy Baker, ScD, MPH, OTR/L, FAOTA
Associate Professor
Department of Occupational Therapy
University of Pittsburgh
Pittsburgh, PA

Skye Barbic, PhD, OT Reg (BC)
Assistant Professor
Department of Occupational Science &
    Occupational Therapy
University of British Columbia
Vancouver, Canada

Kate Barrett, OTD, OTR/L
Associate Professor
Department of Occupational Therapy
St. Catherine University
St. Paul, MN

Sue Berger, PhD, OTR/L, FAOTA
Clinical Associate Professor Emeritus
Department of Occupational Therapy
Sargent College of Health & Rehabilitation Sciences
Boston University
Boston, MA

Christy Billock, PhD, OTR/L
Professor
Occupational Therapy Department
West Coast University
Irvine, CA

Roxie M. Black, PhD, OTR/L, FAOTA
Professor Emerita
Master of Occupational Therapy Program
University of Southern Maine
Lewiston, ME

Bette R. Bonder, PhD, OTR, FAOTA
Professor Emerita
School of Health Sciences
Cleveland State University
Cleveland, OH

Cheryl Lynne Trautmann Boop, MS, OTR/L
Clinical Lead—Clinical Therapies
Homecare
Nationwide Children's Hospital
Columbus, OH

Brent Braveman, PhD, OTR/L, FAOTA
Director
Department of Rehabilitation Services
MD Anderson Cancer Center
Houston, TX

Catana E. Brown, PhD, OTR/L, FAOTA
Professor
Department of Occupational Therapy
Midwestern University
Glendale, AZ

Anita C. Bundy, ScD, OT/L, FAOTA, FOTARA
Professor and Department Head
Department of Occupational Therapy
Colorado State University
Fort Collins, CO
Professor of Occupational Therapy
Faculty of Health Sciences
University of Sydney
Lidcombe, New South Wales, Australia

Paul Carrington Cabell, III
New York, NY

Denise Chisholm, PhD, OTR/L, FAOTA
Professor and Vice Chair
Department of Occupational Therapy
School of Health and Rehabilitation Sciences
University of Pittsburgh
Pittsburgh, PA

Charles H. Christiansen, EdD, OTR(C), FAOTA
Clinical Professor
College of Health Professions
The University of Texas Medical Branch
Galveston, TX

Sherrilene Classen, PhD, MPH, OTR/L, FAOTA, FGSA
Professor and Chair
Department of Occupational Therapy
College of Public Health and Health Professions
University of Florida
Gainesville, FL

Helen S. Cohen, EdD
Professor
Bobby R. Alford Department of Otolaryngology—
    Head and Neck Surgery
Baylor College of Medicine
Houston, TX

Ellen S. Cohn, OTR, ScD, FAOTA
Clinical Professor
EL-OTD Program Director
Department of Occupational Therapy
Sargent College of Health & Rehabilitation Sciences
Boston University
Boston, MA

Susan Coppola, OTD, OT/L, FAOTA
Professor
Occupational Science and Occupational Therapy
University of North Carolina at Chapel Hill
Chapel Hill, NC

Wendy J. Coster, PhD, OTR/L, FAOTA
Professor and Chair
Department of Occupational Therapy
Boston University
Boston, MA

Elizabeth Blesedell Crepeau, PhD, OT, FAOTA
Professor Emerita
Occupational Therapy Department
University of New Hampshire
Durham, NH

Evan E. Dean, PhD, OTR/L
Assistant Professor
Occupational Therapy Education
University of Kansas
Kansas City, KS

Gloria F. Dickerson, BS Psychology
Recovery Specialist
Center for Social Innovation
Newton Centre, MA

Virginia Dickie, PhD, OT, FAOTA
Associate Professor Emerita
Division of Occupational Science and Occupational Therapy
University of North Carolina
Chapel Hill, NC

Regina F. Doherty, OTD, OTR/L, FAOTA
Associate Professor
Program Director
Department of Occupational Therapy
School of Health and Rehabilitation Sciences
MGH Institute of Health Professions
Boston, MA

Julie Dorsey, OTD, OTR/L, CEAS
Associate Professor
Department of Occupational Therapy
Ithaca College
Ithaca, NY

Sanetta H. J. Du Toit, PhD, M Occ Ther, MSc Occ Ther, B Occ Ther
Lecturer, Discipline of Occupational Therapy
Coordinator FHS Abroad
Faculty of Health Sciences
University of Sydney
New South Wales, Australia
Affiliated Lecturer
Department of Occupational Therapy
University of the Free State
Bloemfontein, South Africa

Winnie Dunn, PhD, OTR, FAOTA
Distinguished Professor
Department of Occupational Therapy
University of Missouri
Columbia, MO

Holly Ehrenfried, OTD, OTR/L, CHT
Clinical Specialist
Rehabilitation Services
Lehigh Valley Health Network
Allentown, PA

Mary E. Evenson, OTD, MPH, OTR/L, FAOTA
Associate Professor
Director of Clinical Education
Department of Occupational Therapy
School of Health and Rehabilitation Sciences
MGH Institute of Health Professions
Boston, MA

Cynthia L. Evetts, PhD, OTR
Professor and Director
School of Occupational Therapy
Texas Woman's University
Denton, TX

Janet Falk-Kessler, EdD, OTR, FAOTA
Professor and Occupational Therapy Programs' Director
Assistant Dean of Education, College of Physicians and
    Surgeons
Vice Chair, Department of Rehabilitation and
    Regenerative Medicine
Columbia University
New York, NY

Linda S. Fazio, PhD, OTR/L, LPC, FAOTA
Professor Emerita of Clinical Occupational Therapy
USC Chan Division of Occupational Science and
    Occupational Therapy
University of Southern California
Los Angeles, CA

Denise Finch, OTD, OTR/L, CHT
Assistant Professor
Department of Occupational Therapy
MCPHS University
Manchester, NH

Anne G. Fisher, ScD, OT, FAOTA
Professor Emerita
Division of Occupational Therapy
Department of Community Medicine and Rehabilitation
Umeå University
Umeå, Sweden
Affiliate Professor
Department of Occupational Therapy
College of Health and Human Sciences
Colorado State University
Fort Collins, CO

Kirsty Forsyth, PhD, OTR, FCOT
Professor
Department of Occupational Therapy
School of Health Sciences
Queen Margaret University
Scotland, United Kingdom

Karen Roe Garren, MS, OTR, CHT
Senior Staff Occupational Therapist
Select Physical Therapy
New Milford, CT

Patricia A. Gentile, DPS, OTR/L
Assistant Clinical Professor
Department of Occupational Therapy
Steinhardt School of Culture, Education, and
    Human Development
New York University
New York, NY

Glen Gillen, EdD, OTR/L, FAOTA
Professor and Director, Programs in Occupational
    Therapy
Vice Chair, Department of Rehabilitation and
    Regenerative Medicine
Assistant Dean, Vagelos College of Physicians and
    Surgeons
Columbia University
New York, NY

Kathleen M. Golisz, OTD, OTR, FAOTA
Associate Dean and Professor
School of Health and Natural Sciences
Mercy College
Dobbs Ferry, NY

Glenn David Goodman, PhD
Professor Emeritus
School of Health Sciences
Cleveland State University
Cleveland, OH

Yael Goverover, PhD, OTR/L
Associate Professor
Department of Occupational Therapy
Steinhardt School of Culture, Education, and
    Human Development
New York University
New York, NY

Kay Graham, PhD, OTR/L
Associate Professor and Chair, Gainesville Day Program
School of Occupational Therapy
Ivester College of Health Sciences
Brenau University
Gainesville, GA

Lenin C. Grajo, PhD, EdM, OTR/L
Assistant Professor
Rehabilitation and Regenerative Medicine (Occupational
    Therapy) Columbia University Medical Center
Programs in Occupational Therapy
Columbia University
New York, NY

Lou Ann Griswold, PhD, OTR/L, FAOTA
Associate Professor and Chair
Department of Occupational Therapy
University of New Hampshire
Durham, NH

Sharon A. Gutman, PhD, OTR, FAOTA
Professor of Rehabilitation and Regenerative Medicine
Programs of Occupational Therapy
Columbia University Medical Center
New York, NY

Kristine L. Haertl, PhD, OTR/L, FAOTA
Professor
Department of Occupational Therapy
St. Catherine University
St. Paul, MN

Debra J. Hanson, PhD, OTR/L, FAOTA
Professor
Occupational Therapy Department
University of North Dakota
Grand Forks, ND

Christine A. Helfrich, PhD, OTR/L, FAOTA
Assistant Professor
Department of Occupational Therapy
Boston University
Boston, MA

Clare Hocking, PhD, NZROT
Professor
Department of Occupational Science and Therapy
Auckland University of Technology
Auckland, New Zealand

Barbara Hooper, PhD, OTR, FAOTA
Associate Professor
Director, Center for Occupational Therapy Education
Department of Occupational Therapy
Colorado State University
Fort Collins, CO

Craig W. Horowitz, MS, BS
CW Horowitz Woodworking
York, PA

Laura S. Horowitz, BA
York Content Development
York, PA

Will S. Horowitz
Student, Harrisburg Area Community College
York, PA

Ruth Humphry, PhD, OTR/L, FAOTA
Emeritus Professor
Division of Occupational Science and Occupational Therapy
University of North Carolina
Chapel Hill, NC

Lisa A. Jaegers, PhD, OTR/L
Assistant Professor
Occupational Science and Occupational Therapy,
    Doisy College of Health Sciences
School of Social Work, College for Public Health and
    Social Justice
Director, Transformative Justice Initiative
Associate Director, Health Criminology Research
    Consortium
Saint Louis University
St. Louis, MO

Anne Birge James, PhD, OTR/L, FAOTA
Professor and Associate Director
School of Occupational Therapy
University of Puget Sound
Tacoma, WA

Khalilah Robinson Johnson, PhD, OTR/L
Postdoctoral Fellow
Institute for Inclusion, Inquiry, and Innovation
Department of Occupational Therapy
Virginia Commonwealth University
Richmond, VA

Mary Alunkal Khetani, ScD, OTR/L
Assistant Professor
Departments of Occupational Therapy and Disability and
    Human Development
Program in Rehabilitation Sciences
University of Illinois at Chicago
Chicago, IL

Jessica M. Kramer, PhD, OT, OTR
Associate Professor
Department of Occupational Therapy
Sargent College of Health & Rehabilitation Sciences
Boston University
Boston, MA

Terry Krupa, PhD, MEd, BSc(OT), FCAOT
Professor Emerita
School of Rehabilitation Therapy
Queen's University
Ontario, Canada

Angela Lampe, OTD, OTR/L
Assistant Professor, Director of Distance Education
Occupational Therapy
Creighton University
Omaha, NE

Mary C. Lawlor, ScD, OTR/L, FAOTA
USC Chan Division of Occupational Science and
    Occupational Therapy
Herman Ostrow School of Dentistry
University of Southern California
Los Angeles, CA

Lori Letts, PhD, OT Reg (Ont)
Assistant Dean
Occupational Therapy Program
Professor
School of Rehabilitation Science
McMaster University
Ontario, Canada

Lauren M. Little, PhD, OTR
Assistant Professor
Department of Occupational Therapy
Rush University
Chicago, IL

Helene Lohman, OTD, OTR/L, FAOTA
Professor
Department of Occupational Therapy
Creighton University
Omaha, NE

Rev. Beth Long
Retired Minister
Athens, GA

Catherine L. Lysack, PhD, OT(C)
Professor and Interim Dean
Eugene Applebaum College of Pharmacy and
    Health Sciences
Wayne State University
Detroit, MI

Wanda J. Mahoney, PhD, OTR/L
Associate Professor
Occupational Therapy Program
Midwestern University
Downers Grove, IL

Peggy M. Martin, PhD, OTR/L
Director
Department of Occupational Therapy
University of Minnesota
Minneapolis, MN

Cheryl Mattingly, PhD
Professor of Anthropology
Dana and David Dornsife College of Letters, Arts, and
    Sciences
University of Southern California
Los Angeles, CA

Kathleen Matuska, PhD, OTR/L, FAOTA
Professor and Chair
Department of Occupational Therapy
St. Catherine University
St. Paul, MN

Jane Melton, PhD, MSc
Honorary Professor
School of Health Sciences
Queen Margaret University
Edinburgh, Scotland, United Kingdom

Dawn M. Nilsen, EdD, OTR/L, FAOTA
Associate Professor
Rehabilitation and Regenerative Medicine
    (Occupational Therapy)
Columbia University Medical Center
Department of Occupational Therapy
Columbia University
New York, NY

Angela Patterson, OTD, OTR/L
Assistant Professor
Occupational Therapy
Creighton University
Omaha, NE

Christine O. Peters, PhD, OTR/L, FAOTA
Independent Historian
Indio, CA

Shawn Phipps, PhD, MS, OTR/L, FAOTA
Vice President
American Occupational Therapy Association
Chief Quality Officer
Rancho Los Amigos National Rehabilitation Center
Downey, CA
Adjunct Assistant Professor
University of Southern California
Los Angeles, CA

Noralyn D. Pickens, PhD, OT
Professor, Associate Director
School of Occupational Therapy
Texas Woman's University
Dallas, TX

Nicole M. Picone, OTD, OTR/L
Clinician
Thom Child and Family Services
Boston, MA

Jennifer S. Pitonyak, PhD, OTR/L, SCFES
Associate Professor
School of Occupational Therapy
University of Puget Sound
Tacoma, WA

Susan Prior, Dip, PG Cert, BSc
Senior Lecturer
Occupational Therapy & Arts Therapies Division
Queen Margaret University
Edinburgh, Scotland, United Kingdom

Ruth Ramsey, EdD, OTR/L
Dean, School of Health and Natural Sciences
Professor, Occupational Therapy
Dominican University of California
San Rafael, CA

Emily Raphael-Greenfield, EdD, OTR, FAOTA
Associate Professor
Regenerative and Rehabilitation Medicine
  (Occupational Therapy)
Columbia University Medical Center
New York, NY

S. Maggie Reitz, PhD, OTR/L, FAOTA
Vice Provost of Academic Affairs
Office of the Provost
Towson University
Towson, MD

Panagiotis (Panos) A. Rekoutis, PhD, OTR/L
Adjunct Faculty
Department of Occupational Therapy
Steinhardt School of Culture, Education, and
  Human Development
New York University
New York, NY

Lynn Ritchie, BSc
Lead Occupational Therapist
The WORKS, NHS Lothian
Edinburgh, Scotland, United Kingdom

Patricia J. Rigby, PhD, OT(C)
Associate Professor
Department of Occupational Science and Occupational
  Therapy
University of Toronto
Toronto, Ontario, Canada

Pamela S. Roberts, PhD, OTR/L, SCFES,
  FAOTA, CPHQ, FNAP, FACRM
Executive Director and Professor, Physical Medicine and
  Rehabilitation
Department of Physical Medicine and Rehabilitation
Executive Director, Academic and Physician Informatics
Department of Enterprise Information Services
Cedars-Sinai Health System
Los Angeles, CA

Karen M. Sames, OTD, MBA, OTR/L, FAOTA
Professor
Department of Occupational Therapy
St. Catherine University
St. Paul, MN

Marjorie E. Scaffa, PhD, OTR/L, FAOTA
Professor Emeritus
Department of Occupational Therapy
University of South Alabama
Mobile, AL

Barbara A. Boyt Schell, PhD, OT/L, FAOTA
Professor Emerita
School of Occupational Therapy
Ivester College of Health Sciences
Brenau University
Gainesville, GA
Co-Owner
Schell Consulting
Athens, GA

Winifred Schultz-Krohn, PhD, OTR/L, BCP,
  SWC, FAOTA
Professor and Chair
Occupational Therapy Department
San Jose State University
San Jose, CA

David Seamon, PhD
Professor
Department of Architecture
Kansas State University
Manhattan, KS

Mary P. Shotwell, PhD, OT/L, FAOTA
Professor
Department of Occupational Therapy
Ivester College of Health Sciences
Brenau University
Gainesville, GA

C. Douglas Simmons, PhD, OTR/L, FAOTA
Professor and Program Director
Department of Occupational Therapy
MCPHS University
Manchester, NH

Theresa M. Smith, PhD, OTR, CLVT
Associate Professor
School of Occupational Therapy
Texas Woman's University
Houston, TX

Jo M. Solet, MS, EdM, PhD, OTR/L
Assistant Clinical Professor of Medicine
Division of Sleep Medicine
Harvard Medical School
Cambridge Health Alliance
Department of Medicine
Cambridge, MA

Margaret Swarbrick, PhD, OT, FAOTA
Associate Professor
Rutgers University
Piscataway, NJ
Wellness Institute Director
Collaborative Support Programs of New Jersey
Freehold, NJ

Yvonne Swinth, PhD, OTR/L, FAOTA
Professor, Department Chair
School of Occupational Therapy
University of Puget Sound
Tacoma, WA
Editor, Journal of Occupational Therapy: Schools and
    Early Intervention
CoChair, Washington Occupational Therapy Association
    OT in the Schools (OTIS)

Renée R. Taylor, MA, PhD
Professor and Director of the UIC Model of Human
    Occupation Clearinghouse
Department of Occupational Therapy
University of Illinois at Chicago
Chicago, IL

Linda Tickle-Degnen, PhD, OT, FAOTA
Professor
Department of Occupational Therapy
Tufts University
Medford, MA

Joan Pascale Toglia, PhD, OTR, FAOTA
Professor, Dean
School of Health and Natural Sciences
Mercy College
Dobbs Ferry, NY

Elizabeth A. Townsend, PhD, FCAOT
Professor Emerita
School of Occupational Therapy
Dalhousie University
Nova Scotia, Canada

Barry Trentham, PhD, OT Reg (Ont)
Assistant Professor
Department of Occupational Science and Occupational
    Therapy
University of Toronto
Toronto, Ontario, Canada

Craig A. Velozo, PhD, OTR/L
Division Director and Professor
Division of Occupational Therapy
College of Health Professions
Medical University of South Carolina
Charleston, SC

Anna Wallisch, PhD, OTR/L
Postdoctoral Researcher
Juniper Gardens Children's Project
University of Kansas
Kansas City, KS

Jean Wilkins Westmacott, MFA, BA
Associate Professor and Gallery Director Curator
    (Retired)
Fine Arts Department
Brenau University
Gainesville, GA

Steven D. Wheeler, PhD, OTR/L, CBIS
Professor and Program Director, Occupation Therapy
Department of Rehabilitation, Exercise, and
    Nutrition Sciences
University of Cincinnati
Cincinnati, OH

John A. White Jr., PhD, OTR/L, FAOTA
Professor
School of Occupational Therapy
Pacific University Oregon
Forest Grove, OR

Ann A. Wilcock, PhD, FCOT,
   GradDipPubHealth, BAppScOT
Retired Professor
Occupational Science and Therapy
Deakin University
Victoria, Australia

Jennifer Womack, PhD, OTR/L, FAOTA
Clinical Professor
Division of Occupational Science and Occupational
   Therapy
University of North Carolina at Chapel Hill
Chapel Hill, NC

Wendy Wood, PhD, OTR/L, FAOTA
Professor and Director of Research
Temple Grandin Equine Center
Department of Animal Sciences
Professor
Department of Occupational Therapy
Colorado State University
Fort Collins, CO

Valerie A. Wright-St. Clair, PhD, NZROT
Associate Professor
Department of Occupational Science and Therapy
Co-Director
AUT Centre for Active Ageing
Auckland, New Zealand

Mary Jane Youngstrom, MS, OTR/L, FAOTA
Occupational Therapist and Health Care Management
   Consultant
Overland Park, KS

EDITORIAL REVIEW BOARD

PREFACE

This 13th edition of *Willard & Spackman's Occupational Therapy,* which we are calling the "Centennial Edition," celebrates the 100th anniversary of the founding of the profession. In recognition of that event, we are including two special features in this edition. The first is a special history of the *Willard & Spackman's Occupational Therapy* text itself which details the development of the book as it transitioned from the original edition in 1947 to this edition. Since that 1st edition, this textbook has become an icon in the field. It is the text that welcomes students into the complexities of their newly chosen profession while also serving as a resource to the field by documenting the central knowledge and practices of occupational therapy (OT). It has gained this iconic status in no small part due to the work of previous editors and the many contributors, for which we are thankful.

The second new feature is the addition of "Centennial Notes" to most chapters throughout the book. These snapshots provide insights into the many facets of the field that are difficult to capture in the general history of the profession chapter, which remains in the first unit. Contributors were asked to write something fun or interesting about the history of their topic, how it has changed since the profession's founding and what trajectories can be traced from the past and into the future. This work was greatly aided by the extensive research provided by consulting editor Lori T. Andersen who, along with Barbara Schell, edited and in some cases authored the notes herself. These thumbnail essays serve as postcards from the past and guideposts to the future.

As always, chapters in this text summarize important and complex material in a way that is accessible and which challenges budding practitioners to think deeply about the many facets of occupation that emerge in the daily rounds of life. Furthermore, the process of OT is described across a wide array of practice arenas. This 13th edition continues these traditions, as Barbara A. Boyt Schell continues the role of lead editor, and Glen Gillen continues as a co-editor. Marjorie E. Scaffa and Ellen S. Cohn retire from their respective roles as co-editor and consulting editor but continue as contributors. Joining Schell and Gillen for the first time is a panel of consulting editors including the aforementioned Lori T. Andersen, along with Catana E. Brown and Kristie Patten Koenig. These consultants helped identify contributors, reviewed and edited contributions, and, in general, helped with assuring the high-quality content expected for this text.

This revision of *Willard & Spackman's Occupational Therapy* builds on the successful revisions done in the last edition. To identify needed changes, students and faculty who use the book were surveyed. Several leaders and scholars in the field also graciously provided advice through individual consultations. Although users generally expressed strong satisfaction with the text, some organizational changes were implemented, building on the restructuring done in the 12th edition. This information, in addition to the perspectives of the editors and consulting editors, informed the reorganization of this edition as well as the addition of new chapters and materials. An overall summary of these changes is provided next, followed by an overview of each unit, highlighting the materials included in each.

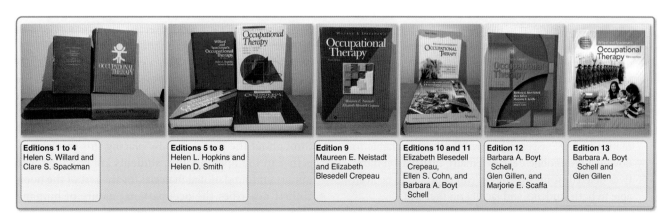

Willard & Spackman's Occupational Therapy, editions 1 to 13, with editors noted.

Overall Changes in the Text and Web-Based Materials

Because feedback on many aspects of the 12th edition was quite positive, *Willard & Spackman's Occupational Therapy* 13th edition retained materials focused on the centrality of occupation as the basis for practice, both as a means and an end of therapy. In this edition, we continue to acknowledge that evaluation and intervention processes are integrated with the theoretical perspectives of practitioners and the influences of the broader social and political environment on the day-to-day lives of practitioners and the clients they serve. Attempts were made to provide a diverse range of examples across cultures, life course, and occupational performance concerns, with particular emphasis on attending to worldwide scholarship within OT.

As in previous editions, we maintain that effective OT requires a collaborative process between or among OT practitioners and the clients they serve. For therapy to be optimally effective, a blending of current best evidence with therapist experience and client preferences must guide the process. Because this process is often complex, contributors were asked to provide many illustrations of the professional reasoning and underlying assumptions that guide practice. Furthermore, contributors were asked to acknowledge the challenges in implementing best practice and suggest approaches for overcoming these challenges.

As authors and editors, we acknowledge the power of language. Throughout this book, we have attempted to use language that is inclusive. That extends to appreciating the many different ways that humans are configured and the ways in which they engage in occupations. We also attempted to be inclusive of international perspectives by acknowledging when content is particularly reflective of U.S. perspectives versus content that appears to be fairly applicable across OT as it is practiced throughout the world.

In addition to the overall guiding principles just described, there were some noticeable changes in the book which include the following:

1. The expansion of expanded Web-based materials. Video resources inaugurated in the last edition were expanded to include children as well as adults. These video cases of clients can be used in conjunction with the book to provide students with opportunities to observe and analyze applications of concepts and techniques. The appendices (which are available on thePoint) related to common conditions affecting occupational performance and OT assessments will both be available for download to mobile devices. Finally, first-person narratives deleted from this edition will continue to be available to both students and faculty on thePoint.
2. Updating of materials to reflect the AOTA's *Occupational Therapy Practice Framework: Domain and Process*, third edition, while retaining an appreciation for broader international perspectives by also relating materials to the World Health Organization (WHO) International Classification of Functioning, Disability and Health (ICF)
3. Expansion of Unit I to include a new chapter on research and scholarship intended to expose students to the importance of that aspect of the profession as well as broadening the chapter on contemporary practice to reflect a more global perspective
4. Addition of four new narratives to Unit III's first-person perspectives to reflect current issues challenging individuals and their families. Narratives deleted from the print version of the text remain available on thePoint.
5. Addition of a new chapter addressing disability in the context of culture in Unit IV and expansion of attention to gender to acknowledge the range of gender identities
6. Tightening of Unit IX Practice Theories to reflect theoretical perspectives for which there is a body of evidence for validity and clinical utility

Unit-by-Unit Summary

The units in this edition were retained as the current general organization seemed to work well for users. We did add some new chapters and, in some cases, renamed chapters to clarify the contents. In the description that follows, new chapters added to the text will be highlighted. Except where noted, all chapters returning from the 12th edition were either updated or completely rewritten; all chapters which were new or were written by new authors were externally reviewed by one of the consulting editors or an external expert, along with reviews by a member of our student reviewer panel.

- Unit I profiles the profession by opening with a chapter on occupation followed by the broad written history of the profession, which places OT history in the context of larger world events. Next, a new chapter on the philosophical assumptions guiding the profession is added to this unit to help students appreciate the core beliefs, which are embedded in the profession. The next chapter in this unit is expanded to profile contemporary practice in from a global perspective. Finally, a new chapter on scholarship and research exposes readers to role of scholarship in all aspects of the profession. The author shares her own journey as she developed her research career and provides specific examples of research throughout the profession. By placing this material together in the opening unit, students are provided with important foundational material for the rest of the book.
- Unit II describes the occupational nature of humans. The opening chapter explores how participation in occupation changes over the course of life. This is followed by

a chapter on the relationships between occupation and health. The final occupational science chapter provides insight into the ongoing research about occupation, with updated examples of how such research informs OT practice.

- Unit III continues to have first-person narratives of people with various occupational challenges after an opening chapter explaining the importance of client narratives to effective practice. A number of new first-person narratives are in the section, including accounts by:

  - Laura and Craig Horowitz as they raised their son Will, a bright young man who is on the autism spectrum. Will describes his childhood and life from toddler days through high school. As a side note, Laura has been the managing editor for *Willard & Spackman's Occupational Therapy* for the last three editions, and she is proud to share that Will graduated from high school this year.
  - A first-person account by Paul Cabell, a veteran who is an actor and comedian challenged by mental illness, substance abuse, and homelessness
  - A narrative by Jean Westmacott, a sculptor and art director who brought her mother, Hildegard Viden Wilkins, home to live with Jean and her husband, in order to care for Hildegard in the final years of her life until her death at over 100 years old
  - An account by Beth Long, a Methodist minister who experienced a stroke while traveling to Ladakh, a northern province of India, who describes her personal and spiritual journey as she recovers, only to find that she has been "retired" from her ministerial position

  We retain the updated narratives of Gloria Dickerson and her successful narrative of her recovery process from the challenges of mental illness, which followed her abusive childhood as well as the collection of narratives of people living with disability in Ecuador.

  Three narratives have been moved from the book but remain available on thePoint. These are Mary Feldhaus-Weber's experience of a head injury, Alex and his parents' views of their child growing up with cerebral palsy, and Donald Murray's poignant description of caring for his wife during her days with dementia. Mary Feldhaus-Weber recently passed away, and Don Murray died before the publication of the last book. We honor their memory and contributions by keeping these narratives available. All of the narratives provide rich opportunities to gain a deeper understanding of how occupation and health challenges interweave in the ongoing lives of real individuals.

- Unit IV on occupations in context contains a number of chapters designed to make a clearer connection with the broad array of contextual factors discussed in the *Occupational Therapy Practice Framework: Domain and Process*, third edition, and the WHO's ICF. The chapter

on "Culture, Diversity, and Culturally Effective Care" includes attention to gender issues, including gender identity. A new author adds an addition to this unit in Chapter 21 entitled "Disability Rights." This replaces Chapter 70 "Disability Rights and Advocacy" that was formerly in Unit XV. Finally, new authors expand the chapter on "Physical and Virtual Environments."

- Unit V focuses on personal factors affecting occupation and continues the inclusion of updated chapters that closely parallel the *Occupational Therapy Practice Framework: Domain and Process*, third edition, as well as the WHO's ICF. The opening chapter on individual factors provides a number of examples to students about how body functions and structures impact performance. The chapter on spirituality and beliefs explains how these individual differences impact the meaning of occupation.
- Unit VI focuses on analyzing occupation, with the first chapter explaining occupational and activity analysis, and a second on performance skills, both of which provide information on ways to consider occupational performance.
- Unit VII contains a number of chapters which explain the OT process. All the chapters from the previous edition return. The introductory chapter to this unit provides an overview of the OT process and outcomes of care. Then, follows a chapter on determining client needs which provides detailed examples of client evaluation in a variety of situations. Next, a chapter on critiquing assessments provides information on how to appraise traditional measurement procedures as well as current psychometric approaches in OT assessments. The process of intervention for individuals and for organizations, communities, and populations is fully explored in the next two chapters. The unit ends a chapter about modifying performance contexts.
- Unit VIII clusters together seven chapters, all of them returning from the last edition. Chapters in this unit address core concepts and skills such as professional reasoning; evidence-based practice; ethical practice; therapeutic relationships and client collaboration; group process and group intervention; professionalism, communication, and teamwork; and documentation in practice.
- Unit IX discusses theories of occupational performance, starting with a chapter examining how theory guides practice. Following this are chapters focused on theories for which there is a body of evidence to support their validity and utility, starting with the Model of Human Occupation. Next is a discussion of Ecological Models in Occupational Therapy which include the Ecology of Human Performance, Person-Environment-Occupation, Person-Environment-Occupational-Performance, and Canadian Model of Occupational Performance and Engagement. This is followed by chapters on Theory of Occupational Adaptation and finally "Occupational Justice." As in all other units, all chapters have been

updated with inclusion of relevant evidence. The emerging theories chapter is omitted in this edition, pending development of further relevant evidence on new theories.

- Unit X retains the chapters of broad theories that inform practice but which are not OT theories per se. These include the Recovery Model, Health Promotion Theories, and Principles of Learning and Behavior Change.
- Unit XI starts with an introductory chapter that provides an overview of evaluation, intervention, and outcomes for the major areas of occupation. Basic and instrumental activities of daily living (BADL and IADL) are discussed in the next chapter, followed by chapters on education, work, play and leisure, rest and sleep, and ending with the chapter on social participation.
- Unit XII provides a survey of focused theories that are commonly used in conjunction with occupational performance theories to guide intervention. All topics from the last edition are retained, including motor control, cognition and perception, and a new chapter on sensory processing in everyday life. The unit ends with a chapter on emotional regulation and one addressing social interaction.
- Unit XIII, entitled *"The Practice Context: Therapists in Action,"* displays therapist decision making as it is implemented in different therapy settings across various continuums of care. The first chapter explains how clients may receive therapy across a wide range of settings, although clusters of settings may be more associated with some health or participation challenges than others. Subsequent chapters each provide a therapist narrative explaining the thinking behind the evaluation and intervention strategies implemented for a particular client. Additionally, each chapter addressed how services commonly occur across different settings. Separate chapters address services for individuals with autism spectrum disorders, traumatic brain injury, and schizophrenia, followed by additional chapters focused on a worker with hand injuries, older adults with changing needs, and disaster survivors. The intent of this unit is to "bring alive" the various theories and intervention approaches by displaying real-world situations.
- Unit XIV contains an updated chapter on Fieldwork, Practice Education, and Professional Entry, and a newly rewritten chapter on Competence and Professional Development.
- Unit XV addresses OT management, supervision, and related topics such as payment for services. The first two chapters focus on management and supervision respectively, with a new co-author contributing to the supervision chapter. Next is a chapter on consultation with a new author and expanded content. The chapter on payment includes the current information on changes in health policy in the United States.
- The glossary contains definitions of key words from chapters and important terminology from other sources such as the WHO's ICF and the AOTA's *Occupational Therapy Practice Framework: Domain and Process*, third edition.

- There are two appendices related to the text, both of which are now on thePoint. The first includes either new or completely updated summaries of resources and evidence related to common conditions for which OT services are provided. The second appendix is an updated table of assessments used in OT.

Special Features

Special features are found both in the text and in the Web materials associated with this text. Special features include the following:

- **Practice Dilemma**: a practice situation related to chapter content with one to three questions designed to challenge students. Answers are not provided to the student.
- **Ethical Dilemma**: a scenario relevant to chapter content which poses an ethical challenge for practitioners
- **Case Study**: an example of OT evaluation and intervention modeling expert practice. Note that these are available both in text and in the form of video vignettes online.
- **Commentary on the Evidence**: a succinct discussion about available evidence to support practice, including identification of where evidence is lacking or inconclusive and where further research is required
- **Centennial Notes**: These notes provide insights into the many facets of the field that are difficult to capture in the general history of the profession chapter. The notes discuss how the topic of the chapter changed since the profession's founding and what trajectories can be traced from the past and into the future.

With this edition, we are pleased to continue to offer specially selected video clips from International Clinical Educators, Inc. These may be found on thePoint (http://thePoint.lww.com/Willard-Spackman13e). Also on thePoint are PowerPoint slides for each chapter, quiz and test banks, additional learning materials, and several professionally developed video clips.

Final Notes

Once again, we are grateful for the guidance provided by many experienced colleagues as we have created this edition. We are particularly thankful for our consulting editors Lori T. Andersen, Catana E. Brown, and Kristie Patten Koenig. It is our hope that this "Centennial Edition" contributes new light on the heritage of this text as it transitioned editors as well as surfacing many less well-known facets of the profession's history. It is our privilege to carry on the tradition of *Willard & Spackman's Occupational Therapy* as a treasury of knowledge and a beacon to light the way for the next generation of OT practitioners.

Barbara A. Boyt Schell
Glen Gillen

ACKNOWLEDGMENTS

This edition of *Willard & Spackman's Occupational Therapy* was accomplished through the collective efforts of the contributors, editors, reviewers, photographers, students, colleagues, friends, and family. We are grateful for their many contributions to this effort and know that their commitment, scholarship, and generosity in sharing these traits have improved the quality of the work presented here.

Editing a book such as this becomes an occupation in and of itself. Like all occupations, it is interwoven within the larger tapestry of activities that comprise our lives. Indeed, there is the "text" and the "subtext" of each edition. The text you see before you. The subtext is hidden behind the scenes. This edition started with a new format of editors, as Marjorie retired from the editorial role and Ellen from the consulting editor role. By the time we were planning this book, Barbara was retiring from her full-time academic and administrative responsibilities. As we complete the book, Glen is stepping up to become program director at his university. As the book progressed, each of our own life stories evolved as well. Health challenges involving ourselves, family members, and colleagues served to personalize many of the concepts in this book as we took turns both supporting and covering for each other. As always, our pets were important reminders of when it was time to eat and play. Barb appreciates Brandy, the 105-lb labrador mix, who is sometimes affectionately referred to as "my little pony." Meanwhile, Glen's dog, Max, continues to spin in circles indicating that he wants attention or has an activity of daily living to attend to.

Barbara thanks her husband John W. Schell, PhD, who is both playmate and professional partner in education and scholarship; photographer extraordinaire; and father/grandfather to our wonderful family, Brad, Trina, Sophie and Izzy Schell, and Alyxius, Marcus, Adrian, Rooke, Akhasa and Samarra Young all of whom give meaning to our lives. Finally, thanks to Helen Clayton for her service in our household.

Glen thanks his parents, Gary and Gail, and nieces and nephews who range from age 3 to 21 years, Julianna, Harry, Avery, and Harper.

Thanks to each of you for your commitment to each of us.

Finally, each of us is very proud of our universities and OT programs, which sustain us in our work and encourage us to greater accomplishments. Our students, faculty, and practitioners in our professional communities provide a background of inspiration for taking on a task such as this. We thank all those who helped us with their insights.

Professional Colleagues and Students

We thank our colleagues for their assistance, support, and insightful feedback. We are grateful for the faculty and students who responded to surveys:

Editorial Review Board
We thank our consulting editors, invited faculty reviewers, and student reviewers who gave generously of their time and knowledge to review chapters in this book to assure that each chapter met our standards for both scholarship and accessibility. They are listed by name earlier in this front matter, but we wish to once again thank them for their service.

Wolters Kluwer/Lippincott Williams & Wilkins
Current and former Lippincott Williams & Wilkins personnel contributed to the development of this book, and we appreciate their ongoing support.

- Mike Nobel, Matt Hauber, Shauna Kelley, Tim Rinehart, and Joan Sinclair
- Harold Medina and his team of Absolute Service, Inc., who once again joined us via the Internet from the Philippines. We appreciate his thoroughness in copy editing and page formatting, willingness to remind us (again!) what he is missing from us, and overall grace in his communications.

York Content Development
Our thanks to Wolters Kluwer for allowing us once again to have the special attentions of this group. This is the third time that Laura and her staff have served to support us in this text, and their contributions are invaluable.

- Laura Horowitz provided overall guidance of the development of the manuscript through the production of the book. Her steady guidance, expertise, patience, and good humor provided significant support to our efforts.
- Gretchen Miller helped us with her careful tracking of contributors, permissions, photos, and all other editorial details needed to bring the book to fruition.

BRIEF CONTENTS

CONTENTS

Available on thePoint (http://thePoint.lww
.com/Willard-Spackman13e)

APPENDIX I
Resources and Evidence for Common
Conditions Addressed in OT

*Katherine Appelbe, Megan Bailey, Gregory Blocki,
Emily Briggs, Ashley Chung, Madeleine Emerson,
Nikoletta Evangelatos, Libby Gross, Colleen Hogan,
Grace Kelso, Ereann Kilpatrick, Jade LaRochelle,
Kristen Layo, Elana Lerner, Estie Martin,
Morgan McGoey, Richard McGuire, Emily Moran,
Nicole Murgas, Rachel Newman, Jack Norcross,
Natalie Petrone, Annie Poole, Casey Primeau,
Alicia Quach, Jeanette Stitik, Nicole Strausser,
Sarah Tuberty, Taryn Wells; edited by Ellen S. Cohn*

APPENDIX II
Table of Assessments:
Listed Alphabetically by Title

Cheryl Lynne Trautmann Boop

APPENDIX III
First-Person Narratives

- *An Excerpt from* The Book of Sorrow,
  Book of Dreams: A First-Person Narrative,
  by Mary Feldhaus-Weber and Sally A. Schreiber-Cohn
- *He's Not Broken—He's Alex: Three Perspectives,
  by Alexander McIntosh, Laurie S. McIntosh, and
  Lou McIntosh*
- *The Privilege of Giving Care, by Donald M. Murray*

FEATURES

Centennial Notes

Commentary on the Evidence

Ethical Dilemma

VIDEO CLIPS

In addition to the features listed above, this edition of *Willard & Spackman's Occupational Therapy* will feature a video library on thePoint (visit http://thePoint.lww.com/Willard-Spackman13e). The videos are from the library of International Clinical Educators, Inc. (http://www.icelearningcenter.com/) and were chosen to supplement various chapters. Although chapter suggestions are listed in the descriptions below, these suggestions are not exhaustive. The videos take place in various contexts (acute care hospitals, home-based services, outpatient services, school-based services, etc.) but are not meant to represent all of the contexts and population that are served by OT practitioners. Video clips are listed by their titles.

Dementia: Part 1: Grooming and Hygiene
This video about the impact of dementia on activities of daily living (ADL) is recommended as a supplement to Chapters 28, 30, 50, 58, and 67.

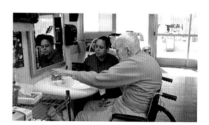

Pediatrics: Fine Motor: Letter Formation and Playdough
This video about improving coordination is recommended as a supplement to Chapters 51 and 57.

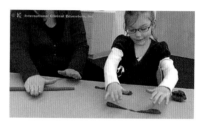

Pediatric Assessment: Administration of the Test of Visual Motor Skills
This video about assessing visual skills is recommended as a supplement to Chapters 23, 28, and 51.

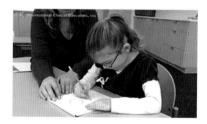

Pediatrics: Sensory Integration/Sensory Processing: Scooterboard and Letter Recognition Activity
This video about sensory interventions is recommended as a supplement to Chapter 59.

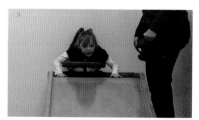

Pediatrics: Mat Activity: Sit to Stand
This video about functional mobility is recommended as a supplement to Chapters 30, 50, and 57.

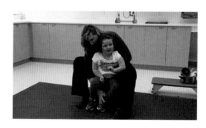

Multiple Sclerosis: Problems Observed in the Home: Part 1
This video about adaptations is recommended as a supplement to Chapters 30, 50, and 52.

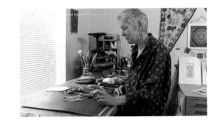

Instrumental Activities of Daily Living: Shining Shoes while Standing
This video about remediating motor function is recommended as a supplement to Chapters 50 and 57.

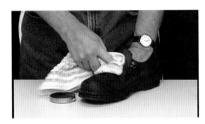

Intensive Care Unit: Treatment Begins, Part 3: Sitting at the Edge of the Bed
This video about early mobilization is recommended as a supplement to Chapters 50 and 62.

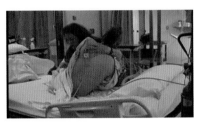

Rotator Cuff Repair, Part 2: Measuring Range of Motion
This video about assessment is recommended as a supplement to Chapters 27, 28, and 29.

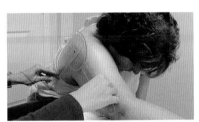

Radial Fracture, 10 Weeks Postsurgery: Paraffin Bath and Scar Mobilization
This video about preparatory interventions is recommended as a supplement to Chapters 30 and 66.

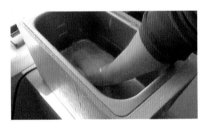

Ventilator: Part 2: Self-care at Edge of Bed
This video about acute ADL training is recommended as a supplement to Chapters 50 and 62.

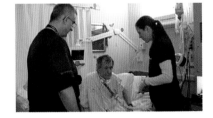

Participation: Expanding Therapy into the Community
This video about community integration is recommended as a supplement to Chapters 55 and 67.

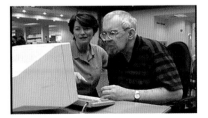

WILLARD & SPACKMAN'S OCCUPATIONAL THERAPY

The Book That Captured a Profession

Peggy M. Martin, Christine O. Peters, Wanda J. Mahoney

The book has "a historical legacy . . . it has taken a broad perspective, and I believe that it has shifted with time." (Cohn, 2017 oral history, lines 430–433)

As readers open the pages of this time-honored book, we challenge you to contemplate the influence of words and ideas not only in this Centennial Edition but also in the prior editions of *Willard & Spackman's Occupational Therapy*. When asked, as in the recent AOTA Centennial celebration, most OT practitioners can quickly name the cover color of their *Willard & Spackman's Occupational Therapy* textbook, placing them in a specific era of OT history. Helen Willard (1894–1980) reported that in 1960, while meeting a group of occupational therapists and students in South Africa, "and one of them looked at us and then broke into broad smiles and said, 'The cover of the book.'" (Willard, 1977 archived oral history, lines 81–82).[1] Clare Spackman (1909–1992) remembered "one of the funniest uses of the book, and there are many which we have collected, is [occupational therapists at] one of the army hospitals had to meet their students at the airport and . . . instructed [the students] to carry a copy of *Willard and Spackman* so they could be picked up." (Willard & Spackman, 1977 archived oral history, lines 91–94).

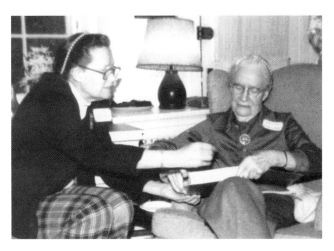

Willard and Spackman signing fifth edition. (Courtesy of AOTA.)

---

[1]The early editions did not have photos of the editors on their covers so it is unknown how the occupational therapists and students recognized the editors.

Today, as in 1947, *Willard & Spackman's Occupational Therapy* is a standard textbook used by many OT programs both in the United States and around the world. The 3rd edition was translated into Japanese, and 4th edition was translated into Japanese and Spanish, noteworthy because of the alignment of the early publications with the development of the World Federation of Occupational Therapists (Mendez, 1986). According to the U.S. National Board for Certification in Occupational Therapy (NBCOT), 76% of occupational therapist curricula in the United States adopted the 12th edition as a required textbook for their students, and it was one of the top 10 textbook references used by NBCOT certification item writers for both OTR and COTA tests (NBCOT, 2016a, 2016b). This edition, now the 13th, continues the legacy.

The Book Begins

Principles of Occupational Therapy started as a book about OT treatment for individuals with physical disabilities, written by Spackman who said she had "gotten so used to writing papers" while studying for her master's degree (Willard & Spackman, 1977 archived oral history, lines 38–40). Spackman explained, "Out of the clear blue sky J. B. Lippincott, Mr. Lippincott himself, invited us to the Union League for lunch. [He] proposed that we edit a book on OT, but he wanted the representatives of all the schools and geographical distribution and the covering of the whole field. So I chucked out most of mine . . . and we put in . . . the whole scope of OT." (Willard & Spackman, 1977 archived oral history, lines 40–45). This collaboration became the first comprehensive OT textbook written by occupational therapists in the United States. Whereas subsequent editions targeted the information to OT students, the first edition was "prepared as a basic text for doctors, nurses, social workers, and occupational therapists, both graduates and students" (Willard & Spackman, 1947, p. viii). Understanding the urgency for a viable book, the founding editors acknowledged the respected reviewers' work to complete the book, "Those who have given

TABLE 1 Editions and Editors of *Willard & Spackman's Occupational Therapy*

Edition	Year	Title	Editors
1	1947	*Principles of Occupational Therapy*	Helen Willard Clare Spackman
2	1954	*Principles of Occupational Therapy*	Helen Willard Clare Spackman
3	1963	*Occupational Therapy*	Helen Willard Clare Spackman
4	1971	*Occupational Therapy*	Helen Willard Clare Spackman
5	1978	*Willard & Spackman's Occupational Therapy*	Helen Hopkins Helen Smith
6	1983	*Willard & Spackman's Occupational Therapy*	Helen Hopkins Helen Smith
7	1988	*Willard & Spackman's Occupational Therapy*	Helen Hopkins Helen Smith
8	1993	*Willard & Spackman's Occupational Therapy*	Helen Hopkins Helen Smith
9	1998	*Willard & Spackman's Occupational Therapy*	Maureen Neistadt Elizabeth Crepeau
10	2003	*Willard & Spackman's Occupational Therapy*	Elizabeth Crepeau Ellen Cohn Barbara A. Boyt Schell
11	2009	*Willard & Spackman's Occupational Therapy*	Elizabeth Crepeau Ellen Cohn Barbara A. Boyt Schell
12	2014	*Willard & Spackman's Occupational Therapy*	Barbara A. Boyt Schell Glen Gillen Marjorie Scaffa *Consulting editor:* Ellen Cohn
13	2019	*Willard & Spackman's Occupational Therapy*	Barbara A. Boyt Schell Glen Gillen *Consulting editors:* Lori T. Andersen Catana E. Brown Kristie P. Koenig

painstaking and helpful criticism . . . have contributed much" (p. viii).[2]

This 1st edition boasted 20 authors and 416 pages expanding to 108 contributors and 1,262 pages by the 12th edition. The book underwent three name changes: from *Principles of Occupational Therapy* (1947, 1954) to *Occupational Therapy* (1963, 1971) to *Willard & Spackman's Occupational Therapy* (1978) with significant practice scope or editorial shifts at each transition.[3] Table 1 lists these editorial shifts along with edition number, publication year, and book title.

---

[2]Prominent physicians Westmoreland, Overholser, Piersol, Krusen, and Phelps reviewed the first edition, as well as recognized occupational therapists Greene, Ackley, Kahmann, and Helmig and administrator Haas, demonstrating the influential power behind the first edition (Willard & Spackman, 1947, p. viii).

[3]Editors state "the title has been changed to *Occupational Therapy* [and] is evidence of the extensive and rapid changes which have been taking place in the profession during the last few years" (Willard & Spackman, 1963, p. v).

The Founding Editors: Willard and Spackman

Helen S. Willard and Clare S. Spackman, experienced OT educators at the Philadelphia School for Occupational Therapy (P.S.O.T.), edited the first book in 1947, calling it *Principles of Occupational Therapy*. Willard, program director at the school, had vast experience as an educator; first teaching English and Latin at college and high school levels following her 1915 graduation from Wellesley College (Willard, 1975). By 1918, Willard was enrolled in a Special War Course for Reconstruction Aides in Physical Therapy where she worked with Dr. Harry E. Stewart as he wrote an early textbook for reconstruction aides (Stewart, 1920; Willard, 1975). One can only surmise that this early professional experience likely influenced her decision 20 years later to edit a book of her own. By 1928, after qualifying as an occupational therapist and practicing in leadership roles, Willard entered academia as the director of the

Curative Workshop and instructor in OT at the P.S.O.T. (Willard, 1975). The next year, Willard met Spackman, a promising student in the 1930 graduating class (Spackman, 1975). By 1931, Spackman was serving as the assistant director for the Curative Workshop of which Willard directed. In 1935, when Willard became director of P.S.O.T., Spackman became director of the Curative Workshop. Spackman's pursuit of advanced degrees in education likely spurred her writing of the first edition. She obtained her bachelor's degree in 1941 and master's degree in 1942, actions that well prepared her to edit a book about OT published 5 years later. Willard and Spackman went on to co-edit three additional editions of the book.

The powerful collaboration between Willard and Spackman fostered the first U.S. book written by occupational therapists, the evolution of educational standards in OT, the beginning of the World Federation of Occupational Therapists, and much more (Mahoney, Peters, & Martin, 2017; Peters, Martin, & Mahoney, 2017). A South African occupational therapist and faculty member at the P.S.O.T. stated, "It was the only textbook we had. And I remember that in South Africa because we had a very small shelf. Most of them were written by physicians. So this was OT." (Cynkin, 1996 oral history, lines 29–36). Willard retired from academia in 1964 followed by Spackman in 1970, and they edited the fourth edition of *Occupational Therapy* in 1971 after their retirements (Spackman, 1975; Willard, 1975). Together, these two women left lasting legacies in OT, including their book whose title remains marked by their names.

Subsequent Lead Editors: Passing the Torch

> [We] worked together very well . . . they [co-editors] had arguments . . . intellectual ones about things in the book and approaches, and . . . I would just sit back and listen . . . basically I synthesized what they were talking about it and would said okay, this is the way forward. (Crepeau, 2017 oral history, lines 501–510)

This book would not exist without the editors' unswerving vision. Editors conceptualized the whole, determined the content that represented exemplar practice, selected highly qualified contributing authors, and "made it happen." The *Willard & Spackman's Occupational Therapy* books are unusual in that different editions had different editorial teams, yet each one was committed to moving the profession forward toward a vision that began with Willard and Spackman (see Table 1). What is noteworthy is that passing the editor role was more than assigning administrative responsibilities; it indicated trust and respect and included mentoring talent. Lead editors and key co-editors, some who became lead editors, joined a well-respected cadre who maintained the standards and legacy of the book.

Each subsequent editorial team retained *Willard & Spackman* in their book's title. The following section describes this series of dedicated editors with a focus on the lead editors. Contributing information was garnered from a series of interviews with most living editors.

The process of selecting the next editors was a weighted and symbolic decision. "Passing the torch" is a leitmotif throughout the 13 editions, be it editors or authors. Editors, moving the book to completion, at times exercised heroic efforts, as captured in the words and remembrances of past and current editors. The "Olympic torch" passed between lead editors four times in the 13 editions: from Willard to Hopkins (5th edition), Hopkins to Neistadt (9th edition), Neistadt to Crepeau (10th edition), and Crepeau to Schell (12th edition). Each successive edition evolved into a seminal compendium book for OT. Former editors noted, "You go to *Willard and Spackman* to find out what you need, it was like an encyclopedia. People referred to it as the OT bible" (Crepeau, 2017 oral history, lines 342–343). "It was used as a reference and a resource book, a go-to book for practitioners and educators. . . . it's so iconic" (Cohn, 2017 oral history, lines 285–287). The book grew in length, depth, and numbers of contributors with increased expertise. Passing the lead editors' torch was traditionally invitational between the 1970s and 2010s, often presented to past co-editors, proven colleagues, sometimes coworkers, and colleagues from professional organizations. Lead editor Schell broke tradition when she put out a competitive call, enlisting the help of academic program directors, to recruit experienced co-editors, attempting to reach a broader geographic and diverse pool.

First Pass: Willard to Hopkins

After three decades of editing the book, Willard and Spackman passed the torch for the fifth edition to their esteemed colleagues, alumnae, and friends, Helen Hopkins (1921–2007) and Helen Smith (1933–2014) (Spackman & Willard, 1978; Willard, 1977 archived oral history, lines 599–601). Hopkins, newly appointed lead editor, graduated from P.S.O.T. in 1947 and then joined Spackman and Willard as an instructor in 1956 to 1959 (AOTA, 1962). Co-editor Smith studied under Willard, Spackman, and Hopkins until she graduated in 1959 when she became assistant director of the Curative Workshop under director Spackman (AOTA, 1962). Spackman and Willard (1978) summarized the first editorial transition in the foreword to the fifth edition, "When thirty-two years ago we agreed to edit what was then called *Principles of Occupational Therapy* it never occurred to us that in 1976 we should at last be passing on the editorship of *Occupational Therapy*" (p. xi). By passing the editorship to such worthy colleagues and friends, Willard and Spackman ensured a well-caste book with a lasting legacy that was retitled *Willard & Spackman's Occupational Therapy* in their honor.

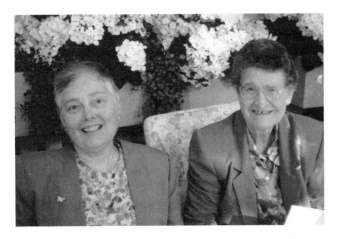

Helen Hopkins and Helen Smith. (Courtesy of H. Hopkins.)

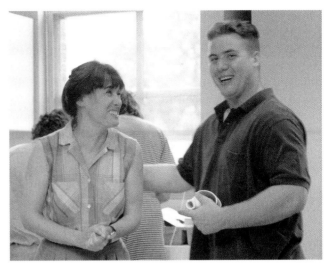

Maureen Neistadt. (Courtesy of G. Samson, Photographic Services, University of New Hampshire, Durham, NH.)

Bringing the team of Hopkins and Smith to life, future editor Crepeau, remembered them.

> The thing I remember most about Hoppy [Helen Hopkins] was how kind and generous she was. . . . But the two of them together [Helen Hopkins and Helen Smith], they were very good friends, and they were always together. They dressed very much alike; they always had blazers on and generally a skirt or slacks. (Crepeau, 2017 oral history, lines 64–72)

Hopkins and Smith edited the fifth through eighth editions of *Willard & Spackman's Occupational Therapy* (1978, 1983, 1988, and 1993). Hopkins, chairperson and founding faculty at Temple University in Philadelphia, retired in 1986. Smith, a faculty member at Tufts University Boston School of Occupational Therapy, retired in 1998. Similar to Willard and Spackman, although retired, "they remained interested in the evolution of the book and supportive of our work as editors" (Crepeau, Cohn, & Schell, 2009, p. vii).

Second Pass: Hopkins to Neistadt

Hopkins and Smith passed the editors' torch to Maureen Neistadt (1950–2000), Smith's former colleague at Tufts University, for the ninth edition which commemorated the 50th anniversary of the first edition of the book. Elizabeth Crepeau, co-editor, remembered, "Maureen was extraordinary, funny, a little salty" (Crepeau, 2017 oral history, lines 133–134). Crepeau recounted how her colleague Neistadt was handed the torch from "the Helens" (Hopkins and Smith) and ultimately how she became involved:

> It turned out the "Helens," Helen Smith and Helen Hopkins, knew Maureen fairly well. Helen Smith and Maureen were colleagues at Tufts. And I knew Hoppy [Helen Hopkins] from various AOTA things. Apparently, they approached Maureen, and said we want you to edit *Willard and Spackman*. But, we also want to approve whoever you ask to co-edit with you. And since they both knew me, I guess it wasn't a problem. (Crepeau, 2017 oral history, lines 43–47)

Crepeau explained the invitation to join the editorial team she received from her coworker, Neistadt, "One night, we both stayed late and met up at the Xerox machine where all important things are decided." She described this meeting as Neistadt asking

> "What would you think about editing *Willard and Spackman* with me?" No preamble or anything, and I thought for a minute. I had recently finished editing SPICES [self-paced instruction for clinical education by AOTA] . . . this is no big deal. "Sure I'll do it." (Crepeau, 2017 oral history, lines 34–42)

Crepeau summarized her sentiments as an editor on this time-honored book, "We were being given both a gift and a huge responsibility to carry on the tradition of *Willard & Spackman*" (Crepeau, 2017 oral history, lines 85–86). The editorial team was gearing up for another transition.

Third Pass: Neistadt to Crepeau

Neistadt and Crepeau began planning the 10th edition of *Willard & Spackman's Occupational Therapy* 1 year after the 9th edition was released. The lead editor, Neistadt, was recovering from treatment for cancer but hopeful about her ability to complete the book (Crepeau, Cohn, & Schell, 2003a). Within 6 months, it was clear that Neistadt would be unable to meet the demands of the lead editor role. Crepeau explained that Neistadt told her, "I know I'm not going to be able to continue editing the book. We need to find somebody else to join you, and the book is too big for just two people" (Crepeau, 2017 oral history, lines 280–281). As co-editors, they recruited their colleagues, Ellen Cohn and Barbara Schell to join the team (Crepeau, 2017 oral history). Sadly, Maureen Neistadt lost her battle to cancer in 2000 after successfully passing the

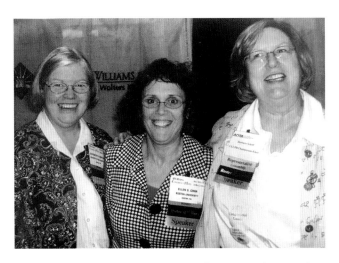

Elizabeth Blesedell Crepeau, Ellen S. Cohn, and Barbara A. Boyt Schell.

editors' torch to another highly competent editorial team, Crepeau, Cohn, and Schell. Displaying fortitude at a time of personal adversity, the 10th edition now meant completing the work begun by Neistadt. Crepeau was characterized in the dedication of the 12th edition as assuming lead editorship "with grace and wit" (Schell, Gillen, Scaffa, & Cohn, 2014, p. v). Crepeau et al. (2003a) wrote, "Maureen [Neistadt]'s spirit has infused and supported our work together. It is our hope that this edition reflects her vision and spirit" (p. xvii). The 10th edition of the book was dedicated to Maureen E. Neistadt (1950–2000). She so valued her editorial role that this activity was prominently described in her obituary, "[Maureen Neistadt] edited a ninth edition textbook in her specialized field, *Willard and Spackman's Occupational Therapy*. The project was completed in 1997 after three years of work" (Vartabedian, 2000). The Crepeau, Cohn, and Schell editorial team of the 10th edition repeated their roles for the 11th edition in 2009. Crepeau explained, "I retired a month or two after 11th edition came out, and I realized I'm not going to be using this . . . I'm not going to be able to assign chapters and see how students respond" (Crepeau, 2017 oral history, lines 491–496). Crepeau's decision to end her tenure as a *Willard & Spackman's Occupational Therapy* editor corresponded with her retirement from academia.

Fourth Pass: Crepeau to Schell

The editorial torch again passed hands between the 11th and 12th editions. Crepeau expressed her confidence in co-editor Schell, "I knew that Barb [Schell] had the stuff to continue with the book and that the book would be in good hands" (Crepeau, 2017 oral history, lines 496–497). Ellen Cohn, the other co-editor, had expressed her desire to retire from the text in order to pursue other academic interests but stayed as a consulting editor, and a new editorial team of Glen Gillen and Marjorie Scaffa were selected by Schell from an open search. Lead editor Schell echoed past editors' sentiments about honor and privilege, "It still certainly felt like an honor" (Schell, 2017 oral history, line 233). "However, by the time I had the opportunity to become the lead editor, I knew what was involved and how to do it" (Schell, 2017 oral history, lines 233–234).

Since its premiere edition, lead editors four times handed the charge to well selected and respected successors. There is a connection in that torch pass, when editors honor their own. In the tradition of transition, editors have dedicated four editions of the book to past editors: Willard (6th edition), Spackman (7th edition), Hopkins and Smith (11th edition), Neistadt (10th edition), Crepeau (12th edition), and now Cohn (13th edition), showing the highest respect. Having their own history, the editors are part of the book's entirety. This book spanned a dozen previous editions, passing from teams of editors who individualistically stepped up to the plate to harness a burgeoning body of knowledge. Current editor Schell summarized, "The book is still such an important resource on so many levels. It also serves to document the history of the profession in many ways" (Schell, 2017 oral history, lines 154–160).

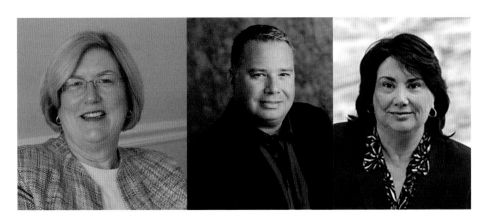

Barbara A. Boyt Schell, Glen Gillen, and Marjorie E. Scaffa.

Capturing a Living History

"You can see the evolution over time, it's the living history of the profession and the embodiment of what we're thinking." (Schell, 2017 oral history, lines 160–161)

Providing a "living history," the book captured OT history. Writing of history is complex, be it a profession or in 12 editions of a book. Screening a progressive timeline in a profession, OT history unfolds in various editions of *Willard & Spackman's Occupational Therapy*. At times, the OT history was the first chapter of the book, giving the past a sense of priority, importance, and introduction to a profession. The foundational cornerstone set forth by physician William Rush Dunton, Jr. (1947) who penned the "History and Development of Occupational Therapy" chapter in the first edition of *Principles of Occupational Therapy* became a model for subsequent editions to organize the profession's history. Dunton (1947) succinctly reviewed OT's history prior to the 20th century, professional growth periods, influence of wars, and training requirements and scholarship, although expanded, renamed, and reworked by other authors. Dunton's historical skeleton has withstood the test of time. This first edition published history of OT was authored by a physician, and although a supportive founder differed from all successive OT history authors who wrote about their own profession. This passing of a torch is seen between chapter authors as well as book editors in the evolution of the book.

Occupational therapy history chapters moved from a chronological descriptive overview to a richer contextual discourse reflecting a more complex interpretation of the remaining record. Most authors were occupational therapists, not schooled historians who wrote about the profession, which can be viewed as a criticism by historical researchers (Barzun & Graff, 1970; Gottschalk, 1969).[4] The occupational therapist as author may have a subjective rather than objective interpretation of a history she or he may have lived or idealized. That said, OT authors presented good historical chronologies, with some authors using sophisticated historical interpretations. Thus, a growing body of historical evidence across the editions occurred.

As different editions were reformatted, the history chapter changed placement in the book. In the premiere edition, Dunton's (1947) "History and Development of Occupational Therapy" was the first chapter and the first page, framing a foundation. The updated chapter in the 2nd edition (1954) was removed in the 3rd and 4th editions of the book. Editors Willard and Spackman (1963) acknowledged the change, noting that the focus was on "achieving optimal usefulness" (p. v) and "because of the deletions . . . it is important that both the previous editions . . . be available to students or to persons who desire more extensive information on occupational therapy" (p. vi). Again, in the 4th edition, editors Willard and Spackman (1971), acknowledged that they were "aware of shortcomings and possible omissions. . . . We present it [the book] with great pride in the past" (p. vi). Editors had already begun the arduous process to select the most pressing information essential for practice. This debate continues as voiced by all editors when interviewed in preparation to write this foreword to the 13th edition.

Lead editor Hopkins had a particular interest in OT history, and after absent history chapters in the previous two editions, she revitalized history by writing "A Historical Perspective on Occupational Therapy" in the fifth edition (1978). Following Dunton's skeleton, Hopkins (1978) expanded themes like "Ancient Origins of Occupation" (p. 3) and "Genesis of Occupational Therapy Profession" (p. 6). By the sixth edition, Hopkins (1983) infused historical critique by citing the work of Greenman's unpublished master's thesis at Tufts who argued that the current status of scientific publication in the profession was "amiss," with journal articles "undocumented, unscientific, and inconclusive" (Hopkins, 1983, p. 12). Hopkins (1983) also cited Bowman's view that OT was not meeting scientific standards, "with abundant unorganized material" (p. 11). By including these alternate views, Hopkins presented plausible and multifaceted interpretations needed when reconstructing the past. Hopkins continued to prioritize history in the sixth (1983), seventh (1988), and eight editions (1993) expanding the foundations section to include philosophy. Hopkins selected Reed (1993) to write the history chapter, which included a wealth of primary sources showing the author's artful ability to find the most hidden information.

Repositioned to the back of the book, Schwartz (1998) skillfully wrote the history chapter for the ninth edition (Chapter 49). Schwartz (1998), a historical scholar, reconceptualized the intellectual foundation of the profession when she analyzed the OT founders and social movements of the time. "The founders' views represent a variety of ideas and movements, some dating back to the 1800s, some during the progressive era 1890 to 1920, including moral treatment, arts and crafts movement, scientific medicine ideology, women's professions and social reform" (p. 854). Schwartz placed the profession in a context of larger history, moving from a descriptive chronology of professional milestones to a complex analysis. Her writing

---

[4]Gottschalk (1969) purports that the historical method is scientific, resulting from verification and intelligent agreement or disagreement among the experts. Barzun and Graff (1970) support the idea that historians, trained in their discipline, are best prepared historical scholars.

was no longer just about OT but about a particular health care profession in American history. Ever dynamic and changing, OT sought a new level of independence at its 50th anniversary, when Schwartz (1998) cited Yerxa's call for autonomy from the medical model and physician prescription. This shift in writing the history of the profession was revolutionary and a change from physician Dunton's frame. Schwartz (2003) further developed her thoughts by delving into the play between social movements in a chapter section called, "A Time of Questioning: Re-evaluating the Direction of the Profession" (p. 9). By addressing the knowledge base of the profession, Schwartz (2003) analyzed the conflict between two paradigms, the founding values or philosophy of OT and the scientific, mechanistic view of the individual. Once again, the history chapter was newly discovered in the opening of the book as the first chapter.

In the 11th edition, Gordon (2009) shifted the focus to include a new view of the emergence of psychotherapy, science, and occupation. Placed as Chapter 21, Gordon's meld of history and science is clear, "The history of occupational therapy itself is also a story of the development of a scientific understanding of occupation" (p. 202). He further states that "the systematic use of occupation was not seen as a continuation of past practice but a truly new endeavor" (p. 205). Gordon's analysis traces current concepts like evidence-based practice as an ideal that resonated with the founding of the profession. This interpretation differs from Schwartz who identified the philosophical values of the founders as different than the scientific and mechanistic framework. This historical debate among different scholars plays out in various editions of the same book.

The 12th edition introduced a new historical writing partnership, led by scholars Christiansen and Haertl (2014) to introduce the key concept that "historical events happen in larger contexts" (p. 10). Using a chronological structure beginning in 1700 until present day, the authors identified a larger worldview of events and seated OT and health care changes into the context. By identifying political, social, and scientific seminal events, the authors presented a historical timeline of change. The extensiveness of the information is noteworthy, and the placement of OT as a part of a greater view is its strength. This chapter was in the first part of the 12th edition, to anchor the introduction of the book.

Occupational therapy history gives insight into professional expansion and maturation as illustrated in successive *Willard & Spackman Occupational Therapy*. Books have documented the history of the profession; anchoring early editions, at times omitted as a formal chapter, relocated to the back or shifted to the front of the book, showing the dilemma of how to place foundational materials in an expanding and futuristic profession.

Expansion of Occupational Therapy Profession: Recurring Motifs

"I didn't realize all the rich resources. It [the book] always gave me a landscape of the profession." (Schell, 2017 oral history, lines 194–195)

As the OT profession expanded, so did the size of *Willard & Spackman's Occupational Therapy*. At times, these researchers questioned whether the book was archiving these changes into written form or if the book translated new approaches, theories, and interventions to practice thereby helping to drive expansion of practice. The series of books capture areas of notable expansion including how OT is practiced and how foundations of practice mature. *Willard & Spackman's Occupational Therapy* books were analyzed for their changes in content, organization, and key themes apparent across the 12 editions.

Occupational therapy has evolved since reconstruction aides practiced in military hospitals and craft teachers facilitated health in state and mental hospitals (Dunton, 1947). Our profession's development narrative is nonlinear, frequently iterative, and always interconnected. We (Martin, Peters, & Mahoney) identified five motifs or themes after analyzing information from all 12 book editions, archived oral histories, oral histories with editors, archival primary and secondary print documents. Resulting themes explained (1) how the definition of OT has evolved; (2) how theorists have organized models to guide OT practice; (3) how professional/clinical reasoning developed; (4) how science has impacted who we are and what we do; and (5) how, more recently, we have grappled with recognizing and addressing diversity within our practice. Each theme is interconnected with others and results in response to the changing historical context of the time. Explanations of each theme follow, asking readers to recognize their interconnectedness despite the linear presentation.

Expanded Definition of Occupational Therapy

Willard & Spackman's Occupational Therapy books archive the evolving definition of OT, effectively transferring current language to practitioners around the world. In 1947, OT was defined in *Principles of Occupational Therapy* as "any activity, mental or physical, medically prescribed, and professionally guided to aid a patient in recovery from disease or injury" (McNary, 1947, p. 10). This definition echoed an earlier 1922 definition,[5] by adding the stipulation that activities be *medically prescribed* and *professionally guided*, documenting OT's alignment with medicine and the desire to be viewed as a professional service. Spackman (1963a) again expanded this definition in the third edition when she wrote, "Occupational therapy is a rehabilitation procedure guided by a qualified occupational therapist who, under medical prescription, uses self-help, manual, creative, recreational and social, educational, pre-vocational and industrial activities to gain from the patient the desired physical function and/or mental response" (p. 2). In this definition, Spackman further medicalized the purpose of OT, adding rehabilitation and the need for therapy to be delivered by skilled therapists to the definition. Eight years later, Spackman (1971a) prominently placed the official 1968 AOTA definition at the beginning of the first page of the fourth edition, "Occupational therapy is the art and science of directing man's response to selected activity to promote and maintain health, to prevent disability, to evaluate behavior and to treat or train patients with physical or psychosocial dysfunction" (Spackman, 1971a, p. 1). This same edition included another definition of OT, written by Gleave (1971), "Occupational therapy is ordered by physicians and administered by registered occupational therapists using work processes and purposeful activities to assist in the improvement, the development and/or the maintenance of mental, social or physical abilities which have been impaired by disease or injury" (p. 33). Gleave prefaced this definition, "A definition of occupational therapy is submitted here for your consideration" suggesting tension regarding how OT was described in the book. Fifth edition (1978) again offered multiple definitions of OT, both definitions originally published by the AOTA, one for the purpose of establishing educational standards (AOTA, 1972) and the other to assist states in obtaining licensure (AOTA, 1977, 1978). Editors positioned the "Occupational Therapy Definition for Purposes of Licensure" in its entirety in the first Appendix to the book (AOTA, 1977, 1978). This placement enabled students and practitioners to readily access the document and demonstrates how the book expanded access to official association documents to students and practitioners. Both definitions expanded the scope of OT beyond medical services to wider ranges of individuals. Five years later, the sixth edition (1983) again favored the AOTA definition for licensure and republished it in Appendix A (AOTA, 1981, 1983, p. 879) where easily retrieved by readers. Of note, the word "occupation" was substituted by "purposeful activity" and expanded to include persons impaired by social structures such as poverty and

culture with more variety of therapy interventions. The 10th edition (2003) marked the next significant expansion when defining OT, incorporating language from the *Occupational Therapy Practice Framework: Domain and Process* (AOTA, 2002). This definition stated, "Occupational therapy is the art and science of helping people do the day-to-day activities that are important and meaningful to their health and well-being through engagement in valued occupations" (Crepeau, Cohn, & Schell, 2003b, p. 28). This definition continued the "art and science" of OT, adding "well-being" while strongly emphasizing the importance of "day-to-day activities" being "meaningful" and "highly valued." The word *occupation* returned to the definition, stating, "The occupation in occupational therapy comes from an older use of the word, meaning people use or 'occupy' their time" (Crepeau et al., 2003b, p. 28). The 12th edition (2014) expanded and validated the currency of the 2003 definition by citing its relationship to two recent professional documents (Schell, Scaffa, Gillen, & Cohn, 2014). Readers can view how OT developed a unique scope of practice defined in meaningful words culturally passed on from one generation of authors to the next.

Expanded Theoretical Approaches

Theory was first introduced by name in the fourth edition (1971), although previous editions alluded to theory in a broad sense. For example, the fourth edition described theoretical approaches to treatment, including psychoanalytic, developmental, interpersonal, milieu, and ego psychological (Gillette, 1971). Early theoretical approaches included psychoanalytic, developmental, sensorimotor, and motor behavior theories not unique to OT. In the late 1970s, when theoretical knowledge in OT expanded, theory filled more pages of text in the fifth edition of *Willard & Spackman's Occupational Therapy*. Theoretical approaches were categorized as developmental, which included sensorimotor and sensory integration, rehabilitative, and occupational behavior (Hopkins & Tiffany, 1978). This structure for theoretical knowledge continued until the eighth edition (1993) when there was a significant expansion to include 11 different theoretical frames of reference including occupation-centered theories, the Model of Human Occupation and Occupational Adaptation (Dutton, Levy, & Simon, 1993). This shift toward occupation in *Willard & Spackman's Occupational Therapy* was consistent with knowledge development at the time. Writing about the history of the profession, Schwartz (2003) noted

> The profession . . . turned its efforts towards promoting occupation-centered theory, research, education and practice. . . . Since the 1980s, the profession has made substantial progress toward developing theoretical models that can guide occupational therapy intervention. (p. 11)

---

[5]Dr. H. A. Pattison presented the following definition for discussion at the 1921 meeting of the National Society for the Promotion of Occupational Therapy: "any activity, mental or physical, definitely prescribed and guided for the distinct purpose of contributing to, and hastening recovery from, disease or injury" (Pattison, 1922, p. 21).

Application of theory to practice and integration of theory into the clinical reasoning process became more explicit in subsequent editions as theory integrated with processes of evaluation and intervention. Current editors recognize the role that *Willard & Spackman's Occupational Therapy* books have played in linking theory to practice. Cohn, co-editor of the 10th and 11th editions and consulting editor to 12th edition, reflected about their effort to properly address theory within the books.

> That was always a very challenging conversation for us because we were looking to represent theories that were well developed. We were constantly trying to determine what kind of theories they were and there were discussions about is it a frame of reference, is it a practice model, is it a theory? . . . We looked at theory from an occupation perspective and then we looked at theories from a learning perspective. (Cohn, 2017 oral history, lines 262–269)

Editors contributed to the theory-building process by selecting which theoretical approaches to include in each edition of the book. They determined the criteria by which theories were sufficiently tested to qualify for entry into the book.

Expanded Professional Reasoning

Professional reasoning, the "process that practitioners use to plan, direct, perform and reflect on client care" (Schell, 2014, p. 384), has changed over the 12 editions of *Willard & Spackman's Occupational Therapy* books. Therapists translate theory to practice when they interpret assessments and implement interventions. The first two editions provided principles for treatment in settings such as general hospitals, mental hospitals, tuberculosis hospitals and sanatoria, children's hospitals, curative and sheltered workshops, home service, and schools for crippled children (McNary, 1947, 1954). At first, books directed therapists to select activities based on the patient's diagnosis. In the 3rd and 4th editions, therapists refined this so that different methods of instruction formed the overarching structure (McNary, 1947, 1954; Spackman, 1963b, 1971b). This changed in the 5th edition when Hopkins and Tiffany (1978) described OT as a problem-solving process using ethical decision making. Ethics continued to ground OT reasoning with ethical dilemmas as examples to guide clinical reasoning in the 9th and 10th editions. In the 9th edition, Schell (1998) named clinical reasoning the "basis for practice" (p. 90), and in the 10th edition, practice was expected to be client centered, occupation centered, and evidence based (Crepeau et al., 2003b). Expert practitioners provided examples of reasoning in the 11th edition, demonstrating the increasing complex and situation-specific nature of professional reasoning.

In the 12th edition, the key components of professional reasoning included research evidence, the client's preferences, and the therapist's experience. Essential components of professional reasoning now included the therapist's experience, including how theory informed expert practice.

Expanded Approach to Diversity

Early editions of *Willard & Spackman's Occupational Therapy* focused on impairments of the person without much direction about how to incorporate the individual's context into therapy. Later editions illustrate how OT expanded its approach to diversity by focusing on the impact of environment and culture on therapy outcomes. As early as 5th edition, readers were exposed to the impact of the environment, including culture and gender, on best practice OT. This edition added the word, "environment" in the glossary as "a composite of all external forces and influences affecting the development and maintenance of the individual" (Hopkins & Smith, 1978, p. 731). The 6th edition added culture as a key factor in the OT process stating, "the need to understand the family and community to which each patient or client belongs" (Hopkins & Tiffany, 1983, p. 93). This edition also introduced concepts of gender identity and gender preference to readers by adding their definitions to the glossary; defining "gender identity" as "the conviction one has about one's gender and its associated role" (Hopkins & Smith, 1983, p. 921) and "gender preference" as "the gender role an individual finds most desirable regardless of compatibility with his/her own core gender identity" (Hopkins & Smith, 1983, p. 921). The 6th edition included a new chapter about human sexuality as an area for functional restoration, and although written from a mainstream heterosexual viewpoint, its presence suggested the profession's openness to previously taboo areas in therapy (Dahl, 1983). In the 8th edition, Mattingly and Beer (1993) introduced the need for collaborative treatment or "the need for the therapist to understand the patient well enough to create a treatment program that the patient values and trusts" (p. 156). This chapter challenged occupational therapists to understand individual differences among their patients in order to provide optimal outcomes. The 9th edition introduced the effect of ethnicity on identity when McGruder (1998) wrote about the importance of using culturally sensitive assessments. Health disparities based on ethnicity were introduced in 10th edition by Sussenberger (2003).

> As the profession of occupational therapy advocates for practice models that are truly client centered and that move away from the institutionalized medical model to community settings and health promotion, it is even more incumbent on us to incorporate and apply knowledge of social, economic, and political factors that affect the health and well-being of people." (p. 108)

In the same edition, editors added xenophobia or "an unreasonable fear or hatred of those different from oneself" to the glossary, again adding words to inform readers about culture and diversity (Spear & Crepeau, 2003, p. 1035). This trend continued in the 11th edition when "homophobia" ("unreasonable fear or hatred of gay or lesbian people," McGruder, 2009, p. 61, 1159) was added to the glossary, providing language to describe the antithesis of cultural sensitivity. By the 12th edition (2014), more pages were devoted to culture, disparity, disability, and diversity than before, including expanded entries to describe different aspects of environment in the glossary. An analysis of the *Willard & Spackman's Occupational Therapy* books over time provides evidence of the expanded depth of understanding in the profession about unique differences of individuals, communities, and populations and the commitment of the editors to introduce language to readers that support this expansion.

Expanded Science

Occupational therapy matured as a profession as its science expanded. From the first two editions (1947, 1954) when Willard and Spackman provoked therapists to prepare themselves to conduct research to the 4 edition (1971) where editors reported increased numbers of authors with advanced degrees, many with PhDs and EdDs. Research, although valued, was tacit and secondary to practice needs for decades and multiple editions of the book. Fish (1947, 1954) cited a need for graduate education and research. In the 3rd edition, editors preferred authors with advanced degrees and research experience to increase the amount and quality of OT research (Willard & Spackman, 1963). Editors Hopkins and Smith reawakened the topic in the fifth edition, when Yerxa (1988) described a new occupational therapist role as consultant and researcher. Promoting opportunity, she stated, "research in OT is in its infancy" (p. 691). Presenting a pioneer spirit of opportunity, therapists answered the call by obtaining advanced degrees, most often in other fields of studies, with limited doctoral options in the 1970s and 1980s in OT (Peters, 2013). Yerxa (1983, 1988), continuing her momentum in the sixth and seventh editions, made a call for self-directed career researchers. Neistadt and Crepeau (1998) added "research notes" throughout the book to inform readers of the "research challenges for our profession" (p. xiii). Then, the 10th edition integrated research with clinical reasoning more explicitly (Crepeau et al., 2003b). These later editions emphasized evidence-based practice over the role of researcher who discovers new knowledge (Schell, Scaffa, et al., 2014).

Occupational science was first mentioned in *Willard & Spackman's Occupational Therapy* 11th edition (1983) in a chapter about OT research. Elizabeth Yerxa promoted descriptive research as a way to increase OT and stated,

"These descriptions would contribute knowledge not only to occupational therapy but to a science of human occupation" (Yerxa, 1983, p. 872). Yerxa is credited with conceptualizing occupational science, and her chapters about research in 1983 and 1988 called for the development of this new science. In the 8th edition, Clark and Larson (1993) wrote a chapter that explained the existence of occupational science as a discipline separate from OT. This chapter exposed occupational science to future and current OT practitioners. The 8th to 10th editions situated occupational science strongly linking ideas to the founding of OT. Occupational science grew to include the construct, occupational justice, which rapidly spread to international audiences. The 11th edition (2009) added a new chapter, written by Australian occupational scientists, Wilcock and Townsend (2009), about occupational justice, a construct from occupational science. Expanding international scholarship of occupational science, the editors invited authors from New Zealand to write the occupational science chapter in the 12th edition (Wright-St. Clair & Hocking, 2014).

This quest for an expanding science started when Willard and Spackman (1947, 1954) rallied young researchers to become autonomous researchers. Since then, some have chosen new vistas like Occupational Science, whereas others remain steadfast to building on OT's early footings.

Conclusion

A panoramic overview of 13 editions of *Willard & Spackman's Occupational Therapy* is spectacular if not daunting. The collective work came with professional sacrifices and a determinism to deliver a lasting addition to the literature. Responding to the call and reflecting a pool of the profession's elite, 29 of 56 (52%) AOTA Eleanor Clarke Slagle lecturers and 37 of 80 (46%) AOTA Award of Merit recipients, including 17 of 26 (65%) combined AOTA Slagle and Merit combined awardees, contributed to the book since its earliest printings. Gillen, a *Willard & Spackman's Occupational Therapy* editor and 2013 Slagle recipient, called the book the "voice of OT."

> The textbook was pretty consistent in editions 1, 2 and 3, the voice of OT and what OT should look like. What OT outcomes should be. I think things started to change in editions 4, 5 and 6 when we were grappling with how sophisticated we were or were not. We were trying to make connections with too many other fields that seemed more scientific. We started to see a loss of the flavor of occupational therapy in certain practice areas. . . . There was a clear shift in terms of not just putting occupation on the back burner, almost not even considering it. . . . I think things started to go back for the better when Betty Crepeau [ninth edition] came on board and things started to shift back. (Gillen, 2017 oral history, lines 133–144)

This historical examination presented a synopsis of the book from the first edition and how it began with a closer look at its namesake editors, Helen Willard and Clare Spackman. Building on their foundation, subsequent editors moved the book forward, similar to passing a torch against trying times. A progression through OT analyzed how OT was presented in the book. As OT grew, the breadth and depth of information in the book expanded. Key elements included a discussion of how OT was defined and changes in OT's knowledge regarding reasoning, theory, science, and culture.

After reviewing this analysis of 13 editions of *Willard & Spackman's Occupational Therapy*, we challenge the reader to contemplate, did the book lead or reflect change in occupational therapy? As you consider your answer to this complex question, know that the answer was debated by editors, "I believe it drove practice because there were really not any specialty textbooks that people were using" (Gillen, 2017 oral history, lines 158–159). "I think we were trying to promote new ideas in the profession, not to create those new ideas necessarily" (Crepeau, 2017 oral history, lines 399–400). Making a case for leading the profession and reflecting, Schell added, "A little bit of both. I think the international perspective, the diversity . . . the book leads by kind of a non-controversial way" (Schell, 2017 oral history, lines 475–478).

What remains relevant above all is how one book captured a profession, withstood the test of time, and remained a staple on many OT bookshelves around the world.

ORAL HISTORIES

Cohn, E. S. (2017). *An oral history with Ellen S. Cohn/Interviewers: Christine O. Peters & Wanda J. Mahoney.*

Crepeau, E. B. (2017). *An oral history with Elizabeth B. Crepeau/Interviewers: Christine O. Peters & Wanda J. Mahoney.*

Cynkin, S. (1996). *An oral history with Simme Cynkin/Interviewer: Rosalie J. Miller.*

Gillen, G. (2017). *An oral history with Glen Gillen/Interviewers: Christine O. Peters & Wanda J. Mahoney.*

Schell, B. A. B. (2017). *An oral history with Barbara Boyt Schell/Interviewers: Christine O. Peters & Wanda J. Mahoney.*

REFERENCES

American Occupational Therapy Association. (1962). *The occupational therapy yearbook 1962.* New York, NY: Author.

American Occupational Therapy Association. (1972). Occupational therapy: Its definition and functions. *American Journal of Occupational Therapy, 26,* 204–205.

American Occupational Therapy Association. (1977, 1978). Occupational therapy definition for purposes of licensure. In H. L. Hopkins & H. D. Smith (Eds.), *Willard & Spackman's occupational therapy* (5th ed., p. 707). Philadelphia, PA: J. B. Lippincott Company.

American Occupational Therapy Association. (1981, 1983). Occupational therapy definition for purposes of licensure. In H. L. Hopkins & H. D. Smith (Eds.), *Willard & Spackman's occupational therapy* (6th ed., p. 879). Philadelphia, PA: J. B. Lippincott Company.

American Occupational Therapy Association. (2002). Occupational therapy practice framework: Domain and process. *American Journal of Occupational Therapy, 56,* 609–639. doi:10.5014/ajot.56.6.609

American Occupational Therapy Association. (2017). *Important events: 1968.* Retrieved from http://www.otcentennial.org/100-events/1968

Barzun, J., & Graff, H. (1970). *The modern researcher: The classic manual on all aspects of research and writing* (Rev. ed.). New York, NY: Harcourt, Brace & World.

Christiansen, C. H., & Haertl, K. (2014). A contextual history of occupational therapy. In B. A. B. Schell, G. Gillen, M. E. Scaffa, & E. S. Cohn (Eds.), *Willard & Spackman's occupational therapy* (12th ed., pp. 9–34). Philadelphia, PA: Lippincott Williams & Wilkins.

Clark, F., & Larson, E. A. (1993). Developing an academic discipline: The science of occupation. In H. L. Hopkins & H. D. Smith (Eds.), *Willard & Spackman's occupational therapy* (8th ed., pp. 44–57). Philadelphia, PA: J. B. Lippincott Company.

Crepeau, E. B., Cohn, E. S., & Schell, B. A. B. (2003a). Acknowledgments. In E. B. Crepeau, E. S. Cohn, & B. A. B. Schell (Eds.), *Willard & Spackman's occupational therapy* (10th ed., pp. xvii–xix). Philadelphia, PA: Lippincott Williams & Wilkins.

Crepeau, E. B., Cohn, E. S., & Schell, B. A. B. (2003b). Occupational therapy practice: Occupational therapy practice today. In E. B. Crepeau, E. S. Cohn, & B. A. B. Schell (Eds.), *Willard & Spackman's occupational therapy* (10th ed., pp. 27–29). Philadelphia, PA: Lippincott Williams & Wilkins.

Crepeau, E. B., Cohn, E. S., & Schell, B. A. B. (2009). Dedication. In E. B. Crepeau, E. S. Cohn, & B. A. B. Schell (Eds.), *Willard & Spackman's occupational therapy* (11th ed., p. vii). Philadelphia, PA: Lippincott Williams & Wilkins.

Dahl, M. R. (1983). Functional restoration: Human sexuality. In H. L. Hopkins & H. D. Smith (Eds.), *Willard & Spackman's occupational therapy* (6th ed., pp. 447–460). Philadelphia, PA: J. B. Lippincott Company.

Dunton, W. R. (1947). History and development of occupational therapy. In H. S. Willard & C. S. Spackman (Eds.), *Principles of occupational therapy* (pp. 1–9). Philadelphia, PA: J. B. Lippincott Company.

Dutton, R., Levy, L. L., & Simon, C. J. (1993). Current basis for theory and philosophy of occupational therapy: Occupational therapy: Introduction. In H. L. Hopkins & H. D. Smith (Eds.), *Willard & Spackman's occupational therapy* (8th ed., pp. 62–63). Philadelphia, PA: J. B. Lippincott Company.

Fish, M. (1947). Educational aims in occupational therapy. In H. S. Willard & C. S. Spackman (Eds.), *Principles of occupational therapy* (pp. 23–39). Philadelphia, PA: J. B. Lippincott Company.

Fish, M. (1954). Educational aims in occupational therapy. In H. S. Willard & C. S. Spackman (Eds.), *Principles of occupational therapy* (2nd ed., pp. 24–42). Philadelphia, PA: J. B. Lippincott Company.

Gillette, N. P. (1971). Occupational therapy and mental health. In H. S. Willard & C. S. Spackman (Eds.), *Occupational therapy* (4th ed., pp. 51–132). Philadelphia, PA: J. B. Lippincott Company.

Gleave, G. M. (1971). Medical records and reports. In H. S. Willard & C. S. Spackman (Eds.), *Occupational therapy* (4th ed., pp. 31–42). Philadelphia, PA: J. B. Lippincott Company.

Gordon, D. M. (2009). The history of occupational therapy. In E. B. Crepeau, E. S. Cohn, & B. A. B. Schell (Eds.), *Willard & Spackman's occupational therapy* (11th ed., pp. 202–215). Philadelphia, PA: Lippincott Williams & Wilkins.

Gottschalk, L. (1969). *Understanding history: A primer of historical method* (2nd ed.). New York, NY: Knopf.

Hopkins, H. L. (1978). An historical perspective on occupational therapy. In H. L. Hopkins & H. D. Smith (Eds.), *Willard & Spackman's occupational therapy* (5th ed., pp. 1–24). Philadelphia, PA: J. B. Lippincott Company.

Hopkins, H. L. (1983). An historical perspective on occupational therapy. In H. L. Hopkins & H. D. Smith (Eds.), *Willard & Spackman's occupational therapy* (6th ed., pp. 3–23). Philadelphia, PA: J. B. Lippincott Company.

Hopkins, H. L., & Smith, H. D. (Eds.). (1978). Glossary. In *Willard & Spackman's occupational therapy* (5th ed., pp. 727–740). Philadelphia, PA: J. B. Lippincott Company.

Hopkins, H. L., & Smith, H. D. (Eds.). (1983). Glossary. In *Willard & Spackman's occupational therapy* (6th ed., pp. 915–930). Philadelphia, PA: J. B. Lippincott Company.

Hopkins, H. L., & Tiffany, E. G. (1978). Occupational therapy: A problem solving process. In H. L. Hopkins & H. D. Smith (Eds.), *Willard & Spackman's occupational therapy* (5th ed., pp. 109–122). Philadelphia, PA: J. B. Lippincott Company.

Hopkins, H.L., & Tiffany, E.G. (1983). Occupational therapy: A problem solving process. In H. L. Hopkins & H. D. Smith (Eds.), *Willard & Spackman's occupational therapy* (6th ed., pp. 89–105). Philadelphia, PA: J. B. Lippincott Company.

Mahoney, W. J., Peters, C. O., & Martin, P. M. (2017). Willard and Spackman's enduring legacy for future occupational therapy pathways. *American Journal of Occupational Therapy, 71,* 7101100020p1–7101100020p7. doi:10.5014/ ajot.2017.023994

Mattingly, C., & Beer, D. W. (1993). Interpreting culture in a therapeutic context. In H. L. Hopkins & H. D. Smith (Eds.), *Willard & Spackman's occupational therapy* (8th ed., pp. 154–161). Philadelphia, PA: J. B. Lippincott Company.

McGruder, J. (1998). Culture and other forms of human diversity in occupational therapy. In M. Neistadt & E. B. Crepeau (Eds.), *Willard & Spackman's occupational therapy* (9th ed., pp. 54–66). Philadelphia, PA: Lippincott-Raven Publishers.

McGruder, J. (2009). Culture, race, ethnicity, and other forms of human diversity in occupational therapy. In E. B. Crepeau, E. Cohn, & B. A. B. Schell (Eds.), *Willard & Spackman's occupational therapy* (11th ed., pp. 55–67). Philadelphia, PA: Lippincott, Williams & Wilkins.

McNary, H. (1947). The scope of occupational therapy. In H. S. Willard & C. S. Spackman (Eds.), *Principles of occupational therapy* (pp. 10–19). Philadelphia, PA: J. B. Lippincott Company.

McNary, H. (1954). The scope of occupational therapy. In H. S. Willard & C. S. Spackman (Eds.), *Principles of occupational therapy* (2nd ed., pp. 11–23). Philadelphia, PA: J. B. Lippincott Company.

Mendez, M. A. (1986). *A chronicle of the World Federation of Occupational Therapists, Part one, 1952-1982.* Jerusalem, Israel: World Federation of Occupational Therapists.

National Board for Certification in Occupational Therapy. (2016a). *COTA® curriculum textbook and peer-reviewed journal report.* Gaithersburg, MD: Author. Retrieved from https://www.nbcot.org/-/media/NBCOT /PDFs/2016-COTA-Curriculum-Textbook-Journal-Report.ashx?la=en

National Board for Certification in Occupational Therapy. (2016b). *OTR® curriculum textbook and peer-reviewed journal report.* Gaithersburg, MD: Author. Retrieved from https://www.nbcot.org/-/media /NBCOT/PDFs/2016-OTR-Curriculum-Textbook-Journal-Report .ashx?la=en

Neistadt, M. E., & Crepeau, E. B. (1998). Preface. In M. E. Neistadt & E. B. Crepeau (Eds.), *Willard & Spackman's occupational therapy* (9th ed., p. xiii). Philadelphia, PA: Lippincott.

Pattison, H. A. (1922). The trend of occupational therapy for the tuberculous. *Archives of Occupational Therapy, 1*(1), 19–24.

Peters, C. O. (2013). *Powerful occupational therapists: A community of therapists, 1950–1980.* New York, NY: Routledge.

Peters, C. O., Martin, P. M., & Mahoney, W. J. (2017). The Philadelphia School of Occupational Therapy: A centennial lesson. *Journal of Occupational Therapy Education, 1*(1), 1–18. doi:10.26681/ jote.2017.010108

Reed, K. L. (1993). The beginnings of occupational therapy. In H. L. Hopkins & H. D. Smith (Eds.), *Willard & Spackman's*

occupational therapy (8th ed., pp. 26–43). Philadelphia, PA: J. B. Lippincott Company.

Schell, B. A. B. (1998). Clinical reasoning: The basis of practice. In M. E. Neistadt & E. B. Crepeau (Eds.), *Willard & Spackman's occupational therapy* (9th ed., pp. 90–102). Philadelphia, PA: Lippincott Williams & Wilkins.

Schell, B. A. B. (2014). Professional reasoning in practice. In B. A. B. Schell, G. Gillen, M. E. Scaffa, & E. S. Cohn (Eds.), *Willard & Spackman's occupational therapy* (12th ed., pp. 384–397). Philadelphia, PA: Lippincott Williams & Wilkins.

Schell, B. A. B., Gillen, G., Scaffa, M. E., & Cohn, E. S. (2014). Dedication. In B. A. B. Schell, G. Gillen, M. E. Scaffa, & E. S. Cohn (Eds.), *Willard & Spackman's occupational therapy* (12th ed., p. v). Philadelphia, PA: Lippincott Williams & Wilkins.

Schell, B. A. B., Scaffa, M. E., Gillen, G., & Cohn, E. (2014). Contemporary occupational therapy practice. In B. A. B. Schell, G. Gillen, M. E. Schaffa, & E. S. Cohn (Eds.), *Willard & Spackman's occupational therapy* (12th ed., pp. 47–58). Philadelphia, PA: Lippincott Williams & Wilkins.

Schwartz, K. B. (1998). The history of occupational therapy. In M. E. Neistadt & E. B. Crepeau (Eds.), *Willard & Spackman's occupational therapy* (9th ed., pp. 854–860). Philadelphia, PA: Lippincott Williams & Wilkins.

Schwartz, K. B. (2003). The history of occupational therapy. In E. B. Crepeau, E. S. Cohn, & B. A. B. Schell (Eds.), *Willard & Spackman's occupational therapy* (10th ed., pp. 5–14). Philadelphia, PA: Lippincott Williams & Wilkins.

Spackman, C. S. (1963a). Co-ordination of occupational therapy with other allied medical and related services. In H. S. Willard & C. S. Spackman (Eds.), *Occupational therapy* (3rd ed., pp. 1–14). Philadelphia, PA: J. B. Lippincott Company.

Spackman, C. S. (1963b). Methods of instruction. In H. S. Willard & C. S. Spackman (Eds.), *Occupational therapy* (3rd ed., pp. 46–54). Philadelphia, PA: J. B. Lippincott Company.

Spackman, C. S. (1971a). Coordination of occupational therapy with other allied medical and related services. In H. S. Willard & C. S. Spackman (Eds.), *Occupational therapy* (4th ed., pp. 1–12). Philadelphia, PA: J. B. Lippincott Company.

Spackman, C. S. (1971b). Methods of instruction. In H. S. Willard & C. S. Spackman (Eds.), *Occupational therapy* (4th ed., pp. 43–50). Philadelphia, PA: J. B. Lippincott Company.

Spackman, C. S. (1975). Curriculum vitae. In *American Occupational Therapy Association Archives (Box 118, Folder 939).* Bethesda, MD: Wilma West Library.

Spackman, C. S., & Willard, H. S. (1978). Foreword. In H. L. Hopkins & H. D. Smith (Eds.), *Willard & Spackman's occupational therapy* (5th ed., p. xi). Philadelphia: J. B. Lippincott Company.

Spear, P. S., & Crepeau, E. B. (2003). Glossary. In E. B. Crepeau, E. S. Cohn, & B. A. B. Schell (Eds.), *Willard & Spackman's occupational therapy* (10th ed., pp. 1025–1035). Philadelphia, PA: Lippincott Williams & Wilkins.

Stewart, H. E. (1920). *Physical reconstruction and orthopedics.* New York, NY: Paul B. Hoeber.

Sussenberger, B. (2003). Socioeconomic factors and their influence on occupational performance. In E. B. Crepeau, E. Cohn, & B. A. B. Schell (Eds.), *Willard & Spackman's occupational therapy* (10th ed., pp. 97–109). Philadelphia, PA: Lippincott Williams & Wilkins.

Vartabedian, T. (2000, October 4). Dr. Maureen E. Purcell Neistadt: She restored many to health, dies at 49. *Haverhill Gazette.* Retrieved from https://www.findagrave.com/memorial/40633716/neistadt

Wilcock, A. A., & Townsend, E. A. (2009). Occupational justice. In E. B. Crepeau, E. S. Cohn, & B. A. B. Schell (Eds.), *Willard & Spackman's occupational therapy* (11th ed., pp. 192–200). Philadelphia, PA: Lippincott Williams & Wilkins.

Willard, H. S. (1975). Curriculum vitae. In *American Occupational Therapy Association Archives (Box 118, Folder 952)*. Bethesda, MD: Wilma West Library.

Willard, H. S. (1977). *Interview by B. Cox* [Video recording]. Bethesda, MD: American Occupational Therapy Association Archives, Wilma West Library.

Willard, H. S., & Spackman, C. S. (1947). Preface. In H. S. Willard & C. S. Spackman (Eds.), *Principles of occupational therapy* (pp. vii–viii). Philadelphia, PA: J. B. Lippincott Company.

Willard, H. S., & Spackman, C. S. (1954). Preface. In H. S. Willard & C. S. Spackman (Eds.), *Principles of occupational therapy* (2nd ed., pp. vii–viii). Philadelphia, PA: J. B. Lippincott Company.

Willard, H. S., & Spackman, C. S. (1963). Preface to the third edition. In H. S. Willard & C. S. Spackman (Eds.), *Occupational therapy* (3rd ed., pp. v–vii). Philadelphia, PA: J. B. Lippincott Company.

Willard, H. S., & Spackman, C. S. (1971). Preface. In H. S. Willard & C. S. Spackman (Eds.), *Occupational therapy* (4th ed., pp. v–vi). Philadelphia, PA: J. B. Lippincott Company.

Willard, H. S., & Spackman, C. S. (1977). *Interview by R. Brunyate Wiemer & B. Cox* [Video recording]. Bethesda, MD: American Occupational Therapy Association Archives, Wilma West Library.

Wright-St. Clair, V. A., & Hocking, C. (2014). Occupational science: The study of occupation. In B. A. B. Schell, G. Gillen, M. E. Scaffa, & E. S. Cohn (Eds.), *Willard & Spackman's occupational therapy* (12th ed., pp. 82–94). Philadelphia, PA: Lippincott Williams & Wilkins.

Yerxa, E. J. (1978). The occupational therapist as consultant and researcher. In H. L. Hopkins & H. D. Smith (Eds.), *Willard & Spackman's occupational therapy* (5th ed., pp. 689–694). Philadelphia, PA: J. B. Lippincott Company.

Yerxa, E. J. (1983). The occupational therapist as a researcher. In H. L. Hopkins & H. D. Smith (Eds.), *Willard & Spackman's occupational therapy* (6th ed., pp. 869–876). Philadelphia, PA: J. B. Lippincott Company.

Yerxa, E. J. (1988). Research in occupational therapy. In H. L. Hopkins & H. D. Smith (Eds.), *Willard & Spackman's occupational therapy* (7th ed., pp. 171–177). Philadelphia, PA: J. B. Lippincott Company.

Occupation Therapy: Profile of the Profession

Meditation on a Calling

To know what a calling truly is
you must discover its soul.
You must see those it has touched
— meet the people who have looked it in the eyes
and trusted in its possibilities.

To fully know what *this* calling is about
you must feel the deep emptiness of not doing,
of unfilled roles, abandoned goals and lost identities.
You must experience the indignities of pity—
how children stare, keenly aware of difference,
how others, more perfect, are offered work.

To be rightly immersed in this calling
you must learn the hymns of its language.
Let the words become notes that inspire you
to occupy fully the landscape its lyrics describe,
and explore its farthest boundaries with those you serve.

Only then can you begin to comprehend its fullness,
to appreciate why strangers once gathered near waters
to unify their vision in the service of others.
Only then can you grasp why their shared ideas endured
despite wars, rivalries and the seductions of simplicity.

Those with shattered bodies and minds appeared.
They came from great battles and daily calamities.
They sought healers with insights and ways for living
who grasped the truth that meaning arises from doing.

You have fully fathomed the depth of this calling
when your understanding starts with each story;
when participation is perceived as a primal need;
and when you recognize that therapy of value is alchemy
that melds science with imagination to enable hope.

Dedicated to the memory of my friend and colleague Gary Kielhofner (1949-2010).

—Charles Christiansen
March, 2017
Used with permission of the author.

What Is Occupation?

Khalilah Robinson Johnson, Virginia Dickie

"MR. JOURDAIN. You mean to say that when I say, 'Nicole, fetch me my slippers' or 'Give me my nightcap' that's prose?
PHILOSOPHER. Certainly, sir.
MR. JOURDAIN. Well, my goodness! Here I've been talking prose for forty years and never known it. . . . "

—MOLIERE (1670)

LEARNING OBJECTIVES

After reading this chapter, you will be able to:

1. Identify and evaluate ways of knowing occupation.
2. Articulate different ways of defining and classifying occupation.
3. Describe the relationship between occupation and context.

Knowing and Learning about Occupation

In the myriad of activities people do every day, they engage in **occupations** all their lives, perhaps without ever knowing it. Many occupations are ordinary and become part of the **context** of daily living. Such occupations are generally taken for granted, and most often are habitual (Aarts & Dijksterhuis, 2000; Bargh & Chartrand, 1999; Wood, Quinn, & Kashy, 2002). Reading blogs, washing hands, gaming on the Internet, walking through a colorful market in a foreign country, and telling a story (in poetry or prose) are occupations people do without ever thinking about them as being occupations.

Occupations are ordinary, but they can also be special when they represent a new achievement such as driving a car or when they are part of celebrations and rites of passage. Preparing and hosting a holiday dinner for the first time and baking the pies for the annual family holiday for the twentieth time are examples of special occupations. Occupations tend to be special when they happen infrequently and carry symbolic meanings such as representing achievement of adulthood or one's love for family. Occupations are also special when they form part of a treasured routine such as reading a bedtime story to one's child, singing "Twinkle, Twinkle, Little Star," and tucking the covers around the small, sleepy body. But even special occupations, although heavy with tradition, may change over time. Hocking, Wright-St. Clair, and

Bunrayong (2002) illustrated the complexity of traditional occupations in their study of holiday food preparation by older women in Thailand and New Zealand. The study identified many similarities between the groups (such as the activities the authors named "recipe work"), but the Thai women valued maintenance of an invariant tradition in what they prepared and how they did it, whereas the New Zealand women changed the foods they prepared over time and expected such changes to continue. Nevertheless, the doing of food-centered occupations around holidays was a tradition for both groups.

To be human is to be occupational. Occupation is a biological imperative, evident in the evolutionary history of humankind, the current behaviors of our primate relatives, and the survival needs that must be met through doing (Clark, 1997; Krishnagiri, 2000; Wilcock, 2006; Wood, 1998). Fromm (as cited by Reilly, 1962) asserted that people have a "physiologically conditioned need" to work as an act of self-preservation (p. 4). Humans also have occupational needs beyond survival. Addressing one type of occupation, Dissanayake (1992, 1995) argued that making art, or, as she describes it, "making special," is a biological necessity of human existence. According to Molineux (2004), occupational therapists now understand humans, their function, and their therapeutic needs in an occupational manner in which *occupation is life itself* [emphasis added]. Townsend (1997) described occupation as the "active process of living: from the beginning to the end of life, our occupations are all the active processes of looking after ourselves and others, enjoying life, and being socially and economically productive over the lifespan and in various contexts" (p. 19).

The Need to Understand Occupation

Occupational therapy (OT) practitioners need to base their work on a thorough understanding of occupation and its role in health and survival. That is, OT practitioners should understand what people need or are obligated to do in order to survive and achieve health and well-being. Wilcock (2007) affirmed that this level of understanding includes how people feel about occupation, how it affects their development, the societal mechanisms through which that development occurs, and how that process is understood. Achieving that understanding of occupation is more than having an easy definition (which is a daunting challenge in its own right). To know what occupation is, it is necessary to examine what humans do with their time, how such activities are organized, what purposes they serve, and what they mean for individuals and society.

Personal experience of doing occupation, whether consciously attended to or not, provides a fundamental understanding of occupation—what it is, how it happens, what it means, what is good about it, and what is not. This way of knowing is both basic and extraordinarily rich. It is the way we learn to participate in the social worlds we inhabit.

Looking Inward to Know Occupation

To be useful to OT practitioners, knowledge of occupation based on personal experience demands examination and reflection. What do we do, how do we do it, when and where does it take place, and what does it mean? Who else is involved directly and indirectly? What capacities does it require in us? What does it cost? Is it challenging or easy? How has this occupation changed over time? What would it be like if we no longer had this occupation? To illustrate, Khalilah (first author) shares her experiences with cooking as she transitioned from home to college (Case Study 1-1).

Between college and the beginning of Khalilah's postgraduate career, cooking took on a different *form* (the need to prepare meals for herself as an independent adult), *function* (family-style meals were no longer reserved for times with family and friends but became a means to forge relationships with strangers), and *meaning* (a way to bridge and create new cultural experiences with her family and friends). These elements—the form, function, and meaning of occupation—are the basic areas of focus for the science of occupation (Larson, Wood, & Clark, 2003).

Khalilah's cooking and communal mealtime example described in Case Study 1-1 illustrates how occupation is a *transaction* with the *environment* or *context* of other people and cultures, places, and tools. It includes the *temporal* nature of occupation—seasonal travel to particular destinations and the availability of specific ingredients based on the season of travel. That she calls herself a cook exemplifies how occupation has become part of her *identity* and suggests that it might be difficult for her to give up cooking.

Basic as it is, however, understanding derived from personal experience is insufficient as the basis for practice. Reliance solely on this source of knowledge has the risk of expecting everyone to experience occupation in the same manner as the therapist. So, although OT practitioners will profit in being attuned to their own occupations, they must also turn their view to the occupation around them and to understanding occupation through study and research.

Looking Outward to Know Occupation

Observation of the world through an occupational lens is another rich source of **occupational knowledge**.

CASE STUDY 1-1 COOKING "SOUTHERN" AT COLLEGE

My first real attempt at cooking a meal independently was my freshman year of college. My dorm had a full kitchen, and I, like many college students, loathed dining hall dinners. I had grown up in a home where my parents prepared dinner nightly and we ate together as a family. My grandparents cooked dinner for our extended family every Sunday, and as Southern culture would suggest, I learned the proper way to braise vegetables, season and smoke meat and fish, concoct gravies, and bake an array of casseroles prior to graduating high school. Meal preparation and meal execution generally adhere to rules and techniques according to the macro culture, local or home culture of the person(s) performing it. Going to college required that I translate that cultural knowledge and adapt those rules to my new environment, understanding that the same products and tools to which I was accustomed would not be available. To build community, I began to cook traditional Southern meals in several kitchens around campus, taking up new ideas and techniques as I "broke bread" with other students. It was not until I received recognition from my peers that I considered myself a true Southern cook. Since that time, I have taken my love of cooking to international spaces, where I learn to prepare traditional meals of the native culture in a local person's home (Figure 1-1).

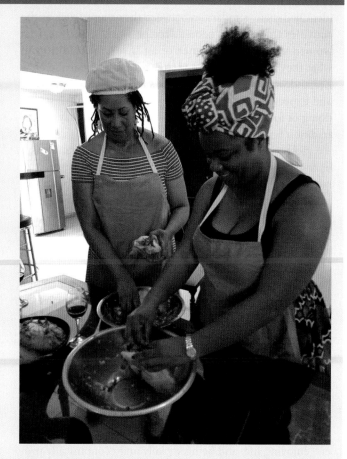

FIGURE 1-1 **Khalilah (on the right) preparing fish.**

Connoisseurs of occupation can train themselves to new ways of seeing a world rich with occupations: the way a restaurant hostess manages a crowd when the wait for seating is long, the economy of movement of a construction worker doing a repetitive task, the activities of musicians in the orchestra pit when they are not playing, the almost aimless tossing of a ball as students take a break from class, texting while engaging in social situations. Furthermore, people like to talk about what they do, and the scholar of occupation can learn a great deal by asking for information about people's work and play. By being observant and asking questions, people increase their repertoire of occupational knowledge far beyond the boundaries of personal interests, practices, and capabilities.

Observation of others' occupations enriches the OT practitioner's knowledge of the range of **occupational possibilities** and of human responses to occupational opportunities. But although this sort of knowledge goes far beyond the limits of personal experience, it is still bounded

by the world any one person is able to access, and it lacks the depth of knowledge that is developed through research and scholarship.

Turning to Research and Scholarship to Understand Occupation

Knowledge of occupation that comes from personal experience and observation must be augmented with the understanding of occupation drawn from research in OT and occupational science as well as other disciplines. Hocking (2000) developed a framework of needed knowledge for research in occupation, organized into the categories of the "essential elements of occupation . . . occupational processes . . . [and the] relationship of occupation to other phenomena" (p. 59). This research is being done within OT and occupational science, but there is also a wealth of information to be found in the work of other disciplines. For example, in anthropology, Orr (1996) studied the work of copy machine repairmen, and Downey (1998) studied computer engineers and what they did. Consumer researchers have studied Christmas shopping (Sherry & McGrath, 1989), motorcycle riding (Schouten & McAlexander, 1995), and many other occupations of consumption. Psychologists have studied habits (Aarts & Dijksterhuis, 2000; Bargh & Chartrand, 1999; Wood et al., 2002) and a wealth of other topics that relate to how people engage in occupation. Understanding of occupation will benefit from more research within OT and occupational science and from accessing relevant works of scholars in other fields. Hocking (2009) has called for more occupational science research focused on occupations themselves rather than people's experiences of occupations.

Defining Occupation

For many years, the word *occupation* was not part of the daily language of occupational therapists, nor was it prominent in the profession's literature (Hinojosa, Kramer, Royeen, & Luebben, 2003). According to Kielhofner and Burke (1977), the founding paradigm of OT was occupation, and the occupational perspective focused on people and their health "in the context of the culture of daily living and its activities" (p. 688). But beginning in the 1930s, OT strove to become more like the medical profession, entering into a paradigm of reductionism that lasted into the 1970s. During that time, occupation, both as a concept and as a means and/or outcome of intervention, was essentially absent from professional discourse. With time, a few professional leaders began to call for OT to return to its roots in occupation (Schwartz, 2003), and since the 1970s, acceptance of occupation as the foundation of OT has grown (Kielhofner, 2009). With that growth, professional debates about the definition and nature of occupation emerged and continue to this day.

Defining occupation in OT is challenging because the word is part of common language with meanings that the profession cannot control. The term *occupation* and related concepts such as *activity*, *task*, *employment*, *doing*, and *work* are used in many ways within OT. It seems quite logical to think of a job, cleaning house, or bike riding as an occupation, but the concept is fuzzier when we think about the smaller components of these larger categories. Is dusting an occupation, or is it part of the occupation of house cleaning? Is riding a bike a skill that is part of some larger occupation such as physical conditioning or getting from home to school, or

is it an occupation in its own right? Does this change over time?

The founders of OT used the word *occupation* to describe a way of "properly" using time that included work and work-like activities and recreational activities (Meyer, 1922). Breines (1995) pointed out that the founders chose a term that was both ambiguous and comprehensive to name the profession, a choice, she argued, that was not accidental. The term was open to holistic interpretations that supported the diverse areas of practice of the time, encompassing the elements of occupation defined by Breines (1995) as "mind, body, time, space, and others" (p. 459). The term *occupation* spawned ongoing examination, controversy, and redefinition as the profession has matured.

Nelson (1988, 1997) introduced the terms **occupational form**, "the preexisting structure that elicits, guides, or structures subsequent human performance," and **occupational performance**, "the human actions taken in response to an occupational form" (Nelson, 1988, p. 633). This distinction separates individuals and their actual doing of occupations from the general notion of an occupation and what it requires of anyone who does it.

Yerxa et al. (1989) defined occupation as "specific 'chunks' of activity within the ongoing stream of human behavior which are named in the lexicon of the culture. . . . These daily pursuits are self-initiated, goal-directed (purposeful), and socially sanctioned" (p. 5). Yerxa (1993) further elaborated this definition to incorporate an environmental perspective and a greater breadth of characteristics. She stated,

> Occupations are units of activity which are classified and named by the culture according to the purposes they serve in enabling people to meet environmental challenges successfully. . . . Some essential characteristics of occupation are that it is self-initiated, goal-directed (even if the goal is fun or pleasure), experiential as well as behavioral, socially valued or recognized, constituted of adaptive skills or repertoires, organized, essential to the quality of life experienced, and possesses the capacity to influence health. (Yerxa, 1993, p. 5)

According to the Canadian Association of Occupational Therapists (as cited in Law, Steinwender, & Leclair, 1998), occupation is "groups of activities and tasks of everyday life, named, organized and given value and meaning by individuals and a culture." In a somewhat circular definition, they went on to state "occupation is everything people do to occupy themselves, including looking after themselves (self-care), enjoying life (leisure), and contributing to the social and economic fabric of their communities (productivity)" (p. 83). More recently, occupational scientists Larson et al. (2003) provided a simple definition of occupation as "the activities that comprise our life experience and can be named in the culture" (p. 16). Similarly, after referencing a number of different definitions of occupation, the Occupational Therapy Practice Framework concluded with the statement that "the term *occupation*, as it is used in the *Framework*, refers to the daily life activities in which people engage (American Occupational Therapy Association [AOTA], 2014, p. S6). The previous definitions of occupation from OT literature help in explaining why occupation is the profession's focus (particularly in the context of therapy), yet they are open enough to allow continuing research on the nature of occupation. Despite, and perhaps because of, the ubiquity of occupation in human life, there is still much to learn about the nature of occupation through systematic research using an array of methodologies (e.g., Aldrich, Rudman, & Dickie, 2017; Dickie, 2010; Hocking, 2000, 2009; Johnson & Bagatell, 2017; Molke, Laliberte-Rudman, & Polatajko, 2004). Such research should include examination of the premises that are built into the accepted definitions of occupation.

At a more theoretical level, such an examination has begun. Several authors have recently challenged the unexamined assumptions and beliefs about occupation of Western occupational therapists (cf. Hammell, 2009a, 2009b, Iwama, 2006; Kantartzis & Molineux, 2011).

These critiques center on the Western cultural bias in the definition and use of occupation and the inadequacy of the conceptualization of occupation as it is used in OT in Western countries to describe the daily activities of most of the world's population. Attention to these arguments will strengthen our knowledge of occupation.

Context and Occupation

The photograph of the two young boys playing in the garden sprinkler evokes a sense of a hot summer day and the experience of icy cold water coming out of the sprinkler, striking, and stinging the boys' faces (Figure 1-2). Playing in the sprinkler has a context with temporal elements (summer, the play of children, and the viewer's memories of doing it in the past), a physical environment (grass, hot weather, hose, sprinkler, cold water), and a social environment (a pair of children and the likelihood of an indulgent parent). Playing in the sprinkler cannot be described or understood—or even happen—without its context. It is difficult to imagine that either boy would enjoy the activity as much doing it alone; the social context is part of the experience. A sprinkler might be set up for play on an asphalt driveway but not in a living room. Parents would

CENTENNIAL NOTES

Occupation: Returning to Our Roots

An enhanced understanding of the contemporary ideas of the profession requires a review of its history. More specifically, this Centennial Notes box aims to review *occupation* as the construct central to our professional identity. Founders of the profession purposefully chose the term *occupation* as it was conceptualized as essential to achieving balance through *doing* or occupying one's time (Dunton, 1917), inherent in human nature, and manifested through in self-care, work, rest, play, and leisure (Meyer, 1922). Adolf Meyer believed engaging in occupations facilitated competence and pleasure in these areas; that is, a blending of work and pleasure—" . . . pleasure in the use and activity of one's hands and muscles . . . " (Meyer, 1922, p. 6). Adopting occupation as the core concept was confirmation and commitment to the profession's original mission and purpose (Evans, 1987). In 1922, Adolf Meyer and Eleanor Clarke Slagle "described a system of 'occupational analysis' as an essential component of the education for occupational therapists" (Bauerschmidt

& Nelson, 2011, p. 339). However, the definition and conceptualization of occupation itself over the last 100 years has been influenced by the evolving climate of health care and scientific research. In their review of OT literature from 1922 through 2004, Bauerschmidt and Nelson (2011) noted that *occupation* was used heavily in the 1920s, replaced in whole or part by the word *activity* during the 1940s through 1960s, was not used much at all in the 1970s and 1980s, and resurged in the 2000s. This coincides with paradigm shifts from the crafts and rehabilitation of the 1920s and 1930s to medicalization mid-century and specialization of therapy services during the 1970s and 1980s. The 1990s and 2000s saw a return to occupation-centeredness. Today, occupation is simply defined in the third edition of the AOTA Occupational Therapy Practice Framework (2014) as the daily life activities in which people perform including activities of daily living (ADL), instrumental activities of daily living (IADL), rest, sleep, work, education, play, leisure, and social participation (AOTA, 2014). This shift now reflects the original values and ideas guiding practice and research.

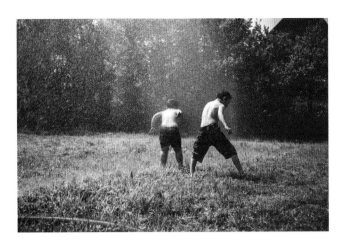

FIGURE 1-2 **Children playing in sprinklers.**

be unlikely to allow their children to get soaking wet in cold weather. The contexts of the people viewing the picture are important, too; many will relate the picture to their own past experiences, but someone who lives in a place where lawn sprinklers are never used might find the picture meaningless and/or confusing, and a person living where drought is a constant would probably find this image upsetting. In this example, occupation and context are enmeshed with one another.

It is generally accepted that the specific *meaning* of an occupation is fully known only to the individual engaged in the occupation (Larson et al., 2003; Pierce, 2001; Weinblatt, Ziv, & Avrech-Bar, 2000). But it is also well accepted that occupations take place in *context* (sometimes referred to as the environment) (e.g., Baum & Christiansen, 2005; Kielhofner, 2002; Law et al., 1996; Schkade & Schultz, 2003; Yerxa et al., 1989) and thus have dimensions that consider other humans (in both social and cultural ways), temporality, the physical environment, and even virtual environments (AOTA, 2014).

Description of occupation as taking place *in* or *with* the environment or context implies a separation of person and context that is problematic. In reality, person, occupation, and context are inseparable. Context is changeable but always present. Cutchin (2004) offered a critique of OT theories of adaptation-to-environment that separate person from environment and proposed that John Dewey's view of human experience as "always situated and contextualized" (p. 305) was a more useful perspective. According to Cutchin, "situations are always inclusive of us, and us of them" (p. 305). Occupation occurs at the level of the situation and thus is inclusive of the individual and context (Dickie, Cutchin, & Humphry, 2006). Occupational therapy interventions cannot be context-free. Even when an OT practitioner is working with an individual, contextual element of other people, the

culture of therapist and client, the physical space, and past experiences are present.

Is Occupation Always Good?

In OT, occupation is associated with health and well-being, both as a means and as an end. But occupation can also be unhealthy, dangerous, maladaptive, or destructive to self or others and can contribute to societal problems and environmental degradation (Blakeney & Marshall, 2009; Hammell, 2009a, 2009b). For example, the seemingly benign act of using a car to get to work, run errands, and pursue other occupations can limit one's physical activity and risk injury to self and others. Furthermore, Americans' reliance on the automobile contributes to urban sprawl, the decline of neighborhoods, air pollution, and overuse of nonrenewable natural resources. Likewise, industry and the work that provides monetary support to individuals and families may cause serious air pollution in expanding economies such as that of China (Facts and Details, 2012).

Personal and societal occupational choices have consequences, good and bad. In coming to understand occupation, we need to acknowledge the breadth of occupational choices and their effects on individuals and the world.

Organizing Occupation

Categorization of occupations (e.g., into areas of activities of daily living [ADL], work, and leisure) is often problematic. Attempts to define work and leisure demonstrate that distinctions between the two are not always clear (Csikszentmihalyi & LeFevre, 1989; Primeau, 1996). Work may be defined as something people *have* to do, an unpleasant necessity of life, but many people enjoy their work and describe it as "fun." Indeed, Hochschild (1997) discovered that employees in the work setting she studied often preferred the homelike qualities of work to being in their actual homes and consequently spent more time at work than was necessary. The concept of leisure is problematic as well. Leisure might involve activities that are experienced as hard work, such as helping a friend to build a deck on a weekend.

Take the two men plating salmon and vegetables (Figures 1-3) for example. Categorizing their activity presents a challenge. They are hovering over a kitchen counter, meticulously placing microgreens on top of the salmon using chef's tweezers. Their activity may be categorized as engaging in work or other productive activity. However, what is not known is whether this is

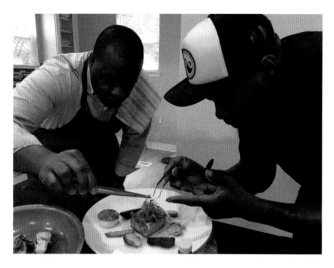

FIGURE 1-3 Two men plating salmon and vegetables.

paid work, caregiving work (e.g., feeding others in the home), or leisure. Both men are dressed in a chef's coat and an apron and utilizing tools that are not commonly used in home kitchens. This may give the appearance that they are engaging in paid work—chefs preparing a meal for paying patrons. But only the gentleman on the left is a chef, which may lead you to interpret the situation as a leisure activity for the gentleman on the right. Categorizing the totality of this occupational situation is complicated. No simple designation of what is happening in the picture will suffice.

Another problem with categories is that an individual may experience an occupation as something entirely different from what it appears to be to others. Weinblatt and colleagues (2000) described how an elderly woman used the supermarket for purposes quite different from provisioning (that would likely be called an instrumental activities of daily living [IADL]). Instead, this woman used her time in the store as a source of new knowledge and interesting information about modern life. What should we call her occupation in this instance?

The construct of occupation might very well defy efforts to reduce it to a single definition or a set of categories. Many examples of occupations can be found that challenge other theoretical approaches and definitions. Nevertheless, the richness and complexity of occupation will continue to challenge occupational therapists to know and value it through personal experience, observations, and scholarly work. The practice of OT depends on this knowledge.

CENTENNIAL NOTES

The Future of Occupation

The use of occupations to optimize engagement in daily life situates OT practice in a unique place in the health care landscape (Rogers, Bai, Lavin, & Anderson, 2017). Occupational therapy has been demonstrated to improve and maximize functional and social needs of clients through cost-effective occupation-based interventions, and the value of occupation is presumed to establish the profession as a health care leader for years to come (Lamb & Metzler, 2014). Within and beyond the health care arena, the challenge practitioners and researchers face is the evolving nature of occupations. Occupations change over time. Consequently, how individuals engage in them also changes over time. Some occupations come and go (e.g., for many, balancing a personal budget now requires access to online banking) or are entirely new (e.g., Khalilah's example of cooking in a local person's home when traveling abroad), and how occupations, in and of themselves, and occupational participation are conceptualized requires perpetual adaption. For instance, technology is so embedded in how occupations are performed every day that it is considered part of performance skills (AOTA, 2016).

In his 2017 Eleanor Clarke Slagle Lecture, Dr. Roger Smith charged OT practitioners to harness the potential of technology as it is inextricably linked to occupation and practice. Tech-driven occupations have changed our capacities for *doing*. That is, how individuals use their hands or bodies for engaging in occupation is not exclusive to the physical but includes virtual and sensorial experiences. Take self-driving vehicles for example. Autonomous driving systems have the potential to change the roles of occupational therapists as driver rehabilitation specialists by shifting focus from the physical capabilities of the person to the cognitive applications of the vehicle. Occupational therapy practitioners utilize technology to meet the needs of their clients, from using the timer function on an iPhone to pace activity to using an app to facilitate motor learning. Thus, incorporating application software technologies into intervention requires practitioners to be flexible, innovative, and knowledgeable of how tech trends impact occupation.

REFERENCES

Aarts, J., & Dijksterhuis, A. (2000). Habits as knowledge structures: Automaticity in goal- directed behavior. *Journal of Personality and Social Psychology, 78,* 53–63.

Aldrich, R., Rudman, D., & Dickie, V. (2017). Resource seeking as occupation: A critical and empirical exploration. *American Journal of Occupational Therapy, 71,* 7103260010p1–7103260010p9. doi:10.5014/ajot.2017.021782

American Occupational Therapy Association. (2014). Occupational therapy practice framework: Domain and process, 3rd edition. *American Journal of Occupational Therapy, 68*(Suppl. 1), S1–S48. doi:10.5014/ajot.2014.682006

American Occupational Therapy Association. (2016). Assistive technology and occupational performance. *American Journal of Occupational Therapy, 70,* 7012410030p1–7012410030p9. doi:10.5014/ajot.2016.706S02

Bargh, J. A., & Chartrand, T. L. (1999). The unbearable automaticity of being. *American Psychologist, 54,* 462–479.

Bauerschmidt, B., & Nelson, D. L. (2011). The terms occupation and activity over the history of official occupational therapy publications. *American Journal of Occupational Therapy, 65,* 338–345. doi:10.5014/ajot2011.000869

Baum, C. M., & Christiansen, C. H. (2005). Person-environment-occupation-performance: An occupation-based framework for practice. In C. H. Christiansen, C. M. Baum, & J. Bass-Haugen (Eds.), *Occupational therapy: Performance, participation, and well-being* (3rd ed., pp. 243–266). Thorofare, NJ: SLACK.

Blakeney, A., & Marshall, A. (2009). Water quality, health, and human occupations. *American Journal of Occupational Therapy, 63,* 46–57.

Breines, E. B. (1995). Understanding "occupation" as the founders did. *British Journal of Occupational Therapy, 58,* 458–460.

Clark, F. A. (1997). Reflections on the human as an occupational being: Biological need, tempo and temporality. *Journal of Occupational Science: Australia, 4,* 86–92.

Csikszentmihalyi, M., & LeFevre, J. (1989). Optimal experience in work and leisure. *Journal of Personality and Social Psychology, 56,* 815–822.

Cutchin, M. P. (2004). Using Deweyan philosophy to rename and reframe adaptation-to-environment. *American Journal of Occupational Therapy, 58,* 303–312.

Dickie, V. A. (2010). Are occupations 'processes too complicated to explain'? What we can learn by trying. *Journal of Occupational Science, 17,* 195–203.

Dickie, V., Cutchin, M., & Humphry, R. (2006). Occupation as transactional experience: A critique of individualism in occupational science. *Journal of Occupational Science, 13,* 83–93.

Dissanayake, E. (1992). *Homo aestheticus: Where art comes from and why.* Seattle, WA: University of Washington Press.

Dissanayake, E. (1995). The pleasure and meaning of making. *American Craft, 55*(2), 40–45.

Downey, G. (1998). *The machine in me.* New York, NY: Routledge.

Dunton, W. R. (1917). History of occupational therapy. *The Modern Hospital, 8*(6), 380–382.

Evans, K. A. (1987). Definition of occupation as the core concept of occupational therapy. *American Journal of Occupational Therapy, 41,* 627–628.

Facts and Details. (2012). *Air pollution in China.* Retrieved from http://factsanddetails.com/china/cat10/sub66/item392.html

Hammell, K. (2009a). Sacred texts: A sceptical exploration of the assumptions underpinning theories of occupation. *Canadian Journal of Occupational Therapy, 76,* 6–22.

Hammell, K. (2009b). Self-care, productivity, and leisure, or dimensions of occupational experience? Rethinking occupational "categories." *Canadian Journal of Occupational Therapy, 76,* 107–114.

Hinojosa, J., Kramer, P., Royeen, C. B., & Luebben, A. J. (2003). Core concept of occupation. In P. Kramer, J. Hinojosa, & C. B. Royeen (Eds.), *Perspectives in human occupation: Participation in life* (pp. 1–17). Philadelphia, PA: Lippincott Williams & Wilkins.

Hochschild, A. R. (1997). *The time bind: When work becomes home and home becomes work.* New York, NY: Metropolitan Books.

Hocking, C. (2000). Occupational science: A stock take of accumulated insights. *Journal of Occupational Science, 7,* 58–67.

Hocking, C. (2009). The challenge of occupation: Describing the things people do. *Journal of Occupational Science, 16,* 140–150.

Hocking, C., Wright-St. Clair, V., & Bunrayong, W. (2002). The meaning of cooking and recipe work for older Thai and New Zealand women. *Journal of Occupational Science, 9,* 117– 127.

Iwama, M. (2006). *The Kawa model: Culturally relevant occupational therapy.* Philadelphia, PA: Churchill Livingstone/Elsevier.

Johnson, K., & Bagatell, N. (2017). Beyond custodial care: Mediating choice and participation for adults with intellectual disabilities. *Journal of Occupational Science, 24,* 546–560. doi:10.1080/14427591.2017.1363078

Kantartzis, S., & Molineux, M. (2011). The influence of Western society's construction of a healthy daily life on the conceptualisation of occupation. *Journal of Occupational Science, 18,* 62–80.

Kielhofner, G. (2002). *Model of human occupation: Theory and application* (3rd ed.). Philadelphia, PA: Lippincott Williams & Wilkins.

Kielhofner, G. (2009). *Conceptual foundations of occupational therapy practice* (4th ed.). Philadelphia, PA: F.A. Davis.

Kielhofner, G., & Burke, J. P. (1977). Occupational therapy after 60 years: An account of changing identity and knowledge. *American Journal of Occupational Therapy, 31,* 675– 689.

Krishnagiri, S. (2000). Occupations and their dimensions. In J. Hinojosa & M. L. Blount (Eds.), *The texture of life: Purposeful activities in occupational therapy* (pp. 35–50). Bethesda, MD: American Occupational Therapy Association.

Lamb, A. J., & Metzler, C. A. (2014). Defining the value of occupational therapy: A health policy lens on research and practice. *American Journal of Occupational Therapy, 68,* 9–14. doi:10.5014/ajot.2014.681001

Larson, E., Wood, W., & Clark, F. (2003). Occupational science: Building the science and practice of occupation through an academic discipline. In E. B. Crepeau, E. Cohn, & B. Schell (Eds.), *Willard & Spackman's occupational therapy* (10th ed., pp. 15–26). Philadelphia, PA: Lippincott Williams & Wilkins.

Law, M., Cooper, B., Strong, S., Stewart, D., Rigby, P., & Letts, L. (1996). The person-environment-occupation model: A transactive approach to occupational performance. *Canadian Journal of Occupational Therapy, 63,* 9–23.

Law, M., Steinwender, S., & Leclair, L. (1998). Occupation, health and well-being. *Canadian Journal of Occupational Therapy, 65,* 81–91.

Meyer, A. (1922). The philosophy of occupational therapy. *Archives of Occupational Therapy, 1*(1), 1–10.

Molineux, M. (2004). Occupation in occupational therapy: A labour in vain? In M. Molineux (Ed.), *Occupation for occupational therapists* (pp. 1–14). Oxford, United Kingdom: Blackwell.

Molke, D., Laliberte-Rudman, D., & Polatajko, H. J. (2004). The promise of occupational science: A developmental assessment of an emerging academic discipline. *Canadian Journal of Occupational Therapy, 71,* 269–281.

Nelson, D. L. (1988). Occupation: Form and performance. *American Journal of Occupational Therapy, 42,* 633–641.

Nelson, D. L. (1997). Why the profession of occupational therapy will flourish in the 21st century. The 1996 Eleanor Clarke Slagle Lecture. *American Journal of Occupational Therapy, 51,* 11–24.

Orr, J. E. (1996). *Talking about machines: An ethnography of a modern job.* Ithaca, NY: Cornell University Press.

Pierce, D. (2001). Untangling occupation and activity. *American Journal of Occupational Therapy, 55*, 138–146.

Primeau, L. A. (1996). Work and leisure: Transcending the dichotomy. *American Journal of Occupational Therapy, 50*, 569–577.

Reilly, M. (1962). Occupational therapy can be one of the great ideas of 20th century medicine. *American Journal of Occupational Therapy, 16*, 1–9.

Rogers, A. T., Bai, G., Lavin, R. A., & Anderson, G. F. (2017). Higher hospital spending on occupational therapy is associated with lower readmission rates. *Medical Care Research and Review, 74*, 668–686. doi:10.1177/1077558716666981

Schkade, J. K., & Schultz, S. (2003). Occupational adaptation. In P. Kramer, J. Hinojosa, & C. B. Royeen (Eds.), *Perspectives in human occupation: Participation in life* (pp. 181–221). Philadelphia, PA: Lippincott Williams & Wilkins.

Schouten, J. W., & McAlexander, J. H. (1995). Subcultures of consumption: An ethnography of the new bikers. *Journal of Consumer Research, 22*, 43–61.

Schwartz, K. B. (2003). History of occupation. In P. Kramer, J. Hinojosa, & C. B. Royeen (Eds.), *Perspectives in human occupation: Participation in life* (pp. 18–31). Philadelphia, PA: Lippincott Williams & Wilkins.

Sherry, J. F., Jr., & McGrath, M. A. (1989). Unpacking the holiday presence: A comparative ethnography of two gift stores. In E. C. Hirschmann (Ed.), *Interpretative consumer research* (pp. 148–167). Provo, UT: Association for Consumer Research.

Smith, R. O. (2017). Technology and occupation: Past, present, and the next 100 years of theory and practice (Eleanor Clarke Slagle Lecture). *American Journal of Occupational Therapy, 71*, 7106150010. doi:10.5014/ajot.2017.716003

Townsend, E. (1997). Occupation: Potential for personal and social transformation. *Journal of Occupational Science: Australia, 4*, 18–26.

Weinblatt, N., Ziv, N., & Avrech-Bar, M. (2000). The old lady from the supermarket—categorization of occupation according to performance areas: Is it relevant for the elderly? *Journal of Occupational Science, 7*, 73–79.

Wilcock, A. A. (2006). *An occupational perspective of health* (2nd ed.). Thorofare, NJ: SLACK.

Wilcock, A. (2007). Occupation and health: Are they one and the same? *Journal of Occupational Science, 14*(1), 3–8.

Wood, W. (1998). Biological requirements for occupation in primates: An exploratory study and theoretical synthesis. *Journal of Occupational Science, 5*, 68–81.

Wood, W., Quinn, J. M., & Kashy, D. A. (2002). Habits in everyday life: Thought, emotion, and action. *Journal of Personality and Social Psychology, 83*, 1281–1297.

Yerxa, E. J. (1993). Occupational science: A new source of power for participants in occupational therapy. *Journal of Occupational Science: Australia, 1*, 3–9.

Yerxa, E. J., Clark, F., Frank, G., Jackson, J., Parham, D., Pierce, D., . . . Zemke, R. (1989). An introduction to occupational science, a foundation for occupational therapy in the 21st century. In J. A. Johnson & E. J. Yerxa (Eds.), *Occupational science: The foundation for new models of practice* (pp. 1–17). New York, NY: Haworth Press.

the**Point**®   *For additional resources on the subjects discussed in this chapter, visit* **http://thePoint.lww.com /Willard-Spackman13e.**

A Contextual History of Occupational Therapy

Charles H. Christiansen, Kristine L. Haertl

LEARNING OBJECTIVES

After reading this chapter, you will be able to:

1. Examine how historical accounts are retrospective attempts to reconstruct and understand the events of the past with the purpose of gaining improved insight into the present.
2. Identify key personalities and events that influenced the founding and development of occupational therapy.
3. Analyze how wars, social movements, and legislation were associated with significant developments in occupational therapy.
4. Evaluate how mind/body dualism and the competition between social and biomedical approaches to health care have been persistent points of tension since occupational therapy's founding.

Introduction

Occupational therapy (OT) has a rich and complex history. It has been influenced, as all professions have, by world events, personalities, and social movements. In this chapter, we identify some of these factors as a way of understanding how OT came into being and evolved as a profession. Industrialization, the civil rights struggles for women and children, world wars, economic shifts, health care legislation, globalization, and the digital age have been major influences on the evolution of the profession. Occupational therapy's history demonstrates Kuhn's contention that science (and science-based professions) do not always progress in logical, uninterrupted, or predictable ways (Kuhn, 1996). Moreover, although OT began in the United States, it is important to remember that many of the factors influencing its development originated in Europe.

What Is a Contextual History?

Historical events happen in larger contexts. History shows that ideas that take hold often benefit from historical timing, the chance good fortune that we sometimes describe as "being in the right place at the right time." Successful ideas also require effective advocates and other conditions (Gladwell, 2002). The conditions that have influenced OT during its history have not always related to health care, yet they shaped attitudes and beliefs that made people and societies more or less amenable to ideas, innovations, and actions. By providing a description of the contexts for events, historians offer *possible* explanations for why events occurred when and how they did. These explanations are of value if people are to derive lessons from the past. To present histories without contexts and without critical examination is to potentially oversimplify events and to miss opportunities to learn from them (Molke, 2009).

The Periods Covered by This Chapter

The periods identified for this chapter include 1700 to 1899 (a prehistory), 1900 to 1919, 1920 to 1939, 1940 to 1959, 1960 to 1979, 1980 to 1999, and 2000 to present. No two eras can claim equivalent impact on the profession because the people, ideas, contexts, and events influencing OT during each time period varied significantly in their importance.

To begin, we draw from Bing (1981), who identified the Age of Enlightenment as an especially fruitful time in the generation of ideas that influenced OT, a period that is appropriately called a "prehistory."

Occupational Therapy Prehistory: 1700 to 1899

Historical Context

During the first hundred years of this time frame (roughly 1700 to 1799), significant social movements sprang up in Western civilization that challenged authority and conventional thinking. This "age of enlightenment" marked the beginning of logical thinking as a trustworthy way of knowing (Paine, 1794). Great artists, composers, and thinkers in history flourished. The concepts of egalitarianism and idealism emerged, and the corruption, abuses, and intolerance of the church and state were challenged. Ideas broadened through intellectual discourse, conducted through regular social gatherings called salons and in academic societies (Sawhney, 2013). With the beginning of the Industrial Revolution, methods of mass production led to the printing and wide distribution of books, helping to spread ideas broadly (Hackett, 1992).

Industrialization brought new opportunities, yet there is evidence that the resulting human migration overwhelmed social infrastructures and created conflict as workers rebelled against exploitation and poor working conditions. Such migration, particularly in Great Britain

and the United States, brought people from rural areas to the cities looking for work, often resulting in overcrowding and unsanitary work environments (Wilcock & Hocking, 2015). Great social change also challenged the ability of people to adapt; many relocated from rural to urban areas, encountered new cultures, and became factory workers.

In the United States, this period also witnessed a collision of moral values and economic traditions that resulted in a great Civil War. Tensions between moral values and economics have recurred at several points in American history, and these tensions are important to OT because the philosophy of the field has such a strong moral core, anchored in concerns for social justice (Bing, 1981).

Nowhere is this moral influence more apparent than in treatment for persons with mental illness. During the late eighteenth century, dramatic changes in how people with mental illness were viewed resulted in more humane treatment, first in Europe and later in the United States (Whiteley, 2004). An emerging belief influencing this change was that the "insane" were people reacting to difficult life situations and therefore must be treated with compassion (Gordon, 2009).

Although often associated with mental illness, **moral treatment** was also applied to physical illness because health and illness had been viewed as related to patient character and spiritual development (Luchins, 2001). This emergence of humanitarian treatment influenced the development of therapeutic communities and the emphasis on engagement of groups in productive activities (Whiteley, 2004).

The ideas of moral treatment also influenced social services, as exemplified by the settlement house movement. The settlement house movement originated in London at Toynbee Hall in 1884, (Harvard University Library, n.d.) a residence where middle class men and women lived collectively with the goal to share knowledge, skills, and resources with the poor and those less educated living nearby (Wade, 2005). It quickly spread to the United States, first at Coit Hall in New York and later at Hull House established in Chicago by Jane Addams and Ellen Gates Starr in 1889 (Harvard University Library, n.d.). Funded through philanthropy, Hull House aimed to create opportunity, participation, and dignity for those served and also became a center for social activism (Carson, 1990). Volunteer workers often lived in the settlement house communities and taught crafts and other practical skills of living. A related and concurrent development, called the arts and crafts movement, also began in Britain and sought to counter the negative consequences of industrialization by encouraging a return to artistic design and the unique and genuine appeal of handmade articles (Levine, 1987). Both the settlement house and arts and crafts movements, originating in Europe, influenced the use of curative occupations in mental illness, and this ultimately led to the birth of OT.

People and Ideas Influencing Occupational Therapy

In his Eleanor Clarke Slagle Lecture, Bing (1981) recounted many of the historical figures and ideas of the eighteenth and nineteenth centuries that he believed influenced the founding of OT. The figures he identified from the eighteenth century were John Locke, Philippe Pinel, and William Tuke. From the nineteenth century, Bing identified Adolf Meyer as a key figure.

John Locke, a physician and philosopher who lived in the late seventeenth century, is credited with advancing many ideas that later influenced the philosophy and practices of OT, including sensory learning and pragmatism (Faiella, 2006).

Philippe Pinel, superintendent of the Bicetre and Salpetriere asylums in Paris, reportedly ordered the removal of chains from some of the inmates held in these places and is widely regarded as a pioneer for more humanitarian treatment. His work emphasized leisure and occupational activities that later formed the foundation for the moral treatment era (St. Catherine University, 2017).

William Tuke, an English philanthropist who founded the York retreat, is credited with being the father of the moral treatment movement. Tuke was appalled by the inhumane conditions he observed in asylums and sought a more compassionate approach to mental health treatment. He eliminated restraints and physical punishment and encouraged conditions where patients could learn self-control and improve self-esteem through participation in leisure and work activities (Digby, 1985; Stanley, 2010).

Adolf Meyer, a Swiss-educated physician who emigrated to the United States in 1892 and became head of an asylum in Kankakee, Illinois, introduced the concept of individualized treatment and began a long career of innovation and leadership in American psychiatry, emphasizing the importance of understanding the key events in the life history of each patient (Figure 2-1) (Christiansen, 2007). While on a trip to the Chicago World's Fair in 1893, Meyer injured his leg and, during a brief convalescence in the city, visited Hull House, and this experience was thought to influence Meyer's thinking about the connections between daily occupations and mental illness. These concepts appeared in an important paper (the philosophy of occupation therapy) he would deliver three decades later at an early meeting of the newly created American Occupational Therapy Association (AOTA) (Lief, 1948; Meyer, 1922).

Influences on the Evolution of Occupational Therapy

During OT's prehistory, the seeds had clearly been planted for the ideas that would lead to the founding of the profession (Box 2-1). However, by 1899, its time had not yet

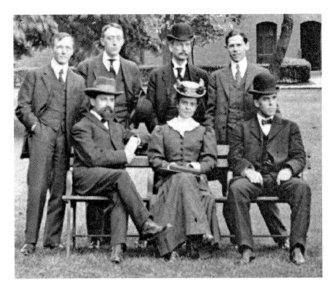

FIGURE 2-1 Dr. Adolf Meyer (seated at far left), a Swiss immigrant known as the father of American Psychiatry, is shown with his staff at the Eastern Illinois Asylum at Kankakee, Illinois, around 1895. Dr. Meyer later became the head of psychiatry at Johns Hopkins University and was a strong advocate for OT after its founding. His philosophy paper on OT, delivered at the Fifth Annual Meeting of the AOTA, continues to be widely cited even today. (Photo credit: Meyer Collection, Allen Chesney Memorial Library, Johns Hopkins University. Used with permission.)

come. In fact, the rise of large public asylums teeming with inmates, the shortage of well-trained physicians, and cost concerns led to a standard of care that fell far short of the individualized treatment and conditions idealized by the moral treatment movement. The ideas that eventually formed the beginning of the Society for the Promotion

---

BOX 2-1   KEY POINTS: PREHISTORY (1700–1899)

- The Age of Reason emphasized logical ways of knowing, ultimately leading to scientific health care and today's evidence-based practice.
- Early roots of social justice led to moral treatment and more humane care for persons with mental illness, ultimately leading to curative treatment involving work.
- Industrialization and technological advances led to global migration and the settlement house movement, a birthplace of many ideas influencing OT.
- Key persons during this period included John Locke, Philippe Pinel, William Tuke, and Adolf Meyer.

of Occupational Therapy would have to be nurtured and applied by several different people in different settings before the profession of OT would take root in the United States.

1900 to 1919

Historical Context

The first two decades of the twentieth century was a period of bold optimism in the United States, driven by rapid innovation and growing prosperity. The century began with the assassination of President McKinley by an anarchist protesting corruption and social inequities tied to industrialization. McKinley was succeeded by his vice president, Theodore Roosevelt, an intelligent and audacious reformer. Although he was from a privileged background, Roosevelt was a populist who supported worker rights and consumer protection, fought cartels, started the Panama Canal project, created a powerful navy, and established a national park system to preserve federal lands (Brinkley, 2009).

This **progressive era** was rounded out by Presidents William Taft and Woodrow Wilson, each of whom was a highly educated and task-oriented leader. Overall, significant social progress, including reforms in education and mental health, occurred during this period; thanks to the influence of John Dewey (an educator) and William James (a psychologist), both of whom were supporters of pragmatism (Schutz, 2011).

The 19th Amendment of the U.S. Constitution, ratified in 1920, afforded women the right to vote, providing a springboard for the advancement of women throughout the culture, particularly in the workplace (Greenwald, 2005). This was significant for OT because its workforce was overwhelmingly dominated by women.

Three years earlier, in 1917, after a period of neutrality and unsuccessful efforts to broker peace, the United States was drawn into the "The Great War," a pointless and horrendous world conflict that began in 1914 and ended on November 11, 1918. Overall, the war resulted in more than 15 million deaths, with 7 million soldiers sustaining wounds resulting in permanent disability (Votaw, 2005). As American soldiers prepared for battle, the War Department, at the request of General John J. Pershing, mobilized plans for the care of wounded soldiers whose disabilities would require rehabilitation and vocational reeducation (collectively called *reconstruction* at the time) to return them to civilian employment (Andersen & Reed, 2017; Quiroga, 1995). Given the horrors of the war, the idea of sending untested occupational and physical therapists, called **reconstruction aides**, to Europe was novel but incongruous, reflecting the sense of unrestrained optimism permeating American culture. Yet, because the war

ended in November 1918, casualties for the American forces were relatively modest in comparison to other countries. Historians generally agree that the timing and fresh troops provided by America's entry, coupled with the attrition of enemy forces, were the primary reasons for the allied victory, not superior training, tactics or bravery per se (Hallas, 2009). Importantly, the reconstruction aide "experiment" was deemed a success, thus assuring that reconstruction aides (and later a field called *rehabilitation*) would have a permanent place within American health care.

People and Ideas Influencing Occupational Therapy (1900 to 1919)

Recall that the assassination of President William McKinley, who died from infection of his bullet wound, began this era. McKinley's preventable death and controversial medical care illustrated the variable quality of American medicine in 1900 (Fisher, 2001). This tragic event was an unfortunate precursor to reform efforts affecting medicine.

Not long thereafter (in 1910), Abraham Flexner completed a report on medical education for the Carnegie Foundation. His critical finding that most medical schools were substandard led to the closing of many "storefront" schools. His report recommended that only medical schools affiliated with large universities be recognized (Beck, 2004). The Flexner report ultimately led to increased emphasis on research and greater public awareness about the connection between science and its application in health care.

These developments set medicine on a firm course that emphasized science to the exclusion of other important factors in health, such as social, psychological, and spiritual influences (Kielhofner & Burke, 1977). It also increased the public standing and political power of organized medicine to an extent insulating it from legitimate criticism (Starr, 1983). Yet, a public that still believed that illness needed to be understood in spiritual and psychological terms did not universally welcome scientific medicine. These sentiments led to social movements that involved patients in the healing process and viewed spiritual and psychological factors as important aspects of healing.

One such movement was *Emmanuelism*, started by an Episcopal minister named Elwood Worcester in Boston (Andersen & Reed, 2017; Quiroga, 1995). The Emmanuel movement was patient-centered, holistic, community-based, and comprehensive, involving social services and lay practitioners. In 1909, public awareness of the movement increased with a series of articles in the widely popular weekly magazine, *Ladies Home Journal*

(Quiroga, 1995). This increased visibility brought criticism from conservative physicians, who questioned its church-based delivery and its use of lay practitioners (Williams, 1909).

During this period, Massachusetts-based physician **Herbert J. Hall** adopted a work-based approach for treating *neurasthenia*, a functional nervous disorder resulting in fatigue and listlessness thought to be caused by the stress of societal change and the new cultural emphasis on productivity and efficiency (Beard, 1880). Hall agreed that the "rest cure" (popular at the time) was the wrong treatment for neurasthenia (Figure 2-2). Instead, Hall's "work cure" at the Marblehead sanatorium in Massachusetts sought to actively engage patients in activities such as weaving, basketry, and pottery, taught by skilled artisans, such as Jessie Luther, who had worked at Hull House in Chicago (S. H. Anthony, 2005). The new "work cure" approach became a suitable response to calls for improved mental health care. The "work cure" was also adopted at the Adams Nervine Asylum in Jamaica Plain, Massachusetts, where nurse **Susan E. Tracy** was hired to train nurses and to develop an active approach for treating patients (Quiroga, 1995).

In 1910, Tracy wrote the first book on therapeutic use of occupations, sometimes referred to as the "work cure approach", called *Studies in Invalid Occupation* (Tracy, 1910). Although primarily a craft book, Tracy's work applied the ideas of William James's pragmatism and led

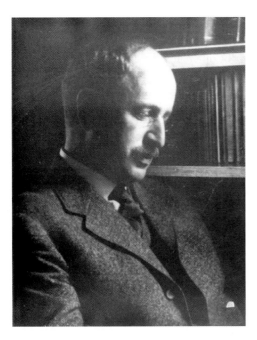

FIGURE 2-2 Dr. Herbert J. Hall, Massachusetts psychiatrist and proponent of curative occupations, played a prominent role in the evolution of OT. (Photo credit: Archives of the AOTA, Wilma L. West Library, AOTF, Bethesda, MD. Used with permission.)

to her involvement in the first course on occupations for patients in a general hospital setting at the Massachusetts General Hospital (Quiroga, 1995).

Tracy's book influenced **William Rush Dunton**, Jr., a psychiatrist practicing at the Sheppard and Enoch Pratt Asylum in Baltimore, to teach his own course on occupations and recreations for nurses working there. In 1912, Dunton was placed in charge of programs in occupation and later wrote his own book on OT (Andersen & Reed, 2017; Bing, 1961). Dunton's enthusiasm was such that he later became a significant advocate and leader in developing the OT profession.

In 1908, **Clifford Beers**, a Yale-educated businessman, wrote *A Mind That Found Itself*, a critical account of his treatment for mental illness in an asylum and his eventual recovery (Beers, 1908). His book spurred reforms in mental health care that led to the creation of the mental hygiene movement. This movement aimed to improve treatment of mental illness by placing emphasis on prevention efforts and providing care outside asylums (Dain, 1980).

As the first decade of the twentieth century ended, many state mental hospitals were using occupations as a regular part of their treatment. Under the auspices of the Hull House in Chicago and influenced by the mental hygiene movement, coursework in occupations and amusements for attendants at public hospitals and asylums began under the newly formed Chicago School of Civics and Philanthropy (Loomis, 1992; Quiroga, 1995).

One of the social work students at the school in a course called *curative occupations and recreations*, **Eleanor Clarke Slagle**, believed that the principles taught there could be applied usefully to idle patients in the state mental hospital at Kankakee, Illinois (Christiansen, 2007; Quiroga, 1995). Slagle's interest in curative occupations gave her impetus to do more study and later develop the curative occupations therapy program with Adolf Meyer at the prominent Phipps Clinic in Baltimore (associated with Johns Hopkins University), where she collaborated with Dr. William Rush Dunton, Jr., at the nearby Sheppard and Enoch Pratt Asylum (Andersen & Reed, 2017; Bing, 1961).

Meanwhile, in 1912, Elwood Worcester of Boston, one of the founders of the Emmanuelism movement, was invited to the Clifton Springs Sanitarium in upstate New York to teach courses to the patients there. One of the patients was an architect, **George Edward Barton**, who was recovering from tuberculosis and hysterical paralysis resulting from his experiences in the Western United States. Barton was so influenced by his personal benefit from the work cure that he became a zealot for using occupations in the recovery of physical illness. Upon his discharge, from the sanitarium, he studied nursing at the facility's school and opened "Consolation House," a convalescence center through which he hoped to apply the ideas of the emerging curative occupation ("work cure") philosophy (Figure 2-3) (Andersen & Reed, 2017; Quiroga, 1995).

Barton began corresponding with prominent advocates for curative occupations, including Susan Tracy, Susan Cox Johnson, and William Rush Dunton, Jr. From 1914 to 1917, Barton wrote articles and developed plans for establishing a profession of caregivers dedicated to the use of occupations in therapy. Dr. Dunton assisted him, but Barton was initially hesitant to use the physician's help, fearing that his lack of medical credentials might diminish his own role. Finally, in mid-March, 1917, the first organizing meeting of the Society for the Promotion of Occupational Therapy was hosted by George Barton at Consolation House in Clifton Springs, New York (Andersen & Reed, 2017; Bing, 1961).

In attendance at that meeting were Barton, Isabel Newton (his secretary and future wife), William Rush Dunton, Jr., Eleanor Clarke Slagle, Thomas Kidner, and Susan Cox Johnson, who had organized many curative occupation programs in New York City. Susan Tracy of Massachusetts had been invited but was not able to attend (Andersen & Reed, 2017). The meeting at Consolation House drew up a charter of incorporation, drafted a constitution for the new society, named committees, planned for an annual conference, and elected officers, with Barton as the inaugural president and Slagle as the vice-president (Andersen & Reed, 2017; Bing, 1961).

The following month, after the loss of American citizens with the sinking of the ocean liner *Lusitania* by German submarines, the United States entered World War I (WWI). The war had begun in 1914, but public opposition to involvement in the United States had remained strong because the casualties wrought by modern weaponry were enormous and neither the Allies (mainly Russia, France, and Great Britain) nor the Central Powers (Germany, Austria-Hungary, and the Ottoman Empire) were making much progress despite these losses. Once public sentiment changed and war was declared, a massive war mobilization effort was undertaken during the ensuing months. Mindful of the war's huge scale and its immense number of casualties, the War Department undertook careful planning to provide assistance to wounded and disabled soldiers who would return from combat (Andersen & Reed, 2017; Quiroga, 1995).

These planning efforts were given a head start through work by the Canadians, who, as part of the British Commonwealth, had been involved in the war since its inception. The vocational secretary for the Canadian Military Hospitals Commission, **Thomas B. Kidner**, a noted expert in manual training and technical education who had experience with vocational rehabilitation in England, was loaned to the U.S. government to assist with vocational rehabilitation efforts (Friedland & Davids-Brumer, 2007; Friedland & Silva, 2008). Then, emerging medical specialties, such as orthopedics, also sought to improve their standing during the war, which created some resistance to the inclusion of an untested group of occupation workers in this effort (Quiroga, 1995, p. 152).

Developments in Occupational Therapy (1900 to 1919)

In the period before WWI, several activities pursued independently by different individuals in different locations would come together in March 1917 during the meeting organized by Barton in Clifton Springs. The organizational meeting establishing OT included discussion about training programs and the need for standards (Andersen & Reed, 2017).

At that time, several programs for training occupation workers had been established in the United States, some of which were organized for nurses and others that were freestanding or organized under the auspices of settlement houses. The need for occupation workers in asylums had received significant impetus from the mental hygiene movement, reform efforts in mental health, and for patients recovering from physical injuries and chronic illnesses such as tuberculosis.

During its mobilization planning for WWI, the United States anticipated the need for a significant number of facilities and rehabilitation workers. Although there were efforts to recruit men to these roles, the military soon realized that women could be recruited and be trained to support the effort (Crane, 1927, p. 57). Some existing programs for curative occupations added courses to meet the anticipated standards of the surgeon general, whereas others were established in large East Coast cities explicitly for the war effort (Figure 2-4) (Andersen & Reed, 2017; Quiroga, 1995).

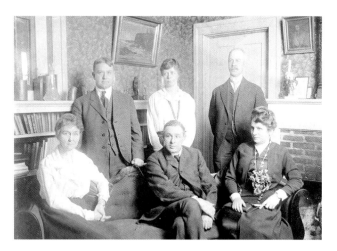

FIGURE 2-3 Society for the Promotion of Occupational Therapy Founders at Consolation House, Clifton Springs, New York, March 1917. Front row (left to right): Susan Cox Johnson, George Edward Barton, and Eleanor Clarke Slagle. Back row (left to right): William Rush Dunton, Jr., Isabel Newton, and Thomas Bessell Kidner. (Photo credit: Archives of AOTA, Wilma L. West Library, AOTF, Bethesda, MD. Used with permission.)

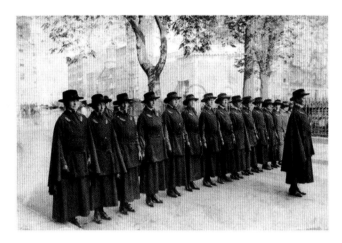

FIGURE 2-4 Reconstruction aides on parade in New York c. 1918. (Photo credit: Image Archive, U.S. Army Medical Department, Office of Medical History.)

Success in quickly establishing these important war training courses for reconstruction aides was made possible through the efforts of committed and prominent individuals who were able to organize the financial and political resources necessary to establish high-quality schools (Andersen & Reed, 2017; Quiroga, 1995). For various reasons, it was decided that a division of roles would be necessary with some reconstruction aides assigned to do orthopedic work, corrective exercise, and massage, whereas others, who became occupational therapists, provided handicrafts and support for "shell shock" which resulted from the stressful conditions of trench warfare, poisonous gas, and constant explosions from artillery (Low, 1992) (Figure 2-5).

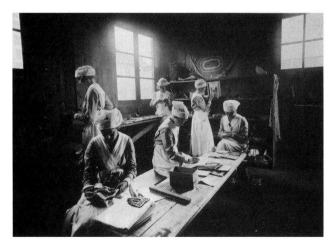

FIGURE 2-5 Reconstruction aides in workshop preparing projects at base Hospital No. 9. Chateauroux, France, during World War I. (Photo credit: Image Archive, History of Medicine Collection, National Library of Medicine.)

Despite the success in recruiting and training qualified reconstruction aides for the war effort, the initial placement of these trained aides proved to be difficult because some physicians continued to view OT as a fad, failing to appreciate that it could have a worthwhile role in the treatment of wounded soldiers. However, after OT reconstruction aides achieved success at base hospitals in France, attitudes began to change (Andersen & Reed, 2017; Low, 1992; Quiroga, 1995).

By November 1918, when Germany and its allies surrendered, at least 200 reconstruction aides were serving in 20 base hospitals in France (Quiroga, 1995). The war ended on November 11, 1918. Between 1917 and January 1, 1920, nearly 148,000 sick and wounded men were treated upon their return to the United States at 53 reconstruction hospitals (Office of the Surgeon General, 1918). The military specifications governing OT for returning soldiers declared that it should have a purely medical function and be prescribed for the early stages of convalescence to occupy the soldier's minds. Even at this early date, there was a lack of clarity and considerable ambiguity in the roles and functions of the reconstruction aides providing OT. However, leadership in the newly formed professional association for OT, which was now known as the AOTA, provided wise advocacy for the recruitment of high-quality trainees. Dr. William Rush Dunton, Jr., succeeded George Barton as president of AOTA in 1917, and his friend Eleanor Clarke Slagle later succeeded him in the role. This provided a period of thoughtful and successful leadership that helped the new profession gain momentum and legitimacy after the war (Quiroga, 1995). See Box 2-2 for a summary of important influences and social movements from this period that impacted OT's development.

1920 to 1939

Historical Context

As the Treaty of Versailles following WWI was negotiated by the allies, President Woodrow Wilson proposed a League of Nations to prevent such wars from recurring. Wilson was successful in getting these terms into the treaty, but he suffered a severe stroke and the U.S. Congress never ratified them reportedly because Wilson refused to compromise on minor details of the ratification (Eubank, 2004). Ironically, the harsh conditions and reparations imposed on Germany at Versailles and the absence of U.S. leadership to organize the League of Nations contributed to political instabilities in Europe, economic shifts, and a rise in nationalism, which led to mistrust between various nations. Eventually, the rise of fascist leadership in Germany and Italy and additional

BOX 2-2   KEY POINTS: EARLY YEARS AND WORLD WAR I (1900–1919)

- A period of progressive movements in the United States brought political and social reform to improve working conditions, advance women's rights, and improve medicine and psychiatry.
- The arts and crafts and curative occupation movements, which were reactions to industrialization and modernization, led to the formation of a formal OT professional society in 1917.

- The U.S. entry into World War I created the need for services to reconstruct wounded soldiers, giving OT an early opportunity to advance its cause.
- Key people during the era included Herbert Hall, George Barton, Eleanor Clarke Slagle, William Rush Dunton, Jr., Susan Tracy, Adolf Meyer, and General J. J. Pershing.

tensions foreshadowed Hitler's decision to invade Poland in September 1939 and begin what was to become World War II (WWII) (Zaloga, 2004).

Within the United States, the period from 1920 to 1939 framed the continuation of significant societal transformations as women asserted their right to vote. The first decade of this period is sometimes called the "roaring twenties" because the advancements of the era in manufacturing, transportation, and communication encouraged a sense of optimism and excess (Cooper, 1990). Profits in industry allowed increased earnings for workers, and the introduction of installment buying led to a very high level of consumerism that fueled a robust economy. Yet, new wealth encouraged widespread and irrational speculation in the stock market, which contributed to the stock market crash of 1929 and a long period of hardship that followed, known as the *Great Depression*.

In rural areas, the economic situation was made more difficult by a persistent drought that was worsened in some areas by poor conservation (Egan, 2006). With unemployment at 25% and family incomes sliced in half, many people were desperate (McElvaine, 1993). President Herbert Hoover, an engineer, humanitarian, and respected administrator, was unable to contend with a crisis made worse by a financial disaster in Europe. In 1932, Franklin D. Roosevelt was elected to the first of four terms, and he quickly moved ahead with economic and social reform programs, collectively called the "New Deal." These included Social Security, higher taxes on the wealthy, new controls over banks and public utilities, and enormous work relief programs for the unemployed, including the Civilian Conservation Corps for rural conservation and environment projects and the Works Progress Administration focusing on constructing or repairing bridges, libraries, and public buildings (Kennedy, 1999). There were also efforts to support artists to create public murals, sculptures, and paintings and writers to produce books and plays. These government-sponsored programs contributed to the public's recognition that creative and productive activities were essential for both economic and social and psychological benefit.

People and Ideas Influencing Occupational Therapy (1920 to 1939)

The founders of the National Occupational Therapy Society had set events in motion for the rapid evolution of their new profession. After George Barton's abrupt resignation in 1917, **Dr. William Rush Dunton, Jr.**, (Figure 2-6) helped to advance the new society, which was then focusing

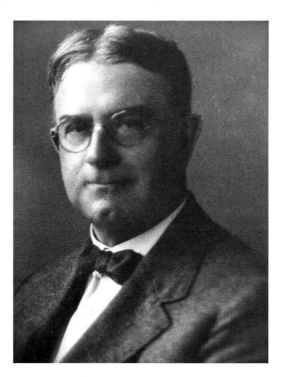

FIGURE 2-6 William Rush Dunton, Jr., MD, a physician at the Shepard and Enoch Pratt Hospital near Baltimore, was a founder of AOTA, an early president of the organization, and a strong proponent of OT. He was a prolific writer of articles and books and served as founding editor of the profession's first journal, *Archives of Occupational Therapy*. (Photo credit: Archives of the AOTA.)

on standardizing educational programs. Dunton embraced Adolf Meyer's theory of psychobiology, which provided a common sense approach to treating mental illness (Christiansen, 2007; Lief, 1948). Psychobiology was holistic and practical, emphasizing that mental disease was reflective of habit disorganization in the lives of those affected. Meyer believed that humans organized time through doing things and that a balance of activities involving work and rest was essential for well-being. More importantly, Meyer and Dunton shared the belief that occupational therapists had an important role in helping patients reorganize their daily habits and regain a sense of optimism. Meyer expressed these ideas in a paper given at the Fifth Annual Meeting of the AOTA held in Baltimore, Maryland, during October 1921 (Meyer, 1922).

Meyer's ideas were consistent with the emerging central beliefs of OT in that it recognized that forced idleness during convalescence was not only morally wrong but also disorienting and physically debilitating. Through engagement in occupations, Meyer asserted that patients could ward off depression and gain a sense of self-confidence that would help motivate them further (Christiansen, 2007). There were also economic motivations to normalize lives by enabling individuals to develop skills that would help them become economically independent of assistance by the state (Figure 2-7).

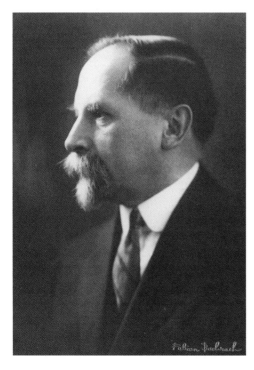

FIGURE 2-7 Dr. Adolf Meyer, a renowned psychiatrist and advocate for OT, shown at the Henry Phipps Clinic at Johns Hopkins University around 1915. (Photo credit: Meyer Collection, Alan Chesney Memorial Library, Johns Hopkins University.)

Within psychiatry, other theoretical perspectives, including the work of Sigmund Freud, overshadowed Adolf Meyer's theory of psychobiology. Freud's emphasis on unconscious drives captured the interest of many psychiatrists as well as the general public (Burnham, 2006). Freudian psychoanalysis remains a contentious topic (Brunner, 2001), and many historians view the distraction it created as a scientific setback (Eysenck, 1985). Moreover, the progress made in general medicine in treating common diseases during that era encouraged pursuit of biological explanations in the treatment of mental illness. One theory held that mental conditions were caused by focal infections in the body and led to unnecessary and sometimes harmful surgeries to some institutionalized mental patients because patient consent was not yet required for experimental procedures (Scull, 2005). Electroconvulsive treatments and lobotomies began to be used with both positive and negative consequences, and these treatments remain controversial (Fink & Taylor 2007; Pressman, 1998).

The trend toward medicalization in OT that occurred in the 1920s and 1930s was purposely influenced by strategic decisions of the profession's leaders. In their quest for professional legitimacy, OT leaders perceived that there would be benefit in allying more closely with organized medicine (Andersen & Reed, 2017). The rise of physical medicine and rehabilitation as a specialty of medicine and the leadership of **Frank H. Krusen, MD**, had a clear influence on the practice of occupational therapists in rehabilitation. Krusen believed that OT was simply a special application of physical therapy and that the two disciplines should merge (Krusen, 1934). This point of view had adherents in Canada, where training programs combined the theory and practices of both professions and produced graduates who could be dually credentialed (Friedland, 2011).

During the 1920s and 1930s, the principles of OT were also viewed as beneficial in the care of persons with tuberculosis, a disease stigmatized through its association with immigrants and poverty. Thomas B. Kidner, the Canadian vocational education expert who had been a member of the American Occupational Therapy Association founder's group at Clifton Springs, decided to remain in the United States after his temporary assignment to advise the surgeon general had concluded. Kidner, who served two separate terms as president of the AOTA, used his role as a vocational expert to plan facilities that included workspaces for OT and vocational training (Friedland & Silva, 2008). Kidner had a keen interest in the relationship between OT and vocational training, yet the formal relationship between these two important areas of social benefit remained distant well beyond his death in 1932. This unresolved issue would reemerge in an area of applied theoretical emphasis 30 years later known as "occupational behavior" (Kielhofner & Burke, 1977; Reilly, 1962).

Occupational Therapy (1920 to 1939)

In OT, the early part of this era was dominated by the continued "reconstruction" of wounded soldiers from WWI, which occurred at more than 50 hospitals established with reconstruction in mind (Quiroga, 1995). These facilities provided employment for occupational therapists in the early 1920s as did the curative occupation programs in place at mental hospitals (Hall, 1922).

The AOTA became an effective organization for promoting the profession through its network of members, annual meetings, and the publication of a journal under three different names (*Archives of Occupational Therapy*, *Occupational Therapy and Rehabilitation*, and *American Journal of Occupational Therapy* [now *AJOT*]) between 1917 and 1925, at which time the association had nearly 900 members listed in its registry (Dunton, 1925) (Figure 2-8).

In order to continue the development and growth of the new profession during the 1920s, Eleanor Clarke Slagle, who served as president and later secretary-treasurer of the new society for 15 years, found creative ways to continue promoting the field through networking among women's clubs and the establishment of a national office in New York City (Figure 2-9) (Andersen & Reed, 2017; Metaxas, 2000; Quiroga, 1995). Attendance in the association and in the society grew steadily during this time so that by 1929, there were 18 state and local OT associations and approximately 1,000 members of the AOTA (Slagle, 1934). The association leadership continued to foster stability and quality in the profession by emphasizing standards for educational programs and their graduates. The profession worked to gain legitimacy through aligning itself with other professionals, especially physicians (Andersen & Reed, 2017; Quiroga, 1995).

In 1935, after several years of negotiation, the accreditation of OT programs was initiated in concert with the American Medical Association (Quiroga, 1995). During this period, male physicians dominated association leadership in OT; still, many more positions for occupational therapists were being created in specialized facilities for physical rehabilitation, mental health, and tuberculosis.

The emergence of physical medicine and rehabilitation in the mid-1930s, which had been influenced by physicians who used physical agents and practiced physical therapy, was reflected in many of the publications during this era (Slagle, 1934). Because occupational therapists assumed roles in rehabilitation units, they adopted goniometry and began adapting tools and equipment to enable patients to gain strength, endurance, and range of motion while doing crafts (Andersen & Reed, 2017).

During this period, polio epidemics and President Franklin Roosevelt's polio-related paralysis brought

OFFICERS
Mr. Thomas B. Kidner, President
370 Seventh Avenue, New York City
Dr. G. Canby Robinson, Vice-President
Johns Hopkins Hospital, Baltimore, Md.
Mrs. Eleanor Clarke Slagle,
Secretary-Treasurer
370 Seventh Avenue, New York City

American
Occupational Therapy
Association
INCORPORATED
370 Seventh Avenue, New York, N. Y.

BOARD OF MANAGEMENT

October 27, 1924

Miss Kinstine Newman,
State Sanatorium for Tuberculosis,
Howell,
Michigan,

My dear Miss Newman,

Enclosed herewith is your membership card for 1925.

We are very glad, indeed, to welcome you as a sustaining member and trust you will attend our annual meetings and enjoy the fellowship of this rapidly growing group of professional workers.

Most cordially yours,

Eleanor Clarke Slagle

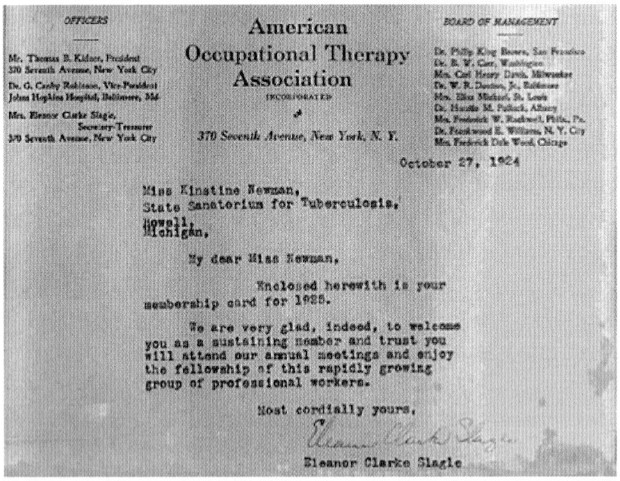

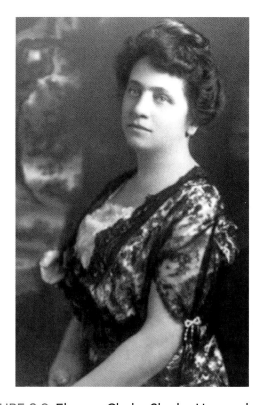

FIGURE 2-8 Letter from Eleanor Clarke Slagle, secretary-treasurer of AOTA, acknowledging dues receipt to a new sustaining member from Michigan (October 27, 1924). (Photo credit: Archives of the AOTA, Wilma L. West Library, AOTF, Bethesda, MD. Used with permission.)

FIGURE 2-9 Eleanor Clarke Slagle. Her work as founder and tireless leader is recognized through a prestigious lectureship named in her honor. (Photo credit: Archives of the AOTA, Wilma West Library, AOTF, Bethesda, MD. Used with permission.)

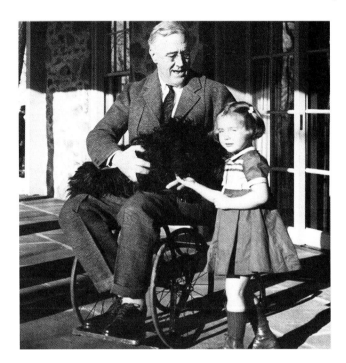

FIGURE 2-10 Franklin D. Roosevelt, president of the United States from 1933 to 1945, pictured with Ruthie Bie (a friend's grand daughter) and his dog Fala at the Roosevelt Cottage in Hyde Park, New York, in 1941. Roosevelt's legs became paralyzed at age 39 after an acute illness. Elected for four terms, he is known for many accomplishments, including the Social Security Act of 1935. (Photo credit: Franklin Delano Roosevelt Library, Library ID 73113:61.)

visibility and public awareness to the disease, leading to treatment facilities and research as well as specialized centers that employed occupational therapists and others for the care of patients (Figure 2-10). Polio epidemics peaked in 1952 and diminished after development of a vaccine by Jonas Salk a decade later (Oshinsky, 2005).

Aided by the advocacy of Thomas B. Kidner, tuberculosis hospitals had also become settings where many occupational therapists assumed roles providing recuperative,

diversional, and vocational therapy for long periods of convalescence (Friedland & Silva, 2008; Kidner, 1922). The principle of activity graded to provide appropriate challenge and physical demand for patients was, by this time, a well-established part of the OT regimen in physical rehabilitation (Laird, 1923). See Box 2-3 for a summary of social challenges and the profession's responses during this period.

1940 to 1959

Historical Context

By 1940, Europe was well embroiled in major turmoil; with Germany having already annexed Austria, it invaded Poland and Czechoslovakia. Those events were followed quickly by declarations of war by Great Britain and France and the invasions of Denmark, Norway, Holland, Belgium, and France. The German army was so dominant that it devastated French and British forces and forced the cross channel retreat of forces from both countries at Dunkirk (Ward & Burns, 2007). Italy joined Germany, and the war soon spread to North Africa. Meanwhile, Adolf Hitler exploited his occupation of the European continent to pursue massive genocide against the Jewish people (Bergen, 2016). Japan then joined the axis powers, further expanding the theater of war to the Pacific (Spector, 1984).

Despite the Neutrality Acts of the 1930s designed to prevent the United States from entering another war, the United States opposed Hitler, and when the Japanese attacked Pearl Harbor in December 1941, the United States entered WWII. With the numbers of men drafted to armed service, the severe unemployment of the late 1930s gave way to a workforce shortage that plagued all areas of industry. This led to an influx of women into the workforce. Many hospitals were understaffed and ill-equipped to meet health care needs of those at home as well as soldiers returning from combat. Health challenges of returning veterans included diseases such as tuberculosis, hepatitis, and rheumatic fever but also war injuries, including amputations and chemical wounds (Richards, 2011).

BOX 2-3   KEY POINTS: POSTWAR GROWTH AND ADVANCEMENT (1920–1939)

- In the aftermath of the treaty ending World War I, advances in manufacturing and great optimism led to consumerism and speculation, leading to a stock market crash and the Great Depression.
- The AOTA, led by wise leaders, focused on allying itself with physicians and hospitals and developing and standardizing its educational programs while

- distinguishing itself from vocational and medical rehabilitation.
- Occupational therapy practice expanded into specialized hospitals treating tuberculosis and polio.
- Key people during the era included Eleanor Clarke Slagle, William Rush Dunton, Jr., Thomas Kidner, and Adolf Meyer.

According to the U.S. Department of Veterans Affairs (2015), WWII killed more people, destroyed more property than previous wars, and was among the most devastating in history, with more than 16 million serving in the armed forces and more than 291,000 American deaths. Total estimates of global fatalities vary, but it is generally accepted that they exceeded 60 million. The economic and social effects of WWII brought changes in health care and the passage of a number of U.S. legislative acts to fund research and services to returning veterans.

The Public Health Service Act gave the National Institutes of Health (NIH) permission to grant awards for nonfederal research, the GI Bill of 1944 funded efforts to aid veterans to transition back to civilian life, and in 1946, President Harry Truman signed the Mental Health Act, which was designed to provide funding for mental health services and research (Harlow, 2007). Rehabilitation expanded to assist veterans to return to work as the amendments in 1943 and 1954 of the Vocational Rehabilitation Act emphasized physical and mental restoration leading to a rise in the development of curative workshops (Gainer, 2008).

The post-WWII era saw the start of the Cold War marked by tensions with Russia that were caused by the conflicting ideals of the democratic philosophies of the United States and the communist beliefs of Russia. Globally, as Japan started to rebuild post-WWII, the Korean War again brought armed forces from the United Nations (including the United States) to support the Republic of Korea (now South Korea). Domestically, post-WWII brought economic growth, and although the United States had only 6% of the world's population, it was producing half of the world's goods (American Machinist, 2000). Yet, despite the economic affluence, more than 36 million Americans remained impoverished, and social concerns were given new political emphasis (Huret, 2010).

As new economic growth and postwar social concerns marked the 1950s, major health care advances took place, including triumph over polio, the discovery of the DNA double helix, the development of the pacemaker, and the formation of the Joint Commission on Accreditation of Health Care Organizations (Gerber, 2007). Yet, despite these advances, there were still areas of health care in dire need of change. Mental health institutions were overcrowded and the rate of alcoholism and juvenile delinquency skyrocketed (Dworkin, 2010). As the stigmatizing effects of mental illness plagued the decade, patients and their families began organizing, and efforts were made to address concerns not only of the clients but also of their families (L. D. Brown, Shepherd, Wituk, & Meissen, 2008). This, paired with the discovery of the antipsychotic effects of chlorpromazine (Thorazine), ushered in a new era of psychiatric treatments for those with mental illness. Although, perhaps helpful, the reliance on pharmaceutical interventions and deinstitutionalization brought a new set of social and health care challenges.

Occupational Therapy (1940 to 1959)

Although occupational therapists didn't serve overseas in WWII, United States-based consultant positions were created along with emergency training programs to provide therapists for the treatment of veterans returning from war (Andersen & Reed, 2017; Hartwick, 1993). This was a time of immense growth and change in OT (Gordon, 2009) because the focus shifted from the use of arts and crafts toward rehabilitation techniques based on scientific methods. Emphasis was placed on reintegrating veterans into society, and therefore, the use of activities of daily living (ADL), ergonomics, and vocational rehabilitation gained favor in therapeutic communities (Gainer, 2008). With battlefield medicine focused on saving severely wounded soldiers, the development of prosthetics and orthotics gained momentum during this period (Ott, Serlin, & Mihm, 2002). Occupational therapists became involved in prosthetic training, which often entailed the use of adapted tools and involved strengthening and conditioning (Figure 2-11).

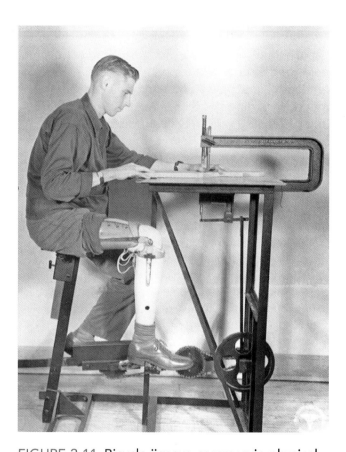

FIGURE 2-11 Bicycle jigsaw, common in physical rehabilitation OT clinics from the 1940s through the 1960s. (Photo credit: Archives of the AOTA, Wilma L. West Library, AOTF, Bethesda, MD. Used with permission.)

With the shift toward hospital-based therapy and the growth of rehabilitation, OT educational programs reorganized their curricula supported by the publication of the first OT textbook written in 1947 in the United States and edited by Helen Willard and Clare Spackman (Mahoney, Peters, & Martin, 2017; Willard & Spackman, 1947). That same year, the first woman and registered occupational therapist, Winifred Kahmann, became president of AOTA (Andersen & Reed, 2017). In 1949, guidelines for OT education were expanded through the Council on Medical Education and Hospitals and the *Essentials of an Acceptable School of Occupational Therapy* were established (Council on Medical Education and Hospitals, 1949).

In 1956, the OT assistant was created to help meet workforce needs, and in 1958, the AOTA took responsibility for accrediting assistant level OT programs (AOTA, 2009). Although the term *certified occupational therapy assistant* did not take hold internationally, countries such as Canada, Australia, and the United Kingdom developed positions similar to the OT assistant in order to augment the workforce demands of the profession (Nancarrow & Mackey, 2005; Salvatori, 2001).

Globally, the number of occupational therapists continued to increase as educational programs expanded, and by 1950, there were seven OT educational courses in England and one in Scotland (Oxford Brookes University, 2011). In 1952, preliminary discussions took place for the eventual formation of the World Federation of Occupational Therapists (WFOT) recognized in 1959 by the World Health Organization, which was at that time just over a decade old (WFOT, 2011). See Box 2-4 summarizing important challenges and the profession's responses from 1940 to 1959.

People and Ideas Influencing Occupational Therapy (1940 to 1959)

Influences on the profession during this period came from OT leaders in the Army as well as from therapists working with individuals having motor paralysis. Here, we include the Bobaths (physiotherapists practicing in England), Ruth Robinson, and Margaret Rood.

Karel and Berta Bobath: Berta Bobath was a German physiotherapist and her husband Karel was a Czech neuropsychiatrist. Together, they jointly developed a popular neurodevelopmental treatment (NDT), originally designed for persons with cerebral palsy but later applied to individuals with stroke or neurodevelopmental conditions. Although the approach originally used manual techniques to control tone and movement patterns, once they noticed a lack of generalization, the Bobaths expanded NDT to use normal play environments and natural contexts to encourage neurological development (Patel, 2005). Although studies question the effectiveness of NDT for various populations, the Bobaths' techniques are still used by occupational and physical therapists throughout the world, and their work encouraged study of the sensory links to motor output (Levin & Panturin, 2011).

Col. Ruth A. Robinson of the U.S. Army helped create OT educational programs for those preparing to serve in the military. Robinson proposed an accelerated training program to meet the needs for expansion during the Korean War (U.S. Army Medical Department, 2012). She continued in leadership positions, serving as the president of AOTA from 1955 to 1958 (Figure 2-12) (Peters, 2011b). During her time in the Army, Col. Robinson became chief of the Army Medical Specialists Corps and served as mentor to Wilma West and Ruth Brunyate (later Ruth Brunyate Wiemer), who later became colleagues and leaders in the AOTA.

Margaret Rood was an occupational and physical therapist credited as one of the earliest theorists on motor control. Rood stressed the importance of reflexes in early development and emphasized the use of facilitation and inhibition techniques, which were soon after used and expanded on by the Bobaths. In addition to clinical work, Margaret Rood took on leadership and educational positions including the development of the Occupational Therapy Department of the University of Southern California (USC), where she served as the first chair (USC, n.d.).

BOX 2-4   KEY POINTS: WORLD WAR II AND CONTINUED DEVELOPMENT (1940–1959)

- World War II, fought in European and Pacific theatres, causes the mobilization of men and material as the United States enters the war in 1941 following the attack on Pearl Harbor.
- Occupational therapy, still influenced greatly by its ties to medical rehabilitation, once again plays a key role in the care of wounded soldiers.
- Developments in prosthetics, assistive technology, neurodevelopmental care, and compensatory techniques for therapy accelerate as part of the war effort.
- Key personalities of the period include Ruth Robinson, Margaret Rood, and Karel and Berta Bobath.

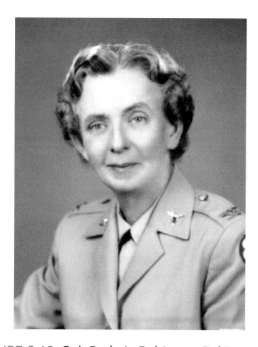

FIGURE 2-12 Col. Ruth A. Robinson. Robinson established accelerated programs in the U.S. Army to train therapists for the Korean War and served several leadership roles in the AOTA, including that of president from 1955 to 1958. (Photo credit: Archives of the AOTA, Wilma L. West Library, AOTF, Bethesda, MD. Used with permission.)

1960 to 1979

Historical Context

During this time frame, Martin Luther King's famous speech, "I Had a Dream," (M. L. King, 1963) symbolized decades of the civil rights movement seeking equality and justice for African Americans. This was also an era of unrest and change marked by the "cold war," a prolonged period of distrust between the Soviet Union (Union of Soviet Socialist Republics [USSR]) and the United States. This political tension led to continued division of Germany and the construction of the Berlin wall, advancements in space science as the two superpowers developed their defense technologies, the Cuban Missile Crisis, and ultimately, a controversial war in Vietnam War. Kennedy's decision to pursue civil rights legislation provided the foundation for President Johnson to sign the **Civil Rights Act** into law in 1964, protecting individual rights and freedom from discrimination in areas such as voting, education, and employment (Andrews & Gaby, 2015). Concerns were raised regarding poverty, access to health care, and quality education for all, leading President Johnson to institute a number of other domestic programs commonly known as the "Great Society" aimed at reducing poverty

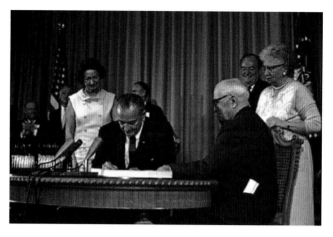

FIGURE 2-13 Lyndon B. Johnson signing the 1965 Medicare and Medicaid Legislation with former President Harry S. Truman, Mrs. Truman, Mrs. Lady Bird Johnson, and members of Congress. (Photo credit: National Archives, photograph collection.)

and providing increased funding in areas such as education and health care (Warner, 2012). Perhaps foremost among these was legislation in 1965, establishing Medicare and Medicaid (Figure 2-13), which provided health care access to millions of seniors and disabled and impoverished American citizens, many of whom previously did not have access to such care (Bakken, 2009). Similar efforts took place elsewhere during this period, with Canada instituting its federal-provincial universal coverage health care system in 1962 and many Western European countries instituting forms of social health insurance in the 1960s and 1970s (Saltman & DuBois, 2004).

By the 1960s, American health care had been modernized greatly with updated equipment, electric beds, advanced communication systems, and innovative laboratories. The demographics of hospitalization shifted because new medicines were discovered and medical advances escalated. With the mass production of antibiotics and other pharmaceutical treatments for physical and mental health conditions, there was a move away from the treatment of acute epidemic illness (e.g., polio and smallpox) toward increased need for care of chronic conditions such as rheumatism, arthritis, and heart conditions (U.S. Department of Health, Education, and Welfare, 1965). The rise of feminism also brought changes domestically and globally bringing new emphasis to women's health and increased representation of women in medical schools (Rosser, 2002). Health planning is increased in order to reduce duplication (Melhado, 2006), and private health insurance was widely provided by employers to compete for workers. Typically, these insurance plans had low deductibles and required little out-of-pocket cost by beneficiaries (Thomasson, 2002). This, alongside the legislation providing government payments under Medicare and Medicaid, contributed to an overuse of services and further stimulated the growth and cost of health care.

A move to close state institutions for the infirmed, particularly those with mental illness, caused additional challenges. The emergence of psychotropic medications paired with the overcrowding and deplorable conditions of many state hospital systems led to the deinstitutionalization movement and subsequent closure of state and psychiatric hospitals both in Canada and the United States (Koyangi, 2007; Sealy & Whitehead, 2004). Although the aim was to contain costs and provide improved care in the community, the development of community mental health services was inadequate to address the demands (Koyangi, 2007). Many of those affected by deinstitutionalization wound up homeless or in the criminal justice systems (McGrew, Wright, Pescosolido, & McDonel, 1999). Efforts to shift the care for those with mental illness to the community have continued globally to the present day, yet challenges remain to provide adequate long-term care and housing.

Occupational Therapy (1960 to 1979)

The decades from 1960 to 1979 brought significant change to OT practice (Box 2-5). During the reorganization of the AOTA in 1964 under the presidency of Wilma West, renewed emphasis was placed on supporting scientific endeavors in OT (Yerxa, 1967b). The board supported the idea of reorganization and expansion, and in 1965, the American Occupational Therapy Foundation (AOTF) was established to advance the science of the field and improve its public recognition (AOTA, 1969). Efforts to emphasize science and theory development led to increased graduate education in the field and later led to a proliferation of models, theories, and frames of references for practice.

Continued emphasis on the legitimacy of the profession increased efforts to regulate practice through state licensure legislation as the U.S. government, concerned about costs for outpatient therapy services, initiated the first caps on payments for services in 1972.

The practice of OT during this period was heavily influenced by medical rehabilitation, which continued the post-WWII mechanistic paradigm emphasizing neuromotor and musculoskeletal systems and their impact on function (Kielhofner, 2009). Advances in neuroscience motivated A. Jean Ayres to expand on the work of the Bobaths and Rood. Ayres used neuroscience to study perceptual motor issues in children and develop and apply a theory of sensory integration (Ayres, 1966, 1972). Influences on practice shifted from the holistic mind–body occupation-based philosophies to those with bottom–up approaches focusing on the underlying source of the problem, often with emphasis on reflex integration and motor function (Figure 2-14).

Various Great Society programs and the *Education for All Handicapped Children Act (1975)* expanded the scope and areas of practice for occupational therapists. Medicare and Medicaid laid the foundation for expanded services to the elderly, those with disabilities, and the poor, and the Education for All Handicapped Children Act mandated access to education for all children, including those with disabilities. These laws, governing provision for health care and educational services to expanded populations, led to expansion of work areas for occupational therapists as the need for therapists in educational systems continued to grow (Coutinho & Hunter, 1988). In 1965, new guidelines were developed for accredited OT programs in the United States, and in 1967, AOTA celebrated the 50th year of OT (Andersen & Reed, 2017).

Internationally, OT was guided by theory-driven clinical models but, similar to the United States, was also driven by the medical profession and the social and health care institutions because these were the main employers of

---

BOX 2-5	**KEY POINTS: FURTHER EVOLUTION OF THE PROFESSION (1960–1979)**

- The civil rights movement and the Great Society lead to historic legislation that influences health care and social justice.
- In OT, educational programs continue to mature and school-based practice gains great momentum with passage of the Education for All Handicapped Children Act; large mental institutions begin to close, affecting the number of therapists employed in longer term mental health settings;

and the American Occupational Therapy Foundation (AOTF) is founded to foster scientific development.
- Increased emphasis is placed on sensorimotor therapies, particularly driven by neurodevelopmental theorists, and occupational behavior emerges as a counterbalance to the medicalization of therapy.
- Key personalities of the period are A. Jean Ayres, Mary Reilly, Gail Fidler, and Wilma West.

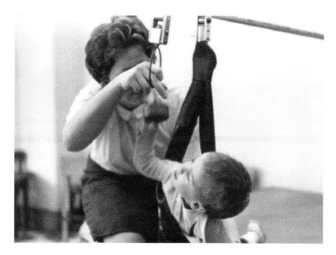

FIGURE 2-14 Therapy for developmental disabilities grew rapidly in the 1980s because therapists applied theories of reflex integration from the neurosciences. In this undated photo from the period, an unidentified therapist works with a young child. (Photo credit: Archives of the AOTA, Wilma L. West Library, AOTF, Bethesda, MD. Used with permission.)

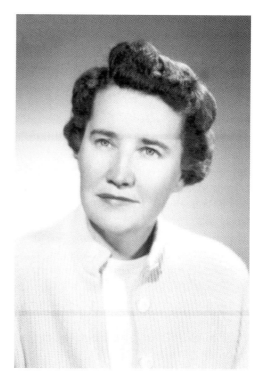

FIGURE 2-15 Dr. Mary Reilly created a frame of reference known as occupational behavior. She was the Eleanor Clarke Slagle lecturer in 1961 and a charter member of the Academy of Research of the American Occupational Therapy Foundation (AOTF). (Photo credit: Archives of AOTA, Wilma L. West Library, AOTF, Bethesda, MD. Used with permission.)

occupational therapists (Clouston & Whitcombe, 2008). The ADL tools and adaptations were developed to accommodate for dysfunctions (Hocking, 2008), and the profession continued to emphasize scientific endeavors. There was also an increase in educational programs throughout the world, fostered in part by international efforts of representatives to the WFOT (Cockburn, 2001).

People and Ideas Influencing Occupational Therapy (1960 to 1979)

Mary Reilly became a distinguished clinician in the U.S. Army Medical Corps during the war (Figure 2-15) (E. J. Brown, 1996) and went on to earn her doctorate in education, serving as the chief of the Rehabilitation Department at the Neuropsychiatric Institute at the University of California, at Los Angeles. She later served as professor and chair in OT at USC, where she became an influential, if controversial, academician. Through her graduate students, she is credited with evolving a theoretical framework known as the "occupational behavior" frame of reference, which emphasized the development of work skills and the societal importance of productive occupations. This work influenced the development of the Model of Human Occupation (MOHO) originally advanced by a team of scholars led by Gary Kielhofner, Janice Burke, and others (Kielhofner & Burke, 1980). In her 1961 Eleanor Clark Slagle lecture, Reilly challenged the profession to reclaim its roots in occupation and famously proclaimed, "Man [sic], through the use of his hands as they are energized by mind and will, can influence the state of his own health" (Reilly, 1962, p. 2).

A. Jean Ayres, an occupational therapist and licensed educational psychologist, applied neuroscience to practice (Figure 2-16). Dr. Ayres was educated at USC, where she served as a student, scientist, practitioner, and educator. Within her research, Ayres developed tools for practice, including assessments of integrated sensory processing, later forming a battery known as the Sensory Integration and Praxis Tests (Ayres, 1989). In 1976, Ayres founded the Ayres Clinic, in which she combined teaching, research, and practice to develop her practice model of sensory integration (Kielhofner, 2009). Her theories and influence continue to present day.

Gail Fidler emphasized the use of occupation as a means for emotional expression (Figure 2-17). Fidler, a teacher and occupational therapist with a background in psychology, was influenced by her studies of interpersonal theory, self-esteem, and ego development (Miller & Walker, 1993). Gail Fidler became a leader in mental health

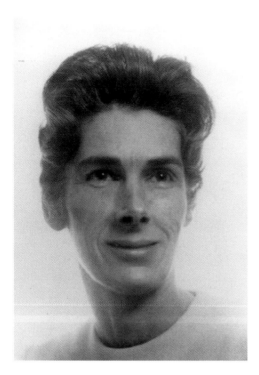

FIGURE 2-16 A. Jean Ayres, PhD, was one of the first occupational therapists to use basic science to develop applied theory in OT. Her area of interest was sensory processing in children with developmental disorders. (Photo credit: Archives of AOTA, Wilma L. West Library, AOTF, Bethesda, MD. Used with permission.)

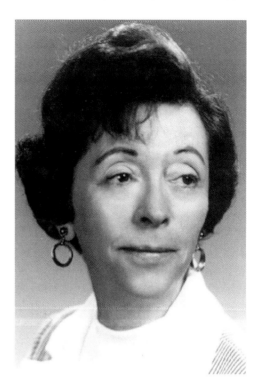

FIGURE 2-17 Gail Fidler was a leading spokesperson for the application of psychodynamic theory in OT, publishing (with her husband, a psychiatrist) one of the first textbooks in the field dedicated to practice in mental health. (Photo credit: Archives of the AOTA, Wilma L. West Library, AOTF, Bethesda, MD. Used with permission.)

OT, studied with her mentor Helen Willard, and worked in a settlement house while a student at the Philadelphia School of Occupational Therapy (Peters, 2011a). She and her husband wrote *Introduction to Psychiatric Occupational Therapy* (Fidler & Fidler, 1954), a groundbreaking book that promoted the application of ego theory and therapeutic use of self in practice. Fidler's contributions include 13 books, numerous articles and service on the executive board of AOTA (Gillette, 2005).

Ann Mosey advanced Fidler's ideas through development of the object relations/psychodynamic frame of reference, which offered concepts integral to understanding the use of activities and groups in therapy (Figure 2-18) (Mosey, 1973). Other prominent theorists emerged at the time, increasing the theory base of OT. *Lorna Jean King* (1974) applied sensory integrative theories to persons with schizophrenia, *Claudia Allen* developed theories of cognition to guide therapy for persons with chronic mental illness (Allen Cognitive Network, 2011), and Kielhofner and Burke (1977) advocated an OT paradigm to refocus on human adaptation and occupation. The core concepts of this work later became the foundation of a widely adopted MOHO (Kielhofner & Burke, 1980).

Wilma L. West, a retired Army colonel who had served with Ruth Robinson during WWII, worked as executive director of the AOTA from 1947 to 1952 and became a powerful influence on the advancement of OT (Figure 2-19). She was a respected and passionate advocate for OT (Gillette, 1996; West, 1991) and served as the president of the AOTF during its key formative years from 1972 to 1982. Among her earnest goals was the promotion of research, and she presided over the creation of the profession's first research journal, *The Occupational Therapy Journal of Research* (*OTJR*), now *OTJR: Occupation, Participation and Health*. The foundation board designated her as its only president emerita, and the Wilma West Library at AOTF is named in her honor (Foto, 1997).

Elizabeth Yerxa, a successor to Mary Reilly, emphasized the importance of advancing theory to the benefit of practice (Figure 2-20). In her 1966 Eleanor Clark Slagle lecture, she asserted the need for occupational therapists to take steps toward professionalism, produce research, and focus on the unique assets of the profession, including purposeful activity and the practice of authentic OT (Yerxa, 1967a). Yerxa later became involved in active promotion of research efforts and in promoting the development of

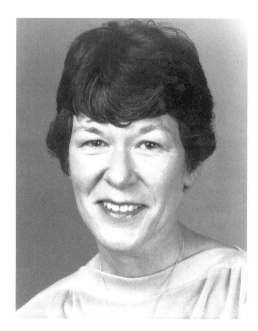

FIGURE 2-18 Ann Mosey, PhD, a widely respected scholar and professor of OT at New York University, published frequently on topics related to the evolution of theory in the field of OT as well as on topics in mental health. (Photo credit: Archives of the AOTA, Wilma L. West Library, AOTF, Bethesda, MD. Used with permission.)

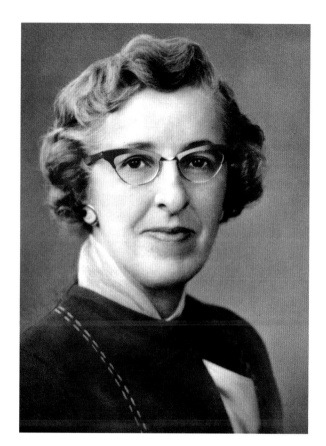

FIGURE 2-19 Wilma West, an Army officer in WWII, served in many important leadership roles in the AOTA and the AOTF. The official library, housing AOTA's archives, is named in her honor, as is a prestigious joint commendation award given by the presidents of the two organizations. (Photo credit: Achives of the AOTA, Wilma L. West Library, AOTF, Bethesda, MD. Used with permission.)

occupational science as an academic discipline and foundation for practice. Yerxa retired in 1988 and is recognized as a distinguished professor emerita at the USC.

Lela A. Llorens became the first person of color awarded the Eleanor Clarke Slagle lecture (Figure 2-21). Her 1970 lecture (Llorens, 1970) emphasized a theory for OT emphasizing the importance of development and its influence on physical, psychosocial, neurophysiological, and psychodynamic facets of development (AOTA, 2017a). Llorens later went on to chair the AOTA–AOTF Research Advisory Council. See Box 2-5 for a summary of the key events and professional developments of this period.

1980 to 1999

Historical Context

The onset of the 1980s brought international change with the end of the Cold War, the collapse of the Soviet Union, and the removal of the Berlin Wall. Internationally, the Treaty of Maastricht was signed in formation of the European Union, later paving the way for the development of the European Free Trade Association. Within the United States, Ronald Reagan took office, and the era of the space shuttle began along with the initiation of an initiative to defend against missile attacks. With the advancement of the scientific age, perhaps one of the most pronounced shifts was the beginning of what was to become a dramatic new era of digital technology.

On January 3, 1983, after a variety of companies, including Commodore, IBM, and Apple, had released versions of interactive personal computers, *Time Magazine* featured a cover naming the home computer the "Machine of the Year" for 1982. Thus, began an era where computer languages and new digital inventions proliferated (Bergin, 2007). As computer use extended to the World Wide Web, the Internet grew in popularity and use, affording unprecedented opportunities for cross-cultural communication and knowledge (Palfrey, 2010). By the late 1990s, computers were becoming integral to all areas of society, including business, education, and health care.

Driven by technological advances, Medicare funding, and the prevalence of chronic diseases, the health

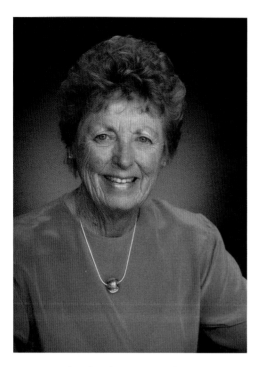

FIGURE 2-20 Elizabeth J. Yerxa led the initial development of the academic discipline of occupational science. Dr. Yerxa received many awards for her work, including the AOTA Award of Merit for her leadership in the profession. (Photo credit: Archives of AOTA, Wilma L. West Library, AOTF, Bethesda, MD. Used with permission.)

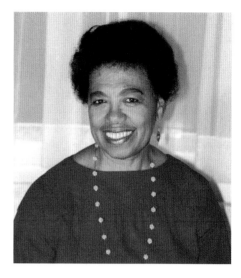

FIGURE 2-21 Lela Llorens served as an educational leader in Florida and California and also provided important leadership within the American Occupational Therapy Foundation (AOTF). Her Eleanor Clarke Slagle lecture on facilitating growth and development provided one of the first comprehensive frameworks for organizing knowledge about OT. (Photo credit: Archives of AOTA, Wilma L. West Library, AOTF, Bethesda, MD. Used with permission.)

care industry expanded greatly. Trends in health concerns shifted during the era as the World Health Organization declared small pox eradicated and the first case of HIV was identified (Hospitals and Health Networks, 2012). Advanced digital imaging technology (such as computed tomography [CT] and magnetic resonance imaging [MRI]) brought increased diagnostic capabilities and costs. Between 1980 and 2000, annual age-adjusted costs per person for health care in the United States nearly tripled (Centers for Medicare & Medicaid Services, 2012).

Hospital stays grew shorter, telemedicine emerged, and increased emphasis was placed on patient choice and participation in health care decisions. Not only did telemedicine provide health professionals the opportunity to extend medical care, but also other digital advances evolved to maintain records and efficiently transfer information from one provider to another. These developments gave rise to concerns about privacy and access to personal health information which could be used by health insurers to deny or restrict coverage, leading to enactment of legislation in 1996 known as the Health Insurance Portability and Accountability Act (known as HIPAA) (Choi, Capitan, Krause, & Streeper, 2006). The public began increasingly to use the Internet to gather information on health care and

medical conditions, providing yet another significant social influence on the delivery of health care (Hernandez, 2005).

Outside of physical medicine, advances in psychiatric rehabilitation were influenced by a paradigm shift away from an expert model toward inclusion of the consumer in treatment decisions. Within mental health, the recovery model emerged (W. A. Anthony, 1993), highlighting the importance of skill training, consumer empowerment, and the development of cooperative alliances in psychiatric rehabilitation. Within this model, concepts of self-determination are emphasized along with empowerment, consumer rights, and community involvement (Tilsen & Nylund, 2008). Goals of mental health recovery included reduced symptoms; enhanced quality of life; and emphasis on personal meaning, purpose, and values (Gagne, White, & Anthony, 2007).

The changing nature of the health care system, along with the renaming and reformulation of the Education for All Handicapped Children Act to the Individuals with Disabilities Education Act (IDEA) and President H. W. Bush's signing of the Americans with Disabilities Act (ADA) in 1990, focused attention on rehabilitation and independent living. Overall, the legislation and trends affecting health care and education during this period influenced areas of OT practice, as increasing numbers of occupational therapists sought employment in school systems (AOTA, 2006b).

Occupational Therapy (1980 to 1999)

During this period, significant public attention was given to health care, especially following the election of William Jefferson Clinton as president. Clinton's health care reform agenda created much discussion but did not result in significant action, primarily due to heavy lobbying by the private health insurance industry, the complexity of the administration's plan, and lack of consensus among members of the majority party in Congress (Birn, Brown, Fee, & Lear, 2003).

In OT, state professional associations continued their lobbying for legislative acts and licensure to regulate the practice of OT and increase the public safety, visibility, and legitimacy of the profession. During this period, emphasis was placed on research, efficacy, and defining the scope of practice for occupational therapists. For example, one significant controversy related to the appropriate use of physical agent modalities by occupational therapists, with some leaders arguing that use of these procedures blurred the distinction between physical therapy and OT (West, 1991).

Also during this time, the AOTF, under the leadership of President Wilma West and Executive Director Martha Kirkland, began a thoughtful series of programs recommended by the Research Advisory Council to advance research and education. The most significant initiatives included the founding of a professional journal *The Occupational Therapy Journal of Research* in 1980 (renamed *OTJR: Occupation, Participation and Health* in 2002) (Classen, 2017) and the creation of the Academy of Research in 1983, an honorary body to recognize outstanding scientists in OT (AOTF, 2012; Christiansen, 1991).

Within the professional association (AOTA), discussions took place regarding the governance of certification activities. In 1986, the AOTA board of directors determined that certification activities and membership functions were not sufficiently independent to avoid potential liability under antitrust legislation. Accordingly, the board voted to create the American Occupational Therapy Certification Board, which later became known as the National Board for Certification in Occupational Therapy (Low, 1997). This action eventually led to a decline in the membership of the AOTA because membership was no longer required for certification purposes.

In addition to activities of the professional association, legislation of the period affecting practicing therapists in the United States included the IDEA (1997), the ADA (1990), and the Balanced Budget Act, enacted August 5, 1997.

In 1997, the IDEA Amendments were signed into law providing strength and accountability for the education of children and adolescents with disabilities. Occupational therapy was one of the specialized services provided for under this Act. The provisions for rehabilitation services in the law gave rise to an increase in therapists practicing in the school system such that by the mid-2000s, education and early intervention was the area with the highest number of practicing therapists (AOTA, 2006b).

The ADA of 1990 became the most comprehensive piece of legislation in U.S. history to provide protection against discrimination for persons with disabilities (Karger & Rose, 2010). The law defined disability and addressed issues of employment accommodation and ensured that persons with disabilities could access public services, transportation, and telecommunications (Hein & VanZante, 1993). The ADA was amended in 2008 to strengthen its provisions and clarify the scope of disabilities protected under the act. Many occupational therapists were well qualified to advocate for clients and consult with organizations seeking to comply with ADA mandates (AOTA, 2000). Yet, despite legislation providing opportunities during this era (such as IDEA and ADA), OT employment growth slowed because of legislation to contain health care costs. The *Balanced Budget Act of 1997* was enacted largely to control Medicare's subacute care costs (Qaseem, Weech-Maldonado, & Mkanta, 2007). However, it reduced positions and led to a decrease in applicants to OT programs, a few of which were eventually closed as a result of low enrollment.

During this era, occupational science was proposed as an academic discipline to provide an underlying foundation for OT (Yerxa, 1990). In 1989, Elizabeth Yerxa and colleagues developed the first occupational science PhD program at USC (Gordon, 2009). Occupational science was developed as a scientific discipline to generate foundational knowledge to inform practice (Clark, Wood, & Larson, 1998; Gordon, 2009). Shortly thereafter, the "occupational science movement" expanded steadily and globally with many academic units changing their names to "occupational science and OT." In Australia, Ann Wilcock and colleagues launched the *Journal of Occupational Science* in 1993 to be followed over the next decade by the creation of societies in several countries dedicated to the study of occupation. In the United States, this body is known as The Society for the Study of Occupation: USA (SSO:USA). There are also Canadian and international societies similarly organized. Refer to Box 2-6 for a summary of important trends during this era.

Individuals during this period who were influential in advancing the study of occupation included Ann Wilcock and Gary Kielhofner. In 1980, Kielhofner and his colleagues published a series of articles on the MOHO (Kielhofner, 1980a, 1980b; Kielhofner & Burke, 1980). Influenced by Mary Reilly's work in occupational behavior and general systems theory, MOHO emphasized motivation, performance, and patterns or routines. Wilcock's book, *An Occupational Perspective of Health,* emphasized the need for promoting health globally through a focus on the occupational nature of humans (Wilcock, 1988). Wilcock's work led to an improved recognition that if engagement in meaningful occupation is necessary for health, a truly just world must ensure human opportunities for such engagement (Stadnyk, Townsend, & Wilcock, 2010).

Additional occupation-based models such as the Person-Environment-Occupational Performance Model (PEOP) (Baum, Christiansen, & Bass, 2015; Christiansen & Baum, 1997), the Ecology of Human Performance Model (Dunn, Brown, & McGuigan, 1994), the Occupational Performance Process Model (Fearing, Law, & Clark, 1997), and the Canadian Model of Occupational Performance (Canadian Association of Occupational Therapists [CAOT], 1997; Townsend, 2002) laid a foundation for the growth of occupation-based practice.

In Canada, the government began programs to help older adults remain independent. In the early 1990s, a 30-month project began to emphasize health prevention and promotion in OT (CAOT, 1993). Soon after, a collaborative group from CAOT, the Client-Centered Practice Committee, met to develop guidelines on consulting, research, education, and practice. Initial representatives included Helene Polatajko, Tracey Thompson-Franson, Cary Brown, Christine Kramer, Liz Townsend, Mary Law, Sue Stanton, and Sue Baptiste. The eventual work resulted in publication of the monograph, *Enabling Occupation: An Occupational Therapy Perspective* (CAOT, 1997; Townsend, 2007).

People and Ideas Influencing Occupational Therapy (1980 to 1999)

Florence Clark completed her PhD in Education at USC and went on to serve as a faculty member, chair, and administrator (Figure 2-22). Clark is a respected scientist in OT and was among a group of faculty who argued that occupational science, the study of humans as occupational beings, is an appropriate academic discipline to serve as a foundation for OT practice. Clark and

colleagues have gained recognition for studying the effect of lifestyle-oriented activity programs for maintaining health and preventing cognitive decline in elders with an aim of helping them remain in their homes and communities (Clark et al., 1997; Clark et al., 2012). Clark was elected president of AOTA in 2012.

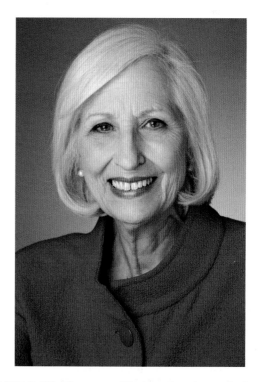

FIGURE 2-22 Florence Clark, scientist, scholar, and association leader, is a strong proponent of science-driven, evidence-based practice. Clark, from the University of Southern California, is a member of the Academy of Research of the American Occupational Therapy Foundation (AOTF). (Photo courtesy of Archives of AOTA, Wilma L. West Library, AOTF, Bethesda, MD. Used with permission.)

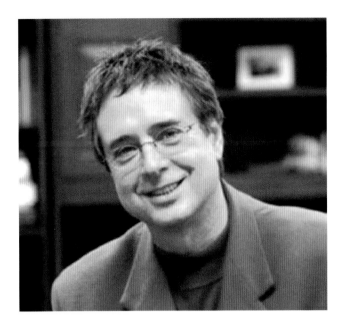

FIGURE 2-23 Gary Kielhofner (1949 to 2010) worked with colleagues in graduate school to develop a Model of Human Occupation, which amalgamated knowledge from the social and behavioral sciences to provide an occupation-based approach to OT practice. During his career, Kielhofner's lectures and publications became internationally known and had a significant influence on practice in Europe, Asia, and South America (Kielhofner, 2008, 2009). (Photo credit: Renee R. Taylor, PhD. Used with permission.)

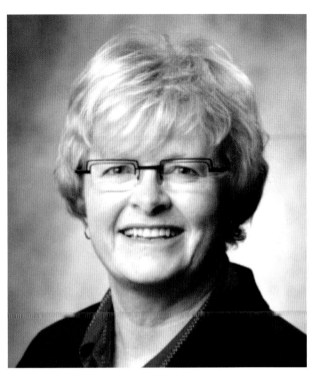

FIGURE 2-24 Mary Law, a Canadian occupational therapist, co-founded an important center in Canada for childhood disability and was co-author of a popular outcome assessment instrument in OT known as the Canadian Occupational Performance Measure (COPM). (Photo courtesy of Mary Law.)

Gary Kielhofner, a graduate of the USC who was influenced by Mary Reilly's occupational behavior model, studied public health at University of California, Los Angeles. He worked with others to propose a MOHO that focused on understanding humans as occupational beings (Figure 2-23). Kielhofner was a prolific writer, publishing more than 19 books and 140 articles (Suarez-Balcazar, 2010). He spent most of his academic career as head of the Department of Occupational Therapy at the University of Illinois at Chicago. Kielhofner spoke and consulted widely and assisted therapists in Sweden, England, and other countries to implement the MOHO in practice. Kielhofner died in 2010 after a brief illness and was described by his colleagues as "extraordinary" in his impact (Christiansen & Taylor, 2011, p. 4) and one of the most "influential and multifaceted OT scholars of the past 30 years" (Braveman, Fisher, & Suarez-Balcazar, 2010, p. 828). For a summary of key events and people during the period 1980 to 1999, see Box 2-6.

Mary Law, a prominent OT clinical scientist in Canada, (Figure 2-24) co-founded the CanChild Centre for Childhood Disability Research at McMaster University in Hamilton, Ontario, and has been a prolific theorist,

researcher, and scholar. Recognized by the AOTF Academy of Research, Law was instrumental in co-developing the Canadian Occupational Performance Measure (COPM) (Law et al., 1990), a widely used outcome assessment tool, and the Person-Environment-Occupation Model (Law et al., 1996), a practice framework used widely in Canada and elsewhere. Law received prestigious recognition from the Canadian government for her career accomplishments when she was named an Officer of the Order of Canada in 2017.

2000 to Present

Historical Context

The dawn of the twenty-first century marked only the second recorded millennium change in documented history, and the transformations that were occurring in the world as the third millennium began were worthy of the occasion. As Thomas Friedman (2006) pointed out, global economic transformation, spawned by digital technology and the Internet, had created a new world that truly was connected economically, so that China, India, and other countries could become significant players in world commerce, both for goods and for services. This increased global connectivity not only created rising middle classes in China and India but also enabled social transformations through the rapid sharing of ideas on social media platforms. The Internet had the potential of influencing large numbers of people in unprecedented ways and at remarkable speed.

Ironically, in the United States, the twenty-first century began with remarkable events that were not related to the Internet. In 2000, the outcome of a historically close presidential election was decided by the Supreme Court, and George W. Bush became the 43rd president under contentious circumstances. Then, on September 11, 2001, during the first year of his presidency, the United States experienced a dramatic terrorist attack on the World Trade Center in New York City. This unprecedented event dominated the news for nearly a year and led to widespread efforts to increase security in ways that permanently changed the way people live their lives. These changes began with passage of the Patriot Act, which suspended some individual liberties in the service of national defense, and extended to creation of a Department of Homeland Security, and the prosecution of controversial wars in Afghanistan and Iraq aimed at eradicating terrorists overseas.

In 2003, President George W. Bush signed legislation that expanded Medicare through provision of a prescription drug plan, known as Medicare Part D (117 Stat. 2066 Pub. L. 108-173).

In his second term in 2008, speculative and unregulated real estate investment led to an economic collapse, which, because of the new global economics, resulted in a serious international market crisis that had profound economic consequences for the United States and most other countries in the world (U.S. Government Printing Office, 2011).

Barack H. Obama, the country's first African-American president, was elected in 2008, inheriting this difficult economic and political situation which required unprecedented legislation to restore market confidence (American Recovery and Reinvestment Act of 2009). In 2010, a significant health care reform bill called the Patient Protection and Affordable Care Act (popularly known as Obamacare) passed without bipartisan support. In addition to its provisions to subsidize premiums so that more people could afford health insurance (resulting in coverage of 30 million more people), the legislation also provided funding for research to promote patient-centered care through creation of the Patient-Centered Outcomes Research Institute, or PCORI (2017). Mr. Obama was elected to a second term, but a divided and partisan Congress continued a legislative stalemate that precluded significant progress on key national issues.

Donald W. Trump, a real estate businessman, was elected president in 2016. Mr. Trump proposed various measures, including immigration restrictions and a repeal of the Affordable Care Act, which was not successful. The Republican-controlled Congress was successful in passing significant tax reform legislation, and the status of health care reform remained uncertain at the end of 2017.

The growth of digital communication accelerated through sales of digital devices such as smartphones, tablets, and e-readers, which made use of cellular and wireless broadband networks. The growth of social networking Websites and Web-based commerce ushered in significant changes in communication and marketing.

Occupational Therapy (2000 to Present)

In the millennium's first two decades, OT practice continued to be influenced in the United States by federal and state legislation and policy changes aimed at achieving cost containment and increasing quality, as determined by measurable outcomes and demonstrated effectiveness. In 2004, the NIH introduced a strategic plan to guide biomedical research called the NIH Roadmap (Zerhouni, 2003). Its purpose was to focus and coordinate biomedical research efforts toward areas deemed important to the health of the nation. This eventually led to the creation of an NIH strategic plan specifically aimed at rehabilitation (Frontera, et al., 2017). Research development in OT was bolstered in this period through NIH-funded training programs aimed at developing clinical scientists in physical and OT.

Increasingly, the federal Centers for Medicare & Medicaid Services and the Agency for Healthcare Research and Quality (AHRQ) began to exert influence on health care practices and research by linking clinical studies of effectiveness to reimbursement through its Effective Health Care Program (Slutsky, Atkins, Chang, & Sharp, 2010).

Increased emphasis of the federal government and private health insurers on cost containment and evidence-based practice led to greater emphasis on research within organized OT. Because hospitals experienced pressures to reduce patient lengths of stay in order to contain costs, the types of procedures offered to inpatients began to focus more on those needed for discharge. More therapy was offered on an outpatient basis or in the home as part of home health services.

Because OT developed globally, existing conceptual models were examined and challenged by the growing numbers of professionals outside North America, particularly in the Asia Pacific region, South America, and the European Union. A key development was the Kawa Model (Iwama, 2006; Iwama, Thomson, & Macdonald, 2009), which offered an alternative view of OT through the lens of Asian Pacific and other collectivist cultures. The influence of international perspectives was also fostered through the emergence of international societies for occupational science. The inaugural organizing meeting of the first SSO:USA was held in Galveston, Texas, in 2002; this was followed by developments in the Asia Pacific region as well as in Canada and the European Community.

In 2004, the AOTA board, under the leadership of Carolyn Baum, charged the vice president, Charles Christiansen, to lead a strategic planning initiative aimed at establishing a Centennial Vision. The aim was to identify goals necessary to position the profession for success beyond 2017 (the 100th anniversary of OT). The Centennial Vision, developed with significant AOTA member input, served as an ongoing goal-setting framework for the AOTA until 2017, emphasizing visibility, influence, research, evidence-based practice, diversity, global connectivity, and attention to the occupational needs of clients as key areas of focus (AOTA, 2006a).

In 2007, the AOTA and the AOTF published the Research Agenda for Occupational Therapy, recommended by a joint panel of OT scientists serving the two organizations (AOTA/AOTF Research Advisory Panel, 2011). This agenda emphasized the importance of providing a strong infrastructure for supporting research in OT that demonstrated the efficacy of services. In 2013, AOTF, in partnership with AOTA, launched a bold research grant program, providing significant funding for projects undertaken by promising emerging scientists with a focus on providing evidence for OT interventions (AOTF, 2014). This initiative was augmented with joint initiatives related to training OT scientists, including workshops and institutes (AOTF, 2015).

Key areas of practice in the United States during 2010 as reflected in association membership data include school-based services and early intervention (27%), hospitals (28%), long-term care facilities (16%), and home health and community (7%), whereas the number of therapists practicing in the United States that reported their primary and predominate area of practice as mental health decreased to 3% (AOTA, 2010). This compares with the 2010 demographics in Canada, where 9,827 occupational therapists held registrations across the provinces, with 11% working in mental health, 46% in hospitals, and 32% working in the community with slightly over 4% employed by residential or assisted living facilities (Canadian Institute for Health Information [CIHI], 2011). By 2014, in the United States, school-based services, mental health, hospitals, home health, and community health settings all showed continued declines, whereas academic settings, freestanding outpatient facilities, early intervention, and long-term care/skilled nursing facilities showed increases (AOTA, 2015). In contrast, across Canada, slight increases in the employment of occupational therapists in mental health, and community settings occurred, whereas there was a slight decline in hospital settings (CIHI, 2015).

During this period, the wars abroad resulted in significant and challenging injuries for many survivors of combat. These returning wounded warriors led to innovations in military OT and called attention to the need for services to reintegrate soldiers sustaining blast injuries that resulted in polytrauma, including brain injuries, severe burns, and amputations (Howard & Doukas, 2006).

In OT education, the growth of clinical doctorate programs escalated during the period. Online and hybrid educational programs also increased, offering a significant portion of curricular content to be delivered over the Internet. This trend accelerated with the growth of online social networking and the development of new digital learning technologies and the advent of mobile wireless smartphones and tablet computing devices.

People and Ideas Influencing Occupational Therapy (2000 to Present)

Ann Wilcock of Australia, one of the first scholars to emphasize the idea of OT as a key contribution to population health (Figure 2-25), and **Elizabeth Townsend**

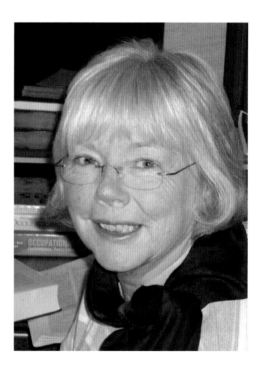

FIGURE 2-25 Ann Wilcock, PhD, DipCOT, BAppSCiOT, GradDipPH of Australia. Dr. Wilcock is the author of *An Occupational Perspective of Health* and other works and is a developer of the concept of occupational justice. (Photo courtesy of Ann Wilcock.)

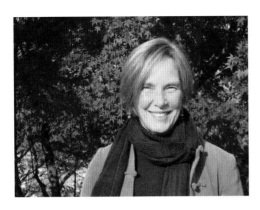

FIGURE 2-26 Elizabeth Townsend, PhD, OT(C), FCAOT, professor emerita of Dalhousie University, Halifax, Nova Scotia, Canada. Dr. Townsend is a coauthor of the Canadian guide to practice known as *Enabling Occupation* and a developer, with Ann Wilcock of Australia, of the concept of occupational justice. (Photo courtesy of Elizabeth Townsend.)

(Figure 2-26), a Canadian who partnered with Wilcock to develop and advance the concept of occupational justice (Townsend & Wilcock, 2004), jointly had a significant global influence on OT. The concept was grounded in the belief that opportunities to engage in meaningful occupation are a prerequisite to health and well-being. Their concept was given additional impetus when the World Health Organization's International Classification of Impairment, Disability, and Handicap was revised to become the International Classification of Functioning, Disability and Health (ICF) (World Health Organization, 2001).

M. Carolyn Baum (Figure 2-27) served as president of the AOTA (for the second time) from 2004 to 2007, emphasizing the important links between practice, education, and research and the need for studies to support evidence based-practice. Baum, a well-recognized leader and scientist, worked with Charles Christiansen to create the PEOP Model in the 1980s and later, as professor and director of OT at Washington University in St. Louis, organized a successful research program, developing innovative assessment tools that focused on cognitive function. As chair of the Research Commission of AOTF, Baum played a key role in advising an important intervention research program.

In 2016, Hawaii became the 50th state to enact the licensure of OT practitioners. In the Spring of 2017, under the leadership of President Amy Lamb, the AOTA board undertook a strategic planning effort to determine goals beyond the Centennial year (AOTA, 2017b, 2017c). These were focused on advocating for the importance of the association and promoting the distinct value of OT. These objectives were undertaken as part of the AOTA board's Vision 2025 initiative, which stated, "Occupational therapy maximizes health, well-being, and quality of life for all people, populations, and communities through effective solutions that facilitate participation in everyday living" (AOTA, 2017b).

In August 2017, the Accreditation Council for Occupational Therapy Education voted to mandate that the level of entry for occupational therapists and OT assistants be at the clinical doctorate (OTD) and bachelor's degree (BS), respectively, by 2027 (AOTA, 2017d).

The international community came together in 2017 as the AOTA hosted the centennial celebration in Philadelphia. It was the largest gathering of occupational therapists in history. Events were hosted throughout the world commemorating the 100th anniversary of OT, and a dedicated Website highlighted OT's history (www.otcentennial.org). For a summary of significant events and people during this era, see Box 2-7.

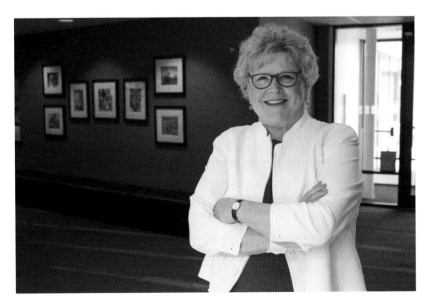

FIGURE 2-27 Carolyn Baum, PhD, is a professor and Elias Michael Director of the Program in Occupational Therapy at Washington University in St. Louis. As a widely recognized leader and scientist, Baum has advocated strongly for the important links between practice, education, and research. (Photo credit: Washington University in St. Louis. Used with Permission.)

CENTENNIAL NOTES

The History of Our History

For much of its first 60 years, records of historical significance were kept in personal files of successive AOTA presidents. When Eleanor Clarke Slagle, AOTA's third president, secured office space in New York City's Flatiron building in 1925, a central file of historical documents was kept. Yet, some documents were likely lost in later office moves.

William Rush Dunton, Jr., MD (1868–1966), a founder and AOTA's second president, wrote many editorials, reports, and obituaries as editor of *the Archives of Occupational Therapy*, the profession's first journal. These writings provide valuable information to historians. Thirty years later, Wilma L. West and Florence Cromwell helped establish the American Occupational Therapy Foundation (AOTF) and encouraged creation of an AOTF library in 1981 (now known as the Wilma L. West Library) to organize and house relevant publications and archival materials. As early as the 1950s, the writing of an official history was discussed, but it was not until historian Virginia Metaxas Quiroga was hired in 1987 that the profession's first official history was started. The first document was published in 1995, nearly 80 years after the profession was founded, and covered only the years from 1900 to 1930 (Figure 2-28).

Dr. Robert K. Bing, who later became an AOTA president, provided personal caretaking for William Rush Dunton, Jr., between 1959 and 1961. During those years, Bing gained access to interviews and personal records for his doctoral dissertation about Dunton. After the association moved its headquarters from New York City to Rockville, Maryland, in 1972, Bing, a devoted historian, was asked to chair a history committee and was able to persuade the association's board to move its aging and poorly organized historical documents and records to the Blocker History of Medicine collection at the University of Texas Medical Branch at Galveston in 1978. There, it could be indexed and preserved under the skillful guidance of dedicated curator Inci Bowman.

The impracticality and cost of maintaining OT's history in Texas led to the return of the archives to AOTA's headquarters in 1992. Since that time, the AOTF has maintained and further developed the collection in the Wilma L. West Library, now in Bethesda, Maryland. Documents are accessible to scholars on site or online through OT Search and the AOTF Website. Access to the archives and official publications has helped support the writing of numerous historical articles and several books, including those by Andersen and Reed (2017), as well as by authors outside the United States, such as Friedland (2011) in Canada and Wilcock and Hocking (2015) of Australia. Access to the archives and official publications has helped support the writing of numerous historical articles and several books. No strategic plan has yet been approved

by the profession's leaders that will assure the preservation of historical documents for future scholars and historians.

Note: Material in this note was compiled through personal correspondence with Lori Andersen, Mary Binderman, Mindy Hecker, Christine Peters, Kathlyn Reed, Ruth Schemm; from various news accounts in AOTA periodicals; and from a January 1998 article by Joel Berg entitled "From Chaos to Archives: The Records of the American Occupational Therapy Association" published in *Perspectives on History*, the news magazine of the American Historical Association.

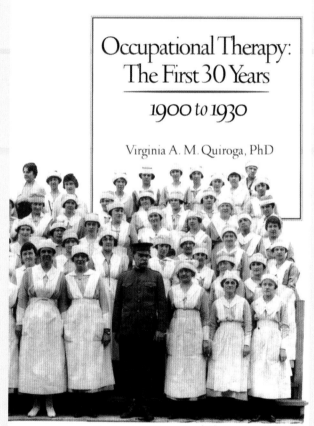

FIGURE 2-28 **Cover of the first official history of OT in the United States. The work documented the profession's first 30 years and was published by the AOTA in 1995. The author was Virginia Metaxas Quiroga. (The photo used in the cover is of reconstruction aides posing with the Army Surgeon General, Major General W. C. Gorgas in 1918. The photo used on the cover is from the Archives of the AOTA, housed in the Wilma West Library of the AOTF.)**

| **BOX 2-7** | **KEY POINTS: THE NEW MILLENNIUM (2000–PRESENT)** |

- Terrorism, globalization, digital technologies, and economic turbulence characterize the early part of the era, leading to dramatic societal changes and political upheaval.
- Occupational therapy expands dramatically in emerging regions, augmented by digital technologies; this leads to models based on different cultural perspectives, the development of online education, and the emergence of clinical doctorates.

- In the United States, practice is increasingly driven by federal reimbursement regulations influenced by cost containment and evidence-based practice, a Centennial Vision is created to guide organized national efforts, research begins to mature.
- Key people during the era included Carolyn Baum, Elizabeth Townsend, and Ann Wilcock.

Summary

In this chapter, more than a century of OT history has been reviewed, beginning with a description of important ideas and personalities prior to the twentieth century that influenced the birth of the profession. For each of five eras, a contextual backdrop was provided to describe the historical circumstances under which different events occurred, with the aim of emphasizing that professions, like individuals, are best understood in situational contexts.

Occupational therapy began during a progressive era that was auspicious for bold ideas and new approaches. Motivated by his own recovery experience and his interest in "the work cure," an ambitious architect and consumer (George Edward Barton) assembled an interdisciplinary group of like-minded advocates together to begin what is now the profession of OT. Within weeks of that meeting, a nation's preparations for war provided a rare opportunity for the fledgling profession to organize around a patriotic cause and demonstrate its value. Because women were just emerging as a political force in the country and still lacked the right to vote, the recruits to OT were uncertain about how to manifest their opportunities. Occupational therapy competed with medical specialties, vocational educators, nurses, and others who believed that they were equally entitled to the use of curative occupations as part of their treatment regimens.

For much of its history, OT practitioners were doers, perhaps insufficiently interested in explaining or proving the theoretical ideas and practical benefits of their actions. This inattention placed the profession at a disadvantage to medicine and other disciplines, where science-based practice had received greater emphasis, until the Centennial Vision led to significant intervention research efforts (AOTF, 2014). Yet, the inherent flexibility of occupations as a therapeutic medium continued to offer creative opportunities for benefiting a wide range of patients and clients. As daunting health problems served by occupational therapists (e.g., tuberculosis, polio) faded into the history books of biomedical success, occupational therapists were able to mobilize in the service of emerging health problems and concerns deemed important by consumers (such as dementia and autism spectrum disorders). Moreover, the cooperative nature of the therapeutic relationship afforded a bridge to connect the body and mind—providing occupational therapists with a rare, important, and enduring place in the lives of their patients—serving as healers as well as technologists.

As OT moves ahead into the twenty-first century, one must ask if these themes will continue to shape the story of the profession. Will the importance of science and theory experience a renaissance? Will therapists reinvent new approaches for serving the emerging diseases of the twenty-first century, and will they preserve and capitalize on their unique position as both technologists and custodians of meaning (Engelhardt, 1983)? Only the histories yet to be written will tell.

REFERENCES

Allen Cognitive Network. (2011). *Brief history*. Retrieved from http://www.allen-cognitive-network.org/

American Machinist. (2000). 1950s. *American Machinist, 144*, 130.

American Occupational Therapy Association. (1969). American occupational therapy organizations. *American Journal of Occupational Therapy, 23*, 519.

American Occupational Therapy Association. (2000). Occupational therapy and the Americans with Disabilities Act (ADA). *American Journal of Occupational Therapy, 54*, 622–625. doi:10.5014/AJOT.54.6.622

American Occupational Therapy Association. (2006a). *The road to the centennial vision*. Retrieved from https://www.aota.org/AboutAOTA/Centennial-Vision.aspx

American Occupational Therapy Association. (2006b). *2006 AOTA workforce and compensation survey: Occupational therapy salaries and job opportunities continue to improve. OT Practice Online, 9-25-06*. Retrieved from https://www.aota.org/~/media/Corporate/Files/Secure/Publications/OTP/2006/OTP%2017%20Sept%2025%202006.pdf

American Occupational Therapy Association. (2009). *History of AOTA accreditation*. Retrieved from https://www.aota.org/Education-Careers/Accreditation/Overview/History.aspx

American Occupational Therapy Association. (2010). Surveying the Profession: AOTA Workforce Study, *OT Practice, 15* (16), 8–11.

American Occupational Therapy Association. (2015). *Salary and workforce survey*. Bethesda, MD: AOTA Press. Retrieved from https://www.aota.org/Education-Careers/Advance-Career/Salary-Workforce-Survey.aspx

American Occupational Therapy Association. (2017a). *100 Influential people: Lela Llorens*. Retrieved from http://www.otcentennial.org/the-100-people/llorens

American Occupational Therapy Association. (2017b). *Fiscal year 2018 board of directors strategic priorities*. Retrieved from https://www.aota.org/AboutAOTA/vision-2025/fiscal-year-2018-board-of-directors-strategic-priorities.aspx

American Occupational Therapy Association. (2017c). Vision 2025. *American Journal of Occupational Therapy, 72*, 7103420010p1. doi:10.5014/ajot.2017.713002

American Occupational Therapy Association. (2017d). *AOTA Board of Directors statement on ACOTE decision (dated 8/21/2017)*. Retrieved from https://www.aota.org/Publications-News/AOTANews/2017/AOTA-board-of-directors-statement-on-ACOTE-decision.aspx

American Occupational Therapy Association/American Occupational Therapy Foundation Research Advisory Panel. (2011). Occupational therapy research agenda. *OTJR: Occupation, Participation and Health, 31*, 52–54. Retrieved from https://www.aota.org//media/Corporate/Files/Practice/Researcher/AOTF-AOTA%20Occupational%20Therapy%20Research%20Agenda.ashx

American Occupational Therapy Foundation. (2012). *Academy of Research in Occupational Therapy*. Retrieved from http://www.aotf.org/awardshonors/forresearch/academyofresearchinoccupationaltherapy.aspxAmerican

American Occupational Therapy Foundation. (2014). *2013 Report to donors*. Bethesda, MD: Author.

American Occupational Therapy Foundation. (2015). *2014 report to donors*. Bethesda, MD: Author.

American Recovery and Reinvestment Act (ARRA) of 2009, Pub. L. No. 111-5, 123 Stat. 115, H.R. 1 (2009).

Americans with Disabilities Act of 1990, 42 U.S.C.A. § 12101 *et seq* (1990).

Andersen, L. T., & Reed, K. (2017). *The history of occupational therapy: The first century*. Thorofare, NJ: SLACK.

Andrews, K. T., & Gaby, S. (2015). Local protest and Federal policy: The impact of the Civil Rights Movement on the 1964 Civil Rights Act. *Sociological Forum, 30*, 509–527. doi:10.1111/socf.12175

Anthony, S. H. (2005). Dr. Herbert J. Hall: Originator of honest work for occupational therapy 1904–1923 [Part I]. *Occupational Therapy in Health Care, 19*, 3–19. doi:10.1080/J003v19n03_02

Anthony, W. A. (1993). Recovery from mental illness: The guiding vision of the mental health system in the 1990's. *Psychosocial Rehabilitation Journal, 16*, 11–23. doi:10.1037/h0095655

Ayres, A. J. (1966). Interrelationships among perceptual-motor functions in children. *American Journal of Occupational Therapy, 20*, 68–71.

Ayres, A. J. (1972). *Sensory integration and learning disorders*. Los Angeles, CA: Western Psychological Services.

Ayres, A. J. (1989). *Sensory Integration and Praxis Tests*. Los Angeles, CA: Western Psychological Services.

Bakken, K. (2009). Health care coverage: The mark of a great society? *Journal of Illinois Nursing, 7–8*.

Balanced Budget Act of 1997, Pub. L. No. 105–33, 111 Stat. 269 (1997).

Baum, C. M., Christiansen, C. H., & Bass, J. D. (2015). The Person-Environment-Occupation-Performance Model. In C. H. Christiansen, C. M. Baum, & J. D. Bass (Eds.), *Occupational therapy: Performance, participation and well-being* (4th ed., pp. 49–56). Thorofare, NJ: SLACK.

Beard, G. M. (1880). *A practical treatise on nervous exhaustion (neurasthenia)*. New York, NY: William Wood.

Beck, A. H. (2004). The Flexner report and the standardization of American medical education. *JAMA, 291*, 2139–2140. doi:10.1001/jama.291.17.2139

Beers, C. (1908). *A mind that found itself: An autobiography*. New York, NY: Longmans, Green and Company.

Bergen, D. L. (2016). *War & genocide: A concise history of the holocaust* (3rd ed.). Lanham, MD: Rowman & Littlefield.

Bergin, T. J. (2007). A history of the history of programming languages. *Communications of the ACM, 50*, 69–74. doi:10.1145/1230819.1230841

Bing, R. K. (1961). *William Rush Dunton, Jr.: American psychiatrist—A study in self* (Unpublished doctoral dissertation). University of Maryland, College Park, MD.

Bing, R. K. (1981). Occupational therapy revisited: A paraphrastic journey. *American Journal of Occupational Therapy, 35*, 499–518. doi:10.5014/ajot.35.8.499

Birn, A., Brown, T. M., Fee, E., & Lear, W. J. (2003). Struggles for National Health Reform in the United States. *American Journal of Public Health, 93*, 86–91.

Braveman, B., Fisher, G., & Suarez-Balcazar, Y. (2010). In memoriam: "Achieving the ordinary things": A tribute to Gary Kielhofner. *American Journal of Occupational Therapy, 64*, 828–831. doi:10.5014/ajot.2010.64605

Brinkley, D. (2009). *The wilderness warrior: Theodore Roosevelt and the crusade for America*. New York, NY: Harper Collins.

Brown, E. J. (1996). Mary Reilly: A true bonafide character. *Advance*, April 1, 1996 edition.

Brown, L. D., Shepherd, M. D., Wituk, S. A., & Meissen, G. (2008). Introduction to the special issue on mental health self-help. *American Journal of Community Psychology, 42*, 105–109. doi:10.1007/s 10464-008-9187-7

Brunner, J. (2001). *Freud and the politics of psychoanalysis*. New Brunswick, NY: Transaction.

Burnham, J. C. (2006). The "New Freud Studies": A historiographical shift. *Journal of the Historical Society, 6*, 213–233. doi:10.1111/j.1540-5923-2006.00176.x

Canadian Association of Occupational Therapists. (1993). *Seniors' health promotion project: Responding to the challenge of an aging population's final report*. Ontario, Canada: Author.

Canadian Association of Occupational Therapists. (1997). *Enabling occupation: An occupational therapy perspective*. Ontario, Canada: Author.

Canadian Institute for Health Information. (2011). *Occupational therapists in Canada—National and jurisdictional highlights and profiles*. Ontario, Canada: Author.

Canadian Institute for Health Information. (2015). *Occupational therapists in Canada series*. Retrieved from https://secure.cihi.ca/estore/productFamily.htm?locale=en&pf=PFC3040

Carson, M. (1990). *Settlement Folk: Social Thought and the American Settlement Movement, 1885–1930*. Chicago, IL: University of Chicago Press.

Centers for Medicare & Medicaid Services. (2012). *Office of the Actuary, National Health Statistics Group, National Health Care Expenditures Data*. Retrieved from https://www.cms.gov/Research-Statistics-Data-andSystems/Statistics-Trends-and-Reports/NationalHealthExpendData/downloads/tables.pdf

Choi, Y. B., Capitan, K. E., Krause, J. S., & Streeper, M. M. (2006). Challenges associated with privacy in health care industry: implementation of HIPAA and the security rules. *Journal of Medical Systems, 30*, 57–64. doi:10.1007/s10916-006-7405-0

Christiansen, C. H. (1991). Nationally speaking: Research: Looking back and ahead after four decades of progress. *American Journal of Occupational Therapy, 45*, 391–392. doi:10.5014/ajot.45.5.391

Christiansen, C. H. (2007). Adolf Meyer revisited: Connections between lifestyles, resilience and illness. *Journal of Occupational Science, 14*, 63–76. doi:10.1080/14427591.2007.9686586

Christiansen, C. H., & Baum, C. (Eds.). (1997). Person-environment occupational performance: A conceptual model for practice.

In *Occupational therapy: Enabling function and well being* (2nd ed., pp. 47–70). Thorofare, NJ: SLACK.

Christiansen, C. H., & Taylor, R. (2011). In memoriam: Gary Wayne Kielhofner (February 15, 1949–September 2, 2010). *OTJR: Occupation, Participation and Health, 31*, 1, 2–4.

Clark, F., Azen, S. P., Zemke, R., Jackson, J., Carlson, M., Mandel, D., . . . Lipson, L. (1997). Occupational therapy for independent-living older adults. A randomized controlled trial. *JAMA, 278*, 1321–1326. doi:10.1001/jama.1997.03550160041036

Clark, F., Jackson, J., Carlson, M., Chou, C. P., Cherry, B. J., Jordan-Marsh, M., . . . Azen, S. P. (2012). Effectiveness of a lifestyle intervention in promoting the well-being of independently living older people: Results of the Well Elderly 2 Randomised Controlled Trial. *Journal of Epidemiology and Community Health, 66*, 782–790. doi:10.1136/jech.2009.099754

Clark, F., Wood, W., & Larson, E. A. (1998). Occupational science: Occupational therapy's legacy for the 21st century. In M. Neistadt & E. Crepeau (Eds.), *Willard & Spackman's occupational therapy* (9th ed., pp. 13–21). Philadelphia, PA: Lippincott Williams & Wilkins.

Classen, S. (2017). OTJR's journey in becoming a world-class journal [Editorial]. *OTJR: Occupation, Participation and Health, 37,* 59–61. doi:10.1177/1539449217699539

Clouston, T. J., & Whitcombe, S. W. (2008). The professionalization of occupational therapy: A continuing challenge. *British Journal of Occupational Therapy, 71*, 314–320. doi:10.1177/030802260807100802

Cockburn, L. (2001, May–June). The professional era: CAOT in the 1950's and 1960's. *Occupational Therapy Now*, 5–9.

Cooper, J. M. (1990). *Pivotal decades: The United States, 1900–1920.* New York, NY: Norton.

Council on Medical Education and Hospitals. (1949). *Essentials of an acceptable school of occupational therapy.* Chicago, IL: Author.

Coutinho, M. J., & Hunter, D. L. (1988). Special education and occupational therapy: Making the relationship work. *American Journal of Occupational Therapy, 42*, 706–712. doi:10.5014/ajot.42.11.706

Crane, A. G. (1927). *The medical department of the United States Army in the World War: Volume XIII: Part One: Physical reconstruction and vocational education.* Washington, DC: U.S. Government Printing Office.

Dain, N. (1980). *Clifford W. Beers, advocate for the insane.* Pittsburgh, PA: University of Pittsburgh Press.

Digby, A. (1985). *Madness, morality, and medicine: A study of the York retreat, 1796–1914.* Cambridge, NY: Cambridge University Press.

Dunn, W., Brown, C., & McGuigan, A. (1994). The ecology of human performance: A framework for considering the effect of context. *American Journal of Occupational Therapy, 48*, 595–607. doi:10.5014/ajot.48.7.595

Dunton, W. R., Jr. (1925). Editorial. *Occupational Therapy and Rehabilitation, 4*, 73–75.

Dworkin, R. W. (2010). The rise of the caring industry. *Policy Review, 161*, 45–59.

Education for All Handicapped Children Act of 1975, Pub. L. No. 94-142, 20 U.S.C. § 1401 (1975).

Egan, T. (2006). *The worst hard time: The untold story of those who survived the great American dust bowl.* New York, NY: Houghton Mifflin.

Engelhardt, H. T. (1983). Occupational therapists as technologists and custodians of meaning. In G. Kielhofner (Ed.), *Health through occupation* (pp. 130–144). Philadelphia, PA: F. A. Davis.

Eubank, K. (2004). *The origins of World War II* (3rd ed.). Somerset, NJ: Wiley-Blackwell.

Eysenck, H. (1985). *Decline and fall of the Freudian empire.* Harmondsworth, United Kingdom: Pelican.

Faiella, G. (2006). *John Locke: Champion of modern democracy.* New York, NY: Rosen.

Fearing, V. G., Law, M., & Clark, J. (1997). An occupational performance process model: Fostering client and therapist alliances. *Canadian Journal of Occupational Therapy, 64*, 7–15. doi:10.1177/000841749706400103

Fidler, G., & Fidler, J. (1954). *Introduction to psychiatric occupational therapy.* New York, NY: McMillan.

Fink, M., & Taylor, M. A. (2007). Electroconvulsive therapy: Evidence and challenges. *JAMA, 298*, 330–332. doi:10.1001/jama.298.3.330

Fisher, J. (2001). *Stolen glory: The McKinley assassination.* La Jolla, CA: Alamar Books.

Foto, M. (1997). Presidential address—Wilma West: A true visionary. *American Journal of Occupational Therapy, 51*, 638–639. doi:10.5014/ajot.51.8.638

Friedland, J. (2011). *Restoring the spirit: The beginnings of occupational therapy in Canada, 1890–1930.* Montreal, Canada: McGill-Queens University Press.

Friedland, J., & Davids-Brumer, N. (2007). From education to occupation: The story of Thomas Bessel Kidner. *Canadian Journal of Occupational Therapy, 74*, 27–37.

Friedland, J., & Silva, J. (2008). Evolving identities: Thomas Bessell Kidner and occupational therapy in the United States. *American Journal of Occupational Therapy, 62*, 349–360. doi:10.5014/ajot.62.3.349

Friedman, T. L. (2006). *The world is flat. A brief history of the 21st century.* New York, NY: Farar, Strauss, and Giroux.

Frontera, W. R., Bean, J. F., Damiano, D., Ehrlich-Jones, L., Fried-Oken, M., Jette, A., . . . Mueller, M. J. (2017). Reports—Rehabilitation research at the National Institutes of Health: Moving the field forward (executive summary). *American Journal of Occupational Therapy, 71*, 7103320010. doi:10.5014/ajot.2017.713003

Gagne, C., White, W., & Anthony, W. A. (2007). Recovery: A common vision for the fields of mental health and addictions. *Psychiatric Rehabilitation Journal, 31*, 32–37.

Gainer, R. D. (2008). History of ergonomics and occupational therapy. *Work, 31*, 5–9.

Gerber, K. M. (2007). Eight decades of health care: The 1950's. *Hospitals & Health Networks, 81*, 10–13.

Gillette, N. P. (1996). Tribute to Wilma West. In R. Zemke & F. Clark (Eds.). *Occupational Science: The evolving discipline* (pp. 403–412). Philadelphia, PA: F. A. Davis

Gillette, N. P. (2005). A tribute to Gail S. Fidler: Our esteemed mentor. *American Journal of Occupational Therapy, 59*, 609–610. doi:10.5014/ajot.59.6.609

Gladwell, M. (2002). *The tipping point: how little things can make a big difference.* New York, NY: Little, Brown, and Company, 2000.

Gordon, D. M. (2009). The history of occupational therapy. In E. B. Crepeau, E. S. Cohn, & B. A. Boyt Schell (Eds.), *Willard & Spackman's occupational therapy* (11th ed., pp. 202–215). Philadelphia, PA: Lippincott Williams & Wilkins.

Greenwald, R. A. (2005). *The triangle fire, the protocols of peace, and industrial democracy in progressive era New York.* Philadelphia, PA: Temple University Press.

Hackett, L. (1992). *The age of enlightenment: The European dream of progress and enlightenment.* Chicago, IL: Chicago Press.

Hall, H. J. (1922). *What is occupation therapy?* Paper written for the General Federation Of Women's Clubs. Chataqua, NY: Official Archives, American Occupational Therapy Foundation, Bethesda, MD.

Hallas, J. H. (2009). *Doughboy War: The American Expeditionary Force in World War I.* Mechanicsburg, PA: Stackpole Books.

Harlow, J. (2007). Eight decades of health care: The 1940's. *Hospitals and Health Networks, 81*, 10–13.

Hartwick, A. M. (1993). *Army Medical Specialist Core: 45th Anniversary.* Washington, DC: Center of Military History, United States Army.

Harvard University Library. (n.d.). *Aspiration, acculturation and impact: Immigration to the United States, 1789–1930.* Retrieved from http://ocp.hul.harvard.edu/immigration/settlement.html

Hein, C. D., & VanZante, N. R. (1993). A manager's guide: Americans with Disabilities Act of 1990. *SAM: Advanced Management Journal, 58*, 40–45.

Hernandez, N. (2005). Telemedicine and the future of telemedicine. *AMT Events, 22*, 74–75; 116–117.

Hocking, C. (2008). The way we were: Thinking rationally. *British Journal of Occupational Therapy, 71*, 185–195.

Hospitals and Health Networks. (2012). *Eight decades of health care*. Retrieved from http://www.hhnmag.com/hhnmag_app/jsp/articledisplay.jsp?dcrpath=HHNMAG/Article/data/07JUL2007/0707HHN_FEA_timeline&domain=HHNMAG

Howard, W. J., III, & Doukas, W. C. (2006). Process of care for battle casualties at Walter Reed Army Medical Center: Part IV. Occupational therapy service. *Military Medicine, 171*, 209–210.

Huret, R. (2010). Poverty in Cold War America: A problem that has no name? The invisible network of poverty experts in the 1950s and 1960s. *History of Political Economy, 2*(Suppl. 1), 53–76. doi:10.1215/00182702-2009-072

Individuals with Disabilities Education Act of 1997, Pub. L. No. 105–117, 20 U.S.C., §614, 672, 20 U.S.C. (1997). Retrieved from http://www2.ed.gov/offices/OSERS/Policy/IDEA/index.html

Iwama, M. (2006). *The Kawa model: Culturally relevant occupational therapy*. Edinburgh, United Kingdom: Churchill Livingstone/Elsevier Press.

Iwama, M., Thomson, N. A., & Macdonald, R. M. (2009). The Kawa model: The power of culturally responsive occupational therapy. *Disability and Rehabilitation, 31*, 1125–1135. doi:10.1080/09638280902773711

Karger, H., & Rose, S. R. (2010). Revisiting the Americans with Disabilities Act after two decades. *Journal of Social Work in Disability & Rehabilitation, 9*, 73–86. doi:10.1080/1536710X.2010.493468

Kennedy, D. M. (1999). 1929–1945. *Freedom from fear: The American people in depression and war*. Oxford, NY: Oxford University Press.

Kidner, T. B. (1922). Work for the tuberculous before and after the cure. *Archives of Occupational Therapy, 1*(5), 363–376.

Kielhofner, G. (1980a). A model of human occupation, part 2. Ontogenesis from the perspective of temporal adaptation. *American Journal of Occupational Therapy, 34*, 657–663. doi:10.5014/ajot.34.10.657

Kielhofner, G. (1980b). A model of human occupation, part 3, benign and vicious cycles. *American Journal of Occupational Therapy, 34*, 731–737. doi:10.5014/ajot.34.9.572

Kielhofner, G. (2008). *Model of human occupation: theory and application* (4th ed.). Philadelphia: Lippincott Williams & Wilkins.

Kielhofner, G. (2009). *Conceptual foundations of occupational therapy practice* (4th ed.). Philadelphia, PA: F. A. Davis.

Kielhofner, G., & Burke, J. P. (1977). Occupational therapy after 60 years: An account of changing identity and knowledge. *American Journal of Occupational Therapy, 31*, 675–689.

Kielhofner, G., & Burke, J. P. (1980). A model of human occupation, part 1. Conceptual framework and content. *American Journal of Occupational Therapy, 34*, 572–581. doi:10.5014/ajot.34.9.572

King, L. J. (1974). A sensory-integrative approach to schizophrenia. *American Journal of Occupational Therapy, 28*, 529–536.

King, M. L. (1963). *I had a dream*. Text of speech delivered August 28, 1963. Washington, DC.

Koyangi, C. (2007). *Learning from history: Deinstitutionalization of people with mental illness as precursor to long-term care reform*. Washington, DC: Kaiser Foundation on Medicaid and Uninsured.

Krusen, F. H. (1934). The relationship of physical therapy and occupational therapy. *Occupational Therapy and Rehabilitation, 13*, 69–77.

Kuhn, T. S. (1996). *The structure of scientific revolutions* (3rd ed.). Chicago, IL: University of Chicago Press.

Laird, A. R. (1923). Occupational therapy and vocational training in the tuberculosis sanitarium. *Archives of Occupational Therapy, 2*(5), 359–367.

Law, M., Baptiste, S., McColl, M., Opzoomer, A., Polatajko, H., & Pollock, N. (1990). The Canadian occupational performance measure: an outcome measure for occupational therapy. *Canadian Journal of Occupational Therapy, 57*, 82–87. doi:10.1177/000841749005700207

Law, M., Cooper, B., Strong, S., Stewart, D., Rigby, P., & Letts, L. (1996). The person-environment-occupation model: A transactive approach to occupational performance. *Canadian Journal of Occupational Therapy, 63*, 9–23. doi:10.1177/000841749606300103

Levin, M. F., & Panturin, E. (2011). Sensorimotor intervention for functional recovery and the Bobath approach. *Motor Control, 15*, 285–301. doi:10.1123/mcj.15.2.285

Levine, R. E. (1987). The influence of the arts-and-crafts movement on the professional status of occupational therapy. *American Journal of Occupational Therapy, 41*, 248–254.

Lief, A. (1948). *The commonsense psychiatry of Adolf Meyer*. New York, NY: McGraw-Hill.

Llorens, L. (1970). Facilitating growth and development: The promise of occupational therapy. *American Journal of Occupational Therapy, 24*, 93–101.

Loomis, B. (1992). The Henry B. Favill School of Occupations and Eleanor Clarke Slagle. *American Journal of Occupational Therapy, 46*, 34–37. doi:10.5014/ajot.46.1.34

Low, J. F. (1992). The reconstruction aides. *American Journal of Occupational Therapy, 46*, 38–43. doi:10.5014/ajot.46.1.38

Low, J. F. (1997). The issue is: NBCOT and state regulatory agencies: Allies or adversaries? *American Journal of Occupational Therapy, 51*, 74–75. doi:10.5014/ajot.51.1.74

Luchins, A. S. (2001). Moral treatment in asylums and general hospitals in 19th-century America. *The Journal of Psychology, 123*, 585–607. doi:10.1080/00223980.1989.10543013

Mahoney, M., Peters, C. O., & Martin, P. M. (2017). Willard and Spackman's enduring legacy for future occupational therapy pathways. *American Journal of Occupational Therapy, 71*, 7101100020p1–7101100020p7. doi:10.5014/ajot.2017.023994

McElvaine, R. S. (1993). *The great depression: America 1929–1941*. New York, NY: Random House.

McGrew, J. H., Wright, E. R., Pescosolido, B. A., & McDonel, E. C. (1999). The closing of Central State Hospital: Long-term outcomes for persons with severe mental illness. *The Journal of Behavioral Health Services & Research, 26*, 246–261.

Melhado, E. M. (2006). Health planning in the United States and the decline of public-interest policymaking. *The Milbank Quarterly, 84*, 359–440. doi:10.1111/j.1468-0009.2006.00451.x

Metaxas, V. A. (2000). Eleanor Clarke Slagle and Susan E. Tracy: Personal and professional identity and the development of occupational therapy in progressive era America. *Nursing History Review, 8*, 39–70.

Meyer, A. (1922). The philosophy of occupation therapy. *Archives of Occupational Therapy, 1*, 1–10.

Miller, R. J., & Walker, K. F. (1993). *Perspectives on theory for practice in occupational therapy*. Gaithersburg, MD: Aspen.

Molke, D. (2009). Outlining a Critical Ethos for Historical Work in Occupational Science and Occupational Therapy. *Journal of Occupational Science, 16*, 75–84. doi:10.1080/14427591.2009.9686646

Mosey, A. (1973). *Activities therapy*. Nashville, TN: Raven Press.

Nancarrow, S., & Mackey, H. (2005). The introduction and evaluation of an occupational therapy assistant practitioner. *Australian Journal of Occupational Therapy, 52*, 293–301. doi:10.1111/j.1440-1630.2005.00531.x

Office of the Surgeon General. (1918). *Carry on: A Magazine on the reconstruction of disabled soldiers and sailors*. Washington, DC: American Red Cross.

Oshinsky, D. M. (2005). *Polio: An American story*. New York, NY: Oxford University Press.

Ott, K., Serlin, D., & Mihm, S. (2002). *Artificial parts, practical lives.* New York, NY: New York University Press.

Oxford Brookes University. (2011). *The Churchill Hospital years.* Retrieved from http://www.brookes.ac.uk/library/speccoll/dorset/dorsethist3.html

Paine, T. (1794).*The age of reason: Being an investigation of true and fabulous theology.* Paris, France: Barras.

Palfrey, J. (2010). Four phases of Internet regulation. *Social Research, 77,* 981–996.

Patel, D. R. (2005). Therapeutic interventions in cerebral palsy. *Indian Journal of Pediatrics, 72,* 979–983. doi:10.1007/BF02731676

Patient-Centered Outcomes Research Institute. (2017). *About us.* Retrieved from the Patient Centered Outcomes Research Insitute Website: https://www.pcori.org/about-us

Peters, C. (2011a). History of mental health: Perspectives of consumers and practitioners. In C. Brown & V. C. Stoffel (Eds.), *Occupational therapy in mental health: A vision for participation* (pp. 17–30). Philadelphia, PA: F. A. Davis.

Peters, C. (2011b). Powerful occupational therapists: A community of professionals, 1950–1980. *Occupational Therapy in Mental Health, 27,* 199–410. doi:10.1080/0164212X.2011.597328

Pressman, J. D. (1998). *Last resort: Psychosurgery and the limits of medicine.* Cambridge, NY: Cambridge University Press.

Qaseem, A., Weech-Maldonado, R., & Mkanta, W. (2007). The Balanced Budget Act (1997) and the supply of nursing home subacute care. *Journal of Health Care Finance, 34,* 38–47.

Quiroga, V. A. (1995). *Occupational therapy: The first 30 years 1900–1930.* Bethesda, MD: American Occupational Therapy Association.

Reilly, M. (1962). Occupational therapy can be one of the great ideas of 20th century medicine. *American Journal of Occupational Therapy, 20,* 61–67.

Richards, E. E. (2011). Responses to occupational and environmental exposures in the U.S. military—World War II to the present. *Military Medicine, 176,* 22–28.

Rosser, S. V. (2002). An overview of Women's health in the U.S. since the 1960's. *History and Technology, 18,* 355–369. doi:10.1080/0734151022000023802

Saltman, R. B., & Dubois, H. F. W. (2004). The historical and social base of social health insurance systems. In R. B. Saltman, R. Busse, & J. Figueras (Eds.), *Social health insurance systems in Western Europe* (pp. 21–32). Berkshire, United Kingdom: Open University Press.

Salvatori, P. (2001). The history of occupational therapy assistants in Canada: A comparison with the United States. *Canadian Journal of Occupational Therapy, 68,* 217–227. doi:10.1177/000841740106800405

Sawhney, H. (2013). Analytics of organized spontaneity: Rethinking participant selection, interaction format, and milieu for academic forums. *The Information Society, 29,* 78–87. doi:10.1080/01972243.2013.758470

Schutz, A. (2011). Power and trust in the public realm: John Dewey, Saul Alinsky, and the limits of progressive democratic education. *Educational Theory, 61,* 491–512. doi:10.1111/j.1741-5446.2011.00416.x

Scull, A. (2005). *Madhouse: A tragic tale of megalomania and modern medicine.* New Haven, CT: Yale University Press.

Sealy, P., & Whitehead, P. C. (2004). Forty years of deinstitutionalization of psychiatric services in Canada: An Empirical Assessment. *Canadian Journal of Psychiatry, 49,* 249–257. doi:10.1177/070674370404900405

Slagle, E. C. (1934). Occupational therapy: Recent methods and advances in the United States. *Occupational Therapy and Rehabilitation, 13,* 289–298.

Slutsky, J., Atkins, D., Chang, S., & Sharp, B. A. (2010). AHRQ series paper 1: Comparing medical interventions: AHRQ and the Effective Healthcare Program. *Journal of Clinical Epidemiology, 63,* 471–473. doi:10.1016/j.jclinepi.2008.06.009

Spector, R. H. (1984). *Eagle against the sun: The American war against Japan.* New York: The Free Press.

St. Catherine University. (2017). *History of the occupational therapy field.* Retrieved from http://otaonline.stkate.edu/blog/how-has-occupational-therapy-changed-over-the-years/

Stadnyk, R., Townsend, E. A., & Wilcock, A. (2010). Occupational justice. In C. H. Christiansen & E. A. Townsend (Eds.), *Introduction to occupation: The art and science of living* (2nd ed., pp. 329–358). Upper Saddle River, NJ: Prentice Hall.

Stanley, J. (2010). Inner night and inner light: A quaker model of pastoral care for the mentally ill. *Journal of Religion and Health, 49,* 547–559. doi:10.1007/s10943-009-9312-4

Starr, P. (1983). *The social transformation of American medicine.* New York, NY: Basic Books.

Suarez-Balcazar, Y. (2010). *OT community mourns the loss of Dr. Gary Kielhofner.* Retrieved from http://www.aota.org/News/AOTANews/Gary-Kielhofner.aspx

Thomasson, M. A. (2002). From sickness to health: The twentieth-century development of U.S. health insurance. *Explorations in Economic History, 39,* 233–253. doi:10.1006/exeh.2002.0788

Tilsen, J., & Nylund, D. (2008). Psychotherapy research, the recovery movement and practiced based evidence in psychiatric rehabilitation. *Journal of Social Work in Disability & Rehabilitation, 7,* 340–354. doi:10.1080/15367100802487663

Townsend, E. (Ed.). (2002). *Enabling occupation: An occupational therapy perspective.* Ontario, Canada: Canadian Association of Occupational Therapists.

Townsend, E. (Ed.). (2007). *Enabling occupation II: Advancing an occupational therapy vision for health, well-being and justice through Occupation.* Ontario, Canada: Canadian Association of Occupational Therapists.

Townsend, E., & Wilcock, A. A. (2004). Occupational justice and client-centered practice. A dialogue in progress. *Canadian Journal of Occupational Therapy, 71,* 75–87. doi:10.1177/000841740407100203

Tracy, S. (1910). *Studies in invalid occupation.* Boston, MA: Whitcomb and Barrows.

University of Southern California. (n.d.). *USC occupational therapy: The 20th century.* Retrieved from the USC Website: http://ot.usc.edu/images/uploads/ot_timeline.pdf

U.S. Army Medical Department. (2012). *Occupational therapy educational programs April 1947–January 1961.* Retrieved from http://history.amedd.army.mil/corps/medical_spec/chapterxv.html

U.S. Department of Health, Education, and Welfare. (1965). *Part I: National trends in health education and welfare trends.* Washington, DC: Author.

U.S. Department of Veterans Affairs. (2015). *Military health history pocket card for clinicians.* Retrieved from http://www.va.gov/oaa/pocketcard/worldwar.asp

U.S. Government Printing Office. (2011). *The financial crisis inquiry report: Final report of the national commission on the causes of the financial and economic crisis in the United States.* Washington, DC: Author. Retrieved from https://www.gpo.gov/fdsys/pkg/GPO-FCIC/content-detail.html

Votaw, J. F. (2005). *Battle orders: The American expeditionary forces in World War I.* New York, NY: Osprey.

Wade, L. C. (2005). *Encyclopedia of Chicago: Settlement houses.* Retrieved from http://www.encyclopedia.chicagohistory.org/pages/1135.html

Ward, J. C., & Burns, K. (2007). *The war: An intimate portrait.* New York, NY: Alfred K. Knopf.

Warner, D. C. (2012). Access to health services for immigrants in the USA: From the Great Society to the 2010 health care reform and after. *Ethnic and Racial Studies, 35,* 40–55. doi:10.1080/01419870.2011.594171

West, W. L. (1991). The issue is: Should the Representative Assembly have voted as it did, when it did, on occupational therapists' use of physical agent modalities? *American Journal of Occupational Therapy, 45*, 1143–1147. doi:10.5014/ajot.45.12.1143

Whiteley, S. (2004). The evolution of the therapeutic community. *The Psychiatric Quarterly, 75*, 233–248. doi:0033-2720/040900/0233/0

Wilcock, A. A. (1998). *An occupational perspective on health.* Thorofare, NJ: SLACK.

Wilcock., A. A., & Hocking, C. (2015). *An occupational perspective of health* (3rd ed.). Thorofare, NJ: SLACK.

Willard, H. S., & Spackman, C. S. (1947). *Principles of occupational therapy.* Philadelphia, PA: J. B. Lippincott.

Williams, T. A. (1909). Requisite for the treatment of psycho-neuroses. *The Kansas City Medical Index-Lancet, 32*, 353–354.

World Federation of Occupational Therapists. (2011). *History.* Retrieved from http://www.wfot.org/AboutUs/History.aspx

World Health Organization. (2001). *International classification of functioning disability and health (ICF).* Geneva, Switzerland: Author.

Yerxa, E. J. (1967a). The 1966 Eleanor Clark Slagle Lecture: Authentic occupational therapy. *American Journal of Occupational Therapy, 21*, 155–173.

Yerxa, E. J. (1967b). The American Occupational Therapy Foundation is born. *American Journal of Occupational Therapy, 21*, 299–300.

Yerxa, E. J. (1990). An introduction to occupational science, a foundation for occupational therapy in the 21st century. *Occupational Therapy in Health Care, 6*, 1–17. doi:10.1080/J003v06n04_04

Zaloga, S. (2004). *Poland 1939: The Birth of Blitzkrieg.* Westport, CT: Praeger.

Zerhouni, E. (2003). Medicine. The NIH roadmap. *Science, 302*, 63–72. doi:10.1126/science.1091867

the**Point**® *For additional resources on the subjects discussed in this chapter, visit* **http://thePoint.lww.com /Willard-Spackman13e.**

CHAPTER 3

The Philosophy of Occupational Therapy

A Framework for Practice

Barbara Hooper, Wendy Wood

LEARNING OBJECTIVES

After reading this chapter, you will be able to:

1. Describe elements of a philosophical framework and their transactions.
2. Explain how a philosophical framework guides practice.
3. Using a comprehensive philosophical framework, articulate occupational therapy's basic philosophical assumptions and their transactions.
4. Given a practice scenario, evaluate the fit of occupational therapy's philosophy with practice.
5. Given a practice scenario, create one or two strategies that could strengthen the congruence between occupational therapy's philosophy and practice.

Introduction

Occupational therapy (OT) has a philosophy, and it may be the most basic element of practice. The profession's philosophy is the foundation upholding all that practitioners, educators, and researchers do; it helps members of the profession to (1) develop clear and coherent professional identities as *occupational* therapists, (2) hone a practice that is unique among health care providers, and (3) explain the hidden and often underestimated complexity of the profession both to themselves and others. Emphasizing how basic philosophy is, Wilcock (1999) stated that "the first essential for each individual in any profession is the acceptance of a philosophy that is the profession's keystone" (p. 192).

Specific influences of many formal philosophies on the field have been carefully detailed elsewhere (Table 3-1) and are beyond the scope of this chapter. Yet, many beliefs, values, principles, and perspectives originally imported from these formal philosophies have melded into a compelling profession-specific philosophy, which is the focus here.

Influential writers have elaborated single elements within this profession-specific philosophy such as beliefs about humans, knowledge, values, and principles for best practice. To our knowledge, however, these elements, often addressed apart from one another, have yet to be assembled into a philosophical framework. Thus, our purpose in this chapter is

TABLE 3-1 Select Resources on the Influences of Formal Philosophies on Occupational Therapy

Formal Philosophy	Select Resources
Pragmatism	Breines, 1986, 1987; Cutchin, 2004; Hooper & Wood, 2002; Ikiugu & Schultz, 2006
Arts and crafts movement	Friedland, 2003; Hocking, 2008; Levine, 1987; Reed, 1986, 2005
European enlightenment	Ikiugu & Schultz, 2006; Wilcock, 2006
Structuralism	Hooper & Wood, 2002
Existentialism	Yerxa, 1967
Humanism	Bruce & Borg, 2002; Devereaux, 1984; Nelson, 1997
Holism	Finlay, 2001
See also	Peloquin, 2005; Punwar & Peloquin, 2000; Reed & Sanderson, 1999; West, 1984

to describe the profession's philosophy using a comprehensive philosophical framework. To do so, we introduce the meaning of philosophy and three elements of a philosophical framework: ontology, epistemology, and axiology. We explore the profession-specific philosophy of OT in relation to these elements, each of which suggests a question as captured in the chapter's headings:

- Ontology: What Is Most Real for Occupational Therapy?
- Epistemology: What Is Knowledge in Occupational Therapy?
- Axiology: What Is Right Action in Occupational Therapy?

We conclude the chapter with a comparison of philosophical and nonphilosophical thinking and practice scenarios to apply the philosophical framework.

The Meaning, Structure, and Use of Philosophy

At its root, the word *philosophy* refers to "love (philo) of knowledge or wisdom (sophia)" ("Philosophy," n.d.). Philosophy is built from a "network" of assumptions and beliefs (Paul, 1995). Assumptions are ideas or principles that are "taken for granted as the basis for argument and action" (http://www.oed.com). **Assumptions** are sometimes referred to as "first principle" that form a bedrock for beliefs (Ikiugu & Schultz, 2006). **Beliefs** are convictions about what is true (Rogers, 1982b; Yerxa, 1979). When assumptions and beliefs are consciously examined and organized, they form a philosophy, which is then used as a *framework for thinking* and a *mode of thinking*. We thus define **philosophy** as (1) a conscious framework of assumptions and beliefs that guides actions and (2) a mode of thinking that actively relies on the framework for processing and responding to experience. A philosophical mode of thinking refers to "thinking with a clear sense of the ultimate foundations of one's thinking" (Paul, 1995, p. 436).

A Philosophical Framework: Ontology, Epistemology, and Axiology

A philosophical framework has at least three categories of assumptions and beliefs. One category, known as ontology, contains beliefs about reality. A second category, epistemology, contains beliefs about knowledge, and the third category, axiology, contains beliefs about appropriate actions (Lincoln, Lynham, & Guba, 2011; Ruona & Lynham, 2004; J. W. Schell, 2018a; Yerxa, 1979). In this section, we define and describe each category and how the three function as a dynamic framework for thinking.

Ontology is concerned with the question *What is most real?* Ontology is defined as the "science or study of being; that branch of metaphysics concerned with the nature or essence of being or existence" (http://www.oed .com). Occupational therapy's ontology can be discerned by examining how the field's scholars and practitioners have addressed the following questions:

- What is OT's view of the human?
- What are the *most* real dimensions of life from an OT perspective?

Yerxa (1979) phrased the question "What is 'really' real in the world?" (p. 26). Other philosophers (e.g., Sire, 2009) have phrased the question "What is prime reality—the really real?" (p. 18). In other words, what aspects of reality are illuminated and foregrounded by one's perspective? Those dimensions of reality that are in the foreground of an OT perspective constitute what is "most" real.

Epistemology asks the question *What is knowledge?* Epistemology is defined as the theory of knowledge (http://www.oed.com). Occupational therapy's epistemology can be discerned by examining how the field's scholars and practitioners have addressed the following questions:

- What knowledge is most important to know and to demonstrate in OT?
- How is knowledge in OT organized?

- How is knowledge acquired and used?
- What is an OT view of the essence or nature of knowledge?

Axiology asks the question *What are right actions?* Axiology is defined as "the study of values including what is good, beautiful, and morally desirable" (Yerxa, 1979, p. 26). Values in turn help "make explicit how we ought to act" (Ruona & Lynham, 2004, p. 154). Thus, axiology entails observable actions that manifest values; such actions are referred to as *methodologies and methods in service to one's values.* A **methodology** is a general approach to practice. **Methods** are the actual processes and procedures used when working within a given methodology. Occupational therapy's axiology can be discerned by examining how the field's scholars and practitioners have addressed the following questions:

- What are OT's enduring values?
- What are the core methodologies and methods that practitioners use in practice that manifest its enduring values?

All three categories of belief—ontology, epistemology, axiology—are fluid, mutually influential, and continually interacting. Ruona and Lynham (2004) accordingly argued that through their dynamic interactions, these categories form "a guiding framework for a congruent and coherent system of thought and action" (p. 154).

To illustrate, we borrow a visual representation from Parker Palmer (2009). Figure 3-1 uses a Möbius strip to depict the dynamic nature and ongoing transactions among OT's ontological, epistemological, and axiological premises. Beliefs about reality and knowledge are commonly more internal to the profession and individual practitioners, sometimes held without full conscious awareness; they are, therefore, depicted on what seems to be the "inside" of the Möbius strip. Beliefs about what actions to take, which are expressed in observable methodologies and methods, are depicted on what seems to be the "outside" of the strip. On closer examination, however, there is no dichotomy between an inside and outside on a Möbius strip. Rather, according to Palmer, the two sides keep coacreating each other.

If Figure 3-1 were made into a three-dimensional object (we encourage readers to do so using instructions found in the Web content), one's finger could continuously move from ontology to epistemology to axiology and so on, indicating that these three elements can be considered one whole. That is, professional beliefs about reality flow into and shape beliefs about knowledge, which flow into and shape actions manifest in practice. In reverse, professional actions and values flow into, reflect, and shape one's beliefs about reality and continue around the Möbius strip.

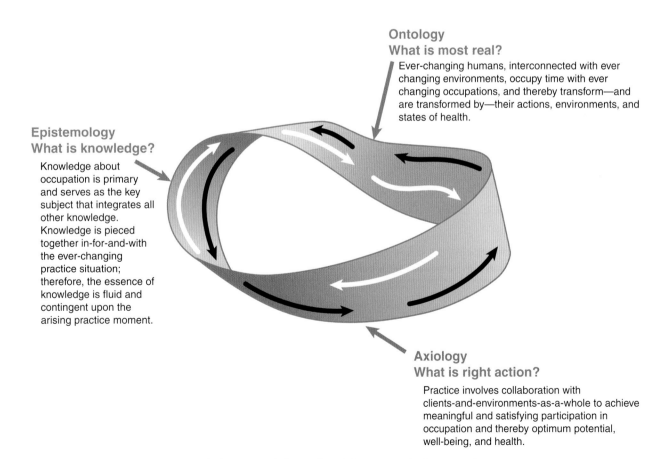

Ontology
What is most real?
Ever-changing humans, interconnected with ever changing environments, occupy time with ever changing occupations, and thereby transform—and are transformed by—their actions, environments, and states of health.

Epistemology
What is knowledge?
Knowledge about occupation is primary and serves as the key subject that integrates all other knowledge. Knowledge is pieced together in-for-and-with the ever-changing practice situation; therefore, the essence of knowledge is fluid and contingent upon the arising practice moment.

Axiology
What is right action?
Practice involves collaboration with clients-and-environments-as-a-whole to achieve meaningful and satisfying participation in occupation and thereby optimum potential, well-being, and health.

FIGURE 3-1 An occupational therapy philosophical framework for practice.

The Relationship of Philosophy to Theory

As argued in Chapter 41, theories help people understand and address something in the world. Theories are, therefore, inextricably linked to ways of seeing the world (ontology), constructing knowledge about the world (epistemology), and acting in the world (axiology) (Ruona & Lynham, 2004). A profession's philosophy consequently underpins its theories. Theory is like an intermediary that helps bind philosophy to practice and research.

The Philosophy of Occupational Therapy

Ontology: What Is Most Real for Occupational Therapy?

In her 1961 Eleanor Clarke Slagle lectureship, Mary Reilly (1962) posed that the most central belief of the profession could be stated in the form of this hypothesis: "That man, through the use of his hands, as they are energized through mind and will, can influence the state of his own health" (p. 6). Influenced by Reilly's hypothesis, and also having considered ideas that have been more recently refined or introduced (as elaborated later), we propose that OT's most central ontological premises can be summarized today as follows (see Figure 3-1):

> Ever changing humans, interconnected with ever changing environments, occupy time with ever changing occupations, and thereby transform—and are transformed by—their actions, environments and states of health.

We next elaborate on each element in this statement, beginning with the ever-changing occupational human.

The Nature of Humans, Ever-Changing Occupational Beings

A profound view of human beings has served as a cornerstone of OT since its inception: Human beings are infused with an innate, biological need for occupation; as humans engage in daily occupations, they seek to meet needs for survival, growth, development, health, and well-being (Wilcock, 2006; Wood, 1993, 1998a; Yerxa, 1998). Dunton (1919) described humans' biological need for occupation quite simply, "Occupation is as necessary to life as food and drink" (p. 17). Reilly (1962) described humans' biological requirement for occupation in neurological terms. If the human organism is to grow and become productive, then there is a vital need for occupation; indeed, in her view, the central nervous system "demands the rich and varied stimuli that solving life problems provides" (Reilly, 1962, p. 5).

Wilcock (2006) likewise argued that occupation activates the integrative functions of the central nervous system, making it possible not only for individuals to develop and experience health and well-being but also for the species to survive. Wilcock and Hocking (2015) further summarized that as humans engage in occupation, they simultaneously meet needs for doing, being, becoming, and belonging.

Embedded in these descriptions of humans' need for occupation is another long-standing belief: Humans are an indivisible whole who possess an "inextricable union of the mind and body" (Bing, 1981, p. 515; Damasio, 1994). Mind, body, and spirit can be united in humans' pursuit of and engagement with occupation (Bing, 1981; Reed & Sanderson, 1999). A core philosophical assumption of the profession, therefore, is that by virtue of our biological endowment, people of all ages and abilities require occupation to survive, grow, thrive, and belong; in pursuing occupation, humans express the totality of their being, a mind-body-spirit union. Yet as noted by Wilcock (2000), saying that humans are occupational beings, or that occupation is indispensable to survival and health, or that mind, body, and spirit are inextricably linked, is much easier than grasping what these complex articles of faith mean. Stopping there, it would be easy to conclude erroneously that these human qualities solely reside within the individual. As next discussed, one must also, therefore, consider how the environment calls forth, develops, and sustains the occupational essence of humans.

The Nature of Humans as Interconnected with Ever-Changing Environments

Being interconnected with the environment does not denote either being in harmony with the environment or being fully determined by the environment. Occupational therapy's view of reality includes simply the belief that human beings, as indivisible wholes, are part and parcel of their daily living environments (Reed & Sanderson, 1999). Kielhofner (1983) posited, for example, that "unity of the human system with the social environment is not a platitude but is an essential part of the human condition" (p. 76). In Yerxa's (1998) words, people are "complex, multileveled (biological, psychological, social, spiritual) open systems who interact with their environments" (p. 413). She maintained that just like "water cannot be reduced to hydrogen and oxygen and still be wet and drinkable," neither can human beings be viewed as separate from their environments nor "be reduced to a single level, say that of the motor system, and retain their richness or identity" (p. 413).

Although an enduring belief of OT is that human beings are best understood in the context of their environments, beliefs about the person–environment relationship have evolved. Earlier conceptions of this relationship have been critiqued for separating the person and environment too much. According to Cutchin (2004), OT historically embraced a view of the environment "as a container" in which an individual carries out occupation. The individual was the focus; the environment the background. This view allowed understandings of people to be too easily separated from understandings of environments as eliciting people's actions and influencing how they perform and experience occupation. As an alternative, scholars advocate for a closer adherence to Dewey's transactionalism, in which the human is viewed as an "organism-in-environment-as-a-whole" (Dickie, Cutchin, & Humphry, 2006, p. 83). Or, as expressed in this chapter, human beings are interconnected with their environments.

The Nature of Transformation and Health

As humans, interconnected with their environments, enact their biological need for occupation, they continuously change. Thus, through occupation, people transform and are transformed by their actions and their environments. Transformation refers to change on both small and grand scales, change for both better and worse, and subtle change such as new manifestations of an unchanging essence. On a small scale, for example, recall a time when participating in a favorite occupation transformed your outlook, emotional state, and body sense. For me (Barb), I can be in the throes of anxiety, feeling out of shape and out of time. Yet, if I can convince myself to go for a bike ride, I am, almost immediately, transformed. My anxiety falls away, joy emerges, strength returns, and time opens. In such fashion, consider how often clients express that they feel much better after working in OT to wash their face and brush their teeth for the first time after surgery. As Hasselkus (2011) persuasively illustrated, these taken-for-granted experiences and interactions reflect small-scale, yet still very important, transformations through occupation; they can even be epiphanous.

Especially prominent in OT is the more grand-scale belief that people's health changes as a function of their occupations over time (e.g., Blanche & Henny-Kohler, 2000; Friedland, 2011; Hasselkus, 2011; Kielhofner, 2004; Meyer, 1922; Peloquin, 2005; Quiroga, 1995; Reed & Sanderson, 1999; Reilly, 1962; West, 1984). In OT, health is not viewed as the absence of disease or pathology but rather as being able to engage in valued occupations. Consequently, health encompasses a dynamic state of thriving and well-being, considerations of human dignity, realization of potential, optimal functional capacities, a good quality of life, and finding meaning and satisfaction in life (Hasselkus, 2011; Peloquin, 2005; Rogers, 1982a; Wood, Lampe, Logan, Metcalfe, & Hoesley, 2017; Yerxa, 1983, 1998). People are viewed as being able to favorably influence these states of their health through occupation. Thus, OT's ontological view of human beings is an optimistic view.

This is not to say that the occupations in which people engage are seen as inevitably positive in either their subjective experiences or consequences. Because engagement in occupation is a biological necessity, when people are blocked from using—for whatever reasons—their powers to act, when they are unable to develop their potentials, when they are thwarted in being able to express their capacities for doing, then the change is toward states of dysfunction, dissatisfaction, poor health, and ill-being. What people do each day can lead to boredom, anxiety, depression, alienation, dysfunction, and ill health. So, too, can what they do lead to excitement, happiness, satisfaction, competence, and good health.

To be clear, we are not claiming a universal, theoretical consensus about occupation, which Hammel (2011) cautioned as "theoretical imperialism" (p. 27). Rather, as Watson (2006) claimed, the profession "unifies around a belief in the power and positive potential of occupation to transform people's lives. This is the profession's 'essence'" (p. 151) even as this belief must be developed in and for people in specific cultural contexts.

Ultimately, changes on a grand scale over time, whether for better or worse, can be understood to result from transformations that occur on a small scale each day. Furthermore, people's persistent "doings" can change not only themselves for both better and worse, but their doings can also change communities, societies, and the health of the planet for both better and worse (Wilcock & Hocking, 2015). Although OT's optimistic view of humans does not deny these realities, it does foreground attention to the inherent potential of all people to experience and cultivate, through occupation, a good life for themselves and others. As well summarized by Peloquin (2005), a core belief of OT is that there is, in occupation, a "capacity to help individuals become hale and whole" (p. 614).

Epistemology: What Is Knowledge in Occupational Therapy?

Occupational therapy's dominant perspective of reality and the nature of humans "sets priorities for knowledge" (Kielhofner & Burke, 1983, p. 43). As shown in Figure 3-1, we propose that the profession's most central epistemological premises today can be summarized as follows:

> Knowledge about occupation is primary and serves as the key subject that integrates all other knowledge and clarifies the desired consequences of action. Toward that end, knowledge is pieced together in-for-and-with the present practice situation that is continuously changing; therefore, the essence of knowledge is both bound and fluid, contingent upon the arising practice moment.

We elaborate on this epistemological premise by discussing each of its elements.

CENTENNIAL NOTES

Adolf Meyer and the Philosophy of Occupation Therapy

Proponents of OT have long been dedicated to articulating and promoting the profession's philosophy, often drawing from established formal philosophies. For example, Adolf Meyer, a psychiatrist, first published "The Philosophy of Occupation Therapy" in 1922 (Figure 3-2). The paper was based on a lecture Meyer gave at the fifth annual meeting of what would become the American Occupational Therapy Association (AOTA). In this classic work, Meyer described the young profession as "a very important manifestation of a very general gain in human philosophy" (p. 4). It is likely that Meyer was addressing how OT was influenced by pragmatism, a formal philosophy of his day that has shaped OT's philosophical foundations to the present day (Breines, 1986; Cutchin, 2004; Hooper & Wood, 2002; Ikiugu & Schultz, 2006).

However, OT historian, Kitty Reed (2017) studied the lecture using the historical research method, source criticism. Reed noted that Meyer did not name prominent pragmatist philosophers John Dewey or William James in his lecture even though they were likely important influences. He did, however, mention 21 other individuals, namely, people with whom he had worked and others whose philosophical ideas—energetics, behaviorism, the Montessori Method, and time-binding—compelled him. Meyer's interesting mix of chronicling his employment, the people he'd met along the way, and some loosely connected philosophical views has made this lecture a difficult read for students and scholars alike. Altogether, the paper is a curious depiction of the philosophy of occupation therapy.

Discussing Adolph Meyer at the 2017 meeting of the Society for the Study of Occupation: USA, Reed shared another finding that could explain the curious structure of Meyer's lecture as we inherited it. The title of the lecture was originally "Evolution and Principles of Occupational Therapy in Personal Reminiscence and Outlook" ("Source in Therapists' Program Ready," 1921). To date, Dr. Reed has not found any correspondence between Meyer and William Dunton, then editor of the *Archives of*

Occupational Therapy, to explain the title change. Reed imagined that perhaps Dunton thought the title was too long. She also noted that the word "occupational" with the "al" on the end appears in the original title but in the *Archives of Occupational Therapy*, the word was spelled "occupation." Like the title change, no explanation for the change in spelling has been uncovered.

Nevertheless, Meyer's classic lecture remains a source whereby students first appreciate the philosophy of OT.

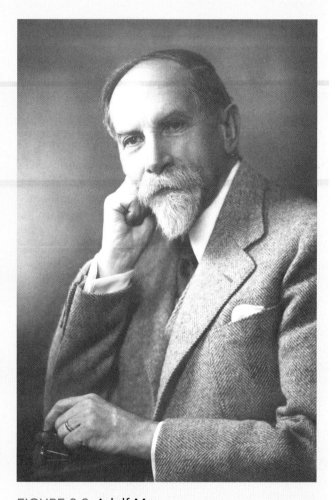

FIGURE 3-2 **Adolf Meyer.**

Knowledge of Occupation Is Primary for Occupational Therapists

Given OT's ontological premises, what is most important to know? Overwhelmingly, the answer is knowledge about occupation. As proclaimed by Weimer (1979), "Ours is, and must be, the basic knowledge of occupation" (p. 43). Reilly (1962) advised that knowledge about anatomy, neurophysiology, personality theory, social processes, and medical conditions that affect these functions, although relevant, are not our unique content. Rather, in Reilly's (1962, 1974) view, the unique knowledge of OT is a deep understanding of the nature of work and productive activity, including the play–work continuum, a belief that she believed aligned with what the founders of OT saw as most central to the new field. That occupation continues to be held today as the foremost subject matter of OT has been corroborated extensively in the official documents of professional associations worldwide (AOTA, 2014, 2017; Craik, Townsend, & Polatajko, 2008; Hocking & Ness, 2002).

As the Primary Subject, Knowledge about Occupation Organizes and Integrates All Other Knowledge

In addition to what's most important to know, epistemology entails questions such as does knowledge have a structure? If so, then how is the structure to be conceptualized? Such questions are of particular interest because knowledge of occupation entails so many, and sometimes seemingly disparate, topics ranging from kinesiology to ethics and culture. Students can feel lost in the field's wide array of topics and, not seeing an organization among them, may mistakenly think that they can pick and choose based on personal interests. It is reassuring, therefore, that scholars have promoted the view that knowledge in OT has a structure.

For example, Kielhofner (1983) conceptualized OT knowledge as a matrix consisting of three integrated and hierarchical domains: biological, psychological, and social knowledge. Neuromusculoskeletal and kinematic knowledge was placed at the bottom of the biological hierarchy, not because it was considered basic knowledge for the field but because it was viewed as being influenced by knowledge at higher levels of the hierarchy, namely, the psychological, social, and symbolic dimensions of occupation. Given this structure, biological knowledge *works* for occupational therapists when it is understood to be regulated by the psychological, social, and symbolic dimensions of occupation. For example, although two people may have an identical injury, "A hand injury to an accountant is not the same as a hand injury to a clock maker" (Kielhofner, 1983, p. 79). In the same way, a hip fracture for a retired, married man is not the same as a hip fracture for a woman who is the caregiver for an ailing spouse. Each situation is unique because of the roles, values, goals, interests, and culture (i.e., psychological, social, and symbolic levels of Kielhofner's structure) into which the injury is introduced and for which it has consequences. Conversely, although two people may have disparate diagnoses, say, schizophrenia or spinal cord injury, they may both share the identical *occupational* diagnosis of limited occupational choice, again due to what is occurring at higher psychological, symbolic, and social levels of each person.

Kielhofner (2004) later modified the relationship between knowledge domains from hierarchical to heterarchical, yet the transactional structure among biological, psychological, social, and symbolic domains remained central to understanding human performance and participation. That is, the arrangements of musculoskeletal components during performance occur in spontaneous dynamic transaction with internal and external components such as intention and contours of an object.

As the Primary Subject, Knowledge about Occupation Clarifies Desired Consequences of Action

What is most important to know and how that knowledge is organized is often linked to a group's vision for society or a set of desired consequences that a group would like to see realized (MacIntyre, 1990). Pragmatist philosophers described knowledge as continually being developed and evaluated in light of "a coveted future" (Hooper & Wood, 2002, p. 42). Thus, knowledge about occupation and how it is structured reflects a future, a set of desired consequences toward which the profession aims. That future is the optimal participation of individuals and populations in health-promoting occupations (Wilcock & Hocking, 2015). This desired future serves as the beacon toward which practitioners aim their knowledge. The exact path for arriving at this distant beacon is discovered through active experimentation that involves piecing OT knowledge together for a given practice situation and evaluating the results in light of how well it contributed to the desired consequence of participation in occupation.

Knowledge Is Pieced Together In-for-and-with the Ever-Changing Practice Situation

Knowledge in OT is bound by subject, structure, and consequence. However, working within that boundary, practitioners continuously compose knowledge domains and modes of reasoning for each practice situation. For example, in Chapter 34, Schell illustrates how practitioners assimilate and use knowledge in multiple domains, including knowledge of (1) their own beliefs, values, abilities, and experiences; (2) professional theories, evidence, and skills; (3) clients' beliefs, values, abilities, and experiences; (4) clients' goals, expectations for therapy, and how health conditions impact their occupations; and (5) the practice culture and its influence on services. Additionally, practitioners shift rapidly among and integrate multiple modes of reasoning including scientific, narrative, pragmatic, ethical, and interactive reasoning (Mattingly & Fleming, 1994; B. A. Schell & Schell, 2018).

Practitioners not only integrate multiple knowledge domains through multiple reasoning processes but also do so again and again with each practice situation. Even if on the surface the situation seems routine, it is likely unique in subtle ways such as the emotional state of the therapist or client, a change in schedule, or a change in the social environment, all of which can make the present practice situation one of a kind. Practitioners recognize that each practice situation is unique and changing even within a single therapy session. Thus, practitioners continuously assemble knowledge with and in response to each practice situation as it presents itself in each moment. Another way of saying this is: Practitioners use OT knowledge by configuring it for and with each practice situation.

The Essence of Knowledge Is Tentative, Fluid, and Contingent with the Arising Practice Moment

The earlier discussion culminates in the central consideration in epistemology: What is the nature of knowledge? In sum, knowledge in OT is bounded by its subject, occupation, and its desired consequence, health-promoting occupational engagement of individuals and populations. Additionally, there are structures for how knowledge about occupation relates to knowledge about its various elements. The subject, structure, and consequence of knowledge serve as boundaries for knowledge in the field. On the surface, these boundaries seem somewhat stable, yet they are always evolving in how we understand and talk about them. Thus, they are paradoxically enduring and tentative. On these seemingly stable foundations, OT knowledge is newly pieced together in-for-and-with each practice situation.

The essence of knowledge in OT is, thus, like a musical score. The practice of music is bounded by notes, music theory, and principles. These seemingly stable boundaries (understood and described in new ways over time) are continuously assembled into new pieces of music, and even the same pieces of music are experimented with and played with, given new interpretations in-for-and-with changing audiences and sociocultural situations.

That knowledge arises from the practice moment in a fluid and contingent manner is important for OT students to understand because it has everything to do with how students learn. That is, along with learning discrete content and skills, students need also to learn how to assemble knowledge, evaluate knowledge, and create knowledge in-for-and-with practice situations. To meet this epistemological challenge, some students find they have to dramatically shift how they have viewed themselves for many years, from a learner who receives knowledge from experts to a learner who thoughtfully and reflectively acquires and integrates knowledge in order to apply it flexibly according to what is needed for a practice situation. This shift can be life-changing (J. W. Schell, 2018b).

Axiology: What Is Right Action in Occupational Therapy?

The profession's axiology answers the questions *Given occupational therapy's central beliefs about reality and knowledge, how then shall we live day to day in practice? What do we value? What will we do?* As illustrated in Figure 3-1, views of reality and of knowledge "shape and direct how we *act* in the world . . . ." (Ruona & Lynham, 2004, p. 154). Coherence between how we act in practice and the other aspects of the field's philosophy is important to work out because as Wilcock (1999) cautioned,

> Skills without a philosophy can be a problem. It allows poaching outside a domain of concern, duplication of skills already available to those being served, the dropping of established skills for different ones when some other discipline changes its direction, or sticking to familiar skills because of no mandate to inform the direction to be taken. (p. 193)

To illustrate links between skills and philosophy, we discuss three key practice methodologies. We do not believe that these methodologies are comprehensive; for example, they do not encompass important values and actions outlined in the Occupational Therapy Code of Ethics (AOTA, 2015). We do believe, however, that these methodologies help to illustrate how actions flow from the field's ontological and epistemological premises as shown earlier in Figure 3-1. In accordance with those premises, we propose that OT's axiology can be summarized as follows:

> Practice involves collaboration with clients-and-environments-as-a-whole to achieve meaningful and satisfying participation in occupation and thereby optimal potential, well-being, and health.

Collaborative Practice

Because ever-changing humans, environments, and occupations are central to OT's beliefs about reality, it follows that entering into a personal collaboration with clients is a fundamental methodology for practice (Taylor, 2008). That is, through collaborative relationships, practitioners explore the occupations and environments with which clients seek to engage. Students will recognize this as client-centered practice but may not have considered how client-centered practice is an outward manifestation of a broader philosophical framework. Considering the philosophical framework in Figure 3-1, collaborative relationships express the profession's ontology. Similarly, if OT's central belief about knowledge involves piecing knowledge together in-for-and-with each situation, it follows that collaboration is necessary for the practitioner to determine which elements of knowledge and experience to assemble for the current situation. Thus, collaborative, relationship-centered practice constitutes a methodology that manifests OT values and beliefs about reality and knowledge.

By using the term, *methodology*, we do not mean to portray collaborative practice as a technical procedure; it is, rather, a long-standing, normative way of practicing OT and exhibiting the profession's values. As Peloquin (2005) stated, "occupational therapy *is* [emphasis added] personal engagement." Watson (2006) elaborated, stating that if we are true to the field's philosophy,

> We will make a personal connection with people in a personal way. The people we are, who we have become . . . and our earnest desire to be of service, will lead us to reach out to the "being" of the "other." (p. 156)

This textbook has much to say about OT's use of collaboration as a methodology in practice. Our purpose here is to highlight how collaborative practice as a methodology stems directly from and manifests the field's views of reality, knowledge, and right action. Collaborative practice can, therefore, serve as a stimulus for reflecting on the congruence between philosophy and practice by asking the following:

- Does this assessment or intervention or my way of being with this client reflect collaborative, relationship-centered care?
- Is collaboration at the center of my actions as an occupational therapist?

Each practitioner will have to work out specific methods for collaborative practice within the parameters of client populations served, cultural contexts for services, and practice setting, among others. But whatever challenges present, collaborative, relationship-centered care is one methodology that naturally expresses the field's core values, ontology, and epistemology.

Occupation-Centered, Occupation-Based, and Occupation-Focused Practice

Because occupation is at the very center of an OT view of reality and what practitioners most need to know, it follows that a core methodology for practice is to help clients participate in meaningful, satisfying, and health-promoting occupations. Since the field's origin, practitioners have provided opportunities for people to engage in occupation and, in so doing, to develop and to transform their skills and potential (see, e.g., Christiansen, Baum, & Bass-Haugen, 2005; Kielhofner, 2004; West, 1984; Wood, 1998b). Students may associate these approaches with being occupation-centered and, therefore, with practicing in an occupation-based or occupation-focused manner. According to Fisher (2013), being occupation-centered means having adopted OT's profession-specific perspective, or "worldview of occupation and what it means to be an occupational being," as a guide to reasoning and action (p. 167). The methodology of occupation-based practice involves using occupation in evaluation and intervention, but this is a complex process that emerges from within

each practice situation through collaborated relationships with clients (Price & Miner, 2007). The methodology of occupation-focused practice involves keeping one's immediate, proximal focus on occupation. From the start of care, therefore, practitioners seek to understand clients' occupations and use those throughout the therapy process. At all times, practitioners make explicit how their therapeutic approaches relate to the occupations that clients want and need to do. Therefore, like collaborative practice, practice that is grounded in occupation manifests beliefs about the occupational nature of humans and about knowledge as continuously being put together in-and-with each situation.

This textbook has much to say about the use of occupation-centered practice as a methodology. Our purpose here is to highlight how occupation-centered practice is a natural right action directly stemming from and manifesting the field's views of reality and knowledge. Occupation-centered practice can, thus, serve as a stimulus for reflecting on the congruence between philosophy and practice by asking the following:

- Does this assessment or intervention or my way of being with this client reflects occupation-centered practice?
- Is occupation at the center of my actions as an occupational therapist?
- Am I making a credible and meaningful connection for clients between occupation and each therapeutic approach that I use?

Once again, although each practitioner will have to work out specific methods for occupation-centered practice within the parameters of client populations served, cultural contexts for services, and practice settings, among others, occupation-centered practice is a methodology that naturally expresses the field's core values, ontology, and epistemology.

Context in Practice: Clients-and-Environments-as-a-Whole

The emphasis in OT's central belief about reality as an essential unity existing between people and environments leads to a third important methodology for practice, referred to here as clients-and-environments-as-a-whole. Occupations that are meaningful to clients—where they occur and with whom, the habits with which occupations are carried out, and the routines that help organize them, and even the musculoskeletal patterns used to perform them—occur in an interconnection between the environment and the client. This is equally true for the environments in which clients live and the environments in which they receive OT services, for example, the hospital, rehabilitation center, outpatient clinic, skilled nursing facility, home, work, school, or community (Cutchin, 2004).

According to Hasselkus (2011), seeing clients as tightly knit together with their environments through memories of places, occupation, meanings, roles, routines, and intentions can positively influence therapy outcomes related to adoption and follow-through with environmental modifications. Conversely, when practitioners view clients as separate from environments, they may overly focus on clients' performance. For example, practitioners may make recommendations for environmental modifications from a template such as widen doorways, put in stair lifts, remove throw rugs, add medical equipment, rearrange furniture, and move items to within easy reach. But because these recommendations have been considered as separate from the clients-and-environments-as-a-whole, the family may refuse to implement them.

Like the other methodologies presented, this textbook has much to say about OT's use of the performance context as a methodology in practice. Our purpose here is to illustrate how clients-and-environments-as-a-whole constitute a natural right action stemming directly from and manifesting the field's views of reality and knowledge. Clients-and-environments-as-a-whole can, therefore, serve as a stimulus for reflecting on the congruence between philosophy and practice by asking the following:

- Does this assessment or intervention or my way of being with this client reflects the unity reflected in clients-and-environments-as-a-whole?

Although each practitioner will, again, have to work out specific methods associated with this methodology within the multiple parameters previously mentioned, clients-and-environments-as-a-whole is a methodology that naturally expresses the field's core values, ontology, and epistemology.

Core Values in Occupational Therapy's Axiology

Lastly, although perhaps most importantly, the methodologies briefly presented earlier uphold and manifest core values of the profession that have been prominent throughout its history (e.g., Bing, 1981; Meyer, 1922; Peloquin, 1995, 2005, 2007; Yerxa, 1983). More specifically, inherent in these methodologies is a distinct valuing of and respect for

- The essential humanity and dignity of all people;
- The perspectives and subjective experiences of clients and their significant others;
- Empathy, caring, and genuine engagement in the therapeutic encounter;
- The use of imagination and integrity in creating occupational opportunities; and
- The inherent potential of people to experience well-being.

Application to Practice: From a Philosophical Framework to a Philosophical Mode of Thinking

Application of the philosophy of OT to practice requires a philosophical mode of thinking. A philosophical mode of thinking is bidirectional. In other words, this mode of thinking requires that a practitioner reflect on OT's philosophical assumptions about reality, knowledge, values, and action and walk those assumptions forward into practices that intentionally manifest them; it also involves reflecting on one's practice and identifying the assumptions about reality, knowledge, values, and action that it seems to manifest. Practicing this mode of thinking will help a practitioner develop a philosophical mind, which may be the most indispensable element of practice.

To further illustrate, consider Paul's (1995) contrast between a philosophical and nonphilosophical mind. The nonphilosophical mind is largely unaware that it thinks within a framework of assumptions and beliefs. Without a clear sense of the foundations that direct it, the nonphilosophical mind cannot critique those foundations; it is, therefore, somewhat trapped or run by its own unconscious, inherited system of thinking. The nonphilosophical mind tends to conform to how things are done, preferring straightforward methods and procedures without realizing that those also stem from systems of thinking. There is little awareness of a broader framework in light of which methods and procedures need to be evaluated.

Conversely, the philosophical mind is aware that all thinking occurs within and from a set of assumptions, beliefs, and values. It is keen on probing those, seeking congruence among them, and realizing them in action. The philosophical mind probes the systems of thinking reflected in methods and procedures and seeks to continuously refine those in light of its chosen broader framework of thinking. Because the philosophical mind does not confuse its own thinking with reality, it continuously considers alternative and refined thinking frameworks.

The two scenarios in the "Practice Dilemma" box (and additional learning activities on the Web) provide opportunities to build a philosophical mode of thinking, hence, to become more philosophically minded. The two scenarios are real, and we have portrayed them as accurately as possible based on direct knowledge of typical practices in each setting. We selected the scenarios because of their contrasts related to application of the philosophy of OT.

Setting A

In Setting A, OT practitioners meet each morning to determine how the client caseload will be distributed and, as opportunities permit, collaborate across the day on intervention ideas. Priorities for self-care are determined with clients and only prioritized activities of daily living (ADL) tasks are addressed. In response to the many priorities of clients beyond basic and instrumental ADL, new occupational spaces have been created in the rehab "gym"; these include an office area with computers and Internet access and a work area in which various mechanical, leisure, or work-related activities occur. The kitchen is in constant use for clients whose priorities involve aspects of home management. After morning ADL, the day is filled with individual sessions, which range from 30 minutes to 1 hour, in addition to one group session. This scheduling approach meets productivity requirements. The occupational therapists played a leadership role in designing the group in which clients commit to completing one realistic occupational project over 3 to 5 days such as, for instance, outdoor picnics for clients and their families, collecting clothing for a women's shelter, and visiting a local flea market. Steps and tasks within these projects are assigned based on clients' interests and the likelihood that they will be both challenged and successful. Although individual sessions may include exercises as a "warm-up," the focus is on either the client's occupational goals or aspects of the group's occupational project. Clients are also often given "occupational homework" for weekends. Significant others are encouraged to take part in both individual and group therapy sessions. When possible, home visits are undertaken to help identify what occupations take place in what spaces and to collaborate with clients and their significant others about acceptable modifications. Discharge planning involves setting up environments and tasks as closely as possible to clients' usual contexts and performance patterns.

Setting B

In Setting B, OT practitioners meet each morning to determine how the client caseload will be distributed and then go about their day largely independent of each other. All clients receive OT for basic ADL in the morning; practitioners emphasize ADL independence and typically complete the same ADL tasks with all clients. The rest of the day consists of consecutive 30-minute individual sessions followed by brief documentation breaks; this way of scheduling sessions is sufficient to meet the high productivity demand of the setting. Sessions emphasize physical components of function such as range of motion, strength, and endurance; prominently used modalities include theraband or putty, the range of motion arc, cones, wrist weights, the upper extremity ergometer, pulleys, dowel exercises, various physical agent modalities, and ball or balloon toss. Also addressed are visual-perceptual and cognitive components of function using modalities such as paper-and-pencil activities, puzzles, pegboards, and computer-based exercises. Intervention seldom varies from client to client, and some clients question why they need to see the occupational therapist because they already had their "therapy," that is, physical therapy that day. There is a kitchen that is used for splinting and staff meetings. Significant others are discouraged from attending therapy so that clients will not be distracted. When a client needs two people to complete a transfer or ambulate, an occupational therapist and a physical therapist may see the client together. Discharge planning may include a kitchen activity such as making a cup of tea to determine safety for returning home. Significant others receive training the last day of service before a client is discharged.

Specifically, the practices in Setting A suggest that practitioners are well grounded in the philosophy of OT and apply a philosophical mode of thinking to how they conceive and deliver services. The practices in Setting B suggest only weak links to the profession's philosophy and little evidence of a philosophical mode of thinking. Despite this divergence, both scenarios are from fast-paced, for-profit hospitals with sub-acute adult neurorehabilitation programs in which demands for productivity are equally high. Also in both settings, clients have various neurological conditions and many have suffered from strokes or other brain injuries. Occupational therapy is provided two or three times daily in both settings and length of stay typically ranges from 3 to 10 days.

As you read each of these practice dilemmas, consider how philosophy contributes to the different practice approaches in each setting. Specifically,

1. Identify both ontological and epistemological assumptions and beliefs that are manifested in how OT is understood and practiced in each scenario.
2. Identify core values that underlie the predominant practice methodologies and methods in each scenario.
3. Guided by Figure 3-1, identify areas of congruence and incongruence with the philosophy of OT in each scenario.
4. For Setting A, identify strategies that practitioners may have used to help them practice in a philosophically minded manner. Do you believe these same strategies might have been possible in Setting B? Why or why not?

Conclusion

As is true of all professions, belonging to and working in OT requires fidelity to its unique philosophy and practice approaches and, additionally, building congruence between those and one's personal philosophies. Wilcock (1999) urged that if such an examination suggests strong *incompatibility* between professional and personal philosophies, then engagement with OT should likely cease for the good of the professional (or student), future clients, and the profession itself. Conversely, Wilcock related congruence between one's personal philosophical and one's professional philosophy with the possibility for meaningful, satisfying, sustaining, and impactful work. Thus are the stakes high for engaging in philosophical modes of thinking.

REFERENCES

American Occupational Therapy Association. (2014). Occupational therapy practice framework: Domain and process, 3rd edition. *American Journal of Occupational Therapy, 68*, S1–S48. doi:10.5014/ajot.2014.682006

American Occupational Therapy Association. (2015). Occupational therapy code (2015). *American Journal of Occupational Therapy, 69*, 6913410030p1–6913410030p8. doi:10.5014/ajot.2015.696S03

American Occupational Therapy Association. (2017). Philosophical base of occupational therapy. *American Journal of Occupational Therapy, 71*, 7112410045. doi:10.5014/ajot.716S06

Bing, R. K. (1981). Eleanor Clarke Slagle Lectureship—1981. Occupational therapy revisited: A paraphrastic journey. *American Journal of Occupational Therapy, 35*, 499–518.

Blanche, E. I., & Henny-Kohler, E. (2000). Philosophy, science and ideology: A proposed relationship for occupational science and occupational therapy. *Occupational Therapy International, 7*, 99–110.

Breines, E. (1986). *Origins and adaptations: A philosophy of practice.* Lebanon, NJ: Geri-Rehab.

Breines, E. (1987). Pragmatism as a foundation for occupational therapy curricula. *American Journal of Occupational Therapy, 41*, 522–525.

Bruce, M. A., & Borg, B. (2002). *Psychosocial occupational therapy: Frames of reference for intervention.* Thorofare, NJ: SLACK.

Christiansen, C. H., Baum, C. M., & Bass-Haugen, J. (Eds.). (2005). *Occupational therapy: Performance, participation, and well-being.* Thorofare, NJ: SLACK.

Craik, J., Townsend, E., & Polatajko, H. (2008). Introducing the new guidelines—Enabling Occupation II: Advancing an occupational therapy vision for health, well-being, & justice through occupation. *Occupational Therapy Now, 10*(1), 3–5.

Cutchin, M. P. (2004). Using Deweyan philosophy to rename and reframe adaptation-to-environment. *American Journal of Occupational Therapy, 58*, 303–312.

Damasio, A. (1994). *Descartes' error: Emotion, reason, and the human brain.* New York, NY: Putnam.

Devereaux, E. B. (1984). Occupational therapy's challenge: The caring relationship. *American Journal of Occupational Therapy, 38*, 791–798.

Dickie, V., Cutchin, M. P., & Humphry, R. (2006). Occupation as transactional experience: A critique of individualism in occupational science. *Journal of Occupational Science, 13*, 83–93.

Dunton, W. R. (1919). *Reconstruction therapy.* Philadelphia, PA: W.B. Saunders.

Finlay, L. (2001). Holism in occupational therapy: Elusive fiction and ambivalent struggle. *American Journal of Occupational Therapy, 55*, 268–276.

Fisher, A. G. (2013). Occupation-centred, occupation-based, occupation-focused: Same, same or different? *Scandinavian Journal of Occupational Therapy, 20*, 162–173.

Friedland, J. (2011). *Restoring the spirit: The beginnings of occupational therapy in Canada, 1890–1930.* Montreal, Canada: McGill-Queen's University Press.

Hammell, K. W. (2011). Resisting theoretical imperialism in the disciplines of occupational science and occupational therapy. *British Journal of Occupational Therapy, 74*, 27–33.

Hasselkus, B. R. (2011). *The meaning of everyday occupation* (2nd ed.). Thorofare, NJ: SLACK.

Hocking, C. (2008). The way we were: Romantic assumptions of pioneering occupational therapists in the United Kingdom. *British Journal of Occupational Therapy, 71*, 146–154.

Hocking, C., & Ness, N. E. (2002). *Revised minimum standards for the education of occupational therapists.* Perth, Australia: World Federation of Occupational Therapists.

Hooper, B., & Wood, W. (2002). Pragmatism and structuralism in occupational therapy: The long conversation. *American Journal of Occupational Therapy, 56*, 40–50.

Ikiugu, M., & Schultz, S. (2006). An argument for pragmatism as a foundational philosophy of occupational therapy. *Canadian Journal of Occupational Therapy, 73*, 86–97.

Kielhofner, G. (1983). *Health through occupation: Theory and practice in occupational therapy.* Philadelphia, PA: F. A. Davis.

Kielhofner, G. (2004). *Conceptual foundations of occupational therapy* (3rd ed.). Philadelphia, PA: F. A. Davis.

Kielhofner, G., & Burke, J. (1983). The evolution of knowledge and practice in occupational therapy: Past, present, and future. In G. Kielhofner (Ed.), *Health through occupation: Theory and practice in occupational therapy* (pp. 3–54). Philadelphia, PA: F. A. Davis.

Levine, R. E. (1987). The influence of the arts-and-crafts movement on the professional status of occupational therapy. *American Journal of Occupational Therapy, 41*, 248–254.

Lincoln, Y. S., Lynham, S. A., & Guba, E. G. (2011). Paradigmatic controversies, contradictions, and emerging confluences, revisited. In N. K. Denzin & Y. S. Lincoln (Eds.), *Handbook of qualitative research.* Thousand Oaks, CA: Sage.

MacIntyre, A. C. (1990). *First principles, final ends and contemporary philosophical issues.* Milwaukee, WE: Marquette University Press.

Mattingly, C., & Fleming, M. H. (1994). *Clinical reasoning: Forms of inquiry in a therapeutic practice.* Philadelphia, PA: F. A. Davis.

Meyer, A. (1922). The philosophy of occupation therapy. *American Journal of Physical Medicine & Rehabilitation, 1*, 1–10.

Nelson, D. L. (1997). Why the profession of occupational therapy will flourish in the 21st century. The 1996 Eleanor Clarke Slagle Lecture. *American Journal of Occupational Therapy, 51*, 11–24.

Palmer, P. J. (2009). *Hidden wholeness: The journey toward an undivided life.* San Francisco, CA: Wiley & Sons.

Paul, R. (1995). *Critical thinking: How to prepare students for a rapidly changing world.* Santa Rosa, CA: Foundation for Critical Thinking.

Peloquin, S. M. (1995). The fullness of empathy: Reflections and illustrations. *American Journal of Occupational Therapy, 49*, 24–31.

Peloquin, S. M. (2005). The 2005 Eleanor Clark Slagle Lecture—Embracing our ethos, reclaiming our heart. *American Journal of Occupational Therapy, 59*, 611–625.

Peloquin, S. M. (2007). A reconsideration of occupational therapy's core values. *American Journal of Occupational Therapy, 61*, 474–478.

Philosophy. (n.d.). In *Online etymology dictionary.* Retrieved from http://www.etymonline.com/index.php?allowed_in_frame=0&search=philosophy&searchmode=none

Price, P., & Miner, S. (2007). Occupation emerges in the process of therapy. *American Journal of Occupational Therapy, 61*, 441–450.

Punwar, A. J., & Peloquin, S. (2000). *Occupational therapy principles and practice* (3rd ed.). Baltimore, MD: Lippincott Williams & Wilkins.

Quiroga, V. A. M. (1995). *Occupational therapy: The first 30 years 1900 to 1930.* Bethesda, MD: American Occupational Therapy Association.

Reed, K. L. (1986). Tools of practice: Heritage or baggage? 1986 Eleanor Clarke Slagle Lecture. *American Journal of Occupational Therapy, 40,* 597–605.

Reed, K. L. (2005). Dr. Hall and the work cure. *Occupational Therapy in Health Care, 19,* 33–50.

Reed, K. L. (2017). Identification of the people and critique of the ideas in Meyer's philosophy of occupation therapy. *Occupational Therapy in Mental Health, 33,* 107–128. doi:10.1080/0164212X.2017.1280445

Reed, K. L., & Sanderson, S. N. (1999). *Concepts of occupational therapy* (4th ed.). Philadelphia, PA: Lippincott, Williams & Wilkins.

Reilly, M. (1962). Occupational therapy can be one of the great ideas of 20th century medicine. *American Journal of Occupational Therapy, 16,* 1–9.

Reilly, M. (1974). *Play as exploratory learning.* Beverly Hills, CA: Sage.

Rogers, J. C. (1982a). Order and disorder in medicine and occupational therapy. *American Journal of Occupational Therapy, 36,* 29–35.

Rogers, J. C. (1982b). The spirit of independence: The evolution of a philosophy. *American Journal of Occupational Therapy, 36,* 709–715.

Ruona, W. E. A., & Lynham, S. A. (2004). A philosophical framework for thought and practice in human resource development. *Human Resource Development International, 7,* 151–164.

Schell, B. A., & Schell, J. W. (2018). Professional reasoning as the basis for practice. In B. A Schell & J. W. Schell (Eds.), *Clinical and professional reasoning in occupational therapy* (2nd ed., pp. 3–12). Philadelphia, PA: Wolters Kluwer.

Schell, J. W. (2018a). Epistemology: Knowing how you know. In B. A. Schell & J. W. Schell (Eds.), *Clinical and professional reasoning in occupational therapy* (2nd ed., pp. 229–257). Philadelphia, PA: Wolters Kluwer.

Schell, J. W. (2018b). Teaching for reasoning in higher education. In B. A. Schell & J. W. Schell (Eds.), *Clinical and professional reasoning in occupational therapy* (2nd ed., pp. 417–437). Philadelphia, PA: Wolters Kluwer.

Sire, J. W. (2009). *Universe next door: A basic worldview catalog.* Madison, WI: Inter-Varsity Press.

Source in therapists' program ready. (1921). *Hospital Management, 12*(4), 42, 76.

Taylor, R. R. (2008). *The intentional relationship: Occupational therapy and use of self.* Philadelphia, PA: F. A. Davis.

Watson, R. M. (2006). Being before doing: The cultural identity (essence) of occupational therapy. *Australian Occupational Therapy Journal, 53,* 151–158.

Weimer, R. (1979). Traditional and nontraditional practice arenas. In *Occupational therapy: 2001 AD* (pp. 42–53). Rockville, MD: American Occupational Therapy Association.

West, W. L. (1984). A reaffirmed philosophy and practice of occupational therapy for the 1980s. *American Journal of Occupational Therapy, 38,* 15–23.

Wilcock, A. A. (1999). The Doris Sym Memorial Lecture: Developing a philosophy of occupation for health. *British Journal of Occupational Therapy, 62,* 192–198.

Wilcock, A. A. (2000). Development of a personal, professional and educational occupational philosophy: An Australian perspective. *Occupational Therapy International, 7,* 79–86.

Wilcock, A. A. (2006). *An occupational perspective on health* (Vol. 2). Thorofare, NJ: SLACK.

Wilcock, A. A., & Hocking, C. (2015). *An occupational perspective of health* (3rd ed.). Thorofare, NJ: SLACK.

Wood, W. (1993). Occupation and the relevance of primatology to occupational therapy. *American Journal of Occupational Therapy, 47,* 515–522.

Wood, W. (1998a). Biological requirements for occupation in primates: An exploratory study and theoretical analysis. *Journal of Occupational Science, 5,* 66–81.

Wood, W. (1998b). Occupation centered practice [Special issue]. *American Journal of Occupational Therapy, 52.*

Wood, W., Lampe, J. L., Logan, C. A., Metcalfe, A.R., & Hoesley, B. E. (2017). The Lived Environment Life Quality Model for institutionalized people with dementia. *Canadian Journal of Occupational Therapy, 84,* 22–33.

Yerxa, E. J. (1967). 1966 Eleanor Clarke Slagle lecture. Authentic occupational therapy. *American Journal of Occupational Therapy, 21,* 1–9.

Yerxa, E. J. (1979). The philosophical base of occupational therapy. In *Occupational therapy: 2001 AD* (pp. 26–30). Rockville, MD: American Occupational Therapy Association.

Yerxa, E. J. (1983). Audacious values: The energy source for occupational therapy practice. In G. Kielhofner (Ed.), *Health through occupation: Theory and practice in occupational therapy* (pp. 149–162). Philadelphia, PA: F. A. Davis.

Yerxa, E. J. (1998). Health and the human spirit for occupation. *American Journal of Occupational Therapy, 52,* 412–422.

thePoint® *For additional resources on the subjects discussed in this chapter, visit* **http://thePoint.lww.com /Willard-Spackman13e.**

Contemporary Occupational Therapy Practice

Barbara A. Boyt Schell, Glen Gillen, Susan Coppola

"People are most true to their humanity when engaged in occupation."
—YERXA ET AL. (1989)

LEARNING OBJECTIVES

After reading this chapter, you will be able to:

1. Define occupational therapy.
2. Explain the focus of the profession using professionally relevant terminology.
3. Discuss the occupational therapy process including core aspects of practice.
4. Describe aspects of the workforce of the profession in the United States and worldwide.
5. Consider possible futures for the profession.

Occupational Therapy in Action

Contemporary occupational therapists work with a vast array of clients in many settings. A selection of clients and settings are outlined in Case Study 4-1. Camila wants to continue to enjoy her friends and her creative activities while dealing with the challenges of aging. Her daughter wants to know that she is safe in a supportive environment. Lydia wants to show that she is responsible so that she can be a good mother, find fulfilling work, and stay a welcome member of her church while avoiding the temptations to start drinking again. Amira wants to be able to work and be competitive so that she can earn as much as possible in her job. Lauro wants to be more autonomous from his parents, use public transportation, live in his own apartment someday, and learn job skills to prepare him for life after high school. Ajay wants to adjust to life after injury while learning to live in his "new body" and cope with the psychological effects of war. And the board members of the history museum want a place that is comfortable to visit for a wide range of people so that it serves to educate all its visitors on the importance of the past. These six scenarios represent the diversity of occupational therapy (OT) intervention for OT clients, be they individuals, groups, organizations, or populations. See Unit VII for more details on the diversity of OT intervention.

CASE STUDY 4-1   EXAMPLES OF CLIENTS AND SETTINGS

Camila

Camila is a retired librarian who lives in a community for older adults. She moved into an apartment there shortly after her husband's death because her sons all lived far away and she didn't feel she could manage the house and garden by herself. Shortly after she moved in, the occupational therapist met with her to help her with her transition to her new home. The occupational therapist encouraged her to volunteer in the community library and to explore the crafts room because quilting and making furnishings for miniature doll houses were long-time hobbies of hers. Over time, Camila became the leader of a crafts group of several women, sharing her files of patterns and showing others how to do needlework.

After about 3 years, some of the women in her group began to notice that Camila was becoming very anxious and forgetful and alerted the nursing staff. Eventually, Camila was diagnosed with multi-infarct dementia. The occupational therapist and the nurse both evaluated Camila and recommended that she be placed on a program where her medications were managed by the nursing staff. Additionally because Camila still had her driver's license, the occupational therapist conducted a screening of key factors related to driving, including vision, cognition, coordination, and reaction time. Camila demonstrated significant deficits in all of these areas. Based on the results of the evaluation, the occupational therapist counseled Camila and her family that she either cease driving or be retested by an on-road driving evaluation. After exploring community mobility alternatives, Camila and her family decided that she would stop driving, and she sold her car. The occupational therapists worked with Camila on using the community van so that she could continue to go on regular outings in town and her family assisted her by driving her when she needed to go shopping.

Lauro

Lauro is a 14-year-old junior high school student with developmental disabilities. He has been successfully included in the public school setting, but he, his family, and his educational team must begin planning for his transition from school to life after graduation. At a recent educational planning meeting, Lauro stated that he would like to take the local bus with his peers to his weekly after-school sports program rather than being driven by his mother each week. Lauro has never used public transportation and has little understanding of how to manage money. He is not sure what he would like to do when he grows up but knows he wants to live in his own apartment someday. Based on these goals, his occupational therapist worked with Lauro on how to manage money. They then started planning short trips on the bus to his sports program, with the occupational therapist going with him and a friend. Once the occupational therapist observed Lauro's performance, she met with the family to

plan how they could support him as he learns to ride the bus and pay for his fare. For now, Lauro is being accompanied by a friend or family member until he gains more confidence and is able to reliably use the bus.

Lydia

Lydia is a 39-year-old mother with a diagnosis of bipolar disorder. She came from a difficult family situation: Her father was abusive, and her mother was addicted to prescription medications. Lydia herself has a history of depression since age 13 years at which time she became withdrawn, started drinking a lot, and even attempted suicide. When she was 23 years old, she sought treatment for alcoholism and has been consistently sober for the past 9 years. Lydia is recently divorced from her husband, and their three surviving children live with their father. Their oldest son was killed last year in a motorcycle wreck. Although she has visitation rights, Lydia rarely sees her children because she does not drive. She doesn't have a regular job but has worked in housekeeping at a local hotel. Although she only went through eighth grade in school, she later obtained her high school diploma by passing the General Educational Development (GED) test.

After her latest episode, Lydia attended a community-based partial hospitalization program called Harborplace, where she was evaluated by an occupational therapist.

The therapist noted that Lydia was pleasant, appeared clean and well groomed, and seemed willing to participate in therapy. Lydia did demonstrate some problematic interpersonal skills such as recognizing and responding to feedback and taking responsibility for her actions. Although Lydia indicated she was interested in many things (i.e., gardening, hiking, cross-stitching, singing, and playing the piano), it was apparent that Lydia did not actually do very much on a daily basis and seemed to have trouble following through on tasks. Her only regular routines were to attend Alcoholic Anonymous (AA) meetings and church on a weekly basis. The occupational therapist worked with Lydia to develop better interpersonal and task skills and to expand her participation in all aspects of life. An important part of therapy was to help Lydia shape some goals for herself related to all her daily activities and to help her problem-solve how to actually follow through on these goals. As a result, Lydia was able to find part-time work in the garden center at a local home improvement store. She participates in several social and charitable church activities and has learned to use public transportation for community mobility and is now able to visit her children.

Amira

Amira works at a textile factory. After a serious hand injury on one of the machines, a surgeon referred her for OT at an out-patient clinic specializing in people with upper body injuries.

(continues)

CASE STUDY 4-1   EXAMPLES OF CLIENTS AND SETTINGS *(continued)*

There, Uri, her occupational therapist, made her a hand splint to protect the areas where she had surgery and showed her the daily wound care routines she would need to do to support healing. He also talked with her about problems she was having managing her activities at home while she recovered and made suggestions on how to manage with one hand. Once her surgeon indicated it was safe for Amira to begin gentle movements, Uri helped Amira regain use of her hand through focused exercise and light activities. Next, Uri talked with the employer to find out her exact duties so that he could gradually have her perform those work activities. From the company he learned that although injuries such as Amira's were less common, there was a relatively larger number of employees at the processing plant experiencing various work-related repetitive trauma injuries. Uri arranged to conduct a worksite assessment to fully understand Amira's job and to arrange for her to return to a modified job until she was able to do her old job. Later, he returned to identify how the various workstations could be changed to avoid repetitive trauma injuries. He also has been working with the work supervisors to develop and implement an employee training program to prevent the onset of these injuries.

Ajay

Ajay is a 26-year-old man who returned from an overseas war after surviving being hit by the shrapnel of a rocket-propelled grenade. He is missing his right upper limb, has burns across his chest wall, and has loss of hearing in his right ear. Prior to deployment, Ajay worked in a supermarket and was living with his girlfriend. Ajay began receiving outpatient OT to prepare for and then train with using his new upper limb prosthesis. While waiting on his new artificial arm, Ajay's occupational therapist taught Ajay how to care for his wounds from the burn and his surgical incisions. Ajay also worked on activities to strengthen his remaining arm and residual limb. Ajay's OT assistant taught him one-handed techniques to perform self-care and introduced assistive devices to help him be more independent in everyday tasks. Ajay was hesitant to accept these devices saying, "I would rather wait for my new arm."

Ajay began missing therapy sessions. When he did attend, he looked fatigued and disheveled. He reported being unable to sleep and concentrate due to reliving the war over and over again in the form of unwanted memories and nightmares. He reported that he and his girlfriend were now fighting and that she was resentful of the assistance that he required. The OT assistant reported these signs of posttraumatic stress disorder (PTSD) to his supervising occupational therapist who, in turn, encouraged Ajay to contact the local veterans' services program for a referral to a mental health worker specialized in treating PTSD. Ajay's occupational therapist worked with him to identify triggers to these unwanted memories and to structure his day so that he

remained active. She suggested that Ajay begin swimming daily (because his wounds had healed) as well as begin journaling activities. Ajay was encouraged to focus on any positive changes/events that occurred from serving in the war and document these changes in his journal. Ajay reported that since his service, he "could face any challenge." This became Ajay's new mantra, as he began the difficult task of working with his occupational therapist on learning to use his new prosthesis. See Figure 4-1 for an example of OT for a wounded soldier.

Isabella

Isabella is an occupational therapist who has been hired by the board of a local history museum as consultant. The board is committed to promoting equality, inclusion, and belonging for all their museum visitors. Isabella began the collaboration by trying to understand the organization's

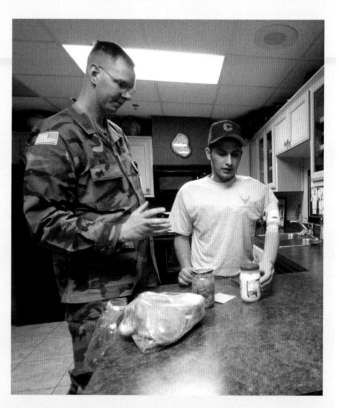

FIGURE 4-1 **Army Capt. James Watt, an occupational therapist, helps Senior Airman Dan Acosta make a sandwich in the life skills area of the amputee rehabilitation clinic at Brooke Army Medical Center in San Antonio. A mock apartment in the center helps patients get used to completing common tasks with their prosthetic limbs. (U.S. Air Force photo/Steve White).**

functioning and desires, needs, and priorities. She met with the director of education, the exhibit design staff, the volunteer coordinator, and the accessibility compliance officer. The director of education identified a need for staff and volunteers to develop a greater appreciation for the range of learning needs of museum visitors with an autism spectrum disorder (ASD). They decided to focus first on the field trip program for elementary schools. The occupational therapist then observed the volunteers guiding the school children through the museum and conducted an extensive activity analysis of the features of the program and how various features of the program may impact the experience of visitors with an ASD. This analysis was presented to the staff. Together, the occupational therapist and staff explored images and stereotypes of ASD in the culture and common behaviors associated with an ASD that might be exhibited in a museum context. They collaborated on a list of recommended tips and strategies for promoting inclusive experiences for visitors with an ASD during their museum experience.

As these scenarios demonstrate, OT practitioners provide services to a variety of clients in many settings, from hospitals and schools to community programs and businesses. These services include direct intervention with individuals to programming for groups to consultation within organizations and public advocacy. In all cases, the overarching goal of OT is to engage people in meaningful and important occupations to support health and to participate as fully as possible in society (Figure 4-2).

Definition of Occupational Therapy

Occupational therapy is a client-centered health profession concerned with promoting health and well-being through occupation. The profession's primary goal is to help people do the day-to-day activities that are important and meaningful to them and those in their lives. Occupational therapy uses a variety of interventions designed to prevent performance problems, promote healthy participation, and reduce the impact of impairment and disability on daily life (American Occupational Therapy Association [AOTA], 2014; World Federation of Occupational Therapists [WFOT], 2017). The *occupation* in OT comes from an older use of the word, meaning how people use or "occupy" their time. Hasselkus (2006) in her Slagle lecture spoke about everyday occupation as something that is so ordinary and embedded in the every day that we may fail to appreciate its complexity and how our occupations constitute an interwoven network of all we do on a daily basis. Occupation includes the complex network of day-to-day activities that enable people to sustain their health, to meet their needs, to contribute to the life of their families, and to participate in the broader society (AOTA, 2014). Finally, occupational engagement is important because it has the capacity to contribute to health and well-being (AOTA, 2017a; Clark et al., 1997; Glass, Mendes de Leon, Marottoli, & Berkman, 1999; Law, Seinwender, & Leclair, 1998). An overview of the concept of occupation is provided in Chapter 1, and aspects of it are more fully described throughout this text.

Occupational therapy draws on the centrality of occupation to daily life. It is concerned with helping clients engage in all of the activities that occupy their time, enable them to construct identity through doing, and provide meaning to their lives (Christiansen, 1999; Zemke, 2004). As the scenarios that opened this chapter illustrate, OT practitioners provide individual and group interventions as well as consultative services that foster community participation, help restore abilities to engage in life, prevent problems affecting participation, and promote the well-being of individuals and populations in a wide range of settings. The desired outcome of OT intervention is that people will live their lives engaged in occupations that sustain themselves, support their health, and foster involvement with others in their social world (Box 4-1).

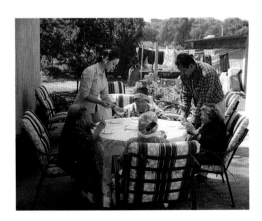

FIGURE 4-2 **Occupational therapy students in Mexico City facilitate participation in a home for older adults.**

BOX 4-1 | DEFINITIONS OF OCCUPATIONAL THERAPY

American Occupational Therapy Association

Excerpts from the AOTA Philosophical Base of Occupational Therapy

The focus and outcome of occupational therapy are clients' engagement in meaningful occupations that support their participation in life situations. Occupational therapy practitioners conceptualize occupations as both a means and an end in therapy. That is, there is therapeutic value in occupational engagement as a change agent, and engagement in occupations is also the ultimate goal of therapy. Occupational therapy is based on the belief that occupations are fundamental to health promotion and wellness, remediation or restoration, health maintenance, disease and injury prevention, and compensation and adaptation. The use of occupation to promote individual, family, community, and population health is the core of occupational therapy practice, education, research, and advocacy (AOTA, 2017b).

World Federation of Occupational Therapy

Excerpt from WFOT Statement on Occupational Therapy

Occupational therapy is a client-centred health profession concerned with promoting health and well-being through occupation. The primary goal of occupational therapy is to enable people to participate in the activities of everyday life. Occupational therapists achieve this outcome by working with people and communities to enhance their ability to engage in the occupations they want to, need to, or are expected to do, or by modifying the occupation or the environment to better support their occupational engagement. (WFOT, 2017, p.1)

Occupational Therapy Process

What is the OT process that supports the provision of services across such a broad array of clients and situations? By understanding occupation and carefully analyzing many factors associated with occupation, practitioners can use this knowledge to turn *occupation* into *therapy*. Occupational therapists must attend to the person or groups doing the occupation, the characteristics of the occupation itself, and the physical and social context in which the occupation occurs. Therapists also appreciate how various occupations interweave and how each support or detract from the other. Therefore, the evaluation process involves careful attention to what the person (or group) wants or needs to do and how both person factors and contextual factors are affecting actual performance. Intervention then involves very carefully selecting those factors that most affect performance and figuring out ways to tip the balance toward performance. Examples of common approaches include the following:

- Collaborating with clients to assess key abilities and problems affecting desired and necessary daily tasks
- Using actual activities embedded in occupations but in a graded or modified form to promote the development or restoration of performance abilities
- Assessing and changing the physical space and equipment to make performance and participation easier, safer, and more effective
- Changing the social context so that adequate support is provided for effective performance and participation

- Teaching alternate ways to perform tasks in order to improve performance and compensate for changes in the person's body functions
- Modifying routines and habits to promote health and participation in meaningful occupations
- Using preparatory activities that help the person be able to perform, such as activities and exercises to increase mobility, cognition, and emotional control (AOTA, 2014)
- Advocating for clients or supporting self-advocacy in order to promote occupational performance and participation

In order to use these approaches, OT practitioners need a wide range of skills related to analyzing and modifying activities and using their own interpersonal skills to encourage and motivate performance as well as engaging in education, consultation, and advocacy to help clients have desired performance opportunities (AOTA, 2014). Ultimately, improved performance in daily tasks and increased participation in life activities is the goal of all OT. See Chapter 27 for more details on the OT process.

Language for Occupational Therapy

As in any profession, OT uses terminology that has evolved to reflect the specific concerns of the profession. There are broad classifications or taxonomies that are useful for understanding the scope of the field and for communication core concerns to wider audiences. Because much of health care is provided in concert with other disciplines, resources described here play an important role in interprofessional communications. Two examples are resources developed by the World Health Organization (WHO) and the AOTA.

World Health Organization International Classifications

The WHO provides several resources for scientists and health care professionals throughout the world. One important document is the International Classification of Diseases (ICD), which provides a standard classification of diseases and health problems (WHO, 2010). This resource is most commonly seen when used in medical records and on billing sheets where the diagnosis is listed. Additionally, it is an important resource for research as well as public health resources. In recent decades, the WHO recognized that the classification of diseases was not adequate to reflect the concerns of people with disabilities. After extensive development, the *International Classification of Functioning, Disability and Health* (ICF) was developed (WHO, 2001). Refer to Box 4-2 for the WHO's description of the ICF. The WHO is in the process of constructing and testing yet another reference entitled the *International Classification of Health Interventions* (ICHI) (WHO, n.d.b). It remains to be seen how the profession's approaches will be reflected in the new document. In the meantime, it is important to appreciate that there is worldwide endorsement (notably in the ICF) of the importance of activities and participation to health. These have long been the core focus of the profession of OT.

International Classification of Functioning, Disability and Health

The ICF provides an organizing framework in which factors related to persons, their performance, and their performance contexts are clustered. In the most basic sense, health occurs when the person is able to participate in activities due to a good "match" between the health status and the context in which the activities occur. At the person level, individuals have body structures (such as bones and nerves) and body functions (such as muscle endurance or the ability to see). At the whole person level, individuals have the capacity to do activities (ride a bike, make dinner). Their actual participation is affected by physical and social aspects of the performance context (safe space to ride the bike, family member's praise for the meal), and thus, actual participation is a function of both personal capacity and the contextual support. So in the example of Camila in the beginning of the chapter, her ability to participate declined partly because of her changing cognitive status (body function), but she was able to continue to participate

---

BOX 4-2   INTERNATIONAL CLASSIFICATION OF FUNCTIONING, DISABILITY AND HEALTH

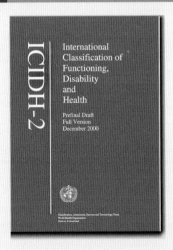

The International Classification of Functioning, Disability and Health, known more commonly as ICF, is a classification of health and health-related domains. These domains are classified from body, individual, and societal perspectives by means of two lists: a list of body functions and structure, and a list of domains of activity and participation. Because an individual's functioning and disability occurs in a context, the ICF also includes a list of environmental factors.

The ICF puts the notions of "health" and "disability" in a new light. It acknowledges that every human being can experience a decrement in health and thereby experience some degree of disability. Disability is not something that only happens to a minority of humanity. The ICF thus "mainstreams" the experience of disability and recognises it as a universal human experience. By shifting the focus from cause to impact it places all health conditions on an equal footing allowing them to be compared using a common metric—the ruler of health and disability. Furthermore, ICF takes into account the social aspects of disability and does not see disability only as a "medical" or "biological" dysfunction. By including contextual factors in which environmental factors are listed ICF allows to records the impact of the environment on the person's functioning.

From World Health Organization. (2001). *International Classification of Functioning, Disability and Health* (para. 1–2). Retrieved from http://www.who .int/classifications/icf/

TABLE 4-1 **International Classification of Functioning, Disability and Health (ICF) Categories with Definitions**

Level of Function	ICF Category	Definition
Person's body or body part	Body structures	Anatomical parts of the body such as organs, limbs, and their components
	Body functions	Physiological functions of body systems (including psychological functions)
	Impairments	Problems in body function or structure such as a significant deviation or loss
Whole person	Activity	The execution of a task or action by an individual
	Activity limitations	Difficulties an individual may have in executing activities
Context	Environmental factors	The physical, social, and attitudinal environment in which people live and conduct their lives
Person in context	Participation	Involvement in a life situation
	Participation restrictions	Problems an individual may experience in involvement in life situations

in community activities because of the environmental supports provided (community bus trips and family members driving her). This WHO document thus provides language that occupational therapists can use to explain their services to a broad audience. Table 4-1 provides a definition of these major classification categories and how each is related to general functioning. See if you can apply these concepts to each of the scenarios at the beginning of the chapter. Notice the impact each has on performance.

Occupational Therapy Practice Framework

In addition to the WHO, OT professional organizations also work to provide resources to practitioners. An important one generated by the AOTA is the Occupational Therapy Practice Framework (OTPF): Domain and Process, 3rd edition (AOTA, 2014). The OTPF presents a "summary of interrelated constructs that describe occupational therapy practice" (AOTA, 2014, p. S1). The current edition represents the evolution of a series of documents in which terminology is listed, definitions provided, and the general scope of practice is described. The authors, working on the behalf of the AOTA, attempt to gather commonly agreed-on terms and concepts. Having this information in one resource promotes more effective communication among OT practitioners as well as to the many others, such as those who pay for OT services and government groups who regulate services. Table 4-2 provides a listing from the Framework of the major domains that OT addresses. Note that there is overlap with the WHO's ICF,

TABLE 4-2 **Aspects of Occupational Therapy Domains**

Areas of Occupation	Client Factors	Performance Skills	Performance Patterns	Context and Environment	Activity Demands
Activities of daily living (ADL)[a]	Values, beliefs, and spirituality	Motor skills	Habits	Cultural	Relevance and importance to client
Instrumental activities of daily living (IADL)	Body functions	Process skills	Routines	Personal	Objects used and their properties
Rest and sleep	Body structure	Social interaction skills	Rituals	Temporal	Space demands
Education			Roles	Physical	Social demands
Work				Social	Sequencing and timing
Play				Temporal Social	Required actions and performance skills
Leisure				Virtual	Required body functions
Social participation					Required body structures

The AOTA notes that all aspects of the domain transact to support engagement, participation, and health, and no hierarchy is intended (AOTA, 2014, p. S4).

[a]Also referred to as basic activities of daily living (BADL) or personal activities of daily living (PADL).

Source: American Occupational Therapy Association. (2014). Occupational therapy practice framework: Domain and process, 3rd edition. *American Journal of Occupational Therapy, 68*, S19–S28.

in that the AOTA adopted some of the same terminology for part of the OTPF (i.e., Body Functions and Structures in the Client Factors list and some of the same categories in Context and Environment). In contrast, careful comparison will show that the AOTA provided a much more nuanced look at the aspects of occupation by including not only major categories or areas of occupation (which are analogous to the WHO's use of the term activities) but also concepts related to the various aspects of occupation and performance (i.e., skills, patterns). This is not surprising because this is the core of the profession's interests. See Figure 4-3, which explores the relationship between the ICF and the OTPF.

In addition to the major domain areas listed, the OTPF goes on to delineate the OT process and major outcomes of intervention. These are described in more detail

in Chapter 27. For now, the important point is to recognize that there is professional language that helps occupational therapists communicate among themselves and with the larger worldwide audience.

Principles That Guide Occupational Therapy Practice

Contemporary OT practice draws on the historical roots of the profession, filtered through current OT, health, and human service research and practice. Meyer (1922/1977), for example, in his oft-quoted address to the National

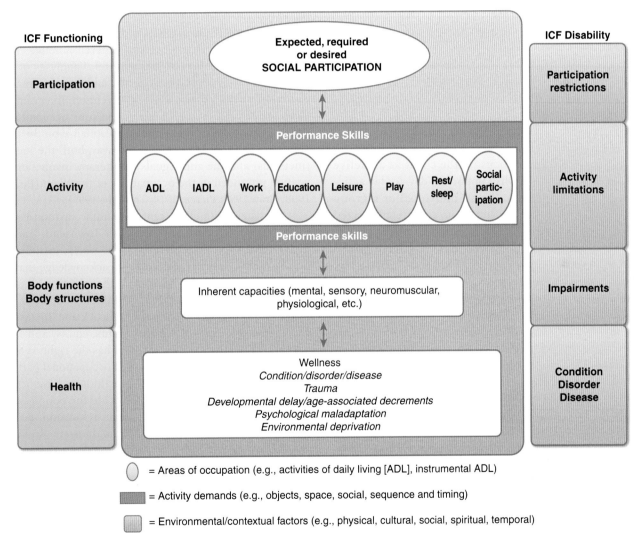

FIGURE 4-3 Connections among the International Classification of Functioning, Disability and Health and the Occupational Therapy Practice Framework. (Modified from Rogers, J. C., & Holm, M. B. [2009]. The occupational therapy process. In E. B. Crepeau, E. S. Cohn, & B. A. B. Schell [Eds.], *Willard & Spackman's occupational therapy* [11th ed. pp. 478–518]. Philadelphia, PA: Lippincott Williams & Wilkins.)

Society for the Promotion of Occupational Therapy asserted, "Our role consists in giving opportunities rather than prescriptions. There must be opportunities to work, opportunities to do, to plan and create, and to use material" (p. 641). Engelhardt (1977), and more recently Pörn (1993), asserted that health is measured by an individual's adaptive capacity and engagement in daily activities. In her Eleanor Clarke Slagle Lecture, Yerxa (1967) explained that authentic OT focuses on clients' humanity and their ability to choose and initiate activities that provide the basis for the discovery of meaning. She further argued that authentic OT requires that the practitioner "in every professional act defines the profession" and, in doing so, enters into a reciprocal relationship characterized by mutual care and that "to care means to be affected just as surely as it means to affect" (Yerxa, 1967, p. 8). Later in her address, Yerxa called for practitioner engagement in research to promote the development of the knowledge base of the profession. These themes translate into four principles that guide contemporary OT.

1. Client-centered practice
2. Occupation-centered practice
3. Evidence-based practice
4. Culturally relevant practice

Client-Centered Practice

At the core of OT is a focus on the client as an active agent seeking to accomplish important day-to-day activities. Note the client can be an individual or a group such as a family whose occupations are interconnected or workers in a company. Occupational therapy practitioners often work with people who are disempowered (Sakellariou & Pollard, 2017; Townsend & Polatajko, 2007). Clients seek care and professional help to "gain mastery over their affairs" (Rappaport, 1987, p. 122). To be client-centered, practitioners must be willing to enter the client's world to create a relationship that encourages the other to enhance his or her life in ways that are most meaningful to that client. Practitioners strive to understand the client as a person embedded in a particular context consisting of family and friends, socioeconomic status, culture, and so forth.

In a client-centered model, practitioner and client collaboratively engage in the therapeutic process (Law, 1998). Mattingly (1991) asserted that this process is narrative in nature, which means that the practitioner and client create an understanding of the client's past, present, and future story. Mattingly further asserted that the future story is co-constructed and constantly revised in the midst of therapy. Practitioners strive to understand human feelings and intentions as well as the deeper meaning of people's lives through what Clark (1993) called occupational storytelling. In contrast, occupational storymaking occurs in the midst of therapy. It is that imaginative process through which clients create and then enact new occupational identities (Clark, 1993).

Occupation-Centered Practice

Contemporary OT emphasizes occupational engagement. Clients seek OT because they need help engaging in their valued occupations. The emphasis on occupational engagement stems from the profession's beliefs, substantiated by emerging research, that people's occupations are central to their identity and that they can reconstruct themselves through their occupations (Jackson, 1998). Occupations are not isolated activities but are connected in a web of daily activities that help people fulfill their basic needs and contribute to their family, friends, and broader community (Hasselkus, 2006). Occupation-centered practice focuses on meaningful occupations selected by clients and performed in their typical settings (Fisher, 1998; Pierce, 1998). Systematic assessment of clients' occupations and priorities are vital to occupation-centered practice. This information—when coupled with careful analyses of the person's capacities, the task's demands, and the performance context—provides the basis for intervention. Intervention goals are directly connected to the person's occupational concerns, and intervention methods capitalize on the person's occupational interests. In this way, both the means (methods) and the ends (goals) of therapy involve intervention grounded in the occupations of the client (Fisher, 1998; Gray, 1998; Pierce, 2014; Trombly, 1995).

Consistent with client-centered and occupation-based practice, Ann Wilcock and Elizabeth Townsend, leaders in OT from two different parts of the world, introduced the concept of occupational justice to acknowledge that all people are occupational beings and that meeting all peoples' need for engagement in meaningful occupation is a matter of justice (see Chapter 45). Wilcock and Townsend equate occupational justice with rights, equity, and fairness and argue that every individual has the right to have equal opportunities for and access to occupational participation. To address injustices, OT practitioners have begun to develop interventions and advocate for people who are disempowered by legislation, war, relocation, political upheavals, dictatorships, or natural disasters. Rudman and colleagues also note that institutional practices, such as those found in biomedical settings, can also create less dramatic forms of injustice through their focus on disease and inattention to important life activities of their patients (Rudman, Stamm, Prodinger, & Shaw, 2014). Although many of the OT initiatives to address instances of occupational injustice have been developed throughout the world, practitioners are still early in the journey to enact the ideals of an "occupationally just" world and develop interventions with these goals in mind.

Evidence-Based Practice

One of the important trends in health care is the increasing demand to base intervention decisions on "the conscientious, explicit, and judicious use of current best evidence" (Sackett, Rosenberg, Muir Granny, Haynes, & Richardson, 1996, p. 71; Straus, Glasziou, Richardson, & Haynes, 2011). This process, called evidence-based practice, entails being able to integrate research evidence and client preferences into the professional reasoning process to explain the rationale behind interventions and predict probable outcomes—or, as Gray asserted, "doing the right things right" (as cited in Holm, 2000, p. 576). Beyond "doing the right things right," evidence-based practice involves being able to explain the evidence and related OT recommendations in a language that the clients will understand (Tickle-Degnen, 2000). Furthermore, intervention based solely on how things have been done in the past no longer meets the ethical requirement that therapists provide therapeutic approaches that are "evidence-based" (AOTA, 2015, p. 2) and for which the client has been provided with "full disclosure of the benefits, risks, and potential outcomes of any intervention" (AOTA, 2015, p. 4).

The challenge for OT practitioners is threefold.

- First, in order to practice evidence-based OT, practitioners must know how to access, evaluate, and interpret relevant research as well as to systematically attend to the data they are obtaining "in the moment" of intervention.
- Second, practitioners must have the capacity to synthesize evidence to support their intervention recommendations.
- Third, once practitioners understand the possible interventions and related outcomes, they need to communicate the probable outcomes to clients and/or their care providers so clients can make informed decisions about their participation in OT.

Not only must practitioners be willing to examine evaluation and intervention practices to see if they are effective but they must also be open to changes in their practice patterns when the evidence suggests more effective approaches than the ones they typically use. There are several sources available to OT practitioners to begin using and critiquing current evidence as shown in Box 4-3. Chapter 35 provides extensive information on how to effectively use evidence for practice.

Culturally Relevant Practice

As the OT profession continues to expand around the world, there is increasing recognition that effective OT practice must fit within the complex social, political, and cultural milieu in which therapy occurs (WFOT, 2010). Not only are there differences across countries but also within various geographical regions, there are cultural differences that impact the practice of OT (Jungersen, 1992). For instance, in the United States, there has long been a focus on promoting independence, a value deeply embedded in the culture (Brown & Gillespie, 1992). Thus, clients are encouraged to learn to do or to regain the abilities to do things by themselves with as little help as possible. However, within the United States as well as throughout the world, there are cultures that place a greater value on interdependence. The goal of therapy in these cultures may be less focused on the complete independence of the individual and more on helping members of the family or social network understand how to care for the person while still promoting meaningful engagement in valued occupations. This is but one example of how attention to the assumptions that are embedded in one's own culture must be carefully examined in light of the client's culture. Effective OT practice involves recognizing that occupations

---

BOX 4-3   EXAMPLES OF RESOURCES FOR EVIDENCE-BASED OCCUPATIONAL THERAPY PRACTICE

- **OTseeker** (http://www.otseeker.com/) is a database that contains abstracts of systematic reviews and randomized controlled trials relevant to OT. The included trials have been critically appraised and rated to assist the readers in evaluating their validity and interpretability. The ratings can be used by the readers to judge the quality and usefulness of the trials to informing clinical interventions.
- **OT Search** (http://www1.aota.org/otsearch/) is a bibliographic database covering the literature of OT and related subject areas, such as rehabilitation, education, psychiatry or psychology, and health care delivery or administration.

- **The McMaster Occupational Therapy Evidence-Based Practice Group** (http://www.srs-mcmaster.ca/Default.aspx?tabid=630) focuses on research to critically review evidence regarding the effectiveness of OT interventions and to develop tools for evaluation of OT programs.
- **The Cochrane Library** (http://www.thecochranelibrary.com/view/0/index.html) is an online collection of databases that brings together, in one place, rigorous and up-to-date research on the effectiveness of health care treatments and interventions including, but not limited to, OT.

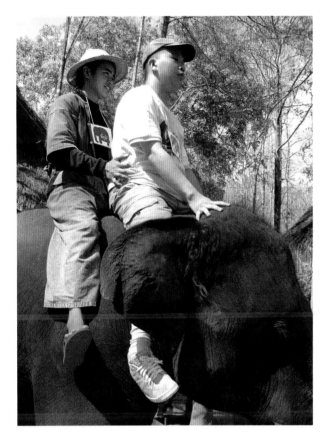

FIGURE 4-4 A child with autism spectrum disorder participates in an elephant camp implemented by occupational therapists in Thailand. Through carefully monitored interactions with the elephants, the outcomes include higher level of adaptive responses and social/communication abilities in the children.

are inherently shaped by culture, and thus, effective OT must attend to the culture of the client (Figure 4-4).

Occupational Therapy Practitioners

Clients are, of course, an essential component of OT intervention, but OT practitioners are also part of the equation. Just as clients have an occupational history, so do practitioners. Each practitioner brings a particular educational background and repertoire of experiences to the therapeutic situation. Occupational therapy education programs vary in level and curricular philosophy while also meeting standards for accreditation or approval. The WFOT Standards require a baccalaureate-level entry for occupational therapists (WFOT, 2016a). In the United States, OT assistants graduate from associate- or baccalaureate-level programs. Occupational therapists enter the

profession in the United States with a graduate degree at the level of master's or clinical doctorate; however, clinical doctorate may become to be the required entry level. Practitioners are also obligated, ethically and in some places legally, to continue their education throughout their career so that clients receive up-to-date, competent practice.

Occupational therapy is a relational practice; thus, practitioners' characteristics and habits enter into practice. Expert practitioners are aware of their own personal, social, and cultural contexts that shape their worldview and endeavor to see the world from the perspective of their clients (Higgs, 2003). Self-awareness, empathy, and professional reasoning abilities combine with preferred theories and interventions as practitioners actualize their knowledge, beliefs, and skills into therapy actions. Also at play in therapeutic situations are the practical realities of their therapy environment and the team members with whom they work (Schell, 2018). Chapter 34 provides an overview of general processes associated with professional reasoning.

Occupational Therapy by the Numbers

Occupational therapy practitioners provide services to clients across a wide range of ages, health concerns, and cultures. The WFOT reports affiliations with more than 95 different national or regional OT professional associations (WFOT, n.d.b). Denmark and Sweden have the highest number of occupational therapists relative to their populations (Denmark 11:10,000; Sweden 10:10,000). In the United States, the reported ratio is 3:10,000, which is only slightly higher than the worldwide average of 2:10,000 (WFOT, 2016b). In many countries where there is a national health service, governmental agencies are the main employers. Throughout the world, women make up an estimated 81% of OT practitioners; in the United States, the AOTA estimates that about 91.6% of both occupational therapists and OT assistants are women (AOTA, 2010).

Practice Areas

In the United States, most OT practitioners work in hospitals (26%), schools (22%), or long-term care/skilled nursing facilities (20%) (AOTA, 2010). Other common practice areas include freestanding outpatient settings (9%), home health (6%), early intervention programs for infants and children (5%), and academic settings (5%). Smaller percentages work in the community, mental health, or other settings. There is a difference between occupational therapists and OT assistants in that proportionately more OT assistants work in long-term care settings.

CENTENNIAL NOTES

Occupational Therapy—An International Idea from the Beginning

Although 2017 marked the centennial of the profession's founding in the United States, OT was an idea that took seed in a number of countries in the 1800s and into the turn of the century. The field's early concepts and approaches benefited from the exchanges of ideas among a variety of social activists and physicians in Europe and the United States. In the United Kingdom and the United States, prior to World War I, the use of occupation was instituted in many psychiatric hospitals, and schools opened to teach productive activities to children with physical and mental handicaps. A number of visits occurred between British, European, and American leaders and reformers committed to improving the daily lives of people with health problems and economic disadvantages (Wilcock, 2002).

The two world wars stimulated growth in the profession on both sides of the Atlantic Ocean. It wasn't long after the conclusion of World War II that OT leaders began to conceive of a formal international organization. The history provided by World Federation of Occupational Therapists (WFOT, n.d.a) notes that initial discussions occurred at a meeting in England in 1951, attended by 28 representatives from a variety of countries. By 1952, 10 OT associations came together to form the WFOT. These included the United States, England, Scotland, Canada, South Africa, Sweden, New Zealand, Australia, Israel, India, and Denmark. Helen Willard of the United States served as temporary chairperson until elections were held. The first elected officers were the following:

- President, Ms. Margaret B. Fulton of Scotland
- First Vice President, Ms. Gillian Crawford of Canada
- Second Vice President, Ms. Ingrid Pahlsson of Denmark
- Secretary-Treasurer, Ms. Clare S. Spackman of the United States
- Assistant Secretary-Treasurer, Mrs. Glyn Owens of England

By 1959, the WFOT became officially affiliated with the World Health Organization (WHO), and in 1963, it was recognized as a nongovernmental organization (NGO) by the United Nations (UN). As of 2017, the WFOT affiliates with over 92 member organizations. Occupational therapists all over the world benefit from the early insights of OT founders and leaders who recognized the importance of international collaboration (Figure 4-5).

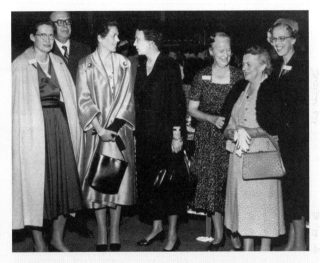

FIGURE 4-5 **Attendees at the 1958 World Federation of Occupational Therapists meeting.**

Vision for the Future

Professional organizations have an important role in setting a vision for the future that guides its work. WFOT's strategic plan for 2013–2018 is aimed at the following vision:

> WFOT will be a cohesive international organisation and the key international representative for occupational therapists and occupational therapy around the world. There will be a WFOT approved occupational therapy programme and an association with an approved constitution in every country of the world. WFOT will be financially viable and rich in resources (financial and human) enabling it to deliver member services to meet its objectives. WFOT will have mechanisms in place to monitor external influences and to measure its performance as an organization. Its members will want to participate in the work of the organisation based on a sound understanding of the organisation and the services it provides. (Pattison, 2014, p. 7)

In anticipation of AOTA's 100th anniversary in 2017, the AOTA created a centennial vision to guide its work. It stated,

> We envision that occupational therapy is a powerful, widely recognized, science-driven, and evidence-based profession with a globally connected and diverse workforce meeting society's occupational needs. (AOTA, 2006, p. 1)

In 2017, the AOTA centennial vision was replaced by Vision 2025, to guide the organizations' strategic priorities. It states,

> Occupational therapy maximizes health, well-being, and quality of life for all people, populations, and communities through effective solutions that facilitate participation in everyday living. (AOTA, 2017c, p. 1)

Pillars of this new Vision emphasize OT's effectiveness in meeting needs of individuals and groups, leadership and advocacy, collaborative processes, and accessibility across cultures. These pillars have relevance to the forces expected to influence the society the future.

- **Effective**: Occupational therapy is evidence-based, client-centered, and cost-effective.
- **Leaders**: Occupational therapy is influential in changing policies, environments, and complex systems.
- **Collaborative**: Occupational therapy excels in working with clients and within systems to produce effective outcomes.
- **Accessible**: Occupational therapy provides culturally responsive and customized services.

In countries and regions throughout the world, OT will continue to grow because of the profession's ability to help solve the problems of daily living and contribute to prevention of disabilities. Forces that will affect the profession include the following:

- Changing systems for delivering and funding care in the United States and throughout the world. As governments change, policies shift between governmental and private control of health care and other services.
- Quest for innovative community-based models of care that are tested and then spread to new regions with consideration for local health care needs, cultural practices, resources, and governmental responses. Primary care is an important focus here.
- Expectation for practitioners to provide evidence supporting evaluation and intervention strategies that lead to important client-centered outcomes (Lin, Murphy, & Robinson, 2010)
- The impact of human genome project on health care approaches and results (Reynolds & Lou, 2009)
- Evidence for the cost-effectiveness and cost savings of OT, such as reducing readmission to the hospital and return to work
- Human rights advancements and losses. Occupational therapy focuses on occupational injustices that limit individuals and groups from their rights to engage in valued occupations (Braveman & Bass-Haugen, 2009; Kronenberg, Pollard, & Sakellariou, 2011).
- The need to respond to individual-, community-, and population-level disruptions and relocations that occur as a result of natural and man-made disasters and armed conflicts (AOTA, 2017a)
- Valuing of assistive technology of all kinds, such as wheelchairs and hearing aids, to enable participation for people with disabilities (WHO, n.d.a)
- Expanding policies for rights of people with disabilities, for resources, and for participation in all aspects of society. This relates to and goes beyond occupational justice.
- Pharmaceutical and surgical advances that reduce impairments that interfere with occupations (e.g., drugs and surgeries for arthritis). These may also increase iatrogenic illnesses and disabilities.

- Proliferation of noncommunicable diseases (NCDs) that are lifestyle-based, chronic, and disabling. Examples are heart disease, diabetes, and pulmonary conditions.
- Aging societies, with a higher percentage of individuals with disabilities; as well, survival of premature and disabled infants. Caregiving needs expand.
- Increasing recognition that problems with mental health and substance abuse are on par with other health conditions with regard to their legitimacy and society's responsibility to provide care
- Occupational science research that can illuminate how change occurs thorough and within occupation
- The rapid development of worldwide technologies, including telehealth (AOTA, 2013), virtual reality, driverless cars, robotics, artificial intelligence, and personal communication devices

These and many more challenges, yet unseen, will continue to shape the profession. With vision and strategic action to advance OT's effectiveness, leadership, collaboration, and accessibility, the profession is preparing to meet society's future needs.

Conclusion

Occupational therapy is a complex process that involves collaborative interaction between the practitioner and the client embedded in the intervention context. Occupational therapy intervention must be grounded in research and focused on the client as an occupational being in a unique life situation. The therapeutic process evolves as the practitioner and client work together to analyze carefully the client's occupations and performance limitations. Because OT involves doing *with* clients and not doing *to* them, there is an improvisational aspect of intervention that requires the practitioner and client to coordinate their actions to achieve the client's goal. The rest of this book delineates the various aspects of OT involved in that process. It emphasizes consistently that best practice involves (1) understanding and respecting clients, (2) collaborating with clients to achieve their occupational goals, (3) using interventions that are supported by research, and (4) tailoring approaches to be consistent with the culture and preferences of the client.

As you start your career, our challenge to you is to strive to achieve the ideals of the profession. First, be aware of the influence of your beliefs and your personal and professional contexts and how these influence your actions. Second, consistently challenge yourself to listen to your clients so that you can facilitate their participation in their desired occupations. Third, use the most effective assessment instruments and interventions to support the progress of your clients. Fourth, advocate for your clients so they can obtain the services they need and learn to advocate for themselves. Finally, systematically evaluate your practice to ensure that your client is getting the most effective care. The people whose scenarios opened this chapter remind us that we have the responsibility to live up to the ideals of the profession. Peloquin (2005), one of our philosophers, concluded her 2005 Eleanor Clarke Slagle with the following statement:

> The ethos of occupational therapy restores our clear-sightedness so that we see what is essential: We are pathfinders. We enable occupations that heal. We co-create daily lives. We reach for hearts as well as hands. We are artists and scientists at once. If we discern this in ourselves, if we act on this understanding every day, we will advance into the future embracing our ethos of engagement. And we will have reclaimed our magnificent heart. (p. 623)

We welcome you to the path of OT.

 Visit thePoint to watch a video about evaluating body structures and functions.

REFERENCES

American Occupational Therapy Association. (2006). *AOTA adopts centennial vision*. Retrieved from http://www.aota.org/News/Media/PR/2006/38538.aspx

American Occupational Therapy Association. (2010). *Occupational therapy compensation and workforce study*. Bethesda, MD: Author.

American Occupational Therapy Association. (2013). Telehealth. *American Journal of Occupational Therapy, 67*, S69–S90.

American Occupational Therapy Association. (2014). Occupational therapy practice framework: Domain and process, 3rd edition. *American Journal of Occupational Therapy, 68*, S1–S48. doi:10.5014/ajot.2014.682006

American Occupational Therapy Association. (2015). Occupational therapy code of ethics (2015). *American Journal of Occupational Therapy, 69*, 6913410030p1–6913410030p8. doi:10.5014/ajot.2015.696S03

American Occupational Therapy Association. (2017a). AOTA's societal statement on disaster response and risk reduction. *American Journal of Occupational Therapy, 71*, 7112410060p1–7112410060p3.

American Occupational Therapy Association. (2017b). Philosophical base of occupational therapy. *American Journal of Occupational Therapy, 71*, 7112410045p1. doi:10.5014/ajot.716S06

American Occupational Therapy Association. (2017c). Vision 2025. *American Journal of Occupational Therapy, 71*, 7103420010p1. doi:10.5014/ajot.2017.7130027103420010p1

Braveman, B., & Bass-Haugen, J. D. (2009). Social justice and health disparities: An evolving discourse in occupational therapy research and intervention. *American Journal of Occupational Therapy, 63*, 7–12.

Brown, K., & Gillespie, D. (1992). Recovering relationships: A feminist analysis of recovery models. *American Journal of Occupational Therapy, 46*, 1001–1005.

Christiansen, C. H. (1999). Defining lives: Occupation as identity: An essay on competence, coherence, and the creation of meaning. *American Journal of Occupational Therapy, 54*, 547–558.

Clark, F. (1993). The 1993 Eleanor Clarke Slagle Lecture—Occupation embedded in a real life: Interweaving occupational science and occupational therapy. *American Journal of Occupational Therapy, 47*, 1067–1078.

Clark, F., Azen, S. P., Zemke, R., Jackson, J., Carlson, M., Mandel, D., . . . Lipson, L. (1997). Occupational therapy for independent-living older adults: A randomized controlled trial. *JAMA, 278*, 1321–1326.

Engelhardt, H. T. (1977). Defining occupational therapy: The meaning of therapy and the virtues of occupation. *American Journal of Occupational Therapy, 31*, 666–672.

Fisher, A. G. (1998). The 1998 Eleanor Clarke Slagle Lecture—Uniting practice and theory in an occupational framework. *American Journal of Occupational Therapy, 52*, 509–521.

Glass, T. A., Mendes de Leon, C., Marottoli, R. A., & Berkman, L. F. (1999). Population based study of social and productive activities as predictors of survival among elderly Americans. *British Medical Journal, 319*, 478–483.

Gray, J. M. (1998). Putting occupation into practice: Occupation as ends, occupation as means. *American Journal of Occupational Therapy, 52*, 354–364.

Hasselkus, B. R. (2006). The 2006 Eleanor Clarke Slagle Lecture—The world of everyday occupation: Real people, real lives. *American Journal of Occupational Therapy, 60*, 627–640.

Higgs, J. (2003). Do you reason like a (health) professional? In G. Brown, S. A. Esdaile, & S. E. Ryan (Eds.), *Becoming an advanced healthcare practitioner* (pp. 145–160). Philadelphia, PA: Butterworth.

Holm, H. B. (2000). The 2000 Eleanor Clarke Slagle Lecture—Our mandate for a new millennium: Evidence-based practice. *American Journal of Occupational Therapy, 54*, 575–585.

Jackson, J. (1998). The value of occupation as the core of treatment: Sandy's experience. *American Journal of Occupational Therapy, 52*, 466–473.

Jungersen, K. (1992). Culture, theory, and practice of occupational therapy in New Zealand/Aotearoa. *American Journal of Occupational Therapy, 46*, 745–750.

Kronenberg, F., Pollard, N., & Sakellariou, D. (2011). *Occupational Therapies Without Borders: Vol. 2. Towards an ecology of occupation-based practices*. St. Louis, MO: Churchill Livingstone/Elsevier.

Law, M. (1998). *Client-centered occupational therapy*. Thorofare, NJ: SLACK.

Law, M., Seinwender, S., & Leclair, L. (1998). Occupation, health, and well-being. *Canadian Journal of Occupational Therapy, 65*, 81–91.

Lin, S. H., Murphy, S. L., & Robinson, J. C. (2010). Facilitating evidence-based practice: Process, strategies and resources. *American Journal of Occupational Therapy, 64*, 164–171.

Mattingly, C. (1991). The narrative nature of clinical reasoning. *American Journal of Occupational Therapy, 45*, 979–986.

Meyer, A. (1977). The philosophy of occupational therapy. *American Journal of Occupational Therapy, 31*, 639–642. (Original work published 1922)

Pattison, M. (2014). World Federation of Occupational Therapists Strategic Plan 2013-2018. *WFOT Bulletin, 69*(1), 7–9.

Peloquin, S. M. (2005). The 2005 Eleanor Clarke Slagle Lecture—Embracing our ethos, reclaiming our heart. *American Journal of Occupational Therapy, 59*, 611–625.

Pierce, D. (1998). What is the source of occupation's treatment power? *American Journal of Occupational Therapy, 52*, 490–491.

Pierce, D. (Ed.). (2014). *Occupational science for occupational therapy*. Thorofare, NJ: SLACK.

Pörn, I. (1993). Health and adaptedness. *Theoretical Medicine, 14*, 295–303.

Rappaport, J. (1987). Terms of empowerment/exemplars of prevention: Toward a theory for community psychology. *American Journal of Community Psychology, 15*, 121–145.

Reynolds, S., & Lou, J. Q. (2009). Occupational therapy in the age of the human genome: Occupational therapists' role in genetics research and its impact on clinical practice. *American Journal of Occupational Therapy, 63*, 511–515.

Rogers, J. C., & Holm, M. B. (2009). The occupational therapy process. In E. B. Crepeau, E. S. Cohn, & B. A. B. Schell (Eds.), *Willard & Spackman's occupational therapy* (11th ed. pp. 478–518). Philadelphia, PA: Lippincott Williams & Wilkins.

Rudman, D. L., Stamm, T., Prodinger, B., & Shaw, L. (2014). Enacting occupation-based practice: Exploring the disjuncture between the daily lives of mothers with rheumatoid arthritis and institutional processes. *British Journal of Occupational Therapy, 77*, 491–498. doi: 10.4276/030802214X14122630932359

Sackett, D. L., Rosenberg, W. M., Granny, J. A., Haynes, R. B., & Richardson, W. S. (1996). Evidence-based medicine. What it is and what it isn't. *British Medical Journal, 312*, 71–72.

Sakellariou, D., & Pollard, N. (Eds.). (2017). *Occupational therapies without borders: Integrating justice with practice* (2nd ed.). Edinburgh, United Kingdom: Elsevier.

Schell, B. A. B. (2018). Pragmatic reasoning. In B. A. B. Schell & J. W. Schell (Eds.), *Clinical and professional reasoning in occupational therapy* (2nd ed., pp. 203–223). Philadelphia, PA: Wolters Kluwer.

Straus, S. E., Glasziou, P., Richardson, W. S., & Haynes, R. B. (2011). *Evidence-based medicine: How to practice and teach it* (4th ed.). Edinburgh, United Kingdom: Elsevier/Churchill Livingstone.

Tickle-Degnen, L. (2000). Communicating with clients, family members, and colleagues about research evidence. *American Journal of Occupational Therapy, 54*, 341–343.

Townsend, E., & Polatajko, H. (2007). *Enabling occupation II: Advancing an occupational therapy vision for health, well-being & justice through occupation*. Ottawa, Canada: Canadian Association of Occupational Therapists.

Trombly, C. A. (1995). The 1995 Eleanor Clarke Slagle Lecture—Purposefulness and meaningfulness as therapeutic mechanisms. *American Journal of Occupational Therapy, 49*, 960–972.

Wilcock, A. (2002). *Occupation for Health*: Vol. 2. *A journey from self health to prescription*. London, United Kingdom: British Association and College of Occupational Therapists.

World Federation of Occupational Therapists. (2010). *Position statement on diversity and culture*. Retrieved from http://www.wfot.org

World Federation of Occupational Therapists. (2016a). *Minimum Standards for the Education of Occupational Therapists revised 2016*. Retrieved from http://www.wfot.org

World Federation of Occupational Therapists. (2016b). *WFOT Human Resources Project*. Retrieved from http://www.wfot.org

World Federation of Occupational Therapists. (2017). *Statement on occupational therapy. Definitions of occupational therapy from member organizations*. Retrieved from http://www.wfot.org

World Federation of Occupational Therapists. (n.d.a). *History*. Retrieved from http://www.wfot.org/AboutUs/History.aspx

World Federation of Occupational Therapists. (n.d.b). *Member organisations of WFOT*. Retrieved from http://www.wfot.org /Membership/MemberOrganisationsofWFOT.aspx

World Health Organization. (2001). *International Classification of Functioning, Disability and Health*. Retrieved from http://www.who .int/classifications/icf/

World Health Organization. (2010). *International Classification of Diseases (10th ed.)*. Retrieved from http://www.who.int /classifications/icd/

World Health Organization. (n.d.a). *Global Cooperation on Assistive Technology*. Retrieved from http://www.who.int/disabilities /technology/gate/en/

World Health Organization. (n.d.b). *International Classification of Health Interventions*. Retrieved from http://www.who.int /classifications/ichi/

Yerxa, E. J. (1967). The 1967 Eleanor Clarke Slagle Lecture—Authentic occupational therapy. *American Journal of Occupational Therapy, 21*, 1–9.

Yerxa, E. J., Clark, F., Frank, G., Jackson, J., Parham, D., Pierce, D., . . . Zemke, R. (1989). An introduction to occupational science: The foundation for occupational therapy in the 21st century. *Occupational Therapy in Health Care, 6*, 1–17.

Zemke, R. (2004). The 2004 Eleanor Clarke Slagle Lecture—Time, space, and the kaleidoscopes of occupation. *American Journal of Occupational Therapy, 58*, 608–620.

the**Point**® *For additional resources on the subjects discussed in this chapter, visit* **http://thePoint.lww.com /Willard-Spackman13e.**

CHAPTER 5

Occupational Therapy Professional Organizations

Shawn Phipps, Susan Coppola

LEARNING OBJECTIVES

After reading this chapter, you will be able to:

1. Examine how member organizations, regulation, and education standards are key elements that form the profession of occupational therapy.
2. Consider the importance of lifelong membership and participation in occupational therapy professional organizations for the individual and the profession.
3. Analyze the structure and function of state, national, and international occupational therapy professional organizations.
4. Determine the purpose and nature of regulatory bodies at state, national, and international levels.
5. Evaluate how professional and regulatory organizations serve the consumers of occupational therapy through standard setting and education.
6. Explain the roles that both volunteer and paid staff members in professional organizations play in developing and supporting all aspects of the occupational therapy profession and the clients served by its members.

Introduction

When students and practitioners from a profession come together to discuss mutual challenges and opportunities, the nucleus of a professional organization (association, society, or federation) is formed (Mata, Latham, & Ransome, 2010). These shared interests and relationships create the core of a profession. **Professional organizations** then work as a formal collective to *define and advance* the interests of practitioners to better serve the public needs. These are typically nonprofit organizations with evolving structures and functions that strengthen and unite the profession around a shared mission and vision and strategic initiatives (Schneider & Somers, 2006). In occupational therapy (OT), these initiatives include setting standards for education and practice, defining and promoting a code of ethics, providing opportunities for professional education and networking, legislative advocacy for practitioners and clients, and promotion of the profession. There is a network of professional organizations, which collectively support OT. Refer to Box 5-1 to see a list of OT organizations and acronyms in USA.

BOX 5-1 | COMMON ACRONYMS IN OCCUPATIONAL THERAPY PROFESSIONAL ORGANIZATIONS (USA)

ACOTE	Accreditation Council for Occupational Therapy Education
AOTF	American Occupational Therapy Foundation
AOTPAC	American Occupational Therapy Political Action Committee
ASAP	Affiliated State Association Presidents
AOTA	The American Occupational Therapy Association, Inc.
ASD	Assembly of Student Delegates
CCCPD	Commission on Continuing Competence and Professional Development
COE	Commission on Education
COP	Commission on Practice
RA	Representative Assembly
EC	Ethics Commission
SIS	Special Interest Sections
NBCOT	National Board for Certification in Occupational Therapy
OT	Occupational Therapy
OTA	Occupational Therapy Assistant
WFOT	World Federation of Occupational Therapists

Another key element of a profession is *regulation* in order to protect the public from harm. Regulatory bodies provide a legal mechanism to ensure that persons who represent themselves as OT practitioners actually are educated, credentialed, ethical, and competent. Most countries with OT associations have a form of regulation. For example, in the United States, there is a national certification process for entry to practice, and each state requires a license to practice. Table 5-1 outlines OT as a profession using Benveniste's (1987) definition of professions as having applied knowledge, education, competency, associations, ethics, and social responsibility.

This chapter explores how elements of the profession, professional organizations, and regulation work together at the local, national, and international levels to make OT a vibrant, valuable, and growing profession. Understanding these elements and the ability to engage with them is essential to being part of the advancement of the profession and to engage in legal and ethical practice in OT. Table 5-2 gives an overview of local, national, and international associations, regulatory bodies, and education standards.

Professional Associations and the Importance of Lifelong Membership

Professional societies have made significant contributions as consultants to governments and academia and have played a major role in establishing the profession and broadening the scope of practice and the scientific body of knowledge (Bickel, 2007). Associations are made up of members who elect individuals to fulfill leadership roles, such as president, vice president, directors, and so forth. If the association has sufficient funds, paid staff enact the administrative functions and strategic priorities. In most cases, volunteers perform many association activities. A strong association enables a profession to be self-defining in standards and scope rather than have other disciplines or policy makers delineate their role. Associations provide coherence and advancement of professions through official documents, publications, professional development activities, educational standards, conferences, linkage to core values, and the profession's code of ethics. Strong associations

TABLE 5-1 | What Makes Occupational Therapy a Profession?

What makes a profession a profession?	What makes occupational therapy a profession?
1. Apply specialized knowledge and skills	OT knowledge, skills and know-how applied to the art and science of practice
2. Have advanced education and training	Accreditation standards for OT education and opportunities for continuing education and professional development
3. Have demonstrated competency and have completed the requirements to be admitted to or maintained in the profession	Certification examination, field-based performance, continuing competence requirements
4. Have the support of a professional association	State, national, and international occupational therapy organizations
5. Are bound by a code of conduct or ethics	National Associations and WFOT have Codes of Ethics
6. Feel a sense of responsibility for serving the public	Individual and collective ethos as well as regulation to protect the public

TABLE 5-2	**Relationship of Associations, Regulatory Bodies, and Education Standards**		
	OT Professional Member Associations	**Regulatory Bodies for OT Practice**	**OT Education Standards**
Purpose	Build and promote the profession to serve societal needs	Protect the public from harm	Establish minimum standards for education in the profession
State/territory/province	OT associations within states, territories, or provinces	State/regional licensure or certification board	
National	Over 85 countries have national associations. Some countries have union membership, whereas others have only regional associations.	62 countries have government regulation. This usually entails a fee and often registration with the Ministry of Health. In the United States, passing the National Board for Certification in Occupational Therapy (NBCOT) Exam is required to enter the profession. Ongoing NBCOT registration is elective for most states.	Some nations have curriculum standards. Others accept the standards from the World Federation. In the United States, AOTA's Accreditation Council for Occupational Therapy Education sets standards for OTA programs, and masters and doctorate entry-level programs for occupational therapists.
International	World Federation of Occupational Therapists (WFOT) Member organizations have a national professional association with a constitution and a code of ethics. Full members of WFOT must also have an approved educational program in their country. Of the 85 member organizations, 67 are full members.	No regulation at the international level	WFOT Minimum Standards for the Education of Occupational Therapists (2016a). As of 2015, there were 778 WFOT Education Programs, and 291 non-approved programs. As of 2016, WFOT education is at the bachelor's level. The WFOT does not approve OTA programs.

promote innovation in practice, monitor societal needs, and advance education standards for entry to the profession and continuing competence.

Opportunities for guided interactions with mentors and professional peers are central to students' professional identity development (Greenwood, Suddaby, & Hinings, 2002). Membership makes available socialization processes by enabling both the acquisition of specific knowledge and skills required for professional practice as well as the internalization of attitudes, dispositions, and self-identity that connect the individual to the larger profession. Members of a professional organization have access to various networks to pursue particular interests and professional goals. These networks are especially important for students or when pursuing a new area of professional interest. Conferences, networking meetings, online practice communities, and professional journals offer guidance and expertise to enhance professional development and ultimately to contribute to the advancement of the profession.

Although each professional organization has its own unique benefits, many professional associations offer "members only" access to a variety of publications, resources, conferences, online communities, scholarships, grants, and professional development opportunities that are not available to nonmembers (Osborn & Hunt, 2007). Member dues are the major source of revenue and political strength of OT associations, although some also are supported by

fees related to publications and continuing education. Lifelong membership can have the benefit of providing students and practitioners with access to knowledge, networks, and resources that can advance one's professional career.

The professional development that occurs through membership and active involvement in professional organizations illustrates the importance of being a lifelong member of state, national, and international professional organizations (Ritzhaupt, Umapathy, & Jamba, 2008). Active participation in professional associations also has the benefit of building leadership in the profession, forming powerful and interconnected collegial networks, and growing OT leaders, education, research, and practice settings. Professional leaders are important to the profession in interacting with a diverse range of stakeholders from both inside and outside the profession while scanning the larger environment for emerging trends and opportunities that can benefit OT and the clients served by the profession. Rather than seeing the future as a minor variation or logical extension of the present, professionals connected to professional organizations see the future as an invention that may require fresh thinking and innovative solutions very different from the current organizational norms.

The next section offers an overview of professional associations at the international, national, and state or province level.

World Federation of Occupational Therapists

The World Federation of Occupational Therapists (WFOT) was created in 1952 as the official international organization for the promotion of OT (Figure 5-1). It is based in Geneva, Switzerland. Since its inception, WFOT has worked to expand OT worldwide to address the needs of an estimated 1 billion persons worldwide who have disabilities (World Health Organization [WHO], 2018). It has more than 85 member countries and seven regional groups around the world, representing more than 480,000 OT practitioners around the globe. The WFOT membership is coordinated through each national association worldwide. The WFOT also interacts with national governments on policy and awareness to build the profession in countries where there is no association.

The WFOT has been in official relations with the WHO since 1959 and is recognized as a nonprofit nongovernmental organization (NGO) by the United Nations (UN) (WFOT, 2018). The WFOT promotes international cooperation for more than 90 member organizations, and advances the international standards for OT practice, education, and research. The WFOT also coordinates with other international groups (Box 5-2).

The WFOT offers support to the international OT community around several important areas:

- *Education*: to increase the number of educational programs relevant to each country's cultural and resource context
- *Human resources*: to increase the number of OT practitioners to provide critical services to clients
- *Standards*: to promote international standards for practice, education, and research; and to governmental support of OT (WFOT, 2018)
- *Scholarship and publications*: to publish the *WFOT Bulletin* twice per year as its official peer-reviewed journal and to organize the WFOT Congress, an international conference that brings together occupational therapists from around the globe every 4 years
- *Policy development*: The WFOT is active in policies at the international level with initiatives such as the WHO's Rehabilitation 2030: A Call for Action, the Global Strategy on Human Resources for Health: Workforce 2030, the World Report on Ageing and Mental Health,

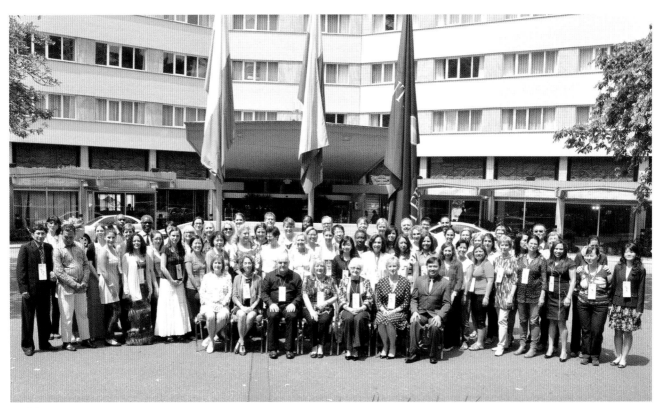

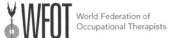 World Federation of Occupational Therapists

World Federation of Occupational Therapists
32nd Council Meeting, Medellin, Colombia – March 2016

FIGURE 5-1 The World Federation of Occupational Therapists' 32nd Council Meeting in Medellin, Colombia, March 2016. (Courtesy of World Federation of Occupational Therapists.)

<table>
<tr><td>

BOX 5-2 **INTERNATIONAL ORGANIZATIONS AND WORLD FEDERATION OF OCCUPATIONAL THERAPISTS**

The World Federation of Occupational Therapy (WFOT) develops and maintains strategic alliances with other international organizations including the following:

- World Health Organization (WHO)
- Handicap International (HI)
- Rehabilitation International (RI)
- International Labour Organisation (ILO)

Regional groups of WFOT are composed of geopolitical regions of the United Nations:

- Confederación Latinoamericana De Terapeutas Ocupacionales (CLATO)
- Association of Caribbean Occupational Therapists (ACOT)
- Asia Pacific Occupational Therapists Regional Group (APOTRG)
- Council of Occupational Therapists for the European Countries (COTEC)
- Occupational Therapy Africa Regional Group (OTARG)
- Kuwait Group
- Arabic Occupational Therapy Regional Group (AOTRG)

</td><td>

BOX 5-3 **COUNTRIES WHERE OCCUPATIONAL THERAPY IS REGULATED**

Argentina[a]	Israel	Seychelles
Australia	Italy	Singapore[a]
Austria[b]	Japan	Slovenia
Belgium	Jordan[a]	South Africa
Bermuda	Kenya[a]	South Korea
Brazil[a]	Latvia	Spain[b]
Canada[a]	Luxembourg	Sri Lanka
Colombia[b]	Madagascar[a]	Sweden
Croatia[a]	Malawi	Switzerland[b]
Cyprus	Malta	Taiwan[a]
Czech Republic	Mexico	Tanzania
Denmark	Namibia	Thailand
France	New Zealand	Trinidad and
Germany	Nigeria	Tobago[a]
Greece	Norway	Tunisia
Hong Kong	Palestine	United
Iceland	Panama	Kingdom
Ireland	Peru[a]	United States[a]
India[b]	Philippines	Venezuela
Indonesia[a]	Portugal	Zambia
Iran[a]	Romania	Zimbabwe

[a]Organized at the state/regional level.
[b]Organized at the national and state/regional levels.

</td></tr>
</table>

World Report on Disability, and Global Cooperation on Assistive Health Technology. Involvement in these initiatives by WFOT helps to ensure that OT perspectives will influence the development of services in many countries.

Information about WFOT's history, current initiatives, as well as information about OT in all member countries can be found at their Website: www.wfot.org.

National Associations

Around the World

In each country, professional organizations are shaped by local cultures and policies. For example, in Denmark, occupational therapists are unionized, and the professional association and the union are linked. Country geography, languages, and business practices influence how decisions are made, the nature of gatherings, and how organizations function. In countries with nationalized health care, OT is primarily delivered through government agencies, and the advocacy approaches differ from countries like the United States where businesses dominate the health care landscape. Box 5-3 identifies the regulation of OT around the world (WFOT, 2016b).

American Occupational Therapy Association

The American Occupational Therapy Association (AOTA) is the national professional organization in the United States that is responsible for guiding and developing professional standards, professional development, and advocacy on behalf of OT practitioners and the clients served by OT (AOTA, 2018a). The AOTA was incorporated in 1917 as the National Society for the Promotion of Occupational Therapy in New York. The name was eventually changed in 1927 to AOTA. The AOTA's membership is composed of individual occupational therapists, OT assistants (OTAs), and students (Box 5-4).

The AOTA members develop and refine AOTA's mission, vision, practice standards, professional development, and code of ethics, all of which shape the future

Students are valued members of AOTA and belong to the Assembly of Student Delegates (ASD). Each educational program may select a student as its delegate to the ASD meeting that takes place during the AOTA Annual Conference and Exposition. The ASD provides a platform for students to share their perspectives on student issues that affect the OT profession (AOTA, 2018b).

success of the OT profession. This is accomplished by individual members working together as volunteers serving the association in various leadership capacities. Members and volunteer leaders are supported by staff employed by AOTA. The staff is supervised by the AOTA executive director, who, in turn, is supervised by the AOTA Board of Directors (BOD). The BOD consists of elected directors, officers, and appointed consumer and public advisors. All board members have voice and vote during official meetings. The Representative Assembly (RA) is the policy-making body of the association that operates as a Congress (AOTA, 2018b). Each representative is elected nationally or by members of their state or jurisdiction. Representatives seek input from their members about policy decisions facing the profession. Policies, such as the proposal for doctoral level entry to the profession, are deliberated and voted upon by the assembly. Practice standards and positions on the role of OT in various specialty areas, such as driving and neonatal intensive care, are ultimately approved by the RA.

The AOTA's federal and state policy departments are active with health care, social, and education policy concerns. The national American Occupational Therapy Political Action Committee (AOTPAC) supports legislation, and many states have formed PACs as well. Evidence-based practice and practice-based evidence are essential to substantiate the efficacy of OT, and thus, member organizations, including the AOTA, actively develop these resources.

Table 5-3 provides profiles of WFOT as an example of the international OT organization and the AOTA as an example of a national association. The selection of the AOTA for this is based in the origins of this text in the United States; however, the authors wish to acknowledge the importance of each national organization in representing and leading the profession.

Associations and Organizations at the State/Region/Territory Level

The municipal structures of each country shape the nature of their organizations, which may have regional bodies. In the United States, each state has a professional organization that serves the regional needs of OT practitioners (AOTA, 2018b). These state organizations are independent from AOTA, and thus, individuals join these state groups directly. State organizations are affiliated with AOTA to advance the profession in that particular state and to advocate for clients who are served by OT (Figure 5-2). For example, AOTA provides model language for state laws and regulations, but the state professional organization must work with the state government directly to get this language into state laws and policies. The president of each state association belongs to the Affiliated State Association Presidents (ASAP), thus supporting a close synergy among

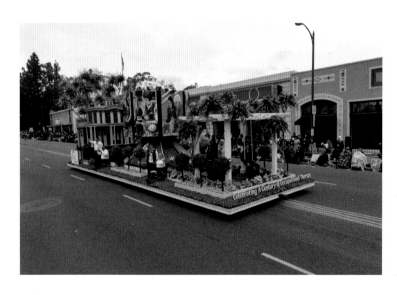

FIGURE 5-2 The Occupational Therapy Centennial Float that the Occupational Therapy Association of California successfully entered in the 2017 Rose Bowl Parade. (Photo credit: Paul Krugman. Photo courtesy of Occupational Therapy Association of California.)

CENTENNIAL NOTES

Starting a National Society

Lori T. Andersen

In the early twentieth century, people interested in the therapeutic use of occupation began to share ideas through publication of books and articles in journals such as *Modern Hospital, Trained Nurse and Hospital Review,* and the *Maryland Psychiatric Quarterly.* They started to correspond with each other and also networked at professional meetings and conferences.

Eleanor Clarke Slagle and William Rush Dunton Jr. established a professional and personal relationship in 1913 when both worked in the Baltimore area. Dunton corresponded with Susan E. Tracy in 1914 about her training program for nurses in invalid occupations and with Herbert Hall about his cement work at Deveraux Mansion, the same year Slagle visited Deveraux Mansion to learn about this work. George Edward Barton and Dunton also struck up a correspondence in 1914. Over the next 2 years, they discussed forming a society of "occupation workers." Their letters made clear that Barton wanted control of the planning and Dunton often deferred to Barton in order to achieve his goal of establishing a society. They disagreed on whether the effort should be directed toward establishing local societies before establishing a national society. Eventually, Barton gave in to Dunton's belief that a national society could serve as a model to establish local societies.

Finally, they set a date for an inaugural meeting. Barton proposed the location—Consolation House, his home in Clifton Springs, New York—as it " . . . is after all one of the most centrally located places in the United States." Barton set the list of invitees, drafted a constitution, suggested specific offices for each founder, and proposed the name of the society—the National Society for the Promotion of Occupational Therapy. He insisted that the word *therapy* be included in the title to emphasize the health-giving side instead of the commercial side of the work involving the sale of patient-made products.

Plans were being finalized when invited guest Susan E. Tracy had to decline due to a prior commitment in Chicago and Eleanor Clarke Slagle requested a 2-week delay to fit her schedule (Figure 5-3). On March 15, 1917, selected participants, George Edward Barton, William Rush Dunton, Jr., Eleanor Clarke Slagle, Susan Cox Johnson, Thomas B. Kidner, and Isabel Newton met at Consolation House to establish and incorporate the new society. The rest is history!

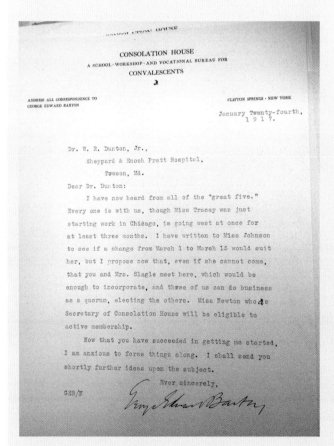

FIGURE 5-3 Letter from George Barton to William Dunton naming March 15, 1917, as the inaugural meeting at Consolation House. (*Source:* Selected letters between founders and early leaders of OT found in *Series 1—Founders and Early History* in the Archives of the AOTA at the Wilma West Library.)

TABLE 5-3 Profiles of American Occupational Therapy Association and World Federation of Occupational Therapists

	American Occupational Therapy Association (www.aota.org)	Word Federation of Occupational Therapists (www.wfot.org)
Volunteer leadership	President, Vice President, Secretary, Treasurer (elected by membership) Board of Directors (elected by membership plus one consumer advisor and one public advisor)	President, Vice President, VP-Finance, Executive Director, Programme Coordinators (elected by council) (WFOT, 2016b)
Staff	Executive Director that oversees a large staff that includes practitioners, attorneys, accountants, policy specialists, and administrative personnel	At this writing, WFOT has two part-time administrative staff and is transitioning to an ex-officio Executive Director and staff.
Headquarters	Bethesda, Maryland	Geneva, Switzerland
Membership	Individual AOTA membership	85 member organizations. Individuals must join through their national association. Some national associations have automatic WFOT individual membership. Others, including United States, have additional WFOT individual membership fees.
Estimated OT practitioners	132,660 practicing occupational therapists 51,600 OTAs	480,000 practicing occupational therapists 63,000 OTAs
Policy-making structure	Representative Assembly (RA) made up of one elected voting delegate from each state and one representing members living outside the United States meets two times per year. Responsible for professional practice policy for professional practice.	WFOT council composed of one voting delegate from each full member organization. All member organizations have alternate delegates but still one vote per country. Meets every 2 years. Executive management team meets annually.
Represents OT to key constituents that set or influence policy (examples)	• Members of congress • Federal government agencies such as the Centers for Medicare & Medicaid, Office of Special Education, Rehabilitation Services Administration, and the Substance Abuse and Mental Services Administration	• National governments • World Health Organization (WHO) • United Nations (UN) • International Labor Organization (ILO)
Publications	• American Journal of Occupational Therapy • OT Practice • Special Interest Section Compendium • AOTA Press publishes books, manuals, consumer guides, and other documents.	• WFOT Bulletin • WFOT Electronic Newsletter • Minimum Standards for the Education of Occupational Therapists • Position statements • Online modules and educational materials
Online networking	AOTA CommunOT https://communot.aota.org/	Occupational Therapy International Online Network (OTION) http://otion.wfot.org/
Conferences	Annual conference, education summit, and specialty conferences	World Congress of Occupational Therapists (held every 4 years)
States/regional groups	Affiliated state associations	Regional groups representing geopolitical regions of the United Nations
Interprofessional collaborations	Collegial professional organizations such as the American Speech and Hearing Association and the American Medical Association	Global Consortium on Rehabilitation to Support, WHO Rehabilitation 2030; UN Sustainable Development Goals
Annual celebrations	April is OT Month.	October 27 is World Occupational Therapy Day.
Structures, organizations, groups	Commissions: • Commission on Practice • Commission on Education • Ethics Commission • Continuing Competence and Professional Development Special Interest Sections (SIS) Assembly of Student Delegates (ASD) Accreditation Council for Occupational Therapy Education (ACOTE)	Programmes: • Executive Programme—Advocacy and Leadership • Research Programme • Practice Development Programme • Education Programme International Advisory Groups (IAG) • Human Rights • Occupational Science • Social Media • International Review Teams
Examples of key current initiatives	• AOTA Evidence-Based Practice Resources • Continuing Competence and Professional Development resources • Public Policy and Advocacy around health care reform • ACOTE educational standards for entry-level practitioners	• Human Resources Project is a demographic analysis of the profession including labor force statistics, regulation, education, and employment trends collected every 2 years. • OT and disaster management • Quality indicators of OT interventions • Development of the profession in countries where it does not exist • Minimum Standards for the Education of Occupational Therapists

BOX 5-5 NATIONAL BOARD FOR CERTIFICATION IN OCCUPATIONAL THERAPY

The OT profession is also supported through the work of the National Board for Certification in Occupational Therapy (NBCOT, 2018). The NBCOT is the credentialing body for occupational therapists and occupational therapy assistants (OTA) practicing in the United States. The NBCOT develops and administers the initial certification examinations that OT practitioners taken after meeting requirements for graduation from an entry-level OT or OTA program. The examinations are comprehensive and are designed to measure the knowledge and skills required for OT practitioners to enter practice. The items in the certification examinations are based on an extensive practice analysis of entry-level practice for both levels of professionals. The certification examination includes items that reflect OT evaluation and intervention with diverse populations in a variety of practice environments. Examination results are shared with individual state licensure boards. Achievement of a passing score on the certification examination is required in all states to be eligible to obtain a license or certificate to practice. Occupational therapists and OTAs from other countries who wish to practice in the United States must successfully complete the certification examination.

state and federal level activities. All affiliated state associations can be accessed via the home page of the AOTA Website. Membership in state organizations is critical for maintaining local networks and for mobilizing advocacy efforts related to state government–funded programs and state policies, including professional licensure.

Each state or jurisdiction regulates OT in some way through a licensure board or regulatory agency (AOTA, 2018a). The definitions and guidelines are enacted by the legislature in that particular state and are intended to protect the citizens of that state. The AOTA is a valued resource for these regulatory agencies, providing information about the profession and assisting with monitoring and advocating for OT in the state legislature. When students complete their academic programs and successfully pass the certification examination of the National Board for Certification in Occupational Therapy (NBCOT), they are eligible to apply for licenses and certificates to practice (Box 5-5). These applications are handled through state government bodies.

How Professional Organizations Support Professional Development

Occupational therapy students, OTAs, and occupational therapists can become members of their state, national, and international professional organizations (Mata et al., 2010). Such involvement builds a sense of professional identity that begins at the point at which an individual chooses OT as a career path and continues to develop throughout a career. Lifelong membership and participation in professional organizations is a key component to a successful OT career trajectory, beginning as an OT student. Professional organizations provide the support needed for professional development, public awareness, **advocacy**, and **standard setting**, making Case Study 5-1 illustrates how OT professional organizations support professional development as an OT student enters the profession.

Benefits of Professional Associations

Continuing Education and Professional Development

Professional organizations often offer continuing education and professional development opportunities, including conferences and continuing education events in person and online often at reduced cost for members (AOTA, 2018a). Occupational therapy state associations typically have an annual conference. The largest event in the United States is the AOTA Annual Conference and Exposition, which includes continuing education, networking, and exhibit hall vendors and employers. The WFOT holds an international conference that rotates among different regions of the world every 4 years. State, national, and WFOT conferences rely on volunteers to peer review conference proposals to select presentations for conferences. Volunteers also help provide the necessary human resources during conferences.

American Occupational Therapy Foundation

The American Occupational Therapy Foundation (AOTF) is a nonprofit organization that was established in 1965 to advance the science and increase public awareness of OT. The AOTF is composed of OT practitioners, corporate

CASE STUDY 5-1 SUMITA ENTERS THE OCCUPATIONAL THERAPY PROFESSION IN THE UNITED STATES

Sumita is recent graduate from an accredited OT program. Based on her academic and fieldwork experiences, she decided to pursue work with children with special needs.

Sumita as a Student

As an OT student, Sumita decided to join the AOTA and on the AOTA membership application, she joined the World Federation of Occupational Therapists (WFOT). She also joined her state association. She attended her first AOTA conference to attend workshops and courses on innovative practice for children with autism and how to make a successful transition from student to practitioner. At the conference, she met students from around the country and found many shared her interests. She also found that the *American Journal of Occupational Therapy*, *OT Practice*, and the *Special Interest Section Compendium* contained interesting articles which she used in various course assignments (AOTA, 2018d). Using OT Connections, a social media site accessible on the home page of the AOTA Website, she read posts from experienced practitioners about their intervention strategies. During her final Level II fieldwork placement, Sumita contacted the National Board for Certification in Occupational Therapy (NBCOT) and applied to take her certification examination near her home after completing her fieldwork.

Getting Ready to Work

Sumita interviewed at clinical sites in South Carolina and close to her home in Texas. Because she was not sure which position she would accept, she contacted the state regulatory boards in both states to apply for licensure. She asked NBCOT to send her examination results to both of them. She anxiously awaited her certification examination results, and was thrilled to learn that she had passed the examination and was now a registered occupational therapist. She accepted the offer from a private pediatric practice group in Texas and began her new job working with children with autism. When her practice obtained a contract to provide telehealth services to clients in Louisiana, Sumita used AOTA's Telehealth advisory resources to find out about licensure there. Later, when a client moved to Mexico and her parents wished to continue intervention, she consulted with the WFOT *Position Statement on Telehealth* (WFOT, 2014).

When Sumita's student memberships expired, she renewed her memberships with the AOTA, WFOT, and her state association and joined both the Developmental Disabilities and the School System Special Interest Sections so that she could communicate with other occupational therapists who worked with this population. In addition, Sumita learned from resources provided by these therapists and by her supervisor and coworkers. She also joined the Autism Society for interdisciplinary networking and conferences.

Practicing Abroad

Sumita was also interested in international practice opportunities, and through her membership with WFOT, she discovered the Occupational Therapy International Online Network (OTION), which facilitated her involvement in OT practice in Haiti. Sumita referred to the WFOT document *Working as an OT in Another Country* to ensure she met regulatory standards for practice in Haiti (WFOT, 2017). She learned of a new Haitian Association of Occupational Therapists, which she joined, and attended a meeting while in Haiti. While she was in Haiti, she was able to attend the regional group conference of the Association of Caribbean Occupational Therapists. There she learned from occupational therapists who provide community-based services on islands with shortages of OT personnel and the efforts to develop OT education programs in the Caribbean region.

Networking and Advocating Back Home

After returning from Haiti, Sumita learned that U.S. federal and state funding for OT services was at risk for children with autism. She immediately went to the AOTA Website to learn about the proposed cuts to services for children with autism and related conditions. Sumita used OT Connections to communicate with other practitioners regarding concerns for declining reimbursement rates and coverage for OT services. She decided to donate to the American Occupational Therapy Political Action Committee (AOTPAC), which provides support to candidates for elected office who support OT services. Sumita also contacted the association to find out how she could get involved with advocating for fair reimbursement and coverage.

Becoming Part of the Solution

Sumita joined an ad hoc committee of practitioners to develop recommendations to the AOTA Board of Directors on strategic priorities for advocating for OT and children with autism. Sumita also scheduled visits with her elected representatives to discuss her concerns regarding the proposed cuts to reimbursement and OT coverage for the children she served. She then invited her elected representatives and their legislative staff to tour her clinic to educate policymakers on the critical role of OT for children with autism. She followed up with each of the legislative representatives with a letter further advocating for reimbursement, and included the AOTA document *Scope of Occupational Therapy Services for Individuals with Autism Spectrum Disorder Across the Life Course* and an AOTA evidence-based practice review article on autism. She then contacted her state association and joined a grassroots advocacy effort to contact state legislators to promote access to OT services for children with autism.

Summary

Through active participation in her state, federal, and international professional associations, Sumita witnessed the power of membership and participation in her professional organizations and committed to maintaining her lifelong state, national, and international professional organizational membership and to actively participate in shaping the future of the OT profession.

partners, and sponsors who support OT education and research. The AOTF is financially supported by private contributions and through sponsors that value OT. Each year, the foundation holds special events at the AOTA annual conference and exposition to raise money to support its work on behalf of OT education and research.

As part of the AOTF mission to advance the science of OT, AOTF publishes a scholarly journal, *Occupational Therapy Journal of Research: Occupation, Participation and Health (OTJR)* (AOTF, 2018). The foundation also maintains the Wilma West Library, a national clearinghouse for OT information. In addition to the excellent library, the foundation maintains OT SEARCH, a comprehensive electronic search engine for literature related to OT.

The AOTF supports students and scholars through educational scholarships and research grants (AOTF, 2018). Small grants are available to graduate students to fund their research. Larger amounts are granted to scholars to fund innovative studies that contribute to the OT body of knowledge and build an understanding of occupational science with a focus on intervention research. Finally, the foundation partners with higher education to fund centers of scholarship and research.

Evidence for Practice

Professional associations can help to link research and practice. A major initiative of the AOTA and the AOTF is building evidence for the practice of OT (AOTA, 2018c). This research generates review articles and evidence-based practice briefs that therapists and students can use to inform and support practice. The AOTA provides links to various publications and virtual resources providing additional information that supports practice.

Public Policy and Advocacy

Professional associations at all levels represent and advocate for the interests of OT practitioners and their clients in the areas of public policy (AOTA, 2018a). This involves communications with government agencies, such as the Ministry of Health and Education in some countries. In the United States, such work involves lobbying with legislators in Congress regarding initiatives that are important to the profession and to the people who are served by OT (Figure 5-4). At the federal level, this may also involve working with the policymakers from the Office of Special Education, the Rehabilitation Services Administration, and other governmental agencies regarding eligibility for service as well as guidelines for reimbursement. The AOTA staff members may provide information and testimony before congressional committees who make recommendations regarding the interpretation and implementation of legislation. State and national associations communicate with members about contacting their representatives

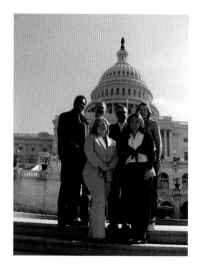

FIGURE 5-4 **Students and practitioners advocating for occupational therapy on Capitol Hill.**

to advocate about legislation affecting the profession and people with disabilities. Even students can get involved (Box 5-6).

The AOTA State Affairs Department and the Federal Affairs Department also support the activities of state OT associations and licensure boards to ensure that language supportive of OT is included in state legislation and that

---

BOX 5-6   HOW TO GET INVOLVED

Did you know there are many ways to get involved in shaping the future of OT through your professional organizations?

- Submit a proposal to present at your state or national conference.
- Write a letter to your legislator on a legislative issue you are passionate about (e.g., increasing access to home health occupational therapy services).
- Visit the advocacy and policy section of the AOTA Website to learn more about how to get involved.
- Join Special Interest Sections that pertain to your interests in OT practice and join the SIS forums on OT Connections from the AOTA Website at www.aota.org.
- Submit an article to *OT Practice*.
- Attend a specialty conference in your area of interest (e.g., school-based practice or mental health).
- Attend AOTA's annual Capitol Hill Day.
- Attend the National Student Conclave, a conference specifically designed for OT and OTA students.
- Join the World Federation of Occupational Therapists Occupational Therapy International Online (WFOT OTION).

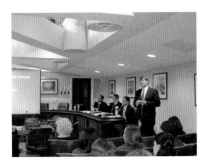

FIGURE 5-5 **Speakers discuss legislative updates and advocacy opportunities to members at a state professional association conference.**

OT is supported and not inappropriately restricted by encroachment by other professions (AOTA, 2018a). The AOTA also provides educational materials and individual support to members and state associations to prepare them to effectively advocate for the profession and those who are served in their area by OT (Figure 5-5).

American Occupational Therapy Political Action Committee

A **political action committee (PAC)** is a committee that provides financial support to candidates that support a profession and its initiatives through private donations from members. The AOTA members can voluntarily donate to the American Occupational Therapy Political Action Committee (AOTPAC) to support candidates for elected office that support OT and the clients served by OT.

Publications

Many professional associations around the world have an official publication. In the United States, the *American Journal of Occupational Therapy (AJOT)* is the peer-reviewed journal with a high-impact factor that demonstrates a rigorous scientific publication (AOTA, 2018c). The association also publishes *OT Practice*, a bimonthly magazine that includes informative articles about the profession. In addition to this magazine and the *AJOT*, AOTA publishes the *Special Interest Section Compendium*, newsletters on state policy initiatives, monthly updates on legislative issues, and biweekly e-mail updates on current events that are of interest to members of the profession. In addition to its periodical publications, AOTA Press publishes books, manuals, and consumer guides that address topics of concern to OT students, practitioners, and consumers.

Some examples of publications from professional associations around the world include the following:

- *Asian Journal of Occupational Therapy*
- *Australian Occupational Therapy Journal*
- *British Journal of Occupational Therapy*
- *Hong Kong Journal of Occupational Therapy*
- *Scandinavian Journal of Occupational Therapy*
- *South African Occupational Therapy Journal*

Conclusion

Occupational therapy professional organizations offer the opportunity to collectively advance the profession in a way that cannot be achieved by an individual student or practitioner alone. Professional organizations are non-profit organizations seeking to further the profession, the interests of individuals engaged in that profession, and the public interest. By building a strong community of students and practitioners that unite the profession around a shared mission and vision, strategies can be developed that advance practice and serve the public interest. These associations represent the interests of students and practitioners through legislative advocacy and public promotion of the profession. As occupational therapists, OTAs, and OT students, we are supported by our state, national, and international OT professional organizations that provide the resources and information that we need to practice effectively. As professionals, we also have the opportunity and responsibility to support and participate in our professional organizations so that we can work toward continually developing, shaping, and promoting the OT profession through lifelong membership and active participation. Regulation of the OT profession is also critical for protecting the public from harm and ensuring that OT practitioners are ethical and competent to practice.

REFERENCES

American Occupational Therapy Association. (2018a). *Accreditation.* Retrieved from http://www.aota.org

American Occupational Therapy Association. (2018b). *Governance.* Retrieved from http://www.aota.org

American Occupational Therapy Association. (2018c). *Publications.* Retrieved from http://www.aota.org

American Occupational Therapy Association. (2018d). *Special interest sections.* Retrieved from http://www.aota.org

American Occupational Therapy Foundation. (2018). *Scholarships.* Retrieved from http://www.aotf.org

Benveniste, G. (1987). *Professionalizing the organization.* San Francisco, CA: Josey-Bass.

Bickel, J. (2007). The role of professional societies in career development in academic medicine. *Academic Psychiatry, 31,* 91–94.

Greenwood, R., Suddaby, R., & Hinings, C. R. (2002). Theorizing change: The role of professional associations in the transformation of institutionalized fields. *Academy of Management Journal, 45,* 58–80.

Mata, H., Latham, T. P., & Ransome, Y. (2010). Benefits of professional organization membership and participation in national conferences: Considerations for students and new professionals. *Health Promotion Practice, 11,* 450–453.

National Board for Certification in Occupational Therapy. (2018). *NBCOT.* Retrieved from http://www.nbcot.org

Osborn, R. N., & Hunt, J. G. (2007). Leadership and the choice of order: Complexity and hierarchical perspectives near the edge of chaos. *Leadership Quarterly, 18,* 319–340.

Ritzhaupt, A. D., Umapathy, K., & Jamba, L. (2008). Computing professional association membership: An exploration of membership needs and motivations. *Journal of Information Systems Applied Research, 1,* 1–22.

Schneider, M., & Somers, M. (2006). Organizations as complex adaptive systems: Implications of complexity theory for leadership research. *Leadership Quarterly, 17,* 351–365.

World Federation of Occupational Therapists. (2014). *Position statement on telehealth.* Retrieved from http://www.wfot.org

World Federation of Occupational Therapists. (2016a). *WFOT Minimum Standards for the Education of Occupational Therapists.* Geneva, Switzerland: Author. Available from www.wfot.org/Store/

World Federation of Occupational Therapists. (2016b). *WFOT Human Resources Project.* Retrieved from http://www.wfot.org

World Federation of Occupational Therapists. (2017). *Working as an OT in another country.* Retrieved from http://www.wfot.org

World Federation of Occupational Therapists. (2018). *History.* Retrieved from http://www.wfot.org

World Health Organization. (2018). *World report on disability.* Geneva, Switzerland: Author. Retrieved from http://www.who.int/disabilities/world_report/2011/en/

the**Point**® *For additional resources on the subjects discussed in this chapter, visit* **http://thePoint.lww.com/Willard-Spackman13e.**

CHAPTER 6

Scholarship in Occupational Therapy

Helen S. Cohen

LEARNING OBJECTIVES

After reading this chapter, you will be able to:

1. Understand what scholarship is.
2. Outline the scholarly activities in which every occupational therapist and occupational therapy assistant can participate.
3. Understand how to incorporate scholarship into clinical practice.
4. Describe the range of occupational therapy scholarship.

Introduction

Early in my career as an occupational therapist and occasionally since then, I have come across an idea, apparatus, or treatment theory that I have known nothing about. Sometimes the new concept or thing has seemed sensible, but sometimes it has not. Sometimes the research literature and standards of practice have provided support, but not always. All new clinicians run across things that were not covered in school. When it happens to you, remember that you are not alone. Something like that happened to me on my first day on my first job.

Since then, I have achieved some success as a clinician/scientist, enough to have been invited to write this chapter for you. On my first day on my new job, however, I had no idea that would happen. I just felt intimidated. You are looking forward to a bright future in an interesting and valuable profession, yet you have no idea what will happen to you, either. Perhaps you, too, feel a little bit intimidated. Don't worry, you are not alone. The editors and chapter authors of this textbook have all been where you are today. So please learn from our experiences.

On that first day of my first job, I had too little self-confidence to ask my supervisor about her support of a treatment method that seemed peculiar to me. In retrospect, I should have asked her for the evidence that supported the treatment method she described. I should have tried to find the facility's (hard copy) library so that I could look up information about that treatment technique, but I did not think that reading research papers was part of my job. Nowadays, going to the digital library is much easier and—many years, many miles, and many patients since that first job—doing, reading about, and even participating in research is part of my job. It is part of your job, too. Scholarship is part of all of our jobs, because being scholarly is an inherent aspect of being a professional.

CENTENNIAL NOTES

The Eleanor Clarke Slagle Lectureship

Lori T. Andersen

In 1953, the American Occupational Therapy Association (AOTA) House of Delegates and Board of Management unanimously passed a resolution hoping to establish one of the traditions of the AOTA.

> *Resolved* That we (the AOTA membership at large) extend the single honor each year at our annual conference of having an "honorary occupational therapy guest lectureship," to be called, out of deference to one of our most outstanding OT pioneers, the "Eleanor Clark Slagle Lectureship." As in other professional scientific fields, this honor would be in recognition of meritorious service to the profession. The lectureship each year would be some outstanding practicing occupational therapist who has made significant contributions to the field. The person selected would give a lecture of his own choosing on the subject of occupational therapy. This candidate will be chosen by the membership at large. (AOTA, 1954a, p. 24)

Originally, the Slagle lecturer was selected by a vote of the membership. The honor of being first was awarded to Florence Stattel of New Jersey in 1954 who presented her lecture at the 1955 AOTA conference in San Francisco. She started her lecture by expressing her appreciation, "It is difficult to find words that would adequately express my feelings and appreciation for the honor which you have extended to me in electing me to present the first Eleanor Clarke Slagle lecture. With deep humility and profound professional pride, I thank you for this privilege" (Stattel, 1956, p. 194). Subsequent Slagle lecturers have conveyed similar sentiments.

Today, lectureship has evolved as a major recognition of scholarship, as shown by the following description from the AOTA:

> The purpose is to honor a member of the Association who has substantially and innovatively contributed to the development of the body of knowledge of the profession through research, education, and/or clinical practice.

Recipients are selected by the AOTA Volunteer Leadership Development Committee, based on nominations from members (AOTA, 2018).

Through the years, many stories have surrounded the Slagle lecture. One story concerns one of the best regarded lectures, the 1961 lecture by Mary Reilly, "Occupational Therapy Can Be One of the Great Ideas of 20th-Century Medicine" (C. O. Peters, 2011, p. 262). As Mary Reilly was a controversial personality, some AOTA leaders tried to talk Reilly out of accepting the lectureship the night before it was awarded to her (C. O. Peters, 2011, p. 262). Imagine if this lecture had not been delivered. Another story relates to Helen Willard. According to the May 1954 House of Delegates newsletter (AOTA, 1954b), Helen Willard led a very preliminary vote to nominate occupational therapists for the first Slagle lecturer. Although this leader never gave a Slagle lecture herself, she did coedit the first four editions of a seminal occupational therapy (OT) textbook now known as *Willard & Spackman's Occupational Therapy*.

Lesson 1: Be Practical

Being a practical occupational therapist or OT assistant, if something strikes you as ridiculous, it probably is! Make an effort to learn about it, however, because someone might have a good reason and good evidence to support what seems weird to you. How do you learn about it? Ask your teachers, your supervisors, your colleagues, and other health care providers; read the literature and ask questions. Ask for the theory, but theory is useless without supporting evidence, so ask for the evidence, too. You can and should read the papers that present that evidence.

Where does evidence come from? Research! People who do research refer to themselves as investigators because they investigate problems or scientists because they do science. Scientists are wonderfully thoughtful, creative, brave, and even fearless sometimes when they are out there on the cutting edge of the research world, living dangerously and subversively in their intellectual lives. By habit, instinct, training, and profession, investigators ask questions every day. Scientists are subversive because they do not accept the status quo. Instead, they look for explanations for phenomena and answers to questions. The results of investigations lead to changes in our understanding of the world, and changes to the world, itself. By using their inquiring minds, occupational therapists who are also scientists have participated in that process. You can, and should, participate in that process, too.

What is it like? It can be lively and crazy in a weirdly sedate sort of way. Published scholarly papers politely describe a problem, the previous research that has been done, the question that must still be answered, the manner in which the author went about asking the question, the actual results of asking the question, and a discussion about what it all means. We use good grammar and are reasonably nice to each other in print.

Listen carefully and you will hear the sounds of science, especially at conferences. Scientific meetings are full of people politely but vigorously challenging each other and the current dogma, saying "Show me the evidence," "What do you mean?" and "What is the evidence for that?" Watch someone point to a particular data point on a graph on a scientific poster and vigorously demand an explanation or provide an answer. Eavesdrop over lunch when some colleagues are arguing about a theory and the data that do or do not support it. Sitting quietly in a hotel lounge or restaurant, drawing on a napkin an electronic device, or finding a data file or figure to illustrate a point, those scientists discuss data, pull the ideas apart and knit them back together, knead them like bread, look at them from different points of view, and gradually approach a greater understanding of their little bits of the world.

Investigators, including clinician/scientists, can be wildly radical and subversive, trying to change things not by shouting slogans and holding up posters while marching in the streets but by politely asking questions and putting up posters in poster halls, showing their data to convince other people of the value of their work. Investigators write scientific papers that may, or may not, support the work that has gone before. They write letters to journals (the letter to the editor, really a letter to the author of a paper); they critique each other's work during the process of peer reviewing other investigators' scientific manuscripts; and as journal and book editors, they decide what work should be presented to the public. As educators, they decide what ideas to pass along to students. Many of the authors in this book have done those things. You can do them, too. The poster sessions at the annual meetings of the state and national professional associations are an excellent way to participate in that effort. We'll return to that point later.

Challenging authority by posing questions and coming up with new, or improved, ideas is a good thing to do. In that way, our society and our profession make progress. When Aristarchus of Samos looked up at the night sky thousands of years ago on the edge of the Mediterranean Sea and realized that the Sun probably did not revolve around the Earth but, instead, the Earth probably revolved around the Sun (Evans, 2017), surely, the gods he worshipped noticed. Few other people noticed, however, and his musings had little effect on the world at the time. Inspired by Aristarchus, but thousands of years later and thousands of miles away, in a small city in Poland, Copernicus described the heliocentric theory after collecting evidence and considering the data (Copernicus, 1543). Because he shared his work with others, waiting until the end of his life to publish for fear of retribution, the world changed profoundly and forever. The Catholic Church punished some investigators who followed Copernicus, but the progress of good ideas cannot be stopped by people who are fearful of change.

In modern times, we accept the heliocentric theory as fact. And a good thing we do, too, because look where it has taken us: to the moon, to Mars, to extraordinary photographs of the giant planets where no people have explored before. Because enlightened people of the Renaissance challenged the accepted dogma of their day and found new points of view, we have the germ theory of disease, vaccines to prevent people from dying from common viruses, and occupational therapists who teach handwashing techniques; we have premature and low-birth-weight babies who survive and occupational therapists who help them thrive; we have patients who survive amputations, strokes, head trauma, cancer, and spinal cord injuries and occupational therapists who help them regain their independence; we have patients with vestibular impairments who learn from their occupational therapists that being sedentary is the worst thing they can do for themselves, and we have patients with low vision who learn from their occupational therapists how to function despite their visual losses; we have computers, smartphones, and other computerized devices and an occupational therapist who gave the 2017 Eleanor Clarke Slagle lecture on the use of technology to help all of those people (Smith, 2017); we have community-dwelling people with chronic mental health problems and occupational therapists who teach them how to function in society; and we have an internationally recognized profession, and we have airplanes, telephones, videoconferences, the Internet, and digital journals so that we can share our ideas and knowledge with occupational therapists around the world. Courtesy of scientists who refused to accept the status quo, who challenged authority with data and reason, we have our modern world with modern health care, including modern OT.

When mental health facilities turned away from prisonlike warehouses to become more therapeutic environments where occupation workers could help the inmates to behave more normally and find meaning in work, the world became a better, healthier place. When the intrepid, young reconstruction aides took their creativity and new profession to the military hospitals to help the shell-shocked soldiers of World War I, despite the new horrors of that war and the social conventions of the day, the world became a better, healthier place. Each time occupational therapists have decided not to keep doing the same old thing but to try something new—to test the efficacy of a new treatment, to build better adaptive equipment, to embrace new technologies, and to expand their practices to new specialties—the world has become a better, healthier place. When people say, "I won't do the same old thing, I want to do it better," or "I'm not going to believe the same old thing just because someone with gray hair said it was true," or "Tell me how you know that this treatment will work," then the world becomes a better, healthier place. Expanding the boundaries of our field by combining the art of therapy with the science supporting it is part of our professional ethos (Peloquin, 2005).

Lesson 2: Embrace New Ideas

Embrace new ideas that are supported by evidence. Change is often uncomfortable and difficult to accept, but change can be good. Changing ideas and practices is a natural result of scholarship. Change your little part of the world for the better, and be proud of yourself for doing that!

Had I, as a young therapist, asked my supervisor for the evidence supporting the treatment that I did not understand, she might have responded thoughtfully and become a better therapist. Had I looked up the evidence myself and presented the lack of research support, all of the therapists might have become better clinicians. That rehabilitation center might have become a better place by the simple act of a staff therapist asking an authority figure to support her assertions. But I was young and felt intimidated, so that opportunity slipped away. Don't be like me in those days. Be brave. Ask your questions. Listen to the answers. Be thoughtful. Be scholarly.

From the earliest days of the occupation workers, acts of inquiry and scholarship have been part of our field. Prior to the official founding of the profession, research supported the ideas on which our work is still based. For example, in the earliest known grant-funded study of OT, Hall studied the use of occupations with psychiatric patients and showed that most patients, especially neurotic patients, benefited from the work cure (Hall, 1910b). The basic findings in that study are still valid today.

Participation in occupation has been shown to be therapeutic in a wide variety of settings as diverse as general rehabilitation in a nursing home (Yoder, Nelson, & Smith, 1989), pain management (Heck, 1988), vestibular rehabilitation (H. Cohen, Kane-Wineland, Miller, & Hatfield, 1995), recovery from substance abuse (Peloquin & Ciro, 2013), handwriting training in children (Chang & Yu, 2017), and upper limb rehabilitation (Hsieh, Lin, Chiu, Meng, & Liu, 2015). In general, skill acquisition in motor learning can be improved with the use of occupation (Ferguson & Trombly, 1997). Early in the profession, crafts activities were used by reconstruction aides (Pettigrew, Robinson, & Moloney, 2017). Although we have largely abandoned crafts work, the principles of therapeutic use of occupation remain valid (Dutton, 1989). As a scholarly occupational therapist, you should be familiar with that literature to know why you do what you do and to be able to explain your rationale to other people. Don't feel intimidated, though. Reading about the great idea that is the basis for our profession is fun and will probably spur your imagination as you consider what you can do with those concepts. In the words of the great OT scholar, Susan Garber (Garber, 2016), "We must acknowledge our past and embrace it!"

As a young occupational therapist, I once attended a continuing education workshop given by a prominent occupational therapist about a type of treatment and the marvelous changes you could accomplish just by manipulating the patient in the correct way. The video was breathtaking, and the ideas enchanting. Everyone in the room applauded loudly. Then, during the 4-hour drive home, while stuck in traffic on the George Washington Bridge with the view of the beautiful Hudson River below, it hit me. That therapist never once told us what happened to the patient an hour after the treatment stopped, a day after the treatment, a week, or a year later. Did it have any short- or long-term effect, or was the effect merely momentary? To this day, I still don't know. Those questions should be posed by all therapists when seated before the so-called experts who teach new treatment techniques, describe new devices that will make people's lives better or new software that will make some tasks possible or easier.

Lesson 3: Ask Questions

Do not take anyone's word for it. Ask your questions: What is the evidence? How do you know? What happens later? How long does the effect last? How does it work? By asking those important questions, you are being scholarly (see Case Study 6-1). As a responsible, ethical clinician, you have the right and even the obligation to ask those questions, to challenge people's assertions, and to know about the evidence that supports your practice. You have the right to know if the latest seating cushion will actually prevent pressure ulcers. Susan Garber, the 2016 Eleanor Clarke Slagle lecturer, built her extraordinary career as a clinician/scientist on that question (Garber, 2016). You have the responsibility to know if that amazing robot really can make dinner, wash the dishes, and clean the floor for your disabled client or if that expensive swing set will make any difference in teaching a developmentally disabled child to sit up and learn to manipulate objects. Because you will be in the position of recommending equipment purchases and planning and implementing treatment, you must practice in a manner that is supported by evidence so that you do not waste money, time, and other resources. Thus, your scope of practice includes asking people to support their assertions, explain their research findings, and convince you that what they want you to do or purchase or recommend is evidence based. In her 2004 presidential address, Carolyn Baum described OT as having three interrelated aspects: clinical practice, education, and research (Baum, 2005). Like a three-legged stool, the profession is most stable when educators teach and clinicians practice based on evidence (Box 6-1). Hence, the editors of this textbook wisely included this chapter.

CASE STUDY 6-1   THE FIRST DAY ON THE JOB

As a scholarly occupational therapist or OT assistant, you are acquainted with some of the research findings, and you have the tools at your disposal to find information as you need it. On your first day on your new job as an occupational therapist on an outpatient neurological rehabilitation unit, your supervisor assigns you to do vacation coverage for another clinician. The caseload includes a patient with cerebral palsy. You read the patient's chart and learn that the goals are to improve functional balance skills and object manipulation with his hands. You learn that the treatment plan includes shining a bright light into the patient's eyes for 3 to 5 minutes twice during the 30-minute visit in preparation to practicing

functional motor tasks. Your supervisor tells you that using the bright light will "stimulate the corpus callosum." You are leery of damaging the patient's vision, and having taken a neuroscience course, you do not understand how this intense light could stimulate anything other than pain receptors in the eyes or how it could lead to improvements in motor skills. What do you do? (This scenario is real. Something similar happened to me when I was a young therapist.)

Being scholarly will help guide your intervention. Explaining the dilemma and the rationale for your treatment plan will help your supervisor and the patient to have confidence in you.

Lesson 4: Be Scholarly

Do not rely solely on experience. Instead, be scholarly: Attend lectures, go to conferences, read the literature, ask your questions, and read the available practice guidelines thoughtfully. The unavoidable biases of the clinician can hide the real phenomena involved. Because clinicians frequently see only one patient at a time and are not able to take an unbiased look at the data from many patients without the presence of potentially confounding variables, such as age, sex, and gender, they may not see the real phenomena that are obscured by factors that may be more evident. Investigators, however, often collect data from groups

of people in controlled studies that eliminate the effects of some variables. Here are two examples:

1. An experienced clinician at a rehabilitation center might tell you that patients recovering from a particular disorder need 2 to 3 months of daily therapy. That clinician might not know, however, that patients who are not sick enough to be admitted for inpatient care often recover within 6 weeks of starting biweekly outpatient therapy. The experienced inpatient therapist's opinion is influenced by his or her experience, which is limited to patients who are relatively more sick.
2. A clinician wants to know if recovery from some disorder is affected by gender. The clinician may receive referrals that are predominantly women, because women might be

BOX 6-1   WHAT THE EXPERTS HAVE SAID: WORDS FROM THE SLAGLE LECTURERS

The Eleanor Clarke Slagle Lectureship honors the memory of one of the founders of our profession. It is awarded to individuals who have made significant contributions to our body of knowledge. Let's consider the opinions of some people who have been lecturers.

In her 1983 lecture, Joan Rogers discussed the relationship between research and clinical reasoning, thus making the connection with clinical care. Supporting that idea in 1986, Kathlyn Reed told us that research results, among several factors, should influence our choices of treatment modalities. In 1989, supporting the work of current and future OT neuroscientists at a time when the need for science in our entry-level curricula was under debate, Shereen Farber reminded the profession of the importance of neuroscience. Margo Holm then told us more concretely how to move toward evidence-based practice (Holm, 2000). Wendy Coster reminded us to select our

research measures carefully (Coster, 2008). In my 2015 lecture, I advised the profession to base our careers in inquiry and to make scholarship an activity of daily living, using the methods described in this chapter (H. S. Cohen, 2015). In 2016, Susan Garber advised us to have open minds to be prepared for the experiences and ideas that come along.

Suzanne Peloquin spoke to the philosophy of our profession and eloquently explained one of our guiding beliefs, that effective therapy combines the art and science of care (Peloquin, 2005). In 2013, Glen Gillen reiterated that idea when he said, "As never before . . . the art and science that is occupational therapy [is] clearly being supported by our scientific methods . . . we need to celebrate it!" (p. 650). He was correct; we should celebrate every day, by including scholarship in our activities of daily living, by having scholarly careers that combine the art and science of OT.

more inclined to seek care for that disorder and perhaps the only men who seek care are relatively more ill or more disabled than the majority of men who have that condition. Therefore, the clinician's opinion might be influenced by that referral pattern. To perform a study correctly, an investigator would recruit approximately equal numbers of men and women with a range of levels of impairment so that the variable of sex can be controlled and evaluated. Otherwise, the investigator might come to the erroneous conclusion that women respond to the treatment better than men simply because more women come for care when, in fact, gender has no influence on the outcome.

Therefore, to be a well-informed clinician, you should not rely solely on experience. You should become familiar with research in the specialty in which you work. The published papers are indexed on PubMed and other online services and are often available online. If you are not sure how to read a research paper, start by reading some papers in the OT journals, which were written to help you (H. Cohen, 1988; Corcoran, 2006; Crocker, 1977; Greenstein, 1980; Worrell, 2000). If you don't understand a paper, consider it carefully, talk to your professors, other professional mentors and colleagues, and find out what they think. Attend a journal club that meets periodically to discuss research papers either on a variety of topics or on a single topic of interest. Practice makes perfect, so the more you read and discuss the literature, the easier it will become. Also, the more you practice reading research, the more habitual it will become. Therefore, reading the current literature will become part of your work routine.

As part of the continuing education that you will pursue throughout your career, you will attend professional conferences and workshops. Sit up front, take notes, and ask questions when you do not understand what the speaker has said. Everyone is allowed to ask questions. Once, after I questioned a speaker, I learned from a friend who had also been there that someone had complained about my questions, until she explained that I do research. Then, the other conference attendee said, "Oh, that's all right, then," as if my career path somehow gives me special privileges. It does not. Asking for clarification and posing questions is a routine part of my work. It should be part of your work, too. Be part of the process, ask questions, request clarification, and demand explanations. Move the field forward!

You can participate in scholarly activities while you are a student. Besides attending classes and completing assignments, you can read thoughtfully and pose questions to your instructors. Some of your instructors are probably doing research. If so, try to get involved by offering to help. If no instructors are doing research, gently encourage them by offering to help. During your fieldwork experiences, you can read the relevant literature and pose questions to your clinical mentors. If a fieldwork site has a journal club, participate. If it does not have a journal club, ask about starting one. If the occupational therapists are engaged in research, try to get involved.

To be scholarly is to be thoughtful and to develop in-depth knowledge. You can be scholarly by doing research, and some occupational therapists are also scientists. Doing research is not the only way to be scholarly, however. You can be scholarly by studying intensively in school and during your fieldwork. You can remain scholarly by attending conferences, going to the poster sessions and podium sessions, reading the literature, and discussing new ideas. You can be scholarly by attending the local meetings of your professional association or by reaching out to other related specialty organizations in whichever specialties you become interested. Think critically about new ideas and feel free to critique them, with questions in person, via a letter to the editor, or e-mail to the investigator. Perhaps an investigator has not considered your unique point of view. Research is never performed in isolation. Ultimately, the consumer of research, the clinician as end user, decides which ideas and research findings are worth keeping and which ones should be discarded. As a consumer of research and other information, you are an essential part of the process (Box 6-2).

CASE STUDY 6-2   GIVING GOOD ADVISE

You work in a large outpatient rehabilitation facility that provides care to patients who have had head trauma. A patient asks your advice about using a cervical collar to restrain her neck movements for several days because she has vertigo every time she moves her head upward or downward. You are not familiar with vestibular rehabilitation so you are not sure what to do. (This is a real scenario. Something similar happens in my clinic several times per year.) What do you do? You could (1) reassure her that the cervical collar won't hurt her, based on no information at all, but you know that option is a poor choice; (2) determine the reason for her vertigo by contacting the physician, reading the chart, or asking a colleague how to evaluate her for vertigo; (3) look on PubMed and find some papers about benign paroxysmal positional vertigo. Options 2 and 3 would be best. Vestibular rehabilitation is within the scope of practice for occupational therapists (H. S. Cohen, Burkhardt, Cronin, & McGuire, 2006), so you may be able to find a colleague who will show you how to assess this patient and will know that many cases of benign paroxysmal positional vertigo occur after head trauma (Baloh, Honrubia, & Jacobson, 1987). Reading the papers that you found on PubMed will inform you that using a cervical collar has no effect on the outcome of treatment with repositioning maneuvers (André, Moriguti, & Moreno, 2010; Stewart, Whelan, & Banerjee, 2017). Therefore, because you are concerned that this patient might lose some cervical range of motion by limiting her head movements, you advise her against using the cervical collar.

BOX 6-2 HOW TO HAVE A SCHOLARLY CAREER

Talk is cheap, but action is more difficult. No one knows that better than a clinician. When you are face-to-face with a patient or client who expects you to help solve a problem, thinking quickly is essential. Part of that process involves knowing what is known, or not known, about the problem confronting you at the moment. How will you know? You should be familiar with the research about that problem. Experience is not a good substitute. Here are two examples of why experience may not be a good guide.

Example 1

Experienced physicians used to advise patients with heart disease to rest after surgery. Now, based on evidence,

cardiologists advise those patients to resume normal activities as soon as possible, even in the intensive care unit (ICU). As a result, occupational therapists now practice in the ICU and are part of the cardiac rehabilitation team.

Example 2

Well into the twentieth century, some people thought that bathing daily, and even washing hands regularly, was a bad practice and might engender sickness. Now, with the germ theory of disease well established, occupational therapists teach handwashing and bathing skills to a wide variety of clients.

Lesson 5: Participate in Research

You are part of the process of research and scholarship. You attend professional presentations. You read professional papers. You purchase equipment and implement treatment plans based on new information. Without you, the consumer

of research and knowledge, the material is meaningless. So, participate as an active, challenging learner. If someone cannot rise to the challenge of answering your questions, then that individual has much to learn from you.

Lesson 6: Develop Research Skills

Occupational therapy investigators do research in a vast universe of specialties. Research and scholarship have been essential to the profession since its inception, when the objectives of the new organization included " . . . the study of the effect of occupation upon the human being and . . . the scientific dispensation of the knowledge" (National Society for the Promotion of Occupational Therapy, 1917). Entry-level OT programs are not designed to prepare therapists to do research, so do not expect to be ready to be an investigator when you finish school. Do expect, however, to develop skills in critical thinking about clinical problems and skills in reading the literature so that you will be a good consumer of research.

Research skills are developed through advanced education in OT and other fields, in programs where research design and specific research skills are taught, and students gain experience in performing research in the specialties of those programs by assisting faculty with their research and eventually performing their own research. More advanced research skills are later developed during the research equivalent of medical residency, that is, during postdoctoral fellowships with other mentors.

Occupational therapists as investigators have always been involved in many different kinds of research. No single source provides a comprehensive list. The following section illustrates the impressive range of research by OT investigators but is not comprehensive.

CASE STUDY 6-3 DECIDING ON NEW EQUIPMENT

You are about to purchase equipment for a new clinic. You attend the AOTA Annual Conference and Exposition. The Exposition has many vendors showing off their latest equipment and other materials. It is colorful, upbeat, and fun. You stop to talk to a vendor at an attractive booth with Post-it Notes for giveaways so that you can take some back for your staff. The vendor tells you that their software will help you plan treatments for children with a wide range of developmental disabilities and do perceptual-motor training on the computer. The price is reasonable. What do you do? (This scenario is real, it happened to me once.) You could (1) take the information and the free Post-it Notes, smile, walk away, and toss the literature in the trash, but doing that would waste paper and would not be ethical; (2) ask for the contact information for some therapists who are already using the software so you can e-mail them and ask their opinions before making a purchasing decision; (3) ask the vendor for a list of publications in peer-reviewed journals where the evidence is published and promise to read and evaluate the research before making a purchasing decision. Option 3 is the best choice, combined with input from therapists in Option 2.

Historical Research

Historians track the development of the profession. Historical research, which has its own peculiar methodology (Schwartz & Colman, 1988), helps us to understand the context of our profession's ideas. Some of those papers have examined brief moments in time, or individual events (Gutman, 1995; Low, 1992; Pettigrew et al., 2017), but some research has been more broad, encompassing the entire history of the profession (Andersen & Reed, 2017; Reed, 1993). Two OT/historians have been honored by the profession with the Eleanor Clarke Slagle Lectureship (Reed, 1986; Schwartz, 2009).

Neuroscience

We have basic neuroscientists such as Sharon Juliano and Sheila Mun-Bryce. Juliano has elucidated the pathways for development of cortical neurons, which are the basis for motor control, and changes in the brain in response to trauma (Abbah & Juliano, 2014; Hutchinson et al., 2016). Mun-Bryce used her understanding of developmental disorders as the basis for research on disorders in the nervous system (Mun-Bryce, Roberts, Bartolo, & Okada, 2006; Mun-Bryce et al., 2004) and, at the end of her life, generously participated as a research subject in clinical trials for the benefit of future patients. Other OT investigators do research directly on the human nervous system (Iyer et al., 2005). Somewhat, more applied behavioral neuroscientists do research at the intersection of neuroscience and motor control (Morin et al., 2017; Pelletier, Higgins, & Bourbonnais, 2015, 2017). More recently, young OT neuroscientists have joined the field (Anglin, Sugiyama, & Liew, 2017; Liew et al., 2016).

Motor Control

Motor control is essential for functional performance. In her 1995 Eleanor Clarke Slagle lecture, Catherine Trombly showed us how some important concepts about occupation are intimately related to concepts about motor control. Occupational therapy investigators have tackled these problems from several points of view. For example, Robert Sainburg has built his scientific career around basic problems in motor control (Coelho, Przybyla, Yadav, & Sainburg, 2013; Mani, Mutha, Przybyla, Haaland, & Sainburg, 2013; Sainburg, Schaefer, & Yadav, 2016; Schaffer & Sainburg, 2017). He has also reached and encouraged other occupational therapists to develop expertise in movement science and to study motor control (Sainburg, Liew, Frey, & Clark, 2017). Other investigators have also examined some problems in motor learning (Giuffrida, Shea, & Fairbrother, 2002; Jarus, 1994; Mathiowetz & Haugen, 1994). Trombly and her colleagues have done some particularly interesting work in motor learning on problems relevant to occupational performance (Ma & Trombly, 2001; Trombly & Wu, 1999; Wu, Trombly, Lin, & Tickle-Degnen, 1998). Some of that work on motor learning has moved into education and fall prevention (Schepens, Panzer, & Goldberg, 2011; Schepens, Sen, Painter, & Murphy, 2012) and stroke rehabilitation (Waddell et al., 2017). In a related area, considerable research is being done on problems related to geriatric rehabilitation with a variety of problems. Cognitive decline caused by stroke affects functional performance in virtually all areas. Fortunately, OT investigators are looking into these problems (Skidmore et al., 2017). Other investigators are also studying problems related to functional performance in older adults (S. Murphy & Tickle-Degnen, 2001; S. L. Murphy, Kratz, & Schepens Niemiec, 2017).

Social Sciences

Other investigators have taken us into social sciences. For example, Jean Spencer, who was anthropologist before she became an occupational therapist, taught us about the use of anthropologic methodology in her research on adaptation to disability (Spencer et al., 2002; Spencer, Krefting, & Mattingly, 1993). In a related area, other OT investigators have studied maintenance of wellness and lifestyle change (Clark et al., 1997; Juang et al., 2018; White, 1998) and problems related to health care utilization and factors affecting admission and discharge rates (Krishnan et al., 2018; C. Y. Li et al., 2018; A. J. Ottenbacher et al., 2014; K. J. Ottenbacher et al., 2014).

Assessments

Having valid and reliable assessments is essential for practice in any specialty. Many OT investigators have developed or normed assessments in specific specialties. Some OT investigators have done research on assessment, in general. For example, Craig Velozo has built his career around asking questions about assessments (Classen, Velozo, Winter, Bédard, & Wang, 2015; Hong, Dodds, Coker-Bolt, Simpson, & Velozo, 2017; McRackan et al., 2017).

Behavioral Health

Mental health was at the heart of our profession at its inception and early research supported the use of occupation as therapy (Hall, 1910a, 1910b). Occupational therapists in behavioral health have moved beyond the limits of crafts, although group work remain important. Occupational therapists are still involved in behavioral health, although the percentage of occupational therapists in that specialty has decreased perhaps partly due to a limited amount of research supporting OT practice in mental health. We do have OT investigators in behavioral health research, however. Mary Donohue's work is an example of a body of scholarly research by an occupational therapist who has pursued a career in inquiry over many years as a clinician, educator, and investigator. Because the ability to function within a group is so important, she has developed and tested an assessment of group functioning and social participation known as the Social Profile (Bonsaksen & Donohue, 2017; Bonsaksen, Donohue, & Milligan, 2016; Donohue, 2003, 2005, 2007, 2013). This body of work is a good example of how an investigator builds a research program around an idea, which the investigator then explores and elaborates with successive studies.

Public Health and Cross-disciplinary Research

Some OT investigators do research in public health and epidemiology (Díaz-Venegas, Reistetter, Wang, & Wong, 2016; Hong, Coker-Bolt, Anderson, Lee, & Velozo, 2016; C. Y. Li et al., 2018; A. J. Ottenbacher et al., 2014; K. J. Ottenbacher et al., 2014). Some of my research has examined vestibular disorders in HIV/AIDS and falls in the HIV/AIDS population (H. S. Cohen, Cox, et al., 2012; Erlandson et al., 2016). Those studies and my research on vestibular screening and rehabilitation led to involvement in another study of falls in children (C. M. Li, Hoffman, Ward, Cohen, & Rine, 2016).

In a wide range of physical disabilities subspecialty treatment areas, OT clinician/scientists have been the principal or coinvestigators in an impressive array of research: hand therapy, driving, Parkinson disease, vestibular rehabilitation, low vision rehabilitation, cardiac care, stroke rehabilitation, arthritis, autoimmune disorders, driving rehabilitation, cognitive rehabilitation, developmental disorders, and many other specialties. Here are two examples of bodies of work by very different investigators.

As described in her remarkable 2016 Eleanor Clarke Slagle lecture, Susan Garber began a career in research by collaborating with a group of physicians and engineers who had developed a device to measure pressure on the ischial tuberosities during sitting but which did not work very well. As an occupational therapist with an interest in function, adaptation to change, and lifestyle redesign, she developed a large body of work that is now the basis for intervention in pressure injury care by nurses, occupational therapists, and other rehabilitation professionals (Carlson et al., 2017; Cogan et al., 2017; Garber, 2014; Garber, Krouskop, & Carter, 1978; Garber, Rintala, Hart, & Fuhrer, 2000; Garber, Rintala, Rossi, Hart, & Fuhrer, 1996; Guihan, Hastings, & Garber, 2009).

As Garber's career path illustrates, a research career may begin with one idea and branch out in other directions. My career took that kind of path, starting in vestibular physiology (H. Cohen, Cohen, Raphan, & Waespe, 1992) and moving to my research on vestibular rehabilitation. Those studies showed that patients with vestibular disorders have functional limitations (H. Cohen, 1992; H. Cohen, Ewell, & Jenkins, 1995;

H. S. Cohen & Kimball, 2000; H. S. Cohen, Kimball, & Adams, 2000; H. S. Cohen, Wells, Kimball, & Owsley, 2003) and improve after intervention with vertigo habituation exercises and activities (H. Cohen, Kane-Wineland, et al., 1995; H. Cohen, Miller, Kane-Wineland, & Hatfield, 1995; H. S. Cohen & Kimball, 2003, 2004) or—for benign paroxysmal positional vertigo—repositioning maneuvers (H. S. Cohen & Kimball, 2005; H. S. Cohen & Murphy, 2007; H. S. Cohen & Sangi-Haghpeykar, 2010). Such a body of work can eventually, and sometimes unexpectedly, lead to research in other areas such as related comorbidities (H. S. Cohen, Kimball, & Stewart, 2004; H. S. Cohen et al., 2010), perception and performance under unusual circumstances (Bloomberg, Peters, Cohen, & Mulavara, 2015; H. Cohen, 1996; Goel et al., 2015; Mulavara et al., 2011), motor learning practice strategies (Batson et al., 2011; H. S. Cohen, Bloomberg, & Mulavara, 2005; Gottshall, Hoffer, Cohen, & Moore, 2006; Roller, Cohen, Kimball, & Bloomberg, 2001), diagnostic testing (Isaacson, Murphy, & Cohen, 2006; Todai, Congdon, Sangi-Haghpeykar, & Cohen, 2014), effects of fatigue on motor performance (Cuthbertson, Bershad, Sangi-Haghpeykar, & Cohen, 2015), and clinical movement screening (H. S. Cohen, Mulavara, Peters, Sangi-Haghpeykar, & Bloomberg, 2012, 2014; H. S. Cohen et al., 2013; H. S. Cohen, Mulavara, Sangi-Haghpeykar, et al., 2014; H. S. Cohen et al., 2017; Mulavara, Cohen, Peters, Sangi-Haghpeykar, & Bloomberg, 2013; B. T. Peters, Mulavara, Cohen, Sangi-Haghpeykar, & Bloomberg, 2012).

You can see from the long lists of papers by Garber, Donohue, Cohen, and their collaborators that a research career generates many papers that seem to go off in a variety of directions but are all focused on a general topic of interest to the investigator. In that way, just like a clinician, the investigator develops specialized expertise. The papers are an investigator's way of sharing his or her ideas and research findings with other people. Think of the ideas in the papers as individual threads that can be woven together to make up the glorious, colorful fabric of science. Each paper adds another thread that can be woven in, changing the pattern ever so slightly and expanding the universe of knowledge.

Occupational therapy investigators are expanding knowledge in a vast array of specialties, from cell biology to clinical care, space medicine, and epidemiology. They are related by the underlying concerns of the investigators for the problems that concern all occupational therapists. This chapter touches on only some of the kinds of research being done by members of our profession to give you some ideas about research. Investigators go where the ideas and questions (and research resources) take them, publishing in journals with "Occupational Therapy" in the title when appropriate, but publishing in other journals, too, depending on the audience that is most appropriate for the individual study. They may be identified as occupational therapists by their credentials or affiliations, but they may not be, depending on the requirements of the journal. Regardless of where

BEYOND ACADEMIA: SCHOLARSHIP IN PRACTICE

Scholarship is a large concept that covers a number of activities, ranging from thoughtful discovery to sharing and application of new knowledge (Hyman et al., 2001–2002). Scholarly thinking and scholarly actions are often discussed in academic settings, as they are central to those institutions (Boyer, 1990; Peterson & Stevens, 2013). However, there are opportunities for scholarship within a broad range of practice roles (see for example, AOTA, 2016; Mahaffey, Burson, Januszewski, Pitts, & Preissner, 2015). Selected examples are shown in the table below.

Professional Role	Examples
Students	• Critical papers • Literature reviews • Appraisals of literature • Research presentations • Thesis • Capstone projects • Dissertations • Presentations, posters, and publication in student and professional organizational venues and journals
Practitioners	• Application of evidence to practice situations • Development of practice protocols within settings • Integration of best practice into documentation protocols • Gaining new knowledge of effective evaluation, intervention, and follow-up methods • New program development • Presentations, posters, and publication of practice knowledge and skills via practice journals, newsletters, and professional organizations • Collaboration with researchers
Fieldwork educators	• Mentorship of students into effective practice • Exploration and implementation of effective teaching practices • Development of fieldwork objectives within setting
Supervisors	• Evaluation of clinical practice skills • Development of practice protocols based on best evidence • Implementation of quality improvement systems • Facilitation of collaboration between researchers and practice setting
Managers and administrators	• Identification and use of professional documents to guide organizational standards and expectations • Development of policies and procedures guiding practice • Development and implementation of quality management systems • Facilitation of research collaboration with universities and employees • Service on institutional review boards • Grant writing
Volunteer leaders	• Development of professional guidelines and standards • Development and implementation of continuing education • Serving as reviewers for journals and conference papers • Serving in leadership roles within professional and consumer organizations

—Barbara A. Boyt Schell

the research papers are published, all of it is accessible to you. Reading those papers is within your scope of practice.

Lesson 7: Follow Your Ideas

Follow your ideas and questions, perhaps into unchartered territory, boldly going where no occupational therapist has gone before. It sounds like *Star Trek* (the movie), doesn't it? Our profession is moving toward the future, where excellence in scholarship and clinical care are taking us—so

the idea of space exploration is not so crazy. In fact, some occupational therapists believe, as I do, that our profession has a role to play in space medicine and health care during and after long duration space flight (H. S. Cohen, Harvison, & Baxter, 2013; Davis, Burr, Absi, Telles, & Koh, 2017). Perhaps you will be the occupational therapist to take us there.

Summary

Scholarship is an inherent part of professional preparation and career-long behavior. Scholarship for all occupational therapists involves reading the literature to be familiar with evidence that is already known; asking astute questions when information is not clear, challenging authorities when necessary; reading journals, attending professional meetings, and otherwise keeping up with new developments in the field; and actively participating in meeting sessions by actively listening and questioning. Some occupational therapists also develop the skills to do research and they develop research portfolios in specific, focused areas.

All occupational therapists can and should have the skills to read, think critically, ask questions, and incorporate new findings and new ideas into practice. Scholarship is one of your activities of daily living. Washing your hands is an activity of daily living that is good for your health, so you should do it frequently. Similarly, scholarship is an activity of daily living that is good for your daily work, good for your career, and good for your profession, so you should do it often, too. Be lively and crazy in a sedate sort of way. Have fun. Move the field forward. Change the world!

Acknowledgments

Many thanks to Susan L. Garber, MA, OTR, FAOTA, and Kathlyn L. Reed, PhD, MLIS, OTR, FAOTA, for their comments.

REFERENCES

Abbah, J., & Juliano, S. L. (2014). Altered migratory behavior of interneurons in a model of cortical dysplasia: The influence of elevated GABAA activity. *Cerebral Cortex, 24,* 2297–2308.

American Occupational Therapy Association. (1954a). Annual reports: Meeting of the House of Delegates. *American Journal of Occupational Therapy, 8,* 24–35.

American Occupational Therapy Association. (1954b). *House of Delegates newsletter: Newsletter no. 6.* New York, NY: Author.

American Occupational Therapy Association. (2016). Scholarship in occupational therapy. *American Journal of Occupational Therapy, 70,* 7012410080p1–7012410080p6. doi:10.5014/ajot.2016.706S07

American Occupational Therapy Association. (2018). *Awards and recognitions.* Retrieved from https://www.aota.org/Education-Careers/Awards

Andersen, L. T., & Reed, K. L. (2017). *The history of occupational therapy: The first century.* Thorofare, NJ: SLACK.

André, A. P. R., Moriguti, J. C., & Moreno, N. S. (2010). Conduct after Epley's maneuver in elderly with posterior canal BPPV in the posterior canal. *Brazilian Journal of Otorhinolaryngology, 76,* 300–305.

Anglin, J. M., Sugiyama, T., & Liew, S. L. (2017). Visuomotor adaptation in head-mounted virtual reality versus conventional training. *Scientific Reports, 7,* 45469.

Baloh, R. W., Honrubia, V., & Jacobson, K. (1987). Benign positional vertigo: Clinical and oculographic features in 240 cases. *Neurology, 37,* 371–378.

Batson, C. D., Brady, R. A., Peters, B. T., Ploutz-Snyder, R. J., Mulavara, A. P., Cohen, H. S., & Bloomberg, J. J. (2011). Gait training improves performance in healthy adults exposed to novel sensory discordant conditions. *Experimental Brain Research, 209,* 515–524.

Baum, M. C. (2005). Presidential address: Building a professional tapestry. *American Journal of Occupational Therapy, 59,* 592–598.

Bloomberg, J. J., Peters, B. T., Cohen, H. S., & Mulavara, A. P. (2015). Enhancing astronaut performance using sensorimotor adaptability training. *Frontiers in Systems Neuroscience, 9,* 129. doi:10.3389/fnsys.2015.00129

Bonsaksen, T., & Donohue, M. V. (2017). Are individual students' characteristics and academic performance associated with group-level functioning in education groups? An exploratory study. *Ergoterapeuten, 2,* 40–49.

Bonsaksen, T., Donohue, M. V., & Milligan, R. M. (2016). Occupational therapy students rating the social profile of their educational group: Do they agree? *Scandinavian Journal of Occupational Therapy, 23,* 477–484.

Boyer, E. L. (1990). *Scholarship reconsidered: Priorities of the professoriate.* Princeton, NJ: The Carnegie Foundation for the Advancement of Teaching.

Carlson, M., Vigen, C. L., Rubayi, S., Blanche, E. I., Blanchard, J., Atkins, M., . . . Clark, F. (2017). Lifestyle intervention for adults with spinal cord injury: Results of the USC-RLANRC Pressure Ulcer Prevention Study. *Journal of Spinal Cord Medicine,* 1–18. doi:10.1080/10790268.2017.1313931

Chang, S.-H., & Yu, N.-Y. (2017). Visual and haptic perception training to improve handwriting skills in children with dysgraphia. *American Journal of Occupational Therapy, 71,* 7102220030p1–7102220030p10.

Clark, F., Azen, S. P., Zemke, R., Jackson, J., Carlson, M., Mandel, D., . . . Lipson, L. (1997). Occupational therapy for independent-living older adults. A randomized controlled trial. *JAMA, 278,* 1321–1326.

Classen, S., Velozo, C. A., Winter, S. M., Bédard, M., & Wang, Y. (2015). Psychometrics of the Fitness-to-Drive Screening Measure. *OTJR: Occupation, Participation and Health, 35,* 42–52.

Coelho, C. J., Przybyla, A., Yadav, V., & Sainburg, R. (2013). Hemispheric differences in the control of limb dynamics: A link between arm performance asymmetries and arm selection patterns. *Journal of Neurophysiology, 109,* 825–838.

Cogan, A. M., Blanchard, J., Garber, S. L., Vigen, C. L., Carlson, M., & Clark, F. A. (2017). Systematic review of behavioral and educational interventions to prevent pressure ulcers in adults with spinal cord injury. *Clinical Rehabilitation, 31,* 871–880.

Cohen, H. (1988). How to read a research paper. *American Journal of Occupational Therapy, 42,* 596–600.

Cohen, H. (1992). Vestibular rehabilitation reduces functional disability. *Otolaryngology—Head & Neck Surgery, 107,* 638–643.

Cohen, H. (1996). Vertigo after sailing a nineteenth century ship. *Journal of Vestibular Research, 6,* 31–35.

Cohen, H., Cohen, B., Raphan, T., & Waespe, W. (1992). Habituation and adaptation of the vestibuloocular reflex: A model of differential control by the vestibulocerebellum. *Experimental Brain Research, 90,* 526–538.

Cohen, H., Ewell, L. R., & Jenkins, H. A. (1995). Disability in Ménière's disease. *Archives of Otolaryngology—Head & Neck Surgery, 121,* 29–33.

Cohen, H., Kane-Wineland, M., Miller, L. V., & Hatfield, C. L. (1995). Occupation and visual/vestibular interaction in vestibular rehabilitation. *Otolaryngology—Head & Neck Surgery, 112,* 526–532.

Cohen, H., Miller, L. V., Kane-Wineland, M., & Hatfield, C. L. (1995). Vestibular rehabilitation with graded occupations. *American Journal of Occupational Therapy, 49,* 362–367.

Cohen, H. S. (2015). A career in inquiry. *American Journal of Occupational Therapy, 69,* 6906150010p1–6906150010p2. doi:10.5014/ajot.2015.696001

Cohen, H. S., Bloomberg, J. J., & Mulavara, A. P. (2005). Obstacle avoidance in novel visual environments improved by variable practice training. *Perceptual and Motor Skills, 101,* 853–861.

Cohen, H. S., Burkhardt, A., Cronin, G. W., & McGuire, M. J. (2006). Specialized knowledge and skills in adult vestibular rehabilitation for occupational therapy practice. *American Journal of Occupational Therapy, 60,* 669–678.

Cohen, H. S., Cox, C., Springer, G., Hoffman, H. J., Young, M. A., Margolick, J. B., & Plankey, M. W. (2012). Prevalence of abnormalities in vestibular function and balance among HIV-seropositive and HIV-seronegative women and men. *PLoS One, 7,* e38419.

Cohen, H. S., Harvison, N., & Baxter, M. F. (2013). *AOTA white paper on NASA's Human Spaceflight Program.* Retrieved from http://www8.nationalacademies.org/aseboutreach/publicview humanspaceflight.aspx

Cohen, H. S., & Kimball, K. T. (2000). Development of the vestibular disorders activities of daily living scale. *Archives of Otolaryngology—Head & Neck Surgery, 126,* 881–887.

Cohen, H. S., & Kimball, K. T. (2003). Increased independence and decreased vertigo after vestibular rehabilitation. *Otolaryngology—Head & Neck Surgery, 128,* 60–70.

Cohen, H. S., & Kimball, K. T. (2004). Decreased ataxia and improved balance after vestibular rehabilitation. *Otolaryngology—Head & Neck Surgery, 130,* 418–425.

Cohen, H. S., & Kimball, K. T. (2005). Effectiveness of treatments for benign paroxysmal positional vertigo of the posterior canal. *Otology & Neurotology, 26,* 1034–1040.

Cohen, H. S., Kimball, K. T., & Adams, A. S. (2000). Application of the Vestibular Disorders Activities of Daily Living Scale. *The Laryngoscope, 110,* 1204–1209.

Cohen, H. S., Kimball, K. T., & Stewart, M. G. (2004). Benign paroxysmal positional vertigo and comorbid conditions. *ORL, 66,* 11–15.

Cohen, H. S., Mulavara, A. P., Peters, B. T., Sangi-Haghpeykar, H., & Bloomberg, J. J. (2012). Tests of walking balance for screening vestibular disorders. *Journal of Vestibular Research, 22,* 95–104.

Cohen, H. S., Mulavara, A. P., Peters, B. T., Sangi-Haghpeykar, H., & Bloomberg, J. J. (2014). Standing balance tests for screening people with vestibular impairments. *The Laryngoscope, 124,* 545–550.

Cohen, H. S., Mulavara, A. P., Peters, B. T., Sangi-Haghpeykar, H., Kung, D. H., Mosier, D. R., & Bloomberg, J. (2013). Sharpening the tandem walking test for screening peripheral neuropathy. *Southern Medical Journal, 106,* 565–569.

Cohen, H. S., Mulavara, A. P., Sangi-Haghpeykar, H., Peters, B. T., Bloomberg, J. J., & Pavlik, V. (2014). Screening people in the waiting room for vestibular impairments. *Southern Medical Journal, 107,* 549–553.

Cohen, H. S., & Murphy, E. K. (2007). An augmented liberatory maneuver for benign paroxysmal positional vertigo for patients who are difficult to move. *Otolaryngology—Head & Neck Surgery, 136,* 309–310.

Cohen, H. S., & Sangi-Haghpeykar, H. (2010). Canalith repositioning variations for benign paroxysmal positional vertigo. *Otolaryngology—Head & Neck Surgery, 143,* 405–412. doi:10.1016 /j.otohns.2010.05.022

Cohen, H. S., Stewart, M. G., Brissett, A. E., Olson, K. L., Takashima, M., & Sangi-Haghpeykar, H. (2010). Frequency of sinus disease in normal subjects and patients with benign paroxysmal positional vertigo. *ORL, 72,* 63–67.

Cohen, H. S., Stitz, J., Sangi-Haghpeykar, H., Williams, S. P., Mulavara, A. P., Peters, B. T., & Bloomberg, J. J. (2017). Tandem walking as a quick screening test for vestibular disorders. *The Laryngoscope.* Advance online publication. doi:10.1002/lary.27022

Cohen, H. S., Wells, J., Kimball, K. T., & Owsley, C. (2003). Driving disability and dizziness. *Journal of Safety Research, 34,* 361–369.

Copernicus, N. (1543). *De revolutionibus orbium coelestium* [On the revolutions of the heavenly spheres]. Nuremberg, Germany: Petreius.

Corcoran, M. (2006). Using the MAARIE framework to read the research literature. *American Journal of Occupational Therapy, 60,* 367–368.

Coster, W. J. (2008). 2008 Eleanor Clarke Slagle Lecture. Embracing ambiguity: Facing the challenge of measurement. *American Journal of Occupational Therapy, 62,* 743–752.

Crocker, L. M. (1977). Linking research to practice: Suggestions for reading a research article. *American Journal of Occupational Therapy, 31,* 34–39.

Cuthbertson, D. W., Bershad, E. M., Sangi-Haghpeykar, H., & Cohen, H. S. (2015). Balance as a measurement of fatigue in postcall residents. *The Laryngoscope, 125,* 337–341.

Davis, J., Burr, M., Absi, M., Telles, R., & Koh, H. (2017). The contributions of occupational science to the readiness of long duration deep space exploration. *Work, 56,* 31–43.

Díaz-Venegas, C., Reistetter, T. A., Wang, C. Y., & Wong, R. (2016). The progression of disability among older adults in Mexico. *Disability and Rehabilitation, 38,* 2016–2027.

Donohue, M. V. (2003). Group profile studies with children: Validity measures and item analysis. *Occupational Therapy in Mental Health, 19,* 1–23.

Donohue, M. V. (2005). Social profile: Assessment of validity and reliability in children's groups. *Canadian Journal of Occupational Therapy, 62,* 164–175.

Donohue, M. V. (2007). Social profile: Interrater reliability in psychiatric and community activity groups. *Australian Occupational Therapy Journal, 54,* 49–58.

Donohue, M. V. (2013). *Social profile. Assessment of social participation in children, adolescents, and adults.* Bethesda, MD: American Occupational Therapy Association Press.

Dutton, R. (1989). Guidelines for using both activity and exercise. *American Journal of Occupational Therapy, 43,* 573–580.

Erlandson, K. M., Plankey, M. W., Springer, G., Cohen, H. S., Cox, C., Hoffman, H. J., . . . Brown, T. T. (2016). Fall frequency and associated factors among men and women with or at risk for HIV infection. *HIV Medicine, 17,* 740–748.

Evans, J. (2017). *Aristarchus of Samos.* Retrieved from https://www .britannica.com/biography/Aristarchus-of-Samos

Farber, S. D. (1989). Neuroscience and occupational therapy: Vital connections. 1989 Eleanor Clarke Slagle lecture. *American Journal of Occupational Therapy, 43,* 637–646.

Ferguson, J. M., & Trombly, C. A. (1997). The effect of added-purpose and meaningful occupation on motor learning. *American Journal of Occupational Therapy, 51,* 508–515.

Garber, S. L. (Ed.). (2014). *Pressure ulcer prevention and treatment following spinal cord injury: A clinical practice guideline for healthcare professionals* (2nd ed.). Washington, DC: Paralyzed Veterans of America.

Garber, S. L. (2016). The prepared mind. *American Journal of Occupational Therapy, 70,* 7006150010p1–7006150010p17. doi:10.5014/ajot.2016.706001

Garber, S. L., Krouskop, T. A., & Carter, R. E. (1978). A system for clinically evaluating wheelchair pressure-relief cushions. *American Journal of Occupational Therapy, 32,* 565–570.

Garber, S. L., Rintala, D. H., Hart, K. A., & Fuhrer, M. J. (2000). Pressure ulcer risk in spinal cord injury: Predictors of ulcer status over 3 years. *Archives of Physical Medicine and Rehabilitation, 81,* 465–471.

Garber, S. L., Rintala, D. H., Rossi, C. D., Hart, K. A., & Fuhrer, M. J. (1996). Reported pressure ulcer prevention and management techniques by persons with spinal cord injury. *Archives of Physical Medicine and Rehabilitation, 77,* 744–749.

Gillen, G. (2013). A fork in the road: An occupational hazard? *American Journal of Occupational Therapy, 67,* 641–652.

Giuffrida, C. G., Shea, J. B., & Fairbrother, J. T. (2002). Differential transfer benefits of increased practice for constant, blocked, and serial practice schedules. *Journal of Motor Behavior, 34,* 353–365.

Goel, R., Kofman, I., Jeevarajan, J., De Dios, Y., Cohen, H. S., Bloomberg, J. J., & Mulavara, A. P. (2015). Using low levels of stochastic vestibular stimulation to improve balance function. *PLoS One, 10*(8), e0136335. doi:10.1371/journal.pone.0136335

Gottshall, K. R., Hoffer, M. E., Cohen, H. S., & Moore, R. J. (2006). Active head movements facilitate compensation for effects of prism displacement on dynamic gait. *Journal of Vestibular Research, 16,* 29–33.

Greenstein, L. R. (1980). Teaching research: An introduction to statistical concepts and research terminology. *American Journal of Occupational Therapy, 34,* 320–327.

Guihan, M., Hastings, J., & Garber, S. L. (2009). Therapists' roles in pressure ulcer management in persons with spinal cord injury. *Journal of Spinal Cord Medicine, 32,* 560–567.

Gutman, S. A. (1995). Influence of the U.S. military and occupational therapy reconstruction aides in World War I on the development of occupational therapy. *American Journal of Occupational Therapy, 49,* 256–262.

Hall, H. J. (1910a). Manual work in the treatment of the functional nervous diseases. *JAMA, 55,* 295–297.

Hall, H. J. (1910b). Work-cure: A report of five years' experience at an institution devoted to the therapeutic application of manual work. *JAMA, 54,* 12–14.

Heck, S. (1988). The effect of purposeful activity on pain tolerance. *American Journal of Occupational Therapy, 42,* 577–581.

Holm, M. B. (2000). The 2000 Eleanor Clarke Slagle Lecture. Our mandate for the new millennium: Evidence-based practice. *American Journal of Occupational Therapy, 54,* 575–585.

Hong, I., Coker-Bolt, P., Anderson, K. R., Lee, D., & Velozo, C. A. (2016). Relationship between physical activity and overweight and obesity in children: Findings from the 2012 National Health and Nutrition Examination Survey National Youth Fitness Survey. *American Journal of Occupational Therapy, 70,* 7005180060p1–7005180060p8.

Hong, I., Dodds, C. B., Coker-Bolt, P., Simpson, A. N., & Velozo, C. A. (2017). How accurately do both parents and health professionals assess overweight in children? *Pediatric Physical Therapy, 29,* 283–285.

Hsieh, H.-C., Lin, H.-Y., Chiu, W.-H., Meng, L. F., & Liu, C. K. (2015). Upper-limb rehabilitation with adaptive video games for preschool children with developmental disabilities. *American Journal of Occupational Therapy, 69,* 6904290020p1–6904290020p5.

Hutchinson, E. B., Schwerin, S. C., Radomski, K. L., Irfanoglu, M. O., Juliano, S. L., & Pierpaoli, C. M. (2016). Quantitative MRI and DTI abnormalities during the acute period following CCI in the ferret. *Shock, 46*(3 Suppl 1), 167–176.

Hyman, D., Gurgevich, E., Alter, T., Ayers, J., Cash, E., Fahnline, D., . . . Wright, H. (2001–2002). Beyond Boyer: The UniSCOPE model of scholarship for the 21st century. *Journal of Higher Education Outreach and Engagement, 7*(1&2), 41–65.

Isaacson, B., Murphy, E. K., & Cohen, H. S. (2006). Does the method of sternocleidomastoid muscle activation affect the vestibular evoked myogenic potential response? *Journal of Vestibular Research, 16,* 187–191.

Iyer, M. B., Mattu, U., Grafman, J., Lomarev, M., Sato, S., & Wassermann, E. M. (2005). Safety and cognitive effect of frontal DC brain polarization in healthy individuals. *Neurology, 64,* 872–875.

Jarus, T. (1994). Motor learning and occupational therapy: The organization of practice. *American Journal of Occupational Therapy, 48,* 810–816.

Juang, C., Knight, B. G., Carlson, M., Schepens Niemiec, S. L., Vigen, C., & Clark, F. (2018). Understanding the mechanisms of change in a lifestyle intervention for older adults. *Gerontologist, 58,* 353–361. doi:10.1093/geront/gnw152

Krishnan, S., Pappadis, M. R., Weller, S. C., Fisher, S. R., Hay, C. C., & Reistetter, T. A. (2018). Patient-centered mobility outcome preferences according to individuals with stroke and caregivers: A qualitative analysis. *Disability and Rehabilitation, 40,* 1401–1409. doi:10.1080/09638288.2017.1297855

Li, C. M., Hoffman, H. J., Ward, B. K., Cohen, H. S., & Rine, R. M. (2016). Epidemiology of dizziness and balance problems in children in the United States: A population-based study. *Journal of Pediatrics, 171,* 240.e3–247.e3.

Li, C. Y., Karmarkar, A., Lin, Y. L., Kuo, Y. F., Ottenbacher, K. J., & Graham, J. E. (2018). Is profit status of inpatient rehabilitation facilities independently associated with 30-day unplanned hospital readmission for Medicare beneficiaries? *Archives of Physical Medicine and Rehabilitation, 99,* 598.e2–602.e2. doi:10.1016/j.apmr.2017.09.002

Liew, S. L., Rana, M., Cornelsen, S., Fortunato de Barros Filho, M., Birbaumer, N., Sitaram, R., . . . Soekadar, S. R. (2016). Improving motor corticothalamic communication after stroke using real-time fMRI connectivity-based neurofeedback. *Neurorehabilitation and Neural Repair, 30,* 671–675.

Low, J. F. (1992). The reconstruction aides. *American Journal of Occupational Therapy, 46,* 38–43.

Ma, H.-I., & Trombly, C. A. (2001). The comparison of motor performance between part and whole tasks in elderly persons. *American Journal of Occupational Therapy, 55,* 62–67.

Mahaffey, L., Burson, K. A., Januszewski, C., Pitts, D. B., & Preissner, K. (2015). Role for occupational therapy in community mental health: Using policy to advance scholarship of practice. *Occupational Therapy in Health Care, 29,* 397–410.

Mani, S., Mutha, P., Przybyla, A., Haaland, K., & Sainburg, R. L. (2013). Contralesional motor deficits after unilateral stroke reflect hemisphere-specific control mechanisms. *Brain, 136,* 1288–1303.

Mathiowetz, V., & Haugen, J. B. (1994). Motor behavior research: Implications for therapeutic approaches to central nervous system dysfunction. *American Journal of Occupational Therapy, 48,* 733–745.

McRackan, T. R., Velozo, C. A., Holcomb, M. A., Camposeo, E. L., Hatch, J. L., Meyer, T. A., . . . Dubno, J. R. (2017). Use of adult patient focus groups to develop the initial item bank for a cochlear implant quality-of-life instrument. *JAMA Otolaryngology—Head & Neck Surgery, 143,* 975–982.

Morin, M., Binik, Y. M., Bourbonnais, D., Khalifé, S., Ouellet, S., & Bergeron, S. (2017). Heightened pelvic floor muscle tone and altered contractility in women with provoked vestibulodynia. *The Journal of Sexual Medicine, 14,* 592–600.

Mulavara, A. P., Cohen, H. S., Peters, B. T., Sangi-Haghpeykar, H., & Bloomberg, J. J. (2013). New analyses of the Sensory Organization Test compared to the Clinical Test of Sensory Integration and Balance in patients with benign paroxysmal positional vertigo. *The Laryngoscope, 123,* 2276–2280. doi:10.1002/lary.24075

Mulavara, A. P., Fiedler, M. J., Kofman, I. S., Wood, S. J., Serrador, J. M., Peters, B., . . . Bloomberg, J. J. (2011). Improving balance function using vestibular stochastic resonance: Optimizing stimulus characteristics. *Experimental Brain Research, 210,* 303–312.

Mun-Bryce, S., Roberts, L., Bartolo, A., & Okada, Y. (2006). Transhemispheric depolarizations persist in the intracerebral hemorrhage swine brain following corpus callosal transection. *Brain Research, 1073–1074,* 481–490.

Mun-Bryce, S., Wilkerson, A., Pacheco, B., Zhang, T., Rai, S., Wang, Y., & Okada, Y. (2004). Depressed cortical excitability and elevated matrix metalloproteinases in remote brain regions following intracerebral hemorrhage. *Brain Research, 1026,* 227–234.

Murphy, S., & Tickle-Degnen, L. (2001). Participation in daily living tasks among older adults with fear of falling. *American Journal of Occupational Therapy, 55,* 538–544.

Murphy, S. L., Kratz, A. L., & Schepens Niemiec, S. L. (2017). Assessing fatigability in the lab and in daily life in older adults with osteoarthritis using perceived, performance, and ecological measures. *The Journals of Gerontology, 72,* 115–120.

National Society for the Promotion of Occupational Therapy. (1917). *Certificate of incorporation.* Clifton Springs, NY: Author.

Ottenbacher, A. J., Snih, S. A., Bindawas, S. M., Markides, K. S., Graham, J. E., Samper-Ternent, R., . . . Ottenbacher, K. J. (2014). Role of physical activity in reducing cognitive decline in older Mexican-American adults. *Journal of the American Geriatrics Society, 62,* 1786–1791. doi:10.1111/jgs.12978

Ottenbacher, K. J., Karmarkar, A., Graham, J. E., Kuo, Y. F., Deutsch, A., Reistetter, T. A., . . . Granger, C. V. (2014). Thirty-day hospital readmission following discharge from postacute rehabilitation in fee-for-service Medicare patients. *JAMA, 311*, 604–614.

Pelletier, R., Higgins, J., & Bourbonnais, D. (2015). Addressing neuroplastic changes in distributed areas of the nervous system associated with chronic musculoskeletal disorders. *Physical Therapy, 95*, 1582–1591.

Pelletier, R., Higgins, J., & Bourbonnais, D. (2017). The relationship of corticospinal excitability with pain, motor performance and disability in subjects with chronic wrist/hand pain. *Journal of Electromyography and Kinesiology, 34*, 65–71.

Peloquin, S. M. (2005). Embracing our ethos, reclaiming our heart. *American Journal of Occupational Therapy, 59*, 611–625.

Peloquin, S. M., & Ciro, C. A. (2013). Self-development groups among women in recovery: Client perceptions of satisfaction and engagement. *American Journal of Occupational Therapy, 67*, 82–90.

Peters, B. T., Mulavara, A. P., Cohen, H. S., Sangi-Haghpeykar, H., & Bloomberg, J. J. (2012). Dynamic visual acuity testing for screening patients with vestibular impairments. *Journal of Vestibular Research, 22*, 145–151.

Peters, C. O. (2011). Powerful occupational therapists: A community of professionals, 1950–1980. *Occupational Therapy in Mental Health, 27*, 199–410.

Peterson, K., & Stevens, J. (2013). Integrating the scholarship of practice into the nurse academician portfolio. *Journal of Nursing Education and Practice, 3*, 84–92.

Pettigrew, J., Robinson, K., & Moloney, S. (2017). The Bluebirds: World War I soldiers' experiences of occupational therapy. *American Journal of Occupational Therapy, 71*, 7101100010p1–7101100010p9.

Reed, K. L. (1986). Tools of practice: heritage or baggage? 1986 Eleanor Clarke Slagle lecture. *American Journal of Occupational Therapy, 40*, 597–605.

Reed, K. L. (1993). The beginning of occupational therapy. In H. L. Hopkins & H. D. Smith (Eds.), *Willard & Spackman's occupational therapy* (8th ed., pp. 26–43). Philadelphia, PA: J. B. Lippincott.

Rogers, J. C. (1983). Eleanor Clarke Slagle Lectureship—1983; clinical reasoning: The ethics, science, and art. *American Journal of Occupational Therapy, 37*, 601–616.

Roller, C. A., Cohen, H. S., Kimball, K. T., & Bloomberg, J. J. (2001). Variable practice with lenses improves visuo-motor plasticity. *Brain Research. Cognitive Brain Research, 21*, 341–352.

Sainburg, R. L., Liew, S. L., Frey, S. H., & Clark, F. (2017). Promoting translational research among movement science, occupational science, and occupational therapy. *Journal of Motor Behavior, 49*, 1–7.

Sainburg, R. L., Schaefer, S. Y., & Yadav, V. (2016). Lateralized motor control processes determine asymmetry of interlimb transfer. *Neuroscience, 334*, 26–38.

Schaffer, J. E., & Sainburg, R. L. (2017). Interlimb differences in coordination of unsupported reaching movements. *Neuroscience, 350*, 54–64.

Schepens, S. L., Panzer, V., & Goldberg, A. (2011). Randomized controlled trial comparing tailoring methods of multimedia-based fall prevention education for community-dwelling older adults. *American Journal of Occupational Therapy, 65*, 702–709.

Schepens, S. L., Sen, A., Painter, J. A., & Murphy, S. L. (2012). Relationship between fall-related efficacy and activity engagement in community-dwelling older adults: A meta-analytic review. *American Journal of Occupational Therapy, 66*, 137–148.

Schwartz, K. B. (2009). Reclaiming our heritage: Connecting the founding vision to the centennial vision. *American Journal of Occupational Therapy, 63*, 681–690.

Schwartz, K. B., & Colman, W. (1988). Historical research methods in occupational therapy. *American Journal of Occupational Therapy, 42*, 239–244.

Skidmore, E. R., Butters, M., Whyte, E., Grattan, E., Shen, J., & Terhorst, L. (2017). Guided training relative to direct skill training for individuals with cognitive impairments after stroke: A pilot randomized trial. *Archives of Physical Medicine and Rehabilitation, 98*, 673–680.

Smith, R. O. (2017). Technology and occupation: Past, present, and the next 100 years of theory and practice. *American Journal of Occupational Therapy, 71*, 7106150010p1–7106150010p15.

Spencer, J., Hersch, G., Shelton, M., Ripple, J., Spencer, C., Dyer, C. B., & Murphy, K. (2002). Functional outcomes and daily life activities of African-American elders after hospitalization. *American Journal of Occupational Therapy, 56*, 149–159.

Spencer, J., Krefting, L., & Mattingly, C. (1993). Incorporation of ethnographic methods in occupational therapy assessment. *American Journal of Occupational Therapy, 47*, 303–309.

Stattel, F. (1956). Equipment designed for occupational therapy. *American Journal of Occupational Therapy, 10*, 194–198.

Stewart, K. E., Whelan, D. M., & Banerjee, A. (2017). Are cervical collars a necessary postprocedure restriction in patients with benign paroxysmal positional vertigo treated with particle repositioning maneuvers? *Otology & Neurotology, 38*, 860–864.

Todai, J. K., Congdon, S. L., Sangi-Haghpeykar, H., & Cohen, H. S. (2014). Ocular vestibular evoked myogenic potentials in response to three test positions and two frequencies. *The Laryngoscope, 124*, E237–E240.

Trombly, C. A. (1995). Occupation: Purposefulness and meaningfulness as therapeutic mechanisms. 1995 Eleanor Clarke Slagle Lecture. *American Journal of Occupational Therapy, 49*, 960–972.

Trombly, C. A., & Wu, C.-Y. (1999). Effect of rehabilitation tasks on organization of movement after stroke. *American Journal of Occupational Therapy, 53*, 333–344.

Waddell, K. J., Strube, M. J., Bailey, R. R., Klaesner, J. W., Birkenmeier, R. L., Dromerick, A. W., & Lang, C. E. (2017). Does task-specific training improve upper limb performance in daily life poststroke? *Neurorehabilitation and Neural Repair, 31*, 290–300.

White, V. K. (1998). Ethnic differences in the wellness of elderly persons. *Occupational Therapy in Health Care, 11*, 1–5.

Worrell, M. B. (2000). Getting started in research. *OT Practice, 5*(16), CE-1–CE-8.

Wu, C., Trombly, C. A., Lin, K., & Tickle-Degnen, L. (1998). Effects of object affordances on reaching performance in persons with and without cerebrovascular accident. *American Journal of Occupational Therapy, 52*, 447–456.

Yoder, R. M., Nelson, D. L., & Smith, D. A. (1989). Added-purpose versus rote exercise in female nursing home residents. *American Journal of Occupational Therapy, 43*, 581–586.

the**Point**® *For additional resources on the subjects discussed in this chapter, visit* http://thePoint.lww.com /Willard-Spackman13e.

UNIT II

Occupational Nature of Humans

Morning Routine

Our talk is made of mundane things,
the dog, the grass, his weight, my car,
but Dad and I keep in touch—
his coastal plain, my foothills joined
by telephone and promise. And he tells me
each time of Mother, too, his latest visit,
her knowing him, or not, her temperament,
her eating, the others at the home.

I use the time to make my bed—the act
a cue to make the call, keep moving
in a useful way, tasks blending into one.
Holding phone to ear, I trot the U from side to side
while I smooth the sheets, rid the bed
of two impressions, tug and tuck the blanket,
square the duvet's rosy border in a manner
less awkward now, one hand learning
to manage without its partner.

—Clela Dyess Reed
from *Bloodline* (Evening Street Press, 2009)
Used with permission of the author.

Transformations of Occupations

A Life Course Perspective

Ruth Humphry, Jennifer Womack

LEARNING OBJECTIVES

After reading this chapter, you will be able to:

1. Apply the principles of a life course perspective to understand how occupational opportunities, people's evaluation of their life situations, and their choices lead to their current pattern of occupations.
2. Explain how communities create occupational opportunities and share normative expectations for certain occupations.
3. Analyze how social participation leads to coordinated occupations supporting acquisition of new or altered occupations.
4. Examine how occupational performance and experiences of meaning emerge from interconnected elements of the occupational situation.
5. Analyze how occupations join people with their life situations, enabling them to participate with others during life transitions.

Introduction

This chapter is about how people acquire occupations and how the things people do change in the course of living their lives. Wilcock (2006) suggested the occupational nature of people evolved simultaneously with sociocultural practices that enabled people to coordinate their actions in occupations for their immediate survival and ultimately sustained survival of the species. Today, researchers study the meaningfulness of participation in groups with common goals and people's sense of being a part of something bigger (Hocking & Wright-St Clair, 2017). This sense of belonging may be to an identified group like a family, workplace, or even a book club. The sense of belonging to a group with shared occupations could be informal situations such as fans of a basketball team. In this chapter, these groups with shared goals and ways of doing things are seen as communities. It is in this type of situation that occupations are acquired and changed. In fact, learning to be part of a community starts before a baby is born as fetuses develop familiarity with the sound of the language of people around them (Choi, Cutler, & Broersma, 2017) and infants only 2 to 3 months of age see patterns in caregiving and want to join in with caregiving routines (Humphry, 2016).

CENTENNIAL NOTES

Evolution in Occupational Therapy Ideas about Child Development

Knowledge is closely linked to the assumptions of disciplines generating the research used to inform occupational therapy (OT). The profession's understanding of changes in how to work with children evolved from common sense and the knowledge of medical doctors to theories put forward by developmental psychology and eventually becoming the understanding of scholars in OT and occupational science.

For example, in the first edition of this text, *Principles of Occupational Therapy* (Willard & Spackman, 1947), the author of the chapter about working with children reflected a common sense form of knowledge, suggesting that therapists speak in a kind voice and try to get to know the pediatric patient. An understanding of children's lives reflected the dominant assumptions in the first half of the 20th century that development is a biological process. Darwin (naturalist), Piaget (biologist), and Gesell and Freud (physicians) contributed to the literature about sequential stages of change. The use of manual crafts, music, and recreation were suggested media for intervention (Figure 7-1).

By the 1960s (when the third edition of this text was published), it was suggested that practitioners' goals were to promote the growth of ill or handicapped children to achieve a healthier adulthood. Occupational therapy practice with children was increasingly informed by neuroscience such as Jean Ayres's attention to sensation, infants' pattern of reflexes, the ontogenetic sequence of motor skills as well as neuromuscular integration theories such as those developed by Bobath and Rood. Content over the next several decades suggested that working with children continued to be informed by knowledge about neuroscience as well as developmental psychology theories. Development of play in the seventh edition was approached as the main modality to enhance function of body capacities.

In the eighth edition (published 1993), information about occupational performance, such as play, was

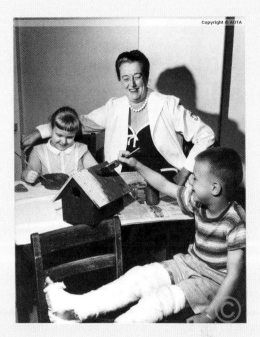

FIGURE 7-1 **The occupational therapist in the photo, Winifred C. Kahmann, was the Director of Occupational Therapy at the James Whitcomb Riley Hospital for Children in Indianapolis, Indiana. Kahmann was the first registered occupational therapist to be elected president of American Occupational Therapist Association.**

included for the first time. In the ninth edition (1998), there was an increasing appreciation that changes in children are not brought about simply by maturation of the nervous system but rather reflect the child interacting and being shaped by the ecological niche the child is raised in—the community, society, and culture. Ultimately, this assumption suggests the type of knowledge to support the acquisition of occupation is multifaceted, not only in children but also across the life course.

Occupational therapists work with people who often need to acquire new occupations or change what and how things are done. These changes accompany a life transition (Blair, 2000). The turning points in life trajectory may be anticipated such as a young person with cerebral palsy who starts college. Or unanticipated turning points can occur like the diagnosis of cardiovascular disease at the early age of 52 years. In this case, people with chronic conditions are encouraged to manage their symptoms by lifestyle changes (Fritz & Cutchin, 2016). This chapter is not about how to practice but offers a framework for understanding how dynamic, multifactorial situations shape changes in occupations.

The ideas presented presume that the reasons people acquire, change, or discontinue occupations goes beyond individual preferences. Instead, these changes represent dynamic transactions among people, situated in a particular place, social, and historical context. As life circumstances change, acquisition of new occupations can occur as well as transformations in what and how things are done to sustain participation. Thus, these dynamic processes challenge us to think beyond conventional views of development of the individual to understand how changes of occupations occur. This dynamic and contextualized perspective asks practitioners to focus on people's evolving occupations as a social process.

The Situated Nature of Changing Occupations

Before discussing what shapes changes in people's occupations, it is important to think about what it means to acquire a new occupation. To explore what it entails, consider Case Study 7-1 in which three generations engage in yoga.

Yoga developed centuries ago in India as an activity for the health of body and mind. This family's occupation reflects both continuity with historic ties and contemporary interest in wellness. It also illustrates how societal changes lead to acquisition of occupation. When Harriet was young, exercise was not part of her generation's expectations of what young women should do. Engagement in occupations is not an individual decision but the choice of what to do is influenced by the practice of others, changing the values of doing it and meaning of belong to the community.

This family scenario also illustrates that taking up new occupations occurs at any point during a lifetime and is not necessarily passed down in a linear manner from older to younger generation. It also shows us that people start doing the same activity for different reasons and learn it different ways. Harriet and Lauren learned yoga in a more structured didactic way which generated procedural knowledge of how to do the poses. Mariah instinctively mimicked the things adults did. For her, the acquisition of the occupation was not a conscious choice.

One can imagine that performance of all family members will undergo changes in their performance of yoga poses over time. Mariah will gain more skills as she appreciates more details of the moves. She will find that there are other things to pay attention to, such as breathing and mental practices. This type of learning does not reflect abstract mental change that occurs out of context of the practice but the active learning as part of being part of a community doing things together (Lave & Packer, 2008; Lave & Wenger, 1991).

For all the family members, their procedural knowledge of yoga reflects **embodied action**. Embodied action assumes that the mind and body are coupled as an entity that experiences the situation as a whole rather than in separate and distinct ways (Overton, Muller, & Newman, 2008). Variability in performance of repeated actions of the same person reflects the **emergent performance** of their occupations. That is, the physical, mental, sensory, and emotional capacities of each person are integrated so people master how to coordinate their occupations with changing body morphology and adapt actions to different environments.

Finally, this case study of a family illustrates how people and their occupations are interdependent elements of a

CASE STUDY 7-1   A FAMILY OCCUPATION

In Figure 7-2, a grandmother, Harriet; her adult daughter, Lauren; and her granddaughter, Mariah, share a morning routine of yoga. Lauren learned the practice of yoga in college from her boyfriend who was attracted to it for the connection between the body/mind and health. After graduation, she took classes and found yoga a great way to be socially active. When she married the man who introduced her to yoga, they exercised together. After Mariah was born, Lauren enrolled her in baby yoga and it became something they shared. When Harriet visited, she became intrigued by the yoga class. She heard about the importance of an active lifestyle and wanted to try yoga. Lauren helped her select poses and practice moves until they became familiar. This picture was taken after Mariah's second birthday when she received yoga pants and a mat. Her parents had not taught her what to do—she seemed to just join in the routines of her mother and grandmother.

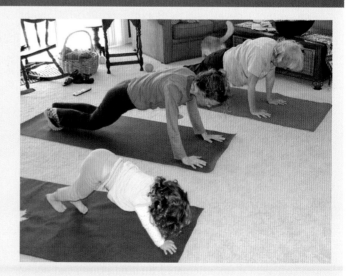

FIGURE 7-2 Engaging in exercise for health and relaxation is an intergenerational occupation for this grandmother, her daughter, and her granddaughter.

larger picture. Focusing on the occupational engagement of one member of a community would lead to an incomplete understanding of how occupations are acquired and performed as a way of joining in something. Doing yoga, or any other occupation, is conceptualized as a **transactional process** where people, the physical space, time, and objects form a functional whole in which the occupation serves to connect people with each other and their life circumstances (Cutchin & Dickie, 2012; Dickie, Cutchin, & Humphry, 2006).

The rest of this chapter is organized around different change models that share a common interest in things people do. The first model, Life Course, is about life-long development linking early life experiences to later adulthood (Elder & Shanahan, 2006). This perspective is relevant because practitioners acknowledge that past experiences inform a person's response to the current situations and occupational challenges. Next, this chapter draws on work of an interdisciplinary group of activity theorists (Hedegaard, 2009; Lave & Wenger, 1991), which has informed a model for developing occupations (Humphry, 2005). Finally, a change model discusses moment-to-moment changes in performance of an occupation (Humphry, 2002; Thelen, 2000).

Life Course Perspective

The life course perspective (Elder & Shanahan, 2006; Johnson, Crosnoe, & Elder, 2011; Mayer, 2009) serves a guiding concept for practitioners working with people of all ages to understand how occupations are acquired in social situations like joining a quilting guild or becoming a patient in a rehabilitation center. These occupations evolve over time as circumstances change. Life course theorists recognize that systematic changes occur from birth to the end of life and move beyond an emphasis on the physical, mental, social, and emotional changes occurring within the individual (Diewald & Mayer, 2009). Rather, life course theorists emphasize that living is a highly situated, socially participatory process in which individuals are part of communities changing social positions and taking up new roles leaving others behind. They recognize that we are born into **birth cohorts** where the sum effects of the times and the people around us serve to create a trajectory or pathway for our lives. Life transitions such as starting a family, emigration, or retirement are seen as turning points that can change the trajectory of people's lives.

A life course perspective as articulated by sociologists orients us to consider the processes shaping people's lives but does not systematically focus on changing occupations. It links context and individuals in life situations in which we believe occupations are implicit. Table 7-1 summarizes principles of a life course (Elder & Shanahan, 2006) and illustrates application to transformations of people's occupations. There are four interdependent factors that alter circumstances, which in turn shape the trajectory of a life course. The first two have already been mentioned. First, there are anticipated changes (like starting kindergarten, moving and meeting new people to go out to dinner with, or a job promotion). The second is unanticipated change (giving birth to twins or being laid off from work) that happens to individual. The third factor occurs at the societal level which also shape people's life course (i.e.,

TABLE 7-1 **Principles of a Life Course Perspective Applied to Changing Occupations**

Life Course Principle	Example
1. Aging and transformations of occupations are lifelong processes; the accumulated experiences with past occupations impact current forms of engagement.	A boy first learns to hike with his family. He joins a hiking club during college and marries a woman he met on a hike. However, they become too busy with careers to continue hiking. However, after retirement they return to hiking as a leisure activity again.
2. People live interconnected lives, and these networks of relationships shape people's occupations.	The director of an assisted living facility retires and a new director changes the schedule to give residents greater freedom in deciding when they want to come to breakfast. Many of the seniors enjoy making decision but a resident with early dementia doesn't remember to come to breakfast for several mornings in a row.
3. Historic times and societal events shape and alter what people do, how they do it, and give it meaning.	During the Afghanistan War, the U.S. military promised veterans' educational benefits. This encouraged a young man to join the army and not the community college as expected. His military experiences made him proud to serve, and he chooses to make being a soldier a career.
4. People make choices about their occupations, which reflect their circumstances and perceived occupational opportunities at that particular time.	A woman accepts a promotion were she supervises people in different parts of the country so it requires travel. Six years later, she and her partner decide to start a family. She leaves the leadership position and takes a job with less responsibility, travel, and pay.
5. Antecedents to an event or life transition and the consequences of such events for a person's occupations vary according to timing in the life course.	A young construction worker was laid off when the housing market crashes. He moves in with his parents and takes a job doing yardwork. An older construction worker also is laid off. He and his wife could not pay their mortgage, and they had to declare bankruptcy.

employment opportunities in renewable energy, the need for active military in the Middle East, changes in funding for health care). Finally, the characteristic of an individual (i.e., gender, ethnicity, race, age, educational, and income levels) which intersects with societal changes to have more or less an effect on what people do and the trajectory of their life course. The life course perspective encourages us to acknowledge the intertwined factors leading to the complexity of any person's changing occupations. It will also determine what occupational opportunities are perceived as available to a person at any point in time.

We start by drawing on a life course perspective of occupation that illustrates what people do is simultaneously individual, interpersonal, social, and historical. We turn to consider the case of Wanda and the importance of incorporating a life course perspective of occupation in light of people's lives and the things they choose to do. Wanda's story will be told in parts throughout the remainder of this chapter and here serves to illustrate the relationship of early life experiences to later occupational behavior.

CASE STUDY 7-2   WANDA, *PART I*

Wanda, a 40-year-old patient in a rehabilitation hospital, has heard the young girl in the room next door crying at night. She overhead the 14-year-old say that she is missing the end of her eighth-grade school year while undergoing rehabilitation after having a stroke. Wanda recalls seeing some costumes and masks in the recreation therapy department and asks her therapist if she can borrow a clown mask and wig to cheer up her young neighbor. That same night, she puts on the costume and asks her nurse to help her across the hall to visit her neighbor. Wanda improvises a mime skit about her own disability and soon has her young neighbor laughing. The two of them continue to support one another through the rehabilitation process and say a tearful goodbye when Wanda is discharged.

How did Wanda become a human being who, despite her own challenges, reaches out to someone else who is struggling? In this brief introduction to her life, we know only that she is a patient in a rehabilitation hospital, that she is 40 years old and has a disability, and that she has reached out to someone younger in a similar circumstance. This snapshot of her life is lacking, however, in social and historical context. What in her background and experience led her to focus on the needs of her young neighbor while facing her own major life transition? As you continue

to read Wanda's story, reflect on how learning about her childhood and family occupations illustrates the value of a life course perspective (Elder & Shanahan, 2006; Johnson et al., 2011) as a lens for understanding the choice to engage in an unanticipated occupations.

CASE STUDY 7-2   WANDA, *PART II*

Wanda was born in the early 1950s with spastic quadriplegic cerebral palsy as the only child of parents whom she describes as "loving, encouraging, and protective." The family lived in a small rural community where they were active church and community members, but there were limited services for Wanda's situation. Her parents traveled with her to regional medical centers for treatment when she was young. Because her birth cohort predated federally mandated accommodation for people with disabilities, her parents sent her at age 8 years to attend a boarding school for children with limited mobility. After 2 years, Wanda and her parents decided she should return to live at home, and she continued living with them through her adult years. Wanda attended the rural public schools when a classroom could accommodate her but primarily received home-based schooling because of limited access of classrooms. Wanda had an aptitude for math; and because writing was difficult, her father helped her learn to use an electric typewriter to organize figures into columns to add and subtract. In her 20s, she began helping a friend of her parents to calculate the income from his truck farming operation; once a week, he brought Wanda receipts and handwritten notes about his cash income, and she would organize the figures by typing them onto a page, calculating the sums, and returning them to the farmer.

One of Wanda's teenage life experiences was helping her parents as volunteers for the county Meals-on-Wheels program. Her father drove the family around their rural county and Wanda handed meals to her mother from the back seat, who then delivered them to the door. Wanda would wave to the person at the door from the back seat of the car. In time, several recipients came to know the family; and eventually, some met the car at the driveway or mailbox so that they could chat with Wanda rather than simply wave to her.

"It was good for them, too," she said. "It gave them some fresh air and a little exercise. And they depended on us showing up for them every day."

Knowing more about Wanda helps to situate her decision to reach out to her young neighbor in the rehabilitation hospital. It had roots in her past experiences when she and her parents entered volunteer roles. Her parents, who valued helping others and including Wanda in their lives, supported Wanda's engagement. When the elderly recipients came out to greet her, volunteering took on additional meaning by connecting her life with theirs. Clearly, this woman's life illustrates the interdependent and situated nature of occupations. Whereas we might, based on a traditional development perspective, have considered a 40-year-old woman with cerebral palsy as never having mastered certain skills, we now see a woman defined not by her disability but by her life experiences, which took place in a given social and historical context.

Wanda's occupations as an informal bookkeeper and volunteer were created not simply by her as an individual but through the relationships within a rural setting and her parents' encouragement. Elements of her circumstance such as the farmer's need for a record of his finances and her father's help in learning to use a typewriter, combined with Wanda's ability to work with numbers, created an occupational opportunity that she readily agreed to do.

The historical time frame in which she was born accounts for differences in disability services and schooling. Wanda and her parents made the choice not to continue at the residential school for students with special needs. By leaving a school that could accommodate her limited mobility, Wanda and her parents relied more on home schooling, which altered her occupations as a student and likely had consequences for her social occupations with peers. Her limited interactions with age mates also increased her contact with adults. One might argue that the choices disadvantaged Wanda, but her later positive social actions seemed shaped by these experiences.

A Life Transition and Occupational Therapy

CASE STUDY 7-2   WANDA, *PART III*

At age 40 years, Wanda wanted to learn to cook and manage the home in which she had lived most of her life. Her mother died when Wanda was 36 years old, and her father passed away 6 months before her 40th birthday. Although Wanda had relatives living nearby who will assist her with household maintenance, she wanted to be able to manage her own life in her home on a day-to-day basis. She and her Medicaid caseworker decided, given Wanda's rural location, that admission into a regional rehabilitation center to maximize her

(continues)

functional skills was the best route to determine her ability to live alone.

The rehabilitation hospital context was a challenge for her as she had to rely on nurses for self-care skills that she has performed independently at home for almost 30 years with the adaptations her parents helped her put in place. Her mobility and speech impairments seemed emphasized in a context where no one was aware of who she was or what she could do. Wanda, however, had two well-developed traits on her side: an outgoing personality that put everyone at ease with her situation and a sense of humor that was soon legendary in the rehabilitation center. Watching her reach out to the young girl crying in the next room made staff aware that Wanda could offer something to her neighbor that staff could not; she was a midlife adult with an understanding of living with disability. Her initiative and actions also brought awareness that Wanda was a person who came into the rehabilitation hospital not to have her disabling condition rehabilitated but to address new challenges brought about by a change in her life situation.

Learning about Wanda's accomplishments throughout her life led her occupational therapist in the rehabilitation center to question why she had never learned to cook or do other things around the house. Wanda laughs when she reports that cooking was one of her mother's favorite things to do, "And she was really good at it! Why would I trade her pot roast for my burned toast?"

Wanda undertook a full range of therapies at the rehabilitation center, but it was in OT that she identified the activities that had prompted her admission. She grew frustrated when emphasis was placed on trying to reduce tone in her lower extremities or correcting some of her long-preferred speech patterns (which Wanda attributed as much to being Southern as to her dysarthria), but in OT, she clearly stated her focus on goals that would allow her to stay in her own home.

Wanda had three primary goals related to cooking: to safely use the microwave, to safely make a "real" pot of coffee, and to find ways to effectively open and close food containers. The first and last goals were met within a few weeks using adaptive strategies and creating adaptive tools that she could manage with stabilized gross motor movements. The coffee-making goal became both her greatest challenge and the mark of her stubborn determination.

Although Wanda had better upper extremity control in a seated position, and she used this strategy to manage the microwave, she refused to move her coffee pot to a table or low counter to use it. A home visit and extensive conversation revealed why this was

(continues)

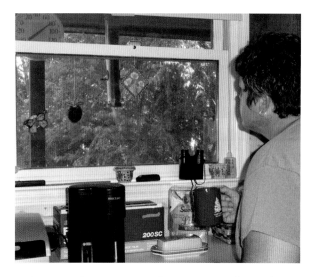

FIGURE 7-3 Patterns of action are shaped over a lifetime as people make choices and develop preferred ways of doing.

the case. In Wanda's home, the family coffee maker sat right beside the kitchen sink (Figure 7-3). Over the sink was a window, and outside the window were three hanging feeders that Wanda and her father placed there to watch the birds each morning. For longer than she could remember, Wanda woke up smelling coffee that her father had put on to brew, made her way into the kitchen in her pajamas, and stood at the sink watching birds with her father and sipping coffee from a covered mug. She wasn't totally stable in that position—she leaned against the sink counter with her hips and held onto the front of the sink with one hand while handling her mug with the other . . . but she was totally content. When she was little, she notes, her mother and father used to have her hold onto the sink in the mornings and stretch out her legs so that she could stand and walk better—sometime in her 20s, the coffee routine was added. Moving the coffee pot from that spot seemed a greater sacrifice than Wanda was willing to make.

In the end, Wanda did successfully make several pots of coffee and pour them into her own mug in a situation simulated to be as much like her home setup as possible. How it happened was a combination of her own bodily stabilization strategies, an adaptation to her coffee pot that allowed her to pivot the canister on a stand rather than lift it to pour, and a stabilizing surface for her mug in front of the pot. Both hospital staff and Wanda's employer participated in crafting the actual modifications she used for this task. Along the way, she also successfully tried a single-cup brewing pot and at the time of discharge was considering asking her aunt for one for her next birthday.

Discussion of Wanda's Success

What does Wanda's story illustrate about the transformation of her occupations in order to live alone at this transition of her life course? In traditional developmental models, the biopsychosocial capacities of the human body are often considered prerequisite for action and certainly for skilled performance. How can we then explain the lack of change in Wanda's body relative to an enormous change in her ability to engage in home making skills? Wanda's spastic movements because of her cerebral palsy did not change during her hospitalization; she did not gain measurable strength or range of motion or endurance beyond that which she had on admission. Yet, Wanda's caseworker was satisfied at the time of discharge that with intermittent help from extended family, she could safely manage in her own home on a day-to-day basis. Her ability to do so was evidence of occupational development through a transactional process between her own life experiences with her body, supports in her physical and social environments, and interaction with a therapist who provided safe opportunities for practice and adaptations for success. Notice the multitude of factors that influence development of skilled occupational performance and the occupational therapist's ability to collaborate in innovative occupation-centered work.

Wanda lived her life as a member of various communities recognized and structured by society such as her family, the residential school, church, rural school, and other organizations including the rehabilitation center. The role of her family and the volunteer work doing meal delivery and the occupational therapist who worked with her are part of circumstances that contribute to transformations of occupations. This chapter turns now to examine how individuals functioning in communities acquire and change their occupations to fulfill the mission of the communities they are part of.

Occupations Embedded in Different Communities

Communities influence the patterns of people's lives, shape their values, and provide structure in the form of opportunities and constraints (Diewald & Mayer, 2009; Elder & Shanahan, 2006; Engeström, 1999). Hedegaard (2009) points out that people move through and participate in many communities during their days. Each community possesses a culture with shared practices and ways of doing things to achieve mutual goals. This does not mean everyone does the same things as there may be different roles but their occupations have meaning, so novices to that community may pay attention to what is being done and the tools being used to achieve the outcome.

Over their life course, people leave and join new communities. The timing of movement between communities and participation within it are often influenced by both informal and structured age-related normative expectations. Within Western society, for example, a woman may informally decide that when the children are self-sufficient, it is time for her to find employment again. On the other hand, leaving the workplace and paid employment to live on retirement income and savings cannot occur until a designated age in many cultures. There is a shared social understanding about what should and should not occur so that opportunities are made available and constraints or consequences put in place. During the life course, we leave and join different communities which change our occupations. To understand how this happens, it helps to consider how these communities and related occupations evolve.

Recall that shared participation is part of our occupational nature to engage with coordinated, interdependent activities which enact the purpose of the community. In this way, they form a variety of communities of practice (Lave & Wenger, 1991). Communities are structured around social positions or roles that may be formal or informal. To sustain the community of doers, there are individuals who fill designated roles as mentors (e.g., teacher, supervisor, older sibling, long-time resident of a retirement community) to orient new members coming to the community. In this way, new members and those less skilled get support in learning to do activities and related practices of the community. The acquisition of occupations specific to the community or how the occupation is done

occurs through this process of collaborative engagement to achieve the common goal.

From this perspective, attention now focuses on social processes that introduce people to new occupations and transform how they do things. Changes in occupations are not unidirectional; new members with emerging skills in doing something have a reciprocal relationship with other members of the community. This defines and shapes the occupations of others in the community. To picture this dynamic process, the reader could reflect on ways a practitioner might promote community and occupational change for a patient whose goals include regaining kitchen skills following a stroke. The therapist might invite a couple other patients at different stages of recovery to join in making coffee and a coffee cake. As they coordinate kitchen activities, they model their adaptation in the social situation and which in turn may promote each other's occupational performance.

Interpersonal Influences Transforming Occupations

As seen in the examples of the family engaged in yoga (Case Study 7-1) and Wanda's volunteer work with her parents (Case Study 7-2), occupations are coconstructed through coordinated actions of participants within social and historical contexts. Various forces or mechanisms bring about changes in how things are done as people engage with an occupation together (Table 7-2). The changes

TABLE 7-2 Proposed Interpersonal Mechanisms Bringing about Change in Occupations

Broad Categories	Proposed Change Mechanisms in Development of an Occupation
Interpersonal influences of occupational engagement	Peripheral participation occurs as novices are part of situations where the occupations occur. As active onlookers, people learn about how things are done, how objects are used, possible outcomes, and what is significant in occupations.
	During coconstructed occupations between two or more people, the performance demands are distributed between participants; people introduce variable situations; and by being engaged with each other, people learn new occupations and alter their understanding about the outcomes and meanings of existing occupation.
	Explicit teaching and scaffolding of the occupation brings a new member's performance to a higher level. The more experienced partner introduces more culturally informed practices and ideas about outcome and meaning.
Engagement in the occupation is transformational for that occupation.	Challenges to familiar ways of doing things lead people to try new combinations of their capacities; variations contribute to discovering new performance strategies. Skilled action occurs when people learn to select performance strategies to fit particular situations.
	Altered experiences of outcome and significance of the occupation leads the person to find new performance strategies.
	Performance and capacities are interrelated with reciprocal influences. As a person uses current abilities in occupations, the repeated practice brings about further refinement of abilities and sustains skill—general skill. These changes in turn transform the occupation.

examined in the remainder of this chapter include not only the acquisition of new occupations but also transformations. These changes include subtle adjustments in performance over time, modifications in performance strategies, and experiences of shared meaning that sustain the occupation as the challenges of new situations are encountered. The cumulative outcome of these changes is notable transformation in occupational performance over time.

Whether young or old, newcomers start as peripheral participants in communities, watching other people and gradually joining elements of the occupations (Lave & Wenger, 1991). People who are familiar with the community's practices expect the novice to watch and acquire the ability to do relevant activities. In this way, learning an occupation is situated where the activity naturally occurs and is carried out by other members of the community. In Figure 7-4, as a relatively new member of his family, this toddler is not familiar with various self-care occupations. Once his teeth started to appear, his parents brush his teeth for him as part of their bedtime routine. In this photograph, he is building on past passive experiences by engaging with the object that is part of the occupation. Grasping the toothbrush by the handle and putting the brush in his mouth suggests that he has been an active learner. This does not suggest that he reflects mentally on the functions of oral hygiene or the steps of brushing his own teeth. Rather, his embodied actions lead to his joining with his father by approximating the actions that he has felt and seen. His father's modeling of more refined grip and action on his front teeth may be more specific than the toddler is capable of doing at this time. The child's attention, though, is focused on his father's mouth where the brush is placed. This picture illustrates that the coconstruction of

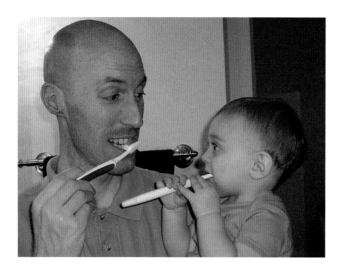

FIGURE 7-4 Father and son's occupation is situated in the bathroom, takes place at certain times of day, and makes use of objects specific to the activity.

occupation takes place at a nonverbal level. People evolved to read the actions of others as purposeful so they attend to how the outcome is achieved (Rosenberg, 2008).

A similar pattern of coconstruction through embodied actions with objects is seen in the case of as an elderly woman with dementia who has been asked to help make coleslaw. Instead of chopping, she just stands looking at the head of cabbage. Although she does not respond to the verbal request, she does join in the activity when she sees someone else shredding cabbage at the chopping block. She can engage in the activity once she is prompted by seeing others do it because those visual cues prompt her body to remember doing something like this in the past. Her dementia limits her ability to understand a verbal request, as words alone are too abstract for her at this stage (Vance, Moore, Farr, & Struzick, 2008). Changes in performance occur through lived bodily experiences of engagement with other people. The point of being able to coordinate actions with the intentional behaviors of others to share an occupation is conceptually important so people of different ages or mental abilities still enter situations when their occupations change.

Recall the second proposed change mechanism in Table 7-2: the coconstruction of occupation that can occur among members of the community at a similar level of proficiency. A social milieu brought about by doing something together ensures continuity of action while also allowing variability and contributing to the construction of meaning. First, shared engagement means that how-to-do-it knowledge is distributed among two or more people, so if one person forgets how to do something, the intentional acts of another person may serve as a cue or substitute so the goal is achieved. The important thing is all participants continue to engage, and it is through this participation that further mastery will occur. Second, doing something with another person inevitably introduces variations in how things are done, which stimulates adaptation and challenges all participants to learn to do things differently. Finally, Lawlor (2003) pointed out that at times, the significance of an occupation rests primarily in the sense of being socially engaged. Even when a person might hesitate to do something, the fact someone else is involved will encourage the beginner to try, which in turn may result in him or her potentially embracing a new occupation and experiencing meaning that makes the activity more appealing the next time the occupational opportunity occurs.

This last point—being drawn into something new for the sake of being socially occupied with someone—illustrates that if new occupations are needed or desired, there are no prerequisites for engagement. In coconstructed occupations, the person with more expertise can fill in missing elements, whereas the beginner experiences participation with occupation at whatever level he or she is able.

CASE STUDY 7-3   PARTICIPATION IN A FESTIVAL

Shufen is 3 years old and has been watching others engage in the Lantern Festival, a traditional celebration in Taiwan. People write their wishes on the paper that are folded into lanterns and released like a hot air balloon, taking their messages up to the Almighty in the sky. It is customary to include people with various abilities because participants believe that the Almighty has the power and wisdom to understand people's wishes. Shufen has seen her family members writing at home and understands many elements of how to write, so she joined in the tradition despite a lack of formal training in writing Taiwanese characters (Figure 7-5).

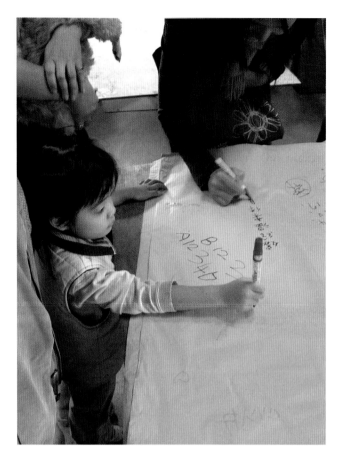

FIGURE 7-5 Social participation enables children to enter situations where they can learn new occupations.

As you can see, Shufen engaged by writing the way she knows; and other people give what she does meaning by writing alongside her in the more traditional characters. They regard her as a cowriter. This suggests that people start being a writer, musician, or playmate by participating with people who write, make music, or play. It also holds true for children with disabilities; engaging in activities that involve writing result in development as a writer, whereas simply addressing underlying skills, like letter recognition or copying geometric shapes, does not lead to the same level of occupational transformation (Hanser, 2010).

Previous examples illustrate that new members of a community like a family or workplace have access to experienced members who already know the routines and cultural practices of the community. When someone new to an occupation has access to more skilled members, the novice often defers to the designated expert. In this way, the power of a shared occupation takes on additional weight as a change process because teaching, scaffolding, or guiding another person's participation becomes part of the situation (Rogoff, 2003). The person with expertise initially adjusts the situation to be consistent with the novice's understanding (Wertsch, 1999). As everyone involved

coordinates his or her actions, facial expressions, words, and actions form the medium for shared meanings and taps in to power of intersubjective feelings (Lawlor, 2012). Once a connection is established by doing the occupation together, the expert introduces new definitions of significance and elaborates on outcomes, giving more information about what is expected and how things are done. Box 7-1 lists ways in which the experienced person contributes to the development of occupation. The evolving definition of the situation includes a shared sense of the

BOX 7-1   HOW AN EXPERIENCED PERSON CAN SUPPORT A NOVICE'S ENGAGEMENT IN A CHALLENGING OCCUPATION

1. Create social opportunities to do the activity with another person.
2. Fill in performance gaps, doing difficult parts of the activity.
3. Suggest or model different ways to do the activity.
4. Introduce and model the use of new objects in the activity.
5. Add relevant information about the activity.
6. Elaborate on alternative outcomes.
7. Bring in more culturally shaped meanings regarding why the activity is significant.

Source: Foot, K. A. (2014). Cultural-historical activity theory: Exploring theory to inform practice. *Journal of Human Behavior in Social Environments, 24*, 329–347.

novice gaining expertise, gradually evolving from a beginner to a more experienced participant.

Note that the strategies suggested previously are part of social engagement in an activity, not the formal instruction that might occur in a patient education session or, for example, in the case of a school therapist asking a child to copy letters on a worksheet. Indeed, Lave and Packer (2008) write, "Both 'socialization' and 'formal instruction' involves extensive mythologies about the mechanisms of learning" (p. 29). Socialization without the dynamics of shared engagement leaves the learner in a passive role of being told what is important to do, whereas formal instruction might be a means of transmitting out of context, abstract information. Neither of these forms of learning explains the phenomenon of a novice functioning on the periphery of a community where engagement in occupations is central to the continuation of that community. This everyday learning of an apprentice takes place in the context of participation by doing accessible parts of the desired occupation and generating an embodied understanding of how to do it.

Having focused on how performance changes over time in communities of practice, we now consider the moment-to-moment changes in performance. Literature about dynamic motor development (Thelen, 2000) and solving problems (Siegler, 2000) speak to emergent performance which is very dependent on bodily action in specific contexts. The concept of emergent performance becomes even clearer perhaps when considering occupational transformations in later adulthood. In contrast to past assumptions about predictable biological changes related to aging, many scholars contend there is more variability than uniformity as humans age (Crosnoe & Elder, 2002; Lachman, 2004; Westerhof, Katzko, Dittmann-Kohli, & Hayslip, 2001). The actual performance of older adults is likely due not only to changing capacities of the individual human being but also to the social and historical contexts in which the person lives. Thus, performance emerges as a result of the person (with his or her own bodily capacities and limitations) acting with the physical and social world, with all its supports for and limitations to performance.

For example, Kaye Tobin is an 81-year-old Californian who travels alone throughout the year—for up to 9 months. She traces her passion for travel to her first trip away from her hometown as a teenager (Lerner, 2011). That we consider Kaye "unusual for her age" is based on our assumptions that a person of 81 years would not typically have an intact repertoire of capacities needed for independent travel abroad. Kaye's travel is not with sponsored tours or with others managing her luggage; on the contrary, she travels with only a backpack and stays in elder or youth hostels so that she can travel more frequently (Lerner, 2011). The entire significance of Kaye carrying out her passion for travel is not simply that she is defying stereotypes about aging. Her independent navigation through new situations speaks to someone with individual capacities that allow her to pursue a favored occupation, but engaging in that occupation in turn helps to maintain those capacities.

Occupations can be transformed also when a person recognizes different outcomes or realizes some new significance in doing it (Humphry, 2002). As discussed earlier, watching other people do things and coconstructing an occupation with others alter the person's experiences about how things are done, what is an expected outcome, and why that matters. People can also discover their own new ideas about their occupations. Even when an occupation seems to be routine, a new meaning changes how it is done or how it is perceived. For the adult who sustains a traumatic injury or loss of functional ability, however, the inability to either temporarily or permanently operate a vehicle imbues the occupation of driving with new importance. The person who is able to resume driving may drive with heightened appreciation for the ability to do so, whereas the person who cannot resume driving comes to view it as a social status rather than simply a functional ability.

Finally, although maturation of capacities does not completely explain changes in occupational performance, capacities do change with use. In a broad biological sense, development of a person occurs simultaneously at several levels, including genetic activity, body structure, the functions of body systems, capacities, and performance (Gottlieb, 2000). Furthermore, there are reciprocal influences across these levels. This means that as people use their capacities, repeated experiences change these levels and directly or indirectly bring their capacities and performance to higher levels of proficiency. Subsequently, more refined capacities become available and occupational performance changes. However, the situated and emergent nature of performance in context needs to also be recognized.

Conclusion

A colleague once observed that occupations are complex and messy. Using a life course perspective, we recognize a range of factors shaping how occupations are acquired and transformed over months and years of living. In looking at the family engaged in yoga in which both the grandmother and granddaughter have recently taken up the practice, we saw that age of the individual is not the primary factor in learning to do something new. They also illustrate that there are multiple reasons for choosing to do something. Whereas the grandmother had reflected on the benefits of exercise and saw yoga offering a desired outcome, the granddaughter, without reflection, joined in as a way to be part of the family. In introducing Wanda and her life course, we illustrate how her choice to engage in clowning around to connect with another patient in a rehabilitation center is best understood as a choice that reflected accumulated experiences in earlier forms of participation with her parents. By reaching out, Wanda also made it easier for the 14-year-old patient to feel part of a community of rehabilitation patients.

Occupational therapy is indicated when a person is unable to do expected or desired occupations that connect that person with desired communities. How OT practitioners conceptualize the change process determines how they practice. We have presented the importance of taking a contextual view regarding what people do and why they do things in a particular way. This is reflected in the modified principles of the life course and illustrated with the case of Wanda. In general, we want to emphasize the interconnected elements of the occupational situation and how occupations serve to connect people with social and physical environments that make up their lives (Cutchin & Dickie, 2012).

This chapter explores how people live their lives as members of a variety of different communities where occupations with specific cultural practices and routines occur. Whether a person enters a new community as student or a patient following an accident, opportunities are created to learn or transform occupations. Over time, the novice is supported in participating by engaging in occupations that others are already familiar with doing. We see that by being brought into coconstructing occupation, the how-to knowledge and what it means is shared between participants. People's performance changes as they learn the occupational form and experience how it is defined as meaningful by others.

Finally, refinement in performance rests on the emergent nature of action where the occupational situation, the person's actual performance, discovery of new strategies, and changing experiences of meaning can all bring about transformations in engagement and understanding about how something is done. Changes in occupational performance and meaning occur over the entire life course and implications of this type of practice for work with people in various life circumstances need further exploration and explication.

REFERENCES

Blair, S. E. E. (2000). The centrality of occupation during life transitions. *British Journal of Occupational Therapy, 63*, 231–237.

Choi, J., Cutler, A., & Broersma, M. (2017). Early development of abstract language knowledge: Evidence from perception–production transfer of birth-language memory. *Royal Society Open Science, 4*, 160660. doi:10.1098/rsos.160660

Crosnoe, R., & Elder, G. H., Jr. (2002). Successful adaptation in the later years: A life course approach to aging. *Social Psychology Quarterly, 65*, 309–328.

Cutchin, M., & Dickie, V. A. (2012). Transactionalism: Occupational science and the pragmatic attitude. In G. Whiteford & C. Hocking (Eds.), *Critical perspectives on occupational science: Society, inclusion, participation* (pp. 23–37). London, United Kingdom: Wiley.

Dickie, V., Cutchin, M. P., & Humphry, R. (2006). Occupation as transactional experience: A critique of individualism in occupational science. *Journal of Occupational Science, 13*, 83–93.

Diewald, M., & Mayer, K. U. (2009). The sociology of the life course and life span psychology: Integrated paradigm or complementing pathways? *Advances in Life Course Research, 14*, 5–14.

Elder, G. H., & Shanahan, M. J. (2006). The life course and human development. In R. M. Lerner (Ed.), *Handbook of person psychology* (6th ed., Vol. 1, pp. 665–715). Hoboken, NJ: Wiley.

Engeström, Y. (1999). Activity theory and individual and social transformation. In Y. Engeström, R. Miettinen, & R.-L. Punamaki (Eds.), *Perspectives on activity theory* (pp. 19–38). Cambridge, NY: Cambridge University Press.

Foot, K. A. (2014). Cultural-historical activity theory: Exploring theory to inform practice. *Journal of Human Behavior in Social Environments, 24*, 329–347.

Fritz, H., & Cutchin, M. P. (2016). Integrating the science of habit: Opportunities for occupational therapy. *OTJR: Occupation, Participation and Health, 36*, 92–98.

Gottlieb, G. (2000). Understanding genetic activity within a holistic framework. In L. R. Bergman, R. B. Cairns, L. Nilsson, & L. Nystedt (Eds.), *Developmental science and the holistic approach* (pp. 179–201). Mahwah, NJ: Lawrence Erlbaum Associates.

Hanser, G. (2010). Emergent literacy for children with disabilities. *OT Practice, 15*(3), 16–20.

Hedegaard, M. (2009). Children's development from a cultural-historical approach: Children's activity in everyday local settings as foundations for their development. *Mind, Culture and Activity, 16*, 64–81.

Hocking, C., & Wright-St. Clair, V. (2017). Editorial: Special issue on inclusion and participation. *Journal of Occupational Science, 24*, 1–4.

Humphry, R. (2002). Young children's occupational behaviors: Explicating the dynamics of developmental processes. *American Journal of Occupational Therapy, 56*, 171–179.

Humphry, R. (2005). Model of processes transforming occupations: Exploring societal and social influences. *Journal of Occupational Science, 12*, 36–41.

Humphry, R. (2016). 2015 Ruth Zemke Lecture in Occupational Science: Joining in, interpretative reproduction, and transformations of occupations: What is "know-how" anyway? *Journal of Occupational Science, 23*, 422–433.

Johnson, M. K., Crosnoe, R., & Elder, G. H. (2011). Insights on adolescence from a life course perspective. *Journal of Research on Adolescence, 21*, 273–280.

Lachman, M. E. (2004). Development in midlife. *Annual Review of Psychology, 55*, 305–331.

Lave, J., & Packer, M. (2008). Towards a social ontology of learning. In K. Nielsen, S. Brinkmann, C. Elmholdt, & G. Kraft (Eds.), *A qualitative stance: In memory of Steinar Kvale, 1938–2008* (pp. 17–47). Aarhus, Denmark: Aarhus University Press.

Lave, J., & Wenger, E. (1991). *Situated learning: Legitimate peripheral participation*. Cambridge, NY: Cambridge Press.

Lawlor, M. (2003). The significance of being occupied: The social construction of childhood occupations. *American Journal of Occupational Therapy, 57*, 424–434.

Lawlor, M. (2012). The particularities of engagement: Intersubjectivity in occupational therapy. *OTJR: Occupation, Participation and Health, 32*, 151–159.

Lerner, N. (2011). Globetrotting grandma: A woman pursues her dreams on solo trips abroad. *AARP The Magazine, 54*(4C), 71.

Mayer, K. U. (2009). New directions in life course research. *Annual Review of Sociology, 35*, 413–433.

Overton, W. F., Muller, U., & Newman, J. L. (Eds.). (2008). *Developmental perspectives on embodiment and consciousness*. New York, NY: Lawrence Erlbaum Associates.

Rogoff, B. (2003). *The cultural nature of human development.* New York, NY: Oxford University Press.

Rosenberg, A. (2008). *Philosophy of social science* (3rd ed.). Boulder, CO: Westview.

Siegler, R. S. (2000). The rebirth of children's learning. *Child Development, 71,* 26–35.

Thelen, E. (2000). Grounded in the world: Developmental origins of the embodied mind. *Infancy, 1,* 3–28.

Vance, D. E., Moore, B. S., Farr, K. F., & Struzick, T. (2008). Procedural memory and emotional attachment in Alzheimer disease: Implications for meaningful and engaging activities. *Journal of Neuroscience Nursing, 40,* 96–102.

Wertsch, J. V. (1999). The zone of proximal development: Some conceptual issues. In P. Lloyd & C. Fernyhough (Eds.), *Lev Vygotsky: Critical assessments* (Vol. 3, pp. 67–78). London, United Kingdom: Routledge.

Westerhof, G. J., Katzko, M. W., Dittmann-Kohli, F., & Hayslip, B. (2001). Life contexts and health-related selves in old age. *Journal of Aging Studies, 15,* 105.

Wilcock, A. A. (2006). *An occupational perspective of health* (2nd ed.). Thorofare, NJ: SLACK.

the**Point**®   *For additional resources on the subjects discussed in this chapter, visit* **http://thePoint.lww.com /Willard-Spackman13e.**

Contribution of Occupation to Health and Well-Being

Clare Hocking

LEARNING OBJECTIVES

After reading this chapter, you will be able to:

1. Describe, in occupational terms, what being healthy means and how that relates to the Ottawa Charter and Healthy People 2020.
2. Explore ways that occupation contributes to the health and well-being of all people in terms of meeting biological needs, developing skills, and using capacities.
3. Drawing on the international literature, describe positive and negative health impacts of people's overall pattern of occupation.
4. Analyze how well-being might be influenced by a person's physical, social, and attitudinal environment.
5. Reflecting on your own community, identify a group whose "belonging through doing" is constrained and outline possible negative health impacts.
6. Analyze how having an impairment might affect well-being, taking environmental barriers into account.

Introduction

When John and Barb visited the farm one Sunday, 6-year-old Alice was excited to show them around. First, they went to feed out hay to the cows. Alice introduced them to the yearlings in one paddock and, up a steep hill leading to the back of the farm, the new calves that had arrived only the week before (Figure 8-1). Mum drove the quad bike with the hay bales, while Barb and Alice walked up. Alice talked all the way, hardly stopping for breath despite the climb. After a lunch of cheese and watercress sandwiches, they all helped clear the table and wash the dishes. Then, leading the way along the farm track, Alice took her visitors to her favorite place, a creek running through the trees. There, moving quietly, she sprinkled breadcrumbs onto the water and waited for her "pet" fish to slip out from the rocks to eat. On the drive back to town that evening, John and Barb reflected on how their day on the farm had dissipated the stress of their busy lives, and laughed again about Alice's book, *The Adventures of John Deere the Tractor*. Most of all, they remembered how Alice's joy in showing them around fostered a sense of belonging. The farm had become a place where they know they are always welcome, and visiting Alice's special place amongst the trees gave them a sense of deep connection with the land.

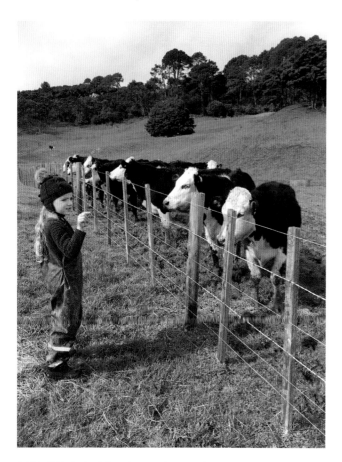

FIGURE 8-1 **Alice introduces the cows.**

Occupation, Health, and Well-Being

Barb and John's day at the farm had many of the elements people in Western societies associate with being healthy. For this couple in their mid-50s, there were physical benefits of fresh air, clean water, and walking from one task to another, some of it up hills and over uneven ground, exercising major muscle groups and maintaining fitness, stamina, and balance. Although John's health condition imposed some limitations, he accepts the World Health Organization's (WHO) view that health is more than the absence of disease (WHO, 2018), gaining a sense of well-being from the sunshine, being able to go at his own pace, and exercising his talents as a photographer. Their nutritious lunch restored energy levels, and they enjoyed the stimulation of answering all Alice's questions and talking with her parents about managing livestock and the effects of the economic downturn. Their day "ticked all the boxes" for health-related quality of life and well-being (Healthy People 2020, 2017b)—physical, mental, emotional, and social functioning. They felt satisfied and engaged, derived • meaning and a sense of accomplishment

from their occupations, and had been interested in what they were doing. Occupational therapists might also note that their **occupations**, meaning all the things they do that occupy their time, fit Wilcock and Hocking's (2015) description of doing, being, belonging, and becoming.

Occupational therapy (OT) is founded on the idea that occupation and health are intimately related. That relationship is also prominent in a WHO document, the Ottawa Charter (WHO, 1986). This influential public health policy document sought to promote broad understandings of the determinants of health. Its key concept, that health is a resource people create in their everyday lives, using their physical capacities and personal and social resources, has taken hold. Both lay people and health professionals refer to health as the ability to do what they want to do, what is important and valuable, and what they have to do, albeit sometimes with assistance (Song & Kong, 2015). That holds true even for people in advanced age, including Medicare members categorized as "at high risk" or "very sick." In a recent study, they described health as "being able to do what and when you want to do" including "enjoying the activities I've always enjoyed," "doing something every day," "being with friends," and being able to go out if they need to (Tkatch et al., 2017). Wellness models also typically include a spiritual aspect (Avera, Zholu, Speedlin, Ingram, & Prado, 2015), which is enacted through religious observances and other occupations in which people find spiritual meaning.

John and Barb's day at the farm with Alice conveys a general sense of well-being, but that is a problematic term because different people define it very differently. A recent large-scale European study supports interpreting **well-being** from an unashamedly occupational perspective, which is "a way of looking at or thinking about human doing" (Njelesani, Tang, Jonsson, & Polatajko, 2014, p. 233). The study, involving 43,000 people, was undertaken to inform governmental efforts to measure well-being. It identified 10 features that combine how people are functioning and how they feel: engagement, meaning, competence, vitality, self-esteem, emotional stability, optimism, positive emotion, positive relationships, and resilience (Huppert & So, 2013). Each of those features can be viewed as referring to the act of doing, or things derived from or sustained by doing. Indigenous people generally also include notions of spiritual well-being and connection to the land (Grieves, 2008). Taking a broader view, the Ottawa Charter asserts that to attain complete well-being "an individual or group must be able to identify and to realize aspirations, to satisfy needs, and to change or cope with the environment" (WHO, 1986, p. 1). In these days of escalating awareness of environmental degradation, we are also reminded that human well-being is inextricably bound to the health of local and global ecosystems (Wilcock & Hocking, 2015).

CENTENNIAL NOTES

Ancient Perspectives on Occupation and Health

Well before any discussion of using occupation for curative purposes, people recognized that what we do—or do not do—affects our health. Volume 1 of Wilcock's (2001) book, *Occupation for Health*, is rich with insights into that history. She describes, for example, how primitive man learned which plants were good to gather and eat and which were harmful by their taste and by observing the effects of eating them. In ancient civilizations, Chinese lore attributed long and healthy lives, in which older people continued to participate in occupation, to lifestyles that followed the seasons and living in a world of relative simplicity. Dating from 2000 BC, the Babylonian calendar also recognized the need for rest, with the 7th, 14th, 21st, and 28th days of the month designated as days when people should be freed from labor. In temples dedicated to Thor, the Egyptian god of medicine, people were encouraged to engage in gymnastics as well as occupations that stimulate the mind and soul: astronomy, mathematics, music, and dancing. These early perspectives of health—eating well, living in harmony with nature, avoiding stress, a balance of rest and exercise, mental stimulation and spiritual contemplation—are implicitly occupational and remain relevant today.

Over the course of more recent history, health advice became more specific. For instance, Ambroise Paré (1510–1590), a military surgeon in France in the 16th century, advised physical exertions including leaping, tennis, and carrying a burden, which should be continued until "the face looks red, sweat beginnes to break forth, we breathe more strongly and quicke" (Johnson, 1634, p. 34) but not so long as to cause stiffness. Idleness, in comparison, was responsible for "goute, apoplexie, and a thousand other diseases" (p. 35). Although we are used to advice about participation in healthy occupations being directed to individuals, there have also been times when occupation was proposed as a cure for societal ills. The Arts and Crafts Movement, which began in Britain around 1880 and spread throughout Europe and North America, was a response to the exceedingly harsh work conditions and social unrest associated with industrialization. In opposition to working with machines, which reduced workers to machinelike components, and making products that had no soul, its proponents exhorted a return to a simple life, an ethos of liberation, and the dignity derived from crafting things by hand. In this history, we can discern both the continuation of ancient advice linking occupation and health, and the philosophy that informed the earliest occupational therapists (Hocking, 2004).

Occupational therapy exists as a profession because, in some circumstances, people experience great difficulty engaging in occupations that support health and well-being. In physical health contexts, knowledge of techniques to restore people to health-sustaining occupation is well developed (Kielhofner, 2009). In other areas, bringing an occupational perspective generates new insights. For example, Sutton, Hocking, and Smythe (2012) revealed how progressive reengagement in occupation at an intensity they can sustain helps people recovering from mental illness to reintegrate a sense of self and reconnect with the environment. As they progress from the disintegrated experience described as nondoing, to half-doing, engaged doing, and, finally, absorbed doing, so they are increasingly able to structure time and space, and future possibilities in the everyday world open up.

As this introduction has shown, the relationship between occupation and well-being is complex. A great number of factors influence the health outcomes of occupation, and knowledge of how the various factors interact is incomplete. To contain the topic and ensure its relevance, priority is given to understandings generated by occupational therapists and occupational scientists. Consistent with those perspectives, the term *occupation* refers to the things people do that they find personally and culturally meaningful, whereas *participation* is used in the more restricted sense of whether a person actually engages in occupation.

To give the discussion depth, evidence reported in literature from around the world is included. The discussion proceeds by considering some of the ways occupation contributes to health and well-being. That includes what can be learned by its absence, when people are deprived of sufficient occupation. To give a balanced account, there is also discussion of the ways in which occupation can be injurious to health. Contextual factors that act as barriers to achieving good health are also described before concluding with a brief summation of the evidence.

How Occupation Contributes to Health and Well-Being

If we are to assert that **participation** in occupation contributes to keeping good health, we need to understand how that comes about. Ann Wilcock, an eminent occupational scientist, considered that question from a biological perspective. She argued that occupation is essential to individual and species survival, because the basic **biological needs** for sustenance, self-care, shelter, and safety are met through the things people do. In meeting those needs and through other occupations of daily life, people develop "skills, social structures and technology aimed at superiority over predators and the environment" (Wilcock, 1993, p. 20). Those skills include growing and cooking nutritious food and constructing warm clothing and dry houses. Also important, although not always achieved, is the skill of living peacefully with neighbors. Depending on the circumstances, many other skills are also relevant to health. Reading and writing, for example, are important means of conveying information relevant to sustaining health and seeking health care in Western societies. It is also important to note that not everyone needs all the skills that are relevant to survival. Rather, health depends on being part of a family or community of people who together have the skills necessary to survive, and perhaps to flourish, as well as access to the resources to put their skills to use.

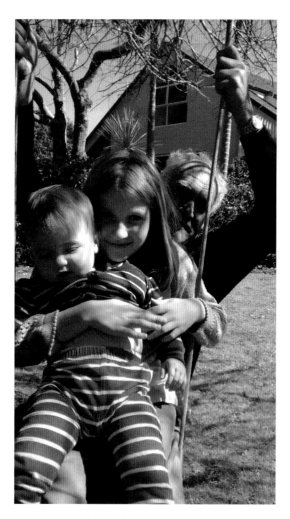

FIGURE 8-2 Gabbe playing on the swing with granddad and Quinn.

Meeting survival needs and becoming skilled are not sufficient to ensure good health; of equal importance is the contribution that occupation makes to developing and exercising personal capacities (Wilcock, 1993, 1995). These **capacities** spring from the biological characteristics shared by all humans: walking upright, opposing thumb and fingers to grasp objects, learning to speak, and so on. People have the capacity to, among other things, carry loads, design new tools and find novel uses for old ones, understand the workings of the universe, accumulate and pass on knowledge, predict what might happen and prepare for the future, form relationships, and express themselves artistically and spiritually. People also have the capacity to play, as Gabbe and her grandfather show us, photographed playing on the swing with little sister Quinn (Figure 8-2).

Each person's capacities reflect this human potential via his or her genetic inheritance, brought into being through the developmental process and a unique life history of occupational opportunities, preferences, choices, and constraints. On the basis of their history of doing things and expectations of what they might do in the future, people are generally aware of the capacities they have: whether they are better at cooking, drawing, or playing sport; whether they find thoughtful or competitive occupations more congenial; and whether they prefer shared or solitary occupations.

What stimulates people to engage in occupations that enhance their chances of survival, develop skills, and exercise capacities is much debated. One suggestion advanced by Wilcock (1993) is that humans experience biological needs that stimulate occupation, which in turn promotes health.

These needs relate, first, to correcting threats to our physiological state, such as being excessively hot or cold or feeling hungry or thirsty. The discomfort of these sensations stimulates us to action: to find some shade, put on more clothing, or seek out food or drink (Figure 8-3).

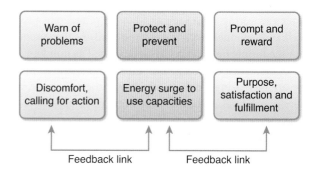

FIGURE 8-3 Biological hierarchy of need for occupation. (From Wilcock, A. [1993]. A theory of the human need for occupation. *Journal of Occupational Science, 1,* 17–24. doi:10.1080 /14427591.1993.9686375.)

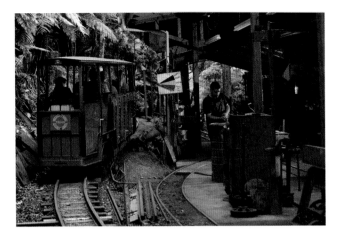

FIGURE 8-4 **Work demanding physical exertion supports cognitive functioning, psychological health, and healthy weight.**

The second set of needs is protective and preventive, such as the need to develop skills and exercise capacities. These are experienced as a surge of energy that propels us to acquire and practice the skills required to solve problems and plan, interact with others, do whatever generates our livelihood, and so on. In so doing, at least before technology removed many of the physical demands of earlier lifestyles, people exercised their capacity for physical, mental, and social functioning. The third and final set of needs prompts and rewards engagement in occupation. Meeting these needs gives a sense of purpose, satisfaction, and fulfillment (Box 8-1).

Evidence that Occupation Affects Health and Well-Being

It is widely acknowledged that occupation benefits health. The Healthy People 2020 report prepared by the U.S. government is one of many authoritative sources asserting that participating in occupations that exercise mental, physical, and social capacities maintains diverse aspects of health and well-being. For instance, it reports that productive occupations support good mental health, whereas, conversely, mental illness often results in people being unable to manage their responsibilities as parents and partners. Occupations that demand physical exertion are a particular focus, as there is good evidence that they support cognitive functioning, psychological health, the strength and agility of older adults, and healthy weight for people of all ages (Healthy People 2020, 2017c) (Figure 8-4). The relationship between weight and being active, however, is not straightforward. For example, data collected for the 2012 National Health and Nutrition Examination Survey National Youth Fitness Survey in the United States confirm a relationship between childhood obesity and lower levels of participation in physically demanding occupations. However, analysis also suggests that despite enjoying such occupations as much as their peers, the risk of being teased

by normal-weight children means that overweight children limit actual participation (Hong, Coker-Bolt, Anderson, Lee, & Velozo, 2016).

Some circumstances encourage participation in physically active occupations. Lifestyle choices such as owning a dog result in community-dwelling older adults living in Britain walking an average of 2,760 additional steps each day, at moderate intensity, compared to non–dog owners, which is a large, potentially health-enhancing difference (Dall et al., 2017). There are also well-documented health consequences of being unemployed. However, analysis of data from the Panel Study of Income Dynamics, a longitudinal study of couples in the United States, indicates that women who become unemployed take advantage of the reduced time demands to be more physically active, which may be beneficial in the long term. In contrast, unemployment is not associated with change in the time men spend exerting themselves physically (Gough, 2017).

Evidence supporting a relationship between participation in occupation and mental health is less prominent, but researchers are beginning to reveal the neurological processes by which physical occupations impact well-being and mood (Tozzi et al., 2016). "Green" physical activities, meaning those undertaken in nature, are thought to be particularly beneficial to emotional and psychological well-being (Yeh et al., 2015). Deciding what to measure to determine the mental health benefits of being physically active is somewhat more complex than determining its physical impact. Taking a direct approach, one group of researchers looked at correlations between happiness and walking, domestic tasks, leisure occupations and vocational pursuits of 11,637 Europeans aged 15 years or older. Overall, the more physically active people were, the higher their level of happiness. That effect was most pronounced for people reporting "a lot" of physical activity associated with their leisure pursuits and domestic life and "some" physical activity related to work (Richards et al., 2015). Importantly, analysis of data from the Chinese Longitudinal Longevity Survey confirms that participation in occupations that exercise physical capacities, such as gardening and housework, and diverse social occupations, including playing cards and attending organized activities, reduces mortality risk. As age increases, however, the beneficial effect of being occupied decreases (Sun, 2017).

Health, Development, and Patterns of Occupation

The overall pattern of people's occupations is also important. Breaking up active participation in occupation with rest contributes to health, whether that is a short break to stretch before returning to computer work, work/rest schedules to enhance the effects of training, or prolonged engagement in restorative leisure occupations. Having a rest confers many benefits, one of which is that it enhances memory, with evidence that preschoolers remember new words better if they have a nap rather than doing something active after learning them (Sandoval, Leclerc, & Gomez, 2017). Rather than resting, however, there is new evidence that going for a fast walk more effectively alleviates the fatigue associated with monotonous work (Aramaki & Hagiwara, 2018). As well as these short-term effects, people's longer term patterns of occupation influence health. For children and youth, both routinely sleeping less than the average (Firouzi, Poh, Ismail, & Sadeghilar, 2014) and excessive screen time, particularly for those with a television in their bedroom (Wethington, Pan, & Sherry, 2013), are strongly associated with obesity. Vocational choices also shape patterns of occupation. The societal and self-imposed expectation that Canadian farmers will be "relentless workers" no doubt contributes to their higher rates of social isolation, distress, and suicide compared with men engaged in other productive roles (Roy, Tremblay, Robertson, & Houle, 2017). Equally, Bangladeshi women are deterred from getting enough exercise by cultural mores that make it unacceptable for them to walk briskly and their husbands' dislike of them going out alone (Khanam & Costarelli, 2008).

Where people live is another powerful influence on occupation. Aesthetically sterile or unsafe urban environments, for example, do not provide spaces for children to be physically active or for older residents to develop community networks, disproportionately affecting people on low incomes (Satcher & Higginbotham, 2008; Semenza & Krishnasamy, 2007) (Figure 8-5). Moreover, environments can change. As the sociodemographic profile of their neighborhood deteriorated, older residents of Detroit

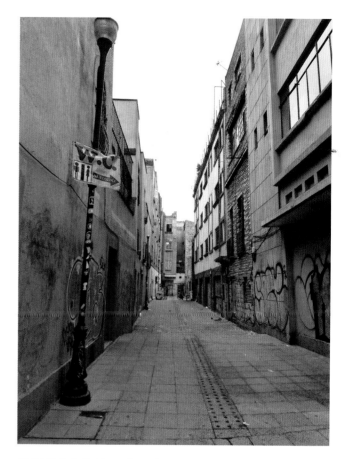

FIGURE 8-5 **Unsafe urban environments restrict engagement in outdoor occupations.**

experienced the loss of shared occupations, such as inviting a neighbor to sit and talk, doing things at different times of the day to avoid going outdoors after dark, and the need for heightened vigilance during daytime occupations (Fritz & Cutchin, 2017). Occupational therapists are also increasingly aware that people's patterns of occupation can be restricted by discrimination, citizenship status, and other circumstances that deprive them of real opportunities to participate in productive, educational, and leisure occupations on an equal footing. Restricted opportunities amounting to occupational injustice are important determinants of health and development. Thus, young people who have experienced homelessness, foster care, or poverty, with its associated housing insecurity, are at risk for poor working memory. In addition, compared to nondisadvantaged peers, those who are homeless or poor are more likely to have deficits in attention and executive functioning (Fry, Langley, & Shelton, 2017).

Ecological and sociopolitical factors also limit or disrupt access to health-giving occupations. Those recently identified in the OT and occupational science literature include unemployment (Aldrich & Callanan, 2011), displacement (Frank, 2011), being a refugee or asylum seeker (Burchett & Matheson, 2010), poverty (Beagan, 2007), and experiences of racism (Beagan & Etowa, 2011). The interdisciplinary literature also recognizes the impact of homelessness, natural disasters such as drought and tornados, lower educational attainment, and displacement (Case Study 8-1). In recognition of the multiple impacts of disadvantageous social conditions that limit equitable access to occupation, the World Federation of Occupational Therapists' (2016) standards for OT education now specify social inclusion as a focus for curricula content, student selection, and lecturers' professional development.

CASE STUDY 8-1   BELONGING THROUGH DOING

Having a sense of belonging is an important aspect of well-being. Belonging means being part of a group or community and feeling connected to particular places. It is enacted by doing things together, helping to look after our homes and other important places and, for some, performing the traditional occupations of their family, culture, or location. To belong means being accepted and enjoying the ease that comes from doing familiar things with people you know and in contexts you understand (Wilcock & Hocking, 2015). Older people who migrated from Finland to Sweden in their youth describe a dual sense of belonging. They are tied to daily life in Sweden by close family, habits, and ways of living while maintaining ties to their homeland by spending time with compatriots, speaking in Finnish, and keeping abreast of the news, exchanging phone calls, and visiting when they can. The prospect of aging in a foreign nation seems daunting only if they were to have difficulty performing their meaningful occupations or expressing their needs and wishes (Arola, Dellenborg, & Häggblom-Kronlöf, 2018).

For young migrants and refugees in Auckland, New Zealand, spending Saturdays at a community arts project is a powerful means of feeling they belong in their new surroundings. Mixing with people from diverse countries, languages, and religions, they sing, dance, play the drums, learn acrobatics, play board games, create graffiti art, and chat together. In summer, they take to the stage to perform a routine they worked on, guided by a professional choreographer who also has an immigrant background. As well as making friends, they learn that this is a place where they can successfully navigate a path between their old life and their new one (Tischler, 2017).

Constraints on Doing and Belonging

Not all migrants are welcome to participate in meaningful occupation in their host country. Lucia, Christina, and Ana worked in professional and service roles before they emigrated from Latin America to Spain. Since the economic crisis, the only work they are offered, when they are offered anything at all, is cleaning and caregiving in private homes (Rivas-Quarneti, Movilla-Fernández, & Magalhães, 2018). There, employers tell them they "have to be at my disposal" (p. 6). Even though they feel enslaved, these immigrant workers have no choice but to accept the low wages and exploitative work situations. Quitting would mean waiting for employment agencies to call them while "the days pass and your need gets sharper, and sharper" (p. 6). Despite restorative occupations like walking on the beach and the support they offer each other, the reality of having no resources beyond "my feet, my back and an attitude of overcoming the struggles to achieve" (p. 7) leaves them feeling frustrated, angry, and endlessly fatigued. The discriminatory attitudes they encounter as women, immigrants, and workers in precarious employment relegate them to the edges of society, with little hope of being truly accepted.

In the United States, undocumented Latin American immigrants similarly experience exploitative employment arrangements that prevent them from belonging through doing. The government's "war on immigration" creates a persistent threat of deportation, leading many to actively withdraw from occupations outside of work and home. Removal of eligibility for a drivers' license, under the REAL ID Act, disrupts not just driving to work but everyday occupations such as joining a library because drivers' licenses are commonly used as identification (Bailliard, 2013). Asylum seekers are also commonly subjected to legal constraints on engagement in educational opportunities and work, even in low paid jobs like the ones Lucia, Christina, and Ana had to accept. The imposed lack of valued and meaningful occupation might last for months or years while they wait to hear the outcome of their asylum application. Having nothing to do and nothing to mark one day from the next has been characterized as suffering. Not surprisingly, it gives rise to mental distress as well as self-harm and suicidal behavior (Crawford, Turpin, Nayar, Steel, & Durand, 2016).

Questions and Exercises

- Research results cited in this case study identify language, attitudinal and legal barriers to occupation, which disrupt people's capacity to do well and derive a sense of belonging to the people and place where they live. In what ways might immigrants, asylum seekers, or other groups living in vulnerable circumstances also experience constraints on their capacity to be and become?

- If you had an opportunity to work with youths living in a community that is new to them, how might you engage them in occupations that would create a sense of belonging?

Too Little and Too Much Occupation

Occupation's contribution to health is evident in accounts of the deleterious effects of not doing enough. Over the last 20 years, occupational scientists have reported the emotional, psychological, and societal harm caused when people experience externally imposed barriers to occupation that limit opportunities to engage in occupations that are meaningful and purposeful (Wilcock & Hocking, 2015). The populations studied include prisoners, people with disabling health conditions, those displaced by armed conflict, immigrants, refugees, and asylum seekers (Hocking, 2017b). However, most international attention has been paid to the increased risk of cardiovascular disease, stroke, cancer, diabetes, osteoporosis, anxiety, depression, and dementia of people who do not regularly engage in physically demanding occupations such as gardening; household chores; swimming; riding a bicycle; planned exercise; and playing sport or games involving running, turning, or jumping.

The scale of international concern and the strength of evidence from research is such that the WHO has published guidelines for the type, duration, frequency, and intensity of physical activities. The guidelines apply to all people aged 5 years and over, irrespective of gender, ethnicity, or income level, albeit with some cautionary advice for postpartum women and people with existing health conditions. Unlike guidelines in the past, these address cardiorespiratory fitness, muscle mass and strength, and bone loading, thus also addressing risk factors for spine and hip fractures and falls attributed to generalized weakness and poor balance (WHO, 2010). With the majority of people in affluent countries failing to meet activity guidelines, the health consequences of too much occupation tend to receive less attention. Nonetheless, one form of occupational imbalance, having too much to do, or doing things at too high intensity over a long time, are also associated with stress disorders, cardiac arrests, stress fractures, and other ill-health outcomes (Wilcock & Hocking, 2015).

It is not always easy to judge what constitutes too much or too little occupation. For example, the many people worldwide who derive psychological and emotional well-being from the engaging and creative work they perform on a computer may simultaneously be described as sitting too much. Even those with active leisure pursuits are at increased risk for obesity because of the many hours spent sitting rather than standing or walking. Clearly, there is a need to "develop approaches to free people from their chairs and render them more active" (McCrady & Levine, 2009), both at home and at work. More broadly, risks inherent in the occupations people need, want and are required to do must be identified, and effective ways of conveying that information to them must be developed (Hocking, 2017a). Achieving risk reduction at the population level will require ongoing action, as new technologies are developed to make virtual leisure pursuits more appealing and work practices more time and cost efficient, often in ways that make us too sedentary but simultaneously too busy to attend to our innate need to be, become and belong.

Disability, Health, and Occupation

Having an impairment associated with a health condition can impede participation in occupations that underpin well-being. Consistent with the *International Classification of Functioning, Disability and Health* (ICF), an **impairment** is defined as any problem with normal psychological or physiological function or with a body structure such as a joint or organ (WHO, 2001). The association between impairments and problems with participation is increasingly recognized in documents shaping health policy. For example, low back pain is the second leading cause of lost work time (Healthy People 2020, 2017a) and decreased vision is recognized to hamper driving, playing sports, using power tools around the home or yard, and maintaining a healthy and active lifestyle into older age (Healthy People 2020, 2017e). Occupational therapists are well aware that having a health condition or impairment can negatively affect occupational performance. Many of the case examples in theory texts, such as those related to the Model of Human Occupation, illustrate that idea. Impairments can mean that people are not sufficiently strong or flexible, unable to focus their thoughts and attention, or too fatigued to participate in occupations that in other circumstances they would choose to do. People also tend to withdraw from occupation if they are hampered by pain, deformity, breathlessness, malnutrition, despair, or the apathy that comes of hopelessness. Accordingly, therapeutic processes to enhance people's engagement in occupations that will "support their physical and emotional well-being" are described (Kielhofner, 2009, p. 3). As people with disabilities readily identify, however, attitudinal barriers and lack of accommodations can limit participation much more than bodily and psychological impairments. Legislative structures to implement universal design and mandate inclusion are helpful. For instance, Norway has a legislative requirement that organized sports be accessible to all children, regardless of disability (Asbjørnslett & Bekken, 2016), but the pace of environmental modifications and changes in people's attitudes is frustratingly slow.

Just as impairments can affect occupation, the ICF makes clear that the relationship can also work the other way; that occupations might threaten health and create impairments. As previously discussed, low-quality work, particularly in the context of discriminatory attitudes or exploitative social arrangements, is associated with poor physical and mental health outcomes. Being bored with what you are doing is unpleasant, but prolonged boredom in the workplace is now known to also be associated with low morale, depression, and engagement in destructive and unauthorized activities (Long, 2004). Many everyday occupations, such as driving a motor vehicle, also have inherent risks to bodily structures and functions. Even leisure occupations can harm us. Skateboarding, for instance, caused more than 125,000 medically treated injuries in the United States in 2015 (National Safety Council, 2018). In the occupational science literature, there has also been some discussion of substance abuse and alcohol consumption as occupations with well-recognized detrimental effects on health (Jennings & Cronin-Davis, 2016). We also know that other people's occupations can pose health threats. For example, exposure to exhaled tobacco smoke increases the risk of children developing respiratory infections and heart disease (Healthy People 2020, 2017d). There is some evidence, however, that when people finally manage to quit smoking, they simultaneously restructure eating habits, take up exercise, and replace smoking with more satisfying occupations to reinforce an identity that is no longer being driven by addiction to nicotine (Luck & Beagan, 2015). Thus, ceasing an occupation that posed a health threat might spur a cascade of health-promoting occupational changes. Societies play a role in health-related occupational adaptations, such as legislation making provisions for smoke-free public places and taxes that make consuming tobacco, alcohol, and sugar increasingly unaffordable.

Conclusion

We do many things to meet our biological needs for sustenance and shelter. Occupation keeps us alive, and occupation in natural environments nourishes us. In the longer term, occupation can provide the physical activity, mental stimulation, and social interaction we need to keep our bodies, minds, and communities healthy. In addition, through participation in occupation, we express ourselves, develop skills, experience pleasure and involvement, and achieve the things we believe to be important. In short, we have opportunities for enhanced levels of well-being, to be, belong, and become what we have potential to be. However, not all people have equal opportunity to engage in health-giving occupations. People with an impairment can experience limitations in their ability to engage in occupation and are known to have lower levels of engagement in physical exercise. People who live in poverty, are displaced by conflict or devastated by natural disasters,

experience unemployment or homelessness, or have lower levels of educational attainment are also likely to experience barriers to participation in occupation that negatively affect health and well-being.

Equally, occupation can threaten or destroy health. Doing too much, doing too little, and doing things that expose us to risk and harm can all have deleterious effects. It is also important to recognize that it is often through having trouble doing things that we become aware of health issues and the full impact of impairments. Furthermore, physical, social, or attitudinal barriers in the environment can exacerbate the impact of a health condition or impairment, sometimes to such an extent that participation in occupation is unsustainable.

REFERENCES

Aldrich, R. M., & Callanan, Y. (2011). Insights about researching discouraged workers. *Journal of Occupational Science, 18,* 153–166. doi:10.1080/14427591.2011.575756

Aramaki, K., & Hagiwara, H. (2018). Effect of walking upon fatigue due to monotonous work. *Advances in Intelligent Systems and Computing, 590,* 171–175. doi:10.1007/978-3-319-60483-1_18

Arola, A., Dellenborg, L., & Häggblom-Kronlöf, G. (2018). Occupational perspective of health among persons ageing in the context of migration. *Journal of Occupational Science, 25,* 65–75.

Asbjørnslett, M., & Bekken, W. (2016). Openness to difference: Inclusion in sports occupations for children with (dis)abilities. *Journal of Occupational Science, 23,* 434–445. doi:10.1080/14427591.2016.1199389

Avera, J., Zholu, Y., Speedlin, S., Ingram, M., & Prado, A. (2015). Transitioning into wellness: Conceptualizing the experiences of transgender individuals using a wellness model. *Journal of LGBT Issues in Counseling, 9,* 273–287. doi:10.1080/15538605.2015.1103677

Bailliard, A. (2013). Laying low: Fear and injustice for Latino migrants to Smalltown, USA. *Journal of Occupational Science, 20,* 342–356. doi:10.1080/14427591.2013.799114

Beagan, B. L. (2007). Experiences of social class: Learning from occupational therapy students. *Canadian Journal of Occupational Therapy, 74,* 125–133.

Beagan, B. L., & Etowa, J. B. (2011). The meanings and functions of occupations related to spirituality for African Nova Scotian women. *Journal of Occupational Science, 18,* 277–290. doi:10.1080/14427591.2011.594548

Burchett, N., & Matheson, R. (2010). The need for belonging: The impact of restrictions on working on the well-being of an asylum seeker. *Journal of Occupational Science, 17,* 85–91. doi:10.1080/14427591.2010.9686679

Crawford, E., Turpin, M., Nayar, S., Steel, E., & Durand, J.-L. (2016). The structural-personal interaction: Occupational deprivation and asylum seekers in Australia. *Journal of Occupational Science, 23,* 321–338. doi:10.1080/14427591.2016.1153510

Dall, P. M., Ellis, S. L. H., Ellis, B. M., Grant, P. M., Colyer, A., . . . Mills, D. S. (2017). The influence of dog ownership on objective measures of free-living physical activity and sedentary behavior in community-dwelling older adults: A longitudinal case-controlled study. *BMC Public Health, 17,* 496. doi:10.1186/s12889-017-4422-5

Firouzi, S., Poh, B. K., Ismail, M. N., & Sadeghilar, A. (2014). Sleep habits, food intake, and physical activity levels in normal and overweight and obese Malaysian children. *Obesity Research & Clinical Practice, 8,* e70–e78. doi:10.1016/j.orcp.2012.12.001

Frank, G. (2011). The transactional relationship between occupation and place: Indigenous cultures in the American Southwest. *Journal of Occupational Science, 18*, 3–20. doi:10.1080/14427591.2011.562874

Fritz, H., & Cutchin, M. P. (2017). Changing neighborhoods and occupations: Experiences of older African-Americans in Detroit. *Journal of Occupational Science, 24*, 140–151. doi:10.1080/14427591.2016.1269296

Fry, C. E., Langley, K., & Shelton, K. H. (2017). A systematic review of cognitive functioning among young people who have experienced homelessness, foster care, or poverty. *Child Neuropsychology, 23*, 907–934. doi:10.1080/09297049.2016.1207758

Gough, M. (2017). A couple-level analysis of participation in physical activity during unemployment. *Population Health, 3*, 294–304. doi:10.1016/j.ssmph.2017.03.001

Grieves, V. (2008). Aboriginal spirituality: A baseline for indigenous knowledges development in Australia. *The Canadian Journal of Native Studies, 28*, 363–398.

Healthy People 2020. (2017a). *Arthritis, osteoporosis and chronic back conditions*. Retrieved from http://www.healthypeople.gov/2020/topicsobjectives2020/overview.aspx?topicid=3

Healthy People 2020. (2017b). *Health-related quality of life & well-being*. Retrieved from https://www.healthypeople.gov/2020/topics objectives/topic/health related quality-of-life-well-being

Healthy People 2020. (2017c). *Physical activity*. Retrieved from http://healthypeople.gov/2020/topicsobjectives2020/overview.aspx?topicid=33

Healthy People 2020. (2017d). *Tobacco use*. Retrieved from https://www.healthypeople.gov/2020/topics-objectives/topic/tobacco-use

Healthy People 2020. (2017e). *Vision*. Retrieved from http://www.healthypeople.gov/2020/topicsobjectives2020/overview.aspx?topicid=42

Hocking, C. (2004). *The relationship between objects and identity in occupational therapy: A dynamic balance between rationalism and Romanticism* (Doctoral dissertation). Auckland, New Zealand: Auckland University of Technology. https://aut.researchgateway.ac.nz/handle/10292/363

Hocking, C. (2017a). Occupation and the risk message recipient. In R. Parrott (Ed.), *The Oxford encyclopedia of health and risk message design and processing* (pp. 1–16). New York, NY: Oxford University Press. doi:10.1093/acrefore/9780190228613.013.357

Hocking, C. (2017b). Occupational justice as social justice: The moral claim for inclusion. *Journal of Occupational Science, 24*, 29–42. doi:10.1080/14427591.2017.1294016

Hong, I., Coker-Bolt, P., Anderson, K. R., Lee, D., & Velozo, C. A. (2016). Relationship between physical activity and overweight and obesity in children: Findings from the 2012 National Health and Nutrition Examination Survey National Youth Fitness Survey. *American Journal of Occupational Therapy, 70*, 7005180060p1–7005180060p8. doi:10.5014/ajot.2016.021212

Huppert, F. A., & So, T. T. C. (2013). Flourishing across Europe: Application of a new conceptual framework for defining well-being. *Social Indicators Research, 110*, 837–861. doi:10.1007/s11205-011-9966-7

Jennings, H., & Cronin-Davis, J. (2016). Investigating binge drinking using interpretative phenomenological analysis: Occupation for health or harm? *Journal of Occupational Science, 23*, 245–254. doi:10.1080/14427591.2015.1101387

Johnson, T. (1634). *The works of that famous chirurgion Ambrose Parey: Translated out of Latin and compared with the French*. London, United Kingdom: Richard Cotes and Willi Du-gard. Retrieved from https://archive.org/stream/workesofthatfamo00par#page/n3/mode/2up

Khanam, S., & Costarelli, V. (2008). Attitudes towards health and exercise of overweight women. *The Journal of the Royal Society for the Promotion of Health, 128*, 26–30.

Kielhofner, G. (2009). *Conceptual foundations of occupational therapy practice* (4th ed.). Philadelphia, PA: F. A. Davis.

Long, C. (2004). On watching paint dry: An exploration of boredom. In M. Molineux (Ed.), *Occupation for occupational therapists* (pp. 78–89). Oxford, United Kingdom: Blackwell.

Luck, K., & Beagan, B. (2015). Occupational transition of smoking cessation in women: "You're restructuring your whole life." *Journal of Occupational Science, 22*, 183–196. doi:10.1080/14427591.2014.887418

McCrady, S., & Levine, J. (2009). Sedentariness at work: How much do we really sit? *Obesity, 1–7*, 2103–2105. doi:10.1038/oby.2009.117

National Safety Council. (2018). *Skateboarding injury can be prevented; Lesson 1: Learn how to fall*. Retrieved from http://www.nsc.org/learn/safety-knowledge/Pages/news-and-resources-skateboarding-safety.aspx

Njelesani, J., Tang, A., Jonsson, H., & Polatajko, H. (2014). Articulating an occupational perspective. *Journal of Occupational Science, 21*, 226–235. doi:10.1080/14427591.2012.717500

Richards, J., Jiang, X., Kelly, P., Chau, J., Bauman, A., & Ding, D. (2015). Don't worry, be happy: Cross-sectional associations between physical activity and happiness in European countries. *BMC Public Health, 15*, 53. doi:10.1186/s12889-015-1391-4

Rivas-Quarneti, N., Movilla-Fernández, M.-J., & Magalhães, L. (2018). Immigrant women's occupational struggles during the socioeconomic crisis in Spain: Broadening occupational justice conceptualization. *Journal of Occupational Science, 25*, 6–18.

Roy, P., Tremblay, G., Robertson, S., & Houle, J. (2017). "Do it all by myself": A salutogenic approach of masculine health practice among farming men coping with stress. *American Journal of Men's Health, 11*, 1536–1546. doi:10.1177/1557988315619677

Sandoval, M., Leclerc, J. A., & Gomez, R. L. (2017). Words to sleep on: Naps facilitate verb generalization in habitually and nonhabitually napping preschoolers. *Child Development, 88*, 1615–1628.

Satcher, D., & Higginbotham, E. J. (2008). The public health approach to eliminating disparities in health. *American Journal of Public Health, 98*, 400–403.

Semenza, J. C., & Krishnasamy, P. V. (2007). Design of a health-promoting neighborhood intervention. *Health Promotion Practice, 8*, 243–256. doi:10.1177/1524839906289585

Song, M., & Kong, E.-H. (2015). Older adults' definitions of health: A metasynthesis. *International Journal of Nursing Studies, 52*, 1097–1106. doi:10.1016/j.ijnurstu.2015.02.001

Sun, R. (2017). Re-examining the role of engaging in activities: Does its effect on mortality change by age among the Chinese elderly? *Ageing International, 42*, 78–92. doi:10.1007/s12126-017-9282-x

Sutton, D. J., Hocking, C. S., & Smythe, L. A. (2012). A phenomenological study of occupational engagement in recovery from mental illness. *Canadian Journal of Occupational Therapy, 79*, 142–150. doi:10.2182/cjot.2012.79.3.3

Tischler, M. (2017). Wendy Preston, Mixit. *Directions*, 24–25.

Tkatch, R., Musich, S., MacLeod, S., Kraemer, S., Hawkins, K., Wicker, E. R., & Armstrong, D. G. (2017). A qualitative study to examine older adults' perceptions of health: Keys to aging successfully. *Geriatric Nursing, 38*, 485–490. doi:10.1016/j.gerinurse.2017.02.009

Tozzi, L., Carballedo, A., Lavelle, G., Doolin, K., Doyle, M., . . . Frodl, T. (2016). Longitudinal functional connectivity changes correlate with mood improvement after regular exercise in a dose-dependent fashion. *European Journal of Neuroscience, 43*, 1089–1096. doi:10.1111/ejn.13222

Wethington, H., Pan, L., & Sherry, B. (2013). The association of screen time, television in the bedroom, and obesity among school-aged youth: 2007 National Survey of Children's Health. *Journal of School Health, 83*, 573–581.

Wilcock, A. (1993). A theory of the human need for occupation. *Journal of Occupational Science: Australia, 1*, 17–24. doi:10.1080/14427591.1993.9686375

Wilcock, A. (1995). The occupational brain: A theory of human nature. *Journal of Occupational Science: Australia, 2,* 68–73. doi:10.1080/14427591.1995.9686397

Wilcock, A. A. (2001). *Occupation for health, volume 1: A journey from self health to prescription.* London, United Kingdom: British Association and College of Occupational Therapy.

Wilcock, A. A., & Hocking, C. (2015). *An occupational perspective of health* (3rd ed.). Thorofare, New Jersey: SLACK.

World Federation of Occupational Therapists. (2016). *Minimum standards for the education of occupational therapists.* Perth, Australia: Author.

World Health Organization. (1986, November). *Ottawa Charter for health promotion, 1986.* Paper presented at the First International Conference on Health Promotion. Ottawa, Ontario, Canada.

World Health Organization. (2001). *International classification of functioning, disability and health: A global model to guide clinical thinking and practice in childhood disability.* Geneva, Switzerland: Author.

World Health Organization. (2010). *Global recommendations on physical activity for health.* Geneva, Switzerland: Author. Retrieved from http://apps.who.int/iris/bitstream/10665/44399/1/9789241599979_eng.pdf

World Health Organization. (2018). *Frequently asked questions.* Geneva, Switzerland: Author. Retrieved from: http://www.who.int/suggestions/faq/en/

Yeh, H.-P., Stone, J. A., Churchill, S. M., Wheat, J. S., Brymer, E., & Davids, K. (2015). Physical, psychological and emotional benefits of green physical activity: An ecological dynamics perspective. *Sports Medicine, 46,* 947–953. doi:10.1007/s40279-015-0374-z

the **Point®** *For additional resources on the subjects discussed in this chapter, visit* **http://thePoint.lww.com/Willard-Spackman13e.**

CHAPTER 9

Occupational Science
The Study of Occupation

Valerie A. Wright-St. Clair, Clare Hocking

LEARNING OBJECTIVES

After reading this chapter, you will be able to:

1. Apply an occupational science evidence-based practice way of thinking about day-to-day practice.
2. Interpret the difference between basic and applied occupational science knowledge underpinning practice.
3. Analyze the observable and phenomenological aspects of occupations.
4. Begin to synthesize occupational science knowledge from diverse studies in order to consider how occupational therapy practice might serve individuals, communities, and society well.
5. Evaluate how well your own practice is guided by the existing and emergent basic and applied occupational science knowledge.

Introduction

This chapter explores how occupational science is informing occupational therapy (OT) practice. First, the discussion looks at occupational science as a basic science underpinning OT knowledge, before recent developments in occupational science are showcased as a way of illustrating its growth as an applied science. Along the way, real-world international examples are offered. Each highlights how the "science" of occupational science is guiding *evidence-based occupational therapy practice*. Each example, in its own way, illustrates occupational science "in play" within the everyday practice worlds of occupational therapists.

Humans as Occupational Beings

India was home for Madhulal and Sadguna Patel until they decided to emigrate to New Zealand in their later years. They followed their adult son and daughter who were already settled and working in their new host country. Madhulal and Sadguna, age 66 and 63 years, respectively, had long contributed to society through their paid employment in India; he as a civil servant and she as a teacher. Yet, their previously productive lives did not prepare them for engaging as older immigrants in a disparate society. Keen to share their story, Madhulal and Sadguna spoke with the "social issues" reporter for a national newspaper. They reflected back on 2 years of abject loneliness after

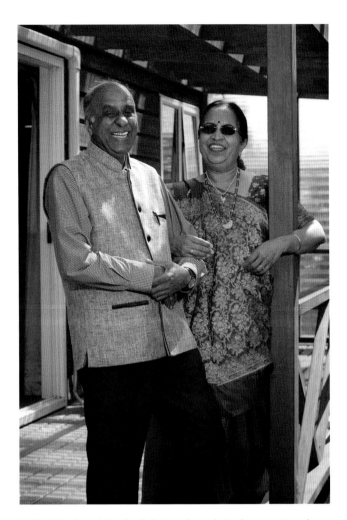

FIGURE 9-1 Madhulal Patel and Sadguna Patel. (Photograph taken by Nick Reed and reproduced with permission by *The New Zealand Herald*/ http://newspix.nzherald.co.nz/.)

their arrival. "We go to the gardens and we take a bench and we cry" (Collins, 2016, p. A9), Sadguna said. Their experience of being socially isolated and lonely changed when they connected with other older Indian immigrants through a not-for-profit organization serving the South Asian community. Now "we dance together, we play together" (Collins, 2016, p. A9), Sadguna happily shared (Figure 9-1).

Madhulal and Sadguna Patel's story (Collins, 2016) reflects what this chapter is about. It reveals how life changes can mean that people, or sometimes communities, need support to learn and successfully engage in new occupations. And it points toward understanding how an in-depth knowledge about *humans as occupational beings* can inform new ways for OT to contribute to healthy families and communities. But first, let's go back to the ideas behind this chapter.

Occupational science opens up new ways to explore the complexities of human engagement in occupations. As a basic science, it aims to build knowledge about the

substrates, **form**, **function**, and **meaning** of what people do (Zemke & Clark, 1996) and the occupational nature of being human (Wilcock & Hocking, 2015). Studying occupation involves building knowledge about its "observable and phenomenological aspects" (Clark & Lawlor, 2009, p. 7). In order to explain the complex ideas behind studying the "observable" and "phenomenological" aspects of occupation, an illustrative tale is offered—Antoine de Saint-Exupéry's (1972) classic story of *The Little Prince*. It opens with the narrator's voice as he reflects back on his boyhood. When only 6 years old, entranced by a picture of a boa constrictor ingesting its prey whole, he produced his first drawing of a boa constrictor having swallowed an elephant. He showed his drawing to the grown-ups and asked if it frightened them. Observing what appeared to be the outline of a hat, the grown-ups said they were not at all frightened. Somewhat puzzled by their response, the boy produced his second drawing. This one left nothing to the imagination; it was a prosection showing the elephant inside the boa constrictor. At this point, the grown-ups advised the boy to give up drawing boa constrictors "whether from the inside or the outside" (de Saint-Exupéry, 1972, p. 8).

In such a simple way, this tale captures the two fundamentally different ways we as occupational therapists can study occupation as a basic science. One way is to study its observable aspects. This way of coming to know things is underpinned by the assumption that, like the boy's second drawing of the elephant inside the boa constrictor, the truth about occupations and the occupational nature of humans exists in the world. Therefore, we can come to know it by gathering data gained through our senses (de Poy & Gitlin, 2016). From this view, through quantitative research, truth or reality can be seen, touched, heard, or measured in some objective way. On the other hand, if we accept there is not one but many truths, or multiple realities about occupations and the occupational nature of humans, this opens the way for studying the **phenomenological aspects of occupation** through qualitative research. This way of coming to know about occupation is underpinned by the assumption that, like the boy's first drawing, people experience their own subjective, contextual reality. In essence, "the what," "the whom," and "the why" of occupations can all be studied as units of analysis within occupational science research.

Building a Basic Knowledge of Occupation

Attempting to give an overview of the knowledge occupational scientists are building is a little like swallowing an elephant; there is no agreed way to go about it and, just as an elephant creates a big bulge in a boa constrictor, the breadth of the field and the diverse methodologies employed make it hard to convey its scope within a few paragraphs. Separating observable from phenomenological perspectives gives some structure, and we have also chosen to focus on the recent literature to give a sense of the whole of the science and its likely future directions.

Observable Aspects of Occupation

Comparatively little occupational science research has addressed the substrates of engaging in occupation: the anatomical structures that we perform with; the neurological functions that direct movement; the physiological functions that maintain homeostasis despite the rigors of performance; and the cognitive functions involved in initiating, monitoring and communicating our actions, and judging the value of the outcome. That is perhaps because many of an occupation's substrates are not directly observable, requiring neuroimaging and other technologies to "see" them. One exception in the recent literature is Williams's (2017) exploration of the sensory processing that occurs as people engage in occupation, which informs the "sense" people make of what they are doing and how they might adapt their actions to achieve a better result. Another is Cogan's (2016) discussion of abnormalities detected in the brain tissue of military personnel with mild brain injuries caused by an explosion, which appear to explain the subtle but pervasive difficulties they experience in everyday occupations.

Observable elements of an occupation's form can often be glimpsed in studies of the experience of engaging in them. Qualitative studies have revealed, for example, that people who build kitset models of aircraft put time and effort into careful construction (Pollard & Carver, 2016) and that the stigma now attached to cigarette smoking has changed the form, leading people to "sneak" a smoke in their car to avoid being observed (Luck & Beagan, 2015). Quantitative measures can also reveal aspects of an occupation's form, such as who does and does not participate in it and the equipment required to do so. For instance, disparities in older adults' access to mobile phones and computers have been noted and identified as contributing to systemic disadvantages for those living in poverty (Kottorp et al., 2016). New understandings of the functions occupations serve are also coming into view. For example, interviews and observational methods revealed that children's sports can function as a means of including children with physical impairments (Asbjørnslett & Bekken, 2016), and shared occupations can function as a site for community members to learn how to help children with brain injuries participate (Jones, Hocking, & McPherson, 2017). The increased use of critical methodologies also reveals aspects of the intersection of occupations and environments, such as how imposed restrictions on the occupations available to asylum seekers in Australia cause high levels of distress (Crawford, Turpin, Nayar, Steel, & Durand, 2016).

Phenomenological Aspects of Occupation

Phenomenally, we can study and come to understand occupation through ideas (de Poy & Gitlin, 2016), which occupational scientists have typically accessed by asking individuals about their lived experiences of doing things. The substrates of occupation are not typically the focus, even though phenomenology encompasses such understandings and is relevant to developing a science of occupation (Lala & Kinsella, 2011). Experiential accounts can generate insights, however, such as the evocative account of turf cutting as "using your legs, you're using your arms, you're using your balance . . . there's a bit of an art to it" (McGrath & McGonagle, 2016, p. 316).

The function of occupation has also been uncovered by studies that asked people about their experiences, such as Bonsall's (2014) narrative phenomenological description of occupations that build and define families, and Beagan and Etowa's (2011) depiction of Canadian women of African descent mediating everyday experiences of racism through prayer and other spiritual and church-related occupations. Finally, insights into the meanings occupations hold for particular people in specific contexts have been generated through studies using a wide range of methodologies. One recently published example used photo elicitation interviews to explore how the declining socioeconomic profile of their neighborhood changed older African Americans' experience of daily occupations, making them more vigilant in monitoring who is about and what is happening around them (Fritz & Cutchin, 2017).

Although we addressed them separately, what is important is not the study of occupation's observable *or* phenomenological aspects but the study of occupation's observable *and* phenomenological aspects. Both dimensions of knowledge are important to studying occupation as a basic science. One informs the other. One exists in accord with the other. It is a synergistic relationship. Beyond these aspects, moral philosophy offers an opportunity to think broadly about living a good life, such as the question of "what counts as an occupationally satisfying life" (Morgan, 2010, p. 217) or, guided by normative ethics, "How ought I practice to enable people to live occupationally satisfying lives?" Such understandings cannot be adequately addressed by observational or phenomenological approaches but may be addressed as the boundaries of occupational science scholarship extend to include more philosophical concerns.

The Occupational Nature of Being Human

Sitting alongside all the studies of observable and phenomenological aspects of occupation, there is an ongoing thread of discussion about the occupational nature of being human and the need to incorporate diverse cultural perspectives. One counterpoint to Western understandings of occupation as active and purposeful is the Greek worldview, which emphasizes balancing periods of hard work with adequate rest, relaxation, and less structured free time (Kantartzis & Molineux, 2011). Alternatively, an **indigenous worldview** frames occupation as deeply spiritual, demanding integrity, respect, and *aroha* (love, compassion) on the part of the performer (Smith, 2017). Critically informed understandings are also increasingly needed to expose the historical, political, and social forces that restrict people's occupational possibilities. This work unmasks misinformed assumptions about what people "choose" to do, when their actions would be more accurately understood to be informed responses to entrenched discrimination (Gerlach, Teachman, Laliberte-Rudman, Aldrich, & Huot, 2017). Over time, such perspectives will propel the development of knowledge of the occupational nature of humans that better represents the implicit relationship between occupation and well-being.

Occupational Science as an Applied Science

Thus far, we have considered occupational science as a basic science, yet it is more than that; it is emergent as an applied science. Applied sciences like biomechanics, ergonomics, and mental health rehabilitation are already familiar to occupational therapists. As a consequence, therapists will be accustomed to using such applied sciences to guide their day-to-day decisions in practice. Applied sciences provide a knowledge base informing what to do and how to go about practice for a given occupational disruption. One helpful resource for practitioners and those seeking OT is the American Occupational Therapy Association's (2014) latest edition of its practice framework for guiding a process for **occupation-focused practice**. Although occupational science may be a new feature within the expansive field of applied sciences, over two decades on from its inception, occupational science's latent potential exists in its capacity to be a "comprehensive translational science" (Clark & Lawlor, 2009, p. 7). Occupational science, as an applied science, is already in the business

of transforming rigorous basic science findings into evidence-based OT. In this way, "occupational science is designed to systematize knowledge about occupation, especially in relation to health and well-being" (Clark & Lawlor, 2009, p. 4). Interpreting this idea further, systematized occupational science knowledge is beginning to guide OT practice at all levels, from individual health to population health approaches. So let's look more closely at what is meant by the systematizing of knowledge.

Systematizing Occupational Science Knowledge

The origins, or etymology, of the word helps us to make sense of what it means to "systematize" occupational science knowledge. "Systema" in Greek was derived from the root words meaning "together" and to "cause to stand"; in other words, *systema* referred to something that stands as one in an "organized whole" (Harper, n.d.). So a process that systematizes occupational science knowledge for OT is a methodical, rigorous way of developing a disciplined, coherent set of rules or methods for application in practice. Systematizing is about identifying, developing, analyzing, and optimizing knowledge for use. It is a translational process—transforming scientific understandings to practice knowledge. As a **translational science**, occupational science is theory-driven research aimed at resolving real-world concerns (Guerra & Leidy, 2010). In reverse, real-world, OT practice-based evidence (PBE) rigorously analyzed from systematized intervention outcomes (Cogan, Blanche, Diaz, Clark, & Chun, 2014; Ghaisas, Pyatak, Blanche, Blanchard, & Clark, 2015) has the potential to inform new ways of theorizing occupational science.

Systematizing occupational science knowledge fits with the international call for health practitioners, including occupational therapists, to use best evidence to guide everyday practice. A methodical way of doing translational occupational science research was put forward by colleagues at the Division of Occupational Science and Occupational Therapy, University of Southern California (USC), in the United States. It is designed as a rigorous way of developing OT practice knowledge from issues about which little is known but which may have an occupational foundation. Figure 9-2 summarizes the process, which begins with identifying and articulating the practice issue and then gathering a first layer of descriptive evidence from which an intervention is derived. The next layers of evidence come from testing how likely the intervention is to bring about the desired outcome, and still further, by measuring the cost-effectiveness of the intervention

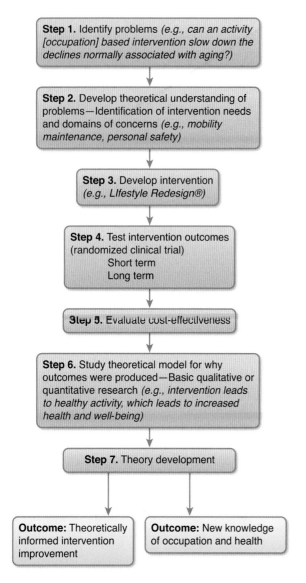

Step 1. Identify problems (e.g., can an activity [occupation] based intervention slow down the declines normally associated with aging?)

Step 2. Develop theoretical understanding of problems—Identification of intervention needs and domains of concerns (e.g., mobility maintenance, personal safety)

Step 3. Develop intervention (e.g., LIfestyle Redesign®)

Step 4. Test intervention outcomes (randomized clinical trial)
Short term
Long term

Step 5. Evaluate cost-effectiveness

Step 6. Study theoretical model for why outcomes were produced—Basic qualitative or quantitative research (e.g., intervention leads to healthy activity, which leads to increased health and well-being)

Step 7. Theory development

Outcome: Theoretically informed intervention improvement

Outcome: New knowledge of occupation and health

FIGURE 9-2 Blueprint for a translational science research program. (Reprinted from Clark, F. A., & Lawlor, M. C. [2009]. The making and mattering of occupational science. In E. B. Crepeau, E. S. Cohn, & B. A. Schell [Eds.], *Willard & Spackman's occupational therapy* [11th ed., pp. 2–14]. Philadelphia, PA: Lippincott Williams & Wilkins. Permission granted by Wolters Kluwer, http://www.lww.com.)

if it is successful. These methodical steps might seem enough in themselves, but for this practice knowledge to "stand together" as an organized whole, understanding why the intervention worked is essential. A coherent body of causal evidence then opens the way to build an explanatory theory, bringing together the research observations with interpretive reasoning to explain outcomes of intervention and add to the body of occupation-based knowledge.

Such a rigorous process shows the symbiotic relationship between the practice and research communities (Blanche, Fogelberg, Diaz, Carlson, & Clark, 2011; Clark et al., 2006; Cogan et al., 2014). That is, in the OT domain, the questions for occupational science research arise from practice-based issues, and the research findings, in return, provide knowledge for practice. Practice and research exist and thrive together. However, implementing the blueprint for generating new knowledge is not for the fainthearted; it takes years to undertake the multiple studies and demands significant funding and researcher commitment. The following examples illustrate how occupational science research can underpin and come to life in the context of OT practice.

Occupational Science Informing Occupational Therapy

Occupational science informing OT is an idea whose time has come (Blanche & Henny-Kohler, 2000; Clark, Jackson, & Carlson, 2004; Molineux, 2004; Pierce, 2011). The following three case studies (Case Studies 9-1, 9-2, and 9-3) show how scientific understandings about human occupation are informing practice across the international OT community. Clark and Lawlor's (2009) blueprint for a systematic program of translational science research (see Figure 9-2) is used explicitly as a way of illuminating the steps involved.

Conclusion

As is already happening in numerous locations internationally, it is time for occupational science to take center stage as a science informing OT practice, alongside other more traditional sciences such as neuroanatomy and biomechanics. You might say that knowledge about the occupations people do, and their capacities and drive to do them, has always informed OT. At one level, this is true; at a far deeper and expansive level, the work done since the 1980s, beginning with researchers and colleagues at USC, is allowing a more profound philosophical, theoretical, and research knowledge base on humans as occupational beings to take root and to flourish. There is a burgeoning amount of high-quality basic science available to practitioners to make sense of in the context of their own practice. Yet, it is occupational science's emergent capacity as a comprehensive applied science informing practice where the future of evidence-based OT lies.

Step 1: Identify the Practice Problem

In the United States, pressure ulcers are a frequent, multifaceted, and costly problem for people with spinal cord injury (SCI). Risk assessment using the existing measurement tools is imprecise. Of particular interest to occupational scientists and therapists is the concern that pressure ulcers could have an occupational foundation and be a recurrent barrier to full participation in everyday occupations (Clark et al., 2006). Everyday occupations are not necessarily mundane. For example, Kerri Morgan's (Figures 9-3 and 9-5) everyday occupations include training for racing in Paralympic events.

Step 2: Identify the Intervention Needs

Occupational scientists at USC and their research collaborators designed a holistic ethnographic, qualitative study, now called the Pressure Ulcer Prevention Study I or PUPS I, to explore the everyday life contexts that contribute to the occurrence of pressure ulcers in men and women from different socioeconomic backgrounds following SCI (Clark, Sanders, Carlson, Blanche, & Jackson, 2007). Through a prolonged, in-depth process of interviewing the study participants and observing them as they went about their usual days, the researchers sought to understand how the complex, dynamic mix of daily circumstances played out as risks for pressure ulcers for each person (Clark et al., 2006). For example, Robert's story is highly illustrative of

how the development of ulcers is affected between an individualized risk profile and th active occupation. Following discharge from a rehab facility to a skilled nursing service, Robert began to dedica a significant "amount of time riding around in his wheelchair with two other young men who lived at the facility" (Clark et al., 2006, p. 1519). He developed two pressure ulcers as a consequence. Just as the researchers came to understand Robert's susceptibility to pressure ulcer development within his occupational world, an individualized and richly contextualized portfolio of occupation in relation to risk emerged for all the study participants. After examining the wider set of stories, the researchers developed a coherent series of pressure ulcer development models. These models incorporated the dynamic balance of liability and buffering factors, individualized risk profiles, a generalized pressure ulcer event sequence (Figure 9-4), and a long-term pressure ulcer event sequence. Although theoretical in nature, the models are grounded in the richness of qualitatively derived, occupational science data.

Among other results, the occupational scientists found that pressure ulcers most commonly occurred, and recurred, for those who (1) had a moderately high-risk profile and (2) experienced a disruptive health or life event. What the findings highlight is the need for preventive interventions to take account of "the unique constellation of circumstances that comprise a person's everyday life" (Clark et al., 2006, p. 1516). The knowledge gained through this preliminary investigative work was ready to be further systematized and tested out in an applied study.

Step 3: Develop the Intervention

Armed with the ethnographic study findings, the occupational scientists now understood how pressure ulcer development was potentially modifiable in the occupational lives of people following SCI. Their next step was to thoughtfully apply this basic knowledge by designing a model for OT intervention to be conducted and tested through an "occupational-science driven clinical trial" (Clark et al., 2004, p. 201). Developing and testing the efficacy of the intervention entailed a process of careful manualization (Blanche et al., 2011) which involved documenting a rigorous therapeutic protocol and determining the outcomes to be measured. Such a practice manual guides the therapist's focus on what matters, articulates the professional reasoning process, and maps out the intervention procedures (Blanche et al., 2011). It was time to put the intervention model to the test.

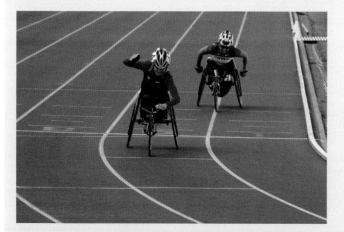

FIGURE 9-3 **Kerri Morgan, United States, racing in the International Paralympic Committee (IPC) World Athletics Championships in Christchurch, New Zealand. (Photograph taken by Karen Boyle. Reproduced with permission.)**

(continues)

Chapter 9 • Occupational Science

129

ULCER RISK: THE USC/
REHABILITATION
N RESEARCH

by the interplay
e quest for
ilitation
te

PRESSURE ULCER RISK: THE USC/
OS NATIONAL REHABILITATION
ULCER PREVENTION RESEARCH
ued)

Pressure Ulcer Ris...
Specific instantiation of
risk-relevant influences
stemming from individualized
risk profile, change event, and
ongoing contextual
situation/response

↓

Skin Contact Event
Interface of physical pressure (weight/force;
duration of contact; qualities of contact
surface; nature of force of contact [e.g.,
shear, injury] and skin susceptibility (general
skin integrity; current state)

↓

Pressure Ulcer Outcome → No Ulcer

↓

Ulcer

↓

Response to Ulcer

FIGURE 9-4 Overview of generalized pressure
ulcer event sequence. (Reprinted from Clark,
F. A., Jackson, J. M., Scott, M. D., Atkins, M. S.,
Uhles-Tanaka, D., & Rubayi, S. [2006]. Data-based
models of how pressure ulcers developing daily-
living contexts of adults with spinal cord injury.
Archives of Physical Medicine and Rehabilitation,
87, 1516–1525. doi:10.1016/j.apmr.2006.08.329.
Copyright [2006], with permission from Elsevier.)

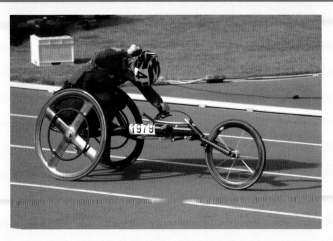

FIGURE 9-5 **Kerri Morgan, United States, winning
at the 2011 IPC Athletics World Championships in
Christchurch, New Zealand. (Photograph taken by
Karen Boyle. Reproduced with permission.)**

Step 4: Test the Intervention

In conducting the occupational science–based randomized
controlled trial (RCT) referred to as PUPS II, the researchers
set out to systematically assess whether the lifestyle
intervention, termed the Pressure Ulcer Prevention Program
(PUPP), was more effective than standard care in preventing
medically serious (i.e., stage 3 or 4) pressure ulcers (Clark
et al., 2014). One hundred and seventy men (144) and women
(26) who had sustained an SCI at least 6 months earlier, were
nonambulatory, and had experienced at least one previous
serious pressure ulcer were enrolled in the study. They were
randomly assigned into either the 12-month occupation-
based PUPP intervention group or a standard care group.
The intervention included participants' self-selected goals,
active problem solving, and engagement in motivational
interviewing. The incidence rate of new serious pressure
ulcers was the primary outcome measured (Clark et al., 2014)
before intervention, at 12 months and at a 24-month follow-
up. Although the study was complete, the unanticipated
challenges of conducting an RCT in the real world, such
as insufficient statistical power and the participants'
unpredictable chaotic life circumstances (Ghaisas et al.,
2015), meant the researchers' ability to determine how
much the lifestyle intervention *caused* positive change was
compromised and the results of the intent-to-treat analysis
were inconclusive (Carlson et al., 2017). However, it was still

CASE STUDY 9-1   OCCUPATIONS AND PRESSURE ULCER RISK: THE USC/ RANCHO LOS AMIGOS NATIONAL REHABILITATION CENTER PRESSURE ULCER PREVENTION RESEARCH PROGRAM *(continued)*

possible to examine the *relationship* between participants' lifestyle changes and pressure ulcer status. A secondary analysis of the intervention group participants' treatment notes, as of December 2011, showed four patterns to the relationship between lifestyle changes and pressure ulcer development. The resulting case profiles can inform occupational therapists working in the field (Ghaisas et al., 2015) who use **occupation-focused lifestyle interventions**.

In addition, these occupational scientists codesigned a comprehensive set of evidence-based, readily available online resources that can be employed by occupational therapists or consumers. For example, one provides guidance on pressure ulcer prevention techniques to families or carers. Perhaps most important, another provides information for people with SCI on the importance of everyday occupations as well as the risks associated with engagement in them (USC, 2013). More recently, the researchers published a practice-based evidence framework for methodically customizing the lifestyle intervention manual for therapy with a different group, U.S. veterans (Cogan et al., 2014).

Systematizing occupational science knowledge for application by occupational therapists means everyone wins: the clients, their families and friends, the health care funders and providers, the greater community, and of course, the occupational therapists.

Step 5: Evaluate the Cost-Effectiveness

There is work still to be done to determine the efficacy and cost-effectiveness of the PUPP. The planned between-groups comparison of costs and net health benefits was not possible from the initial RCT because of the inconclusive results.

Step 6: Study Why the Outcomes Were Produced

The secondary analysis of the PUPS II results (Ghaisas et al., 2015) allowed the researchers to examine the relationship between lifestyle and behavior changes and alterations in participants' pressure ulcer status. Therapists are likely to find the case studies used to illustrate the resulting four-pattern typology useful in their practice.

Step 7: Develop the Theory

The PUPS research program has already generated considerable theory development. For example, its qualitative arm produced overarching principles of pressure ulcer risk and data-based models therapists can employ to more comprehensively understand the elements that contribute to pressure ulcer risk (Clark et al., 2006; Jackson et al., 2010). Furthermore, a conceptual model was developed from the clinical trial. The model depicts how adherence to the lifestyle intervention and utilization of its components can have positive effects on recipients' self-efficacy, knowledge and social support, which, in turn, can mediate pressure ulcer prevention (Clark et al., 2014). Two additional papers are currently being prepared that provide insights on (1) why certain participants in the intervention nevertheless incurred medically serious pressure ulcers and (2) on the protective factors that enabled others to counteract developing any. Ultimately, the goal of this research program is to provide occupational therapists with a theoretically guided, scientifically grounded, and evidence-based intervention approach for lessening pressure ulcer risk in people with SCI.

CASE STUDY 9-2   PARTICIPATION FOR CHILDREN WITH PHYSICAL DISABILITIES: THE *CANCHILD* CENTRE FOR CHILDHOOD DISABILITY RESEARCH PROGRAM

In a position statement to the Canadian Standing Senate Committee on Human Rights, Mary Law (2011) made the case that the exclusion from everyday occupations, such as play (Figure 9-6), and school occupations, such as reading (Figure 9-7), is a human rights issue for young people with physical disabilities. But, the capacity to influence good public policy did not start there. It began over a decade ago when the *CanChild* team embarked on a research journey of generating and translating occupational science knowledge for use in OT practice. As is the case for applied research in OT, it started with understanding the problem.

Step 1: Identify the Practice Problem

Like many other places, young people with disabilities in Canada make up approximately 5% of the country's population (Law, 2011). Of particular concern to the *CanChild* team was knowledge indicating that these children are often excluded from engaging in age-appropriate occupations, especially leisure and sporting activities (Law, 2011). For example, research with the newly developed Participation and Environment Measure for Children and Youth (PEM-CY) (Coster et al., 2011) indicated that "24% of children and youth with disabilities never take part in unstructured physical activities in the community in comparison to only 2% among their typically developing peers" (Law, 2011, p. 3). In spite of research proposing children's occupational development occurs as a process (Wiseman, Davis, & Polatajko, 2005) and understanding

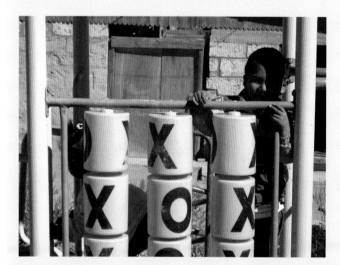

FIGURE 9-6 **Young children at play. (Photograph taken by Valerie Wright-St Clair.)**

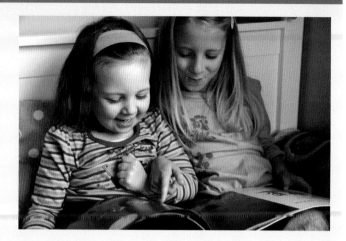

FIGURE 9-7 **Children reading together. (Photograph taken by Andrea Casey. Reproduced with permission.)**

children's play as an occupation (Waldman-Levi & Bundy, 2016), new ideas were emerging about play as a quality of occupational engagement rather than a type of activity (Pollock et al., 1997). Further exploration was warranted.

Step 2: Identify the Intervention Needs

Beginning with a qualitative interview-based study, 10 adolescents with congenital disabilities and 10 age- and gender-matched peers were asked about their play experiences. Both groups said play occupations needed to be self-chosen and be "playful" or fun in nature. Nevertheless, those with disabilities mentioned more barriers to participation, such as needing to develop the motor skills for engaging, being limited by the physical environment, and feeling different to peers or not belonging (Pollock et al., 1997). Where these qualitative findings hinted at some of the occupational needs faced by young people with disabilities, the *CanChild* longitudinal Participate Study (Law, 2011) provided stronger descriptive evidence. With the aim of determining the factors that enhance participation in childhood occupations for those with physical disabilities, Law and her team observed 427 6- to 16-year-olds over time. Although activity preferences (Imms et al., 2017) and supportive family relationships were significant contributors, the contextual environment was "one of the most important factors influencing participation of children and youth with disabilities" (Law, 2011, p. 4). The strength of these findings suggested that one approach to improving participation could be modifying the contextual factors.

CASE STUDY 9-2 PARTICIPATION FOR CHILDREN WITH PHYSICAL DISABILITIES: THE *CANCHILD* CENTRE FOR CHILDHOOD DISABILITY RESEARCH PROGRAM *(continued)*

Step 3: Develop the Intervention

The *CanChild* team partnered with colleagues at the University of Alberta to design an RCT to compare the efficacy of two different therapy approaches aimed at promoting children's participation in everyday occupations (Law et al., 2007). One group of children would receive **"context-focused" therapy** aimed at modifying the occupations and environment found to hinder goal-directed participation. The other group would get "child-focused" therapy aimed at identifying and remediating impairments, such as muscle tone, to improve movement patterns and improving a child's skills. By repeating chosen outcome measures over time, the researchers would be able to evaluate the functional gains made between the two intervention groups.

Step 4: Test the Intervention

For the study, 128 children with cerebral palsy received either the context-focused or child-focused weekly intervention for a period of 6 months (Law et al., 2011). Standardized measurements of the children's level of disability, gross motor function, range of motion, and participation in everyday occupations beyond school activities, as well as family empowerment, were conducted at the beginning and end of the intervention period and then repeated 3 months later. Interestingly, children in both groups made similar significant gains in their functional and participation outcomes. This important finding means that therapy focusing on changing the occupation and the environment is just as effective as therapy aimed at changing the child's impairments and improving abilities through practice of functional activities.

Step 5: Evaluate the Cost-Effectiveness

Future research can determine the cost-effectiveness of interventions focused on changing the occupation and environment. Observations made during the trial suggest that environmental changes can lead to improved participation very quickly, but this observation needs to be tested.

Step 6: Study Why the Outcomes Were Produced

Both the child-focused and context-focused interventions identified goals for therapy intervention. With the child-focused approach, specific problems with performance

were identified for intervention. In the context-focused approach, the Canadian Occupational Performance Measure (COPM) (Law et al., 2005) was used to identify individualized child goals. Goal setting has been shown to improve the effectiveness of therapy (Löwing, Bexelius, & Brogren Carlberg, 2009; Ostensjø, Oien, & Fallang, 2008). Through changing the occupation and/or environment, barriers to participation are eliminated to enable the child to perform the occupation using his or her current skills and abilities (Lim, Law, Khetani, Pollock, & Rosenbaum, 2016b).

Step 7: Develop the Theory

Thanks to Law's *CanChild* research program focused on children's occupations, therapists have several evidence-based, *participation-focused assessment* tools to use in practice: the Assessment of Preschool Children's Participation (APCP), the Children's Assessment of Participation and Enjoyment (CAPE), and the Preferences for Activities of Children (PAC) (*CanChild* Centre for Childhood Disability Research, 2011). These robust tools continue to be used in contemporary research in Canada and other countries (Imms et al., 2017). The team's commitment to a comprehensive program of research related to children with disabilities' participation means they continue to develop and test measures such as the PEM-CY and the Young Children's Participation and Environment Measure (YC-PEM). Knowing that the cultural relevance of measures used by occupational therapists matters, the research team developed and tested a culturally equivalent Singaporean YC-PEM (Lim, Law, Khetani, Pollock, & Rosenbaum, 2016a; Lim et al., 2016b). Therapists can have confidence in shifting their focus from impairments to occupations and the environment in order to promote participation of children with physical disabilities (Pashmdarfard, Amini, & Hassani Mehraban, 2017). At the population level, therapists have grounds for promoting public policies that promote "child and youth participation in community settings" (Law, 2011, p. 5). Furthermore, by making the research findings and resources available on their Website (http://www.canchild.ca/en/), the *CanChild* Center for Childhood Disability Research ultimately benefits the community as a whole (Law et al., 2005).

CASE STUDY 9-3   EVERYDAY OCCUPATIONS AND AGING WELL: THE LIFE AND LIVING IN ADVANCED AGE COHORT STUDY NEW ZEALAND: *TE PUĀWAITANGA O NGĀ TAPUWAE KIA ORA TONU* (MĀORI TRANSLATION)

At the School of Population Health, University of Auckland, New Zealand, a multidisciplinary team led by geriatrician Dr. Ngaire Kerse conducted the Life and Living in Advanced Age Cohort Study New Zealand (LiLACS NZ) prospective cohort study to establish the determinants of aging well for older New Zealanders (Hayman et al., 2012). In particular, the study aimed to understand the relative importance of medical, cultural, functional, activity (occupational), social, and economic factors to relevant health and longevity outcomes. Following a preliminary feasibility study with 112 participants to test the extensive, interview-based questionnaire, 937 older adults were enrolled during 2010 from selected urban and rural regions: 516 non-Māori turning 85 years and 421 Māori age 80 to 90 years (extended age criterion to get adequate numbers). The first wave of data gathering was completed by the end of 2011 and the sixth and final wave in 2016. So, let's look more closely at the occupational science research strand.

Step 1: Identify the Practice Problem

As in most other countries, New Zealand's population is aging. The number of older adults, people age 65 years and over, is projected to double between 2013 and 2038 (Statistics New Zealand, 2015a). Of this population sector, those age 85 years and older make up the fastest growing subgroup, with a predicted 600% increase in the first half of this century (Dunstan & Thomson, 2006). Similar to current proportions of older indigenous American Indian and Alaska natives (Turner Goins et al., 2015), older *Māori*, New Zealand's indigenous peoples, constituted less than 6% of the country's older adult population in 2013 (Statistics New Zealand, 2015a). The projected doubling of the older Māori population to 12% of all those age 65 years and over by 2038 is good news for Māori families and communities as well as wider society (Statistics New Zealand, 2015b). Overall, this means many more people of diverse ethnicities will be living into their late 80s and beyond. Accordingly, understanding what helps people age well and live well in advanced age is important. The consensus so far is that engaging in occupations of some sort is positively associated with aging well and/or longevity (Agahi, Silverstein, & Parker, 2011; Fushiki, Ohnishi, Sakauchi, Oura, & Mori, 2012; Glass, Mendes de Leon, Marottoli, & Berkman, 1999; Katz, 2000; Menec, 2003). However, findings as to what kind of occupations lead to greater health and well-being are mixed and, at times, inconclusive (Wright-St Clair et al., 2017). Furthermore, little is known about how older New Zealanders prefer to use their time

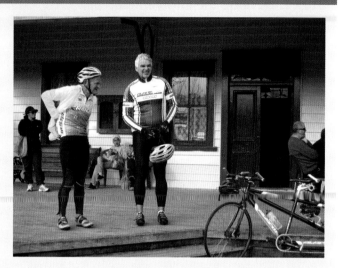

FIGURE 9-8 Leisure time use for Garth Barfoot and Steve Kingdon includes preparing for a club cycle race to the top of the Waitakere Ranges, Auckland, New Zealand, June 2011. (Photograph taken by Valerie Wright-St Clair. Reproduced with permission.)

(Figure 9-8). Occupational therapists designing community- and individual-level interventions for older adults have little culturally specific knowledge to draw on.

Step 2: Identify the Intervention Needs

Two basic research projects are informing this step of the research program. Initially, a qualitative, hermeneutic phenomenological study was conducted in 2006 to explore older New Zealanders' experiences of being in their everyday lives. Community-dwelling elder Māori and non-Māori of European descent, age 71 to 97 years, were interviewed about their everyday life with a focus on particular events (Wright-St Clair, Kerse, & Smythe, 2011; Wright-St Clair & Smythe, 2012). Several phenomena stood out in the findings. In advanced age, "doing the things ordinarily attended to, in accustomed ways, holds things steady" (Wright-St Clair et al., 2011, p. 93) and keeps things going in the context of getting older. Paradoxically, this accustomed comfortableness in doing things, when it was suddenly lost, revealed potential transition points in life. Such sudden discomforts amid doing usually deeply familiar occupations announced change.

To illustrate, 97-year-old Ferguson, who lived alone with help from his daughter, only came to know his rapidly fading strength when putting his dressing gown on a few days earlier. It was a task usually so easy, so familiar, he ordinarily did not notice doing it. He said he "had a hell of a time. And when I did get it on, it was too heavy and yet I have worn it all my life" (Wright-St Clair et al., 2011, p. 92). A few weeks later, Ferguson was admitted to an aged care facility. In addition, the findings suggested that **compelling occupations**, the things that brought a deep purposefulness to being in the everyday, were not only wellness-promoting but essentially different for Māori and non-Māori. Elder Māori spoke more of doing things with and for the collective Māori community. These phenomenological findings justified the case for testing an open question about people's most important occupations in the LiLACS NZ feasibility study.

Māori participants who chose to be interviewed in their native language were asked, "Ko ēhea ki a koe ngā mea nui rawa atu e toru ka mahia e koe?" Those interviewed in English were asked, "Of all the things you do, which three are the most important to you?" (Wright-St Clair et al., 2012; Wright-St Clair et al., 2017). Participants were invited to begin with their first-in-importance thing. In total, 315 open responses were recorded verbatim. They were coded using the *International Classification of Functioning, Disability and Health* (ICF) (World Health Organization [WHO], 2001) "activities and participation" items then collapsed into the highest level domain codes. The feasibility study showed the ICF was, overall, a useful tool to classify the participants' self-nominated important things they do. However, some culturally specific things named by the elder Māori needed careful interpretation to fit under the standardized ICF items (Wright-St Clair et al., 2012). Acknowledging this limitation, the researchers included the open question about important things people do in the main cohort study (Wright-St Clair et al., 2015).

Six hundred and forty-nine of the 937 cohort study participants answered the question about important occupations; 252 were Māori and 397 non-Māori, of whom 286 were men and 363 were women (Wright-St Clair et al., 2017). The Māori and non-Māori data were examined separately in order to honor each group's cultural heritage. In all, 580 important things done were self-nominated by Māori and 968 by non-Māori. The two datasets were analyzed by ethnicity and gender for those things nominated first in priority and all things named as important. A summary of the findings is presented showing the ICF item codes in speech marks and examples of participants' responses in italics. Across all Māori data, "taking care of plants, indoors and outdoors" was most common for first in importance. The things named included *gardening* and *keeping my grounds tidy*. Next was "reading," such as *reading the newspaper*, then "'Extended family relationships,' such as *communicating with family*, *sharing games with family* and *whānau* (the extended family)" (Wright-St Clair et al., 2017, p. 439). Māori men self-nominated "walking" and "managing diet and fitness" by *continuing to be physically active* or *cycling* as being of primary importance to them. In comparison, Māori women most often nominated *gardening* or "taking care of plants" as the most important thing they did, followed by things such as keeping a *clean and tidy house* or "cleaning the living area." Looking at what non-Māori said, as for Māori, "taking care of plants" like *gardening* and *mowing* were first in importance, followed by "reading." Non-Māori men named things like *boating*, *bowling*, or *golf* or "sports" as being of primary importance, whereas non-Māori women said it was "reading" (Wright-St Clair et al., 2017).

A glimpse at some of the other wave I results suggests participants spent most of their time doing the things that were important to them. For example, in the previous 4 weeks, spending time on a hobby or handicraft every day was something 34% of the elder Māori said they did, compared with 80% of non-Māori; whereas twice as many elder Māori than non-Māori said they visited, or were visited by, family or friends daily. At an interpretive level, the differences may point to spiritual and cultural differences, related to the traditional collective nature of the Māori and the more individualistic focus of non-Māori society.

The next stage of analysis will be examining the relationship between doing important occupations and people's health and longevity outcomes. These data will not show cause and effect; however, they might show that doing particular occupations, that are important to the person, is associated with health and longer life.

Step 3: Develop the Intervention

Because this is a longitudinal study, it will be several years before intervention needs for community-dwelling older adults as well as those living in aged care can be fully identified. What is exciting about the occupational thread in New Zealand's largest cohort study of aging well is the potential to explore the predictive qualities of everyday occupations for health, quality of life, and survival outcomes. Several possible applied research projects are

(continues)

CASE STUDY 9-3   EVERYDAY OCCUPATIONS AND AGING WELL: THE LIFE AND LIVING IN ADVANCED AGE COHORT STUDY NEW ZEALAND: *TE PUĀWAITANGA O NGĀ TAPUWAE KIA ORA TONU* (MĀORI TRANSLATION) *(continued)*

envisioned, such as designing and testing an occupation-based screening tool to identify community-based older adults who are at risk for an acute hospital or aged care facility admission; examining whether enabling participation in valued occupations promotes aging well for older New Zealanders; and testing whether an OT program that enhances participation in occupations that are self-chosen as being important promotes living well for those in aged care facilities. Such questions will only be able to be answered in the context of a systematic program of translational science research. To support translation into practice, the LiLCS NZ Research Program (Ministry of Health, 2017) researchers are making information about the study and summaries of the findings freely available to New Zealanders living in advanced age, their whānau/families, and health practitioners on the Ministry of Health website. Fourteen short reports were publicly available as of May 2017, including "Extra help with daily activities in advanced age," "Participation in Māori society in advanced age," and "Independence in daily activities in advanced age."

Occupational therapists can apply the results by taking older people's diverse preferences into account when working with indigenous and nonindigenous populations. In particular, "participation preferences should be assessed using open questions rather than measures using pre-itemised lists that may exclude personally-, culturally-, gender-important activities" (Wright-St Clair et al., 2017, p. 444).

CENTENNIAL NOTES

Engaging Hearts and Hands: From Seeds to Science

Looking back, the seeds for a science that came to be called "occupational science" were planted by innovative practitioners nearly a century ago. Ora Ruggles's methods for helping soldiers disabled during World War I through engaging of their hearts and hands doing craft-based hobbies were transformative and considered somewhat magical by onlookers (Peloquin, 1995). About the same time, Adolf Meyer (1922/1977) used "occupation—including recreation and any form of helpful enjoyment—as the leading principle" for providing just forms of "treating" the incarcerated.

Although OT as a profession formally began in 1917, it wasn't until the 1980s that a number of scholars proposed that occupational science become a formal academic discipline. The proposal for a doctor of philosophy (PhD) in occupational science was approved at the USC, Los Angeles, in 1989 (Clark et al., 1991). Within a couple of years, word spread that a new science of occupation was being developed somewhere in America. Just hearing the term *occupational science* was sufficient to fire Ann Wilcock's imagination. In rapid succession, she introduced occupational science to Australasia and, in 1993, established the *Journal of Occupational Science: Australia* (Wilcock & Hocking, 2015). Along with conferences, seminars and articles in OT journals, the journal has helped to disseminate knowledge of humans as occupational beings and thus promote acceptance of occupational science among a number of OT scholars as well as those from other disciplines. As the journal's international reach was realised, *Australia* was dropped from the title.

In 1999, the first "meeting of International Society for Occupational Science (ISOS), originally called the International Interdisciplinary Group for the Promotion of Occupational Science, took place in a forum at the OT Australia National Conference in Canberra" (International Society for Occupational Science, n.d.). Shortly after, in 2002, the first U.S.-based Society for the Study of Occupation was formed by a group of scholars meeting in Galveston, Texas (Society for the Study of Occupation: USA, n.d.). Australasia (Australia and New Zealand), Brazil, Canada, Chile, Europe, Ireland, Japan, South Africa, the Republic of China, and the United Kingdom, for example, have since established formal groups to further occupational science knowledge development, research, and practice. The science's global spread is evident in the growing number of OT education providers including "occupational science" in the program and/or school titles. See Wicks (2012) for a comprehensive global history of the field.

Acknowledgments

The authors thank Florence Clark, Jeanine Blanchard, and Mary Law for their commitment to reviewing and contributing essential detail to the case studies.

REFERENCES

Agahi, N., Silverstein, M., & Parker, M. G. (2011). Late-life and earlier participation in leisure activities: Their importance for survival among older persons. *Activities, Adaptation & Aging, 35,* 210–222. doi:10.1080/01924788.2011.596758

American Occupational Therapy Association. (2014). Occupational therapy practice framework: Domain and process (3rd edition). *American Journal of Occupational Therapy, 68*(Suppl. 1), S1–S48. doi:10.5014/ajot.2014.682006

Asbjørnslett, M., & Bekken, W. (2016). Openness to difference: Inclusion in sports occupations for children with (dis)abilities. *Journal of Occupational Science, 23,* 434–445. doi:10.1080/14427591.2016.1199389

Beagan, B. L., & Etowa, J. B. (2011). The meanings and functions of occupations related to spirituality for African Nova Scotian women. *Journal of Occupational Science, 18,* 277–290. doi:10.1080/14427591.2011.594548

Blanche, E. I., Fogelberg, D., Diaz, J., Carlson, M., & Clark, F. (2011). Manualization of occupational therapy interventions: Illustrations from the Pressure Ulcer Prevention Research Program. *American Journal of Occupational Therapy, 65,* 711–719.

Blanche, E. I., & Henny-Kohler, E. (2000). Philosophy, science and ideology: A proposed relationship for occupational science and occupational therapy. *Occupational Therapy International, 7,* 99–110.

Bonsall, A. (2014). "This is what we do": Constructing post-modern families through occupations. *Journal of Occupational Science, 21,* 296–308. doi:10.1080/14427591.2014.914459

CanChild Centre for Childhood Disability Research. (2011). *Measures of participation: CAPE & PAC.* Retrieved from https://www.canchild.ca/en/resources/43-measures-of-children-s-participation-and-enjoyment-cape-pac

Carlson, M., Vigen, C. L. P., Rubayi, S., Blanche, E. I., Blanchard, J., Atkins, M., . . . Clark, F. (2017). Lifestyle intervention for adults with spinal cord injury: Results of the USC–RLANRC Pressure Ulcer Prevention Study. *Journal of Spinal Cord Medicine.* Advance online publication. doi:10.1080/10790268.2017.1313931

Clark, F. A., Jackson, J. M., & Carlson, M. (2004). Occupational science, occupational therapy and evidence-based practice: What the Well Elderly Study has taught us. In M. Molineux (Ed.), *Occupation for occupational therapists* (pp. 200–218). Oxford, United Kingdom: Blackwell.

Clark, F. A., Jackson, J. M., Scott, M. D., Atkins, M. S., Uhles-Tanaka, D., & Rubayi, S. (2006). Data-based models of how pressure ulcers develop in daily-living contexts of adults with spinal cord injury. *Archives of Physical Medicine and Rehabilitation, 87,* 1516–1525. doi:10.1016/j.apmr.2006.08.329

Clark, F. A., & Lawlor, M. C. (2009). The making and mattering of occupational science. In E. B. Crepeau, E. S. Cohn, & B. A. Schell (Eds.), *Willard & Spackman's occupational therapy* (11th ed., pp. 2–14). Philadelphia, PA: Lippincott Williams & Wilkins.

Clark, F. A., Parham, D., Carlson, M. E., Frank, G., Jackson, J., Pierce, D., . . . Zemke, R. (1991). Occupational science: Academic innovation in the service of occupational therapy's future. *American Journal of Occupational Therapy, 45,* 300–310.

Clark, F. A., Pyatak, E. A., Carlson, M., Blanche, E. I., Vigen, C., Jay, J., . . . Azen, S. P. (2014). Implementing trials of complex interventions in community settings: The USC-Rancho Los Amigos Pressure Ulcer Prevention Study (PUPS). *Clinical Trials, 11,* 218–229. doi:10.1177/1740774514521904

Clark, F. A., Sanders, K., Carlson, M., Blanche, E., & Jackson, J. (2007). Synthesis of habit theory. *OTJR: Occupation, Participation and Health, 27*(Suppl. 1), 7S–23S.

Cogan, A. (2016). White matter abnormalities in blast mild traumatic brain injuries in the military. *Journal of Occupational Science, 23,* 339–351. doi:10.1080/14427591.2015.1113494

Cogan, A. M., Blanche, E. I., Diaz, J., Clark, F. A., & Chun, S. (2014). Building a framework for implementing new interventions. *OTJR: Occupation, Participation and Health, 34,* 209–220. doi:10.3928/15394492-20141009-01

Collins, S. (2016, September 30). Arrivals face burden of loneliness. *The New Zealand Herald,* p. A9.

Coster, W., Bedell, G., Law, M., Khetani, M. A., Teplicky, R., Liljenquist, K., . . . Yao, K. C. (2011). Psychometric evaluation of the Participation and Environment Measure for Children and Youth (PEM-CY). *Developmental Medicine and Child Neurology, 53,* 1030–1037.

Crawford, E., Turpin, M., Nayar, S., Steel, E., & Durand, J.-L. (2016). The structural-personal interaction: Occupational deprivation and asylum seekers in Australia. *Journal of Occupational Science, 23,* 321–338. doi:10.1080/14427591.2016.1153510

de Poy, E., & Gitlin, L. N. (2016). *Introduction to research: Understanding and applying multiple strategies* (5th ed.). St. Louis, MO: Elsevier.

de Saint-Exupéry, A. (1972). *The little prince* (K. Woods, Trans.). London, United Kingdom: Penguin Books.

Dunstan, K., & Thomson, N. (2006). *Demographic aspects of New Zealand's ageing population.* Wellington, New Zealand: Statistics New Zealand.

Fritz, H., & Cutchin, M. P. (2017). Changing neighborhoods and occupations: Experiences of older African-Americans in Detroit. *Journal of Occupational Science, 24,* 140–151. doi:10.1080/14427591.2016.1269296

Fushiki, Y., Ohnishi, H., Sakauchi, F., Oura, A., & Mori, M. (2012). Relationship of hobby activities with mortality and frailty among community-dwelling elderly adults: Results of a follow-up study in Japan. *Journal of Epidemiology, 22,* 340–347. doi:10.2188/jea.JE20110057

Gerlach, A. J., Teachman, G., Laliberte-Rudman, D., Aldrich, R. M., & Huot, S. (2017). Expanding beyond individualism: Engaging critical perspectives on occupation. *Scandinavian Journal of Occupational Therapy, 25,* 35–43. doi:10.1080/11038128.2017.1327616

Ghaisas, S., Pyatak, E. A., Blanche, E., Blanchard, J., & Clark, F. (2015). Lifestyle changes and pressure ulcer prevention in adults with spinal cord injury in the Pressure Ulcer Prevention Study Lifestyle Intervention. *American Journal of Occupational Therapy, 69,* 6901290020p1–6901290020p10. doi:10.5014/ajot.2015.012021

Glass, T. A., Mendes de Leon, C., Marottoli, R. A., & Berkman, L. F. (1999). Population based study of social and productive activities as predictors of survival among elderly Americans. *BMJ, 319,* 478–483.

Guerra, N. G., & Leidy, M. S. (2010). Conducting translational research on child development in community settings: What you need to know and why it is worth the effort. In V. Maholmes & C. G. Lomonaco (Eds.), *Applied research in child and adolescent development: A practical guide* (pp. 155–173). New York, NY: Psychology Press.

Harper, D. (n.d.). *Online etymology dictionary.* Retrieved from http://www.etymonline.com/index.php?search=system&searchmode=none

Hayman, K., Kerse, N., Dyall, L., Kepa, M., Teh, R. O., Wham, C., . . . Jatrana, S. (2012). Life and living in advanced age: A cohort study in New Zealand—Te Puāwaitanga o Nga Tapuwae Kia Ora Tonu, LILACS NZ: Study protocol. *BMC Geriatrics, 12,* 33. doi:10.1186/1471-2318-12-33

Imms, C., King, G., Majnemer, A., Avery, L., Chiarello, L., Palisano, R., . . . Law, M. (2017). Leisure participation–preference congruence of children with cerebral palsy: A Children's Assessment of Participation and Enjoyment International Network descriptive study. *Developmental Medicine & Child Neurology, 59,* 380–387. doi:10.1111/dmcn.13302

International Society for Occupational Science. (n.d). *ISOS history, 1999*. Retrieved from http://isos.nfshost.com/history.php

Jackson, J., Carlson, M., Rubayi, S., Scott, M. D., Atkins, M. S., Blanche, E. I., . . . Clark, F. A. (2010). Qualitative study of principles pertaining to lifestyle and pressure ulcer risk in adults with spinal cord injury. *Disability and Rehabilitation, 32*, 567–578.

Jones, M., Hocking, C., & McPherson, K. (2017). Communities with participation-enabling skills: A study children with traumatic brain injury and their shared occupations. *Journal of Occupational Science, 24*, 88–104. doi:10.1080/14427591.2016.1224444

Kantartzis, S., & Molineux, M. (2011). The influence of Western society's construction of a healthy daily life on the conceptualisation of occupation. *Journal of Occupational Science, 18*, 62–80. doi:10.1080/14427591.2011.566917

Katz, S. (2000). Busy bodies: Activity, aging, and the management of everyday life. *Journal of Aging Studies, 14*, 135–152.

Kottorp, A., Nygård, L., Hedman, A., Öhman, A., Malinowsky, C., Rosenberg, L., . . . & Ryd, C. (2016). Comment: Access to and use of everyday technology among older people: An occupational justice issue—but for whom? *Journal of Occupational Science, 23*, 382–388. doi:10.1080/14427591.2016.1151457

Lala, A. P., & Kinsella, E. A. (2011). Phenomenology and the study of human occupation. *Journal of Occupational Science, 18*, 195–209. doi:10.1080/14427591.2011.581629

Law, M. (2011). *Participation of children and youth with disabilities in recreation and leisure activities*. Hamilton, Ontario, Canada: CanChild Centre for Childhood Disability Research.

Law, M., Baptiste, S., Carswell, A., McColl, M. A., Polatajko, H., & Pollock, N. (2005). *Canadian Occupational Performance Measure* (4th ed.). Ottawa, Ontario, Canada: Canadian Association of Occupational Therapists.

Law, M., Darrah, J., Pollock, N., Rosenbaum, P., Russell, D., Walter, S. D., . . . Wright, V. (2007). Focus on function—a randomized controlled trial comparing two rehabilitation interventions for young people with cerebral palsy. *BMC Pediatrics, 7*, 31. doi:10.1186/1471-2431-7-31

Law, M., Darrah, J., Pollock, N., Wilson, B., Russell, D. J., Walter, S. D., . . . Galuppi, B. (2011). Focus on function: A cluster, randomized controlled trial comparing child- versus context-focused intervention for young people with cerebral palsy. *Developmental Medicine & Child Neurology, 53*, 621–629. doi:10.1111/j.1469-8749.2011.03962.x

Law, M., King, G., Rosenbaum, P., Kertoy, M., King, S., Young, N., . . . Hurley, P. (2005). *Participate Study: Final report to families and community partners on the Participate Study findings*. Hamilton, Ontario, Canada: CanChild Centre for Childhood Disability Research.

Lim, C. Y., Law, M., Khetani, M., Pollock, N., & Rosenbaum, P. (2016a). Establishing the cultural equivalence of the Young Children's Participation and Environment Measure (YC-PEM) for use in Singapore. *Physical & Occupational Therapy in Pediatrics, 36*, 422–439. doi:10.3109/01942638.2015.1101044

Lim, C. Y., Law, M., Khetani, M., Pollock, N., & Rosenbaum, P. (2016b). Participation in out-of-home environments for young children with and without developmental disabilities. *OTJR: Occupation, Participation and Health, 36*, 112–125. doi:10.1177/1539449216659859

Löwing, K., Bexelius, A., & Brogren Carlberg, E. (2009). Activity focused and goal directed therapy for children with cerebral palsy—do goals make a difference? *Disability Rehabilitation, 31*, 1808–1816.

Luck, K., & Beagan, B. (2015). Occupational transition of smoking cessation in women: "You're restructuring your whole life." *Journal of Occupational Science, 22*, 183–196. doi:10.1080/14427591.2014.887418

McGrath, M., & McGonagle, H. (2016). Exploring 'wicked problems' from an occupational perspective: The case of turf cutting in rural Ireland. *Journal of Occupational Science, 23*, 308–320. doi:10.1080/14427591.2016.1169437

Menec, V. H. (2003). The relation between everyday activities and successful aging: A 6-year longitudinal study. *The Journals of Gerontology. Series B, Psychological Sciences and Social Sciences, 58*, S74–S82.

Meyer, A. (1977). The philosophy of occupation therapy. *Archives of Occupational Therapy, 31*, 639–642. (Original work published 1922)

Ministry of Health. (2017). *The LiLACS NZ Research Programme*. Retrieved from http://www.health.govt.nz/our-work/life-stages/health-older-people/lilacs-nz-research-programme

Molineux, M. (Ed.). (2004). *Occupation for occupational therapists*. Oxford, United Kingdom: Blackwell.

Morgan, W. J. (2010). What, exactly, is occupational satisfaction? *Journal of Occupational Science, 17*, 216–223. doi:10.1080/14427591.2010.9686698

Ostensjø, S., Oien, I., & Fallang, B. (2008). Goal-oriented rehabilitation of preschoolers with cerebral palsy—a multi-case study of combined use of the Canadian Occupational Performance Measure (COPM) and the Goal Attainment Scaling (GAS). *Developmental Neurorehabilitation, 11*, 252–259.

Pashmdarfard, M., Amini, M., & Hassani Mehraban, A. (2017). Participation of Iranian cerebral palsy children in life areas: A systematic review. *Iranian Journal of Child Neurology, 11*(1), 1–12.

Peloquin, S. M. (1995). The fullness of empathy: Reflections and illustrations. *American Journal of Occupational Therapy, 49*, 24–31.

Pierce, D. (Ed.). (2011). *Occupational science for occupational therapy*. Thorofare, NJ: SLACK.

Pollard, N., & Carver, N. (2016). Building model trains and planes: An autoethnographic investigation of a human occupation. *Journal of Occupational Science, 23*, 168–180. doi:10.1080/14427591.2016.1153509

Pollock, N., Stewart, D., Law, M., Sahagian-Whalen, S., Harvey, S., & Toal, C. (1997). The meaning of play for young people with physical disabilities. *Canadian Journal of Occupational Therapy, 64*, 25–31.

Smith, V. (2017). Energizing everyday practices through the indigenous spirituality of haka. *Journal of Occupational Science, 24*, 9–18. doi:10.1080/14427591.2017.1280838

Society for the Study of Occupation: USA. (n.d.). *Society information: History*. Retrieved from https://ssou.memberclicks.net/history

Statistics New Zealand. (2015a). *2013 Census QuickStats about people aged 65 and over*. Retrieved from http://www.stats.govt.nz

Statistics New Zealand. (2015b). *How is our Māori population changing?* Retrieved from http://www.stats.govt.nz/browse_for_stats/people_and_communities/maori/maori-population-article-2015.aspx

Turner Goins, R., Schure, M. B., Crowder, J., Baldridge, D., Benson, W., & Aldrich, N. (2015). *Lifelong disparities among older American Indians and Alaska Natives*. Washington, DC, AARP Public Policy Institute.

University of Southern California. (2013). *USC/Rancho Lifestyle Redesign® pressure ulcer prevention project*. Retrieved from http://pups.usc.edu

Waldman-Levi, A., & Bundy, A. (2016). A glimpse into co-occupations: Parent/caregiver's support of Young Children's Playfulness Scale. *Occupational Therapy in Mental Health, 32*, 217–227. doi:10.1080/0164212X.2015.1116420

Wicks, A. (2012). The International Society for Occupational Science: A critique of its role in facilitating the development of occupational science through international networks and intercultural dialogue. In G. Whiteford & C Hocking (Eds.), *Occupational science: Society, inclusion, participation* (pp. 163–183). Oxford, United Kingdom: Blackwell.

Wilcock, A. A., & Hocking, C. (2015). *An occupational perspective of health* (3rd ed.). Thorofare, NJ: SLACK.

Williams, K. (2017). Understanding the role of sensory processing in occupation: An updated discourse with cognitive neuroscience. *Journal of Occupational Science, 24*, 302–313. doi:10.1080/14427591.2016.1209425

Wiseman, J. O., Davis, J. A., & Polatajko, H. J. (2005). Occupational development: Towards an understanding of children's doing, *Journal of Occupational Science, 12,* 26–35. doi:10.1080/14427591.2005 .9686545

World Health Organization. (2001). *International classification of functioning, disability and health.* Geneva, Switzerland: Author.

Wright-St Clair, V. A., Kepa, M., Hoenle, S., Hayman, K., Keeling, S., Connolly, M., . . . Kerse, N. (2012). Doing what's important: Valued activities for elder New Zealand Māori and non-Māori. *Australasian Journal on Ageing.* Retrieved from http://onlinelibrary.wiley.com /journal/10.1111/%28ISSN%291741-6612/earlyview

Wright-St Clair, V. A., Kerse, N., & Smythe, L. (2011). Doing everyday occupations both conceals and reveals the phenomenon of being aged. *Australian Occupational Therapy Journal, 58,* 88–94. doi:10.1111/j.1440-1630.2010.00885.x

Wright-St Clair, V. A., Rapson, A., Kepa, M., Connolly, M., Keeling, S., . . . Kerse, N. (2017). Ethnic and gender differences in preferred activities among Māori and non-Māori of advanced age in New Zealand. *Journal of Cross-Cultural Gerontology, 32*(4), 433–446. doi:10.1007/s10823-017-9324-6

Wright-St Clair, V. A., & Smythe, E. A. (2012). Being occupied in the everyday. In M. Cutchin & V. Dickie (Eds.), *Transactional perspectives on occupation* (pp. 25–37). New York, NY: Springer.

Zemke, R., & Clark, F. (1996). Preface. In R. Zemke & F. Clark (Eds.), *Occupational science: The evolving discipline* (pp. vii–xviii). Philadelphia, PA: F. A. Davis.

the**Point**® *For additional resources on the subjects discussed in this chapter, visit* **http://thePoint.lww.com /Willard-Spackman13e.**

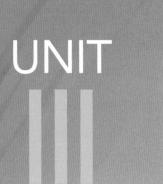

UNIT III

Narrative Perspectives on Occupation and Disability

Roll-in Shower

Phil and me in the roll-in shower
both getting totally soaked
as I wash his hair and skinny boy body.
Hot steam roiling up around us
as we look out the windows of the basement,
we're not caring how much snow is piled up
out there in Minnesota this sunny day.

This house on the bluff, each section built
with love by Phil's traveling dad.
He sketched and planned every detail
of this barrier-free shower
for his well-loved, wheelchair-bound,
youngest son.

> —Pat Adams, Mother to three sons, two of
> whom had muscular dystrophy
> Used with permission of the author.

Narrative as a Key to Understanding

Ellen S. Cohn, Elizabeth Blesedell Crepeau

LEARNING OBJECTIVES

After reading this chapter, you will be able to:

1. Explain the relationship between experience, narrative, and the interpretive process.
2. Identify ways to begin to think about narratives and how they may influence clients' experience and occupational therapy intervention.
3. Analyze the role of narratives in occupational therapy practice.
4. Explain why listening to clients' stories is an essential component of occupational therapy practice.

Introduction

Think back over the past few days. How many times have you told a story about an experience you had? How many times have you listened to a story told you by a friend or family member? We tell stories all the time about the things that we did or that happened to us and to others as a way to share and interpret our experience. In fact, we could be called *Homo narratus* rather than *Homo sapiens* because of the centrality of storytelling to human experience (Fisher, 1984). Some people are better storytellers than others. Good storytellers can infuse their narratives with tension, drama, and suspense, but regardless of how well the story is told, it is human nature to tell or listen to stories (Figure 10-1). The capacity to understand the world through stories can begin early in life. For example, some children learn to listen to stories even before they can speak (Figure 10-2). Consequently, it is not surprising that occupational therapy (OT) clients and their family members have stories to tell about their experiences with injury, disease, or disability. This unit is devoted to these stories, written by the people themselves, their family members, or by an occupational therapist who listened to, translated, and interpreted stories of people living with disabilities. Because stories of OT practitioners are also important to understand, the narrative perspective of practitioners from various practice contexts is included in Unit XIII. That two units are devoted to these narratives indicates the importance of the narrative perspectives of the people who seek and provide OT and how essential narrative is to the entire OT process.

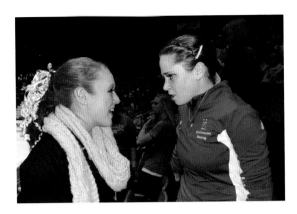

FIGURE 10-1 Stories can be filled with drama and surprise. (Photo courtesy of Ellen S. Cohn.)

In the 1980s, social scientists were rediscovering the significance of narrative to understand human experience, and there was a tremendous growth of interest in patients' stories in the health care fields (J. A. Clark & Mishler, 1992; Kleinman, 1980; Mishler, 1984; Polkinghorne, 1988). The interest in patients' stories of living with illness emerged from a "dehumanized" and highly technological approach to health care that lacked sufficient attention to the personal aspects of experience. This "narrative turn" in OT occurred in the mid-1980s when an anthropologist, Cheryl Mattingly, directed a clinical reasoning study, an ethnographic study of occupational therapists in a large teaching hospital (Mattingly & Fleming, 1994). In her observations of therapists throughout their work day, Mattingly noted that therapists used different forms of talk to discuss their work with clients. Therapists used what Mattingly referred to as "chart talk," a formal reporting register that typically occurred during team meetings and

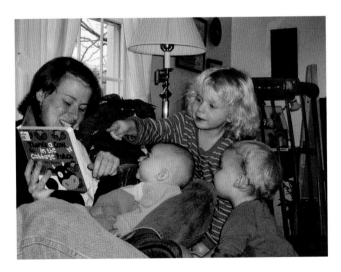

FIGURE 10-2 Reading to children orients them to the power of stories. (Photo courtesy of Elizabeth Blesedell Crepeau.)

other structured situations to describe the technical and reimbursable aspects of practice. In contrast, therapists told stories during lunch and other times to describe the rich, more interpretive aspects of their meaningful interactions with clients. These stories had all the elements that we have come to expect from a story: a plot, drama, suspense, action, and a moral or lesson.

Mattingly's work legitimized the telling of stories as an interpretive process that helped therapists to make sense of their experience. This influential work also focused attention on the value of OT practitioners listening to clients' stories, for it is through storytelling that clients convey the meaning of their experiences. Moving beyond listening and telling stories, Mattingly noted that clients and OT practitioners collaboratively create new or different "meaningful" life narratives in the context of living with disease or disability. She introduced the idea that OT intervention involved a "narrative" process in which the therapy involved a dramatic plot transforming therapy into a path of recovery that instilled hope, healing, and a new future (Mattingly, 2010). In addition, the importance of narrative during the OT assessment process has been recognized (Franits, 2005; Simmons, Crepeau, & White, 2000).

Since then, a significant amount of research in OT has examined narrative from the perspective of clients (Alsaker & Josephsson, 2010; Howie, Coulter, & Feldman, 2004), their families (Cohn, 2001; Isaksson, Josephsson, Lexell, & Skär, 2008), students (Pizzi, 2015), and therapists (Labovitz, 2003; Mattingly, 1991). The narrative turn has influenced research on how storytelling influences the clinical reasoning of team members (Crepeau, 2000), how health care students experience and process ethical dilemmas (Monrouxe, Rees, Endacott, & Ternan, 2014), and how people with HIV experience stigma (Winskell et al., 2015). Finally, narrative research has helped us understand the importance of the alignment of practitioner and client stories (Cohn et al., 2009; Crepeau & Garren, 2011).

Narrative and Story

There are numerous ways to define *narrative* and *story*. In some traditions, particularly literary theory, *narrative* and *story* refer to distinct phenomena. However, in this chapter, we will use *narrative* and *story* equivalently (as do Mattingly & Garro, 2000; Polkinghorne, 1988; Riessman, 2008). In everyday speech, stories are quite common, perhaps so natural that they do not need explaining. Stories are told from the perspective of the speaker. They may be told and retold because they provide a way of understanding and interpreting experience—sharing what is meaningful and important at a moment in time rather than a mere accounting of some objective truth (Leight, 2002). Stories are temporally and contextually situated, and although we think a story may be finished, stories are open for new tellings, new interpretations, and new meanings. Consequently, the same story may vary in relation to who tells the story, when it is told, the way it is told, or its purpose for the intended audience (Bruner, 1991). Although common, stories are incredibly complex and quite difficult to describe. Nonetheless, as Gorman (2008) argues, it is through storytelling that we gain the capacity to understand those who seek our care and to use their stories to guide our clinical decision making. In a very fundamental way, stories concern action and offer a way to make sense of experiences. By linking narrative, act, and consequence, stories offer us windows on social life and human character.

In this chapter, we will draw on Mattingly's definition: "Stories are about someone trying to do something, and what happens to her and others as a result" (Mattingly, 1998, p. 7). Consider an excerpt from Gloria Dickerson's chapter (see Chapter 13). Gloria's story has numerous features that make stories especially appealing for understanding her experiences in living with severe mental illness and trauma. Gloria's story is event-centered, concerns human action and interaction, and includes the social aspects of human behavior.

As the narrator of these stories, Gloria carefully selects the relevant details to direct our attention to her multiple plot lines. Her stories illustrate how enduring family stories, told and retold, can shape our identities. Gloria, now a 64-year-old woman, starts her stories by orienting us to the characters and setting, placing herself in the context of her family. The "early years" stories serve a referential function. In telling about the things that happened to her, she provides a retrospective glance at past events. She narrates the sequence of events in a way to convey her message and ultimately communicates to the reader that she has amazing endurance and hope and that feeling connected and valued as an adult is vital to who she is as a person. She tells and comments on her stories at the same time, as if she is talking directly to you, the reader, to emphasize her view. And her stories have a deep moral message: Gloria's stories teach us that recovery is not an end but a continuing process, an ongoing story. That is, interpretations and reinterpretations of stories are always possible.

Gloria's stories are dialectical, they move back and forth between cyclical pain-filled struggles and endurance and survival. Two seemingly conflicting plot lines are both essential. In these stories, Gloria tells what happened in her life and how she and her mother shared an unspoken pride of being defiant and resilient. Yet, the same mother who shared her survivor legacy with Gloria was the source of incredibly painful life experiences and actions that Gloria did not understand as a child. These dialectical stories highlight the value of listening for multiple plot lines to gain an understanding of the whole.

Listening for Meaning

Frank (1995, 2002) argues that in listening to patients' stories, health care practitioners bear witness to suffering as well as to personal strengths and triumphs. Listening enables practitioners to "seeing, feeling, and hearing life differently" (Kirkpatrick, 2008, p. 63). Kirkpatrick (2008) urges health care practitioners to listen to and strive to understand narratives at multiple levels, being sensitive to the narrative types from the culture that might frame the stories. Although client narratives represent the client's

NOTES

Narrative as a Window to Lived Experience

Telling, listening to, and interpreting stories is our way of making sense of human experience. The profession's focus on engagement in occupation requires an appreciation of the lived experience of the performer and an investigation of human motives. The first edition of what we now call *Willard & Spackman's Occupational Therapy* reflected the medical and rehabilitation models that predominated health care while simultaneously recognizing the importance of the patient's needs (Gleave, 1947) and psychological response to disability (Spackman, 1947). In subsequent editions, understanding patient perspectives included being encouraging, friendly, and courteous, not showing racial, religious, or political prejudices (Fay & Kellogg, 1954), maintaining "continuous and systematic" reciprocity in communication, and considering the person as a whole "not merely as a case" (Spackman, 1971, p. 154). Tiffany's (1978) discussion of the interview process in a mental health setting expands the initial interview to include more social factors such as the person's living situation, work or school history, social supports, and hopes for the future. The eight edition reflects the emerging influence of the narrative reasoning (Fleming, 1993; Mattingly & Beer, 1993). Subsequent editions have further articulated the centrality of narrative in OT (Hamilton, 2008).

past and current perspectives, they are also shaped by dominant narratives in the culture (Kirkpatrick, 2008). Consequently, although the same diagnosis may confer similar experiences to individuals, these individuals are quite likely to tell very different stories based on their life history, including their socioeconomic status, ethnicity, religion, and other individual attributes and the cultural narratives available to them. For example, until very recently, the cultural narrative available to girls and young women was very narrow and focused mainly on finding a husband and raising a family limiting the view of girls to envision a different future (Coontz, 2011).

Narrative as an Interpretive Process

Creating stories or narratives is an interpretive process that involves selecting aspects of past experience and representing that experience to others in the present (Bruner, 1991). Because storytelling is interpretive, the way in which an individual interprets the past may be strongly influenced by present circumstances (Figure 10-3). This does not mean that storytelling is a fabrication; rather, stories are constructed to present a coherent interpretation of the past in light of the present.

There are two ways of interpreting stories. The first focuses on types of illness narratives delineated by Frank. The second takes a more cultural perspective. Frank (1995) listened to illness and disability stories of others and read personal accounts of illness and disability. Through this process, he identified three types of illness narratives: restitution, chaos, and quest narratives. These narrative types might not be the only types of illness narratives, but Frank

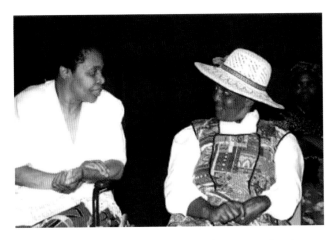

FIGURE 10-3 Storytelling provides a mechanism for shared understanding. (Photo courtesy of Theresa Lorenzo.)

reported that they presented themselves in many of the stories he listened to and read. Individuals may use one or more of the types in one story or may shift narrative types depending on the standpoint from which they are telling the story.

Clients telling a restitution story show how medicine has resolved their problems to return them to health (Frank, 1995). Clients often tell restitution stories retrospectively, but they might also use this story form to project themselves into the future. A plotline might involve a major surgical intervention, such as a joint replacement, followed by rehabilitation and ultimate return to former occupational pursuits. These stories are easy to listen to because they represent the triumph of Western medicine. In contrast, Frank (1995) asserts that chaos narratives are the most difficult to hear because, unlike the restitution narrative, they are not sequenced by a plotline that we are socialized to follow. Chaos narratives represent an out-of-control life with no obvious solutions. They are characterized by events that are connected by phrases such as "and then . . . and then . . . and then . . . ." This lack of causal ordering or plot renders the telling hard to understand because the person is still enmeshed in the experience. Quest narratives, in contrast, show the personal transformation that can occur when clients confront serious illness and disability and, as a result, make fundamental changes in their lives. Simi Linton's book (2006), *My Body Politic: A Memoir*, is an example of a quest narrative. Now, 35 years after a car accident, this disability rights activist recounts her "coming out"—a transformation from early challenges with paraplegia and the marginalization of people with disabilities to promoting the contributions of people with disabilities to society. Her book invites the reader to consider the negative stereotypes attributed to people with disability, particularly its negative representation in society and the arts. This negative representation of people with disabilities is an example of the prejudicial master narrative Kirkpatrick (2008) asserts is so disempowering to those without power.

Master narratives represent the values of a culture, which may reflect the power of the dominant members of society and the prejudices held by them (Kirkpatrick, 2008). These master narratives may become stereotypes, which suppress the individuality of people and convey negative attitudes and prejudices. People who lack power—the poor, disabled, or racial or ethnic minority members—are particularly vulnerable to negative narratives that oppress and deprive them of opportunities. Kirkpatrick (2008) proposes three levels of narratives: personal stories, community narratives, and dominant cultural narratives. Kirkpatrick, drawing on the work of Clandinin and Connelly (2000), argues that personal stories incorporate (1) individual experience as it is reflected through a temporal lens of past, present, and future; (2) the social interaction that occurs during the storytelling and how this process shapes the story; and (3) place, which provides the social and environmental context containing either opportunities or barriers to the individual. Second, community narratives reflect the communal stories of a group of people. For example, family stories can reflect positive or negative aspects about an individual within the family structure. These stories can be shaped and reshaped over time, both at the level of the family and by the individual. Third, dominant cultural narratives present master narratives of different groups of people. These are stereotypes that provide a shorthand way of characterizing a group. Although master narratives may present those without power in a negative fashion, counter-narratives such as Linton's have the power to reshape these negative narratives and provide more positive master narratives for individuals and communities. Gloria's story offers a counterstory to a master narrative.

We learn about Gloria's experiences of living in the Southern United States in the 1950s and how she constructs her sense of self in the context of social and economic inequalities. The subjective experience of people who have been marginalized is often denied in the dominant culture and exploring such narratives may help us engage with patients as socially positioned people (Stone-Mediatore, 2003). Holland and colleagues' integration of identity theories and cultural studies directs our attention to the idea that "identities are lived in and through activity and must be conceptualized as they develop in specific social situations from the cultural resources at hand" (Holland, Lachiotte, Skinner, & Cain, 1998, p. 4). The field of cultural studies advocates exploring identity in the flow of historically, socially, culturally, and physically constructed lives as well as examining the impact of social positioning in the process of self-identification. Gloria's stories remind us that understanding the historical context of her childhood is essential. She also reminds us that behavior is mediated by senses of self, which implies that there is no presumption that a person has only one sense of self or a consistency of self across contexts. Gloria's story is situated in an African-American cultural experience which includes a legacy of mistrust. We recognize the heterogeneity in African Americans as cultures are dynamic processes, constantly being interpreted and reinterpreted, consciously and unconsciously. Consideration of the sociohistorical situatedness of Gloria's narrative, however, offers the potential for a particular understanding. Thus, we read Gloria's narrative in the context of this historical legacy. She places her experiences within the context of the grand narratives of racism and sexism within U.S. culture and ultimately shows readers how she shapes her future actions by reflecting on her experience to rewrite and live out a new life story.

Gloria, in telling her individual story, also illustrates how we may compose stories by adopting the narratives available in our culture. Her story is also situated in a paradigm shift within the mental health field over the past two decades (Farkas, 2007). The recovery movement in mental health has done much to help rewrite the master narrative about mental illness and has provided ways for individuals and programs to use these narratives to foster recovery. Community or shared narratives within a group of people can influence members' view of themselves. Health care systems or OT departments, as a form of community narrative, can influence and shape our experience in either empowering or constraining ways. The community narrative of the Boston University Center for Psychiatric Rehabilitation influenced Gloria's recovery by providing context in which she could recognize her options and develop a valued role in life. In this way, the community narrative can be an important element in the change process. In an important and powerfully reciprocal manner, individual stories can impact the community narrative. For example, Gloria's story is a moving account of her recovery and can be instrumental in influencing the community narrative to embrace a strengths-based recovery perspective rather than a disease- and deficit-oriented community narrative.

Gloria's story is worth telling because it conveys to the reader a unique recovery process that she feels is important for us to understand. We can share in Gloria's gratitude that she is proud of how far she has come in her life. We have learned a lot about Gloria. We know she is an intelligent woman who finds it healing to focus on what she can accomplish. She is an effective storyteller who can incorporate drama and irony into her storytelling. By listening to our clients' stories, we can understand their interpretation of their experience and begin to discern who they are as individuals, their illness or disability experience, and how this experience has shaped their daily occupations. The interpretive process of storytelling helps to differentiate our clients from each other, even those with very similar medical and social histories. Although we may work with many clients with the same diagnosis, their lived experience and the stories they tell about their lives will be as important as their particular occupational problems in shaping the way in which we work with them to plan and implement their OT intervention.

Understanding Client Narratives

Drawing on Riessman's (1993) delineation of the multiple levels of representation of experience in narrative analysis, we propose that the chapters in this unit have several levels of representation. These levels are (1) the author's attention to the experience in the moment, (2) the telling of this experience in the writing of the chapter, (3) the editorial process, and (4) the interpretation derived from reading the chapter. First of all, just as Gloria was selective, other storytellers select what is important or meaningful to them at that moment. Second, the editors of *Willard & Spackman's Occupational Therapy* asked the chapter authors to tell their story to make it accessible to you. In doing so, the authors have ordered and interpreted events to create a coherent account that you, as the reader, can understand. Because they were asked to write about their experience for OT students, their stories are told from that standpoint. Their chapters might have a different focus if they were writing for a different audience. In this sense, the chapters are "constructed" for a certain purpose, to convey their experience to readers who will someday be working with people who might have had similar experiences with illness or disability. Thus, the chapters are positioned to reflect experience from a particular interpretive lens: "Let me tell you my story so that you will understand the experience of your future clients." In fact, some authors end their chapters by addressing you directly as future occupational therapists to be sure that you understand the importance of their message. The third level of the process involves editing the chapter, which may further shape the story. The editors of these chapters tried to sustain the perspective of the authors while helping them to bring clarity and order to their writing. This is a delicate process because in editing, there is always the risk of changing the representation of their experience by shaping of it. Finally, you will bring your own interpretive process to your reading of these chapters. How you react to these powerful stories will teach you much about your worldview.

The Role of Narrative in Occupational Therapy Practice

Storytelling

Occupational therapy practice provides many opportunities to listen to and elicit stories from clients and to tell clients' stories as a form of motivation or to help them see themselves in therapeutic plots (Mattingly, 1998). Occupational therapists also tell stories to each other while socializing and during team meetings and other interdisciplinary forms of communication (Crepeau, 2000). They might tell puzzling stories to each other to make sense of what happened or determine how they should proceed with a client. They may also use stories to persuade others of a point of view or insight about a client. For example, an occupational therapist used a very persuasive account of a patient in a geropsychiatric unit to reformulate the patient's problem from one of refusal to participate in the milieu to one of an inability to participate. The occupational therapist's interpretation of the client's story proved to be a turning point for the team in planning care for this person (Crepeau, 2000). Consequently, the therapist's interpretation of the client's behavior reconstructed the team's view and plans for the client's care.

Storymaking

Although this chapter has focused on storytelling as a way to interpret and share experience, stories do not simply look back and interpret past events in light of the present. Mattingly proposed that narratives can shape action and that OT intervention involves a prospective "therapeutic emplotment" in which clients and therapists create new narratives; that is, new "stories are created in clinical time" (Mattingly, 2000, p. 183). She argued that therapists and clients create a collaborative intervention process to understand and enable clients to move from where or who they are to where or who they want to be (Mattingly, 1991, 1998). Elaborating on Mattingly's argument, F. Clark (1993) introduced the term *occupational storymaking* to describe how occupational therapists engage people in desired occupations to rewrite, revise, or recreate their life story and imagine new possibilities. As clients engage in desired occupations and experience their potential to participate in desired activities, a new story is enacted in the intervention process. F. Clark described her intervention with Penny Richardson, a colleague who experienced a cerebral aneurysm at the age of 47 years. Because F. Clark listened to Penny and understood her life story, F. Clark and Penny were able to identify Penny's challenges to engagement in desired occupations and rewrite potential solutions to occupational problems. In one example of the process, F. Clark and Penny identified the walker as a constant reminder of Penny's continued balance problems and a symbol of disability. Before the aneurysm, Penny enjoyed outdoor activities, was an avid hiker, and pushed herself to be physically competent. Recycling her familiar story lines and attending to her motives to remove stigmatizing barriers, Penny began what she called "cane hiking" to transition from walking with a walker to using a cane. This and other redefined occupations enabled Penny to connect her former self to her new self.

Conclusion

Our purpose in writing this chapter is to give you a very brief overview of the importance of narrative to OT practice. Our hope is that you will read the chapters in this unit and will approach working with others with a respect

BOX 10-1   NARRATIVES: QUESTIONS TO CONSIDER

1. What is the plot of the chapter and what is the moral of the story?
2. What are major themes represented in the story?
3. What insights have you gained from the stories in these chapters?
4. If you were an occupational therapist for these individuals, how would their narratives shape your work with them?
5. Whose stories get heard?
6. How could the story be told another way?
7. Identify the elements of hope in the story you read and consider how you might integrate hopefulness into your interactions and interventions.

for the importance of narrative to understand how people interpret their experience and how storytelling and storymaking can be used as part of the therapeutic process. By seeking client stories, you will discover the richness of their lives, their fears, and their hopes and dreams. This deeper understanding of their unique perspective will help you create with them a story filled with hope for the future. As you read the following chapters, consider the questions listed in Box 10-1.

REFERENCES

Alsaker, S., & Josephsson, S. (2010). Occupation and meaning: Narrative in everyday activities of women with chronic rheumatic conditions. *OTJR: Occupation, Participation and Health, 30,* 58–67.

Bruner, J. (1991). The narrative construction of reality. *Critical Inquiry, 18,* 1–21.

Clandinin, D. J., & Connelly, F. M. (2000). *Narrative inquiry: Experience and story in qualitative research.* San Francisco, CA: Jossey-Bass.

Clark, F. (1993). Occupation embedded in a real life: Interweaving occupational science and occupational therapy. 1993 Eleanor Clarke Slagle Lecture. *American Journal of Occupational Therapy, 47,* 1067–1078.

Clark, J. A., & Mishler, E. G. (1992). Attending to patients' stories: Reframing the clinical task. *Sociology of Health & Illness, 14,* 344–372.

Cohn, E. S. (2001). From waiting to relating: Parents' experiences in the waiting room of an occupational therapy clinic. *American Journal of Occupational Therapy, 55,* 167–174.

Cohn, E. S., Cortés, D. E., Hook, J. M., Yinusa-Nyahkoon, L. S., Solomon, J. L., & Bokhour, B. (2009). A narrative of resistance: Presentation of self when parenting children with asthma. *Communication & Medicine, 6,* 27–37.

Coontz, S. (2011). *A strange stirring: The feminine mystique and American women at the dawn of the 1960s.* New York, NY: Basic Books.

Crepeau, E. B. (2000). Reconstructing Gloria: A narrative analysis of team meetings. *Qualitative Health Research, 10,* 766–787.

Crepeau, E. B., & Garren, K. (2011). I looked to her as a guide: The therapeutic relationship in hand therapy. *Disability and Rehabilitation, 33,* 872–881.

Farkas, M. (2007). The vision of recovery today: What it is and what it means for services. *World Psychiatry, 6,* 68–74.

Fay, E. V., & Kellogg, I. M. (1954). Occupational therapy in general hospitals. In H. S. Willard & C. S. Spackman (Eds.), *Principles of occupational therapy* (2nd ed., pp. 117–137). Philadelphia, PA: Lippincott.

Fisher, W. R. (1984). Narration as a human communication paradigm: The case of public moral argument. *Communication Monographs, 51,* 1–22.

Fleming, M. H. (1993). Aspects of clinical reasoning in occupational therapy. In H. L. Hopkins & H. D. Smith (Eds.), *Willard & Spackman's occupational therapy* (8th ed., pp. 867–880). Philadelphia, PA: Lippincott.

Franits, L. E. (2005). Nothing about us without us: Searching for the narrative of disability. *American Journal of Occupational Therapy, 59,* 577–579.

Frank, A. W. (1995). *The wounded storyteller: Body, illness, and ethics.* Chicago, IL: University of Chicago Press.

Frank, A. W. (2002). "How can they act like that?" Clinicians and patients as characters in each other's stories. *The Hastings Center Report, 32,* 14–22.

Gleave, M. (1947). Occupational therapy in children's hospitals and pediatric services. In H. S. Willard & C. S. Spackman (Eds.), *Principles of occupational therapy* (pp. 141–174). Philadelphia, PA: Lippincott.

Gorman, G. (2008). An exploration and invitation: Narrative healthcare. *Substance Use & Misuse, 43,* 2172–2174.

Hamilton, T. B. (2008). Narrative reasoning. In B. A. Boyt Schell & J. W. Schell (Eds.), *Clinical and professional reasoning in occupational therapy* (pp. 125–126). Baltimore, MD: Lippincott Williams & Wilkins.

Holland, D., Lachicotte, W., Skinner, D., & Cain, C. (1998). *Identity and agency in cultural worlds.* Cambridge, MA: Harvard University Press.

Howie, L., Coulter, M., & Feldman, S. (2004). Crafting the self: Older persons' narratives of occupational identity. *American Journal of Occupational Therapy, 58,* 446–454.

Isaksson, G., Josephsson, S., Lexell, J., & Skär, L. (2008). Men's experiences of giving and taking social support after their wife's spinal cord injury. *Scandinavian Journal of Occupational Therapy, 15,* 236–246.

Kirkpatrick, H. (2008). A narrative framework for understanding experiences of people with severe mental illnesses. *Archives of Psychiatric Nursing, 22,* 61–68.

Kleinman, A. (1980). *Patients and healers in the context of culture: An exploration of the borderland between anthropology, medicine, and psychiatry.* Berkeley, CA: University of California Press.

Labovitz, D. R. (Ed.). (2003). *Ordinary miracles: True stories about overcoming obstacles and surviving catastrophes.* Thorofare, NJ: SLACK.

Leight, S. B. (2002). Starry night: Using story to inform aesthetic knowing in women's health nursing. *Journal of Advanced Nursing, 37,* 108–114.

Linton, S. (2006). *My body politic: A memoir.* Ann Arbor, MI: University of Michigan Press.

Mattingly, C. (1991). The narrative nature of clinical reasoning. *American Journal of Occupational Therapy, 45,* 998–1005.

Mattingly, C. (1998). *Healing dramas and clinical plots: The narrative structure of experience.* New York, NY: Cambridge University Press.

Mattingly, C. (2000). Emergent narratives. In C. Mattingly & L. C. Garro (Eds.), *Narrative and the cultural construction of illness and healing* (pp. 181–211). Berkeley, CA: University of California Press.

Mattingly, C. (2010). *The paradox of hope: Journeys through a clinical borderland.* Berkeley, CA: University of California Press.

Mattingly, C., & Beer, D. W. (1993). Interpreting culture in a therapeutic context. In H. L. Hopkins & H. D. Smith (Eds.), *Willard & Spackman's occupational therapy* (8th ed., pp. 154–160). Philadelphia, PA: Lippincott.

Mattingly, C., & Fleming, M. H. (1994). *Clinical reasoning: Forms of inquiry in a therapeutic practice.* Philadelphia, PA: F. A. Davis.

Mattingly, C., & Garro, L. C. (2000). *Narrative and the cultural construction of illness and healing.* Berkeley, CA: University of California Press.

Mishler, E. G. (1984). *The discourse of medicine: Dialectics of medical interviews.* Norwood, NJ: Ablex.

Monrouxe, L. V., Rees, C. E., Endacott, R., & Ternan, E. (2014). 'Even now it makes me angry': Health care students' professionalism dilemma narratives. *Medical Education, 48,* 502–517.

Pizzi, M. A. (2015). Hurricane Sandy, disaster preparedness, and the recovery model. *American Journal of Occupational Therapy, 69,* 6904250010p1–6904250010p10.

Polkinghorne, D. E. (1988). *Narrative knowing and the human sciences.* Albany, NY: State University of New York Press.

Riessman, C. K. (1993). *Narrative analysis.* Thousand Oaks, CA: Sage.

Riessman, C. K. (2008). *Narrative methods for the human sciences.* Newbury Park, CA: Sage.

Simmons, D. C., Crepeau, E. B., & White, B. P. (2000). The predictive power of narrative data in occupational therapy evaluation. *American Journal of Occupational Therapy, 54,* 471–476.

Spackman, C. S. (1947). Treatment for the limitation of motion of joints, flaccid paralyses and industrial injuries. In H. S. Willard & C. S. Spackman (Eds.), *Principles of occupational therapy* (pp. 175–190). Philadelphia, PA: Lippincott.

Spackman, C. S. (1971). Occupational therapy for the restoration of physical function. In H. S. Willard, & C. S. Spackman (Eds.), *Occupational therapy* (4th ed., pp. 151–215). Philadelphia, PA: Lippincott.

Stone-Mediatore, S. (2003). *Reading across borders: Storytelling and knowledge of resistance.* New York, NY: Palgrave Macmillan.

Tiffany, E. (1978). Psychiatry and mental health. In H. L. Hopkins & H. D. Smith (Eds.), *Willard & Spackman's occupational therapy* (5th ed., pp. 269–334). Philadelphia, PA: Lippincott.

Winskell, K., Holmes, K., Neri, E., Berkowitz, R., Mbakwem, B., & Obyerodhyambo, O. (2015). Making sense of HIV stigma: Representations in young Africans' HIV-related narratives. *Global Public Health, 10,* 917–929.

the**Point**® For additional resources on the subjects discussed in this chapter, visit **http://thePoint.lww.com /Willard-Spackman13e.**

Who's Driving the Bus?

Laura S. Horowitz, Will S. Horowitz, Craig W. Horowitz

1999 to 2005, by Laura

The First Year or So

Will was born on a hot August morning in 1999. He weighed 10 lb, 1 oz, and was almost 24 inches long—he was already tall and skinny. He was a much-longed-for child, born to me, Laura, at age 41, and his dad, Craig, at 50. We were truly blissfully happy. We were all lacking sleep, and I was perpetually hot and sticky nursing a very hungry 10-lb baby in humid weather, but we had lots of help from family and friends, and we all enjoyed my maternity leave (Figure 11-1).

From the beginning, it was clear that Will was very sensitive to sound. The chiming of the grandfather clock delighted him, but the sound of the doorbell terrified him. He was also very sensitive to temperature. He disliked warm bottles and baths, preferring both to be room temperature. Sunlight bothered him as well, and he happily wore hats his whole first year whenever we were outside.

Will did not sleep a lot during the day, and when he was awake, he was happy only when being held. He hated "tummy time" and learned to turn himself over at 8 weeks old so that he wouldn't have to lie facing down. He loved the crystal chandelier in our dining room, and he would happily lie on the table while we ate dinner, staring up at the light. Will met all of his developmental milestones on time or early, ate well, grew quickly, and started sleeping through the night at 10 weeks.

I went back to work full-time when Will was 6 months old, and Craig became the stay-at-home parent. As the first year went by, he loved stroller rides, playing peek-a-boo, and flying high in his swing outdoors. And every day, Craig and Will went out and did the errands, with Craig carrying Will in a sling (Figure 11-2). At 7 months, he developed acute separation anxiety and had a hard time warming up to new people. He never did crawl, but at exactly 1 year, he took his first steps. He started babbling late, which we discussed with his pediatrician, but his gestural speech was great, and we had no trouble understanding what he wanted. He started talking at 14 months (first words: "light," "hot," and "woof-woof"), and by 16 months, he spoke his first full sentence ("I see a balloon").

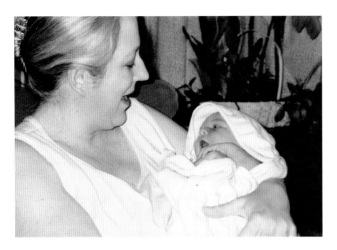

FIGURE 11-1 Will at 1 week. He was a very cuddly baby who bonded with us very quickly.

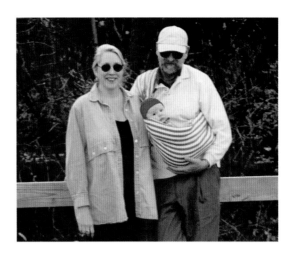

FIGURE 11-2 Will at 3 months in his beloved sling. It was his preferred mode of transportation until he could walk, at which point he refused to use it any more.

Toddlerhood

As Will started his second year of life, he was walking, running, talking, and playing. He loved clocks, pinwheels, cars, and trains—anything that contained something round that spun—especially his huge collection of Hot Wheels cars, which he lined up in precise rows (Figure 11-3). We thought that was odd and mentioned it to his pediatrician, who assured us that it was normal and not to worry.

At 22 months, he started attending day care. We knew it would be a tricky transition. Will had never outgrown his separation anxiety, and he had a hard time being away from us and accepting new people. So we eased him into day care. For the first week or so, either Craig or I would take him to the day care and stay with him in the "toddler room" for an hour or two, just playing and letting him get used to the teachers and children. After many days, we left him there for an hour, then 2 hours, and so on. Eventually, we were able to bring him in at 9:00 in the morning and pick him up at 4:00. It was a fantastic day care with caring, educated teachers who took great care of him. But every morning was a tearful separation, and every afternoon, he was waiting at the playground, peeking through the fence slats to see my car pull up.

As he turned 3, he was moving up to the "threes" room at the day care, along with children from the toddler room and his teachers, who would "loop" with him for his entire time there. One afternoon, the senior teacher, Heather, pulled me aside and said that she was concerned about Will because he wasn't "blossoming socially the way the

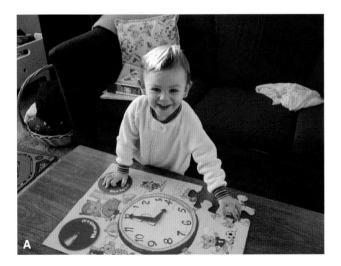

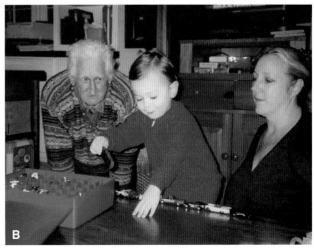

FIGURE 11-3 Will developed a love of clocks at an early age (**A**) and loved lining up his Hot Wheels (**B**) (with his grandpa and mom as audience), which his pediatrician dismissed as "normal."

other 3-year-olds are." She said that the Child Find team was coming in to assess a few children and asked whether we would consent to have Will evaluated. We said yes.

A few weeks later, a speech-language therapist came to the day care. She met Will and took him to a quiet spot. She asked him a few questions, which he answered, and then he proceeded to tell her all about the clock museum in a nearby town, describing every grandfather clock they had and naming the various kinds of escapements each used. I found a handwritten note in Will's cubby that afternoon. It said that he was a delightful child, clearly bright and well-mannered. It said that his receptive and expressive language skills were right on target but that his pragmatic skills were lacking, so he qualified for speech therapy.

I didn't know what to think. I knew what receptive and expressive language skills were, but I had never heard the term *pragmatic skills*. So I went online, typed in that phrase, and received 10,000 hits about autism. I thought something was wrong. My happy, healthy, loving little boy didn't have autism. What is wrong with this Google thing? So I tried again. Same results. I opened the first link and started reading. Within 3 links, I was terrified. Within 10 links, I was sobbing. It was suddenly clear to me that Will did indeed have some form of autism.

The Therapy Years

Will started speech therapy right away. His speech-language therapist, Miss Marcia, was wonderful. She encouraged me and Craig to sit in on the therapy sessions, answered all of our questions, gave great advice, and clearly enjoyed her time with Will. She explained that his thinking was rigid and that her job was to help his thinking become more flexible. We saw her every week for a ½ hour for a few months while we were waiting for a full evaluation from the Child Find team.

That happened when Will was 3 ½. A speech-language therapist, a psychologist, and an occupational therapist spent an afternoon with Will, putting him through all kinds of play-based assessments. At the end of the day, they said, "We aren't qualified to diagnose, but we suspect he is on the autism spectrum and most likely has Asperger syndrome. We recommend that he continue with speech therapy and also receive occupational therapy and social skills therapy."

And so we went home. And we waited for someone to tell us what to do. I was devastated and sad. I cried a lot. Slowly, it dawned on me that no one was going to tell us what to do. We were going to have to figure that out for ourselves. A friend said to me "you are going to have to drive the bus." So I did. I got his therapies lined up. I started reading everything I could find. I bought books, joined an online forum, attended lectures, and helped start a local support group for parents of children with Asperger syndrome. I asked everyone what services would help Will, what was available, what I needed to know and do.

By the time Will was 4 years old, the following were in place:

- 1 hour of speech-language therapy every week
- ½ hour of occupational therapy every week
- 2 hours of social skills therapy every week
- 2 hours of an aide in his day care classroom every day to help him socialize
- Monthly meetings with the day care and special education team to keep us all on the same page
- Quarterly meetings with the agency that provided the classroom aide
- Quarterly meetings with the agency's psychologist to requalify for the help
- Yearly paperwork for Medicaid, which paid for the classroom aide and some of the special ed therapy

"The bus" was pretty full, and I was driving it. All of that was on top of regular doctor appointments, play dates, and the normal errands that all parents run. And I worked full time, as did Craig. I had a huge three-ring binder that held all of the paperwork, test results, ideas, and plans. I coordinated the efforts of the team. For example, we decided that we would all work on the same goal at the same time. One month, it was "greetings." So the day care teachers, all three therapists, and the classroom aide all made it a point of saying "Good morning Will" and helping him to reply appropriately. After a month, he mastered that, and we were able to move on to another goal.

I learned about writing Social Stories, a technique for helping children realize what's going to happen (e.g., at school, when mom has a business trip, when visitors are coming, when there's a long list of errands to do, when you're last in line), what their choices are during the event, and what their options are if they start to get upset. Writing social stories and schedules for Will made his life much easier.

Craig was much calmer about Will's diagnosis, and he reminded me often that Will was a happy, healthy child and that he would be fine. Will was very attached to Craig, and they enjoyed each other's company. Craig could often understand what Will needed based on his actions and gestures. Craig says that "while Laura became focused on the future—learning everything she could about Asperger syndrome and what help Will needed—I focused on the present." Craig and Will went for long walks, watched movies, drove around looking for trains, and continued to do a lot of our errands, visiting their usual round of friendly local businesses.

Our lives revolved around Will's needs and our work. There wasn't much time left over for anything else. And that was ok. We were well past the age when we felt the need to see every movie that came out or upgrade our wardrobes each season. Will was always a good sleeper, so we had our evenings free to enjoy a glass of wine and watch TV. And we were lucky to have good friends (most with much older children) who accepted Will and included him in invitations whenever it was appropriate. But Will's separation anxiety was still very high, so when he was home, he was glued to my side. By the time he was about 4, I did need some "me" time, so I took an occasional weekend trip with girl-friends, which was always a nice treat. And Craig and Will indulged their passion for steam trains by taking day trips, and sometimes even overnight trips to give me a break. Craig continued to be the calm center of our family. He wasn't bothered at all by Will's diagnosis, and he happily took Will to social skills or speech therapy if I was busy. He worried more about me than about Will in those days.

We continued to support Will's passions, which at that point were steam trains, clocks, the planets, and U.S. presidents. We visited museums, read books, and watched videos. We tried to introduce him to new topics, branching off of his existing passions. We figured out that he was a visual learner, so any time he had to do something new, like going to the dentist or flying in an airplane for the first time, we would find a video that showed him what it was like, and then he would be ok when the new event took place.

Slowly but surely, Will grew more trusting of the world around him and in his ability to navigate through it. His language skills grew. He learned to recognize when he was feeling anxious and to ask an adult for help when he needed it. He learned how to dress himself, ride a bike, tie his shoes, and kick a ball. He knew the alphabet and loved counting way up into the hundreds. He made friends, attended play dates, and loved birthday parties.

I often say that all of the therapy Will received would benefit any child, and he was lucky to receive all that help. All of his therapists worked hard to teach Will the skills he would need to be successful. But still, I worried. I think worry was my predominate state of mind from the moment Will was diagnosed. Luckily, Craig was more calm and hopeful, so we had a good balance.

2005 to 2018, by Will

Elementary School

After all the therapy I had received, it was time for the ultimate test, school. I had recently turned 6 years old, and mom told me I was to attend Country Day School and

start kindergarten. Since I was born in August, she wanted me to start school later so I could be older than most. In any case, I was welcomed to this new place, but I was a tad uneasy. I had already met two of my future classmates, Nicholas, who lived four houses down the street, and Luke, who I met only briefly. To my delight, there were only six kids in my class: Nicholas, Luke, Ben D., Ben J., William F., and me. Mrs. Lears, our teacher, was the only female in the room.

It was all fun, but some days, I could have been considered one of the more difficult kids to be around. For starters, I was the oldest which may or may not have gone to my head. I never wanted to be last, and it was not too hard to make me cry. My dislike of being last changed slowly over time, but my intense emotional states did not. This would carry on from kindergarten to first grade where two changes occurred, the obvious being a new classroom and teacher. The other was the total amount of students changed from 6 to 15. This was due to the fact that there were two kindergarten classes, and now, we were combined. My emotional problems did not vanish, instead they got worse. Even though I don't remember this part, I was told I cried at least once a week, and often every day. I needed help, some of my classmates were afraid to come near me, and mom was worried. She sought help from my pediatrician who referred us to a child psychiatrist who prescribed anti-anxiety medications, which lowered my anxiety levels dramatically. After 1 week on the medication, I told my mom "I feel new." Now, I barely ever cried, and I was regaining trust, which lasted the rest of first grade and into the second. By third grade, I was having trouble focusing on schoolwork, and the psychiatrist added a medication for attention-deficit/hyperactivity disorder (ADHD), which helped a lot. During this time, I had three magnetic resonance imaging (MRI) sessions at Johns Hopkins in Baltimore, Maryland, as part of a brain study on Asperger syndrome.

However, at the end of third grade, the largest change in my 9 soon-to-be 10 years of life, we moved houses. We only moved about a quarter of a mile away, but it meant we were moving into another township with a good public school district. So I transferred to another school, Indian Rock Elementary. My nerves were at the apex, I didn't know anyone in my class, or so I thought. But this change actually reunited me with my old friends from day care as well as some other friends who had transferred to Indian Rock from Country Day previously. This change also was good for my education since apparently I could barely read at all, but that all changed rapidly with the help of the reading specialist. Nothing really happened that was significant took place after that, and I graduated fifth grade at age 11 in 2011.

Middle School

Elementary school was finished and off to middle school I went. Like anyone who was going to be in the sixth grade and going to the middle school, I was nervous. A big change was the students of the two different elementary schools would combine into one middle school. But if you talk to someone who has been through middle school, you'll hear pretty negative views. And that's not far off. I mean yes, there were some highlights, but basically middle school was bad. My having Asperger only made it worse.

I was harassed on an almost daily basis. It ranged from kids walking past me in the hall saying "trains are stupid" to having pencils thrown at me to having my laptop stolen. Having Asperger I had a tendency to react to any comment that I heard. That would turn out to be a wrong move since my reaction would fuel their interest to push my buttons. I was constantly seeking help from my guidance counselor, my mom, and my teachers. Once or twice, I even tried to fake being sick, just so I wouldn't get picked on.

Continuing into seventh grade, three things changed, and they gave me something to look forward to. The first of them was the musical, "Fame Jr." I was part of the chorus. It was sometimes hard dealing with all the commotion and noise level, but in the end, it was a ton of fun and I found out I really enjoy being on stage. Second, I began to really trust my school counselor, Mr. Show, and didn't hesitate to go to him if I needed help. The third was in the summer of 2013, both my dad and I became volunteers for the nonprofit organization Steam Into History—a tourist railroad—as flaggers at the railroad crossings. This helped keep my mind off of all the negativity there was in middle school, and it also kind of gave me something to brag about. The same story basically applies to my eighth grade year, I did the musical again, this time it was "Cinderella" where I had a small speaking role; I volunteered at Steam Into History, and I got through the painful 3 years of middle school, graduating from eighth grade at age 14 years in 2014.

As you can see, I find school very stressful, but I have great summers. I work at the railroad, I travel with my parents, and every year for 6 years in a row, I attended a full week of railroad camp in Tennessee.

Note from the bus driver: We are lucky to live in a school district that works hard to eliminate bullying or harassment in any form. Will's school counselors were instrumental in helping Will understand what was "just joking around" versus bullying (it was and is hard for him to tell the difference). They always believed Will when he was upset and always took steps to rectify the problem. For example, the time that two kids were throwing their pencils at Will during English class when the teacher's back was turned, the counselor called in both boys, the assistant principal, and the boys' parents. Within 2 hours, both boys has been assigned school and home punishment and had apologized to Will. Within a few days, Will and I each received handwritten letters from the boys apologizing again. When Will's laptop was stolen, the counselor scrolled through the security videos and retrieved the laptop within an hour. The counselors were very helpful to me as well. It was so good to know there was someone at each school who would help me with anything needed. One of my favorite things about Will is that once someone apologizes to him, he forgives them completely and never mentions the bullying again—even the pencil throwers, who Will now claims are very nice boys (I have my doubts!).

High School

The transition from the middle school to high school was a day I won't forget. The high school basically greeted the incoming freshmen with open arms. Also as time went on, there was a decrease in the harassing. I had heard tales that the sophomores, juniors, and seniors would give hell to the ninth graders, but I was wrong. However, my struggles with my Asperger continued. Freshman year started out fine—all my teachers were great except for one. My history teacher talked at such a rapid pace that I could not process what he was saying. It was so bad that my mom and my counselor switched me out of that class. Even if my history class was a bust, I made up for it by doing 200 hours of volunteer work at Steam Into History, earning myself an additional 1.5 credits. But after that debacle, everything was sorted out, and I went from freshman year into sophomore year.

Sophomore year was basically the same story as freshman, except I was in history again (with a different teacher), and I tried out for the musical again, this time it was "The Little Mermaid." Again, this was a lot of fun and I actually played three small parts, one with a few lines. Also, I sat with really good friends during lunch that year, and I am really thankful they are my friends. Same setup applied to junior year except I was sitting at lunch with a different, and quite frankly, less pleasant group, but I had a bigger role in "The Pajama Game," speaking 18 lines of dialogue. Now I am in my senior year. I started driving to school, I have senior privileges, I have a speaking role in "Shrek: The Musical," and I am applying for college (Figure 11-4).

Note from the bus driver: The reduction in bullying from eighth to ninth grade was remarkable, and after ninth grade, it almost completely disappeared. Maturity is a wonderful thing! Over the high school years, my level of worrying has gone steadily down and my hopeful thoughts have gone steadily up.

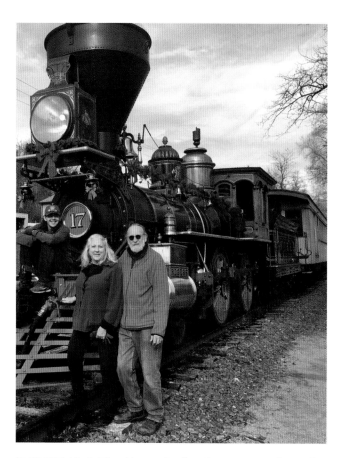

FIGURE 11-4 The Horowitz family in December of 2017 on the railroad where Craig and Will volunteer.

2019 and Beyond, by Craig

Our alarm goes off every morning at 6:00 a.m., and I often have had only a few hours of sleep. While Laura worries less as Will gets older, I worry more.

Will has a long and deep involvement with trains—all things trains. Anyone who knows Will knows that he has an encyclopedic knowledge of trains and that all he has ever wanted to do is be a train engineer. But it's a hard job with a high rate of injury. Trains are large and unforgiving. People who get hurt by trains lose body parts and end up in wheelchairs, so I worry. It does not require a college degree to be a train engineer, but we feel Will needs another 4 years at least to mature to the level of being able to get and keep a job with a railroad. Because of that, we have encouraged Will to go to college, and we are suggesting he go to one of the local schools so that we can help him adjust to a college schedule. We know it won't be an easy transition.

Laura and I think Will would be a great elementary school teacher. He is kind and wonderful with young children, and they love him. If he were to become a teacher, we

think he would enjoy it and be good at it, and in addition, he would have summers off so he could work on a tourist railroad. But Will doesn't like that idea and will likely start college with an undeclared major, so I worry.

I want Will to be self-sufficient. I want Will to have a successful career. I want him to have a good marriage. All parents want those things for their children, but I worry. Luckily, at this point, Laura is more hopeful, so we still have a good balance. Time will tell, and we have a few more years of helping Will mature and decide on a path for his adulthood. Wish us luck!

Epilogue, by Laura and Craig

We want to emphasize that along with worry and hope, we had a lot of very good luck. We were lucky that Will was diagnosed at such a young age. That happened because of his educated, alert, caring day care teachers and a speech-language therapist who did her job well. We're lucky that Asperger disorder was a diagnosis. It was included in the fourth edition of the *Diagnostic and Statistical Manual of Mental Disorders* (*DSM-IV*) of the American Psychiatric Association in 1994, and Will was diagnosed in 2003. When the *DSM-5* came out in 2013, Asperger disorder was no longer a separate diagnosis—it is now included as part of the autism spectrum disorders, and we'll never know if Will would have qualified for an ASD diagnosis at age 3.

We were lucky that we had chosen an excellent day care for Will, that we believed his teachers when they said they were concerned, that we had the wherewithal to figure out what Will needed and the resources to take him to all his therapies, the ability to put him in private school for his early years, and the finances to allow us to move into a better school district when the private school was no longer working out.

We are lucky that Will has always been an even-tempered child. He had meltdowns many times when he was little, but he was never violent, and returned to his usual mellow state once the meltdown was over.

We were lucky to be able to move into an excellent public school district that has always helped and supported Will. And we are lucky to have had supportive family and friends and colleagues (like the editors of *Willard & Spackman's Occupational Therapy*) who helped us along the way. Most families don't have that much luck. We are grateful.

the**Point**® *For additional resources on the subjects discussed in this chapter, visit* **http://thePoint.lww.com /Willard-Spackman13e**. *See* **Appendix I, Resources and Evidence for Common Conditions Addressed in OT** *for more information on autism spectrum disorder.*

Homelessness and Resilience

Paul Cabell's Story

Paul Carrington Cabell III, Sharon A. Gutman,
Emily Raphael-Greenfield

Early Years—The Black Sheep of the Family

Hello, my name is Paul Cabell, and I'm telling you my story so that you can gain a better idea of how someone can slip through the cracks and become homeless. I was born April 22, 1951, in Birmingham, Alabama. I was the second child born to my parents and had an older sister and a younger brother and sister. My parents were very strict, and there was a lot of drinking, smoking, and arguments in the house. We moved a lot because my father was always looking for work. There were a couple of years when my father worked for Alcoa Aluminum in Alabama, and we had money during this time, but he left that job and we moved every few years. We must have moved about eight times in my childhood and teen years.

I guess that my parents were the strictest with me of all my siblings because they viewed me as the black sheep of the family. My father beat me with a belt from age 4 until 13 and when he beat me, he didn't know when to stop. When I was older, he and I got into physical fights, too. I got into a lot of trouble as a kid, and I think that my parents didn't know how to deal with me, so they tried to control me through rules and regulations and physical punishment. For example, when I was a toddler I got into rat poison, and they had to take me to the hospital and pump out my stomach. When I was 7, I remember that my mother drove us to the bakery to buy my birthday cake. It was a big cake with cowboys on it, and my sister said something mean, and instead of hitting her, I smashed the cake. I knew I would get into trouble if I hit her, so I hit the cake instead. But then my mother got so mad at me that we couldn't have my party and I was punished.

I remember in 1953, we moved to Florence, Alabama, and then a few years later to Lynchburg, Virginia. By then, I was 9 and the day we moved, I remember that I pulled my bicycle off the moving van and road it up and down our new block. But I hit a rock, and the bike did a somersault and I broke my leg. We didn't know I broke my leg that day, but I knew that it hurt badly. But my parents said that they couldn't take me to the hospital because they had to take the furniture off the moving van and then return the truck. They told me it was just a sprain. The next day, my leg was much worse, and they took me to a doctor who said that I broke my leg. But the doctor set my leg wrong, and I've had a limp ever since.

Here's a photo of me when I was almost 7 in February of 1957 (Figure 12-1). My mother took this photo, and I remember putting my Mickey Mouse guitar over my head and impersonating Elvis Presley. I loved rock and roll music since I was a kid. I knew all of Elvis's songs, and I could sing them by heart for hours. Like I said, my parents were so strict with me probably because they didn't know how to deal with me. I thought I had a learning disability, but no one identified it. I have memories of teachers making fun of me and children laughing at me in class. I had to teach myself how to write because we moved so much that I was always behind in school. They said that I was slow to learn and I didn't comprehend history, words, or math. But I knew that wasn't true. I was only given extra help when I was in high school. But by then, I was far behind compared to the other kids. I took a speed reading course later in my life and learned how to read faster and with better comprehension. But in high school, I felt like a failure and a loser in school. I thought that I didn't have what it takes to be successful. My father tried to motivate me to work harder in school by paying his children for grades. He used to give $1.00 for As and 50 cents for Bs. I tried hard but I wasn't getting As like my older sister and brother. So I said, "Forget it. I don't want your money. I'll just do without it."

In high school, I was a loner and I didn't have many friends. I remember when a girl asked me to the junior prom. I thought I'd never go because I was afraid to ask any girl. In high school, my parents brought me to a psychiatrist for depression, which I suffer from to this day. He told my mother that I wouldn't amount to anything more than an auto mechanic. I didn't like him. I saw him

for about a year and then I told my mother that I wanted to stop because he wasn't helping me. He gave me white pills that made me itch and pink pills that made me break out in hives. They were antidepressants. I was feeling down because my siblings were getting good grades, and they were popular in school and I wasn't. I was bullied in school. I went to the toughest high school in Tulsa, Oklahoma, with thugs and hoodlums. They used to pick on me and steal my money, but I never told my parents because I knew they wouldn't help me.

In 1963, I was 12, and I was hanging out by the railroad, throwing rocks at the trains and putting rocks on the tracks to derail them. I got caught by two policemen, and my father beat me with a belt. I still have scars from it. He would take his handkerchief and shove it down my throat. In 11th grade I left high school and went to work for my father's brother, my uncle, in Texas. He was working on an oil rig making good money and he got me a job making $100 a week. But I blew it all on Texas restaurants and baseball games. He said that I was goofing off on the job so I got fired. So I went back home. I was good in sports, and I was a boxer and won a couple of fights but not enough to make a living.

Homeless as a Teenager

So one day, I left my parent's home—they were in Kansas now—and went to California to pursue a movie career. I guess that all of the moving around in my childhood and teens made me feel like I could go anywhere and start over. So I got on a bus and went to Los Angeles. Later, I went to San Francisco and it was cold, and I wasn't prepared for the weather, and I walked around all day until I met up with some hippies and they let me crash with them. I lived with them for a few months, sleeping on their floor, and I worked at Chicken Delight. I tried to go back to high school there, and I worked all day and then went to school at night. I had no real place to stay. I met up with a convict who had been at San Quentin prison, and I started sleeping on his floor. That didn't last too long when the landlord found out, and I got pitched out and was homeless again. So, my homelessness started when I was a teenager.

I was trying to make any money that I could to survive and I started selling porn books even though I was underage. If I had gotten caught I would've been thrown in the slammer. In Los Angeles, I met someone from my hometown, and he gave me a place to stay. He'd been in the Army and was a few years older than me, but he played me for a sucker. He stole my driver's license, my bus ticket back to Kansas, my money, and my radio.

Then I got a job delivering telephone books and then selling papers on Hollywood Boulevard. One night, a gang stole all of the money I made from selling papers,

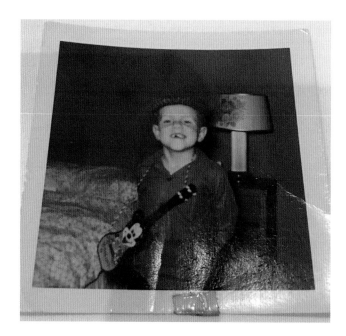

FIGURE 12-1 Paul at age 6 impersonating Elvis Presley.

and they ripped off my high school ring and watch. I'd call my parents every once in a while and they said, "Well, if that's where you want to be and you can support yourself, that's fine. We're not gonna send you money anymore." They did send me money a few times when I was robbed but then they stopped. I went to meet an acting agent and she said, "Do you have a portfolio? Do you have an actor's union card?" And I realized that Hollywood wasn't what I thought it would be. So I went to San Francisco. Then I went back home to Hutchinson, Kansas, and my mother told me that I'd have to pay her $20 a month to iron my clothes and cook my food because when I was out on my own I took care of myself, so I'd still have to do it.

When I was in San Francisco, I met up with a guy who had been in Vietnam and he told me that I should think about going into the service. That's the first time that I started thinking about the military. I tried to get into the Navy but I flunked the Armed Forces Qualification Test twice. So I went to Hutchinson Junior College and got my GED there—this was when I moved back into my parent's home after my first stay in San Francisco. I got a job at a family restaurant as a cook. I was doing okay, but I didn't like living with my parents, and they had the same strict rules for me, and their drinking and arguing got on my nerves. So, one day a friend and I drove up to Santa Monica, California, and I took a bus to San Francisco and started hanging out with the same old low-lifes—selling whatever I could, drinking, doing drugs. It was stupid. I stayed there for several months.

One day, I lost my job, and I decided to go to Chicago. I had no friends, no job, but hoped that my life would be better. I was 19 years old, and I got a job as a day laborer. Then I started delivering telephone books on the East, West, and North Sides of Chicago. In those days, the North Side of Chicago was a Spanish community and I knew Spanish from the time my family moved to Puerto Rico when I was a kid. Part of the job was to deliver new telephone books and bring back old ones for recycling. I brought back a lot of old telephone books and got good money for it. And my coworkers used to say, "Hey man, how come you can bring back so many old books?" Because no one else could bring back as many as I could. And I said, "Because I know Spanish." I used to talk to the Dominican people in Spanish and we got to know each other. So when I came around, they always had their old phone books for me!

But one day, when I went to the South Side of Chicago, there was a gang of teens who threw rocks at me, and I got badly hurt and shook up. And I told my boss that I couldn't work there anymore. I was staying in a flop house [a cheap rooming house] for $2.25 a night then and I couldn't find another job. That's when I became homeless again. I was out on the street, this time in the cold weather of Chicago. It was the winter of 1971, and I was using the rest room at the bus station and they threw me out. I tried to find shelter in the back lot of a restaurant and they called the police. I was stealing candy bars from Woolworth's to survive. Every night, I went to a mission to try to eat. They gave me a ham sandwich and a cup of coffee and that was it. But I was grateful for it. I slept in the train station. They didn't throw me out of there. It was cold and raining and I had pneumonia. A guy came and asked me if I wanted to meet five alcoholics, and they would pay me $50 for five hours of company. So he said, "Follow me," and took me a few streets away. It was a dead end alley and he began to beat me really bad. I tried to defend myself but I couldn't [*Paul begins to cry*]. Finally, a man came and said he was gonna call the police unless we both got out of there, so we ran away and I was able to shake him off.

I went back to the train station. One night I went to the police station seeking help to get off the streets, and a cop asked me if I wanted to see a doctor and I said yes. He handcuffed me because of my disorganized speech and conduct and put me in the wagon and took me to the hospital. He took my bible, which my mother gave to me when I was 10, and he forgot to give it back. And I still tear up when I think that I lost the one gift that I had from her. But he said to me, "You'll be alright now." He took me to a psychiatric hospital and I stayed there for several months until I got well. And when I got out, I went back home to my parents. They lived in Albia, Iowa, then and after a while I went to Des Moines because there were no jobs in Albia where they lived.

I got jobs in restaurants and went through about three restaurant jobs until I worked in one where the boss liked me. I worked hard setting up five to seven party rooms every night. And then I stayed for the parties and bussed the tables. I was at work by 9:00 a.m. and went home each night at 1:00 a.m., 6 days a week. I was living at the YMCA for $18.30 a week, working all the time and making nothing. So I starting thinking about the Army recruiter that I had heard about and decided I was gonna go see him. I told him that I wanted to get into radar and technology and he said, "Okay, if you want radar and technology, that's what we'll get for you." This was 1971 during the Vietnam War, and in 1972, I was sworn into the United States Army in Des Moines, Iowa. I was 20 years old.

I Join the Army

I was in the Army for a little over 2 years but after the first 3 weeks, the Army psychiatrist came to see me and said, "You're not really working out so good son, do you want to get out of the Army?" I was having trouble learning all of the drills and the sequences of firing a rifle. But the Army was the first time in my life that I felt safe and had a purpose. So I said, "No, I want to stay." I passed basic training and I went to advanced training in Fort Harrison, Indiana, in May of 1972. They had me working with the first early computers and taught me how to run wiring. I flunked after the first 5 weeks and I cried all night long because I thought I was gonna lose something that had become important to me for the first time in my life. I got recycled and had to take the training again. But in the second 5 weeks I knew what was going on, and it was a breeze for me and I passed. I had the memories of Chicago—the homelessness and violence that I was constantly exposed to. And I felt safe in the Army. At least I had a roof over my head, a place to sleep, and three meals a day. And I was learning a trade for myself. I volunteered to work for the Criminal Investigator of Drugs and I let them know who was selling drugs in the Army. Drugs were all over the place then and many guys were doing drugs. I didn't like it. I admit that I was drinking alcohol but I didn't do drugs.

In July 1972, I went home on a 30-day leave and then reported to Fort Dix, New Jersey. From there, I got sent overseas to Germany but the drugs were bad there, too, maybe worse. In 1972, I met a Mormon man who was also in the Army. He was clean and a good person, and he didn't drink or smoke. And it was really the first time that I was ever around anyone like him. So I said, "Can I room with you? I drink and smoke, but I'll do it behind the door." And he said "yes" and that was my first exposure to Mormonism and a different way of life than I had been used to. Meeting him began to change my life. The drugs were bad in the Army base in Germany and one night the Army busted the whole unit. So they sent me to the psychiatric hospital both for my protection—because I had turned the unit in—and for my depression, which was severe. In a few months, they transferred me back to the states and I said that I wanted to go to the psychiatric hospital in San Francisco, Letterman Army Hospital. I was there for 6 months and then I got out of the Army. I was diagnosed with depression and substance use disorder.

After the Army

When I got out of the Army, I went to work in the Dutch Kitchen restaurant in St. Francis Hotel in San Francisco making $24 a day plus tips. And I lived in a room that was so small I could barely walk in it. The bathroom was down the hall and I shared it with the other people who lived in the building. My depression was so bad that I wouldn't get out of bed to shower or shave. I'd wear the same clothes for weeks at a time. I was smelly and my boss would say, "You gotta get clean," but I wouldn't. One day, a customer left a big steak on his plate, and I took it into a back room and I ate it. And the boss caught me and gave me a pink slip. I didn't care because I hated the job, but then I was unemployed for a while. It took me a year to adjust from being in the military in Germany to being a civilian in the U.S.

Everything was different when I got out. The people were different, the stores had changed, the jobs were gone. I got only one payment from the Army when I was discharged even though I was legally entitled to monthly benefits.

The Road to Hollywood

So I became a manager at McDonald's during the night and I went to school during the day for broadcasting and acting at San Francisco City College. Being a manager was easy, because McDonald's had a manager's manual and I would read it, and it told me exactly what to do and say. And I did well and got promoted. And again, I was working all night and going to school in the day on my GI Bill. Then I started working in a factory, and in 1975, a plastic surgeon fixed my nose. And then in 1978, I got my first movie part from a Hollywood studio called *Mr. Too Little*. I got $25! And then I started getting acting parts as an extra in teenager beach movies. In 1979, I was on the *Dating Game*. I didn't win, but I got paid $179.80. And in the meantime, I was doing stand-up comedy at the Comedy Store. I wasn't homeless in this period of my life, but it was still a struggle to make ends meet and pay the rent.

I started working in Las Vegas and did comedy shows there, but I got behind in my rent at the hotel where I was staying and they were gonna kick me out. So I started working as a maintenance man from 2:30 a.m. in the morning til 10:30 a.m., five nights a week. I cleaned the slot machines, floors, and the bars. Finally one night, I went to the manager and said, "This Vegas life isn't for me. I'm sick of the fights and drinking. I'm going back to LA." It was hard work, and I resigned from the job and returned to Hollywood, California. When I was on welfare in Hollywood, one night I put on a suit and pretended I was an attendant in a parking lot. No one asked me any questions—they just assumed I was the parking lot manager. I parked cars and told other people where to park cars, and I made $18 in tips that night so that I could eat. But I never did it again because I didn't want to get caught.

The King of Extras

Back in LA, I became king of the extras in Hollywood. I did movies like *Raging Bull* and *The Idolmaker*. I worked on the *Merv Griffin Show* cleaning the set, and that's where I met a lot of Hollywood celebrities. Joan Rivers said she'd put me in her next movie but never made the movie. Joey Bishop sent me an autographed glossy photo and wrote to me five times while I was in the Army. When I got out of the Army and met him, he treated me like I was a member of the family. But a lot of stars blew me off, like Mel Tillis and Don Rickles. When I tried to talk to them, they told me to get the hell out of here. I had a passion to act and do comedy, but it was a roller coaster because it wasn't steady work and I had to get odd jobs to exist. One day, I was in the Beverly Hills Hotel and I was so hungry that when room service was delivered to a hotel guest, I ate their food. I can't imagine what the guests thought when they lifted up their dish trays and saw an already eaten meal.

I was in California from 1976 to 1982 and then I went to New York. I started doing comedy in New York City and my first show was as an extra in Ghost Busters in 1983. I took classes at the NY Comedy Store, but they said my stuff was too weak. For example,

> "The pilgrims came over on the Mayflower ship. My relatives came over on the Mayflower moving van." Ba dum bum.
>
> "A guy on the street said to me, 'Mister, can I borrow $20 bucks until pay day?' I said, 'When's pay day?' He said, 'I don't know, you're the one who's working.'"
>
> "A guy on the street asked me for spare change. I said, 'Today's Tuesday. Pay day's Friday. What do you want me to do, lend on credit?'"
>
> "I ate at a restaurant and said that I wanted to speak to the manager. I said, 'This is the worst meal I ever had. I'm going to report you to the Better Business Bureau.' He said, 'Good, we could use better business.'"

New York, Salt Lake City, and the Mormons

I stayed in NY from 1982 to 1986, and then I went to Salt Lake City. They put me in the psych ward in Salt Lake because I was walking around asking "Where are the subways, where are the old buildings?" And I met a woman who was raised in the Mormon Church and we got engaged. I went back to NY, and she was living in Salt Lake. We wrote letters back and forth and had long distance phone calls. And then one day she called me up and said, "I'm pregnant and I have two children that I want you to be the father of." And I said, "What? Forget about it!"

When I lived in NY, I lived all over the place. I was so poor that once I lived in someone's closet. I lived in all kinds of dives and dumps. When I was working in LA, a summer job came up at a restaurant in Yellowstone National Park. And I really wanted it because I wanted to get away from the city with all the pollution, drinking, smoking, and violence. This second photo that I have (Figure 12-2) was taken June 5, 1982, at Yellowstone National Park in Wyoming. I had a job there in a hamburger shop—I made hamburgers, burritos, fries, and shakes for tourists. That's when I became baptized by the Mormon Church in June 1982. They baptized me right there in the river in Yellowstone National Park and when I came up from the river I felt alive and rejuvenated. And the man asked me if I wanted to join the Church and I said that

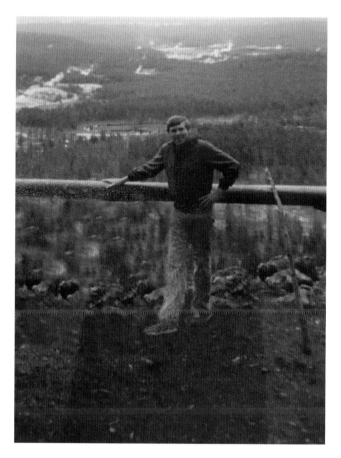

FIGURE 12-2 Paul at about age 30 at Yellowstone National Park.

I had to get cleaned up first—I had to stop drinking and smoking and eating bad. And I did clean up and then I joined. I was 31 and it was a new way of life for me—a new leaf that I turned over.

So I stayed in NY and people would call me, and I would work here and there. And I did a movie called *Perfect* in 1984 with John Travolta. Then I went on tour in 1985 with the Robin Hood Players in Phoenix, Arizona. We rehearsed for a month to go on the road and do educational theater in schools. And the following year I worked in NYC at the Schubert Organization and did really well. I made decent money as a ticket agent for three and a half years, and the big boss promoted me to mailroom supervisor in the executive offices and I got good reviews. To this day, I still get two free house seats at some of the Shubert Theaters. But while working there, I started having panic attacks and anxiety, and the depression came back.

Depression Hits Again

I went into the Manhattan VA hospital for a year. After being discharged, I stayed in my room in East Harlem because it was too dangerous to go outside, so I just vegetated.

They took me to Manhattan State Psychiatric Hospital on Wards Island and I was there for three and a half years for depression. The other patients were abusive and assaulted me. They punched me in the face and kicked me in my gut [*begins to cry*]. And then I attempted suicide with a butter knife but that didn't work. My depression was so bad that I couldn't get out of bed in the morning and all I wanted to do was sit in a chair and sleep all day.

Then they sent me to a mentally ill chemically addicted (MICA) residence in Crown Heights, Brooklyn, and I started learning how to take care of myself. That's when I met Larry Deemer, my occupational therapist at the Brooklyn VA. His day programs were so important to me that I didn't want to leave at the end of the day, and I didn't want to go back to the residence every night to do chores. There were four people in my residence room, and it was noisy and I could never sleep. I would tell Larry that I didn't want to go home and I'd ask him, "Larry, what else can I do for you?" So I did all kinds of projects for him. He taught me how to manage on my own with my finances and take care of myself and my apartment room better. When I was attending the VA Program in Brooklyn, a veteran representative helped me do the paperwork necessary to secure the monthly veteran benefits, which I continue to receive today. My difficulties in getting those benefits left me facing homelessness and extreme poverty for many years.

One day Emily Weinstein, another occupational therapist at the VA, brought in all kinds of old records and she put us on teams and we had to guess the songs and artists. I knew all of the artists' names, the song titles, the year they came out, and the record companies! No one could believe it! But I've loved music since I was 6 years old and watched American Bandstand every day—I even met Dick Clark and his wife on the *Merv Griffin Show*!

Safety with the VA and the Mormons

The Brooklyn VA Program became a safe place for me. One day when I was in my residence in Crown Heights, Brooklyn, as I was coming down the street, the leader of a gang stopped me when I was going to deposit money in the bank and he said, "You ain't going nowhere!" And he hit me over the head and split my head open, and there was blood all over and I had to go to the hospital [*becomes teary eyed*]. He stole all my money. A Mormon Church family helped me get the apartment that I'm living in now which is much safer. I've been there 14 years now. It's like a palace compared to every other place I've lived. It's a Dominican community, but I speak Spanish so I fit right in. I've been in the Church since 1982. I've been a Church

librarian, a bookkeeper, a ward coordinator, I teach a religion class once a month, and on Friday nights, I go to the Boy Scout meetings and help out. And on Saturdays I help out in the Bishop's Storehouse to give groceries to people who don't have money for food. And I speak every year at New York University to the occupational therapy students. So giving back is very important to me now. I haven't had coffee, alcohol, or smoked a cigarette for 35 years.

The Church called me for missionary work, and from 2011 to 2013, I helped students find apartments and jobs when they came to New York City from Idaho. And I'm much happier doing this than when I was in show business. That was a rough roller coaster ride, but I wanted to be an actor at that time and I'm glad that I tried because if I hadn't, I would have always kicked myself for not trying. I still have a passion and love for acting. In 2016, I became a member of the WFDU Radio Station in Teaneck, New Jersey. It's a public radio station that Fairleigh Dickinson owns. I made a donation to keep the radio station on the air. One of the DJs invited me to go on the air with him, and I brought in 10 songs and knew all of the artists' names and the date when each song came out. I know music artists and dates from 1956 to 1975. I can go like this [*snaps fingers*] and rattle off the names, titles, dates, and lyrics. I'm like a walking encyclopedia. Everyone always comments about my incredible memory. When I meet people, I ask them what state they're from. I can name all of the cities in America. Music has always been a passion and held great meaning for me. I know the country music songs, too. I've been in the station twice on the air with the DJs, but I mostly call in from home and they put me on the air with them.

My Life Today

And I'm eating healthy now for the first time in my life. I had bariatric surgery on November 2, 2016, and now I can't have any more burgers or French fries. No fried foods. There's a restaurant in my neighborhood that lets me eat on credit because I'm a Church member and they know that I always pay them back. So they cook for me sometimes. And sometimes other Church member families invite me to their homes to have dinner. And I have Meals on Wheels 7 days a week. I'm learning to take care of my body in a way I never understood before. I've had skin cancer three times. My appendix, gallbladder, and tonsils have all been taken out. I've had shingles, athlete's foot, and in 1999 I had a heart attack in the Brooklyn VA.

My father died on his 87th birthday in 2007 and my mother passed away in 2012 only a week after the anniversary of my father's death. In the last years of their lives, we had a relationship, but we weren't really close. I was closer with my mom. She and I wrote to each other from time to time over the years. They knew that I was stable and I remember them saying that, "We have all good children, we don't have any bad children." That made me feel good and proud. My brother and sister don't care about me at all. They don't care if I live or die. They don't call or e-mail me. They won't come here and I have no reason to go there. My younger sister died of anorexia in 1988. The Mormon Church is my family now. They help me with everything—food, money, company, whatever I need. And I help them back.

My greatest strength has been the Church. They helped me get rid of my bad habits, like alcohol and porn, and hanging out with the wrong people. The programming at the VA has also helped me—occupational therapy, nutrition, counseling, and social work. My doctors are great, too, at the James J. Peters VA Medical Center in the Bronx where I am getting all of my medical and psychiatric care now. The depression isn't that bad anymore. Regularly taking my medication helps. And if I feel down, the old rock and roll music is another thing that keeps me going. I'm happy when I hear the old songs over and over again—I never get tired of them. Listening to the radio station and talking with the DJs help. Attending the Young Men's and Young Women's Hebrew Association of Inwood and Washington Heights Senior Center twice a week has also been helpful. I take Spanish, Wellness, and Life Reflection classes. I also know everyone in my apartment building which consists of six floors of families, Church members and non-Church members. I worked hard to get a bench for the lobby so that I have a place to sit and other people can join me for a visit. And I work hard at serving the Church and not thinking about myself. When I feel bad, I help someone else out. That's the best thing—to do some kindness for others.

When I was homeless on the streets of Chicago, it was the saddest time of my life. I learned true hardship from this experience and saw firsthand how homelessness can happen. I learned that everyone has to have food and a roof over their head to survive. From homelessness, I learned that people can be mean and cold hearted. One day, I was delivering telephone books in the snow and I fell down and all the phone books went all over the street. No one would even stop to help me. Being homeless taught me the importance of being kind to others—especially those who need help. The most important things I've learned in life are to respect myself

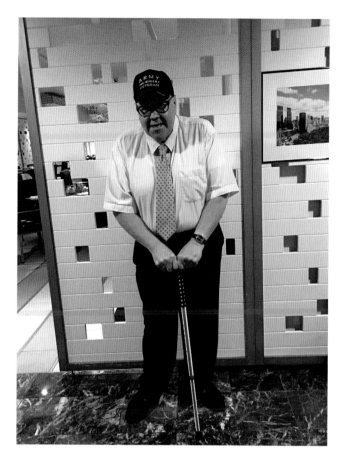

FIGURE 12-3 **Paul in September, 2017.**

and others, and acknowledge my strong work ethic and ability to be resilient through any hardship. I also learned that homelessness can come and go, but by being clean—no alcohol, drinking, or porn, eating healthy, and believing in myself—I could keep myself stable and out of homelessness forever (Figure 12-3)! My early experiences did not provide me with a trusted support system but I did discover as an adult the value of friendship and a safety net in the Mormon Church and Veteran's Administration.

thePoint® *For additional resources on the subjects discussed in this chapter, visit* **http://thePoint.lww.com /Willard-Spackman13e**. *See* **Appendix I, Resources and Evidence for Common Conditions Addressed in OT** *for more information on homelessness.*

CHAPTER 13

While Focusing on Recovery I Forgot to Get a Life

Focusing on My Gifts

Gloria F. Dickerson

Prologue

Hello! My name is Gloria. I am now a 64-year-old Black woman living in Boston. I first wrote this chapter about 10 years ago for the 11th edition of *Willard & Spackman's Occupational Therapy*. I was very concerned that my reliance on therapeutic relationships and focus on recovering from trauma led me to forget to "get a life." I realized that I wasn't developing valued relationships in a community of my choice. The focus on my resilience and life hardiness was a substitute for any confidence or plan to make needed changes. This is a legacy of trauma and the resulting lifetime of fears for my safety which led me to cope by living in isolation.

Most of my life, I have meandered along within the bubble of mental health treatment under a variety of designated attributes of being ill. My sole primary and trusted relationships are with providers and colleagues within health services. At age 15, I was introduced to the mental health system as a patient. Now I look back and revisit my journey through a life of treatment in the light of today. From this vantage point, my life seems to have been an initiation into the land of never good enough, never quite arrived, filled with cyclical pain-filled struggles and some rays of sun. My birth seems to have hurled me into a predesignated life sentence of less than and a never-ending journey of repetitive bouts of trying to rise.

In 2013, I updated the chapter to tell you about who I am and where I have been. I attempted to explain how I learned who I was and how this has affected every aspect of my being, from my excess weight to my choices of occupations and even to my dress. My present gifts and my abilities, my pain and my hope, as well as my deficits and despair can be traced back to events during the first few years of my life. As with everyone on the planet, every event and experience, good or bad, has shaped me and culminated in making me the person that I am. After learning the facts of my life, people who have come to know me are surprised and astonished that I have survived with my intellect and hope intact. After hearing what I have lived through, most people react with jaw-dropping awareness and awe and silence. As people get to know me, they recognize that my life has been filled with extreme horror and that my endurance and survival are amazing.

By the time I came to update this version, I realized that I had learned to accept my limitations and focus on my gifts. As you will see, I am proud of who I am and who I have been able to become.

1951 to 2008

The Early Years

I begin with accounts of memories about my family of origin and my early years. My first years in the South as a young girl were riddled with incidents of trauma. I consider myself to be a Southerner because, up to the age of 5, my ancestral roots, my psyche, and consciousness spring from events that occurred within a small town in Alabama. The family relationships and life in this small town caused essential disconnections within myself, with others, and with the world. My experiences include parental abuse resulting in the birth of my daughter, long inpatient stays in mental hospitals, graduation from college, more hospitalizations, suicide attempts, five different postcollege graduate programs, work throughout the human services field, and 39 years of therapy. These are only a few of the most influential and important experiences that dot the course of my life.

For years, I was the only girl child of my parents. My daddy (James) was born in 1925. My ma (Stella) was born in 1927. My brother Andrew is 1 year older and was born in 1949. I was the oldest girl and was born in 1951. My brother Roger was born 11 months later, in 1952. We often joked that this close proximity in our birth made us almost twins. We have always felt closest to each other. My brother Junior was born in July 1953, and he was the baby for many years. My brother Donnie was born in 1955. He died tragically and suddenly, and his existence has been erased from all family accounts. My sister Daisy was born in 1958. Her birth was my dream come true. I always thought she was a personal gift from God. Her choice to become and to remain estranged from me has been one of the greatest losses of my life. My brother George was born in 1962. Amazingly, he still fails to be recognized as a valued and independent person by my family system. My brother David was born in 1967. Although he is nearly 40, his life continues to affirm his status as my mom's "baby." As a Black man with untreated dyslexia, he makes do and escapes all aspects of being an adult, except procreation, and he lives without income on his relationships with others.

As for most of our neighbors, Black and White, life in the South meant Sundays in church, life as a sharecropper, and extremes of joy, violence, calmness, and pain. The residues of lives touched by violent, chaotic nights and the hard-fought-for appearance of calm, peaceful days set the stage for a culture of fear. The minister was pivotal in helping individuals caught in the maze of violence

find meaning and maintain hope necessary for endurance. There are at least two types of ministers. Some ministers believe in, are motivated by, and love "God" and all the things that a good "God" stands for. A minister operating from powerful needs to nurture "a loving and hopeful life-affirming world" will make mistakes, but her or his intention is to promote relationships between people that rest on ideals of love and hope. The conscious actions of a good minister start from deep-seated basic beliefs such as "Love your neighbor as you would yourself" and "Do no intentional harm." Other ministers beam out their fears of confronting feelings and thoughts that they deem evil and project negative intentions and motivations onto others. My grandfather was the second type: a fire and brimstone type minister. He could not have designed a better-suited context (the ministry) in which he could hide and insinuate his personal brand of fear and pain. Under the cover of the prevailing myths of goodness, high praise, and quality attributes of a minister, he operated unquestioned. He could do no wrong. His motives were never questioned. His actions were revered. His destruction is immeasurable.

My mother's and my father's children can be understood by looking at my parents' life context. Knowing how we learned to be the people we are is not an excuse for our failures and our deficits. It teaches us how to make meaning and find understanding. The meanings we make tell us how to understand our "self," others, and our relationships in the world. This is the foundation from which we begin to act or not act, choose or not choose, know or not know. We learn what it is to be a human being early. We learn about relationships from those around us. We learn what is important, what our value is, and what is right and what is wrong from our early relationships. They form the lens through which we see and know everything. What follows are some of the experiences that make up my lens. This is my beginning.

My mother was 23 years old and my father 25 years old when I was born. My mother tells a story about my birth and early days of life that has been critical to forming my vision of myself, my character, and my strength that has at different times both supported and diminished my assessment of my worth in my own eyes. I have heard this story since . . . well . . . the beginning. She said,

> When you were born, you weighed 4 pounds and 10 ounces. Your father came to see you. He said you were so small that he was scared to hold you. When he first saw you he looked at you and said, "God, she's so hairy and looks just like a little rat." And while you were in the hospital you lost down to three pounds. Everyone thought you were going to die. You stayed in the hospital for one month in a makeshift incubator. Dr. Everage was so good. He made an incubator from odds and ends and pumped oxygen into it to keep you alive. But you were not gaining weight so they sent you home. I think they thought you were going to die. I was so scared and I put you in a dresser drawer with a hot

water bottle. I had to stay up all night with you and I kept pinching you to make you cry because I was so afraid you were going to die. I had to struggle and work so hard to keep you alive. You put me through so much.

My mother has reminded me of this story periodically and with precision throughout my life, reiterating the fact that my father thought I looked like a rat and keeping the wounds of this image alive and potent. Her pronouncements of her great sacrifice and the extreme imposition and burden of my birth have weighed heavily and occasionally tipped the scales in favor of trying to secure my early demise through serious suicide attempts. Often, to make a point during times I "got too big for my britches" or became "too full of myself" by thinking that I was smart or worthy of high praise or love, she would remind me of my botched entrance into the world, reducing me to the reality of her perception that I was "filthy and less than dirt." Her spiel often concluded with pronouncements that the debt I owed her could never be repaid and I was lucky to be alive. The picture my mother painted about how she and my father greeted me and her feelings about me combine with the full weight of subsequent events leave me with profound feelings of guilt and terror and periods of dissociated pain and thoughts that plunged me into depths of despair and my own personal brand of hell all my life.

My mother's family worked as sharecroppers on a farm in Alabama in 1954. My grandfathers on both sides of the family were ministers. As a minister's family, we had some social status among other poor Black families in the area. Yet, my grandmother's predicament seemed to be no different from that of other Black women in the area. Most of the women of the South lived as silent subjects in the land of domineering husbands. But Black women that I grew up with had the additional burden of being alternately longed for, sexually desired, while at the same time their essence as beings was despised, sometimes by their husbands and most of the time by all men and women within this slice of society.

I learned at a very early age that a woman's safety depended on the repertoire of defensive maneuvers of women and on the emotional state, whims, and actions of men. Unfortunately for my mom, she grew up with men who became enraged and physically abusive to any woman who dared think and act as if she was as intelligent and entitled to rights as any other human being, particularly a man. My mom tells stories that show her radical insistence on saying what she wanted, when she wanted, relentlessly voicing her opinions, and naming what was unacceptable. To my great despair, her tales of bravery often concluded with epic depictions of her getting "beat down to the ground." Yet to my amazement, she took great delight in the struggle—in the standing up. The defeat seemed to be incidental. The pride she beamed out every time she tossed her head back and recounted her defiance, blow after blow, left its mark on my heart and mind. I resonate with her physical strength and resilience but mostly with her pride of being defiant. This defying of "the beat down" reminds me that I come from a long line of survivors. The need to fight injustice has often thrilled me, motivated me. Overall, my mother's life taught her that she was inferior. She learned that her pain and terror were caused because she was Black and a female. Depending on the context, her Blackness, her womanhood, or both got her mercilessly victimized. She had to endure, cajole her way out of, and fight against rape and verbal and physical assault from early childhood by her father, brother, and other male relatives. Later, as a woman, she entered the world of having to fight off White men in the households where she worked. These are the things that infiltrated my mother's heart, made my mother who she was, and caused her to hate that which came from her: her firstborn girl.

It is as if every time my mother looked at me, she saw a girl with all the qualities and characteristics that she imagined that every person saw that led them to hurt and hate her. My face was a mirror. She looked into my face at 1 week, at 1 year, and for the rest of my life, and she could only see the vile, filthy little girl that got her beat and brutalized and kept her from the life she wanted. I have always felt hated by my mother. I could see that when she looked at me, she felt tremendous hatred and rage. There was no escaping the consequence of my meaning for her. I was everything that she thought others saw that made them hurt her. And I was gonna pay!

The life context in which my family lived overwhelmed their human potential and capacity for being hopeful. In this context, their actions can be understood, though it can never be a justification. The context shows how I learned to make meanings that sustain my life throughout recovery from devastating and unimaginably hurtful events in my life.

Keeping Time in Chaos

The phrase *keeping time in chaos* adequately describes my life during and for years after the emergence of my mental illness. My first 5 years of daily life in the South contained moments of exquisite pleasure, of running through the fields, pulling up peanuts when I wanted, and finding buried treasure by digging deep in the ground and pulling up unsuspecting sweet potatoes or carrots. Sitting by the water at one of the only swimming and fishing areas near our house, I often watched ants. My eyes went back and forth as I followed them as they went scurrying. I remembered wondering what they could possibly be thinking about.

I have always settled for the basic tenets of life, making lemonade out of lemons. Knowing that I missed out on love from a family and from friends, I lacked a viable self that is based on knowing that one is safe and loved.

I am left knowing that I substituted therapy for a life and therapeutic relationships for love. My having a mental illness, posttraumatic stress disorder (PTSD) and depression, could not have been avoided. Life circumstances and early relationships made this inevitable. I was lucky and unlucky—lucky because I got mental health treatment. I was unlucky because my disorders are PTSD and dissociative identity disorder (DID). The emergence of DID was a lifesaving technique. I learned that I could live through overwhelming experiences by "turning around inside myself," and soon I had a host of friends and loved ones of my own creations. Having DID allowed me to compartmentalize my life—the tasks, developmental stages, reactions, feelings, thoughts, and reality. I learned to put away what I could not deal with so that I could get through the day and keep functioning with a modicum of sanity. DID, my prize possession, was a great skill. I could, in my mind, change myself to fit any situation, provide for other people's needs, avoid threats, and as for the chameleon, change was a great tool for functioning.

This survival technique, like all maneuvers to change reality, became a double-edged sword. The downside of dissociation, like all actions to change internal states by various techniques of avoidance, was that it took on a life of its own. My style of "functioning" was based on using "magical thinking" and the appearance of functioning well to drift through my life. Changing my state by magical thinking replaces my adult consciousness with a child's-eye view, a child's reactions, and a child's feelings, which are out of place. Yesterday's solution is a barrier now. Along with magical shifts in my consciousness come the pain and horror images, thoughts, and feelings and my deep immersion in "memory hell." Being in memory hell is like being locked in a closet full of feelings and thought patterns from the most torturous times in my life. Themes of abandonment, terror, humiliation, pain-filled body states, and loss fill my vision and cloud my judgment. I walk through life in a 60-year-old body pretending—pretending so well that even I am not aware of the incongruence between being 60 and acting like I am 5 years old.

As a young adult, I had only a few vague recollections about my past. I never knew when or how my dissociation began. Even a month ago, I did not understand the implication of my trauma reaction and how it affected my perceptions, thoughts, feelings, and daily life. I have great shame and humiliation about being in a 60-year-old body with no ability to monitor lapses in time and no way to place things in chronological order. When asked to remember when an event occurred, confusion and embarrassment erupt, and I usually respond by saying, "Well, I believe it was a couple of weeks ago." Often, I wake up to find that I have been able to justify using an abusive tone and questioning of my allies' commitment, integrity, and moral stance because I was triggered.

The ability to divide my consciousness and convince myself that the shift is real began early in my life. I remember witnessing my brother getting shot by my mother. Later, I saw the rape and brutal murder of my best friend. I experienced sexual abuse and torture at the hands of my mother and father. I witnessed the lynching of my uncle. This all occurred before I turned 6 years old. After my baby brother was killed, before my friend died, and before my uncle was killed, my family left our home in Birmingham. We went to live in my grandfather's home in Alabama. I believe my family was running away from questions about the death of my baby brother.

Starting Over

Life had started over. My brothers, my parents, and I never mentioned the name or existence of my brother again. I became best friends with a little White girl, named Paula. We both knew that we could never be seen together. One day, we were playing in the barn, and Paula, my best friend in the world, was killed. Her slaying was brutal, and today my mother's words still haunt me: "See what happens to your friends." I have come to believe that her death occurred because she was White and a needed target for sexual abuse. After Paula was killed, one night while sleeping, I was awakened by yelling and loud bangs on the door. My family was hauled out into the dark and beaten. I was raped before my family. My uncle was tortured and lynched and eviscerated. My heart was broken as a child. As an adult, I get to relive every gut-wrenching episode, try to metabolize that pain, and free myself from the memory by knowing what it was like through the repetition compulsion and then the frantic attempts to undo that come with hypervigilance.

I believe that the level of trauma my parents experienced and their demoralization are directly responsible for the abuse they heaped on my siblings, on me, and on others in their world. My father and mother gave words to high spiritual values and had a core work ethic that informed them. My father worked in construction, and my mother worked as a presser in a laundry and, in her later life, as a home health aide. My mother demonstrated that maintaining your life is the prime task of life. I am a survivor, and I come from a long line of survivors. We survived physically—some of us with hope and love intact but most often not. Like other victims of racism and genocide, I believed that traumatic and abusive relationships were the only model of how to live. Racism and postslavery oppression created a caustic environment, showing my parents that hope for a better future and rights of Americans to full citizenship seemed bound to remain a theoretical illusion simply because of the color of their skin. The illusion of freedom and acceptance of all within society made the reality all the harder to bear. Like a knife twisting and distorting their soul, words of freedom, equality, and acceptance remained great high-sounding values that never seemed to make their way into their lives.

No Hope for Safety

I came to Boston when I was approaching my sixth birthday, leaving behind my maternal step-grandmother. On arriving in Boston, I became more immersed in living in my head because I believed that my step-grandmother was all that stood between my death and me. When I entered school, I lost all hope of being safe in the world. School was terrifying because I was never allowed to be around White people in the South, especially after the murder of my best friend on the farm where my grandfather was a sharecropper. Terror interfered with my functioning as I entered school and I saw my teachers and met the principal. They were all White people, and all the kids were Black.

I was basically nonverbal but had a great imagination. Living in my head created an oasis from chaos, terror, and pain created by adults who were sexually abusive and often enraged for reasons that I could not understand. During September of that year, I heard my birth name, "Gloria," for the first time when my mother took me to kindergarten. On entering kindergarten, I already knew how to write my name. My older brother taught me how to make letters and write my name. He was teaching me that the letters meant something. He would say, "Now Fay," because they all called me "Fay," "make a straight line down, like a pole. Now, make a line on the top of the pole like a hat. That is how you make a 'T.'" I learned to hate messing up because my brother was good at everything. My mother loved everything he did. My father liked what he did. My grandparents thought he was so smart. He was everything to all of them. After all, he was lucky. He was a boy. The difference between how my mother looked at him and how she looked at me made me work harder to overcome my primordial defect of being a girl. So I learned I would have to work extra hard to be liked, to become, to finally deserve to be alive. My prized secrets were that I really was better than my brother and that I could do anything as well as my older brother and any boy or man. This notion that I was deemed inferior by all those I loved was critical to my development. I have lived a life of striving and overcoming. I was going to show everyone that I was as good as a boy. Anyone who stated or indicated in any way that I was inferior to a boy because of my gender could count on my angry protestation. Any authority figure making such accusations could count on my secret retribution for what I felt was a most heinous assault against my very being. I tried to do everything that a boy could do. I rebelled against my lot in life because of the unalterable fact that I happened to be a girl.

As the teacher discovered my skills, she made a decision, and I was placed in first grade. Then the tide turned. The teacher's enthrallment with my gifts was short-lived,

and I was demoted and returned to kindergarten. This event precipitated seeds of doubt about my intelligence that has followed me all my life. It is not every child who can say she or he was demoted in first grade. My teacher's explanation was that I was extremely "immature." My persistent hysterical crying, flailing about, and screams for my mother led them to conclude that I was very babyish. This first entry into school began to show that my sorrow and pain were deeply entrenched.

Unprotected Prey

When I was 15, my mother and father fought over money, accusations of extramarital affairs, infidelity, and alcohol-related distress. They also fought over my father's excessive attention and sexual abuse of me. I had been an A student, and up until age 15, I had found school to be a sanctuary. At 15, I became terrified of school. I slept little. During the night, I would literally run out of my house to Boston City Hospital. I would sit in the lounge area with sick people who were waiting to see a doctor. I only went to the hospital because I was aware that as a young girl on the streets of Boston, I was still unprotected prey. Every night for months, I ran away after becoming frightened while trying to sleep. Each night, I envisioned that as soon as I fell asleep, a man would come and stand over me. He would wait until my sleep was deep, and when terror peaked and fear of surprise was imminent, I knew he would spring upon me. I knew as sure as I can see the words on this page that he would end my life in torturous ways. It became safer to stay up all night in the emergency room. I slept during the day. I missed a lot of school. I was able to forge notes from my mom and escaped consequences of unexcused absences for almost a year. My physical and emotional state became unmanageable and my distress apparent. I cried for days. I felt so alone, trapped, and abandoned. There was no one I could tell without getting into trouble. I went to school one day and collapsed on the gym floor. I had a miscarriage. My friend Wanda recently told me that I was curled up in a ball on the floor. I was whispering to her, "Wanda, please don't let them come and get me . . . please . . . please!" She cites this as my introduction to the mental health system. All I know is that in 1966, at age 15, I had my first visit with a psychiatrist.

The Promise of Caring

The psychiatrist was a woman who came from another country. She had a heavy accent. I was too shy to tell her that often I did not understand a word she was saying. I wanted to trust her. I immediately acted as if she loved and cared about me even though I did not really know. I was starved for affection and love. I was so lonely I could die. I wanted someone to trust and love so much that any semblance of trustworthiness and any inquiry into what I wanted passed for love and caring. Simple courtesy and proximity with another human being who asked me questions was soothing. These simple acts of kindness and professionalism were the salve and balm that soothed my wounds emanating from torture, abandonment, and neglect. I learned to glean hope and security from her gestures, pseudotrust, and questions that I thought were enough for me to prove that she loved me. The professionals became surrogate family with all the attending loyalties and conflicts, and later, therapeutic relationships were enough.

At age 16, I entered a public psychiatric institution and started on my path of receiving professional services in lieu of mutual loving nurturing relationships, with the goal of reducing pain and fear. I was terrified on entering Boston State Hospital, but from the first moment that adults asked me what I thought, what had hurt me, and what I needed, I was hooked on treatment. The focus was on me, and people said they wanted to help me feel better. I have stayed in mental health treatment for 39 years because I settled for the promise of caring. Professional caring was, and still is, the only caring that has felt safe enough for me to allow in my life. This is the only caring that I felt I could get.

My treatment for symptoms of mental illness has been successful in that it allowed me to go to Tufts University and learn from five graduate programs, even though I have not completed a master's degree. I have been able to work and live on the periphery of life, settling for the love of my therapist and an apartment, and substituting work and getting well for getting a life. If appearance was the test of having fully recovered, I often passed with flying colors. As for most of us with a mental illness, recovery is full of relapses and recurrences of illness. The journey of recovery is full of moratoriums and plateaus in between mountains and valleys. The journey becomes less tumultuous for most, but eruptions of symptoms can never be ruled out. Life with mental illness is precarious and a terrible predicament in which to find oneself.

Believe Me

Think of what I have told you about my early life: the accounts of witnessing the death of my brother before age 6, the murder and rape of my best friend, the sexual abuse and torture I experienced, and the lynching of my uncle. Some doctors find my statements unbelievable and preposterous. One doctor even chided me saying, "Now Gloria, think about what you are saying. Don't you believe that the police would have intervened?" I would laugh except I know that his thinking is caused by the fact that most people have forgotten what life was like for Black people in 1955. This lack of historical knowledge, paired with a pervasive need to "not know" the pain of racism and family dysfunction, is extremely prevalent in our society. It always feels like a personal affront when helpers replace my real-life experiences with their theories

of what "really" went on. This not being believed simply because what happened to me is out of the experience of my professional friends continually causes me the most pain in my life. The questioning of the truth of my experience occurs because my professional friends believe in the severity of the impact of my trauma and because their training requires them to dissect every statement I make in an attempt to find the errors in my thinking and judgment. This sophisticated way of "nulling" and "voiding" my experience and replacing it with theoretical guessing is really based only on the fantasy in their heads. These interactions always leave me feeling isolated, discriminated against, and demoralized, leaving me hopeless to ever gain credibility when my life experience is diminished because it is so radically different from that of most people.

I realize that once I entered into the contract of therapy and treatment—like a binding contract with the devil—it is perpetual, and its course is certain. It is rare that anyone who enters mental health treatment will ever escape or ever lose the devastating moniker and attributes associated with the status of being a "mental patient." After years of faithful immersion in and commitment to therapeutic treatment, I find myself left feeling tricked, deceived, and abandoned. I believe these feelings are primarily the result of my feelings of being hurt by powerful administrators within the mental health system and worsened when my brother Junior, at age 46, died unnecessarily because of the negligence of staff within a vendor agency of the mental health system.

My interface with medical health providers has added an additional burden to my recovery. I am older and require medical care from doctors who stigmatize and humiliate me because I have been diagnosed as "mentally ill," then react with anger, hostility, and retribution to my complaints about their hurtful behavior. My other professional helpers have not responded to my pleas to help me access basic rights to humane and decent treatment in medical settings. All these factors culminate in leaving me with profound feelings of despair. I missed out on structuring a life that supports and sustains me after the 9-to-5 professional friends go home. My previous therapists all said that my past traumas were too devastating for me ever to marry. Therapy and the psychiatric hospitals have created a cocoon that kept me in isolation, with a fear of living. The stigma of being an older mental patient now fills me with sadness.

My lot in America meant that my life was going to be difficult. The additional burden of abuse, 39 years of mental health treatment, and an active, curious, and generally very fine mind left me disillusioned. With the awareness of what could have been, my losses test my resilience, hope, and faith. I now exist without my many disguises, my alternate selves, and without the benefit of a loving support system. This life of having to make lemonade out of lemons created habitual responses of resilience that now keep me on the planet, however unhappy, and striving for better. My personal existential crisis is how do I endure, do no harm, and wait—after all I have been through. I still have hope in the goodness of people.

An Equal Playing Field

At Boston University Center for Psychiatric Rehabilitation Center, I met people who happened to be professionals. They were outrageously radical professionals. Their theories of how to help were not based on seeking out what is wrong with me. They did not think that it was impossible that I was their equal. They did not label me defective or tell me how sick I was. They spoke of my having options and a valued role in life. They told me that my inability to succeed was caused by barriers. They had requirements and expectations. They made plans based on my needs, wants, and preferences, requiring me to make choices. They believed that I would achieve and grow. They inspired me and sided with my resilience, leaving me feeling energized, ready to act in my own behalf, and hopeful for a better outcome. Dr. Spaniol mentored me and gave me a valued role facilitating recovery groups and cofacilitating statewide workshops. He provided knowledge and skills to increase my competence, and pairing this with doable expectations, he increased my overall life functioning and satisfaction exponentially.

I now have a newly found identity of educator. This was a dream of mine when, as a little girl, I played school with my childhood friends. These experiences allowed me a glimpse into the land of being accepted and well respected. And now, I am forever changed, and giving up is simply harder because of them. Their use of the universal concept that difficulties are caused by barriers took me out of the land of a defective human being failing to function and placed me squarely back in the land of human beings striving to overcome environmental obstacles without judgments about my intellect, character, or motivation. I was on an equal playing field with all others. I was a person who needed help, knowledge, skills, and support. I am not an inferior being treated by superiors. Many of the conflicts and power struggles embedded in traditional therapy are no longer an issue. This subtle and exquisite shift in perspective allows practitioners to have a better chance of greeting a real live person rather than a collection of symptoms.

I am an equal partner with responsibilities to participate to ensure a good outcome. As a partner with the practitioner, I do not sit passively by, awaiting my rescue. The knowledge that my counselors at Boston University cared created a feeling in me that their theories about me, their interventions, and the specific treatment outcomes were never as healing as their personhood, their stated desire, and intention. Without their genuine curiosity that allowed

BOX 13-1   EFFECTIVE THERAPY

Effective therapy is only as good as the quality of the relationship between the therapist and the consumer, paired with a "goodness of fit" between the need of the consumer and the specific therapeutic tools used. My therapy was effective or "good" only when there was collaboration between my therapist and myself. My most effective therapist knew the difference between her intention to help and my perception of being helped. She understood that my perception of being helped is a subjective state of feeling helped that can be discerned only by me.

My therapist is extremely respectful. She knows that any attempts to help me must be based on my stated wishes, desires, and needs. She allows me to choose, to take risks, and sometimes even to fail. The intention to "help," "being helpful," or "giving help" is only one part of the helping process. *The "end" of the helping process is achieved when the person being helped feels "helped."*

them to listen, their respect that kept them from judging, and the high regard for my individualism that allowed them to tolerate me being me, I could not have withstood facing my woundedness and despair. The words "I don't always know how to help but I really want to help you" feel like balm on an open sore and soothe me in ways that I can only approximate by saying, "It healed my soul." This is one of the many supreme gifts of human connection that I have found only in my relationship with my therapist and my counselors at Boston University (Box 13-1).

The Phoenix Rising

I have had a lot of experiences that showed me how to "make meaning" and transform injury and devastation into hopeful scenarios. Routinely affirming hopefulness and habitually responding to devastation with resilience are skills that helped me to transform evil and rise from the ashes. "The phoenix rising" is my life metaphor. As life plunges me into the depths of despair, I look inside and find a light of hope to try and live well. I have repeatedly risen from the ashes, and with my faith intact, I can envision no other response. The latest series of life challenges have come in medical treatment settings.

After 10 years of struggle to find a physician who would not attribute my symptoms of shortness of breath and periods of rapid irregular heartbeat to PTSD and anxiety, I was able to get medical treatment because of a diagnosis of atrial fibrillation and congestive heart failure. Three brothers have died before the age of 60 years old for similar symptoms. My hope is that one day health care disparities will be nonexistent and professionalism is demonstrated routinely in health care settings.

The anonymity of health care providers when they are alone in the room with patients reveals that a great chasm exists between providers who value their role as healers and life-support people and those who are in this position of privilege for all the wrong reasons. My life is a great journey with many challenges and a huge number of inspiring people who go the extra mile and make every day a welcoming experience for people with histories similar as mine. I have learned to be vigilant, a skeptic and despite all attempts to act counter to fear-based reactions in the presence of others, fear and feeling done too are my default settings. This makes trusting others too fragile. Eventually, even the most trusted individuals in my life have their actions and their motives processed through my feelings of being victimized or potentially hurt. This level of skepticism is very hard on relationships. This default is something I live with and in periods of renewal, I challenge. My dreams of friends, love, and connections that are genuinely felt as reliable and predictable are deferred and hoped for. I don't mind this. My hope springs eternal and is part of my life force that makes the journey more worthwhile than anticipated endpoints. I truly wish that you can reframe your disappointments in life's lot in ways that keep you on the planet in the pursuit of dreams.

2008 to 2013

Safety versus Change

The need for safety still outweighs my desire to make needed changes. This is my lot. I feel resigned and still harbor hope for a miracle, some altered state where relationships do not strike the fear of God in my soul and mind. I hope that I can place my trauma in a context that allows the past to be a foundation, a springboard into my future even at such a late date.

I have endured a life of injustice and mistreatment that was made bearable by my religious upbringing and years of therapy. My religious upbringing was both extremely painful and exquisitely inspiring. The deep, profound hope that is embedded in the words and concepts of the Black Church and Bible gave me a foundation of hope that serves as a compass and, although sorely tested, has never been destroyed. The idea that we are all connected, obligated, and encompassed in a mission greater than each of us gives my life purpose and meaning. I have tried to turn away from my faith and connectedness many times, but life always brought me back to center (Figure 13-1).

The ability to make choices has been critical to my relearning skills of self-reliance and safety when engaging with others. Engagement and building trust have always

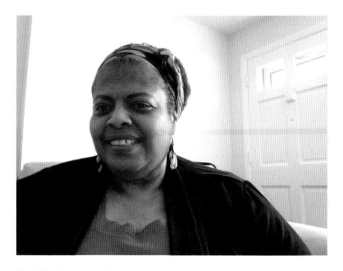

FIGURE 13-1 Gloria Dickerson.

been elusive concepts. For me, trusting a therapist begins with warm greetings, kindness, and acknowledgment of my rights as an adult. I can endure conflicts, misgivings, errors, hurts, and slights if I feel connected and valued as an adult.

Life Is Bigger Than Therapy

My therapy, though freeing, was very concentrated and focused. Unfortunately for me, all of us forgot one little thing: a therapeutic relationship is an assist to learning to establish other relationships that become a source of primary sustenance. Therapeutic relationships should never become a substitute for intimate, loving family, and friends. Life is bigger than the therapy relationship. Stabilization and maintenance are great goals to awaken hurt souls. However, once an individual grasps and mourns the losses and pain that brought her or him into therapy, then what? We need to remember that the primary pain associated with having severe mental illness and trauma often comes out of failed and abusive relationships. My primary "disconnect" emerged over time. Like a stealth bomber, silent at first, it soared in the night and then swooped down, blowing my insides into shards, simply changing the course of my life forever.

In addition to religion, therapy and now sustainable work are primary sources for hope in the goodness of people, for staying alive, and for trying to find a way to live well. Work has become a huge life support. During times of severe depression and feelings of depletion, I rely on my work and my success as the recovery specialist at the Center for Social Innovation in Needham to inspire me to embrace my legacy of responding to impending defeat with resilience and tenacious hold on life. I get to create all day long. I write recovery curriculum and Web site articles and facilitate national training on moving from consumer involvement to integration and social inclusion. The expert help of my therapist has helped to reduce the effects of parental mistreatment, torture, and sexual and physical abuse (Box 13-2).

BOX 13-2	ESSENTIAL QUALITIES OF EFFECTIVE THERAPISTS

There are some basic and essential qualities of all effective therapists regardless of theoretical orientation. Therapists must like people, access the ability to personally censor, be curious, respect difference, create a repertoire of skills, and have the ability to maintain commitment over time. Therapists must learn to acknowledge personal biases, avoid harm, and use their personal self-knowledge to educate for change. Skilled therapists use all of their knowledge, skills, and personal gifts and deficits gleaned from their own life journey and operate from the position of being a change agent and healer. It is not enough to be correct theoretically. Therapists must be skilled human beings who care about and like others. The therapists I love have all these qualities.

2013 to 2017

Focusing on My Gifts

This third update finds me in acceptance of my limitations and losses and focusing on my gifts. Looking back, I see the huge impact of trauma in my life. Intimate, nonprofessional, and lasting relationships have been almost impossible to maintain. When speaking of the impact of trauma, it has become almost trite to speak of mistrust as a barrier to intimacy. My life attests to the need for early interventions after trauma that focus on repairing the wounds to self and trust.

My mistrust and fears were masked by my outgoing gestures when engaging others. Doubts about the intentions of others were always just below the surface. I am okay with what I have! It has been healing to focus on what I have been able to accomplish given the difficulties in my early years. The past is over. The present is a great gift! Every day I have an opportunity to behave in ways that make me proud of how far I have come in my life. From this stance my life looks great! I am happy and grateful . . . what more can I ask!

thePoint® *For additional resources on the subjects discussed in this chapter, visit* **http://thePoint.lww.com /Willard-Spackman13e.**

Mom's Come to Stay

Jean Wilkins Westmacott

Warning Signs

The day after Labor Day in 1999, my cousin, Bob Chalfant, called me at work to tell me that my mom had fallen and was in the hospital. She had tripped on a strip of metal joining two areas of linoleum at a doorway in her home in Surf City, New Jersey. Fortunately, Bob and his mother, Jean, my mother's sister, were there for their annual visit and called for an ambulance. Bob cancelled his flight and stayed with her until I could get to New Jersey from Georgia, where my husband, Richard, and I live. Mom had fractured the upper part of her femur near the hip joint. The break was serious enough to require three titanium screws to secure the bone. The surgeon asked about her last bone density tests, as she definitely had osteoporosis. He then gave Mom a prescription for Fosamax. Apparently, her general practitioner (GP), Dr. P, had never tested her bone density or recommended calcium supplements, despite being her doctor for 20 years. After her hospitalization, Mom was moved to a nearby rehab facility. This incident was a wakeup call for me.

Hildegard Viden Wilkins, my mom, was an incredibly healthy woman for most of her long life. The only times she'd been hospitalized, prior to her last couple years of life, were to give birth to me and for two bouts of poison ivy, to which she was extremely allergic. She did wear glasses, bifocals, and her hearing had been deteriorating for several years, to the point that she began wearing hearing aids. She had trouble adjusting to caring for her hearing aids and changing the batteries, a task that later devolved on me. Although she was exceedingly clever with handcrafts, she was often flummoxed by electronic devices.

After the surgery to pin her femur, her surgeon told me he wanted her to stay in rehab for several weeks and that I should return to Georgia until she was ready to move back to her house. Within 3 days of that return, the rehab facility called to say they were going to release my mother to return home. With the help of the surgeon and the minister from her church, we were able to stall her release by requesting a home inspection. That bought us time: for Mom to make more progress, for a social worker to check out her house, and for me to organize my family and job responsibilities in order to return to New Jersey and to make the necessary changes at Mom's house in order for her to function safely with a walker. This was the beginning of my education as a caregiver and "health advocate" for an elderly person.

The changes needed at her home were mainly cosmetic, to make it easier for her to move about with her walker. We removed scatter rugs,

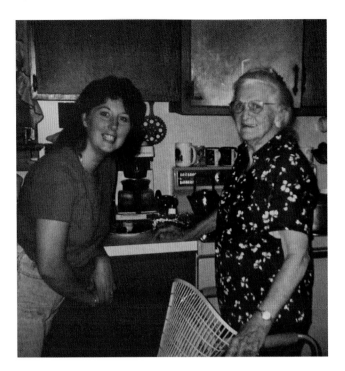

FIGURE 14-1 Mom with her great niece, Wendy Copenhaver, and her adapted walker.

rearranged frequently used items in the kitchen and bath to be within easy reach, checked for loose flooring and thresholds, installed a safety bar by the shower/tub, and had railings added by entry steps. We also attached a small basket to the front of her walker so she could carry things (Figure 14-1). One of the other actions we took was to sign her up for a medical alert system, recommended by the hospital social worker. Mom was given a discreet looking alert device designed as a necklace. It had a button to press if she needed help, which was linked to the phone system. Someone from the alert system would answer and contact the appropriate person/agency for assistance. They also had a weekly check-in call system with trained personnel. Mom enjoyed their calls and often spoke to the same people who were friendly and chatty. Try as we might, we could not convince her that it was ok to wear her alert necklace in the shower, that it was completely waterproof and safe. In fact, it was even more critical an area for her to wear it as so many home accidents happen in the bathroom!

At a follow-up meeting, the surgeon wanted to know why Dr. P had not renewed the Fosamax prescription as ordered in his letter to Dr. P. We discovered that she was supposed to stay on Fosamax for the foreseeable future to counter her osteoporosis. Although pleased the surgeon took such care with the details of Mom's condition, these meetings with him tended to lack the simple courtesy that ought to be part of medical care. Because my mother was 89 and wore a hearing aid, the surgeon behaved as if she

was invisible and directed his attention to me when discussing my mother's medical situation. Despite asking him to direct what he was saying to her, he continued to ignore her. I realized that as important it was for me, as her advocate, not to miss important information or instructions, it was just as important not to intrude on her interactions with medical people. And to remind insensitive medical personnel that my mom was their patient, not me.

Remarkably, Mom had been driving the 800 plus miles to and from Georgia for part of the winter every year since we'd moved there in 1977 until she was 90, except the year she'd had the fractured femur. The next few years, she flew south to stay with us for the holidays, and I would take her to stay for a month with her sister, Jean, who lived in Columbia, South Carolina. Without any pressure from me, Mom decided to give up driving and sold her car when she was 93. She'd had a small fender bender and realized that her reaction times were slowing. Our son, Jesse, who lived near her, was a godsend by doing her grocery shopping and ferrying her to doctors' appointments. She also had a wonderful group of friends who supported each other. They played bridge, had game nights, went out for meals and cultural events, worked as volunteers, and enjoyed various community and church activities. They kept each other engaged in living.

Fortunately, Mom was also comfortable spending time alone. She loved reading, doing crossword puzzles and other word games, was an excellent knitter, and made all sorts of handcrafts. These activities kept both her mind and fingers nimble. As she was no longer driving, it was a blessing that the local library had a service of bringing books to people who were homebound.

The Time Is Coming

Richard and I live in a very rural area about 20 miles from Athens, Georgia. Richard taught in the landscape architecture program at the University of Georgia. I am a sculptor and have a number of works in public areas in Georgia. During this time, I worked as the gallery director/curator for Brenau University in Gainesville, Georgia, and taught in the fine arts department. We could see Mom would not be able to live on her own for many more years, and the long trek between New Jersey and Georgia made it difficult to keep tabs on her. She dreaded the idea of having to move to a nursing home, and I never considered putting her in one. My parents set an example of care for me when they moved Mom's father to our home when I was in high school. He lived with us for 2 years before he died. Also, Mom had talked about her mother and the care she had needed dealing with the effects of diabetes. My grandmother had most of one leg removed and used a wheelchair for the last years of her life. Mom gave Grandma her insulin shots and helped Granddad care for her. When my parents married, Mom's widowed elder brother, Al, took over helping with Grandma's care. Perhaps because I was an only child, Mom and I were very close, and except for the usual teen year spats, we enjoyed each other's company. I knew I would take her to our home when the time came.

We Make a Place

Richard and I decided to build an addition to our home that would create an area for Mom as well as a TV room and office for us. Her area, on the first floor, consisted of a bedroom/sitting area, bathroom, closet, mini-kitchen, and dining area. Richard retired from teaching in the College of Environment and Design at the University of Georgia in 2001. He was a skilled carpenter and a self-taught plumber, and so he did most of the work himself. I pitched in by doing the electrical work, finishing sheetrock, prepping and sealing the floor, and painting.

Knowing that she would eventually be living with us, I gradually furnished her space with some of her furniture, pictures painted by her and her sister, an extra set of her dishes and silverware, and familiar ornaments—much of which she'd not been able to fit into the small house in Surf City when she'd moved from Reading, Pennsylvania. Reading was where my parents lived when my father, Spencer Wilkins, worked as a heating and air engineer and where they raised me. Summers and many weekends were spent by the ocean in Surf City. A couple of years after my father's death in 1970, Mom sold their Reading house and lived in an apartment in the same area until she was 75. At that point, she decided to move full time to Surf City. She was an eminently practical person and dealt rationally with whatever circumstances and her finances required. As an example, my parents wanted me to be able to go to college. My father had a 2-year associate's degree and eventually felt stymied in his career by not having a college degree. My mother had gone to work right after her high school graduation for the Penn Mutual insurance company in Philadelphia. It was during the Depression and my grandfather was sometimes laid off from his drafting jobs, so Mom's contribution was needed. When my mother and father married, she had to leave her position. At that time, like many companies, Penn Mutual had a policy to employ only women who were unmarried. When I was in the seventh grade, Mom realized that college would not be affordable on my father's salary, so she went back to work as a bookkeeper for a firm in Reading. Her decision made it possible for me to get my undergraduate degree at Temple University.

Perhaps because of her experience as a bookkeeper or just her pragmatic attitude to life, she contacted an estate planning firm when she was in her early 90s. She had them create a revocable living trust, a pour-over will (that would automatically put all of her assets into the trust upon her death), and a living will, plus papers making me her agent with durable general power of attorney and durable health care power of attorney. In the event of my death or incapacitation, Jesse was listed as my back up. I am grateful that she did all this under her own initiative and while she was still in good mental and physical shape. It allowed me to act on and in her behalf as she gradually became less able to deal with financial matters such as paying bills and doing her tax returns as well as making some medical decisions. Discussing medical options was not easy or comfortable to face, but I admired the way she handled everything so sensibly.

While visiting Mom in the early summer of 2005, I took her to her Dr. P for a checkup; he was worried about her sudden loss of weight since her last visit. Also, a visit to the eye doctor revealed that she had macular degeneration, the type that could not be treated. When I cleaned out her refrigerator, I found spoiled food that she thought was ok. Arthritis in her hands made it difficult for her to lift heavy pans in the kitchen, and arthritis in her knees was making walking and climbing stairs more difficult. It was time for Mom to come to stay with us in Georgia.

The Move

I stayed with Mom for most of the summer of 2005 in Surf City and, after hosting our annual neighborhood Labor Day potluck dinner, we packed up and moved her to Georgia. Our plan was to bring her back to Surf City for long stays so she could remain connected with her friends there and family who lived in South Jersey and Delaware. Jesse would make sure Mom's house would be taken care of while she was with us.

As I was working at Brenau University during the week, Richard took care of my mother through the 2005/2006 academic year. She was able to walk, although increasingly with the aid of a walker, and her mind was good. He made her meals and took her to weekly bridge games in Athens and to doctors' appointments. Richard's and my friends were very thoughtful to include Mom in most social invitations, several of them becoming her good friends, too. The bridge games provided a place where she met and became friends with people closer to her generation and interests. All these new friendships were invaluable to her life in Georgia. We didn't want her to feel marooned.

Given that Richard and my mother did not have an easy relationship, he was a saint to help so much with her care that year. However, by midwinter, I realized that it was expecting too much of him and decided to hand in my resignation and retire by August 2006. The summer of that year became a transition period for all of us.

I Retire Early

In June of 2006, Mom and I drove to New Jersey. She spent the next few months reconnecting with her New Jersey friends. Toward the end of the summer, I had to return to Georgia for 2 weeks to complete a grant report for Brenau University Galleries before my official retirement. (It was a task that would have been unfair to leave for my successor to complete.) I worried about how Mom would manage during my absence. Two dear friends of mine had been using an agency to provide health care workers for their mother, who lived across the street from Mom. I contacted the agency, and they sent a wonderful, experienced woman named Adwoa. She arrived by bus from the Bronx and moved in to help while I was gone. She was friendly, no-nonsense, and understood everything that needed to be done. As this was the first time hiring someone to help with Mom's care, I was glad Adwoa and I were able to overlap a couple of days before I had to leave for Georgia. Mom was uneasy about the arrangement initially, thought it unnecessary, but by the time I left, she and Adwoa were getting on like old friends.

Mom's arthritis was getting pretty painful, especially in her knees. A veterinarian friend of ours suggested trying Hyalgan (hyaluronic acid) shots. She said it was developed for use with racehorses and had been very effective, and the U.S. Food and Drug Administration (FDA) had approved its use for humans. The summer of 2005, we made an appointment with Dr. K, an orthopedic doctor in nearby Manahawkin. He gave her a series of three injections in both knees. She experienced a significant reduction in pain and increased mobility in her knees that lasted nearly 6 months and was followed up by our Georgia doctor that winter. We continued to alternate these injections for the next several years in New Jersey and Georgia. The Hyalgan treatments were so successful for Mom's knees that Dr. K suggested trying some shots in her hip during the summer of 2006. That procedure had to be done at the local hospital under X-ray by Dr. Y. She received three injections, spaced by a week between each procedure. These were even more long lasting in reducing the arthritis pain in her hip, above the site of her femur fracture from 1999. Unfortunately, the orthopedic doctor we later visited in Georgia refused to continue the hip injections as prescribed by her New Jersey orthopedist, suggesting prescription drugs to control pain and inflammation. As she was already taking pain medication, we waited until we returned to New Jersey for her to receive another course of these injections in 2008.

She also received some treatments from a local chiropractor, Dr. T, who was quite honest about the limits of what he could do to alleviate her joint pain and the scoliosis in her back. Mom had a few sessions with him spaced over a couple of years. He did make several useful suggestions, such as having her wear bras with broad straps that fastened in the front and experimenting with various pillow designs. He was very personable with Mom, one of the best. Dr. T and his staff sent Mom birthday and holiday cards long after her visits to him had ceased. He and Dr. G, Mom's GP in Georgia, were the only two doctors who sent condolence cards after her death.

Poor Mom, I think she felt a bit like a human guinea pig. When she started developing numbness in her legs from peripheral neuropathy, she was even willing to try acupuncture. She had a couple sessions with a recommended doctor in Watkinsville, Georgia, not too far from our home. He gave her some homeopathic pills to try as well. Acupuncture did not really work for her neuropathy problems, and later, when I was packing her things to move her to Georgia, I found all the pills hidden unused in her underwear drawer!

Our New Routine

Through the rest of 2006 and 2007, Mom and I settled into a comfortable routine. First thing in the mornings, I'd work with her doing some light exercises, including Kegel exercises to help with some bladder leakage issues. Then she would get washed and dressed while I made breakfast. Later in the day, she did other exercises such as lifting some 2- and 3-lb hand weights and using a "Sit n' Stroll" foot peddle machine or lifting ankle weights to keep her leg muscles active. During this time, she was capable and happy enough to be left on her own for short periods of time in our house in Georgia while I spent a couple hours in my studio or worked on rental house renovation projects on our property with Richard. Mom liked to be of use. She would help dust, polish silver, and wash or dry dishes. When I was preparing dinner, there was always some task for Mom like grating cheese or setting the table. In good weather, she enjoyed sitting outside with me while I worked in the garden. Otherwise, she spent time knitting or reading. In the evenings, we all watched TV shows, or she and I would play board games. Scrabble was her particular favorite, followed by Yahtzee and Parcheesi. Dominoes was a new game we added to our repertoire. Until her eyesight became too diminished, we loved to put together jigsaw puzzles, too. Whenever we had three or more people, she loved to play "May I," a sort of additive Rummy game using two or even three decks of cards depending on the number of players.

To keep her from feeling shut in, I usually took her with me shopping, to the library, or out to lunch with friends. She continued playing bridge with the group in Athens. At first, I would drop her off so I could run some errands. Then Jackie, the woman organizing the bridge games, started asking me to join them when they were short of participants. I wondered why I'd avoided learning bridge all my life as I finally learned to play and enjoy the game, thanks to Jackie's patient instruction. Mom was delighted to have me share something she had always loved doing. As her eyesight, hearing, and memory diminished, some of the women we played with became impatient. I was asked to sit with Mom to help with her playing, which I was happy to do.

A year or so later, another woman took over from Jackie to organize the bridge games at the church. She told me Mom's playing was no longer "good enough to continue playing with them." This was very hurtful for Mom, who was still pretty sharp although uneven in her playing. Jackie was quite upset as the point of these gatherings was to provide fun, social occasions, especially for older participants, not to be competitive. To lift Mom's spirits and keep her playing, Jackie and I organized bridge games at our homes twice a month.

Managing Mom's Medical Care: Medications and Doctors

In mid-May of 2007, Mom and I drove to Surf City to spend the summer at her home there. We checked in with Dr. P, who prescribed Lyrica, a medication he thought would help with her peripheral neuropathy. By this time, Mom was taking about 10 prescription medications prescribed by three different doctors: a blood thinner, two pain medications, something for bladder control, a sleep medication, something for peripheral neuropathy (not Lyrica), and three medications for her heart arrhythmia. Every time we went to any of her doctors' visits, we had to hand in a list of her medications. I kept a current list on my computer to have ready for each visit. Over the next couple of weeks, Mom's legs and feet started to swell and then to seep fluid. Dr. P arranged for a home health care worker to come by to bath and bandage Mom's legs. This continued through the summer, with no improvement, and no suggestions from Dr. P about the cause, despite continued checkups.

As my stay in New Jersey was going to be quite long, I planned two return trips to Georgia to spend some time with Richard. In June, I hired another caretaker, Beatrice, from the agency we'd used before. Beatrice cared for Mom

beautifully while I was away. It gave Richard and me a wonderful breather. In August, I planned another 2-week visit to Richard inGeorgia. Unfortunately, neither Adwoa nor Beatrice was available. The person sent by the agency gave me qualms this time, mainly because her English was not very good. But Evelyn seemed nice and convinced me she understood Mom's needs. I left detailed written instructions for her and for Jesse, who promised to check on Mom frequently while I was away. About a week after I was in Georgia, Jesse called to say he thought there were problems. He said Mom was acting strangely, didn't understand whatever he talked to her about and didn't look well. I cut short my stay and returned immediately to New Jersey. I found Mom looking unkempt and in a very confused and disoriented state. Evelyn had completely misunderstood Mom's medication regime and had either forgotten medicines or had given her double or triple the dose of others. I realized she could not read English well at all. Also, she hadn't cleaned or changed the batteries in Mom's hearing aids as I'd demonstrated. When I walked in the door, days early, she dropped to the floor apologizing. She was terrified about losing her job, but I couldn't risk Mom's health. I called the agency to cancel the caretaker's stay and asked someone to come pick her up. The agency was more annoyed with me than concerned about the caretaker's mistakes. Mom rebounded as soon as she was back on her correct medicine schedule and had new batteries in her hearing aids. It was a very sad and disappointing experience.

When I took Mom for her annual vision check that same summer, the ophthalmologist found cataracts in both her eyes. The macular degeneration was less obstructive in one eye than the other, and he suggested she see an eye surgeon about cataract surgery for the better eye. After examining Mom's eyes, the eye surgeon, Dr. E, concurred and scheduled the surgery. However, he wanted the condition with Mom's legs to be cleared up first and to have her GP and a heart doctor give written approval for the cataract surgery.

We made an appointment to see Dr. P and pick up the approval letter, but when we arrived, we were told that he had gone on vacation without giving his approval. Instead, he had arranged for Mom to meet with a new doctor who had just joined the practice. This turned out to be a blessing. Dr. S was wonderful. It turned out he had experience in geriatric medicine. He checked Mom's feet and legs and then really looked over her medication list. He said the dosage for Lyrica was too high for her and was the probable cause of swelling in her legs and feet. He took a couple other medications off her list and said he'd reduce the number of heart medications after she'd had her eye surgery. Dr. S said it was often the case that elderly patients were on too many or conflicting medications or the dosages were too high. After getting his approval, Mom then saw a heart doctor who signed off on the eye surgery. Within a week of the Lyrica adjustment, the swelling and seepage in Mom's legs and feet disappeared, and by the next week, all lesions had healed. What a relief!

The cataract surgery was a complete success. Mom recovered quickly and was so pleased to realize how much her vision was improved. Dr. E said Mom set the record as his oldest cataract surgery patient. The improvement in her vision was so good that she could read and knit again for another 2 years. Even then, it was more the problems with memory loss that diminished her reading, knitting, and game playing skills. When her ability to follow and remember story lines in books began to falter, friends of ours in Georgia loaned us their Aladdin Ultra Telesensory machine, a sort of "reading machine," which they had bought for one of their parents. We could place a book, magazine, or other reading material on a flatbed, and the exposed page would appear enlarged on a screen above. I had hoped this would enable Mom to read more on her own, but she couldn't get the hang of operating the machine. We began reading books together, aloud. I would read a few pages and she followed the words on the screen, then she would read while I operated the machine for her. Reading or watching the words on the screen and listening followed by us talking about the story or subject seemed to enhance her ability to remember characters and plot in a novel or retain information from a magazine or newspaper article.

Sharing the Care

When we returned to Georgia in the fall of 2007, I decided to hire someone to stay with Mom a couple days a week so I could work more in my studio. I had to complete a sculpture commission for Brenau University that was going too slowly. At first, Mom was offended and thought she would be fine on her own. I tried having her in the studio with me but found it difficult to concentrate. After interviewing a couple of people, we found Bessie, who lived in a nearby town and came highly recommended. Mom was actually quite rude to and about her at first—just because she didn't think she needed a "babysitter." Bessie handled Mom's rebuffs with great patience and aplomb. Gradually, Mom grew to like her very much.

Bessie took care of some meals, laundry, light cleaning in Mom's area, and best of all, played games—cards, dominoes, Yahtzee, etc.—while I worked in my studio. Mom was a very modest person. As her ability to care for herself diminished, she needed help with personal care such as bathing, washing her hair, nail care, dressing, etc. It was a bit awkward at first, but she grew used to being undressed in front of me. It was more difficult getting her used to having someone else help her. The care she needed in the hospital, then in rehab, did help prepare her to submit to other people's assistance with more intimate tasks. Bessie

was very sensitive to Mom's feelings and helped her relax. Bessie was so responsible; when she was unable to work because of illness or family emergencies, she would arrange for her daughter, Anita, her daughter-in-law, Tasha, or her friend, Annette, to fill in for her. What a wonderful group of people!

Mom was often restless at night. When her walking became more uncertain, a friend loaned us a baby monitor to keep in her area with a receiver in our bedroom so I could hear her getting up at night. I would rush downstairs to make sure she didn't fall while going to the bathroom. If she couldn't get to sleep, she would often rock on the side of the bed, and sometimes slipped off onto the floor. I borrowed an aluminum U-shaped "handle" that had two rods that slid under the mattress and bent up next to the bed to prevent Mom from accidentally rolling off the bed and provide something she could hold onto as she stood up. After a year or so with the baby monitor, I realized that she needed someone to be with her during the night. We got a hospital bed via Medicare but kept her old bed for me to use. Caring for Mom most days and then every night began to wear on me. By 2009, I realized that I was occasionally getting cranky with Mom and my husband due to lack of sleep. Sometimes, Bessie would stay a night to spell me, but she had family responsibilities that limited how often she could come. Bessie's sister, Paulette, worked in a nursing home during the day but wanted to earn more money. She offered to help with nighttime care. The occasional night grew to a regular three nights a week: usually Monday, Wednesday, and Friday from 8 p.m. to 8 a.m. She and Mom really hit it off. They loved playing games before Paulette helped Mom get ready for bed. In the morning, Paulette would make sure Mom did some exercises, put in her dentures, dressed her in a robe and slippers, and sat her at the table ready for me to serve breakfast. Getting those three nights of good sleep a week made a huge difference for me.

From the fall of 2007 until Mom's death on April 3, 2011, Bessie, Anita, Tasha, and Paulette's help made it possible for me to continue my studio work, completing three fair-sized sculpture commissions plus several smaller works. One commission was especially meaningful for Mom and me. The commission was for Anne's Garden being installed outside the Northeast Georgia Medical Center in Gainesville by the Fockele Garden Company. The donors wanted it to be a "healing garden" for patients and visitors to enjoy. They also wanted a sculpture with the theme of "healing" to be commissioned and placed in the garden. I was delighted to be the chosen sculptor for the project.

Healing is not a static thing; it is a transition from illness to health. Inspired by classical works such as Bernini's Daphne and Apollo, where Daphne is changing into a tree to escape Apollo's unwanted attentions, or the ancient

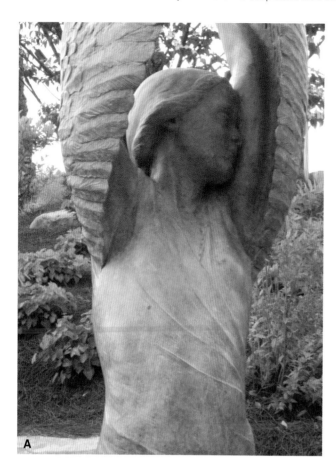
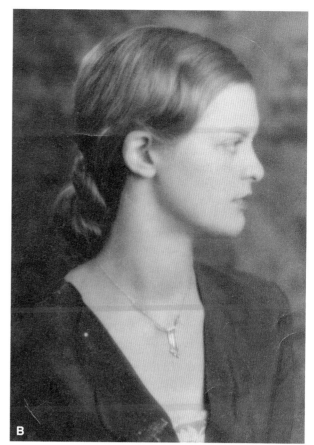

FIGURE 14-2 **A.** Close up of "Elpida." (Photo by Stephanie Olson Gordon.) **B.** Mom at age 20.

Greek nikes, winged women symbolizing victory, I chose to do a "transforming" image. The cast bronze sculpture, named *Elpida*, from the Greek meaning "hope for," was of a woman rising from an amorphous base with root-like shapes becoming folds of a dress. Raised arms changing into wings enfolded above and around her head. Mom was especially beautiful as a young woman. There were several wonderful photographs of her when she was about 20 that looked like Hollywood studio shots! I used these photos to model Elpida's face (Figure 14-2). Thankfully, Mom was able to attend the dedication of the completed sculpture in Anne's Garden in May of 2010, a month after her 100th birthday.

Toward the End

In the last 2 to 3 years of her life, Mom used a wheelchair to get around. It was an adjustment for both of us. Although it meant we could move faster, we also had more obstacles to surmount—stairs, curbs, rough ground, etc. Home health care workers were very helpful in demonstrating how to move Mom: from her chair into bed, into

and out of the shower, into and out of easy chairs or sofas, and in and out of the car. They introduced me to two simple but ingenious pieces of equipment. The first was a broad belt secured by Velcro to put around Mom's waist to help lift her. The second was a smooth birch sliding board about 3 ft long with an opening near one end for a handle. The board worked like a charm, allowing me to slide Mom from her wheelchair to the car, or bed, or easy chair without having to actually lift her. What a life and back saver!

Although it was an effort to take Mom places and to travel long distances with her, she appreciated our trips. In addition to our journeys up and down the East Coast for our summer/fall stays in New Jersey, I tried to make sure Mom got to see her family as often as possible—a brother, his children, and their families in southern New Jersey; her sister in Columbia, South Carolina; and another brother and his wife in Wilmington, Delaware. We also made trips to see a mutual friend in southern Alabama, a couple of trips to see old friends in Reading, Pennsylvania, and we even drove to upstate New York a couple of times to stay with a good friend of mine, who Mom loved visiting. Mom was always "game" for an adventure, and she valued family above anything. By the summer of 2010, I realized I needed help to make the long trip to and from New Jersey. Paulette came with us for the drive north and stayed for 1 week and then took the train back to Georgia. It was a wonderful trip with her; she was so enthusiastic. She had never traveled more than once or twice outside the state of Georgia and kept calling her husband every time we crossed a state line to tell him where she was! I managed to care for Mom on my own until the end of the summer when Bessie took a train north, stayed with us the last week in New Jersey, and then we drove south together. Those sisters really made it possible for Mom to have that last time in Surf City. I think making the effort to stay in touch with family and friends kept Mom enjoying life, and it was definitely worth the effort on my part to make that happen.

We had big birthday celebrations for Mom's 99th birthday and an even bigger one for her 100th. Both occasions drew a crowd. A lifetime of small and large kindnesses endeared Mom to all her nieces and nephews and their families as well as many of our friends. For her 100th birthday in the spring of 2010, we had over 40 people at our home in Georgia. We set up tables outside, everyone contributed food and brought presents, and neighbors provided places to stay for our overflow guests from out of town (some had driven all the way from South Carolina, New Jersey, and Maryland). Mom received a card from President Obama that really dazzled her. We celebrated all the afternoon and evening. Mom opened presents and talked with everyone there. She had such a good time (Figure 14-3). Even when her dementia got pretty bad later that year, she always remembered her 100th birthday party!

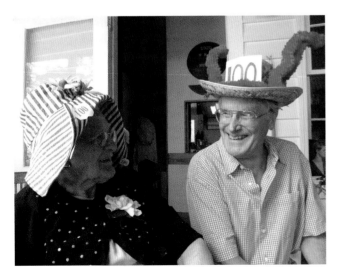

FIGURE 14-3 **Mom and friend, Devereaux Weeks, at her 100th birthday party. (Photo by Jamie Derevere.)**

In the winter of 2011, Mom developed an abscess under her right arm. A course of treatment ordered by a dermatologist we visited seemed to backfire. Instead of "bursting open," the abscess became more and more inflamed and infected. After a month, Mom's dementia increased dramatically, she developed a fever and was very weak. A home health care nurse who was checking on her became alarmed and called an ambulance. Mom stayed in the hospital for about a week. A surgeon checked the abscess and decided not to operate. They brought the fever down, opened and cleaned out the abscess and treated her with antibiotics, and then sent her home. I had instructions on how to keep the wound clean, and increased home health care nursing visits were scheduled for the next couple weeks. During this time, we added another caretaker, Mary, as Bessie was having problems with her knees. Mary was a great help and very well trained and experienced. She really had a calming effect on Mom. "It takes a village" sometimes to care for those you love. Mom's mental and physical health improved, but the abscess never seemed to completely heal.

In mid-March, Mom had another episode of delirium, fever, and weakness and another ambulance trip to the hospital. This time, she kept refusing to eat, so she received fluids and some nourishment intravenously. Her behavior was so erratic. She would cry out when nurses came to turn her, change the sheets, or clean and bath her. Inserting a catheter was a nightmare. She tried to pull out tubes and refused to swallow medicines. Much of the time, she did not know me. The hospital set up a bed for me in her room so I could keep an eye on her. For 2 weeks, I stayed with her day and night. The doctor in charge of coordinating her care was incredibly good. She brought in a specialist to check the abscess. He gave Mom a topical anesthetic and cleaned out the wound. We had a contretemps with the surgeon (the same one who had seen her during her previous stay). The surgeon suddenly, without having seen Mom, or met with me, ordered that Mom be prepped for surgery to remove the abscess. He wanted her under total anesthesia with a tube inserted down her throat. The surgeon had never talked with Mom's coordinating care doctor or the specialist who checked the abscess. They both were alarmed and felt Mom should not be put under total anesthesia or have a tube inserted and thought the procedure did not have to be done in the operating room. They delayed the prescribed surgery, met with the surgeon, and came to a compromise. The surgeon would use a "twilight" anesthesia and scrap inserting the tube, but the procedure would be done in the operating room. The surgery was successful. By the time Mom was brought back to her room, she obviously felt much better. She ate the chicken broth and Jell-O brought for her dinner, the first food she had willingly taken in 2 weeks!

The next morning, her eyes were bright; she greeted me by name cheerily and ate all her breakfast. The doctor was impressed by the change in her condition and said she could have semisoft foods that day and perhaps more solid foods the day after. The improvement was quite dramatic. We talked, I took her for a "walk" in her wheelchair (the first time out of bed during her stay), she got a good wash, and I "styled" her hair. The doctor and I talked about arranging for Mom to be released in 2 days to a rehab facility, in the same nursing home where Paulette worked. The next day, I arranged for Mary to stay with Mom for the night at the hospital, as we thought Mom was out of the woods. I decided to join Richard and some friends for a concert that evening and spend the night at home. During that afternoon, Mom and I had some good conversations. She talked about how she looked forward to coming back to our home to sit on the back porch and look out over the garden. We said how much we loved each other, and she told me how much she appreciated all Richard and I had done for her. She thanked me for taking such good care of her. I stayed until Mary arrived, while Mom ate her dinner. When I left, she was tucking into her dessert of ice cream, probably her favorite food. That night, we got a call from Mary at 2:30 a.m. that Mom had died peacefully in her sleep. Her heart had simply stopped beating a week and a half before her 101st birthday.

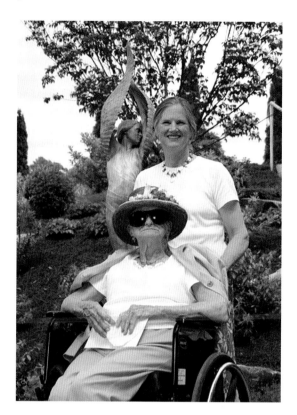

FIGURE 14-4 Jean with her Mom at the dedication of Elpida. (Photo by Christie Hudson.)

Final Thoughts

The years caring for Mom were difficult but some of the most meaningful of my life. Caring for Mom was so different than caring for our son Jesse. With Jesse, we looked forward to each new development, acquired skills, and interests. We took delight in his growing curiosity about the world. With Mom, we dealt with loss of abilities, skills, and a diminishing horizon (Figure 14-4). Caring for her expanded my capacity to anticipate needs, learn new coping skills, and sympathize more deeply with how we all must face mortality. I am very grateful for our time together and all she taught me. Thanks, Mom.

thePoint®   *For additional resources on the subjects discussed in this chapter, visit* http://thePoint.lww.com /Willard-Spackman13e. *See* **Appendix I, Resources and Evidence for Common Conditions Addressed in OT** *for more information on orthopedic conditions, arthritis, visual impairments, and peripheral nerve injury.*

Journey to Ladakh

Beth Long

Introduction

My name is Beth Long. I was married for almost 20 years before being amicably divorced in 2009. I have no children. In 2006 and again in 2013 had had cardiothoracic surgery to replace a defective mitral valve. I have been ordained a priest in the Episcopal Church since 1992. On August 21, 2015, when I was 63 years old, I traveled to Ladakh, a very northern province in India, once known as little Tibet, to celebrate the opening of the Pangong Cashmere Center (Figures 15-1 and 15-2).

I expected to return to my home in Georgia on September 5 and to my work as the rector [a priest who is the head pastor] of an Episcopal Church where I had served since May of 2006. I suffered a stroke on August 30 during that trip.

My Stroke in India

Although I am told I that I did not lose consciousness, I have no memory of most of the first week after the evident onset of the stroke. Those next 3 weeks, during which my family endeavored to bring me back to the United States with the help of the Episcopal Church Pension Group, seemed like an eternity, fraught with terrors of being left in India, and profound spatial and temporal disorientation. It took me some months to realize, with tears, awe, and even laughter, how compromised was my brain function in those early days. Many people contributed to a fund to cover the expenses of bringing Jeanne Long and Pat Coller to India to accompany me home and to help with alterations to Eric's house where I would spend most of my recovery. I am unspeakably grateful for the generosity of so many persons on my behalf. My family, who lives in the Maryland suburbs of Washington, DC, determined that they could best provide ongoing support as I recovered to the point of independent living (Figure 15-3). Although doctors and therapists were very optimistic for my long-term recovery, the next 9 months until I returned to Athens, Georgia, unfolded at a seeming snail's pace. I am told that nerves regenerate a millimeter a month, and truly, that is how it felt. New limitations in agility, ability, resilience, and independence were unwelcome challenges. In addition, not even the country seemed the same one I had inhabited before the stroke. It was as if I went on a trip, fell asleep, and wakened to wonder if my fellow Americans had also suffered brain damage!

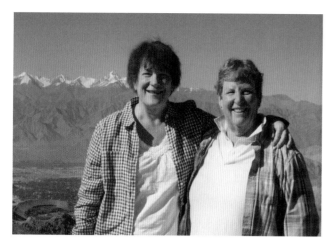

FIGURE 15-1 Beth Long and Donna Cazagnac at Khardungla Top (elevation 1,830 ft—the highest motorable road in the world). (Photographer Linda Cortwright/Fiber Tours 2015.)

Hope for a Return to Work

The neuropsychologist who evaluated my vocational/intellectual abilities determined that I would be able to resume my work, as a parish priest, with accommodations according to American Disabilities Act (ADA) guidelines, which included returning to full-time work over a period of 10 to 12 weeks of gradually increasing the hours and days of work while maintaining good sleep, nutrition, and exercise hygiene. I required additional time for processing and preparing. I couldn't do things in a hurry as I had been used to before the stroke. My emotions were more on the surface than before. I am to this day deeply moved by the care and tenderness extended to me since the stroke and my feelings about that are at times inconveniently accessible!

I had no plans to retire and was expecting to return to work. Alas, the parish was not willing to risk receiving me back to work with accommodations. Worse, the leadership would not communicate to the congregation that this was their decision, not mine. I wanted to return to work. Essentially, I was fired. We negotiated severance and I sought disability retirement with the Church Pension Group, who also assisted me with pursuing Social Security Disability Insurance since I was not yet 65. I cannot begin to describe what a deep loss this was for me and do not wish to revisit that grief here.

Rebuilding My Life

Since May 2016, I have done what I can to find a new life following involuntary retirement and am still discovering what is next and not sure how long or whether

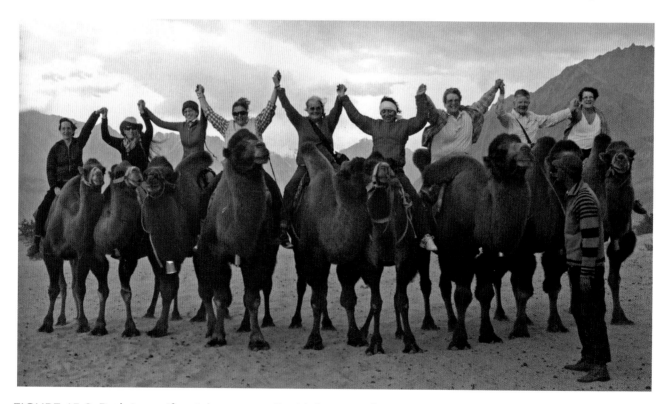

FIGURE 15-2 Beth Long (far right on camel) with her traveling companions—Fiber Arts Tour group. (Photographer Linda Cortwright/Fiber Tours 2015.)

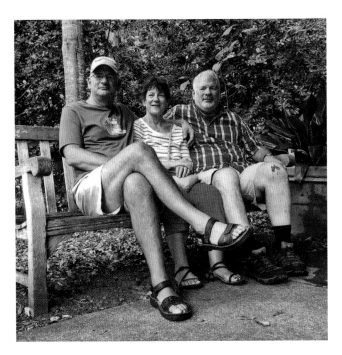

FIGURE 15-3 Beth with her brother Larry Long (left) and Eric Long (right). She stayed with Eric during her rehabilitation. (Photographer Pat Coller. Used with permission.)

which I experienced some profound healing and freedom around the grief of the way my parish ministry came to an end. I know that I can stay in Athens, and I can start a new life elsewhere if I desire. I believe that our most important life decisions are not so much "decided" as they are "revealed." What is next is not yet clear so I am taking my time and living each day with whatever presents itself from moment to moment. After all, we never have more than what is right here and right now in just "this." And fortunately, all the fullness and grace of everything is nowhere other than right here and right now in "this."

I will close with the sermon I preached on October 2, 2016, on the occasion of my last service at St. Gregory the Great, where I had been rector since May 2006 and which tells more of the story of the first year following the stroke.

I will stay in Athens. I am able to live comfortably on my pension here. Driving is relatively easy here. Since leaving parish ministry, I have canvassed door-to-door for the presidential and now local elections. I have continued in a biblical Hebrew class in which I participated before the stroke. I stumbled upon a bobbin lace-making group in which I have participated for a year, thanks to their generous encouragement and patient teaching. I learned recently that one of the teachers was deliberate in her outreach to me believing that this demanding craft would be "good for me." I often wondered why I kept doing this difficult and often frustrating activity, but now, I am finally getting the hang of it and experiencing the satisfaction of that. I'm sure some of these things have been a kind of occupational therapy. Indeed, life itself is occupational and physical therapy! I have done more sewing than I ever did while working and recently have begun to volunteer in an afterschool program with elementary, middle, and high school girls learning to sew for business and pleasure (Figure 15-4). I enjoy a seat in the back row of another congregation of another denomination on Sunday mornings.

Nevertheless, I am drawn to be geographically nearer my brothers with whom I am very close and to their families (Figure 15-5). All of my nieces and nephews live in the DC metropolitan area along with numerous cousins. A few months ago, I went on a weeklong retreat during

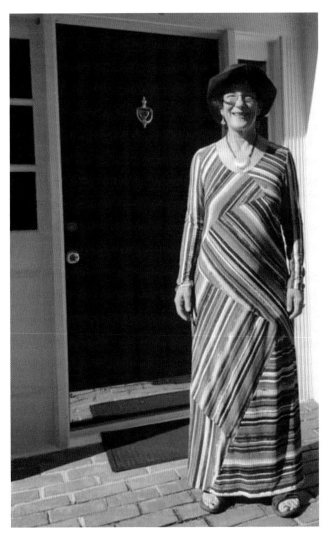

FIGURE 15-4 Beth wearing a dress she made herself as part of her new activities in life after her retirement.

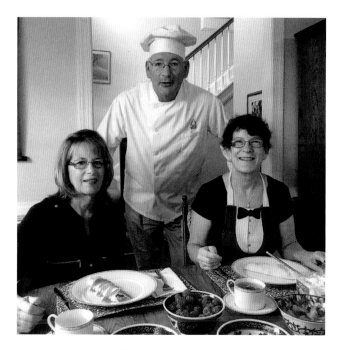

FIGURE 15-5 Beth, her brother Larry Long, and friend the Rev. Patricia Coller at a celebratory breakfast before her last service. (Photographer Eric Long. Used with permission.)

The Sermon

And when I comes to die, give me Jesus, nobody but Jesus.
You can have all of this world; give me Jesus.

My husband Bill used to say that we can never know what is best for us, not really. Even when we think we know, even when mistakes have been made. He was right.

On August 30, 2015, while traveling with a group led by Linda Nesbit Cortright of Wild Fibers Magazine and Konchuk Stobgais of Ladakh, India, I succumbed to a stroke. A genetic skin disorder I suffered on and off for 30 years was in an extreme flare. Inflamed and infected, the infection got into my blood stream. I also have a prosthetic mitral valve, and the septic emboli acted like a blood clot and hence the stroke. I was on intravenous antibiotic until Halloween, starting in India and continuing at MedStar Health and Rehabilitation Center in Washington, DC. I came home to my brother Eric's house to continue with outpatient recovery and therapy. My sister-in-law Kathy worked from home 2 days a week and other family members, nieces, cousins, neighbors, and friends helped with transportation, meals, and many kinds of support. My brothers did most of the driving to appointments. Every other Friday, Larry took me to therapies and then to his house for dinner with Diane and sometimes their sons and families. Since I am an ordained Episcopal priest in parish ministry, for 25 years, I have never been able to celebrate the high holy days with family except

for twice when they joined me at Easter time where I was serving. This was the first Thanksgiving and Christmas I spent with them since I was ordained.

For more than 20 years, I have had a love affair with the Ladakhi people after reading about them in the book, *Ancient Futures*, by Helena Norberg-Hodge. I told stories about them in sermons. I believed that if Jesus had grown up there, he wouldn't have been murdered. They already live what he teaches.

So when Donna, from my first parish, invited me to go on this trip last summer because she heard me tell the stories many years ago, I couldn't resist. Never did I imagine I would enjoy the amazing privilege of meeting these people I had so long admired.

We went to celebrate the opening of a Cashmere Center, which will help local women work and profit from the cashmere wool crop that they supply. That's right, think of Ladakh when you wear cashmere. Those goats only thrive in the harsh conditions like the foothills of the Himalayas. Without the indigenous people who tend them, this fiber would cease to be available to us.

As the time drew closer, I became apprehensive. Some of you were aware of my unease. I secretly hoped one of my docs would tell me not to go. Instead, they said the opposite. And I saw them all! It turned out that my body was in no shape to be going anywhere, but no one, not even the professionals knew that. On some level, my inner wisdom was sending an alarm. For a long time, I had deep regret for not listening and thereby doing such harm.

But here is the great irony. Had I stayed home or had access to state-of-the-art care at the very outset of the stroke, the clot-busting treatment, which is standard, might have killed me or maimed me far worse than I am.

These people to whom I had been drawn for so many years and their primitive little hospital in the far north of India saved my life.

And they saved my soul too.

I experienced the good shepherd simply in the way they live and move and have their being. Even before I was sick, I experienced this in small and subtle gestures, which had a profound effect, then and since. Yes, we recognize the shepherd's voice, the shepherd's very being. Christianity has nothing to do with it. It is more deeply imprinted on us than any words or doctrine from anyone or anywhere.

This people, not of my tribe, my language, my culture, or even my religion never left me alone in those first days. They brought their friends and family in to sing to me or be with me. Apparently, the singing was one thing that lessened my anxiety. They even brought their Buddhist monks in to chant. The Muslim proprietor of the hotel found a way to provide the necessary cash for the air ambulance to transport me to a better hospital in Delhi. Not the Western travel insurance, oh no; a Muslim Ladakhi. A Jewish traveler with us, an EMT nurse in her former life was the one who said after assessing my normal vital signs, "Something else is wrong with her. I think it might be a stroke." Today is Rosh Hashanah, the Jewish New year. Happy New Year Amy, and thank you for helping me to get to this one.

I received love and care and tenderness that I never could have imagined and from people from whom I had no reason to expect it, and with such lavish extravagance as I will never recover from for the rest of my days. Three of them [Eric and Larry Long, and the Reverend Patricia Coller] are here with me, and you, today and represent not only themselves but also their families. Another one of them has been among you all this last year.

And there were my nieces who barely saw me for most of their lives and go to no church. Jeannie came to India to retrieve me; she was there for 2 weeks. Sarah defended me from the vagaries of insurance bureaucracies. My friend Pat was the good shepherd who flew to the Indian wilderness to retrieve this lost sheep and bring her safely to the arms of her brothers and their families.

Today, I stand before you for one reason: to give thanks for love that is real.

Not words in a book, or words about words in a book. The day before Christmas, I was afraid I had wrecked Eric's Christmas with all my oddball spiritual ideas. I said, and I mean this, what good is it if Jesus lived and died and rose again 2000 years ago. But you, Eric, show me Jesus, you are being Jesus to me now and you don't even know it.

You can have all of this world:
Give me Jesus.

I thought I wanted everything, even to know the dark night of the soul, since all the great saints and mystics seemed to know it. But truly I tell you, no, you do not want that. Deluded spiritual materialism is what that is. For so many years, I despaired of ever losing those extra pounds that have accumulated since I was ordained, only to wish that one day I could again be hungry for breakfast.

You can have all of this world.
Give me Jesus.

When the days were dark and sleep was full of terrors, I knew that This One knows the wilderness, knows the darkness, the emptiness, the vast expanse of grey and nothing. (This is the one, like the farmer's wife in a mountain song I used to frail on the banjo, who goes down to hell and comes back again.)

The song that Kendall sang just now, "Give Me Jesus," was how I put myself to sleep in those early days. It was my lullaby. The Shema, which we read, was a passage I knew without having a bible to read and I remembered that the Jews hope to be saying it as they die.

I learned that you will sell all you own and follow Jesus when all this world is nothing. Buying the field for the treasure or the pearl of great price is not a choice. It's not a reasoned action. You can do nothing else.

You can have all of this world.
Give me Jesus.

The more I became aware, the more I feared what worse things could happen that were dreadful. I was so gripped with fear I could hardly bear to let Larry leave the hospital one night when he came to visit. My friend Ann came from Canada and she sang to me. I especially wanted to hear Christmas hymns. I found the darkness, the silence, the wilderness, to be as much present in the birth as in the crucifixion. Suddenly, I saw that as much as terrible things can happen, so too, goodness cannot be stopped or prevented. If a child is to be born into the world that will turn the world upside down, it cannot be stopped. And if people want to know this Jesus, they will not be prevented.

I keep in my heart and have new appreciation for prisoners of war and persons on death row or unjustly imprisoned who do not know if anyone will ever come for them or help them. I am deeply grateful for the work that Bryan Stevenson does, [in the Equal Justice Initiative—see his book, *Just Mercy*] and for people who work to rescue the trapped, the lost, the endangered, and the unjustly imprisoned.

My life was saved by people who offered hospitality to the stranger in their midst.

I am challenged by their witness not to turn away from the stranger my own body had become.

Finally, a day came when I was actually glad to be alive. Life is hard. There are no good enough reasons for that.

Love also has no reasons, no reasons at all.

The enormity of that swallows up everything.

The Reverend Beth L. Long
St. Gregory the Great Episcopal Church
Athens, Georgia

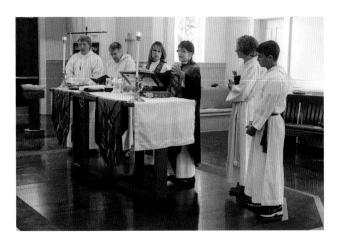

FIGURE 15-6 The Rev. Beth Long celebrating Eucharist at the last service she officiated at St. Gregory the Great Episcopal church, one year after her stroke. (Photographer Eric Long. Used with permission.)

CHAPTER 16

Experiences with Disability

Stories from Ecuador

Kate Barrett

LEARNING OBJECTIVES

After reading this chapter, you will be able to:

1. Analyze how different aspects of culture and context influence the experience of disability.
2. Explore the potential power of storytelling in the context of occupational therapy.
3. Challenge predisposed assumptions about the dynamic nature of disability and roles of therapist and client.

Gracias

As the listener, interpreter, and translator of these narratives, I would like to begin by expressing my deepest gratitude to Maria, Horacio, Maura, and Don Ulvio for sharing their stories with me. I am in awe of how willing each was to share his or her story in order to contribute to the education of the occupational therapy (OT) profession. Each has a moving story; each offers a unique perspective and teaches us something about the experience of living with disability in Ecuador. I traveled to Ecuador to learn from people with disabilities and listen to their stories. These four individuals were chosen because they represent different life stages, different disabilities, and were willing and wanting to share their stories. I listened; wrote what I heard; and, because these are their stories, provided each with an opportunity to provide additions, deletions, and corrections to ensure that these stories honestly and accurately represent their experience. Each narrative below has been read and approved by the person or family described. They are the true authors of this chapter.

Introduction

Statistics about Ecuador

Ecuador is located in South America on the west coast, just north of Peru and south of Colombia (Figure 16-1). The capital of Ecuador is Quito, which is a World Heritage Site because of its well-preserved authentic historic center. With a population of almost 15 million, 38% of the population

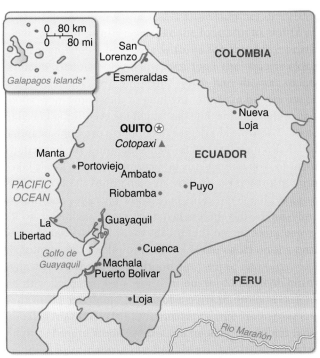

Islands not shown in true geographical position.

FIGURE 16-1 **Map of Ecuador.**

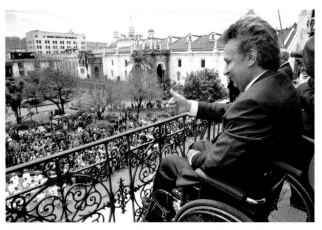

FIGURE 16-2 **Lenin Moreno, President of Ecuador.**

charitable model. Slowly, since the 1950s, the models have been shifting away from charity and toward a rights-based model (CONADIS, n.d.).

Narratives

Maria: Mother of Samantha

> My daughter is normal, she just happens to have cerebral palsy.

Maria, age 49 years, is the mother of 11-year-old Samantha. She begins. . . .

My story is long. I come from the Oriente [the rural jungle area of Ecuador]. I traveled from the Amazon to get my daughter help. My daughter is my everything, I love my daughter, she was my only child at the time. I had an older daughter, but I lost her to the streets. She left home and was running around with men.

My daughter, Samantha, was born healthy. At 9 months she became ill with pneumonia which led to meningitis, which led to seizures. I brought her to the hospital in Tena, the nearest hospital to where we lived in the jungle. She was there for a month, but they were unable to cure her. She continued to have seizures.

I decided to take her to Quito (8 hours by bus). At this point, she was being fed through a nasogastric tube and on oxygen as well. On the way to Quito, Samantha ran out of oxygen and had a seizure. I felt so helpless, I did not know what to do. She could not breathe well on her own and we still had a far way to go. I prayed hard, and I convinced the bus driver to call an ambulance. God got us to Quito in an ambulance. I have never been so sure of His existence and presence in my life.

We arrived at the children's hospital in Quito at 11:00 p.m. at night. By 2:00 in the morning, the doctors told me that Samantha would not live. They told me to leave her

lives below the national poverty line. Most people speak the official language, Spanish, yet many indigenous also or only speak Quichua, the Ecuadorian dialect of Quechua. The population is made up of a mix of mestizo, indigenous, Afro-Ecuadorian, and European descendants. Sixty percent of the population live in urban areas. The Amazon tropical forest is sparsely populated, with only 3% of the population living there (U.S. Department of State, n.d.).

In the late 1990s, Ecuador moved from using its own money, the sucre, to using the U.S. dollar in order to avoid extreme inflation. This caused an economic crisis, and many Ecuadorians emigrated to the United States and Europe between 2000 and 2001. It is estimated that there are 1 to 2 million Ecuadorians living abroad (U.S. Department of State, n.d.).

According to Consejo Nacional para la Igualdad de Discapacidades (CONADIS, n.d.) (the National Advisory Council for Persons with Disabilities in Ecuador), as many as 13.2% of the total population of Ecuador have some type of disability (as defined by the World Health Organization). Interestingly, Lenin Moreno, President of Ecuador as of 2017, uses a wheelchair (Figure 16-2). He is the world's only head of state to use a wheelchair. Moreno was nominated for the 2012 Peace Prize for his advocacy for people with disabilities. Since his election, he has worked to increase the resources for persons with disabilities inclusive of advocating for better access to voting, housing, wheelchairs, and assistive devices. Historically, assistance for persons with disabilities was dependent on a to die. But I have a strong character, a very strong character, and I was not going to leave my daughter in a hospital to die. I stayed with her, I did not leave. And then, Samantha did die. I went crazy, I tried to resuscitate her myself. I begged them to give her medicine. I knew that God would not take her from me. The doctors gave me tranquilizers to calm me down, but it did not work. I fought the medicine. I kept blowing into Samantha's mouth, and she came back to life. A mother cannot leave her child, we hold on until the end, until we end up where we end up. Some people do not understand, it is hard to explain, but when you are a mother of a sick child, you understand.

Samantha spent 3 years in the hospital. When she came home I put her in therapy from 8:00 in the morning until 4:00 in the afternoon. I worked while she was in therapy to pay for it. By that point, any money I had was gone; it is expensive to have a child with disabilities. I am a single mother. My husband left me when I was 5 months pregnant with Samantha. He left me with nothing. I was a chef for tourists in the jungle, I made a comfortable living, but when he left me, he took everything, all of our savings, all of my jewelry. In order to pay for Samantha's therapy, I spent no money on myself. I did not buy food or clothing for myself. I would only eat food that was free and wear only clothes that were given to me. All of the money went to Samantha and her therapy; that is what a mother does.

My older daughter, who I lost to the streets, abandoned her two children. I took them in. I take care of them now also, they are ages 6 and 7 (Figure 16-3). We live in a two-room apartment; there is the kitchen, and the bedroom, that is it. The boys have their bed and I sleep with Samantha. She cannot sleep unless I am at her side. We go outside to use the bathroom and bathe. It is what I can afford.

I take care of Samantha, I do everything for her. When she needs to be suctioned, I suction her, when she needs injections, I do that too. I know how to move her, position

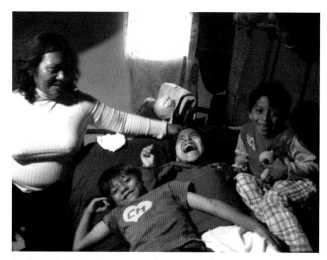

FIGURE 16-3 Maria with Samantha and her two grandsons.

her, feed her, work with her. I know everything there is to know about her. I manage everything for her, like a doctor. But I don't have a degree, and I don't have a big fancy vocabulary. I get mad when professionals, doctors, nurses, and therapists don't treat me well. When they talk at me like I don't know anything or they know more about Samantha than me. Life has taught me everything I need to know. I don't need a degree to be able to care for Samantha.

I also fight like hell for her. Sometimes, the buses don't want to stop and pick us up because her wheelchair takes up extra room on the bus, or sometimes the bus drivers want to charge me more, but I know my rights and I know the law. The bus drivers just don't know any better, so it's my job to educate them. I let them know what the law says—Samantha's ticket is half, and mine is discounted. If they continue to treat me poorly, I simply don't pay anything. When they argue with me, I ask to speak with an official who can help me educate the bus drivers. Now they know me, and they know the law. I have quite a reputation with the bus drivers in our community. We need to think and communicate. I used to just fight, but now I understand. We all need to be thinking and communicating with one another about how we collaborate with people with disabilities. As mothers of children with disabilities, it is hard, very very hard, we need to be strong. I ask God for help to be strong every day. I know that nobody else is going to open their eyes up to our children, that it is up to us as mothers. No one knows the life of another. We need to have compassion and work with one another. We should go out of our way to help, rather than discriminate and treat one another as lesser.

I don't know what I will do when she passes. I know she is quite ill, I can hear it when she breathes. We have been through so much together. I can have things planned in my head, but not in my heart. And when I go, what will happen to the boys? Who will feed them? They have suffered alongside me.

My daughter is perfectly normal, she just has cerebral palsy; other than that, she is like the rest of us. Samantha is my fight, she is my purpose, she is my everything.

My Reflection: My Home Visit

I traveled with Maria and Samantha to their home by bus. Maria manages Samantha in her wheelchair up and down the bus stairs. Once on the bus, she put the brakes on and held on to the chair. We then walked a few blocks to reach their home; her boys were waiting for us and greeted us with large smiles, and they chanted Samantha's name. After climbing the full flight of stairs up to their home, we entered the two-room apartment. It struck me as very clean, organized, and humble. Inside the home, there were beds, a refrigerator, and a stove. There was neither a bathroom nor a shower inside; those were down the stairs and outside and shared with neighbors.

I thought about how strong Maria is, the love and energy she must possess to wake each day, change, bathe, and dress Samantha to travel 1½ hours by bus to get Samantha to therapy on time. In comparison to my routines of getting up and ready for the day . . . How does she change Samantha's diapers? Where do they do laundry? Because of where she lives, a simple task such as bathing takes on a whole new meaning, is more time consuming, requires more planning, and takes more energy. I have the ease of doing all of these activities in my own home, and at the pace I choose for myself. How would it change if I had a child in a wheelchair and all of the facilities were a flight downstairs and outside? Maria chooses this life every day, she chose to love Samantha back to life and care for her abandoned grandchildren. She chooses to bathe, dress, and get Samantha to therapy every day. She is incredibly resilient and is living out her values of love and family.

Horacio: Disability Is Not the Same as Incapacitated

My name is Horacio, I was an engineer. I have congenital spinal stenosis in my cervical spine. The medulla is compressed between C2 through C5. My sickness started 2 years ago with pain in my arms, my stomach, and my back. I then started to have very painful headaches accompanied by a hissing sound between my ears. My pain worsened until I almost could not walk. As the pain worsened, I also became very depressed. I started looking for help; the doctors told me that I would need to have surgery. This worsened my depression because I was convinced that I would die in surgery because of where they would have to operate.

I started to see a psychologist who prescribed antidepressive medication. With the help of the therapy and medicine, my fear of the surgery lessened. I tried alternative medicine such as chiropractics, homeopaths, and herbal medicine. These did not seem to help me. I then visited many different neurologists to help understand if a surgery was indeed the best answer. Finally, I spoke with my wife, and together we agreed to pursue the operation.

I found a neurosurgeon with the best experience and reputation for my surgery. I entered surgery at 3:00 p.m. At 7:00 p.m. that same day, I woke up and the surgeon asked me to try to move an arm or leg. Not only could I not move, I could not feel a thing. I immediately went back into surgery, woke up again, and still there was no movement or sensation whatsoever. I had become a quadriplegic.

I was transferred to a different hospital and they said that they could do nothing for me there because the first surgeon had done so much damage to the medulla. Fifteen days later, a doctor specializing in trauma, agreed to try surgery. After a 5-hour surgery, I woke with a neck collar and IV medicine to decrease the inflammation of the medulla. Again, they put me on antidepressant medication. The doctor told me that I would never walk again. Then they sent me home. My wife looked at the doctors and asked them, "Now what do I do?" The doctor's response was "Go and pray. He will be able to move something eventually." In my mind, this was very poor medical practice regarding my health. I wanted to kill myself, but I couldn't; I couldn't move from the neck down.

After that surgery, my life changed. I went from having all the physical and professional capacity a person can have to nothing. I was 49 years old and my life had changed so definitively. I was no longer the Horacio who only knew life through a materialistic lens and who never did anything to help out someone in need.

When I came home, my wife hired a nurse to help care for me. She would turn me every hour to make sure I did not get bedsores. To calm myself, I needed antidepressants. The experience of being turned like that was very scary. I never knew what was going to happen; I couldn't feel anything.

A week later, my wife hired a therapist to come to the house. My wife was the only one who believed that one day I might be able to move on my own. The therapist spent 4 to 6 hours a day lifting my legs, my arms, moving me, but I did not feel a thing. I didn't want to feel because I was afraid I would feel pain.

Then it dawned on me. I thought about everything I had accomplished in life; nothing had happened to my cognition or intelligence. If I could do what I had done, why could I not rehabilitate? Someone told me that before I could heal, I would have to forgive myself as well as others. I did not know how to do this. I was not familiar with the concept of faith.

I did not have a relationship with my father. When people would ask me about my father, I would respond, "He is dead to me." I knew that in order to heal, I needed to forgive my dad and ask for his forgiveness. I started to forgive myself. My dad forgave me. I put a picture of my dad on my ceiling and would look at it as I did my exercises from my bed. I would ask my dad for the strength I needed to do the exercises.

In the middle of the night, I could not sleep. I found myself praying to God, asking him to give me another opportunity to live, to not just leave me in the bed, unable to move. I promised to help others with disabilities recuperate if I could be healed. I imagined what it would feel like to move. With that, my foot moved, then my body moved. My therapist came the next morning and I told him what had happened. As the therapist started to move me, I could feel the movement; I knew I was on my way to recovery.

Three months after wanting to commit suicide, I stood in a walker. I started to see, feel, and love strength

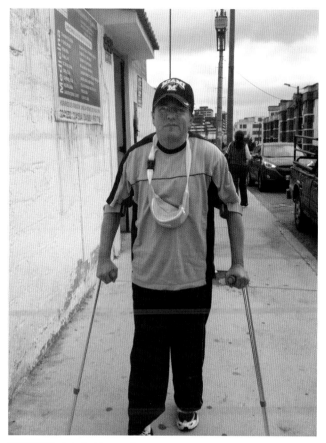

FIGURE 16-4 **Horacio.**

within my body. I promised myself I would never give up on myself, not my mind or my body, from that day forward.

Today, I can move all of my limbs (Figure 16-4). I can use the bathroom independently. So far, I still can't write, get up from the floor, or bathe or dress myself, but I think those things will come with time. I am a man that understands what disability means. But disability is not the same as incapable. *Disability does not mean incapacitated.* People with disabilities have the capacity to do things. I accept that I am a person with a disability, and I will learn how to live my life with these added challenges.

I hope to write a book, telling all of my stories about my rehabilitation. I want to serve the society and give an example of how to be patient, consistent, and strong. For now, each day I come to therapy, I try to make it better for my peers. I want to be the center of happiness, strength, and hope for those who arrive to therapy sad, scared, tired, and who are still questioning "Why me?" When therapy is done right, people leave feeling better and more hopeful than when they arrived.

On the outside, I appear a clown to help other people feel better, but don't let me fool you; I have a lot of tears on the inside. I still have very hard days, very sad days, I feel a lot of sadness. If you can't recuperate your body, you can recuperate your mind. It is very difficult to understand,

but the first thing the mind wants to do is to quit. Every day is a fight to not quit. Only when one is truly dead, is it impossible to live. Every day, I choose to live.

My Reflection: Walking with Horacio on the Street

When I met Horacio in the clinic, he was telling jokes and laughing with the therapist and other clients in the room. It was clear that everyone thought he was funny and enjoyed his company. I was a bit intimidated by the thought of interviewing him. I wondered if I would understand his use of humor or if he would take the process seriously. When we started the interview, his entire demeanor changed. He spoke slowly and intentionally, he made sure I understood every word. For Horacio, sharing his story with me was very important and serious. I came to understand his sudden change in demeanor as his story unfolded.

After listening to Horacio's story, I walked out to the street with him. He walked very carefully and slowly with two sling crutches. He told me that he wanted to show me something "very big." After crossing over a small incline, Horacio placed both crutches in one hand, and slowly, step-by-step, walked without assistance. He asked me to videotape his walking so that he could appreciate the progress he would make in the next year. The following day Horacio arrived walking with just one crutch. When I asked him about the other crutch, he replied, "Kate, telling my story to you has given me renewed strength and energy for my recovery. Thank you." Storytelling is indeed powerful.

Don Ulvio Lopez Arquello: The Power of Family and Community

To begin, getting to a life where one can feel tranquility is difficult. I feel like I was close, until the accident. I was hit by a drunk driver, and broke my neck. I can't move my legs; I can move my arms a little, that is getting better. So, my hope for tranquility is gone, but I have to continue to move forward. Medicine will not help me; I have to help myself through therapies. I ask God for help every day. I thank God every day for my family, my beautiful family, my wife, my kids, and everyone who cares for me (Figure 16-5).

The hardest part of being disabled for me is not being able to work. I was a hard worker. I started selling shoes, but I realized I could make shoes to sell, so that is what I did. I started making shoes to sell. They were good shoes too; people could see the quality in them. I would make shoes in the morning; and in the afternoon, I would work on building my house. I built this house, everything you see here, I built. But ultimately, my income was dependent

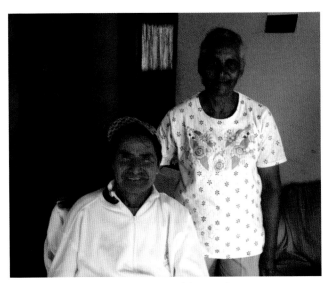

FIGURE 16-5 Don Ulvio and his wife.

on how many shoes I could sell. My goal was to have a job that paid a salary, a job where I made the same amount of money each month. I wanted a more stable life to provide for my family. So, I started to work for the municipality. They paid a salary; I was very happy with that. Then I decided I wanted to work for myself, so I got a car and started using it as a taxi. I was very contented working for myself. I was a hard worker. Before the accident, I did everything around the house. If the roof needed fixing, I fixed it. I built, I fixed, I did it all. But now, I can do nothing. [He looks at Maura, his daughter-in-law.] She does everything for me now. Sometimes I lose my patience. When I am alone, I start thinking about all of my life. It makes me sad to think that I can't do the things that were so important to me.

I am motivated to keep going by my grandchildren. I want to see them grow up. When I was in the hospital, they were all I could think about. The doctor told me that in order to return home, I needed to be able to breathe and eat on my own. Well, that was all I needed to hear, I would do anything to go home. So, I practiced eating and swallowing until I could do it. Then, we tried to take the oxygen off, and I was OK. I did not want to be on oxygen at home, it is too big and invasive. The only thing I wanted to do when I was in the hospital was to go home and see my children and grandchildren.

When I returned home, I realized that life would never be the same. It was difficult for me to fit into my home in a wheelchair. My neighbors came and made changes to the home so that my family could move me around in it. They also came to visit and brought food with them. I am so blessed. My son is an engineer. He created a pulley system so that my wife can put me to bed by herself. [Note: His son created a Hoyer lift in his bedroom.] I never knew how many people in my life care about me. In order to pay for my wheelchair and bath chair, I had to sell my chickens

and my truck. What if I had had nothing to sell? That is a sad reality for many people. My mind is weak and fragile. I have to remind myself to give God thanks every day for the people who surround me. I feel lucky, I have people in my life to help me organize my life and take care of me. I choose to feel grateful. Everything happens for a reason.

Maura Lucas: Don Ulvio's Caretaker

We live a couple of hours outside of Quito. Don Ulvio was a normal guy. He was a hard worker. He had his own car out of which he worked. His wife also worked in agriculture. He and his wife had four children. They were a poor family but saw to it that their children pursued education and entered a profession. Each child moved to different towns within 2 to 3 hours of home to pursue their careers. Each would return home every 15 days or so to visit their parents. Although Don Ulvio and his wife lived alone, they were happy, they were contented. Although poor, the couple was well known for helping out their neighbors when they were in need.

Just 1 year ago, Don Ulvio was in an accident. He was driving with his son when a drunk driver hit them. Don Ulvio took the impact of the accident, his son was not hurt. Don Ulvio was taken to a hospital, where they found out that he had fractured his cervical spine. All of his children gathered in Quito to discuss the news and support their mother.

Don Ulvio was a smoker, he already had bad lungs. In addition to being paralyzed, he would need to be on oxygen as well. He was also unable to eat independently due to dysphasia, so he had a feeding tube put in. After 3 months in the hospital on oxygen and with a feeding tube, the doctors suggested that we try to take him home without oxygen for a month. If it went well, he could stay home off of oxygen. If it did not go well, he would need oxygen at home.

He came home like a baby, he needed help for everything, he could not move from his neck down. But because he had helped so many people in the past, his neighbors and family all gathered to help support Don Ulvio and his wife. People really came through for us; they came with food, clothes, and their time to help us.

We moved our family to Quito to help with his care. I left my mother, who is on dialysis. It was so hard for me to leave her. When we received the phone call that Don Ulvio had been in a car accident, our entire lives changed. Sometimes I just want to throw in the towel. This is not the life I imagined for myself, taking care of my mother and then my father-in-law and not pursuing my professional career. But where God is, it is immense, and He is here with us. I have to keep going, I have to focus on the positive: He did not lose his mind, his sight, or his hearing. He is still here with us today. We have to grab hold of the love and continue to move forward.

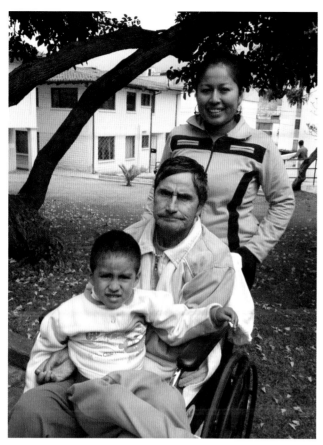

FIGURE 16-6 Maura, Don Ulvio, and Maura's son.

He had his time to enjoy his life, he worked hard to contribute to his community and help those in need. He also put all four children through school and saw to it that they were prepared to become self-sufficient adults. Now is his time to rest and receive care.

For now, this is my life. I visit my mom every month. I care for Don Ulvio. And I take care of my son (4 years old) (Figure 16-6). My life is about taking care of delicate people. Sometimes it makes me mad and sad; it is not what I imagined my life to be. I don't have what I want now, but I think God will look down on me one day and see that I am deserving of what I want and He will provide. I ask God for strength and I ask Him for love. We don't have our own home; we live in very tight quarters with my husband's parents. I want to work; I want to be able to send money to my mom. When my son starts school, I hope I can find a job.

My Reflection: Visiting Don Ulvio and Maura in Their Home

I walked out of therapy with Don Ulvio and Maria to the truck in which they had come. They lifted Don Ulvio into the bed of the truck, which was covered overhead and open in the back. Don Ulvio rode in the back of the pick-up truck with his wheelchair. They put him on top of a mattress and covered him with blankets. Don Ulvio travels for 2 hours each way to get to therapy.

I asked Don Ulvio if I could visit him in his home, he smiled and invited me along with the three occupational therapists from the center to visit him. We all gratefully accepted the invitation. As we took the 2-hour bus drive, we thought about Don Ulvio making the same trip in the back of the truck. When we arrived, Don Ulvio was outside waiting for us in the sun. As we pulled up to his home, he was grinning from ear to ear. His smile spoke a thousand words. While I was at Don Ulvio's home, his cousin stopped after church for a visit and brought fruit with him for the family. I also was able to see the Hoyer lift that his son made. It was clear that Don Ulvio experienced a lot of family and community support. The occupational therapists and I commented with one another on how positive the experience was for us and how much we enjoyed getting to know Don Ulvio in his home. The occupational therapists commented that they had not met his wife before because she is unable to make the trip to therapy, nor had they appreciated the vast countryside in which he lives. They observed that the amount of community involvement seemed much stronger than what they had seen in the city of Quito. We discussed the role of context in therapy and how the clinical setting can influence how and what we come to know about the people with whom we work.

Interpreting Narratives

I have been truly humbled by my experience. When I was initially asked to gather stories for this chapter, I could not imagine the power, emotion, and tenderness I would find in each story. I experienced the power of storytelling firsthand.

It is clear that there are common threads throughout these narratives that I believe are shared experiences of disability across cultures. The first is that having a disability is very expensive. Maria, Horacio, Don Ulvio, and Maura Lucas each have experienced loss of employment and many extra costs in order to access therapy, care, equipment, and transportation. The second theme throughout the stories is spirituality. Each person turned to a higher power for strength, patience, gratitude, and/or hope. The third theme found in each of the stories is a transformed sense of self. See Box 16-1 to consider ways each person developed this new sense of self.

Discussion

Each of these stories offers a powerful message. Each also demonstrates how both culture and socioeconomics impact the experience of having a disability. Maria's

---

BOX 16-1   TRANSFORMED SENSE OF SELF

Think about times in each of the stories in which people experienced and accepted a different and new sense of self and answer the following questions:

- What led to those experiences?
- What or who helped to facilitate the acceptance process?

---

story teaches us lessons about how to interact with people, how to work with family members, and the importance of respecting the knowledge of the family members. Maria has had negative experiences with health care workers speaking down to her. However, even more powerful is how she has fought for her daughter at every turn. She has gone without food and clothing herself to provide for her children. Without a formal education, she has been an advocate, a nurse, a doctor, a therapist, and a social worker for her daughter.

Horacio's story teaches us about faith. He told a story about forgiveness and hope and how each played an important role in his healing and rehabilitation process. Horacio was so incredibly proud to tell his story, he would sometimes pause to think of the reader and what he wanted them to know. The very act of telling his story was therapeutic for Horacio.

Don Ulvio's story was about the power of love he experienced from family and community after his accident. Don Ulvio's sense of self changed drastically from self-sufficient worker and provider for family to feeling dependent and needing to accept help. His story also teaches us about the significant role that community plays in one's experience of disability. After his accident, it was Don Ulvio's family and friends that were his drive to return home to the countryside, where it is quiet, peaceful, tranquil, and familiar. Maria's story as Don Ulvio's caretaker teaches us about selflessness and family expectations in the Ecuadorian culture.

The four people in these stories are full of warmth and resilience. Their willingness to open up and share their stories of heartbreak, challenge, and acceptance touched something deep inside of me. Reflect on the stories of Maria, Horacio, Don Ulvio, and Maura. Use the following questions to discuss the role of narrative in OT. As a profession, how can we better understand people's stories?

- How can we take the time to listen, to understand, and to know the people with whom we work?
- How would what we do be different if we knew people's stories?
- How do stories change based on who is telling them, who they are being told to, where they are told, and why they are being told?
- How might we use stories of transformation to understand what it is we do as occupational therapists?

REFERENCES

Consejo Nacional para la Igualdad de Discapacidades. (n.d.). *CONADIS: Consejo Nacional para la Igualdad de Discapacidades.* Retrieved from http://www.consejodiscapacidades.gob.ec/

U.S. Department of State. (n.d.). *Ecuador.* Retrieved from https://www.state.gov/p/wha/ci/ec/

the**Point**® *For additional resources on the subjects discussed in this chapter, visit* http://thePoint.lww.com /Willard-Spackman13e.

UNIT IV

Occupation in Context

Taking the Beach Home

Collect what we will
There's no bringing it home.
That hard-edge
two-color painting
half tan sand
half several blues
(mainly indigo chasing turquoise)
And particulars
to break the heart:
seaweed on rock
parting like drowned girls' hair;
pebbles shellacked by water,
subtle-hued as lentils,
beach glass

satined aqua, white,
amber, green;
a bit of pottery stamped France
We should know by now
What context demands
and how
things are all outdone by memory,
but we're still intent on
taking details home,
arriving
with only the sand in our sandal straps,
two shells chipped beyond repair,
stones and beach glass
dried dull as driveway gravel.

Eleanor Risteen Gordon
Used with permission of the author.

Family Perspectives on Occupation, Health, and Disability

Mary C. Lawlor, Cheryl Mattingly

LEARNING OBJECTIVES

After reading this chapter, you will be able to:

1. Identify ways to understand family occupations and the implications for collaborating with families.
2. Explore how family members might experience illness and disability and how these experiences are situated in family life.
3. Analyze knowledge, skills, and behaviors that facilitate effective "partnering up" and collaboration.
4. Acknowledge the expertise that family members have and bring to health care encounters, including occupational therapy sessions.
5. Examine the health care encounter as a complex social arena in which perceptions and decisions about care are created, contested, and negotiated by multiple social actors.

Introduction

Many of us have deep understandings of family life drawn from our first-hand, experiential knowledge of family, whether from family of origin or family created through our engagements in interpersonal worlds. The word **family** itself often evokes a complex array of thoughts, emotions, and embodied actions. The phrase "you are family" marks a belonging to a particular social world. In some ways, it could be said we know family. So how is it that forming effective partnerships with families in our clinical practices can be both so complicated and so essential?

Occupational therapy (OT) sessions as well as other health care encounters are key sites for facilitating partnerships, addressing needs and concerns, and supporting family life. Health care encounters are not only specific events but also episodes in the histories of client and family life and, conceivably, also episodes that are embedded in practitioners' lives and institutional cultures. Encounters such as OT sessions, particularly ones in which significant experiences happen, are events in longer illness and developmental trajectories. Significant moments in therapy sessions may resonate across time to other moments in one's life and across place to the extent that the impact is felt in other contexts, such as life at home, school, or work. Collaborative partnerships with families afford opportunities for salient moments in home and family life to be taken up in ways that influence the happenings that occur in OT sessions and their mattering in people's lives. Such partnerships generate deep learning for therapists who often have compelling narratives about how their engagements with families have transformed their practices and influenced their lives.

When I (first author) started to study how therapists work with families, I would ask them to tell me a story about a time when they felt they had a particularly successful and positive experience with families and, alternatively, a time when they wished things would have gone very differently. And it probably is not a big surprise that I found that the stories were very similar, revealing the complexity of engagements with families. It is hard to tell a story without some kind of trouble, so even stories of great success often contained reparations, rethinking, changing course, dilemmas, and tensions. These stories, and subsequent research described later in this chapter, also reveal that the mattering of OT is grounded in family life.

The purpose of this chapter is to provide an overview of family life, introduce family occupations, and discuss how understandings of family experiences related to illnesses and disabilities shape health care encounters including OT practices. This chapter concludes with a discussion of family-centered care and a case study example to illustrate how occupational therapists collaborate with families. We draw on a longitudinal, urban ethnographic research program entitled Boundary Crossings: Re-Situating Cultural Competence that we describe later in this chapter and conducted at the University of Southern California (USC) with funding from 1997 to 2011.[1] We also draw on findings from Autism in Urban Context: Linking Heterogeneity with Health and Service Disparities (AUCP), a 3-year study with a cohort of African American children with autism, their families, and practitioners who served them.[2]

The heart of this chapter moves from general considerations of family life to the intricacies, dilemmas, surprises, and riches of therapeutic work that take seriously the illness and disability experiences of families. Processes related to "partnering up" between practitioners and family members are also examined.

Understanding Family Life

Family life is dynamic, often compelling, complicated, and multifaceted. Although the term *family life* may imply a unitary construct, understanding family life involves the recognition of its heterogeneity and diversity. Family life is situated in broader sociocultural contexts as well as intergenerational and historical contexts. Family life is constituted through an array of cultural and social practices and lived through engagements in occupations (Figure 17-1). The particularities or details of life within families often reveal the relationships, social networks, activities, values, beliefs, priorities, occupations, history, resources, and challenges inherent in families. Family life is enacted through the interplay of the ordinary routines of daily life and the extraordinary experiences of family life, events, and unexpected happenings. The ordinary or everyday occupations reflect the ways that habits and routines give structure and meaning to our lives, but the surface sense of ordinariness often obscures their complexity and particularity in

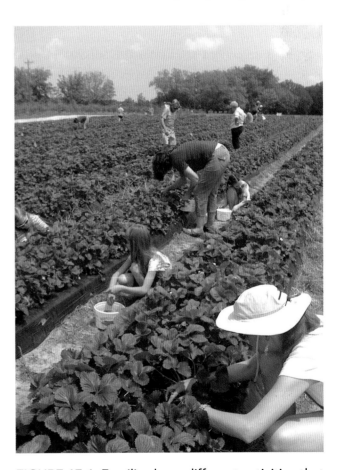

FIGURE 17-1 Families have different activities that they share. Here, cousins and their parents pick strawberries while visiting the grandparents—an annual summer event.

[1]This research program comprised three research grants: MCJ-060745, Maternal and Child Health Program, Health and Services Administration, Department of Health & Human Services; Boundary Crossing: A Longitudinal and Ethnographic Study (#R01 HD 38878); and Boundary Crossings: Re-Situating Cultural Competence (#2R01 HD 38878), funded by National Institute of Child Health and Human Development (NICHD), National Institutes of Health (NIH). Pseudonyms are used to provide greater confidentiality.
[2]This research project entitled Autism in Urban Context: Linking Heterogeneity with Health and Service Disparities was funded by the National Institute on Mental Health, National Institute of Health (# R01 MH089474), principal investigator: Dr. Olga Solomon.

terms of individual and family life (Hasselkus, 2006). For some families who have family members with illnesses or disabilities, the achievement of a sense of routine everydayness or ordinariness can, in fact, be an extraordinary achievement (Mattingly, 2010).

Family life is marked by the interdependency of family members (Bandura, Carprara, Barbaranelli, Regalia, & Scabini, 2011). As Glen Elder (1998) reminds us, lives are *linked* through our engagements in social worlds. Longer life expectancies have contributed to greater opportunities for intergenerational relationships, including those of grandparents and grandchildren, often supported by the parents or middle generation (Swartz, 2009). Relationships with family members permeate our life course and are understood to be both enduring and changing (Swartz, 2009). Families often work to make sure that current family members have an appreciation of family members who are not in proximity due to death, illness, geographic distance, deployment, or other factors. Photographs, family stories, naming conventions, and artifacts such as a grandmother's ring or recipes are all cultural resources to infuse contemporary family life with a sense of roots, history, and connectedness.

Understanding family also involves an appreciation of how culture relates to family life. Families have their own cultures (Fitzgerald, 2004; Lawlor & Elliot, 2012; Lawlor & Mattingly, 2009), and family life is constituted through cultural beliefs, practices, and occupations that are both particular to any family and illustrative of broader sociocultural influences on family life. For example, birthday parties in Joe's family might always include the cooking of the favorite meal of the celebrant, the wearing of a "Happy Birthday" crown, being seated at the head of the dinner table, and being relieved of any household chores for the day. This cluster of actions might not only be unique to Joe's family but also has resonances of broader sociocultural influences related to mealtime, birthday events, and family life. For many, the implicit nature of family culture is revealed when a potentially new family member—such as a date, fiancé, partner, or in-home caregiver—first enters family life. Such questions as "Is your family always like this?" or comments like "I don't get your family" mark the particularity of family cultures.

Contemporary studies of human development and conceptual models in sociocultural psychology have reinforced our appreciation for how family life serves as a particularly potent context for learning, especially for infants and young children (Rogoff, 2003). As Hanks (1991) argues, "Learning is a process that takes place in a participation framework, not in an individual mind" (p. 15). Families constitute the primary social unit by which children first learn about the world and occupations (Fitzgerald, 2004). Learning within the occupations and activities of family life incorporates understandings of

a family's beliefs, routines, culture, and cultural practices as well as skill development (Kellegrew, 1998). Family routines provide a naturally occurring social context and organizing structure to promote learning (Rabb & Dunst, 2004). Occupational therapists have studied family routines and challenges and described a number of intervention approaches designed to support family routines (e.g., Ausderau & Juarez, 2013; Boyd, McCarty, & Sethi, 2014; Dunn, Cox, Foster, Mische-Lawson, & Tanquary, 2012; Segal, 2004).

Family Occupations

There are many ways to conceptualize occupations within family life. In a general sense, family occupations can be understood as the occupations conducted with more than one family member that contribute to the health, well-being, and interrelationships among family members. Like the occupations of individuals, family occupations represent meaningful engagements in which family members invest energy, skills and talents, and physical and emotional resources to support family life and the ongoing development of family members. These occupations include routine daily practices, such as caregiving, cooking, and driving children to school, as well as family practices that reflect family culture, intergenerational transmission of values and priorities, and the creation of significant experiences and events such as a visit from the tooth fairy or maintaining a memento box of the artifacts of childhood.

The term *co-occupation* has been used to describe when more than one person is engaged in an occupation. Other terms to describe occupations that are not individual and are more collective include *shared occupations*, *joint occupations*, *joint endeavors*, and *co-created occupations* (Lawlor, 2003). The theoretical basis for these terms is not yet well theorized but reflects recent attempts to develop a more social, dynamic, and transactional approach to understanding occupation (Dickie, Cutchins, & Humphry, 2006; Lawlor, 2003). Other approaches to categorizing family occupations have included designations like mothering, parenting, fathering, and caregiving occupations (e.g., Bonsall, 2014a, 2014b; Esdaile & Olson, 2004).

Family Perspectives on Health and Disability

When individuals experience illness or disability, family members also have illness and disability experiences (Lawlor & Mattingly, 2009; Mattingly & Lawlor, 2003). Most people who come to OT live in social worlds that include families of some kind. Families, in various forms and partnership arrangements, matter for most people who experience illness or disability, no matter what the age, ethnicity, socioeconomic status, or geographical location. Even when people live apart from their families, it is very likely that some family members will be instrumental in healing, recovery, caregiving, and participation in occupations. How clients experience disability and how it affects their functioning in the world often depend heavily on the clients' relationships with family members and other significant people in their social worlds. Family life also influences participation, and family participation and occupations can be affected when one or more family members have disabilities or special health care needs (Law, 2002).

Attempts to understand illness and disability experiences have been facilitated by the "narrative turn" in medicine (Charon, 2006; Garro & Mattingly, 2000; Hurwitz, Greenhalgh, & Skultans, 2004). Literature in anthropology, particularly medical anthropology, occupational science and therapy, medicine, and other health-related fields is increasingly drawing on narrative approaches to (1) enhance understanding of illness and disability from the perspectives of the individuals and their families who are living with illnesses or disabilities (e.g., Bluebond-Langer, 1978; A. Frank, 1995; G. Frank, 2000; Kleinman, 1988, 2006; Lawlor & Solomon, 2017; Monks & Frankenberg, 1995; Murphy, 1990), (2) analyze how narrative modes of reasoning or narrative-based ethics influence health and therapeutic practices (e.g., Becker, 1997; Cain, 1991; Charon & Montello, 2002; Fleming & Mattingly, 1994; Hurwitz et al., 2004; Mattingly, 2014), and (3) recognize narrative as a structure for creating significant experiences in therapeutic practices (Clark, 1993; Mattingly, 1998).

Occupational therapists have also found it helpful to read and reflect on first-person or family accounts of illness and disability experiences, such as those provided in Unit III. An extensive listing of written narratives can be found on thePoint (e.g., Bauby, 1997; Greenfeld, 1978, 1986; Hockenberry, 1995; Jamison, 1996; Park, 1982, 2001; Peete, 2010; Williams, 1992). At times, popular media, including films and television shows such as *Parenthood* can generate insights that support practitioners' reflections on their clinical practices. Even films or television shows that present portrayals of illnesses or disabilities or health and therapeutic practices that may be disturbing, demeaning, or inaccurate can provide important experiences for clarifying beliefs and philosophies.

Family-Centered Care

So, what I did is, I became very personal with my therapist. She just wasn't a lady I saw once a week; she was adopted into my family. And I brought my family to therapy with me. I brought children. I brought my grandma [*laughs*],

so that she could be in on what it is that we would be trying to achieve. What it was that we need my daughter to accomplish. I brought children, aunties, uncles, close neighbors—everybody that was a part of my close daily surroundings, went to therapy. And that's just the way it was. So that the therapy was not just once a week, it was seven days a week. It was from the minute we woke up to the minute we went to bed.

The aforementioned quote is an excerpt from a transcribed interview with a mother who was telling a story about her daughter's OT program. It is drawn from an ethnographic research study conducted by the authors and an interdisciplinary research team that will be described in more detail later in this chapter. The family-centered care movement, cost containment initiatives, and technological advancements in care delivery have fundamentally altered the expectations of families and practitioners, the nature of health care and caregiving practices, and outcomes of interventions. Health care encounters, once characterized by dyadic communication between a patient and doctor, are now complex social arenas in which multiple social actors, including family members, convene. The adoption of new technologies such as computer-based documentation also can affect communication and interactions (Solomon, Angell, Yin, & Lawlor, 2015). Health care encounters involving family members are sites of intense **boundary crossing** where families and practitioners create, negotiate, contest, and/or modify perceptions, perspectives, and caregiving and treatment practices. Multiple perspectives on health care events are both anticipated and managed within often relatively brief moments of interaction. Some of the interesting dilemmas and opportunities that emerge when practitioners involve families actively in the therapeutic process are highlighted in this chapter.

Although the development of services that center on the needs and values of families began in early childhood programs through family-centered care initiatives (Hanft, 1991; Lawlor & Mattingly, 1998), many of the principles apply to services for people of all ages (Humphry, Gonzales, & Taylor, 1993), and expansion of family-centered care principles are evident in new areas such as care coordination (Moyers & Metzler, 2014). As human service systems moved into the community and family members began providing more home care, practitioners developed a deeper appreciation of the centrality of families in healing, recovery, and adaptation. Practitioners also recognized that family members often had different perspectives from those of the professionals about the needs, priorities, and strengths of the client. This recognition led to a shift from perceiving family members as people who will carry out the doctors' and practitioners' orders to perceiving family members as people who are most knowledgeable about the client and who are partners in decision making. Family members' perspectives about how the client is doing, what

CENTENNIAL NOTES

Involvement of Family Members

Mary C. Lawlor, Barbara A. Boyt Schell

In the sixth edition of *Willard & Spackman's Occupational Therapy* (Hopkins & Smith, 1983), there is only one indexed item related to families, which is qualified as "family, in mental retardation programs." The text includes the following: "Involvement of family members must continue to increase" (Sebelist, 1983, p. 348). Such a call appears quite modest today in view of the emphasis on supporting family-centered care across the life course. Comparisons to more recent editions reveal considerable expansion of the attention to families and family-centered care.

Many of the key themes in this chapter have resonances in the earlier history of OT. The implementation of federal initiatives related to providing services for children with special health care needs and their families was documented as early as 1912, with the establishment of the United States Children's Bureau. Julia Lathrop was recommended by Jane Addams of Hull House to become the first director of the bureau, and on April 17, 2012, President Taft named Lathrop as chief (Figure 17-2). Julia Lathrop became the first woman ever to be appointed head of a federal bureau. This same Julia Lathrop worked at Hull House, developed a course called "Invalid Occupations" at the Chicago School of Civics and Philanthropy, and apparently was a mentor of Eleanor Clarke Slagle. According to the government history of this agency, Julia Lathrop took the reins with a small budget of just over $25,000 but a grand vision. She selected infant mortality as the Bureau's first area of focus: conducting research, advocating comprehensive birth registration, and publishing advice for parents. Later in its first decade, with a budget 10 times its initial appropriation, the Bureau expanded its efforts to include research and standard setting in the areas of child labor, juvenile delinquency, mothers' aid, illegitimacy, child welfare, and child health (Children's Bureau, U.S. Department of Health & Human Services, n.d.).

Fifty years later, Tate (1974) underscored the importance of students understanding the life situations of their patients.

> Students of occupational therapy must be exposed to whole life situations of the aged, the disabled and the chronically ill and not just see them in hospital or rehabilitation centre as they do now. They must be able to recognize and understand the influence of cultural patterns, economic conditions, environmental stress, in order to identify the unmet needs and problems in their fullest implication. They must then be able to define the role of the occupational therapist and bring to bear an analytical, problem solving approach to help the individual in the resolution of his problems, acting as a collaborator rather than instructor in the process. (p. 8)

Although much of the language around family participation has changed, many of the earlier principles have been retained. Contemporary practice calls for an even closer attention to supporting families in their daily lives due to knowledge generated through developmental science, expanding accounts of lived experiences, pressing societal needs, and the changing landscape of health care and education.

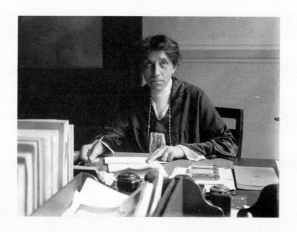

FIGURE 17-2 Julia Lathrop, the first director of the United States Children's Bureau.

the client needs, what the family needs, and what is most important and meaningful in everyday life have become part of the clinical dialogue.

Family-centered care involves much more than thinking of adding family members into the therapy session; OT practice is fundamentally altered when family members are brought into the therapeutic process in a central way (Lawlor & Mattingly, 1998). Family members, including parents, often have powerful roles in the creation of significant experiences in therapy (Lawlor, 2009; Mattingly & Lawlor, 2001). The challenge for the OT practitioner is to collaborate with clients, their families, and other team members in designing a program that builds on strengths and addresses needs (Figure 17-3). When done successfully, intervention services are individualized to each family and reflect their unique cultural world. Drawing on the work of Dunst, Trivette, and Deal (1988), we have defined **family-centered care** as "an experience

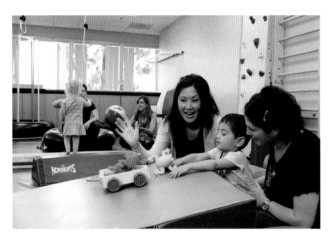

FIGURE 17-3 Family members are an integral part of therapy. (Photo courtesy of University of Southern California.)

that happens when practitioners effectively and compassionately listen to the concerns, address the needs, and support the hopes of people and their families" (Lawlor & Cada, 1993; Lawlor & Mattingly, 1998).

Family-centered care is enacted through the collaborative efforts of family members and practitioners (Edelman, Greenland, & Mills, 1993; Lawlor & Mattingly, 1998) and typically is provided through multidisciplinary and interdisciplinary team structures. Partnerships are created on the basis of the establishment of trust and rapport as well as respect for family values, beliefs, and routines (Hanft, 1989). Additional elements of successful collaboration include clarity and honesty in communication, mutual agreement on goals, effective information sharing, accessibility, and absence of blame (McGonigel, Kaufmann, & Johnson, 1991). Successful collaboration occurs when practitioners and family members form relationships that foster a shared understanding of the needs, hopes, expectations, and contributions of all partners (Lawlor & Cada, 1993). This type of engagement is often described as a means of enabling and empowering families (Deal, Dunst, & Trivette, 1989).

The Processes of "Partnering Up" and Collaboration

Occupational therapists draw on their own life experiences of family as well as professional and theoretical concepts of families when collaborating with families (Fitzgerald, 2004). Collaboration is much more than being "nice" (Lawlor & Mattingly, 1998; Mattingly, 1998). **Collaboration** involves complex interpretative acts in which the practitioner must understand the meanings of interventions, the meanings of illness or disability in a person and family's life, and the feelings that accompany

these experiences. Collaboration is also dependent on the development of a quality of interrelatedness that is evident in many therapy sessions that is not merely a question of establishing good rapport, eliciting cooperation, or prompting a client or patient to buy into a particular agenda in order for him or her to perform required tasks (Lawlor, 2003). The central question for practitioners and clients and their families is "How can we come to know enough about each other to effectively partner up?" (Lawlor & Mattingly, 2001). For therapists, the nature of the work in collaboration is not merely technical in the sense that a procedure is done or a therapy or other intervention is provided, nor does the work just entail drawing on clinical expertise. Rather, "partnering up" requires skilled relational work and involves the drawing on a range of social skills including intersubjectivity, communication, engagement, and understanding (Lawlor, 2004, p. 306).

Assumptions about race, culture, ethnicity, social status, economic level, and education (and frequently the contesting of these assumptions) often powerfully influence the process of partnering up between families and professionals. Family members and practitioners live and operate in a multiplicity of cultural domains that are shaped by their profession, economic class, ethnicity, and community affiliations. When practitioners and family members interact, their values, assumptions, and perceptions about the interaction are shaped by their membership in these cultures. See Chapters 19 and 20 for more information.

Partnering up also involves bridging differences, establishing points of common interests and mutuality, and capitalizing on complementarities. This aspect of collaboration is particularly important when family members and practitioners perceive that they come from seemingly differently lived worlds. Mattingly (2006), drawing on reconceptualizations of culture that are prevalent in current anthropology, argues that health care encounters are like border zones, where there is often heightened engagement related to marking differences, finding commonalities, and creating understanding. Families in many ways are the consummate travelers in border zones with the daunting task of coming to understand biomedical, institutional, and practitioner cultural worlds and practices and participating in these practices in such a way that their nonbiomedical conceptualizations of their children, their families, and illness and disability can shape health care encounters.

We have come to conceptualize partnerships with families as grounded in complementarity such that all parties contribute expertise, understandings, practical reasoning, desires and hopes, and problem-solving strategies. **Complementarity** has been defined as *the quality or state of being complementary*, with a secondary definition of *completing* (http://www.dictionary.com), meaning both parties together make a whole. Parallels with the term reciprocity add to our selection of this term described as how *one thing supplements or depends on the other* (https://thefreedictionary.com) or as *combining in such a way as to enhance or emphasize the qualities of each other or another; a relationship or situation in which two or more different things improve or emphasize each other's qualities* (https://en.oxforddictionaries.com). The most effective partnerships are built on mutual respect and reciprocity but draw on the different perspectives, knowledge, and strengths of all the partners. Like most relationships, collaborative partnerships work best with a degree of differentiation and difference among the partners. In other words, most people who seek advice and care from health care practitioners want the practitioners to offer expertise and decisions that are different from what they already know.

Troublesome Assumptions about Disability, Illness Experiences, and Families

Over the past 20 years, there has been considerable attention toward understanding the ways in which family members participate in health care practices, (e.g., Hinojosa, Sproat, Mankhetwit, & Anderson, 2002; Law, Hanna, King, Hurley, King, Kertoy, & Rosenbaum, 2003; Lawlor & Mattingly, 1998; Schreiber, Benger, Salls, Marchetti, & Reed, 2011), but much additional knowledge and reflection are needed (Cohn, 2001; Ochieng, 2003). Many practitioners who work in multicultural settings recognize the complexity of organizing health care and therapy practices in such a way as to understand and address the specific needs of family members and capitalize on their strengths. The following sections illustrate how problematic or flawed assumptions about the illness and disability experiences of family members can affect care.

The Disability Belongs to the Individual

One of the most pervasive assumptions in biomedicine is that the professional's task is to treat the individual who has the illness or medical condition. Sometimes, this is narrowly interpreted among health professionals as "treating the pathology," but OT practitioners usually try to remember that they are also treating a whole person who has a condition that results in challenges. Put differently, practitioners try to treat what anthropologists speak of as *the illness experience* rather than simply the disease (Good, 1994; Good

& Good, 1994; Kleinman, 1988; Luhrmann, 2000). In the context of OT, another term used is *the disability experience*, for it is certainly possible to have a disability, even one that requires therapy, without being ill. Practitioners try to attend both to the disability, or illness, as a physiological condition and to the meaning this particular condition carries for the person who has the disability as well as his or her family (Mattingly, 1998, 2000; Mattingly & Fleming, 1994). If a practitioner knows that a client wants to relearn how to drive, dress independently, eat out at restaurants, or continue to work as an auto mechanic, the practitioner may be able to organize therapeutic tasks that aid the client in carrying out these activities.

Therapeutic approaches should also situate these goals in an understanding of the family and social worlds that impact on these occupations. This is especially true for goals that concern the client's social world and the connection between functional skills and social relationships. It is artificial to treat only narrowly defined functional skills as though they were unrelated to a client's social world because a key aspect of the meaning of a condition is how it affects an individual's personal relationships and participation. By contrast, with such goals as learning how to dress oneself and learning wheelchair mobility, goals and concerns that are connected to family relations are much more difficult to define, and they are certainly likely to be hard to measure. Helping a client to reclaim his identity as a good father to his 5-year-old daughter even though he has a spinal cord injury, for example, is harder to translate into discrete, skill-based goals than is learning how to increase upper body strength or learning how to eat independently. However, learning what family members hope for—what they would like to see happen—is critical to the development of collaborative therapy practices with families. As Cohn, Miller, and Tickle-Degnan (2000) found in their qualitative study of parents of children with sensory modulation disorders, skillful listening to parents' perspectives can generate insights that promote therapy that is meaningful in terms of family goals and values.

Family-oriented goals are likely to be tied to outcomes that are diffuse, complex, subtle, and difficult to measure, even when they are deeply significant to the client and family. When a client's goals and concerns are tied to shifting family relationships, these might seem out of professional bounds for the OT practitioner. Despite the many difficulties in trying to understand how a condition affects a client's role in the family, ignoring this aspect often means being blind to the most significant aspects of the illness (or disability) experience. Ignoring family-oriented goals or the meaning of a disability as it ties to family concerns and family relationships can mean ignoring the person altogether.

Occupational therapy holds deep values for supporting individuals, and it is possible that some might interpret this family emphasis as competing with or diminishing a person-centered approach. This is a misread of family-centered care in which the needs of individuals are met within the context of their family and community life. Patient-centered care principles incorporate family involvement as a key component to the collaborative processes that undergird care, coordination, and planning (Mroz, Pitonyak, Fogelberg, & Leland, 2015).

As one therapist who participated in the Boundary Crossings project expressed,

> I just love to see the process of therapy and what it can bring to a person who has the need for it. And especially what it can bring to a family. And I think that's what's so rich with children is you have this family unit. And I've learned over the years that it doesn't matter what I do with that child, it's what I do with that family. . . . And I love it.

There Is Only One Perspective per Family

Although much of the literature on family-centered care presumes that practitioners come to know all members of the family, we have found that often, one member of the family, typically a mother or spouse, serves as the primary contact for the practitioner. It is this individual's perspective that practitioners come to know. However, this might be only one of several perspectives held by family members. Practitioners sometimes get to know other family members, but in many settings, the primary contact is the family member who brings the child to therapy or accompanies an adult or parent to therapy. Often, the family member who comes to the therapy session has a complicated culture-brokering role in which the person needs to both represent home, family, and community life in the clinic world and represent the clinic and institutional world back in home and family life. Such questions as "So, what happened?" are indicative of the information requests that spouses, significant others, grandparents, and other family members might ask.

Family members may also have quite divergent perspectives on the nature of the problem, priorities for intervention, and meanings of illness and disability in daily life (see Figure 17-3). These within-family differences often generate within-family negotiations and a kind of partnering up within family life that will influence family–practitioner partnerships. The dynamics of these multiple perspectives and within-family negotiations will likely change over time and be influenced by changes in illness trajectories, developmental agendas, household configurations, and constellation of household resources and needs. In addition, illness and disability might only be one subplot or drama in family life, competing with other pressing concerns and needs.

Illness and Disability Generate Only Negative Experiences

The following quote is from a father in AUCP excerpted from a collective narrative group with families.[3] He is describing his experiences with his son.

> . . . a very energetic kid it's been a, a blessing to have Bryce. He's, um, taught us and me a lot about oh so many things, mostly about his perception of the world, how we began to notice he sees things differently and because he sees things differently, you know, often the saying it goes, "Kids see the world through their parents' eyes," you got the, inverse is also true sometimes, a parent can begin to see the world through their children's eyes—it's very enlightening.

There has been, and continues to be, an assumption that all of the effects of illness and disability on a family are negative. This belief leads to the erroneous conclusion that family reactions to illness and disability are both predictable and shared. In other words, the practitioner might presume to know about the effect of an illness or disability on the family without fully understanding a particular family. These notions get dismissed once one listens to families talk about their experiences. We have been struck by the incredible richness of their stories and the difficulty people have in reducing their complex reactions to a few discrete categories such as stress, grief, or acceptance.

Much of the research that has been conducted that relates to the response of family members to illness or disability has been conducted with parents of children who have special health care needs. Parents and other family members have offered critiques of this body of research (e.g., Lipsky, 1985), citing the failure of researchers to recognize positive outcomes from these experiences. Researchers have tended to measure such predetermined variables as maternal depression and stress. Critics note that personal reports of other effects, including positive changes in family life, have been discounted. Advocates of the family-centered care movement note the failure of many researchers and practitioners to understand the unique features of family adaptation and coping and assert the need for further research that is grounded in the perspectives of family members. Although it is beyond the scope of this chapter to summarize this body of literature, the assumption that the effects of disability are unilateral and negative must be challenged as both simplistic and inadequate.

Practitioners need to seek understanding of the effects of illness and disability on the families of the people

---

[3]Based on our narrative inquiry methods, we developed a form of group narrative interviewing that we described as Collective Narratives (Jacobs, Lawlor, & Mattingly, 2011; Lawlor & Mattingly, 2001; Mattingly, Lawlor, & Jacobs-Huey, 2002; Solomon & Lawlor, 2013).

who come to them for assistance. These effects will likely change over time, and the perceptions of the relative stress of families will be shaped by other events in the family and the availability of resources. The presumption that the entirety of a family's experience can be summarized as stressful often leads to misunderstandings and lost opportunities to promote any positive aspects and celebrate successes (Lawlor & Cada, 1993; Lawlor & Mattingly, 1998; Mattingly & Lawlor, 2000).

Having a family member with illnesses and/or disabilities can substantially impact family life including participation, routines, priorities, practices, and identity (Law, 2002; Werner DeGrace, 2004). Although much of the literature emphasizes potentially negative influences such as stress, decreased economic resources, or excessive time demands, the picture is far more complicated. On the Boundary Crossings research program at USC, described briefly later in this chapter, families have worked to make sure that we understand and appreciate the positive elements that having a family member with special needs brings to family life. These include the cultivation of strengths and skills; love; "blessings" and renewed or enhanced spirituality; positive affects on siblings; and adoption of new career paths, advocacy, or social activism. Our intent is not to romanticize family life but rather to point toward the range of possible experiences of families when managing illness or disability trajectories. We have come to understand that strengths and challenges are intimately interrelated and perhaps can best be understood as relational aspects of family experience. Families have often used phrases such as "strengths beget strengths" or "God only gives me what he knows I can handle" to convey their lived experiences of the co-relations of strengths and challenges.

The Professional Is the Expert

Practices steeped in Western biomedical traditions frequently adopt professional–client relationships that are based on hierarchical models or expert-driven models. The expert model remains prevalent in early childhood practices despite increasing recognition that elements of this model create barriers to developing collaborative partnerships and understanding family life. The expert model tends to promote dependence within recipients of services, to limit opportunities for families to contribute insights and have their specific concerns and needs addressed, to burden the professional with the unrealistic expectation of always having the expertise to respond to all issues (Cunningham & Davis, 1985), and to organize services in ways that are self-serving to the expert (Howard & Strauss, 1975).

It is not surprising that reliance on expert models fosters relationships between practitioners and family members that could incorporate compliance and coercion strategies. This leads to considerable confusion about whether the "story" is one of collaboration, coercion, or compliance (Lawlor & Mattingly, 1998). The issue is not merely a semantics problem. Each approach to working relationships creates distinctly different experiences for all parties. Practitioner judgments that a person is noncompliant, or in the terms used by family members—"bad parent," "bad daughter," and the like, divert energies away from more reflective analysis or direct attempts to understand alternative perspectives (Trostle, 1988). Comments such as "They are just in denial" often indicate a breach in understanding, a dismissal of family or personal perspectives. Families typically have tremendous expertise and knowledge related to their family members, family life, the illness or disability of their family member, and the ways in which treatment recommendations can most likely be implemented in the home (Egilson, 2010). As Bedell, Cohn, and Dumas (2005) note, parents are well situated to promote and support their child's development in home and community life and able to modify or develop effective strategies. Perhaps the most troubling dimension of a hierarchical model of expertise is that family expertise is not acknowledged and taken up in meaningful ways. In fact, in some health care encounters, family expertise remains quite invisible.

Perhaps the most important consideration in understanding expertise is the understanding and recognition of the expertise that individuals and families develop. The cultivation of expertise related to managing a health or developmental condition, navigating the health care and educational arenas, appraising the meanings of illness and disability in daily life, and achieving desired outcomes is often experienced as a deep moral imperative (Lawlor & Solomon, 2017; Mattingly, 2014). Effective collaborative partnerships require that all parties including practitioners capitalize on the expertise of the other partners and create a working relationship that fosters sharing of information (Harrison, Romer, Simon, & Schulze, 2007). The legacy of hierarchical models of expertise must be overcome so that families feel respected for their knowledge, ideas, and perspectives, and practitioners do not feel their own expertise is under threat (Silverman & Brosco, 2007).

Expanding Opportunities for "Partnering Up" with Families

So far, we have emphasized ways in which a family-centered approach can support family life. Family life does not occur just within homes, it also is embedded in community life. It is anticipated that as OT practitioners expand their approaches designed to facilitate participation and inclusion for individuals with challenges and their families, practitioners will strengthen family-centered approaches to address challenges in community life that affect participation (Gibbs & Toth-Cohen, 2011). Participation in community life has been identified as a primary area of concern for families (Khetani, Cohn, Orsmond, Law, & Coster, 2013; Woodgate, Edwards, & Ripat, 2012).

The following data excerpt from the AUCP illustrates the complexities families may encounter.

> Yeah I've had people give me dirty looks in stores because and you know we were at an amusement park once and he just put his head and he dropped to the ground and just put his head down because he was so overwhelmed it was just too much stimulation for him. And people are looking walking by and you know they didn't understand but you know they had comments like "Uh she don't even know how to control her kids" and if that was my kid you know that type of thing. "Oh what's wrong with him?" . . . But my focus has to be you know . . . I have to shift my focus from them to him. And realizing that at some point he's overwhelmed so I either need to change the venue or go to a more quiet place because that's my cue and it has nothing to do with him wanting you know to misbehave but I have to remember my child has special needs and this is one of those times.

This mother's story points toward the ways in which occupational therapists might use their knowledge of sensory processing and sensory strategies to support family engagements in community settings. A number of occupational therapists are also working at the level of community institutions, such as museums, to identify ways they can use their expertise to support environmental, attitudinal, and behavioral changes to promote full engagement and inclusion.

Many of the stories we have heard as part of our research projects also point toward the importance of participating in the activities of the extended family, often outside of the family's home (e.g., Lawlor & Solomon, 2017). In the excerpt below, also from the AUCP study, a mother talks about how her extended family members engaged in providing supports for her sons with autism.

> I think probably either last Thanksgiving or the Thanksgiving before that, yeah it was the Thanksgiving before . . . He [referring to the relative who was hosting the extended family dinner] went out and I had told him some things that the boys like and everything, so he went out and Angie [the host's partner] made a big deal of [he] went out and picked these things up and I had nothing to do with it, and [he] picked up some toys to keep the boys occupied at their house. And he got some stuff that would be like flashing lights and I would think, oh my God they're gazing . . . great toys, thanks. So yeah, but they were happy, they were not ruining dinner and their sensory needs were met. That was one of the best Thanksgivings we've ever had because the boys weren't destroying dinner.

Family Experiences and Occupational Therapy Practice

This chapter addresses the need to attend to family perspectives in providing services to people with chronic illnesses or disabilities and the experiences of family members that are related to their participation in OT services. We have spent many hours watching OT practices, primarily with children. In addition, we have interviewed many parents and other family members and practitioners. These data have been gathered as part of a longitudinal, urban, ethnographic research project currently entitled Boundary Crossings: Re-Situating Cultural Competence. We have followed a cohort of African American children with illnesses and/or disabilities, their primary caregivers, family members, and the practitioners who serve them for approximately 15 years. This is a multifaceted study that included analysis of meanings of illness and disability in family and clinical worlds; cross-cultural communication in health care encounters; health care practices including OT; health disparities; and processes of partnering up and how illness and disability, family life, health care, and development are interrelated (e.g., Lawlor, 2003, 2004, 2009, 2012; Mattingly, 2006, 2010, 2014). The conceptual framework for the study draws heavily on narrative, interpretive, and phenomenological approaches to understanding human experience.

One of our most striking discoveries is the way in which seemingly casual conversation, brief moments of social engagement, attention to connectedness, and shared moments in the course of therapy sessions can deeply affect the experiences of family members and practitioners and, perhaps most important, the outcomes of therapy. These moments can be quite subtle and appear to be a kind of backdrop to the real work in therapy time or in health care encounters. Their seemingly mundane nature can belie their impact. As is illustrated later in this chapter, there are also times of heightened engagement in which there is intensity around the learning or insights to understanding that are unfolding.

In the following passages, we provide examples of family experiences related to illness and disability and their interactions with practitioners, including occupational therapists. Occupational therapists have shared many stories that relate to how they or their practice has been influenced by their experiences with families. We will begin by returning to the quote that was used to introduce family-centered care. In that quote, this mother shared her strategy for ensuring that her family, including extended members, was knowledgeable about her child's therapy program and the clinical world in which therapy

COMMENTARY ON THE EVIDENCE

Twenty years ago, we (Mary Lawlor and Cheryl Mattingly) published a chapter in the ninth edition of *Willard & Spackman's Occupational Therapy* (Neistadt & Crepeau, 1998) entitled "Disability Experience from a Family Perspective." Since that time, we have continued to study practices with children and families including OT, meanings of illness and disability in family life, engagement and participation, health disparities, and processes of "partnering up" to facilitate collaboration and outcomes. Our ethnographic, narrative, longitudinal, and phenomenological methods have enabled us to be with children and families in home, clinical, educational, and community worlds and develop understandings of their lived experiences over time. We have also been privileged to spend many hours with therapists and other practitioners in their practice settings to learn how they "come to know" enough about the families with whom they are engaged to address the needs, listen to the concerns, and support the hopes of families in such a way that they are able to capitalize on strengths and deliver care that is experienced as family-centered. Such work has deepened our appreciation for the complexity of family-centered practices, the almost inevitable emergence of challenging dilemmas, and the transformative nature of the interrelationships cultivated through exemplary collaborative processes.

With dilemmas and challenges in our practice come many opportunities for growth and strengthening our impact. There is a great deal of variability in the conceptualization of family-centered care (Barnard-Brak, Stevens, & Carpenter, 2017) and the nature and dosage of family-centered OT services (American Occupational Therapy Association [AOTA], 2015). We have yet to adequately answer the key question of which collaborative processes with particular, real-life families produce which outcomes at what point in time. Increased attention to the need for tailorization and customization of interventions should yield more intense efforts to build our evidence base for family-centered practices across the life course, a call that extends to many disciplines (e.g., Dempsey & Keen, 2008). Opportunities to expand our family-centered services are widely evident and include the creation and evaluation of community- and strength-based interventions, health self-management for caregivers, enhanced utilization of available technologies for participation and health, and development and testing of new approaches to address burgeoning unmet needs such as holistic programs for adolescents and adults with autism spectrum disorder (ASD) and their families (Kuhaneck & Watling, 2015).

takes place. The following passages, excerpted from interviews with the occupational therapist, provide insights into her experiences related to meeting this family and her deep appreciation for lessons learned through this partnership. The occupational therapist credits this mother, whom we will call Leslie, with helping her to learn how to engage with Leslie's daughter, a toddler, who initially would not let the therapist come near her to work with her. As the following quote reveals, this successful partnership began with a rather precarious start:

And it, it was just such a nice relationship, building of a relationship and then to come back and have her do her therapy with me was a really nice thing. But the first, um, 4 months of therapy I couldn't touch her. And that was interesting. I think that almost was successful because I had to work through Leslie. Leslie did all the therapy and I sort of sat . . . It was really funny [*laughter*]. I wish we could have some videotape, this was so funny. In the room I would sit in the corner. I had . . . I even couldn't approach her [the child] or she would start to cry. And I would sit a certain distance, which got closer and closer each session and I would direct Leslie what to do. And I think that that taught her so much about what she needed to do and gave her that physical, um, experience that just doing something with her daughter and knowing what it was, what the goals were, rather than sitting back and watching it. That might have been . . . I don't know. 'Cause I just see her as so successful with that and I wonder sometimes if that wasn't part of it. . . . 'Cause she had to, to do her daughter's therapy [*laughter*]. I, I couldn't. I couldn't get . . . you know. Then finally, and it was Leslie's idea and my idea, too, to bring her other children in because we couldn't get her to move. She wouldn't . . . she was terrified . . . climb up in things or any normal things that would . . . a normal child would explore. She was terrified. So when you see her today, it's like not the same. It was really, really interesting.

At another time, the therapist elaborated on what she had learned from this mother:

And so she taught me a lot about that. And she also—what happens when you work with a mother like that, they, they teach you about the power of negotiation and respecting an individual's rights. Because sometimes as a therapist, when the therapist doesn't have children, I can take more of the teacherly role and put my foot down and push through. And, and I can do that. And as a mother, I don't think that works so much in a household. You just get confrontation. You don't have that kind of power over your kids like a teacher. And she has the most incredible way of negotiating with the personality and she actually taught me how to do that with her daughter. So if I, there were situations where I would kinda be more teacherly and put my foot down and this is the rules and here we go. And Leslie would sort of pull me into a more productive understanding of how she raises her kids and that was really helpful.

The therapist, whom we will call Megan, further clarifies how knowledge about family life facilitates the therapeutic process. Leslie's strategy to bring family members into the therapy world not only enabled the family members to understand more about therapy but also provided Megan with information that helped her to picture possibilities of family life. Megan also skillfully incorporated stories into therapy conversations that further illuminated life outside the clinic world. In one interview, she commented,

> But it's not like in Leslie's case where you just get this just fabulous, you know, understanding of what's going on here. And this sort of communication and commitment and feedback about what's happening there in this other world. Like I have such a knowledge of what's happening in Leslie's world. I mean, I feel like I almost have pictures of their family life and I imagine, you know, she'll tell me a story about the Christmas tree and how Kylie's [the child], you know, she's making her put ornaments in this one section high up because then she has to use her arm in that way. And I can just see the family and I, I . . .

As part of our research, we are trying to understand more about how practitioners and families do come to know and understand enough about each other to effectively partner up and what attributes influence partnerships. Leslie shares her perspective as follows:

> It has nothing whatsoever to do with how much schooling you've had. It's just all from your life experience. And that makes a difference. Because I think my experience that I had with Megan as far as us having to communicate with one another. . . . I don't know a lot—I don't know and I didn't know an awful lot about her personal life. Okay, but I knew enough to know that whatever has happened to her in her life has either made her stronger, or, I don't know if that's what I'm looking for—it gave her a sense of caring about people. Whether it was something that really bad, that she said, "Okay I'm not gonna be like that," or something that was really good because she was brought up in a nurturing environment, it just made her personality care. And, and that made a big difference. 'Cause that's what she brought to the table. You know? And, my strong sense of family, and 'course, that's my baby we're talking about, you know. And you have those two, us two bringing back to the table . . . when we sit down to discuss what is best for a child. I think that made a big difference. If—if Megan would have been more of just all business, keep it very technical . . . you know, I think the outcome would have been different. And I probably would have told somebody, I don't want her to be my therapist for my baby. You know, I mean 'cause I wouldn't have felt that, that nurturing that's within her. That's needed as far as I'm concerned; to deal with every child, not just mine. But, oh it's, oh, that is so great!

We now want to just briefly describe a portion of an OT session that illustrates the often subtle but highly effective participation of family members in therapy sessions. The moment that we describe in Case Study 17-1 occurred partway through a session in which an occupational therapist was working with a young boy with a brachial plexus injury. The activity that she planned provided an opportunity to evaluate his sensation, fine motor abilities, and bilateral coordination. This vignette shows the narrative structuring of therapy sessions and the ways in which family members can contribute through both co-narration and their participation as social actors in the therapy scene (Lawlor, 2003, 2009, 2012; Mattingly, 1998). Even though we are describing only several minutes within a therapy session here, we are excerpting key aspects. Therapy time, particularly sessions with heightened engagement and family participation, is too rich and too complex to provide all the detail and description.

It is always a bit difficult in written text to convey social action among engaged social actors. In the brief passages in the case study, we have attempted to evoke the kinds of animation, attunement, engagement, enjoyment, and joint coordination that marked these moments. These family members and this therapist created a therapeutic experience that addressed Micah's challenging clinical needs while affording an opportunity for engaging moments. These moments were engaging enough that this family was actively designing ways to replicate the experience at home to recreate this event in the clinic as a family experience at home.

Conclusion

In this chapter, we highlighted many of the challenges that are involved in attempting to respond to the needs of clients and their families. Challenges are coupled with opportunities. As practitioners discover ways of getting to know families and understanding their perspectives, opportunities emerge for practitioners to construct richer, more meaningful experiences. The more meaningful the experience is, the more likely it is that treatment will be efficacious.

We have found that discussions of opportunities must be tempered with specific cautions. Approaches to getting to know families must be noninvasive, sensitive, nonjudgmental, and respectful of the parameters for privacy and disclosure that individuals indicate. Understanding a perspective does not presume that as an OT practitioner, you are responsible for intervening in every dimension of that perspective. Family-centered care is implemented most effectively in situations in which interdisciplinary efforts are well coordinated and effectively communicated. In situations in which practitioners are working in relative isolation, care must be exercised to ensure that they are practicing within the bounds of their expertise and appropriately facilitating access to other resources as needed.

One of the greatest challenges for practitioners is to understand how their own lived experience shapes their interactions with family members in the course of providing services. Conceptual models of practice and theory

CASE STUDY 17-1   THE MAGIC BOX

The therapist, whom we will call Georgia, announces a guessing game and presents a rather elaborately decorated box, approximately 9 inches square and 12 inches tall. Micah, who is approximately 4 years old his brother Damian, who is several years older; and his mother Sheana are all present along with one of the authors who is videotaping. Sheana, who is sitting off to the side, says, "Oooh," with dramatic intonation. Georgia further proclaims that it is a "magic box." The two brothers join her in a fairly tight circle on the floor mat. Georgia instructs Micah that he must reach into the box without peeking and find things (these things are small objects that are buried among beans). By touching his left arm, she cues him that this is the arm she wants him to use. (Micah's brachial plexus injury is on his left side.) "See if you can find anything. Move your arm in there. I'll tell you when you have something. No. [whispers] It's a secret box. No, you cannot peek. It's a secret. Find anything in there?" Micah has tried to look under the lid of the box as an adaptive strategy, as he is apparently having trouble feeling the objects buried in the beans. Micah whines a bit in frustration and slips his right hand into the box and quickly retrieves an object. Georgia says, "No, no this hand may not . . . ," and his mother says, "Only lefty can, Micah," thus supporting the therapist's agenda that he use his left arm. Georgia takes the retrieved object and places it in Micah's left hand. She then asks him to show and give the object to his brother, thus smoothly incorporating Micah's older brother into this therapy activity that clearly has potential for further intrigue.

The activity unfolds with continued skillful co-narration and participation of Sheana and Damian. The brothers are highly engaged, and Damian at times seems to scaffold for his brother, thus heightening Micah's potential for success. For example, as Micah reaches into the box, Damian comments, "They might be all the way down," thus facilitating Micah's attempts to move deeper into the box. Sheana, at times, skillfully co-manages the session, seemingly vigilant that Damian does not take over or become too involved, thus disrupting Micah's session or become disengaged in a way that limits his ability to support the therapeutic activity. For example, she calls out

Damian's name when she wants him to pull back a bit or, conversely, to pay more attention.

The action that all four of these actors produce is almost seamless, almost choreographed in its fluidity, but also obviously spontaneous and organized in the flow of therapy. The work that the mother, brother, and therapist do to help make this session so effective is not merely related to promoting the desired behavior, although this is important. Both mother and brother skillfully use changes in tone of voice to support Micah's efforts. The transcript of the session is peppered with comments such as "You did it!" and "Oooh," a kind of quieter admiration. They also seem to be heightening the engagement in the doing, making the "guessing game" more appealing, more dramatic. For example, Damian becomes a kind of announcer about the characters that are retrieved from the box. What seemed initially to be a box of farm animals becomes a box with oddities such that Mickey Mouse, lions, and gorillas appear with considerable puzzlement and humor. As Damian comments when Mickey is found, "What's he doing here?"

At other times in this session, Damian was given many of the same tasks as his brother, such as swinging on the trapeze or picking up the beans that had been strewn on the floor while Micah was digging in the "magic box." Damian's inclusion not only helped to make the session more fun but also provided many opportunities for reciprocity, turn taking, and sharing between these two brothers. Sheana's careful attention to the session and her sons' behaviors, as well as her skillful co-narration, further added to the perception that this was a family event.

Near the end of the activity, Sheana comments, "It's a very cute thing." Georgia responds with both a smile and the comment, "It's something you really could enjoy at home." This is a replay of a conversation that occurred partway through the game when Damian had said, "Let's take it home" in the midst of his enjoyment, after his mother's comment "That's a cute little idea—I like that." A brief exchange follows about whether beans or rice would be better. Interspersed throughout this activity had been comments from Georgia related to the ways in which this was a therapeutic activity for Micah.

regarding family systems and human development, ethics, and public and institutional policies all contribute to our framework for family-centered interventions. However, practitioners, as the instruments for intervention, bring their own selves and their cultural views of families into clinical interactions.

We intuitively recognize that such things as our ethnicity, nationality, geographical home, and perhaps even religion provide us with powerful cultural worlds. These aspects of our background help to make us who we are,

culturally speaking. We are often not fully aware that our profession and our family also offer cultural worlds that shape some of our deepest assumptions, beliefs, and values. This chapter concerns a kind of cultural intersection between the practitioner (acting as a member of a professional culture) and a client (acting as a member of a family culture). Practitioners, of course, have families, and clients often have professions. However, when practitioners and clients meet during OT intervention, the practitioner's professional and institutional cultures are particularly significant in shaping how the practitioner defines good intervention and a good professional–client relationship.

Occupational therapy practitioners come to their profession with life experiences of being a member of a family. This lived experience of growing up in a family significantly shapes who we are as practitioners, particularly in situations in which practitioners are getting to know a family and seeking to understand their needs, priorities, values, hopes, and resources. These assumptions about family life tend to be quite tacit, and we are often not aware of their influence unless we actively reflect on our actions. Guided reflection through mentorship and supervision as well as discussions with other team members concerning beliefs about specific families are essential components of intervention planning and implementation with clients and their families.

Acknowledgments

This chapter was supported by work related to four research projects. One study was supported by grant MCJ-060745 from the Maternal and Child Health Program (Title V, Social Security Act), Health Resources and Services Administration, Department of Health & Human Services. Appreciation is expressed to the American Occupational Therapy Foundation for their support of pilot work related to that study. Research was also supported by Boundary Crossing: A Longitudinal and Ethnographic Study (#R01 HD 38878) and Boundary Crossings: Re-Situating Cultural Competence (#2R01 HD 38878) funded through the NICHD, NIH. In addition, we acknowledge the research project entitled Autism in Urban Context: Linking Heterogeneity with Health and Service Disparities, funded by the National Institute on Mental Health, NIH (# R01 MH089474), principal investigator: Dr. Olga Solomon. The contents of this chapter are solely the responsibility of the authors and do not necessarily represent the official views of any of these agencies. We also would like to express our appreciation to the many children, families, therapists, and practitioners who have participated in these research efforts and who have willingly shared their experiences. We would also like to specifically thank Olga Solomon, Emily Ochi, Kevin Casey, Karen Crum, Michelle Elliot, Melissa Park, Beth Crall, Cristine Carrier, Kim Wilkinson, Jesus Diaz, Lisa Hickey, Cynthia Strathmann, Emily Areinoff, Claudia Dunn, and Aaron Bonsall for their contributions and assistance in preparing this chapter.

REFERENCES

American Occupational Therapy Association. (2015). *Autism spectrum disorder: Critically appraised topic (CAT)*. Bethesda, MD: Author.

Ausderau, K., & Juarez, M. (2013). The impact of autism spectrum disorders and eating challenges on family mealtimes. *Infant, Child, and Adolescent Nutrition, 5*, 315–323.

Bandura, A., Carprara, G. V., Barbaranelli, C., Regalia, C., & Scabini, E. (2011). Impact of family efficacy beliefs on quality of family functioning and satisfaction with family life. *Applied Psychology: An International Review, 60*, 421–448.

Barnard-Brak, L., Stevens, T., & Carpenter, J. (2017). Care coordination with schools: The role of family-centered care for children with special health care needs. *Maternal and Child Health Journal, 21*, 1073–1078.

Bauby, J. D. (1997). *The diving bell and the butterfly*. New York, NY: Random House.

Becker, G. (1997). *Disrupted lives: How people create meaning in a chaotic world*. Berkeley, CA: University of California Press.

Bedell, G. M., Cohn, E. S., & Dumas, H. M. (2005). Exploring parents' use of strategies to promote social participation of school-age children with acquired brain injuries. *American Journal of Occupational Therapy, 59*, 273–284.

Bluebond-Langer, M. (1978). *The private worlds of dying children*. Princeton, NJ: Princeton University Press.

Bonsall, A. (2014a). Fathering occupations: An analysis of narrative accounts of fathering children with special needs. *Journal of Occupational Science, 21*, 504–518. doi:10.1080/14427591.2012.760423

Bonsall, A. (2014b). "This is what we do": Constructing postmodern families through occupations. *Journal of Occupational Science, 21*, 296–308. doi:10.1080/14427591.2014.914459

Boyd, B. A., McCarty, C. H., & Sethi, C. (2014). Families of children with autism: A synthesis of family routines literature. *Journal of Occupational Science, 21*, 322–333. doi:10.1080/14427591.2014.908816

Cain, C. (1991). Personal stories: Identity acquisition and self-understanding in Alcoholics Anonymous. *Ethos, 19*, 210–253.

Charon, R. (2006). *Narrative medicine: Honoring the stories of illness*. New York, NY: Oxford University Press.

Charon, R., & Montello, M. (2002). *Stories matter: The role of narrative in medical ethics*. New York, NY: Routledge.

Children's Bureau, U.S. Department of Health & Human Services. (n.d.). *The children's bureau legacy: Ensuring the right to childhood*. Retrieved from https://cb100.acf.hhs.gov/CB_ebook

Clark, F. (1993). Occupation embedded in real life: Interweaving occupational science and occupational therapy: 1993 Eleanor Clarke Slagle Lecture. *American Journal of Occupational Therapy, 47*, 1067–1078.

Cohn, E. S. (2001). From waiting to relating: Parents' experiences in the waiting room of an occupational therapy clinic. *American Journal of Occupational Therapy, 55*, 167–174.

Cohn, E. S., Miller, L. J., & Tickle-Degnan, L. (2000). Parental hopes for therapy outcomes: Children with sensory modulation disorders. *American Journal of Occupational Therapy, 54*, 36–43.

Cunningham, C., & Davis, H. (1985). *Working with parents: Frameworks for collaboration*. Philadelphia, PA: Open University Press.

Deal, A., Dunst, C., & Trivette, C. (1989). A flexible and functional approach to developing individualized family support plans. *Infants and Young Children, 1*, 32–43.

Dempsey, I., & Keen, D. (2008). A review of processes and outcomes in family-centered services for children with a disability. *Topics in Early Childhood Special Education, 28*, 42–52.

Dickie, V., Cutchins, M. P., & Humphry, R. (2006). Occupation as transactional experience: A critique of individualism in occupational science. *Journal of Occupational Science, 13*, 83–93.

Dunn, W., Cox, J., Foster, L., Mische-Lawson, L., & Tanquary, J. (2012). Impact of a contextual intervention on child participation and parent competence among children with autism spectrum disorders: A pretest–posttest repeated-measures design. *American Journal of Occupational Therapy, 66*, 520–528. doi:10.5014/ajot.2012.004119

Dunst, C., Trivette, C., & Deal, A. (1988). *Enabling and empowering families: Principles and guidelines for practice.* Cambridge, MA: Brookline.

Edelman, L., Greenland, B., & Mills, B. (1993). *Building parent professional collaboration: Facilitator's guide.* St. Paul, MN: Pathfinder Resources.

Egilson, S. T. (2010). Parent perspectives of therapy services for their children with physical disabilities. *Scandinavian Journal of Caring Sciences, 25,* 277–284.

Elder, G. (1998). The life course as developmental theory. *Child Development, 69,* 1–12.

Esdaile, S., & Olson, J. (Eds.). (2004). *Mothering occupations: Challenge, agency, and participation.* Philadelphia, PA: F. A. Davis.

Fitzgerald, M. H. (2004). A dialogue on occupational therapy, culture, and families. *American Journal of Occupational Therapy, 58,* 489–498.

Fleming, M., & Mattingly, C. (1994). *Clinical reasoning: Forms of inquiry in therapeutic practice.* Philadelphia, PA: F. A. Davis.

Frank, A. (1995). *The wounded storyteller: Body, illness, and ethics.* Chicago, IL: University of Chicago Press.

Frank, G. (2000). *Venus on wheels: Two decades of dialogue on disability, biography, and being female in America.* Berkeley, CA: University of California Press.

Garro, L., & Mattingly, C. (2000). Narrative turns. In C. Mattingly & L. C. Garro (Eds.), *Narrative and the cultural construction of illness and healing* (pp. 259–269). Berkeley, CA: University of California Press.

Gibbs, V., & Toth-Cohen, S. (2011). Family centered occupational therapy and telerehabilitation for children with Autism Spectrum Disorders. *Occupational Therapy in Health Care, 25,* 298–314.

Good, B. (1994). *Medicine, rationality, and experience.* Cambridge, United Kingdom: Cambridge University Press.

Good, B., & Good, M. J. (1994). In the subjunctive mode: Epilepsy narratives in Turkey. *Social Science in Medicine, 38,* 835–842.

Greenfeld, J. (1978). *A place for Noah.* New York, NY: Henry Holt.

Greenfeld, J. (1986). *A client called Noah: A family journey continued.* New York, NY: Henry Holt.

Hanft, B. E. (1989). *Family-centered care: An early intervention resource manual.* Rockville, MD: American Occupational Therapy Association.

Hanft, B. E. (1991). Impact of public policy on pediatric health and education programs. In W. Dunn (Ed.), *Pediatric occupational therapy: Facilitating effective service provision* (pp. 273–284). Thorofare, NJ: SLACK.

Hanks, W. (1991). Foreword. In J. Lave & E. Wenger, *Situated learning: Legitimate peripheral participation* (pp. 13–34). Cambridge, United Kingdom: Cambridge University Press.

Harrison, C., Romer, T., Simon, M. C., & Schulze, C. (2007). Factors influencing mothers' learning from paediatric therapists: A qualitative study. *Physical & Occupational Therapy in Pediatrics, 27,* 77–96.

Hasselkus, B. R. (2006). 2006 Eleanor Clarke Slagle Lecture—The world of everyday occupation: Real people, real lives. *American Journal of Occupational Therapy, 60,* 627–640.

Hinojosa, J., Sproat, C. T., Mankhetwit, S., & Anderson, J. (2002). Shifts in parent-therapist partnerships: Twelve years of change. *American Journal of Occupational Therapy, 56,* 556–563.

Hockenberry, J. (1995). *Moving violations: War zones, wheelchairs, and declarations of independence.* New York, NY: Hyperion.

Hopkins, H. L., & Smith, H. D. (Eds.). (1983). *Willard & Spackman's occupational therapy* (6th ed.). Philadelphia, PA: J. B. Lippincott.

Howard, J., & Strauss, A. (1975). *Humanizing health care.* New York, NY: Wiley.

Humphry, R., Gonzales, S., & Taylor, E. (1993). Family involvement in practice: Issues and attitudes. *American Journal of Occupational Therapy, 47,* 587–593.

Hurwitz, B., Greenhalgh, T., & Skultans, V. (2004). Introduction. In B. Hurwitz, T. Greenhalgh, & V. Skultans (Eds.), *Narrative research in health and illness* (pp. 1–20). Malden, MA: Blackwell.

Jacobs, L., Lawlor, M., & Mattingly, C. (2011). I/we narratives among African American families raising children with special needs. *Culture, Medicine, and Psychiatry, 35,* 3–25.

Jamison, K. R. (1996). *An unquiet mid: A memoir of moods and madness.* New York, NY: Vintage Books.

Kellegrew, D. H. (1998). Creating opportunities for occupation: An intervention to promote the self-care independence of young children with special needs. *American Journal of Occupational Therapy, 52,* 457–465.

Khetani, M. A., Cohn, E. S., Orsmond, G. I., Law, M. C., & Coster, W. (2013). Parent perspectives of participation in home and community activities when receiving Part C early intervention services. *Topics in Early Childhood Special Education, 214,* 234–245.

Kleinman, A. (1988). *The illness narratives: Suffering, healing, and the human condition.* New York, NY: Basic Books.

Kleinman, A. (2006). *What really matters: Living a moral life amidst uncertainty and danger.* New York, NY: Oxford University Press.

Kuhaneck, H. M., & Watling, R. (2015). Occupational therapy: Meeting the needs of families of people with autism spectrum disorder [Editorial]. *American Journal of Occupational Therapy, 69,* 6905170010. doi:10.5014/ ajot.2015.019562

Law, M. (2002). Participation in the occupations of everyday life. *American Journal of Occupational Therapy, 56,* 640–649.

Law, M., Hanna, S., King, G., Hurley, P., King, S., Kertoy, M., & Rosenbaum, P. (2003). Factors affecting family centred service delivery for children with disabilities. *Child: Care, Health & Development, 29,* 357–366.

Lawlor, M. C. (2003). The significance of being occupied: The social construction of childhood occupations. *American Journal of Occupational Therapy, 57,* 424–434.

Lawlor, M. C. (2004). Mothering work: Negotiating health care, illness and disability, and development. In S. Esdaille & J. Olson (Eds.), *Mothering occupations: Challenge, agency, and participation* (pp. 306–322). Philadelphia, PA: F. A. Davis.

Lawlor, M. C. (2009). Narrative, development, and engagement: Intersections in therapeutic practices. In U. Jensen & C. Mattingly (Eds.), *Narrative, self, and social practices* (pp. 199–220). Aarhus, Denmark: Philosophia Press, Aarhus University.

Lawlor, M. C. (2012). The particularities of engagement: Intersubjectivity in occupational therapy practice. *OTJR: Occupation, Participation and Health, 32,* 151–159.

Lawlor, M. C., & Cada, E. (1993). Partnerships between therapists, parents, and children. *OSERS News in Print, 5*(4), 27–30.

Lawlor, M. C., & Elliot, M. L. (2012). Physical disability and body image in children. In T. Cash (Ed.), *Encyclopedia of body image and human appearance* (pp. 650–656). Oxford, United Kingdom: Elsevier Press.

Lawlor, M. C., & Mattingly, C. F. (1998). The complexities in family-centered care. *American Journal of Occupational Therapy, 52,* 259–267.

Lawlor, M. C., & Mattingly, C. F. (2001). Beyond the unobtrusive observer. *American Journal of Occupational Therapy, 55,* 147–154.

Lawlor, M. C., & Mattingly, C. F. (2009). Understanding family perspectives on illness and disability experiences. In E. Crepeau, E. Cohn, & B. Schell (Eds.), *Willard & Spackman's occupational therapy* (11th ed., pp. 33–44). Philadelphia, PA: Lippincott Williams & Wilkins.

Lawlor, M. C., & Solomon, O. (2017). A phenomenological approach to the cultivation of expertise: Emergent understandings of autism. *Ethos, 45,* 232–249. doi:10.1111/etho.12162

Lipsky, D. K. (1985). A parental perspective in stress and coping. *American Journal of Orthopsychiatry, 55,* 614–617.

Luhrmann, T. M. (2000). *Of two minds: The growing disorder of American psychiatry.* New York, NY: Knopf.

Mattingly, C. (1998). *Healing dramas and clinical plots: The narrative structure of experience.* Cambridge, United Kingdom: Cambridge University Press.

Mattingly, C. (2000). Emergent narratives. In C. Mattingly & L. C. Garro (Eds.), *Narrative and the cultural construction of healing* (pp. 181–211). Berkeley, CA: University of California Press.

Mattingly, C. (2006). Pocahontas goes to the clinic: Popular culture as lingua franca in a cultural borderland. *American Anthropologist, 106,* 494–501.

Mattingly, C. (2010). *The paradox of hope: Travels in clinical border-lands.* Berkeley, CA: University of California Press.

Mattingly, C. (2014). *Moral laboratories: Family peril and the struggle for a good life.* Berkeley, CA: University of California Press.

Mattingly, C., & Fleming, M. (1994). *Clinical reasoning: Forms of inquiry in a therapeutic practice.* Philadelphia, PA: F. A. Davis.

Mattingly, C., & Lawlor, M. C. (2000). Learning from stories: Narrative interviewing in cross-cultural research. *Scandinavian Journal of Occupational Therapy, 7,* 4–14.

Mattingly, C., & Lawlor, M. C. (2001). The fragility of healing. *Ethos, 29,* 30–57.

Mattingly, C., & Lawlor, M. C. (2003). Disability experience from a family perspective. In E. Crepeau, E. Cohn, & B. Schell (Eds.), *Willard & Spackman's occupational therapy* (10th ed., pp. 69–79). Philadelphia, PA: Lippincott Williams & Wilkins.

Mattingly, C., Lawlor, M., & Jacobs-Huey, L. (2002). Narrating September 11: Race, gender, and the play of cultural identities. *American Anthropologist, 104,* 743–753.

McGonigel, M. J., Kaufmann, R. K., & Johnson, B. H. (Eds.). (1991). *Guidelines and recommended practices for the individualized family service plan.* Bethesda, MD: Association for the Care of Children's Health.

Monks, J., & Frankenberg, R. (1995). Being ill and being me: Self, body, and time in multiple sclerosis narratives. In B. Ingstad & S. R. Whyte (Eds.), *Disability and culture* (pp. 107–134). Berkeley, CA: University of California Press.

Moyers, P. A., & Metzler, C. A. (2014). Interprofessional collaborative practice in care coordination. *American Journal of Occupational Therapy, 68,* 500–505. doi:10.5014/ajot.2014.685002

Mroz, T. M., Pitonyak, J. S., Fogelberg, D., & Leland, N. E. (2015). Client centeredness and health reform: Key issues for occupational therapy. *American Journal of Occupational Therapy, 69,* 6905090010. doi:10.5014/ajot.2015.695001

Murphy, R. F. (1990). *The body silent.* New York, NY: Norton.

Neistadt, M. E., & Crepeau, E. B. (Eds.). (1998). *Willard & Spackman's occupational therapy* (9th ed.). Philadelphia, PA: J. B. Lippincott.

Ochieng, B. M. N. (2003). Minority ethnic families and family-centered care. *Journal of Child Health Care, 7,* 123–132.

Park, C. C. (1982). *The siege: The first eight years of an autistic child.* Boston, MA: Little, Brown.

Park, C. C. (2001). *Exiting Nirvana: A daughter's life with autism.* Boston, MA: Little, Brown.

Peete, R. (2010). *Not my boy: A father, a son and one family's journey with autism.* New York, NY: Hyperion.

Rabb, M., & Dunst, C. (2004). Early intervention practitioner approaches to natural environment interventions. *Journal of Early Intervention, 27,* 15–26.

Rogoff, B. (2003). *The cultural nature of human development.* Oxford, United Kingdom: Oxford University Press.

Sebelist, R. M. (1983). Mental retardation. In H. Hopkins & H. Smith (Eds.), *Willard & Spackman's occupational therapy* (6th ed., pp. 335–351). Philadelphia, PA: J. B. Lippincott.

Segal, R. (2004). Family routines and rituals: A context for occupational therapy interventions. *American Journal of Occupational Therapy, 58,* 499–508.

Schreiber, J., Benger, J., Salls, J., Marchetti, G., & Reed, L. (2011). Parent perspectives on rehabilitation services for their children with disabilities: A mixed methods approach. *Physical & Occupational Therapy in Pediatrics, 31,* 225–238.

Silverman, C., & Brosco, J. P. (2007). Understanding autism: Parents and pediatricians in historical perspective. *Archives of Pediatrics & Adolescent Medicine, 161,* 392–398.

Solomon, O., Angell, A. M., Yin, L., & Lawlor, M. (2015). "You can turn off the light if you'd like": Pediatric health care visits for children with autism spectrum disorder as an interactional achievement. *Medical Anthropology Quarterly, 29,* 531–555.

Solomon, O., & Lawlor, M. C. (2013). "And I look down and he is gone": Narrating autism, elopement and wandering in Los Angeles. *Social Science & Medicine, 94,* 106–114.

Swartz, T. T. (2009). Intergenerational family relations in adulthood: Patterns, variations, and implications in the contemporary United States. *Annual Review of Sociology, 35,* 191–212.

Tate, S. W. (1974). The scope for occupational therapists in the community in the future. *Canadian Journal of Occupational Therapy, 41,* 7–9.

Trostle, J. A. (1988). Medical compliance as an ideology. *Social Sciences in Medicine, 27,* 1299–1308.

Werner DeGrace, B. (2004). The everyday occupation of families with children with autism. *American Journal of Occupational Therapy, 58,* 543–550.

Williams, D. (1992). *Nobody nowhere: The extraordinary autobiography of an autistic.* New York, NY: Avon Books.

Woodgate, R. L., Edwards, M., & Ripat, J. (2012). How families of children with complex needs participate in everyday life. *Social Science & Medicine, 75,* 1912–1920.

thePoint® *For additional resources on the subjects discussed in this chapter, visit* **http://thePoint.lww.com /Willard-Spackman13e.**

Patterns of Occupation

Kathleen Matuska, Kate Barrett

LEARNING OBJECTIVES

After reading this chapter, you will be able to:

1. Examine roles, routines, rituals, and habits and their influence on health and well-being.
2. Compare/contrast measures of roles, routines, habits, and life balance and their usefulness for occupational therapy assessment.
3. Discuss intervention approaches that address problems in occupational patterns.
4. Analyze a theoretical model of life balance and its application to occupational therapy.

Introduction

This chapter discusses performance patterns and how they contribute to or detract from health and well-being. Other chapters in this book describe occupational therapy (OT) assessment and intervention for personal and environmental factors influencing occupational performance (the *what*, *why*, and *where*), and this chapter explores the patterns of occupations (the *how*) and how those patterns influence health and well-being. The Occupational Therapy Practice Framework: Domain and Process, 3rd edition (American Occupational Therapy Association [AOTA], 2014) identifies performance patterns as habits, routines, roles, and rituals used in the process of engaging in occupations or activities that can support or hinder occupational performance. This chapter also includes life balance, a holistic view of **occupational patterns** in the context of living.

Roles

Occupational roles are normative models for behavior shaped by culture and society (Crepeau & Schell, 2009). Examples of roles in life are student, friend, worker, and mother. Roles are dynamic throughout the life course because new roles are learned and old roles are replaced. Individuals experience a sense of purpose, identity, and structure when carrying out roles (Kielhofner, 2009) and are learned through a process of socialization and acculturation.

NOTES

Use of Social Media—A New Occupational Pattern of the Twenty-First Century

The twentieth century brought new technology that changed the occupational patterns for most people in developed countries. For example, instead of spending time handwashing clothes, people loaded a washing machine and pushed a button. Then, they were free to engage in other occupations as the machine did the work for them. Clothes washing machines and dryers, dishwashers, microwaves, calculators, cell phones, and many other time-saving devices reshaped occupational patterns in the twentieth century and contributed to more discretional time for leisure or other pursuits.

The new technology in the twenty-first century brought the Internet, Wi-Fi technology, and an explosion of social media that has and will continue to have a most profound influence on how we use our time. As few as 20 years ago, people couldn't imagine that a significant part of their daily routines would include talking to friends on social media from their phones, reading the daily news from their tablets, or sending videos of their activities to friends through computers. Now, 84% of American households contain at least one smartphone, 80% of households contain a desktop or laptop computer, and 68% own a tablet computer, and many households have multiple devices (Olmstead, 2017).

Social media use has become the most popular daily activity for the majority of emerging adults (18 to 29 years old) in the United States. Ninety percent of U.S. emerging adults use social media every day (Perrin, 2015). Similarly, for teens, text messaging is the preferred form of peer communication with 24% of teens using it "almost constantly" and the majority using two or more social networking sites each day (Figure 18-1) (Lenhart, 2015). For many, being online is so pervasive that it is a constant condition of waking life (Scott, Bay-Cheng, Prince, Collins, & Nochajski, 2017). Clearly, the occupational patterns in modern life have shifted, and it is new enough that the long-term effects on health and well-being are still emerging.

Young people use social media as a central conduit to information, advice, and relationships, and it expands their sphere of associations. These attributes promote a sense of belonging and self-disclosure, two important peer processes that support identity development (Davis, 2012). On the other hand, there is a growing concern about the physical and mental health effects of overuse of social media. Does the overdependence on social media diminish other important autonomy or social skills? Parents complain that their children do not contribute to family conversations because they are always looking at their phones. Overuse is a related to poor glycemic control for youth with diabetes (Galler, Lindau, Ernert, Thalemann, & Raile, 2011), poor sleep quality (Nuutinen, Ray, & Roos, 2013), anxiety (Davis, 2012), and increased risk for distracted driving and automobile accidents (National Highway Traffic Safety Administration, 2017).

Given this new and pervasive occupational pattern that will rapidly grow and change, occupational therapists need to be attentive to its effect on individual and population health and well-being. Occupational profiles need to include use of media as part of an overall lifestyle assessment. How can it contribute to well-being? How does it distract from other important occupations?

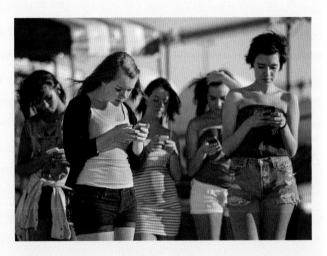

FIGURE 18-1 According to the Pew Research Center, 92% of U.S. teens report going online daily with more than half going on several times a day (Lenhart, 2015).

Roles can be disrupted, altered, or ended by the presence of a disability. For example, a study by Davies Hallet, Zasler, Maurer, and Cash (1992) found that roles change significantly after traumatic brain injury (TBI). The study found that many persons with TBI experienced important role changes such as loss of a worker role, which resulted in feelings of anger, frustration, apprehension, confusion, boredom, and fear. Young adults who had a stroke also reported a disrupted sense of self because of altered worker and friendship roles (Lawrence, 2010). These effects of stroke are "invisible" but have significant impact on quality of life.

Caregiving can also disrupt valued roles. Caregivers of children or family members with disabilities influence how and which roles are performed (Crowe, VanLeit, Berghmans, & Mann, 1996). The increased demands of caregiving can result in altered social roles, underemployment, and low levels of well-being (Bainbridge & Broady, 2017).

Occupational therapists help people to construct or reconstruct their roles when they have experienced a lack of engagement in desired roles or an unexpected/undesired loss or change in their roles.

While understanding a person's roles, we must be cautious to not overgeneralize their meaning. Roles do not easily translate from culture to culture and may limit us to singular or normative expectations of behavior and meaning (Jackson, 1998). Expectations of roles change from culture to culture, and therefore, role assessments cannot always be used across cultures. When considering a person's roles, it is important for the OT practitioner to listen carefully to the client for his or her own interpretation of the meaning and responsibilities associated with his or her roles.

Assessment of Roles

There are several assessments commonly used in OT to learn about a client's roles. See Table 18-1 for a review of common role assessments.

Habits

Habits are specific, automatic behaviors; performed repeatedly; relatively automatically; and with little variation. Because they can be performed in different contexts, they are not necessarily performed in exactly the same way each time (Clark, 2000). Habits can be useful, dominating, or impoverished and can be difficult to break (Clark, 2000).

An example of a useful habit is brushing teeth before bed every night. It is performed consistently without planning, and when barriers arise (such as when stranded overnight at an airport), the loss is noticed but is not incapacitating. Useful habits can help organize time and resources so that less cognitive energy is needed throughout the day. For example, with a habit of putting car keys on a hook by the door when entering the house, less time and energy are spent trying to find the keys when needed. Or when appointments are immediately recorded on a calendar, the cognitive load to remember the date is reduced. These useful habits reduce fatigue because they require less effort, free attention for other things, and allow novel actions without having to recall or attend to the specific details (Clark as cited in Young, 1988). Simple, useful habits may be developed to manage time and reduce the stress that interferes with daily performance. For example, an occupational therapist may help a client with spinal cord injury (SCI) develop useful habits in the morning routine so that time and energy is not wasted on locating and setting up supplies before going to work.

When people have difficulty learning new useful habits because of a dysfunctional internal state, they may have impoverished habits. People with Alzheimer disease, depression, or attention-deficit/hyperactivity disorder may not be able to develop new useful habits that help them adjust to their disability (Clark, 2000). Instead, the occupational therapist will consult with the caregivers for ways to modify the environment or the activity for optimal performance. For example, teaching the caregiver to have all lunch supplies available and in one place every day can cue the individual with Alzheimer disease to make a sandwich.

Dominating habits are those that are consistently performed even if they interfere with optimal performance. Over time, some habits can become addicting and affect one's health, such as the need to smoke a cigarette when driving or consuming snacks when watching TV. Occupational therapy intervention may assist individuals to identify and practice alternative habits that are less harmful. Other dominating habits create stress or anxiety if they cannot be performed, such as needing to wash hands after touching anything. The anxiety from performing the handwashing and/or not being able to handwash make it difficult to carry on with the other tasks in a day. Habit domination can occur with obsessive-compulsive disorder (OCD), autism, or other mental health disorders. These can be very difficult to change and are sometimes managed with medication.

Assessment of Habits

Structured interview with the client, family member, or caregiver is a useful assessment of habits. Questions should address how the individual performs activities of daily living (ADL) and instrumental activities of daily living

TABLE 18-1	Common Role Assessments				
Assessment Tools	**Developers**	**Purpose**	**Method**	**Comment**
Role Checklist	Oakley, Kielhofner, Barris, & Reichler (1986)	To assess a person's perception of participation in 10 major life roles (i.e., worker, caregiver, volunteer) and the value placed on these roles	The client identifies and rates the roles that he or she has done in the past and is currently engaged in as well as roles that he or she would like to have.	It is a relatively easy and quick way to assess how someone feels about the roles that he or she holds and to see changes in role patterns over time.
The Adolescent Role Assessment	Black (1976)	To assess four domains: developing aspirations, developing interpersonal competencies, developing self-efficacy, and developing autonomy	A semistructured interview that provides both narrative and quantitative information regarding worker role development	It is based on the idea that during adolescence, one explores interests, assumes increased responsibility, and develops values and goals that influence occupational choice and work attitudes necessary for entering an occupation.
The Role Activity Performance Scale	Good-Ellis, Fine, Spencer, & DiVittis (1987)	To assess a person's role performance in 12 major roles over a period of 18 months. The role activities assessed include work, education, home management, family of origin relationships, extended family relationships, partner/spouse relationship, social relationships, leisure, self-management, hygiene and appearance, and health care.	Interview process that allows for information to be collected from the client as well as other sources including family, medical record, and the health care team	It is used in mental health settings and is designed to guide intervention planning as well as be used as a research tool to measure intervention outcomes.
The Role Change Assessment	Jackoway, Rogers, & Snow (1987)	To assess the level of engagement and satisfaction experienced in these roles and how they have changed over time	A semistructured interview format to examine 48 roles in family and social, vocational, self-care, organizational, leisure, and health care categories for older adults	The interview format allows the OT practitioner to assess both role stability as well as change.
Worker Role Interview (WRI)	Braveman et al. (2005)	To assess psychosocial capacity in injured workers for readiness to return to work; to address both psychosocial and environmental factors that impact return to work	Semistructured interview formats for recently injured workers and persons who are chronically disabled	The information gathered complements other work/physical capacity assessments to ensure a well-rounded picture of the client and his or her needs that should be addressed to ensure return to work.

(IADL) and the specific habits used during performance of each activity. For example, "Describe the steps you take in the morning to get ready for the day." It is important to determine if these habits are a help or hindrance to performance. See Table 18-2 for a summary of the LIFE-H 3.0 habit assessment.

Routines

Routines are "a type of higher-order habit that involves sequencing and combining processes, procedures, steps, or occupations and provide a structure for daily life" (Clark, 2000, p. 128S). An example of a health-promoting routine is following a predictable series of stretches and exercises followed by a nutritious breakfast before going to work every day. For someone with a disability, a healthful routine may include taking care of medical equipment and setting up medications for the next day before going to bed. Older adults typically embed cues to take their medications into daily routines of mealtime and wake-up or sleep times (Sanders & Van Oss, 2013). People who have hired caregivers will be most efficient at managing their care if they have a predictable routine to teach their caregiver. Occupational therapists must help clients embed their newly learned strategies into everyday activities and routines to ensure greater compliance with recommendations (Radomski, 2011).

TABLE 18-2   Assessments of Habits or Routines

Assessment Tools	Developers	Purpose	Method	Comment
The Assessment of Life Habits (LIFE-H 3.0)	Fougeyrollas, Noreau, & St-Michel (2001)	To evaluate social participation of people with disabilities, regardless of the type of underlying impairment; to measure level of difficulty and type of assistance needed	Self- or therapist-administered; ratings for 12 life habit categories (nutrition, fitness, personal care, communication, housing, mobility, responsibility, interpersonal relationships, community, education, employment, and recreation)	Fits well in the International Classification of Functioning, Disability and Health (ICF) participation domains; measuring a person's involvement in a life situation
The Model of Human Occupation Screening Tool (MOHOST) Version 2.0	Kielhofner et al. (2007); Parkinson, Forsyth, & Kielhofner (2006)	To measure the Model of Human Occupation (MOHO) concepts of volition, habituation, communication/interaction skills, motor skills, process skills, and the environment	One of the six subscales measures performance patterns related to routines, adaptability, roles, and responsibility. Scoring reflects whether the individual's performance patterns facilitate, allow, inhibit, or restrict optimal performance.	The MOHOST has initial validity evidence for use as an overview of occupational performance and for use of the six subscales representing the MOHO concepts.
The Family Routines Inventory	Boyce, Jensen, James, & Peacock (1983); Jensen, James, Boyce, & Hartnett (1983)	To measure the predictability of routine in the daily life of a family. It measures 28 positive, strength-promoting family routines and has demonstrated validity and reliability.	Scoring is based on the number of routines endorsed by the family (they do the routine), frequency of adherence to the routine (how often they do it), and how important the routine is to them.	Examples of items include "family eats at the same time each night," "each child has some time each day for playing alone," "family regularly visits with the relatives," and "parents and children play together some time each day."
The Scale of Older Adults' Routine (SOAR)	Zisberg, Young, & Schepp (2009)	To measure stability in activities on a daily and weekly basis for older adults. SOAR provides information about the stability or disruption of routine.	It is administered by in-person interview and includes 42 routine activities in five domains (basic, instrumental, leisure, social, and rest) measured on four dimensions (frequency, timing, duration, and sequence).	This assessment may be useful for occupational therapist in exploring altered routines during transitions such as from home to a retirement community, independent living to assisted living, or a nursing home.
The Social Rhythm Metric (SRM-5)	Monk, Flaherty, Frank, Hoskinson, & Kupfer (1990); Monk, Frank, Potts, & Kupfer (2002)	To quantify daily lifestyle regularity (routines) with respect to event timing	Diary-like tool where participants record the timing of five daily events over the course of 1 week: when they get out of bed, have first contact with a person, start of work, school, volunteer or family care, have dinner, and go to bed	This measure was developed from the theory that social rhythms (i.e., eating and sleeping schedules) are important for structuring individuals' days and for maintaining circadian rhythms, and alterations in these rhythms lead to disentrainment and poor health.

Because routines provide a useful daily structure, the loss of routines can also be disruptive. People who have chronic diseases may find it difficult to maintain a steady routine because managing their disease symptoms is challenging and often unpredictable. Dressing, for example, is typically done in a sequential way with similar steps and procedures used from day to day. However, research on women with rheumatoid arthritis (RA) and diabetes showed they altered their dressing routines because they had much more difficulty performing the steps (Poole & Cordova, 2004). Women with fibromyalgia who reported high levels of order and routine in their lives gained greatly from actively coping with their illness compared to women who did not have high levels of routine (Reich, 2000).

Routines can be a very important component of managing one's overall health but can also be damaging (Friese et al., 2002; Segal, 2004). Sometimes, people with chronic diseases avoid making future plans and limit social engagements to minimize potential discomfort. This pattern of avoidance leads to a vicious cycle of less positive social engagements (Zautre, Hamilton, & Yocum, 2000). Long-term patterns of sedentary or isolative behavior such as watching television every night for several hours can have a negative effect on health or well-being.

Performance patterns are disrupted with acute or chronic diseases or conditions. Several diseases have fatigue as one of the primary symptoms, and often, the additional requirement of managing disease symptoms taps into available energy reserves. Occupational therapists address performance patterns and help people create new habits or routines that maximize their available energy. For example, people who had an SCI recognized different levels of energy at different times of the day or week and learned to organize their time so that they were doing the most when they felt the best. This type of planning was viewed as a very useful strategy for participating in the activities that were important to them (Chugg & Craik, 2002).

Chronic diseases such as multiple sclerosis, chronic fatigue syndrome, or fibromyalgia include symptoms of severe fatigue that interfere with routines and participation in everyday life.

Fatigue is often unpredictable and severe, making it difficult to follow desired routines or to make future plans. People who experience this type of fatigue are forced to make choices about how they are going to expend their limited energy and make reductions in the number and type of activities in which they participate (Matuska & Erickson, 2008).

Occupational therapists teach principles of energy conservation that address the importance of health-promoting routines in managing fatigue. Common energy conservation strategies include analyzing and modifying activities to reduce energy expenditures, balancing work and rest, delegating some activities, examining and modifying standards and priorities, using the body efficiently, organizing workspaces, and using assistive technologies to conserve energy (Matuska, Mathiowetz, & Finlayson, 2007). All of these strategies create positive changes in daily routines, and when individuals integrate them into their lives, there has been an associated reduced fatigue impact and improved quality of life (Mathiowetz, Finlayson, Matuska, Chen, & Luo, 2005; Mathiowetz, Matuska, & Murphy, 2001).

Family Routines

Family routines are important to address because they have been shown to be important in individual and family well-being (Denham, 2003; Friese, 2007; Friese et al., 2002). Family routines are observable and repetitive patterns involving family members that occur with predictable regularity in family life (Denham, 2002). Routines can help family members arrange everyday life in a way that helps them cope with illness or stress. When families are stressed, interventions are most effective when the new health routines are aligned with family values, meaningful, and applicable to family needs and when resources were available (Denham, 2002).

Assessment of Routines

Several assessment tools are available to assess routines. See Table 18-2 for a summary of common assessments for routines.

Rituals

Rituals are different from routines in that they include strong elements of symbolism (Crepeau, 1995). Rituals often are a reflection or enactment of one's culture. A strong sense of meaning and identity is experienced when a person feels engaged and included in a ritual. Many people associate the word *ritual* with religious activities such as a baptism, bar mitzvah, pilgrimage to Mecca, or other religious ceremony. Rituals can also be secular such as a holiday parade, high school graduation, or initiation into a group of people (gang, sorority, fraternity, etc.). Rituals often signify to a community of people a transition from one state of being to another, such as from child to adult, single to married, or student to graduate.

Rituals also exist in the context of families. Family rituals contain symbolic and affective components that serve to construct and affirm family identity (Segal, 2004). Examples of family rituals could include Sunday afternoon picnics, family reunions, or how families greet one another. Rituals occur at regular intervals or on special occasions. They may occur daily (kissing one another hello), weekly (family dinner), annually (reunion), or only once in a lifetime (bar mitzvah). Figure 18-2 shows a group of extended family members making a traditional Irish recipe that brings them together every year.

Rituals offer individuals and groups of people an opportunity to carry out identified roles and to feel a sense of belonging and meaning. Although we do not have a formal way of assessing rituals in OT, it is important for occupational therapists to be aware that what may appear as "routine" may actually be experienced as a ritual by the person engaged. Rituals may also be thought of as a tool to be used in OT as we acknowledge the significant transitions one experiences in therapy: from nonacceptance to acceptance of a disability, meeting therapeutic goals, or transitioning off of a unit.

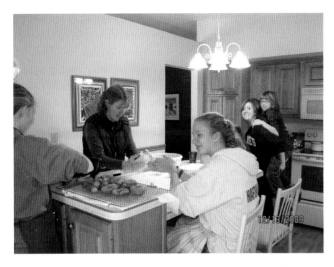

FIGURE 18-2 Extended family members in their annual ritual of making traditional Irish potato donuts.

Occupational Balance

Occupational therapy was founded on the idea that practicing a kind of balanced rhythm between work, play, rest, and sleep leads to wholesome living (Meyer, 1977). Occupational therapy is an important profession for addressing lifestyles in both preventive and restorative ways because of the expertise and understanding of occupational patterns. Lifestyles are unique patterns of everyday occupations including roles, habits, routines, and rituals and can lead to an overall life balance or imbalance with long-term consequences on health, well-being, and quality of life. *Occupational balance* refers to a perception that one's patterns of everyday occupations are satisfactory and include a range of meaningful occupations. *Life balance* is similar but uses words more commonly understood outside of the OT profession (Matuska, 2012b; Matuska & Christiansen, 2009). **Life balance** is defined as "a satisfying pattern of daily activity that is healthful, meaningful, and sustainable to an individual within the context of his or her current life circumstances" (Matuska & Christiansen, 2008, p. 11).

The Life Balance Model (Matuska, 2012b) depicts the relationships between occupational patterns, life outcomes, and the environment (Box 18-1). Occupational patterns should enable people to meet important needs such as supporting biological health and physical safety (i.e., exercise, rest, medication management), contributing to positive relationships (i.e., friends and family), feeling engaged and challenged (i.e., hobbies, stimulating work), and creating a positive personal identity (i.e., caregiving, volunteering) (Matuska & Christiansen, 2008). The extent people are able to engage in patterns of occupations that address all of these needs, they will perceive their lives as more

satisfying, less stressful, and more meaningful, or *balanced*. People also need to have the skill to organize their time and energy in ways that enable them to meet their important personal goals and renewal (Matuska, 2012b). In other words, life balance requires the skill to create a match between how much time one *desires* to engage in activities and *actually* engages in the activities that meet important needs.

It is conceivable that the constraints of the environment could make it difficult to engage in a satisfactory pattern of occupations. Matuska (2012b) found that life balance was lower for people of a racial minority and was negatively affected by employment and having children at home. A highly supportive environment could improve life balance. For example, having enough financial security to create a satisfactory life was also viewed as important for life balance among Swedish men and women (Wagman, Håkansson, Matuska, Björklund, & Falkmer, 2011).

Even though there is increasing evidence that life balance is related to lower stress and higher psychological well-being (Matuska, 2012b; Matuska, Bass, & Schmitt, 2013; Sheldon, Cummins, & Khamble, 2010), creating balanced lives is challenging for most people. It may be even more challenging for people who have chronic illnesses such as multiple sclerosis or parents of children with autism spectrum disorder (Stein, Foran, & Cermak, 2011). Being obese or having a medical condition that limits participation is related to higher stress and lower life balance (Matuska & Bass, 2016). These and other chronic health conditions can influence what people are able to do and whether or not they can create a satisfactory balance of occupations in their lives. For example, women with multiple sclerosis expressed how managing their health needs became a major factor in their lives and how they needed to make daily adaptations in order to continue doing things that were important to them (Matuska & Erickson, 2008). Their disease often dictated what their activity options were in a given day. Occupational therapists have an important contribution to fostering life balance in preventative and restorative modes for individuals and families with or without chronic illnesses.

Assessment of Life Balance and Occupational Patterns

The Life Balance Inventory (LBI) was created to measure life balance as conceptualized in the Life Balance Model (Matuska, 2012a). The 53-item LBI measures perceived balance across the four need-based dimensions in the Life Balance Model (health, relationships, challenge, identity) and was designed to allow unique configurations of daily occupations for each person within each of those dimensions. The scoring is based on the idea that imbalance could result from spending too little or too much time in

BOX 18-1	THE LIFE BALANCE MODEL

Figure 18-3 is a visual depiction of the Life Balance Model. The two ovals in the center represent activity configurations. Oval A represents activity configuration *congruence*, which reflects the match between desired and actual time engaged in valued activities. In other words, people are spending the right amount of time doing the things they want. Oval B represents the *equivalence* of satisfaction across the four need-based dimensions in the Life Balance Model (health, relationships, challenge, and identity). The overlap of ovals A and B represents life balance, where people are satisfied with the time spent in activities across the four need areas. Life balance has associated positive outcomes such as lower perceived stress, higher personal well-being, and need satisfaction (Matuska, 2012a). On the other hand, if people are dissatisfied with the amount of time spent in activities or they are not meeting all four need areas, then the model depicts this situation as life imbalance with associated negative health consequences. The model is surrounded by a large oval representing the environment and its influence on life balance.

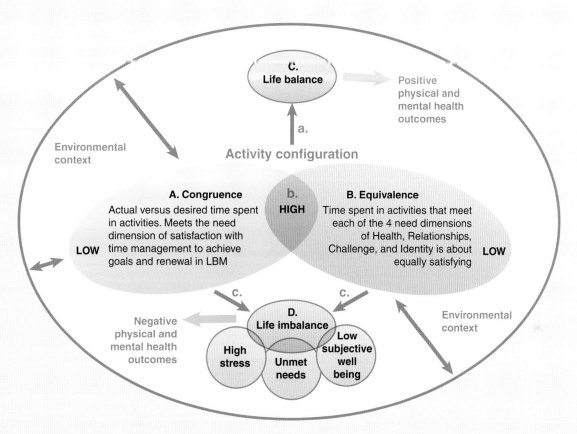

FIGURE 18-3 The Life Balance Model. (From Matuska, K. [2012]. Validity evidence for a model and measure of life balance. *OTJR: Occupation, Participation and Health, 32,* 229–237. Copyright 2012 by the American Occupational Therapy Foundation. Reprinted with permission.)

any activity. The LBI has demonstrated acceptable internal consistency and content validity as a measure for life balance (Matuska, 2012a).

The LBI can be accessed online at http://minerva.stkate.edu/LBI.nsf, and the output consists of an overall life balance score and balance scores in each subscale.

Daily activity logs are another method of examining occupational patterns. The purpose of activity logs is to have an accurate record of what occurs in peoples' lives by recording activities at regular intervals. The length of the intervals and what is recorded varies. For example, an activity log could be a 24-hour record divided into 30-minute intervals, and an individual is asked to fill it out for three consecutive 24-hour periods. Individuals could be asked to simply record what they were doing every 30 minutes, or contextual information could be included such as "what

I was doing, where it occurred, who I was with, and how I felt." Activity logs help the person to be more aware of how time is spent and can be a first step in making healthy lifestyle changes. Occupational therapy practitioners may coach clients when life imbalances are evident.

Life imbalance is when patterns of daily occupations are perceived to be unsatisfactory (there is not a good match between desired and actual engagement in valued activities), increasing the risk for physical and mental health problems. Life imbalance means that occupational patterns limit or compromise participation in valued relationships; are incongruent for establishing or maintaining physiological health and a satisfactory identity; or are mundane, uninteresting, or unchallenging (Matuska & Christiansen, 2009). People who have disabilities experience life imbalance when they cannot participate in valued occupations because of physical or environmental barriers.

People who do not have disabilities also experience life imbalance, and addressing this problem is an emerging role for OT practitioners. For example, people who are transitioning into retirement, caring for children and aging parents (sandwich generation), single parents, and workaholics may benefit from coaching by an OT

practitioner who could help them create more balanced patterns of occupation. See Case Study 18-1 for an example of an occupational therapist helping a patient with life imbalance.

Summary

Roles, habits, routines, and rituals create the framework of people's lives and together make up lifestyles that are unique to each person. Life balance should be a consideration in any OT intervention. Are current lifestyle patterns contributing to a sense of overall well-being or taking away from a sense of well-being? When occupational patterns are dysfunctional, health and well-being are at risk. In turn, adapting or establishing satisfactory roles, habits, routines, and rituals may be used as tools in therapy to help a person improve life balance. Occupational therapy practitioners can use the tools described in this chapter to identify unhealthy patterns of occupation and help their clients create new patterns that are more satisfactory and healthy. The desired outcome for any OT intervention is life satisfaction and improved quality of life.

CASE STUDY 18-1   LIVING WITH MULTIPLE SCLEROSIS

SJ is a 45-year-old woman who was diagnosed with multiple sclerosis 7 years ago. She is married and has a son who is 14 years old. Twice a week she works as a dental hygienist in a clinic that is 30-minute drive from her home. SJ has intermittent weakness and tingling sensation in her right arm, and she complains that fatigue is her most disabling symptom.

Performance Patterns

SJ has the most energy in the morning, and she uses that time to shower, groom, and prepare breakfast for herself and family. After breakfast, she tries to capitalize on her energy by doing other household work. Typically, she crashes in the afternoon and evening, however. On workdays, she is usually so fatigued in the evenings that she cannot get off the couch, and sometimes, the fatigue lasts through the next day.

SJ has gained 20 lb and she wants to have a regular exercise routine, but when she works out for 20 minutes, she feels fatigued the rest of the day. She used to go out with her husband and friends, but now, she won't make plans because she doesn't know if she'll feel well enough to go. SJ is very dissatisfied with her life because her fatigue disrupts her social opportunities and fulfilling her roles.

Occupational Therapy Assessment

The occupational therapist asked SJ to complete a daily activity log for 1 week where she wrote down what she did every hour and how she felt during that activity, including physical symptoms. Together, they examined the activity log to determine patterns and create an activity plan. SJ discovered that she felt tired after her morning shower but ignored it in order to accomplish more. The 30-minute drive to and from work was also problematic, and she noticed much more fatigue on the days after she worked. The occupations that SJ prioritized were continuing to work 2 days a week, doing the laundry, cooking at least two meals a week, working out at least 2 days a week, attending at least one of her son's soccer/basketball games each month, and going out with her husband and friends once or twice each month.

Occupational Therapy Intervention

The occupational therapist discussed with SJ the principles of energy conservation: Plan your day; rest before fatigue; spread activities throughout the day; and prioritize, delegate, simplify, and use proper body mechanics.

Morning Routine

She tried showering in the evening right before bed and found that she was less fatigued after her grooming routine in the

CASE STUDY 18-1   LIVING WITH MULTIPLE SCLEROSIS *(continued)*

morning. A 10-minute rest period was built in immediately after breakfast, which helped her feel more energetic the rest of the morning.

Rest throughout the Day

She decided to build a routine of rest into her schedule to prevent the severe disabling fatigue. Every 2 hours, she rested for 15 to 30 minutes. She discussed her fatigue with her employer, and she was allowed to bring an easy chair into the back room for resting during her breaks. Instead of doing paperwork over the lunch break, she rests 30 minutes and has more energy at the end of the day to stay a few minutes later to do the paperwork.

Proper Body Mechanics

The occupational therapist discussed principles of body mechanics and restful positioning regarding her 30-minute drive to and from work. SJ repositioned the driver's seat to be more upright and created an armrest out of a shoebox

that she placed next to her. She also decided to choose mellow and restful music for the drive home.

Delegate and Simplify

SJ and her occupational therapist discussed the energy conservation strategies with her husband and son. Together, they prioritized the activities where help was needed and ways to simplify activities that SJ wanted to keep. For example, cleaning was delegated to her family, and for SJ to continue doing the laundry, they decided to bring the washer and dryer to the main floor to save energy-draining trips to the basement. SJ agreed to cook dinner on 2 days when she didn't work and to plan the menu ahead so her husband could have the ingredients available. Foods that required less preparation time such as precut vegetables and bag salads would be used regularly. The family planned to rest 10 to 15 minutes after meals before beginning the cleanup. SJ liked this plan because her family spent more time together.

REFERENCES

American Occupational Therapy Association. (2014). Occupational therapy practice framework: Domain and process, 3rd edition. *American Journal of Occupational Therapy, 68*, S1–S48. doi:10.5014/ajot.2014.682006

Bainbridge, H. T. J., & Broady, T. R. (2017). Caregiving responsibilities for a child, spouse or parent: The impact of care recipient independence on employee well-being. *Journal of Vocational Behavior, 101*, 57–66. doi:10.1016/j.jvb.2017.04.006

Black, M. M. (1976). Adolescent Role Assessment. *American Journal of Occupational Therapy, 30*, 73–79.

Boyce, W. T., Jensen, E. W., James, S. A., & Peacock, J. L. (1983). The family routines inventory: Theoretical origins. *Social Sciences Medicine, 17*(4), 193–200.

Braveman, B., Robson, M., Velozo, C., Kielhofner, G., Fisher, G., Forsyth, K., & Kerschbaum, J. (2005). *Model of occupational therapy clearinghouse.* Retrieved from http://www.uic.edu/depts/moho/assess/wri.html

Chugg, A., & Craik, C. (2002). Some factors influencing occupational engagement for people with schizophrenia living in the community. *British Journal of Occupational Therapy, 65*, 67–74.

Clark, F. (2000). The concepts of habit and routine: A preliminary synthesis. *OTJR: Occupation, Participation and Health, 20*, 123S–137S.

Crepeau, E. B. (1995). Rituals. In C. B. Royeen (Ed.), *The practice of the future: Putting occupation back into therapy* (pp. 5–23). Bethesda, MD: American Occupational Therapy Association.

Crepeau, E. B., & Schell, B. A. B. (2009). Analyzing occupations and activity. In E. B. Crepeau, E. S. Cohn, & B. A. B. Schell (Eds.), *Willard & Spackman's occupational therapy* (11th ed., pp. 359–374). Baltimore, MD: Lippincott Williams & Wilkins.

Crowe, T. K., VanLeit, B., Berghmans, K. K., & Mann, P. (1996). Role perceptions of mothers with young children: The impact of a child's disability. *American Journal of Occupational Therapy, 51*, 651–661.

Davies Hallet, J., Zasler, N. D., Maurer, P., & Cash, S. (1992). Role change after traumatic brain injury in adults. *American Journal of Occupational Therapy, 49*, 241–246.

Davis, K. (2012). Friendship 2.0: Adolescents' experiences of belonging and self-disclosure online. *Journal of Adolescence, 35*, 1527e1536. doi:10.1016/j.adolescence.2012.02.013

Denham, S. A. (2002). Family routines: A structural perspective for viewing family health. *ANS Advances in Nursing Science, 24*, 60–74.

Denham, S. A. (2003). Relationships between family rituals, family routines, and health. *Journal of Family Nursing, 9*, 305–330. doi:10.1177/1074840703255447

Fougeyrollas, P., Noreau, L., & St-Michel, G. (2001). *Life Habits measure—shortened version (LIFE-H 3.0).* Quebec, Canada: Canadian Society and Quebec Committee on the International Classification of Impairments, Disabilities, and Handicaps.

Friese, B. H. (2007). Routines and rituals: Opportunities for participation in family health. *OTJR: Occupation, Participation and Health, 27*, 41S–49S.

Friese, B. H., Tomcho, T., Douglas, M., Josephs, K., Poltrock, S., & Baker, T. (2002). A review of 50 years of research on naturally occurring family routines and rituals: Cause for celebration. *Journal of Family Psychology, 16*, 381–390.

Galler, A., Lindau, M., Ernert, A., Thalemann, R., & Raile, K. (2011). Associations between media consumption habits, physical activity, socioeconomic status, and glycemic control in children, adolescents, and young adults with type 1 diabetes. *Diabetes Care, 34*, 2356–2359. Retrieved from http://go.galegroup.com.pearl.stkate.edu/ps/i.do?p=EAIM&sw=w&u=clic_stkate&v=2.1&it=r&id=GALE%7CA280004198&asid=4ec1028825da06160e0315f74d09a2df

Good-Ellis, M. A., Fine, S. B., Spencer, J. H., & DiVittis, A. (1987). Developing a Role Activity Performance Scale. *American Journal of Occupational Therapy, 41*, 232–241.

Jackoway, I. S., Rogers, J. C., & Snow, T. L. (1987). The Role Change Assessment: An interview tool for evaluating older adults. *Occupational Therapy in Mental Health, 7*, 17–37.

Jackson, J. (1998). Is there a place for role theory in occupational science? *Journal of Occupational Science, 5*, 48–55.

Jensen, E. W., James, S. A., Boyce, T., & Hartnett, S. A. (1983). The Family Routines Inventory: Development and validation. *Social Science Medicine, 17*(4), 201–211.

Kielhofner, G. (2009). *Conceptual foundations of occupational therapy practice* (4th ed.). Bethesda, MD: American Occupational Therapy Association.

Kielhofner, G., Fogg, L., Braveman, B., Forsyth, K., Kramer, J., & Duncan, E. (2007). A factor analytic study of the Model of Human Occupation Screening Tool of hypothesized values. *Occupational Therapy in Mental Health, 25*, 127–137.

Lawrence, M. (2010). Young adults' experience of stroke: A qualitative review of the literature. *British Journal of Nursing, 19*, 241–248.

Lenhart, A. (2015). *Teens, social media & technology overview 2015*. Retrieved from http://www.pewinternet.org/2015/04/09/teens-social-media-technology-2015/

Mathiowetz, V., Finlayson, M. L., Matuska, K., Chen, H. Y., & Luo, P. (2005). Randomized controlled trial of an energy conservation course for persons with multiple sclerosis. *Multiple Sclerosis, 11*, 592–601.

Mathiowetz, V., Matuska, K., & Murphy, M. (2001). Effectiveness of an energy conservation program for fatigue in multiple sclerosis. *Archives of Physical Medicine and Rehabilitation, 82*, 449–456.

Matuska, K. (2012a). Development of the Life Balance Inventory. *OTJR: Occupation, Participation and Health, 32*, 220–228.

Matuska, K. (2012b). Validity evidence for a model and measure of life balance. *OTJR: Occupation, Participation and Health, 32*, 229–237.

Matuska, K., & Bass, J. (2016). Life Balance and stress in adults with medical conditions or obesity. *OTJR: Occupation, Participation and Health, 36*, 74–81.

Matuska, K., Bass, J., & Schmitt, J. (2013). Life balance and perceived stress: Predictors and demographic profile. *OTJR: Occupation, Participation and Health, 33*, 146–158.

Matuska, K., & Christiansen, C. (2008). A proposed model of lifestyle balance. *Journal of Occupational Science, 15*, 9–19.

Matuska, K., & Christiansen, C. (Eds.). (2009). *Life balance: Multidisciplinary theories and research*. Bethesda, MD: American Occupational Therapy Association.

Matuska, K., & Erickson, B. (2008). Lifestyle balance: How it is described and experienced by women with multiple sclerosis? *Journal of Occupational Science, 15*, 20–26.

Matuska, K., Mathiowetz, V., & Finlayson, M. (2007). Use and effectiveness of energy conservation strategies for managing multiple sclerosis fatigue. *American Journal of Occupational Therapy, 61*, 63–70.

Meyer, A. (1977). The philosophy of occupational therapy. *American Journal of Occupational Therapy, 31*, 639–642.

Monk, T. H., Flaherty, J. F., Frank, E., Hoskinson, K., & Kupfer, D. J. (1990). The Social Rhythm Metric: An instrument to quantify the daily rhythms of life. *Journal of Nervous and Mental Disease, 178*, 120–126.

Monk, T. H., Frank, E., Potts, J. M., & Kupfer, D. J. (2002). A simple way to measure daily lifestyle regularity. *Journal of Sleep Research, 11*, 183–190.

National Highway Traffic Safety Administration. (2017). *Distracted driving*. Retrieved from https://www.nhtsa.gov/risky-driving/distracted-driving

Nuutinen, T., Ray, C., & Roos, E. (2013). Do computer use, TV viewing, and the presence of the media in the bedroom predict school-aged children's sleep habits in a longitudinal study? *BMC Public Health, 13*, 684.

Oakley, F., Kielhofner, G., Barris, R., & Reichler, R. (1986). The Role Checklist: Development and empirical assessment of reliability. *OTJR: Occupation, Participation and Health, 6*, l57–l70.

Olmstead, K. (2017). *A third of Americans live in a household with three or more smartphones*. Retrieved from http://www.pewresearch.org/fact-tank/2017/05/25/a-third-of-americans-live-in-a-household-with-three-or-more-smartphones/

Parkinson, S., Forsyth, K., & Kielhofner, G. (2006). *The Model of Human Occupation Screening Tool (MOHOST) Version 2.0*. Retrieved from http://www.uic.edu/depts/moho/assess/mohost.htm

Perrin, A. (2015). *Social media usage: 2005-2015*. Retrieved from http://www.pewinternet.org/2015/10/08/social-networking-usage-2005-2015/

Poole, J., & Cordova, J. S. (2004). Dressing routines in women with chronic disease: A pilot study. *New Zealand Journal of Occupational Therapy, 51*, 30–35.

Radomski, M. V. (2011). More than good intentions: Advancing adherence to therapy recommendations. *American Journal of Occupational Therapy, 65*, 471–477. doi:10.5014/ajot.2011.000885

Reich, J. W. (2000). Routinization as a factor in the coping and mental health of women with fibromyalgia. *OTJR: Occupation, Participation and Health, 20*, 41S–51S.

Sanders, M. J., & Van Oss, T. (2013). Using Daily Routines to Promote Medication Adherence in Older Adults. *American Journal of Occupational Therapy, 67*, 91–99. doi:10.5014/ajot.2013.005033

Scott, C. F., Bay-Cheng, L. Y., Prince, M. A., Collins, R. L., & Nochajski, T. H. (2017). Time spent online: Latent profile analyses of emerging adults' social media use. *Computers in Human Behavior, 75*, 311–319. doi:10.1016/j.chb.2017.05.026

Segal, R. (2004). Family routines and rituals: A context for occupational therapy interventions. *American Journal of Occupational Therapy, 58*, 499–508.

Sheldon, K., Cummins, R., & Khamble, S. (2010). Life balance and well-being: Testing a novel conceptual and measurement approach. *Journal of Personality, 78*, 1093–1134.

Stein, L., Foran, A., & Cermak, S. (2011). Occupational patterns of parents of children with autism spectrum disorder: Revisiting Matuska and Christiansen's model of lifestyle balance. *Journal of Occupational Science, 18*, 115–130.

Wagman, P., Håkansson, C., Matuska, K., Björklund, A., & Falkmer, T. (2011). Validating the model of lifestyle balance on a working Swedish population. *Journal of Occupational Science, 4*, 1–9.

Young, M. (1998). *The metronomic society*. Cambridge, MA: Harvard University Press.

Zautre, A. J., Hamilton, N., & Yocum, D. (2000). Patterns of positive social engagement among women with rheumatoid arthritis. *OTJR: Occupation, Participation and Health, 20*, 21S–40S.

Zisberg, A., Young, H. M., & Schepp, K. (2009). Development and psychometric testing of the Scale of Older Adults' Routine. *Journal of Advanced Nursing, 65*, 672–683. doi:10.1111/j.1365-2648.2008.04901.x

the**Point**® *For additional resources on the subjects discussed in this chapter, visit* **http://thePoint.lww.com/Willard-Spackman13e.** *See* **Appendix I, Resources and Evidence for Common Conditions Addressed in OT** *for more information about the conditions discussed in this chapter.*

CHAPTER 19

Culture, Diversity, and Culturally Effective Care

Roxie M. Black

"An individual has not started living until he can rise above the narrow confines of his individualistic concerns to the broader concerns of all humanity."

—MARTIN LUTHER KING, JR.

LEARNING OBJECTIVES

After reading this chapter, you will be able to:

1. Differentiate between culture, race, and ethnicity.
2. Analyze how a client's culture may affect occupational choice and performance.
3. Discuss the impact of culture on the occupational therapy evaluation and intervention process.
4. Analyze the need for cultural awareness and culturally effective skills in occupational therapy.
5. Compare and contrast individualistic and collectivistic cultures.

Introduction

World demographics are rapidly changing. Each country has its own blend of cultures and ethnicities. In the United States, population statistics indicate ever-increasing ethnic and social diversity in rates that surpass any other generation. Additionally, swiftly developing technology connects us to people, places, and news anywhere in the world. This is now the world of occupational therapy (OT). Examples of how these realities affect practice are presented in the three scenarios presented next (see Practice Dilemmas 19-1, 19-2, and 19-3).

Although books related to culture and diversity in health care have proliferated in the past decade (Black & Wells, 2007; Bonder & Martin, 2013; Edberg, 2012; Spector, 2016; Wells, Black, & Gupta, 2016), a recognition of the need to understand the unique culture of a client was first cited in professional publications in 1968 (Committee on Basic Professional Education, Council on Standards, as cited in Black, 2002). A few of the main reasons that occupational therapists have been concerned about diversity for so long is their belief about the uniqueness of each individual and the profession's emphasis on client-centered practice (Mroz, Pitonyak, Fogelberg, & Leland, 2015). **Client-centered practice** focuses on the individual clients with whom we work, attempting to understand their beliefs, values,

CENTENNIAL NOTES

Culture and Diversity Awareness in Occupational Therapy

Over the past century, the world has changed significantly, and although the profession of OT has developed and grown, the emphasis on treatment and care for the individual has remained constant. A century ago, the language of culture and diversity was not found in OT literature, but early recognition of and sensitivity to client uniqueness found in the first set of standards for the profession (1920) set the foundation for today's focus on culturally effective care. At the third annual meeting of the National Society for the Promotion of Occupational Therapy, when developing the guidelines and standards for the education, the committee stated that OT students "should know a little about the different racial groups, their habits, customs, beliefs, etc., in order to work with them more sympathetically and intelligently" (National Society for the Promotion of Occupational Therapy, 1919, p. 23). Although working with diverse clients and practitioners was not a focus in the early years of the profession, the foundation for the development of so was written in the very earliest U.S. documents. Additionally, with the inception of the World Federation of Occupational Therapists in 1951 (World Federation of Occupational Therapists [WFOT], 2012) learning about and from a variety of countries and people continued to expand the worldview of U.S. OT practitioners, educators/scholars, and scientists.

PRACTICE DILEMMA 19-1

Susan, a Caucasian OT student entered the clinic of a large urban hospital, knowing that the first patient of the day was Peter, a 54-year-old African American man who was a day laborer on the piers. Peter is being followed after his hand surgery for tendon repairs following a crush injury. Although his wounds are now closed, he continues to need activities to obtain full mobility and dexterity in his right hand, so he can return to work. She greeted him warmly and because it was near the holidays, she offered him the opportunity to join in making some holiday cookies. Susan was a technically knowledgeable student and knew cutting out cookie dough and manipulating the decoration materials would be good for his dexterity.

Peter was cooperative during the session, but as Susan was reflecting on the interaction following their session together, she recalled the little shake of his head prior to the task and the sardonic little grin Peter wore as he seemed to indulge her choice of intervention. "I wonder what that was all about?" she thought.

Questions

1. What should Susan have considered when choosing an activity for Peter?
2. Even though Susan knew Peter's diagnosis and intervention goals, what other information should she have sought from him?
3. Considering Peter's cultural and work history, what other occupational activities might have been more appropriate for this patient?

and dreams in order to collaboratively develop appropriate and meaningful interventions. In order to do this well, OT practitioners must learn about a person's culture as a means of understanding his or her unique characteristics and how that culture impacts the person's occupational choices and behaviors. This also applies in a broader sense to our work with communities, populations, as discussed elsewhere in this text (see Chapter 31), although this chapter focuses on interventions with individuals and their families.

In Practice Dilemma 19-1, the enthusiastic OT student chose an activity (cookie making) that did achieve the results she wanted (tendon stretching) but had no meaning for the client with whom she was working. As a result, the client would more than likely not repeat this activity outside of the OT clinic. Had the student learned a little of this man's culture and interests, together they may have collaborated in determining an intervention activity that not only achieved the physical results they were aiming for but would also excite the client in a way that he may choose to repeat the activity often for its therapeutic and cultural value. Let's begin to further explore this with an examination of culture.

Culture

Definition of Culture

The story in the preceding text indicates the significance of the examination of issues of culture for the OT practitioner. It is important to understand what we mean by the term. Each person is a cultural being, and each has a distinct cultural makeup. *Culture* is a broad term that encompasses many aspects about an individual and has been defined in many ways. Iwama (2004) states that culture is a "slippery concept, taking on a variety of definitions and meanings depending on how it has been socially situated and by whom" (p. 1); yet, OT students and practitioners alike must have an understanding of what culture means. Black and Wells (2007) define culture as

> the sum total of a way of living, including values, beliefs, standards, linguistic expression, patterns of thinking, behavioral norms, and styles of communication that influence the behavior(s) of a group of people [and] is transmitted from generation to generation. It includes demographic variables such as age, gender, and place of residence; status variables such as social, educational, and economic levels; and affiliation variables. (p. 5)

One can see by this definition that the concept of culture is all-encompassing and quite complex. It incorporates all those aspects of a person that make him or her unique. Historically, anthropologists and others have determined that a large part of a person's identity is determined by his or her cultural allegiances (La Fontaine, 1985). If identity is determined at some level by one's culture, then it is imperative that OT practitioners learn about a client's culture in order to truly understand that person. Interrelated with the concept of culture are the concepts of race and ethnicity.

Race and Ethnicity

Race

Often, people think of race when asked about culture. Even though the United States Census Bureau and many other organizations and countries ask people to check a certain box to indicate their race, scientists today question the validity of the biological concept of race (Haney Lopez, 1994; Marks, 1996). The term *biological race* is used by those who believe that "there exist natural, physical divisions among humans that are hereditary, reflected in morphology, and roughly but correctly captured by terms like Black, White, and Asian" (Haney Lopez, 1994, p. 6). In other words, race is recognized by physical attributes. Marks (1996) believes that dividing the human population among these discrete groupings is "arbitrary, not natural" (p. 124). Additionally, scientists have proven that identifying a group of people by their skin color (which often typifies the concept of race) does not represent a distinct cultural group; rather, "greater genetic variation exists *within* [emphasis added] the populations typically labeled Black and White than between these populations" (Haney Lopez, 1994, p. 13). In contrast to this biological definition, Haney Lopez (1994) believes that race is a social construction and that "terms like Black, White, Asian, and Latino are social groups, not genetically distinct branches of humankind" (p. 14), whereas Relethford (as cited in Nittle,

2011) characterizes race as "a concept of human minds, not of nature." Within each of these social groupings are many different ethnic and cultural groups with different beliefs and values, languages, and behaviors.

What these arbitrary distinctions of race have accomplished is to separate people and support racism (Abizadeh, 2001). **Racism** "is most fundamentally the assessment of individual worth on the basis of real or imputed group characteristics. Its evil lies in the denial of people's right to be judged as individuals, rather than as group members, and in the truncation of opportunities or rights on that basis" (Marks, 1996, p. 131). Yet, more current authors found that there continues to be wide agreement that the concept of race "is important to consider in clinical care" (Hunt, Truesdell, & Kreiner, 2013). But there is much controversy among health professionals. Some argue that "taking racism/ethnicity into a patients' genetic heritage . . . can provide convenient insight into a patients' genetic heritage, behavioral habits, and socioeconomic status" (Nawaz & Brett, 2009; Wolinsky, 2011). Others argue that these practices may "increase disparities by promoting stereotyping" (Acquaviva & Mintz, 2010; Ncayiyana, 2007).

Racism remains a social problem that affects the OT profession. Although some countries such as New Zealand seem to be actively working to find ways to honor and work within perspectives of their native tribal groups, systematic and institutionalized racism in the United States (and likely other places as well) impacts access to exemplary education to minority populations (Rothenberg, 1998). This, in turn, limits the number of ethnically diverse students who are academically prepared for OT education which results in a limited multicultural workforce, which is a detriment to our profession. Pittz (2005) believes that racism results in health disparities, limiting health access and service to people of color and those otherwise marginalized.

Ethnicity

As with the concept of culture and race, the term *ethnicity* has multiple definitions, many of which indicate that ethnicity is a social grouping of people who share cultural or national similarities (Figure 19-1). The most common characteristics of an ethnic group include "kinship, family rituals, food preferences, special clothing, and particular celebrations" (Srivastava, 2007, p. 12). Many people who are White or Caucasian living in the United States can identify with an ethnic background such as Italian American, Franco American, or Irish American. People who consider themselves Black or Asian also come from differing ethnic groups, such as Ethiopian or Filipino. Abizadeh (2001) discusses the impact that a common descent has on one's ethnicity. Although he speaks of the myth of common descent, he states, "people share a common ethnicity insofar as they share a myth of common descent—that is, insofar as they *believe* themselves to be

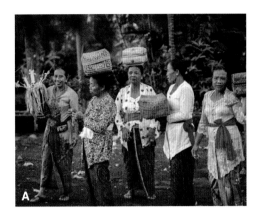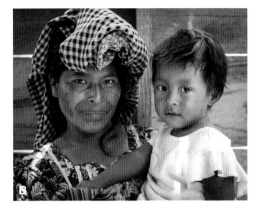

FIGURE 19-1 **A.** Balinese women in traditional clothes on their way to their temple. **B.** Guatemalan mother with traditional headwear. (Courtesy of R. Andrew Hamlin, photographer.)

descended from common ancestors" (p. 25). Leininger (2002), however, goes on to remind us that although ethnicity may reflect a shared culture, the terms *ethnicity* and *culture* cannot be used interchangeably. One must remember, however, that as OT students and practitioners, acknowledging the importance of a client's ethnicity and/or culture is a vital aspect and function of client-centered care. Other important client issues are noted subsequently.

Cultural Differences Not Related to Race and Ethnicity

The majority of cultural differences that an OT practitioner may face are not related to race and ethnicity. Some of these include differences in class or socioeconomic status, education, religion, sexual orientation, age, and political views, all of which impact occupational choices and behaviors. Many of these characteristics are personalized by the client and have great meaning to him or her, just as they do for the practitioner. Therefore, these factors are often emotionally laden for both. The inability to recognize and address cultural differences may become problematic in client–practitioner interactions due to of issues of prejudice, stereotyping, and discrimination.

Prejudice and Discrimination

Prejudice

Most OT practitioners in the United States have grown up in this country and culture where racism, sexism, heterosexism, ageism, and many other -isms are prevalent, leading to (often subconscious) prejudice against certain groups of people. Most practitioners do not want to characterize people in a negative way, and many may not even be aware that they are doing so; yet, many do. **Prejudice** has

---

🛐 PRACTICE DILEMMA 19-2

The OT practitioner was on his first home visit with an older woman who had been discharged from the rehabilitation center following a stroke. He was there to evaluate the home, meet the woman's family, and provide education about activities of daily living (ADL) strategies specific to the home environment. When he arrived, the client introduced the practitioner to her wife. The practitioner realized he was dealing with a lesbian couple and was personally uncomfortable in this situation. He decided to "grin and bear it" and went on to evaluate the home and educate the two women, although he knew he wasn't his usual relaxed self.

Questions

1. What might the practitioner have done to avoid the "surprise" that awaited him in the client's home?
2. Given his discomfort, what action might the practitioner take to help reflect on his reaction?
3. Because of his discomfort with the client's lifestyle and his concern that he might not be able to provide unbiased and effective therapy, should the practitioner request to be taken off this case?

---

been defined as "preconceived ideas and attitudes—usually negative about a particular group of people, often without full examination of the facts" (Black & Wells, 2007, p. 86). Hecht (1998) expands that definition by discussing four major metaphors for prejudice as shown in Table 19-1.

Reviewing Practice Dilemma 19-2, one can recognize that the practitioner may be feeling some discomfort because of unrecognized prejudice against people who are homosexual. In that story, his stilted interaction with the couple impacts his client-centered approach, which

TABLE 19-1   Metaphors for Prejudice

Metaphor	Basis for Prejudice
Difference as a threat	A fear of difference or the unknown
Difference as aversive	A dislike of difference or the unknown
Difference as competition	Competition with difference for scarce resources
Difference due to hierarchy	Beliefs that are hierarchical and structured

Adapted from Hecht, M. L. (Ed.). (1998). *Communicating prejudice* (p. 3). Thousand Oaks, CA: Sage.

may result in less than effective intervention planning and implementation. This story may exemplify one of the first two of Hecht's (1998) metaphors as shown in Table 19-1 (difference as a threat or as aversive). Have you ever noticed prejudice caused by competition or hierarchy, the last two metaphors?

Stereotyping and Ethnocentrism

Prejudice is often the result of stereotyping and ethnocentrism. **Stereotyping** occurs when one attributes certain characteristics to an entire group of people, or what Herbst (1997) defines as "an exaggerated image of their characteristics, without regard to individual attributes" (p. 212). These can be thoughts about people related to age, race, gender, sexuality, occupation, ethnicity, and physical and mental abilities. Some common stereotypes that have been heard by the author include

- All Black people can dance.
- Obese people are lazy.
- Feminists are man-haters.
- Old people are grumpy.
- Gay men are promiscuous.

Many of us have been raised in a society that teaches us stereotypical concepts. Although we often cannot control these thoughts, which may come unbidden to our consciousness, it is important to be aware of them and then choose not to listen to or act on them. This kind of thinking, which negates the importance of recognizing the uniqueness of each individual, may develop into prejudicial beliefs. **Ethnocentrism**, on the other hand, is the "tendency of people to put their own group (*ethnos*) at the center; to see things through the narrow lens of their own culture and use the standards of that culture to judge others" (Herbst, 1997, p. 80). This is a common human response to difference. Instead of looking at someone who is different from oneself as unique, interesting, and someone to learn about and from, a person with an ethnocentric viewpoint would judge the other person to be less

than, not as good as, or inferior to oneself. It is apparent that this combination of stereotyping and ethnocentrism can promote prejudice which can lead to discrimination.

Discrimination

If prejudice is related to one's thoughts and beliefs, discrimination is the action or behavior associated with those beliefs. **Discrimination** "denies equal treatment to people because of their membership in some group" (Herbst, 1997, p. 185) and can occur at many levels including individual, institutional or organizational, and structural (Rothenberg, 1998). Individual discrimination may occur when an immigrant woman is shunned in her community by other residents who believe she is "stealing" welfare support from them. It may also be observed when a Caucasian client or patient refuses to be treated by a practitioner of color. Organizational discrimination reinforces individual discrimination by "instituting rules, policies, and practices that have an adverse effect on nondominant groups such as minorities, women, older people, people with disabilities, and people with varying sexual identities" (Black & Wells, 2007, pp. 88–89). This may be seen in social clubs that disallow women or people of color to join. Another example is the inability of same-sex couples to be married or recognized as family in some states, disallowing partners to have access to one another's insurance coverage for medical care. The highest level of discrimination, structural discrimination, is that which reproduces itself among the fields of employment, education, housing, and government as described by Rothenberg (1998):

> Discrimination in education denies the credentials to get good jobs. Discrimination in employment denies the economic resources to buy good housing. Discrimination in housing confines minorities to school districts providing inferior education, closing the cycle in the classic form. (p. 140)

This systematic level sustains poverty and health disparities, resulting in lack of access to other goods and services to those who are discriminated against. Because of its systematic nature, this level of discrimination is very difficult to change. One area of discrimination still apparent in the United States is that of obesity which has been labeled as the "last bastion of prejudice" (Flanagan, 1996). Although there has been much effort in the last decade regarding the recognition of obesity as a social as well as a health issue, not much has changed since Flanagan made the statement in the preceding text. There is more about this later in this chapter.

As OT practitioners, we may not be able to be free of prejudicial thoughts and beliefs, but we can and must monitor and manage our behaviors. In order to avoid discriminating against others, we must be aware of our beliefs and values. The development of discrimination is outlined in Figure 19-2.

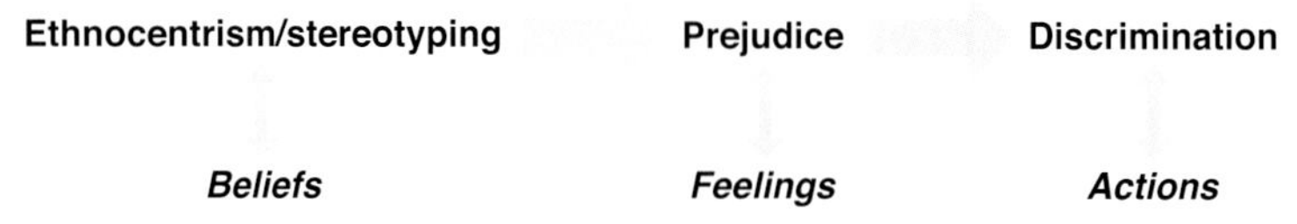

Ethnocentrism/stereotyping   Prejudice   Discrimination

Beliefs   *Feelings*   *Actions*

FIGURE 19-2 The development of discrimination.

PRACTICE DILEMMA 19-3

Sally, a 57-year-old woman, entered a local hospital for a routine hip replacement surgery. She is a college professor with a warm, engaging personality. Additionally, she is 5 ft 3 in tall and weighs 389 pounds. As she began to fall asleep under anesthesia, she heard a member of the surgical team say, "How in the world are we ever going to move and position her without killing ourselves."

Following the surgery, Sam, the contracted occupational therapist came to Sally's bedside to help her learn the correct safety procedures in the hospital and as she prepared to be transferred to the small rehabilitation center in her community. While communicating with the nursing staff, Sam realized that most of the nurses did not want to treat Sally, and no one had attempted to help her mobilize at bedside because they did not have a lift to assist her.

When Sally finally arrived at the local rehabilitation center, Sam realized the center did not have any bariatric equipment either, including wheelchairs and commodes, and Sally waited a few days for them to order the correct equipment. She confided with Sam that she "felt terrible," shamed and embarrassed that people had to "go out of their way" because of her weight to help her out. As a result, the total experience was not a good one for Sally, and it hindered her progress in healing as well as her independence, whereas Sam was frustrated that he couldn't assist Sally the way he wanted to.

Questions

1. What do you think Sam's role should have been in this situation?
   a. With the patient?
   b. With the nursing director or hospital staff?
   c. With the rehabilitation director?
2. Have you ever been discriminated against because of your weight, or do you have friends or family members who have been?
3. If you or others that you know have been discriminated against because of your (their) weight, what might you do to try to improve the situation?

Culture and Occupational Therapy

Culture and OT are inextricably intertwined. Occupational therapy is founded on the recognition of the uniqueness of each individual with whom we work and sustained by

a belief in client-centered care. Additional elements that indicate the importance of and mandate the examination of culture for the OT profession include the American Occupational Therapy Association (AOTA) Centennial Vision (AOTA, 2012), the Occupational Therapy Practice Framework (OTPF) (AOTA, 2014), AOTA's official document on *Occupational Therapy's Commitment to Nondiscrimination and Inclusion* (AOTA, 2004), and many occupation-based models of practice.

Client-Centered Care

One of the major tenets of OT, client-centered or person-centered care, is based on the profession's belief in the worth of and respect for each individual. Client-centered care is rooted in Carl Rogers's (1959/1989) notion of providing clients with "unconditional positive regard." Client-centered care supports the premise that a client is capable of leading the therapy process and making decisions about his or her health care, and that therapy is a collaborative process between the client and the practitioner. This requires the OT practitioner to understand the client's condition through the client's eyes, not his or her own (Sumsion, 1993). Every client who engages in OT brings his or her own cultural lens and worldview to each session. In order to interact effectively, the OT practitioner must carefully listen to and understand the client's cultural values and beliefs about health and well-being. In other words, as described earlier, effective client-centered care must include an awareness of and knowledge about clients' culture (Black, 2005) and their unique expression of that culture. More information about client-centered care is available in Units VI and VIII.

Practice Guidelines

Occupational therapy organizations throughout the world are guided by statements regarding the scope of OT practice. Those reviewed for this chapter included the AOTA OTPF (AOTA, 2014), Canada's Profile of Practice (Canadian Association of Occupational Therapists, 2012), New Zealand's Code of Ethics (Occupational Therapy Board of New Zealand, 2015), and Australia's Scope of Practice Framework (Occupational Therapy Australia, 2017). Each clearly addresses the importance of cultural awareness and knowledge for providing effective care.

In AOTA OTPF (AOTA, 2014), the domain and practice of OT are described, presenting "a summary of interrelated constructs that define and guide occupational therapy practice" (p. 625). Through this document, the profession identifies and establishes the breadth of OT practice and the ways in which we may work with our clients. One specific area the OTPF identifies as part of the domain of OT practice is the context and environment within which clients engage in occupation and that influences their occupational performance. The multiple contexts of a person's life identified in the OTPF include cultural, personal, temporal, physical, social, and virtual. A client's cultural context is defined as customs, beliefs, activity patterns, behavior standards, and expectations accepted by the society of which the client is a member. "[It] includes ethnicity and values as well as political aspects, such as laws that affect access to resources and affirm personal rights. [Cultural context] also includes opportunities for education, employment, and economic support" (AOTA, 2014, p. S28).

Because cultural context greatly impacts occupational choice and occupational behaviors based on beliefs, values, and societal expectations, it is necessary and imperative that OT practitioners incorporate cultural knowledge of their clients during their evaluation and intervention planning.

Official Documents on Nondiscrimination and Inclusion

The AOTA recognizes the importance and value of a multicultural or pluralistic society. **Multiculturalism** has been defined as "an ideal in which diverse groups in a society coexist amicably, retaining their individual cultural identities" (Herbst, 1997, p. 154). The United States is progressing toward that goal. The AOTA's official document on *Occupational Therapy's Commitment to Nondiscrimination and Inclusion* (AOTA, 2004) clearly speaks to the importance of valuing individuals for all of their unique characteristics and treating everyone fairly and equitably. The authors state, "when we do not discriminate against others and when we include all members of society in our daily lives, we reap the benefits of being with individuals who have different perspectives, opinions, and talents from our own" (AOTA, 2004, p. 668).

The WFOT is the key international representative for occupational therapists and OT around the world and the official international organization for the promotion of OT. In 2009, WFOT published an informative document supporting occupational therapists, OT organizations, OT educational programmes, and OT researchers in their consideration, and understanding of incorporating the principles of diversity and culture into their daily practice and business. This document is a pragmatic tool for all OT personnel who are seeking information about how to become more culturally effective in practice.

Occupation-Based Models of Practice

Kielhofner and Burke (1980) developed one of the earliest occupation-based models of practice, the *Model of Human Occupation*. From its inception, this model incorporated the analysis of a client's culture and its impact on occupational choice. Subsequently developed models of practice, many of which is more thoroughly described in Unit IX of this book, also recognize the importance of understanding a client's culture as a necessary focus of analysis in the provision of client-centered care (Baum & Christiansen, 2005; Dunn, Brown, & McGuigan, 1994; Iwama, 2006; Law et al., 1996; Schkade & Schultz, 2003). These practice models provide theoretical and practical approaches for OT intervention, all of which consider the importance of recognizing how a client's culture may impact his or her occupations.

The Impact of Culture on Occupation

Think about all of the activities or occupations you engaged in yesterday. Why did you choose these? **Occupational choice** is determined by one's values; interests and beliefs; social situation; gender; age; sexual identity; and physical, cognitive, and emotional abilities. Many of these factors are characteristics of one's culture. For example, when considering what leisure pursuits to engage in, an African American, 65-year-old educated woman from the northeastern part of the United States may choose activities such as snowshoeing with her grandchildren or meeting friends in a nearby shopping mall for lunch. These activities would meet the expectations of her family, friends, and community and her own beliefs about the appropriate role of women from her society and culture. Across the world, another 65-year-old working-class Chinese woman from a small city in China might choose to exercise on one of the numerous pieces of equipment found in the many small parks near her neighborhood before sharing a cup of tea with a neighbor as they sit together on the stoop of their urban *hutong*. Each of these women values exercise and has chosen socially and culturally appropriate activities that support her beliefs and lifestyle. Figure 19-3 shows some culturally determined occupational choices from Bali and Guatemala.

In an OT setting, it is important that OT choices be focused on the client's interests and values and that the activity holds cultural meaning for him or her. For example, it is common for OT practitioners to focus on helping individuals gain self-care skills after they have survived strokes. However, if an older Latino man does not want to engage in practicing donning shoes and socks with adaptive equipment in the OT clinic because his wife and his grown daughter will insist on doing it for him when he is back home, should the OT practitioner continue to focus on that activity? What would be a client-centered approach to this issue?

Not only is the choice of occupation determined by one's cultural beliefs and expectations but how one's

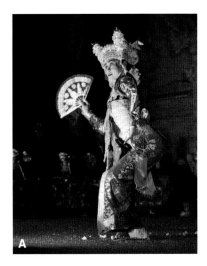 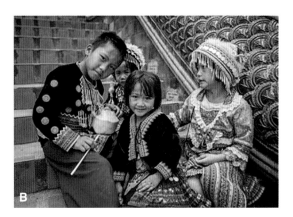

FIGURE 19-3 Culturally determined occupations. **A.** Balinese woman performing a ceremonial dance. **B.** Guatemalan children begging for money from tourists in the marketplace. (Courtesy of R. Andrew Hamlin, photographer.)

occupational performance is also influenced by culture. Occupational performance is defined as "the act of doing and accomplishing a selected action (performance skill), activity of occupation that results from the dynamic transaction among the client the context and the activity" (AOTA, 2014, p. S43). Cultural context certainly impacts one's performance of an activity. For example, eating a meal is an important occupation in many cultures; yet, mealtime activities are performed differently all around the world. People in the United States and many other Western countries may sit in chairs at a table at most meals, whereas someone from another culture and place in the world may sit on the ground around an open hearth. Children in most Western cultures are taught to use utensils such as forks, knives, and spoons to eat their food, whereas East Asian

children deftly use chopsticks to get their food into their mouths, and many Africans use their hands and fingers to accomplish the same task. Even within each culture, there are variances as in the children shown eating in Figure 19-4.

Family beliefs reflect those of their society's culture and will determine whether everyone eats at the same time, sits around a designated eating space, eats in front of the television and other electronic games, or eats alone in their rooms. Therefore, an OT student or practitioner working with a client on mealtime activities must understand exactly what activities that client engages in during a typical mealtime. One cannot assume that all occupations are performed in the same way at the same time and being sensitive to cultural differences will help a practitioner, in collaboration with the client, to develop appropriate and

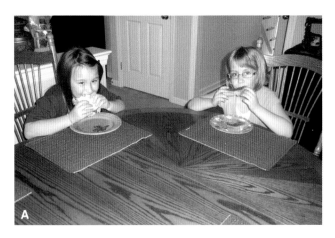 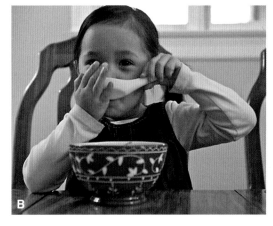

FIGURE 19-4 Diverse mealtime occupational performances. **A.** American children at lunch in York, Pennsylvania, United States. **B.** A Chinese child at lunch. (Photographs courtesy of [A] Gretchen Miller and [B] Art Hsieh.)

meaningful interventions. Besides these examples, there are many other cultural issues that may impact effective cross-cultural interactions in OT.

Cultural Issues That May Impact Cross-Cultural Interactions in Occupational Therapy

Cultural differences sometimes result in discord in cross-cultural interactions, particularly when they impact one's values, and there is little understanding between the participants. It is important to remember that each person within a therapeutic relationship enters that interaction with his or her own cultural lens and worldview, beliefs and values, and preferred behaviors. Therefore, every interaction between an OT practitioner and his or her client could be considered a cross-cultural interaction. There are many specific characteristics of culture that may impact a therapeutic relationship including self-concept, perceptions of power and authority, and the beliefs about and use of time (Black, 2010). The following are examples of issues that may result in discomfort or misunderstanding if the OT practitioner and client are from different cultures.

Beliefs about Health, Well-being, and Illness

Concepts of health, and beliefs about what constitutes well-being and what causes illnesses, or a group's explanatory model of health and illness are culturally determined and influenced (Bonder & Martin, 2013). One learns about healthy and nonhealthy practices from family, peers, and the media. In the United States and many other Western countries, the biomedical model, or allopathic medicine, prevails. The **biomedical model** is based on scientific knowledge that "attributes health and illness to physiological, biological, and scientifically explainable changes in one's body" (Lattanzi & Purnell, 2006, p. 137). Typical of an individualistic society, the biomedical model "emphasizes the treatment of the individual's body and minimizes the links to households, communities or the supernatural" (Lattanzi & Purnell, 2006, p. 138). Health, according to this model, is the absence of disease and pharmaceutical intervention is typical, often neglecting the psychological, behavioral, and social dimensions of illness (Srivastava, 2007). However, there has recently been an increased interest in health promotion and wellness and disease prevention, which shifts the way people view health and illness. Reitz (2010) avers that occupation has been used in multiple cultures to promote well-being and health for centuries. As a result of the current emphasis on health and wellness, many people are more health conscious and are changing their occupational behaviors to support a healthier lifestyle.

There are many groups of people, however, who view health and the cause of illness in a far different manner than the biomedical model. Some may believe that illness is caused by evil and is eradicated through the use of spiritual or magical intervention. One of the most common beliefs is that of the *evil eye*. The concept of the evil eye is that someone can "project harm by gazing or staring at another's property or person" (Spector, 2016, p. 83). Khalifa, Hardieb, Latifc, Jamild, and Walkere (2011) suggest that the evil eye is related to envy. This widespread belief was brought to the United States by immigrants from Southern Europe, the Middle East, and North Africa (Mahoney, 1976) and is still practiced by some of their descendants. Some of the common understandings of the evil eye are that the injury or sickness happens suddenly and the victim may not know the source, and the injury or sickness may be prevented or cured with rituals or symbols (Mahoney, 1976). Someone with a strong belief in the evil eye may not accept medical or OT intervention or follow through on suggested activities but may require a healer from their own culture to provide a ritual before participating in therapy.

Traditional and Folk Practices

Folk practices are common for many cultures (Bonder & Martin, 2013), and it is important for practitioners to be familiar with them. **Folk practices** are traditional home remedies used by certain family, ethnic, and cultural groups to counteract illness and support wellness. In my family, my mother would string a whole nutmeg around my neck when I had the croup as a young child and would pour warm oil in my ears for an earache. I'm not sure that these home remedies actually made me better, but she believed they did. Many of you will be able to recall other practices used in your own family and may chuckle at these approaches; yet, how many of us can deny how good chicken soup makes us feel when we are sick.

Folk practices, however, are very different than health care practices in the Western world and have been problematic when immigrants and others have sought out health care. *Coin rubbing*, for example, is the practice of rubbing a coin, which is sometimes heated or used with oil, vigorously over the body in order to draw out illness. The red welts this causes is evidence to the person doing the rubbing that the sickness has come to the surface of the body. This approach to healing is practiced by many people from Asia, including Cambodians, Chinese, Korean, and Vietnamese (Galanti, 2004; Lattanzi & Purnell, 2006). A similar approach is called **cupping** where a heated glass is placed on the back, causing a vacuum that raises and reddens the skin. Users of this practice, including many Asians, Latin Americans, and some Europeans, believe that the hot glass will equalize the coldness in one's body caused by the disease or condition; they also may believe that the cupping will draw out an evil spirit (Galanti, 2004; Lattanzi & Purnell, 2006). Because these practices result in lesions on the skin, health care professionals may misunderstand the cause and may falsely accuse the family of abuse or treat the patient with disrespect. These alternate health occupations and practices must be understood by the OT practitioner in order to provide appropriate information, culturally sensitive conversation, and effective therapy.

Many groups of people who use folk healing also prefer to use a folk healer as part of their health care practices. A **folk healer** is a person who is recognized within the culture who uses traditional magico-religious practices and rituals to help heal the sick. Latino individuals may seek out a *curandero* (spiritual healer) or a *yerbera* (herbalist) to treat their symptoms because they believe a medically based health system alone is insufficient for their needs (Galanti, 2004; Lattanzi & Purnell, 2006; Spector, 2016), whereas a Native American Cherokee woman may search for a shaman or medicine man or woman for adjunctive therapy. Determining how these other health specialists become part of the diverse client's treatment is the job of the intervention team, which may include the OT practitioner.

Gender and Family Roles

Another cultural characteristic that may impact OT practice is the way different cultures determine gender and family roles. Most people have strong personal values and beliefs about gender roles as well as family interactions and expectations. When people with differing beliefs or lifestyles are compelled to interact with one another, such as in a health care setting, these differences may become a barrier to effective communication.

Gender

In the United States and much of the Western world, the women's movement of the 1970s began the process to eliminate restrictive gender roles. Although the system is not perfect, women in these societies have moved much closer to equality with men economically and in the areas of education, the workplace, and sometimes the family. However, there are many cultures and societies that do not share this value, and gender roles and expectations are more conservatively practiced. In many traditional cultures, women are seen as mothers, wives, and housekeepers, some with dominance over decisions made for the home, whereas men continue to hold the power and authority both in public settings and sometimes within the family, acting as

---

🧘 PRACTICE DILEMMA 19-4

The young Somali man didn't seem very friendly. He didn't shake the hand of the experienced therapist and seemed to respond to her in an imperious manner. Although the occupational therapist tried many ways to get him to tell her his story and how he understood his mental illness, he did not respond, finally standing up and saying that he did not want to talk with her. He would only discuss these issues with a male doctor. She described him as uncompliant in his chart and suggested that his behavior was part of his symptomology.

Questions

1. Given the patient's response to her, should the OT practitioner continue to try to work with him or should she ask one of the male therapists to take over the case?
2. If she continues to work with him, how should she approach him at their next scheduled appointment?

---

spokesman and decision maker (Galanti, 2004). In a health care situation, a man may speak and answer for his wife, even if she is the client. Although this kind of interaction may feel uncomfortable for a Western health provider who values a woman's independence, understanding why this occurs and responding appropriately for that culture will facilitate the therapeutic relationship with both the client and her spouse. In many cultures, strict rules are followed regarding public contact between men and women. This is particularly true in some Asian, Middle Eastern, and African communities. If the therapist in Practice Dilemma 19-4 had sought out more information regarding gender role behavior within the Somali culture, where traditional men will not touch a woman outside of his family, she may have understood the young man's refusal to shake her hand rather than labeling him as being uncompliant.

Family Structure

One cannot examine gender roles without understanding the family structure and dynamics within which these roles are enacted. In many countries, a traditional family is composed of a male father, female mother, and their children. However, there are many alternative or nontraditional family structures today. There are increasingly more families with same-sex parents (Lev, 2004), grandparents acting in the parent role (American Association of Retired Persons, n.d.), or one-parent households. Regardless of the structure, however, family cultural issues must be considered in OT practice. Galanti (2004) stated that when nurses were asked what was the most common problem when dealing with non-Anglo ethnic groups, they responded, "Their families!" (p. 76). When an OT practitioner does not understand the cultural values of a particular family and has a difficult time getting the client to say what she expects from therapy until she talks with her father or grandfather, or has trouble effectively treating another client because her room is always filled with extended family members, the OT practitioner might agree with the nurses' sentiment earlier. Many Western health care systems are based on the premise that individuals can make their own health care decisions and that independence is a valued goal for all. However, many cultures perceive the family as a unit, and as part of the values of solidarity, responsibility, and harmony, the entire family makes the health care decisions for one of its members (Srivastava, 2007). These cultures, which include traditional Asian (Srivastava, 2007) and many Latino families (Galanti, 2004), among others, are considered collectivist societies, whereas the United States and many other Western societies are considered individualistic.

Collectivist versus Individualistic Societies

Despite the rhetoric in the U.S. media about family values and despite the importance placed on their families, in general, U.S. society is considered individualistic in nature. **Individualistic societies**, found in North America, Sweden (Lattanzi & Purnell, 2006), and many other European and Western nations, believe in individual rights, and each person within the family or work unit is viewed as a separate entity. Individualistic societies value self-expression, personal choice, autonomy, individual responsibility, and independence (Srivastava, 2007) and may even expect children to voice their opinions and make simple decisions for themselves. Clients from these societies will share many values with most of their Caucasian, U.S.-born OT practitioners and may respond best if the therapist

- Recognizes that illness threatens the client's independence,
- Collaborates with the client on all decisions so he or she feels more in control,

- Encourages the client to "work hard" toward his or her recovery and health,
- Respects the client as a unique individual, and
- Sets individual goals toward independence (Black, 2010).

In contrast, people from **collectivist societies** tend to put more value on the family as a unit than on the individual. *Inter*dependence is valued and the focus is on the "we" as opposed to the "I" of individualistic groups. Decisions are made by the family, who considers what is good for the entire group before focusing on the individual. Health may even be measured by how well one can function within the group (Black, 2010). Because these values may differ from those of some Western occupational therapists, there may be more chance of misunderstanding or miscommunication. Although not necessarily considered a collectivist society, research indicates that many African American individuals also rely heavily on closely knit groups of friends and family and are therefore less likely to welcome strangers such as home health care therapists into their homes and health care networks (Gordon, 1995). Table 19-2 outlines aspects of individualistic and collectivist societies.

It is important for the OT practitioner who is interacting with someone who has a collectivist worldview to

- Work closely with family and group members when the client needs to make health care decisions,
- Be aware that you may be viewed as an outsider and that you may have to work hard to establish trust with the client and his or her family or group,
- Recognize that the client's family and friends may stay with the client much of the time, and
- Emphasize the team approach for safe and effective care (Black, 2010).

Having an awareness of gender and family roles and expectations as well as an understanding about where the client falls on the collectivist–individualist continuum will assist the OT student and practitioner in communicating

TABLE 19-2 Aspects of Collectivist and Individualistic Societies

Collectivist	Individualistic
Priority to needs of the group	Focus on needs of individual
Motivated by group norms	Promotion of self-realization
Group-imposed duties	Individual goals and desires
Harmony and cooperation	Competition
Family is primary unit	Individual is primary
Interdependence	Independence
Family makes decisions for children	Children given many options and encouraged to make own decisions
Rarely have advanced directives	Advanced directives are valued
People more important than time constraints	Time constraints are often strictly adhered to

Adapted from Lattanzi, J. B., & Purnell, L. D. (Eds.). (2006). *Developing cultural competence in physical therapy practice*. Philadelphia, PA: F. A. Davis; Srivastava, R. H. (2007). *The healthcare professional's guide to clinical cultural competence*. Toronto, Ontario, Canada: Mosby.

well and providing effective client-centered care with diverse clients. Another cultural characteristic that may impact therapeutic interactions is the use of touch and space.

The Use of Touch and Space (Proxemics)

Touch

Each person has an inherent natural need to touch and be touched. As occupational therapists, we have learned that the tactile (touch) system is the first sensory system to develop in utero (Montagu, 1986; Soderlund, 2017) and that touch is one of the main systems used to learn about one's own body space and how one "fits" within one's environment (Figure 19-5). Gardner (2010) describes the complex and fascinating neuroscience that occurs when someone touches an object or person or is touched by someone or something in their environment. She summarizes the process by stating, "The sensory and motor components of touch are connected anatomically in the brain, and are important functionally in guiding skilled behaviors" (para. 1). Soderlund (2017) states, " . . . it is likely that touch lays the foundation for the parent-child bond" (para. 1) and that touch "is a powerful tool for connection, calming and nurturing" (para. 5). Ashley Montagu (1986), the author of the seminal book, *Touching*, states that touching is also "our first medium of communication" (p. 3). Although this may be true, as a child develops, he or she learns the unspoken and overt rules about touch in his or her society; when to touch, how to touch, and who

you may touch. The use of touch is culturally determined. Societies may be seen as "high touch" or "low touch" with individuals from each sociocultural group falling somewhere on the continuum between the two. People from **low-touch societies** tend to avoid touch between adults, especially in public, except in prescribed situations such as the handshake during a greeting. Generally, touching between young children and adults is accepted, even in public. For many, a casual touch between members of the opposite sex may be interpreted as a sexual overture and should be avoided (Lattanzi & Purnell, 2006). In many Muslim societies, even a handshake between men and women is forbidden. Figure 19-6 shows touching among Guatemalan family members, a high-touch society.

People from **high-touch societies**, however, may seek out touch as a means of communication and are comfortable with casual touch. As OT students or practitioners, we are often expected to touch our clients, but touching may be viewed as personal or intrusive. It is vitally important to understand the meaning of touch for each client and to carefully explain the necessity for touch in the therapeutic intervention process.

Proxemics

Closely associated with touch is the concept of proxemics. Anthropologist Edward T. Hall (1966/1990) first coined the term in 1966, defining it as "the measureable distance between people as they interact" (p. 114) and addressed how it may affect cross-cultural exchanges. Hall developed the delineation of physical distance as intimate distance (for embracing, touching, or whispering), personal

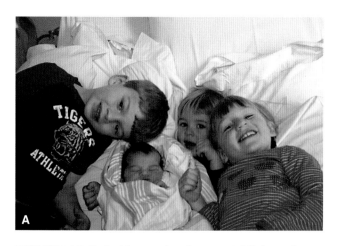
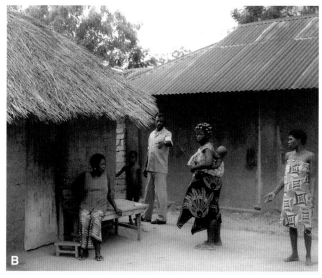

FIGURE 19-5 **A.** The author's grandchildren demonstrating the importance of touch in some cultures. **B.** A mother and baby in South Africa spend much of their time touching. (Photographs courtesy of [**A**] Roxie Black and [**B**] Virginia Skinger.)

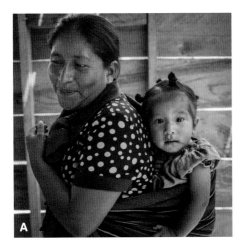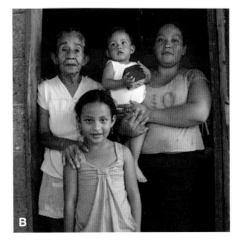

FIGURE 19-6 Touching among Guatemalan family members. (Courtesy of R. Andrew Hamlin, photographer.)

distance (interactions between good friends and family members), social distance (interaction among acquaintances), and public distance (used for public speaking), as shown in Table 19-3 (Hall, 1966/1990).

Various cultures hold different norms about personal space, which they practice unconsciously in order to feel comfortable when interacting with others. For example, people in the United States, Canada, and Great Britain tend to keep about 18 in between themselves when conversing (Lattanzi & Purnell, 2006), whereas some Latinos, who prefer closer contact during conversations, perceive Anglos as being distant and unapproachable (Juckett, 2005).

Additionally, people from Arab countries are more comfortable standing very close to one another when conversing. Their practice of social space is more like North Americans' intimate space (Sheppard, 1996), often resulting in a sense of discomfort for the partner from the United States. I had an opportunity to observe this in a work situation in the United States. I have a Moroccan friend and colleague who often stands very close to others when he speaks, making large gestures as part of his communication style. Several of the women at the facility spoke to me about being nervous or uncomfortable around him and tried to avoid him. This example indicates how cross-cultural interactions can be negatively impacted if participants do not understand the differences in standards related to proxemics and how important it is to have this knowledge when working with people from diverse cultures. Understanding cultural differences and practicing effective cross-cultural interactions is part of being culturally effective, or culturally competent, an important skill for OT practitioners.

TABLE 19-3	Edward T. Hall's Delineation of Physical Distance
Phase	**Distance**
Intimate Distance: For Embracing, Touching, Whispering	
Close phase	Less than 6 in
Far phase	6–18 in
Personal Distance: For Interactions among Good Friends and Family Members	
Close phase	1.5–2.5 ft
Far phase	2.5–4 ft
Social Distance: For Interactions among Acquaintances	
Close phase	4–7 ft
Far phase	7–12 ft
Public Distance: Used for Public Speaking	
Close phase	12–25 ft
Far phase	25 ft or more

Adapted from Hall, E. T. (1990). *The hidden dimension.* New York, NY: Knopf Doubleday. (Original work published 1966)

Culturally Effective Occupational Therapy Practice

Cultural Competence

What is culturally effective practice? Is it **cultural competence**? Can it be called something else? Over the past decade, there has been much published about the need for and importance of cultural awareness and cultural competence in OT practice (Black & Wells, 2007; Bonder, Martin, & Miracle, 2002; Mu, Coppard, Bracciano,

Doll, & Matthews, 2010; Odawara, 2005) as well as the impact of culturally focused curriculum offerings in OT education on the development of cultural competence in OT students and practitioners (Murden et al., 2008; Rasmussen, Lloyd, & Wielandt, 2005; Steed, 2010). Cultural competence is the ability to effectively interact with those who differ from oneself and is often described in the literature as encompassing cultural awareness and attitudes, cultural knowledge of self and others, and cultural skill, which includes effective communication (Callister, 2005; Dillard et al., 1992; Saldana, 2001; Wells & Black, 2000). Developing cultural competency is a somewhat complex process and has been represented as a developing continuum by several theorists (Campinha-Bacote, 2002; Cross, Bazron, Dennis, & Isaacs, 1989; Purnell & Lattanzi, 2006).

Developing the skills and attitudes for cultural competence is not easy, however. Hoops (1979) speaks of the difficulty of moving to cultural competency because of the natural resistance of allowing oneself to be vulnerable and the threat of probing one's identity, which may occur in the process of developing cultural self-awareness. Yet, the importance of developing effective cross-cultural interactions with one's OT clients is essential. Culturally competent care has been found to improve health status among vulnerable populations (Callister, 2005; Lynn-McHale & Deatrick, 2000; Majumdar, Browne, Roberts, & Carpio, 2004) and to increase quality and effectiveness of health care as well as decrease costs (Fortier & Bishop, 2004; Suh, 2004). The results of cultural incompetence may be distrust and miscommunication, lack of adherence to therapeutic recommendations, frustration for both the client and the therapist, and decreased quality of intervention and client/therapist interaction.

Although cultural competence has been described as "a journey rather than an end . . . [and] a lifelong process" (Black & Wells, 2007, p. 31), Gupta (2008) states that it "inadvertently implies that a hypothetical endpoint exists that can be reached by acquiring the right knowledge and skills and attitudes needed to work with persons of different cultures" (p. 3). Supporting Gupta's words, I've had my own students ask, "How can anyone ever achieve cultural competence? There is so much to learn." Perhaps, the terminology itself is a misnomer with the word *competence* misleading people to think that one does have to reach a certain (very high) level in order to achieve this rare state. Other terms used in OT and other health professions to address cross-cultural interactions include culturally responsive caring, cultural emergent, and cultural congruence. Muñoz (2007) has coined the term **culturally responsive caring** which he states "communicates a state of being open to the process of building mutuality with a client and to accepting that the cultural-specific knowledge one has about a group may or may not apply

to the client they were currently treating" (p. 274). Bonder, Martin, and Miracle (2004) use the term **cultural emergent** to describe a model that "suggests that the symbolic aspects of culture and cultural identity emerge in interaction and are displayed primarily through talk and through action" (p. 162). Bonder and her colleagues believe that culture is uniquely expressed by individuals and that it constantly changes, based on the person's context and experiences. **Cultural congruence**, a term used by Schim and Doorenbos (2010), is used to describe how health professionals think and act in ways that fit with a person or group's beliefs and cultural style. This can occur only when one knows and uses in appropriate and meaningful ways the values, expressions, practices, and patterns of various cultural groups. Although the language and meaning of these terms are subtly different, they all encompass basic similarities when talking about effective cross-cultural interactions; one must be culturally self-aware, respect people as individuals, learn about the culture of our diverse clients, and actively engage in the process of developing cultural competence.

Culturally Effective Care

The aforementioned definitions help determine specific ways of interacting with clients who are culturally different that we are. Wells et al. (2016) has added to the dialogue by extending and renaming this practice as Culturally Effective Care. Although this model incorporates the philosophy of cultural competence, it also emphasizes the importance of deep reflection both while interacting with the client and following the intervention in the manner of Schon's (1983) concept of reflection in action and reflection on action. Additionally, the examination of the impact of the context within which the intervention occurs is also an important aspect of this model. See Wells and colleagues' reference earlier for a more detailed explanation. Occupational therapy practice must include a more encompassing thoughtfulness and consideration of one's environment and context to be truly effective.

Conclusion

Occupational therapy practice is based on the premise that humans are occupational beings and that occupation, or meaningful activities, are necessary for health. The purpose of OT intervention is to achieve "the end-goal of supporting health and participation in life through engagement in occupations" (AOTA, 2008, pp. 646–647). Although OT's "clients" may include individuals, organizations, and populations, the OT process remains the same: to examine and evaluate the transaction between the client, the environment or context, and the activities in which the client engages in order to collaboratively and effectively choose an intervention plan that supports the client in his or her participation in life activities. Because each person with whom we work is a culturally unique individual, it is vital that therapy practitioners understand how a person's [-client's] values, beliefs, and interests influence and impact his or her occupational choices and performance. The profession of OT has identified the need to examine a client's cultural context, stating that "[c]ultural contexts often influence how occupations are chosen, prioritized, and organized" (AOTA, 2008, p. 646). In fact, the awareness and use of culture in OT theory and practice is ubiquitous and cannot be ignored.

As has been said earlier, every client/therapist interaction can be considered a cross-cultural interaction. Given this statement and the increasing cultural diversity in client populations, providing effective cross-cultural or culturally competent OT care is imperative. Learning to provide this kind of care may be challenging, but it can also leave you impassioned and energized—outstanding traits of highly competent occupational therapists. Although only a brief examination of the importance of culture and culturally effective care is provided in this chapter, there are numerous resources available that can guide you in your quest for further information, both written and online, some of which are included in the reference list.

Acknowledgments

I'd like to thank my son, Andrew Hamlin, who is a travel photographer, for collaborating with me on this chapter and for providing many of the images.

REFERENCES

Abizadeh, A. (2001). Ethnicity, race, and a possible humanity. *World Order, 33,* 23–34.

Acquaviva, K. D., & Mintz, M. (2010). Perspective: Are we teaching racial profiling? The dangers of subjective determinations of race and ethnicity in case presentations. *Academic Medicine, 85,* 702–705.

American Association of Retired Persons. (n.d.). *GrandFacts state fact sheet for grandparents, relatives raising grandchildren.* Retrieved from http://www.aarp.org/relationships/friends-family/grandfacts-sheets/?CMP=KNC-360I-GOOGLE-RELFRI&HBX_PK=grandparents_as_parents&utm_source=GOOGLE&utm_medium=cpc&utm_term=grandparents%2Bas%2Bparents&utm_campaign=G_Grandfacts&360cid=SI_308824831_10641909541_1

American Occupational Therapy Association. (2004). AOTA position paper: Occupational therapy's commitment to nondiscrimination and inclusion. *American Journal of Occupational Therapy, 58,* 668.

American Occupational Therapy Association. (2008). Occupational therapy practice framework: Domain & process, 2nd edition. *American Journal of Occupational Therapy, 62,* 646–647.

American Occupational Therapy Association. (2012). *AOTA's centennial vision.* Retrieved from http://www.aota.org/News/Centennial.aspx

American Occupational Therapy Association. (2014). Occupational therapy practice framework: Domain and process, 3rd edition. *American Journal of Occupational Therapy, 68*(Suppl. 1), S1–S48. doi:10.5014/ajot.2014.682006

Baum, C., & Christiansen, C. (2005). Person-environment-occupation-performance: An occupation-based framework for practice. In C. Christiansen & C. Baum (Eds.), *Occupational therapy: Performance, participation and well-being* (3rd ed., pp. 242–267). Thorofare, NJ: SLACK.

Black, R. M. (2002). Occupational therapy's dance with diversity. *American Journal of Occupational Therapy, 56,* 140–148.

Black, R. M. (2005). Intersections of care: An analysis of culturally competent care, client centered care, and the feminist ethic of care. *Work, 24,* 409–422.

Black, R. M. (2010). Culture and meaningful occupation. In K. Sladyk, K. Jacobs, & N. MacRae (Eds.), *Occupational therapy essentials for clinical competence* (pp. 11–22). Thorofare, NJ: SLACK.

Black, R. M., & Wells, S. A. (2007). *Culture and occupation: A model of empowerment in occupational therapy.* Bethesda, MD: American Occupation and Therapy.

Bonder, B., & Martin, L. (2013). *Culture in clinical care: Strategies for competence* (2nd ed.). Thorofare, NJ: SLACK.

Bonder, B., Martin, L., & Miracle, A. (2002). *Culture in clinical care.* Thorofare, NJ: SLACK.

Bonder, B., Martin, L., & Miracle, A. (2004). Culture emergent in occupation. *American Journal of Occupational Therapy, 58,* 159–168.

Callister, L. C. (2005). What has the literature taught us about culturally competent care of women and children? *American Journal of Maternal/Child Nursing, 30,* 380–388.

Campinha-Bacote, J. (2002). The process of cultural competence in the delivery of health-care services: A model of care. *Journal of Transcultural Nursing, 13,* 181–184.

Canadian Association of Occupational Therapists. (2012). *Profile of practice of occupational therapists in Canada 2012.* Nepean, Ontario, Canada: Author.

Cross, T. L., Bazron, B. J., Dennis, K. W., & Isaacs, M. R. (1989). Towards a culturally competent system of care: A monograph on effective services for minority children who are severely emotionally disturbed. Washington, DC: Child and Adolescent Service System Program Technical Assistance Center, Georgetown University Child Development Center.

Dillard, M., Andonian, L., Flores, O., Lai, L., MacRae, A., & Shakir, M. (1992). Culturally competent occupational therapy in a diversely populated mental health setting. *American Journal of Occupational Therapy, 46,* 721–726.

Dunn, W., Brown, C., & McGuigan, A. (1994). The ecology of human performance: A framework for considering the effect of context. *American Journal of Occupational Therapy, 48,* 595–607.

Edberg, M. C. (2012). *Essentials of health, culture and diversity: Understanding people, reducing disparities.* Burlington, MA: Jones & Bartlett.

Flanagan, S. A. (1996). The last bastion of prejudice. *Obesity Surgery, 6,* 430–437. doi:10.1381/096089296765556520

Fortier, J. P., & Bishop, D. (2004). *Setting the agenda for research on cultural competence in health care, final report.* Rockville, MD: Agency for Healthcare Research and Quality. Retrieved from http://www.ahrq.gov/research/cultural.htm

Galanti, G. A. (2004). *Caring for patients from different cultures* (3rd ed.). Philadelphia, PA: University of Pennsylvania Press.

Gardner, E. P. (2010). Touch. In *Encyclopedia of Life Sciences.* Chichester, United Kingdom: Wiley. doi:10.1002/9780470015902.0000219.pub2

Gordon, A. K. (1995). Deterrents to access and service for blacks and Hispanics: The Medicare Hospice Benefit, healthcare utilization, and cultural barriers. *The Hospice Journal, 10,* 65–83.

Gupta, J. (2008). Reflections of one educator on teaching cultural competence. *Education SIS Quarterly, 18,* 3.

Hall, E. T. (1990). *The hidden dimension.* New York, NY: Knopf Doubleday. (Original work published 1966)

Haney Lopez, I. F. (1994). The social construction of race: Some observations on illusion, fabrication, and choice. *Harvard Civil Rights-Civil Liberties Law Review, 1*, 11–17.

Hecht, M. L. (Ed.). (1998). *Communicating prejudice*. Thousand Oaks, CA: Sage.

Herbst, P. H. (1997). *The color of words: An encyclopaedic dictionary of ethnic bias in the United States*. Yarmouth, ME: Intercultural Press.

Hoops, D. (1979). Intercultural communication concepts and the psychology of intercultural experiences. In M. Pusch (Ed.), *Multicultural education: A cross-cultural training approach* (pp. 9–38). Yarmouth, ME: Intercultural Press.

Hunt, L. M., Truesdell, N. D., & Kreiner, M. J. (2013). Genes, race, and culture in clinical care: Racial profiling in the management of chronic illness. *Medical Anthropology Quarterly, 27*, 253–271.

Iwama, M. (2004). Meaning and inclusion: Revisiting culture in occupational therapy [Guest Editorial]. *Australian Occupational Therapy Journal, 51*, 1–2.

Iwama, M. (2006). *The KAWA model: Culturally relevant occupational therapy*. Toronto, Ontario, Canada: Churchill Livingstone.

Juckett, G. (2005). Cross-cultural medicine. *American Family Physician, 72*, 2267–2274.

Khalifa, N., Hardieb, T., Latifc, S., Jamild, I., & Walkere, D. (2011). Health beliefs about Jinn, black magic and the evil eye among Muslims: Age, gender and first language influences. *International Journal of Culture and Mental Health, 4*, 68–77.

Kielhofner, G., & Burke, J. (1980). A model of human occupation, part one: Conceptual framework and content. *American Journal of Occupational Therapy, 34*, 572–581.

La Fontaine, J. S. (1985). Person and individual: Some anthropological reflections. In M. Carrithers, S. Collins, & S. Lukes (Eds.), *The category of the person: Anthropology, philosophy, history* (pp. 123–140). Cambridge, United Kingdom: Cambridge University Press.

Lattanzi, J. B., & Purnell, L. D. (Eds.). (2006). *Developing cultural competence in physical therapy practice*. Philadelphia, PA: F. A. Davis.

Law, M., Cooper, B., Strong, S., Stewart, D., Rigby, P., & Letts, L. (1996). The person-environment-occupation model: A transactive approach to occupational performance. *Canadian Journal of Occupational Therapy, 63*, 9–23.

Leininger, M. (2002). Essential transcultural nursing care concepts, principles, examples and policy statements. In M. Leininger & M. R. MacFarland (Eds.), *Transcultural nursing: Concepts, theories, research and practice* (3rd ed., pp. 45–70). New York, NY: McGraw-Hill.

Lev, A. I. (2004). *The complete lesbian and gay parenting guide*. New York, NY: Berkley.

Lynn-McHale, D. J., & Deatrick, J. A. (2000). Trust between family and health care providers. *Journal of Family Nursing, 6*, 210–230.

Mahoney, C. (Ed.). (1976). *The evil eye*. New York, NY: Columbia University Press.

Majumdar, B., Browne, G., Roberts, J., & Carpio, B. (2004). Effects of cultural sensitivity training on health care provider attitudes and patient outcomes. *Journal of Nursing Scholarship, 36*, 161–166.

Marks, J. (1996). Science and race. *American Behavioral Scientist, 40*, 123–133.

Montagu, A. (1986). *Touching: The human significance of the skin* (3rd ed.). New York, NY: Harper and Row.

Mroz, T. M., Pitonyak, J. S., Fogelberg, D., & Leland, N. E. (2015). Client centeredness and health reform: Key issues for occupational therapy. *American Journal of Occupational Therapy, 69*, 6905090010p1–6905090010p8. doi:10.5014/ajot.2015.695001

Mu, K., Coppard, B. M., Bracciano, A., Doll, J., & Matthews, A. (2010). Fostering cultural competency, clinical reasoning, and leadership through international outreach. *Occupational Therapy in Health Care, 24*, 74–85.

Muñoz, J. (2007). Culturally responsive caring in occupational therapy. *Occupational Therapy International, 14*, 256–280.

Murden, R., Norman, A., Ross, J., Sturdivant, E., Kedia, M., & Shah, S. (2008). Occupational therapy students' perceptions of their cultural awareness and competency. *Occupational Therapy International, 15*, 191–203.

National Society for the Promotion of Occupational Therapy. (1919). *Minutes from the third annual meeting*. Towson, MD: Author.

Nawaz, H., & Brett, A. S. (2009). Mentioning race at the beginning of clinical case presentations: A survey of US medical schools. *Medical Education, 43*, 146–154.

Ncayiyana, D. J. (2007). Racial profiling in medical research: what are we measuring? *South African Medical Journal, 97*, 1225–1226.

Nittle, N. K. (2011). *Scientific and social definitions of race: Debunking the ideas behind this construct*. Retrieved from http://racerelations.about.com/od/understandingrac1/a/WhatIsRace.htm

Occupational Therapy Australia. (2017). *Position paper: Occupational therapy scope of practice framework*. Fitzroy, Victoria, Australia: Author.

Occupational Therapy Board of New Zealand. (2015). *Code of ethics for occupational therapists*. Wellington, New Zealand: Author.

Odawara, E. (2005). Cultural competency in occupational therapy: Beyond a cross-cultural view of practice. *American Journal of Occupational Therapy, 59*, 325–334.

Pittz, W. (2005). *Closing the gap: Solutions to race-based health disparities*. Retrieved from http://cchonline.org/sites/default/files/ClosingGap.pdf

Purnell, L. D., & Lattanzi, J. B. (2006). Introducing steps to cultural study and cultural competence. In J. B. Lattanzi & L. D. Purnell (Eds.), *Developing cultural competence in physical therapy practice* (pp. 21–37). Philadelphia, PA: F. A. Davis.

Rasmussen, T. M., Lloyd, C., & Wielandt, T. (2005). Cultural awareness among Queensland undergraduate occupational therapy students. *Australian Occupational Therapy Journal, 52*, 302–310.

Reitz, S. M. (2010). Historical and philosophical perspectives of occupational therapy's role in health promotion. In M. E. Scaffa, S. M. Reitz, & M. A. Pizzi (Eds.), *Occupational therapy in the promotion of health and wellness* (pp. 1–21). Philadelphia, PA: F. A. Davis.

Rogers, C. (1989). A theory of therapy, personality, and interpersonal relationships as developed in the client-centered framework. In H. Kirschenbaum & V. Henderson (Eds.), *The Carl Rogers reader* (pp. 236–262). Boston, MA: Houghton Mifflin. (Reprinted from *Psychology: A study of science, Vol. 3. Formulations of the person and the social context*, pp. 184–256, by S. Koch, Ed., 1959, New York, NY: McGraw-Hill.)

Rothenberg, P. S. (1998). *Race, class, and gender in the United States: An integrated study* (4th ed.). New York, NY: St. Martin's Press.

Saldana, D. (2001). *Cultural competency: A practical guide for mental health service providers*. Austin, TX: University of Texas at Austin, Hogg Foundation for Mental Health.

Schim, S. M., & Doorenbos, A. Z. (2010). A three-dimensional model of cultural congruence: Framework for intervention. *Journal of Social Work in End-of-Life and Palliative Care, 6*, 256–270. doi:10.1080/15524256/2010/529023

Schkade, J. K., & Schultz, S. (2003). Occupational adaptation. In E. Crepeau, E. Cohn, & B. A. B. Schell (Eds.), *Willard and Spackman's occupational therapy* (10th ed., pp. 200–203). Philadelphia, PA: Lippincott Williams & Wilkins.

Schon, D. A. (1983). *The reflective practitioner: How professionals think in action*. New York, NY: Basic Books.

Sheppard, M. (1996). *Proxemics*. Retrieved from http://www.cs.unm.edu/sheppard/proxemics.htm

Soderlund, A. (2017). *What is the first sensory system to develop in babies?* Retrieved from https://www.livestrong.com

Spector, R. E. (2016). *Cultural diversity in health and illness* (9th ed.). Norwalk, CT: Pearson.

Srivastava, R. H. (2007). *The healthcare professional's guide to clinical cultural competence*. Toronto, Ontario, Canada: Mosby.

Steed, R. (2010). Attitudes and beliefs of occupational therapists participating in a cultural competency workshop. *Occupational Therapy International, 17,* 142–151. doi:10.1002/oti.299

Suh, E. E. (2004). The model of cultural competence through an evolutionary concept analysis. *Journal of Transcultural Nursing, 15,* 93–102.

Sumsion, T. (Ed.). (1993). *Client-centered practice in occupational therapy: A guide to implementation.* New York, NY: Churchill Livingstone.

Wells, S. A., & Black, R. M. (2000). *Cultural competency for health professionals.* Bethesda, MD: American Occupational Therapy Association.

Wells, S. A., Black, R. M., & Gupta, J. (2016). *Culture and occupation: Effectiveness for occupational therapy practice, education, and research.* Bethesda, MD: American Occupational Therapy Association.

Wolinsky, H. (2011). Genomes, race and health: Racial profiling in medicine might just be a stepping stone to personalized health care. *EMBO Reports, 12,* 107–109.

World Federation of Occupational Therapists. (2009). *Guiding principles on diversity and culture.* London, United Kingdom: Author.

World Federation of Occupational Therapists (2012). *History.* Retrieved from http://www.wfot.org/AboutUs/History.aspx

the**Point**® *For additional resources on the subjects discussed in this chapter, visit* **http://thePoint.lww.com /Willard-Spackman13e.**

Social, Economic, and Political Factors That Influence Occupational Performance

Catherine L. Lysack, Diane E. Adamo

LEARNING OBJECTIVES

After reading this chapter, you will be able to:

1. Distinguish between socioeconomic status, social class, and social inequalities.
2. Discuss how health is related to an individual's position in the social hierarchy.
3. Outline how individual and community level socioeconomic factors impact health.
4. Explain how socioeconomic disadvantages experienced in childhood affect the occupational performance of clients as adults.
5. Describe three actions that occupational therapy practitioners can take to reduce the negative impact of social inequalities and health disparities in clients' lives.

Introduction

The focus of this chapter is on the social, economic, and political forces that affect health and occupational performance across the life course. The bottom line is this—higher socioeconomic status (SES) is associated with better health and more numerous opportunities for engagement in, and benefit from, meaningful occupations. There is overwhelming evidence in the scientific literature of the robust relationship between health and wealth, for which SES is a marker. This relationship suggests that it is not only the poor who tend to be sick, whereas the rich are healthy, but also that there is a continual gradient from the top to the bottom of the SES ladder. Status, related to income and wealth, has been linked to chronic stress, heart disease, ulcers, type 2 diabetes, rheumatoid arthritis, certain types of cancer, and premature aging (Evans, Barer, & Marmor, 1994; U.S. Department of Health and Human Services [USDHHS], Office of Minority Health, 2011; R. Wilkinson & Marmot, 2003; R. Wilkinson & Pickett, 2009b, 2017). Although it is true that at very high wealth levels, the health gains become much smaller and incremental, there is no debate that at low, middle, and even upper middle-class levels the "health-wealth" gradient is significant (Lynch et al., 1998).

CENTENNIAL NOTES

The Social, Political, and Economic Challenge of Immigration

Lori T. Andersen

The second half of nineteenth century and beginning of twentieth century saw a significant influx of immigrants from Europe. During that time, the social, political, and economic problems facing the United States were compounded with the arrival of these immigrants. Coming with little more than the clothes on their backs, the immigrants were often forced to live in poverty in overcrowded, unsanitary urban areas. The immigrants were looked on with suspicion because they were competing with Americans for jobs; they had different values, customs, habits, political beliefs, and, in many cases, spoke only a foreign language. The Americans believed that Europe did not send their best but rather those who were diseased and insane (Luchins, 1988). As such, many of these immigrants had difficulty adjusting to life in a new country—socially, politically, and economically.

The wave of immigration corresponded to an increase of foreign-born people admitted to insane asylums. The percentage of foreign-born first admissions to Worcester State Hospital, Massachusetts, ranged from 45% to 56% between the years of 1903 and 1933 (Bockoven, 1963, p. 24). From 1895 to 1912, the total number of admissions to Newberry State Hospital (formerly Upper Peninsula Hospital for the Insane in Michigan) was 2,612 patients, of which 1,843 patients or 70% were foreign-born (Figure 20-1) (Board of Trustees of Newberry State Hospital, 1913, p. 51).

NEWBERRY STATE HOSPITAL. 51

TABLE No. 8.—*Nativity of patients admitted.*

	Period ending June 30, 1912.			Since opening.		
	Men.	Women.	Total.	Men.	Women.	Total.
Total admissions	235	168	403	1,596	1,016	2,612
*Born in Michigan	24	18	42	249	192	441
*Born in United States	48	44	92	342	248	590
Foreign born	163	106	269	1,151	692	1,843
Unascertained	2	3	5	57	35	92
Assyria	0	1	1	0	1	1
Austria	10	6	16	58	18	76
Bulgaria				1	0	1
Bohemia	3	1	4	6	4	10
Belgium				4	1	5
Canada	29	22	51	235	149	384
Denmark	6	0	6	9	9	18
England	16	3	19	88	51	139
France	1	0	1	1	2	3
Finland	45	36	81	308	172	480
Germany	9	5	14	78	52	130
Holland	0	1	1	1	2	3
Hungary	0	1	1	5	2	7
Italy	5	1	6	29	15	44
Ireland	13	4	17	66	42	108
Norway	3	1	4	29	32	61
Persia				2	0	2
Poland	0	3	3	16	13	29
Prussia				0	1	1
Russia	4	0	4	13	3	16
Sweden	16	17	33	182	115	297
Roumania				1	0	1
Switzerland				3	2	5
Scotland	1	1	2	14	3	17
Turkey				1	0	1
Unascertained	2	3	5	57	35	92

*Those born in the United States, also include those born in Michigan.

FIGURE 20-1 Eleanor Clarke Slagle, newly graduated from the Chicago School of Civics and Philanthropy, spent 3 months at this hospital in 1911 to help set up a program in occupations and amusements.

(continues)

The Progressive and Settlement House Movements developed in the late nineteenth century to address some of the social and economic problems of the times. The goals of these movements were to promote social justice, to improve quality of life for all, and, specifically in the case of one of the best known settlement houses, Hull House, to help immigrants gain the knowledge and skills to adapt to American life and culture and earn a living (Quiroga, 1995, pp. 37, 38). The Progressive and Settlement House Movements influenced the evolution of occupational therapy (OT), and of course, the connection between Jane Addams, founder of Hull House, and Eleanor Clarke Slagle is legendary.

It is not difficult to see how higher education, higher income and wealth, and status could be related to better health. In general, well-educated adults tend to get better jobs than those with little or no education. Those with paid work are also more likely to have health insurance that helps to secure more reliable access to quality health care as compared to the unemployed or those working for an hourly wage. Yet, there is more to wealth–health story. In a recent analysis of this gradient in 16 countries, researchers showed that the positive association between wealth and health held in all countries even after controlling for demographic attributes like education and household income (Semyonov, Lewin-Epstein, & Maskileyson, 2013). Thus, even if you do have a stable job and a middle-class income, your health is not as good as someone in the wealthiest 1%. There is something very fundamental about social stratification that matters and has a real impact on health.

The challenge that remains is to understand the impact of the wealth–health gradient in context of acute care and rehabilitation treatment, overall habilitation, and health maintenance. The literature is replete with studies that document how inequality translates into **toxic stress** that harms human health (B. S. McEwen, 2012; Shonkoff, 2011). There is no longer any doubt, for example, that early-childhood trauma resulting from adverse social structures and relationships negatively influences children's bodily systems and brain development through recurrent stress (C. McEwen & McEwen, 2017). Research in human development is showing direct links between childhood misfortune (e.g., poverty, trauma) and elevated rates of obesity, depression, and heart disease for example (Loucks, Almeida, Taylor, & Mathews, 2011). For occupational therapists, it is important to become more familiar with this scientific literature and think about how the social and economic status of their patients shapes their opportunities for health.

It is beyond the scope of this chapter to review the literature on toxic stress and the extent to which its deleterious effects can be mitigated by social support and interventions that prevent or compensate for the early biological effects of toxic social environments. It is essential, however, for occupational therapists to recognize in basic terms what this means for their patients. For example, adults with lower SES experience more stressful life events and tend to have fewer psychological resources (e.g., self-confidence, self-control, delayed gratification) to deal with life's challenges (Kawachi & Berkman, 2003; Schulz et al., 2006; Williams, 1997). Research shows that the harms associated with lower SES begin even before birth (e.g., a mother's prenatal nutrition, a safe family context), which can influence health even into the final years of life (Barker, 1998; Lynch et al., 1994; Schulz et al., 2006; Shonkoff, 2011). There is research to show that low SES increases the risk for developing psychiatric and chronic medical disorders (Adler, Marmot, McEwen, & Stewart, 1999). Research by Gianaros and colleagues (2007) using MRI studies of brain structures reveals that even one's perception of oneself as holding a low social standing may result in smaller brain structures with less neuronal circuits and thus, lower function. More public health and brain research is needed, but there is no longer any doubt that health tracks a socioeconomic gradient.

The remainder of this chapter explores the consequences of these powerful relationships and their impact on occupational performance across the life course. To illustrate these issues, consider the case study of Annie and Desmond and the role that social and economic forces have played in shaping their family's health (Case Study 20-1).

Many possible disparities are suggested in this case. Annie's deceased husband Desmond may have contracted his illness on the job. Living in the inner city near an industrial area, the entire family may have been exposed to unsafe levels of environmental pollutants that are adversely affecting their health now. Now, Annie is struggling to regain mobility and live safely and independently at home after her fall, but her physical impairments are not the primary barrier. Rather, the material and social resources matter most.

In this chapter, the focus is on groups of people who are systematically disadvantaged—those rendered most vulnerable by underlying social structures and political and economic systems. Disadvantaged groups in this sense include, for example, the elderly, the poor, ethnic and racial minorities, and people with disabilities. It has been noted that OT practitioners as a group are overwhelmingly White and middle class (Sladyk, Jacobs, & MacCrae, 2010; Wells & Black, 2000) and live more privileged lives than most of their clients. Competent and ethical practitioners need to recognize their social position relative to their clients and actively reflect on how these differences create assumptions, unfounded judgments, and biases in the

CASE STUDY 20-1   I HOPE THE GOOD LORD WILL SEE ME THROUGH

Annie is 72 years old and spent 2 weeks in the hospital. As Annie described it, she "took a spell" and tumbled down her basement steps. She fractured a hip and two ribs. Annie uses a wheelchair now and hopes it is temporary, but she is worried about managing at home alone. She is also coping with the consequences of a mild stroke 2 years ago. Annie lives in Detroit. Her house has two small bedrooms and a bathroom on the second floor, with laundry facilities in the basement. She is a widow, and her only surviving child, a son, lives in Chicago. For most of her life, Annie stayed home to raise three children while her husband Desmond worked at an automotive supply company. After 31 years of work, Desmond was laid off, and shortly afterward, he became ill with lung cancer and died. Desmond was a nonsmoker. Des and Annie and other plant workers who lost their family members wondered if their jobs had made them sick. Unfortunately, the plant Des worked for went out of business and this meant Annie lost the small pension she received as a surviving spouse. Now, she gets by on her social security check and Medicare. Her income is just over $21,000 per year.

Just before being discharged from the hospital, Annie was assessed by an occupational therapist who gave her recommendations for bathing and dressing. She received information about Dial-a-Ride, a transportation service for older adults and people with disabilities, and the name of a senior center where she could take exercise classes and join social activities. Annie was disappointed that she would not receive an in-home evaluation like another woman did. According to Annie, this lady got "a nice solid bath-seat and grab bars and even a fancy ramp." Annie's insurance covered none of this—not even the raised toilet seat her therapist told her would help prevent another fall.

After 3 weeks at home, Annie is worried about the slowness of her recovery and her mounting out-of-pocket expenses for medications. Occasionally, her church friends drop in with a meal and help with groceries, but Annie is anxious to be more self-sufficient. Still, she doesn't trust her legs "not to buckle." In a phone call to her son, she expressed fear about going out in her neighborhood, saying that she felt vulnerable, like "a sitting duck." Annie wonders whether the woman she met weeks ago in the hospital is faring better than she is and how different it would be if she could get more help. Although she calls her friends her "lifeline," she is also praying "the good Lord will see [her] through."

delivery of care. Therapists must take great care to analyze the context of their clients, too, to ensure the patients are not blamed for relatively poorer health status that is often deeply rooted in social and economic structures, not individual traits of motivation and compliance.

Defining the Social Causes of Health and Illness

Socioeconomic Status, Class, and Social Mobility

Several terms are used to signal the influence of social and economic factors on health and each has a different meaning. One of the most familiar terms is **socioeconomic status** or SES. Socioeconomic status refers to the occupational, educational, and income achievements of individuals or groups. Krieger (2001, 2010) has argued that SES may overemphasize social prestige and underemphasize the role of material resources in shaping one's life chances related to health, an idea we return to in later sections of this chapter.

The term **class** is also used to indicate social differences between groups, as in *lower class*, *working class*, *middle*

class, and *upper class*. The Online Dictionary of the Social Sciences (2017) defines class as a group of individuals sharing a common situation within a social structure, usually their shared place in the structure of ownership and control of the means of production. In land-based economies, this means class structures are based on one's relationship to the ownership and control of property. Ownership of property brings with it wealth and power, which means resources are available to be used to achieve better health. It is important to recognize that the degree to which one moves up or down the social ladder of society, something sociologists call social mobility, is in large part dictated by class status.

Class and SES also affect health, occupational performance, and participation. In 2009, Bass-Haugen reviewed the literature and showed how the activity profiles, home and work environments, experiences in health systems, and outcomes of health care services differ based on SES and class. She concluded that occupational performance deficits are most notable for non-White and low-income Americans through mechanisms related to restricted activity and participation. For example, when neighborhood quality is poor, it is difficult for children to find safe places to play, and for older adults to walk in an environment that allows them to exercise and socialize (Schulz et al., 2006; Yen, Michael, & Perdue, 2009). In a study of college students, MacPhee and colleagues (2013) showed that women and minorities perceive their academic self-efficacy more poorly than other groups, despite similar academic standing. Over time, these disadvantages accumulate so that by later adulthood, the gap between those who have had rich opportunities to learn, develop, work, and contribute to society and those who have not is wide.

Social Inequalities and Health Disparities

The terms *social inequalities* and *health disparities* come to us from the public health literature and are related to characteristics such as class, gender, age, race, ethnicity, and sexual orientation, among others. **Social inequality** refers to a situation in which individual groups in a society do not have equal social status. Social inequality is linked to racial inequality, gender inequality, and wealth inequality. Social inequality is the portion of the unequal opportunities and rewards that accrue to these subgroups that are *unfair, unjust, avoidable,* and *unnecessary* (Krieger, 2001, 2010).

A major problem arises when social inequalities lead to difficulty accessing medical care and treatment. A **health disparity** is a gap in access to health care, treatment provided, and health outcomes that are unfair and may be the direct result of either underlying social inequalities or improper actions by professionals within the health system (USDHHS, 2017a). For example, studies have found that even after controlling for symptoms and insurance coverage, U.S. doctors are more likely to offer White patients life-preserving treatments, including angioplasty and bypass surgery for cardiac disease, and are more likely to offer people of color various less desirable procedures such as amputations for diabetes (Institute of Medicine [IOM], 2002). This research indicates that clinical encounters between minorities and health care professionals may be the source of additional poor treatment. Stereotyping and institutional racism are widely recognized as unjust forces in the health care environment that must change (Clark, 2004).

The second reason why social inequalities are of great concern to health professionals is that social inequalities put people at risk for poorer health. Life expectancy is shorter, and most diseases are more common farther down the social ladder. Decades of research have shown this is true in both rich and poor societies (Marmot & Wilkinson, 1999). In a set of famous studies commonly referred to as the Whitehall studies, Marmot, Shipley, and Rose (1984) studied British civil servants for more than three decades and found that men in the lowest levels of the civil service and office support workers had a mortality rate 4 times greater than that of men in the highest administrative jobs. The mechanisms for this are complex, but increasing

numbers of studies are pointing to stress as the fundamental mechanism.

Stressful life experiences and impoverished environments contribute to poorer health in many ways. It means low-income families will live in neighborhoods that have fewer resources like playgrounds, libraries, parks, and good schools. Low-income families may not have easy access to affordable and quick transportation that makes attending rehabilitation appointments more difficult and missing appointments more likely that, in turn, can be linked to poorer functional outcomes. This cannot be seen to be the fault of the client but rather a very real contextual issue of practice that must be part of the therapists' problem-solving process if those with reduced SES are to have the best chance possible to benefit from therapeutic interventions.

Unfortunately, "upward mobility," that is, doing better and having more than our parents, is not happening as much as in the past. Some researchers have questioned if it has all but disappeared in the United States (Surowiecki, 2014). As occupational therapists consider the real-life circumstances of their clients, it is important to appreciate how large economic trends impact lives and opportunities for good health. Today, more than 40% of Americans born in the bottom wealth quintile remain stuck there as adults (Braveman & Gottlieb, 2014). Evidence in the United States overall points to a shrinking middle class and growing income and wealth inequalities which further challenge health (Pew Charitable Trust, 2015). The growing gap between rich and poor portends a future where the wealthiest achieve health and the poorest do not. Research by Saez and Zucman (2014) shows that, astoundingly, America's wealthiest 1% of the population holds more than 50% of the nation's wealth, whereas the bottom 90% of the population hold three-quarters of the nation's debt. With such pronounced inequality, how we can we possibly expect that those with much more limited financial resources to do as well in anything, including health? Although the United States is not the only developed country that has seen wealth inequality rise over the past three decades, it is an extreme outlier. The wealthiest 5% households in the United States have almost 91 times more wealth than the median American household, the widest gap among 18 of the world's most developed countries (Organisation for Economic Co-operation and Development [OECD], 2015). The next highest is the Netherlands, which has a ratio less than half that (OECD, 2015).

The mechanisms by which income and wealth inequality negatively affect health are many. Bass-Haugen (2009) cites research that documents the link between SES and occupational performance differences in children and adults seen by occupational therapists shows that poor adults are two to three times more likely to report that general and specific physical activities are difficult or impossible to perform. Poor adults also had the highest percentage of limitations in activities and need for special equipment as well as the lowest percentage of participation in physical exercise and activities. A plethora of more recent research confirms the wealth–health gradient, and unhealthy levels of stress are much higher for those with fewer financial resources (American Psychological Association [APA], 2015; New America, 2017).

The Intersections of Gender, Ethnicity, Age, Disability, and Sexual Orientation

Other factors that influence health and occupational performance are inextricably linked to the social categories individuals belong to, including gender, ethnic heritage, age, sexual orientation, and whether they are disabled or not (America's Children, 2017; Krieger, 2010; USDHHS, Office of Minority Health, 2011). Individuals often belong to more than one of these categories. As occupational therapists, we must constantly ask ourselves if we make assumptions about our clients based on the social categories they occupy, or do we truly see the person behind the category and practice client-centered OT?

Gender Inequalities

For some women, the experience of being a woman continues to be one of inequality. Research shows that, on average, women's pay is still only 80 cents for every 1 dollar a man earns (Institute for Women's Policy Research, 2017). The gender pay gap is partly explained by the number of women compared to men who perform the kinds of jobs with lower salaries but that does not explain the entire difference.

Women face more systemic barriers to workplace advancement. The Pew Research Center (2017) reports that 4 out of 10 women experience gender discrimination in the workplace, a rate twice that of men. The most common barrier is receiving less pay for the same job, but there is evidence that employers tend not to hire and promote women at the same rates as men because women will step out of the workforce to have a family (Pew Research Center, 2017). There is truth to this. A survey earlier this year of America, Australia, Britain, France, Germany, and Scandinavian countries by The Economist and YouGov, a pollster, gauged how children affected working hours. Of women with children at home, 44% to 75% had scaled back after becoming mothers, by working fewer hours or switching to a less demanding job, such as one requiring less travel or overtime. A critical problem is that the United States is only 1 of 8 United Nations' 193-member states without a paid parental leave policy. Although some women are in jobs covered by the Family Medical Leave Act that provides up to 12 weeks of unpaid leave, lower wage workers cannot afford unpaid absences from work. The situation around the world is much different. In Sweden, for example, new parents are entitled to a total of 16 months of paid leave to split between them as they see fit (New America, 2017). Business Insider (2017) reports that United States continues to suffer from lagging economic growth because of the absence of paid leave for new parents and the high cost of child care. In America, the only rich country without legal entitlement to maternity leave, a quarter of women return to work within 10 days of giving birth. But many never return because they cannot bear the thought of leaving a newborn in child care or because paying for it would wipe out all or most of what they earn (The Economist, 2017).

Gender also exerts a strong influence on health. Currently, within much of the Western world, women enjoy a longer average life expectancy than men (OECD, 2017). However, once the patterns of illness and disability are examined by gender, the picture is more ambiguous. Although men die earlier than women, women have higher rates of chronic illness at every age. For example, women account for two-thirds of all people diagnosed with arthritis (National Center for Health Statistics [NCHS], 2015). Similarly, depression is nearly twice as common in women as it is in men. Some of these gender differences are accounted for by biological differences between the sexes; others are related to differences in gender roles that may increase stress for women (Adams, Martinez, & Vickerie, 2010). Stress is known to worsen arthritic conditions and depression (USDHHS, 2017b). Practitioners must recognize that gender differences may lead to health inequalities and, unfortunately, sometimes disparities in the treatment women receive.

Ethnic Inequalities

Ethnicity affects life chances for health but also for a range of other societal opportunities like education and work. The term *ethnicity* is used here rather than *race* to signal cultural rather than biological explanations for differences in social and economic opportunity.

Research shows that discrimination negatively influences educational attainment. Roscigno and Ainsworth-Darnell (1999), for example, suggest there may be differences in the treatment of students that account for educational attainment differences based on ethnic group. They cite studies that show teachers give affluent students more attention, assistance, and higher expectations than their less affluent students (Kau & Thompson, 2003). This is a subtle mechanism whereby teachers, consciously or not, do not invest time and energy in students if they think the return on their investment will not pay optimal dividends.

Education is a critical factor in life because employment opportunities and income are tied to early educational attainment (Miringoff & Miringoff, 1999; Shonkoff

& Phillips, 2000), but neither educational opportunities nor their quality is equally distributed (America's Children, 2017). The U.S. government recognized this fact as early as the 1950s when it established the Head Start program, a national network of comprehensive child development programs that targeted low-income families and their communities (U.S. Census Bureau, 2016). Poor minority children are at an educational disadvantage because they grow up in poor neighborhoods, which have poorer quality schools, staffed by teachers with fewer resources to enrich the learning environment (Young, 1997). This example highlights the intersection of ethnicity and economic status. Individuals with diminished chances in the early years seldom catch up. A sad fact is that in the United States in 2015, 21% of all children ages 0 to 17 years lived in poverty. In 2015, the federal poverty threshold for a family of four with two children was $24,036—not very much money for extras (America's Children, 2017). The challenge is similar around the world, as low-income citizens struggle to achieve a standard of economic well-being that ensures good health. A lack of resources affects health in so many different ways. United States data show, for example, that nearly 8% of the population do not take their medications as prescribed because they do not have the money (Cohen & Villarroel, 2015). Still, as a relatively wealthy country and with the per capita health care spending more than twice the average of other developed nations (OECD, 2017), Americans should have better health.

Poverty affects health and so does ethnicity, and these factors are often found together. Census data show, for example, that the prevalence of hypertension is about 40% higher in African Americans than in non-Hispanic White Americans, and African Americans are 10% less likely to have it under control (USDHHS, Office of Minority Health, 2011). Infant mortality rates indicate a similar pattern. The U.S. average is 5.8 infant deaths per 1,000 live births, but for African Americans, the figure is twice that (NCHS, 2016). International comparisons are available. The OECD (2017) ranks the United States 23rd in the world for infant mortality. Rates are half that in countries like Norway, Iceland, Japan, Spain, France, Italy, and Australia and other countries which all have more equal access to health care.

Age Inequalities

Age is another factor that is closely related to health and occupational performance. All societies have some shared cultural expectations of its members based on age. **Ageism** is the term used to describe discrimination based on age (Estes, 2001). Although it is against the law in the United States to discriminate in hiring based on age, the 60-year-old who wants or needs to find a new job does not find many open doors regardless of his or her work experience (AARP, 2017; J. Wilkinson & Ferraro, 2002). However, there

are indications this is changing. The AARP (2015) reports that older workers are becoming much more sought after in recent years because of an upward spike in the economy since the Great Recession in 2009. The stereotype is that older workers are less creative and less productive, but the reality is that when it comes to actual performance, research confirms older workers surpass younger workers, scoring high in leadership, commitment, and workplace wisdom—that is, they have learned how to get along with people, solve problems without drama, and call for help when necessary. Older works are also able to take new ideas and connect those ideas to other knowledge, helping companies be more successful overall.

Yet, health and aging are tightly intertwined. Not surprisingly, "age is the single most important predictor of mortality and morbidity" (Weitz, 2004, p. 52). Because age and illness are so closely tied, when the average age of the population increases, so does the prevalence of health problems. The U.S. population 65 years and older will increase from 35 million in 2000 to 74 million in 2030. People 65 years and older are expected to grow to be 21% of the population by 2030 (U.S. Administration on Aging [USAoA], 2016). The health problems associated with aging populations and the financial costs of meeting those needs are anticipated to be an enormous financial and political challenge for which the United States may not be well prepared to handle given that it is a relatively young country. For example, Japan, the oldest country in the world, currently has 26% of its population over age 65 years; the comparable U.S. figure is 15%. Other old countries like Italy and Greece and Germany have had several more decades to adjust to these quickly changing demographics and may provide lessons for younger countries as they prepare for a society with fewer workers and fewer tax dollars to offset the costs of illness that are associated with older age.

Inequalities due to Disability

Disability is associated with disadvantage regardless of individual skills or financial resources. According to the U.S. Census Bureau (2016), more than 40 million people or 12.8% of the population have a disability. This represents nearly 20% of the population aged 5 years and older living in the community. The World Bank (2013) reports that 1 billion people or 15% of the world's population experience some form of disability, with disability prevalence higher for developing countries. Employment rates vary by type of disability. Employment rates are highest for people with hearing (51.0%) and vision disabilities (41.8%) and lowest for people with self-care (15.6%) and independent living disabilities (16.4%) (Institute on Disability, 2016). The consequences for those who experience multiple inequalities are noteworthy. Women with disability are said to face the cumulative disadvantage or "double jeopardy" of being female and disabled (Chappell & Havens, 1980; Pentland, Tremblay, Spring, & Rosenthal, 1999). Medical and technological advances have enabled people to live longer and be more independent, but full social inclusion and community participation have not been realized. The actions that led to the passage of the Americans with Disabilities Act reflect the long-standing efforts of the disability rights movement and its allies (including OT practitioners) to improve life conditions for people with disabilities (Colker, 2005; Hurst, 2003).

People with disabilities also have poorer health than nondisabled people. Higher rates of diabetes, depression, elevated blood pressure and blood cholesterol, obesity, and vision and hearing impairments are all reported (USDHHS, 2017a). Lower rates of positive and recommended health behaviors such as cardiovascular fitness have been found too, as have low rates of patient education and treatment for mental illness.

Inequalities Based on Sexual Orientation

Understanding the inequalities faced by individuals as a function of their sexual orientation is a significant challenge given the tremendous lack of knowledge about the experiences and specific health needs of the lesbian, gay, bisexual, transgender, questioning, and intersex (LGBTQI) populations. The IOM (2011), in its report *The Health of Lesbian, Gay, Bisexual, and Transgender People: Building a Foundation for Better Understanding*, has noted that despite the increased visibility of these groups in society, almost nothing is known about their social experiences across the life course, how their health needs may be similar or different from the heterosexual population, and how interventions to address health needs of LGBTQI individuals should best be tailored.

It must be recognized that the experiences of LGBTQI individuals are not uniform and are shaped by factors of race, ethnicity, SES, geographical location, and age, any of which can have an effect on health-related concerns and needs. Individuals in same-sex relationships who are also older, or are visible minorities, may face a similar type of "double disadvantage" mentioned earlier. The combined negative effects of occupying two stigmatized statuses may be greater than occupying either status alone (Fredriksen-Goldsen, Kim, & Barkan, 2012). Research with visible minorities has documented the deleterious effects of persistent racial discrimination on health through mechanisms of chronic stress (Clark, 2004), and it appears that a similar mechanism may be implicated for LGBTQI individuals. Fredriksen-Goldsen and colleagues (2012) found that lesbian and bisexual women experience higher rates of chronic diseases such as lifetime asthma, arthritis, and obesity. Higher mental distress prevalence among all of the groups and higher poor physical health among gay men and bisexual women and men are also significant indicators of disability.

Research is also needed that goes beyond the individual level. Lesbian, gay, bisexual, transgender, questioning, and intersex individuals are in relationships and many have children. When the child in an LGBTQI family encounters the medical system, how do occupational therapists respond? Many of the same issues arise as in other cases of patient diversity. However, there can be unique challenges that more closely resemble those of new immigrants or migrant workers or even prison populations where a range of legal rights and statuses are relevant to the process of seeking care and being well. For example, children raised in same-sex households may not receive adequate health care if the parents' nontraditional partnership is not recognized as legal (Hacker, Anies, Folb, & Zallman, 2015). The U.S. Census shows that same-sex couples are raising children in nearly every U.S. state. Nationwide, approximately 1 in 8 same-sex partner households had children younger than the age of 18 living with them (U.S. Census Bureau, 2011), whose needs may be ignored. This is similar to most developed countries like Canada and other European countries. Yet, despite several resolutions by the American Medical Association targeted to reduce health care disparities based on sexual orientation, legislative challenges persist, particularly in those states banning same-sex civil unions and marriages (Grossberg, 2006). Such restrictions impose health disparities based on sexual orientation that can negatively affect the family at many points across the life course.

The inequalities and ill effects by race and sexual orientation are now being experienced by another minority group, undocumented immigrants. Whether consider "illegal" or not, individuals living in any country without proper care is a significant factor in respect to life opportunities that span education and employment but also health which many see as a basic human right. United States Colleges have recently been inserting themselves into the conversation on Deferred Action for Childhood Arrivals (DACA), the Obama-era program shielding undocumented immigrants brought to the United States as children from deportation and allowing them to work legally in the country. The popular press reports that university leaders have condemned the Trump administration's decision to end the program, arguing that DACA recipients are strong students and productive members of the workforce (The Atlantic, 2017). Irrespective of a fundamental discussion about the right to health, given that this group of nearly 1 million students is poised to enter university, there may be at minimum a deleterious effect of unrealized tuition dollars on American institutions of higher learning and a loss of young talent to the nation's economy.

The Intersection of Multiple Inequalities

In summary, regardless of OT's professed beliefs in equal opportunity and despite legislation intended to prevent discrimination, life choices, opportunities, and access to health and meaningful occupations are not equal; they are mediated by an array of powerful social and economic forces that dictate the fate of individuals and ultimately health. These factors are not easily changed or overcome through individual desire and effort, either our own or that of our clients. Much larger forces, including the health system, play an integral role. Previously, we have discussed how inequalities based on gender, age, ethnicity, poverty, and sexual orientation alone shape the activity profiles and occupational experiences of children, working age adults, and the elderly. Also raised was the notion of double jeopardy, that is, the more than additive experience of living with multiple inequalities.

The Political Economy of the Health Care System

To fully appreciate the influence of social and economic factors in the lives of individuals and families, these factors must be set against the backdrop of national health care systems. For instance, the U.S. approach to health care is certainly the most expensive system in the world. Health expenditures in the United States in 2009 represented 17.6% of the country's gross domestic product, by far the highest share of any country in the OECD and more than 8% higher than the OECD average of 9.5% (OECD, 2017). The United States spent $8,233 on health per capita in 2015, the most of any single OECD country and two-and-a-half times the OECD average of $3,223 (OECD, 2017). The United States spends more than twice as much per capita on health care as relatively rich European countries such as France and Germany, and as the section that follows highlights, the investment is not providing a strong return.

Comparisons between the United States and Other Countries

Despite the huge amount spent, the United States ranks low on many health indicators (World Health Organization, 2010), and there is mounting evidence that the system is plagued with serious problems at all levels (Moss, 2000; Rylko-Bauer & Farmer, 2002). Life expectancy in the United States stands at 78.2 years, 1 year less than the average for the 30 developed countries that belong to the OECD (2017). Japan, Italy, Spain, and Australia all have life expectancies above 81.5 years. Infant mortality in the United States is worse, too: 5.8 deaths per 1,000 live births in 2016, above the OECD average of 4.4.

Nordic countries (Iceland, Finland, and Sweden), Japan, Greece, Portugal, and Korea all have lower infant mortality rates than the United States rate, and these countries spend a fraction of what the United States spends on health care (OECD, 2017). This focus on population health outcomes is important because social and environmental context shapes health and opportunities for occupational engagement and participation in society. Preventative care, such as childhood vaccinations and cancer screening, saves lives and significantly reduces the burden of secondary health conditions. In a system where financial resources are the means to access key screening tests as well as expensive medical interventions, then those with low SES are at a distinct disadvantage. Without this care, low-SES patients will come to OT in worse health and with fewer opportunities to benefit from our interventions and recommendations than their high-SES counterparts.

The Role of Health Insurance in the United States

Health insurance (or, more accurately, medical insurance) is important because access to health care in the mostly private U.S. system requires either a job with health benefits or the financial means to pay out of pocket. A substantial number of U.S. citizens lack both. However, the number of uninsured has decreased considerably. Currently, 28.1 million residents are uninsured (U.S. Census Bureau, 2016) compared to 50.7 million in 2009 due largely to the implementation of the Affordable Care Act. Since the Affordable Care Act became law in 2010, the uninsured rate has declined by 43%, from 16.0% in 2010 to 9.1% in 2015, primarily because of the law's reforms (Obama, 2016). In 2016, non-Hispanic Whites had the lowest uninsured rate among race and Hispanic origin groups at 6.3%. The uninsured rates for Blacks and Asians were higher than for non-Hispanic Whites at 10.5% and 7.6%, respectively. Hispanics had the highest uninsured rate at 16.0% (U.S. Census Bureau, 2016). Although these findings are encouraging, inequalities still exist. Health care providers must be aware of the political controversies surrounding access to care and health insurance and thus require continued vigilance to be aware of how the status of health care insurance influences coverage and what the course of action should be for the uninsured or underserved ethnic and racial minority groups.

There is no question that there is a need to care about the uninsured and rising costs of health care whether based on social justice or simply as a matter of dollars and cents. Kawachi and Berkman (2003) warn that the least fortunate in society must be cared for, or spillover effects will adversely affect everyone. Wide income disparities lead to stress, family disruption, and mass frustration, which in turn lead to violence and crime. Research shows that the distribution of household income, for example, in the United States is becoming increasingly unequal. In 2015, the top 10% of Americans earned 51% of the nation's income (Saez, 2016).

Mechanisms of Disadvantage across the Life Course

There is an untested assumption that health inequalities arise from inadequacies in health care. Of course, there is a gap in this logic. The fact that there are problems with a medical system does not mean that the system caused the problems. So why do differences in health status exist across different groups in society? As a reader of this chapter, you already appreciate that a significant part of the problem is poverty and income and wealth inequality. Figure 20-2 illustrates the many pathways by which SES factors at both the individual and community levels can influence health.

Economic Disadvantage and Health

Poverty is bad for health. The term *poverty* refers to the lack of material resources that are necessary for subsistence.

Poverty increases exposure to factors that make people sick, and it decreases the chances of having high-quality medical insurance (and thus care) when the person needs it. Children, older adults, new immigrants, persons with disabilities, and members of ethnic minorities are at greatest risk of poverty (U.S. Census Bureau, 2016). An alarming fact is that the poverty rate in the United States in 2016 was 12.7%. In 2016, 40.6 million Americans were living in poverty (U.S. Census Bureau, 2016).

Economics and health policy experts are asking whether these pronounced levels of income inequality are taking a toll on health and the fabric of society (R. Wilkinson & Pickett, 2017). Perhaps this has fueled the entry of two new terms into the popular lexicon: *the working poor* and *the new poor*. The working poor are people who work full-time but whose wages do not raise them above the poverty line. In 2010, 72.9 million U.S. workers aged 16 years and older were paid hourly rates, representing 58.8% of all wage and salary workers. Among those paid by the hour, 1.8 million earned the federal minimum wage of $7.25 an hour (U.S. Department of Labor, 2011). Critics ask how the working poor manage to survive (Ehrenreich, 2001; Shipler, 2005). The **new poor** are those people who have fallen into poverty because of sudden or unexpected circumstances such as serious illness, divorce, or sudden job layoffs related to changes in the structure of our economy, including technology which continues to replace human workers.

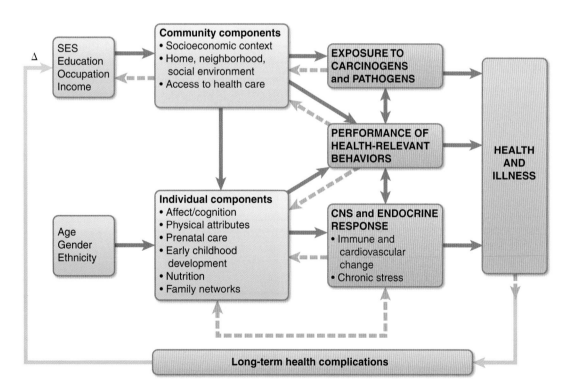

FIGURE 20-2 A model of socioeconomic status (SES) influences and interactions on health. *CNS*, central nervous system.

Money can buy health services, but it provides safe neighborhoods and pays for better food and for costs related to participating in sports and staying fit. Money is also necessary to pay college and university tuition fees that will provide the education needed to compete successfully for a well-paid job. In addition, a lack of financial resources can produce prolonged stress, which in turn negatively affects health. Proponents of a "social determinants" or "fundamental causes" perspective argue that to solve these problems will require greater redistribution of wealth (R. Wilkinson & Pickett, 2009a, 2009b). Health care experts and economists alike are increasingly suggesting that fixing the health care system by addressing disparities in access and medical treatment is only part of the solution (R. Wilkinson & Pickett, 2009a, 2009b). If improvement in the health of the most disadvantaged in society is desired, reducing the social inequalities that exist in society is imperative. This would need to begin in early childhood and continue throughout life.

Effects over a Lifetime

A plethora of observational research and intervention studies show that the foundations of adult health are laid in early childhood, even before birth (Brown et al., 2004; Hackman, Farah, & Meaney, 2010; Young, 1997). Low SES influences prenatal care and the health of the unborn child/fetus. Compared to women with high SES, women with low SES experience higher levels of stress, higher infection rates, and poorer nutrition during pregnancy that, in turn, lead to low birth weight and premature delivery (Spencer, Bambang, Logan, & Gill, 1999). Increased stress may also lead to poor health practices, such as smoking and choosing foods of low nutritional value (Kramer et al., 2001). Indirectly, but no less importantly, SES determines the access one has to financial resources to purchase adequate food. Healthier foods also cost more and are often less available and more costly in low-income neighborhoods. Researchers have concluded that the negative mental health consequences are highest for those most vulnerable, including young children, the elderly, and particularly older adults in racial and ethnic minority groups (Byrnes, Lichtenberg, & Lysack, 2006).

The combination of a poor start and slow growth "become embedded in biology during the processes of development, and form the basis of the individual's biological and human capital, which affects health throughout life" (R. Wilkinson & Marmot, 2003, p. 14). Studies have demonstrated that as cognitive, emotional, and sensory inputs program the brain's responses, insecure emotional attachment and poor stimulation can lead to low educational attainment, problem behavior, and the risk of social marginalization in adulthood (Barker, 1998). Higher rates of depression, anxiety, attention problems, and conduct

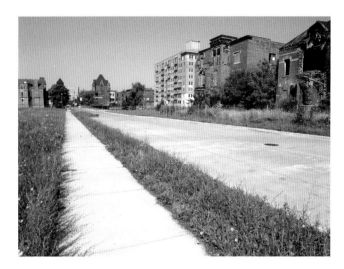

FIGURE 20-3 **Unsafe neighborhoods.**

disorders plague children and adolescents from lower SES backgrounds (Merikangas et al., 2010). Slow physical growth in infancy is also associated with reduced cardiovascular, respiratory, pancreatic, and kidney function, which increases the risk of serious illness in adulthood (Shonkoff & Phillips, 2000).

Children learn and develop through play. Not only does play help them to learn about themselves as individuals, but it also helps them to acquire their fundamental social interaction and motor and cognitive skills (Case-Smith, 2000). Yet, the playing field is not equal. Kozol (1991, 1995) describes neighborhoods overrun by poverty, crime, and economic neglect. In such neighborhoods, parents are afraid to let their children play outdoors because of high rates of violence and exposure to environmental toxins (Brown et al., 2004; Surkan et al., 2007) that place them at risk for injuries and disease (Figures 20-3 and 20-4). Living in an impoverished home

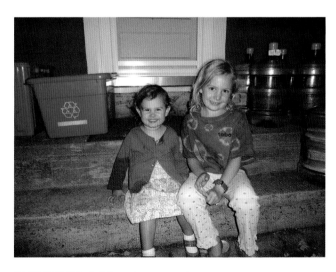

FIGURE 20-4 **No place to play.**

environment when younger impedes normal development (Martin, McCaughtry, Flory, Murphy, & Wisdom, 2011; C. McEwen & McEwen, 2017). The lack of early stimulation from books, computers, and parental communication inhibits the development of language skills such as acquiring vocabulary and interpreting verbal cues. Compromised memory function, executive function, and neural processing of emotions are far more evident in low-SES children (Loucks et al., 2011; Waber et al., 2007), with far-reaching effects as one grows older. Occupational therapists are trained to identify the smallest opportunities for functional improvement, to facilitate occupational engagement, and to bring tremendous skill in identifying motivational features of the child's interests and environment (Parham & Primeau, 1997). Hutton, Tuppeny, and Hasselbusch (2016) argue in the British context that significant inroads to improve the long-term health prospects of children with disabilities living in chronic poverty could be achieved with only small changes to health legislation. President Obama (2016) in reference to the United States and the world stated that income inequality "may be the defining challenge of our time."

Social inequalities over the life course contribute to occupational performance deficits in adults as well. This occurs in all areas of occupational performance from social relationships to work. Rates of anxiety, substance abuse, and depression are all higher in populations in which unemployment is high (USDHHS, Office of Minority Health, 2011). For those who are employed, there are other stress-related problems; research has shown that lack of personal autonomy and control in one's work (often characteristic of low-paying, low-skilled jobs) is significantly related to cardiovascular disease (Bosma, Peter, Siegrist, & Marmot, 1998). Chronic stress has deleterious effects on the human body that weaken the immune system and, in turn, place individuals at greater risk for heart disease, stroke, cancer, and other chronic illnesses (Goode, 2002).

Despite clear evidence that stress is bad for health, workers in the United States workplace have less time for rest and recreation. A recent international travel survey by Expedia.com (2016) found that adults in the United States work the most hours of any affluent country, yet only earn 15 vacation days annually on average, the fewest of any developed country. This lags behind countries like Germany and France and Italy for example, with 30 vacation days offered. The second problem is that the United States is also the only industrialized nation in the world where paid vacation is not mandatory (Expedia.com, 2016). It is estimated that 1 in 4 workers in the United States accrue no vacation time. This may be taking a toll because a full 25% of Americans report feeling "very vacation deprived."

The Role Occupational in Addressing H Disparities

Townsend and Wilcock (2003) asserted that it is an occupational injustice to ignore the social and economic determinants of health. We argue here that these factors affect opportunities for and engagement in occupation. Others have called on occupational therapists to address the segregation of groups of people based on lack of meaningful participation in daily life occupations, something that Kronenberg and Pollard (2005) have provocatively called **occupational apartheid**. There is little doubt that social and economic factors are real and exert a powerful influence on health and occupational performance, but what can occupational therapists do in the face of what appears to be intractable problems on a very large scale? After developing greater awareness of the influence of social inequalities on health and the extent of health disparities among the clients OT practitioners serve, what are the next practical steps?

First, occupational therapists can apply the small but growing body of research evidence available that focused interventions early in a vulnerable child's life can produce lasting benefits throughout their life. For example, OT can effectively address sensory motor performance deficits, lack of peer-play relationships (Tanta, Deitz, White, & Billingsley, 2005), and maladaptive family interactions (Bedell, Cohn, & Dumas, 2005), which all may be more prevalent in socioeconomically disadvantaged families. Occupational therapists can also support parents to better understand their children's emotional and cognitive needs and modify school and home environments to facilitate occupational performance (Letts, Rigby, & Stewart, 2003). All gains realized during childhood will positively affect the individual throughout their life.

Second, occupational therapists are experts at person–environment fit and recognize the centrality of meaningful occupations to good health. Yet, there are serious gaps in knowledge. For example, little is known about meaningful occupational engagement for chronically unemployed people and what kinds of interventions might be effective. Even less is known about occupational deprivation due to immigration, geographical isolation, and incarceration (Whiteford, 2000). More research and stronger advocacy is needed to ensure OT and its benefits are part of the health care system and accessible to all marginalized populations (Creek, 2011).

Third, a unique strength of the profession is its appreciation for the person. This means therapists must learn

...s,

say

...018)

...ioners

...al differ-

...ual thera-

...s needed to

...and daily rou-

...endations rele-

...tional deprivation

...at therapists become

...nd other institution-

...nent and fair allocation

...e is growing research in

...the world to show that OT

...251

a...

of reha...

the United S...

services are not eq... ...buted (Fiorati & Elui, 2015). Simply put, clients who... ...k financial resources will not access needed services, or they will receive a lower quality of services unless they are able to access alternative private pay or charity. Therapists regularly identify socioeconomic barriers in the home that impact occupational performance but may be less attentive to the adequacy of their client's neighborhood and availability of accessible transportation, nutritious foods, and quality housing, for example (Figure 20-5). As stated earlier in this chapter, occupational therapists must focus some of their efforts on effecting change at the level of organizations (e.g., schools, hospitals, housing administrators, transportation authorities) and systems (e.g., health insurers, employers).

Finally, occupational therapists must leverage their position in the health care system to reduce the negative consequences of SES and social conditions on their clients' health and occupational performance. For example, therapists can enlighten insurance payers about the needs of their low-income clients by recommending the ideal OT

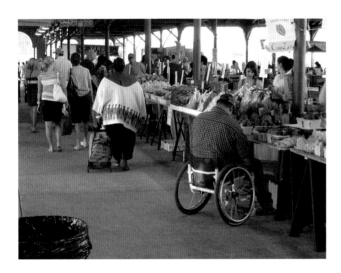

FIGURE 20-5 Farmer's market.

services for their clients in addition to the documentation required for services currently eligible for reimbursement. Another obvious and imperative step is to use standardized measures more consistently to evaluate treatment effectiveness (Velozo & Woodbury, 2011). More recently, Stover (2016) spoke to the issue of patient and client advocacy and suggested specific ways to document medical necessity to increase the quality of care. If we employ the specific rules and language of insurance companies including Medicare and Medicaid OT interventions, we will have the best chance of being accepted by payers (Lohman & Brown, 1997; Stover, 2016; Uili & Wood, 1995). With persistence, these efforts can be effective and worthwhile because successful changes in policy can benefit thousands of clients.

Conclusion

Client-centered care emphasizes listening, asking the right questions, and truly understanding and empathizing with the client (Law, 1998; Lawlor, 2003; Wood, 1996). Although listening to and learning from individual clients are paramount to effective OT interventions, this approach individualizes the underlying problems of health disparities and inequalities that are fundamentally social in nature. Occupational therapists who work with socioeconomically disadvantaged clients are well acquainted with this tension. In the OT literature, Dr. Sandra Galheigo (2011) has spoken boldly about the need to prepare the new generation of occupational therapists to engage in social transformation, not only individual change, and to address issues of invisibility and lack of access to human rights. In her work with orphans in an institutional environment, she has urged therapists to shift their therapeutic attention to working with the children and staff as a collective to create an environment that provides more and better opportunities for occupational engagement.

In a similar vein, Jennifer Creek, in her 2011 Hanneke van Bruggen Lecture, challenges occupational therapists to ask themselves what they are really doing to help their clients. She states,

> We think that we want to hear what the client has to say but, in reality, we fear that we will not be able to understand or cope with a diversity of needs. It is safer to carry out a procedure or fill in a checklist than to confront our own inadequacy in the face of another's distress.

Although some experts have argued that the path forward lies in large-scale professional coalitions aimed at major transformations of the health care system (Cutler, 2004), this takes time to achieve. In the meantime, occupational therapists must work in a system that is imperfect, knowing that it does not meet many of their clients' most pressing needs.

Recall once more Annie's struggle to recover from a lifetime of social and economic disadvantage. There are many "Annies" who you will meet in OT practice. To accomplish the true promise of OT undoubtedly requires better knowledge of the communities from which our clients come and the socioeconomic, historical, and political forces that have shaped their lives and their health. Identifying inequalities and disparities where they exist as well as working to ameliorate them is one of our ethical responsibilities as health care professionals. This is the only way to advance health for all.

REFERENCES

AARP. (2015). *The surprising truth about older workers.* Retrieved from https://www.aarp.org/work/job-hunting/info-07-2013/older-workers-more-valuable.html

AARP. (2017). *Age discrimination goes online.* Retrieved from https://www.aarp.org/work/working at 50 plus/info 2017/age discrimination-online-fd.html?intcmp=AE-WOR-W50-AD-R2-C1

Adams, P. F., Martinez, M. E., & Vickerie, J. L. (2010). Summary health statistics for the U.S. population: National Health Interview Survey, 2009. *Vital Health Statistics, 10,* 1–115.

Adler, N. E., Marmot, M., McEwen, B., & Stewart, J. (Eds.). (1999). *Socioeconomic status and health in industrialized nations: Social, psychological, and biological pathways* (Vol. 896). New York, NY: Academy of Sciences.

American Psychological Association. (2015). *Stress in America: Paying with our health.* Retrieved from https://www.apa.org/news/press/releases/stress/2014/stress-report.pdf

America's Children. (2017). *Child poverty and family income.* Retrieved from http://www.childstats.gov/americaschildren/eco1.asp

Barker, D. (1998). *Mothers, babies and disease in later life* (2nd ed.). Edinburgh, United Kingdom: Churchill Livingstone.

Bass-Haugen, J. (2009). Health disparities: Examination of evidence relevant for occupational therapy. *American Journal of Occupational Therapy, 63,* 24–34.

Bedell, G. M., Cohn, E. S., & Dumas, H. M. (2005). Exploring parents' use of strategies to promote social participation of school-age children with acquired brain injuries. *American Journal of Occupational Therapy, 59,* 273–284.

Board of Trustees of Newberry State Hospital. (1913). *Report of Board of Trustees of Newberry State Hospital for the period ending June 30, 1912.* Lansing, MI: Wynkoop Hallenback Crawford Co. State Printers.

Bockoven, J. S. (1963). *Moral treatment in American psychiatry.* New York, NY: Springer.

Bosma, H., Peter, R., Siegrist, J., & Marmot, M. (1998). Two alternative job stress models and risk of coronary heart disease. *American Journal of Public Health, 88,* 68–74.

Braveman, P., & Gottlieb, L. (2014). The social determinants of health: It's time to consider the causes of the causes. *Public Health Reports, 129*(Suppl 2), 19–31.

Brown, B., Bzostek, S., Aufseeser, D., Berry, D., Weitzman, M., Kavanaugh, M., . . . Auinger, P. (Eds.). (2004). *Early child development in social context: A chartbook.* New York, NY: The Commonwealth Fund. Retrieved from http://www.commonwealthfund.org/usr_doc/ChildDevChartbk.pdf

Business Insider. (2017, September 7). *Here's how much paid leave new mothers and fathers get in 11 different countries. Maternity leave in 11 countries.* Retrieved from http://www.businessinsider.com/maternity-leave-worldwide-2017-8

Byrnes, M., Lichtenberg, P., & Lysack, C. (2006). Environmental press, aging in place, and residential satisfaction of urban older adults. *Journal of Applied Sociology, 23,* 50–77.

Case-Smith, J. (2000). Effects of occupational therapy services on fine motor and functional performance in preschool children. *American Journal of Occupational Therapy, 54,* 372–380.

Chappell, N., & Havens, B. (1980). Old and female: Testing the double jeopardy hypothesis. *The Sociological Quarterly, 21,* 157–171.

Clark, R. (2004). Significance of perceived racism: Toward understanding the ethnic group disparities in health, the later years. In N. Anderson, R. Bulato, & B. Cohen (Eds.), *Critical perspectives on racial and ethnic differences in health in late life* (pp. 540–566). Washington, DC: National Academies Press.

Cohen, R., & Villaroel, M. (2015). Strategies used by adults to reduce their prescription drug costs: United States, 2013. *NCHS Data Brief,* (181), 1–8.

Colker, R. (2005). *The disability pendulum: The first decade of the Americans with Disabilities Act.* New York, NY: New York University Press.

Creek, J. (2011, November). *2011 ENOTHE Inaugural Hanneke van Bruggen Lecture "In praise of Diversity."* Paper presented at the 2011 annual meeting of the European Network of Occupational Therapy in Higher Education (ENOTHE) in Ghent, Belgium. Retrieved from http://www.enothe.eu/activities/meet/ac11/Appendix3.4.pdf

Cutler, D. (2004). *Your money or your life: Strong medicine for America's health care system.* New York, NY: Oxford University Press.

Ehrenreich, B. (2001). *Nickel and dimed: On (not) getting by in America.* New York, NY: Henry Holt.

Estes, C. (2001). *Social policy and aging: A critical perspective.* Thousand Oaks, CA: Sage.

Evans, R. G., Barer, M. L., & Marmor, T. L. (Eds.). (1994). *Why are some people healthy and others not? The determinants of health of populations.* New York, NY: Aldine de Gruyter.

Expedia.com. (2016). *Vacation deprivation survey.* Retrieved from https://viewfinder.expedia.com/news/work-life-imbalance-expedias-2016-vacation-deprivation-study-shows-americans-leave-hundreds-millions-paid-vacation-days-unused/?mcicid=social.vf

Fiorati, R. C., & Elui, V. M. C. (2015). Social determinants of health, inequality and social inclusion among people with disabilities. *Revista Latino-Americana de Enfermagem, 23*(2), 329–336. doi:10.1590/0104-1169.0187.2559

Fredriksen-Goldsen, K. I., Kim, H. J., & Barkan, S. E. (2012). Disability Among Lesbian, Gay, and Bisexual Adults: Disparities in Prevalence and Risk. *American Journal of Public Health, 102,* e16–e21. doi:10.2105/AJPH.2011.300379

Galheigo, S. M. (2011). What needs to be done? Occupational therapy responsibilities and challenges regarding human rights. *Australian Occupational Therapy Journal, 58,* 60–66.

Gianaros, P. J., Horenstein, J. A., Cohen, S., Matthews, K. A., Brown, S. M., Flory, J. D., . . . Hariri, A. R. (2007). Perigenual anterior cingulate morphology covaries with perceived social standing. *Social, Cognitive and Affective Neuroscience, 2,* 161–173.

Goode, E. (2002, December 17). The heavy cost of chronic stress. *The New York Times.* Retrieved from http://www.nytimes.com/2002/12/17/science/the-heavy-cost-of-chronic-stress.html?pagewanted=all&src=pm

Grossberg, P. M. (2006). An evidence-based context to address health care for gay and lesbian patients. *Wisconsin Medical Journal, 105*(6), 16–18.

Hacker, K., Anies, M., Folb, B. L., & Zallman, L. (2015). Barriers to health care for undocumented immigrants: A literature review. *Risk Management and Healthcare Policy, 8,* 175–183. doi:10.2147/RMHP.S70173

Hackman, D. A., Farah, M. J., & Meany, M. J. (2010). Socioeconomic status and the brain: Mechanistic insights from human and animal research. *Nature Reviews Neuroscience, 11,* 651–659.

Hurst, R. (2003). The international disability rights movement and the ICF. *Disability and Rehabilitation, 25*, 572–576.

Hutton, E., Tuppeny, S., & Hasselbusch, A. (2016). Making a case for universal and targeted children's occupational therapy in the United Kingdom. *British Journal of Occupational Therapy, 79*, 450–453.

Institute for Women's Policy Research. (2017). *The gender wage gap: 2015*. Retrieved from https://iwpr.org/issue/employment-education-economic-change/pay-equity-discrimination/

Institute of Medicine. (2002). *Unequal treatment: Confronting racial and ethnic disparities in health care*. Washington, DC: National Academies Press.

Institute of Medicine. (2011). *The health of lesbian, gay, bisexual, and transgender people: Building a foundation for better understanding*. Washington, DC: National Academies Press.

Institute on Disability. (2016). *2016 Disability Statistics Annual Report*. Retrieved from https://disabilitycompendium.org/sites/default/files/user-uploads/2016_AnnualReport.pdf

Kau, G., & Thompson, J. S. (2003). Racial and ethnic stratification of educational achievement and attainment. *Annual Review of Sociology, 29*, 417–442.

Kawachi, I., & Berkman, L. (2003). *Neighborhoods and health*. New York, NY: Oxford University Press.

Kozol, J. (1991). *Savage inequalities: Children in America's schools*. New York, NY: HarperCollins.

Kozol, J. (1995). *Amazing grace: The lives of children and the conscience of a nation*. New York, NY: Crown.

Kramer, M. S., Goulet, L., Lydon, J., Séquin, L., McNamara, H., Dassa, C., . . . Koren, G. (2001). Socio-economic disparities in preterm birth: Causal pathways and mechanism. *Paediatric and Perinatal Epidemiology, 15*(Suppl. 2), 104–123.

Krieger, N. (2001). A glossary for social epidemiology. *Journal of Epidemiology and Community Health, 55*, 693–700.

Krieger, N. (2010). Social inequalities in health. In J. Olsen, R. Saracci, & D. Trichopolous (Eds.), *Teaching epidemiology: A guide for teachers in epidemiology, public health, and clinical medicine* (3rd ed., pp. 215–239). Oxford, NY: Oxford University Press.

Kronenberg, F., & Pollard, N. (2005). Overcoming occupational apartheid: A preliminary exploration of the political nature of occupational therapy. In F. Kronenberg, S. Algado, & N. Pollard (Eds.), *Occupational therapy without borders: Learning from the spirit of survivors* (pp. 58–86). New York, NY: Elsevier.

Law, M. (1998). *Client-centred occupational therapy*. Thorofare, NJ: SLACK.

Lawlor, M. (2003). Gazing anew: The shift from a clinical gaze to an ethnographic lens. *American Journal of Occupational Therapy, 57*, 29–39.

Letts, L., Rigby, P., & Stewart, D. (Eds.). (2003). *Using environments to enable occupational performance*. Thorofare, NJ: SLACK.

Lohman, H., & Brown, K. (1997). Ethical issues related to managed care: An in-depth discussion of an occupational therapy case study. *Occupational Therapy in Health Care, 10*, 1–12.

Loucks, E. B., Almeida, N. D., Taylor, S. E., & Matthews, K. A. (2011). Childhood family psychosocial environment and coronary heart disease risk. *Psychosomatic Medicine, 73*, 563–571. doi:10.1097/PSY.0b013e318228c820

Luchins, A. S. (1988). The rise and decline of the American asylum movement in the 19th century. *The Journal of Psychology, 122*, 471–486.

Lynch, J. W., Kaplan, G. A., Cohen, R. D., Kauhanen, J., Wilson, T. W., Smith, N. L., & Salonen, J. T. (1994). Childhood and adult socioeconomic status as predictors of mortality in Finland. *Lancet, 343*, 524–527.

Lynch, J. W., Kaplan, G. A., Pamuk, E. R., Cohen, R. D., Heck, K. E., Balfour, J. L., & Yen, I. H. (1998). Income inequality and mortality in metropolitan areas of the United States. *American Journal of Public Health, 88*, 1074–1080.

MacPhee, D., Farro, S., & Canetto, S. (2013). Academic self-efficacy and performance of underrepresented STEM Majors: Gender, ethnic, and social class patterns. *Analyses of Social Issues and Public Policy, 13*, 347–369.

Marmot, M., Shipley, M., & Rose, G. (1984). Inequalities in death—specific explanations of a general pattern? *Lancet, 1*, 1003–1006.

Marmot, M., & Wilkinson, R. (Eds.). (1999). *Social determinants of health*. London, United Kingdom: Oxford Press.

Martin, J., McCaughtry, N., Flory, S., Murphy, A., & Wisdom, K. (2011). Using social cognitive theory to predict physical activity and fitness in underserved middle school children. *Research Quarterly for Exercise and Sport, 82*, 247–255.

McEwen, B. S. (2012). Brain on stress: How the social environment gets under the skin. *Proceedings of the National Academy of Sciences of the United States, 109* (S2), 17180–17185. Retrieved from http://www.pnas.org/content/109/Supplement_2/17180.full

McEwen, C., & McEwen, B. S. (2017). Social structure, adversity, toxic stress, and intergenerational poverty: An early childhood model. *Annual Reviews of Sociology, 43*, 445–472.

Merikangas, K., He, J., Brody, D., Fisher, P., Bourdon, K., & Koretz, D. (2010). Prevalence and treatment of mental disorders among U.S. children in the 2001–2004 NHANES. *Pediatrics, 125*, 75–81.

Miringoff, M., & Miringoff, M. (1999). *The social health of the nation: How America is really doing*. New York, NY: Oxford University Press.

Moss, N. (2000). Socioeconomic disparities in health in the US: An agenda for action. *Social Science & Medicine, 51*, 1627–1638.

National Center for Health Statistics. (2015). *Health, United States, 2015, with chartbook on trends in the health of Americans*. Hyattsville, MD: Author.

National Center for Health Statistics. (2016). *Infant mortality and African Americans*. Retrieved from https://minorityhealth.hhs.gov/omh/browse.aspx?lvl=4&lvlid=23

New America. (2017). *Paid family leave: How much time is enough?* Retrieved from https://www.newamerica.org/better-life-lab/policy-papers/paid-family-leave/#

Obama, B. (2016). United States Health Care Reform Progress to Date and Next Steps. *JAMA, 316*, 525–532. doi:10.1001/jama.2016.9797

Online Dictionary of the Social Sciences. (2017). *Online resource*. Retrieved from http://bitbucket.icaap.org

Organisation for Economic Co-operation and Development. (2015). *In It Together: Why Less Inequality Benefits All*. Paris, France: Author. Retrieved from http://dx.doi.org/10.1787/9789264235120-en

Organisation for Economic Co-operation and Development. (2017). *OECD health data 2017: How does the United States compare*. Retrieved from http://www.oecd.org/els/health-systems/health-data.htm

Parham, L. D., & Primeau, L. (1997). Play and occupational therapy. In L. D. Parham & L. Fazio (Eds.), *Play in occupational therapy for children* (pp. 2–22). St. Louis, MO: Mosby Year Book.

Pentland, W., Tremblay, M., Spring, K., & Rosenthal, C. (1999). Women with physical disabilities: Occupational impacts of ageing. *Journal of Occupational Science, 6*, 111–123.

Pew Charitable Trust. (2015). *The American middle class is losing ground: No longer the majority and falling behind financially*. Retrieved from http://www.pewsocialtrends.org/2015/12/09/the-american-middle-class-is-losing-ground/

Pew Research Center. (2017). *Gender discrimination comes in many forms for today's working women*. Retrieved from http://www.pewresearch.org/fact-tank/2017/12/14/gender-discrimination-comes-in-many-forms-for-todays-working-women/

Purtilo, R., Haddad, A., & Doherty, R. (2018). *Health professional and patient interaction* (8th ed.). Philadelphia, PA: Saunders.

Quiroga, V. A. M. (1995). *Occupational therapy: The first 30 years: 1900 to 1930*. Bethesda, MD: American Occupational Therapy Association.

Roscigno, V. J., & Ainsworth-Darnell, J. W. (1999). Race, cultural capital, and educational resources: Persistent inequalities and achievement returns. *Sociology of Education, 72*, 158–178.

Rylko-Bauer, B., & Farmer, P. (2002). Managed care or managed inequality? A call for critiques of market-based medicine. *Medical Anthropology Quarterly, 16,* 476–502.

Saez, E. (2016). *Striking it richer: the evolution of top incomes in the united states.* Retrieved from https://eml.berkeley.edu/~saez/saez-UStopincomes-2015.pdf

Saez, E., & Zucman, G. (2014). *Wealth Inequality in the United States since 1913: Evidence from Capitalized Income Tax Data* (NBER Working Paper No. 20625). Retrieved http://www.nber.org/papers/w20625

Schulz, A., Israel, B., Zenk, S., Parker, E., Lichtenstein, R., Shellman-Weir, S., & Klem, A. (2006). Psychosocial stress and social support as mediators of relationships between income, length of residence and depressive symptoms among African American women on Detroit's eastside. *Social Science & Medicine, 62,* 510–522.

Semyonov, M., Lewin-Epstein, N., & Maskileyson, D. (2013). Where wealth matters more for health: The wealth health gradient in 16 countries. *Social Science & Medicine, 81,* 10–17.

Shipler, D. (2005). *The working poor: Invisible in America.* New York, NY: Knopf.

Shonkoff, J. (2011). Protecting brains, not simply stimulating minds. *Sciences, 333,* 902–903.

Shonkoff, J., & Phillips, D. (Eds.). (2000). *From neurons to neighborhoods: The science of early childhood development.* Washington, DC: National Academies Press.

Sladyk, K., Jacobs, K., & MacCrae, N. (Eds.). (2010). *Occupational therapy essentials for clinical competence.* Thorofare, NJ: SLACK.

Spencer, N., Bambang, S., Logan, S., & Gill, L. (1999). Socioeconomic status and birth weight: Comparison of an area-based measure with the Registrar General's social class. *Journal of Epidemiology and Community Health, 53,* 495–498.

Stover, A. (2016). Client-centered advocacy: Every occupational therapy practitioner's responsibility to understand medical necessity. *American Journal of Occupational Therapy, 70,* 7005090010p1. doi:10.5014/ajot.2016.705003

Surkan, P. J., Zhang, A., Trachtenberg, F., Daniel, D. B., Mckinlay, S., & Bellinger, D. C. (2007). Neuropsychological function in children with blood lead levels of <10μg/dl. *Neurotoxicology, 28,* 1170–1177.

Surowiecki, J. (2014, March 3). The mobility myth. *The New Yorker.* Retrieved from https://www.newyorker.com/magazine/2014/03/03/the-mobility-myth

Tanta, K., Deitz, J., White, O., & Billingsley, F. (2005). The effects of peer-play level on initiations and responses of preschool children with delayed play skills. *American Journal of Occupational Therapy, 59,* 437–445.

The Atlantic. (2017, September 18). *What DACA's end could mean for colleges.* Retrieved from https://www.theatlantic.com/education/archive/2017/09/what-dacas-end-could-mean-for-colleges/540024/

The Economist. (2017, October 7). *The gender pay gap.* Retrieved from https://www.economist.com/news/international/21729993-women-still-earn-lot-less-men-despite-decades-equal-pay-laws-why-gender

The World Bank. (2013). *Disability inclusion.* Retrieved from http://www.worldbank.org/en/topic/disability

Townsend, E., & Wilcock, A. (2003). Occupational justice. In C. Christiansen & E. Townsend (Eds.), *Introduction to occupation: The art and science of living* (pp. 243–273). Upper Saddle River, NJ: Prentice Hall.

Uili, R. M., & Wood, R. (1995). The effect of third-party payers on the clinical decision making of physical therapists. *Social Science & Medicine, 40,* 873–879.

U.S. Administration on Aging. (2016). *Older Americans: Key indicators of well-being.* Retrieved from https://agingstats.gov/docs/LatestReport/Older-Americans-2016-Key-Indicators-of-WellBeing.pdf

U.S. Census Bureau. (2011). *Same-sex households with children in the United States.* Retrieved from https://www.census.gov/prod/2011pubs/acsbr10-03.pdf

U.S. Census Bureau. (2016). *Income, poverty, and health insurance coverage in the United States: 2016.* Retrieved from https://census.gov/content/dam/Census/library/publications/2017/demo/P60-259.pdf

U.S. Department of Health and Human Services. (2017a). *Healthy people 2020.* Retrieved from http://www.healthypeople.gov/2020/topics-objectives/topic/social-determinants-of-health

U.S. Department of Health and Human Services. (2017b). Disability and health. In *Healthy People 2020.* Retrieved from https://www.healthypeople.gov/2020/topics-objectives/topic/disability-and-health

U.S. Department of Health and Human Services, Office of Minority Health. (2011). *Infant mortality and African Americans.* Retrieved from http://minorityhealth.hhs.gov/templates/content.aspx?lvl=2&lvlID=51&ID=3021

U.S. Department of Labor. (2011). *Employment standards administration wage and hour division.* Retrieved from http://www.dol.gov/dol/topic/wages/minimumwage.htm

Velozo, C., & Woodbury, M. (2011). Translating measurement findings into rehabilitation practice: An example using Fugl–Meyer Assessment–Upper Extremity with patients following stroke. *Journal of Rehabilitation Research and Development, 48,* 1211–1222. doi:10.1682/JRRD.2010.10.0203

Waber, D., De Moor, C., Forbes, P., Almli, C., Botteron, K., Leonard, G., … Rumsey, J. (2007). The NIH MRI study of normal brain development: Performance of a population based sample of healthy children aged 6 to 18 years on a neuropsychological battery. *Journal of the International Neuropsychological Society, 13,* 729–746.

Weitz, R. (2004). *The sociology of health, illness, and health care.* Belmont, CA: Wadsworth.

Wells, S., & Black, R. (2000). *Cultural competency for health professionals.* Bethesda, MD: American Occupational Therapy Association.

Whiteford, G. (2000). Occupational deprivation: Global challenge in the new millennium. *British Journal of Occupational Therapy, 63,* 200–204.

Wilkinson, J., & Ferraro, K. (2002). Thirty years of ageism research. In T. Nelson (Ed.), *Ageism: Stereotyping and prejudice against older persons* (pp. 339–358). Cambridge, MA: Massachusetts Institute of Technology Press.

Wilkinson, R., & Marmot, M. (Eds.). (2003). *Social determinants of health: The solid facts* (2nd ed.). Copenhagen, Denmark: World Health Organization, Regional Office for Europe.

Wilkinson, R., & Pickett, K. (2009a). Income inequality and social dysfunction. *Annual Review of Sociology, 35,* 493–511.

Wilkinson, R., & Pickett, K. (2009b). *The spirit level: Why equality is better for everyone.* London, United Kingdom: Penguin Books.

Wilkinson, R., & Pickett, K. (2017). The enemy between us: The psychological and social costs of inequality. *European Journal of Social Psychology, 47,* 11–24.

Williams, D. R. (1997). Race and health: Basic questions, emerging directions. *Annals of Epidemiology, 7,* 322–333.

Wood, W. (1996). Delivering occupational therapy's fullest promise: Clinical interpretations of "life domains and adaptive strategies of a group of low-income, well older adults." *American Journal of Occupational Therapy, 50,* 109–112.

World Health Organization. (2010). *The world health report 2010.* Geneva, Switzerland: Author.

Yen, I. H., Michael, Y. L., & Perdue, L. (2009). Neighborhood environment in studies of health of older adults: A systematic review. *American Journal of Preventive Medicine, 37,* 455–463.

Young, M. E. (1997). *Early childhood development.* Washington, DC: The World Bank Development.

Disability, Community, Culture, and Identity

John A. White Jr.

LEARNING OBJECTIVES

After reading this chapter, you will be able to:

1. Explore how disability is one of many differences on the continuum of human experience and one that each person will likely experience.
2. Analyze the components of the social construct of disability.
3. Identify barriers to social participation for people with disabilities and generate strategies for deconstructing those barriers.
4. Compare and contrast the models of disability and relate these to occupational therapy practice paradigms.
5. Describe the disability rights movement in the United States and its history as an example of a social movement's framing of the disability experience from within.
6. Critically reflect on the sociopolitical, economic, and cultural perspectives that influence your practice as an occupational therapist.

Pl-ease

Clive Blake

Don't see only our disability-ease,
Don't deny us basic facility-ease,
Don't ignore our many ability-ease,
Don't compound our varied difficult-ease,
Deal head-on with the harsh realit-ease.

You never know what life has in store,
You may fall one day and rise no more,
You may join our ranks, afraid, unsure,
You may write words to plead; implore.

We are not an alien race,
We have a voice, we have a face,
We have our part to play; a place.

Let us join life's lively dance,
Let us have an equal chance.

Pl-ease.

Introduction

Imagine a world in which people of all abilities participate equitably in society with adequate opportunities for economic stability, housing, work, leisure, health care, and a range of meaningful occupations. Such a socially and occupationally just world would provide for these basic needs, which many consider as basic human rights. This is perhaps a utopian vision, but in a country with such a high percentage of the world's wealth and consumption, the United States could certainly move closer to this goal. And there are countries that we can look to that have been much more successful at integrating people with disabilities into society than in the United States. Although no country can be considered to be ideal in supporting equitable participation of disabled citizens, those that are recognized as doing it well (e.g., most Nordic countries and Germany) are those that provide health care, housing supports, public transportation, financial supports, and educational opportunities that foster full community inclusion (Penketh et al., 2015).

In this chapter, we explore the concepts related to disability and disability rights to frame an understanding of why people with disabilities[1] were considered by early disability scholars as second-class citizens (Eisenberg, Griggins, & Duval, 1982; Falconer, 1982; Sims & Manley, 1982), a categorization that is still made today (Duckworth, 2017; Meikle, 2016). They are second-class in that they are frequently deprived of opportunities for social participation by a society structured to systematically exclude them from participation. To better understand the source of this exclusion, we examine the social construct of disability (Berger & Luckmann, 1966; Berkowitz, 1987; Bogdan & Taylor, 1992; Bumiller, 1988; Davis, 1997a; Liachowitz, 1988; Smart, 2009; Wolfensberger, 1972) and analyze the attitudinal, political, economic, institutional, and architectural barriers that contribute to that construct. As we build that understanding, we describe the role of the occupational therapist as a change agent who can prepare their disabled clients for success in dealing with the barriers to their participation created by the social construct. This is work that goes beyond the typical rehabilitation approach that focuses on improving activities of daily living (ADL) and instrumental activities of daily living (IADL) independence. It is work that assures clients learn skills for self-advocacy in societies where although laws grant

---

[1]Although the term *people with disabilities* often appears in the literature as recommended people-first language, *disabled people* and other "disability-centered" terms are increasingly preferred and used by many activists and scholars who promote positive disability identity as an act of resistance against disability oppression (e.g., the focus is not on the deficit in the individual but on the society that imposes disability on disabled people as a collective minority group).

BOX 21-1	INITIAL LEARNING ACTIVITY

Take out a piece of paper and jot down what you think about when you hear the words *disability* and *independence*. What do these words mean to you? How are they defined and constructed in society (e.g., by the public or in the media)? How does the profession of OT view disability and independence?

civil rights for people with disabilities, social attitudes and physical and economic barriers continue to hold them in a second-class citizen status. Whether as an occupational therapy (OT) practitioner you choose to work individually, organizationally, or at the population level to improve opportunities for people with disabilities to pursue their definition of a meaningful life, you will learn strategies for working toward this vision of a much more equitable, inclusive, and diverse world.

In previous chapters, you have read accounts by people with disabilities or their family members that provide insights to the experience of life with a disability. In many ways, it is like any other life, filled with a need to do, to relate to others, and to contribute to the social good. However, pursuing those life goals is complicated by both the medical condition that impairs function and especially by the way society perceives the person with the condition. The facts of bodily impairment cannot be denied, but it is the interaction of the person in disabling environment that is repeatedly shown to be the stronger handicapping factor (Box 21.1).

What Is Disability?

In some ways, there are as many definitions of **disability** as there are people with disabling conditions. This is because each person experiences the condition in a way unique to their personality, culture, physical body, and environmental context. However, to support our discussion, several widely accepted definitions are presented that show views of disability from various perspectives. The examples here come from U.S. policymaking, health care, welfare, and economics.

A definition that highlights the socially constructed nature of disability (Nagi, 1991) and brings in task and role function is

> Disability refers to social rather than organismic functioning. It is an inability or limitation in performing socially defined roles and tasks expected of an individual within a sociocultural and physical environment. (p. 315)

The definition presented in the Americans with Disabilities Act (ADA) (Pub. L. 103-336) is perhaps the best known.

> The term "disability" means, with respect to an individual—(A) a physical or mental impairment that substantially limits one or more of the major life activities of an individual; (B) a record of such an impairment; or (C) being regarded as having such impairment. (§ 12102, [2])

The focus of the ADA definition on "major life activities" indicates the important role that OT should play in evaluating and recording these effects on major life activities. For example, an occupational therapist is well equipped to participate in the process that helps determine whether or not a person's disability qualifies for accommodations under the ADA, or the occupational therapist might serve as an expert witness (DeMaio-Feldman, 1987) in a disability discrimination case. Occupational therapists are often called on to apply their skills in activity analysis to document the "essential functions" (Canelón, 1995) of a job to better determine whether or not people with disabilities can perform the job "with or without accommodation." The last component (C) of the ADA definition points toward the effects of stigma and attitudes toward the idea of disability, even in the absence of functional limitations, and suggests an advocacy role for the therapist.

In a similar role, occupational therapists are well equipped to participate in the disability determination process (Marfeo et al., 2016) that helps determine whether or not a person's disability qualifies for benefits from the Social Security Administration (SSA), such as Social Security Disability Insurance (SSDI) and Supplemental Security Income (SSI), and that affect eligibility for health insurance through Medicare or Medicaid (SSA, 2018a). This definition of disability focuses solely on the person's ability to work for pay. Therefore, an economically derived definition of disability under the Social Security Act (Act) is

> A person is disabled under the Act if he or she can't work due to a severe medical condition that has lasted, or is expected to last, at least one year or result in death. The person's medical condition must prevent him or her from doing work that he or she did in the past, and it must prevent the person from adjusting to other work. (SSA, 2018b)

An example of how definitions can affect an individual who was determined as disabled by the SSA and then returned to gainful employment is about Scott (Case Study 21-1), a man with complete tetraplegia. After completing a probationary employment period, Scott received a letter from the SSA that declared " . . . you are no longer disabled . . . " to which he replied with a wry smile—so I guess I can sell my wheelchair now that I'm no longer disabled!

The World Health Organization (2008), through a document called The *International Classification of Functioning,* *Disability and Health* (ICF) in an attempt to include social influences, acknowledges the impairments related to disabling conditions and provides some attempts to bridge many of these definitions by considering disability as an umbrella term for *impairments*, *activity limitations*, and *participation restrictions*. An **impairment** results from problems with body function or structure, and an **activity limitation** occurs when a person has trouble executing a task or action, whereas a **participation restriction** indicates a person's difficulty engaging in a "life situation" (engaging in roles or occupations). Although the ICF provides a common language for discussion of the concepts related to disability, operationalizing this framework for use across multiple countries, agencies, and institutions is no simple task, although the ICF is helpful for us to understand disability from a more universal perspective and provides language that is familiar related to its adoption into the *Occupational Therapy Practice Framework* (OTPF) (American Occupational Therapy Association [AOTA], 2014b). The ICF acknowledges the social and medical contexts of health and disability as experiences of all human beings. These experiences are shaped by interactions with both environmental and personal factors. The unique interaction of these factors with an individual affects how the person can engage in essential life activities and participate in society.

In summary, the lens through which one defines disability shapes perspectives about the person or population that is considered to have the disability. Therefore, whether one uses a medical, legal, or social definition will shape one's attitudes and actions toward and with disabled people. This leads us to consider various models of disability in order to better understand the full implications of the social construct of disability.

The Social Construct of Disability[2]

With OT's adoption of practice models that rely on the person-environment-occupation (PEO) interaction that results in occupational performance, it may be useful to trace the foundations of the PEO models that support our understanding of the social construct of disability. It has been well established that the experience of disability is directly related to barriers that have been socially constructed. The earliest suggestion of the social construct of disability arose out of what Kurt Lewin (1935) proposed as a person-in-environment interaction and was elaborated

---

[2]Much of the content in this section is from White, J. A. (1999). *Occupation and adaptation: An ethnographic study of people with disabilities using the ADA to fight employment discrimination* (Unpublished doctoral dissertation). University of Southern California, Los Angeles.

CASE STUDY 21-1   SCOTT: ADVOCACY, OCCUPATION, AND POLICY

Recently graduated from high school and looking for his next life experience, Scott signed up to join the Marines to do his patriotic duty. However, on his 19th birthday while celebrating with friends at the river, Scott dove into too shallow water and sustained a C5–C6 fracture resulting in complete tetraplegia. After spending the next 7 years living with his parents on their farm, "looking out the window at the cows or watching TV" and intermittently trying community college courses, Scott emerged from his depression and the "mental fog" created by medications to treat it and his spasticity and pursued education. Using work incentives like the Plan to Achieve Self-Support (PASS; https://www.ssa.gov/pubs/EN-05-11017.pdf) and vocational rehabilitation funds to pay for tuition, books, and a computer, he had much success, graduating magna cum laude and earning two Bachelor of Arts degrees (in Psychology and Computer Science) and eventually his Master of Business Administration (MBA). During college, Scott became very active in and eventually headed the campus for disabled student union, and he became a strong disability rights advocate and a consultant on navigating the complex disability benefit system. These roles helped him land a reasonably paid position with the state, supervising the office of disability affairs. After working there for 2 years, he was considered no longer disabled by Social Security Administration and received health insurance through his employer and had managed to maintain Supplemental Security Income (SSI) support for his personal care assistant (PCA). However, he was about to get a $300 per month raise, but unfortunately, this increase in income would have eliminated his eligibility for Social Security Administration funds that he paid for his part-time PCA and so he felt compelled to quit work due to what are called "work disincentives." In having to pay for his health care, PCA, and other disability-related expenses (catheters, wheelchair maintenance, etc.) out of his salary, he would have

less discretionary income than the approximately $100 per month he had on his SSDI check (that also made him eligible for Medicare and the PCA supplement). Thus, he chose to quit a job that he enjoyed and was successful in for not only because of the added income it provided but also because he had built a more active social life with coworkers and felt he was finally giving back to society rather than just taking support through disability programs. As he said, "The work disincentives won!"

Through his frustrations, Scott was motivated to become more active in disability rights policymaking and with the help of his local congressional representative, introduced the Work Incentive Network (WIN) legislation in 1990, which recommended changes in Social Security Administration policy to decrease work disincentives. The legislative effort stalled related to funding challenges, and an assumption that the ADA which passed that year, would make the recommendations moot. However, his work did find success when the state vocational rehabilitation office eventually adopted a unit called the WIN that counsels people with disabilities on getting work while optimizing benefits. Also, elements of Scott's WIN bill eventually appeared in the "Ticket to Work and Work Incentives Improvement Act" in 1999. Disappointingly, the "Ticket" act fell short of the ambitious plan that would have guaranteed health care benefits for permanently disabled individuals in regardless of employment status. Nor did the Ticket assure essential supports like transportation and supplemental funds to pay PCAs regardless of employment status, benefits that some disability advocates are still promoting. However, Scott took pride in having moved the balance a little closer to improved policy for persons with disabilities and reveled in his identity as a disability rights advocate and activist, occupational roles that helped him find his meaningful place in the world.

---

by psychologist Roger Barker (1948) and his colleagues (Barker, Wright, & Gonick, 1946). They recognized that the problems and barriers faced by people with disabilities were not so much related to an individual's physical impairments but constructed through social attitudes as well as perceptions of those impairments as different and incapacitating.

For instance, Scott (1969) points out that "blindness itself is a learned social role" (p. 23) in which the blind learn "how to be blind" through socialization in American culture. Blind men depicted in Scott's study learned a dependent role, with a certain degree of social isolation from the sighted population. This construction of the role for blind men in mid-century America contrasted to that found among Native American men in a rural New Mexican village (Gwaltney, 1970). In that village, men who were blind

held important community roles. The blind men traveled from village to village guided by boys or young men, and begged for their sustenance. In this capacity, they simultaneously served as intervillage communicators, advisors to the younger generation, and were even imbued with special powers to interpret dreams (Gwaltney, 1970). This example can show "how our apparently objective perceptions of handicaps as socially incapacitating biological conditions are the perceptual products of a prior—and unconscious—social construction" (Gleidman & Roth, 1980, p. 30).

> But most able-bodied people remain the prisoners of traditional misconceptions about disability. Here it seems obvious that the disease-like characteristics of handicaps can use the disabled person's deviance-especially when the stigmas of disability are genuine medical conditions like paraplegia.

It requires great effort of the imagination to recognize that the judgement of deviance comes first. The disease-like condition, the handicap, dominates our perception of the person's social nature only because we have already decided that he is a deviant. (p. 25)

Another perspective on the social construction of disability is by Claire Liachowitz (1988) who wrote that people with impairments are disabled by a process of devaluation and segregation. The impairment represents a deviation from acceptable physical norms which is translated into an assignment of social inferiority by the "normal" (i.e., dominant) social group. Attitudes like this contribute to the phenomenon of *ableism*, a term that summarizes the discrimination and prejudice experienced by people with disabilities and in favor of the able-bodied. Ableists view people with disabilities as having or being a defect that needs to be fixed as opposed to a more liberated view of disability as a dimension of difference. These views of inferiority and devaluation have had a profound impact on the creation and implementation of public policy toward people with disabilities (Liachowitz, 1988; Minow, 1990) and have led to a form of institutionalized dependency and social isolation for this population. To help dismantle this construct and ableists' discrimination, it is important to advocate against at least six forms of ableism as outlined in Box 21-2 (Zeilinger, 2015).

The tendency to place people with disabilities into categories or classes is a natural human phenomenon. Categorization is an essential cognitive strategy that allows humans to cope with the vast amount of information available to them (J. A. White, 1999). Unfortunately, this categorizing process can also lead to negative stereotyping and labeling based on the most easily observed characteristics of a person (Gleidman & Roth, 1980; Minow, 1990). For people with disabilities who are easily placed in a category of difference from the norm, it is common for the "normal" group to exclude those with the difference from everyday social discourse. The social cues emitted by the person with a physical difference tend to set certain expectations within those of the normal group. For example, a person may drool, which is a trait associated with infancy, or demonstrate inarticulate speech that may imply stupidity or drunkenness, when these traits may be caused by a neurological condition unrelated to development or cognition (Gleidman & Roth, 1980). Similarly, just because a person uses a wheelchair doesn't mean that he or she cannot participate in competitive sports or experience courtship, marriage, or parenthood (Figure 21-1) (Strother, 1992). This tendency to stigmatize people with disabilities due to their apparent or imagined disabilities is compounded by the phenomenon of internal oppression. Internal oppression (associated with "self-hate") occurs in at least two ways. One is when a person within an oppressed group has adopted beliefs about and embraces stereotypes commonly held toward the group and may identify so strongly with the oppressor that they attempt to assimilate into the oppressing group. A way that internalized oppression works in relation to disability is when an

---

BOX 21-2 FORMS OF ABLEISM THAT OCCUPATIONAL THERAPISTS SHOULD RESIST

1. Failing to offer a full range of accessibility options, beyond that for wheeled mobility, such as for sensory impairments related to low vision, hearing loss, or sensory processing disorders
2. Using discriminatory (ableist) language in pejorative ways such as crazy, retarded, crip, gimp, or deaf and dumb
3. Acknowledging that many **temporarily able-bodied individuals (TABs)** rarely, if ever, check their privilege such a parking in disability-only parking spaces or using accessible bathroom stalls without thinking, and failing to acknowledge the value of universal design such as the benefit of a curb cut when using a stroller or hand truck, or activating power door opener when hands are full.
4. The assumption that the disabled have no agency or autonomy by automatically assuming that they need help. Although a person challenged by a steep incline might appreciate help pushing their wheelchair up the hill, or a blind individual may value a guiding hand to navigate a crowded space, it is always appropriate to ask and not assume that the person is helpless or without motivation to meet those challenges.
5. The assumption that it's OK to ask how a person's disability occurred. This is considered by many people with disabilities as an unnecessary and unwanted intrusion into their personal lives and space. Although it is easier to forgive children that ask this question, it inadvertently teaches them that it's justified to ask of people with disability-related differences.
6. Assuming that disability is obvious and apparent. This enables TABs to discriminate in subtle and not-so-subtle ways against people with mental health conditions, autism, learning disabilities, or chronic illnesses (e.g., tragic encounters of people with mental illness being incarcerated or killed due to a lack of police understanding of the effects and behaviors associated with mental illness [Myers, 2017]).

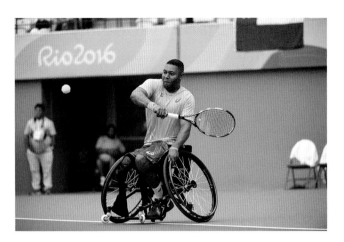

FIGURE 21-1 The first Paralympic Games were held in 1960 and they are now the second biggest sporting event in the world.

able-bodied person sustains a chronically disabling condition and his or her previously held biases and discriminatory behaviors toward people with disabilities persist against themselves (David & Derthick, 2014). This creates intense internal conflict and distress and significantly slows the person's responses to recovery and rehabilitation. This might lead the person to focus on rehabilitation with intense effort to get back to being normal and, although commendable and understandable, may slow his or her acceptance of oneself in this identity (see Chapter 13, "While Focusing on Recovery I Forgot to Get a Life").

When these patterns of categorization and discrimination lead to exclusion, the results, as in racism, are often confused with the effects of biology (Williams, 1991). Although people with disabilities are showing up in public in slowly growing numbers, there is still a dearth of people with disabilities in jobs, as political leaders, and visible in the community. This absence reinforces the stereotypical attitude held by many people without disabilities that they cannot, and should not, participate in social roles (Gleidman & Roth, 1980).

These classifications can develop into socially ingrained patterns of discrimination such as architectural or employment barriers. When an entire class of people with disabilities is then excluded from social participation due to these barriers, they, in essence, form a layer in a "socially constructed caste system" (Funk, 1987, p. 24). Hahn (1985a, 1985b) has shown how such a caste system has developed through public policy, particularly over the last century, and contends that "disability is defined by public policy" (Hahn, 1985a, p. 294). Using political–historical analysis, Hahn has emphasized how people with disabilities constitute a minority group in the American political landscape. His analysis has helped move the conceptualization of disability away from an inherent characteristic of the person to one that emphasizes its politically and

socially constructed nature (Hahn, 1985a, 1985b, 1987). This is a phenomenon that Higgins (1992) calls "policy(ing) disability." Higgins also notes how institutionalization (and later, ill-supported de-institutionalization), disability-targeted charities (see controversies over Jerry Lewis's Muscular Dystrophy Telethons [Phillips, 1990; Shapiro, 1993]), economic utility analyses of disability, and civil rights laws have all contributed to the "making of disability" in America.

In addition to how public policy has contributed to the social construct of disability, health care professionals have played an important role as they "interpret the meaning of disability to society at large" (Gleidman & Roth, 1980, p. 35) and to their patients through the process of *medicalization* (Illich, 1976) and *professionalization* (Berkowitz, 1987). Medicalization occurred as medical and rehabilitation professionals assumed more and more responsibility for the treatment, goal setting, training, equipment provision, and even policymaking for people with disabilities (DeJong, 1983; Funk, 1987; Liachowitz, 1988). Within the medical model, the person with a disability is cast as a "patient," perpetuating the dependency and nonparticipation (Funk, 1987) expected of people in the "sick role" (Parsons, 1951; 1975). Medicalization offers a perspective of disability as illness that interacts with disability laws to limit social participation and options for productivity (Gleidman & Roth, 1980). The relative idleness of people forced into this role of nonparticipation and nonproductivity is a dilemma that forces them into second-class citizenship (Eisenberg et al., 1982).

To conclude this section on socially constructed employment barriers affecting people with disabilities, I offer a selection from the work of sociologist and feminist, Rosemarie Thomson. She has written a critique of images of disability in American culture and literature that focuses on "extraordinary bodies" and how they "figure" in American culture. "People deemed disabled are barred from full citizenship because their bodies do not conform with architectural, attitudinal, educational, occupational, and legal conventions based on assumptions that bodies appear and perform in certain ways" (Thomson, 1997, p. 46). People with mental health conditions or developmental disabilities face similar exclusion (P. E. Deegan, 1996).

As these constructs became more clearly defined and more widely examined during the late 1960s and 1970s, people with disabilities (primarily led by men and women with mobility impairments) took action that would lead to the creation of the independent living movement and the disability rights movement, which is described later in this chapter. Their goals were to increase opportunities for equal participation in society, politics, and employment (DeJong, 1979). In order to accomplish these goals, they set out to restructure common perspectives of disability.

Therefore, a fundamental theme that underscored pursuit of each of the aforementioned goals was to show that the disabling effects people with disabilities experienced resides primarily in the relationship between the person with an impairment and a given environment and not within the person. Although OT practitioners have the potential to be powerful allies in the effort to significantly improve this person–environment interaction (AOTA, 2014b; Frieden, 1992; Frieden & Cole, 1985), this chapter shows how OT professionals sometimes contribute to this disabling construct as evident in several ethnographic accounts of OT services (Clark, 1993; McCuaig & Frank, 1991; Price-Lackey & Cashman, 1996) and provides tools and knowledge to assure that your practice is one that breaks down these barriers and does not contribute to them.

Models of Disability: Shaping the Worldview of Disability

Models, similar to theories, are tools for thinking (Miller, 1988). Models provide shortcuts for categorizing and symbolizing a more complex set of ideas that explain phenomena; in this case, the phenomenon of interest is disability. The models presented here are intended to explain worldviews of disability and to help you understand various conceptualizations of disability and related sources of attitudes and barriers that limit activities and social participation of people with disabilities. These models or worldviews, not only affect people with disabilities but also affect anyone touched by them, including you as a world citizen, and especially you as an occupational therapist or OT assistant. Disability models do not exist in isolation but interact with each other to add to the complexity of the disability experience and of building a comprehensive understanding of disability. There are whole books written on each of these models: Our brief review of them will provide enough information to provide you with a context for understanding their effects on the construct of disability. For more information on most of the models and a compelling view of the social construct of disability, consider reading insider perspectives in *A New Disability History* (Longmore & Umansky, 2001) or the earlier *Making Disability* (Higgins, 1992) which details the sources and effects of the models, or *Disability as a Social Construct* (Liachowitz, 1988).

As you read here about these models, consider how they interact with your own understandings and attitudes about disability. Also reflect on how you have seen people with disabilities treated in a public context or in health care settings and how various models may have shaped those interactions, with special attention to the medical and social models.

Moral or Charity Model of Disability

Some of the earliest conceptions of disability fit into what is called either the moral model of disability or the charity model. Within the *moral model of disability*, handicap and impairment are explained as results of divine action to provide the person with a challenge to overcome and demonstrate moral worthiness, or as a punishment for offenses against the moral order, an order often defined by religious institutions. The *charity model of disability* is considered to have arisen out of the moral model as a recognition that the faith-based organizations, civic community, or both have a responsibility to care for those less capable of caring for themselves by extending some form of assistance to help sustain the disabled person's life (Longmore & Umansky, 2001). Unfortunately, support motivated by morality or charity may also reflect a belief that the recipient deserves pity. Others, or even the recipients may express contempt for individuals or lack of respect for individuals who are not financially independent (Shapiro, 1993).

Welfare and Economic Models of Disability

The charity model contributed to the evolution of what is considered the *welfare model of disability*. This model is still prevalent, especially in developed countries that have financial and other benefits intended to support people whose disabilities prevent them from earning a living that is adequate to support themselves (Oliver, 1996). In the welfare model, particularly through the 1950s, but with lingering influences today, people with disabilities are considered part of the "worthy poor" (Berkowitz, 1987; Scheer & Groce, 1988). The "worthy," including the disabled, are people who through no fault of their own are worthy to receive government support through cash supplements and benefits that support their existence, even if it means grouping them together with needy others such as the sick, poor, or frail in institutions. For example, young people with severe chronic disabilities are sometimes still housed in nursing homes that are typically considered for the sick and frail elderly (e.g., in 2013, 14.2% of nursing home residents were below age 65 years [Cleek, 2013]).

Major dilemmas of the welfare model in the United States are in how it has created work disincentives that tend to erect barriers to employment for disabled individuals desiring to work and invoke pity or contempt by the able-bodied. They legitimately qualify for the benefits if they remain unemployed but lose access to essential social, health care, and daily life supports as their income rises but doesn't rise enough for them to adequately purchase the services they lose (Berkowitz, 1987; Longmore, 2003). This quandary is often referred to as a "catch-22" and arises out of the dilemma of difference (Minow, 1990). Minow defined the dilemma of difference as the situation one faces when he or she has a difference (e.g., based on race, gender, disability, or other category) and face discrimination. The difference entitles him or her to a legal right through policy like the ADA or the Civil Rights law, but claiming the right further highlights his or her difference and/or limits his or her options for social participation. Such a catch-22 led disability scholar Paul Longmore to protest his dilemma by burning the book he had labored to publish. He burned it because royalties from the book caused him to lose health insurance and the personal care assistant (PCA) that were necessary conditions for his continued employment as a university professor and researcher (*Why I Burned My Book and Other Essays on Disability*, Longmore, 2003).

For those people with disabilities who do have the capability to work and earn a living and to pay taxes, their economic value to society increases. Programs like Vocational Rehabilitation and Workers' Compensation emerged in the early 20th century to support their employment or lack of it, respectively. Such programs define and quantify various forms of impairment, especially physical disability as having specific economic value. The values vary by state worker compensation laws, but a worker with a newly amputated arm could receive between $48,000 and $439,000, depending on their state of residency at the time of the loss (Grabell & Berkes, 2015). These institutions and the people they serve are influenced by the *economic model of disability*. In the economic model, the worth of the person is related to either their ability to work and earn money on which they would pay taxes, or their inability to work and their cost to society (Berkowitz, 1987).

Medical Model of Disability

About the time that OT was emerging as a profession in the early twentieth century, disability became more of a focus of the medical community as the rehabilitation of people with physical and mental disabilities became possible. This "medicalization" (Illich, 1976) of disability has several benefits such as attention to medical cures for disabling illnesses, treatments that mitigate impairments, and equipment that substitutes for lost function. However, a purely biomedical lens on disability tends to highlight the impairment of the person. This individualizes disability as residing within the person versus an acknowledgment that disability is an interaction of the person, impairment, and environmental context as is the hallmark of the *social model of disability*. In starkest terms, medicine views sickness as something that must be fixed so that the person can

return to fulfilling normative social roles and functions. Medicine is traditionally focused on helping sick people get well and so when the "sickness" is a chronic condition affecting person, that person is viewed as incurable and thus permanently occupying the "sick role" (Parsons, 1951; 1975). Sociologist Talcott Parsons described the expectations of a person in the sick role as being temporarily excused from social obligations, is not responsible for their condition, and is obligated to comply with the healer's ministrations in the effort to be healed. The challenge of applying this to a person with a chronic disability is that in strict medical terms, they can't get well. This places them in a liminal (i.e., neither here nor there) position (R. Murphy, Scheer, Murphy, & Mack, 1988; Turner, 1977) that clouds self-identity and leaves one in deviance to social norms and expectations. Therefore, in spite of the benefits derived from a medical model approach, many in the disability rights community have criticized the medical model as being a barrier to full participation by people that are disabled because it fails to recognize the limiting barriers imposed by the social structure.

Social Model of Disability

In ways that most occupational therapists will recognize, the *social model of disability* focuses on the interaction of the person with their environment and the resulting effect on what the disabled person can do to participate in society (i.e., a parallel to the PEO-based OT models) (Kielhofner, 2009). These social alternatives to the economic, charity, and medical models have been proposed that highlight the role of the sociocultural and physical environment in creating many of the participation barriers faced by people with disabilities. These models are grouped into the social model of disability (Oliver, 2013).

One such approach was coined the *minority group model* (Hahn, 1985b, 1987) as it conceived of people affected by a wide range of disabilities having in common the experience of systematic oppression, marginalization, alienation, and social and political isolation. It also identified the strengths of the group as having power to influence policy, pride in a common identity of resilience and adaptability, and innovative ways of living. The minority group model was partially inspired by how other minority groups (e.g., based on race, gender, or sexual identity) in mid-century America had fought for their rights through political advocacy and activism. The minority model also helped establish a common point of identification across the many varied sources and categories of disability (e.g., physical, mental, and developmental) and pointed toward political solutions to breaking down barriers to social and political participation. This model incorporated terms and concepts from other rights campaigns that emerged as *disability culture*, *disability pride*, and *disability identity* that helped lay the groundwork for passage of the ADA.

The minority group model is one of many models that fall within the family of social models of disability such as the *Nordic relational model* (society must adapt to support participation of the disabled), *the sociopolitical model* (a precursor to the minority group model), *the equal environmental accommodations model* (Hahn, 1993) (similar to the Nordic model), *the British or United Kingdom social model*, and others (Shakespeare, 2006c). These approaches are commonly lumped together as the *social model of disability* and often presented in contrast to the medical model (Table 21-1). The social model views disability as an inevitable human experience that with proper environmental accommodations and social supports should not limit a person's ability to accomplish common life goals and fully participate in social, economic, and political life. There are critiques of the social model that point out ways in which it fails to fully explain the experience of disability and account for certain inconsistencies (Shakespeare, 2006a; Stoltzfus & Schumann, 2011); however, the social models are widely embraced as the best available way to understand disability.

Social model proponents describe how the built environment is both a product of discriminatory attitudes and a reinforcer of those attitudes (Goodley, 2017; Oliver, 2013; Shakespeare, 2006a). Therefore, one remedy for disability exclusion is to change the physical environment. For example, adapting the environment and objects that serve a wide variety of people is a concept built into a universal design

---

TABLE 21-1 • Comparison of Disability and Independence Constructions

	Medical Model	Rehabilitation Model	Minority Group/Social Model
What is disability?	Disability is deficiency or abnormality.	Disability is loss or inability to functionally perform everyday activities independently or in a socially expected way (e.g., timely, safely, efficiently).	Disability is difference. (Some would argue for saying that *impairment* is difference, whereas *disability* occurs only when societally imposed barriers limit people.)
How is disability constructed?	Being disabled is negative.	Being disabled is negative and something to overcome or to accept/adjust or adapt to its negative consequences within one's life.	Being disabled is neutral; negative constructions occur when society imposes barriers and oppresses participation; positive constructions occur when the personal and social world own difference and support and validate people.
Where is disability located?	Disability is in the individual body.	Disability is in the individual or in the interaction between the individual and the immediate environment.	Disability derives from the interaction between the individual and society. Disability is located in societal structures and practices that oppress.
What is the mechanism for change?	The remedy for disability-related problems is cure or normalization.	The mechanism for change for disability-related problems is to rehabilitate or remediate to normal and/or to become as physically/cognitively independent in everyday activities as possible.	The mechanism for change is changing the interaction between the individual and society.
What are examples of change strategies?	Examples are surgery, medication, medical technology, and intervention.	Examples are individual remediation and person/environment compensation or adaptation.	Examples are systems and social action change; collective activism; and disability identity, pride, and culture.
Who/what are the agents of change?	The agent of remedy is the professional.	The agent of change is the professional in collaboration with the individual client and/or people in client's immediate social world (e.g., client-centered approach).	The agent of change can be the individual; an advocate or ally; any person or group of people that changes the interaction; the community; the society's sociopolitical structure and systems; and art, culture, and media.
What is independence?	Independence is individual physical, cognitive, and mental ability to perform and capacity to make decisions.	Independence is individual physical and cognitive ability to perform everyday activities safely and in a reasonable amount of time.	Independence is the freedom to do what you want to do, when, where, and with whom you want; choice; power over life decisions; and control over everyday life and resources to support it.

Adapted by Joy Hammel and Access Living from Gill, C. (1999). *Models of disability*. Chicago, IL: Chicago Center for Disability Research; Linton, S. (1998). *Claiming disability: Knowledge and identity*. New York, NY: New York University Press; Longmore, P. K. (1995). The second phase: From disability rights to disability culture. *Disability Rag and Resource, 16*, 4–11; Oliver, M. (1996). *Understanding disability from theory to practice*. New York, NY: St. Martin's Press: Macmillan; Rioux, M. (1997). Disability: The place of judgment in a world of fact. *Journal of Intellectual Disability Research, 41*, 102–112.

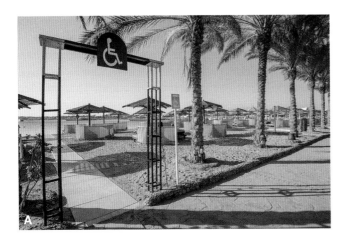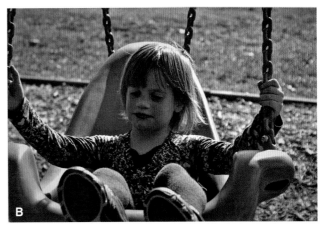

FIGURE 21-2 Universal design principles were employed at a beach to allow everyone access to the ocean (**A**) and at a playground to allow all children to participate (**B**).

approach and is an essential tool of the occupational therapist (Figure 21-2). Imagine the value of universal design principles (Letts, Rigby, & Stewart, 2003) applied to everyday life and social interaction. Envision a worker delivering goods with a hand truck, parents with baby strollers, and travelers with roll-aboard luggage as they all benefit from ramps, sidewalk curb cuts, elevators, and automatic door openers (Figure 21-3). Consider the simple change from a round door knob to a lever-operated door and how many people benefit from the ease of use of the lever. As you move about your environment, look for these "facilitators of function" and consider the range of individuals that benefit from these often taken-for-granted adaptations. Not all environments can be adapted for everyone, such as a steep, uneven mountain trail or the soft sand of seaside beach; however, technological advances are making travel in these areas increasingly available to those with

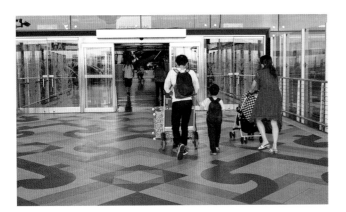

FIGURE 21-3 Universal design benefits the able-bodied as well as those with disabilities. Imagine this family trying to get through the doors of the airport if they didn't open automatically.

sensory or physical disabilities. Students and therapists are encouraged to learn about and use comprehensive checklists of universal design principles and features available at no cost, such as that developed by occupational therapists under the brand *SafeScore* (Pruett & Pruett, 2018).

Oppressive attitudes about disability have proven even harder to change than the environmental barriers, and this is an area of intense work by supporters of the social model. Oppression becomes even more pronounced when the disabled person's status intersects with other minority traits such as race, gender, or sexual orientation that creates a double or triple handicap for the person to negotiate (M. J. Deegan & Brooks, 1984; Fawcett, 2000; Gerschick, 2000; Hillyer, 1993). In this case, the social model has been influenced by perspectives shared with feminism, and the sociopolitical views of race, and gender activists. That is, societal beliefs, attitudes, practices, and ideologies must undergo structural change in order for the oppressed group to move freely, and participate equitably, within society.

Summarizing the key points of this section on models, we see contrasting views of where disability is located and how to minimize the effects of its disablement. From the classic medical model perspective, the individual with an illness or impairment is deficient and abnormal. A professional or team of professionals is required to heal, fix, or cure the deficiency in the individual's body through medication, surgery, and technology; and independence is the ultimate goal and measure of success. From a social model viewpoint, disability is simply another type of difference on the human continuum of difference (skin color, gender, size, ethnicity, etc.) and disablement is a result of oppressive social structures. Like all differences, especially those attributed to minority groups, there are positive and negative aspects of the lived experience, many of which are heavily influenced by social policies, practices, attitudes, and other constructs. Rather than change the individual through medical intervention to improve their ability to function toward professionally determined goals, needed change will come about in the social practices and structures that shape the individual's life experience. A welcoming and accessible society will promote opportunities for social participation by all people affected by disability (Oliver, 2013; Shakespeare, 2004) and we'll be that much closer to our utopian vision of full inclusion.

The Case for an Occupational Therapy Focus on Interdependence

History has shown that the most significant positive change for the disability minority has come about through direct activism and advocacy of people with disabilities (and their allies) as they have demanded their rights to equal treatment and participation (Berkowitz, 1987; Scotch, 1984). Independence is also a goal of activism, and its measure is in one's control over everyday life decisions and options. However, the way that independence is expressed has a much wider range of functioning across the disability spectrum and will frequently highlight the *interdependent* nature of human existence. The concept of interdependence is one that has only scant attention in the OT literature (Gage, 1997; Haywood & Lawlor, 2017; Levin & Martinez, 2016; N. Murphy et al., 1999; Reed, 2015) and has only slightly more attention in the disability studies field (Abrams, 2011; Grills, 2015; Levin & Martinez, 2016; Reindal, 1999; G. W. White, Simpson, Gonda, Ravesloot, & Coble, 2010) but will hopefully become a greater focus of research in both fields.

All humans are interdependent, and true independence from other human contact or endeavor is rarely achieved. Imagine the life of a fully independent person. They live off the grid; have no tools that they haven't made themselves out of raw materials they've assembled; eat only what they kill, forage, or grow; and have shelter and the ability to make fire. This independent person has no health care unless he or she creates it out of natural materials and his or her own knowledge of healing, and this person is content socializing and finding entertainment with oneself and nature.

Although at times in our technology-drenched lives, this existence may be momentarily attractive; its luster quickly fades when we realize all that we would trade in exchange. So why has independence taken on such a huge role in rehabilitation and in our U.S. society and

culture? The answer lies deeper than we can plumb in this chapter, but Reindal (1999) proposes that the roots lie in Enlightenment philosophy. In an oversimplification of history, the eighteenth century enlightenment period realized the development of the scientific method. That enabled early scientists to explain natural phenomena that offered independence from deeply held traditions of religious beliefs or supernatural explanations. Truth, as it had been handed down mostly by religious leaders and was unquestioned, became malleable and subject to discovery through careful observation and experimentation (Reindal, 1999). Humans were free to learn new secrets of nature to question infallible truths like the earth is round, not flat, and the moon is not a spirit, goddess, or divine light but solid sphere more like earth than something ethereal. The independent spirit was born.

If human independence was born in the Enlightenment, it was refined and perfected through the stories and images of the American pioneer. The early pioneers did have to build a great deal of self-reliance but with few exceptions even the most remote settler in the new country's wilderness probably had a manufactured weapon, flint and steel for fire, and an axe and a few tools made by others obtained through purchase or barter. Independence, economic self-sufficiency, and self-reliance became life goals and through America's evolution was strengthened by tales of men (women rarely featured in these stories) who "pulled themselves up by their bootstraps" or "went from rags to riches" or followed in the footsteps of the fictional heroes of stories by Horatio Alger (Scharnhorst, 1980). In the Horatio Alger myths, Alger's protagonists started life in rather deprived circumstances and through strong moral character, good deeds, and a wealthy benefactor that recognized the young man's (women were not Alger's protagonists) good work and work ethic, the protagonist rose into the ranks of the middle class, or even better. These influences became dominant cultural themes that further contributed to negative attitudes, whether of pity or disgust, toward people who were assumed incapable of pursuing this "American Dream" of independence.

Reindal (1999), a sociologist, writes that the disability rights movement could benefit from adopting a stronger focus on interdependence. The benefits would come from identifying, promoting, and educating the members and the general public on the interdependent nature of human life. Doing so would help deemphasize the importance of independence and lessen the stigma on dependence that people with disabilities experience as the general population realizes how much the seemingly most independent individuals among us are actually interdependent on others.

As you move into practice, consider how the typical focus of intervention on your clients becoming independent may in fact be setting them up for failure with a goal that is unattainable even by "normal" people. How might you use the language and concepts of interdependence to give them permission and affirmation in their reliance on adaptive equipment, PCAs, assistive technology, and medical treatments like medications and ongoing therapies? By stressing to your clients that we all need a supportive circle of social connections, friends, and family, you may help them learn how shared occupational interests often brings people together. Following are some examples of this approach:

- People with mental health conditions were provided with arranged social support, such as paid companions who checked in on them regularly by phone and shared social engagements like dining out or attending the cinema. The people with mental health conditions who had these interdependent relationships showed decreased symptomology and acute episodes, and some were able to decrease medication usage (Davidson, 2007).
- Equipping your client not only with the skills to brush their teeth by themselves but also by helping them to develop strategies to ease a new acquaintance's **existential anxiety**. Such anxiety is believed to stem from fear and anxiety of one's own disablement when confronted by people with disabilities (Frank & Stein, 2004).
- Developing interventions to prepare clients for the structural barriers they will face in their goal to live an engaged and participatory life. This can be challenging, especially in medical model settings. But if we are to truly serve our clients' best interests, our practice should be informed by the social model and concepts like interdependence, self-advocacy, and empowerment.

Disability Rights History, Policy, Empowerment, and Relationship to Occupational Therapy

Knowing the history of the **Disability Rights Movement (DRM)** and related **Independent Living Movement (ILM)** is useful for occupational therapists for two reasons. First, there are parallels to the evolution of our own profession, and understanding the intertwined history can provide useful insights into our place in the larger health care system. Secondly, this historical knowledge helps one identify both the sources of discrimination and oppression of people with disabilities as well as the source of empowerment gained through the events of that history. What follows is a condensed version of that history; for history enthusiasts, there are a number of excellent accounts that are presented from various perspectives, and although written in the midst of the early evolution of the movements, capture

history up to the publication date quite effectively. A list of some of them is available on thePoint.

Gary Kielhofner has described the evolution of the OT profession as a series of paradigmatic transitions (Kielhofner, 2009). He called the first transition that of preparadigm to the *paradigm of occupation* that began in 1917 with the OT founders' promotion of the innovative use of occupation as a healing agent. They conceptualized the use of occupation to combat the alienating and disabling forces of industrialization, war, and poor quality mental health. This revolutionary approach to supporting people not only with primarily mental but also physical disabilities acknowledged that people with disabilities had agency, dignity, and potential for meaningful lives. Occupational therapy's embrace of these more humane attitudes toward the disabled was part of a wave of activity in civic, political, and health care institutions that marked significant milestones in the march toward civil rights for people with disabilities. However, our history is not untarnished in the fact that the eugenics movement's ideas (a philosophy between 1880 and 1940 promoting genetic cleansing by sterilizing those with negative traits—such as congenital, developmental, or physical impairments) were embraced by Adolf Meyer, an innovative psychiatrist and strong proponent of the use of occupation in mental health treatment (Dowbiggin, 1997). This fact should be weighed in relation to Meyer's many contributions to OT and psychiatry such as his theory of psychobiology (Meyer, 1931/1957), the importance of collecting a patient's life history for best intervention (Frank, 1996), and powerful hypotheses about the mechanisms and applications of occupation (Gordon, 2009).

By the time OT was officially established, the U.S. federal government had instituted supports for disabled and blind veterans as early as the Revolutionary War of 1776 (Liachowitz, 1988; Shapiro, 1993) and funded the publication of braille books by 1879 (Oberman, 1965). However, there was actually very little political and social recognition of the plight of people with disabilities. States had begun developing worker compensation laws in 1911 that recognized the impact of on-the-job injuries to productivity when a person sustained a disabling injury (Berkowitz, 1987). Mutual aid societies, what we now called self-help, self-empowerment, or special interest groups, first formed in the United States at this time. The Disabled American Veterans (DAV) formed in 1920 to support the many soldiers injured in World War I (WWI), and the National Federation for the Blind (NFB) was established in 1921 (Scotch, 1984). These early aid societies were often formed by nondisabled supporters of these populations but eventually the disabled people themselves claimed more control as with the DAV or formed their own organizations such as the Paralyzed Veterans of America did in 1946 and as blind people formed the American Federation for the Blind in 1940.

Not all activity was progress for people with disabilities. A powerful example is the eugenics movement that eventually gained legislation first passed in the Commonwealth of Virginia that allowed forced sterilization of people shown to be "feebleminded, insane, depressed, mentally handicapped, epileptic and other" with alcoholics, criminals, and drug addicts subject to being legally sterilized (Dowbiggin, 1997, p. 76). When contested, the U.S. Supreme Court upheld this law with Chief Justice Holmes equating sterilization to vaccination. Eventually 27 states legalized wholesale sterilization programs that by 1970 had affected 60,000 "undesirables" (Dowbiggin, 1997; Scotch, 1984).

When Congress passed the landmark Social Security Act of 1935, it recognized the need for the federal government to provide support to a range of citizens with benefits including old age pensions, more supports for the blind, new programs for disabled children, and expansion of existing vocational rehabilitation programs that supported disabled workers. Perhaps the country's mood that supported this type of legislation helped embolden a group of people with disabilities in New York City that formed the League for the Physically Handicapped (LPH) to protest discrimination by the Works Progress Administration (WPA, a grand federal employment program). In what was likely to be considered the first civil disobedience protest by people with disabilities, members of the LPH held a sit-in at the Home Relief Bureau for 9 days and another at the WPA headquarters to protest discriminatory treatment in job hiring. These actions eventually led to the creation of 1,500 jobs for people with disabilities in New York City before the end of the decade (Longmore, 2003).

The carnage and impact on soldiers fighting in World War II (WWII) had an effect of accelerating medical and rehabilitative science and was an impetus for significant growth in the OT profession. Whereas WWI had been a powerful motivator in the development of "reconstruction aides" a core of women from whose work evolved the professions of OT and physical therapy (see Figures 2-4 and 2-5 in Chapter 2, "A Contextual History of Occupational Therapy"), military and health care leaders saw the need for more rehabilitation providers. This prompted the development and growth of several short-course OT training programs at a time when OT enrollments had been steadily falling through the 1930s (Gritzer & Arluke, 1985). This new generation of therapists was encouraged to embrace medical science and its technological advances. Occupational therapy and medical leaders urged therapists to adopt a more scientific approach to practice by breaking down essential therapeutic tasks into the core units. The OT would see the patient in a more machine-like way that could be fixed with the proper application of prescribed therapy units (e.g., a weighted arm to stack so many cones or application of psychodynamic concepts versus engagement in meaningful occupation). This period of the

"second paradigm of internal mechanisms" is commonly referred to as the mechanistic or reductionistic period of OT evolution (Kielhofner, 2009).

Occupational therapists practicing from the reductionistic paradigm were less likely to focus on the patient's larger life goals and instead seek interventions and goals that could more easily be quantified. Many benefits to the profession accrued from the reductionistic paradigm such as improved research methods, new understandings of neurophysiological underpinnings of performance and behavior, and development of technological solutions to dysfunction (e.g., adaptive equipment, assistive technology, and aids to function) as well as greater validation by our medical colleagues (Kielhofner, 2009). Medical approval was an important consideration since at that time, the American Medical Association was in charge of accrediting OT schools and had a role in certification of practitioners (Gritzer & Arluke, 1985).

The relevance for disability history of this transition to reductionism is that OT professionals were more likely to dictate predetermined goals to their patients than it was that they would collaborate to establish personally meaningful life goals. In this way, therapists became part of what has been called the *professionalization of disability* (Berkowitz, 1987; Gritzer & Arluke, 1985; Higgins, 1992). Professionalization occurs when medical and rehabilitation professionals take an inordinate degree of control over the fates of those they serve. Although well intended, a result to the person with a disability that experiences professionalization is disempowerment and overdependence on systems he or she relies on for his or her treatment. This might occur in medical and vocational rehabilitation systems that make pronouncements from professionals of when one is fully rehabilitated (regardless of patient satisfaction with that goal), how disabled they are (related to employment), or how successfully, or not, they completed the treatment team's goals. Disability scholars attribute the relatively slow progress of disability rights through the roughly 30 years following WWII to overprofessionalization because of how disabled people in physical or mental rehabilitation systems were thus disempowered (Berkowitz, 1992; Higgins, 1992; Scotch, 1984; Shapiro, 1993).

The three decades between 1940 and 1970 were not bereft of change that benefitted people with disabilities; however, the disabled themselves were less often a direct actors in those changes. Beneficial policy and health care practice improvements were most often implemented by temporarily able-bodied allies (Shapiro, 1993). A number of legislative and administrative policies were adopted that improved life for people with disabilities such as improvements to social security. For example, provisions for SSDI that provided cash and other assistance to disabled workers passed in 1956. Also, vocational rehabilitation benefits and services were extended to the severely disabled such as PCAs, homemaker services, and job training (Thomson, 1997).

However, disability policy through this period viewed disability " . . . as a loss to be compensated for, rather than difference to be accommodated. Disability then becomes a personal flaw, and disabled people are the 'able-bodied' gone wrong. Difference thus translates into deviance" (Thomson, 1997, p. 49). This perceived deviance continued the stigmatization and marginalization of this second-class citizenry.

Recognizing the very low percentage of people with disabilities who were working, President Harry Truman initiated the President's Committee on Employment of the Physically Handicapped (PCEH) in 1952. The PCEH was charged with promoting work opportunities for the handicapped and monitoring national rehabilitation programs (Scotch, 1984). Decades later, this committee was renamed the President's Committee on Employment of People with Disabilities, or PCEPD (Worklife, 1989), a group that helped build support for passage of the ADA (Shapiro, 1993). In spite of decades of work by these committees, unemployment rates over that time period for working-age adults who would like to work are typically twice as high as the nondisabled. Among some populations with more severe disabilities (e.g., severe schizophrenia or people with major wheelchair reliance), unemployment can be as high as 70% (International Center for the Disabled, 1986; Kessler Foundation/National Organization on Disability, 2010; National Organization on Disability, 1998).

Unemployment continues to be a significant problem among people with disabilities. In general, the unemployment rate of working-age people with disabilities who would like to work is double that of the temporarily able-bodied population. This statistic has been fairly stable for the past 30 years, through both good economic times and bad (e.g., the recession that began in 2008). Although the ADA has improved work options for the disabled slightly since its passage in 1990, for example, by improving physical access to many workplaces. People with disabilities put crucial benefits at risk once their income rises to a level considered a living wage what the SSA calls "substantial gainful activity (SGA)". In 2018, the SGA figure was $1,180 for nonblind people with disabilities and $1,970 for a blind person (SSA, 2018a), figures that point out inequities built into the SSA system. That is, due to SSA limitations and caps, a disabled work will lose dependable health care benefits and other social security benefits like paid personal care assistance once their earnings rise above the SGA. Although tweaks to both the ADA and SSA policies over the last 20 years have been more supportive of disabled workers, the bottom line is that once a person achieves a stable work and earnings record (30 months of continuous employment with pay above the SGA), they lose access to federal and state provided health care and to other cash benefits like the supplement to pay for PCA.

During the postwar years, momentum was growing for oppressed groups, especially Black Americans, to work toward and eventually demand their civil rights through civil protest and other activist strategies. The history of the black civil rights movement is highly relevant to the evolution of disability-related civil rights for it provided a template for how minority groups gain a powerful voice in civic and policy dialogue (Liachowitz, 1988; Scotch, 1984). Years of struggle led to passage of The Civil Rights Act (Pub. L. 88-352), signed July 2, 1964 by President Lyndon Johnson (see Figure 2-13), that prohibited discrimination on the basis of race, religion, ethnicity, national origin, and creed (gender was added later). This Act outlawed discrimination on the basis of race in public accommodations and employment as well as in federally assisted programs. In drafting the provisions of the Act, then Senator Hubert Humphrey attempted to include people with disabilities in the groups protected under this law. However, other supporters of the civil rights bill feared that addition of the ill-defined class of the handicapped would dilute civil rights gains and decrease the chances for passage (Scotch, 1984). It would be over 25 years before a similar law was enacted to grant similar rights to people with disabilities in the form of the ADA (Pub. L. 103-336).

Several factors emerging in the 1960s forward converged to lay the foundation for the Disability Rights Movement and Independent Living Movement. Those factors included powerful activists with disabilities, adoption of nonviolent protest tactics, a failure of prior legislation (e.g., the Rehabilitation Act of 1973 with its Section 504 [Pub. L. 93-112]) to achieve equal access, frustration by disabled people with limited life options, deinstitutionalization of people with mental health conditions, and a growing recognition that all people with disabilities share the experience of marginalization and oppression (Shapiro, 1993; Winter, 2003). Although the ILM and the DRM are often considered distinct movements, many of their goals are overlapping, and therefore for our purposes here, we will consider them synonymous. The DRM is a worldwide, member-driven sociopolitical movement dedicated to the acquisition of full and equal opportunities for people with disabilities to enjoy full social participation without discrimination in housing, transportation, leisure, education, and civic participation (Figure 21-4) (Shakespeare, 2006b; Winter, 2003). These activities can be summed up using the OTPF term of the *occupation of social participation* (AOTA, 2014a). In summary, "disability rights movements seek to replace oppression with empowerment, and, marginalization with full inclusion" (Winter, 2003, p. 32).

People with severe disabilities and primarily physical conditions such as quadriplegia and cerebral palsy were attempting to work, live more independently, or attend college and found attitudinal and structural barriers blocking their access. Their advocacy and activism informed government entities and public businesses that they deserved a "place at the table" and they would not accept no for an answer. These soldiers in the fight for

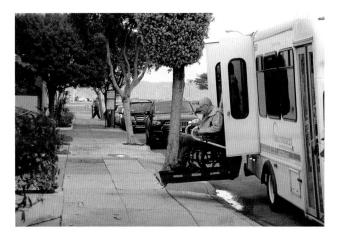

FIGURE 21-4 Access to public transportation is a focus of the Disability Rights Movement (DRM).

disability rights started using nonviolent methods like sit-ins, picketing, marches, and, most effectively, the occupation of congressional offices and federal agencies that had the most influence on policy change (Figure 21-5). The DRM emerged as a true movement following a series of civil disobedience actions to pressure Joseph Califano Jr.,

President Jimmy Carter's Secretary of Health, Education, and Welfare, to sign regulations to implement the provisions of the Rehabilitation Act of 1973 (Pub. L. 93-112). The Rehabilitation Act, as it's often called, included Section 504 which granted civil rights in programs, employment, and services offered by the federal government to people with disabilities through language adopted from the original Civil Rights Act. Califano was refusing to sign the regulations and disability activists coordinated a nationwide protest of sit-ins and occupations. One such occupation of the New York Health Education and Welfare (HEW) office, led by Judy Heumann, lasted 25 days and helped push Califano to finally sign the regulations. This action played out in newspapers and on television news stories, and was such a dramatically different image of people with disabilities that it took many by surprise, and challenged the notion of the disabled as pitiable and helpless victims. It was a major step toward empowerment of people with disabilities and strengthening the coalition of what had been disparate groups.

As promising as Section 504 was for people with disabilities to be able to come out of the shadows of their marginalization, it had only very limited impact on the

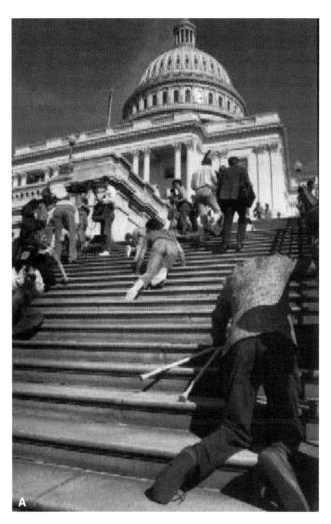

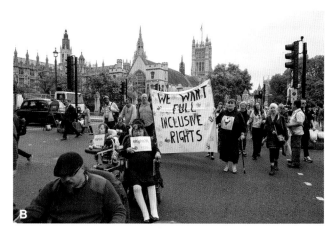

FIGURE 21-5 Collective activism was used by persons with disabilities during the fight to pass the Americans with Disabilities Act in 1964 (**A**) and is still used today (**B**) where activists from Disabled People Against Cuts (DPAC) marched on Downing Street in London to protest the closing of the Independent Living Fund in the United Kingdom.

disabled gaining their rights. Also, in the mid-1970s Congress, recognized the impact of discrimination in public schools in which children with disabilities were often segregated in "handicapped schools" or not educated at all. The Education for All Handicapped Children Act (Pub. L. 94-142), later modified and renamed the *Individuals with Disabilities Education Act* (IDEA), granted the right to a "free appropriate education" for all children with disabilities. The IDEA also provides for services to infants and children. Through the empowerment realized through the DRM and increased visibility in public, employment, and in education, disability advocates continued to pressure Congress to take action and by the late 1980s, a broad coalition of individuals, disability organizations, and able-bodied allies drafted language for the ADA. Lex Frieden, an educator, activist, researcher, and disability policy expert, is considered a primary architect of the ADA and one of the founders of the ILM. Frieden also co-authored an article with occupational therapist Jean Cole

Spencer that outlined the OT role in the ILM (Frieden & Cole, 1985) as well as a statement about how the profession could support the success of the ADA (Frieden, 1992).

The conditions were growing for evolution of the third Contemporary Paradigm of Occupation (Kielhofner, 2009), although wider acceptance would not occur in the profession until the 1990s and beyond. Although some therapists (Reilly, 1962; West, 1989; Yerxa, 1967) never abandoned a belief in the healing power of occupation as the force that made OT unique and gave it the promise of making highly innovative contributions to health care and society, their voices did not find a substantial audience until the 1980s. The current of reductionism continued flowing strongly in the final decades of the twentieth century and into the twenty-first century. However, factors introduced into research, education, and practice such as disability scholarship, the growth of disability studies programs (Jarman & Kafer, 2014), systems theory (von Bertalanffy, 1968), and ecological theories (Bronfenbrenner, 1979) laid

CENTENNIAL NOTES

Leading Disability Advocates and Founders of the Disability Rights Movement

Some of the leading disability advocates include the following. These prominent disability advocates either directly or indirectly had a significant effect on the evolution of occupational therapy perspectives on topics such as independence, interdependence, and social participation by claiming their place in society and helping expand the roles that PWD could play in society:

- Ed Roberts, who had total quadriplegia from polio, founded the Center for Independent Living (CIL), a consumer-run (i.e., people with disabilities) advocacy and resource service to promote independent living. After suing for admission to college and to live in the dorm versus a nursing home, Ed graduated and was soon denied services by Vocational Rehabilitation for being "too disabled." Years later, he was appointed as the head of the California Vocational Rehabilitation (VR) Department.
- Judy Heumann, also with a polio-related disability, had to fight to earn her educational degrees and right to work as a teacher. Heumann founded Disabled in Action and eventually was appointed assistant secretary of Education for Special Education and Rehabilitative Services in the Clinton administration.
- Wade Blank, founder of American Disabled for Attendant Programs Today (ADAPT), was an able-bodied ally of the movement who could not tolerate the neglectful circumstances for young disabled

people that he saw in his job as a nursing home manager. He led ADAPT in successful protests against the Denver public transportation system for not having accessible buses and later focused on more independent, and less costly housing options to move people of all ages out of nursing homes (The Ragged Edge, 1993).
- Lex Frieden was a teenager when he broke his neck in a diving accident. He eventually became a congressional staff member and helped create the National Institute on Disability and Rehabilitation Research (NIDRR), a unit of the U.S. Department of Education and later on the National Council on Disability (NCD) in the mid-1980s. His work there and later as a staffer for another Congress member positioned him to contribute significantly to the writing and passage of the Americans with Disabilities Act (ADA). President George H. W. Bush appointed him to serve as the executive director of the NCD in 2002. In that capacity, he directed a study of the implementation of the ADA and used the results to gain passage of the ADA Improvements Act of 2008. He went on to teach and research about rehabilitation and independent living at Baylor University and has been the director of the Independent Living Research Utilization (ILRU) program there.

Alliances such as the one struck between occupational therapists Jean Cole Spencer and Lex Frieden (Frieden & Cole, 1985) helped reflect another paradigmatic change in the profession of OT that supported a return to the roots of the profession.

a fertile ground for a revised look at occupation that could still retain the technological advances obtained from the mechanistic period (Kielhofner, 2009). Another factor was recognition by people with disabilities that they should be treated as *people* for whom mechanistic prescriptions in rehabilitation would improve aspects of functioning but would not support a fuller recovery. In order to recover their challenged identities (Christiansen, 1999; J. A. White, 1999) and dignity, rehabilitation patients needed a more holistic approach that acknowledged their agency, supported their own understanding of their conditions, and prepared them more effectively for independent and interdependent living (Bachelder, 1985; Bowen, 1993; Crewe & Zola, 1983; DeJong, 1979; Frieden, 1983). These and other factors made it easier for occupational therapists to adopt new ideas such as the one presented through the operationalization of a client-centered approach to collaborative goal setting with the Canadian Occupational Performance Measure (COPM) (Law et al., 1990). The COPM was grounded in the *Canadian Model of Occupational Performance*, an early OT model emphasizing the PEO interaction and identifying a spiritual component of the person that represents the motivation and meaning in life that's derived from, and shaped by, their engagement in occupations—the doing in life (Law, Baptiste, & Mills, 1995; Law et al., 2005; Townsend, De Laat, Egan, Thibeault, & Wright, 1999).

The introduction of the innovative scientific discipline of *occupational science* in 1989 at the University of Southern California, also propelled the evolution of the contemporary paradigm of occupation. Derived from a recognition that OT would be strengthened by growth in knowledge of the profession's primary therapeutic tool-occupation, occupational science extended an in-depth look at the form, function, and meaning of occupation (Clark, 1993; Yerxa, 1989). This research into occupation has gone well-beyond typical ways and topics of research in the practice profession of OT. The study of occupation has expanded and is now well established in many countries, further building an international and intercultural perspective on occupation as well as views on the disability experience around the world, and how this knowledge is used in practice.

The expanded boundaries of our understanding of occupation contributed significantly to the third paradigm as evidenced in guiding practice documents like the OTPF (AOTA, 2014a) and provided a foundation for new concepts that expand how OT can be applied. An idea that emerged in the late 1990s is *occupational justice* (Townsend & Whiteford, 2005) that recognizes the *occupational deprivation* that is caused by the social exclusion of persons with disability (PWD). Another newly interpreted concept is the identification of the importance of an individually determined balance of creative, productive, self-maintaining, and leisure activities called *occupational*

balance (Matuska & Christiansen, 2009). This balance is a state that is more difficult for high numbers of PWD to achieve when precluded from employment by discriminatory barriers. Recognition that political practices and policies systematically oppress populations led to the identification of *occupational apartheid*, a term related to the experience of black South Africans only in that they experienced systematic deprivation of occupational opportunity that readily applies to circumstances that marginalize PWD (Kronenberg & Pollard, 2005). A final example of third paradigm influences comes from Australian occupational therapist Anne Wilcock, an early occupational scientist who traced evolutionary views of occupation (Wilcock & Hocking, 2015). Her history provides evidence for the essential need that humans, across the ability spectrum, have for occupation and supported an OT view of a population as a client (AOTA, 2014a). When we view the population of 56 million PWD (SSA, 2018b) as a client, it makes it easier for us to see how advocacy for disability rights can be an appropriate focus of our practices. When we practice in this way we are engaging in what Frank Kronenberg and colleagues call pADL or *political activities of daily living* (Kronenberg & Pollard, 2005; Pollard, Kronenberg, & Sakellariou, 2008; Whiteford, 2007a).

This type of pADL practice benefits from awareness of the social construct of disability, knowledge of legislative practices, policy development, and a commitment to the population being served by your pADL practices. However, one can incorporate pADL in many smaller ways such as participating in a national or state OT legislative day, writing to your legislator about disability-related needs in your community, joining AOTA and your state OT association to support lobbying for the profession and disability issues, or speaking out when you see discriminatory behavior in your community. Many stories exist about how occupational therapists have practiced pADL in traditional and unique settings (Agner, 2017; Boggis, 2009; Smith & Hilton, 2008; Whiteford, 1997, 2014). A fascinating example of how pADL practices helped identify the potentially disabling effects of the pollution, water contamination, and occupational disruption and deprivation caused by mountaintop mining was conducted by students and faculty at Eastern Kentucky University (A. Marshall, 2003). Sabriye Tenberken is a blind woman (not an occupational therapist but who used occupation effectively) who challenged the socially constructed nature of blindness in Tibet to bring blind children out of isolation and seclusion. In her story "The Right to Be Blind without Being Disabled" (Tenberken & Kronenberg, 2005), she developed a school for the blind and provided students with education and employable skills. However, first she had to advocate and argue for the blind children's potential against traditional views that their disability was supernatural retribution for past misdeeds of family members. Families dealt with the stigma and shame that resulted by hiding away the children from public exposure (Tenberken & Kronenberg, 2005). Some years after founding the school Braille Without Borders, Tenberken co-led, with Erik Weihenmayer, the first blind climber to summit Mt. Everest, a party of former students who were blind, on a high altitude climbing expedition featured in the documentary film *Blindsight* (Orr & Walker, 2008).

The fact that the evolution of the DRM and the social model coincided with the third paradigm in OT was not just coincidence because they emerged from the influence of several forces such as a new appreciation of human agency through human rights campaigns, growing recognition and appreciation of narrative research methods that revealed more about a person's experience and meaning, and a realization that medicine, surgery, and technology can only take a person so far in their recovery. Plus, disability scholarship was contributing a new perspective that was influencing OT and occupational science scholars to consider a more ecological view of the OT intervention process (Kielhofner, 2009). As the value of occupation became more apparent through the work of occupational scientists and occupational therapists embracing the social model and considering the influence of environments on disability and occupation, it became easier to build alliances with the DRM. As part of this movement into the contemporary paradigm of occupation, researchers moved from reductionistic quantitative methods into more phenomenological (i.e., what happened and what does it mean) and ethnographic (description of lives and culture) methodologies grouped under qualitative research. These more narrative accounts highlighted the life stories of people's experience in and out of therapy and when combined as mixed methods (quantitative and qualitative approaches), provided meaning to the numbers and statistics (Denzin & Lincoln, 2018).

Spirituality, client centeredness, and occupation, the doing of life, became a central focus within OT practice (Kielhofner, 2009). These ideas and methods supported by an occupational justice framework opened up new possibilities for occupational therapists to work in new ways and with new populations to reach underserved groups of people with disabilities, for example, individuals who are incarcerated (Cesaroni & Peterson-Badali, 2010; Duncan, Munro, & Nicol, 2003; Farnworth, Morgan, & Fernando, 1987; Hamilton, 2007; Whiteford, 2007b) or homeless (C. A. Marshall, Lysaght, & Krupa, 2017; Tryssenaar, Jones, & Lee, 1999), especially those with co-occurring disorders of mental illness and addiction, and people with HIV/AIDS (Bedell & Kaplan, 1996; Clark & Jackson, 1990; Ramugondo, 2005), and to work in collaboration with public health practitioners and methods toward prevention of disabling conditions (Braveman, 2016). Other practice and research projects that are part of this paradigm have addressed the needs of community-dwelling elders to mitigate or prevent disability (Clark et al., 1997; Mandel, Jackson, Zemke, Nelson, & Clark, 1999). The third paradigm of OT supported expansion of our understanding of occupation and its applications to innovative practices and populations. What steps can you take as a student and new therapist to reach groups of people who have limited access to health intervention in ways that can support their social participation and dismantle barriers to health and participation inherent in the social construct of disability?

Key Legislation and Policy Affecting People with Disabilities

Although many consider the United States a leader in pioneering civil rights laws for people with disabilities based on passage of Section 504 of the Rehabilitation Act in 1973 and the ADA in 1990, as early as 1968, African countries of Zambia (Handicapped Persons Act) and South Africa (Blind Persons Act) adopted laws assuring nondiscrimination and/or disability-related rights. Many other countries were developing laws related to disability rights and benefits to services before or almost simultaneous to the ADA (Disability Rights Education and Defense Fund [DREDF], 2018). For a comprehensive and up-to-date list of disability related laws in all other countries, visit the DREDF Website https://dredf.org.

Disability rights, as a subset of civil rights, are somewhat unique. We usually think that civil rights apply to classes of people that are based on fixed characteristics such as gender, skin color, race, or, perhaps the most changeable, religion. Although a minority of U.S. citizens (17%; Kraus, Lauer, Coleman, & Houtenville, 2018) to whom disability rights apply are born with an impairment that qualifies them to be considered disabled, the majority of the 1 billion people in the world with a disability (15% of world population) acquire the disabling condition, through injury, illness, or accident (World Health Organization, 2011). As such, one might think that civil rights for people with disabilities would be the easiest to move into policy and law, that these would be the rights that everyone would strive for and uphold, because everyone is only one concussion, car accident, or disabling illness away from falling into that class. This potentially temporary status of able-bodiedness is why some in the disability community refer to people without disabilities as TAB or the Temporarily Able-Bodied (Goodley, 2017; "To: The Temporarily Able-Bodied," 2007). One hypothesis as to why there is not stronger support for disability rights and law is that when TABs see people with impairments, disfigurements, or incapacities, they are reminded in an unpleasant way, of their own frailty, and potential disablement. This existential anxiety (Frank & Stein, 2004; Hahn, 1988) leads the person so affected to at the least turn away and attempt to ignore the offending party, at worst, the able-bodied person takes actively hostile or discriminatory action toward the disabled person or population in general.

Even in the face of the strong bipartisan passage of the ADA (Pub. L. 103-336) and almost 30 years to implement its purpose to "assure equality of opportunity, full participation, independent living, and economic self-sufficiency for such individuals" (Pub. L. 103-336, § 2[8]), we have fallen far short of this aim.

People who experience difference due to psychological, physical, or developmental disabilities have typically been treated in ways that tend to push them to the margins of society and limit their choices of occupations and roles, thus constraining their social participation. Although these occupational deprivations tend to occur less frequently for those with less visible disabilities, their social participation is also limited. Recognition of these limitations across the disability spectrum is what finally moved the scale of justice to favor granting civil rights to citizens with disabilities in the form of the ADA.

ADA

The ADA (Pub. L. 103-336) is a comprehensive civil rights law that mandates equal opportunities for people with disabilities in American society in the areas of employment, public services, public accommodation, transportation, and telecommunication. This Act was signed into law by President George Bush on July 26, 1990. It reflected the culmination of strong bipartisan Congressional action as prompted by a grassroots lobbying effort of diverse disability and civil rights groups. Activists of the DRM had worked for over two decades to show the American people and government that more than 43 million people with disabilities (at that time) constituted a minority group which had been systematically excluded from social participation based solely on his or her disability status. That exclusion had persisted in spite of the Section 504 law that had made some inroads into these discriminatory practices but only in a limited way in the federal agencies and some contractors. The efforts of the DRM in passing the ADA were aided by a coalition of supporters for disability and civil rights that included the American Coalition of Citizens with Disabilities, Reverend Jesse Jackson, the Leadership Conference on Civil and Human Rights, and even corporate support from Dupont, IBM, and Marriott (Altman & Barnartt, 1993).

However, in spite of such a broad coalition of support, and although the final ADA version contained the essential titles of earlier drafts, the law was enacted with a number of weakening compromises. A few examples of those compromises are that the Act required less stringent compliance deadlines and placed a limit on the size of business to be affected (15 or more employees) (Shapiro, 1993). Also, instead of the requirement for *all* buildings to be made accessible, only new construction and buildings undergoing major renovation would need to comply with accessibility guidelines (Shapiro, 1993; Watson, 1993). There were no provisions covering health care policies in the enacted law perpetuating one of the most significant work disincentives affecting PWD seeking employment (DeJong & Batavia, 1990) or was there an affirmative action policy to encourage hiring qualified job candidates (Nosek, 1992; Watson, 1993).

The ADA as enacted had few provisions for enforcement of its regulations, and those that were specified divided enforcement among various federal agencies (e.g., Equal Employment Opportunity Commission, Department of Justice, Department of Transportation). There are no ADA requirements for affected entities to report compliance, and it is the individual's obligation to challenge discrimination when it is encountered—a significant barrier to enforcement due to the complex and intimidating nature of litigation, especially against employers who typically have more resources with which to engage in litigation. Therefore, refinement and definition of the law has evolved through the interpretation and testing of specific legal cases in court. Unfortunately, the courts have most often taken the narrow interpretation of the law that has made it harder for PWD to realize full benefit of the rights granted. However, based on these challenges, Congress passed the ADA Amendment Act of 2008 (Pub. L. 110-325) and some of these weaknesses in the law were addressed. The primary changes broadened the definition of disability and clarified accessibility guidelines for public and government facilities. The Amendments also placed more responsibility on the courts to determine if disability-based discrimination has occurred rather than the prior emphasis on whether or not the individual meets the criteria of that definition. The ADA proposed a new focus on access, ability, and accommodation. This policy stance is stated clearly in the "Findings and Purposes" of the Act.

> The continuing existence of unfair and unnecessary discrimination and prejudice denies people with disabilities the opportunity to compete on an equal basis and to pursue those opportunities for which our free society is justifiably famous, and costs the United States billions of dollars in unnecessary expenses resulting from dependency and nonproductivity. (42 U.S.C. § 12101 [a][8])

This statement recognizes that from an economic as well as socio-political perspective, discrimination based solely on the basis of a person's disability must be eliminated. Congress further acknowledged that such discrimination is based on "stereotypic assumptions" about people with disabilities that do not adequately consider the abilities of such people to contribute to society. And by including in their definition of disability people who may be "perceived as having" a disability, even if they don't (42 U.S.C. § 12101 [a][2]), Congress made clear the desire to eliminate the attitudinal component of the social construct of disability (J. A. White, 1999). The tenets of the law and subsequent amendments that are useful for the OT practitioner to know are, beginning with the definition of an "otherwise qualified individual" (someone who fits the definition). In some circumstances, the definition includes parents associated with an individual known to have a disability and employees who are retaliated against for assisting others who assert his or her rights under the ADA (Pub. L. 103-336).

Occupational therapy implication: Regarding "a limitation in a major life activity," OT has an important opportunity, considering occupational therapists are the experts in assessing occupational performance across the range of life activities. This also opens opportunities for occupational therapists to serve as expert witnesses in court or to assess performance capacity for another's testimony. Learn a basic overview of this role in "*The Occupational Therapist as an Expert Witness*" (DeMaio-Feldman, 1987).

The ADA has five "titles" or subsections that describe who and what is affected by the law, and what compliance means for the "covered entities" (e.g., depending on the title, it might be a public or private employer, government agency, public accommodation such as a cinema, restaurant, or retail business, and transportation companies).

Title I (42 U.S.C. § 12111), the employment antidiscrimination section, covering recruitment to discharge for employers with 15 or more employees. It is useful to know the terms in quotes as they apply to OT across a wide spectrum. Employers must offer "reasonable accommodations," an adaptation that helps the individual meet the "essential functions" of the job (a list of all the tasks and physical and cognitive demands of the work). The accommodations must be "readily achievable" and will not present an "undue hardship" on the employer (i.e., will not cost the employer a disproportionate amount relative to the value the typical worker produces and the size of the business) and providing that the work of the individual does not pose a "direct threat" to the health or safety of others in the workplace (meaning, coworkers or clients can't be put at risk). Due to the disability myth that people with mental health conditions are violent, many employers have used this stigmatizing defense for not hiring disabled applicants.

Enforcement is handled by the Equal Employment Opportunity Commission (EEOC). The onus of enforcement is on the person experiencing discrimination. The person must file a charge against the employer who the EEOC considers. If EEOC deems discrimination was likely in the case, they issue a letter for the "right to sue." In cases of grievous discrimination, EEOC may pursue litigation against the employer to help build case law supporting Title I. Litigation is emotionally and financially costly for both sides, and many PWD put up with discrimination rather than sue until the discrimination ends the job, or becomes too intolerable (J. A. White, 1999). However, in 2 years following passage of the ADA Amendment Act, litigation increased 20% (Heathfield, 2018) related to improvements in the law for PWD.

Occupational therapy implication: With the knowledge that occupational therapists have about activity analysis, task grading, and adaptation, they are well-suited to help determine essential functions, develop reasonable accommodations, and assess a person's occupational performance capacities needed to meet the essential functions with or without accommodation.

Title II (42 U.S.C. § 12131) *Subtitle A* affects publicly funded services and agencies such as municipal, county, and state, most public schools (the federal government is covered by Section 504 of the Rehabilitation Act of 1973). *Subtitle B* of Title II applies to public transportation agencies that were not previously covered (e.g., air carriers were covered by Air Carrier Access Act of 1986). (1) "Fixed route," the typical type of urban bus service; (2) "demand responsive," paratransit services; (3) commuter rail service; and (4) inter-city rail services will have to fully accessible by 2020.

Occupational therapy implication: Similar services as provided for Title I could be provided to public entities for employment-related services. As described next under Title III implications, occupational therapists could consult with public transportation entities, but there's more complexity to the public transportation access guidelines related to various conveyances and multiple laws addressing each type of transport.

Title III (42 U.S.C. § 12181) covers public accommodations and services that are operated by private entities such as theaters, hotels, private schools, retailers, and restaurants. This title extends Section 504 provisions to the private business sector to have an accessible physical structure. This provision requires that buildings and services be made fully accessible when "readily achievable," or if this poses an "undue burden" on the business or entity, then making reasonable accommodation to provide access or services to the patron with a disability. All new construction and major renovations after 1992 would need to comply with the ADA Accessibility Guidelines (ADAAG) with the troubling exception that 2-story buildings do not need elevators but 3 or more story buildings do. Yet, the language and spirit of Title III is intended to provide a "vision of an inclusive public world" (Parmet, 1993, p. 128) that truly belongs to all of us.

The key provision reads

> No individual shall be discriminated against on the basis of disability in the full and equal enjoyment of the goods, services, facilities, privileges, advantages, or accommodations of any place of public accommodation by any person who owns, leases (or leases to), or operates a place of public accommodation (42 U.S.C. 12182 § 302[a]).

Occupational therapy implication: The ADAAG compliance regulations are extensive but well-worth knowing to support consultation with businesses that want to improve access, and for identifying noncompliant businesses. This offers a chance to practice pADL by offering education to clients on the guidelines. Additionally, OT practitioners can advocate on a local level by respectfully encouraging the business to improve access and compliance, consult with them on the standards, or in severe cases, report the infraction.

Title IV: Independent use of telecommunication services is the focus (42 U.S.C. 12201 § 401) in support of people with hearing and speech impairments and actually is an amendment to Title II of the Communications Act of 1934. Private telecommunication carriers must provide relay services or appropriate equipment so that people with disabilities can have full use of the national telecommunications system. A TT or TTY (i.e., text telephone), that allows sound or graphic communication, is the most likely device to be used, and often replaces the more traditional TDDs (telecommunication devices for the deaf). Advances in the internet since 1990, cellular phones, and software applications such text messaging, social media, and email have lessened the importance of this Title, but there are still people in need of these communication aids related to lack of internet access, low income, or preference (Maiorana-Basas & Pagliaro, 2014). The prevalence of closed captioning is partially due to this Title (42 U.S.C. 12201 § 402), although the law only requires television providers to caption the verbal content of public service announcements. Closed captioning is a good example of Universal Design because it enables most TV viewers to know what is happening on screen by reading, even in noisy areas or when the sound is turned off.

Occupational therapy implication: Primarily for therapists working with the deaf or hard of hearing who may need these services.

Title V (42 U.S.C. § 12201) includes various "Miscellaneous Provisions" which describe the relationship of the ADA to other laws such as the Rehabilitation Act of 1973. This title states that the ADA would not hold precedent over a law with stricter standards, for example, Sections 501 and 504 of the Rehabilitation Act of 1973 or the same for any state or local law, which provides greater or equal protection for the targeted individuals. This title allows the collection of attorney's fees that result from

action related to the ADA and calls for the development of Technical Assistance Guides (TAGs) by appropriate agencies: to facilitate implementation of the various titles. Also in Title V, Congress included itself as being subject to the antidiscrimination provisions of the ADA. Title V further amended the Rehabilitation Act of 1973 to clarify that only drug addicts and alcoholics whose job performance is not impaired by the use of such drugs can be considered as disabled under this law (i.e., they must not be actively using). Finally, Congress uses Title V to encourage "alternative dispute resolution" (i.e., means other than full litigation) to settle conflicts of discrimination whenever possible. Using language from the title, transvestitism, homosexuality, and pedophilia as not being impairments that are considered disabilities for the purpose of the Act.

Occupational therapy implication: The most significant aspect of this section for OT practitioners is the provision that drug addiction and alcoholism be considered disabilities as long as the addict is in recovery. This information could be useful for those working in addiction services, particularly in relation to teaching advocacy skills to overcome discrimination.

Enforcement for Titles II, III, and V is carried out by the Department of Justice (DOJ), and similar to Title I, there is little active enforcement (i.e., the DOJ doesn't actively seek out noncompliance). Therefore, it is up to people with disabilities and his or her allies (like occupational therapists) to call out this discrimination when it appears and support the decision of the people experiencing it to follow his or her conscience in filing charges or not.

Other Disability Policies

The *Section 504 of Rehabilitation Act of 1973* was hastily added to the annual vocational rehabilitation funding authorization bill and was the section that prohibits discrimination against PWD in federal agencies, contractors, and those receiving federal grants, including universities (Watson, 1994). Language and provisions in Section 504 laid the foundation for framing the ADA. However, prior to passage of this law, individuals with severe disabilities had previously been excluded from vocational rehabilitation due to the expectation that the disabilities would prevent them from successful employment (Berkowitz, 1987; Shapiro, 1993), and gaining access to employment and education services through this law was a substantial improvement for people with severe disabilities (e.g., tetraplegia, severe cerebral palsy, chronic schizophrenia), although there is a history of people with mental health conditions being underserved compared to those with physical disabilities (Berkowitz, 1987). However, as a force for change, it was more symbolic than pragmatic in changing the social construct of disability for at least three reasons. It only applied to the federal government and it had no "teeth" for enforcement. Last, it had no guidelines for implementation until 1977 (recall that Califano did not sign the implementation regulations until pressured by disability protests that provided impetus for the DRM).

The failure of the Rehabilitation Act of 1973 to substantially change participatory options for people with disabilities is an instructive case for the importance of effective implementation. Recall that Section 504 was a rather sudden inclusion in the Rehabilitation Act. The rapid action involved in attaching it to the law apparently involved little forethought of how it would be implemented. Occupational therapy practitioners involved with federal agencies, contractors, or universities receiving federal grants should know the distinction of which law, Section 504 or ADA, applies to clients served.

Genetic Information Nondiscrimination Act of 2008 (GINA): As genetic information and technology has advanced, this law was passed to prohibit discrimination based on genetic information about or related to an individual in employment or access to insurance services. Because some disabilities are inherited, there have been successful disability discrimination cases won based on this law (http://www.ginahelp.org/GINAhelp.pdf).

Work Disincentives

Many laws have been passed and regulations adopted to support people with disabilities to gain or return to work. Although each has had at least a small impact on the problem of disability unemployment, the net result is what Edward Berkowitz (1987) calls a patchwork of policies and programs many of which create *work disincentives*. These disincentives create dilemmas for PWD who want to work but have to wade through a complex set of rules and regulations. Often, the rules are related to several different state and federal agencies and the person is juggling a fragile set of financial and daily living benefits that may disappear or be reduced with long-term successful employment. A work disincentive is anything that discourages a person to work and more specific to our purpose, a governmentally provided benefit that makes it more attractive not to work.

The primary disincentives that occur in the U.S. welfare and disability insurance programs are related to access to cash payments, health care insurance, and disability-related services. Cash payments most often come to PWD through SSI, SSDI, and sometimes through private disability insurance. Health care insurance may come through a family member's employment health care plan or for the wealthy, a privately paid policy, but most PWD rely on Centers for Medicare & Medicaid Services (CMS) programs. The CMS has one of two ways to insure the poor and disabled. Medicare is for people over retirement age and certain younger people with disabilities. Most PWD

who are under the age of retirement (minimally age 65 years) get insurance through Medicaid. Medicaid is cofunded by each state in partnership with federal funds through CMS; some states are fairly generous with these benefits, and others are not. As such, the amount that any state provides for health care for a disabled person varies widely. The Affordable Care Act (ACA or Obamacare) was passed to help minimize those variances, but for political reasons, a number of typically more conservative states rejected the ACA, and these states usually have less Medicaid funding for all their citizens. Disability-related services include supports such as PCA (a person hired to provide individualized home care for person unable to care for their own needs like dressing, bathing, and transfers), transportation assistance, and adaptive equipment including wheelchairs.

A person with a disability that has a work history is likely to be paid through SSDI and the amount will depend on lifetime earnings before the disability and averages $1,200 per month in 2018 ($700 to $2,800 range). However, without the work history, the person will receive cash assistance through SSI, a total of $733 per month for a single person, and that person can earn up to $785 beyond the payment (SSA, 2018a). If the person's income should rise above the threshold, they will either have their SSI payment reduced or may have to return overpaid funds to the SSA. Unfortunately, SSI recipients may not be informed of the overpayments for several months and they may have a large lump sum payment due to the SSA. See Case Study 21-1 on Scott's challenges with juggling his resources and trying to minimize the effect of work disincentives while maximizing the incentives such as the Plan for Achieving Self-Support (SSA, 2018b), vocational rehabilitation funds for work-related expenses (some of which counted toward his income, and some that did not). As you can see, part of the disincentive in returning to work for a person on SSI is the complexity of resource juggling and interpreting the many rules governing income and benefits, and this example in Scott's story is actually quite oversimplified.

The implication for OT is that it can be useful to understand the interrelationships of these programs and be aware that with possible fluctuations in health care coverage, your clients may not be able to attend therapy for fear of incurring bills that they can't pay. It would also be useful to know where you can refer newly disabled clients to for assistance with applying for, managing, and optimizing their benefit options. Most CILs provide resource and referral information and counseling that typically includes a specialist in social security and health care benefits. Scott served in that capacity as a volunteer in his local CIL and enjoyed sharing his hard won knowledge of the system. Actions that occupational therapists can take to advocate for disability rights are outlined in Box 21-3.

BOX 21-3   ADVOCATING FOR DISABILITY RIGHTS

Actions to take to learn more about and become involved in advocacy for disability rights and practice political activities of daily living include the following:

- Visit your local Center for Independent Living and offer to volunteer.
- Learn about disability services on your local campus and see if there are ways that you can provide paid (e.g., work-study) or volunteer support for students with disabilities on your campus.
- Know the Americans with Disabilities Act (ADA) basics and accessibility guidelines and speak up when you see architectural barriers that shouldn't be there or discriminatory behaviors toward the disabled.
- Assure that your employer is "disability friendly" for patrons, for clients, and in hiring.
- Be prepared to teach your clients who face chronic disability about their rights and assure that your

interventions go beyond activities of daily living (ADL) to prepare them to self-advocate against the social construct of disability.

- Practice political ADL in a way that is comfortable to you from the simple act of staying informed about disability issues to the role of activist or politician.
- Celebrate the anniversary of the ADA every July 26th by advocating in small or large ways for improved access to full civic and social participation for people with disabilities.
- Have a movie break with *When Billy Broke His Head* (Golfus & Simpson, 1994) or *Lives Worth Living* (Neudel, 2011) or other disability focused documentaries such as *Blindsight* (Orr & Walker, 2008) and discuss the implications for you as an occupational therapist.
- Choose titles from a reference list of disability-related books and films that feature autobiographies, biographies, documentaries, and scholarly texts (see a list on thePoint).

Summary

This chapter provides insights into the challenges that people with disabilities face in negotiating the barriers imposed by the social construct of disability and the complexities of social welfare systems intended to support but sometimes serve as yet another barrier to their participation in important occupations like work. Through our examination of the models of disability, you may have reflected on which models, or worldviews of disability, have influenced your perception of disabled people. You may have even considered whether or not you experience existential anxiety in your encounters with PWD. If you do, dig deeper in your reflections to consider the source of that anxiety and discuss with peers, faculty members, therapists, and ideally with acquaintances with disabilities what this all means, especially in relation to how you will manage those emotions when working with PWD in practice. As we've traced the intertwined history of the DRM and the paradigmatic progression of OT, we've built a case for

why a client-centered, occupation-based, and collaborative approach to practice. Hopefully, you've seen how that approach is likely to yield better treatment outcomes and set your clients better prepared to succeed on their path to recovery. Through a brief exposure to the evolution of the disability policy, you've seen examples of how even well-intended laws and practices can sometimes fail to effectively serve the end goal. You've learned or been reminded about the role of pADL in everyday practice and how occupational justice can be a part of every occupational therapist's professional life. As you integrate these many elements that contribute to the disability experience, you'll have a question to consider in your encounters with clients and especially those facing a life of chronic disability. That question is, "Will the service I provide today serve not only the short-term goals for their rehabilitation program but also more importantly serve their long-term recovery of a place in the world that is meaningful and prepared for the many challenges that lie ahead, well-past discharge?"

REFERENCES

Abrams, K. (2011). Performing interdependence: Judith Butler and Sunaura Taylor in the Examined Life. *Columbia Journal of Gender and Law, 21,* 474–491.

Agner, J. (2017). Understanding and applying empowerment theory to promote occupational justice. *Journal of Occupational Science, 24,* 280–289. doi:10.1080/14427591.2017.1338191

Altman, B. M., & Barnartt, S. N. (1993). Moral entrepreneurship and the promise of the ADA. *Journal of Disability Policy Studies, 4,* 21–40.

American Occupational Therapy Association. (2014a). Occupational therapy practice framework: Domain and process (3rd edition). *American Journal of Occupational Therapy, 68,* S1–S48. doi:10.5014/ajot.2014.682006

BOX 21-4   SUMMATIVE LEARNING ACTIVITY

Take out a piece of paper again and reflect back on your replies to the questions at the start of this chapter. How would you change your responses? How would you change your actions as an individual, as a member of society, and as an occupational therapist?

American Occupational Therapy Association. (2014b). Occupational therapy's commitment to nondiscrimination and inclusion. *American Journal of Occupational Therapy, 68*, S23–S24. doi:10.5014/ajot.2014.686S05

Americans with Disabilities Act of 1990, Pub. L. No. 101-336, § 12101 (1990).

Bachelder, J. (1985). Independent living programs: Bridges from hospital to community. *Occupational Therapy in Health Care, 2*, 99–107.

Barker, R. G. (1948). The social psychology of physical disability. *Journal of Social Issues, 4*, 28–38.

Barker, R. G., Wright, B. A., & Gonick, M. R. (1946). *Adjustment to physical handicap and illness: a survey of the social psychology of physique and disability.* New York, NY: Social Science Research Council.

Bedell, G., & Kaplan, M. (1996). Position paper: Providing services for persons with HIV/AIDS and their caregivers. *American Journal of Occupational Therapy, 50*, 853–854.

Berger, P., & Luckmann, T. (1966). *The social construction of reality: A treatise in the sociology of knowledge.* New York, NY: Anchor Books.

Berkowitz, E. D. (1987). *Disabled policy: America's programs for the handicapped—A twentieth century fund report.* Cambridge, MA: Cambridge University Press.

Berkowitz, E. D. (1992). Disabled policy: A personal postscript. *Journal of Disability Policy Studies, 3*, 1–16.

Bogdan, R., & Taylor, S. J. (1992). The social construction of humanness: Relationships with severely disabled people. In P. M. Ferguson, D. L. Ferguson, & S. J. Taylor (Eds.), *Interpreting disability: A qualitative reader* (pp. 275–294). New York, NY: Teachers College Press.

Boggis, T. (2009). Enacting political activities of daily living in occupational therapy education: Health care disparities in Oregon. In N. Pollard, D. Sakellariou, & F. Kronenberg (Eds.), *A political practice of occupational therapy* (pp. 145–153). Oxford, United Kingdom: Elsevier/Churchill Livingstone.

Bowen, R. (1993). Statement: The role of occupational therapy in the Independent Living Movement. *American Journal of Occupational Therapy, 47*, 1079–1080.

Braveman, B. (2016). Health policy perspectives—Population health and occupational therapy. *American Journal of Occupational Therapy, 70*, 7001090010. doi:10.5014/ajot.2016.701002

Bronfenbrenner, U. (1979). *The ecology of human development: Experiments by nature and design.* Cambridge, MA: Harvard University Press.

Bumiller, K. (1988). *The civil rights society: The social construction of victims.* Baltimore, MD: Johns Hopkins University Press.

Canelón, M. F. (1995). Job site analysis facilitates work reintegration. *American Journal of Occupational Therapy, 49*, 461–467. doi:10.5014/ajot.49.5.461

Cesaroni, C., & Peterson-Badali, M. (2010). Understanding the adjustment of incarcerated young offenders: A Canadian example. *Youth Justice, 10*, 107–125.

Christiansen, C. (1999). The 1999 Eleanor Clarke Slagle Lecture. Defining lives: Occupation as identity: An essay on competence, coherence, and the creation of meaning. *American Journal of Occupational Therapy, 53*, 547–558.

Clark, F. (1993). Occupation embedded in real life: Interweaving occupational science and occupational therapy. *American Journal of Occupational Therapy, 47*, 1067–1078.

Clark, F., Azen, S. P., Zemke, R., Jackson, J., Carlson, M., Mandel, D., . . . Lipson, L. (1997). Occupational therapy for independent-living older adults. *JAMA, 278*, 1321–1326.

Clark, F., & Jackson, J. (1990). The application of the occupational science negative heuristic in the treatment of persons with human immunodeficiency infection. *Occupational Therapy in Health Care, 6*, 69–91.

Cleek, A. (2013). *Young, disabled and stuck in a nursing home for the elderly.* Retrieved from http://america.aljazeera.com/articles/2013/10/2/young-disabled-andstuckinnursinghomes.html

Crewe, N. M., & Zola, I. K. (Eds.). (1983). *Independent living for physically disabled people.* San Francisco, CA: Jossey-Bass.

David, E. J., & Derthick, A. O. (2014). What is internalized oppression, and so what? In E. J. David (Ed.), *Internalized oppression: The psychology of marginalized groups* (pp. 1–30). New York, NY: Springer.

Davidson, L. (2007). Habits and other anchors of everyday life people with psychiatric disabilities may not take for granted. *OTJR: Occupation, Participation and Health, 27*, 60S–68S.

Davis, L. J. (1997a). Constructing normalcy: The bell curve, the novel, and the invention of the disabled body in the nineteenth century. In L. Davis (Ed.), *The disability studies reader* (pp. 9–28). New York, NY: Routledge.

Deegan, M. J., & Brooks, N. A. (1984). Women and disability: The double handicap. In M. J. Deegan & N. A. Brooks (Eds.), *Women and disability: The double handicap* (pp. 1–5). New Brunswick, Canada: Transaction Books.

Deegan, P. E. (1996, September). *There's a person in here* [Abstract]. Paper presented at the the Sixth Annual Mental Health Services Conference of Australia and New Zealand, Brisbane, Australia. Retrieved from https://www.patdeegan.com/pat-deegan/lectures/conspiracy-of-hope

DeJong, G. (1979). *The movement for independent living: Origins, ideology, and implications for disability research.* East Lansing, MI: University Center for International Rehabilitation, Michigan State University.

DeJong, G. (1983). Defining and implementing the independent living concept. In N. M. Crewe & I. K. Zola (Eds.), *Independent living for physically disabled people* (pp. 4–27). San Francisco, CA: Jossey-Bass.

DeJong, G., & Batavia, A. I. (1990). The American with Disabilities Act and the current state of U.S. disability policy. *Journal of Disability Policy Studies, 1*, 65–75.

DeMaio-Feldman, D. (1987). The occupational therapist as an expert witness. *American Journal of Occupational Therapy, 41*, 590–594. doi:10.5014/ajot.41.9.590

Denzin, N. K., & Lincoln, Y. (2018). *Handbook of qualitative research* (5th ed.). Thousand Oaks, CA: SAGE.

Disability Rights Education and Defense Fund. (2018). *International Laws for Disability Rights.* Retrieved from https://dredf.org/legal-advocacy/international-disability-rights/international-laws/

Dowbiggin, I. R. (1997). *Keeping America sane: Psychiatry and eugenics in the United States and Canada 1880–1940.* Ithaca, NY: University of Cornell Press.

Duckworth, T. (2017, October 17). Congress wants to make Americans with disabilities second-class citizens again. *Washington Post.* Retrieved from https://www.washingtonpost.com/opinions/congress-is-on-the-offensive-against-americans-with-disabilities/2017/10/17/f508069c-b359-11e7-9e58-e6288544af98_story.html?noredirect=on&utm_term=.df070c885808

Duncan, E. A., Munro, K., & Nicol, M. M. (2003). Research priorities in forensic occupational therapy. *British Journal of Occupational Therapy, 66*, 55–64.

Education for All Handicapped Children Act, Pub. L. No. 94-142, 773 Stat. 773-796 (1975).

Eisenberg, M., Griggins, C., & Duval, R. J. (Eds.). (1982). *Disabled people as second class citizens.* New York, NY: Springer.

Falconer, J. (1982). Health care delivery: Problems for the disabled. In M. Eisenberg, C. Griggins, & R. Duval (Eds.), *Disabled people as second class citizens* (pp. 137–151). New York, NY: Springer.

Farnworth, L., Morgan, S., & Fernando, B. (1987). Prison based occupational therapy. *Australian Occupational Therapy Journal, 34*, 40–46.

Fawcett, B. (2000). *Feminist perspectives on disability*. Essex, United Kingdom: Pearson Education.

Frank, G. (1996). Life histories in occupational therapy clinical practice. *American Journal of Occupational Therapy, 50*, 251–264.

Frank, G., & Stein, C. (2004). The meaning of self-care occupations. In C. H. Christiansen & K. Matuska (Eds.), *Ways of living: Adaptive strategies for special needs* (3rd ed., pp. 21–36). Bethesda, MD: American Occupational Therapy Association.

Frieden, L. (1983). Understanding alternative program models. In N. Crewe & I. Zola (Eds.), *Independent living for physically disabled people* (pp. 62–72). San Francisco, CA: Jossey-Bass.

Frieden, L. (1992). The Americans with Disabilities Act of 1990—Will it work? (Pro). *American Journal of Occupational Therapy, 46*, 468–469.

Frieden, L., & Cole, J. A. (1985). Independence: The ultimate goal of rehabilitation for spinal cord-injured persons. *American Journal of Occupational Therapy, 39*, 734–739.

Funk, R. (1987). Disability rights: From caste to class in the context of civil rights. In A. Gartner & T. Joe (Eds.), *Images of the disabled, disabling images* (pp. 7–30). New York, NY: Praeger.

Gage, M. (1997). Muriel Driver Lectureship. From independence to interdependence: Creating synergistic health care teams. *Canadian Journal of Occupational Therapy, 64*, 174–183.

Gerschick, T. J. (2000). Toward a theory of disability and gender. *Signs, 25*, 1263–1268.

Gleidman, J., & Roth, W. (1980). *The unexpected minority: Handicapped children in America*. New York, NY: Harcourt Brace Jovanovich.

Golfus, B., & Simpson, D. (Directors.). (1994). *When Billy broke his head* [Movie]. United States: Independent Television Service.

Goodley, D. (2017). *Disability studies: An interdisciplinary introduction* (2nd ed.). San Francisco, CA: Sage.

Gordon, D. (2009). The history of occupational therapy. In E. B. Crepeau, E. S. Cohn, & B. B. Schell (Eds.), *Willard & Spackman's occupational therapy* (11th ed., pp. 202–215). Philadelphia, PA: Lippincott Williams & Wilkins.

Grabell, M., & Berkes, H. (2015, March 5). How much is your arm worth? Depends on where you work. *ProPublica*. Retrieved from https://www.propublica.org/article/how-much-is-your-arm-worth-depends-where-you-work

Grills, N. (2015). Interdependence: a new model for the global approach to disability. *Christian Journal for Global Health, 2*(2), 1–4.

Gritzer, G., & Arluke, A. (1985). *The making of rehabilitation: A political economy of medical specialization, 1890–1980*. Berkeley, CA: University of California Press.

Gwaltney, J. (1970). *The thrice shy: Cultural accommodation to blindness and other disasters in a Mexican community*. New York, NY: Columbia University Press.

Hahn, H. (1985a). Introduction: Disability policy and the problem of discrimination. *American Behavioral Scientist, 28*, 293–318.

Hahn, H. (1985b). Toward a politics of disability: Definitions, disciplines, and policies. *The Social Science Journal, 22*, 87–105.

Hahn, H. (1987). Civil rights for disabled Americans: The foundation for a political agenda. In A. Gartner & T. Joe (Eds.), *Images of the disabled, disabling images* (pp. 181–203). New York, NY: Praeger.

Hahn, H. (1988). Can disability be beautiful. *Social Policy, 18*, 26–32.

Hahn, H. (1993). Equality and the environment: The interpretation of "reasonable accommodations" in the Americans with Disabilities Act. *Journal of Rehabilitation Administration, 17*, 101–106.

Hamilton, T. B. (2007, April). *Community reentry from a correctional halfway house*. Paper presented at the AOTA Annual Conference, St. Louis, MO.

Haywood, C., & Lawlor, M. (2017). Understanding complex relationships among transition-age youth with spinal cord injury and their caregivers. *American Journal of Occupational Therapy, 71*, 7111505072p1. doi:10.5014/ajot.2017.71S1-RP302A

Heathfield, S. M. (2018). *Prevent employment discrimination lawsuits*. Retrieved from https://www.thebalancecareers.com/prevent-employment-discrimination-and-lawsuits-1917923

Higgins, P. C. (1992). *Making disability: Exploring the social transformation of human variation*. Springfield, IL: Charles C. Thomas.

Hillyer, B. (1993). *Feminism and disability*. Norman, OK: University of Oklahoma Press.

Illich, I. (1976). *Medical nemesis: The expropriation of health*. New York, NY: Pantheon.

International Center for the Disabled. (1986). *The ICD survey of disabled Americans: Bringing disabled Americans into the mainstream: A nationwide survey of 1,000 disabled people. Study No. 854009*. New York, NY: Harris and Associates.

Jarman, M., & Kafer, A. (2014). Guest editors' introduction: Growing disability studies: Politics of access, politics of collaboration. *Disability Studies Quarterly, 34*(2), 1–7.

Kessler Foundation/National Organization on Disability. (2010). *The 2010 Survey of Americans With Disabilities*. Retrieved from http://www.2010DisabilitySurveys.org

Kielhofner, G. (2009). *Conceptual foundations of occupational therapy* (4th ed.). Philadelphia, PA: F. A. Davis.

Kraus, L., Lauer, E., Coleman, R., & Houtenville, A. (2018). *2017 Disability statistics annual report*. Durham, NH: University of New Hampshire.

Kronenberg, F., & Pollard, N. (2005). Overcoming occupational apartheid: A preliminary exploration of the political nature of occupational therapy. In F. Kronenberg, S. Simó-Algado, & N. Pollard (Eds.), *Occupational therapy without borders: Learning from the spirit of survivors* (pp. 58–86). London, United Kingdom: Elsevier/Churchill Livingstone.

Law, M., Baptiste, S., Carswell, A., McColl, M., Polatajko, H. J., & Pollock, N. (2005). *The Canadian Occupational Performance Measure* (4th ed.). Ontario, Canada: Canadian Association of Occupational Therapists.

Law, M., Baptiste, S., McColl, M., Opzoomer, A., Polataijko, H., & Pollock, N. (1990). The Canadian Occupational Performance Measure: an outcome measure for occupational therapy. *Canadian Journal of Occupational Therapy, 57*, 82–87.

Law, M., Baptiste, S., & Mills, J. (1995). Client-centred practice: What does it mean and does it make a difference? *Canadian Journal of Occupational Therapy, 62*, 250–257.

Letts, L., Rigby, P., & Stewart, D. (Eds.). (2003). *Using environments to enable occupational performance*. Thorofare, NJ: SLACK.

Levin, S., & Martinez, C. (2016). Is independence overrated? Conceptualization of familial interdependence in the Latino population. *American Journal of Occupational Therapy, 70*, 7011505152p1. doi:10.5014/ajot.2016.70S1-PO5022

Lewin, K. (1935). *A dynamic theory of personality*. New York, NY: McGraw-Hill.

Liachowitz, C. H. (1988). *Disability as a social construct: Legislative roots*. Philadelphia, PA. University of Pennsylvania Press.

Longmore, P. K. (2003). *Why I burned my book and other essays on disability*. Philadelphia, PA: Temple University Press.

Longmore, P. K., & Umansky, L. (Eds.). (2001). *The new disability history: American perspectives*. New York, NY: New York University Press.

Maiorana-Basas, M., & Pagliaro, C. M. (2014). Technology use among adults who are deaf and hard of hearing: A national survey. *The Journal of Deaf Studies and Deaf Education, 19*, 400–410. doi:10.1093/deafed/enu005

Mandel, D., Jackson, J. M., Zemke, R., Nelson, L., & Clark, F. (1999). *Lifestyle redesign: Implementing the well elderly program*. Bethesda, MD: American Occupational Therapy Association.

Marfeo, E., Ni, P., Meterko, M., Marino, M., Peterik, K., McDonough, C., . . . Jette, A. (2016). Development of a new instrument to assess work-related function: Work Disability Functional Assessment Battery (WD-FAB). *American Journal of Occupational Therapy, 70,* 7011500012p1. doi:10.5014/ajot.2016.70S1-RP402B

Marshall, A. (2003, October). *Water quality and the contextual nature of occupation.* Paper presented at the SSO: USA 2nd Annual Research Conference, Park City, Utah.

Marshall, C. A., Lysaght, R., & Krupa, T. (2017). The experience of occupational engagement of chronically homeless persons in a mid-sized urban context. *Journal of Occupational Science, 24,* 165–180. doi:10.1080/14427591.2016.1277548

Matuska, K., & Christiansen, C. (2009). *Life balance: Multidisciplinary theories and research.* Thorofare, NJ: SLACK.

McCuaig, M., & Frank, G. (1991). The able self: Adaptive patterns and choices in independent living for a person with cerebral palsy. *American Journal of Occupational Therapy, 45,* 224–234.

Meikle, J. (2016, July 19). People with disabilities treated like second-class citizens, says watchdog. *The Guardian.* Retrieved from https://www.theguardian.com/society/2016/jul/19/people-with -disabilities-treated-like-second-class-citizens-says-watchdog

Meyer, A. (1931/1957). *Psychobiology: A science of man.* Springfield, IL: Charles C. Thomas.

Miller, R. J. (1988). What is theory, and why does it matter? In B. R. J. Miller, K. W. Sieg, F. M. Ludwig, S. D. Shortridge, & J. Van Deusen (Eds.), *Six perspectives on theory for the practice of occupational therapy* (pp. 1–16). Rockville, MD: Aspen.

Minow, M. (1990). *Making all the difference: Inclusion, exclusion, and American law.* Ithaca, NY: Cornell University Press.

Murphy, N., Messina, W., Getter, E., Gutterman, L., Martin, T., Rincon, P., & Zimmerman, I. (1999). The Village AIDS Day Treatment Program: A model of interdisciplinary and interdependent care. *American Journal of Occupational Therapy, 53,* 561–565. doi:10.5014/ajot.53.6.561

Murphy, R., Scheer, J., Murphy, Y., & Mack, R. (1988). Physical disability and social liminality: A study in the rituals of adversity. *Social Science & Medicine, 26,* 235–242.

Myers, C. A. (2017). Police violence against people with mental disabilities: The immutable duty under the ADA to reasonably accommodate during arrest. *Vanderbilt Law Review, 70,* 1393–1425.

Nagi, S. Z. (1991). Disability concepts revisited: Implications for prevention. In A. M. Pope & A. R. Tarlov (Eds.), *Disability in America: Toward a national agenda for prevention* (pp. 309–327). Washington, DC: National Academy Press.

National Organization on Disability. (1998). *The 1998 N.O.D./Harris Survey of Americans with Disabilities.* New York, NY: Harris and Associates.

Neudel, Eric (Writer). (2011). Lives worth living [video]. In A. Gilkey (Producer). New York, NY: Storyline Motion Pictures & Independent Television Service (ITVS).

Nosek, M. A. (1992). The issue is: The Americans with Disabilities Act—Will it work? (Con). *American Journal of Occupational Therapy, 46,* 466–467.

Oberman, C. E. (1965). *A history of vocational rehabilitation in America.* Minneapolis, MN: T. S. Denison and Co.

Oliver, M. (1996). *Understanding disability: From theory to practice.* New York, NY: St. Martin's Press.

Oliver, M. (2013). The social model of disability: Thirty years on. *Disability & Society, 28,* 1024–1026. doi:10.1080/09687599.2013 .818773

Orr, S. R. (Producer), & Walker, L. (Director). (2008). *Blindsight* [Movie]. United Kingdom: Robson Entertainment.

Parmet, W. E. (1993). Title III: Public accommodations. In L. O. Gostin & H. A. Beyer (Eds.), *Implementing the Americans with Disabilities Act: Rights and responsibilities of all Americans* (pp. 123–136). Baltimore, MD: Paul H. Brookes.

Parsons, T. (1951). Illness and the role of the physician: A sociological perspective. *American Journal of Orthopsychiatry, 21*(3), 452–460. doi:10.1111%2Fj.1939-0025.1951.tb00003.x

Parsons, T. (1975). Illness and the role of the physician reconsidered. *Health and Society: Milbank Memorial Fund Quarterly, 53*(3), 257–278. doi:https://doi.org/10.1111/j.1939-0025.1951.tb00003.x

Penketh, A., Connolly, K., Kirchgaessner, S., McDonald, H., McCurry, J., Crouch, D., . . . Bawden, A. (2015, April 15). Which are the best countries in the world to live in if you are unemployed or disabled? *The Guardian.* Retrieved from https://www.theguardian.com/politics/2015/apr/15 /which-best-countries-live-unemployed-disabled-benefits

Phillips, M. J. (1990). Damaged goods: Oral narratives of the experience of disability in American culture. *Social Science & Medicine, 30,* 849–857.

Pollard, N., Kronenberg, F., & Sakellariou, D. (2008). A political practice of occupational therapy. In N. Pollard, D. Sakellariou, & F. Kronenberg (Eds.), *A political practice of occupational therapy* (pp. 3–22). London, United Kingdom: Elsevier.

Price-Lackey, P., & Cashman, J. (1996). Jenny's story: Reinventing oneself through occupation and narrative configuration. *American Journal of Occupational Therapy, 50,* 306–314.

Pruett, S., & Pruett, S. (2018). *Safescore: Universal design checklist.* Retrieved from https://safescore.org/checklists

Ramugondo, E. L. (2005). Unlocking spirituality: Play as a health-promoting occupation in the context of HIV/AIDS. In F. Kronenberg, S. S. Algado, & N. Pollard (Eds.), *Occupational therapy without borders: Learning from the spirit of survivors* (pp. 313–325). London, United Kingdom: Elsevier.

Reed, K. L. (2015). Key occupational therapy concepts in the Person-Occupation-Environment-Performance Model: Their origin and historical use in the occupational therapy literature. In C. H. Christiansen, C. M. Baum, & J. D. Bass (Eds.), *Occupational therapy: Performance, participation, and well-being* (4th ed., pp. 559–641). Thorofare, NJ: SLACK.

Rehabilitation Act of 1973, Pub. L. No. 93-112, 355 Stat. (1973).

Reilly, M. (1962). Occupational therapy can be one of the great ideas of 20th century medicine. *American Journal of Occupational Therapy, 16,* 1–9.

Reindal, S. M. (1999). Independence, dependence, interdependence: Some reflections on the subject and personal autonomy. *Disability & Society, 14,* 353–367. doi:10.1080/09687599926190

Scharnhorst, G. (1980). *Horatio Alger Jr.* New York, NY: Twayne.

Scheer, J., & Groce, N. (1988). Impairment as a human constant: Cross-cultural and historical perspectives on variation. *Journal of Social Issues, 44,* 23–37.

Scotch, R. K. (1984). *From good will to civil rights: Transforming federal disability policy.* Philadelphia, PA: Temple University Press.

Scott, R. (1969). *The making of blind men: A study of adult socialization.* New York, NY: Russell Sage Foundation.

Shakespeare, T. (2004). Social models of disability and other life strategies. *Scandinavian Journal of Disability Research, 6,* 8–21. doi:10.1080/15017410409512636

Shakespeare, T. (2006a). Critiquing the social model. In T. Shakespeare & P. Harper (Eds.), *Disability rights and wrongs* (pp. 29–53). London, United Kingdom: Routledge.

Shakespeare, T. (2006b). *Disability rights and wrongs.* London, United Kingdom: Routledge.

Shakespeare, T. (2006c). The family of social approaches. In T. Shakespeare (Ed.), *Disability rights and wrongs* (pp. 85–102). London, United Kingdom: Routledge.

Shapiro, J. P. (1993). *No pity: People with disabilities forging a new civil rights movement.* New York, NY: Times Books.

Sims, B., & Manley, S. (1982). Keeping the disabled out of the employment market. In M. Eisenberg, C. Griggins, & R. J. Duval (Eds.), *Disabled people as second class citizens* (pp. 123–136). New York, NY: Springer.

Smart, J. (2009). *Disability, society, and the individual* (2nd ed.). Austin, TX: Pro-ed.

Smith, D. L., & Hilton, C. L. (2008). An occupational justice perspective of domestic violence against women with disabilities. *Journal of Occupational Science, 15,* 166–172.

Social Security Administration. (2018a). *Disability determination process.* Washington, DC: Author.

Social Security Administration. (2018b). *The faces and facts of disability.* Retrieved from https://www.ssa.gov/disabilityfacts/facts.html

Stoltzfus, M. J., & Schumm, D. Y. (2011). Beyond models: Some tentative Daoist contributions to disability studies. *Disability Studies Quarterly, 31*(1).

Strother, W. G. (1992). Where's disability (wo)man? *Quill, 12*(5), 6–19.

Tenberken, S., & Kronenberg, G. (2005). The right to be blind without being disabled. In F. Kronenberg, S. S. Algado, & N. Pollard (Eds.), *Occupational therapy without borders: Learning from the spirit of survivors* (pp. 31–39). London, United Kingdom: Elsevier.

The Civil Rights Act of 1964, Pub. L. No. 88-352, 241 Stat. (1964).

The Ragged Edge. (1993). Wade Blank 1940-1993, Disability Rights Movement advocate remembered. *The Ragged Edge.*

To: The temporarily able-bodied [Editorial]. (2007, May 1). *New York Times,* p. A22. Retrieved from https://www.nytimes.com/2007/05/01/opinion/01tue1.html

Thomson, R. G. (1997). *Extraordinary bodies: Figuring physical disability in American culture and literature.* New York, NY: Columbia University Press.

Townsend, E., De Laat, D., Egan, M., Thibeault, R., & Wright, W. A. (1999). *Spirituality in enabling occupation: A learner-centered workbook.* Ottawa, Canada: Canadian Association of Occupational Therapists.

Townsend, E., & Whiteford, G. (2005). A participatory occupational justice framework. In F. Kronenberg, S. S. Algado, & N. Pollard (Eds.), *Occupational therapy without borders: Learning from the spirit of survivors* (pp. 110–126). London, United Kingdom: Elsevier.

Tryssenaar, J., Jones, E. J., & Lee, D. (1999). Occupational performance needs of a shelter population. *Canadian Journal of Occupational Therapy, 66,* 188–196.

Turner, V. (1977). Variations on a theme of liminality. In S. F. Moore & B. G. Myerhoff (Eds.), *Secular ritual* (pp. 36–52). Amsterdam, The Netherlands: Van Gorcum.

von Bertalanffy, L. (1968). *General system theory: Foundations, development, applications.* New York, NY: George Braziller.

Watson, S. D. (1993). A study in legislative strategy: The passage of the ADA. In L. O. Gostin & H. A. Beye (Eds.), *Implementing the Americans with Disabilities Act: Rights and responsibilities of all Americans* (pp. 25–34). Baltimore, MD: Paul H. Brookes.

Watson, S. D. (1994). Applying theory to practice: A prospective and prescriptive analysis of the implementation of the Americans with Disabilities Act. *Disability Studies Quarterly, 5*(1), 1–24.

West, W. L. (1989). Perspectives on the past and future, part 1. *American Journal of Occupational Therapy, 43,* 787–790.

White, G. W., Simpson, J. L., Gonda, C., Ravesloot, C., & Coble, Z. (2010). Moving from independence to interdependence: A conceptual model for better understanding community participation of Centers for Independent Living consumers. *Journal of Disability Policy Studies, 20,* 233–240. doi:10.1177/1044207309350561

White, J. A. (1999). *Occupation and adaptation: An ethnographic study of people with disabilities using the ADA to fight employment discrimination* (Unpublished doctoral dissertation). University of Southern California, Los Angeles.

Whiteford, G. (1997). Occupational deprivation and incarceration. *Journal of Occupational Science, 4,* 126–130.

Whiteford, G. (2007a). Autonomy, accountability, and professional practice: contemporary issues and challenges. *New Zealand Journal of Occupational Therapy, 54,* 11–14.

Whiteford, G. (2007b). Occupational deprivation and incarceration in New Zealand. *Journal of Occupational Science, 4,* 126–131.

Whiteford, G. (2014). Enacting occupational justice in research and policy development: Highlighting the experience of occupational deprivation in forced migration. In D. Pierce (Ed.), *Occupational science for occupational therapy* (pp. 169–179). Thorofare, NJ: SLACK.

Wilcock, A. A., & Hocking, C. (2015). *An occupational perspective of health* (3rd ed.). Thorofare, NJ: SLACK.

Williams, P. J. (1991). *The alchemy of race and rights: Diary of a law professor.* Cambridge, MA: Harvard University Press.

Winter, J. A. (2003). The development of the disability rights movement as a social problem solver. *Disability Studies Quarterly, 23*(1), 33–61.

Wolfensberger, W. (1972). *The principle of normalization in human services.* Ontario, Canada: National Institute on Mental Retardation.

Worklife. (1989). Justin Dart: New President's Committee chairman. *Worklife, 2*(4), 19–23.

World Health Organization. (2008). *International Classification of Functioning, Disability and Health (ICF).* Geneva, Switzerland: World Health Organization.

World Health Organization. (2011). *World report on disability.* Geneva, Switzerland: Author.

Yerxa, E. J. (1967). 1966 Eleanor Clarke Slagle lecture. Authentic occupational therapy. *American Journal of Occupational Therapy, 21,* 1–9.

Yerxa, E. J. (1989). An introduction to occupational science, a foundation for occupational therapy in the 21st century. *Occupational Therapy and Health Care, 6,* 1–15.

Zeilinger, J. (2015). *6 Forms of ableism we need to retire immediately.* Retrieved from https://mic.com/articles/121653/6-forms-of-ableism-we-need-to-retire-immediately#.dWG18gsXb

the**Point**® *For additional resources on the subjects discussed in this chapter, visit* http://thePoint.lww.com/Willard-Spackman13e.

CHAPTER 22

Physical and Virtual Environments

Meaning of Place and Space

Noralyn D. Pickens, Cynthia L. Evetts, David Seamon

LEARNING OBJECTIVES

After reading this chapter, you will be able to:

1. Explain why and how qualities of the physical environment and place are important dimensions of human life and experience.
2. Describe what a phenomenological approach to human experience entails and how it can be used to examine the human experience of environments and places.
3. Define place in terms of human experience using the concepts of insideness and outsideness.
4. Define the phenomenological concepts of lived body and environmental embodiment and discuss their relevance for occupational therapy.
5. Apply the concepts of home and at-homeness to people's lives and explain how home and at-homeness can be strengthened or undermined by physical features of dwellings and neighborhoods.
6. Explain the relevance of virtual worlds and virtual places and apply to occupational therapy conditions and contexts for engagement in occupation.
7. Explain the critical importance of environment and place for effective occupational therapy practice.

Environments, Places, and Occupational Therapy

Physical and virtual environments influence human health, well-being, and productive occupations (Dunn, Haney McClain, Brown, & Youngstrom, 2003; Gitlin, 2009; Hasselkus, 2011; Rowles, 2003; Stewart et al., 2003; Ulrich et al., 2008). How human beings *experience* environments, places, and spaces is central to understanding occupational therapy (OT). **Phenomenology** is the description and interpretation of human experience (Finlay, 2011; Seamon, 2000; van Manen, 1990). In this chapter, the phenomenological approach is briefly described and four environmental themes important for occupational therapists and scientists are considered including (1) place, (2) environmental embodiment, (3) home and at-homeness, and (4) virtual technology and place.

CENTENNIAL NOTES

The Concepts of Place and Space

Famous innovative architect Frank Lloyd Wright attended meetings of the Chicago Arts and Crafts Society at Hull House during the early years of the formulation of occupational therapy (Bryan & Davis, 1990). George Barton, another architect, experienced disconnectedness and uneasiness while a patient recovering from tuberculosis. Barton served as the first president of the National Society for the Promotion of Occupational Therapy (NSPOT) (now American Occupational Therapy Association [AOTA]) and went on to design spaces for individuals with disabilities to live, learn, and work (Andersen & Reed, 2017).

Although the physical environment has always been integral to OT, the concepts of place and space come from our colleagues in humanistic geography who study human experience and action in relation to the geographical environments. Occupational scientists, such as Betty Hasselkus (1998, 2011), engaged the writings of Yi-Fu Tuan (1977), Graham Rowles (1999, 2006), and David Seamon (2002), among others, who provide a depth of understanding through phenomenological and ethnographic research.

In 2001, the World Health Organization published the International Classification of Functioning, Disability and Health (ICF) with a fresh emphasis on holistic well-being rather than disease and illness. This perspective included an acknowledgment that context and environment play a significant role in the disablement of individuals. A short time later, AOTA published the first version of the Occupational Therapy Practice Framework in 2002, including context as one of six major aspects within the domain of practice. When AOTA developed the Blueprint for Entry-Level Education in 2008, environment-centered factors were included as one of four sections of curriculum content (Andersen & Reed, 2017).

Occupational therapists today work with architects and contractors to design spaces that are accessible and that encourage occupational participation and facilitate occupational performance. All areas of OT practice include consideration of the impact of environmental and contextual factors on functional outcomes of persons, groups, and populations. Whether socially and culturally constructed, natural or built, and actual or virtual, the environment is inextricably linked to occupation and function.

Phenomenology and Occupational Therapy

To study human beings phenomenologically is to study human experiences, behaviors, situations, and meanings as they arise in the world of everyday life. For OT and occupational science, one significant phenomenological topic is the **lifeworld**—a person or group's everyday world of *taken-for-grantedness* normally unnoticed and thus hidden as a phenomenon (Finlay, 2011; Seamon, 1979; Toombs, 2001; van Manen, 1990). One aim of phenomenological research is to disclose and describe the various lived structures and dynamics of the lifeworld—for example, the mostly unnoticed but crucial importance of places in people's daily lives. An understanding of a client's lifeworld is central for occupational therapists because, typically, the taken-for-grantedness of his or her world has shifted or disappeared, including occupational dimensions (Clarke, 2009; Cronin-Davis, Butler, & Mayers, 2009; Finlay, 2006; Padilla, 2003).

Most of the time in everyday life, the lifeworld is *transparent* in the sense that day-to-day life *just happens*, grounded in predictable spatiotemporal patterns (Seamon, 1979). An integral part of this lived transparency is good health, which is lived as a kind of tacit attunement normally not given direct attention (Carel, 2008; Stefanovic, 2008; Svenaeus, 2001; van Manen, 1998). In contrast, illness and disability activate a resistance to the usual lifeworld in that they transform its transparency into awkwardness, unease, or discomfort. Daily life that, before, simply unfolded and happened without the need for self-conscious awareness, is now a continual event to be faced, whether because of pain, inconvenience, or inability to perform as usual. In this sense, one task of occupational therapists is to understand the client's former mode of "being at home" and to locate pathways whereby he or she can reaccess and recover that mode in the same or related fashion (Svenaeus, 2001). As the next sections demonstrate, qualities of places and physical environments can help facilitate this return to "being at home."

Place and Occupational Therapy

One integral dimension of the lifeworld is **place**, which can be defined as any environmental locus that gathers individual or group meanings, intentions, and actions spatially (Casey, 2009; Relph, 1976/2008). A place can range in scale from a furnishing or room to a building, neighborhood, city, or region (Manzo, 2005; Relph, 1976/2008). One of the most accessible phenomenologies of place is geographer Edward

Relph's *Place and Placelessness* (Relph, 1976/2008). Relph (1976/2008) argued that the existential crux of place experience is *insideness*—in other words, the more deeply a person or group feels themselves inside an environment, the more so does that environment become, existentially, a place. The deepest experience of place attachment and identity is what Relph termed *existential insideness*—a situation where the person or group feel so much at home and at ease in place that they have no self-conscious recognition of its importance in their lives, unless the place or the client in it changes in some way—for example, a home is destroyed by flood or a client is no longer able to walk because of an auto accident. In one sense, a major aim of occupational therapists is working with a client in ways whereby, as much as possible, they might help him or her reestablish existential insideness.

In his phenomenology of place, Relph (1976/2008) described several other modes of place insideness and its lived opposite, *outsideness*—a situation where the person or group feels separate or alienated from place in some way. These modes of place experience (Table 22-1) are useful for the occupational therapist because they provide an accessible language through which particular place experiences can be identified in terms of the intensity of meaning and intention that a person and place hold for each other. Through illness or accident, for example, a person's taken-for-granted sense of existential insideness can be ruptured, and he or she falls into a particular mode of existential outsideness in which the lifeworld as it was before is now different, often strangely or uncomfortably so.

Relph's modes of insideness and outsideness offer a flexible means for distinguishing the lived experience of place from its material or assumed qualities. In domestic abuse, for example, the home, typically a place of existential insideness, becomes a place of existential outsideness.

The environmental themes discussed in this chapter are illustrated by the lifeworld of man who experienced polio in two life periods (Case Study 22-1). For students learning to become occupational therapists, this story can be a powerful example of how occupation is transacted through environment and context.

Themes of place, insideness, and outsideness can offer occupational therapists valuable insights. In his research on rural older people, gerontological geographer Graham Rowles (2003) emphasized that their lifeworlds typically involve strong emotional attachments to place. Rowles identified three dimensions of place related to Relph's theme of existential insideness: first, *physical insideness*, a sense of being physically entwined with the environment; second, *social insideness*, whereby people feel an integral part of their community through social relationships and exchanges; and, third, *autobiographical insideness*, the ways in which places and place qualities coalesce into an environmental mosaic relating to and marking out one's personal and communal history in relation to those places (Rowles & Watkins, 2003, pp. 78–79). Rowles (1999) emphasizes that understanding place experience is important for occupational therapists because it reveals "the role of the person's experienced spatiotemporal environment in conditioning his or her response

TABLE 22-1 Modes of Insideness and Outsideness

Mode	Description
Existential insideness	Feeling completely at home and immersed in place, to such a degree the experience is not usually noticed unless the place dramatically changes in some way (e.g., one's home and community are destroyed by natural disaster). The mode of place experience most human beings strive for; typically, the mode of place experience that occupational therapists work toward recovering for their clients.
Existential outsideness	Feeling alienated or separate from place, which may seem oppressive or unreal (e.g., the experience of homesickness or the deep sense of disjunction one feels, having suddenly become disabled because of an accident). The mode of experience that many people fall into after a disabling accident or after becoming ill or learning they are ill. A major task of the occupational therapist is to help clients shift, as much as possible, out of existential outsideness back toward existential insideness.
Objective outsideness	A dispassionate attitude of separation from place, which becomes an object of study or directed attention (e.g., designing a hospital using measurable criteria like size of potential patient pool, square footage based on functional needs, building layout determined by staff efficiency).
Incidental outsideness	The experience in which place is a background or mere setting for activities (e.g., the short-term patient's limited relationship with the hospital environment in which she finds herself temporarily).
Behavioral insideness	A deliberate attending to the appearance of place (e.g., using environmental cues like landmarks and signage to find one's way around a place). The first stage in becoming an insider to a new place (e.g., mastering the layout of a hospital complex where one has just started working).
Empathetic insideness	Being open to place and attempting to understand it more deeply (e.g., the occupational therapist's effort to see and to understand the client's lifeworld as it *really is* and not as the occupational therapist supposes it to be).
Vicarious insideness	Deeply felt secondhand involvement with place (e.g., learning about worlds of illness or disablement through films, novels, or autobiographical accounts) (e.g., Bauby, 1997; A. W. Frank, 2002; Hockenberry, 1995; Hull, 1990).

From Relph, E. (2008). *Place and placelessness.* London, United Kingdom: Pion. (Original work published 1976)

CASE STUDY 22-1   VINNIE'S LIFEWORLD

As a child born in the 1940s in the midwest United States, Vinnie experienced childhood in a small third floor apartment above a butcher shop with his parents. His mother was a factory worker, and his father was an electrician. His father had trouble keeping work due to heavy drinking, and the family often had financial challenges. The family never owned a home or a car, renting apartments and relying on the public transportation. Their apartment was centrally located in the city, close to Vinnie's schools and their church. Vinnie's neighborhood was bound by three busy streets, creating an island of sorts. This island had a large group of children of all ages. Small "gangs" of kids grouped together to play handball, kickball, or jump rope. Vinnie experienced *existential insideness*, taking for granted the sense of place and people. It was a community of people who knew each other well. Parents watched out for each other's children and disciplined the group when needed. As teens graduated high school, they most often moved away from the neighborhood to new apartments, work, and lives. Their return to the neighborhood, full of stories from their new life, was a source of excitement for the children, especially the older teens like Vinnie.

Then, polio struck the neighborhood: a disease that put fear in families and the tight-knit community. Children were kept inside; a few were stricken with the disease. It felt random and threatening. An *existential outsideness* crept into the lives of the people there. The social connectedness of the neighborhood became a series of concerned whispers. Children began to be hospitalized. At 14 years old, Vinnie was one of the older children who became ill. He went from the freedom of his neighborhood to the confines of a hospital and eventually into an iron lung. His mother spent every afternoon with him after her shift ended. She felt helpless as she saw her son become increasingly weaker, unable to do the simplest activities for himself. Although the hospital staff attempted to create comfort and routine, the *incidental outsideness* of the clinical "home" was distressing. Volunteer groups attempted to provide some sense of normalcy for the children by offering school lessons and activities (Figure 22-1). As Vinnie improved, and when the hospitals became too full, Vinnie's parents brought him back to their apartment. His mother quit her job to help him rehabilitate at home. She moved his limbs and exercised his body by encouraging him to do as much for himself as he could. Working toward independence was not hard for a now 15-year-old teen. He was embarrassed that his mother had to bathe him and dress him. His father drank more, and Vinnie was frustrated by not being in school and moving forward with his life as his friends were doing. A long year passed and the children began to play outside again. Vinnie's polio affected him with crossover body weakness from his left shoulder, chest (back and abdomen), and right hip/upper leg. At 15 years old, Vinnie was in a growth period. His right leg was to be always 1 inch

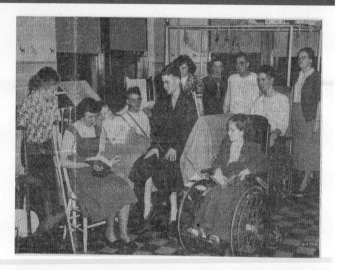

FIGURE 22-1 Vinnie's lifeworld recovering in hospital (Vinnie, age 14 years, in center of photo).

shorter than his left, and his left arm weaker than his right. None of Vinnie's close friends were affected by polio; they went on with their schooling and plans for work or college. Even the insideness of the neighborhood felt alienated. His rooted patterns with friends were gone. Having missed a year of school and seeing his friends move on without him, Vinnie and his parents decided he would go to the seminary to complete his high school education.

Seminary was a common option for a good education for boys like Vinnie. It was *regenerative*, opening new opportunities for socialization and activities that were less physically demanding. Vinnie took up choir and journalism, writing for the seminary newsletters. He regained an "*at-easeness*," content in his new surroundings and satisfied with his occupations. His future was not in the priesthood, so upon graduation, he went to college majoring in journalism. He met his future wife, graduated, and married, and with a new job, they bought a home together in the city. Within 5 years, three children were born to them. Vinnie started his own business. The marriage was not strong, and his long work hours, along with a pattern of heavy drinking, caused his marriage to end in divorce when the children were teens. He remarried and lived in the city running his small business.

In his 50s, Vinnie began to experience weakness and found he had post-polio syndrome. The business climate was not good for his industry, and by his 60s, he sold the company to retire early and move to a rural northern community with a home overlooking a lake. The one-story home was a refuge. He and his wife filled it with craft and art from friends and local artisans. The small town community suited him as he became a local fixture at coffee shops, cafes, parks, and library (Figure 22-2).

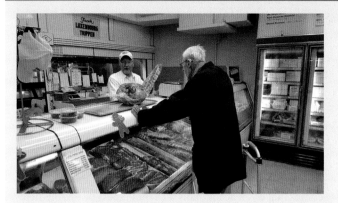

FIGURE 22-2 Vinnie's lifeworld in his local community.

Insideness was short-lived when Vinnie found his balance was a problem in the community as he became weaker in his legs and core muscles. He started using a cane—a stylized cane with eagle's head handle, and happily noted that people treated him with more respect, "Now people hold doors for me and call me Sir!" He and his wife continued to socialize with close friends and family, but Vinnie increasingly became less interested in going out in the community. His rooted routine of stopping by shops gradually went away. He now used a rollator walker and needed help getting in and

out of chairs, which embarrassed him. The winter snow and ice made many months of the year impossible to navigate outside without fear of falling. On the recommendation of an occupational therapist, his family put in a bench and grab bars in the shower and rails at the toilet. He worked with a physical therapist on a home exercise plan to maintain strength. He maintained strong vision and cognition.

He spent his days preparing "snacks" for the birds, meditating, watching sports on television, surfing and video calling family with his computer, and reading books. He read over 100 books a year, with the local library holding books from the best-seller lists for him to read first. Just as a teen with his mother, he was embarrassed that his wife had to assist him with bathing and dressing but knew this time he would not be getting stronger and began to accept assistance from a care aide twice a week. He joked he created a better nest than his bird friends, with his homemade quilts, bowls made of pottery by his friends, and his beloved books. He created place with three rooms of the house—bed, bath, and living rooms. His routines were comforting, and he was at ease with his life. After a bout with pneumonia, he accepted using oxygen intermittently and then continuously. The noise of the oxygen machine and tubing kept him now mostly in his bedroom. His view overlooking the lake, his birds, and books became his world. One more bout of pneumonia took his strength, and Vinnie died in his sleep, at home, in his bed, with a book on his lap.

to dysfunctions and to intervention strategies meant to remedy them" (p. 270). Vinnie's story provides clear rendering of place, at-homeness, and environmental embodiment as expressed in Vinnie's everyday experience across his life course. He worked to create a sense of place in his physical environment, both in his community and at home. Routine occupation both organized and regenerated his lifeworld. Use of film and books in OT programs create opportunities for students to develop *vicarious insideness* (Figure 22-3).

Environmental Embodiment, Home, and At-Homeness

The Lived Body, Body-Subject, and Environmental Embodiment

In exploring human experience, phenomenologists emphasize that humans are *bodily* beings, a lived fact important for

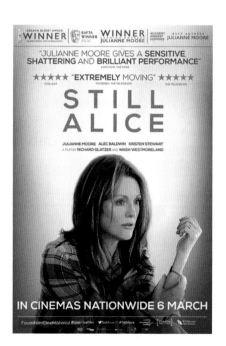

FIGURE 22-3 Vicarious insideness is a sense of knowing that is felt when watching Alice try to navigate her once-familiar lifeworld.

OT's central focus on the well-being of the *whole person*. A phenomenological perspective claims that bodily being is more than physical corporeality: "The body is our basic mode of being in the world, consciousness is embodied consciousness, and a person is embodied being, not just the possessor of a body" (Madjar & Walton, 1999, p. 4). Phenomenologists speak of the **lived body**—a body that simultaneously experiences, acts in, and is aware of a world that, normally, responds with immediate pattern, meaning, and contextual presence (Finlay, 2006; Seamon, 2002; Simms, 2008b; Toombs, 2001). The lived body is the primary means of being in, experiencing, and encountering the world. The lived body falls ill, it experiences pain, it fails to heal, it heals badly, it becomes older, it remains impaired, it returns to good health, and it learns new ways to cope with illness or disablement.

In considering the environmental and place dimensions of the lived body, phenomenologists focus on **environmental embodiment**—the various ways, both sensorially and movement wise, that the lived body engages and coordinates with the world at hand, especially its environmental aspects (Seamon, 2002; Simms, 2008a, 2008b). A key thinker is French phenomenologist Maurice Merleau-Ponty (1962), who emphasized what he termed **body-subject**—the innate awareness of the body in habitual movement and response to the environment in which the action unfolds. Body-subject experiences change in temporal and environmental as expressed in more complex bodily movements and patterns extending over time and space (Allen, 2004; Cole, 2004; Hill, 1985; Seamon, 1979). One can speak of at least two such ensembles: first, **body routines**—sets of coordinated corporeal actions sustaining a specific task or aim, for example, driving, cooking, or lawn mowing; and second, **time-space routines**—sets of more or less habitual bodily actions that extend through a considerable portion of time, for example, a getting-up routine, a going-to-the-gym routine,

or a going-to-church-and-lunch routine (Seamon, 1979, 2002). Clearly, many occupational activities involve such *taken-for-granted* bodily ensembles.

For teaching OT, body-subject and its extended habitual patterns are an important dimension of everyday human experience that can be explored through firsthand phenomenological exercises—for example, having OT students move a thing that has a place in their home to a different place or setting oneself to go to a destination by a route other than the one he or she normally travels (Seamon, 1979). It is important that students *really see* and understand the significance of the lived presence of body-subject dynamics in their own daily experiences so that they are better able to empathize with the lifeworld changes, distortions, and difficulties that often accompany a client's illness or disablement.

Phenomenological illustrations are important for OT and occupational science because they provide detailed, experience-grounded depictions of specific modes of illness and disability (Table 22-2).

One exemplary study is movement educator Maureen Connolly's (2010) efforts to embed meaningful movement into the everyday school activities of children with autism spectrum disorder (ASD). Recognizing that children with ASD do best when everyday routines and schedules are highly predictable, Connolly aimed, through environmental alterations and movement education, to help children "gradually learn to accept greater levels of variation and unpredictability" (Connolly, 2010, p. 114). For example, Connolly created a classroom environment incorporating subdued lighting; thick, absorptive, unstable surfaces; contrasts in ceiling height; and different places within the classroom for different tasks and functions. These design elements slowed and organized the movements of the children and provided a means, through physical contact, for them to experience a more placid and bodily grounded engagement with their surroundings.

TABLE 22-2   Illness and Disability Phenomenology Examples

Title of Paper	Author(s) (Date)
"'Transforming' Self and Worth: A Phenomenological Study of a Changing Lifeworld Following a Cochlear Implant"	Finlay & Molano-Fisher (2007)
"'My Own Way of Moving'—Movement Improvisation in Children's Rehabilitation"	Bjorbækmo & Engelsrud (2011)
"'Frustrating Disability': The Lived Experience of Coping with the Rehabilitation Phase Following Flexor Tendon Surgery"	Fitzpatrick & Finlay (2008)
"Persons Who Are Dependent upon Technologies for Care: Lived Experience of Being Cared for Following Lower Limb Amputation"	Koszalinski & Locsin (2015)
"Complexities During Transition to Adulthood for Youth with Disabilities: Person-Environment Interactions"	Stewart et al. (2014)
"Lifeworld Perspectives Utilizing Assistive Devices: Individuals, Lived Experience Following a Stroke"	Pettersson, Appelros, & Ahlström (2007)
"Recovery as the Re-fabrication of Everyday Life: Exploring the Meaning of Doing for People Recovering from Mental Illness"	Sutton (2010)
"Occupational Experiences of Older Patients on Hospital Wards"	Martin & Stack (2015)

As Connolly's (2010) teaching efforts suggest, an integral component of environmental embodiment is the physical and spatial environment in which the lived body finds itself. Sometimes, drawing on **universal design** (fabricating products and environments that work well for almost everyone), occupational therapists and other professionals have considered how architecture and environmental design can sustain and enhance patients' and clients' lifeworlds (Preiser & Smith, 2011; Rickerson, 2009; Söderback, 2009; Ulrich et al., 2008). Brooks and colleagues (2011), for example, examined how patients in assisted-living and rehabilitation settings made use of bedside-table devices and then designed three improved "smart stand" prototypes that were more efficient in terms of object reach, placement, storage, and mobility. In a study that examined assisted-living residents' walking behaviors, Lu (2010) developed design recommendations to improve residential walkability, including looped indoor and outdoor walkways; hallways with furnished alcoves usable by residents who otherwise might obstruct corridors; and windowed interior walkways that offer residents a visual connection to the world outside, especially the natural environment (Ulrich et al., 2008, pp. 87–91).

Home and Universal Design

Another important aspect of the lifeworld is *home* and *at-homeness* (Blunt & Dowling, 2005; Gitlin, 2003; Mallett, 2004; Manzo, 2003; J. Moore, 2007; Rioux & Werner, 2011; Seamon, 2010). These studies indicate that home has specific physical, personal, social, cultural, and political dimensions but, experientially, is lived as a human and environmental whole that incorporates and facilitates a wide range of existential significances. Home is not only a physical place but also a locus of activities, an anchor of identity, a repository of memories bonding past and present, and a center of stability and continuity (Figure 22-4). This literature also emphasizes that some homes can involve a "shadow side" of discomfort, distress, and trauma—for example, homes where there is domestic violence (Anthony, 1997; Blunt & Dowling, 2005; Manzo, 2003).

For OT, one key conceptual and lived division is home as a physical environment versus home as a locus of human life and meaning (Rowles, 2006). In studying the former, one considers the home as a dwelling incorporating the equipment, things, and spaces of daily living. One important question is how the dwelling's design and construction sustain or interfere with environmental embodiment, especially if residents are ill, older, or dealing with impairments (Kopec, 2006; Rosenfeld & Chapman, 2008). With regard to aging, for example, research demonstrates that older people typically spend more time in the residence and increasingly centralize their home by setting up "control centers"—for instance, a favorite chair and side table that allow the older person an easy reach to many of his or her daily needs

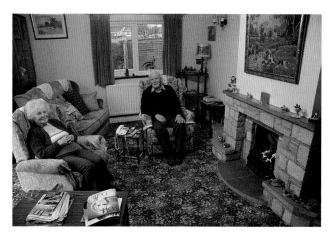

FIGURE 22-4 An older couple at home in their living room in northern England. One's home is not only a physical environment but also a place of activities, an anchor of identity, a repository of memories, and a center of stability and continuity. A major task for the occupational therapist is helping clients to recover as much as possible their sense of home and at-homeness. (Photograph by Walter Lewis and used with permission. © 2011 Walter Lewis.)

(Figure 22-5) (Rosenfeld & Chapman, 2008; Schaie, Wahl, Mollenkopf, & Oswald, 2003). In addition, older people may rearrange furniture and other home furnishings to remove obstacles to mobility or to provide sturdy anchors so they are less likely to fall when walking (Rowles, 2006).

There is also the question of how, through design, existing houses and dwelling units can be modified to

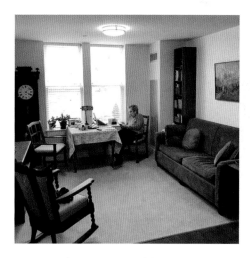

FIGURE 22-5 This 90-year-old woman just moved into an independent living apartment in a new facility. She brought her own furniture and set up her kitchen table in the window where she likes to drink coffee, read her Kindle, and open her mail.

match more closely the lifeworld needs of residents as they age or become ill or less abled (Kopec, 2006). Occupational therapists and other professionals have been actively involved in working out effective ways, through environmental interventions and assistive technology, to make home environments more accommodating—for example, widening doors, installing grab bars, adding entrance ramps, providing intercom systems, and so forth (Cook McCullagh, 2006; Corcoran & Gitlin, 1997; Iwarsson, 2009; Söderback, 2009; Steinfeld & Danford, 1999; Trefler & Hobson, 1997). In some situations, however, environmental interventions and assistive technology in the home can disrupt residents' lives, as A. J. Moore, Anderson, Carter, and Coad (2010) demonstrate in their study of the medical equipment and technology that many children with complex needs depend on in their homes: "The home space becomes an appropriated landscape—no longer a family landscape but a landscape of care, 'like a mini hospital,' with some parents feeling this particularly keenly" (A. J. Moore et al., 2010, p. 4).

Home as place offers a sense of well-being, safety, and comfort (Hasselkus, 2011). Healy-Ogden (2014) explored the meaning of place and dwelling in home care, finding that her participants dwelled in play space, creative space, nature's space, and spiritual space. When health care providers support well-being, they move beyond a simplistic view of a patient's house to understand the home as a meaning-filled dwelling. The experience of spaces may overlap. Pleasurable occupations such as gardening or table games with family and friends occur in play space. Play and creative spaces are nurturing and positive. Inside and outside spaces facilitate creative expression. Nature's space can be experienced inside or outside the home (Figure 22-6).

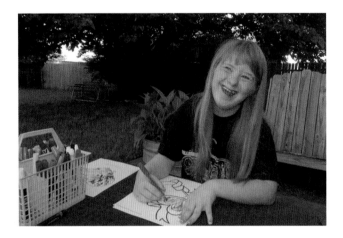

FIGURE 22-6 Addi Jo enjoys working at a back-yard picnic table. Extending activity outside into the natural environment makes participation joyful, one way to create *warmth* in setting the stage for a just-right challenge.

Dwelling in spiritual space involves a connection through prayer or creative expression (Healy-Ogden, 2014). Being mindful of home care patient and family member's sense of dwelling place opens possibilities of using the environment therapeutically to foster well-being.

Drawing on the principles of universal design, architects and interior designers have made major efforts to envision housing and other environments that accommodate the needs of users, whatever their age or degree of impairment (Cook McCullagh, 2006; Jennings, 2009; Preiser & Smith, 2011; Steinfeld & Danford, 1999; Steinfeld & White, 2010). This work is grounded partly in understanding how people function at different stages of life and in regard to different degrees of ableness and disablement (Kopec, 2006). One aim is homes that support **aging in place**—in other words, dwelling units that residents, if they so choose, can occupy from childhood to old age unless illness or impairment come into play (Rosenfeld & Chapman, 2008; Steinfeld & White, 2010; Young, 2011). As indicated by the dwelling design illustrated in Figure 22-7, this **universal housing** includes such features as stepless entrances with flush thresholds; kitchen and laundry appliances at convenient heights; bathing fixtures allowing multiple bathing options; and clear sight lines and adequate space for wheelchair use, including wide hallways, pocket doors, roll-under sinks, and wheelchair-height fixtures. See Box 22-1 for principles of universal design.

An important social aspect of place incorporates participation in community life through visiting others at home. Building and remodeling homes with *visitability* creates home as a place to gather others. Designers developing universal housing emphasize that issues of convenience, mobility, accessibility, and visitability are not limited to the dwelling alone but extend to the realm of the dwelling's immediate surroundings and larger neighborhood (Steinfeld & White, 2010). The concept of visitability supports the social value of the home. Three requirements need to be met for a home to be "visitable": (1) one zero-step entrance, (2) doors with 32 inches of clear passage space, and (3) one bathroom on the main floor accessible by wheelchair (Scovel & Lichter, 2016). (See http://www.visitability.org for more information.)

If a universal dwelling is located in a car-dependent neighborhood, it cannot provide wider scale accessibility for residents who cannot drive—an increasingly important group as the populations of countries age. Many architects and planners today favor compact, human-scaled communities providing easy access to a wide range of functions, services, and activities (Seamon, 2002; Steinfeld & White, 2010). Such walkable, handicap-accessible neighborhoods might motivate residents to be more physically active and thus provide valuable health benefits (L. D. Frank, Engelke, & Schmid, 2003). In addition, the higher densities and a

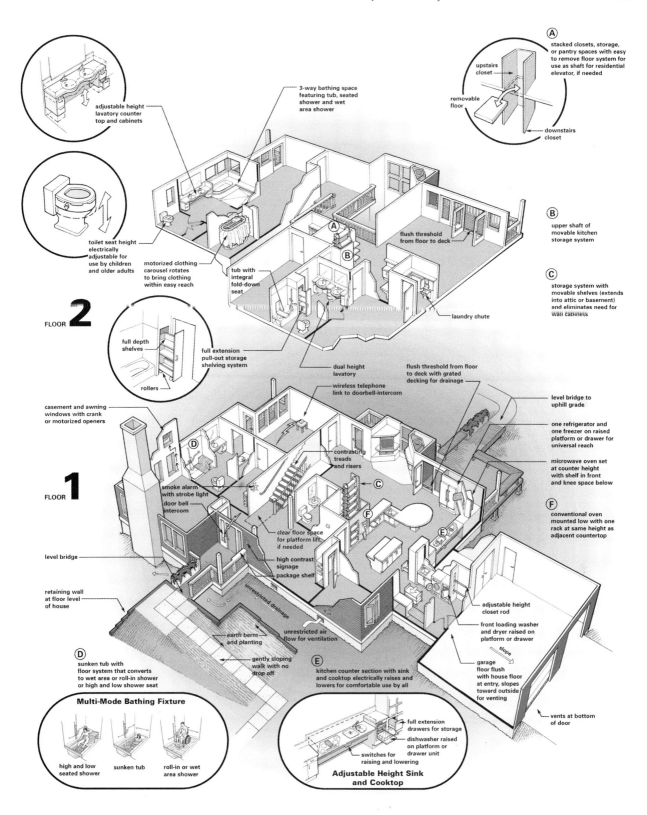

FIGURE 22-7 Two-story universal house. (Source: Preiser, W. F. E., & Smith, K. H. [Eds.]. [2011]. *Universal design handbook* [2nd ed.]. New York, NY: McGraw-Hill, p. 24.6. Illustration by Ron Mace and Rex Pace, Center for Universal Design, North Carolina State University, Raleigh; used with permission of the Center for Universal Design.)

BOX 22-1   UNIVERSAL DESIGN

Principles of Universal Design

1. **Equitable use**: The design does not disadvantage or stigmatize any group of users.
2. **Flexibility in use**: The design accommodates a wide range of individual preferences and abilities.
3. **Simple, intuitive use**: Use of the design is easy to understand regardless of the user's experience, knowledge, language skills, or current concentration level.
4. **Perceptible information**: The design communicates necessary information effectively to the user regardless of ambient conditions or the user's sensory abilities.
5. **Tolerance for error**: The design minimizes hazards and the adverse consequences of accidental or unintended actions.
6. **Low physical effort**: The design can be used efficiently and comfortably and with a minimum of fatigue.
7. **Size and space for approach and use**: Appropriate size and space is provided for approach, reach, manipulation, and use regardless of the user's body size, posture, or mobility.

Universal Design Resources

- Institute for Human Centered Design—Principles of Universal Design: https://www.humancentereddesign.org/universal-design/principles-universal-design
- Center for Universal Design (NC State University): https://projects.ncsu.edu/ncsu/design/cud/
- Center for Excellence in Universal Design—The 7 Principles of Universal Design: http://universaldesign.ie/What-is-Universal-Design/The-7-Principles/#p2
- Center for Excellence in Universal Design—10 Things to Know About UD (which could be summarized in a paragraph or two): http://universaldesign.ie/What-is-Universal-Design/The-10-things-to-know-about-UD/

more active street life might motivate residents to feel responsible for their neighborhood and be more willing to look out for each other (Gardner, 2011; Mehta & Bosson, 2010; Rosenbaum, Sweeney, & Windhorst, 2009). The occupational therapist plays a pivotal role in regard to housing needs because he or she has an intimate knowledge of clients' home requirements, restrictions, and possibilities. He or she can serve as an important go-between for helping clients articulate their environmental situation and needs to architects, interior designers, and contractors. Knowing clients' limitations firsthand, the occupational therapist can play a central role in "design teams" that plan aging in place or impairment-accommodating housing (Gitlin, 2003) and community centers or environments (Figure 22-8).

One way to document accessibility in a neighborhood is to use the Walkability Checklist (available at https://www.nhtsa.gov/sites/nhtsa.dot.gov/files/walkingchecklist.pdf). This resource is provided by the National Highway Traffic Safety Administration. It provides a checklist to guide a survey of safety for pedestrians in a particular area. For each problem identified, specific potential short-term and long-term solutions are suggested. Short-term actions are aimed at immediate safety; actions that may require more time include ways to advocate for safe neighborhoods and communities. The Health by Design assessment looks at neighborhoods as places in which goods and services should be walkable. Its developers were interested in building strong communities and interaction. After safety is evaluated, the rater determines what common destinations, such as grocery store, dry cleaners, salons, banks, medical clinics, and parks, are within a 10-minute walk (available at http://www.healthbydesignonline.org/documents/WalkabilitySurvey_HbD.pdf). Lastly, the Workplace Walkability Audit (Dannenberg, Cramer, & Gibson, 2005) is another resource that addresses not only safety but also aesthetics and shade around the workplace, where people spend considerable time when away from home.

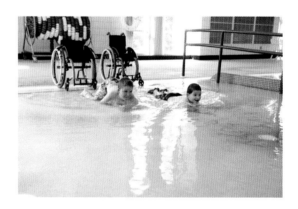

FIGURE 22-8 This recreation center, designed with an *objective outside* perspective, provides a space where all people can participate without segregation. An *empathic inside* understanding emerges among those who witness Simon and Manuel in an environment in which they are equally equipped to participate without restrictions or barriers. (Source: Reprinted with permission from http://committoinclusion.org/universal-design/)

At-Homeness and Occupational Therapy

Besides being a physical dwelling that founds a particular mode of daily living, the home is also a constellation of experiences, meanings, and situations that relates to residents' personal and communal sense of identity and belonging (Manzo, 2003; Percival, 2002; Rowles, 2006; Rowles & Chaudhury, 2005; Stafford, 2009). One phenomenological concept that helps integrate the lived dimensions of home is **at-homeness**, which can be defined as the taken-for-granted situation of feeling completely comfortable and intimately familiar with the world in which one lives his or her everyday life (Oldenburg, 1999, pp. 39–41; Seamon, 1979, p. 78). For the clients of occupational therapists, at-homeness has often been disrupted or eroded; a delineation of the lived dimensions of at-homeness provides one means for considering the client's residential needs more precisely and thinking through routines they might be restored or better accommodated.

Table 22-3 depicts the existential structure of at-homeness in terms of five lived qualities that can support

TABLE 22-3   Aspects of At-Homeness: Sustaining and Undermining Dimensions

Sustaining Aspect	Description	Spatial Expression	Undermining Aspect	Implications for Occupational Therapy
Rootedness	Organizes the habitual, bodily stratum of a person's life; intimately related to environmental embodiment and body-subject.	Concentrated in places, paths, and points of use, especially favorite places within and around the home; undeveloped in unused portions.	Disconnectedness: involves spatial disorientation, bodily discomfort, or loss of mobility and accessibility.	Ensure meaningful daily occupations can be maintained through retraining and environmental supports. Focus on the client's bodily "doing" and "being" in and around the home, especially bodily routines and actions.
Appropriation	Involves feeling a sense of autonomy and control in regard to home and immediate surroundings; typically includes a sense of privacy.	Roughly concentric and generally strongest for most important "centers" in the home; intensity in proportion to use and attachment; relates to "centers," paths, places for things, and things themselves.	Imposition: includes loss of autonomy; dependence on external assistance, whether human, environmental, or technological.	Provide adequate human help and assistive technologies to support personal autonomy and self-worth (e.g., installing appropriate bathing equipment so client can maintain independence).
At-easeness	Involves "freedom to be" and contentment; relates to inner mood and sense of well-being; things and situations that give everyday satisfaction are readily available.	Usually strongest in the home but possible in other places outside the home (i.e., third places) where person feels comfortable and relaxed.	Uneaseness: involves a situation where comfortableness of lifeworld called into question by personal, social, or environmental changes.	Enable satisfying occupations that can be engaged in alone or with others (e.g., working to maintain client's valued hobbies).
Regeneration	Relates to restorative powers of home and at-homeness; home not only as a site of relaxation and rest but also as a place of psychological recuperation and rejuvenation.	Generally associated with the home but possible in other places with restorative powers (e.g., the route a person walks his or her dogs each day).	Degeneration: relates to disruption in rest and regeneration due to personal, social, or environmental changes.	Enable relaxing occupations through environmental modifications (e.g., incorporating more appropriate lighting or changing room use). Consider how such modifications may shift daily activities (e.g., if a living area is converted to a bedroom, where will the client go to relax and engage in leisure?)
Warmth	Relates to supportive ambience of sustenance and well-being; invokes positive emotions like kindness, cheerfulness, good will, and camaraderie.	Most common in interior spaces and expressed by decoration, sense of order, and interpersonal harmony; also present in cared-for outside environments like gardens.	Coldness: relates to an unpleasant or hostile environmental ambience; spirit of place devolves into raw material space.	Work with client's values and find compromises (e.g., managing a level of cleanliness that is acceptable or decluttering a space but preserving what is most meaningful for client).

Adapted from Seamon, D. (1979). *A geography of the life world*. New York, NY: St. Martin's Press.

or undermine a sense of familiarity and comfort (Seamon, 1979, 2010). First, *rootedness* refers to the quality of at-homeness to organize the habitual, bodily stratum of a person's life and is intimately related to environmental embodiment and body-subject. Literally, the home roots the person spatially, sustaining a physical center for departures and returns. In cases of impairment, illness, or aging, rootedness may be displaced by *disconnectedness*, which can include spatial disorientation, bodily discomfort, or loss of mobility and accessibility. Second, *appropriation* refers to a resident's feeling a sense of autonomy and control in regard to his or her home and immediate surroundings. At least in the modern Western context, appropriation typically includes a sense of privacy, whereby residents and family can readily be alone. Compromised through disablement or illness, appropriation devolves into *imposition*, a situation where the resident is less autonomous and more dependent on external assistance, whether human, environmental, or technological.

A third quality of at-homeness is *at-easeness*, which refers to the "freedom to be." In a situation of at-homeness, residents can be who they most comfortably are and do what they most wish to do, a situation that can shift into *uneasiness* when a lifeworld is upset in some way. Unlike appropriation, which relates more to physical and psychological control of the home, at-easeness relates to inner mood and sense of well-being. To be at ease is to have readily available the things and situations that give one everyday satisfaction and sustain the lifeworld's transparency and taken-for-grantedness. Fourth, *regeneration* refers to the restorative powers of home and at-homeness. Regeneration involves the home not only as a site of relaxation and rest but also as a place of psychological recuperation and rejuvenation. In a disrupted lifeworld, regeneration becomes *degeneration* due to stress, worry, or physical difficulties associated with sleeping and resting. Finally, *warmth* speaks to an intangible atmosphere of sustenance and well-being that often involves positive emotions like joy and happiness. Sometimes, the warmth of home life perseveres in times of illness or impairment, or it can disappear or devolve into *coldness*. A sense of place becomes spiritless space.

These five lived qualities of at-homeness are heuristic and broadly diagnostic in that they provide one way to think through a particular client's home situation in terms of daily occupations (A. J. Moore et al., 2010, pp. 4–5). Different clients' everyday worlds will involve different combinations and intensities of the five qualities of at-homeness. Their potential value is that each points toward a different set of possibilities and means for transforming a quality's negative pole into its positive opposite. For example, rootedness is grounded in the lived body, and one occupational aim is to find ways, through environmental intervention, assistive technology, and the client's

rehabilitation efforts, to return his or her lifeworld to its former taken-for-grantedness in terms of bodily actions and routines. Or, in regard to at-easeness, the occupational therapist works to learn a client's daily pleasures and satisfactions and find ways whereby they might be reincorporated in his or her everyday life, although sometimes in revised or partial ways. The central aim in using at-homeness as a diagnostic focus is to envision the client's abled and impaired lifeworlds from a multidimensional perspective that might spur creative interventions not imagined otherwise (see Case Study 22-1).

There are other ways to create a sense of at-homeness for clients who are displaced temporarily (i.e., inpatient in hospital or rehabilitation centers) or who have experienced a permanent move yet have lost a feeling of being at-home (i.e., assisted living, long-term care facilities, refugees, and homeless individuals and families). Simple tasks of daily living can feel foreign until one *adopts* a new location by *adapting* to change. Fischer and Hotchkiss (2008) proposed a Model of Occupational Empowerment that can be applied in such cases. They identified that *disempowering environments* can lead to *occupational deprivation* which reinforces *learned helplessness*. Further, they assert that *occupational therapy programs can empower* individuals through occupation to *promote positive change* (Fischer & Hotchkiss, 2008, p. 60).

Empowering occupations have positive outcomes. For example, a despondent new resident of a nursing home was not dressing or engaging in daily hygiene, nor leaving her room for any reason. After a conversation revealed that she did not at all feel at home and was not even aware of what personal possessions had been moved to this new place, the therapist and resident set about to explore her new space. Over the course of several sessions, they emptied her closet, assessed the contents, and rearranged it to suit her taste and ability to access what she wanted and needed. They did the same to the dresser, nightstand, and bathroom cabinets. Now familiar with this place through **behavioral insideness**, she could readily engage in familiar routines for self-care and as a result began to venture out to the dining area, chapel, and dayroom for activities. Although not yet an insider, she was beginning to feel more at home.

Real Places, Virtual Places, and Occupational Therapy

There is considerable indication that virtual technologies are dramatically reshaping human life in the twenty-first century (Friesen, 2011; Relph, 2007). Currently, we can envision only glimpses of what robotics, virtual realities, and **information and communication technologies (ICT)** might mean for occupations and OT (Fok, Miller Polgar, Shaw, Luke, & Mandich, 2009; Mihailidis & Davis, 2005; Rakoski, 2013). The desire of older and less able individuals to live independently has spurred development of the **smart house**, which incorporates robotics, networked appliances, and other digital devices connecting residents with their home and wider community (Sanchez, Taylor, & Bing-Jonsson, 2017). This integration of home services with technology is called **domotics**, which works to "improve safety, security, comfort, communication, and technical management in the home" (Rosenfeld & Chapman, 2008, p. 25). One example is digital lighting that automatically provides residents moving through their home with an illuminated pathway, helping to reduce falls. Also significant are domestic robotic devices that include telerehabilitation, robotic pet therapy, and robotic assistants, the last of which can provide, among other home services, therapy and mental stimulation (Bedaf, Gelderblom, & De Witte, 2015; Broekens, Heerink, & Rosendal, 2009; Cherry, et al., 2017; Sicurella & Fitchsimmons, 2016). In addition, these robotic devices can monitor health and behaviors and connect residents to health care providers and to friends and relatives living elsewhere (Bedaf et al., 2015).

More transformative technological possibilities for occupational activities involve innovations in the **brain-computer interface (BCI)**, which allows objects and images to be manipulated via sensory devices registering brain waves or facial movements (Graham-Rowe, 2011). By shifting the eyes or picturing an action or symbol cognitively, the user can direct a robotic assistant, activate networked appliances, or manipulate items on a computer screen (Corralejo, Nicolas-Alonso, Alvarez, & Hornero, 2014; Miralles et al., 2015). For many older and impaired individuals, this technology could well be life changing because they gain the mental and physical autonomy to control computers, wheelchairs, assistive technologies, and other aspects of their everyday environment. Perhaps even more compelling is the coupling of BCI with virtual reality technology, which allows people with impairments to generate and participate in online virtual worlds like "Second Life," where users (called "residents") meet other residents, socialize, create virtual homes and other virtual places, offer virtual goods and services, and so forth (Graham-Rowe, 2011).

Virtually connected homes are infusing place with technologies that link home dwellers to outside communities and supports for cognitive assistance, safety, and simple information. The concept of *at-homeness* will evolve as families and individuals weigh the functional and ethical balance of privacy and monitoring (Sanchez et al., 2017). The term *aging-in-place* suggests a continuous habitation of one's home in older years regardless of health impairment. Virtual monitoring of older adults comes at a cost

of privacy and loss of connectedness to important others; that external monitoring would lessen the need for physically present social visits. Virtual monitoring reduces a sense of place by bringing "outsiders" in to the home; the boundary created for privacy of inhabitants is lost. To bring care closer is to bring the stranger in (Lopez & Sanchez-Criado, 2009).

Virtual worlds and virtual places may provide a radically innovative means for occupational therapists to assist clients in recovering and recreating what was called, at the start of this chapter, "being at home." In this sense, occupational therapists will contribute fabricating virtual places that allow clients to become involved in virtual occupations unlikely or impossible in the clients' real worlds. Clearly, virtual realities will create a new world of occupations in a dynamic context.

REFERENCES

Allen, C. (2004). Merleau-Ponty's phenomenology and the body-in-space encounters of visually impaired children. *Environment and Planning D: Society and Space, 22,* 719–735.

Andersen, L. T., & Reed, K. L. (2017). *The history of occupational therapy: The first century.* Thorofare, NJ: SLACK.

Anthony, K. H. (1997). Bitter homes and gardens: The meanings of home to families of divorce. *Journal of Architectural and Planning Research, 14,* 1–19.

Bauby, J. D. (1997). *The diving bell and the butterfly* (J. Leggart, Trans.). New York, NY: Vintage International.

Bedaf, S., Gelderblom, G. J., & De Witte, L. (2015). Overview and categorization of robots supporting independent living of elderly people: What activities do they support and how far have they developed. *Assistive Technology, 27,* 88–100. doi:10.1080/10400435.2014.978916

Bjorbækmo, W. S., & Engelsrud, G. H. (2011). "My own way of moving"—Movement improvisation in children's rehabilitation. *Phenomenology & Practice, 5,* 27–47.

Blunt, A., & Dowling, R. (2005). *Home.* New York, NY: Taylor & Francis.

Broekens, J., Heerink, M., & Rosendal, H. (2009). Assistive social robots in elderly care: A review. *Gerontechnology, 8,* 94–103.

Brooks, J. O., Smolentzov, L., DeArment, A., Logan, W., Green, K., Walker, I., . . . Yanik, P. (2011). Toward a "smart" nightstand prototype: An examination of nightstand table contents and preferences. *Health Environments Research & Design Journal, 4,* 91–108.

Bryan, M. L. M., & Davis, A. F. (Eds.). (1990). *100 Years at Hull House.* Bloomington, IN: Indiana University Press.

Carel, H. (2008). *Illness: The cry of the flesh.* Stocksfield, United Kingdom: Acumen.

Casey, E. S. (2009). *Getting back into place: Toward a renewed understanding of the place-world* (2nd ed.). Bloomington, IN: Indiana University Press.

Cherry, C. O., Chumbler, N. R., Richards, K., Huff, A., Wu, D., Tilghman, L. M., & Butler, A. (2017). Expanding stroke telerehabilitation service to rural veterans: A qualitative study on patient experiences using the robotic stroke therapy delivery and monitoring system program. *Disability and Rehabilitation: Assistive Technology, 12,* 21–27. doi:10.3109/17483107.2015.1061613

Clarke, C. (2009). An introduction to interpretative phenomenological analysis: A useful approach for occupational therapy research. *British Journal of Occupational Therapy, 7,* 37–39.

Cole, J. (2004). *Still lives: Narratives of spinal cord injury.* Cambridge, MA: MIT Press.

Connolly, M. (2010). Constructing a curriculum of place: Embedding meaningful movement in mundane activities for children and youth with autism spectrum disorder (ASD). In M. Barber, L. Embree, & T. J. Nenon (Eds.), *Phenomenology 2010: Vol. 5. Selected essays from North America, Part I* (pp. 107–134). Bucharest, Romania: Zeta Books.

Cook McCullagh, M. (2006). Home modification. *American Journal of Nursing, 106,* 54–63.

Corcoran, M., & Gitlin, L. (1997). The role of the physical environment in occupational performance. In C. Christiansen & C. M. Baum (Eds.), *Occupational therapy: Enabling function and well-being* (pp. 336–360). Thorofare, NJ: SLACK.

Corralejo, R., Nicolas-Alonso, L. F., Alvarez, D., & Hornero, R. (2014). A P300-based brain computer interface aimed at operating electronic devices at home for severely disabled people. *Medical & Biological Engineering & Computing, 52,* 861–872. doi:10.1007/s11517-014-1191-5

Cronin-Davis, J., Butler, A., & Mayers, C. A. (2009). Occupational therapy and interpretative phenomenological analysis: Comparable research companions? *British Journal of Occupational Therapy, 72,* 332–338.

Dannenberg, A. L., Cramer, T. W., & Gibson, C. J. (2005). Assessing the walkability of the workplace: A new audit tool. *American Journal of Health Promotion, 20,* 39–44.

Dunn, W., Haney McClain, L., Brown, C., & Youngstrom, M. J. (2003). The ecology of human performance. In E. B. Crepeau, E. S. Cohn, & B. A. B. Schell (Eds.), *Willard & Spackman's occupational therapy* (10th ed., pp. 223–227). Philadelphia, PA: Lippincott Williams & Wilkins.

Finlay, L. (2006). The body's disclosure in phenomenological research. *Qualitative Research in Psychology, 3,* 19–30.

Finlay, L. (2011). *Phenomenology for therapists: Researching the lived world.* Chichester, West Sussex: Wiley-Blackwell.

Finlay, L., & Molano-Fisher, P. (2007). "Transforming" self and world: A phenomenological study of a changing lifeworld following a cochlear implant. *Medicine, Health Care, and Philosophy, 11,* 255–267.

Fischer, G. S., & Hotchkiss, A. (2008). A Model of Occupational Empowerment for marginalized populations in community environments. *Occupational Therapy in Health Care, 22,* 55–71. doi:10.1300/J003v22n01_05

Fitzpatrick, N., & Finlay, L. (2008). "Frustrating disability": The lived experience of coping with the rehabilitation phase following flexor tendon surgery. *International Journal of Qualitative Studies on Health and Well-Being, 3,* 143–154.

Fok, D., Miller Polgar, J., Shaw, L., Luke, R., & Mandich, A. (2009). Cyberspace, real place: Thoughts on doing in contemporary occupations. *Journal of Occupational Science, 16,* 38–43.

Frank, A. W. (2002). *At the will of the body: Reflections on illness.* New York, NY: Houghton Mifflin Harcourt.

Frank, L. D., Engelke, P. O., & Schmid, T. L. (2003). *Health and community design: The impact of the built environment on physical activity.* Washington, DC: Island Press.

Friesen, N. (2011). *The place of the classroom and the space of the screen: Relational pedagogy and Internet technology.* New York, NY: Peter Lang.

Gardner, P. J. (2011). Natural neighborhood networks—Important social networks in the lives of older adults aging in place. *Journal of Aging Studies, 25,* 263–271.

Gitlin, L. N. (2003). Conducting research on home environments: Lessons learned and new directions. *The Gerontologist, 43,* 628–637.

Gitlin, L. N. (2009). Environmental adaptations for older adults and their families in the home and community. In I. Söderback (Ed.), *International handbook of occupational therapy interventions* (pp. 53–62). London, United Kingdom: Springer.

Graham-Rowe, D. (2011, July). Control your home with thought alone: The latest brain-computer interfaces meet smart home technology and virtual gaming. *NewScientist, 2819.* Retrieved from http://www.newscientist.com/issue/2819/

Hasselkus, B. R. (1998). Occupation and well-being in dementia: The experience of day-care staff. *American Journal of Occupational Therapy, 52,* 423–433.

Hasselkus, B. R. (2011). *The meaning of everyday occupation* (2nd ed.). Thorofare, NJ: SLACK.

Healy-Ogden, M. J. (2014). Being "at home" in the context of home care. *Home Health Care Management Practice, 26,* 72–79.

Hill, M. (1985). Bound to the environment: Towards a phenomenology of sightlessness. In D. Seamon & R. Mugerauer (Eds.), *Dwelling, place and environment: Towards a phenomenology of person and environment* (pp. 99–111). Dordrecht, The Netherlands: Martinus-Nijhof.

Hockenberry, J. (1995). *Moving violations: A memoir. War zones, wheelchairs, and declarations of independence.* New York, NY: Hyperion.

Hull, J. M. (1990). *Touching the rock: An experience of blindness.* New York, NY: Vintage.

Iwarsson, S. (2009). Housing adaptations: Current practices and future challenges. In I. Söderback (Ed.), *International handbook of occupational therapy interventions* (pp. 63–69). London, United Kingdom: Springer.

Jennings, M. B. (2009). Hearing accessibility and assistive technology use by older adults: Application of universal design principles to hearing. In L. Hickson (Ed.), *Proceedings of the second international adult conference: Hearing care for adults 2009—The challenge of aging* (pp. 249–254). Staefa, Switzerland: Phonak AG.

Kopec, D. (2006). *Environmental psychology for design.* New York, NY: Fairchild.

Koszalinski, R. S., & Locsin, R. C. (2015). Persons who are dependent upon technologies for care: Lived experience of being cared for following lower limb amputation. *International Journal for Human Caring, 19,* 38–43.

Lopez, D., & Sanchez-Criado, T. (2009). Dwelling the telecare home: Place, location, and habitability. *Space and Culture, 12,* 343–358. doi:10.1177/1206331209337079

Lu, Z. (2010). Investigating walking environments in and around assisted living facilities: A facility visit study. *Health Environments Research & Design Journal, 3,* 58–74.

Madjar, I., & Walton, J. (Eds.). (1999). *Nursing and the experience of illness: Phenomenology in practice.* London, United Kingdom: Routledge.

Mallett, S. (2004). Understanding home: A critical review of the literature. *The Sociological Review, 52,* 62–89.

Manzo, L. C. (2003). Beyond house and haven: Toward a revisioning of emotional relationships with place. *Journal of Environmental Psychology, 23,* 47–61.

Manzo, L. C. (2005). For better or worse: Exploring multiple dimensions of place meaning. *Journal of Environmental Psychology, 25,* 67–86.

Martin, M., & Stack, C. (2015). Occupational experiences of older patients on hospital wards. *British Journal of Occupational Therapy, 78,* 43–44.

Mehta, V., & Bosson, J. K. (2010). Third places and the social life of streets. *Environment and Behavior, 42,* 779–805.

Merleau-Ponty, M. (1962). *The phenomenology of perception.* New York, NY: Routledge & Kegan Paul.

Mihailidis, A., & Davis, J. (2005). The potential of intelligent technology as an occupational enabler. *Occupational Therapy Now, 7*(1), 22–23.

Miralles, F., Vargiu, E., Dauwalder, S., Solà, M., Müller-Putz, G., Wriessnegger, S. C., . . . Howish, H. (2015). Brain computer interface on track to home. *The Scientific World Journal, 2015*, 623896. doi:10.1155/2015/623896

Moore, A. J., Anderson, C., Carter, B., & Coad, J. (2010). Appropriated landscapes: The intrusion of technology and equipment into the homes and lives of families with a child of complex needs. *Journal of Child Health Care, 14*, 3–5.

Moore, J. (2007). Polarity or integration? Toward a fuller understanding of home and homelessness. *Journal of Architecture and Planning Research, 24*, 143–159.

Oldenburg, R. (1999). *The great good place: Cafés, coffee shops, bookstores, bars, hair salons, and other hangouts at the heart of a community* (3rd ed.). New York, NY: Marlowe & Company.

Padilla, R. (2003). Clara: A phenomenology of disability. *American Journal of Occupational Therapy, 57*, 413–423.

Percival, J. (2002). Domestic spaces: Uses and meanings in the daily lives of older people. *Ageing & Society, 22*, 729–749.

Pettersson, I., Appelros, P., & Ahlström, G. (2007). Lifeworld perspectives utilizing assistive devices: Individuals, lived experience following a stroke. *Canadian Journal of Occupational Therapy, 74*, 15–26. doi:10.2182/cjot.0605

Preiser, W. F. E., & Smith, K. H. (Eds.). (2011). *Universal design handbook* (2nd ed.). New York, NY: McGraw-Hill.

Rakoski, D. R. (2013). The virtual context of occupation: Integrating everyday technology into everyday practice. *OT Practice, 18*(9), CE1–CE8.

Relph, E. (2007). Spirit of place and sense of place in virtual realities. *Techné: Research in Philosophy and Technology, 10*, 1–8.

Relph, E. (2008). *Place and placelessness*. London, United Kingdom: Pion. (Original work published 1976)

Rickerson, N. (2009). Universal design: Principles and practice for people with disabilities. In I. Söderback (Ed.), *International handbook of occupational therapy interventions* (pp. 159–165). London, United Kingdom: Springer.

Rioux, L., & Werner, C. (2011). Residential satisfaction among aging people living in place. *Journal of Environmental Psychology, 31*, 158–169.

Rosenbaum, M. S., Sweeney, J. C., & Windhorst, C. (2009). The restorative qualities of an activity-based, third place café for seniors: Restoration, social support, and place attachment at Mather's— More than café. *Seniors Housing & Care Journal, 17*, 39–54.

Rosenfeld, J. P., & Chapman, W. (2008). *Home design in an aging world.* New York, NY: Fairchild.

Rowles, G. D. (1999). Beyond performance: Being in place as a component of occupational therapy. *American Journal of Occupational Therapy, 45*, 265–271.

Rowles, G. D. (2003). The meaning of place as a component of self. In E. B. Crepeau, E. S. Cohn, & B. A. B. Schell (Eds.), *Willard & Spackman's occupational therapy* (10th ed., pp. 111–119). Philadelphia, PA: Lippincott Williams & Wilkins.

Rowles, G. D. (2006). Commentary: A house is not a home: But can it become one? In H. W. Wahl, H. Brenner, H. Mollenkopf, D. Rothenbacher, & C. Rott (Eds.), *The many faces of health, competence and well-being in old age: Integrating epidemiological, psychological and social perspectives* (pp. 25–32). Dordrecht, The Netherlands: Springer.

Rowles, G. D., & Chaudhury, H. (Eds.). (2005). *Home and identity in late life.* New York, NY: Springer.

Rowles, G. D., & Watkins, F. (2003). History, habit, heart, and hearth: On making spaces into places. In K. W. Schaie, H. W. Wahl, H. Mollenkopf, & F. Oswald (Eds.), *Aging independently: Living arrangements and mobility* (pp. 77–96). New York, NY: Springer.

Sanchez, V. G., Taylor, I., & Bing-Jonsson, P. C. (2017). Ethics of smart house welfare technology for older adults: A systematic literature review. *International Journal of Technology Assessment in Health Care, 33*, 691–699. doi:10.1017/S0266462317000964

Schaie, W. K., Wahl, H. W., Mollenkopf, H., & Oswald, F. (Eds.). (2003). *Aging independently: Living arrangements and mobility.* New York, NY: Springer.

Scovel, G., & Lichter, M. (2016). Come on in. *Paraplegic News, 70*(1), 29–33.

Seamon, D. (1979). *A geography of the lifeworld.* New York, NY: St. Martin's Press.

Seamon, D. (2000). A way of seeing people and place: Phenomenology in environment-behavior research. In S. Wapner, J. Demick, T. Yamamoto, & H. Minami (Eds.), *Theoretical perspectives in environment-behavior research—Underlying assumptions, research problems, and methodologies* (pp. 157–178). New York, NY: Plenum.

Seamon, D. (2002). Physical comminglings: Body, habit, and space transformed into place. *OTJR: Occupation, Participation and Health, 22*, 42S–51S.

Seamon, D. (2010). Gaston Bachelard's topoanalysis in the 21st century: The lived reciprocity between houses and inhabitants as portrayed by American writer Louis Bromfield. In L. Embree (Ed.), *Phenomenology 2010: Vol. 5. Selected essays from North America, Part I* (pp. 225–243). Bucharest, Romania: Zeta Books.

Sicurella, T., & Fitzsimmons, V. (2016). Robotic pet therapy in long-term care. *Nursing, 46*(6), 55–57. doi:10.1097/01.NURSE.0000482265.32133.f6

Simms, E. (2008a). Children's lived spaces in the inner city: Historical and political aspects of the psychology of place. *The Humanistic Psychologist, 36*, 72–89.

Simms, E. (2008b). *The child in the world.* Detroit, MI: Wayne State University Press.

Söderback, I. (2009). Adaptive interventions: Overview. In I. Söderback (Ed.), *International handbook of occupational therapy interventions* (pp. 39–51). London, United Kingdom: Springer.

Stafford, P. B. (2009). *Elderburbia: Aging with a sense of place in America.* Westport, CT: Praeger.

Stefanovic, I. (2008). Holistic paradigms of health and place: How beneficial are they to environmental policy and practice? In J. Eyles & A. Williams (Eds.), *Sense of place, health and quality of life* (pp. 45–57). Burlington, VT: Ashgate.

Steinfeld, E., & Danford, G. S. (1999). *Enabling environments. Measuring the impact of environment on disability and rehabilitation.* New York, NY: Kluwer Academic.

Steinfeld, E., & White, J. (2010). *Inclusive housing: Design for diversity and equality.* New York, NY: Norton.

Stewart, D., Law, M., Young, N. L., Forhan, M., Healy, H., Burke-Gaffney, J., & Freeman, M. (2014). Complexities during transitions to adulthood for youth with disabilities: Person-environment interactions. *Disability and Rehabilitation, 36*, 1998–2004.

Stewart, D., Letts, L., Law, M., Cooper, B. A., Strong, S., & Rigby, P. J. (2003). The person-environment occupation model. In E. B. Crepeau, E. S. Cohn, & B. A. B. Schell (Eds.), *Willard & Spackman's occupational therapy* (10th ed., pp. 227–233). Philadelphia, PA: Lippincott Williams & Wilkins.

Sutton, D. (2010). Recovery as the re-fabrication of everyday life: Exploring the meaning of doing for people recovering from mental illness. *New Zealand Journal of Occupational Therapy, 57*(1), 41.

Svenaeus, F. (2001). The phenomenology of health and illness. In S. K. Toombs (Ed.), *Handbook of phenomenology and medicine* (pp. 87–108). Dordrecht, The Netherlands: Kluwer Academic.

Toombs, S. K. (Ed.). (2001). *Handbook of phenomenology and medicine.* Dordrecht, The Netherlands: Kluwer Academic.

Trefler, E., & Hobson, D. (1997). Assistive technology. In C. Christiansen & C. M. Baum (Eds.), *Occupational therapy: Enabling function and well being* (pp. 482–506). Thorofare, NJ: SLACK.

Tuan, Y. (1977). *Space and place: The perspective of experience.* Minneapolis, MN: University of Minnesota Press.

Ulrich, R. S., Zimring, C., Zhu, X., DuBose, J., Seo, H., Choi, Y., . . . Joseph, A. (2008). A review of the research literature on evidence-based healthcare design. *Health Environments Research & Design Journal, 1*, 61–125.

van Manen, M. (1990). *Researching lived experience: Human science for an action sensitive pedagogy.* Albany, NY: State University of New York Press.

van Manen, M. (1998). Modalities of body experience in illness and health. *Qualitative Health Research, 8*, 7–24.

Young, L. C. (2011). Universal housing: A critical component of a sustainable community. In W. Preiser & K. H. Smith (Eds.), *Universal design handbook* (2nd ed., pp. 24.3–25.13). New York, NY: McGraw-Hill.

thePoint®   *For additional resources on the subjects discussed in this chapter, visit* **http://thePoint.lww.com/Willard-Spackman13e**.

UNIT V

Client Factors and Occupational Performance

So Much Depends

on a tumor smaller than a pin head.
Any smaller, it would be invisible.
They'll remove it, sew you up, send it for biopsy.

So small, but more than nothing.
A few weeks of radiation therapy.
Nothing you can't handle.

But oh, you've tested positive for The Gene.
Now they want to take nothing from you
that makes you human, but everything
that makes you woman
except this

              eleven-year-old
with his passion for trains, whose smile
could make angels stand in line
to dance on the head of a pin.

For Laura

Addy Robinson McCulloch
Used with permission of the author.

CHAPTER 23

Individual Variance

Body Structures and Functions

Barbara A. Boyt Schell, Glen Gillen, Marjorie E. Scaffa, Ellen S. Cohn

LEARNING OBJECTIVES

After reading this chapter, you will be able to:

1. Consider how personal characteristics and factors are related to occupations and occupational performance.
2. Discuss how knowledge of personal factors is used in occupational therapy evaluation and intervention.
3. Identify examples of body functions and structures that are considered in the occupational therapy process.

Introduction

Throughout this text, there is recognition that occupation is a function of the individual performing within a specific context. How that occupational performance occurs, then, is a reflection of all the unique characteristics of the person doing the acting as well as the specific context in which the action occurs. In Unit IV, important contextual factors were discussed. In this unit, we examine the personal factors that influence occupational performance.

This chapter provides an overview of the various personal characteristics and factors that affect occupational performance. **Personal factors** is a broad term used here to encompass several aspects of the human condition. Different professional groups, such as the American Occupational Therapy Association (AOTA, 2014) and the World Health Organization (WHO, 2001), organize these descriptors of individuals in different ways. The AOTA Practice Framework uses the term *client factors* (AOTA, 2014, p. S7) to encompass many aspects of the person, the WHO uses the term *body structures and body functions* (WHO, 2001, p. 10), and other international models may use the term *performance components* or *occupational performance components* (Chapparo, Ranka, & Nott, 2017) to refer to many aspects of personal factors.

Regardless of the specific terminology used, occupational therapy (OT) requires close attention to the many ways that individuals are unique. Examples include basic information such as the person's age, gender, and ethnicity. People also vary in body structures, or anatomical parts, such as bones and organs and body functions, or physiological processes of the body, including psychological function (WHO, 2001). For instance, people may vary physically in terms of height, weight, and bodily strength; they may

CASE STUDY 23-1 CYNDE: PERSONAL FACTORS REQUIRED TO BE A NATURALIST ON A WHALE-WATCHING BOAT

Cynde is a naturalist on a whale-watching boat. In this description, some of the personal factors affecting her performance are noted. Refer to Tables 23-1, 23-2, and 23-3 to see if you can pinpoint the specific terms. Additionally, try to match other terms that connect to the many personal factors affecting her performance.

Cynde has been passionate about whales for as long as she can remember, and she is deeply committed to preserving the ocean habitat to ensure their survival (values and beliefs). Her job requires that she orient tourists to the whale boat safety rules, educate tourists about whales, and help them understand what they are seeing when they observe whale surface behavior. Because of her commitment to sustainability, she also tries to explain how personal actions in daily life can impact marine life many miles away from home.

Cynde starts each trip by standing on the dock, going over boat safety rules, and also explaining a bit about whales (Figure 23-1). Note that she has to hold (body function—musculoskeletal) the microphone with one hand (body structure—nervous system, movement-related structures) while demonstrating with another. She had to memorize (body function—long-term memory) what she needs to say (body function—language expression and working memory) and deliver her talk in a certain amount of time (body function—organization, planning, self-monitoring) while the boat is being readied for departure. She demonstrates enthusiasm and humor (body function—range of emotion, appropriate level of excitement) during her presentation. Once on the boat, she has to climb a steep ladder to get to the captain's area, where she will again use the microphone to call attention to the whales and their behavior. She works with the boat captain to detect whales at a long distance, using her visual skills. When she gets closer, she recognizes the distinctive patterns on the whale tails (called flukes), as

this is important to tracking individual whales. While she is providing commentary, she is also photographing whales and supervising science interns as they collect scientific data about whale sightings and surface behavior.

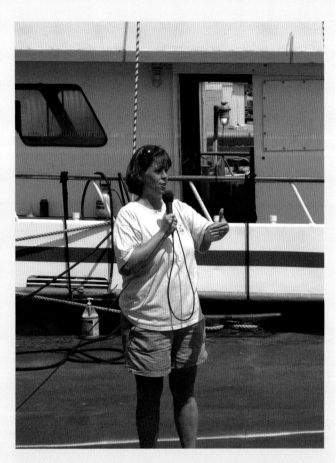

FIGURE 23-1 **Cynde is going over boat safety rules and also explaining a bit about whales.**

vary in their responses to different sensory experiences such as a preference for spicy food or cold drinks, and they may vary in their emotional responses to specific situations. Furthermore, these differences may or may not impact the person's occupational performance, depending on the demands and challenges the individual experiences in life. See Case Study 23-1 as an illustration of the many personal factors affecting individual occupational performance. Later in the chapter are tables listing many of the personal factors that may be considered by occupational therapists.

The Whole Is Greater Than the Sum of the Parts

Personal factors do not operate in isolation. Anyone who has tried to maneuver in unfamiliar space in the dark (such as finding the bathroom in a dark hotel room in the middle of the night) can attest to the importance of vision to movement. All bodily factors work synergistically, which is why it is

BOX 23-1   OBJECTIVE AND SUBJECTIVE REPORTS OF BODY FUNCTIONS AND STRUCTURES

"I Didn't Have a Clue"

In a study seeking to understand the subjective experience of regaining self-care skills after a stroke or spinal cord injury, Guidetti, Asaba, and Tham (2007) reported numerous examples of what it felt like for the study participants to attempt familiar tasks with various impairments. For instance, one participant who was recovering from a stroke appears to have had what objectively might be documented as a sensory loss, along with neglect of the affected upper extremity. She described her experience this way: "I didn't have a clue where it [her hand] was, it was behind my back and like this, so the first night it could have been anybody's hand" (Guidetti et al., 2007, p. 306).

"When You're Sitting There by Yourself, You're Just Eating"

In a study examining supported socialization for people with mental illness, Davidson and his colleagues (2004) argued that people with persistent mental illness are lonely and isolated, not by choice (or objective impairments) but because of lack of opportunity and encouragement. When viewed solely from an objective perspective, people with persistent mental illness have been described as having impairments in volition, self-awareness, or coping (affective and cognitive impairments) and are thought to no longer desire human connection, with a preference for being alone. In a randomized control trial of supported socialization intervention, Davidson and colleagues (2001) found that people with mental illness desire friendships. One participant in the study commented that eating with her friend was better than eating alone at Burger King: "I'm alone. I sit down at the table, I eat a hamburger. But when I go with somebody else, and I'm sitting there at the table and eating it, she'll say 'Oh, is your hamburger good?' Then it becomes, the hamburger becomes noticeable, and then your mind starts to think about the taste. But when you're sitting there by yourself, you're just eating" (Davidson et al., 2001, p. 380).

This woman's description of eating with a friend illustrates the importance of considering clients' subjective experience. Without consideration of the subjective experience, intervention may not address aspects of occupational performance that were meaningful to this woman.

---

difficult to generate a definitive list of factors to which practitioners should attend. That is the case in this chapter as well, and the selected lists of factors and descriptions are presented to prompt your thinking. The categorizations that are presented here are not, nor can they be, a complete list of all the factors that affect human behavior. They are, at best, suggestions of factors to consider in analyzing occupational performance.

Practitioners can consider all of these factors from an objective standpoint or as subjectively experienced by the client. When considering personal factors objectively, therapists typically start by carefully observing occupational performance. If more information is needed to understand why the person is acting in a particular way, the therapist may evaluate body functions and structures using standardized approaches that other observers can replicate. Examples include muscle testing, sensory testing, and cognitive testing in relation to occupational performance. Chapters 28 and 29 address the use of objective assessments and the importance of using reliable and valid measures to obtain objective data. Although objective approaches are undeniably useful for informing professional reasoning, the client's subjective experience is also important. For example, objective measurement may indicate impairment; however, the person may not consider this limitation problematic in terms of daily life. Consequently, there may not be a need for intervention. Alternatively, comparison of objective and subjective findings may show that a client is unaware of safety concerns that are observed by the therapist.

Therefore, skilled practitioners consider both the client's perspective and the objective information during the OT process. Box 23-1 provides some examples of objective and subjective reports related to body functions and structures.

Our job as OT practitioners is twofold. First, we must carefully observe occupational performance so as to understand which personal factors support occupational engagement and which ones are limiting engagement. Additionally, we must go beyond the generic labeling and understandings of diagnostic conditions to a deeper and more personal understanding of how clients perceive and experience their specific situations.

Reasoning about Personal Factors: Occupational Therapy as a Bridge

Occupational therapy practitioners like to say that they treat the whole person. Whereas other professions (such as nursing) legitimately make a similar claim, OT is unique in its focus on how daily occupations are the synergistic product of the personal factors within the individual and factors that are external to the person in the larger context.

Another way to think about OT and how we consider the factors under discussion is to contrast OT with other professions. Think of OT as a bridge between the medical world and the lifeworld. In the medical world, there are many professions that focus on particular sets of body structures and functions. The field of medicine has obvious examples, with specialties in dermatology, endocrinology, gynecology, psychiatry, ophthalmology, and the list goes on and on. But other professions can also be examples. For instance, nutritionists focus on the digestive system, physical therapists focus on the neuromuscular and musculoskeletal systems, and speech-language pathologists focus primarily on the cognitive and oral-motor systems as they relate to communication. Although all of these professionals are interested in improving an individual's function, their contribution is very specific, and their knowledge about body functions and structures within their specific scope is typically quite extensive.

In contrast, other professions organize themselves around major roles or tasks of life. For instance, vocational evaluators and rehabilitation counselors focus on work-related concerns, educators focus on helping people learn to become productive citizens, recreation professionals focus on play and leisure, and social workers focus on family and community life. These professionals may attend to the impact of personal factors. So, for example, vocational rehabilitation practitioners know a great deal about job demands, employer requirements, and government standards related to work. Special education teachers are particularly aware of the impact of cognitive abilities and limitations for students in the classroom. Similarly, recreation therapists are quite knowledgeable about recreational spaces and places, the value of leisure in life, and the kinds of equipment that individuals might use to pursue leisure interests. However, for the most part, these professionals are very different from those in the medically oriented fields in that they typically have little or no background related to anatomy, physiology, and the specific impact of different health conditions on performance. Additionally, these professions typically are less likely to attend to the full array of social and psychological factors affecting performance. Rather, they have broad working knowledge about the skills and social demands that are required for their area of interest.

Occupational therapists have the education and ability to understand and address the impact of body structures and functions on life roles and tasks. This is done with full appreciation of the interconnected nature of occupations as well as how occupations are learned and change over the life course. In addition, OT practitioners recognize the transactions among personal factors and the environments in which the person must function (AOTA, 2015). As a result, OT as a profession provides information that bridges the clients' personal factors with the roles and task competencies required in daily life.

Complexity: An Asset and a Challenge

Occupational therapy is unique as a profession in its willingness to consider all the client's personal factors along with all contextual factors as they shape engagement in the daily activities and routines of life. It is this appreciation of the transactional nature of occupational performance that makes OT so customized and effective for helping to solve complex problems of daily life. This uniqueness is a tremendous asset. However, for new practitioners and even some experienced ones, it can be challenging not to get absorbed in one aspect and thus lose sight of the larger picture. Practitioners who focus on one area of function may refer to themselves as hand therapists, cognitive therapists, or vision therapists and lose sight of the totality of our work as occupational therapists. Depth of knowledge about the personal factors is very important to expert practice; however, clients are best served when these factors are viewed in relation to the use of occupation as a means for intervention. Further, occupational engagement is the desired outcome regardless of how individual differences affect the ways in which this outcome is achieved. For example, as opposed to "doing hand therapy," our focus should be stated as "improving occupational performance after a hand injury." Examples of such reasoning are provided through the therapist narratives in Unit XIII. All of the practitioners in Unit XIII indicate a deep understanding of body functions and structures that are relevant to their clients, but they view these factors in relation to occupational performance. Furthermore, OT practitioners grade their use of interventions in a way that is mindful of each person's individual characteristics, development, impairments, potential for recovery, and/or need for adaptive approaches. Practitioners also are very cognizant of how social and cultural contexts influence their clients' lives. *Thus, OT practitioners specialize not in body parts or body functions but in achieving health, well-being, and participation in life through engagement in occupation* (AOTA, 2014).

Intertwining Knowledge and Theories

For OT practitioners to work effectively with people who have impairments or developmental conditions that affect their performance, practitioners must intertwine knowledge about occupation with knowledge about the client's particular health problems. As noted earlier, this chapter provides only a topical overview of the many person factors that practitioners may consider. Knowing what to do requires in-depth appreciation of relevant theories and research in order to assure effective intervention.

Unit XII provides the reader with examples of how theories guide practice to improve occupational performance in the focused areas of motor control, cognition and perception, sensory processing, emotional regulation, and communication/social interaction. The therapists' narratives in Unit XIII provide examples of using different theories to guide practice. Readers are encouraged to look at those chapters for examples of how to integrate theories about body functions and structures into an OT intervention.

Personal Factors That Are Commonly Considered

In this section, we provide several tables that readers might find helpful to prompt consideration of one or more personal factors (Tables 23-1, 23-2, 23-3, and 23-4). Readers will likely find the language useful in communicating about personal factors. As was discussed earlier, there is no practical way to make a comprehensive list, so we make no claim that the tables are all inclusive. Information for these tables was drawn primarily from the *International Classification of Functioning, Disability and Health* (WHO, 2001), the Occupational Therapy Practice Framework (AOTA, 2014), and topical areas that are addressed in this unit as well as chapters from Unit IV.

Clues to personal factors that could be affecting performance are gained from at least three sources:

- **Reason for referral.** Referral information may contain a medical, psychological, or educational diagnosis and sometimes precautions to consider during intervention. Even when precautions, symptoms, or other descriptors are not included, knowledge about typical body structures and functions that are affected by the condition can guide practitioners regarding factors to consider.

  Example: Diagnosis—rotator cuff tear. Knowledge of the body structure will lead practitioners to evaluate for the *impact* that pain, weakness, and limited shoulder range of motion may have on identified limitations in occupational performance. Limitations may include inability to perform self-care (e.g., shampooing hair), inability to fulfill a homemaker role (e.g., putting groceries away, washing windows), inability to engage in leisure activities (e.g., fly fishing), inability to perform job responsibilities (e.g., writing on a blackboard), and/or inability to fulfill child-care responsibilities (e.g., lifting a toddler into a high chair).

| TABLE 23-1 | Examples of Personal Factors (Excluding Body Functions and Structures) That Are Considered in Occupational Therapy |

Factor	Common Categories or Descriptors
Age	Historical cohort (e.g., people who lived through the depression and how that experience affects their worldview) Internalization of societal expectations regarding development and achieving a particular developmental milestone at a given time in the life course Personal expectations about age-related behavior
Gender	Personally adopted social/cultural norms and roles regarding gender
Values	Meanings associated with physical and social spaces Importance of family Standards of conduct Qualities considered desirable Principles considered worthwhile
Beliefs	Knowledge that is held to be truth Beliefs about causes and interventions related to illness Perceived locus of control Cognitive content held as truth
Spirituality	Beliefs about the meaning of life Quest to understand ultimate life questions Religious and sacred beliefs
Family and significant others	Internalized family experiences that shape worldview Internalized expectations about relationships
Socioeconomic status	Financial status Work status Educational attainment
Ethnicity	Internal beliefs about membership in groups of common descent; can include race, culture, language, religion, and politics
Sexual orientation	An individual's sexuality, usually related to an individual's romantic, emotional, and/or sexual attraction to persons of a particular gender

TABLE 23-2	Examples of Body Structures Considered in Occupational Therapy
Structure	**Common Categories or Descriptors**
Nervous system	Brain (cortical, subcortical including brain stem) Spinal cord Spinal nerves Sympathetic and parasympathetic systems
Eye and ear	Eye (retina, cornea, lens) External ocular muscles Ear (inner, middle, outer)
Voice and speech	Mouth (lips, cheek, tongue, teeth, palate) Nose Pharynx (nasal and oral) Larynx (vocal cords)
Cardiovascular, immunological, respiratory	Heart Veins Arteries Lungs Trachea Bronchial tubes Muscles of respiration Lymphatic system
Digestive, metabolic, endocrine	Esophagus Stomach Intestine Many glands
Genitourinary, reproductive	Bladder, ureters, urethra Reproductive structures
Movement-related structures (head/neck, upper and lower extremities, trunk, pelvic region)	Bones Joints Muscles Tendons Ligaments Fascia
Skin and related structures	Skin layers Skin glands Hair Sensing organs in skin

Source: American Occupational Therapy Association. (2014). Occupational therapy practice framework: Domain and process, 3rd edition. *American Journal of Occupational Therapy, 68,* S1–S48; and World Health Organization. (2001). *International classification of functioning, disability and health (ICF).* Geneva, Switzerland: Author.

- **Client self-report.** Clients themselves, their families, and other key people in their social environments (e.g., teachers, employers, caregivers) often give practitioners information about factors that they believe are affecting client performance.

  Example: A third-grade teacher reports to the occupational therapist that Alicia is highly distractible in class, requires multiple prompts and cues to stay on task, and is falling behind her classmates in reaching educational objectives. Alicia expresses a desire to play with other girls during recess but doesn't quite know how to join the group.

- **Observation of client.** Observations of the client engaging in occupations often prompt practitioners to consider one or more factors that are affecting performance.

  Example: During an evaluation of meal preparation skills, the OT practitioner notes that Mr. Brown is unable to independently complete a task as he did prior to his recent decline in cognitive function. He now requires step-by-step cues to sequence and organize the process of making a soup and salad.

  Example: Coleman attends a residential school for adolescents with traumatic brain injury. Since his accident, Coleman becomes fatigued, withdrawn, and apathetic by mid-afternoon. Every week, six teenage boys plan a Thursday evening community outing to relax and have fun together. The occupational therapist observes that Coleman does not offer suggestions for outings and rarely interacts with his peers during the outing. To accommodate for Coleman's personal factors and engage during a time of day when his performance is optimal, the practitioner plans to change the community outings to Saturday morning.

Skillful intervention requires that practitioners respond to these cues and then use credible resources to obtain needed objective information. This information, combined with

TABLE 23-3   Examples of Body Functions Considered by Occupational Therapists

ICF	Category	Examples
Global mental functions (affective, cognitive, perceptual)	Consciousness	Alertness, arousal level, continuity of wakeful state
	Orientation	Person Place Time Self Others Past Present
	Intellectual functions	Understanding Integration of cognitive functions
	Psychosocial functions	Interpersonal skills Social interactions
	Temperament/personality	Emotional stability Disposition Confidence
	Energy and drive	Energy level Motivation Impulse control Appetite
	Sleep functions	Amount and onset of sleep Quality Sleep cycle functions
Specific mental functions (affective, cognitive, perceptual)	Attention	Selectivity Sustainability Shifting Divided
	Memory	Short term Long term Working
	Perception	Auditory Visual Olfactory Gustatory Tactile Visuospatial
	Sensory processing	Reception Organization Assimilation Integration
	Thought	Ideation Pace of thought Content
	Higher level cognitive functions	Volition Organization/planning Purposeful action Self-awareness Self-monitoring Decision making Problem solving Judgment Time management Coping
	Emotional	Behavioral regulation Range of emotion
	Psychomotor functions	Appropriate affect Response time Level of excitement/agitation Speed of behavior

TABLE 23-3   Examples of Body Functions Considered by Occupational Therapists *(continued)*

ICF	Category	Examples
	Mental functions of language	Reception of language (spoken, written, and sign)
		Expression of language (spoken, written, and sign)
	Mental functions of sequencing complex movement	Praxis
Sensation and pain	Taste	Quality
		Intensity
	Smell	Quality
		Intensity
	Touch	Light
		Deep pressure
	Temperature	Hot
		Cold
	Pain	Sharp
		Stabbing
		Aching
		Burning
	Proprioception	Quick
		Sustained
	Vestibular	Linear
		Angular
	Visual	Acuity
		Intensity
		Contrast
	Auditory	Acuity
		Intensity
		Contrast
		Rhythm
Neuromuscular and movement	Joint mobility	Passive ROM
		Active ROM
	Muscle strength	Pinch
		Grip
		Force
	Muscle tone	Quality
	Voluntary motor control	Coordination (dexterity, gross motor, bilateral integration)
		Motor execution (mobility)
	Involuntary motor control	Reflexes
		Unconscious movement
	Posture	Alignment
		Orientation
		Stability
		Control
		Balance
		Adaptation
Cardiovascular, immunological, respiratory	Heart rate	Tension
	Blood pressure	Rate
	Respiration	Rhythm
		Depth

ICF, International Classification of Functioning, Disability and Health; ROM, range of motion.

From American Occupational Therapy Association. (2014). Occupational therapy practice framework: Domain and process, 3rd edition. *American Journal of Occupational Therapy, 68,* S1–S48; Dunn, W. (2011). *Best practice occupational therapy: In community service with children and families* (2nd ed.). Thorofare, NJ: SLACK; and World Health Organization. (2001). *International classification of functioning, disability and health (ICF).* Geneva, Switzerland: Author.

TABLE 23-4 Examples of Impaired Body Functions and Potential Impact on Occupational Performance

Impairment of Body Function	Potential Difficulty with Daily Life Occupations
Impaired visuospatial processing	Inability to orient clothing to self Misjudging distance when reaching for a utensil Inability to align car in parking space Spilling juice when pouring from carton into glass Difficulty finding the way in new environments and fear of getting lost results in self-imposed participation restrictions (Árnadóttir, 2016)
Decreased shoulder range of motion	Inability to manage hair care Unable to tuck shirt into back of pants Inability to retrieve book from high shelves at the library Inability to change a light bulb Difficulty holding and playing with one's children or grandchildren Role strain from inability to perform job responsibilities and inability to fulfill role of primary financial provider
Poor emotional regulation	Poor performance at job interview Inability to cope during finals week at college, resulting in poor test performance Social isolation due to inappropriate affect Difficulty initiating, developing, and maintaining interpersonal relationships Inability to make decisions due to overwhelming anxiety
Sensory loss in feet	Increased incidence of falls during community outings Inability to walk on rough terrains (beach, hiking trails, etc.) Inability to drive a car Decreased participation in social/leisure activities due to fear of falling
Decreased attention	Difficulty attending to one conversation at a time at a dinner party Unable to attend to school lectures/lessons Inability to cook toast and tea at the same time Difficulty following verbal and written instructions on the job Experiences of relationship strain as a partner may perceive a lack of interest due to easy distractibility (Gillen, 2009).

the subjective data provided by the client, is then synthesized to develop interventions that enable the client's occupational performance. It is important to remember that the "presence or absence of specific body functions and body structures do not necessarily ensure a client's success or difficulty with daily life occupations" (AOTA, 2014, p. S7). A person with memory loss may be able to fully participate in most aspects of life using compensatory strategies such as memory notebooks/diaries, electronic paging systems, written reminder lists posted in the environment, and/or smartphone alarm

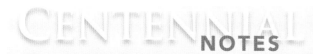

NOTES

Body Structures, Functions, and Occupational Performance

Occupational therapy practitioners have long been concerned with how body structures and functions support or limit occupational performance. Indeed, many chapters in the first edition of Willard and Spackman's (1947) text on OT are organized around body functions and structures as well as impairments related to them. In Chapter 2, McNary (1947) discusses what she calls the "types of problems presented to OT" and goes on to explain:

> The human problems to be benefitted by occupational therapy can be of a physiologic or a psychologic or nature, or both. The complex elements of a human being

vary with the individual's relation to his environment and when one or more of these factors are abnormal or lacking, normal functioning of the individual as a member of society is disturbed. (p. 11)

Examples of types of conditions that were listed in the first edition included cardiac conditions, metabolic disorders, skin conditions, and respiratory conditions, among others. The authors further described OT for special conditions of the eye, ear, nose, throat, blood and skin. It is interesting to note that McNary (1947) kept attention on how abnormality or dysfunction was also influenced by its interaction with the environment, presaging focus of today's OT practitioners on occupational performance and participation.

reminders. Optical aids, text-to-speech translators, and the use of guide dogs can provide a person with vision loss with the ability to live life fully and independently.

Conclusion

Occupational therapy practitioners routinely consider body functions, structures, and other personal factors during intervention. By integrating knowledge and theories about these personal factors with theories that relate to occupation and occupational contexts, practitioners provide a unique contribution to society and to the clients they serve.

 Visit thePoint to watch a video about evaluating body structures and functions.

REFERENCES

American Occupational Therapy Association. (2014). Occupational therapy practice framework: Domain and process, 3rd edition. *American Journal of Occupational Therapy, 68*, S1–S48.

American Occupational Therapy Association. (2015). Occupational therapy's perspective on the use of environments and contexts to support health, well-being, and participation in occupations. *American Journal of Occupational Therapy, 69*, 6913410050p1–6913410050p13.

Árnadóttir, G. (2016). Impact of neurobehavioral deficits on activities of daily living. In G. Gillen (Ed.), *Stroke rehabilitation: A function-based approach* (4th ed., pp. 573–611). St. Louis, MO: Elsevier.

Chapparo, C., Ranka, J., & Nott, M. (2017). The Occupational Performance Model (Australia): A description of constructs, structure and propositions. In M. Curtin, M. Egan, & J. Adams (Eds.), *Occupational therapy for people experiences illness, injury or impairment* (7th ed., 134–147). Edinburgh, United Kingdom: Elsevier.

Davidson, L., Shahar, G., Stayner, D. A., Chiman, M. J., Rakfeldt, J., & Tebes, J. K. (2004). Supported socialization for people with psychiatric disabilities: Lessons from a randomized control trial. *Journal of Community Psychology, 32*, 453–477.

Davidson, L., Stayner, D. A., Nickou, C., Styron, T. H., Rowe, M., & Chinman, M. L. (2001). "Simply to be let in": Inclusion as a basis for recovery. *Psychiatric Rehabilitation Journal, 24*, 375–388.

Dunn, W. W. (2011). *Best practice occupational therapy: In community service with children and families* (2nd ed.). Thorofare, NJ: SLACK.

Gillen, G. (2009). *Cognitive and perceptual rehabilitation: Optimizing function.* St. Louis, MO: Elsevier/Mosby.

Guidetti, S., Asaba, E., & Tham, K. (2007). The lived experience of recapturing self-care. *American Journal of Occupational Therapy, 61*, 303–310.

McNary, H. (1947). The scope of occupational therapy. In H. S. Willard & C. S. Spackman (Eds.), *Occupational therapy* (pp. 10–22). Philadelphia, PA: J. B. Lippincott.

Willard, H. S., & Spackman, C. S. (Eds.). (1947). *Occupational therapy.* Philadelphia, PA: J. B. Lippincott.

World Health Organization. (2001). *International classification of functioning, disability and health (ICF).* Geneva, Switzerland: Author.

thePoint® *For additional resources on the subjects discussed in this chapter, visit* **http://thePoint.lww.com/Willard-Spackman13e.**

CHAPTER 24

Personal Values, Beliefs, and Spirituality

Christy Billock

"Spirituality looks like folding the towels in a sweet way and talking kindly to the people in the family even though you've had a long day."

—SYLVIA BOORSTEIN (2016)

LEARNING OBJECTIVES

After reading this chapter, you will be able to:

1. Develop an understanding of the meaning of personal values, beliefs, and spirituality as related to occupational therapy practice, including definition, related themes, and distinction from religion.

2. Recognize the relationship between spirituality, occupation, health, and well-being.

3. Identify the relationship of spirituality to occupational therapy's history.

4. Understand the relevance of individual experiences of spirituality through occupation by examining important factors, such as context, reflection, intention, and mindfulness, and occupational engagement.

5. Describe strategies to integrate personal values, beliefs, and spirituality into occupational therapy practice.

6. Explore how personal values, beliefs, spirituality, and occupation might intersect in your own life experiences.

Introduction

Founded on principles of holism, the occupational therapy (OT) profession emphasizes the importance of helping clients experience meaning in their lives through daily occupational participation. Understanding the rich interconnections of personal values, beliefs, and spirituality as experienced through occupation provides OT practitioners the opportunity of enhancing the profession's unique heritage of a holistic approach to health and wellness. This chapter serves as an introductory resource for understanding personal values, beliefs, and spirituality in OT practice. The exploration begins by looking at the interconnections of values, beliefs, and spirituality as important facets of occupation. Second, this chapter discusses the multiple ways in which spirituality is experienced through occupation. Third, it provides strategies for integrating values, beliefs, and spirituality into OT practice.

Framing Personal Values, Beliefs, and Spirituality from an Occupational Therapy Perspective

Occupational therapy thrives within a holistic context of care where "in pursuing occupation, humans express the totality of their being, a mind-body-spirit union" (Hooper & Wood, 2014, p. 38). The transactions of mind, body, and spirit through occupational engagement help answer the question—what do you live for? At the heart of those answers lie a person's values, beliefs, and spirituality. **Values** can be understood as "principles, standards, or qualities considered worthwhile by the client who holds them" (American Occupational Therapy Association [AOTA], 2014, p. S7). The notion of **beliefs** closely relates to values and can be defined as "cognitive content held as true" (AOTA, 2014, p. S7). Both values and beliefs often influence a person's subjective experience of occupation because of the qualities of individualized meaning and centrality in the person's life. Values and beliefs can derive from multiple sources including personal experience, friends and acquaintances, family, culture, religion, and politics, among others.

The multidimensional and complex nature of spirituality defies simple definition and a consideration of how the concept relates to occupation further complicates the pursuit. The Occupational Therapy Practice Framework (AOTA, 2014) refers to Puchalski et al.'s (2009) definition of spirituality as "the aspect of humanity that refers to the way individuals seek and express meaning and purpose and the way they experience their connectedness to the moment, to self, to others, to nature, and to the significant or sacred" (p. S45). Another way to understand spirituality in the context of occupational experience is as follows—**spirituality** is a deep experience of meaning brought about by engaging in occupations that involve the enacting of personal values and beliefs, reflection, and intention within a supportive contextual environment (Billock, 2005). For example, a person might experience spirituality through the occupation of walking her dog through a neighborhood park while reflecting on how much she loves her dog and regard the relationship as a vital and meaningful part of her life (Figure 24-1).

Occupational therapy places meaning as a central tenet of the profession, and meaning-making, in its essence, is a spiritual process that seeks expression through occupation (Peloquin, 1997). Wilcock and Townsend (2014) put forth meaning-making, experiencing meaning, and self-expression as the "activist element of human existence" (p. 542). People often experience spirituality

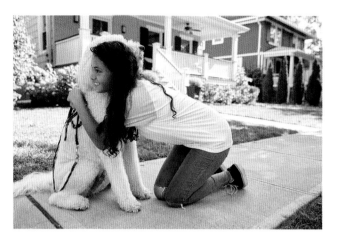

FIGURE 24-1 **This young girl might experience spirituality through the occupation of walking her dog through a neighborhood park while reflecting on how much she loves her dog.**

through engagement in everyday activities; consequently, occupation creates meaning and purpose in life and helps to answer larger existential questions of the meaning of life (Christiansen, 1997; Frankl, 1959). Spirituality thrives on actual experiences of occupations that provide the opportunity to bring one's values and beliefs to life.

Religious participation and spiritual experience can occur together; however, the two are not synonymous. **Religion** can be defined as a set of shared beliefs and attendant practices used to relate to the sacred. As individual and communal practices, religion permeates many people's daily experiences of spirituality through participation in rituals and occupations such as prayer, meditation, reading theological books, and attending religious services. Not only do religions provide followers with practices directly relating to theological beliefs, but religious beliefs often ascribe spiritual meaning to daily occupations such as food preparation, work, and intimacy, especially if "understood as commanded by God" (Frank et al., 1997, p. 201). Although many people use religion as a tool for framing spirituality in their lives, individual spiritual experience does not depend on religious affiliation or practice.

Evidence suggests that practicing spirituality and religion positively influences health through the physiological processes of the immune, neuroendocrine, and cardiovascular systems (Aldwin, Park, Jeong, & Nath, 2014; Seeman, Dubin, & Seeman, 2003). Spiritual health takes on many definitions but generally connotes being able to experience meaning, fulfillment, and connection with self, others, and a higher power or larger reality (Hawks, Hull, Thalman, & Richins, 1995). Experiences of occupational alienation (Townsend & Wilcock, 2004), that is, an inability to create meaning and express one's spirit through occupation, demonstrates a lack of spiritual

CENTENNIAL NOTES

Personal Values, Beliefs, and Spirituality: From Moral Treatment to Now

Exploring founding principles of OT reveals traces of personal values, beliefs, and spirituality as important to the work of the profession. Moral treatment influenced the founders of OT in the early twentieth century (Bockhoven, 1971). Advocates of moral treatment valued ideals such as holism, humanism, and a recognition that engagement of the mind, body, and spirit through occupation promoted health and brought meaning to life (Meyer, 1922/1977). In the 1920s and 1930s, the medical establishment criticized OT for its lack of theory grounded in scientific principles (Gritzer & Arluke, 1989). In an attempt to legitimize the profession, occupational therapists adopted reductionistic models through the 1950s, thereby minimizing the emphasis on recognition of the human spirit and subjective experience as expressed in occupation (Yerxa, 1992). In 1962, Reilly expressed concern that reductionistic views of OT could not capture the role that occupation could play in facilitating health. Reilly's words proved to be a catalyst for the reemergence of a holistic perspective valuing spirituality and personal beliefs as central concepts of OT (Atler, Fisher, Moret, & White, 2000).

In the late twentieth century, the Canadian Association of Occupational Therapy (CAOT) explicitly integrated spirituality into theories about client-centered practice and occupational engagement, placing spirituality at the center of theoretical constructs of occupation guiding OT practice (CAOT, 1997; Polatajko, Townsend, & Craik, 2007). In the United States, the AOTA in 1997 devoted an entire issue of the *American Journal of Occupational Therapy* to the topic of spirituality. Spirituality gained inclusion in the Occupational Therapy Practice Framework as a context for occupation (AOTA, 2002) and then as a client factor as interpretations of spirituality's relationship to OT practice evolved (AOTA, 2008, 2014). As AOTA's Vision 2025 looks toward the future of the profession by maximizing health, well-being, and quality of life through participation in everyday life, consideration of values, beliefs, and spirituality will necessarily continue to play an important role in the holistic heritage of the profession.

health or well-being for a person (Simó-Algado, Mehta, Kronenberg, Cockburn, & Kirsh, 2002). Mental and physical wellness, as nurtured by occupational participation, necessarily involves inclusion of a perspective involving spirit, along with mind and body.

At the heart of OT beats a strong reminder that clients need something to live for—purpose in life, meaning, connection, coping with challenges, and/or hope for the future. Occupational therapy practitioners tenaciously seek to understand which occupations will spark motivation in their clients to maximize engagement and participation in life and facilitate health and well-being. Figuring out such occupations and facilitating participation in them essentially provides a glimpse into the spirit of a person, thereby representing some of the best benefits OT can uniquely offer.

Experiencing Spirituality through Occupation

Personal values, beliefs, and spirituality can come to life through occupational engagement. Although spirituality can be experienced outside of occupation, participating in occupation is the most common and effective mechanism for making spirituality a real, tangible reality in daily life. Peloquin (1997) refers to occupation as an act of making that represents an extension and animation of the human spirit:

> To see such radical making in the acts that we commonly name *doing* purposeful activities, *performing* life roles and tasks, *adapting* to the environment, *adjusting* to disability, and *achieving* skills or mastery, is to discern the spiritual depth of occupation. (p. 167)

Linking occupation and spirituality together with the notion of "making" implies a fluid and active approach to the phenomenon. In making, a person expresses tangibly the intangible yet vital realities of life. These internal representations of values and beliefs about the meaning of reality and the world drive people to orchestrate occupations to express those meanings (Kroeker, 1997). Therein lies the importance of finding occupations that make clients' faces light up and motivate them to get out of bed in the morning.

From 2007 to 2014, the number of people within the United States identifying as religiously unaffiliated jumped from 16.1% to 22.8% (Pew Research Center, 2014). The trend away from religion appears to cross geographic regions, gender, race and ethnicity, age groups, and educational levels. Other identified trends point toward a greater number of people creating a personal construction of practices for the foundation of spiritual life (Wuthnow, 1998, 2010). McColl (2002) contends that given the erosion of meaning in work from industrialization and the prevalence of secular

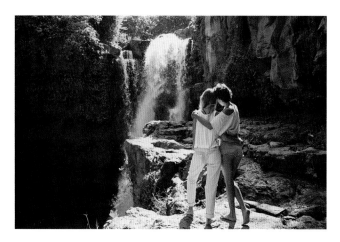

FIGURE 24-2 Taking a hike might serve the vitally important role of facilitating experiences of spirituality.

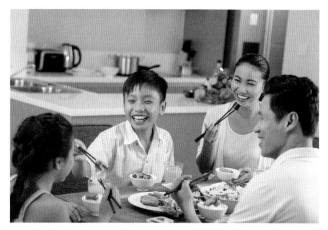

FIGURE 24-3 Gathering to share a meal can be an occupation with spiritual potential.

pluralism in modern society, occupation "may be the most effective medium available through which individuals can affirm their connection with the self, with others, with the cosmos, and with the divine" (p. 352). Orchestration of and engagement in everyday occupation holds the potential of helping people to meet the fundamental need for spiritual expression. For example, the busy executive's attending a yoga class, receiving a massage, or taking a hike might serve the vitally important role of facilitating his or her experiences of spirituality due to the especially meaningful nature of such occupations to the person (Figure 24-2).

Contextual Factors

Spiritual experiences through occupation depend on and are vulnerable to transactions with several contextual factors, including physical and social worlds (Billock, 2005). The physical world can serve to potentially facilitate or block spiritual experiences (Jackson, 1996). Some experience spirituality through occupations in nature such as hiking in the mountains, fly fishing in a stream, or walking along the beach. Built spaces such as churches, houses, and other structures serve to refine and make more vivid human feeling, perception, and comprehension of reality (Tuan, 1977). Out of experiencing those spaces and the objects within them, a person draws a sense of place that is "an organized world of meaning" (Tuan, 1977, p. 179). For example, a home filled with memories of family gatherings and decorated with special pieces of art and pictures of loved ones can provide support for experiencing spirituality through occupational participation. Gathering around a table appointed with grandmother's linens and pottery made by friends, then lighting candles when friends come to share a meal, mark the event as one with special meaning, personal value, and spiritual import (Figure 24-3). Whereas home can support one person's experiences of

spirituality, for another, home might be a place of strained memories and relationships. For a woman physically abused by her partner in the privacy of their home, experiences of occupation within the home may show less potential for spiritual experience.

The social world can significantly influence spiritual experience because meaning is both personally and socially constructed (Hasselkus, 2011). Therefore, attempts to understand spiritual experience involve looking at the doer of the occupation in reference to the social and cultural worlds of engagement. Engaging in occupations with others, or co-occupation (Zemke & Clark, 1996), can potentiate the likelihood of a spiritual experience—a deep experience of meaning and connection. As a growing public health concern, loneliness and lack of social connection can increase mortality and a range of disease morbidities and points to the necessity for helping people find ways to connect with others (Holt-Lunstadt, Robles, & Sbarra, 2017; Holt-Lunstadt, Smith, Baker, Harris, & Stephenson, 2015). Religions recognize the importance of believers practicing their faith with others as a means of mutual support and affirmation of belief and provide the context for many shared occupations and ways for parishioners to connect (Howard & Howard, 1997). Beyond religious occupations, communal occupations such as attending sporting events, concerts, or political protests as well as family celebrations such as weddings or graduations can be rich environments for spiritual experience, the enacting of personal values and beliefs, and the fundamental human need for connection.

Reflection, Intention, and Mindfulness

Personal reflection, intention, and mindfulness enhance spiritual experience (Billock, 2005). All three of these supporting factors involve a focused, attentive engagement of the mind. *Reflection* refers to the exploration of one's inner world and necessarily involves recognition of feelings, emotions, and motivations to act. Reflection also becomes a tool of interpretation that can lead to a setting apart of spiritual experiences as different from everyday life, something special or transcendent (Bell, 1997). *Intention* involves using a value, belief, or ideology to guide one's occupational engagement, thereby changing the meaning of the experience.

Mindfulness has emerged in recent years as supportive to well-being and health and as a way to mitigate the stress of everyday life and counter mindless and distracted modes of living. *Mindfulness* can be understood as a "flexible state of mind where we are actively engaged in the present, noticing new things and sensitive to context" (Langer, 2000, p. 220). Mindfulness can be both a cognitive trait and a meditative practice (Elliot, 2011). Some people utilize mindfulness activities such as meditation or yoga as an intentional part of their spiritual life. Mindful awareness, reflection, and intention can be active while participating in a wide array of varied occupations from hiking to drinking a cup of tea, thereby potentiating experiences of spirituality.

Occupations engaging a person's creativity offer the opportunity for deep levels of reflection, intention, mindful awareness, and ultimately spiritual experience. Kidd (1996), speaking of creativity and spirituality, says, "My creative life is my greatest prayer" (p. 123). In her classic work, *The Artist's Way: A Spiritual Path to Higher Creativity*, Cameron (1992) shares a similar view of the intertwining of spirituality and creativity:

> Creativity is an experience—to my eye, a spiritual experience. It does not matter which way you think of it: creativity leading to spirituality or spirituality leading to creativity. In fact, I do not make a distinction between the two. (p. 2)

Infusing occupation with creativity allows for expression of internal states innately spiritual in nature and can translate into enhanced modes of coping (Corry, Lewis, & Mallett, 2014; Simó-Algado et al., 2002). Whereas artistic occupations such as painting, making pottery, or writing poetry show high potential for spiritual experience, other everyday occupations can be filled with creativity as well (Hasselkus, 2011). Occupations such as cooking, conversing with others, playing an instrument, or planning a party, along with countless others, can be occupations in which creativity is expressed (Figure 24-4).

Occupational Participation

Not all occupations are experienced as spiritual, but all occupations hold the potential to be spiritual. Although people often name occupations stemming from religious traditions as spiritual, the lived experience might feel rote or disconnected to self and might not necessarily be

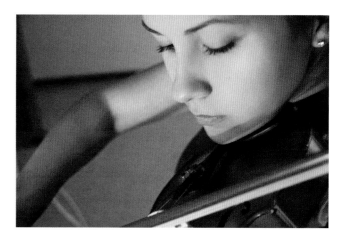

FIGURE 24-4 An occupation that engages creativity can offer the opportunity for a spiritual experience.

spiritual for the person at that point in time. Everyday occupations such as work, walking the dog, or gardening might be experienced as spiritual but might not be named as religious (Howard & Howard, 1997; Unruh, 1997). Occupations that are deeply meaningful to the person, imbued with personal reflection and intention, and carried out within a supportive contextual environment offer the highest potential for spiritual experience (Billock, 2005). Kidd (1996) stated, "In a way all sacred experience and all journeys of soul lead us to the smallest moment of the most ordinary day" (p. 221). The line between secular and sacred becomes blurry with thoughtful examination of lived experiences of occupation. For the immigrant who left behind a homeland with limited resources, even the quotidian act of brushing her teeth with a toothbrush, toothpaste, and clean running water can spark a deep experience of meaning and gratitude.

People frequently experience rituals as spiritual, and throughout history, many ordinary activities such as serving food have been used in ritual (Bell, 1997). Rituals can be understood as "symbolic actions with spiritual, cultural, or social meaning" (AOTA, 2014, p. S8). Common to understandings of ritual are the notions of repetition, fixedness, and predictability and are often embedded in the doing of religion (Hasselkus, 2011). Outside of religion, any occupation can take on ritualistic characteristics of formalism, tradition, invariance, sacral symbolization, and performance. It is these characteristics that differentiate sacred experience from the more mundane aspects of life (Bell, 1997). Depending on an individual's engagement, an occupation such as taking a bath could be experienced as spiritual owing to ritualized characteristics. Bell (1997) recognizes the importance of ritual-like performances because they "communicate on multiple sensory levels, usually involving highly visual imagery, dramatic sounds, and sometimes even tactile, olfactory, and

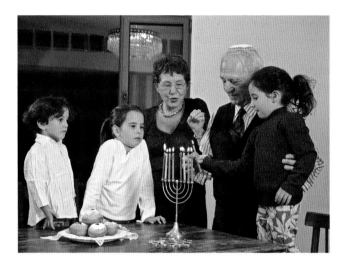

FIGURE 24-5 Engagement in the occupations of a holiday celebration with its attendant ritual practices offers the possibility of spiritual experience in bringing together personal, familial, social, religious, and cultural aspects of life.

gustatory stimulation" (p. 160). For example, engagement in the occupations of a holiday celebration with its attendant ritual practices involving food and particular actions offers the possibility of spiritual experience in bringing together personal, familial, social, religious, and cultural aspects of life (Luboshitzky & Gaber, 2001) (Figure 24-5).

Integrating Personal Beliefs, Values, and Spirituality into Occupational Therapy Practice

As a profession rooted in holistic and humanistic values, OT holds a unique opportunity to help clients restore meaning to their lives, a vitally important and essentially spiritual task. Although most OT practitioners recognize spirituality as an important aspect of life, integrating a client's personal beliefs, values, and spirituality into OT practice proves problematic because of breadth of definitions, large diversity of practitioners' understanding of the notions, and need for more extensive or further education (Enquist, Short-DeGraff, Gliner, & Oltjenbruns, 1997; Johnston & Mayers, 2005; Morris, et al., 2014). These challenges can lead to role ambiguity and a lack of confidence in addressing spirituality in practice in spite of a recognized need for its inclusion (Belcham, 2004). As Howard and Howard (1997) indicate, "occupational therapists need not

look beyond the tools, theories, and values of the profession to provide a context for acknowledging the spiritual in the clinic" (p. 185). If spirituality is a deep experience of meaning effectively experienced through occupational engagement, then OT intervention strategies that uphold holism through occupation-based and client-centered techniques will likely promote clients' spiritual health and well-being.

Recognizing the difficulty of integrating spirituality into practice, Egan and Swedersky (2003) identified several strategies used by occupational therapists who successfully achieve this integration. Two strategies include addressing clients' religious concerns and assisting clients in dealing with suffering. Addressing clients' religious concerns can include talking about the accessibility of the clients' place of worship, practicing transfers to the type of seating in the religious setting which might also involve kneeling down on a bench or the floor. Working with a Muslim client could involve practicing floor to stand transfers to be able to assume the traditional prayer posture or discussing adaptations for completing the five times daily occupation. Understanding various religious beliefs in relation to illness and suffering also proves important. For example, in the Buddhist tradition, pain and suffering are viewed as tools for spiritual insight or enlightenment. Often, OT practitioners work with clients and families dealing with a major life event or transition that demands coping and being able to find meaning and purpose to move forward—an important role that spirituality can play (Jones, Topping, Wattis, & Smith, 2016; Maley, Pagana, Valenger, & Humbert, 2016). Spiritual beliefs and personal values can inform the type of coping intervention and could include occupations such as prayer, meditation, or writing a note of gratitude to a friend. Also, leisure occupations such as gardening can be experienced as spiritual and support living and coping with stressful life events (Unruh & Hutchinson, 2011).

Integrating spirituality into practice necessarily involves a reflective process of the OT practitioner (Townsend, DeLaat, Egan, Thibeault, & Wright, 1999). Practitioners must consider their own understanding of spirituality and how their spirituality plays out in their occupations and experiences. Additionally, this self-reflective process may lead to the recognition of personal biases, values, or beliefs that could interfere with the crucially needed openness to clients' diverse beliefs and experiences. Self-reflection also aids in the ethically important need for therapeutic interventions to be consistent with the client's spiritual life, not the therapist's (Rosenfeld, 2001). Those who practice therapeutic use of self through active listening, empathy, tolerance, unconditional acceptance, and flexibility toward the client's desires and needs demonstrate a spiritual approach to therapeutic interaction. A spiritual perspective within OT can lead the practitioner to view his or her work as deeply meaningful and transformative (Egan & Swedersky, 2003).

Several approaches and tools assist in the integration of spirituality for all the phases of the OT process. Many consumers of OT experience disruptions to and loss of the occupations through which they experience spirituality and meaning. By honoring the subjective experiences of clients in the evaluation, goal-setting, and intervention-planning processes, the practitioner moves toward integrating spirituality into practice and will likely increase the client's motivation (Townsend et al., 1999). Tools such as the Canadian Occupational Performance Measure allow for a client-centered and occupation-based approach that can address spiritual needs through actively integrating the client into the phases of evaluation and intervention (Law et al., 2014). Conducting an occupational profile gathers relevant information about important and meaningful occupations and builds a client-centered foundation for intervention (AOTA, 2014).

Multiple health care professions utilize spiritual assessment tools as a practical method for including spirituality in practice (Koenig, 2007; Puchalski & Romer, 2000). Occupational therapy practitioners have found spiritual assessments FICA and HOPE as practical and convenient for gathering vital information about their clients' spiritual lives (Anandarajah & Hight, 2001; Bouthot, Wells, & Black, 2011). However, these tools do not uniquely focus on OT concerns. The OT-QUEST (Schulz, 2008) is an OT spiritual assessment with a combination of Likert scale and open-ended questions.

Another spiritual assessment specifically tailored to OT is the Occupational Therapy Spiritual Narrative Assessment (OTSNA) (Box 24-1). The OTSNA consists of

---

BOX 24-1 OCCUPATIONAL THERAPY SPIRITUAL ASSESSMENT

Personal Values and Beliefs
What activities do you do to express your personal values or beliefs?
Other Ways to Explore the Question:

- Tell me about a time when you did an activity that made you feel connected to your personal values or beliefs.
- What do you most look forward to doing each day or week?
- What activities are you most passionate about participating in?
- What do you notice about yourself when you are connected to passions in your life?
- What activities make you feel most like yourself?
- Tell me about any beliefs that might influence your wellness, medical care, and/or recovery process.

Coping
Tell me about how you cope with difficulties in life.
Other Ways to Explore the Question:

- Tell me about a time when you successfully managed a hardship in your life.
- What gives you hope for the future?
- When times are tough, what gets you through the day?
- What helps you feel peaceful?
- Who do you turn to when you need help?

Community
Tell me about your participation with a spiritual, religious, or other group.
Other Ways to Explore the Question:

- Tell me about a memorable experience spending time with a spiritual, religious, or other group.

- Do you have a group that you spend time with regularly?
- What do you like to do with your spiritual/religious community or other group?
- Tell me about your connections within your spiritual/religious community or group.
- If you attend services in a spiritual or religious setting now or in the past, how do you participate?

Connection
How do you experience connection in your life?
Other Ways to Explore the Question:

- Tell me about a time where you did an activity that made you feel connected to other people, the world, or a higher power.
- What do you do to connect with other people, the world, or a higher power?
- How do you feel when you are doing things you love?
- Who do you love most and who loves you?
- How do you experience love?

Referral
Would you like to talk with someone about any spiritual or religious concerns?
Other Ways to Explore the Question:

- Tell me about a time when someone was able to help you through a difficult time.
- Who do you speak with about your spiritual or religious concerns?
- Who do you talk with when life gets hard?
- Tell me how your present concerns might be shared.
- Would you like to talk with a chaplain?
- Would you like to talk with your clergyperson?

© 2018 Christy Billock, PhD, OTR/L; with special thanks to Michelle Elliot, PhD, OTR.

guiding qualitative narrative interview questions designed to better understand a client's lived experiences of spirituality to help enable integration of holistic spiritual care in OT. The tool's design strives to facilitate a meaningful conversation between OT practitioner and client about areas of deep meaning relating to occupational participation and is meant to be flexible according to client needs. The five core categories of personal values and beliefs, coping, community, connection, and referral all have a primary question with other optional exploratory questions. Questions can be skipped, reordered, or modified as needed. Facilitation takes between 5 and 10 minutes and can be utilized with adult clients, family members, or caregivers.

After spiritual assessment, bringing spirituality into intervention proves important. A client-centered OT approach that draws spirituality into practice requires close attention to the client's culture, personal values, and beliefs (Simó-Algado et al., 2002). Practitioners sometimes feel uncomfortable integrating clients' religious occupations into practice. If a client names these occupations as important in daily life, religious occupations such as prayer or reading sacred texts can be integrated into intervention sessions as deeply meaningful occupations. Addressing culture might call for learning more about rituals and religious traditions different from the practitioner's own religious experience or exposure. Clergy from the client's religion as well as family members can serve as resources for the practitioner to increase cultural and religious competence (Rosenfeld, 2001). For clients dealing with emotional trauma, occupations encouraging reflection and expression of internal states, such as artistic pursuits and storytelling, can provide opportunity for spiritual insight and coping (Simó-Algado et al., 2002). Last, engaging in mindful awareness practices may facilitate a sense of connection for clients and open the door to spiritual experience.

Conclusion

The rich concepts of personal beliefs, values, and spirituality provide occupational therapists with valuable tools for understanding the deep meaning of engaging in occupation. Although OT demonstrates substantial strides in integrating spirituality into practice, there is still room for growth. Future growth areas include strengthening education both in the preparation of and continuing education for practitioners, gaining a deeper understanding about children's experience of spirituality (Harrison & Cox, 2017), and exploring the intersections of disability and spiritual experience (do Rozario, 1997) to name a few. Important to clients' health and well-being, integrating spirituality into OT practice proves relevant to the profession's goal of providing holistic occupation-based and client-centered care now and into the future.

REFERENCES

Aldwin, C. M., Park, C. L., Jeong, Y., & Nath, R. (2014). Differing pathways between religiousness, spirituality, and health: A self-regulation perspective. *Psychology of Religion and Spirituality, 6,* 9–21.

American Occupational Therapy Association. (2002). Occupational therapy practice framework: Domain and process. *American Journal of Occupational Therapy, 56,* 609–639.

American Occupational Therapy Association. (2008). Occupational therapy practice framework: Domain and process, 2nd edition. *American Journal of Occupational Therapy, 62,* 625–683.

American Occupational Therapy Association. (2014). Occupational therapy practice framework: Domain and process, 3rd edition. *American Journal of Occupational Therapy, 68,* S1–S48.

Anandarajah, G., & Hight, E. (2001). Spirituality and medical practice: Using the HOPE questions as a practical tool for spiritual assessment. *American Family Physician, 63,* 81–89.

Atler, K., Fisher, C., Moret, S., & White, J. (2000, March). *Combining spirituality and storytelling: Changing lives and enhancing practice.* Paper presented at the annual meeting of the American Occupational Therapy Association, Seattle, WA.

Belcham, C. (2004). Spirituality in occupational therapy: Theory in practice? *British Journal of Occupational Therapy, 67,* 39–46.

Bell, C. (1997). *Ritual: Perspectives and dimensions.* Oxford, United Kingdom: Oxford University Press.

Billock, C. (2005). *Delving into the center: Women's lived experience of spirituality through occupation* (Doctoral dissertation). Available from ProQuest Dissertations and Theses database. (Accession Order No. AAT 3219812).

Bockhoven, J. S. (1971). Legacy of moral treatment: 1800's to 1910. *American Journal of Occupational Therapy, 25,* 223–226.

Bouthot, J., Wells, T., & Black, R. (2011). Spirituality in practice: Using the FICA spiritual history assessment. *OT Practice, 18*(3), 13–16.

Cameron, J. (1992). *The artist's way: A spiritual path to higher creativity.* New York, NY: Penguin Putnam.

Canadian Association of Occupational Therapy. (1997). *Enabling occupation: An occupational perspective.* Ontario, Canada: Author.

Christiansen, C. (1997). Nationally speaking: Acknowledging a spiritual dimension in occupational therapy practice. *American Journal of Occupational Therapy, 51,* 169–172.

Corry, D. A. S., Lewis, C. A., & Mallett, J. (2014). Harnessing the mental health benefits of the creativity-spirituality construct: Introducing the theory of transformative coping. *Journal of Spirituality in Mental Health, 16,* 89–110.

do Rozario, L. A. (1997). Spirituality in the lives of people with disability and chronic illness: A creative paradigm of wholeness and reconstitution. *Disability and Rehabilitation, 19,* 427–434.

Egan, M., & Swedersky, J. (2003). Spirituality as experienced by occupational therapists in practice. *American Journal of Occupational Therapy, 57,* 525–533.

Elliot, M. L. (2011). Being mindful about mindfulness: An invitation to extend occupational engagement into the growing mindfulness discourse. *Journal of Occupational Science, 18,* 366–376.

Enquist, D. E., Short-DeGraff, M., Gliner, J., & Oltjenbruns, K. (1997). Occupational theorists' beliefs and practices with regard to spirituality and therapy. *American Journal of Occupational Therapy, 51,* 173–180.

Frank, G., Bernardo, C. S., Tropper, S., Noguchi, F., Lipman, C., Maulhardt, B., & Weitze, L. (1997). Jewish spirituality through actions in time: Daily occupations of young orthodox Jewish couples in Los Angeles. *American Journal of Occupational Therapy, 51,* 199–206.

Frankl, V. (1959). *Man's search for meaning.* New York, NY: Washington Square Press.

Gritzer, G., & Arluke, A. (1989). *The making of rehabilitation: A political economy of medical specialization: 1890–1980*. Los Angeles, CA: University of California Press.

Harrison, L., & Cox, D. (2017). Myth or reality? How do occupational therapists address the spirituality of children with disabilities? *British Journal of Occupational Therapy, 80,* 40–41.

Hasselkus, B. R. (2011). *The meaning of everyday occupation* (2nd ed.). Thorofare, NJ: SLACK.

Hawks, S. R., Hull, M. L., Thalman, R. L., & Richins, P. M. (1995). Review of spiritual health: Definition, role and intervention strategies in health promotion. *American Journal of Health Promotion, 9,* 371–378.

Holt-Lundstadt, J., Robles, T. F., & Sbarra, D. A. (2017). Advancing social connection as a public health priority in the United States. *American Psychologist, 72,* 517–530.

Holt-Lundstadt, J., Smith, T. B., Baker, M., Harris, T., & Stephenson, D. (2015). Loneliness and social isolation as risk factors for mortality: A meta-analytic review. *Perspectives on Psychological Science, 10,* 227–237.

Hooper, B., & Wood, W. (2014). The philosophy of occupational therapy: A framework for practice. In B. A. B. Schell, G. Gillen, & M. Scaffa (Eds.), *Willard & Spackman's occupational therapy* (12th ed., pp. 35–46). Philadelphia, PA: Lippincott Williams & Wilkins.

Howard, B. S., & Howard, J. R. (1997). Occupation as spiritual activity. *American Journal of Occupational Therapy, 51,* 181–185.

Jackson, J. M. (1996). Living a meaningful existence in old age. In R. Zemke & F. Clark (Eds.), *Occupational science: The evolving discipline* (pp. 339–361). Philadelphia, PA: F. A. Davis.

Johnston, D., & Mayers, C. (2005). Spirituality: A review of how occupational therapists acknowledge, assess, and meet spiritual needs. *British Journal of Occupational Therapy, 68,* 9.

Jones, J., Topping, A., Wattis, J., & Smith, J. (2016). A concept analysis of spirituality in occupational therapy practice. *Journal for the Study of Spirituality, 6,* 38–57.

Kidd, S. M. (1996). *Dance of the dissident daughter: A woman's journey from Christian tradition to the sacred feminine.* San Francisco, CA: HarperCollins.

Koenig, H. G. (2007). *Spirituality in patient care: Why, how, when, and what* (2nd ed.). West Conshohocken, PA: Templeton Press.

Kroeker, T. (1997). Spirituality and occupational therapy in a secular culture. *Canadian Journal of Occupational Therapy, 64,* 122–126.

Langer, E. (2000). Mindful learning. *Current Directions in Psychological Science, 9,* 220–223.

Law, M., Baptiste, S., Carswell, A., McColl, M. A., Polatajko, H., & Pollock, N. (2014). *Canadian Occupational Performance Measure* (5th ed.). Ontario, Canada: Canadian Association of Occupational Therapists.

Luboshitzky, D., & Gaber, L. B. (2001). Holidays and celebrations as a spiritual occupation. *Australian Occupational Therapy Journal, 48,* 66–74.

Maley, C. M., Pagana, N. K., Valenger, C. A., & Humbert, T. K. (2016). Dealing with major life events and transitions: A systematic literature review on and occupational analysis of spirituality. *American Journal of Occupational Therapy, 70,* 7004260010p1–7004260010p6.

McColl, M. A. (2002). Occupation in stressful times. *American Journal of Occupational Therapy, 56,* 350–353.

Meyer, A. (1977). The philosophy of occupation therapy. *American Journal of Occupational Therapy, 31,* 639–642. (Original work published 1922)

Morris, D. N., Stecher, J., Briggs-Peppler, K. M., Chittenden, C. M., Rubira, J., & Wismer, L. K. (2014). Spirituality in occupational therapy: Do we practice what we teach? *Journal of Religion and Health, 53,* 27–36.

Peloquin, S. M. (1997). Nationally speaking: The spiritual depth of occupation: Making worlds and making lives. *American Journal of Occupational Therapy, 51,* 167–168.

Pew Research Center. (2014). *2014 Religious landscape study.* Retrieved from http://www.pewforum.org/2015/05/12/americas-changing-religious-landscape/

Polatajko, H. J., Townsend, E. A., & Craik, J. 2007. Canadian Model of Occupational Performance and Engagement (CMOP-E). In E. A. Townsend & H. J. Polatajko (Eds.), *Enabling Occupation II: Advancing an occupational therapy vision of health, well-being, & justice through occupation* (pp. 22–36). Ottawa, Canada: Canadian Association of Occupational Therapists.

Puchalski, C., Ferrell, B., Virani, R., Otis-Green, S., Baird, P., Bull, J., . . . Sulmasy, D. (2009). Improving the quality of spiritual care as a dimension of palliative care: The report of the Consensus Conference. *Journal of Palliative Medicine, 12,* 885–904.

Puchalski, C., & Romer, A. (2000). Taking a spiritual history allows clinicians to understand patients more fully. *Journal of Palliative Medicine, 3,* 129–137.

Reilly, M. (1962). Eleanor Clarke Slagle Lecture: Occupational therapy can be one of the great ideas of 20th century medicine. *American Journal of Occupational Therapy, 16,* 1–9.

Rosenfeld, M. S. (2001). Exploring a spiritual context for care. *OT Practice, 6*(11), 18–26.

Schulz, E. (2008). OT-QUEST Assessment. In B. J. Hemphill-Pearson (Ed.), *Occupational therapy assessment in mental health* (2nd ed., pp. 263–289). Thorofare, NJ: SLACK.

Seeman, T. E., Dubin, L. F., & Seeman, M. (2003). Religiosity/spirituality and health: A critical review of the evidence for biological pathways. *American Psychologist, 58,* 53–63.

Simó-Algado, S., Mehta, N., Kronenberg, F., Cockburn, L., & Kirsh, B. (2002). Occupational therapy intervention with children survivors of war. *Canadian Journal of Occupational Therapy, 69,* 205–215.

Townsend, E., DeLaat, D., Egan, M., Thibeault, R., & Wright, W. A. (1999). *Spirituality in enabling occupation: A learner-centered workbook.* Ottawa, Canada: Canadian Association of Occupational Therapists.

Townsend, E., & Wilcock, A. (2004). Occupational justice and client-centered practice: A dialogue in practice. *Canadian Journal of Occupational Therapy, 71,* 75–85.

Tuan, Y. (1977). *Space and place: The perspective of experience.* Minneapolis, MN: University of Minnesota Press.

Unruh, A. M. (1997). Spirituality and occupation: Garden musings and the Himalayan blue poppy. *Canadian Journal of Occupational Therapy, 64,* 156–160.

Unruh, A. M., & Hutchinson, S. (2011). Embedded spirituality: Gardening in daily life and stressful life experiences. *Scandinavian Journal of Caring Sciences, 25,* 567–574.

Wilcock, A. A., & Townsend, E. A. (2014). Occupational justice. In B. A. B. Schell, G. Gillen, & M. Scaffa (Eds.), *Willard & Spackman's occupational therapy* (12th ed., pp. 541–552). Philadelphia, PA: Lippincott Williams & Wilkins.

Wuthnow, R. (1998). *After heaven: Spirituality in America since the 1950's.* Los Angeles, CA: University of California Press.

Wuthnow, R. (2010). *After the baby-boomers: How twenty- and thirty-somethings are shaping the future of American religion.* Princeton, NJ: Princeton University Press.

Yerxa, E. J. (1992). Some implications of occupational therapy's history for its epistemology, values, and relation to medicine. *American Journal of Occupational Therapy, 46,* 79–83.

Zemke, R., & Clark, F. (1996). Section V: Co-occupations of mothers and children: Introduction. In R. Zemke & F. Clark (Eds.), *Occupational science: The evolving discipline* (pp. 213–215). Philadelphia, PA: F. A. Davis.

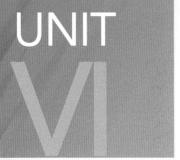

UNIT VI

Analyzing Occupation

"How we spend our days is, of course, how we spend our lives.
What we do with this hour, and that one, is what we are doing."

—Annie Dillard
The Writing Life

CHAPTER 25

Analyzing Occupations and Activity

Barbara A. Boyt Schell, Glen Gillen, Elizabeth Blesedell Crepeau, Marjorie E. Scaffa

LEARNING OBJECTIVES

After reading this chapter, you will be able to:

1. Describe approaches to analyzing occupations and activities in occupational therapy.
2. Compare activity analysis and occupational analysis.
3. Discover how occupational performance is the result of skilled transactions between the person and the performance context.
4. Explain the concept of occupational orchestration.
5. Analyze occupations in order to understand factors that promote or limit performance and participation.
6. Analyze activity in general and as experienced by an individual.

Introduction

Think about all the things you have to or will do today as you go about your daily rounds. Perhaps you started your day with a bath or shower. Did you do that? Or do you prefer to bathe at night? Are you someone who prefers to bathe every other day? If you did bathe or shower, did you wash your hair? If you washed your hair, did you shampoo it once or twice? Did you apply a conditioner? Did you wash your hair before or after you washed the rest of your body? Were you standing in a shower, sitting in a tub, or leaning over a basin? How hot was the water? Did your arms get tired? Did you dry your hair with a towel or just comb it and let it dry itself? Or did you style your hair with a hair dryer? Did you use a pick, comb, or brush? What physical functions would you say are critical to doing your hair? What mental functions? Where was the place where you bathed? Did you have to go very far to get to the bathing area? Was it inside or outside? Did you have to carry your supplies or are they stored in the bathing area? Was it a private place or were others bathing at the same time? Were you afraid while you bathed? Now that you think about it, what do you take for granted about bathing? Do you think this is the same for others?

Answering questions such as these are part of the daily thinking processes that occupational therapy (OT) practitioners consider when they go about planning and implementing care for their patients and clients. Whether the attention is on self-maintenance activities, such as bathing and hair care, or on work activities, such as driving a bulldozer or planting crops, practitioners require systematic frameworks to understand exactly what each person wants or needs to do. Application of these systematic frameworks is called **occupational analysis** and **activity analysis**. Occupational analysis refers to systematically analyzing what and how a person or groups of people actually do an activity. Activity analysis refers to considering a more general idea of how things are usually done.

Occupational therapy practitioners analyze **activities** to understand their component parts, the setting in which the activity commonly occurs, their possible meaning to clients, and their therapeutic potential. For instance, a therapist who sees a lot of clients from a local chicken-processing factory may wish to do an activity analysis to have a good idea of what is usually involved in working in that setting. If the assembly work typically involves reaching up to get the poultry item and then placing it in a container before sending it down the line, then the therapist may wish to create a simulated portion of that activity back in the outpatient clinic using the same sorts of containers at the same work height.

Practitioners analyze the specific **occupations** of clients as they engage in them to gain an appreciation of specific performance strengths and potential problems clients are encountering and to notice how the context affects the performance. Using the example of the chicken plant, a practitioner may observe a particular worker who is very short to see what specific aspects of the usual factory routine are aggravating a back or hand condition. In a different therapy situation, the therapist may be interested to see how a client manages money. Observing the client while shopping may reveal no problems related to the physical manipulation of money but an inability to calculate money (acalculia). The problems of money management may be worse when the person has no calculator available to compensate. Such a problem can interfere with the occupations of household management, shopping in the mall, or online shopping and banking. Occupational analysis is used to design therapeutic interventions intended to enable clients to engage or reengage in those occupations that have particular meaning and value.

Practitioners also analyze how clients orchestrate their occupations across a day, week, and longer periods of time. **Occupational orchestration** reflects the capacity of individuals to enact their occupations on a daily basis to meet their own needs and the expectations of the many environments in which they are required to function. This may include attention to habits and routines and the interface of these with the needs and expectations of others. Orchestration, a musical term, implies a rhythmic, harmonious composition of daily life that has habitual or routine components but is also responsive to changes in demands from day to day (Larson, 2000). Occupational therapy intervention consists of engaging clients in meaningful occupations to enable or improve their ability to meet their goals and participate in daily life. The occupations may be focused, such as taking a shower, or more complex, such as the orchestration of the array of daily occupations necessary to live a full and satisfying life. For example, making up an agenda for the next meeting of the pastoral care committee of the church or cooking dinner for the family may each be very feasible for an individual to perform. However, performing these tasks in a timely and effective manner while working full-time and caring for other family needs requires skillful planning and coordination of multiple activities.

The analytic processes practitioners bring to their work are at the core of OT practice. This chapter describes these processes and links them to professional reasoning as it occurs throughout the therapeutic process.

CENTENNIAL NOTES

Analyzing and Prescribing Occupation

Lori T. Andersen

The first thing to be done, as we believe and are at work upon, is for occupational therapy to provide an occupation which will produce *a similar therapeutic effect to that of every drug in materia medica. An exercise for each separate organ, joint and muscle of the human body. An exercise? An occupation! An occupation? A useful occupation!* Then it can fill the doctor's prescriptions, yes, even his prescriptions *written in the terms of materia medica.* (Barton, 1915, p. 139)

With that statement, George Edward Barton proposed that a specific occupation could be prescribed for a specific occupational illness if one knew the characteristics of the occupation, just as a pill could be prescribed for a specific medical illness. A series of Round Table discussions at early American Occupational Therapy Association (AOTA) conferences focused on determining "which occupation was best for a specific diagnosis" based on the different attributes of the activity. In 1928, the AOTA Committee on Installations and Advice wrote a number of articles analyzing different craft activities to help occupational therapists select appropriate occupations for patients (Robeson et al., 1928a, 1928b, 1928c). These articles provided the initial basis for activity analysis in OT.

Two Perspectives on Analysis: Occupation and Activity

Occupational therapy practitioners approach the process of activity analysis from two different perspectives—occupational analysis and activity analysis. In the first approach, practitioners are concerned with understanding the specific situation of the client and therefore must understand the specific **occupations** the client wants or needs to do in the actual context in which these occupations are performed. We refer to this as occupational analysis because the term *occupation* connotes personally experienced performance (Pierce, 2001). This is a customized approach that is embedded in the entire OT process. Occupational analysis attends carefully to the specific details of the client's occupations within a specific context. Indeed, it is this customized approach that differentiates the OT perspective from that of many other professions who do activity analysis, such as vocational educators and industrial engineers. In the bathing example provided in the opening paragraph, your answers to how you specifically perform the process of bathing represent part of an occupational analysis in that it helps describe the way that you actually do a particular occupation in your own life. See Box 25-1 for the rationale for the specific terms we are using in this chapter.

The second approach is commonly called activity analysis. In activity analysis, the practitioner considers an activity in the abstract or general sense, as it might typically be done within a given culture (Pierce, 2001). Practitioners do this sort of activity analysis for at least two reasons. First, the practitioner may wish to anticipate possible areas of concern in working with clients with different kinds of health conditions or occupational performance challenges. Second, practitioners often need to generate activities, sometimes called "**purposeful activities**," which are "designed and selected to support the development of performance skills and performance patterns to enhance occupational engagement" (AOTA, 2014, p. S29). Examples include practicing transfers in and out of the tub on the rehabilitation unit, practicing shoe tying using one hand, and filling out a mock job application. These activities can be effectively designed or graded to help a client develop functional capacities, recover from impairment, or learn an adaptive approach. For instance, if a practitioner thinks about what is typically involved in bathing or showering for many people in the United States, then he or she might be able to anticipate possible problems for someone with a partial paralysis (e.g., difficulty stepping over the tub wall, risk of fall, inability to reach the faucets) or difficulty remembering how to sequence activities (e.g., applying soap prior to wetting the body, beginning to dry off before rinsing off soap). Alternatively, while at a toy store or hardware store, the practitioner might notice and mentally consider how various toys or objects lend themselves to helping individuals develop or improve various skills or bodily capacities. For example, the practitioner might analyze how the video games can be used to challenge postural control, eye–hand coordination, motor planning, endurance, self-confidence, and problem solving. Having these ideas in the practitioner's mental "toolbox" makes it easier to generate therapy possibilities for working with clients. Such consideration of activity possibilities is a *decontextualized approach* because it is an abstract or general idea of what the practitioner thinks typically occurs. It is not what any one particular person actually experiences. To summarize, the term **activity** is used in this chapter to represent the *general idea* about the kinds of things individuals do and the way they typically do them in a given culture (Pierce, 2001). The term *occupation*(s) is used to denote the *personal activities* that individuals choose or need to engage in and the ways in which each individual actually experiences them. Practitioners must be able to analyze both the general idea of how an activity typically occurs within a culture as well as the actual occupations as they are performed by particular individuals. These perspectives can also be applied to groups of people (e.g., members of a choir or workers in a plant), organizations (e.g., the local recreation center), and populations (e.g., the homeless urban campers, middle school students, or elders in a community). This chapter focuses primarily on analysis of activity and occupation at the individual level because the application to groups builds on these core analytic approaches. Other chapters later in the text provide illustrations of how occupational analysis can be used in relation to groups, organizations, and populations. Readers are also encouraged to deepen their understanding of occupational analysis and how occupational science informs OT practice (Pierce, 2014).

Performance Contexts and Environments

Occupational performance is by nature embedded within a social and physical environment, situated in a performance context (AOTA, 2014; Dunn, Brown, & Youngstrom, 2003; Pierce, 2001). *Environment* includes the external physical and social environments in which clients perform their occupations. The physical environment includes "the natural and built nonhuman surroundings," including the objects in them (AOTA, 2014, p. S28) The social environment is constructed by the presence, relationships, and expectations of persons, groups, or populations with whom the client has contact" (AOTA, 2014, p. S28). **Context** includes the external physical, social, economic, political, and cultural environments in which people function (Kronenberg, Pollard, & Ramugondo, 2011) as well as the internal or

BOX 25-1   WORDS MATTER: DEFINING ACTIVITY AND OCCUPATION

Words matter because they shape the way we think and the meanings we ascribe to their underlying concepts (Hymes, 1972). Words also matter because there is an essential link between terminology and theory (Bauerschmidt & Nelson, 2011). Occupational therapy, like many other professions and disciplines, engages in ongoing debates about the meaning of specific terms as they relate to the profession. This debate can become confusing because professional jargon may or may not parallel the way the same words are used in everyday speech (Reed, 2005). Occupation and activity are two such words with everyday meanings and specialized professional meanings. The use of these terms has fluctuated greatly even in our profession's official documents. An analysis of 90 years of documents found that "the term occupation appeared dominant in the 1920s, but it appeared to be replaced in whole or in part by the word activity in the 1940s, 1950s, and 1960s. Neither term received much use in the 1970s and 1980s, and the term task, although used to some extent, did not replace them. The use of both occupation and activity—especially occupation—surged in the 2000s" (Bauerschmidt & Nelson, 2011, p. 342). The authors interpreted this shift "to indicate a widespread resurgence in occupational terminology after an extended period during which the term occupation was rarely used" (Bauerschmidt & Nelson, p. 344). Because these terms are so central to our field, many scholars have attempted to articulate precise meanings. The abundance of these definitions can be confusing, especially to OT students who are new to the field and seeking to understand it.

Definitions of *occupation* typically include a combination of the following concepts[a]:

- Is personally experienced and goal directed
- Reflects culture and cultural values
- Provides meaning
- Involves pursuits that extend over time
- Involves multiple tasks
- Provides organization and structure to living
- Meets needs of the individual and others in the social world
- Fills/occupies time
- Uses abilities and skills
- May have a physical and/or mental component
- Is recognized by the culture

- Provides pleasure and enjoyment
- Contributes to family and broader community
- Contributes to health and well-being
- Aligns with development of the individual

Definitions of *activity* typically share a mix of the core concepts listed below. Activity is frequently modified with terms such as *purposeful*, *occupational*, or *functional* to give it more specific meaning. In these cases, the term *activity* itself is not defined but assumed to be common knowledge. The core concepts[b] for most definitions of activity include the following:

- Incorporates small units of behavior
- Includes use of objects
- Involves action
- May or may not result in a product
- Is goal directed
- Is required for development, maturation, and use of sensory-perceptual, motor, social, psychological, and intellectual functions

In contrast, Pierce (2001) has defined *activity* as

" . . . an idea held in the minds of persons and in their shared cultural language. An activity is a culturally defined and general class of human actions. . . . An activity is not experienced by a specific person; is not observable as an occurrence; and is not located in a fully existent temporal, spatial, and sociocultural context" (p. 139).

For the purpose of this chapter, we have chosen to adopt Pierce's definition of activity because this definition enables us to make the distinction between the general ideas we have about a particular activity for activity analysis; for example, swimming—versus the engagement in swimming as an occupation that is dependent on the way or ways a particular person swims, where the person swims, with whom, and the meaning he or she ascribes to it. Consequently, throughout this chapter when you read *activity*, you should remember that this reflects the general decontextualized concept and *occupation* is the way a particular person enacts this activity in a specific context. In other chapters in this book, you will find terminology used differently. You need to look behind the terminology to understand the intent of the authors in their word choice.

[a]Adapted from Christiansen & Baum (2005); Clarke et al. (1991); Hinojosa & Kramer (1997); Law, Polatajko, Baptiste, & Townsend (1997); Nelson & Jebson-Thomas (2003); Spear & Crepeau (2003)
[b]Adapted from Allen (1987); Cynkin (1995); Hinojosa & Kramer (1997); Llorens (1986); Mosey (1981); Reed (2005); Trombly (1995).

personal aspects, such as age, gender, socioeconomic status, education level, and motivation of the person (AOTA, 2014). Additionally, occupations are located in a temporal context in terms of stage of life, the specific amount of time involved, and the history and projected future related to occupation. Finally, some occupations occur in virtual contexts, such as Web-based blogs and spaces, social networking sites, text messaging, and online gaming. Paralleling the distinction just made between activity and occupation, many aspects of the environment and context can be considered in abstract or as the client actually experiences them.

Arenas and Settings

Lave (1988), an anthropologist, makes a distinction between the potential uses of environmental contexts and the ways people actually interact with them. She used the term **arena** to describe the places in which activities occur, such as a library, school, or hospital. In contrast, she used the word **setting** to describe those aspects of the arena to which the person attends. This distinction is useful in that it, once again, illustrates the twin ideas of actual experience versus abstract conceptualizations. For example, a library is an arena, and many of us conjure up an idea of what a library is. In fact, some of us may think of a particular library as a physical place in our community and others a virtual place to obtain music and books. Whether physical or virtual, each individual will use the library in different ways and construct different meanings from their experiences. For instance, a man entering a local community library with his young child will most likely go to the children's section to look at colorful picture or chapter books. He is likely to sit on a small chair or a pillow while reading to his child. Later, he may help the child select books to take home. In contrast, another person may go to the computer section in the same library to access online materials related to a job search. Alternatively, a college student may only interact with a university or global library via online searches of journals and books for research. A retired woman may go to the library as a volunteer to help in the gift shop. Thus, although the library as an arena remains the same, the library as a setting differs from person to person. The distinction Lave makes between arena and setting is similar to the distinction made earlier between activity and occupation. Like activity, arena is an abstract or general idea, whereas setting is where the occupational activity is specifically performed.

Roles: Social Constructions versus Personally Enacted

Role theory has had an influence on the development of theory within the profession. For instance, the Model of Human Occupation described in Chapter 42 uses role as a way of articulating how individuals see themselves and the multiple aspects of a person's life. The concept of role is translated into assessments such as the Role Checklist and Worker Role Interview. In sociological and psychological theories, roles are seen as social positions (Hagedorn, 2000; Jackson, 1998a). As Fisher (1998) noted in her Slagle lecture, "the role dimension pertains to the relationship between one's roles and the related collection of task performances that must unfold in a logical, timely, and socially appropriate manner. We must understand the person's perceived roles and any incongruities between his or her role behavior and the role behavior that is expected by society or desired by the person" (p. 514). Thus, roles can be thought of as normative

models shaped by the culture. For example, they help articulate expectations for what constitutes being a "good" mother, father, or student, and the activities and occupations people in these positions are supposed to perform. Individuals within roles may adopt these normative expectations or may interpret the expectations to fit their own values and beliefs.

Jackson (1998a, 1998b) argued that our concern should be on the occupations individuals engage in, not their roles, because the concept of role is problematic from several perspectives. First, roles may overlap. For example, it is often impossible to distinguish children's "student" roles from their "friend" roles. When someone is cooking, is it in the role as mother or father, church volunteer, or chef? In both instances, our concern is in the occupation, the person's ability to engage in the occupation, and the meaning the person ascribes to it, not the role to which the occupation connects. Second, although the concept of role provides a shorthand way of understanding the occupational world of an individual, Jackson (1998a) argued that this approach is risky because inherent in the concept of role are the power issues embedded in many cultural models. For example, who decides what a "good mother" is? Who says the mother is the one to do the cooking for the family?

Still, role is not easy to ignore because it is such a widely held concept. For example, Trombly Latham (Trombly, 1995; Trombly Latham, 2014) uses role as an organizing construct; however, she cautions that roles should be considered from the definitional perspective of the individual rather than from the normative expectations of society. But how does one get to this definitional perspective except through understanding the occupations the individual attaches to a particular role? By focusing on occupations people engage in, we can see what people do, what the occupation means to them, how they feel about their performance, and how they organize their occupations to meet their needs and the needs of the people around them. Our analysis begins with occupation and may result, if needed, in clustering these occupations into the individual's personal definition of the occupations associated with the roles. Once again, we see the contrast between the abstract notion of role and the personally experienced situation of the individual, sometimes called **occupational role**.

Jackson's (1998a, 1998b) cautions about the use of roles are important because it is easy to unconsciously slip into normative expectations or use one's personal experience to frame the expectations for others. Practitioners bring unarticulated personal assumptions to the therapy process (see Chapter 34 on Professional Reasoning). Consequently, the concept of role was not chosen as an organizational construct for this chapter because we want to focus on those occupations that are most important to an individual regardless of what role or roles to which that person might be involved. Instead, the orchestration of occupations as they are enfolded and integrated in the course of daily life is examined.

Occupational Analysis and Meaning

Over and over again, practitioners need to remind themselves that meaning is individually constructed and interpreted and is central to human existence (Bruner, 1990; Frankl, 1959; Hasselkus, 2002; Peloquin, 2005, 2007). A practitioner is obligated to understand the meaning of occupations from the client's perspective. Using the library example discussed previously, it is possible if one talked to the father about the meaning of going to the library with his child that he might mention the pleasure he derives from instilling in his child the value and enjoyment of reading and the quiet time they share together. He might recall his childhood and the times he went to the library with one of his parents. Alternatively, he might explain that he never had the opportunity to go to the library with his father because his father had abandoned the family. The latter experience would create an entirely different meaning and motivational structure for **co-occupation** of this father–child dyad. *Co-occupation* is defined as an occupation that implicitly involves two or more individuals (Zemke & Clark, 1996).

As this example illustrates, the different experiences, values, and beliefs of clients make the interpretation of meaning a particularly complex aspect of practice. This challenge is exacerbated by potential cultural and socioeconomic differences between practitioners and their clients. These make it more challenging for practitioners to fully understand the experiences of their clients and the meanings they ascribe to their occupations (Crepeau, 1991; Kielhofner & Barrett, 1998; Payne, DeVol, & Dreussi Smith, 2001; see also Chapters 19, 20, 21, and 22, which address culture, socioeconomics, place, and spirituality, respectively). It is the practitioner's responsibility to develop therapeutic relationships that foster an understanding of clients and their world (Crepeau & Garren, 2011; Peloquin, 1995; see also Chapter 37, which addresses client-centered collaboration and the therapeutic relationship). Activity analysis and occupational analysis are tools that practitioners can use to achieve this understanding. Table 25-1 provides a quick reference of concepts that are tied to the person's subjective experience versus what terms are more related to practitioners' general understanding of typical demands.

TABLE 25-1	Terms: From the Abstract/General to the Particular/Specific	
	Abstract Concept	Real Experience
What is done	Activity	Occupation
Where and with whom	Arena	Setting
How it is organized	Social role	Occupational orchestration

Activity and Occupational Analysis in Practice

Occupational therapy practitioners draw on their education, knowledge of activities, and professional experience when analyzing activities (Neistadt, McAuley, Zecha, & Shannon, 1993). This analysis may be so automatic that it is often ignored or unappreciated, becoming another aspect of the tacit nature of the reasoning process used by practitioners (Mattingly & Fleming, 1994; Schell & Cervero, 1993). Practitioners analyze activities from the perspective of practice theories to understand problems in performance and intervention strategies appropriate from that theoretical perspective. Their analysis is also based on access to particular activities and the degree to which they are willing to engage in trial and error or experimentation to understand activities more fully (Schell, 2018).

Studies that have attempted to make activity analysis an objective process have demonstrated that the number of variables is so great that the goal of objectivity would be exceedingly difficult to achieve (Llorens, 1986; Neistadt et al., 1993; Trombly, 1995). Adopting the distinction between activity analysis and occupational analysis renders this concern moot. If the outcome of activity analysis is to understand the *potential* demands of an activity, objectivity is not the goal. Rather, identifying the multiple skills typically required and the potential meanings the activity may have enable practitioners to have a deeper understanding of this activity in general.

In contrast to the consideration of activities for their therapeutic implications, occupational analysis is a highly individualized process because it is embedded in the particular perspective of the person, the person's occupational performance, and the performance context. Occupational analysis occurs when attempting to understand the person as an occupational being in concert with identifying occupational performance skills and barriers to effective performance (Coster, 1998; Fisher & Jones, 2014; Hocking, 2001; Polatajko, Mandich, & Martini, 2000; Trombly, 1995; Trombly Latham, 2014). Client-centered evaluation models examine the ability of a person to engage in a valued occupation and the transaction among actual performance, activity demands, and context (Law, 1998). Box 25-2 provides examples of the various degrees of focus that practitioners use to consider occupations.

Both occupational and activity analysis are required for effective practice. By blending these analytic models, practitioners can gain an understanding of the particular ways in which clients relate to their occupations and can then use their knowledge of activity and practice theories to use those occupational activities for therapeutic purposes. This understanding is achieved through both forms of analysis. Table 25-2 summarizes the questions addressed in both activity and occupational analysis. Box 25-3 shows how practitioners weave analysis of occupational

BOX 25-2   OCCUPATIONAL SCALE: A QUESTION OF FOCUS

Just as there is little agreement in the field about the definition of activity, there is little agreement about the scope or scale of what actually constitutes an occupation. Hinojosa captured this dilemma eloquently when he shared his personal reflections about occupation:

> I am uncomfortable with the current trend in the profession to call everything we do as occupation. I personally cannot believe that brushing my teeth or being able to effectively use toilet paper in the bathroom is an occupation. I do believe that they are important purposeful activities. I have come to realize that the combination of these two activities is fundamental to complete personal hygiene occupations. (Hinojosa, Kramer, Royeen, & Luebben, 2003, p. 8)

Hinojosa's concern could be restated as follows:

Is an occupation a collection of tasks within a broad scope of one's life (cooking) or some of the subtasks within this category (making a meal) or even smaller units (preparing vegetables for the salad)?

There is little agreement in the field on this issue with scholars proposing a variety of ways to nest the subunits of occupations within the broader category. These include the following:

- Trombly Latham (2014) nests activities within tasks which constitute life roles.
- Polatajko et al. (2000) break down occupations into tasks that contain segments, units, and subunits.
- Baum and Christiansen (2005) start with roles, tasks, and actions.
- Fisher (1998) considers the role dimensions of an individual's occupations and places tasks (what the person does) within this category but notes the importance of starting with a person's goals.

The purpose here is to point out the lack of agreement and say that we have no solution to the problem. It is important to recognize that there are varying ways to consider analyzing occupations. Crabtree (1998) uses a metaphor comparing the OT reasoning process to a camera lens. Sometimes it is important to zoom out to see the big picture, and sometimes it is necessary to zoom in to capture the fine details. The depth and scope of analysis is directly related to the client's goals for intervention and the practitioner's reasoning process in responding to these goals, as noted in the example above.

Lens	Example: Cooking	Analytical Questions
	Making a meal 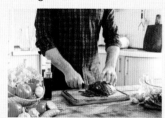	Why does this person cook? What does this person cook? In what settings does the person cook (i.e., home, community center, homeless shelter kitchen)? How often does the person cook? How does it overlap or enfold within other occupations (i.e., is it important in the person's job) or to duties to his or her spouse or partner? Can the person do the planning and organization necessary? Does the person have skills to prepare the food? Does the person cook safely? Does the person get each part of the meal done in a timely manner? Is the quality of the result satisfactory to the person and significant others?
	Preparing a salad 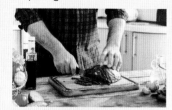	Can the person get the salad ingredients from the refrigerator? Does the person remember to get all of the ingredients and supplies he or she needs? Can the person use a knife safely with different ingredients? Can the person use a knife effectively with all the ingredients? Can the person get the salad to the table? Does the person season it to his or her own standards and that of those sharing the salad?
	Slicing cabbage 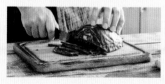	Does the person choose the right utensil to cut the cabbage? Can the person grasp the cabbage? Does the person hold it too tightly or too loosely? Can the person hold the knife by the handle? Can the person coordinate both hands while holding and cutting the cabbage? Does the person know to hold the handle as opposed to the blade? Can the person generate enough force to cut the cabbage? Does the person position the knife correctly relative to the cabbage? Is the person at risk of being cut? Does the person cut the cabbage in the desired shape? Do the cabbage slices meet the person's own standards and that of others eating the salad?

TABLE 25-2   Analysis Format for Activities and Occupations

Scenario: James, a 32-Year-Old Single Male, Making a Sandwich

Activity Analysis	Occupational Analysis	Example of Occupational Analysis
Description		
Describe the activity in one to two sentences.	Briefly describe the occupation. How does the person usually do this occupation and in what settings?	James typically makes a cold cut sandwich with cheese and mayonnaise each weekday morning to bring to work.
Objects Used and Their Properties		
Describe the tools, materials, and equipment typically used. Note the potential symbolism/meaning of the objects in the relevant culture.	Describe the tools, materials, and equipment actually used. Note the symbolism/meaning of the objects to this person.	James uses fresh cold cuts, prepackaged cheese slices, mayonnaise, a store-purchased loaf of bread, a butter knife, a plastic bag, and a paper bag to make and store his lunch. He uses a damp sponge to clean his work space.
Space Demands		
Describe the physical environment in which the activity being analyzed is usually performed. Include key aspects, such as the following: • Does this occur in a natural or built environment? • What are the major natural or built structures? • Describe the placement of any furnishings and equipment. • What is the light level? Does it change or is it constant? • Describe the kind and level of noise. How might it impact the activity to be performed? • Describe any other features which may impact the senses (e.g., smell, humidity, texture, temperature) and affect performance. • Is this the typical context for this activity? If not, what other contexts might be appropriate? Briefly describe them, with emphasis on how the other contexts are different.	Describe the actual physical environment in which the occupation will be performed. Consider how the physical environment supports or impedes performance. Include key aspects, such as the following: • Does this occur in a natural or built environment? • What are the major natural or built structures? • How do structures, furnishings, and equipment affect the person's performance? • What is the light level and does it change? How does lighting affect performance? • Describe the kind and level of noise and how it affects performance. • Describe any other features that affect the person's performance (e.g., smell, humidity, texture, temperature). • In addition to the context just described, where else does this person engage in this occupation? Briefly describe all additional contexts, with emphasis on how they are different from the first one described.	James always makes his sandwich in the galley kitchen of his one-bedroom apartment. He keeps the cold cuts and cheese in a bottom left refrigerator drawer and the mayonnaise in the door of the refrigerator. He stores the bread on top of the refrigerator. The knife and storage bags are in adjacent drawers under the counter where he works. The sink, including the sponge, is directly behind James as he faces his work counter. Due to the small size of his kitchen, all objects are within reach of his countertop work surface. His kitchen is lit by a fluorescent fixture. He keeps the TV on while he does his morning routine to listen to the news.
Social Demands		
Describe the social and cultural demands or the range of demands that may be required by this activity or elicited by engagement in this activity using the categories listed below. • Describe other people involved in the activity. What is their relationship to each other? What do they expect from each other? • Describe the typical rules, norms, and expectations involved in doing this activity. • Describe the cultural and symbolic meanings typically ascribed to this activity. • Speculate about other social contexts in which the activity might be performed. How might the rules, expectations, and meanings vary from this setting?	Describe the social and cultural demands as the person engages in this occupation using the categories listed below. • Describe other people involved in the occupation. What is their relationship to each other? What do they expect from each other? • Describe the rules, norms, and expectations of this person as he or she engages in this occupation. • Describe the cultural and symbolic meanings that this person and his or her significant others ascribe to this occupation. • Consider all the other social contexts in which the occupation might be performed. How do the rules, expectations, and meanings vary from this setting?	James lives by himself and most typically performs his morning routine alone. Occasionally, a friend may sleep over. On these days, James simultaneously makes a pot of coffee for his guest. If a guest is present, he keeps the TV off so that he can converse with his guest. The kitchen is not conducive to two people working simultaneously, so James takes on full responsibility for the food and drink preparation.

(continues)

TABLE 25-2   Analysis Format for Activities and Occupations (continued)

Activity Analysis	Occupational Analysis	Example of Occupational Analysis
Sequence, Timing, and Patterns		
List the sequential steps (no more than 15) of the activity. Include any timing requirements, such as waiting for glue to dry, bread to rise, etc. • How much flexibility exists in the sequence and timing of the steps of this activity? • Does this activity typically occur or reoccur at a specific time of day? With what frequency (i.e., daily, weekly, monthly)?	List the sequential steps (no more than 15) of the occupation as the person does it. Include any timing requirements, such as waiting for glue to dry, bread to rise, etc. • How much flexibility exists in the sequence and timing of the steps of this occupation? • Does this occupation typically occur or reoccur at a specific time of day? When and with what frequency (i.e., daily, weekly, monthly)?	James only makes a lunch sandwich on weekdays because on weekends, he prefers to go out to brunch. Steps include retrieving the bread and placing it on the counter; retrieving the cheese, cold cuts, and mayonnaise from the refrigerator and placing them on the counter; opening the packages and container; retrieving the knife from the drawer; spreading the mayonnaise on both sides of the bread; placing three slices of cold cuts and two slices of cheese on the bread; folding and cutting the sandwich in half; retrieving the storage bags; placing the sandwich in the plastic bag followed by the paper bag; and restoring and cleaning his workspace by wiping the counter down with a damp sponge.
Required Skills (Observable Actions/Performance Skills)		
Using the Occupational Therapy Practice Framework, or other published list of skills, identify 5–10 skills critical to activity performance. • Consider skills which demand from the person movement, cognition, sensory, and emotional perception as well as communicative and social actions. • Consider skills typically demanded from the applicable environment (physical, social, and virtual).	Using the Occupational Therapy Practice Framework, or other published list of skills, identify 5–10 skills critical to this person's occupational performance. • Consider skills which demand from the person movement, cognition, sensory, and emotional perception as well as communicative and social actions. • Consider skills typically demanded from the applicable environment (physical, social, and virtual).	Examples of the skills that James requires include *initiating* the task, *searching for* and *locating* the needed objects, *choosing* the correct objects, *using* the objects appropriately, *bending* and *reaching* for the objects, *manipulating* the objects, *continuing* the task, and knowing when to *terminate* the task.
Required Body Structures and Functions		
Consider the underlying capacities of the person that are typically required when doing this activity. • Briefly list the body structures (anatomical parts of the body) typically used. • Briefly list the essential body functions (physiological and psychological).	Consider the underlying capacities of the person that are required when doing this occupation in the contexts just identified. • Briefly list the body structures (anatomical parts of the body) the person uses. • Briefly list the essential body functions (physiological and psychological).	Examples of required body structures include all extremities and trunk, including bones, joints, muscle, tendon, eyes, and central and peripheral nervous systems. Examples of body functions include arousal, working memory, sustained attention, praxis, visual acuity, interpreting spatial relationships, problem solving (e.g., if missing an ingredient), tactile feedback, active joint range of motion, muscle strength, and postural alignment and control.
Safety Hazards		
List potential safety hazards for this activity. Think especially of children, people with cognitive and judgment problems, people with diminished sensation, etc.	List potential safety hazards for this person as he or she performs this occupation. Consider cognitive and judgment problems, diminished sensation, etc.	Potential hazards include choosing the incorrect knife, using/holding the knife incorrectly (e.g., holding the blade), cutting himself due to poor vision or tactile sensation, falling, leaving the refrigerator open allowing food to spoil, leaving the sink running, and having the water overflow.

TABLE 25-2	Analysis Format for Activities and Occupations *(continued)*	
Activity Analysis	**Occupational Analysis**	**Example of Occupational Analysis**
Adaptability to Promote Participation		
How much flexibility exists for people to do this activity in different ways? Consider the following: • Person-based variables (e.g., personal context, impairments) • External contextual variables (physical, social, temporal, virtual, cultural)	How much flexibility exists for this person to do this occupation in different ways? How willing is the person and key stakeholders to consider doing it differently? Consider the following: • Person-based variables (e.g., personal context, impairments) • External contextual variables (physical, social, temporal, virtual, cultural)	James refers to himself as a "creature of habit." His tendency is to make a similar sandwich each day. However, there are days when he does not engage in this occupation but instead buys his lunch on the way to work at his local delicatessen.
Grading		
List three ways to make the task easier in relation to an identified personal or contextual variable.	List three ways to make the occupation easier in relation to an identified personal or contextual variable.	This occupation can be made less challenging regarding organization and sequence skills and/or from an endurance perspective via presetting the work space (e.g., placing the bread, knife, and storage bags on the counter prior to beginning the meal preparation, providing James with a list of the necessary steps, labeling the environment, e.g., "silverware drawer").
List three ways to make the task more challenging in relation to an identified personal or contextual variable.	List three ways to make the occupation more challenging in relation to an identified personal or contextual variable.	This occupation can be made more challenging via placing increased demands on balance/postural control, reaching abilities, ideation and organization skills, and selective attentions skills via respectively placing the needed objects out of James's arm span (e.g., paper bags under the sink), placing more objects in the refrigerator to serve as distractors, and providing more environmental stimuli (e.g., turning up the television and discussing current events while James is making the sandwich).

Adapted from American Occupational Therapy Association. (2002). Occupational therapy practice framework: Domain and process. *American Journal of Occupational Therapy, 56,* 609–639; American Occupational Therapy Association. (2008). Occupational therapy practice framework: Domain and process, 2nd edition. *American Journal of Occupational Therapy, 62,* 625–683; American Occupational Therapy Association. (2014). Occupational therapy practice framework: Domain and process, 3rd edition. *American Journal of Occupational Therapy, 68,* S1–S48.

performance throughout the therapy process. Box 25-4 lists some of the ways that these analyses inform practice decisions.

Activity Analysis

Activity analysis is a way of thinking about activities. Practitioners must perform quick analyses while working with clients. In addition, OT practitioners may also think about activities for their therapeutic potential, for instance, by sizing up new games, cooking gadgets, technology, and other objects or activities. Activity analysis addresses the typical demands of an activity, the range of skills involved in its performance, and the various cultural meanings that might be ascribed to it. The goal of activity analysis is to understand as much as possible about an activity, including the particular skills required to do it competently and its relation to participation in the world at large (Cynkin, 1995).

It is this knowledge of activities, their properties, and their potential cultural meanings that sensitize practitioners to the occupations of their clients and helps practitioners know which particular activities to suggest to their clients. Through activity analysis, practitioners gain an understanding of the therapeutic potential of a wide range of activities. Because practitioners routinely analyze activities, they develop the capacity to quickly analyze a wide range of activities for their therapeutic or evaluation potential.

Activity Analysis Format

The activity analysis format shown is based on the organization of the Occupational Therapy Practice Framework (AOTA, 2014) and the International Classification of Functioning, Disability and Health (ICF) (World Health Organization, 2001) as well as information from various chapters within this text. The Occupational Therapy Practice Framework is designed to reflect the current practice of OT and its concern for

BOX 25-3   ANALYSIS OF OCCUPATIONAL PERFORMANCE

Occupational performance is the accomplishment of the selected occupation or activity resulting from the dynamic transaction among the client, the context and environment, and the activity (AOTA, 2014, p. S43). Evaluation of occupational performance involves the following:

- Synthesizing information from the occupational profile to focus on specific areas of occupation and contexts that need to be addressed
- Observing the client's performance in desired occupations and activities, noting effectiveness of the performance skills and performance patterns
- Selecting and using specific assessments to measure performance skills and patterns as appropriate
- Selecting assessments, as needed, to identify and measure more specifically contexts or environments,

activity demands, and client factors that are influencing performance skills and performance patterns
- Interpreting the assessment data to identify what supports performance and what hinders performance
- Developing and refining hypotheses about the client's occupational performance strengths and limitations

Following the evaluation of occupational performance, the practitioner then engages in the following:

- Creating goals in collaboration with the client that address the desired outcomes
- Determining procedures to measure the outcomes of intervention
- Delineating potential intervention approach or approaches based on best practice and available evidence

---

occupational engagement to support health and participation of people in society. Activity analysis focuses on the identification of activity demands and performance skills. Activity demands include aspects of the activity such as amount of effort, the objects typically used, the space, and social demands of the activity. The analysis format also includes consideration of the typically required body structures (e.g., cardiovascular, psychological, and neurological structures) and functions (e.g., attention processes, temperament, joint mobility, gait pattern, emotional regulation) as they relate to the skills often used in the activity. Also included in the analysis are the expected skills that represent the interface between the person and the performance setting (Fisher & Jones, 2014). See Chapter 26 for an in-depth discussion of performance skills.

As part of activity analysis, practitioners may consider the use of the activity as viewed through different

theoretical lenses. For instance, a therapist who is working with a population of people with biomechanically related impairments (i.e., hand injuries, back injuries) may analyze activities in terms of the typical strength, range of motion, and endurance required to complete them. Alternatively, someone who is concerned about supporting interpersonal skills in clients with mental illnesses may look primarily at the complexity of social interactions which the activity typically demands (Davidson, 2003). By using the principles of a particular practice theory, OT practitioners analyze activities as they think about performance strengths and problems addressed by the particular theory. The potential therapeutic intervention should be consistent with the theory and will likely entail the grading and adaptation of the occupations chosen by the client. Table 25-2 presents a format for analysis of activities.

BOX 25-4   WAYS ACTIVITY AND OCCUPATIONAL ANALYSIS INFORM PRACTICE

Practitioners analyze activity in the abstract for the following reasons:

- To understand the therapeutic potential of a wide range of activities
- To identify activities which lend themselves to

    a. Improving client performance through acquiring new skills or learning adaptive strategies
    b. Restoring a skill or client factor that impacts performance skills
    c. Prevention of future problems by changing or adapting activity demands or performance context

Practitioners analyze the occupations of their clients to

- Evaluate the quality of current performance in valued occupations and the client's effectiveness in orchestrating their occupations
- Determine the impact of personal factors (including health condition) on current performance
- Determine the impact of contextual factors on current performance
- Prognosticate future performance in identified contexts
- Identify ways to grade or adapt occupations to foster improved performance

Occupational Analysis

In contrast to activity analysis, occupational analysis *places the person in the foreground* by taking into account the particular person's life experiences, values, interests, and goals. Occupational analysis attends to *the actual* body functions and structures, the actual performance skills within an *actual* performance setting, including physical and social contexts along with the demands of the occupation itself. These considerations shape the practitioner's efforts to help the person reach his or her goals through carefully designed evaluation and intervention. Practitioners vary the scope of the occupational analysis depending on the nature of the client's concerns, occupational performance challenges, health problems, and the nature of the intervention setting.

As discussed earlier, occupational analysis may be focused on a particular occupation, such as using a keyboard on the computer or brushing one's teeth, or it may be focused on a broader scope of how individuals orchestrate numerous aspects of occupational performance into daily life, such as being an effective worker. Two approaches to analyzing occupations which vary by the scope of the client's concerns are illustrated.

- **Occupational analysis:** Analysis of occupations parallels activity analysis, with the important difference that it is examining an actual occupation that the person does in his or her own unique way. Questions used for occupational analysis are found in the middle column of Table 25-2.
- **Analysis of occupational orchestration:** Table 25-3 illustrates ways to consider how individuals engage and manage their multiple occupations.

Analysis of Occupational Performance Skills

Occupational therapy practitioners apply the analytic processes just described when observing individuals as they engage in their desired occupations. This may range from

TABLE 25-3 Analysis of Orchestration of Occupations

Analysis of Orchestration of Occupations	
Occupations	Identify the occupations that are central to the person's identity. List these occupations.
Meaning	• How meaningful are these occupations to the individual? • How central are the occupations to the person's identity? • How important are the occupations to the individual? • How important is the occupation to others in the person's social world (family, friends, coworkers, etc.)?
Purpose	What purpose(s) does each occupation serve in the individual's life (e.g., self-maintenance, health, support to family, support to friends or others, contribution to community, play or leisure, work)?
Level of Skill and Efficiency	For each occupation, does the individual believe that he or she is able to do this occupation at an appropriate level of skill within the expected timelines? • If not, what are the problems/concerns from the individual's perspective? • If not, what are the problems/concerns from the perspective of people in the individual's social world?
Routines	Identify the pattern in which the individual engages in these occupations. • What occupations occur daily? • What occupations occur weekly? • What occupations occur monthly and annually? • Describe a typical day. • Describe a typical week.
Organization of Routines	To what extent is the daily and weekly pattern of occupations routinized (patterns of behavior that are observable, regular, repetitive, and provide structure for daily life; routines and occupations with established sequences)? • Is the individual satisfied with this level of organization? If not, why not? • To what extent do these routines meet the expectations of family, friends, and coworkers? • Are these expectations reasonable given the person's physical and emotional capacities, and expectations from the context, family, friends, and employers? • Describe the degree to which these routines are disorganized, stable, or hyperstable.
Adaptability to Promote Participation	To what extent are the occupations and/or routines flexible based on • Individual-based variables: personal context, impairments, openness to change? • Expectations from social environment (family, friends, coworkers)? • Environmental adaptability (potential to change physical environment to promote increased participation)?
Needs	Describe the extent to which the occupational routine is sufficient to meet the person's needs and the needs of those in his or her social world. This might include attention to occupational deprivation or overload. Describe the changes required to meet the individual's needs: • Changes in the individual (skill development) • Changes in the social environment (expectations for performance) • Changes in the occupation (adapting or grading to promote more effective performance)

observing a student in the classroom or on the playground, a person working in an office or factory, an older adult in a leisure setting or an assisted living facility, or a homeless person at a shelter. In all these situations, the practitioner's attention is on the dynamic transaction of the person's occupational performance within the performance environment and context. Although the practitioner must be concerned with the quality of the results, the major focus is on the process of engagement. Thus, practitioners become adept at carefully observing skills associated with occupational performance. These performance skills are the smallest observable units of occupational performance, goal-directed actions a person carries out one by one during naturalistic and relevant daily life task performances (Fisher & Jones, 2014). See Chapter 26 for an in-depth discussion of performance skills.

Analysis of Personal Factors That Impede or Support Performance

Occupational therapy practitioners may also analyze chosen occupations from a micro perspective in terms of how the presence, absence, or impairment of body functions support or limit occupational performance. Árnadóttir (2016) suggests that the therapist can use occupational analysis to detect occupational errors via skilled observation of occupational

performance. She further states that these errors may indicate the effect of neurobehavioral deficits on task performance. Subsequently, the therapist can hypothesize about the impaired body functions that caused the error. "Therapists can benefit from detecting errors in occupational performance while observing activities of daily living and thereby gain an understanding of the impairments affecting the patient's activity limitation. Therapists can use the information based on observed task performance in a systematic way as a structure for clinical reasoning to help them assess functional independence related to the performance and to subsequently detect impaired neurologic body functions" (Árnadóttir 1990, p. 462). The approach suggested by Árnadóttir can be expanded to include musculoskeletal impairments, psychological impairments, and so forth (Table 25-4). See Chapter 23 for in-depth discussion of personal factors.

Conclusion

This chapter describes two types of analyses: activity analysis and occupational analysis. Use of these analyses requires practitioners to understand the following:

- The general properties and demands of activities as they are customarily performed in given arenas and cultures
- How to select activities that are occupationally relevant to clients
- How to use occupations valued by clients to achieve their goals as occupational beings

TABLE 25-4   **Analysis of Personal Factors That May Support or Impede Performance**

Activity to Be Analyzed: *Morning Self-Care*		
Body Function	**Support for Effective and Efficient Occupational Performance**	**Impairment of Body Function Resulting in Occupational Error**
Praxis	Understands the concept of a morning routine, knows how to use tools (comb, razor, socks, etc.), is able to organize and sequence the steps of the task and to plan movements	Apraxia: uses the comb to brush teeth; improperly sequences the steps of dressing (socks on top of shoes); unable to plan movements related to donning pants, resulting in clumsy and inefficient movements
Visuospatial processing	Judges depth and distance, orients clothing properly to body, differentiates foreground from background such as finding a bar of white soap on a white sink	Spatial relations impairment: spills toothpaste when attempting to squeeze it on to the brush, dons shirt backward, unable to differentiate sleeves from the body of shirt
Arousal/ attention	Alert, stays on task, disregards irrelevant environmental stimuli, attends to stimuli in both the right and left attentional fields	Arousal/attention deficits: falls asleep, gets distracted by television and stops dressing before completing the task, does not attend to clothing hanging on the left side of the closet
Motor control	Controls posture to stand at the sink, bends to retrieve shoes from the floor, reaches into the closet for a tie, coordinates movements to brush teeth	Impaired motor control: leans to the left while standing at the sink, loses balance while bending or reaching for clothing, trembles while reaching for brush, can't reverse movements for efficient toothbrushing
Affect	Motivated to engage in tasks, able to tolerate frustrations that arise, show affect appropriate to situation and task	Affective disturbance: requires coaxing and encouragement to participate in and continue morning care, easily frustrated and terminates task, moods shift rapidly during performance

Data from Árnadóttir, G. (1990). *The brain and behavior: Assessing cortical dysfunction through activities of daily living.* St. Louis, MO: Elsevier/Mosby; and Árnadóttir, G. (2016). Impact of neurobehavioral deficits on activities of daily living. In G. Gillen (Ed.), *Stroke rehabilitation: A function-based approach* (4th ed., pp. 573–611). St. Louis, MO: Elsevier/Mosby.

These core skills are critical for effective OT evaluation and intervention. Both processes ultimately center on occupation and its capacity to motivate people to act and to create meaning in their lives. Brockelman (1980), a philosopher, recognized the importance of occupation in the following statement: "The tools of our minds and the tools of our hands are of meaningless use without deep and personal reasons of the heart to set their purpose and guide their use" (p. 24). It is through practitioners' deep understanding of people as occupational beings that effective OT intervention occurs.

 Visit thePoint to watch a video about occupations that can be analyzed.

REFERENCES

Allen, C. K. (1987). Activity: Occupational therapy's treatment method. 1987 Eleanor Clarke Slagle lecture. *American Journal of Occupational Therapy, 41,* 563–575.

American Occupational Therapy Association. (2002). Occupational therapy practice framework: Domain and process. *American Journal of Occupational Therapy, 56,* 609–639.

American Occupational Therapy Association. (2014). Occupational therapy practice framework: Domain and process, 3rd edition. *American Journal of Occupational Therapy, 68,* S1–S48. doi:10.5014/ajot.2014682006

Árnadóttir, G. (1990). *The brain and behavior: Assessing cortical dysfunction through activities of daily living.* St. Louis, MO: Elsevier/Mosby.

Árnadóttir, G. (2016). Impact of neurobehavioral deficits on activities of daily living. In G. Gillen (Ed.), *Stroke rehabilitation: A function-based approach* (4th ed., pp. 573–611). St. Louis, MO: Elsevier/Mosby.

Barton, G. E. (1915). Occupational therapy. *The Trained Nurse and Hospital Review, 54,* 138–140.

Bauerschmidt, B., & Nelson, D. L. (2011). The terms occupation and activity over the history of official occupational therapy publications. *American Journal of Occupational Therapy, 65,* 338–345.

Baum, C. M., & Christiansen, C. H. (2005). Person-environment-occupation-performance: An occupation-based framework for practice. In C. H. Christiansen, C. M. Baum, & J. Bass-Haugen (Eds.), *Occupational therapy: Performance, participation, and well-being* (3rd ed., pp. 243–266). Thorofare, NJ: SLACK.

Brockelman, P. T. (1980). *Existential phenomenology and the world of ordinary experience: An introduction.* Lanham, MD: University Press of America.

Bruner, J. (1990). *Acts of meaning.* Cambridge, MA: Harvard University Press.

Christiansen, C. H., & Baum, C. M. (2005). The complexity of human occupation. In C. H. Christiansen, C. M. Baum, & J. Bass-Haugen (Eds.), *Occupational therapy: Performance, participation, and well-being* (3rd ed., pp. 4–23). Thorofare, NJ: SLACK.

Clarke, F. A., Parham, D., Carlson, M. E., Frank, G., Jackson, J., Pierce, D., . . . Zemke, R. (1991). Occupational science: Academic innovation in the service of occupational therapy's future. *American Journal of Occupational Therapy, 45,* 300–310.

Coster, W. (1998). Occupation-centered assessment of children. *American Journal of Occupational Therapy, 52,* 337–344.

Crabtree, M. (1998). Images of reasoning: A literature review. *Australian Occupational Therapy Journal, 45,* 113–123.

Crepeau, E. B. (1991). Achieving intersubjective understanding: Examples from an occupational therapy treatment session. *American Journal of Occupational Therapy, 45,* 1016–1025.

Crepeau, E. B., & Garren, K. R. (2011). I looked to her as a guide: The therapeutic relationship in hand therapy. *Disability and Rehabilitation, 33,* 872–881.

Cynkin, S. (1995). Activities. In C. B. Royeen (Ed.), *AOTA self-study series: The practice of the future: Putting occupation back into therapy* (Module 7; pp. 1–52). Bethesda, MD: American Occupational Therapy Association.

Davidson, L. (2003). *Living outside mental illness: Qualitative studies of recovery in schizophrenia.* New York, NY: New York University Press.

Dunn, W., Brown, C., & Youngstrom, M. J. (2003). Ecological model of occupation. In P. Kramer, J. Hinojosa, & C. B. Royeen (Eds.), *Perspectives in human occupation: Participation in life* (pp. 222–263). Philadelphia, PA: Lippincott Williams & Wilkins.

Fisher, A. G. (1998). Uniting practice and theory in an occupational framework. 1998 Eleanor Clarke Slagle Lecture. *American Journal of Occupational Therapy, 52,* 509–521.

Fisher, A. G., & Jones, K. B. (2014). *Assessment of motor and process skills: User manual* (8th ed.). Fort Collins, CO: Three Star Press.

Frankl, V. E. (1959). *Man's search for meaning: An introduction to logotherapy.* New York, NY: Pocket Books.

Hagedorn, R. (2000). Glossary. In R. Hagedorn (Ed.), *Tools for practice in occupational therapy: A structured approach to core skills and processes* (pp. 307–312). Edinburgh, United Kingdom: Churchill Livingstone.

Hasselkus, B. R. (2002). *The meaning of everyday occupation.* Thorofare, NJ: SLACK.

Hinojosa, J., & Kramer, P. (1997). Statement—Fundamental concepts of occupational therapy: Occupation, purposeful activity, and function. *American Journal of Occupational Therapy, 51,* 864–866.

Hinojosa, J., Kramer, P., Royeen, C. B., & Luebben, A. J. (2003). Core concept of occupation. In P. Kramer, J. Hinojosa, & C. B. Royeen (Eds.), *Perspectives in human occupation* (pp. 1–17). Philadelphia, PA: Lippincott Williams & Wilkins.

Hocking, C. (2001). Implementing occupation-based assessment. *American Journal of Occupational Therapy, 55,* 463–469.

Hymes, D. (1972). Toward ethnographies of communication: The analysis of communicative events. In P. P. Giglioli (Ed.), *Language and social context* (pp. 21–44). New York, NY: Pelican.

Jackson, J. (1998a). Contemporary criticisms of role theory. *Journal of Occupational Science, 5,* 49–55.

Jackson, J. (1998b). Is there a place for role theory in occupational science? *Journal of Occupational Science, 5,* 56–65.

Kielhofner, G., & Barrett, L. (1998). Meaning and misunderstanding in occupational forms: A study of therapeutic goal setting. *American Journal of Occupational Therapy, 52,* 345–353.

Kronenberg, F., Pollard, N., & Ramugondo, E. (2011). Introduction: Courage to dance politics. In F. Kronenberg, N. Pollard, & D. Sakellariou (Eds.), *Occupational Therapies Without Borders: Vol. 2. Towards an ecology of occupation-based practices* (pp. 1–16). New York, NY: Churchill-Livingstone Elsevier.

Larson, E. A. (2000). The orchestration of occupation: The dance of mothers. *American Journal of Occupational Therapy, 54,* 269–280.

Lave, J. (1988). *Cognition in practice: Mind, mathematics and culture in everyday life.* Cambridge, United Kingdom: Cambridge University Press.

Law, M. (Ed.). (1998). *Client-centered occupational therapy.* Thorofare, NJ: SLACK.

Law, M., Polatajko, H., Baptiste, W., & Townsend, E. (1997). Core concepts of occupational therapy. In E. Townsend (Ed.), *Enabling occupation: An occupational therapy perspective* (pp. 29–56). Ottawa, Canada: Canadian Association of Occupational Therapists.

Llorens, L. A. (1986). Activity analysis: Agreement among factors in a sensory processing model. *American Journal of Occupational Therapy, 40,* 103–110.

Mattingly, C., & Fleming, M. H. (1994). *Clinical reasoning: Forms of inquiry in a therapeutic practice*. Philadelphia, PA: F. A. Davis.

Mosey, A. C. (1981). *Occupational therapy: Configuration of a profession*. New York, NY: Raven Press.

Neistadt, M. E., McAuley, D., Zecha, D., & Shannon, R. (1993). An analysis of a board game as a treatment activity. *American Journal of Occupational Therapy, 47*, 154–160.

Nelson, D. J., & Jebson-Thomas, J. (2003). Occupational form, occupational performance, and a conceptual framework for therapeutic occupation. In P. Kramer, J. Hinojosa, & C. B. Royeen (Eds.), *Perspectives in human occupation: Participation in life* (pp. 87–155). Philadelphia, PA: Lippincott Williams & Wilkins.

Payne, R. K., DeVol, P., & Dreussi Smith, T. (2001). *Bridges out of poverty: Strategies for professionals and communities* (Rev. ed.). Highland, TX: aha! Process.

Peloquin, S. M. (1995). The fullness of empathy: Reflections and illustrations. *American Journal of Occupational Therapy, 49*, 24–31.

Peloquin, S. M. (2005). Embracing our ethos, reclaiming our heart. *American Journal of Occupational Therapy, 59*, 611–625.

Peloquin, S. M. (2007). A reconsideration of occupational therapy's core values. *American Journal of Occupational Therapy, 61*, 474–478.

Pierce, D. (2001). Untangling occupation and activity. *American Journal of Occupational Therapy, 55*, 138–146.

Pierce, D. (2014). *Occupational science for occupational therapy*. Thorofare, NJ: SLACK.

Polatajko, H. J., Mandich, A., & Martini, R. (2000). Dynamic performance analysis: A framework for understanding occupational performance. *American Journal of Occupational Therapy, 54*, 65–72.

Reed, K. L. (2005). An annotated history of the concepts used in occupational therapy. In C. H. Christiansen, C. M. Baum, & J. Bass-Haugen (Eds.), *Occupational therapy: Performance, participation, and well-being* (3rd ed., pp. 567–626). Thorofare, NJ: SLACK.

Robeson, H. A., Dunton, W. R., Haas, L. J., Kidner, T. B., Lindberg, B., Sample, G., . . . Tompkins, A. B. (1928a). Analysis of crafts: Continuation of the report of Committee on Installations and Advice. *Occupational Therapy and Rehabilitation, 7*, 131–136.

Robeson, H. A., Dunton, W. R., Haas, L. J., Kidner, T. B., Lindberg, B., Sample, G., . . . Tompkins, A. B. (1928b). Analysis of crafts: Continuation of the report of Committee on Installations and Advice. *Occupational Therapy and Rehabilitation, 7*, 211–216.

Robeson, H. A., Dunton, W. R., Haas, L. J., Kidner, T. B., Lindberg, B., Sample, G., . . . Tompkins, A. B. (1928c). Report of Committee on Installations and Advice: Making a physical analysis of crafts. *Occupational Therapy and Rehabilitation, 7*, 29–43.

Schell, B. A. (2018). Pragmatic reasoning. In B. A. B. Schell & J. W. Schell (Eds.), *Clinical and professional reasoning in occupational therapy* (pp. 203–224). Philadelphia, PA: Wolters Kluwer.

Schell, B. A., & Cervero, R. M. (1993). Clinical reasoning in occupational therapy: An integrative review. *American Journal of Occupational Therapy, 47*, 605–610.

Spear, P. S., & Crepeau, E. B. (2003). Glossary. In E. B. Crepeau, E. S. Cohn, & B. A. Boyt Schell (Eds.), *Willard & Spackman's occupational therapy* (10th ed., pp. 1025–1035). Philadelphia, PA: Lippincott Williams & Wilkins.

Trombly, C. A. (1995). Occupation: Purposefulness and meaningfulness as therapeutic mechanisms. *1995 Eleanor Clarke Slagle Lecture. American Journal of Occupational Therapy, 49*, 960–972.

Trombly Latham, C. A. (2014). Conceptual foundations for practice. In M. V. Radomski & C. A. Trombly Latham (Eds.), *Occupational therapy for physical dysfunction* (7th ed., pp. 1–20). Baltimore, MD: Lippincott Williams & Wilkins.

World Health Organization. (2001). *International classification of functioning, disability and health (ICF)*. Geneva, Switzerland: Author.

Zemke, R., & Clark, F. (1996). *Occupational science: The evolving discipline*. Philadelphia, PA: F. A. Davis.

thePoint® *For additional resources on the subjects discussed in this chapter, visit* http://thePoint.lww.com/Willard-Spackman13e. *See* **Appendix II, Table of Assessments** *for more information on Role Checklist and Worker Role Interview.*

Performance Skills

Implementing Performance Analyses to Evaluate Quality of Occupational Performance

Anne G. Fisher, Lou Ann Griswold

LEARNING OBJECTIVES

After reading this chapter, you will be able to:

1. Describe the difference between (1) performance skills and (2) body functions.
2. Implement an analysis of performance skills (performance analysis) and document a person's baseline quality of occupational performance.
3. Describe how the results of a performance analysis are used to collaboratively establish client-centered goals.

Introduction to Performance Skills

Performance skills are the smallest observable actions or units of occupational performance that we can observe as a person carries out his or her daily life tasks. Noting the degree of performance skill that can be observed is critical for evaluating the quality of a person's occupational performance. Consider, for example, what Karla observes as she watches Maurice perform daily life tasks (see Case Study 26-1).

In Case Study 26-1, Karla evaluated the quality of Maurice's occupational performance by observing the small goal-directed actions Maurice enacted one by one as he engaged in relevant and meaningful daily life task performances. More specifically, she observed the quality of his occupational **performance skills** (Fisher, 2009; Fisher & Kielhofner, 1995; Kielhofner, 2008). Kielhofner (2008) referred to these observable performance skills as "discrete purposeful actions [that] can be discerned" (p. 103). Performance skills are links in a larger chain of actions, which link by link, action by action, become the whole chain—the task performance (Fisher, 2009; Figure 26-2).

The term *performance skills* has been used to refer to these smallest observable units of occupational performance because each person we evaluate demonstrates more or less occupational skill when he or she completes (i.e., "constructs") a daily life task performance. These small units of observable actions were first conceptualized in the mid-1980s (Fisher, 2006), and they have now been incorporated into major occupational therapy (OT) models of practice, including the Model of Human Occupation (Kielhofner, 1995, 2008) and the Occupational Therapy Intervention Process

CASE STUDY 26-1   PERFORMANCE SKILLS—OBSERVABLE CHAINS OF GOAL-DIRECTED ACTIONS

Karla, Maurice's occupational therapist, observes him as he is engaged in preparing himself a glass of orange juice and a bowl of cereal. As she observes his occupational performance **motor skills**, she observes that he momentarily props (*stabilizes*) on the kitchen counter as he *walks* to the refrigerator. He then *bends* forward, *reaches* out, and grasps (*grips*) the handle on the door of the refrigerator without any evidence of clumsiness or increased physical effort. When he attempts to open the door of the refrigerator (*moves*), he does not pull hard enough (*calibrates*)—the door does not open. She then observes him as he pulls again (*moves*, *calibrates*) on the handle of the refrigerator door and, this time, she sees the refrigerator door open. Karla then observes that Maurice effectively *reaches* in, *grips* a container of orange juice, *lifts* it, and takes it out of the refrigerator, but that he is somewhat unstable (*stabilizes*) when he *walks* and *transports* the container of juice over to the counter where he has placed a glass. See Figure 26-1.

As Karla observes Maurice as he is engaged in preparing his breakfast, she also observes his occupational performance **process skills**. For example, Karla observes that although Maurice *initiates* most task actions without a delay, he pauses momentarily before reaching for the handle of the refrigerator door. She also sees that he *continues* each action through to completion without any unnecessary pauses (e.g., continuing pulling on the refrigerator door until it is open, continuing walking until the orange juice is transported to the counter). As Maurice *initiates* pouring orange juice into the glass on the counter, he again pauses. Moreover, Karla observes that he does not *terminate* pouring the orange juice before some orange juice spills over the rim of the glass. She also observes that Maurice performs task actions in a logical order (*sequences*). For example, she observes that he opens the lid of the orange juice container and then pours juice into the glass and not vice versa. Finally, she observes Maurice as he *searches* for and *locates* the orange juice container in the refrigerator, *chooses* orange juice, *gathers* the orange juice container to the same workspace where he has placed the glass, and *organizes* his workspace effectively—not too crowded, not too spread out.

Later, as Karla observes Maurice as he is engaged in a social exchange with his care provider, Joyce—planning the weekly meals and making a shopping list—she observes Maurice's **social interaction skills**. More specifically, she observes that he readily *approaches* his social partner and *starts* a conversation. As he does so, and throughout the social exchange, Maurice *turns toward*, but frequently does

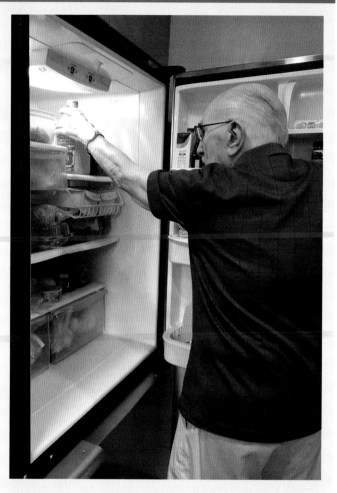

FIGURE 26-1 **Maurice reaching into refrigerator to get the bottle of orange juice.**

not *look* at his social partner when they are talking to each other. As Maurice is talking, she observes that he *produces speech* that is clearly audible and that he *gesticulates* by nodding his head and smiling in a manner that is socially appropriate. She also observes that Maurice often stammers and pauses during his spoken messages (*speaks fluently*), and that he occasionally starts messages but leaves them "hanging in the air" and never finishes them (*times duration*). When Joyce asks Maurice questions (e.g., "What would you like to eat this week?"), he frequently *replies* with messages that are markedly irrelevant to the ongoing conversation (e.g., "My son called me last night."). Finally, Karla observes Maurice as he *takes turns* with his social partner, and that he frequently "talks over" and interrupts his social partner (*times response*).

Occupational performance
A chain of small actions

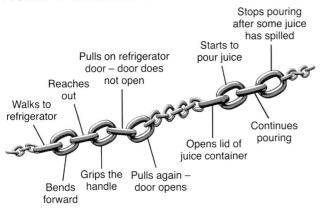

FIGURE 26-2 Performance skills: smallest observable units of occupational performance—links in a chain of ongoing actions that a person performs one by one as he or she "constructs" the overall daily life task performance. (Adapted from Fisher, A. G. [2009]. *Occupational Therapy Intervention Process Model: A model for planning and implementing top–down, client-centered, and occupation-based interventions*. Fort Collins, CO: Three Star Press. Reprinted with permission.)

Model (Fisher, 1998, 2009). They were also included in the first and third editions of the *Occupational Therapy Practice Framework* (American Occupational Therapy Association [AOTA], 2002, 2014). The smallest observable actions of occupational performance have been variously referred to as *performance skills* (AOTA, 2002, 2014; Fisher, 2006; Fisher & Kielhofner, 1995), *performance units* (Hagedorn, 2000), *units* or *subunits of occupational performance* (Fisher, 2006; Polatajko, Mandich, & Martini, 2000), *occupational skill* (Kielhofner, 2008), and *actions of performance* (Fisher, 1998). Within the *International Classification of Functioning, Disability and Health* (ICF; World Health Organization [WHO], 2001), performance skills are analogous to the smaller discrete actions that are part of larger task performances defined within the "Activities" and "Participation" domains. In all of these instances, performance skills have been clearly differentiated from underlying body functions.

Differentiation between Performance Skills and Body Functions

Body functions pertain to *what the person's body systems do* (see Chapter 23). Examples of body functions include memory, motor planning and praxis skill, perceptual skill, joint mobility, muscle power, fine motor coordination, and emotional regulation. In contrast, performance skills pertain to *what the person does* as he or she interacts with task objects (e.g., *swing* a baseball bat and *hit* a baseball, *jump* rope, *choose* a pencil and *use* it to *write*) in the context of engagement in meaningful occupation (playing baseball with friends, jumping rope with classmates, completing a schoolwork task; Figure 26-3). When a person is engaged in occupation that includes social interaction with others, it also becomes possible to observe social interaction skills (*greet* one's friends, *laugh* at a friend's joke; see the Commentary on the Evidence box).

As shown in Figure 26-3, person factors and body functions are not the same thing as performance skills. Although body functions (as well as task and environmental demands) can support or hinder quality of occupational performance, body functions and performance skills represent different constructs. Swinging a bat and hitting a ball may be supported by the person having strength and coordination, but being strong and coordinated does not mean that the person can skillfully swing a bat and hit a ball. Moreover, people can demonstrate occupational skill despite having impairments of their body functions.

In Case Study 26-1, we note that when Karla observed Maurice as he attempted to open the refrigerator door, he did not pull hard enough and the door did not open. From the perspective of occupational performance (what Maurice did), Karla observed that Maurice did not pull with enough force to open the refrigerator door. When Karla began to reason as to why Maurice might not have pulled with enough force to open the door, her first thought was that he might have diminished strength in his upper limb.

In such instances, occupational therapists may think they "see" decreased strength, but in fact, they do not. Rather, they observe the person to perform some action that has an underlying demand for strength and therefore reason that diminished strength is the cause of the occupational performance problem observed. But Karla has not observed diminished strength because strength cannot be directly observed, nor was diminished strength necessarily the reason Maurice did not open the refrigerator door.

When Karla reasoned as to why did Maurice not open the door on his first attempt, she actually considered many possibilities besides diminished upper limb strength, such as "Is the seal on the refrigerator door unusually tight?" "Is he unfamiliar with this particular refrigerator and more familiar with one that opens more easily?" She could not determine the answer based solely on what she had observed. She needed to use her professional reasoning skills to speculate about possible reasons or causes for Maurice's observed problem with occupational performance and then evaluate further to determine why Maurice did not open the door on his first attempt. Karla also was aware that the reasons or causes may be

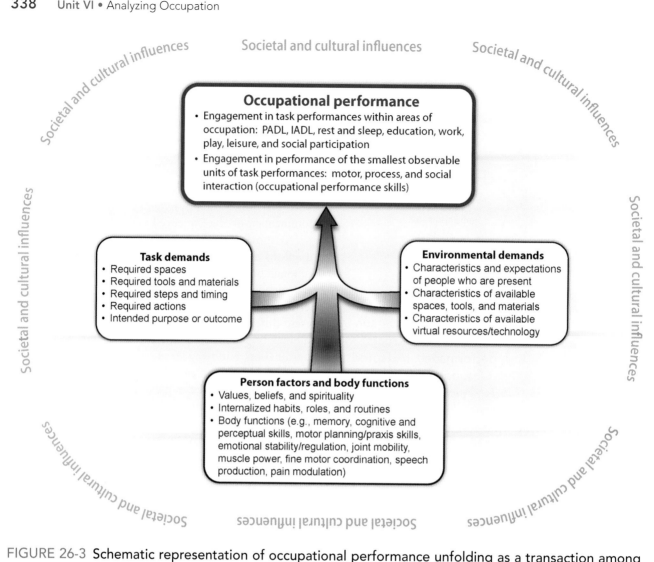

FIGURE 26-3 Schematic representation of occupational performance unfolding as a transaction among person factors and body functions, task demands, environmental demands, and societal and cultural influences. *IADL,* instrumental activity of daily living; *PADL,* personal activity of daily living. (Adapted from Fisher, A. G. [2009]. *Occupational Therapy Intervention Process Model: A model for planning and implementing top–down, client-centered, and occupation-based interventions.* Fort Collins, CO: Three Star Press. Reprinted with permission.)

related not only to body functions but also to person factors, task demands, environmental demands, and/or societal and cultural influences (see Figure 26-3).

Universal versus Task-Specific Performance Skills

Universal Performance Skills

Performance skills can be viewed as being *universal* or more *task specific.* The brief definitions of universal motor, process, and social interaction performance skills

included in Table 26-1 are based on the operational definitions of each skill within three standardized tests of occupational performance skill: the *Assessment of Motor and Process Skills* (AMPS; Fisher & Jones, 2012, 2014), the *School Version of the Assessment of Motor and Process Skills* (School AMPS; Fisher, Bryze, Hume, & Griswold, 2007), and the *Evaluation of Social Interaction* (ESI; Fisher & Griswold, 2015). They are considered to be universal because they can be observed in virtually any daily life task performance and, in the case of social interaction skills, virtually any daily life task performance involving social interaction. As we will discuss next, these universal performance skills can be complemented by an endless number of task-specific occupational performance skills.

Using the AMPS as an example, Figure 26-4 helps to clarify the concept of *universal skills.* As the AMPS is a test

COMMENTARY ON THE EVIDENCE

Performance Skills Cannot Be Equated with Body Functions

Many respected authors within OT equate performance skills with body functions. That is, (1) process skills are sometimes referred to as cognitive skills, and/or (2) motor planning, executive functions, and perceptual skills are considered to be performance skills. One such example is the second edition of the *Occupational Therapy Practice Framework* (AOTA, 2008). Within the framework, performance skills are described as including motor and praxis skills, sensory-perceptual skills, emotional regulation skills, cognitive skills, and communication and social skills. When compared to Figure 26-3, one can readily see a discrepancy. In both Figure 26-3 and within the ICF (WHO, 2001), praxis skill (i.e., motor planning), perceptual skill, cognitive skill, and emotional regulation are viewed as underlying body functions, not performance skills.

What is the evidence to support the differentiation between performance skills and these underlying body functions? One such resource comes from Rexroth, Fisher, Merritt, and Gliner (2005) who implemented a study where they compared the level of motor and process skill between 1,939 persons with right hemispheric strokes and 1,939 persons with left hemispheric strokes. If we compare these two groups, persons who have had right hemispheric strokes are much more likely to demonstrate visual perceptual impairments and unilateral neglect, whereas persons who have had left hemispheric strokes are much more likely to demonstrate aphasia and apraxia (Bartels, Duffy, & Beland, 2016). These are impairments of body functions.

If performance skills, specifically motor and process skills, are to be equated with praxis and perceptual skill, it should follow that persons with right versus left hemispheric stroke will differ significantly in terms of their levels of motor and/or process skill. Yet, Rexroth et al. (2005) found that there was no significant difference between the two groups in any of the 36 motor and process skills studied. These results indicate that performance analysis, focused on performance skill (i.e., the person's observed quality of doing), is very different from assessment methods focused on underlying body functions (see Table 26-1 for a list of the 36 performance skills they compared).

TABLE 26-1 Universal Performance Skills

Universal Performance Skills	Description
Motor Skills	
Stabilizes	Moves through task environment and interacts with task objects without *momentary* propping or loss of balance
Aligns	Interacts with task objects without evidence of *persistent* propping or *persistent* leaning
Positions	Positions self an effective distance from task objects and without evidence of awkward body positions
Reaches	Effectively extends the arm and, when appropriate, bends the trunk to effectively grasp or place task objects that are out of reach
Bends	Flexes or rotates the trunk as appropriate to the task when bending to grasp or place task objects that are out of reach or when sitting down
Grips	Effectively pinches or grasps task objects such that the task objects do not slip (e.g., from the person's fingers, from between the teeth)
Manipulates	Uses dexterous finger movements, without evidence of fumbling, when manipulating task objects (e.g., manipulating buttons when buttoning)
Coordinates	Uses two or more body parts together to manipulate, hold, and/or stabilize task objects without evidence of fumbling task objects or objects slipping from one's grasp
Moves	Effectively pushes or pulls task objects along a supporting surface, pulls to open or pushes to close doors and drawers, or pushes on wheels to propel a wheelchair
Lifts	Effectively raises or lifts task objects without evidence of increased effort
Walks	During the task performance, ambulates on level surfaces without shuffling the feet, instability, propping, or use of assistive devices
Transports	Carries task objects from one place to another while walking or moving in a wheelchair
Calibrates	Uses movements of appropriate force, speed, or extent when interacting with task objects (e.g., not crushing task objects, pushing a door with enough force that it closes)
Flows	Uses smooth and fluid arm and wrist movements when interacting with task objects
Endures	Persists and completes the task without *obvious* evidence of physical fatigue, pausing to rest, or stopping to "catch one's breath"
Paces	Maintains a consistent and effective rate or tempo of performance throughout the entire task

(continues)

TABLE 26-1 **Universal Performance Skills** *(continued)*

Universal Performance Skills	Description
Process Skills	
Paces	Maintains a consistent and effective rate or tempo of performance throughout the entire task
Attends	Does not look away from what he or she is doing, thus interrupting the ongoing task progression
Heeds	Carries out and completes the task originally agreed on or specified by another
Chooses	Selects necessary and appropriate type and number of tools and materials for the task, including the tools and materials that the person was directed to use or specified he or she would use
Uses	Employs tools and materials as they are intended (e.g., using a pencil sharpener to sharpen a pencil, but not to sharpen a crayon) and in a hygienic fashion
Handles	Supports or stabilizes tools and materials in an appropriate manner, protecting them from damage, slipping, moving, or falling
Inquires	(1) Seeks needed verbal or written information by asking questions or reading directions or labels and (2) does *not* ask for information in situations where the person had been fully oriented to the task and environment and had immediate prior awareness of the answer
Initiates	Starts or begins *the next* action or step without hesitation
Continues	Performs single actions or steps without interruptions, such that once an action or task step is initiated, the individual continues on without pauses or delays until the action or step is completed
Sequences	Performs steps in an effective or logical order and with an absence of (1) randomness or lack of logic in the ordering and/or (2) inappropriate repetition of steps
Terminates	Brings to completion *single actions* or *single steps* without inappropriate persistence or premature cessation
Searches/Locates	Looks for and locates tools and materials in a logical manner, both within and beyond the immediate environment
Gathers	Collects together *related* tools and materials into the same workspace and "regathers" tools or materials that have spilled, fallen, or been misplaced
Organizes	Logically positions or spatially arranges tools and materials in an orderly fashion within a single workspace and between multiple appropriate workspaces, such that the workspace is not too spread out or too crowded
Restores	Puts away tools and materials in appropriate places and ensures that the immediate workspace is restored to its original condition
Navigates	Moves the arm, body, or wheelchair without bumping into obstacles when moving in the task environment or interacting with task objects
Notices/Responds	Responds appropriately to (1) nonverbal task-related cues (e.g., heat, movement), (2) the spatial arrangement and alignment of task objects to one another, and (3) cupboard doors or drawers that have been left open during the task performance
Adjusts	Effectively (1) goes to new workspaces; (2) moves tools and materials out of the current workspace; and (3) adjusts knobs, dials, or water taps to overcome problems with ongoing task performance
Accommodates	Prevents ineffective task performance
Benefits	Prevents problems with task performance from recurring or persisting
Social Interaction Skills	
Approaches/Starts	Approaches and/or initiates interaction with the social partner in a manner that is socially appropriate
Concludes/Disengages	Effectively terminates the conversation or social interaction, brings to closure the topic under discussion, and disengages or says goodbye
Produces speech	Produces spoken, signed, or augmentative (i.e., computer generated) messages that are audible and clearly articulated
Gesticulates	Uses socially appropriate gestures to communicate or support a message
Speaks fluently	Speaks in a fluent and continuous manner, with an even flow (not too fast, not too slow), and without pauses or delays *during* the message being sent
Turns toward	Actively positions or turns the body and the face toward the social partner or the person who is speaking
Looks	Makes eye contact with the social partner
Places self	Places oneself at an appropriate distance from the social partner during the social interaction
Touches	Responds to and uses touch or bodily contact with the social partner in a manner that is socially appropriate
Regulates	Does not demonstrate irrelevant, repetitive, or impulsive behaviors that are not part of social interaction

TABLE 26-1	**Universal Performance Skills** *(continued)*

Universal Performance Skills	Description
Questions	Requests relevant facts and information and asks questions that support the intended purpose of the social interaction (e.g., asking about the social partner's opinions)
Replies	Keeps conversation going by replying appropriately to questions and comments
Discloses	Reveals opinions, feelings, and private information *about oneself* or *others* in a manner that is socially appropriate
Expresses emotion	Displays affect and emotions in a way that is socially appropriate
Disagrees	Expresses differences of opinion in a socially appropriate manner
Thanks	Uses appropriate words and gestures to acknowledge receipt of services, gifts, and/or compliments
Transitions	Smoothly transitions the conversation and/or changes the topic without disrupting the ongoing conversation
Times response	Replies to social messages without delay or hesitation and without interrupting the social partner
Times duration	Speaks for reasonable time periods given the complexity of the message sent
Takes turns	Takes one's turn and gives the social partner the freedom to take his or her turn
Matches language	Uses a tone of voice, dialect, and level of language that is socially appropriate and matched to the social partner's abilities and level of understanding
Clarifies	Responds to gestures or verbal messages signaling that the social partner does not comprehend or understand a message and ensures that the social partner is "following" the conversation
Acknowledges/Encourages	Acknowledges receipt of messages, encourages the social partner to continue interaction, and encourages all social partners to participate in social interaction
Empathizes	Expresses a supportive attitude toward the social partner by agreeing with, empathizing with, or expressing understanding of the social partner's feelings and experiences
Heeds	Uses goal-directed social interactions that are focused toward carrying out and completing the intended purpose of the social interaction
Accommodates	Prevents ineffective or socially inappropriate social interaction
Benefits	Prevents problems with ineffective or socially inappropriate social interaction from recurring or persisting

Adapted from Fisher, A. G. (2009). *Occupational Therapy Intervention Process Model: A model for planning and implementing top–down, client-centered, and occupation-based interventions.* Fort Collins, CO: Three Star Press. Reprinted with permission.

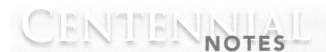

NOTES

The Origin of Performance Skills and Performance Analysis

Unlike task analysis and activity analysis, methods that date from the founding of OT (cf. Barton, 1917; Gilbreth & Gilbreth, 1919), the concepts of performance skills and performance analysis are relatively new. The concept of performance skills—the goal-directed actions a person carries out one by one during naturalistic and relevant daily life task performances—first emerged in the late 1980s (Fisher, 1989) as a result of an ongoing dialog between persons from different OT traditions who were struggling to better understand the difference between underlying body functions and performance skills. One of those persons was Anne Fisher, the first author of this chapter, an occupational therapist with a background in sensory integration, neuropsychological disorders, neurological disorders, and motor control theories. The other was Gary Kielhofner who came from a background within the occupational behavior tradition. The focus of their struggle was to understand

if motor and process skills were small observable units of occupation, something the person does, or underlying body functions, something within the person that the person's brain–body does. In the end, Fisher and Kielhofner (Fisher, 1998; Fisher & Kielhofner, 1995; Kielhofner, 1995) concluded that performance skills are the smallest observable units of occupational performance, not body functions. What enabled Kielhofner and Fisher to come to this conclusion was the realization that as occupational therapists, we often think we can observe impairments of underlying body functions, but what we actually observe are "errors" of occupational performance. These occupational performance errors, however, reflect diminished occupational performance skill, not impairments of body functions. The concept of performance analysis emerged somewhat later as the name of the type of analysis an occupational therapist performs when observing a person's performance skills in order to assess a person's quality of occupational performance (Fisher, 1998).

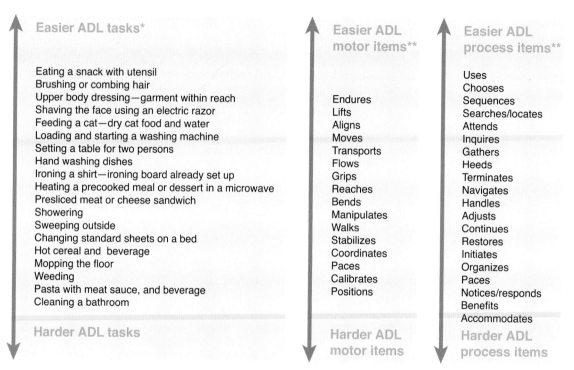

Easier ADL tasks*

Eating a snack with utensil
Brushing or combing hair
Upper body dressing—garment within reach
Shaving the face using an electric razor
Feeding a cat—dry cat food and water
Loading and starting a washing machine
Setting a table for two persons
Hand washing dishes
Ironing a shirt—ironing board already set up
Heating a precooked meal or dessert in a microwave
Presliced meat or cheese sandwich
Showering
Sweeping outside
Changing standard sheets on a bed
Hot cereal and beverage
Mopping the floor
Weeding
Pasta with meat sauce, and beverage
Cleaning a bathroom

Harder ADL tasks

Easier ADL motor items**

Endures
Lifts
Aligns
Moves
Transports
Flows
Grips
Reaches
Bends
Manipulates
Walks
Stabilizes
Coordinates
Paces
Calibrates
Positions

Harder ADL motor items

Easier ADL process items**

Uses
Chooses
Sequences
Searches/locates
Attends
Inquires
Gathers
Heeds
Terminates
Navigates
Handles
Adjusts
Continues
Restores
Initiates
Organizes
Paces
Notices/responds
Benefits
Accommodates

Harder ADL process items

* Each person evaluated using the AMPS chooses to perform, from among over 120 ADL tasks included in the AMPS manual, two ADL tasks that are meaningful, perceived as presenting a challenge, and prioritized for intervention.

** The 16 ADL motor and 20 ADL process items (universal performance skills) that can be observed during any ADL task performance and are scored based on the person's quality of performance of each of the two chosen ADL tasks.

FIGURE 26-4 Selected standardized tasks included in the Assessment of Motor and Process Skills (AMPS) and each of the activities of daily living (ADL) motor and ADL process items (task actions, performance skills) that are scored based on the person's quality of performance of each ADL task action (degree of skill as indicated by lack of observable clumsiness or physical effort, inefficiency, safety risk, and/or need for assistance).

of a person's ability to perform personal activities of daily living (PADL) tasks and instrumental activities of daily living (IADL) tasks (collectively, activities of daily living [ADL]), the motor and process performance skills included in the AMPS are referred to as ADL skills. There are more than 120 standardized ADL tasks in the current edition of the AMPS (Fisher & Jones, 2014). No matter which of these ADL tasks a person is observed performing, the occupational therapist can observe the person's degree of occupational performance skill as the person *lifts* tasks objects, *moves* objects, *walks* within the task environment, *chooses* needed tools and materials, *initiates* task actions, and so on. Moreover, when performing ADL tasks, easier performance skills (e.g., *endures, lifts, uses, chooses*) are likely to be easier actions to perform in a skilled manner no matter which ADL task the person performs. Which ADL motor and ADL process skills are harder or easier and the extent to which the challenge of an ADL task can affect the degree of observed occupational performance skill has been based on a many-facet Rasch analysis

of more than 148,000 people who are currently included in the international standardization sample of the AMPS (Fisher & Jones, 2012). These same principles also apply to the school motor and school process skills included in the School AMPS and the social interaction skills included in the ESI.

Task-Specific Performance Skills

Although the occupational therapist can use the existing taxonomies of universal motor, process, and social interaction skills listed in Table 26-1 in either a standardized or a nonstandardized manner, the occupational therapist is never restricted to these taxonomies. Rather, the occupational therapist may observe and evaluate the quality of any motor, process, or social action that is part of the observed occupational performance (i.e., the observable links in the chain of task actions). Moreover, many daily life task performances involve the performance of motor, process, and social actions that are more unique to the particular task performed. For example, when Michaela watches José as he is playing baseball, she observes him *throw* the ball to the first baseman, and she observes the first baseman *catch* the ball. Later, when José is up to bat, she observes him *swing* the bat, *drop* the bat, *run*, and *slide* into first base. Finally, she observes José's mother *smile* and the audience *cheer*.

A Rationale for Implementing Performance Analyses

There are several interrelated advantages of implementing a **performance analysis**, either standardized or nonstandardized. The first is that by implementing performance analyses, we, as occupational therapists, focus our evaluation on occupational performance, not person factors and body functions or environmental demands that may underlie or cause the ineffective performance (see Figure 26-3). The second advantage is that we make explicit which performance skills the person performed effectively and which were performed ineffectively (i.e., errors of occupational performance). The result is that we become better able to differentiate between occupational performance skill and underlying body functions and describe to others—including the client, team members, and third-party payers—using "everyday language," the person's observed problems of occupational performance. The final two advantages may be the ones that are most important. That is, if we use "everyday language" in describing quality of occupational performance, the result will be that we more readily (1) work collaboratively with the client to establish occupation-focused goals and plan and implement occupation-based interventions and (2) use "occupation-first" language in our documentation and in our communication with others. The advantage is that people will better understand that occupation is the important focus of our profession.

Advantages and Disadvantages of Standardized and Nonstandardized Performance Analyses

Although standardized performance analyses such as the AMPS, School AMPS, and ESI have several advantages, they also have a number of disadvantages. One major advantage is that the use of standardized performance analyses allows the trained occupational therapist to generate an objective linearized measure (Bond & Fox, 2007) of the person's quality of occupational performance that can be used to document outcomes and implement evidence-based practice. The second advantage is that evaluation practices become more consistent, which promotes the ability to compare results across occupational therapists, clients, and settings (e.g., hospital vs. community). Another important advantage is that the person's linear performance measure can be compared to established criterion measures and normative values that enable the interpretation of the person's results from a criterion-referenced and a norm-referenced perspective. The final advantage is that formal training in standardized performance analysis methods facilitates the occupational therapist's ability to perform nonstandardized performance analyses and avoid common misperceptions that performance skills can be likened to body functions.

An important disadvantage of existing standardized performance analyses is that formal training and rater calibration often is required. Another disadvantage is that standardized assessments sometimes lack the flexibility needed to observe virtually any daily life task performance. For example, the AMPS is a test of ADL, and the School AMPS is a test of schoolwork task performance (e.g., cutting, writing, drawing, computing). Neither can be used to assess the quality of task performance in the areas of work or play.

Obviously, the major advantage of nonstandardized performance analyses is their flexibility. That is, the occupational therapist can implement an informal evaluation of performance skills based on the observation of performance of any daily life task. The only requirements are that the occupational therapist and the person observed must have a clear idea of what the person plans to do, or, if directed by another, what the person has been directed to do. For example, if the occupational therapist plans to observe a child in a classroom setting, he or she must know what the teacher has asked the students to do and what tools and materials they are expected to use. Then, after observing the person's performance, the occupational therapist must systematically rate each universal or task-specific motor skill, process skill, and (when relevant) social interaction skill observed. For example, the occupational therapist can subjectively judge whether the observed actions were skilled, and if not, if the actions (i.e., performance skills) were mildly, moderately, or markedly ineffective. The occupational therapist can also note the frequency or duration of any observed occupational performance errors (Fisher, 2009).

Differentiating Performance Analyses from Task, Activity, and Occupational Analyses

Performance analysis should not be confused with **task analysis** or **activity analysis**, which are intended for purposes of identifying (1) the underlying impairments of body functions as well as other person-related, environmental, task-related, and/or societal and cultural factors that underlie or cause the person's observed problems with occupational performance or (2) the inherent therapeutic value of a task for remediating underlying impairments, respectively (Hagedorn, 1995; Llorens, 1993; Mosey, 1986; Piersol, 2014; Watson, 1997) (Table 26-2). An example of a standardized *task analysis* is the Neurobehavioral (NB) scale of the ADL-focused Occupation-based Neurobehavioral Evaluation (A-ONE; formerly, Árnadóttir OT-ADL Neurobehavioral Evaluation) (Árnadóttir, 1990, 2016; Árnadóttir, Fisher, & Löfgren, 2009). The NB scale of the A-ONE was designed to be used to evaluate the underlying neurobehavioral impairments that cause diminished ADL task performance based on direct observation within the natural context of those ADL task performances. More specifically, scoring of the A-ONE requires that the trained occupational therapist use the operational definitions of the NB items, combined with his or her professional reasoning skills and knowledge of neurology and neuropsychology, to formulate hypotheses related to interpreting the observed errors of ADL task performance. The goal is to identify what underlying neurobehavioral impairments are speculated to be the cause of the person's diminished occupational performance (Árnadóttir, 2016; Árnadóttir et al., 2009; Árnadóttir, Löfgren, & Fisher, 2010).

Standardized task analyses such as the NB scale of the A-ONE; Kitchen Task Assessment (KTA) (Baum & Edwards, 1993); Children's Kitchen Task Assessment (CKTA) (Rocke, Hays, Edwards, & Berg, 2008); Executive Function Performance Test (EFPT) (Baum et al., 2008; Baum, Morrison, Hahn, & Edwards, 2007); the Perceive, Recall, Plan, and Perform (PRPP) System of Task Analysis (Aubin, Chapparo, Gélinas, Stip, & Rainville, 2009; Nott, Chapparo, & Heard, 2009); and the visual motor, fine motor, and gross motor scales of the Miller Function and Participation Scales (M-FUN) (Miller, 2006) were all designed to fulfill an important need within OT for more ecologically relevant assessments of underlying body functions (e.g., cognition, including executive functions and information processing; gross and fine motor coordination; motor planning; visual motor skills) based on professional reasoning about the causes of observed occupational performance errors. They fulfill, however, an important need that is very different from the one that is filled by standardized or nonstandardized performance analyses. Performance analyses are used at the stages of the OT intervention process where the occupational therapist (1) observes the person perform prioritized daily life tasks and (2) identifies what task actions (performance skills) the person performed effectively or ineffectively. In contrast, task analyses are used to help the occupational therapist clarify the cause of the ineffective actions (Figure 26-5).

| TABLE 26-2 | Comparison among Different Types of Occupational Analyses: Performance Analyses, Task Analyses, and Activity Analyses |

Occupational Analyses		
Performance Analysis—Analysis of What We Observe	**Task Analysis ("Explanatory Analysis")—Analysis of Why We Observed What We Have Observed**	**Activity Analysis ("Solution Analysis")—Analysis of How Could We Minimize the Person's Problem**
• *Occupation-focused*: Focus is on quality of occupational performance skills	• *Not occupation-focused*: Focus is on how client factors, body functions, task demands, and/or the environment impact occupational performance	• *Not occupation-focused*: Focus is on how to make changes to client factors, body functions, task demands, and/or the environment to design therapeutic occupation
• *Occupation-based*: The occupational therapist must always observe the person performing a task	• *Occupation-based*: The occupational therapist must always observe the person performing a task	• *Not occupation-based*: The occupational therapist does *not* observe the person performing a task; sometimes done as an decontextualized "academic exercise"
• The occupational therapist asks, "During the observation, what do *I know*, what did I actually see?"	• The occupational therapist asks, "Now that I have observed, what do *I hypothesize* might be the reasons I saw what I did?"	• The occupational therapist asks, "What do *I think* might be some good possibilities for intervention?"

Adapted from Fisher, A. G. (2009). *Occupational Therapy Intervention Process Model: A model for planning and implementing top–down, client-centered, and occupation-based interventions.* Fort Collins, CO: Three Star Press. Reprinted with permission.

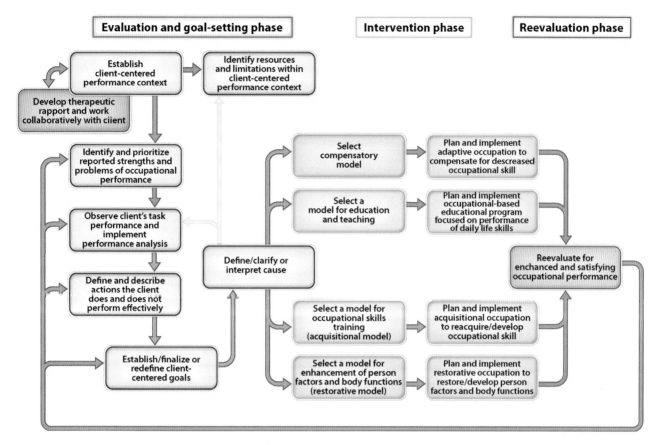

FIGURE 26-5 Schematic representation of the occupational therapy intervention process. (Adapted from Fisher, A. G. [2009]. *Occupational Therapy Intervention Process Model: A model for planning and implementing top–down, client-centered, and occupation-based interventions*. Fort Collins, CO: Three Star Press. Reprinted with permission.)

Performance analyses also should not be confused with the term **occupational analysis** as described in Chapter 25. An occupational analysis includes steps in the OT intervention process that precede as well as follow the actual performance analysis. Thus, performance analysis can be viewed as one part of the more global occupational analysis.

Implementing Performance Analyses: Evaluations of Occupational Performance Skill

With this background information related to performance skills and performance analysis, we will turn to discussing in more detail how an occupational therapist implements

a performance analysis. Our focus, and the case example, will be on implementing nonstandardized performance analyses.

When an occupational therapist implements a performance analysis, the evaluation always occurs within the context of observing the person as he or she is engaged in the performance of a prioritized task. That is, each task performance observed should be one that the client has identified as a concern and prioritized as a potential target for intervention. Which tasks to observe are typically determined based on a thorough OT interview where the occupational therapist comes to understand the client from the client's perspective, what resources and limitations exist within the context of the client's task performances, and what task performances the client views as occupational strengths or problems of occupational performance (see Figure 26-5).

Once the client and the occupational therapist have collaboratively determined which task performances to prioritize, the occupational therapist introduces the idea of observing the person perform prioritized tasks and initiates one or more performance analyses. Each performance analysis progresses over four steps:

- **Step 1:** Observe the person perform a chosen and prioritized daily life task in his or her usual manner and take observational notes of observed occupational performance errors.
- **Step 2:** Rate the person's observed level of occupational performance skill. Either the universal performance motor, process, and social interaction skills shown in Table 26-1 or more task-specific motor, process, and social interaction skills can be evaluated. Each performance skill is rated in terms of ease (physical effort and/or clumsiness), efficiency (time and space organization), safety (risk of harm to person or damage to task objects), independence, or, in the case of social interaction skills, social appropriateness. The occupational therapist can use standardized scoring criteria outlined in the respective test manual or he or she can use a nonstandardized qualitative scale (e.g., no problem, mild problem, moderate problem, or severe problem) to rate the observed quality of each performance skill (Fisher, 2009).
- **Step 3:** Make a list of all of the ineffective performance skills observed and select up to 10 motor and process skills and/or 10 social interaction skills that best capture the person's diminished quality of occupational performance. In a similar manner, the motor, process, and/or social interaction skills that best capture the person's strengths of occupational performance also should be identified.
- **Step 4:** Create clusters of interrelated performance skills and write summary statements that can be used to document the person's quality of occupational performance.

In Figure 26-5, step 1 is shown as *Observe client's task performance and implement performance analysis.* Steps 2 through 4 are all part of the phase in the OT process where the occupational therapist is to *define and describe actions the client does and does not perform effectively.*

Once the occupational therapist has completed the performance analysis and determined which performance skills most reflect and best describe the person's quality of occupational performance, the occupational therapist has progressed to the phase in the OT intervention process where he or she and the client work collaboratively to establish and document client-centered goals (see Figure 26-5). The summary statements developed in step 4 of the performance analysis represent the person's baseline level of occupational performance. They provide the foundation for collaboratively developing observable and measurable client-centered and occupation-focused goals.

Finally, the occupational therapist considers the reasons or "causes" for the person's diminished quality of occupational performance (see Figure 26-5). The various factors that may be contributing to and influencing the quality of the person's occupational performance are the internal and external factors that comprise the context of the observed occupational performance: person factors and body functions, task demands, environmental demands, and/or more overarching societal or cultural influences (see Figure 26-3). This phase most often involves the implementation of standardized or nonstandardized task analyses. The process of implementing a performance analysis, preceded by a thorough OT interview and followed by establishing client-centered goals, is illustrated in Case Study 26-2.

CASE STUDY 26-2   IMPLEMENTING NONSTANDARDIZED PERFORMANCE ANALYSES

Background: Referral and Occupational Therapy Interview

Maurice is 78 years of age and lives in his own home. Until recently, Maurice was considered a healthy aging adult, but over the past 6 months, he has fallen on several occasions and was hospitalized for observation and treatment of severe lacerations on the back of his head. These falls and hospitalizations have taken their toll; Maurice has become increasingly frail. His doctor has spoken to Maurice and his family, and he has recommended that they consider some form of alternative housing for Maurice, somewhere where he would have 24-hour supervision.

Maurice, however, is determined to continue living at home. He already pays for a woman, Joyce, to come in each day and help him with his daily chores. Because his family wants to support Maurice's wishes, they have requested an OT evaluation to ensure Maurice's safety, particularly during the time that Joyce is not with him. When they contacted Karla, the occupational therapist, they mentioned not only Maurice's recent falls but also that he often seems to be "a bit confused." They feel that his confusion, combined with moderate hearing loss, has led to increasing challenges when they are trying to communicate with him. They expressed concern that Maurice and Joyce may also be having similar problems when discussing his desires and needs.

With this background information gathered during the referral process, Karla contacted Maurice and made arrangements for a visit. Karla began her OT interview by introducing herself and telling Maurice that she was an

CASE STUDY 26-2   IMPLEMENTING NONSTANDARDIZED PERFORMANCE ANALYSES *(continued)*

occupational therapist and that her role was to help him do the things that he wanted to do, such as dressing, doing activities around the house, going out in the community, and engaging in leisure activities. She then transitioned to asking Maurice to tell her about what he currently does during a typical day, what he would like to do, and what are his concerns and priorities.

During this OT interview, Karla learned that Maurice is satisfied overall with his current living situation. He has a supportive family with whom he has daily telephone contact and biweekly visits. He explained that Joyce comes in 8 hours a day, 6 days a week to prepare his lunch and dinner, clean, take him on errands, and spend time with him. Maurice has daily routines that include getting dressed, preparing his breakfast, and reading the newspaper, all of which he performs before Joyce comes for the day. He also showers twice each week before Joyce arrives. During the day, he watches television, uses his computer, talks to family on the phone, and reads. He likes to go to town two or three times a week to go to the bank, post office, and grocery store. Joyce drives him to town and accompanies him, but Maurice takes care of his own errands. He has had his bathroom adapted to include grab bars, a raised toilet seat, and a shower bench, enabling him to remain independent in personal activities of daily living (PADL).

As the interview progressed, Karla guided the discussion to learn about tasks that Maurice currently does that are challenging for him and to hear about other tasks that Maurice does not currently do but might want to do. Maurice stated that he is satisfied with most of the tasks he is doing and does not have others that he wants to do at this time. He said that he is having difficulty putting on his shoes and socks. He also said that preparing his breakfast (orange juice and cold cereal) has gradually become more difficult and that he wants to be able to keep doing that for himself each morning. When she focused in on other aspects of dressing and showering, tasks Karla reasoned also were likely to be challenging, Maurice denied any problems.

Desiring to maintain a client-centered focus and to ensure that Maurice is safe in doing the two tasks that he identified as more challenging and important to him, Karla and Maurice decided that she would observe him perform these. She told Maurice that after she observed his performance, she would be able to make suggestions to help him do these tasks more easily. As Maurice had also acknowledged that he does not always "follow conversations" when he is interacting with others, he also agreed that Karla could observe him when he and Joyce would be deciding on meals for the week and writing a shopping list for the grocery store.

Implementing a Performance Analysis: Step 1— Observe the Person Perform Chosen Daily Life Tasks

When Karla observed Maurice perform the two activities of daily living (ADL) tasks and the social interaction with Joyce, she ensured that he performed each task in his usual manner and she remained an unobtrusive observer. During each of his task performances, she took notes of any occupational performance errors that reflected diminished quality of Maurice's occupational performance.

Implementing a Performance Analysis: Step 2— Rating the Person's Quality of Performance

After Karla had observed Maurice perform the two ADL tasks and engage in social interaction with Joyce, she proceeded to rate Maurice's quality of performance in relation to each of the motor, process, and social interaction skills shown in Table 26-1. When she did her rating, she used a four-category qualitative scale: no problem, mild problem, moderate problem, and marked problem.

Implementing a Performance Analysis: Step 3— Defining the Actions of Performance That Were Effective/Ineffective

After scoring both of the observed ADL tasks and the social exchange, Karla transitioned to making a list of all of the motor and process skills and all of the social interaction skills that she had observed to be ineffective. When she did this, she first listed each performance skill and then she made note of what behavior she had observed that led to her rating. Finally, Karla put a check mark (✓) by those performance skills that she reasoned best captured Maurice's diminished quality of occupational performance (Tables 26-3 and 26-4 show Karla's lists for *Putting on socks and shoes* and *Planning the weekly meals and making a shopping list*). As she also wanted to capture Maurice's relative strengths, she made similar lists of the motor, process, and social interaction skills that most supported his occupational performance.

Implementing a Performance Analysis: Step 4— Identifying Clusters of Interrelated Skills and Writing Summary Statements for Use in Documentation

Karla's next step was to create clusters of performance skills that she judged to be interrelated. Once she created each cluster, she wrote a summary statement that she used to document Maurice's baseline level of occupational performance. For example, she created three clusters of motor and process skills related to the task of *Putting on shoes and socks* and

(continues)

CASE STUDY 26-2 IMPLEMENTING NONSTANDARDIZED PERFORMANCE ANALYSES (continued)

TABLE 26-3 Maurice's Motor and Process Skills That Most Reflected His Diminished Quality of Activity of Daily Living Task Performance— Putting on His Socks and Shoes

ADL Motor Skills	Behavior Observed	Rating
✓ Stabilizes	• Risk of a fall—standing and bending down to get shoes	• Marked
✓ Reaches	• Increased effort and risk for fall—reaching down to get shoes	• Marked
	• Increased effort and audible shortness of breath—reaching forward to pull leg up over opposite knee	• Moderate
✓ Bends	• Increased effort and risk of a fall—bending down to get shoes	• Marked
	• Increased effort and audible shortness of breath—bending forward to pull leg up over opposite knee	• Moderate
Grips	• Grip slips from socks when pulling them up	• Mild
Manipulates	• Fumbles shoelaces	• Mild
✓ Moves	• Increased effort and audible shortness of breath—pulling leg up over opposite knee and pulling up socks	• Moderate
✓ Lifts	• Increased effort and risk of a fall—lifting shoes from the floor	• Marked
Walks	• Walks using a walker	• Mild
✓ Endures	• Audible shortness of breath	• Moderate
ADL Process Skills	**Behavior Observed**	**Rating**
Initiates	• Occasional short pauses before initiating task steps	• Mild
Continues	• Starts to pull up sock, pauses, returns to pulling up sock	• Mild
✓ Accommodates	• Demonstrates risk of a fall (reaches, bends, lifts); he did not prevent his problems	• Marked
✓ Benefits	• Audible shortness of breath persisted (reaches, bends, moves, endures)	• Moderate

ADL, activity of daily living.

TABLE 26-4 Maurice's Social Interaction Skills That Most Reflected His Ineffective Quality of Social Interaction—Planning Weekly Meals and Making a Shopping List Together with Joyce

Social Interaction Skills	Behavior Observed	Rating
✓ Concludes/Disengages	• J starts to bring discussion to a close, but M continues to talk about what he will eat	• Mild
Speaks fluently	• Speaks in a hesitant manner, with short pauses and stammering, "I think w-we . . . should . . . buy some apples"	• Mild
	• On two occasions, M pauses 3–4 seconds in the middle of a message	• Moderate
✓ Looks	• Frequently looks down and away from J	• Mild
✓ Regulates	• Occasionally fidgets with pencil and notepad used for shopping list	• Mild
✓ Replies	• Replies with markedly irrelevant responses (e.g., when asked what he wants to eat, he replies, "My son called")	• Marked
✓ Transitions	• Transitions to a markedly irrelevant topic (e.g., abruptly changes topic to getting a phone call from his son)	• Marked
✓ Times response	• M interrupts J as she is speaking; occasionally delays before replying to J's questions	• Moderate
✓ Times duration	• Starts messages, but leaves two messages "hanging in the air"	• Moderate
✓ Clarifies	• J asks M to clarify what he meant, "Let's buy some scapple"; he does not clarify; his reply is markedly irrelevant, "I need to make a doctor's appointment"	• Marked
✓ Heeds	• When engaged in a social interaction with an intended purpose of making a shopping list, M begins to discuss his son and a doctor's appointment	• Moderate
✓ Accommodates	• Demonstrated markedly inappropriate Replies, Transitions, and Clarifies skill; he did not prevent his problems	• Marked
✓ Benefits	• Several of M's moderately inappropriate social interaction skill deficits persisted	• Moderate

J, Joyce; M, Maurice.

CASE STUDY 26-2   IMPLEMENTING NONSTANDARDIZED PERFORMANCE ANALYSES *(continued)*

four clusters related to social interaction skills. Those clusters and her summary statements were as follows:

Putting on Socks and Shoes

- *Stabilizes, Reaches, Bends, Lifts:* Maurice demonstrated marked fall risk when standing and bending to reach down and lift his shoes up from the floor.
- *Reaches, Bends, Moves, Endures:* He also demonstrated moderate increase in effort and audible shortness of breath when reaching forward to pull his leg up over his opposite knee and when pulling up his socks.
- *Accommodates, Benefits:* Maurice did not anticipate and prevent problems from occurring, and his problems persisted throughout the task performance.

Planning Weekly Meals and Making a Shopping List Together with Care Provider

- *Looks, Regulates:* He frequently looked down and away from his social partner and occasionally "fidgeted" with task objects (e.g., pencil and note pad).
- *Speaks Fluently, Times Duration:* More importantly, he frequently paused "mid-message." On two occasions, these pauses were 3 to 4 seconds in length, and on two additional occasions, he began but never finished sending his messages.
- *Replies, Transitions, Clarifies, Heeds:* Moreover, on two occasions, his replies were markedly irrelevant to the intended purpose of the social exchange.
- *Accommodates, Benefits:* Finally, Maurice did not modify his social interactions to prevent these problems from occurring, and his problems often reoccurred during the ongoing social exchange.

When Karla actually documented Maurice's baseline level of occupational performance, she wanted to place her summary statements in the context of her overall observation. Therefore, she began with an introductory phrase to clarify what it was that Maurice had done (e.g., put on his socks and shoes) and incorporated into that a global baseline statement that would document his overall quality of ADL task performance. Then, she added her summary statements to document his specific baseline. For example, her final documentation for *Putting on socks and shoes* was as follows:

> While Maurice was independent when putting on his shoes and socks, he demonstrated marked safety risk and moderate increase in physical effort. More specifically, Maurice demonstrated marked fall risk when standing and bending to reach down and lift his shoes up from the floor. He also demonstrated moderate increase in effort and audible shortness of breath when reaching forward to pull his leg up over his opposite knee and when pulling up his socks. Maurice did not anticipate and prevent problems from occurring, and his problems persisted throughout the task performance.

Progressing from Implementing a Performance Analysis to Establishing Client-centered Goals

When Karla documented his baseline level of occupational performance, she also discussed with Maurice her observations and engaged him in a discussion of how he felt about his performance and what might be his desired outcomes of OT services. For example, she pointed out to Maurice that even though he was holding onto his rollator, he almost fell when he bent down and picked up his shoes from the floor. Maurice acknowledged that falling has been a major issue and is one of the reasons his doctor does not want him living at home anymore. Maurice indicated that he wanted to be able to perform tasks without fall risk.

Karla, therefore, discussed with him his baseline statement related to putting on socks and shoes—*marked fall risk when standing and bending to reach down and lift his shoes up from the floor*—and engaged Maurice in determining what was his desired goal. As Maurice specified that he did not want to have a fall risk, Karla and Maurice decided that his goal would be *no fall risk when putting on socks and shoes*. Karla did not refer to Maurice's standing, bending down, or lifting his shoes as she wanted to leave open the option for introducing compensatory strategies that would enable Maurice to avoid fall risk. Karla engaged Maurice in similar collaborative discussions related to his obvious increased physical effort and shortness of breath when putting on his socks and shoes as well as the challenges he faced with preparing his breakfast and engaging in social interaction with his care provider.

Questions to Prompt Professional Reasoning

1. Given that Maurice likely has problems with balance, would you have been inclined to use a different assessment approach than was described in this chapter?
2. How does conducting a performance analysis contribute to the role of OT in an interprofessional team?
3. How might intervention have changed had Karla focused on evaluating body functions rather than analyzing performance skills observed during desired task performances?
4. What was the benefit of Karla's separately describing the quality of each of Maurice's task performances, based on her analysis of his observed level of occupational performance skill, when she wrote her documentation?
5. How does conducting a performance analysis support a collaborative process between the occupational therapist and client?
6. Three visits from OT are not many. Karla decided to use one visit for evaluation, leaving her with only two more visits. Discuss the benefit of spending time doing a performance analysis for Maurice.

Visit thePoint to watch a video that demonstrates performance skills.

REFERENCES

American Occupational Therapy Association. (2002). Occupational therapy practice framework: Domain and process. *American Journal of Occupational Therapy, 56,* 609–639.

American Occupational Therapy Association. (2008). Occupational therapy practice framework: Domain and process 2nd edition. *American Journal of Occupational Therapy, 62,* 625–683.

American Occupational Therapy Association. (2014). Occupational therapy practice framework: Domain and process (3rd edition). *American Journal of Occupational Therapy, 68*(Suppl. 1), S1–S48. doi:10.5014/ajot.2014.682006

Árnadóttir, G. (1990). *The brain and behavior: Assessing cortical dysfunction through activities of daily living.* St. Louis, MO: Mosby.

Árnadóttir, G. (2016). Impact of neurobehavioral deficits on activities of daily living. In G. Gillen (Ed.), *Stroke rehabilitation: A function-based approach* (4th ed., pp. 573–609). St. Louis, MO: Mosby.

Árnadóttir, G., Fisher, A. G., & Löfgren, B. (2009). Dimensionality of nonmotor neurobehavioral impairments when observed in the natural contexts of ADL task performance. *Neurorehabilitation & Neural Repair, 23,* 579–586.

Árnadóttir, G., Löfgren, B., & Fisher, A. G. (2010). Difference in impact of neurobehavioural dysfunction on activities of daily living performance between right and left hemispheric stroke. *Journal of Rehabilitation Medicine, 42,* 903–907.

Aubin, G., Chapparo, C., Gélinas, I., Stip, E., & Rainville, C. (2009). Use of the Perceive, Recall, Plan, and Perform System of Task Analysis for persons with schizophrenia: A preliminary study. *Australian Occupational Therapy Journal, 56,* 189–199.

Bartels, M. N., Duffy, C. A., & Beland, H. E. (2016). Pathophysiology, medical management, and acute rehabilitation of stroke survivors. In G. Gillen (Ed.), *Stroke rehabilitation: A function-based approach* (4th ed., pp. 2–45). St. Louis, MO: Mosby.

Barton, G. E. (1917). Movies and the microscope. *The Trained Nurse and Hospital Review, 58,* 193–197.

Baum, C. M., Connor, L. T., Morrison, T., Hahn, M., Dromerick, A. W., & Edwards, D. F. (2008). Reliability, validity, and clinical utility of the Executive Function Performance Test: A measure of executive function in a sample of people with stroke. *American Journal of Occupational Therapy, 62,* 446–455.

Baum, C. M., & Edwards, D. F. (1993). Cognitive performance in senile dementia of the Alzheimer's type: The Kitchen Task Assessment. *American Journal of Occupational Therapy, 47,* 431–436.

Baum, C. M., Morrison, T., Hahn, M., & Edwards, D. F. (2007). *Test protocol booklet: Executive Function Performance Test.* St. Louis, MO: Washington University School of Medicine.

Bond, T. G., & Fox, C. M. (2007). *Applying the Rasch model: Fundamental measurement in the human sciences* (2nd ed.). Mahwah, NJ: Lawrence Erlbaum Associates.

Fisher, A. G. (1989). *Assessment of Motor and Process Skills.* Fort Collins, CO: Three Star Press.

Fisher, A. G. (1998). Uniting practice and theory in an occupational framework: 1998 Eleanor Clarke Slagle lecture. *American Journal of Occupational Therapy, 52,* 509–521.

Fisher, A. G. (2006). Overview of performance skills and client factors. In H. M. Pendleton & W. Schultz-Krohn (Eds.), *Pedretti's occupational therapy: Practice skills for physical dysfunction* (6th ed., pp. 372–402). St. Louis, MO: Mosby.

Fisher, A. G. (2009). *Occupational Therapy Intervention Process Model: A model for planning and implementing top–down, client-centered,* *and occupation-based interventions.* Fort Collins, CO: Three Star Press.

Fisher, A. G., Bryze, K., Hume, V., & Griswold, L. A. (2007). *School AMPS: School Version of the Assessment of Motor and Process Skills* (2nd ed.). Fort Collins, CO: Three Star Press.

Fisher, A. G., & Griswold, L. A. (2015). *Evaluation of social interaction* (3rd ed., Rev. ed.). Fort Collins, CO: Three Star Press.

Fisher, A. G., & Jones, K. B. (2012). *Assessment of Motor and Process Skills: Development, standardization, and administration manual* (7th ed., Rev. ed.). Fort Collins, CO: Three Star Press.

Fisher, A. G., & Jones, K. B. (2014). *Assessment of Motor and Process Skills: User manual* (8th ed.). Fort Collins, CO: Three Star Press.

Fisher, A. G., & Kielhofner, G. (1995). Skill in occupational performance. In G. Kielhofner (Ed.), *A model of human occupation: Theory and application* (2nd ed., pp. 113–137). Baltimore, MD: Williams & Wilkins.

Gilbreth, F. B., & Gilbreth, L. M. (1919). *Applied motion study: A collection of papers on the efficient method to industrial preparedness.* New York, NY: MacMillan.

Hagedorn, R. (1995). *Occupational therapy: Perspectives and processes.* Edinburgh, United Kingdom: Churchill Livingstone.

Hagedorn, R. (2000). *Tools for practice in occupational therapy: A structured approach to core skills and processes.* Edinburgh, United Kingdom: Churchill Livingstone.

Kielhofner, G. (1995). *A model of human occupation: Theory and application* (2nd ed.). Baltimore, MD: Williams & Wilkins.

Kielhofner, G. (2008). *Model of human occupation: Theory and application* (4th ed.). Baltimore, MD: Lippincott Williams & Wilkins.

Llorens, L. A. (1993). Activity analysis: Agreement between participants and observers on perceived factors in occupation components. *Occupational Therapy Journal of Research, 13,* 198–211.

Miller, L. J. (2006). *Miller Function and Participation Scales.* San Antonio, TX: PsychCorp.

Mosey, A. C. (1986). *Psychosocial components of occupational therapy.* New York, NY: Raven Press.

Nott, M. T., Chapparo, C., & Heard, R. (2009). Reliability of the Perceive, Recall, Plan and Perform System of Task Analysis: A criterion-referenced assessment. *Australian Occupational Therapy Journal, 56,* 307–314.

Piersol, C. V. (2014). Occupation as therapy: Selection, gradation, analysis, and adaptation. In M. V. Radomski & C. A. Trombly Latham (Eds.), *Occupational therapy for physical dysfunction* (7th ed., pp. 360–393). Philadelphia, PA: Lippincott Williams & Wilkins.

Polatajko, H. J., Mandich, A., & Martini, R. (2000). Dynamic performance analysis: A framework for understanding occupational performance. *American Journal of Occupational Therapy, 54,* 65–72.

Rexroth, P., Fisher, A. G., Merritt, B. K., & Gliner, J. (2005). Ability differences in persons with unilateral hemispheric stroke. *Canadian Journal of Occupational Therapy, 72,* 212–221.

Rocke, K., Hays, P., Edwards, D., & Berg, C. (2008). Development of a performance assessment of executive function: The Children's Kitchen Task Assessment. *American Journal of Occupational Therapy, 62,* 528–537.

Watson, D. E. (1997). *Task analysis: An occupational performance approach.* Bethesda, MD: American Occupational Therapy Association.

World Health Organization. (2001). *International classification of functioning, disability and health (ICF).* Geneva, Switzerland: Author.

*the*Point® *For additional resources on the subjects discussed in this chapter, visit* **http://thePoint.lww.com /Willard-Spackman13e.**

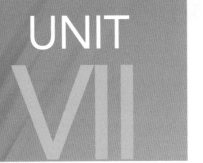

UNIT VII

Occupational Therapy Process

"Occupational therapy practitioners will ask
'what matters to you'
not 'what's the matter with you?"

—Ginny Stoffel
Past president of the American Occupational
Therapy Association (AOTA)

Overview of the Occupational Therapy Process and Outcomes

Denise Chisholm, Barbara A. Boyt Schell

LEARNING OBJECTIVES

After reading this chapter, you will be able to:

1. Explain the components of the occupational therapy process.
2. Examine how evidence from research and practice is integrated in the occupational therapy process.
3. Analyze the professional reasoning typically associated with components of the occupational therapy process.
4. Apply the occupational therapy process to client cases.

Introduction

This chapter provides an overview of the occupational therapy (OT) process in preparation for understanding the more detailed information regarding assessing client needs as well as the provision of intervention services presented in the following chapters in this unit. First, we describe the general process of service delivery and its relationship with OT. In the second section of this chapter, an illustration or "map" of the OT process is provided to assist you in visualizing the essential components and their dynamic and interactive relationships. Each component of the OT process—evaluation, intervention, reevaluation, and continuation/discontinuation of services based on client outcomes—will be expanded on in subsequent sections. Our hope is that the OT process map will direct the services you provide as an OT practitioner. Evidence and professional reasoning have been embedded in the process map as essential markers to assure accuracy in planning the most effective OT services. Case studies have been woven throughout this chapter to give you the opportunity to apply the OT process map.

Occupational Therapy as a Process

Occupation is the central focus of OT services. The general process used in the delivery of OT services parallels the process used by other health-related professionals (e.g., nurses, physical therapists, physicians, dietitians). It provides a structure for practitioners to employ therapeutic professional reasoning based on evidence in order to address the client's health-related problems. The process is neither diagnosis-specific (i.e., disease, disorder, condition, syndrome) nor age-specific, and it can be applied in any practice setting—hospital, outpatient clinic, school, workplace, or client's home. Occupational therapy practitioners customize the process with the end goal of "achieving health, well-being and participation in life through engagement in occupations" (American Occupational Therapy Association [AOTA], 2014, p. S2). Occupational therapy services incorporate the therapeutic use of occupation as a primary means for promoting the client's engagement in and performance of his or her preferred daily activities. The use of occupation as both an end goal and a means to achieve the goal is OT's unique application of the service delivery process. Occupational therapy practitioners must deliver services that are occupation centered. In the words of Fisher (2009), if we are to practice as OT practitioners, we must use *occupation* as our primary form of therapy; that is, we must implement OT (p. 10).

The Occupational Therapy Process Map

Embarking on a trip without a map increases the risk of getting lost, which in turn results in confusion and frustration. This is analogous to what can occur when an OT practitioner provides therapy services without the guidance of a process "map." Just as when someone takes a trip, OT practitioners need a clear diagram illustrating the road for traveling from the starting point—that is, evaluation—to the final destination or outcome of the therapy journey. We need to become competent in reading the markers that provide us with the evidence that supports taking the best route in both the evaluation and intervention portions of the trip. Our competency in "map reading" is reliant on our professional reasoning, which is used to calculate and recalculate or problem-solve the best route options, assuring sound therapy decisions. With a thorough understanding of the process map, you can effectively educate your clients about their OT services. When clients "know where they are going," they can actively and collaboratively participate in the process to support their health, well-being, and participation in life through engagement in occupation.

There are many different interpretations and illustrations of the OT process (AOTA, 2014; Christiansen & Baum, 1997; Christiansen, Baum, & Bass-Haugen, 2005; Fearing, Law, & Clark, 1997; Fisher, 1998, 2009; Law, Baum, & Dunn, 2005; Reed & Sanderson, 1999; Rogers & Holm, 1989, 2009). Our OT process map (Figure 27-1) is an adaptation of the process outlined in the "occupational therapy practice framework" (AOTA, 2014).

Although the OT process is highly dynamic and cyclical, it does have a definitive starting point and

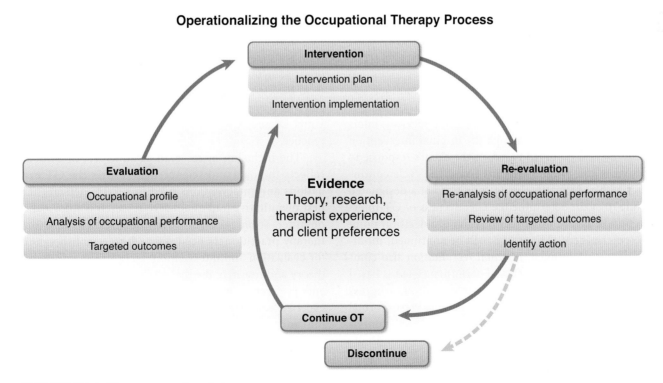

FIGURE 27-1 **The occupational therapy process.**

important milestones along the way. These are evaluation, intervention, reevaluation, and therapy outcomes.

- **Evaluation** is the systematic collection and analysis of data needed to make decisions. Occupational therapy practitioners use the evaluation results and conclusions to plan and implement interventions to assist clients in positively changing their occupational performance. Sometimes, the terms *evaluation* and *assessment* are used interchangeably; however, consistently using these terms based on distinct definitions can increase OT's efficacy (Hinojosa, Kramer, & Crist, 2010). We will delineate the terms as follows: evaluation is the comprehensive process of obtaining and interpreting data necessary to understand the person, system, or situation for intervention (AOTA, 2010, p. S107; AOTA, 2015, p. 2), and assessment refers to specific tools, instruments, or systematic interactions (e.g., observation of performance and context, interview with the client and significant others, record review, and direct assessment of specific aspects of performance) used during the evaluation process (AOTA, 2010, p. S107; AOTA, 2014, p. S14; AOTA, 2015, p. 2).
- **Intervention** is the implementation of skilled actions directed at facilitating the client's engagement in occupation related to health and participation (AOTA, 2010, p. S107; AOTA, 2015, p. 2). In order to determine the effectiveness of OT interventions, another evaluation or reevaluation must be conducted.
- **Reevaluation** can be conducted both *formally* and *informally*. *Formal reevaluation* compares the client's occupational performance data obtained during evaluation with the client's occupational performance after having received a phase of intervention. Based on the formal reevaluation results, the occupational therapist makes one of two decisions—to continue or to discontinue OT services. If the decision is to discontinue services, intervention is ended and the client is discharged from OT. If the decision is to continue services, intervention is resumed, although the original intervention plan may be modified based on the client's response to services and progress toward goals. The cycle continues with reevaluation being conducted at a designated time to again determine the effectiveness of OT interventions. Each formal reevaluation is a decision point to determine if OT services will be continued, modified, or discontinued. *Informal reevaluation* also compares the client's occupational performance but is based on the client's response to the intervention, progress toward goals, and attainment of outcomes versus formal reevaluation results. The subsections for each component (evaluation, intervention, reevaluation, and outcomes) of the process are described in more detail later in this chapter.

The consideration of **outcomes** is inherent in every phase of the process. Outcomes are specifically identified results of OT interventions (AOTA, 2014). In OT therapy, outcomes include improved performance and participation in desired and meaningful occupations as well as increased abilities to adapt to occupational challenges. Additional outcomes include engaging in activities designed to prevent future limitation or to promote well-being, improve quality of life and role competence, and increase self-advocacy. As markers of achievement, outcomes guide the therapy process and help clients and therapists decide if OT is effective, completed, or needs to be modified to either achieve different or additional outcomes or if approaches need to be changed to improve progress.

Evidence provides the background that supports the OT process. The process is influenced and guided by a collection of evidence that includes theory, research, the therapist's experience, and the client's preferences (AOTA, 2014). This facilitates evidence-informed practice, which combines the best current published evidence with practitioner expertise and client preferences (Bannigan & Moores, 2009; Law & Baum, 1998; Sackett, Straus, Richardson, Rosenberg, & Haynes, 2000). Chapter 35 in Unit VIII specifically addresses evidence-based practice.

Occupational therapy, like most health professions, is a multitheory profession with occupational therapists applying one or more theories to examine and explain the occupational performance strengths and needs of each client. Theory reflects the operating assumptions that direct and guide the delivery of skilled services. Theories are a collection of concepts, definitions, and hypotheses that help occupational therapists make predictions about relationships between events (Hinojosa et al., 2010). Theory is one piece of evidence that is important in the selection of assessment tools and interventions. In this chapter, the term *theory* is used synonymously with *frame of reference* and *model of practice*, which are other terms you may see. Units IX and X address broad and specific theories of practice.

The inclusion of research as an aspect of evidence reflects the data and science that verifies the OT evaluations and interventions used in service delivery. The best quantitative and qualitative research is information obtained from peer-reviewed journals. Occupational therapy practitioners need research to establish validity for evaluation and intervention decisions. In addition to theory and research, the therapist's experience and the client's preferences are important sources of evidence. Your experience as an OT practitioner—your knowledge, training, and competencies—supports your implementation of the OT process. The experience of the OT practitioner provides evidence that the right professional is providing the right service in the right way, in the right place, and at the right time, which should then result in the right outcome (Graham, 1996; Gray, 1997; Holm, 2000; Sackett et al., 2000; Silverman, 1998).

The OT process is accomplished through a collaborative relationship between clients and practitioners. Note that the term *client* can be an individual, group, or population (AOTA, 2014). For individuals, the term includes not only the person with the occupational performance problem but also their advocates (e.g., family members, significant others, caregivers, care managers, community members). Clients that are groups are a collective of individuals (e.g., families, workers, students), and populations are a collective of groups or individuals with the same or similar concerns (e.g., veterans, people with mental illness). Client preferences are based on life experiences, values, choices, needs, and priorities and are an integral piece of evidence supporting the OT process. Occupational therapists need to consciously and systematically integrate the client's preferences into all components of the OT process because they can significantly influence the outcomes. The best available evidence, including theory, research, therapist experience, *and* client preferences, must be used to achieve the best outcomes. Of significance is the choice of the word *and* in the previous sentence versus *or*. *All* available aspects of evidence must be used, including the client's preferences, for clients to gain maximum benefit from OT services (Holm, 2000; Law, 1998; Lee & Miller, 2003).

Just as each component of the OT process is supported by evidence, each component also requires professional reasoning. Professional reasoning, sometimes referred to as *clinical reasoning*, includes therapy decisions and problem solving. Chapter 34 discusses the nature of

professional reasoning. In this chapter, in addition to taking a closer look at the details of the OT process, we describe the professional reasoning and evidence focus for each component of the process. Subsequent chapters in this unit will provide further and more in-depth examination of evaluation and intervention and factors that connect with and shape the OT process.

Evaluation

Evaluation is the beginning of the OT process journey (Figure 27-2). The data occupational therapists collect and analyze is information about the client's occupational performance—strengths and problems. The occupational therapist is responsible for evaluating the client; however, the OT assistant can contribute to the evaluation. For example, the OT assistant, under the supervision of the occupational therapist, may administer a standardized assessment, perform an activities of daily living (ADL) evaluation, and/or other elements of the evaluation that do not require the professional judgment or skills of an occupational therapist during the actual administration of the assessment. Occupational therapists are always responsible for the interpretation of assessment results and synthesis of those results into a full evaluation. There are professional guidelines to assist occupational therapists in determining when it is appropriate to delegate to OT assistants (see Chapters 70 and 72 for further discussion of these).

The primary question or therapy decision the occupational therapist has to make during evaluation is "Who is my client and does my client need occupational

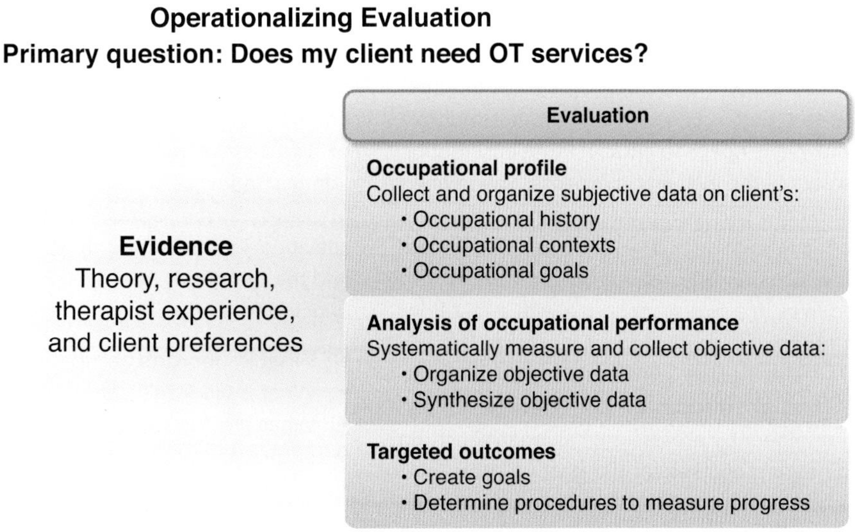

Operationalizing Evaluation
Primary question: Does my client need OT services?

Evidence
Theory, research, therapist experience, and client preferences

Evaluation

Occupational profile
Collect and organize subjective data on client's:
- Occupational history
- Occupational contexts
- Occupational goals

Analysis of occupational performance
Systematically measure and collect objective data:
- Organize objective data
- Synthesize objective data

Targeted outcomes
- Create goals
- Determine procedures to measure progress

FIGURE 27-2 Operationalizing evaluation.

therapy services?" In order to decide if the client needs OT services, we must first obtain information that will assist us in problem solving answers to several secondary questions. These include but are not limited to the following:

- What is the client's occupational history and experience?
- What is the client's pattern of ADL?
- What are the occupations the client needs, wants, and is expected to perform?
- What is/are the client's problem(s)?
- Can OT assist in resolving the client's problem(s)?
- What are the client's priorities?
- What are the client's environmental issues?
- What occupations is the client able to and unable to perform?
- What occupations, skills, patterns, and aspects of context and environment affect the client's performance?
- What measurable and objective goals can address the client's targeted outcomes?

In order to effectively problem solve the answers, we need to complete the occupational profile, perform an analysis of occupational performance, and identify targeted outcomes.

Occupational Profile

A profile describes and summarizes information related to the client's history, resources, and performance. Because the focus of our skilled services is on occupation, we need to create an occupational profile of our clients that describes their occupational performance collecting and organizing data on the client's occupational history, occupational contexts, and occupational goals (AOTA, 2014). It is important to gather the client's perceptions about his or her occupations and related performance strengths and concerns as this information may or may not be consistent with what others might say who observe the client's performance. Remember that the client may include not only the person with an occupational performance concern but also others important in the client's life, such as spouses or partners, family members, caregivers, as well as those who are concerned about the client's performance, such as employers or teachers.

The historical information collected from and about clients' needs to relate to the performance of their life activities, that is, ADL, instrumental ADL, rest and sleep, education and work, play and leisure, and social participation (AOTA, 2014). The contextual information collected needs to describe the physical and social environments where the client performs his or her preferred occupations and illustrate contextual issues (i.e., cultural, personal, temporal, virtual) relevant to the client. The occupational profile also needs to include information related to the client's occupational goals. Occupational therapists need to know why their clients are seeking services; what their occupational performance concerns are; and what daily occupations they need, want, and are expected to perform. And finally, it is imperative that we know the outcomes the client wants and expects to attain through OT. Refer to Case Study 27-1 to see how an occupational profile emerges during the evaluation process.

CASE STUDY 27-1   OCCUPATIONAL PROFILE: WHO IS GEORGE?

Susan, an occupational therapist, receives a new client on her caseload. Based on the information she received with the referral for OT services, she knows his name is George, he is on the acute care unit, is 62 years old, and has multiple sclerosis. Susan knows she needs to find out more information about George as part of the evaluation process. She reviews George's medical record and learns that George is married, has three children, is a semiretired teacher, has had recent falls without injury, uses a cane, has type 2 diabetes and hypertension, and lives in a two-story house with a first floor bedroom and bathroom. Susan introduces herself to George and describes OT (refer to Box 27-1 to see approaches to describing OT). Through discussion with George, Susan finds out he is an engineer by profession, has been teaching college-level engineering courses for the past 15 years, and is currently an adjunct instructor, co-teaching two courses each year. George has four grandchildren (ages 4, 7, 8, and 11 years—all girls) and enjoys attending their school and sport events. He plays the violin and volunteers as an usher for symphony events. George enjoys cooking and playing cards. He has an office and music room on the second floor of his house, and there are 12 steps to enter the front door of his house and 2 steps to enter the back door. Through administration of the Canadian Occupational Performance Measure, Susan obtains data on George's priority daily activities—participating in volunteer activities at his church and the symphony, teaching, cooking, bathing, and ballroom dancing with his wife.

- What is George's occupational history and experience?
- What is George's pattern of activities of daily living?
- What are the occupations George needs, wants, and is expected to perform?
- What are George's priorities?
- What additional information would be beneficial for Susan to add to George's occupational profile?

BOX 27-1   DESCRIBING OCCUPATIONAL THERAPY

Each OT practitioner has his or her own individual therapeutic style when describing the OT process to a client. Additionally, the description is tailored to make it relevant to the client. Although there is not a cookbook for what to say to your client, the following are some helpful hints when describing OT.

- Say occupational therapy, occupational therapist, and occupational therapy assistant versus "OT."

  Hello George. My name is Susan. I am your occupational therapist. My job as your occupational therapist is to help you do the things that you need and want to do throughout your day.

- Use examples of relevant daily occupations based on what you know about your client.

  Examples for George might include safely getting dressed and showered, doing activities in your home such as making meals and yard work, and visiting with family and friends.

  Examples for Nicholas might include tying shoes, using a pencil, throwing a ball, organizing his desk and backpack, and playing board games.

- Engage your client in a dialogue—ask questions and follow up on responses by asking additional questions to obtain more information.

  Have you ever heard of occupational therapy or known someone who had occupational therapy? If the person

says, "Yes," ask them to tell you about the experience to determine if it is similar to or different from the services they will have.

Ask the person about his or her daily routine:
Describe your daily routine to me.
Tell me about what you do at home.
Tell me about what you do at school.
Tell me about what you do at work.
Tell me about the daily activities you need or want to do.
Ask your client if they have questions.

- Don't use medical or health care buzzwords, acronyms, or abbreviations—they are likely meaningless to your client and can be confusing.

- Emphasize that the OT process is collaborative.

  George, we are going to work together to help you get back to your volunteer activities at church and the symphony.

  Nicholas, you and I are a team; together we are going to make your school activities easier and more fun.

- Practice makes perfect. Practice describing OT . . . to your family, friends, colleagues, and to your clients. What did you say? Did you use person-centered communication? Did you address occupation? Did you customize your comments? How did you engage the person in the collaborative process?

As a reminder, the occupational profile is a "summary" of information, so although there is a wide range of data options, the occupational therapist collects what is most relevant to the specific client's occupational performance. Additionally, although we collect much of the data during the first session with the client, we also add to the data over sessions while working with the client.

Occupational Performance Analysis

Whereas the occupational profile addresses the collection and organization of primarily *subjective data* based on the client's perceptions, the analysis of occupational performance addresses the collection, organization, and synthesis of primarily *objective data* regarding the client's occupational performance (AOTA, 2014). Objective data are descriptions that can be easily replicated by others observing the same phenomenon. In order to collect objective data, we have clients perform selected activities important to their

occupations—that is, activities the client wants or needs to perform or that others expect him or her to perform. Ideally, clients perform the priority occupations in their usual manner, with the objects and equipment they usually use, in the setting(s) in which they typically perform the occupation (Rogers & Holm, 2009). The ideal performance situation reflects the client's real-life situation. However, attainment of the real-life or ideal performance situation is dependent on the practice setting and may not always be feasible. Practitioners attempt to replicate real-life performance contexts and environments as closely as possible given the constraints of the practice setting. Practitioners need to understand that in the contrived setting of the OT clinic, the performance demands are different and thus may not fully reflect actual performance in the natural setting. Dr. Joan Rogers, well known for her research in task performance, highlights this issue well when she would challenge practitioners by saying "if you want to understand the importance of context, try going home and making dinner in your neighbor's kitchen . . . see how much longer it takes and whether you are able to do things as well."

CASE STUDY 27-2   EVALUATION: DOES NICHOLAS NEED OCCUPATIONAL THERAPY SERVICES?

Nicholas is 7 years old and was referred for school-based OT services because he has sloppy handwriting, difficulty sitting still in class, and easily becomes frustrated. Gina, the school occupational therapist, meets with Nicholas's first grade teacher, his father, and Nicholas to describe OT services (see Box 27-1) and to obtain information for Nicholas's occupational profile. Gina finds out the following information: Nicholas has recently been diagnosed with attention-deficit/hyperactivity disorder; his father and mother wish to try behavior strategies before considering medications; he has three older teenage siblings and a 5-month-old brother; has difficulty following rules at home and in the classroom; enjoys gym class; takes swimming lessons and is a cub scout; and is slow to complete schoolwork, dress himself, and do his chores. Gina analyzed Nicholas's occupational performance by observing him in the classroom, administering standardized assessment tools to Nicholas, and requesting his parents and teacher complete standardized questionnaires. The data indicated

that Nicholas has problems with fine motor skills (difficulty holding and manipulating everyday objects—pencil, fork, toothbrush), dressing (difficulty fastening and adjusting clothes, unable to tie shoes), and cognitive skills (difficulty following directions and organizing himself and his environment and limited attention span). The data also indicated that Nicholas has strengths in gross motor activities (swimming, running, and kicking and throwing balls), motivation (wants to do well in school and at home and please his parents and teacher), and social skills (gets along well with his siblings and peers).

- What are Nicholas's problems?
- Do Nicholas's problems relate to his occupational performance?
- What outcomes would be appropriate for Gina to target in OT services in the school setting?
- Can OT assist in resolving Nicholas's problems?
- What goals can address Nicholas's targeted outcomes?

In order to collect objective data, therapists need to rely on valid and reliable assessment tools specifically designed to measure factors that support and restrict occupational performance. Chapters 28 and 29 provide in-depth discussions about the importance of effective assessment tools. Performance may be impacted by the person's body structures and functions, by the context of the performance, or by the transaction among them in the form of skills and patterns of performance. Therefore, depending on the client's needs, assessment tools may be used to measure client factors, contexts and environments, activity demands, performance skills, and performance patterns in one or more areas of occupation (AOTA, 2014). As a reminder, although the occupational profile and analysis of occupational performance are presented sequentially, they are dynamic in nature and are typically integrated when evaluating a client. Data, both objective and subjective, should be collected about the client's strengths as well as limitations. See Case Study 27-2 to apply the concepts about evaluation discussed so far.

Targeted Outcomes

Once the data are collected and organized, the final task is to synthesize the data in order to define the performance problems that OT interventions can appropriately target.

As part of the synthesis, the occupational therapist develops hypotheses about the client's occupational performance (Rogers & Holm, 1989, 2009). The hypotheses explain why the problem is occurring based on the subjective and objective data. Well-defined and highly specific problem statements and hypotheses are needed to develop relevant targeted outcomes. Creating short-term (i.e., goals achieved in the near future—in a few days, week, or month) and long-term goals (i.e., ones achieved over a longer period of time—in 2 months to a year) and determining procedures to measure progress toward goal attainment are in the final aspect of evaluation—targeted outcomes (AOTA, 2014).

Goal establishment is done in collaboration with the client and needs to reflect occupational performance problems relevant to the client's desired outcomes. Goals need to be written as objective, measurable statements with an identifiable time frame and predetermined objective methods to measure progress. Whether the problem limiting the client's performance is related to a client factor; performance skill; or pattern, context, or environment, the goal statement needs to be connected with an occupation in addition to addressing the performance problem.

In practice, short-term goals represent small steps along the way toward the long-term goals related to occupational engagement. They may address aspects of body functions, sets of skills or important contextual factors. For instance, a short-term goal may be to work effectively getting food to the mouth through therapeutic strategies such as engaging in graded eye-hand coordination activities as well as using adaptive feeding equipment. Long-term goals reflect performance of the client's meaningful and important daily occupations. Thus, a long-term goal in this example would be independence in all aspects of feeding and eating. The targeted outcomes, including long- and short-term goals, help predict what the client will achieve through OT intervention. See chapter 40 for more information on documentation and goal writing.

Evidence Focus during Evaluation

The evidence focus for evaluation requires the therapist to use evidence-based information that supports the acquisition of information needed for the occupational profile, analysis of occupational performance, and targeted outcomes. For evaluation, we need to consider what theory or operating assumptions are most relevant for the client and clinical setting. We need to identify and integrate the available *research* regarding the validity and reliability of appropriate assessment tools. Examples of relevant evidence for evaluation include studies addressing the use of a theoretical perspective with clients similar to your client and studies reporting the reliability of assessment tools appropriate to use with your client. The *therapist experience* is an essential consideration. The occupational therapist needs to reflect on the following questions: "What is my experience in evaluating this type of client?" and "What is my experience in administering the appropriate assessment tools?" Your responses to these questions are important in determining what your needs are in order to best evaluate your client. And finally, but very important in conducting the evaluation, is the evidence related to the *client's preferences*. Your client is central to the OT process, so the evidence indicating his or her preferred occupations has to be systematically and meticulously collected because it provides the foundation for a client-centered, occupation-focused evaluation. The therapist must reason in a manner that considers

- The client's preferred occupational outcomes,
- The therapist's analysis of the factors affecting performance, and
- The agreed-on target outcomes.

The results of the therapist's professional reasoning in turn affect the transition into the next component of the OT process—intervention.

⚖ ETHICAL DILEMMA

Raul has just started his first job as an occupational therapist. He is working in a fast-paced outpatient clinic that specializes in rehabilitation for individuals with orthopedic conditions. Raul learns during orientation to his job responsibilities that the clinic has evidence-based protocols for evaluations and interventions based on diagnosis. The protocol lists the specific assessment tools that are to be administered and the problems that are to be addressed for clients with that diagnosis. Raul notices that the protocols do not include creating an occupational profile of the client. He also notices that the therapists do not seem to ask their clients questions about their occupational history, occupational contexts, or occupational goals. Based on his observation, Raul feels that the therapists follow the protocols and that all clients with the same or similar diagnosis receive the same evaluation process, have the same targeted outcomes, and engage in the same interventions. Raul learned (and believes) that the focus of OT services is on occupation and that in order to best understand a client's occupational performance that occupational therapists need to create an occupational profile, conduct an individualized evaluation, and provide customized interventions that support the client's goals. Raul asks some of the other therapists why they do not create an occupational profile for clients. The responses were "It's not on the protocol," "It takes too much time," and "Everyone has the same problems."

Questions

1. What is the problem/issue in Raul's situation?
2. Is it an ethical, legal, or practical problem or a combination of these?
3. If an ethical problem/issue – what are the values and/or principles relevant to the ethical concern?
4. What resources could Raul access to help address the problem/issue?
5. What are potential courses of action that Raul can take? (Brainstorm as many as possible)
6. What are the potential consequences of each possible course of action?
7. Which course of action is best for Raul to take?
8. Once Raul implements the best course of action, what are some ways he might evaluate his course of action?
9. How can Raul follow up to determine the outcomes of his course of action and see if further action is necessary?

Intervention

Intervention follows evaluation in the OT process (Figure 27-3). The data collected and analyzed about the client's occupational performance during the evaluation provide navigational information for determining the

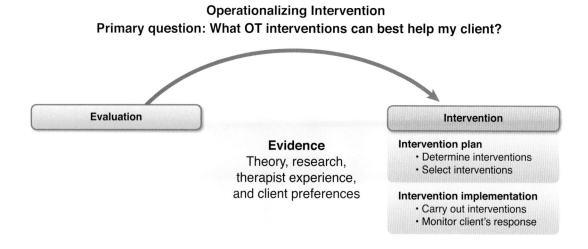

FIGURE 27-3 Operationalizing intervention.

best therapeutic route for the planning and implementation of intervention services. The primary question or therapy decision the OT practitioner has to make during intervention is "What occupational therapy interventions can best help my client?" In order to decide the appropriate intervention course, we must consider information obtained from problem-solving answers to secondary questions relevant to intervention planning and implementation. These include but are not limited to the following:

- What is the range of appropriate interventions based on the evidence?
- Which interventions would the client prefer performing?
- Which interventions are most effective?
- Which interventions can be implemented given the environment parameters of the therapeutic setting?
- How does the client respond to the interventions?
- Are the interventions addressing the client's occupational performance problems?
- Are the interventions promoting the client's engagement in and performance of his or her preferred daily activities?

Occupational therapy practitioners need to repeatedly ask themselves these questions throughout the intervention phase of the OT process. Discussing possible answers with colleagues can assist in increasing the breadth and depth of one's professional reasoning. Think of these questions as road markers and billboard announcements directing you toward your destination of OT interventions that best help your client. Making therapy decisions based on answers to these questions will help focus your interventions on your clients' occupational performance needs.

The **intervention** component of the OT process includes the intervention plan and intervention implementation (AOTA, 2014). In order to develop an intervention plan, we need to consider the client's current occupational performance and envision what the client will achieve through OT interventions. The results of the client's occupational profile and analysis of occupational performance provide subjective and objective information about the client's current occupational performance, and the targeted outcomes predict what the client will achieve through OT interventions. Therefore, although intervention is a separate component in the OT process, it is fully dependent on and explicitly interconnected with evaluation.

Intervention Plan

The intervention plan determines the selection of specific OT activities used to address the client's targeted outcomes (AOTA, 2014). The intervention plan is developed in collaboration with the client. Although the occupational therapist is responsible for the development of the plan, it is the *client's* intervention plan, not the occupational therapist's intervention plan. The first step in developing the plan is to determine the range of interventions appropriate to address the client's occupational performance problems. Occupational therapy interventions can be categorized as occupations and activities or preparatory methods and tasks (AOTA, 2014). Occupations selected as interventions focus on the client engaging in client-directed daily life activities that match and support the client's targeted outcomes. Activities used as interventions are often components of occupations and engage clients in practicing activities related to occupations. Additional activities may be specifically selected to help clients to develop skills that enhance occupational performance. Preparatory methods and tasks are techniques used to prepare the client for or are used concurrently with occupations and activities. Chapters 30 and 31 provide detailed information on OT interventions with individuals and for groups and populations.

Once the range of interventions appropriate to address the client's occupational performance problems is identified, the OT practitioner selects the interventions that have the greatest potential to improve performance and that are the best match with the client's occupational profile. The final decision to include a selected intervention is made in collaboration with the client. Doing so maximizes the client's understanding of the relationship between the selected interventions and his or her preferred daily occupations.

Intervention Implementation

Once the plan is established, the next step is to put the plan into action. Intervention implementation includes the process of carrying out the interventions and monitoring the client's response (AOTA, 2014). The interventions clients engage in need to be appropriate to address their targeted outcomes related to their occupational performance problems. Although monitoring of the client's response to his or her performance of interventions is listed separate from carrying out the interventions, both occur concurrently. The OT practitioner is observing and examining the client's performance while the

client engages in the intervention. The practitioner adjusts aspects of the intervention as needed to better accommodate or challenge the client's occupational performance in order to achieve the targeted outcomes. Monitoring the client's response is part of the informal reevaluation described earlier in the chapter. See Case Study 27-3 for a clinical example of the intervention component of the OT process.

Evidence Focus during Intervention

Theory, research, the therapist's experience, and the client's preferences influence and guide intervention as much as they do evaluation but with a different focus. The focus for evidence to support intervention is on planning and implementation of intervention services. Examples of relevant information would be studies about the relative benefits of one approach versus another, studies about common occupational challenges for clients in a similar place in their life, and medical and educational information about the client's condition. Occupational therapists need to consider how each intervention identified within the range of interventions relates to the theory or operating assumptions most relevant for the client and the clinical setting. In addition, practitioners need to reflect on personal competencies relative to the intervention, along with experiences administering them for this type of client. And last but certainly not least, we must identify the evidence related to the client's preferences. As during evaluation, the

---

CASE STUDY 27-3   INTERVENTION: WHAT OCCUPATIONAL THERAPY INTERVENTIONS CAN BEST HELP ROSA?

Suraj, an OT assistant on an orthopedic rehabilitation unit, is assigned a new client, Rosa, on his caseload by the occupational therapist he works with. Rosa is 72 years old and was just transferred from the acute care unit where she had surgery to replace her hip. She is a widow; lives in an apartment building with elevator access; uses the public bus system; enjoys gardening; plays bingo at the local senior citizen center three nights a week; and does all of her own shopping, cooking, laundry, and cleaning of her apartment. The laundry facilities are in the basement of her apartment building; her bathroom has a tub with a shower—she prefers baths; she has season tickets to the local theater with her sister; she is an avid reader of mystery novels, retired as a bank teller 7 years ago, and loves to travel—she and her sister have plans to go on a

cruise to Alaska in a month. Rosa is currently using a walker; however, she anticipates only needing a cane when she is discharged. Her upper extremity strength is limited, and she fatigues easily. Rosa has some pain in her hip and is fearful of falling. Rosa's priority is to be able to go on the cruise with her sister.

- What is the range of appropriate interventions Suraj might include in Rosa's intervention plan?
- Which interventions do you think Rosa will prefer performing?
- Which interventions would be most effective for Rosa?
- How do the interventions promote Rosa's engagement in and performance of her preferred daily activities?
- How do you think Rosa will respond to the interventions?

occupational therapist must systematically and meticulously integrate the client's preferred daily occupations into the plan and delivery of OT interventions. The combined evidence assists the occupational therapist in problem solving and making therapeutic decisions that result in the selection and implementation of appropriate interventions. These therapeutic decisions reflect informal aspects of the next component of the OT process—reevaluation. The occupational therapist informally reevaluates the client's response to each intervention and effectiveness in assisting the client in achieving his or her goals.

Reevaluation

The third component of the OT process is reevaluation (Figure 27-4). The formal reevaluation is basically a return to the evaluation component of the process. Data about the client's occupational performance is again collected and analyzed. As with evaluation, reevaluation provides navigational information for determining the best therapeutic route for the planning and implementation of intervention services. During reevaluation, the targeted outcomes established during evaluation are assessed using the same measures employed during the original or initial evaluation. Ultimately, the occupational therapist is determining

if the best therapeutic intervention route was taken previously along with identifying the best therapeutic route to take from this point forward.

The primary question or therapy decision the occupational therapist has to make during reevaluation is "How has occupational therapy affected my client's occupational performance?" As with the other components of the OT process, in order to make the therapeutic decision about the continued need for services, we must first obtain information that will assist us in problem solving answers to the following secondary questions. These include but are not limited to the following:

- How has the client's occupational performance changed when comparing assessment findings upon admission to present status?
- What occupations are the client now able to perform?
- What occupations are the client still unable to perform?
- Can OT continue to assist in resolving the client's occupational performance problem(s)?
- How do the client's measurable and objective goals need to be modified to address the client's targeted outcomes?

In order to effectively problem solve the answers, we need to reanalyze the client's occupational performance, review the client's targeted outcomes, and identify the appropriate action to take regarding the continuation of OT services.

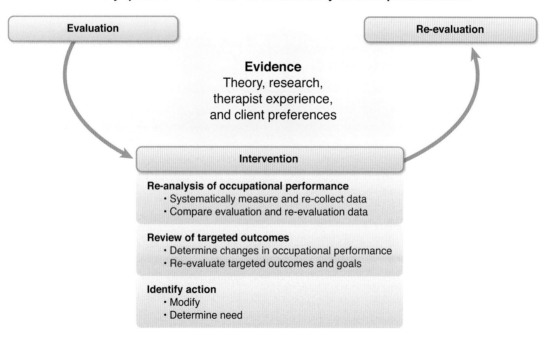

FIGURE 27-4 Operationalizing reevaluation.

Reanalysis of Occupational Performance

Occupational therapists systematically measure and recollect data as the first step in the reanalysis of occupational performance. The next step in the reanalysis is to compare the data obtained during the original evaluation with the current data obtained during reevaluation. As with any comparison, occupational therapists need to ensure that they are comparing equivalent items. Therefore, it is imperative that we use the same measures during reevaluation that were used during the evaluation phase. Doing so is the only dependable way through which the occupational therapist can measure change accurately. If we do not use the same measures, then we are not measuring comparable aspects of occupational performance. And if we are not measuring comparable aspects of occupational performance, we are not able to accurately and with valid evidence determine how OT has affected the client's performance. The comparison of data directly impacts the review of the targeted outcomes. The timing of the reevaluation is based on the occupational therapist's prediction of how long OT interventions will take to achieve the client's targeted outcomes. Additionally, some practice settings and payers have standard requirements for the timing of reevaluations.

Review of Targeted Outcomes

Changes in occupational performance are used to determine whether OT interventions achieved the intended targeted outcomes through goal attainment. Review of the targeted outcomes requires the occupational therapist to determine change in the client's occupational performance relevant to the measureable goals established during evaluation (AOTA, 2014). The degree of goal attainment can be determined by comparing the client's performance measured at evaluation with performance measured at reevaluation. The targeted outcomes and goals are then reviewed and reevaluated in order to identify the appropriate action (AOTA, 2014).

Action Identification

After reevaluation, the therapist considers whether to continue therapy, refer the client to another service or specialty, or discontinue services. Continuation of services is justified if the client is making progress toward the overall goals or if there is reason to believe alternate approaches might work to improve progress. Additionally, new or altered targeted outcomes and goals may emerge as a result of the therapy process. In some cases, it may be apparent that the client could benefit from the services of other professionals, in addition to OT, or that a different specialty intervention within OT is warranted. In those cases, the occupational therapist refers the client to the appropriate resources. Services are terminated when the client has reached targeted outcomes or there is evidence to suggest that further intervention will not substantially improve occupational performance. When therapy services are terminated, the client is often provided with aftercare or follow-up recommendations in order to maintain and build on their therapy gains.

Reevaluation should be ideally scheduled at the end of the anticipated time for the OT intervention to have an effect on the client's occupational performance. Determining the "just right" time for reevaluation is a challenge (Rogers & Holm, 1989, 2009). If reevaluation occurs too early, a course of intervention may be prematurely considered unsuccessful because the client hasn't had enough time to show change in performance. In contrast, if reevaluation occurs too late, the client may have already achieved a targeted outcome and progression in occupational performance is not continuing because the targeted outcomes, measurable goals, and intervention plan have not been appropriately modified to accommodate the positive change.

There are other factors external to the occupational therapist's professional reasoning that determine the time for reevaluation. These factors include third-party payment sources, health organization policies and procedures, and practice guidelines. The evidence focus for reevaluation requires occupational therapists to consider the available research regarding reevaluation for the specific type of client and the assessment tools administered at evaluation. Evidence for reevaluation combines relevant information from studies supporting evaluation decisions with those addressing intervention options. Although we would hope that the external factors impacting decisions regarding reevaluation are based on evidence, occupational therapists need to be aware that this is not always the case. We need to be advocates for the use of evidence-based decisions regarding all aspects of OT services, including reevaluation. See Case Study 27-4 for a clinical example of the reevaluation component of the OT process.

Outcomes: Continue or Discontinue

Outcomes are integrated throughout the OT process (Figure 27-5). As previously stated, "achieving health, well-being and participation in life through engagement in occupations" is the all-encompassing goal of the OT services (AOTA, 2014). Occupational therapy's unique focus on occupation is a primary focus in this inclusive outcome. As previously addressed in evaluation, targeted outcomes are identified that reflect the client's occupational performance problems. Measurable goals with an identifiable time frame and predetermined objective method to

CASE STUDY 27-4   REEVALUATION: HOW HAS OCCUPATIONAL THERAPY AFFECTED TIM'S OCCUPATIONAL PERFORMANCE?

Tim is 24 years old and sustained a traumatic brain injury 2 months ago due to a car accident. One month ago, he was discharged from the hospital and referred for OT at the outpatient center. The data Mark, Tim's occupational therapist, collected during the evaluation indicated that Tim requires moderate physical assistance for putting on lower and upper body clothing due to decreased right arm strength and sequencing problems; Tim needed moderate physical and cognitive assistance to perform money management and meal preparation tasks; he required constant supervision for safety when performing tasks due to impulsivity; and he easily became frustrated, exhibiting angry outbursts. Mark predicted that it would take 4 weeks to achieve the goals addressing the targeted outcomes he and Tim identified. Mark administered the same measures to Tim during the formal reevaluation that he had administered to him during the initial evaluation in order to accurately compare his past and current occupational performance and to determine progress. The following is Tim's current occupational performance: his right arm strength is now adequate for him to put on and off his clothing; however, he is unable to fasten his clothing (buttons/zippers); Tim is able to independently sequence dressing tasks with the use of a written outline; he requires minimal assistance to physically perform money management and meal preparation tasks; however, he continues to require moderate cognitive assistance and supervision for safety in the kitchen environment; and Tim is now able to ask Mark for assistance when he becomes frustrated without display of anger.

- How has Tim's occupational performance changed since evaluation?
- What occupations is Tim now able to perform?
- What occupations is Tim still unable to perform?
- Can OT continue to assist in resolving Tim's occupational performance problems?
- How do Tim's goals need to be modified to address his targeted outcomes?

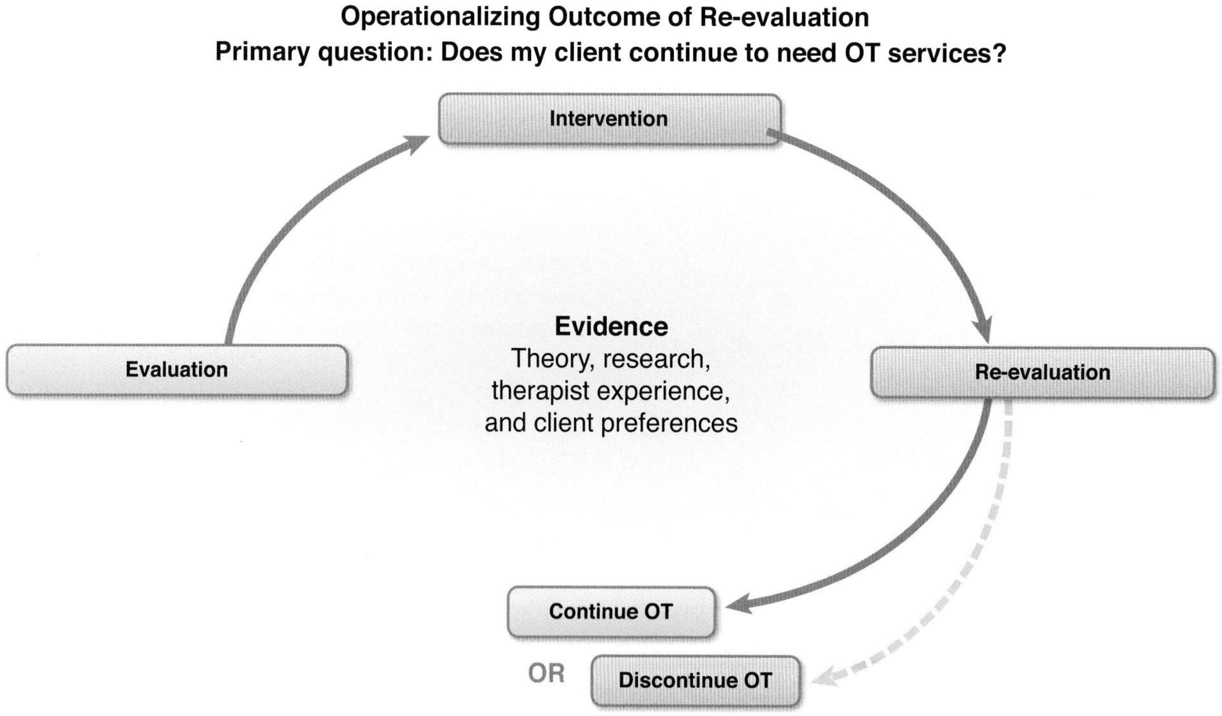

FIGURE 27-5 Operationalizing outcome of reevaluation.

measure progress are essential in determining the attainment of targeted outcomes. The occupational therapist carefully considers the client's targeted outcomes when developing an intervention plan and implementing interventions. The targeted outcomes are revisited formally during reevaluation to address progress.

The primary question the occupational therapist must answer is "Does my client continue to need occupational therapy services?" As with all previous aspects of the process, the occupational therapist must obtain information to problem-solve secondary questions. These include the following:

- Has OT positively impacted the client's ability to perform daily occupations?
- Can OT continue to assist in resolving the client's occupational performance problems?
- Has the client achieved as much benefit as possible from OT services?
- Does the client want to continue receiving OT services?
- Is there sufficient justification for continuing OT services?

The occupational therapist uses information from evaluation, intervention, and reevaluation to determine the answers in order to conclude if OT services should be continued or discontinued.

As with all other aspects of the OT process, evidence provides the foundation for determining whether the client needs continued OT services. The *evidence focus* requires the identification of the available research regarding the duration of services for this type of client based on evaluation and reevaluation results. Additionally, theoretical perspectives, the therapist's experience with the intervention route and attainment of targeted outcomes for similar clients, and the specific client's preferences in addition to his or her evaluation and reevaluation data must be considered when making the therapy decision. If the evidence supports that the client would benefit from continued OT services, then the targeted outcomes, goals, and intervention plan are modified as needed and intervention is resumed. At a predetermined time, another reevaluation is completed to systematically measure and to recollect data using the previously administered assessment tools. Based on the new reevaluation results, a therapeutic decision is made based on the evidence—both prior and new evidence—that either supports the continuation or discontinuation of OT services, and intervention and reevaluation is repeated until ideally, the targeted outcomes are attained and the evidence supports the discontinuation of OT services. The more frequently the process is navigated, the more observant we are of the markers directing us to the evidence that supports our professional reasoning throughout all aspects of the OT process. See Case Studies 27-5 and 27-6 for clinical examples of the outcomes component of the OT process.

CASE STUDY 27-5   OUTCOMES: DOES MARGARET CONTINUE TO NEED OCCUPATIONAL THERAPY SERVICES?

Margaret is 57 years old and sustained a right wrist fracture. She has been receiving OT services at an outpatient center since her cast was removed 3 weeks ago. When Pam, her occupational therapist, completed her initial evaluation, she had limited range of motion in her left wrist; decreased strength; experienced increased pain with movement; and reported difficulty performing her work activities (typing, mouse use, filing), opening doors, washing dishes, unloading/loading the washer/dryer, lifting objects (pots, bags of groceries), driving, and engaging in leisure activities (needlepoint, tennis). Upon reevaluation, Margaret's range of motion is within functional limits; her strength has increased and she is able to lift medium-weight objects—prefers using two hands for heavy objects; Margaret is able to perform her work activities using the strategies that Pam taught her—taking breaks, performing stretching exercises, varying her activities, and so on; she is able to open doors and drive; she has resumed doing her needlepoint for short periods of time and just yesterday started practicing hitting a tennis ball. Margaret reports minimal pain and only when lifting heavy objects. Margaret is able to perform her home activity and exercise program independently and is able to use the strategies that Pam instructed her in to upgrade her activities and exercises. Margaret reports that she feels that her wrist has improved and that she is able to do almost all of her daily activities.

- Has OT positively impacted Margaret's ability to perform her daily occupations?
- Can OT continue to assist in resolving Margaret's occupational performance problems?
- Has Margaret achieved as much benefit as possible from OT services?
- Does Margaret want to continue receiving OT services?
- Is there sufficient justification for continuing Margaret's OT services?

CENTENNIAL NOTES

The Occupational Therapy Process

The OT process has been a focus of the profession from its earliest days. In 1923, Louis Haas, the Director of Therapeutic Occupations at Bloomingdale Hospital in White Plains, New York, discussed the importance of careful attention to the patient's progress and the need to change the therapy plan in response to that patients progress.

"Does the carefully planned and controlled machinery of therapeutic occupation, having been set in motion, run smoothly, with little further attention, the desired result being slowly attained? Experience does not show that the problem begins and ends with the successful introduction of the new case to occupational treatment. What it does show is that the planning of the treatment begins then, continues throughout the patient's stay in the hospital, and perhaps ends in the discharge of the case. This being true, it is readily understood that various changes must be made from time to time, in the treatment applied in the form of occupation therapy to mental and nervous cases. This is not surprising; the same continuous changing of plans of treatment would appear to follow throughout the entire field of therapeutics. Those prescribing or planning various forms of treatment must be ever alert to observe and record the patient's progress, expressed in reactions. These reactions, or indications of progress are carefully read weighing the information contained. This guides and moulds further treatment, which in the light of these observations, can be planned and applied with more precision" (Haas, 1923, p. 277).

Sixty years later, Pelland suggested a model which she stated was a modification of the case-based approach for problem solving (Figure 27-6). Notice how many of the major areas are related to the steps described in this chapter.

Models such at Pelland's Conceptual Model and the Occupational Therapy Practice Framework (AOTA, 2014) (which informed much of this chapter) are based on consensus findings of experts which are validated by broad input from the profession. In the future, models of the OT evaluation and intervention process are likely to be further enhanced by clinical research which speaks to the effectiveness of these models.

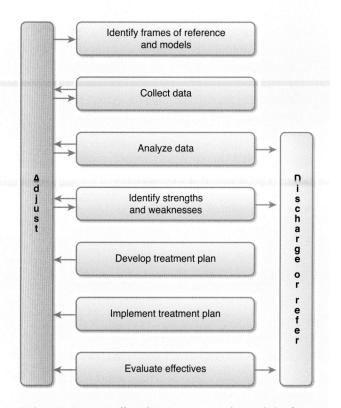

FIGURE 27-6 Pelland's Conceptual Model of Treatment Planning (Pelland, 1987, p. 353). (Reproduced with permission from *American Journal of Occupational Therapy.*)

CASE STUDY 27-6   OUTCOMES: DOES CHENG CONTINUE TO NEED OCCUPATIONAL THERAPY SERVICES?

Cheng is 27 years old with schizophrenia. He currently lives in a group home. Cheng's most recent hospitalization was 6 months ago, and since that time, he has been working with Bonnie, his occupational therapist, one time a week. His OT sessions have primarily focused on his work-related goal to maintain a part-time job. Cheng's OT interventions have addressed appropriate grooming and hygiene for the work setting; interpersonal skills with coworkers and customers; time management; work skills and patterns; initiation, sustaining, and completing work tasks; and compliance with work norms and procedures. Cheng recently began working part-time at a local grocery store stocking shelves in the evening. Bonnie has continued seeing Cheng for OT sessions to assure continuation of his work performance;

however, because he has achieved his goal, he may be appropriate for discharge in the next few weeks. During Cheng's last session, he said that because he is now working and has an income that he would like to pursue living in his own apartment.

- Has OT positively impacted Cheng's ability to perform his daily occupations?
- Can OT continue to assist in resolving Cheng's occupational performance problems?
- Has Cheng achieved as much benefit as possible from OT services?
- Does Cheng want to continue receiving OT services?
- Is there sufficient justification for continuing Cheng's OT services?

Summary

Occupation is fundamental to the OT process and is embedded with both the best available and comprehensive evidence and the individual occupational therapist's professional reasoning. In this chapter, we have provided a map of the primary components of the OT process—evaluation, intervention, reevaluation, and continuation/discontinuation of services—to assist you in successfully navigating the OT services you provide to your clients. As you gain experience in map reading and navigation, we are confident that your use of the evidence and professional reasoning will correspondingly develop, assuring sound therapy decisions and successful outcomes in the therapy journey you take with your clients.

 Visit thePoint to watch a video about the occupational therapy process.

REFERENCES

American Occupational Therapy Association. (2010). Standards of practice for occupational therapy. *American Journal of Occupational Therapy, 64,* S106–S111. doi:10.5014/ajot.2010.64S106-64S111

American Occupational Therapy Association. (2014). Occupational therapy practice framework: Domain and process, 3rd edition. *American Journal of Occupational Therapy, 68*(Suppl. 1), S1–S48. doi:10.5014/ajot.2014.682006

American Occupational Therapy Association. (2015). Standards of practice for occupational therapy. *American Journal of Occupational Therapy, 69*(Suppl. 3), 6913410057p1–6913410057p6. doi:10.5014/ajot.2015.696S06

Bannigan, K., & Moores, A. (2009). A model of professional thinking: integrating reflective practice and evidence based practice. *Canadian Journal of Occupational Therapy, 76,* 342–350.

Christiansen, C. H., & Baum, C. M. (Eds.). (1997). *Occupational therapy: Enabling function and well-being.* Thorofare, NJ: SLACK.

Christiansen, C. H., Baum, C. M., & Bass-Haugen, J. (Eds.). (2005). *Occupational therapy: Performance, participation, and well-being.* Thorofare, NJ: SLACK.

Fearing, G., Law, M., & Clark, J. (1997). An occupational performance process model: Fostering client and therapist alliances. *Canadian Journal of Occupational Therapy, 64,* 7–15.

Fisher, A. G. (1998). The 1998 Eleanor Clarke Slagle lecture. Uniting practice and theory in an occupational framework. *American Journal of Occupational Therapy, 52,* 509–521.

Fisher, A. G. (2009). *Occupational therapy intervention process model: A model for planning and implementing, top-down, client-centered, and occupation-based interventions.* Fort Collins, CO: Three Star Press.

Graham, G. (1996, June). Clinical effective medicine in a rational health service. *Health Director,* 11–12.

Gray, J. A. M. (1997). *Evidence-based healthcare: How to make health policy and management decisions.* New York, NY: Churchill Livingstone.

Haas, L. J. (1923). Observations of patients' reactions, the guide to further treatment. *Archives of Occupational Therapy, 2*(4), 277–286.

Hinojosa, J., Kramer, P., & Crist, P. (Eds.). (2010). Evaluation: Where do we begin? In *Evaluation: Obtaining and interpreting data* (3rd ed., pp. 1–20). Rockville, MD: American Occupational Therapy Association.

Holm, M. B. (2000). The 2000 Eleanor Clarke Slagle lecture. Our mandate for the new millennium: Evidence-based practice. *American Journal of Occupational Therapy, 54,* 575–585.

Law, M. (1998). *Client-centered occupational therapy.* Thorofare, NJ: SLACK.

Law, M., & Baum, C. M. (1998). Evidence-based occupational therapy. *Canadian Journal of Occupational Therapy, 65,* 131–135.

Law, M., Baum, C. M., & Dunn, W. (2005). *Measuring occupational performance: Supporting best practice in occupational therapy* (2nd ed.). Thorofare, NJ: SLACK.

Lee, C. J., & Miller, L. T. (2003). The process of evidence-based clinical decision making in occupational therapy. *American Journal of Occupational Therapy, 56,* 344–349.

Pelland, M. J. (1987). A conceptual model for the instruction and supervision of treatment planning. *American Journal of Occupational Therapy, 2,* 351–359.

Reed, K. L., & Sanderson, S. N. (1999). *Concepts of occupational therapy* (4th ed.). Baltimore, MD: Lippincott Williams & Wilkins.

Rogers, J. C., & Holm, M. B. (1989). The therapist's thinking behind functional assessment. In C. Royeen (Ed.), *Assessment of function: An action guide* (pp. 1–29). Rockville, MD: American Occupational Therapy Association.

Rogers, J. C., & Holm, M. B. (2009). The occupational therapy process. In E. B. Crepeau, E. S. Cohn, & B. A. Schell (Eds.), *Willard & Spackman's occupational therapy* (11th ed., pp. 478–518). Baltimore, MD: Lippincott Williams & Wilkins.

Sackett, D. L., Straus, S. E., Richardson, W. S., Rosenberg, W., & Haynes, R. B. (2000). *Evidence-based medicine: How to practice and teach EBM* (2nd ed.). New York, NY: Churchill Livingstone.

Silverman, W. A. (1998). *Where's the evidence? Debates in modern medicine.* New York, NY: Oxford University Press.

the**Point**® *For additional resources on the subjects discussed in this chapter, visit* http://thePoint.lww.com/Willard-Spackman13e.

CHAPTER 28

Evaluating Clients

Mary P. Shotwell

LEARNING OBJECTIVES

After reading this chapter, you will be able to:

1. Differentiate screening, assessment, and evaluation.
2. Apply the Occupational Therapy Practice Framework (OTPF) to the evaluation process.
3. Identify strategies for interviewing about, observing, and assessing occupational performance.
4. Explain personal and contextual factors that influence the evaluation process.

Introduction

This chapter reviews the process of client evaluation. The first section of the chapter defines terminology and discusses components of the evaluation process, including review of documentation/referral, interview and occupational profile, specific assessment measures, interpretation and findings, and recommendations for intervention. The second part of this chapter explores models that might be used to guide client-centered evaluation, including the Occupational Therapy Intervention Process Model (Fisher, 2009) and the use of the Occupational Therapy Practice Framework (OTPF) 3rd edition (American Occupational Therapy Association [AOTA], 2014a) as a guide for the evaluation process. The third part of this chapter considers factors that influence the evaluation process such as practice environment, therapist experience, tools and documentation used in the evaluation process, and ethical issues in evaluation.

Terms Relevant to Evaluation

In a discussion of the evaluation process, it is important to clarify relevant terms such as *screening*, *evaluation*, and *assessment* because they each have specific meaning as used in this chapter and common professional documents in the United States (Hinojosa, Kramer, & Crist, 2014).

Screening

Screening is often the first part of the occupational therapy (OT) process and consists of a quick review of the client's situation to determine if an OT evaluation is warranted. It may occur when a referral is made or may be a routine activity that a therapist does any time a new client enters a given practice setting (Hinojosa et al., 2014). For example, in long-term care settings, it is a routine practice for newly admitted residents to be screened for potential to benefit from OT services. Once the therapist determines that the client might be a candidate for OT, and it is agreed that the client may benefit from OT services, the evaluation process begins.

Evaluation

Evaluation is the term used for the whole process of obtaining and interpreting information needed for intervention planning and effectiveness review. This includes planning for and documenting both the evaluation process and the results (AOTA, 2013; Hinojosa et al., 2014). Niestadt (2000) posited that "occupational therapy evaluation is both a set of procedures and a thought process" (p. 1).

According to the OTPF, evaluation consists of an "Occupational Profile" as well as an "Analysis of Occupational Performance" (AOTA, 2014a, p. S10). The "Occupational Profile" typically uses an interview process to understand the history and life experience of the client along with patterns of engagement in meaningful occupation. An "Analysis of Occupational Performance" uses observations as well as formal and informal assessment strategies to identify the client's strengths and challenges related to engagement in occupation (AOTA, 2014a). The AOTA has a template available on their Website for completing an Occupational Profile (AOTA, 2017a).

The procedural part of the OT evaluation can consist of performing interviews, observations, assessments, and hands-on strategies to understand the client's strengths and challenges in occupational performance. In reality, it is not possible to ever fully separate evaluation from intervention because practitioners maintain an evaluative view of clients throughout the OT process (screening to discharge). The thought process of evaluation uses all types of professional and clinical reasoning as the therapist considers medical, social, and/or educational diagnoses; contextual factors in the client's world; and pragmatic factors that influence the client and the intervention process (Hinojosa et al., 2014).

Closely related to evaluation, **reevaluation** is defined by the AOTA Standards of Practice as the "Reappraisal of the client's performance and goals to determine the type and amount of change that has taken place" (AOTA, 2015a, p. 2). As discussed in Chapter 27, reevaluation enables the therapist to assess the client's response to intervention and to collaborate with the client to determine changes to the intervention plan.

Assessment

As part of the evaluation, therapists may need to gather specific information via the use of assessment tools. Hinojosa and colleagues (2014) describe an **assessment** as " . . . a specific tool, instrument or systematic interaction used to collect occupational profile and occupational performance areas during the evaluation process" (p. 3). An assessment can be informal in that the therapist uses a given situation to obtain data or it may involve using a standardized interview or observation tool. Standardized assessments typically involve a process in which the client performs specific actions that are graded or rated by the therapist according to a predetermined set of criteria. Assessments can be *criterion-referenced* where the client is graded in terms of some behavioral standard or *norm-referenced* where the client is compared to a group of other people who have taken the same measure. In today's practice environment, it is often not practical to perform numerous assessments; therefore, it is critical that therapists carefully choose assessment tools when measuring occupational performance. Chapter 29 provides guidance about factors to consider in choosing tools to assess client performance.

Professional Standards Related to Evaluation

Because the occupational therapist is educated at the professional level, he or she is responsible for all aspects of the evaluation process. The AOTA Standards of Practice (AOTA, 2015a) state: "An occupational therapist, in collaboration with the client, evaluates the client's ability to participate in daily life tasks, roles, and responsibilities by considering the client's history, goals, capacities, and needs; analysis of task components; the activities and occupations the client wants and needs to perform; and the environments and context in which these activities and occupations occur" (p. 3). Using appropriate and relevant assessment strategies or tools, the therapist gathers and synthesizes data from the occupational profile and the assessment of occupational performance. The therapist interprets information and makes recommendations for OT intervention and/or referral to other services from which the client might benefit.

Occupational therapy practitioners must respond to referrals and procedures in a manner that complies with regulatory, financial, and ethical requirements. Verbal and/or written communication of evaluation findings should be provided within time frames as specified by practice settings, legal/regulatory, accreditation, and payer requirements. All communication regarding clients should be conducted within boundaries of ethics related to client confidentiality (AOTA, 2015b).

Occupational therapists may ask OT assistants (OTAs) to contribute to the evaluation process. Under the supervision of an occupational therapist, OTAs may perform and report findings from selected assessments for which they have service competency (AOTA, 2014b). Chapter 70 provides more information about the process of establishing competence, and Chapter 72 discusses the overall differences in practice roles between the professionally educated occupational therapist and the technically educated OTA.

NOTES

Evaluation and Intervention: Shifting Paradigms

Kielhofner (2004) describes three periods in history for OT: (1) the occupation period, (2) the mechanistic period, and (3) the contemporary period. In the occupation period in our history, the terms *assessment* and *evaluation* do not appear in our founding documents, although these documents do mention the necessity of finding out meaningful occupations for each "client." For example, Adolf Meyer (1922) notes, "It takes, above all, resourcefulness and the ability to respect at the same time the native capacities and interests of the patient" (p. 7). In her discussion of how "aides" should be trained, Slagle (1922) asserts that an important part of training should be a system of "occupational analysis" (p. 16). Faulkes (1923) contends that clinicians should observe clients " . . . for a period in order to ascertain what they can and cannot do. When, what they can do has been determined, the task becomes one of getting their interest in doing one of those things; unless the interest can be obtained, the training and placement that follows will, in all probability, be only temporary" (pp. 114, 115).

As our profession progressed into the mechanistic period (1940 to 1970s), the focus of care was on remediating client factors with frequent mention of equipment such as standing tables, braces, etc. (Kielhofner, 2004). In terms of evaluation, this is where occupational therapists began using assessment tools such as range of motion, perceptual tests, and more standardized assessments of activities of daily living (ADL) to comprise the OT evaluation.

Kielhofner (2004) contends that the mechanistic period led to the contemporary period where we questioned our roots in occupation. Fisher (1998) describes the crisis of questioning when she states: " . . . they [occupational therapists] often use evaluation and intervention methods that are so similar to those of their colleagues in physical therapy, neuropsychology, social work, and nursing that any distinctions between OT and these professions became blurred and even abolished" (p. 558). She further notes,

"If we are to remain a viable profession and avoid the risk of being viewed as redundant, we must continue the move away from the mechanistic paradigm and reconnect to our philosophical foundations" (Kielhofner, 2004, p. 561). This contemporary period led to a search for evaluation strategies that would help us focus on occupation. Fisher's Occupational Therapy Intervention Process Model (2009) and the Canadian Model of Occupational Performance (Townsend & Polatajko, 2007) led to the development of assessment tools as well as philosophy about evaluation that focuses on measuring occupation rather than a strict focus on component skills or client factors. For example, some of these occupation-based assessments include the Assessment of Motor and Process Skills (Fisher, 1998) and the Canadian Occupational Performance Measure (COPM) (Law et al., 2005).

Pizzi and Richards (2017) note that a paradigm shift is necessary to direct focus onto well-being as well as quality of life (QOL) as a primary outcome of OT services delivered to individuals, communities, and populations. To that end, they advocate for evaluation strategies that focus on measurement of QOL. Some would argue that we have moved from the contemporary period to a pluralistic or postmodern period. Powers Dirette (2013) as well as Hinojosa (2017) posit a more pluralistic approach to evaluation and intervention, noting that we should select the best guideline for intervention that meets a client's as well as the practitioners' circumstances. Arguing against an exclusive focus on occupation, Powers Dirette states, "If we go back to the past, however, we must not forget what we have learned along the way. For example, if we only evaluate and treat a person's ability to perform occupations following an acquired brain injury, we dissociate from what we have learned about the underlying neurological causes and process of recovery. We must instead build on our body of knowledge through a careful and constant critique of our ideas" (p. 4). Powers Dirette as well as Hinojosa argue that it is not an "either/or" proposition but rather an approach we consider both client factors "and" occupation in our evaluation and intervention.

Occupational Therapy Evaluation as Choreography

The practice of OT, like that of many service professions, is an art as well as a science. The science is evident in the methodical processes used by therapists as they explore client challenges and collaborate with the client to develop strategies for dealing with problems in daily living. The artistry in OT comes from the relationship or the connectedness with the client and his or her situation in order to generate individualized and creative solutions to help enhance the client's quality of life (QOL). Part of the artistry in practicing OT is the ongoing dance that happens between evaluation and intervention throughout the OT process. Typically, throughout the evaluation phase, the therapist may be incorporating intervention strategies. Similarly, when implementing intervention, therapists gather data to evaluate the client's response and modify therapy accordingly. Evaluation does not only happen at the beginning and at the end of intervention; it should be happening throughout the OT process to explore effectiveness of intervention. In recent years, the AOTA has published practice guidelines in many practice areas (e.g., Children and Youth; Productive Aging; Mental Health; Driving and Community Mobility) that give practice specific suggestions for evaluation and assessment strategies.

The metaphor of dance provides a helpful way to examine the process; because in order to provide effective client-centered services, occupational therapists must choreograph the whole OT process (Figure 28-1). The process of

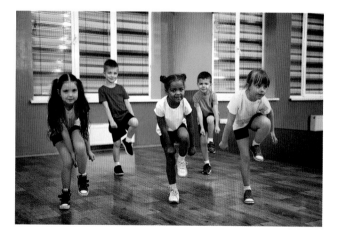

FIGURE 28-1 Just as these young dancers must attend carefully to each other in order to create an effective performance, occupational therapists must work with their clients to choreograph an evaluation that results in effective intervention.

choreography includes several components such as sources of inspiration, collaboration with others, entering the studio, elements of creation, making movement, composing the piece, and performing the piece (Canadian National Centre for the Arts, n.d.). Table 28-1 demonstrates parallels between choreographing a dance and the OT process.

Throughout the process of composing a dance, the choreographer must always keep in mind the "end product," which is the dance that will be performed before an audience. The choreographer considers all elements such as use of space, costume, set, and lighting, for example. Similarly, the occupational therapist must simultaneously consider evaluation, intervention, and discharge planning in light of client and contextual factors. Skilled practitioners carefully choose interview and assessment strategies that will help gather the most valuable information to guide intervention. Novice therapists might not consider discharge planning until they are well into the intervention process, but more experienced practitioners know to treat each client visit as though it might be the last visit before discharge or transfer to another setting. The OT evaluation typically follows a sequence that includes screening and referral, document review, interview and occupational profile, specific assessment measures, interpretation and findings, and recommendations for intervention.

Much like a beginning dancer, the novice OT practitioner is often somewhat clumsy and mechanical in interviewing, observing client performance, and in administering standardized assessments. Inexperienced therapists may be so concerned with their own performance (especially when being closely supervised) that they have limited ability to engage or enjoy the artistry of their practice. Focusing on the mechanics of performing an evaluation may result in limited mental reserves available for interpretation, synthesis, and documentation of findings. An expert occupational therapist seems to effortlessly flow through the dance of evaluation as he or she carefully chooses interview questions and observes relevant performance factors. The seasoned therapist can demonstrate skilled reasoning to select appropriate assessment tools, seemingly knowing what questions to ask, what assessment tools to use, and when the evaluation is completed. Taking the metaphor of determining client needs as choreography a little further, foundational texts on choreography tells us that in order to compose a dance, there are factors that influence the outcome. These elements are our guide for the rest of this chapter.

Screening and Referral: Prelude to the Dance

In many practice settings, screening for services often occurs prior to referral for OT. In some settings, occupational therapists screen new clients as a matter of course,

TABLE 28-1	Comparing Choreography of Dance to Occupational Therapy Process

Element of Choreography in Dance	Related Concept in the Occupational Therapy Process	Pragmatics with Clients in Occupational Therapy
Collaboration Even the solo performer is dependent on stage people to adjust environmental factors including lighting, music, and costumes. The end product is a collaboration between the dancer and many other people.	Working "with" the client rather than "doing for" the client. Occupation therapists should also be aware of practitioners in other disciplines who might be working with the client and ensure collaboration in the best interest of the client.	Occupational therapist must ask the client what he or she wants to accomplish. Client must participate in goal setting rather than merely agree with goals you generate.
Studio The place where the dance is crafted, but the ultimate test is to perform the dance on a stage in front of an audience.	The place where you do therapy (which may not be the place in which the skill is generalized).	Occupational therapist must provide opportunities for skills to generalize to different settings, times, social situations, etc.
Elements The who, what, and where of the dance. What is the story the dance is trying to tell? Where will the dance be performed? What will the backdrop look like? What costumes will be worn?	Clients come with a multitude of factors that influence occupational performance. Similarly, therapists have their context that they bring to the OT process.	Occupational therapist's job is to figure out what needs to be emphasized during the OT process.
Making movement Deciding at what point in the music the dance will begin. Dancers must consider elements of timing, space, and props.	Typically, time must be spent on developing therapeutic rapport with the client, especially when dealing with sensitive or personal information. Therapists need to have some degree of logical flow through an assessment or an intervention session. In medicine, the physical assessment begins at the head and ends with private parts so as not to invade one's most intimate area at the beginning of the assessment.	Occupational therapist must consider time, tools, and therapist skills available for assessment.
Composition How does the piece flow from beginning to end? Are there "movements" in the piece that signify "chapters" in the story?	The more smoothly the assessment process flows, the more confidence the client has in the therapeutic relationship and in the potential outcomes of intervention. There needs to be some degree of transparency in the assessment process.	Occupational therapist must use time during an assessment wisely, often intertwining interviewing with other assessment measures.
Final step Any composition needs closure that signifies the conclusion and interpretation of the piece.	Clients typically expect some interpretation to be made at the end of the assessment session. Therapists are cautioned not to be too quick to make firm conclusions about the client's source of occupational performance problems; however, they should give some indication of possible sources and thus goals that might be used to address the occupational challenge.	Occupational therapist has to know when to close the assessment.

whereas in other settings, occupational therapists only screen clients as requested by other professionals such as nurses or teachers. In many long-term care settings, for example, all new residents are screened for their potential to benefit from therapy services as a way of potentially helping the client to transition to this new living environment. In school system practice, the therapist often engages with the teacher or a support team to screen students (often via observation or work samples) and makes recommendations (often in the form of adaptations) that the teacher might implement to see if problems can be abated.

Should the child not respond to the support team recommendations, there is often a referral for an OT evaluation.

Screening involves gathering preliminary data about a client's challenges in occupational performance and determining whether or not the client may benefit from skilled OT services or perhaps referral(s) to other professionals. Screening is viewed as a "hands-off" approach where there is limited interaction between the client and the therapist, often taking the form of consulting with staff members or reviewing intake information on clients who are new to a facility or an agency. *The key things that the occupational*

CASE STUDY 28-1 AMANDA: SCREENING AN ADOLESCENT IN AN ALTERNATIVE SCHOOL

When I started working in a residential and alternative school setting for adolescents, I was asked to screen each of the students. For a week, I went into the facility and met each of the adolescents one at a time, getting to know them and performing screenings and requesting OT evaluation orders where appropriate. Amanda was a resident who I began "screening" the first day I started working at this facility. The first thing one of the staff said was, "I don't know whether or not you can help her (Amanda), but she needs something . . . " Amanda noted that I hadn't "picked her" yet and yelled across the day room: "Hey OT lady, aren't you going to work with me? . . . Probably not, they say I'm too much trouble."

Throughout my few days there, I had noticed that Amanda seemed to seek attention from staff and from male students. She seemed to impose herself on groups during unstructured time, and according to the staff, she often "stirred up trouble" between students, particularly if two girls were interested in one boy. Upon reviewing her records, I noted that she had been in three different residential facilities in the past year and a half. Apparently, she was discharged from these facilities due to fighting with other female students. Without more information, I wasn't sure what I might be able to do with her, but it seemed clear that she was having some occupational performance concerns, so I asked for an OT order to evaluate the student.

therapist should look for in intake information are recent changes in living environment, health status, or occupational performance. For example, in a long-term care environment, the client's records might be screened for recent history of falls or declines in performance of activities of daily living (ADL). In school system settings, screenings often take place after the student support team has recommended that the occupational therapist observe a student in a classroom and has given suggestions for the teacher to implement to enhance a child's classroom performance.

The mere presence of a diagnosis or clinical condition should not dictate whether a client is screened for or receives OT services; clients should be screened when they are experiencing challenges in occupational performance. When dealing with caregivers, organizations, or populations, screening can be done by using results of surveys, incident reports, and population statistics that might influence occupational performance. Some examples of documents that might be used for determining if OT screenings might be needed for a group or population might be the number of falls in a facility, the causes of back injuries to staff members, or national health statistics about secondary disability in a population of people with spinal cord injury.

Once it is determined that an OT evaluation is warranted, the therapist receives the appropriate written referral as per agency policies and procedures. For example, in most medical settings, a physician order is necessary for an OT evaluation. In a school system setting, the referral for an OT evaluation usually comes from the student support team, the special education staff, or the school psychologist. Occupational therapists in the United States typically have the legal ability to enter a case without a referral from another professional, so clients can self-refer for OT services and they can self-pay; however, more

often, agency or payment requirements and mere pragmatics often supersede self-referral or self-payment. See Case Study 28-1 for an example of how a screening might result in a referral.

Clients: The Source of Inspiration

In the arts, there are many sources of inspiration. In OT, the client, the group, or the population is the source that inspires our evaluation process. Fisher (2009) categorizes the client in three ways: (1) The "client" can be a "person" who seeks or is referred for OT services, (2) a "client constellation" that includes both the individual who seeks or was referred for services and others who are closely connected to that individual, and (3) a "client group" that includes people who share similar problems in occupational performance (p. 3). Table 28-2 gives examples of terms and strategies for assessing different types of clients.

Regardless of the way in which we define the term *client*, a collaborative focus on occupation is critical in the OT process. This is true even when the therapist feels the client goals are unrealistic. Consider Len in Case Study 28-2.

When working with Len (Man with a Mission), I was working in a rehabilitation setting that placed a high value on the use of the Functional Independence Measure (FIM) (Uniform Data System, 2010) as one of the main outcome tools to determine whether a "patient" was making adequate progress. Given that Len had severe pain and discomfort along with requiring total assistance for ADL, I initially viewed him as an inappropriate candidate for rehabilitation because he only wanted to do therapy while he was in his hospital bed. By being hyper focused on the FIM scale, I couldn't see that being independent in

	Client	Client Constellation	Client Group/Population
Terms used to describe	• Patient • Student • Consumer • Resident • Member • Customer	• Family members • Caregiving staff • Teachers • Church groups • Support circle	• Class • Support group • Community • Staff • Organization or agency
Strategies for assessing needs	• Interview • Observation • Performance measures	• Interview • Self-efficacy surveys • Observation of performance	• Focus groups • Surveys • Reports • Performance measures
Considerations	• Must be able to articulate needs	• Being a caregiver does not necessitate OT involvement; caregivers must face challenges in their caregiving role to warrant intervention.	• Individual or group making the OT referral may have different opinions about the occupational performance challenges than do the individuals with whom you are directly working.

TABLE 28-2 Terms and Assessment Strategies for Working with Different Types of Clients

self-care was not nearly as important to this client as was his returning to productive employment.

Len taught me that if I was to be an effective practitioner, I had to listen to my clients and to trust rather than question their wishes and desires. Instead of focusing on his performance of basic activities of daily living (BADL), I eventually began to explore his level of pain and possible strategies to reduce pain. Additionally, because of his strong desire to return to using a computer, I realized that I could use computer use as a valued occupation to promote movement and pain reduction. I was able to figure out how to use a sip and puff interface for Len to be able to use his computer. We started slowly by just playing solitaire to learn the mechanics of operating a computer in a new way. After 1 day of using the computer, Len was able to reduce his pain level and he began to have the desire to sit up for longer periods and to learn to transfer to a

wheelchair to attend therapy sessions. I used his strong values of "work" as being critical to his identity and used as a motivator to guide therapeutic intervention.

Document Review: Understanding the Backdrop for the Dance

In many settings, there are client records that can provide useful information, such as demographic information, and often some type of history about the recent events or challenges experienced by the client. For example, in a medical or long-term care environment, the patient's record will discuss the reason for coming to the facility, procedures performed, and results of tests. In the educational setting, the student records may have reports from

CASE STUDY 28-2 LEN: A MAN WITH A MISSION

While working in a rehabilitation facility, I encountered Len, a 46-year-old man who was diagnosed with Guillain-Barre syndrome after being ill with a flu-like illness for about 2 weeks prior to admission. In my prior experience, I had worked with people who had made rapid recovery from this condition, so I expected a similar situation. When I went in Len's room and asked him what he would like to accomplish, he stated that his main goal was to return to work as a project manager for a defense agency. He stated, "I don't care about getting dressed, just figure out a way that I can use my computer from my bed."

My initial bedside evaluation revealed that Len had no cognitive or perceptual difficulties, but he had severe pain

that limited my ability to perform sensory or motor testing. When I moved his extremities to check passive range of motion (he was quadriplegic at this point), he screamed out in pain. He told me to stop moving him and to reposition him so he was comfortable. This activity took about 20 minutes as we could not find the right spot for his pillow where he was comfortable for me to leave the room. At this point, he was completely dependent in all self-care and mobility. How could I help him use his computer if he couldn't even move his body?

1. Consider what else you might want to know?
2. Read through to the chapter to see options to consider.

various professionals, results of educational testing, and an Individualized Education Plan (IEP) or a 504 Plan (student accommodations in educational settings) where appropriate. In the case of groups or populations, documents may include personnel files, incident reports, survey results, and statistics about a concern or health condition. For new practitioners, as well as those new to a particular practice area, it can be difficult to identify which documents and what information should be the focus of the record review. Table 28-3 gives suggestions of potentially important documents to review by practice setting.

In medical settings, records will contain a history and physical, which reviews the systems in the body and the past medical history and provides consultation reports. The medical report, specialist consultation reports,

progress notes, and results of testing can provide information vital to the OT evaluation, such as reason for admission (i.e., stroke or admission for a surgical procedure), and it provides information about body systems/functions that might have an impact on occupational performance. A key understanding of the results of a history and physical can guide the therapist's choice of evaluation strategies as well as guide intervention. For example, a history and physical that lists sensory awareness as impaired would guide the therapist to interview and observe performance related to safety in the home environment. The history and physical, as well as sections regarding orders and test results, may guide the therapist to a particular action or precaution that may be indicated for a specific client. For example, when test results are indicative of a blood clot, the client may be on bed rest, or when electrolytes are

TABLE 28-3 Types of Documents Helpful in the Records Review Process

Setting	Types of Documents Available	Important Notes	Tests and Lab Results
Medical	• Demographic sheet • Doctors' orders/precautions • Consultation reports • Daily progress notes	• Nurses • Specialist notes • PT/SLP notes	• X-rays • Blood work • Cardiac/respiratory
Long-term care/skilled nursing	• Demographic sheet • Doctors' orders • MDS/RUGs • Therapy plan of care • Daily notes	• Nurses • Specialist notes • PT/SLP notes	• X-rays • Blood work • Cardiac/respiratory
Educational	• Demographic sheet • Educational testing • Specialist reports • IEP/RtI (in public school systems)	• Teacher reports • Psychologist reports • Educational testing	• Hearing and vision screening • Psychological evaluation • Standardized testing
Outpatient/home health	• Demographic sheet • Discharge notes from medical setting • Initial evaluation from intake coordinator • Therapy plan of care • IFSP (early intervention) • Progress notes	• Nurses • Specialist notes • PT/SLP notes	• X-rays
Mental health	• Demographic sheet • Doctors' orders • Consultation • Reports • Care plan	• Psychiatrist • Neuropsychology • Nursing • Mental health technician • Behavioral specialist	• Blood work (may be important to determine therapeutic levels of medications)
Group/organization	• Reports of prior intervention • Incident reports • In-service logs • Meeting minutes • Survey or observation results	Must know who is requesting OT intervention. If the recipients are not the same people who requested the service, they may have mistrust that the organization is employing OT services to find problems with individuals or groups.	Tests and lab results may be reported for groups and population, but these are typically reported by means and standard deviations and may not always be valuable in planning a group- or population-based intervention.
Population	• Request for proposal • Health statistics or community data		

IEP/RtI, Individualized Education Plan/response to intervention; IFSP, Individual Family Service Plan; MDS, minimum data set; PT, physical therapy; RUGs, resource utilization groups; SLP, speech-language pathologists.

imbalanced, the therapist might notice the client to be mentally confused. When in doubt about anything in a client's records, the clinician should seek clarification prior to working with a client.

The first thing that the OT practitioner should review is the reason for the OT referral. Often, the referral will read, "OT Eval and Treat," which is short for "perform an evaluation and treat per OT guidelines." On the one hand, this open-ended language is good for our profession in that we have opportunity to be client-centered, but for the novice practitioner, it provides little guidance about why the referral source believes this individual or group may need the services of an occupational therapist. The occupational therapist is cautioned against merely assuming that the diagnosis is the reason for the referral. For example, a client might be admitted to the hospital for a hip fracture but have a former diagnosis of a left hemiplegia due to a stroke that might be impeding use of a walker, which in turn may affect self-care. In this case, the occupational therapist may need to assist the client to compensate for inability to use their left upper extremity.

Once the clinician reviews the reason for the referral, the next step is to understand basic demographic information about the client. In many contexts in which individual services occur, there is a *face sheet* or some other introductory information sheet about the client that includes name, age, address, names of family members or guardians, diagnosis/diagnoses, education level or grade in school, and, in some settings, religious or spiritual preferences. This information can be used to more efficiently get to know the client by providing a starting point in the OT interview questions. For example, the client's *demographic sheet* in a medical setting might say that she is a retired teacher who lives with her sister in a large metropolitan area. These demographic characteristics might be used to ask the client about the sister's ability to help in the home or the availability of public transportation when the client returns home. In educational settings, there are often reports of the student's progress along with testing that also might be used to interview the student, teacher, or family member(s) about the student's strengths and challenges in the educational setting. In this way, the occupational therapist can begin to build an occupational profile of the client as well as anticipate possible occupational performance needs and challenges.

After reviewing the demographic information, the therapist then focuses on important data within a client's documentation that might be pertinent to the client, the setting, and the OT process. Particular attention should be paid to issues related to client safety that might include factors such as unstable medical status (vital signs, blood chemistry, seizures, presence of an infection, precautions, response to medication, etc.), history of falls or other injuries, unpredictable behavioral changes, and response to

intervention thus far. *In short, the therapist wants to know what to expect regarding potential adverse events that might influence evaluation and intervention.* The therapist might also use information about medical status to anticipate any potential communication difficulties in interviewing the client. For example, if the client is on a ventilator, it may be difficult or at least time-consuming to obtain verbal responses. Similarly, if the record says that the client has unpredictable behavioral changes, the therapist might want to modulate the initial interview so as not to agitate the client.

Understanding Client Precautions: Dancing Safely

The therapist should review and note any precautions in the physician's order or documentation that should be attended to during evaluation and intervention. Precautions may include those related to diet and swallowing, neurological and orthopedic conditions (such as a lack of sensation or motion and weight-bearing restrictions), seizures, behavioral or cognitive impairments (particularly nighttime confusion in elderly clients), infection control (particularly important with clients who are immunosuppressed), open wounds or surgical sites, precautions related to medical devices, general cautions related to medications or blood chemistry (such as patients taking blood thinners need to take extra caution when shaving), and preparation for a procedure (such as restriction of water or food prior to testing).

Critical Pathways: Script for the Dance

In many rehabilitation settings, therapists employ the use of interdisciplinary critical pathways as a guide for evaluation and intervention. Commonly used in settings with patient populations who have orthopedic impairments or strokes, rehabilitation teams generate typical pathways or "care maps" that guide clinicians about what evaluation and intervention activities should be done by each clinical discipline for each day or week of care. Novalis, Messenger, and Morris (2000) reviewed data across multiple organizations that used care plans for clients with hip fractures finding that OT practitioners were most commonly involved in evaluation and intervention for self-care activities as well as transfers and mobility. For example, a care plan for an elderly woman with a hip fracture in an acute care setting might include tasks to be accomplished on each day for the 3 days after an open reduction and internal fixation. Table 28-4 gives a sample of what might be included in the OT portion of a care plan.

TABLE 28-4   Sample of Occupational Therapy Aspects of a Care Plan

	OT Assessment and Intervention
Day 1	1. OT assessment completed within 24 hours after admission. a. Assessment includes measurement of ROM and strength in UE. b. Assessment of BADL. c. Interview regarding discharge plan and home environment.
Day 2	1. Client will sit up in chair. 2. Client will engage in and demonstrate use of long-handled equipment for dressing. 3. Client will be able to ambulate into bathroom with walker and transfer on and off commode with minimum assist.
Day 3	1. Preparation for discharge home. 2. Reassessment of neuromusculoskeletal factors, areas of occupation. 3. Client will be able to perform transfers to and from toilet and tub bench with SBA. 4. Client will adhere to orthopedic precautions while performing mobility and ADL tasks.

ADL, activities of daily living; BADL, basic activities of daily living; ROM, range of motion; SBA, stand by assist; UE, upper extremities.

Interview and Occupational Profile: Collaborating in the Dance

Once the "preparation" for the evaluation is completed, the therapist then meets the client and performs an interview to ascertain the client's perspective. Brown (2009) states, "The usefulness of interview and observation should not go unmentioned. . . . An interview can be invaluable in determining underlying factors that are interfering with performance" (p. 164). Depending on the practice setting, the interview may take many different forms. It can be structured in terms of using a standard agency-based form in which therapists ask questions and fills out a form. Conversely, there may be no guidance for the interview, and the therapist follows the client conversation to guide the interview questions. Just as we might learn about a dance partner while dancing with him or her, the interview is often interspersed with occupation-based assessment strategies. Regardless of the interview format, the therapist must ascertain some degree of information regarding the client's perceptions about occupational performance. Recent changes in the American Medical Association CPT evaluation codes for OT include the completion of an occupational profile (AOTA, 2017b). As mentioned before, AOTA has a template available for completing an occupational profile (AOTA, 2017a).

Depending on the practice setting, therapists often find key questions that help them understand the occupational life of the client. Table 28-5 gives some typical questions asked in various practice settings along with typical spaces in which evaluations occur. A question such as "Tell me about a typical day?" often elicits information about what the client needs, wants, or is expected to do. The client response guides the therapist in knowing the occupations in which the client typically engages. To understand more about occupational challenges, therapists can ask the question "What is the most stressful/least stressful time of day?" That

may help the therapist know about activities that have different levels of demand for the client. Depending on the client's response to this question, the therapist may wish to probe further about why the client sees this time of day or a particular activity as challenging. For example, if you were to ask me the two times of day that I find particularly challenging, I would say (1) getting myself and my two adolescent children out of the house each morning and (2) coming home and deciding what to fix for dinner. My response might lead you to generate several hypotheses about my occupational challenges, which might include home or time management as well as caring for my children, not to mention cooking.

A skilled therapist can quickly ascertain multiple patient factors while asking the patient simple, yet "high yield" interview questions. High-yield questions are those few questions that will help us gather the most data. For example, knowing with whom a client lives or the type of housing that they anticipate returning to might be critical to discharge planning. The interview is an excellent opportunity to discover what the patient needs or wants to do when he or she leaves the hospital setting. The therapist gathers information about typical activities in which the client engages as well as the client's "home" environment and potential support the patient has, which may be critical factors in discharge planning. The interview is an excellent tool for gaining an overall picture of the patient's cognitive status (and is frequently the best and only method required, thus limiting embedding a cognitive evaluation). Finally and most important, the interview helps establish rapport with clients. *A word of caution is advised about interviewing clients with cognitive impairment who may not have accurate insights about their performance or needs. In this case, the clinician may also interview family, friends, or staff who can offer insights about the client's occupational challenges.* At the same time, one should still obtain the client's perspective because the presence of cognitive impairment doesn't negate the need to understand and respond to the client's concerns.

TABLE 28-5 Potential Assessment Strategies in Various Practice Settings

	Occupational Profile Questions	Focused Questions that may Elicit Rich Responses to Guide the OT Process	Observation Environments/Items Needed	Common Assessment Tools	Key Forms of Documentation	Important Considerations for This Setting
Acute care medical setting	• Before you came to the hospital, what was your typical day like? • What do you think a typical day will be like during the weeks after you are discharged from here?	What things might hinder you from going home?	Client's bed/ chair and bathroom Wash basin, toothbrush, comb, etc.	• COPM • ROM • MMT • BADL	• Standard evaluation form • Critical pathway • Daily progress notes	• Medical stability and necessary precautions • Relationships with medical/ nursing personnel
Adult rehabilitation/ long-term care setting	• Tell me about a typical day for you. What do you need, want, or are required to do? In your home? In the community?	What things might hinder you from going home?	Client's bed/chair and bathroom, therapy area, ADL suite	• COPM • ROM/MMT • FIM • Cognitive-perceptual • BADL/IADL	• Standard evaluation form/ plan of care • Daily/weekly progress notes	Medicare Part A requirements for clients' ability to tolerate therapy hours appropriate to the setting
Home health	• Tell me about a typical day for you. What do you need, want, or are required to do?	What do you need to be able to do to continue living at home?	Client's living, dining, and bedroom as well as kitchen BP cuff, gait belt, adaptive ADL equipment as needed	• COPM • BADL/IADL	• Standard evaluation form/ plan of care • Daily/weekly progress notes	With Medicare funding, occupational therapists may not have permission to "open" a case; must be opened by nurse or physical therapist
Community mental health	• Tell me about a typical day for you. What do you need, want, or are required to do? In your home or at work/ school?	Tell me about your daily chores. Do you cook? Clean? Do laundry, etc.? With whom do you eat and/or socialize? Tell me about your work/ transportation situation.	Home, group/day treatment setting; work environment Pencil, paper, IADL activities (e.g., making a grocery list; steps to do laundry)	• COPM • Cognitive-perceptual • BADL/IADL • Prevocational or career assessments	Documentation may not be standardized.	May have to educate agency on potential services of OT

(continues)

TABLE 28-5   **Potential Assessment Strategies in Various Practice Settings** *(continued)*

	Occupational Profile Questions	Focused Questions that may Elicit Rich Responses to Guide the OT Process	Observation Environments/Items Needed	Common Assessment Tools	Key Forms of Documentation	Important Considerations for This Setting
School system	To teacher: What is the student expected to do? To student: What kinds of things do you have to do at school? Like to do?	What subject is your (most/least) favorite? Who do you play with at recess? What games do you play at recess?	Classroom, playground, cafeteria, bathroom Pencil, paper, seating adaptations, visual and fine motor activities	• School function assessment • Quick neurological screening test	• IEP; RtI • Daily or weekly progress notes • 6-month or annual reports • Handwriting assessment tools • Visual perceptual and visual-motor assessment tools	OT services are related and must be educationally relevant to educator-generated IEP goals.
Private pediatric setting	To parent: Tell me about your child and their role in your family. What things do you want them to be able to do?	For the parent: What is the worst/best time of day for you with your child? Tell me about your child's friends. Child: If you could do any play activity right now, what would it be?	Clinic, suspended equipment, table top activities, floor mobility activities, fine motor manipulatives	• Sensory Integration and Praxis Tests • Peabody Developmental Motor Scales • Bruininks-Oseretsky Test of Motor skills • Sensory Profile	• Initial evaluation report • Plan of care • Daily/weekly progress notes	Services often require prior authorization; therefore, therapists must estimate number of visits requested.
Work-based setting	Tell me about your job. Tell me about your responsibilities at home. What do you do in your free time since you haven't been able to work?	What did you like best/ least about your job? Your coworkers? Your boss? What do you see needing to happen in order for you to return to work or be retrained for another job? If you had a choice, would you return to your job or train for another job?	Actual or simulated work environment; work hardening setting/clinic	• Career interest inventories • Career aptitude measures • Focus on barriers to work performance, environment, body functions, performance skills	• Initial evaluation report • Plan of care • Daily/weekly progress notes	In order to delineate OT from other services, focus on the interaction of person-task-environment. Significant interaction with case managers.

ADL, activities of daily living; BADL, basic activities of daily living; BP, blood pressure; COPM, Canadian Occupational Performance Measure; FIM, Functional Independence Measure; IADL, instrumental activities of daily living; IEP, Individualized Education Plan; MMT, manual muscle testing; OT, occupational therapy; ROM, range of motion; RtI, response to intervention.

In order to facilitate occupation-based practice, the therapist should begin with a client-centered interview. Chisholm, Dolhi, and Schreiber (2004) state that "putting occupation into your practice is often easier said than done" (p. 5). They recommend doing a client-centered interview by asking a client to list five occupations in three key areas—(1) occupations I need to do, (2) occupations I want to do, and (3) occupations I am expected to do—and then having the client circle the five most important occupations that they want to address. Once these five important occupations are identified, the performance factors contributing to these occupations would be further evaluated. This occupational performance analysis helps the therapist target the appropriate behaviors the client needs to perform desired occupations.

The COPM (Law et al., 2014) is a standardized semistructured client-centered interview to explore the client's perceptions about his or her current level of function in self-care, productivity, and leisure. The client is asked to identify the five most important problems in occupational performance. Using a visual analog scale ranging from 1 to 10, the patient is then asked to take each of these five problems and rate the importance and level of satisfaction with activity performance. The value in using the COPM is that patient's perception can be used as an objective measure of progress, which may be particularly valuable when progress is slower than expected or in cases where a client seems to be "higher functioning" but is having QOL concerns.

Roberts and colleagues (2008) used the COPM throughout the United Kingdom and found that there was an increase in mean scores of satisfaction with occupational performance. This same study found that both clients and physicians were more satisfied with the services of OT after implementing the use of the COPM. Roberts and colleagues saw patterns of responses when using the COPM, whereby older adults reported more concerns regarding self-care and younger people tended to report more difficulties with productivity, which confirms that a "one-size-for-all" approach to evaluation may not be appropriate. It is therefore critical to ascertain each client's concern about his or her occupational performance.

Therapists often intersperse observation of occupational performance or client factors with the interview. The most difficult part of this "dance" is knowing what questions to ask and when to ask them because clients may not be able to focus on action and answering questions at the same time. It is also helpful to the client if the interview questions relate to the actions being performed. For example, the therapist may be asking the client to sit at the edge of the bed, and while the client is moving or resting after performing this action, the therapist may ask an interview question about anticipated difficulties getting in and out of bed when they go home. Brown (2009) notes that where possible, observation of a client in their natural environment can yield valuable information about the client's

method of doing a particular occupation and can also help identify barriers to performing an occupation.

The Occupational Therapy Practice Framework: Backdrop for the Dance

The OTPF (AOTA, 2014a) notes the interview and occupational performance analysis to be effective tools to identify factors such as body functions that may be influencing occupational performance. During the interview, the therapist should ask clients about the following:

- Performance patterns, including habits, roles, and routines
- Contexts for occupational performance that include cultural, personal, physical, social, temporal, or virtual
- Activity demands that take into account objects used, space demands, social demands, sequencing, required actions, and body functions or structures that the patient typically performs in his or her daily life activities

Occupational therapists from the Cardinal Hill Healthcare System (Skubik-Peplaski, Paris, Boyle, & Culpert, 2006) attempted to operationalize the 2002 version of the OTPF and worked across all practice areas in their organization to incorporate occupation into services and OT documentation. Using the framework, they developed forms and structured interview protocols to be able to understand the client's occupational needs. Interview protocols that they developed typically ask clients about a typical day and about activity demands, objects, space, and timing of daily life occupations. They assert that therapists should ask clients about areas beyond basic self-care, such as work and leisure. They also advocate asking interview questions about context, particularly social support. The online resources listed on the Willard and Spackman Website provide a sample evaluation form, which is adapted from a sample evaluation by Shotwell, Johnson, and Flecha (2017) containing ideas similar to those in the Cardinal Hill application of the OTPF.

Strategies for Assessment: Adding Elements to the Dance

Tables 28-6 to 28-13 provide examples of how a practitioner might incorporate concepts described in the OTPF (AOTA, 2014a). The evaluation should begin with the client's perception of his or her own performance in areas of occupation. Clients should be asked about a typical day to understand the areas of occupation in which the client engages. In addition to interview and understanding client perceptions, the evaluation should also include the use of

TABLE 28-6   Strategies for Evaluation of Areas of Occupation

	Examples of Standardized Measures	Interview/Observational Strategies
Overall areas of occupation	• Canadian Occupational Performance Measure (COPM) • Occupational Performance History Interview II	• Ask client about a typical day.
Basic activities of daily living (BADL)	• Functional Independence Measure (FIM/WeeFim) • Barthel Index	• Observe client dressing, bathing, feeding, etc.
Instrumental activities of daily living (IADL)	• Kohlman Evaluation of Living Skills • Milwaukee Evaluation of Daily Living Skills	• Observe client doing a shopping, budgeting, or cooking task.
Education/work	• School Function Assessment • School Assessment of Motor and Process Skills • Worker Role Interview	• Observe client doing a work-related or school-related task.
Play/leisure	• Transdisciplinary Play-Based Assessment • Leisure Assessment Inventory	• Observe child on the playground.
Social participation	• Social Interaction Scale of the Bay Area Functional Performance Evaluation (BaFPE)	• Note interaction during interview. • Ask client about his or her social life. • Observe in structured and nonstructured social environments.
Rest/sleep	• National Institutes of Health Activity Record	• Do you have difficulty with sleeping?

standardized assessment tools for areas in which the therapist seeks further information. The use of standardized assessment tools also contributes to the goal of our profession to provide evidence to support our practice.

In evaluating the areas of occupations, the therapist is trying to find out about basic or personal ADL (BADL or PADL) as well as instrumental ADL (IADL) that are necessary to "run our lives." Some of the IADL occupations include managing one's finances, cleaning one's home, shopping for goods and services, and so forth. Therapists need to ascertain if the client is having difficulties with sleep, rest, work, school, or participation in leisure activities. In acute medical situations, clients may not think about ADL or functional performance and may assume that these skills will immediately return once the body functions or body structures are restored to health. Although this may be true in some cases, occupational therapists can often ease the process and reduce the time that it takes a client to engage in desired occupations. In many cases, this can alleviate the need to stay in a congregate care facility (e.g., hospital, nursing home, or assisted living facility) and help to enhance the individual's QOL. In institutional environments, it may be difficult to have the client engage in some of the IADL tasks during the

evaluation process; so many times, information is gathered via interview rather than actual occupational performance. Table 28-6 gives some strategies for assessment of areas of occupation.

Assessing Overlapping Occupational Concerns: Composition of the Dance

To say that occupation is complex seems to be an understatement. Many times, it is not one occupation that is problematic, but, often, the interface among various occupational demands may be causing difficulty in occupational performance. This orchestration of various occupational demands can be challenging just as it can be challenging for dancers to combine different dance elements. For example, I am quite capable of cooking and cleaning, but my role of worker and of parent often supersede my engagement (or motivation) to engage in these tasks necessary for the "job of living." Case Study 28-3 provides an example of an individual who was working in a sheltered workshop setting. Although this client was successful in performing work-related tasks, the client had difficulty transitioning

TABLE 28-7   Strategies for Evaluation of Client Factors—Values, Beliefs, and Spirituality

	Examples of Standardized Measures	Interview/Observational Strategies
Values, beliefs, spirituality	• Canadian Occupational Performance Measure (COPM) • Quality of Life Inventory • Health-Related Quality of Life • Multidimensional Measurement of Religiousness/Spirituality for use in Health Research.	• Tell me about your life . . . Family? Work? Social? • For some people, their religious or spiritual beliefs act as a source of comfort and strength in dealing with life's ups and downs; Is this true for you? • Do you engage in any practices that enhance your spirituality? • What is the most important (occupation) for you to be able to do?

TABLE 28-8   Strategies for Evaluation of Client Factors—Body Functions

Body Functions	Examples of Standardized Measures	Interview/Observational Strategies
Specific mental functions	• Allen Cognitive Level Screen • Toglia Category Assessment	• Have you noticed a change in your ability to remember, to pay attention, or to follow directions?
Global mental functions	• Mini-Mental State Examination • Cognitive Assessment of Minnesota	• Have you noticed a change in your mental abilities?
Sensory functions and pain	• Sensory Profile (all ages) • McGill Pain Questionnaire • Vision or hearing screening	• Do you have numbness or tingling anywhere in your body? • Do you have pain? Where? Type? Duration? What makes it better? • Do you have difficulty tuning out specific sensory things in the environment (noise, visual distractions, and things next to your body)? • Do you have difficulty getting aroused or calmed down?
Neuromusculoskeletal and movement-related functions	• Quick Neurological Screening • Range of motion or manual muscle testing • Berg Balance Scale	• Notice coordination, strength (effort), or difficulty moving. • If you notice difficulty in the above you might ask this: • Do you have a history of falls? • Do you have difficulty bending, reaching, or grasping?
Voice and speech functions	• Usually done by observation rather than formal assessment, which is typically done by a speech-language pathologist	• During the interview, note particularly soft or loud voice, ability to articulate words, or difficulties in expressive or receptive language. • Ask client to talk after eating or drinking (a "wet" sounding voice may be indicative of swallowing problems).
Organ system function (cardiovascular, respiratory, hematological, immunological, digestive, metabolic, endocrine, genitourinary, and reproductive functions)	• Pulse oximetry, blood pressure; pulmonary function test. Occupational therapists may be involved in a modified barium swallow study, which is designed to view the swallowing functions or they may administer the Swallowing Ability and Function Evaluation (SAFE).	• When working with clients who are on digital monitor, therapist can note changes in these numbers during the occupational therapy session. For example, a client may be comatose but have changes in heart rate or blood pressure when the therapist moves an extremity during fabrication of a splint. OT practitioners should be keenly aware by looking, feeling, and listening to changes in body functions as evidenced by changes in sweating, color of skin, respiration patterns, and so forth, because these may be signs of organ system changes.

TABLE 28-9   Strategies for Evaluation of Client Factors—Body Structures

Body Structures	Evaluation Method	Interview/Observational Strategies
• Nervous system • Eyes, ear, and related structures • Structures involved in voice/speech • Structures related to movement • Skin and related structures • Organ system structures (cardiovascular, respiratory, immunological, digestive, metabolic, endocrine, genitourinary, and reproductive systems)	Not typically evaluated by an occupational therapist because occupational therapists do not evaluate structures independent of a functional/purposeful activity. Many of the diagnostic procedures that physicians request would be used to assess body structures. An example might be an X-ray, an angiogram, or a magnetic resonance imaging, which are all designed to view structures and any potential abnormalities.	Much of this information can be found in clients' records. Look for history and physical that details prior injuries, procedures, and tests that the client may have undergone. Although the questions below are not necessarily indicative of a structural problem, positive client responses may be indicative of potential difficulties with body structures (and certainly warrant further evaluation and/or referral). • Do you have numbness, tingling, or difficulty moving? • Do you have any trouble with your eyes or hearing? • Do you have any wounds right now? Difficulty with skin healing? • Have you had any procedures for your heart, lungs, stomach, or reproductive system? Why?

TABLE 28-10   Strategies for Evaluation of Performance Skills

Performance Skills	Examples of Standardized Measures	Interview/Observational Strategies
Overall performance	• Assessment of Motor and Process Skills	Watch a client engage in activities of daily living (ADL) that involves neuromusculoskeletal, cognitive, and social interaction, which may give some overall picture of performance.
Sensory/ perceptual	• Developmental Test of Visual Perception • Motor-Free Visual Perception Test	Observe client as he or she engages in tasks in his or her environment. Does client tend to miss things on one side of his or her world? Does client have evidence of poor visual acuity?
Motor/praxis	• Jebsen Hand Function Test • Peabody Developmental Motor Scales	Observe client as he or she engages in occupational tasks. Does he or she have a tremor? Slowness or problems with speed of movement? Is the accuracy of movement impaired? Does the client seem to have difficulty executing movements necessary for functional tasks?
Emotional regulation	• Coping Inventory/Early Coping Inventory • Tennessee Self-Concept Scale	When presented with a task that challenges a client's competence, does he or she become frustrated or defeated? Is the client's response to his or her situation proportional to the magnitude of client's challenges?
Cognitive	• Executive Function Performance Test • Routine Task Inventory • Performance Assessment of Self-Care Skills	Does the client seem to have difficulty initiating, sequencing, terminating, problem solving, and so forth, during occupational performance?
Communication/social skills	• Assessment of Communication and Social Interaction • Vineland Adaptive Behavior Scales	Is the client able to communicate his or her needs, wants, desires?

TABLE 28-11   Strategies for Evaluation of Performance Patterns

Performance Patterns	Examples of Standardized Measures	Interview/Observational Strategies
• Habits • Roles • Routines/rituals	• Role Checklist • Adolescent Role Assessment • Self-Discovery Tapestry • Worker Role Interview • National Institutes of Health Activity Record • OPHI; OCAIRS	• Tell me about a typical day for you. • May have to structure questions into categories for self-care, homemaking, work/school, social/leisure activities.

OCAIRS, Occupational Circumstances Assessment-Interview Rating Scale; OPHI, Occupational Performance History Interview.

TABLE 28-12   Strategies for Evaluation of Context and Environment

	Interview/Observational Strategies	Examples of Standardized Measures
Cultural	• Are there special rituals, foods, practices in which you engage?	• Alberta Context Tool
Personal	• Where do you live? Work? Engage in leisure? With whom? • Do you prefer to do things alone or with others?	• Work Environment Impact Scale • School Setting Interview • Classroom Environment Scale
Physical	• Tell me about your home. . . . Try to identify potential barriers/strengths.	• Safety Assessment of Function and the Environment for Rehabilitation (SAFER) • Person–Environment Fit • In-Home Occupational Performance Evaluation (I-HOPE)
Social	• With whom do you live? Other sources of social support?	• Alberta Context Tool • World Health Organization (WHO) Quality of Life-BREF
Temporal	• What is the best/worst time of day for you or your family?	• National Institutes of Health (NIH) Activity Record
Virtual	• Do you use the Internet, e-mail, cell phone, etc.? • For what purposes? Shopping, communicating?	• WHO Quality of Life-BREF

TABLE 28-13   Strategies for Evaluation of Activity Demands

Activity Demand	Interview/Observational Strategies
Objects used and their properties	• Do you have all of the tools needed to do the activity? • Weight, size, amount of resistance of various objects/tools
Space demands	• Environmental considerations (social, cultural, physical, etc.). • Organization of space and materials
Social demands	• Do you "have" to do this task or "want" to do it? • Is this a task that you enjoy? If not, have you tried to get someone else to help you with the task?
Sequencing and timing	• Frequency; repetitions and duration of a task/subtask • Temporal components of the task (speed, sequencing, flow) • Is this a task that could be broken up into parts? Do all the steps of the task need to be done in one time period?
Required body functions	• Neuromusculoskeletal: difficulty in bending, reaching, gripping, stiff or effortful movement; apparent lack of awareness of body in space • Does it involve climbing, stooping, and frequent bending or prolonged body position? • Perceptual/cognitive: missing one aspect of the visual field on a consistent basis; forgetting the steps to a task; doing the task inaccurately or incorrect sequence; forget what you were doing during this or other tasks? • Do you lose your tools/objects or forget what you were doing while engaging in this activity? • Social/emotional: easily frustrated; tends to work alone; does not share materials; becomes easily discouraged; seeks constant reinforcement or never asks for help; passive; disinterested; hyperfocused; and lack of ability to transition
Required body structures	• Required strength, joint mobility, respiratory status, etc.? • Do you need to sit or rest during this activity? Do you become short of breath or fatigued?

from sheltered to community-based employment because of occupational performance concerns regarding hygiene and clothing management.

After understanding the client's areas of occupational engagement, the therapist begins to try to understand various factors that may facilitate or hinder occupational performance. Client factors include values, beliefs, and spirituality; body functions; and body structures. In many settings, the focus of OT evaluation and intervention is on body functions, such as cognition, sensory, and neuromusculoskeletal functions, but therapists are cautioned to recognize the importance of values, beliefs, and spirituality on both the therapeutic relationship and the whole OT process.

A point worth mentioning in terms of client factors is that the term *spirituality* is meant in the broadest sense rather than religiosity. Although religion may provide a sense of spirituality, people may have many factors that influence their sense of inner peace and focus. When I interview a client, I sometimes ask what activities give

CASE STUDY 28-3   TRAVIS: COMBINING WORK AND SELF-CARE FOR EFFECTIVE PARTICIPATION

Travis was a 47-year-old man who I encountered while working in a vocational program that included community placements as well as "sheltered workshop" employment. The goal of the agency was that all clients eventually be employed in community-based settings, but the staff was concerned about Travis not because of his work skills but more because of his hygiene. Travis had been involved with this agency for the past 2 years, and the staff reported that he was capable of learning new jobs and could perform simple one- to two-step work tasks such as placing labels on boxes or repackaging materials for store display. The staff was concerned that they could not move Travis into a community-based position because he needed constant cueing to brush his teeth and take a shower. When picking Travis up on the facility bus each morning, the bus driver stated that at least once or twice a month, she did not allow Travis to get on the bus because of his poor personal hygiene (which is a requirement for participating in the program). When told that he needed to go back into his home to shower, Travis would do so, but he seemed to have limited insight regarding why personal hygiene was necessary for successful work performance.

1. Why do you think that Travis has difficulty with his habits of self-care?
2. What environmental factors might be influencing Travis's difficulties in self-care?

them a sense of peace and calm, and client responses are often indicative of spirituality. Typical answers from clients might be "prayer," "meditation," "being out in nature," "petting my dog," and "being with family." Table 28-7 lists some possible measures and questions a therapist might attend to regarding values, beliefs, and spirituality (see Chapter 24).

In many practice settings, the focus of evaluation and intervention is on client factors such as the body functions of cognitive, sensory processing, or neuromusculoskeletal factors that influence occupational performance. Body functions can be evaluated via the use of standardized assessment tools or through interview and observation. In medical or rehabilitation settings, typically, body functions such as sensory functions and neuromusculoskeletal functions are emphasized, but the therapist should always keep in mind that impairments in these functions do not necessitate dysfunction in occupation. Table 28-8 gives potential strategies for evaluating body functions.

In addition to understanding the client's body functions, therapists must have some appreciation for body structures that might have potential to influence occupational performance. Although these are not typically evaluated in a formal manner, therapists (particularly those working with clients with more acute medical concerns) must have awareness of these areas. Information about body structures can be gathered via test results such as the laboratory reports or X-rays. Many of the diagnostic procedures performed by medical specialists are designed to evaluate body structures. Table 28-9 lists potential strategies for evaluation of body structures.

Ultimately, it is the goal of OT to help a client enhance occupational performance. Therapists must assess how clients use body functions and structures to perform given skills that comprise occupations. In other words, I could have the body "structures" necessary to see and to move my fingers to type this chapter and I could have the body "functions" such as global and specific mental functions necessary to organize my thoughts for ideas to write this chapter, but I could have great difficulty in enacting this occupation of "professional writing." My difficulties could be in performance skills (initiating, attending, or problem solving to find good references) or with performance patterns (e.g., not making the time to write or conflicting roles between that of writer and parent). Tables 28-10 and 28-11 give potential strategies for how a therapist might evaluate occupational performance skills and performance patterns that may include both standardized assessment tools as well as interview.

Our job as therapists is to identify which components of occupation (client factors, performance skills, performance patterns, or context) are causing the greatest challenge and to remediate or compensate for these challenges to enable performance.

Assessing the Environment and the Demands: The Setting for the Dance

The choreographer must know the setting for the dance and the type of dance to be performed. If the stage has a different type of flooring or lighting on which the dancers are not familiar, the rehearsal period may need to be extended. Additionally, if a dance requires a high degree of lifting or athleticism, the choreographer or director will choose dancers who excel in strength and endurance because of the demands of the piece to be performed. Similarly, the occupational therapist needs to understand the context in which occupations are performed and how those tasks are typically performed. When it is not possible to be in the real environment, the therapist asks questions about the environment and the ways in which the client typically performs tasks. This may include asking questions about location, surfaces, heights of various objects or surfaces, tools used, and social or cognitive aspects of task performance.

Table 28-12 gives strategies for evaluation of context and environment. Although many occupational therapists tend to focus on the physical environment, one must also consider the other aspects of the environment that can influence occupational performance. Consider the case of Harlan (Case Study 28-4) who was gainfully employed but underproductive in his work environment. In this case, my main interest was in a contextual evaluation of his work area(s), tools, tasks, and social and cultural aspects involved in productive employment as a grocery store employee.

Factors Influencing the Evaluation Process

Just as the choreographer may be influenced by the potential audience, the space, the budget, and the artistic desires of various stakeholders, so, too, is the occupational therapist influenced by ethics, reimbursement, organizational factors, and requirements for documentation. First is the Occupational Therapy Code of Ethics, in which all principles seem to apply to evaluation and intervention. Beneficence and non maleficence apply to safety and doing what is in the best interest of the client. Autonomy and confidentiality related to respecting the rights and privacy of clients throughout the OT process. The ethical principle of duty relates to maintaining professional competence and using the best evidence available to provide client care. Procedural justice relates to evaluation and intervention in that the occupational therapist must comply with laws and policies guiding the OT profession.

CASE STUDY 28-4   HARLAN: CONTEXTUAL AND ACTIVITY DEMANDS

As I observed Harlan in the grocery store, I noticed that the store had several employees with disabilities of varying types. Additionally, there were posters around the break room that supported the company's efforts to promote diversity, which might be indicative that the cultural context of this organization was to support diversity practices including the hiring of people with disabilities. I noticed that all of the associates took time to speak with each other, particularly the employees with disabilities to "make them feel special." Although this culture of social acceptance of people with disabilities was desirable, I also noticed that there seemed to be "lower" expectations of the employees with disabilities, that is, until Harlan's manager noticed and questioned that his productivity and accuracy was not consistent with nondisabled employees in the same position. I observed him take at least 15 minutes to empty one trash can, and he took 30 minutes to sweep a small area near the pharmacy section. I also noticed that most workers seemed to be hurried about their work and that the temporal context of the workplace was to enable customers to get out of the store as efficiently as possible. Harlan's slowness in work performance was not consistent with the temporal demands of the environment.

In order to provide a "complete" picture of a client's occupational performance, the therapist must also have understanding of activity demands. Table 28-13 lists some possible strategies for exploration of activity demands. In reviewing the "activity demands" of Harlan's position at this grocery store, I reviewed the job description used for all people in his same position. Job descriptions can provide some guidance about the tools, space, and body functions required for a specific job. In the workplace, this may be easy as locating job descriptions, which often have lists of "essential functions"; however, for many other occupations, such as homemaking or hobbies, the activity demands are evaluated by interviewing the client about the task demands. For example, one client may do laundry by going to a commercial laundry facility, whereas another client has to go to the basement in his or her home to do laundry (Figure 28-2). The fact that the demand for one person may require driving or walking a distance to access a laundry facility may be a barrier for the first client, whereas ascending and descending steps to do laundry may provide a barrier for the second individual.

Typically, after the client has identified their top five valued activities, the therapist can probe further about the activity demands of these tasks because people vary greatly in task demands based on all of the other factors involved in analysis of occupation. Therapists are cautioned about making judgments about the "right or wrong" way to perform an occupation. If we are to help clients with occupational performance, we need to help them learn or resume occupations in ways that they are most comfortable rather than using our preferred method of occupational engagement.

Another strategy for understanding the activity demands is to observe a client engaging in his or her valued occupation.

The ability to see the client actually performing a task in his or her own environment using his or her own tools and space is most optimal, although this may not be possible in clinical settings. Therapists are encouraged to try to simulate occupational performance to best analyze the fit between the "person" (client factors, performance skills, performance patterns), the "environment" (cultural, physical, temporal, social, etc.), and the "task" (activity demands). In the case of Harlan, I wanted Harlan to stay gainfully employed; however, I questioned the match between the person, the task, and the environment. My report and my recommendations for intervention would have to take person, task, and environment into account if I was to help Harlan be successful in his employment.

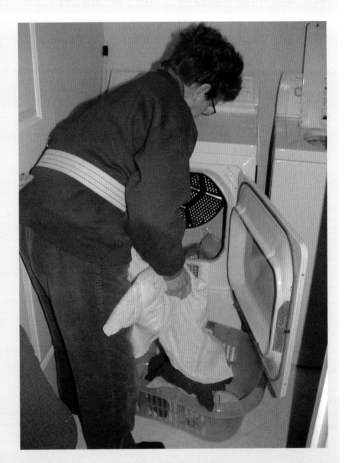

FIGURE 28-2 As part of the evaluation process, clients are observed performing tasks that are important to their daily routines. This requires attention to safety as well as the quality of performance. This client is wearing a gait belt because she has problems with balance when she bends over. In this way, the therapist can observe her routine performance but be ready to support her if needed. (Photo courtesy of Mary Shotwell.)

In terms of complying with laws and policies, occupational therapists speak to many audiences in their communication regarding evaluation and intervention. Not only do facilities have specific requirements for what should be included in evaluation and progress reports but accreditation agencies as well as funding organizations often require specific factors be attended to in OT practice. This being said, occupation therapists need to be mindful in preventing non-OT personnel dictating what should be included in OT evaluation and intervention planning as well as documentation. In order to advocate for OT, practitioners are advised to keep abreast of laws, policies, and the professional evidence regarding our practice.

Interpretation and Intervention Planning: Doing the Dance

Practitioners use their professional reasoning to interpret results of interview, observation, and assessment(s). Typically, the interpretation involves making some judgment about the client's strengths and challenges regarding occupational performance. The therapist makes a statement about the client's ability to benefit from therapy and predicts the duration, frequency, and type of intervention strategies that will likely be used. In some organizations, the use of a "critical pathway" may guide these decisions; however, one must keep in mind that critical pathways are based on statistical means and may not apply to all individuals.

Once the therapist determines that the client may benefit from OT services, long- and short-term goals are formulated in collaboration with the client. Long-term goals may be accomplished in days, weeks, or months depending on the intervention context. Therapists must estimate the number of visits that a client will require so they must have some idea about typical lengths of stay or the number of visits that a client might need for their specific concerns. In the acute care setting, the length of stay can be as short as 1 day, so the evaluation, intervention, and discharge plan may all occur within the same day. For example, a client with an orthopedic condition may have an evaluation, receive adaptive equipment and education in its use, and be ready to go home. In this situation, the therapist may believe that the client will need follow-up OT services in his or her own home.

Client goals should be behaviorally oriented in terms of what the client will do. For example, the goal might read, "Client will participate in education regarding . . . " rather than "therapist will educate client about . . . " Goals should be timed and measureable, which is often a challenge for the novice therapist who has little experience knowing how long it will take a client to achieve a goal; let alone being able to identify the benchmark for successful outcome(s) of services. When generating individualized goals and intervention plans, the therapist must consider person, task, and environment. Intervention plans typically consider a multitude of factors such as medical stability of the client, home environment, available social support, and task/activity demands.

Summary

In this chapter, we have reviewed the OT process of determining client needs. The therapist must be good at interspersing interviews with assessment and maximizing the time allotted to complete an evaluation in order to best reflect the client's concerns regarding occupational performance. Like well-planned choreography, effective evaluation requires attention to multiple factors. When done well, the "dance" of therapy flows from evaluation into intervention. In this process, the clinician is challenged to consider contextual factors of the client as well as the practice setting and to incorporate the use of interviews, observation, and standardized assessment tools where possible. Using guides for evaluation such as the AOTA Practice Framework (AOTA, 2014a) and *The Guide to Occupational Therapy Practice* (Moyers & Dale, 2007) and the AOTA Practice Guidelines may aid the occupational therapists' reasoning by providing the range of factors affecting occupational performance.

 Visit thePoint to watch a video about evaluating clients.

REFERENCES

American Occupational Therapy Association. (2013). Guidelines for documentation of occupational therapy. *American Journal of Occupational Therapy, 67,* S32–S38. doi:10.5014/ajot.2013.67S32

American Occupational Therapy Association. (2014a). Occupational therapy practice framework: Domain and process, 3rd edition. *American Journal of Occupational Therapy, 68,* S1–S48. doi:10.5014/ajot.2014.682006

American Occupational Therapy Association. (2014b). Guidelines for supervision, roles, and responsibilities during the delivery of occupational therapy services. *American Journal of Occupational Therapy, 68,* S16–S22. doi:10.5014/ajot.2014.686S03

American Occupational Therapy Association. (2015a). Standards of practice for occupational therapy. *American Journal of Occupational Therapy, 69,* 6913410057. doi:10.5014/ajot.2015.696S06

American Occupational Therapy Association. (2015b). Occupational therapy code of ethics (2015). *American Journal of Occupational Therapy, 69,* 6913410030. doi:10.5014/ajot.2015.696S03

American Occupational Therapy Association. (2017a). *Occupational profile template.* Retrieved from https://www.aota.org/~/media/Corporate/Files/Practice/Manage/Documentation/AOTA-Occupational-Profile-Template.pdf

American Occupational Therapy Association. (2017b). *The new evaluation codes: What are performance deficits?* Retrieved from https://www.aota.org/~/media/Corporate/Files/Advocacy/Federal/coding/Performance-Deficits-new-CPT-evaluation-codes.pdf

Brown, C. (2009). Functional assessment and intervention in occupational therapy. *Psychiatric Rehabilitation Journal, 32*, 162–170.

Canadian National Centre for the Arts. (n.d.). *The choreographic process.* Retrieved from http://artsalive.ca/en/dan/make/process/chprocess.asp

Chisholm, D., Dolhi, C., & Schreiber, J. (2004). *Occupational therapy intervention resource manual: A guide for occupation-based practice.* Clifton Park, NY: Delmar Learning.

Faulkes, W. F. (1923). Restoration of the crippled. *American Journal of Occupational Therapy, 3*, 113–116.

Fisher, A. G. (1998). Uniting Practice and Theory in an Occupational Framework. 1998 Eleanor Clarke Slagle Lecture. *American Journal of Occupational Therapy, 52*, 509–521.

Fisher, A. G. (2009). *Occupational therapy intervention process model: A model for planning and implementing top-down, client-centered, and occupation-based interventions.* Fort Collins, CO: Three Star Press.

Hinojosa, J. (2017). "How society's philosophy has shaped occupational therapy practice for the past 100 years." *The Open Journal of Occupational Therapy, 5*(2), Article 12. doi:10.15453/2168-6408.1325

Hinojosa, J., Kramer, P., & Crist, P. (2014). Evaluation: Where do we begin? In J. Hinojosa & P. Kramer (Eds.), *Evaluation: Obtaining and interpreting data* (pp. 1–18). Bethesda, MD: AOTA Press.

Kielhofner, G. (2004). *Conceptual foundations of occupational therapy* (3rd ed.). Philadelphia, PA: F. A. Davis.

Law, M., Baptiste, S., Carswell, A., McColl, M., Polatajko, H., & Pollock, N. (2005). *Canadian occupational performance measure.* Ottawa, Canada: Canadian Association of Occupational Therapists.

Law, M., Baptiste, S., Carswell, A., McColl, M. A., Polatajko, H., & Pollock, N. (2014). *The Canadian Occupational Performance Measure* (5th ed.). Ontario, Canada: Canadian Association of Occupational Therapists.

Meyer, A. (1922). Philosophy of occupation therapy. *Archives of Occupational Therapy, 1*(1), 1–10.

Moyers, P. A., & Dale, L. M. (2007). *The guide to occupational therapy practice* (2nd ed.). Bethesda, MD: American Occupational Therapy Association.

Niestadt, M. E. (2000). *Occupational therapy evaluation for adults: A pocket guide.* Philadelphia, PA: Lippincott Williams & Wilkins.

Novalis, S. D., Messenger, M. J., & Morris, L. (2000). Occupational therapy benchmarks within orthopedic (hip) critical pathways. *American Journal of Occupational Therapy, 54*, 155–158.

Pizzi, M. A., & Richards, L. G. (2017). Promoting health, well-being, and quality of life in occupational therapy: A commitment to a paradigm shift for the next 100 years. *American Journal of Occupational Therapy, 71*, 7104170010p1. doi:10.5014/ajot.2017.028456

Powers Dirette, D. (2013). Trading in our paradigm shifts for a staircase. *The Open Journal of Occupational Therapy, 1*(4), Article 1. doi:10.15453/2168-6408.1067

Roberts, A. E. K., James, A., Drew, J., Moreton, S., Thompson, R., & Dickson, M. (2008). Measuring occupational performance and client priorities in the community: The COPM. *International Journal of Therapy and Rehabilitation, 15*, 22–29.

Shotwell, M., Johnson, K. R., & Flecha, I. M. (2017). Evaluation of acute care patients. In H. Smith-Gabai & S. E. Holm (Eds.), *Occupational therapy in acute care.* Bethesda, MD: American Occupational Therapy Association.

Skubik-Peplaski, C., Paris, C., Boyle, D., & Culpert, A. (2006). *Applying the occupational therapy practice framework: The Cardinal Hill occupational therapy participation process.* Bethesda, MD: American Occupational Therapy Association.

Slagle, E. C. (1922). Training aides for mental patients. *Archives of Occupational Therapy, 1*(1) 11–17.

Townsend, E. A., & Polatajko, H. J. (2007). *Enabling occupation II: Advancing an occupational therapy vision for health, well-being & justice through occupation.* Ontario, Canada: Canadian Association of Occupational Therapists.

Uniform Data System. (2010). *About the FIM system.* Retrieved from http://www.udsmr.org/WebModules/FIM/Fim_About.aspx

the Point *For additional resources on the subjects discussed in this chapter, visit* **http://thePoint.lww.com/Willard-Spackman13e.**

Critiquing Assessments

Sherrilene Classen, Craig A. Velozo

LEARNING OBJECTIVES

After reading this chapter, you will be able to:

1. Discuss the application and importance of measurement theory relative to occupational therapy assessment.
2. Describe traditional versus modern testing approaches as they relate to occupational therapy practice.
3. Describe and apply a framework to evaluate assessments by type and structure.
4. Recognize the uses of standardized versus nonstandardized tests.
5. Define and apply the concepts of reliability to occupational therapy assessments.
6. Identify the components of validity and apply that knowledge to assessments.
7. Describe the basic components of item response theory (IRT).
8. Discuss factors important in critiquing IRT-based assessments.

Introduction

This chapter provides students and occupational therapy (OT) practitioners with the basic knowledge necessary for critiquing assessment tools used in practice. As noted in Chapter 28, the use of assessment tools is inherent in the OT evaluation process because they are important sources of evidence to inform effective decision making for both therapists and clients. Additionally, the prediction and measurement of occupational performance is a cornerstone for developing evidence to enhance therapy services. Therapists must critically evaluate which assessments are best to use in a given situation, and this in turn requires an understanding of the concepts of measurement and the process of using assessment tools. Key information covered includes the concepts of measurement theory, how to evaluate potential assessment tools and their psychometric properties (including reliability, internal consistency, and validity), information on the implications of using standardized versus nonstandardized assessments, and the need to be aware if any cut points exist to understand the sensitivity and specificity of measures used. To help readers apply this information, an ongoing case study is provided featuring an occupational therapist, Karen, as she seeks to evaluate a client who is at risk in terms of driving safety.

CASE STUDY 29-1   KAREN EVALUATES A CLIENT FOR DRIVING

Karen is an occupational therapist working in a regional medical center. She needs to evaluate Mr. Patel, a patient with Parkinson disease (PD). One concern is whether Mr. Patel should continue driving. For many individuals in the United States and similar countries, the ability to drive has a far-reaching impact on community participation. Thus, Karen has to carefully select and administer the best possible assessments in order for her to make an informed recommendation to Mr. Patel, his family, and the appropriate medical and legal authorities.

Foundational to understanding measurement issues is an understanding of **classical test theory (CTT)** as well as generalizability theory approaches, which are part of traditional measurement. However, because measurement theory is advancing, Karen should also appreciate a more "revolutionary" way to think about assessing and more specifically "measuring" her client. Traditional measurement approaches continue to have a prominent role in our understanding of assessment, but modern approaches are having a significant impact on how Karen and others will assess clients, especially in the future. Therefore, this chapter includes information on both classical and modern approaches to critiquing assessments. The more modern approaches include presentations of a comparison of item response theory (IRT) to traditional test theory, advantages of IRT (efficiency and precision), linking assessments, computerized adaptive testing, and a modern approach to psychometric assessment. In this way, the chapter provides foundational information for occupational therapists to critique assessments used in everyday practice.

Traditional Approach to Critiquing Assessments

Measurement, in its simplest form, is defined as the rules for quantifying a classification of certain attributes or characteristics (Law, 1987). For example, occupational therapists use measures to reflect a child's performance in school tasks or an adult's ability to perform self-care or community living skills. The assignment of a number makes it possible to mathematically evaluate the attributes that are being measured in a standardized way. This allows comparisons about performance or capacity across individuals or groups of individuals. It also provides a way to document how an individual's performance has changed over time and across performance contexts. Because occupational therapists make judgments that affect the lives of our clients, it is an ethical responsibility to understand the strengths and limitations of any measure used as part of the evaluation process. The OT practitioner must understand aspects related to the types of assessments; their structural characteristics; and basics about construction, standardization, reliability, and validity.

Nonstandardized versus Standardized Assessments

As noted in Chapter 28, many OT evaluations include a blend of standardized and nonstandardized assessments. Although standardized assessments bring confidence in validity and reliability when used appropriately, nonstandardized assessments were, are, and will continue to be an important source of information gathering during the OT process. Luebben and Royeen argue that "every standardized assessment begins its life as a non-standardized test" and that "a new assessment moves along non-standardized continuum toward the standardize end as a result of rigorous development . . . " (as cited in Hinojosa, Kramer, & Crist, 2005, p. 125).

Nonstandardized assessments, as the name implies, do not follow a standard approach or protocol. For instance, they may not involve a consistent set of questions, directions, or conditions for administration, testing, or scoring. Such assessments may contain data collected from observations or interviews (e.g., with the referring physician, the client, or the family member) as well as during the OT evaluation via questionnaires (e.g., demographic, health, or medication) and observation of performance. Data obtained from this method are most effective when they reflect attention to the issues raised in Box 29-1 (Hinojosa et al., 2005). Additionally, this data is most useful when combined with the following approaches.

BOX 29-1   QUESTIONS TO ASK IN CRITIQUING NONSTANDARDIZED ASSESSMENTS

- Is it guided by theoretical frameworks and/or models of practice?
- Does it inform further clinical reasoning and decision making?
- Is it client centered?
- Is it a means to an end and not an end in itself?
- Is it based on having a good rapport with the client?
- Does it acknowledge the diversity of clients?

A **standardized assessment** is developed using prescribed procedures. It is administered and scored in a consistent manner under the same conditions and test directions. The standardization of test questions, directions related to performance, conditions of testing, and scoring is needed to make test scores comparable and to assure, as much as possible, that clients have equal, unbiased opportunities to demonstrate what they know and can do (Association of American Publishers, n.d.). Standardized assessments have typically undergone extensive development. Usually, the developers of such assessments provide a user manual detailing the process of development, protocol for administration, procedure for scoring, rules for interpretation, criteria or norms for performance, and the psychometric properties of the assessment. Research on the development of the assessment should be available in peer-reviewed journals to demonstrate that the quality of the assessment has been critically appraised. Box 29-2 provides a list of the different aspects of a standardized test that need to be considered in choosing an assessment, each of which is defined in the sections the follow, along with issues to consider regarding each of these factors.

Types of Assessments

Generally, assessments can be classified as descriptive, evaluative, or predictive. An assessment can be used to meet the demands of both a descriptive and an evaluative tool, for example, but for illustrative purposes, we provide examples of each type.

Descriptive Assessments

Descriptive assessments use items to describe individuals within groups and to characterize the differences between individuals on the attribute being measured. This information can be used by the therapist to assess the specific characteristics of an individual to determine if and what type of intervention is needed. An example of a descriptive assessment is the Clinical Dementia Rating, a clinical staging assessment for dementia (Morris, 1993). Broadly, it characterizes six domains of cognitive and functional performance: memory, orientation, judgment and problem solving, community affairs, home and hobbies, and personal care. The information to make each rating is obtained through a semistructured interview with a client

---

BOX 29-2 COMPONENTS TO CONSIDER WHEN CRITIQUING STANDARDIZED ASSESSMENTS

1. Type
   a. Descriptive
   b. Evaluative
   c. Predictive

2. Structural
   a. Format
   b. Cost
   c. Orientation
   d. Clinical utility

3. Construction
   a. Levels of measurement
      i. Nominal
      ii. Ordinal
      iii. Interval
      iv. Ratio

4. Psychometric evaluation
   a. Reliability (classical test theory vs. generalizability theory)
      i. Measurement error
         1. Random
         2. Systematic
         3. Sources

   ii. Type
      1. Test–retest
      2. Rater (interrater and intrarater)
      3. Internal consistency (split-half, Cronbach's alpha, Kuder-Richardson formulas)

   b. Validity (evidence to support the construct)
      i. What the instrument looks like
         1. Face
         2. Content

      ii. How the instrument acts
         1. Construct (convergent, discriminant)
         2. Criterion (concurrent, predictive)

   c. Screening
      i. Sensitivity
      ii. Specificity
      iii. Positive predictive value
      iv. Negative predictive value

   d. Item response theory
      i. Unidimensionality (fit statistics/factor analysis)
      ii. Local independence
      iii. Precision
      iv. Person-item match

5. Summary of strengths and weaknesses of the assessment

CASE STUDY 29-2   ASSESSING MR. PATEL'S DRIVING PERFORMANCE— NONSTANDARDIZED ASSESSMENT

Before selecting assessments to measure Mr. Patel's driving ability, Karen first wants to know a little more about him. Karen reviews the personal and medical history available from his chart and decides that her first step is to interview Mr. Patel to get his self-report on potential problems that may impact his driving ability. Karen also interviews his wife, asking her about his driving performance to form a more comprehensive approach of his driving abilities. As a result of her nonstandardized assessments (chart review and interviews), she finds that Mr. Patel is a 72-year-old man who is retired from business and lives in the community with his wife. He has some college after high school graduation.

Mr. Patel has had PD for 17 years and is on antiparkinsonian drugs. He also has arthritis in his knees and neck and wears trifocals to see well. He was referred by a neurologist from a movement disorders center with a concern about his continued safe driving. Mr. Patel tells Karen that he feels sleepy during the day, and she notes that he demonstrates a flat affect during the interview. He has a driver's license, drives about 3 to 4 days per week, mainly with his wife. His wife adds that he has had two citations in the last 3 years and a fender bender. Karen is now ready to think through which standardized evaluations she wishes to use to complete her initial evaluation.

and a reliable collateral source, such as a caregiver or family member. The Clinical Dementia Rating table provides descriptors that guide the clinician in making appropriate ratings based on interview data and clinical judgment. In addition to ratings on a 5-point scale for each domain (except personal care, which is rated on a 4-point scale), an overall Clinical Dementia Rating score is derived. This score is useful for globally staging the level of impairment: 0 = no impairment, 0.5 = very mild dementia, 1 = mild dementia, 2 = moderate dementia, and 3 = severe dementia (Morris, 1993).

Evaluative Assessments

Evaluative assessments use criteria or items to measure an individual's trait or attribute over time. The most appropriate characteristics included in an evaluative assessment are those that can be sensitive to change within an individual. The Simulator Sickness Questionnaire (SSQ) (Kennedy, Lane, Berbaum, & Lilienthal, 1993), used to quantify simulator sickness symptoms as a result of being exposed to a driving simulator, is an example of an evaluative measure. The SSQ can be administered at various time points during the simulator drive so that comparisons can be made to assess whether simulator sickness symptoms are increasing. This is important clinically to determine whether the client will be able to tolerate use of the simulator without becoming ill. Essentially, the SSQ rates 16 symptoms across three domains, which include the oculomotor, disorientation, and nausea domains. Clients report the degree to which they experience each symptoms on a scale from 0 to 3, with 0 = none, 1 = slight, 2 = moderate, 3 = severe. The total SSQ score is derived by using a weighted scale and a standard algorithm (a step-by-step procedure for calculations). By comparing the scores after

the first 5 minutes of driving with the scores obtained after 15 minutes of driving, the OT practitioner may be able to intervene with clients who show an increase in simulator sickness symptoms. For a description of the use of the SSQ and clinical application with returning combat veterans with mild traumatic brain injury (TBI), please see Classen and Owens (2010).

Predictive Assessments

Predictive assessments use criteria to classify individuals to predict a certain trait in comparison to set criteria. For example, a predictive tool can measure skills underlying driving performance to predict whether an older adult will be able to successfully return to driving. The Useful Field of View (UFOV), a computer-based assessment of visual attention (subtest 1), divided attention (subtest 2), and selective attention (subtest 3), is an example of a predictive assessment (Edwards et al., 2006). The first UFOV subtest involves identifying a single object (either a car or a truck) presented centrally on the touch screen. Subtest 2 (divided attention) required the client to identify a peripheral target while still attempting to correctly identify the central target (car or truck). Subtest 3 (selective attention) involves the same procedure as subtest 2, with the exception of distracter triangles being present surrounding the peripheral target. After completion, threshold scores are provided as well as a risk index (low, moderate, and high) for all tasks. Higher scores indicate longer times to process the information and thus, poorer performance. The UFOV is one of the best predictors of crash involvement and poor on-road performance for drivers with Alzheimer disease (Owsley & McGwin, 1999). The divided attention component (subtest 2) is rated as the best predictor of (at-fault) crash involvement among older adults (Owsley, McGwin, & Ball, 1998).

CASE STUDY 29-3   ASSESSING MR. PATEL'S DRIVING PERFORMANCE—SELECTING STANDARDIZED ASSESSMENTS

Knowing that advanced stages of PD can also affect cognition, especially the executive functions, Karen decides that she will have to assess Mr. Patel's general cognition. Recently, she has also read in one of her journals that divided attention, a critical important function for driving, may be affected in people with neurological disorders. Thus, Karen decides to use the Mini-Mental State Examination (MMSE) (Folstein, Folstein, & McHugh, 1975) to assess Mr. Patel's general cognition and the Trail Making Test Part B (Trails B) (Reitan, 1958) to assess Mr. Patel's divided attention, which is also known as set shifting. She is also concerned about visual changes that may have occurred as a result of the chronic neurological progression of PD as well as his impaired range of motion (ROM) due to the

arthritis in his neck and trunk. Karen decides to also include a comprehensive visual battery using the Optec 2500 visual analyzer (registered trademark of Stereo Optical Co., Inc. that measures visual acuity, peripheral vision, contrast sensitivity, depth perception, lateral and vertical phorias, and color discrimination). Finally, she used her knowledge of ROM and Manual Muscle Testing (MMT) to assess the corresponding functions in Mr. Patel's neck and trunk. All of these assessments are considered standardized, but Karen is aware that she must delve a bit deeper into the published literature as well as the assessment manuals to be sure that she has identified good measures that she is justified in using to make a reasonable fitness-to-drive recommendation for Mr. Patel.

Structure of Assessments

The previous section introduced the reader to the types of assessments. We next discuss the structure of the assessments as it pertains to its characteristics, clinical utility, and basic information on constructing items. Characteristics of the assessments may include the format, cost, and orientation of the test.

CASE STUDY 29-4   DESCRIPTIVE, PREDICTIVE, AND EVALUATIVE ASSESSMENTS

After reviewing the nature of the assessments she has selected, Karen is convinced that the Trails B is a *predictive assessment*, especially after reading in a recent article that Trails B was highly correlated with passing/failing an on-road test in people with PD (Classen et al., 2009). In the same study, Karen also read that the MMSE was moderately correlated to on-road outcomes. She is not sure if the MMSE is sufficiently predictive or not. Knowing that using the Optec 2500 visual analyzer to determine Mr. Patel's visual function can characterize his visual acuity, peripheral visual fields, contrast sensitivity, ocular movements, and depth perception, Karen decides that these assessments fit the *descriptive* criteria well. Certainly, the ROM tests as well as the MMT tests can be considered *evaluative tools*, especially because Karen can expect changes (improvements) in Mr. Patel's measures based on interventions to improve his neck and trunk mobility and strength.

Format

Assessments may appear in a paper-and-pencil format, for example, the Mini-Mental State Examination (MMSE), or as a computerized test, for example, the UFOV. Paper-and-pencil tests are very common in state, national, and international organizations, but computer-based testing (CBT) is gaining ground quickly. Some advantages of CBT include reduced administration time, fewer data entry errors, worldwide testing via the Web, and quick results (Kraut et al., 2004; Streiner & Norman, 2008a). However, limitations of CBT include questionable reliability and validity, apprehension for individuals not skilled with computers, and security of test materials.

Cost

Cost of the assessment is an important consideration because some assessment tools may be available free of charge, for example, the Craig Handicap Assessment and Reporting Technique (CHART) (Whiteneck et al., 1998). Others, such as a driving simulator, may be very expensive in terms of equipment and training costs.

Orientation

Knowledge about the *orientation*, whether the assessment is invasive or not and insight into how much cooperation from the client and/or other stakeholders is needed, must be considered. Therefore, the OT practitioner must also consider the *clinical utility* of the test.

Clinical Utility

Clinical utility refers to how *acceptable* the assessment will be among OT practitioners when used in the clinic. As such, acceptability may be influenced by the clinical

CASE STUDY 29-5   KAREN CONSIDERS ASSESSMENT CHARACTERISTICS

Karen knows that the assessment tools she has selected use paper-and-pencil method for scoring (MMSE, Trails B), with the exception of Optec 2500 visual analyzer, which is computer based. The cost of all the assessments, with the exception of the Optec 2500 visual analyzer machine, is reasonably low. Luckily, Karen's facility has invested in the Optec to measure the visual function of the low-vision clients; thus, no further financial expenses are incurred for her to use this assessment. She also realizes that the ROM and MMT may be a little invasive because they require hands-on testing, but it is important to assess whether such functions are impaired in Mr. Patel because they are important for neck and trunk movement during driving, especially during backup

functions. She doesn't think that it will pose a problem and thus is satisfied that she has identified tools that are feasible to use in her setting.

Karen is confident that all the assessments that she has chosen will help her clinical reasoning to assess Mr. Patel's abilities important for driving performance. She has calculated that it will take her about 28 minutes to assess Mr. Patel's visual (15 minutes with the Optec), cognitive (5 minutes for the MMSE and 3 minutes for Trails B), and physical abilities (gross MMT and ROM for 5 minutes). True to following a client-centered approach, she discusses the type of assessments with Mr. Patel, and he concurs to participate as she conducts this part of her evaluation.

applicability of the assessment (usefulness of the assessment for making interpretations to facilitate interventions), time demands (time to complete the assessment, time allocated to scoring of the test, and time required to be trained to administer the assessment), and acceptability of the assessment to the clients (Rudman & Hannah, 1998).

In general, OT practitioners need to make decisions regarding which test to use (descriptive, evaluative, or predictive) based on the specific purpose of the assessment, characteristics of the assessment, and clinical utility of the tool, including the practical steps in administering the tool.

Construction

Construction of a test pertains to devising or writing the items in such a way that they will match the purpose of the assessment. For a more detailed discussion on aspects of construction, please go to thePoint and see the document entitled "Constructing Assessments." Items can be constructed to include different levels of measurement, discussed next in detail. Refer to Box 29-3 for a summary of measurement levels and scales. These are important because they dictate the kinds of statistical analyses that can be done using the assessment results across clients. It is helpful to realize that measurement exists on different levels and that the scale itself limits or determines the analysis of the data. For example, if ordinal data are to be analyzed, then the scale from which these data are derived must contain defined ranks and intervals to approximate rank order. Moreover, critiquing measures must be pursued with knowledge of its rules, the nature of the trait being measured, and a consideration of the purpose of measuring.

In addition to how a test is constructed, a psychometric evaluation or an empirical way to evaluate the quality of the assessment tool must include testing related to **reliability** (Does the test yield the same or similar scores consistently?), **external validity** (Can generalizations be made to the general population?), **internal validity** (Does the assessment measure what it is supposed to measure [i.e., a specific trait, behavior, construct, or performance?]), **sensitivity** (predictor test's ability to obtain a positive test when the condition really exists), and **specificity** (predictor test's ability to obtain a negative test when the condition does not exist). Each of these components of the psychometric evaluation is discussed next.

Reliability—Traditional Approaches

Reliability pertains to the reproducibility of test results and the amount of variation measured that is real and not due to error. Reliability, generally, is based on a correlation coefficient or a measure of agreement and referred to as a reliability coefficient, which can range from 0 to ± 1 (0 = no reliability and 1 = perfect reliability). Two theoretical concepts related to reliability are CTT and generalizability theory.

Classical test theory, also called classical reliability theory, centers around the notion that each observation or test score has a single true score and yields a single reliability coefficient (Nunnally & Bernstein, 1994). Classical test theory postulates that a test score has two components: the true score and the measurement error score. Although many sources of error exist, only one source (e.g., either the rater or the assessment itself) is estimated; meaning

BOX 29-3   SCALES OF MEASUREMENT

Assigning numbers to traits results in measurement scales. The four scales of measurement are nominal, ordinal, interval, and ratio (Portney & Watkins, 2009).

- **Nominal.** The nominal scale represents the first level of measurement. This involves mutually exclusive categories (e.g., female vs. male, driving vs. nondriving). Assigned numbers are simply used as labels or means of identification with no attempt to quantify or order the differences.
- **Ordinal.** A second level is the ordinal scale. In this scale, the numbers represent the relative rank order of the trait under investigation. For example, driving evaluators often use a Global Rating Scale, indicating whether a client who has taken an on-road test should fail = 1, fail with options for remediation = 2, pass with recommendations = 3, or pass = 4 (Justiss, Mann, Stav, & Velozo, 2006). The assigned numbers merely indicate the rank order; they do not represent absolute quantities, and the intervals between the ranks cannot be presumed equal. In this example, someone who is passing the on-road test is not twice as competent as someone who is passing with recommendations. Thus, no inference can be made about the magnitude of the difference between scores.
- **Interval.** The interval scales represent the third level. The intervals between scores are equal so that comparisons can be made between individuals. Also, characteristic of an interval scale is that there is no true zero value.

An example of an interval scale that is commonly used in OT surveys is the bipolar (goes in both directions) Likert scale (e.g., 0 = strongly disagree, 1 = disagree, 2 = agree, 3 = strongly agree) and the unipolar (goes in one direction) adjectival scale, (e.g., 0 = cannot do, 1 = very difficult, 2 = somewhat difficult, 3 = a little difficult, 4 = not difficult).[a] Although a client can get the lowest value (a zero) on a driving assessment that uses the adjectival scale, there is no true "absence of driving safety." Although not having an absolute zero limits some mathematical operations, most psychometric operations such as calculations of means and standard deviations are commonly performed on interval scales.

- **Ratio.** The ratio scales reflect the fourth and highest level scale in measurement. It has equal distances but, in addition, has a meaningful zero point. The zero point indicates a total absence of whatever trait is being measured. To use these scales, absence of the attribute being measured must be meaningful. Range of motion (ROM) measurements assessed by a trained clinician with standardized equipment, such as a goniometer, will yield ratio data. All mathematical operations can be accomplished with a ratio scale data (addition, subtraction, multiplication, division) and statistical (means, standard deviations, and standard errors) calculations. In this case, it is correct to indicate that a person has gained twice as much movement between measurements of 20° elbow flexion and 40° elbow flexion.

[a]Some measurement experts believe that Likert scales are not interval scales. Although Likert scales look like they are interval in nature, for example, the distance between a value of 1 to 2 and 2 to 3 are equal, we cannot be assured that there are equal distances between the qualifiers that these numbers represent (e.g., maximum assistance, moderate assistance, and minimum assistance) (Bond & Fox, 2007).

that the difference therefore between the observed score and the true score is due to random error (Portney & Watkins, 2009). This model is overly restrictive and often unrealistic in situations where there may be multiple sources of error. Examples of multiple error sources include differences among raters (see interrater reliability) and differences in testing context (e.g., driving assessed in one's own car or driving assessed in an evaluator's car). Additionally, measures themselves are heterogeneous (e.g., driving can be operationalized, and therefore measured, in various ways such as driving awareness, driving behaviors, driving confidence, driving habits, driving fitness, driving performance, and/or driving safety).

Generalizability theory provides a framework for conceptualizing, investigating, and designing reliable observations. It was originally introduced by Cronbach and colleagues (Cronbach, Gleser, Nanda, & Rajaratnam, 1972; Cronbach, Nageswari, & Gleser, 1963) in response

to the limitations of CTT. Generalizability theory recognizes different sources of error and attempts to quantify the sources from those various errors. So, not all variations in the administration of an assessment are attributed to random error. Relevant testing conditions that may influence test scores are identified (e.g., time of day such as driving in the midmorning vs. driving in peak traffic where there are many more demands from the driving environment). In identifying the different sources of error, one may be better able to identify why an assessment score changes and thus provide additional explanations beyond the assumption of random error (Portney & Watkins, 2009).

Measurement Error

Measurement error arises when there is a difference between the true value, such as one's absolute weight measured with a precise scale (e.g., an electronic scale in a doctor's office), and the observed value (e.g., weight as measured by a spring-based bathroom scale). The observed value (X) is therefore a function of two components: a true score (T) and an error component (E), expressed as

$$\text{Observed Score} = \text{True Score} \pm \text{Error}$$
$$X = T \pm E$$

Error can appear as random error or systematic error. *Random error* is represented by inconsistencies that cannot be predicted, for example, fatigue or mechanical inaccuracy of the measurement assessment, causing the error. *Systematic error* refers to predictable fluctuations occurring during measurement. Systematic error may occur in design flaws such as subject selection, for example, recruiting from a pool of clients that includes individuals only from low socioeconomic backgrounds. Usually, systematic errors occur in one direction and consistently overestimate or underestimate the true score. When the error is identified, it may be easier to manage or correct the systematic error compared to when random error occurs as outlined in Box 29-4.

BOX 29-4	SOURCES OF SYSTEMATIC MEASUREMENT ERROR

- The individual taking the measurements (e.g., raters or evaluators that are biased in expecting the client to have improved due to driving training)
- The measurement assessment (e.g., poorly calibrated mechanical parts of a driving simulator)
- The variability of the characteristics being measured (e.g., ROM when measured early in the morning may be different than when measured late in the day)

Types of Reliability

There are several different types of reliability that reported related to assessments. See Table 29-1 for a synopsis of reliability testing.

TABLE 29-1	Reliability by Type, Use, Source or Error, and Method of Testing

Type	Use	Sources of Error	Method to Test
Test–retest reliability	Test is given to the same people after a period of time.	How time, changes in the construct, reactivity, over or underestimation, and changes in the environment effect the reliability of a measure.	Intraclass correlation coefficient (ICC)[a]
Rater reliability	To illustrate the stability of data collected.		ICC or kappa
• *Intrarater reliability*	To illustrate the stability of data collected by one rater on two or more trials over time.	Tool administration procedures, calibration of instrument, untrained rater, recall, or other forms of bias	ICC or kappa
• *Interrater reliability*	To determine rater variability between two or more raters who measure the same clients.	The effect of time, rater interaction with the client, or variables that may influence observation skills of the raters	ICC or kappa
Internal consistency	To determine the degree of agreement between the items in a test that measure an underlying trait or construct.		Cronbach's coefficient alpha
• *Alternate form*	Tests the same group of people on two separate occasions using two distinct but parallel forms of the test.	Length of the test	ICC
• *Split-halves*	The same group of people partakes in the test where the total set of items in the test is divided in half.	Method of splitting	Spearman-Brown Prophecy statistic
• *Cronbach's alpha or Kuder-Richardson formulas*	To estimate the reliability of scales or commonality of one item in a test with other items in a test.	Consistency of content of test	Cronbach's coefficient alpha

[a]A perfect correlation is indicated by a correlation coefficient expressed as $r = 1.0$, $p \leq .05$. A strong correlation is indicated if $r \geq 0.75$, a moderate correlation if $r = 0.50$ but < 0.75, and weaker correlation if $r < 0.50$ when $p \leq .05$. Also note that acceptability of correlation strength may vary according to the purpose for reliability testing. For example, one may tolerate lower reliability estimates to indicate differences/similarities of groups, but values required for making accurate predictions in terms of diagnoses will need to have a high correlation coefficient. Correlations can be conducted with various methods, such as kappa and ICC through Cronbach's coefficient alpha (Portney & Watkins, 2009).

Test–Retest Reliability

The test–retest method estimates the reliability or stability of measurements when the same test is given to the same people after a period of time. One obtains a correlation between scores on the two administrations of the same test. It is presumed that responses to the test will correlate because they reflect the same true score; however, the correlation of measurements across time will be less than perfect. This may occur because of *instability* of measurements taken over various time points. For example, a client may be distracted, have a bad (or a good) day, or be influenced by the test administrator (Carmines & Zeller, 1979; Portney & Watkins, 2009). Other factors that can influence (increase or decrease) test–retest reliability are the following:

- *A construct may change*, such as the influence of environmental changes, for example, the use of in-vehicle technology, on the driving task and thus the fitness to drive construct (please see detailed discussion under "Construct Validity" section).
- *Reactivity*, or change in the measured trait or behavior occurring as a result of the testing. For example, drivers may alter their performance due to their awareness of being observed. Therefore, drivers may perform more optimally when driving with a driving evaluator than when they drive by themselves under natural conditions.
- *Overestimation or underestimation*. It is well known in the driving literature that older drivers (and most other drivers) overestimate their driving ability as they report that they are better drivers than what they really are when compared to their performance on a road test. Similarly, older drivers may underestimate number of citations received when their self-report data are compared to official citation records.

Rater Reliability

Intrarater reliability refers to the stability of data collected by one rater on two or more trials over time. The objective nature of scientific inquiry demands that even when experts are used, that intrarater reliability should be tested. Error in this type of reliability can be reduced by training the rater in the use of the tool(s), using the tool administration procedures, calibrating measurement assessments, training rater skills to avoid deterioration over time, and assessing the rater for bias based on memory, training, views, and/or assumptions. Developing objective grading criteria may be conducive to limiting measurement error occurring as a result of intrarater reliability (Hinojosa et al., 2005; Portney & Watkins, 2009).

Interrater reliability concerns detecting rater variability between two or more raters who measure the same clients (Portney & Watkins, 2009). To establish interrater reliability, it is best for the raters to view the same clients at the same point in time. In driving research, for example, the use of a driving simulator, which allows for video playback versus on-road testing, is particularly helpful for raters to rate a subject and useful for researchers to establish interrater reliability. Not only can one include a wide variety of raters with this testing method but also disagreements among the raters may be resolved through consensus and rewatching the video. Should the raters test the client during an on-road driving test, their scores may be influenced by their seating position in the vehicle as well as the interaction of the evaluator with the tester. For example, the optimal seating position for the driving evaluator is the right front seat and the worst seating position is the back left seat because observation of many driver responses, such as eye movements or positioning of the vehicle, may be restricted as a result of the seating position. Likewise, the evaluator that is providing travel directions to the driver may rate the driver differently than the raters without any interaction with the driver.

Internal Consistency

Internal consistency determines the degree of agreement between the items in a test that measure an underlying trait or construct. It is essentially an estimation of the *homogeneity* of the test. Ways to test for internal consistency are alternate form, split-halves, Cronbach's alpha, or Kuder-Richardson formulas.

- *Alternate form* tests the same group of people on two separate occasions using two distinct but parallel forms of the test. Although more expensive and time consuming, because two forms of the test need to be developed, this method is obviously superior to test–retest method. Specifically, it reduces the effect to which the individual's memory can bias the results (i.e., result in improved score due to recall of the test questions) and therefore also the strength of the correlation.
- In contrast to the alternate form method, the *split-halves method* can be conducted in one time period. Specifically, the same group of people partakes in the test wherein the total set of items in the test is divided in half. The scores on the halves are then correlated to obtain an estimate of reliability. One limitation is that the manner in which the items are subdivided will affect the reliability coefficient (Carmines & Zeller, 1979; Portney & Watkins, 2009; Streiner & Norman, 2008b). The Spearman-Brown prophecy formula, a statistical method, can be used to correct for such incongruent results (Carmines & Zeller, 1979).
- *Cronbach's alpha* (also referred to as *coefficient alpha*) and *Kuder-Richardson formulas* are used to estimate

the reliability of scales or commonality of one item in a test with other items in a test. The difference is that Cronbach's alpha is used when the test scale is composed of *nondichotomous* responses (i.e., rating scale), whereas the Kuder-Richardson formulas is used for *dichotomously* scored items (e.g., correct/incorrect). Essentially, the purpose of applying these formulas is to identify the items that do not contribute to the overall construct that are being measured and therefore, such items may be lowering a test's reliability. The reader is referred to select references (Carmines & Zeller, 1979; Portney & Watkins, 2009; Streiner & Norman, 2008a) for more information on these methods.

Validity—Traditional Approaches

Validity is defined as the extent to which any assessment measures what it is intended to measure. The definition of validity is straightforward, but it is imperative to realize that although an assessment may yield valid data when being used to measure certain population traits under certain conditions, the same assessment may not be replicated if traits of a different population are being measured. Likewise, the same assessment may not be replicated if the same population is being measured under different conditions. For example, the Driving Habits Questionnaire has been developed and tested psychometrically for use among older adults in a research setting (Owsley, Stalvey, Wells, & Sloane, 1999). As such, if this tool is being used in a group of novice drivers (different population), or used to record the history of night driving in older drivers (different conditions), the validity may be impacted. The question then becomes *if the assessment is still valid when measuring attributes of different populations or the same population but under different conditions*. The practitioner need to cautiously consider these aforementioned points before using an assessment.

To determine the accuracy of a measurement tool, one may ask what the assessment *looks* like and also how it *acts*. The "look" pertains to whether the assessment has *face validity* (e.g., Does it overall look like the assessment is measuring what it is supposed to measure?) and/or *content validity* (e.g., Do expert raters rate the items in that they are comprehensively represent the content area?). The "act" pertains to a more rigorous process in assessment development that includes *construct validity*, or how the assessment compares to other assessments measuring the same construct (*convergent*) or different (*divergent*) constructs, as well as *criterion validity*, which may be *concurrent* (measured at the same point in time) or *predictive* (measured at some point in future). See Table 29-2 for a synopsis of validity.

| TABLE 29-2 | **Validity by Type, Use, and Method to Test and Strength of Estimate** |

Type	Use	Method to Test	Strength of Estimate
Face validity	Is the measure testing what it is supposed to measure? Are the items plausible?	Peer review	No statistical inference testing
Content validity	Does the measurement instrument reflect a specific domain of content?	Content validity index (CVI)	CVI ≥ 80%
Construct validity	Does the assessment measure a construct and the theoretical components underlying the construct?	Tests of correlation	Higher correlation coefficients are better, thus $r \geq 0.80$, $p \geq .05$.
• *Convergent validity*	Is the level of agreement between two tests that are being used to measure the same construct acceptable?	Tests of correlation	Higher correlation coefficients are better, thus $r \geq 0.80$, $p \leq .05$.
• *Discriminant validity*	Is the level of disagreement (poor or zero correlation) when two tests measure a trait, behavior, or characteristic acceptable?	Tests of correlation	Higher correlation coefficients are better, thus $r \geq 0.80$, $p \leq .05$.
Criterion validity	Can the outcome of one assessment be used as a substitute test to the established *gold standard criterion* test?	Prediction methods	See below
• *Concurrent validity*	Do the results of a criterion measure and a target test, given at the same relative time point, concur with one another?	Receiver operating characteristics (ROC) curves	Area under the curve (AUC) ≥ 0.70, with $p \leq .05$
• *Predictive validity*	Does the outcome of a target test predict a future criterion score or outcome?	Prediction methods, for example, regression analyses	The higher the R^2 in the prediction model, the better the validity.

NOTE: The above statistical tests are examples to illustrate the points raised. To evaluate validity, other methods may be explored with biostatistician or psychometrician colleagues because the reader gets more accomplished in applying principles of validity testing.

Face Validity

Face validity indicates that a measure is testing what it is supposed to and that the items are viewed as plausible. No statistical manipulation of the data is involved in this process, and the measure is peer reviewed (i.e., reviewed by experts in the field) to determine plausibility of the items. For example, in the development of the items of the Safe Driving Behavioral Measure (SDBM), face validity was tested by asking a group of doctoral students and researchers to evaluate the chosen items based on ease of reading, content, clarity, appropriateness, and time that it took to answer the items. Recommendations from the peer review were followed in refining the items prior to content validity testing (Classen et al., 2010).

Content Validity

Fundamentally, **content validity** depends on the extent to which an empirical measurement reflects a specific domain of content. Following the guidelines of Lynn (1986), Classen and colleagues (2010) invited four expert raters to complete a *content validity index* (CVI)—an index of consensus related to the relevance of the items—on each of the items in the SDBM. Apart from rating each SDBM item on a 4-point Likert scale (1 = not relevant, 2 = relevant with major revisions, 3 = relevant with minor revisions, and 4 = very relevant), the experts also gave feedback on item accuracy, purpose, organization, clarity, appearance, understandability, and adequacy (Grant & Davis, 1997). Usually, content validity can be claimed if the rater agreement on the item relevance is 80% or higher (House, House, & Campbell, 1981).

Construct Validity

Construct validity establishes whether the assessment measures a construct and the theoretical components underlying the construct. A construct is an abstract idea that we cannot observe directly. Many, if not all, occupational assessments measure abstract ideas that we can only indirectly observe through behaviors. For example, we cannot directly observe job satisfaction but can indirectly assess it by direct observation (e.g., watching an individual in a job situation) or through questionnaires (e.g., asking the client his or her satisfaction with different aspects of his or her job). Two different types of construct validity can be established, *convergent* and *discriminant*.

• **Convergent validity** is the level of agreement between two tests that are being used to measure the same construct. For example, if one wants to determine if *lane maintenance* is challenging for a novice driver, one may test the driver on a driving simulator and on the road. Should there be a high correlation between lane maintenance under these two testing conditions (simulator and

on road), one may infer construct validity pertaining to the lane maintenance aspect of driving.

• **Discriminant validity** is the level of disagreement (poor or zero correlation) when two tests measure a trait, behavior, or characteristic. Let's assume that community-dwelling older drivers are screened before taking an on-road test. The driving rehabilitation specialist will administer an MMSE to assess cognitive functioning and a visual acuity test to assess distant vision before participating in an on-road test (Folstein et al., 1975; Folstein, Folstein, White, & Messer, 2010). A successful evaluation of discriminant validity will show that the test of cognition (MMSE) is poorly correlated with a test of visual acuity because these tests are designed to measure different concepts.

The process of establishing construct validity involves at least three steps (Carmines & Zeller, 1979):

1. Determine the theoretical relationship between the concepts themselves.
2. Determine the empirical relationship between the measures of the concepts.
3. Interpret the empirical evidence to clarify the construct validity of a measure.

This is a challenge to researchers as a construct, for example, safe driving is an *abstract* idea and is *multidimensional* (e.g., includes aspects of the driver, the vehicle, and the environment). Testing the construct is an ongoing process, and statistical methods used may include factor analysis or hypothesis testing, next described.

• **Factor analysis** is based on the idea that a construct contains one or more dimensions or theoretical components. As such, thinking about safe driving, one may assume that at least three dimensions are involved to execute a driving maneuver such as exiting a ramp and merging with traffic. Those are the person dimension (e.g., vision, cognition, and motor functions), the environment dimension (e.g., highway ramp, lanes on highway, traffic, weather, light), and the vehicle dimension (e.g., roadworthiness of vehicle and working status of all vehicle controls). Factor analysis helps to tease out the underlying dimensions of an assessment by grouping variables or items that correlate highly with one another.

• **Hypothesis testing** can be used to determine if an assessment can distinguish between people at different levels of safe driving. For example, one may postulate that older women who resume driving after the death of a spouse may have a greater number of errors related to driving skills when compared to older men who are the primary drivers in a family. If the assessment is able to detect such differences and affirm the hypothesis, one may infer construct validity pertaining to the population for the given test conditions.

Challenges to construct validity may include *changes in the environment or society over time* which influences the construct of the measurement tool. For example the Fitness-to-Drive Screening Measure (FTDS), developed from 2008 to 2015 (Classen, Velozo, Winter, Bédard, & Wang, 2015) included items reflective of fitness to drive, prior to the onset of the semiautonomous or autonomous revolution currently evolving in the automobile industry (Denaro, Zmud, Shladover, Walker Smith, & Lappin, 2014). These days, many vehicles are equipped with in vehicle technologies such as advance driver assistance systems (ADAS) or in-vehicle information systems (IVIS) (Alvarez & Classen, 2017). *ADAS,* for example, a collision avoidance system, are integrated systems that can directly help drivers with vehicle control, especially in high-risk situations (Wilschut, 2009). *IVIS, such as* a lane departure warning system with haptic (vibration) feedback, are technologies that provide information or warnings to drivers but do not assume functions related to driving tasks such as steering, accelerating, or braking. The use of such technologies may impact fitness to drive abilities. The absence of including items that accurately reflect a presence of ADAS or IVIS may compromise the construct validity and the stability of the FTDS. This (not having items reflective of ADAS or IVIS) is no small matter as this screening tool is making *predictions* on the risk probability of older adults' fitness to drive abilities. The construct validity of an instrument (in this case using items reflective of the fitness to drive construct) contributes to the ability to predict the risk associated with fitness to drive. Because construct validity is a key factor in prediction of an outcome, systematic measurement error may be introduced if the FTDS does not reflect inclusion of ADAS and IVIS items.

Criterion Validity

Criterion validity implies that the outcome of one assessment can be used as a substitute test for the established gold standard criterion test. Criterion validity can be tested as concurrent validity or predictive validity.

- *Concurrent validity* is inferred when two measures, the criterion measure and a target test, are given at relatively the same point in time and the results of the two tests concur with one another. Most often, when proven more efficient and/or cost-effective than the criterion test, the target test may be used as a substitute for the gold standard test. Currently, a comprehensive driving evaluation (CDE) conducted by a driving rehabilitation specialist is considered the industry or gold standard to determine driving ability (Di Stefano & Macdonald, 2005). However, the CDE is expensive, time consuming, offers limited access (i.e., presently, there is a shortage of driving rehabilitation specialists), and invites an element of risk because it is conducted in the real world. To overcome many of these challenges, researchers are investigating the concurrent validity between the driving simulator and the CDE (Bédard, Parkkari, Weaver, Riendeau, & Dahlquist, 2010; Shechtman, Classen, Awadzi, & Mann, 2009).

- *Predictive validity* establishes that the outcome of a target test can be used to predict a future criterion score or outcome. For example, in a review of vision impairment and driving, the UFOV was shown to be one of the best predictors of crash involvement as tested in a simulator and on road (gold standard criterion) in drivers with Alzheimer disease (Owsley et al., 1998). Thus, one may infer that the UFOV has predictive validity with the criterion (on-road testing) for the population under study.

Ecological Validity

Ecological validity implies that the outcome of an assessment can "hold up" in the real-world circumstances. For example, if Mr. Patel, our case study participant, is deemed to be able to drive based on the findings of an assessment, one must ask if that assessment outcome will also hold true in the real world. If so, one can infer ecological validity.

Screening Tools

Many assessments are specifically developed for the purposes of being used as a *screening* tool. A screening is a brief measure that tests the presence or absence of a disease, condition, or an outcome. Because screening tools are often used by clinicians to determine if a client will require further treatment, it is very important to verify their validity (see Box 29-5 and Figure 29-1 for an example).

Sensitivity and Specificity

Sensitivity is defined as the predictor test's ability to obtain a positive test when the condition really exists (a true-positive). For example, when a predictor test suggests that the client will fail an on-road test, and this prediction is then verified by the actual outcome of the on-road test, sensitivity is evident. **Specificity** is defined as the predictor test's ability to obtain a negative result when the condition is really absent (a true-negative). An example here is if the predictor test suggests that the client should pass, and this result is then verified by the client passing the on-road test (Portney & Watkins, 2009).

Positive and Negative Predictive Value

Positive predictive value is the probability of the client, given a certain cut point on the predictor test to fail in the actual situation (e.g., the on-road test). **Negative predictive value** is the probability of the client, given a cut point on the predictor test, to pass (in this case to pass the on-road test). It is important to note that the number of false-positives (those who receive a failing score but pass the road test) and false-negatives (those who receive a passing score but fail the road test) and thus the sensitivity and specificity

CASE STUDY 29-6   KAREN CRITIQUES HER ASSESSMENTS AND COMPLETES HER EVALUATION

Karen is ready to critique her assessments. She has developed a matrix displayed in Table 29-3 and included information from the published studies that she has read to assess if she is on the right track.

Karen has chosen assessments with a structure that is conducive to Mr. Patel's needs. Two of the assessments (Trials B, ROM) provide interval-level data, two more (MMSE, Vision) ratio data, and the other (MMT) ordinal data. Even though not all the components of reliability and validity are known (through the publications that she has read), the overall psychometrics of the tools are acceptable and suggesting that Karen's decision to use these tools is evidence based.

Karen proceeds to assess Mr. Patel using the MMSE and Trails B. She also assesses his vision with the Optec 2500 along with selected ROM and MMT pertinent to driving. From these results, she finds that he is demonstrating some mild difficulty with divided attention, impaired contrast sensitivity, and limitations in his neck and trunk mobility. All these impairments may affect Mr. Patel's ability to continue to drive. Based on these results, she recommends an on-road driving evaluation to be conducted by a certified driving rehabilitation specialist, both to determine a baseline for his driving performance and to make recommendations for any modifications, adaptations, compensatory strategies, or referrals (e.g., to an ophthalmologist) needed to assure appropriate fitness-to-drive abilities.

TABLE 29-3   Matrix to Critique Assessments

| | Structure | | | | Level of Measurement | | | | Psychometrics | | | | | | |
| | | | | | | | | | Reliability | | | Validity | | | |
Assessment	Format	Cost	Orientation	Clinical Utility	Nominal	Ordinal	Ratio	Interval	Test-retest	Rater Reliability	Internal Consistency	Face	Content	Construct	Criterion
MMSE	x	x	x	x			R		x	x	?	x	x	x	x
Trails B	x	x	x	x				I	x	x	x	x	x	x	x
Vision	x	x	x	x			R		x	?	?	x	x	x	x
ROM	x	x	x	x				I	x	x	?	x	x	x	?
MMT	x	x	x	x		O			x	x	?	x	x	x	?

NOTE: The "x" indicates a positive response to reflect that the component of the assessment that is being rated is acceptable. The "?" indicates that the component of the assessment being rated is not known.
I, interval; R, ratio; O, ordinal; MMSE, Mini-Mental State Examination; MMT, Manual Muscle Testing; ROM, range of motion.

values, change with the cutoff value. Ultimately, one wants the false-positives and false-negatives to be as close to zero as possible. The formulas for calculating these values are well described in many of the texts cited in this chapter.

Modern Approaches to Critiquing Assessments

Although most OT clinicians and researchers have been trained on traditional psychometric methods (CTT and generalizability theory), unfortunately, these approaches have several shortcomings. First, traditional assessments generate *scores* versus *measures*. Scores are simply the sum of the frequency of answers marked as "correct" or if using a Likert or adjectival scale, the sum of the ratings of each item. Although our scores on our assessments may look more sophisticated when converted into a percentage of the total score, in essence, they still simply reflect a frequency count. Second, the traditional analyses are specific to the sample from which they were derived. That is, although most researchers report on the reliability and validity of an assessment as if it is a stable characteristic, it is not. Reliability and validity are *sample dependent*. That is, reliability and validity values are unique to the

BOX 29-5   USING EVIDENCE TO EVALUATE SCREENING TOOLS: AN EXAMPLE FROM THE LITERATURE

Occupational therapists are encouraged to make decisions regarding screening tools by examining the evidence that the tool is effective to predict the relevant criterion outcome. For example, in a pilot study with 19 drivers with Parkinson disease (PD) who underwent a clinical battery of tests and an on-road driving test, the researchers wanted to determine which of the screening tests were most predictive of those clients who failed the on-road test. Figure 29-1 demonstrates how to calculate sensitivity, specificity, positive predictive value, and negative predictive value for the Useful Field of View (UFOV) Risk Index in 3-point cutoff value ($N = 19$ drivers with PD). The researchers determined that the sensitivity (true-positives or those drivers with PD who really failed the road test and who were predicted to fail by the UFOV) was 87%. The specificity (true-negative or those drivers with PD who really passed the road test and who were predicted to pass by the UFOV) was 82%. The positive predictive value (probability of the driver with PD, given a cut point of 3 on the UFOV Risk Index to fail the on-road test) was 78%. The negative predictive value (probability of the PD drivers, given a cut point of 3 on the UFOV Risk Index to pass the on-road test) was 90%. In this study, the authors concluded that among this sample of drivers with PD tested and compared to other clinical measures of disease, cognition, and vision, the UFOV was a superior screening measure for predicting on-road outcomes (Classen et al., 2009).

Global rating scale (fail/pass)

	+ (FAIL)	− (PASS)
+ (UFOV ≥3)	a true-positives (hits) [n=7]	b false-positives (misses) [n=2]
− (UFOV ≤3)	c false-negatives (false alarms) [n=1]	d true-negatives (correct rejections) [n=9]

(UFOV risk index)

FIGURE 29-1 Calculating sensitivity, specificity, positive predictive value, negative predictive value, and error for the Useful Field of View (UFOV) Risk Index value of 3 ($N = 19$ drivers with Parkinson disease). Sensitivity = $a / (a + c)$ [$7 / (7 + 1) = 0.87$]; specificity = $d / (b + d)$ [$9 / (2 + 9) = 0.82$]; positive predictive value = $a / (a + b)$ [$7 / (7 + 2) = 0.78$]; negative predictive value = $d / (c + d)$ [$9 / (1 + 10) = 0.90$]; total error = $1 - $ sensitivity $ + 1 - $ specificity [$0.13 + 0.18 = 0.31$].

particular sample from which they were derived. Although impractical, every time we use an assessment for a clinical population or research study, we should reevaluate the reliability of that assessment.

Third, scores are *test dependent*. That is, a score on one assessment cannot be readily translated to a score on a second assessment. For example, a score of 50 on one road test does not carry the same meaning as a score of a 50 on any other road test. Test scores are dependent on the difficulty of the items (tasks or questions) of the assessment. An individual with a particular level of ability (e.g., who can drive well only in his or her home town) will get a low score on a challenging driving assessment (e.g., one that only involves complex driving situations such as negotiating traffic in peak traffic hours) and a high score on an easy driving assessment (e.g., one that only involves simple driving situations such as putting the car in gear and pulling out of the driveway). Finally, in most cases, traditional assessments require the client to take all items of the assessment. Obviously, if a client takes fewer of the items and the items are summed for a total score, he or she will get a lower score on the assessment, even though his or her ability has not changed.

In recent years, there have been dramatic advances in measurement theory in health care. Modern test theory (MTT), more commonly referred to as IRT and Rasch measurement theory, which emerged from the field of education, has had dramatic impact on clinical assessments in OT and health care (Cella & Chang, 2000). For purposes of this chapter, we use the term *item response theory*. Several OT assessments have been developed using IRT methods, as shown in Box 29-6. The purpose of this part of the chapter is to introduce IRT or Rasch measurement theory and its applications in critiquing OT assessments.

Item Response Theory

In contrast to traditional psychometrics that focuses on the entire "test," IRT, as the name implies, focuses on the items of the test. As a measurement theory, IRT addresses many limitations of traditional test theory. First, IRT is *sample free*. That is, one should expect that the results from an IRT analysis should be the same no matter what sample is chosen from a population. Second, IRT is *test free*. The basis of an assessment being test free is that in IRT, the items of an

EXAMPLES OF OCCUPATIONAL THERAPY ASSESSMENTS USING ITEM RESPONSE THEORY METHODS

- Assessment of Motor and Process Skills (AMPS) (A. G. Fisher, 1993)
- School AMPS (Munkholm, Löfgren, & Fisher, 2012)
- Fitness-to-Drive Screening Measure (Classen et al., 2015)
- Occupational Performance History Interview (Kielhofner, Dobria, Forsyth, & Basu, 2005)
- Pediatric Evaluation of Disability Inventory (Haley, Ludlow, & Coster, 1993)
- School Function Assessment (Coster, Deeney, Haltiwanger, & Haley, 1998).
- DriveSafe and DriveAware (Kay, Bundy & Clemson, 2009)

assessment measure a latent trait. A *latent trait* is a hypothesized construct or attribute that is not directly observed but is inferred from responses on an assessment (Smith, 2000). For example, driving, as assessed by a specific driving assessment, is represented by the particular items from that assessment. Tasks such as stopping at stoplights, turning at an intersection, and passing another vehicle on a highway only represent a small sample of the almost infinite number of driving tasks that can represent the latent trait of driving. Finally, in contrast to scores (frequency counts) generated from traditional assessments that are only ordinal in nature, the measures generated for some IRT models are interval in nature. Note that we are using the term *scores* to refer to the numbers obtained from traditional assessments and the term *measures* for values derived from IRT-based assessments. That is, measures have equal intervals between their values (i.e., there are equal "distances" between a one and two, two and three, etc.). Interval-level data are necessary for any level of mathematics, from the simplest addition of two numbers to complicated statistical analyses.

The aforementioned unique characteristics of IRT offer advantages of measurement that have not been achievable with traditional psychometric approaches. First, because IRT is sample free, norms are not *necessary* for measurement. That does not mean that norms are unimportant in OT. On the contrary, for example, developmental norms are extremely important in determining if a client is within the range of what is "normal" or "typical," as for instance, for a developing child. But norms are not necessary for measurement (i.e., norms are not necessary to determine if you have more or less of something). Because IRT is sample

free, an assessment should perform the same way for every sample from a particular population. That is, the relative challenge of the items on an instrument should have the same difficulty for every sample taken from a population. For example, for the population of elder drivers, predriving skills (e.g., opening a car door, inserting a key into the ignition) will always be easier than on-the-road driving skills (e.g., taking left-hand turns against traffic, merging onto a highway), independent of whether they have low or high driving ability. When using IRT, one should be confident that measures are replicable across different samples.

Advantages of Item Response Theory

Because IRT is test free, two important advantages arise. First, it is unnecessary to use all the items from an assessment to measure a client. Although typically, when using traditional assessments, one sums the responses on all the items of the assessment to determine the "ability" of the client, with IRT, instead of using all the items or an assessment, one can use only the most relevant items to measure a particular client. Figure 29-2 shows items of different challenge for driving. Items to the far left (obey traffic lights and stay in proper lane) represent easy driving items, and items to the far right (drive at night and drive in heavy wind and rain) represent hard items. For example, if an individual is capable of driving in heavy wind and rain, he or she is very likely to be capable of obeying traffic lights and staying in proper lane. If a client is successful at a more challenging task, it is unnecessary to test them on a very easy task. This feature of IRT provides considerable efficiency for both the client and therapist. Clients do not have to be burdened by taking all the items of an assessment, and therapists can save time by only assessing items that are most relevant to a client.

The second advantage of the test-free nature of IRT is communication between assessments. With traditional assessments, the scores generated from one assessment are not readily comparable to the scores generated from another assessment. For example, even though most activities of daily living (ADL) assessments have similar items (e.g., eating, grooming, dressing, bathing), the scores generated from each assessment carry different meanings (i.e., a score of 50 on the Functional Independence Measure [FIM™] has a different meaning than a 50 on the Barthel ADL Index). When using an IRT-based assessment, the concept of the individual assessment fades. Instead, all assessments measuring a particular latent trait represent subsets of the "infinite" number of items that can represent that latent trait. If specific assessments represent subsets of items from the same latent trait (e.g., ADL), then measures from one assessment should be readily translatable to another assessment. Fisher and colleagues used this principle to translate measures

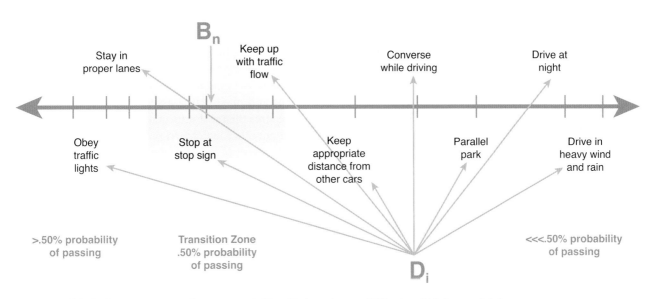

FIGURE 29-2 Comparison of person ability (B_n) to item difficulty (D_i) for a driving assessment.

between two ADL scales, the FIM and the Patient Evaluation Conference System (PECS) (Fisher, 1995). Velozo, Byers, and Joseph (2007) have also used this principle to translate measures between the FIM and the ADL items of the Minimum Data Set (MDS). Because different assessments are often used in different facilities (e.g., FIM in inpatient rehabilitation facilities and MDS in skilled nursing facilities), linking assessments provides the capability of monitoring a client's progress as he or she move from facility to facility even when those facilities use different assessments.

Basic Formula Underlying Item Response Theory

As noted previously, there are several IRT models with the most basic IRT models being the one-parameter Rasch model. In spite of their complexity, all IRT models compare *person ability* to *item difficulty*. If it is a math test, it is whether or not the student (person ability) can pass the question (item), "8 + 8 = ?" If the person is more able than the question, he or she gets it correct, but if the person is less able than the question, he or she gets it wrong. This basic principle works for all assessment situations, even the assessment of clients in OT. If someone is assessed on driving, the critical question is whether the client (person) can pass the driving task (item). For example, is the client successful in taking a left-hand turn against traffic? If the client is more able than the task, he or she passes the task, but if the client is less able than the task, he or she fails the task.

A basic statistical formula that expresses this comparison of person ability and item difficulty is the one-parameter IRT or Rasch formula (Figure 29-3). The left side of the

formula represents the probability of the person passing a specific item (P_{ni}) divided by the person failing an item ($1 - P_{ni}$). The right side of the equation represents the comparison of person ability versus item difficulty ($B_n - D_i$).

Figure 29-2 presents how this formula "works" when assessing someone on a driving assessment. B_n from the formula is represented by B_1, a person with a "low" driving ability level. D_i from the formula is represented by nine driving items of different difficulty levels. To the far left are easy items, represented by predriving activities such as opening a car door and adjusting mirrors. To the far right are difficult items, such as driving at night, driving in complex situations, and driving in heavy rain and wind. The client B_1 will have a higher than .50 probability of passing the easy items such as opening a car door and a much lower than .50 probability of passing the difficult items such as driving in heavy rain and wind. But for the items that are close to his or her ability level (e.g., staying in the proper lane when turning), he or she will have a .50 probability of passing. These items are at "just the right" challenge for the individual.

$$\log [P_{ni}/1\text{-}P_{ni}] = B_n - D_i$$

P_{ni} = probability of person n passing item i
$1\text{-}P_{ni}$ = probability of person n failing item i
B_n = ability of person n
D_i = difficulty of item in i

FIGURE 29-3 Rasch one-parameter item response theory formula.

This IRT model of relating a person's ability to item difficulty can be applied to assessing any client on any assessment. If we can think of our assessments as a series of items or tasks that have different challenges, we would expect that our client would have a high probability of being successful with items that were "below" his or her ability (the easiest items). These items could be "easy" ADL tasks such as eating and grooming, easy motor development items such as being able to roll from prone to supine, or easy upper extremity movement tasks such as moving one's arm in a gravity-eliminated position. We would expect that our client would have a low probability of being successful on items that were above his or her ability level. Challenging ADL tasks could be bathing or walking up the stairs, challenging motor development items could be running and jumping, and challenging upper extremity movement tasks can be lifting one's arm while extended holding a 10-lb object. As an occupational therapist, a major interest is determining the ability of a client. From a clinical perspective, IRT can

be described as finding the "just right" challenge for a client. That is, not what is too easy or too hard, but the tasks that are appropriately challenging for a client.

One of the advantages of an IRT perspective for critiquing an assessment is that it provides solutions to increasing assessment efficiency (reducing respondent burden) and maximizing assessment precision. Because one acquires the most information from an assessment by using items that match a client's ability, it is logical that all of the items of an assessment are not necessary. Items that are too easy or too hard provide fairly little information about a client. This leads to the concept of "efficiency," assessing clients on only the most relevant items. This has the advantage of reducing respondent (client) burden and therapist assessment time. The IRT perspective also allows for maximizing measurement precision. A client's improvement can be measured by including items that he or she can do now but could not do previously. For example, referring to Figure 29-4, if prior to

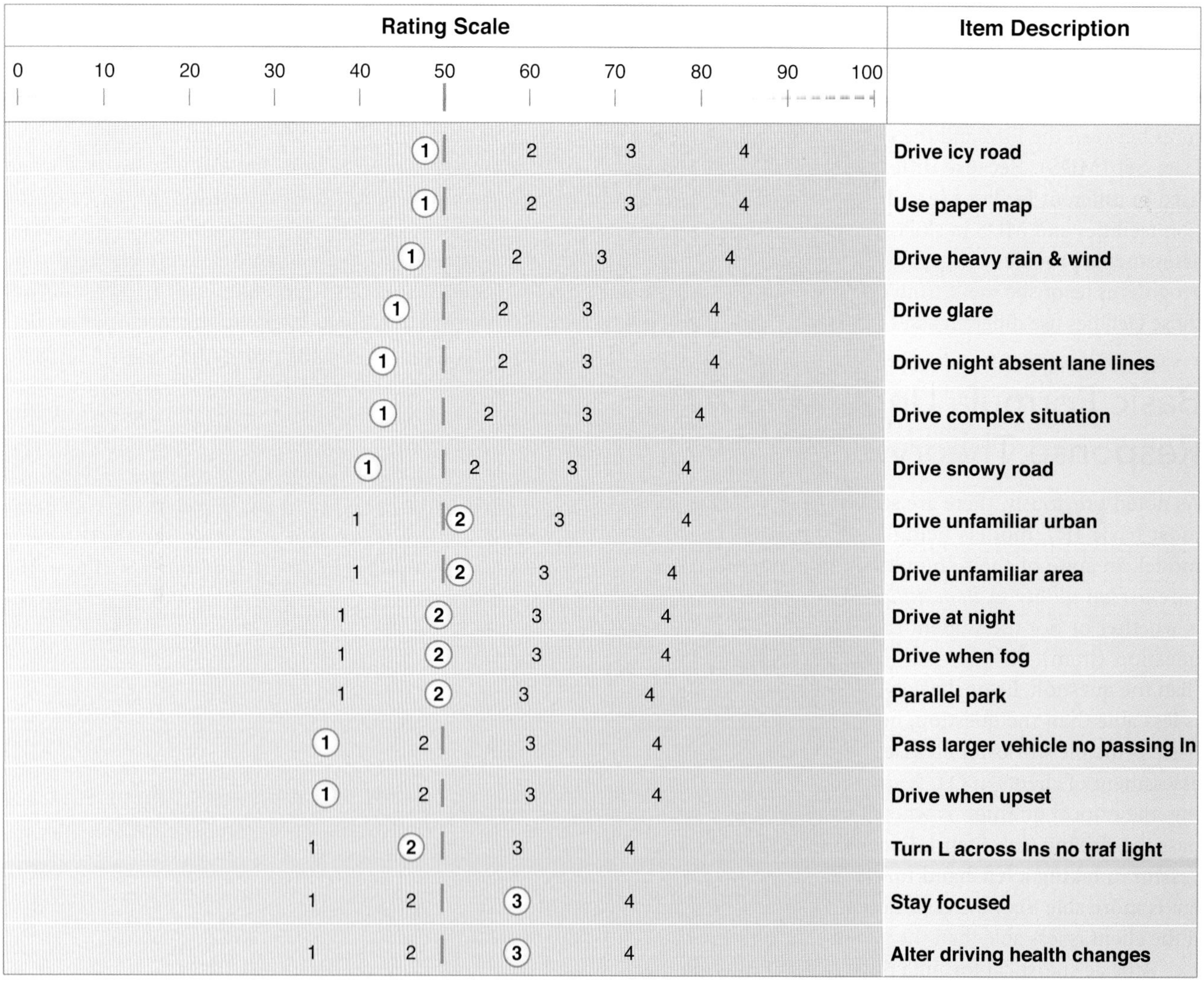

Rating Scale											Item Description
0	10	20	30	40	50	60	70	80	90	100	
					① 2	3	4				Drive icy road
					① 2	3	4				Use paper map
				①	2	3	4				Drive heavy rain & wind
				①	2	3	4				Drive glare
				①	2	3	4				Drive night absent lane lines
				①	2	3	4				Drive complex situation
				①	2	3	4				Drive snowy road
			1		② 3	4					Drive unfamiliar urban
			1		② 3	4					Drive unfamiliar area
			1	②	3	4					Drive at night
			1	②	3	4					Drive when fog
			1	②	3	4					Parallel park
		①	2		3	4					Pass larger vehicle no passing ln
		①	2		3	4					Drive when upset
			1	②	3	4					Turn L across lns no traf light
			1	2	③	4					Stay focused
			1	2	③	4					Alter driving health changes

FIGURE 29-4 Part of the Fitness-to-Drive Screening Measure key form.

rehabilitation, a client could only accomplish predriving activities (e.g., opening car door and adjusting mirrors) but through rehabilitation can now do some basic driving skills (e.g., maintain lane when turning, stop at stop sign), improvement will be detected by including these basic driving tasks. This logic can also be used to eliminate floor effects (the inability of the assessment to discriminate among clients of low ability) and ceiling effects (the inability of the assessment to discriminate among clients of high ability). To remove a floor effect, easy items can be administered (e.g., more predriving tasks), and to remove a ceiling effect, hard items can be administered (e.g., challenging driving tasks). Although this approach is logical, the obvious question is "How do I find the most relevant assessment items for an individual?" If an assessment has a logical hierarchy in terms of the difficulty of items, such as a motor development test, this can be quite easy to find the most appropriate items. This can be accomplished by starting with easy items and progressively administering more difficult items until the client fails several items (e.g., DENVER II, previously known as the Denver Developmental Screening Test; Frankenburg et al., 1992).

Item response theory–based assessments are also effectively designed for goal setting and treatment planning. As indicated in Figure 29-2, the client ability measure (B_n) is associated with the client having a .50 probability of being successful with items at his or her ability level (e.g., maintaining a lane when turning), and he or she has a lower probability of being successful for items above his or her ability level (e.g., stopping at a stop sign, merging on the highway, driving in a complex situation). Logical short-term goals would be to increase the client's success on items at his or her ability level, and logical longer-term goals would be to increase the client's success on items above his or her ability level.

A useful way to demonstrate a client's performance on an IRT-based measure is through a key form which presents the responses on individual items of the instrument. Figure 29-4 presents part of the key form of the FTDS. The top of the key form presents the scale of the instrument from 0 to 100 with the dashed vertical line representing the measure of a client (about 51). The right side of the key form presents the items of the key form with the easier items at the bottom (e.g., altering driving after health changes, stay focused) and the harder items at the top (e.g., drive icy road, use paper map). The numbers 1 to 4 which stair-step to the right are the ratings of the instrument (i.e., 1 = very difficult, 2 = somewhat difficult, 3 = a little difficult, and 4 = not difficult). The typical pattern shows higher ratings on easier items and lower ratings on more difficult items. Key forms can be used to set treatment goals. For example, short-term goals could be for the client to improve on items that

are rated 2 to 3 to ratings of 3 to 4, and long-term goals could be for the client to improve on items that are rated with 1's to ratings of 2 to 3. Coster, Deeney, Haltiwanger, and Haley (1998) show how key forms which include the item ratings on the School Function Assessment, can be used to set realistic goals (e.g., moving from a rating of a 3, inconsistent performance, to 4, consistent performance, on more challenging items). Velozo and Woodbury (2011) have used similar key forms of the Fugl-Meyer Assessment of upper extremity to suggest short- and long-term goals for clients recovering from upper extremity movement impairments following stroke.

Computerized Adaptive Testing

For assessments in which we do not have a clear item difficulty order, paper-and-pencil administration techniques may be ineffective. We would have to search through our assessment for the most appropriate items for our client. For example, if we find our client failing items, we would have to locate easier items. Similarly, if we found our client passing items, we would have to locate harder items. Unfortunately, for many of our assessments, the item difficulty order is not clear, thus making the selection of the most relevant items for a client even more challenging. In those cases, computer technology provides the solution. Computer software programs can be programmed to select items, even from hundreds of items (often referred to as an item bank), to administer the most relevant items to a client.

Item response theory, in combination with computer application of assessment items, can be used to automate both efficiency and precision in measurement. Computers can be programmed with algorithms (i.e., sets of rules) to direct only the most appropriate items to the client to maximize efficiency (use the fewest number of items) and maximize precision (use those items that differentiate one client from another or differentiate a client from one stage of progress to another) (Figure 29-5). In general, computerized adaptive testing involves presenting questions to a client until a desired level of precision (reduced error) is reached. At the beginning of the assessment, before we present any items, we have little idea of the client's ability (e.g., he or she could be a poor driver or could be an excellent driver), our error is large, and we have a large confidence interval. But every time we assess the client on an item or task, we get more information on the client, reduce our error of measurement, and get a smaller confidence interval. A simple computerized adaptive testing algorithm can be described in six steps (see Figure 29-5). At the beginning of an assessment, we have little idea of the client's ability (ADL, driving, depression, etc.);

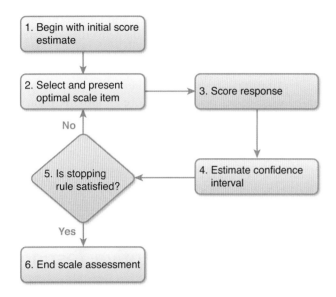

FIGURE 29-5 Computer adaptive test algorithm. (Adapted from Wainer, H., Dorans, N. J., Eignor, D., Flaugher, R., Green, B., Mislevy, R. J., . . . Thissen, D. [2000]. *Computerized adaptive testing: A primer* [2nd ed.]. Mahwah, NJ: Lawrence Erlbaum Associates.)

therefore, we typically estimate the client's ability to be at the "middle difficulty" of the items. Steps 2 through 5 represent the item administration process. The computer presents the item that most closely matches the client's initial ability estimate and/or the item that provides the most information about a client (e.g., "Do you stop at stop signs?") (step 2), and the client is scored on the item (step 3). That is, they either pass or fail (successfully stop or fail to stop) or get a particular rating (1 = failed to stop, 2 = partially stopped, 3 = stopped completely). After answering each question, the computer algorithm estimates a confidence interval or amount of precision we have in our measurement of a client (step 4). Upon answering each question, we get a smaller confidence interval and more precision. The computer continues to administer questions until we have reduced the confidence interval to a designated level (step 5); we then end the assessment and provide the client with a final assessment measure (step 6).

Presently, there are few specific OT computerized adaptive tests available for clinical use. This is probably because most assessments in OT are performance-based and computerized adaptive tests are typically self-report (often referred to as patient-reported) or proxy-report assessments. In pediatrics, a popular OT assessment, the Pediatric Evaluation of Disability (PEDI), has a CAT administration for parent responses (Allen, Ni, & Haley,

2008). Patient-reported outcomes (PROs) are gaining considerable attention in health care area and several of these measures exist in the broader area of rehabilitation (e.g., Activity Measure for Post Acute Care [AM-PAC], Computer Adaptive Measure of Functional Cognition for Traumatic Brain Injury [CAMFC-TBI]) (Donovan et al., 2011; Haley et al., 2006). The National Institutes of Health invested in several PRO computerized adaptive measures for chronic disease, including the Patient Reported Outcomes System (PROMIS) (Cella et al., 2007). As these assessments become readily available via the Web, occupational therapists and other rehabilitation professionals are likely to incorporate these assessments in clinical practice.

Critiquing Item Response Theory–Based Assessments

Item response theory, being a different psychometric theory than CTT and generalizability theory, demands a different set of methods for evaluation. Item response theory is based on a set of strong psychometric assumptions or requirements. Although most of these methods are beyond the scope of the masters-level occupational therapist practice, we generally describe them here. There are four general areas in which IRT is typically critiqued: unidimensionality, local independence, precision, and person-item match.

Unidimensionality

Unidimensionality is the determination of whether an assessment measures a single trait. Although it is often argued that human beings are multidimensional, assessing multiple dimensions at the same time often leads to confusion. For example, ADL assessments often involve both physical function and cognitive items when evaluating a total score on the assessment; it is difficult to know what combination of attributes makes up that total score. Does the score reflect equal amounts of physical function and cognition items? Does the score represent a person with a lot of physical function ability and little cognitive ability or a lot of cognitive ability and little physical function ability? This becomes more complex interpretation following treatment of the client. Let's say that a client improves in his or her overall ADL score from admission to discharge. Has he or she improved in both physical and cognitive functioning? Improved just in physical functioning or improved just in cognitive functioning? Measuring a single or unidimensional trait is less confusing.

There are several psychometric methods to determine unidimensionality. One method is "item fit." This statistic determines how well items fit the IRT model. Items that do not fit the IRT model may be measuring a second trait (Bond & Fox, 2007). A second, more preferred method of determining unidimensionality is factor analysis. In general, factor analysis groups items that correlate with each other. An indication of unidimensionality is when all assessment items show a high correlation, or "load" on a single factor (e.g., all load on physical functioning). An indication of multidimensionality is when items load on separate factors (e.g., physical functioning and cognitive functioning).

Local Independence

Local independence is an indication of whether the items of an assessment independently contribute to the measurement of a particular trait. That is, are some items redundant or not adding anything new to the measuring of a particular trait? This can be a particularly confusing concept and may seem in conflict with an objective of assessing a client. For example, from a *qualitative* perspective, one would want to know every aspect of a client's driving ability (e.g., can he or she insert a key into the ignition, open the window, and press the gas pedal?). But some of these items may be redundant in terms of measuring driving ability. For example, pressing the gas pedal may be essentially equivalent to pressing the break or doing some other lower extremity activity. Turning a key may be essentially equivalent to adjusting a car mirror. If this is the case, then one can remove items that are redundant. Fairly sophisticated analyses, such as polychloric correlations or the correlation of item residuals, identify that items are redundant and can be removed from an assessment (Reeve et al., 2007).

Precision

Precision of an assessment is a critical feature of measurement in IRT. Obviously, we would like to have assessments that are as precise as possible because we would expect that the more precise assessment will be more effective in differentiating our patients from one another and, more importantly, be effective in detecting change in our clients following OT intervention. There are several indices of precision used in IRT. Two important indicators of precision are error and information. Although in traditional testing, one gets only one value of error for an assessment in IRT, error can be plotted across the range of an assessment (across easy to hard items). Typically, we find that the error of an assessment increases at the extremes of the assessment. That is, there is usually more error at the easy and hard items of an assessment. Information is the reciprocal or inverse of error; therefore, the more information provided by an assessment, the more precise it is.

Person-Item Match

Person-item match, as noted earlier, characteristic of all IRT models is the comparison of person ability to item difficulty. This relationship can tell us how well the items of our assessment match the abilities of the clients under study. This can be exemplified by ceiling and floor effects in our assessments. Ceilings effects are when an assessment cannot differentiate the most able clients (i.e., clients are more able than what our assessment can assess), and floor effect are when an assessment cannot differentiate the least able clients that (i.e., clients are less able than what our assessment can assess). Based on IRT models, this is related to whether or not we have items that match a client's ability. For ceiling effects, we do not have items that differentiate the most able clients. For example, if we have good drivers in our sample and our hardest item is driving in our hometown, it is likely that all of these clients will get "perfect" measures on our assessment. The reality may be that if we tested these clients on more challenging items, for example, merging onto a highway, we would then be able to differentiate these clients of high ability. Similarly, a floor effect suggests that we do not have items that differentiate the lowest ability-level clients and likely indicates that we do not have easy enough items to differentiate these clients. For example, if we do not have predriving tasks on our assessment, we may not be able to differentiate those individuals who cannot do on-the-road driving. If one has a good conceptual model for an assessment, that is, an understanding of the relative challenge of the items of our assessment, resolving these problems can be easy. Ceiling effects can be eliminated by creating more challenging items, and floor effects can be eliminated by creating easy items.

Summary

The purpose of this chapter is to provide an overview on the many methods used to critique assessments. As evident by the number of areas covered in this chapter, critiquing assessments is not an easy task. It requires both clinical knowledge of one's specialty area and statistical knowledge on reliability and validity. Critiquing assessments becomes more daunting with the addition of new measurement theories such as IRT and new test administration methods such as computerized adaptive testing. Obviously, the practicing therapist cannot be up to date on all OT assessments. But as a practicing occupational therapist, it is essential that one is able to critique the assessments that one uses in daily practice.

CENTENNIAL NOTES

Measurement and Changing Technology in Occupational Therapy

Attention to effective assessment processes in OT date back to the early days of the profession. One of the core principles for the newly developing profession that was recommended by William Rush Dutton, Jr., MD, was an assertion that the "only reliable measure of the value of the treatments is the effect on the patient" (Maryland Psychiatric Society, 1919, p. 72). Furthermore, it was recognized that in order for the profession to become better recognized, scientific approaches to measuring effectiveness were required, as noted by a Ms. Manning at the fifth American Occupational Therapy Association (AOTA) House of Delegates meeting (AOTA, 1922): "We have thousands of cases available, but we haven't a scientific measure of improvement as contrasted to what would have happened if they had not had occupational therapy" (p. 350).

Currently, the profession has many more such scientific methods available. However, occupational therapists must continually and critically appraise properties of measurement tools to determine how to most reliably and accurately assess occupational performance. This process is dependent on an understanding of measurement principles. Measurement principles, derived from classical test theory and/or item response theory, are generally used to inform the occupational therapist's critical appraisal skills. With the emergence of new technologies such as robotics (Smith, 2017), artificial intelligence or machine learning (Mihailidis & Hoey, in press), and vehicle automation (Alvarez & Classen, 2017), we propose that occupational therapists will experience challenges measuring their clients' performances in the next decades. For example, in-vehicle technologies related to driving may influence the construct validity of previously validated instruments related to driving assessment. As our clients continue to engage in everyday life activities with the assistance of technologies, we also propose that many of the standardized assessments generally used in OT, may not hold up to be valid or reliable. As such, besides critically appraising the existing assessments, an additional challenge for occupational therapists will be to perhaps help develop, test, and refine new measurement tools to adequately reflect the emergence of the advance technologies that are becoming standard use in everyday life.

REFERENCES

Allen, D. D., Ni, P., & Haley, S. M. (2008). Efficiency and sensitivity of multidimensional computerized adaptive testing of pediatric physical functioning. *Disability and Rehabilitation, 30*, 479–484.

Alvarez, L., & Classen, S. (2017). In-vehicle technology and driving simulation. In S. Classen (Ed.), *Driving simulation for assessment, intervention, and training: A guide for occupational therapy and health care professionals* (pp. 265–278). Bethesda, MD: AOTA Press.

American Occupational Therapy Association. (1922). Proceedings of the Fifth Annual Meeting of the National Society for the Promotion of Occupational Therapy. *Archives of Occupational Therapy, 1*, 51–85.

Association of American Publishers. (n.d.). *Standardized assessment: A primer* (Rev. ed.). Washington, DC: Author.

Bédard, M., Parkkari, M., Weaver, B., Riendeau, J., & Dahlquist, M. (2010). Assessment of driving performance using a simulator protocol: Validity and reproducibility. *American Journal of Occupational Therapy, 64*, 336–340.

Bond, T. G., & Fox, C. M. (2007). *Applying the Rasch model: Fundamental measurement in the human sciences.* Mahwah, NJ: Lawrence Erlbaum Associates.

Carmines, E. G., & Zeller, R. (Eds.). (1979). *Reliability and validity assessment.* Thousand Oaks, CA: Sage.

Cella, D., & Chang, C. H. (2000). A discussion of item response theory and its applications in health status assessment. *Medical Care, 38*(Suppl.), II66–II72.

Cella, D., Yount, S., Rothrock, N., Gershon, R., Cook, K., Reeve, B., . . . Rose, M. (2007). The Patient-Reported Outcomes Measurement Information System (PROMIS): Progress of an NIH roadmap cooperative group during its first two years. *Medical Care, 45*(Suppl. 1), S3–S11.

Classen, S., McCarthy, D. P., Shechtman, O., Awadzi, K. D., Lanford, D. N., Okun, M. S., . . . Fernandez, H. H. (2009). Useful field of view as a reliable screening measure of driving performance in people with Parkinson's disease: Results of a pilot study. *Traffic Injury Prevention, 10*, 593–598.

Classen, S., & Owens, A. B. (2010). Simulator sickness among returning combat veterans with mild traumatic brain injury and/or post-traumatic stress disorder [Special Issue]. *Advances in Transportation Studies, 2010*, 45–52.

Classen, S., Velozo, C. A., Winter, S. M., Bédard, M., & Wang, Y. (2015). Psychometrics of the Fitness-to-Drive Screening Measure. *OTJR: Occupation, Participation and Health, 35*, 42–52. doi:10.1177/1539449214561761

Classen, S., Winter, S. M., Velozo, C. A., Bédard, M., Lanford, D., Brumback, B. A., & Lutz, B. J. (2010). Item development and validity testing for a safe driving behavior measure. *American Journal of Occupational Therapy, 64*, 296–305.

Coster, W., Deeney, T., Haltiwanger, J., & Haley, S. (1998). *School Function Assessment user manual.* San Antonio, TX: The Psychological Corporation.

Cronbach, L. J., Gleser, G. C., Nanda, H., & Rajaratnam, N. (1972). *The dependability of behavioral measurements: Theory of generalizability for scores and profiles.* New York, NY: Wiley.

Cronbach, L. J., Nageswari, R., & Gleser, G. C. (1963). Theory of generalizability: A liberation of reliability theory. *The British Journal of Statistical Psychology, 16*, 137–163.

Denaro, R. P., Zmud, J., Shladover, S., Walker Smith, B., & Lappin, J. (2014, May). Automated vehicle technology: Ten research areas to follow. *TR News, 292,* 19–24.

Di Stefano, M., & Macdonald, W. (2005). On-the-road evaluation of driving performance. In J. M. Pellerito (Ed.), *Driver rehabilitation and community principles and practice* (pp. 255–274). St. Louis, MO: Mosby.

Donovan, N. J., Heaton, S. C., Kimberg, C. I., Wen, P. S., Waid-Ebbs, J. K., Coster, W., . . . Velozo, C. A. (2011). Conceptualizing functional cognition in traumatic brain injury rehabilitation. *Brain Injury, 25,* 348–364.

Edwards, J. D., Ross, L. A., Wadley, V. G., Clay, O. J., Crowe, M., Roenker, D. L., & Ball, K. K. (2006). The Useful Field of View test: Normative data for older adults. *Archives of Clinical Neuropsychology, 21,* 275–286.

Fisher, A. G. (1993). The assessment of IADL motor skills: An application of many-faceted Rasch analysis. *American Journal of Occupational Therapy, 47,* 319–329.

Fisher, W. P., Jr. (1995). Rehabits: A common language of functional assessment. *Archives of Physical Medicine & Rehabilitation, 76,* 113–122.

Folstein, M. F., Folstein, S. E., & McHugh, P. R. (1975). "Mini-mental state." A practical method for grading the cognitive state of patients for the clinician. *Journal of Psychiatric Research, 12,* 189–198.

Folstein, M. F., Folstein, S. E., White, T., & Messer, M. A. (2010). *Mini-Mental State Exam: User's guide* (2nd ed.). Lutz, FL: PAR.

Frankenburg, W. K., Doods, J., Archer, P., Bresnick, B., Maschka, P., Edelman, N., & Shapiro, H. (1992). *DENVER II training manual.* Denver, CO: Denver Developmental Materials.

Grant, J. S., & Davis, L. L. (1997). Selection and use of content experts for instrument development. *Research in Nursing & Health, 20,* 269–274.

Haley, S. M., Ludlow, L. H., & Coster, W. J. (1993). Pediatric Evaluation of Disability Inventory: Clinical interpretation of summary scores using Rasch rating scale methodology. *Physical Medicine and Rehabilitation Clinics of North America, 4,* 529–540.

Haley, S. M., Siebens, H., Coster, W. J., Tao, W., Black-Schaffer, R. M., Gandek, B., . . . Ni, P. (2006). Computerized adaptive testing for follow-up after discharge from inpatient rehabilitation: I. Activity outcomes. *Archives of Physical Medicine & Rehabilitation, 87,* 1033–1042.

Hinojosa, J., Kramer, P., & Crist, P. (Eds.). (2005). *Evaluation: Obtaining and interpreting data* (2nd ed.). Bethesda, MD: AOTA Press.

House, A. E., House, B. J., & Campbell, M. B. (1981). Measures of interobserver agreement: Calculation formulas and distribution effects. *Journal of Behavioral Assessment, 3,* 37–57.

Justiss, M. D., Mann, W. C., Stav, W., & Velozo, C. (2006). Development of a behind-the-wheel driving performance assessment for older adults. *Topics in Geriatric Rehabilitation, 22,* 121–128.

Kay, L., Bundy, A., & Clemson, L. (2009). Predicting fitness to drive in people with cognitive impairments by using DriveSafe and DriveAware. *Archives of Physical Medicine & Rehabilitation, 90,* 1514–1522. doi:10.1016/j.apmr.2009.03.0118

Kennedy, R. S., Lane, N. E., Berbaum, K. S., & Lilienthal, M. G. (1993). Simulator Sickness Questionnaire: An enhanced method for quantifying simulator sickness. *The International Journal of Aviation Psychology, 3,* 203–220.

Kielhofner, G., Dobria, L., Forsyth, K., & Basu, S. (2005). The construction of keyforms for obtaining instantaneous measures from the Occupational Performance History Interview rating scales: Empirical quantitative study. *OTJR: Occupation, Participation and Health, 25,* 23–32.

Kraut, R., Olson, J., Banaji, M., Bruckman, A., Cohen, J., & Couper, M. (2004). Psychological research online: Report of Board of Scientific Affairs' Advisory Group on the Conduct of Research on the Internet. *The American Psychologist, 59,* 105–117.

Law, M. (1987). Measurement in occupational therapy: Scientific criteria for evaluation. *Canadian Journal of Occupational Therapy, 54,* 133–138.

Lynn, M. R. (1986). Determination and quantification of content validity. *Nursing Research, 35,* 382–385.

Maryland Psychiatric Society. (1919). National Society for the Promotion of Occupational Therapy. *Maryland Psychiatric Quarterly, 72,* 68–74.

Mihailidis, A., & Hoey, J. (in press). *Machine learning in assistive technology.* Manuscript submitted for publication.

Morris, J. C. (1993). The Clinical Dementia Rating (CDR): Current version and scoring rules. *Neurology, 43,* 2412–2414.

Munkholm, M., Löfgren, B., & Fisher, A. G. (2012). Reliability of the school AMPS measures. *Scandinavian Journal of Occupational Therapy, 19,* 2–8. doi:10.3109/11038128.2010.525721

Nunnally, J. C., & Bernstein, I. H. (1994). *Psychometric theory* (3rd ed.). New York, NY: McGraw-Hill.

Owsley, C., Ball, K. K., McGwin, G., Jr., Sloane, M. E., Roenker, D. L., White, M. F., & Overley, E. T. (1998). Visual processing impairment and risk of motor vehicle crash among older adults. *JAMA, 279,* 1083–1088.

Owsley, C., & McGwin, G., Jr. (1999). Vision impairment and driving. *Survey of Ophthalmology, 43,* 535–550.

Owsley, C., McGwin, G., Jr., & Ball, K. K. (1998). Vision impairment, eye disease, and injurious motor vehicle crashes in the elderly. *Ophthalmic Epidemiology, 5,* 101–113.

Owsley, C., Stalvey, B. T., Wells, J., & Sloane, M. E. (1999). Older drivers and cataract: Driving habits and crash risk. *Journal of Gerontology: Series A: Biological Sciences & Medical Sciences, 54,* M203–M211.

Portney, L., & Watkins, M. P. (2009). *Foundations of clinical research: Applications to practice* (3rd ed.). Upper Saddle River, NJ: Prentice Hall.

Reeve, B. B., Hays, R. D., Bjorner, J. B., Cook, K. F., Crane, P. K., Teresi, J. A., . . . Cella, D. (2007). Psychometric evaluation and calibration of health-related quality of life item banks: Plans for the Patient-Reported Outcomes Measurement Information System (PROMIS). *Medical Care, 45*(Suppl. 1), S22–S31.

Reitan, R. M. (1958). Validity of the Trail Making Test as an indicator of organic brain damage. *Perceptual and Motor Skills, 8,* 271–276.

Rudman, D., & Hannah, S. (1998). An instrument evaluation framework: Description and application to assessments of hand function. *Journal of Hand Therapy, 11,* 266–277.

Shechtman, O., Classen, S., Awadzi, K. D., & Mann, W. (2009). Comparison of driving errors between on-the-road and simulated driving assessment: A validation study. *Traffic Injury Prevention, 10,* 379–385.

Smith, R. (2000). Fit analysis in latent trait measurement models. *Journal of Applied Measurement, 1,* 199–218.

Smith, R. O. (2017). *Eleanor Clarke Slagle lecture: Technology and occupation: Past 100, present and next 100 years.* Retrieved from https://www.aota.org/Publications-News/AOTANews/2017/Videos-2017-Annual-Conference-Available.aspx

Streiner, D. L., & Norman, G. R. (Eds.). (2008a). Devising the items. In *Health measurement scales: A practical guide to their development and use* (4th ed., pp. 17–36). Oxford, NY: Oxford University Press.

Streiner, D. L., & Norman, G. R. (Eds.). (2008b). *Health measurement scales: A practical guide to their development and use* (4th ed.). Oxford, NY: Oxford University Press.

Velozo, C. A., Byers, K., & Joseph, B. (2007). Translating measures across the continuum of care: Using Rasch analysis to create a crosswalk between the functional independence measure and the minimum data set. *Journal of Rehabilitation Research and Development, 44,* 467.

Velozo, C. A., & Woodbury, M. L. (2011). Translating measurement findings into rehabilitation practice: An example using Fugl-Meyer assessment-upper extremity with patients following stroke. *Journal of Rehabilitation Research and Development, 48,* 1211–1222.

Wainer, H., Dorans, N. J., Eignor, D., Flaugher, R., Green, B., Mislevy, R. J., . . . Thissen, D. (2000). *Computerized adaptive testing: A primer* (2nd ed.). Mahwah, NJ: Lawrence Erlbaum Associates.

Whiteneck, G., Brooks, C. A., Charlifue, S., Gerhart, K. A., Mellick, D., Overholser, D., & Richardson, G. N. (1998). *Craig Handicap Assessment and Reporting Technique 1998.* Retrieved from http://www.craighospital.org/repository/documents/Research%20 Instruments/CHART%20Manual.pdf

Wilschut, E. S. (2009). *The impact of in-vehicle information systems on simulated driving performance: Effects of age, timing and display characteristics* (Unpublished doctoral dissertation). University of Groningen, The Netherlands.

the**Point®** *For additional resources on the subjects discussed in this chapter, visit* **http://thePoint.lww.com /Willard-Spackman13e.**

Occupational Therapy Interventions for Individuals

Glen Gillen

LEARNING OBJECTIVES

After reading this chapter, you will be able to:

1. Understand the overarching themes that occupational therapists embrace when choosing interventions for their clients.
2. Differentiate between interventions that are categorized as "occupation as ends" and "occupation as means."
3. Develop and choose interventions for clients that combine the principles of occupation as ends and occupation as means.
4. Compare and contrast a variety of specific intervention approaches that are used for clients receiving occupational therapy services.
5. Begin to understand when to choose one type of intervention over another, combine interventions, and/or switch the intervention plan.
6. Understand the concept of grading interventions.

Introduction

When developing intervention plans for clients, occupational therapists work under the guidance of three overarching and interrelated themes. Interventions must be client centered, evidence based, and chosen based on sound professional reasoning. The term *client-centered practice* has been defined as

> an approach to providing occupational therapy, which embraces a philosophy of respect for and partnership with people receiving services. It recognizes the autonomy of individuals, the need for client choice in making decisions about occupational needs, the strengths clients bring to an occupational therapy encounter and the benefits of client-therapist partnership and the need to ensure that services are accessible and fit the context in which a client lives. (Law, Baptiste, & Mills, 1995, p. 253)

Sumsion and Law (2006) have reviewed and analyzed subsequent definitions of client-centered practice and concluded that the various definitions share many similar components including " . . . a strong emphasis on a collaborative approach or partnership, respect for the client, facilitating choice and involving the client in determining the occupational goals that emerge from his or her choices" (p. 154). The reader is referred to Chapter 37 for a further discussion on this topic.

CENTENNIAL NOTES

World Health Organization Classifications

When plans for the United Nations were developing in 1945, the desire for an international health organization surfaced, which resulted in the formation of the World Health Organization (WHO) in 1948 (WHO, n.d.a). One of the early efforts of the WHO was to work on a method for countries around the world to share data about diseases. Medical statisticians had worked for over a century to establish methods to classify diseases. In the 1900s, those efforts led to the International Classification of Causes of Death (WHO, n.d.b). In 1946, the International Health conference asked the Interim Commission of the World Health Organization to prepare a sixth revision of the International Lists of Diseases and Causes of Death (WHO, n.d.c). These early efforts were the beginning of several important international classification systems widely used today in many health professions, including OT: the International Classification of Diseases (ICD) and the International Classification of Functioning, Disability and Health (ICF).

International Classification of Diseases

Currently in its 10th edition and being revised for the 11th edition, this listing of diseases is the basis for many of the diagnostic coding systems used in documenting and billing medically based services (WHO, 2010). Occupational therapists are affected by these systems as

these classifications are used by insurance companies, governments, and other payors as a way to describe what is considered a "covered" condition for service.

International Classification of Function

The ICF (WHO, 2001) was initially developed in an attempt to classify the outcomes of diseases. The first attempt to tackle this problem by the WHO was the International Classification of Impairment, Disability and Handicap (WHO, 1980). This document recognized that disability involved not only body functions and structures but also activities and the context in which those activities were being performed. Over time, this document evolved into the ICF (WHO, 2001), in which the ICF has moved away from being a "consequences of disease" classification (1980 version) to become a "components of health' classification" (WHO, 2001, p. 4).

Occupational therapists quickly adopted much of the language of the ICF. The American Occupational Therapy Association [AOTA] Practice Framework (AOTA, 2014) adopted the terminology of the body functions/body structures section as part of the client factors section. Additionally, the notion of participation and the increase attention to environmental, social, and political barriers all resonated well with OT. Although not without its critics (Hemmingsson & Jonsson, 2005), the ICF has proved to be an important resource in articulating OT's unique contributions to health and well-being.

Sumsion and Law (2006) further point out that development of the literature regarding client-centered practice parallels the development of our understanding of evidence-based practice. Sackett, Strauss, Richardson, Rosenberg, and Haynes (2000) define evidence-based practice as "the integration of best research evidence with clinical expertise and patient values" (p. 1). Client values include "the unique preferences, concerns and expectations each patient brings to a clinical encounter" (Sacket et al., 2000, p. 1). A major component of evidence-based practice is the clear message that we, as occupational therapists, must use evidence to inform our intervention choices (Bennett et al., 2003). Bennett and Bennett (2000) summarize that the research literature can provide guidance concerning the effectiveness and choices of occupational therapy (OT) interventions, the way in which interventions are best implemented, and whether there are any associated difficulties related to the intervention. They conclude that "occupational therapists can use this sort of research evidence to help clients understand, plan and cope with their situation" (Bennett & Bennett, 2000, p. 173). See Chapter 35 for more detail regarding evidence-based practice.

The literature regarding evidence-based decision making has consistently emphasized that research evidence alone is not adequate to guide the choice of interventions. Rather, clinicians must apply their clinical expertise and professional reasoning to assess the patient's deficits while at the same time incorporating the research evidence (Haynes, Devereaux, & Guyatt, 2002). Bennett and Bennett (2000) also stress that evidence needs to be integrated with clinical expertise and reasoning so that the practitioner can decide if valid and potentially useful results from a research study can apply to the individual that he or she is working with. They proposed the following questions to guide the application of evidence:

1. "Do these results apply to my client? (i.e., is my client so different from those in the study that its results cannot help me?)
2. Does the treatment fit in with my client's values and preferences?
3. Are there resources available to implement the treatment?" (Bennett & Bennett, 2000, p. 177)

In addition to these questions, the occupational therapist must consider how or if the evidence relates to our profession's underlying assumptions and philosophy (AOTA, 2014). It is important to remember that just because an intervention is deemed effective does not automatically mean that it is an appropriate OT intervention. The reader is further referred to Chapter 34 for detailed information regarding the professional reasoning process. Case Study 30-1 was developed to provide the reader with insight into the OT intervention process that is described in detail in this chapter. As you read, note that the various interventions were developed based on the clients' needs and desire to maintain access to their community. The interventions were planned based on the findings of a variety of evaluation techniques. Finally, note that the combinations of interventions were used to meet client-centered goals. More case studies are provided at the end of this chapter to further illustrate intervention processes.

CASE STUDY 30-1   BENJAMIN: A MARRIED OLDER MAN WHOSE FAMILY IS CONCERNED ABOUT HIS DRIVING ABILITIES

Occupational Profile

Benjamin is a 79-year-old male who lives with his wife Bess in a retirement community. Benjamin and Bess have always enjoyed visiting their children and grandchildren who live in neighboring towns. Benjamin had a myocardial infarction about 7 years ago and underwent bypass surgery. Although Benjamin remains independent in his basic activities of daily living (ADL), plays cards with his longtime buddies, and enjoys walks about the community's gardens, he can get short of breath with exertion. One year ago, Bess experienced a mild/moderate stroke with residual left-sided weakness and a visual field cut. She has not driven since the stroke, needs assistance with transfers, and uses a scooter except for short distances, thus making road trips more stressful due to mobility and vision issues. Up until a year ago, Benjamin and Bess shared driving responsibilities, functioning as a team for navigation. Since Benjamin assumed full responsibility for driving and navigation, Bess has reported several "near misses" while driving, but Benjamin is quick to report that these incidents were the fault of other drivers. Recently, they both were upset after a "fender bender" that Benjamin insisted was the fault of a driver who "came out of nowhere." Bess tearfully admits that she struggles to assist in navigation and there have been some tense moments as they struggled to find their way home when returning from a trip to see their grandchildren. She relies on her husband for transportation, so she waffles back and forth with her concerns. The adult children are now worried for both of their parents' safety and discussed the issue with Benjamin and Bess's physician. The physician referred Bess to a general practice occupational therapist to address her mobility issues, and Benjamin was referred to an occupational therapist who is a driver rehabilitation specialist for a comprehensive driving evaluation.

Assessment Findings

Benjamin, Bess, and their adult children were interviewed by the driver rehabilitation specialist to review Benjamin's medical and driving history as well as to understand the environmental context for community mobility resources. The occupational therapist reviewed Benjamin's medications and cardiac history and administered an array of clinical assessments to cover his cognitive, motor, and visual abilities. Specifically, assessments included (1) functional range of motion and strength of the neck, arms, and legs; (2) visual acuity; (3) contrast sensitivity; (4) visual fields and tracking; (5) Short Blessed cognitive exam; (6) Trail-Making Test A and B; (7) the Useful Field of View (UFOV) (computer-based screen for selective attention); (8) clock drawing; (9) brake reaction timer; and the occupational therapist observed Benjamin making a meat and cheese sandwich and coffee. Benjamin wore his glasses for the vision testing and demonstrated very poor contrast sensitivity and vision that was 20/70. When asked, Benjamin had not had a vision evaluation for more than 10 years. There were no field cuts or difficulty tracking visually. Benjamin's cognitive abilities did not show any sign of significant dementia, but his processing speeds were slow with the Trail-Making Test, UFOV, and brake reaction timer. He also had some range of motion restrictions with his neck. The behind the wheel (BTW) evaluation was delayed until Benjamin was able to see an optometrist. After the optometrist evaluated Benjamin's vision and prescribed new glasses, his visual acuity increased to 20/30. However, the contrast sensitivity remained poor, not unusual for his age. The BTW assessment demonstrated that Benjamin follows the rules of the road, did not make any significant errors, but was slow in making decisions at unprotected turns and drove significantly slower than other traffic on the highway component of the evaluation.

Goal

Several goals were established: (1) Their automobile would be modified with a swing front seat for improved transfer for Bess; (2) Benjamin would remain independent in driving with a recommended restricted license; and (3) Benjamin, Bess, and their children would make plans for alternative transportation when needed and eventual driving retirement.

(continues)

CASE STUDY 30-1   BENJAMIN: A MARRIED OLDER MAN WHOSE FAMILY IS CONCERNED ABOUT HIS DRIVING ABILITIES (continued)

Intervention

Bess was seen by an occupational therapist generalist who recommended that their motor vehicle be modified with a scooter lift as well as a swing-out seat for ease of transfers from the scooter to the front passenger seat to decrease the physical toll when using their automobile (adaptation). Both Benjamin and Bess would be educated on the proper use. The therapist also evaluated Bess's instrumental ADL (IADL) in the home and assisted her in modifying the kitchen and bathroom to improve her independence (environmental modifications).

Using a prevention approach, the driver rehabilitation specialist made the recommendation to restrict Benjamin's license to daytime driving only due to the poor contrast sensitivity because evidence demonstrates the relationship of contrast sensitivity and crashes (Owsley & McGwin, 1999; Owsley, Sekuler, & Siemsen, 1983; Owsley, Stalvey, Wells, & Sloane, 1999). The therapist also recommended that highway driving be eliminated as well as planning local routes to avoid unprotected turns or yield signs because evidence shows that risk of crashes of these types of intersections increase significantly with slowed processing (Stutts, Martell, & Staplin, 2009). The driving rehabilitation specialist reviewed Benjamin and Bess's community mobility needs and planned routes that posed less risk for crashes, including right-hand turns and intersections with signals. Meeting with the adult children, Benjamin, and Bess, alternative transportation plans included the children picking up their parents when an activity might involve nighttime driving, and the grandchildren would alternate in picking their grandparents up for a visit. Both began to use the retirement community's transportation for some events. Three months later, Bess and Benjamin indicated that traveling had become much easier with the scooter lift and transfer seat. No further "close calls" were reported, and Benjamin and Bess reported it was sometimes delightful to be chauffeured by their grandchildren.

Occupation as Therapy

As occupational therapists, our outcomes are focused on improving occupational performance. We achieve this goal by using occupation as a therapeutic change agent. Therefore, we believe in the therapeutic value of occupational engagement and that engagement in occupations is also the ultimate goal of therapy (AOTA, 2017). The therapeutic occupations we use are ideally both *meaningful* and *purposeful*. Meaningful suggests that the task at hand is motivating and has some level of significance (Trombly, 1995). The task may be something the person wants to do, has to do, or needs to do throughout the day. The purposeful component may serve to organize and enhance performance as it pertains to the client's aim, reason for doing, or personal goal (Fisher, 1998; Trombly, 1995). Interventions may involve changing occupations in ways that either foster development or improvement in desired performance or allow for participation in spite of limitations. Based on the intervention choices that are outlined in the following discussion, occupations can be graded to create "just the right challenge." The term *grading* refers to systematically increasing the demands of an occupation to stimulate improved function or reducing the demands to respond to client difficulties in performance.

When grading, the OT practitioner increases the demands of the task at hand to potentially reduce an underlying impairment or performance skill deficit. In other cases,

the OT practitioner may downgrade the demands so that the task can be achieved despite a client's limitations. A person who is recovering from cardiac transplant surgery that was preceded by a long period of bed rest may be engaged in occupations that are systematically graded to improve strength and endurance as to foster participation in meaningful occupations. The therapist may grade therapeutic occupations based on the posture assumed while performing tasks (standing as opposed to sitting), duration of the task, number of rest breaks, use of adaptive equipment, and vanishing physical assistance by the therapist to complete the task. Occupational therapists may also downgrade demands and modify the task or the environment so that a client can still participate despite persistent impairments. A therapist may work with an adult who is living with schizophrenia to circumvent daily life problems by teaching use of a daily planner to help organize and complete home and work tasks. The therapist may grade the number of verbal cues required for organization and sequencing when teaching the client to use the planner to create a grocery list.

Fisher (1998) describes occupation as a "noun of action" that has the power to enable people "to perform the actions they need and want to perform so that they can engage in and 'do' the familiar, ordinary, goal directed activities of every day in a manner that brings meaning and personal satisfaction" (p. 511). She further outlines groups of activities and their attributes that can be implemented as OT (Table 30-1).

TABLE 30-1	Intervention Methods Potentially Used by Occupational Therapy Practitioners				
Activity Type	Examples	Focus of Therapy	Source of Meaning and Purpose	How Real or Natural	OT Practice Framework Classification
Exercise: rote exercise or practice	Elastic bands, weight lifting, practice line drawing for eye–hand coordination	Remediation of impairments	Practitioner-chosen for therapy benefits Client expected to "comply"	Contrived— typically only done in therapy situation	Preparatory method
Contrived occupation: exercise with added purpose and occupation with a contrived component	Practice picking up balls from the floor and placing them in a bucket, placing cones on a shelf pretending they are dishes, hammering nails into wood, throwing bean bags at a target	Remediation of impairments or skill development	Practitioner-chosen for therapy benefits Client expected to "comply"	Contrived, therapy using culturally common objects	Purposeful activity
Therapeutic occupation[a]: graded occupations to treat impairments, direct intervention of impairments in the context of occupation	Challenging balance skills via organizing library book shelves for a client who loves to read, working on social skills during a group focused on adolescents making a cake for one of their mothers, using a favorite card game to improve attention	Remediation of impairments or skill development	Chosen collaboratively for meaning to client and therapy potential	More naturalistic, uses authentic aspects of occupation (tools, context)	Occupation-based intervention
Adaptive/ compensatory occupation[a]: assistive devices, teach compensatory strategies, modify physical or social environments	Adapting a shopping task to compensate for poor endurance Learning to drive again after an orthopedic injury Working in a job for person with developmental disabilities	Improved occupational performance	Chosen collaboratively based on occupations, with therapy processes selected to support performance	Naturalistic activity in natural contexts	Occupation-based intervention

Note that current trends in the field suggest that occupation-based approaches (indicated by [a]) are often most effective and provide a clearer external reflection of OT profession's contribution to health care. Additionally, interventions may involve a mix of methods in order to both minimize effects of impairment and promote occupational functioning.

Data from Fisher, A. G. (1998). Uniting practice and theory in an occupational therapy framework, 1998 Eleanor Clarke Slagle lecture. *American Journal of Occupational Therapy, 52*, 509–522.

Occupation as Ends as Intervention

In her Eleanor Clarke Slagle Lecture, Catherine Trombly (1995) described **occupation as ends** as being "not only purposeful but also meaningful because it is the performance of activities or tasks that a person sees as important" (p. 963). Occupation as ends refers to engaging your client in occupations that constitute the end product of therapy (i.e., the occupations to be learned or relearned). Occupation as ends has been described by Trombly as the following:

- Directly teaching the activity or task
- Using whatever abilities a client has at his or her disposal to learn a task
- Providing adaptations to learn a task or activity
- A rehabilitative approach

- A skills training approach
- An approach in which the therapist serves as teacher or adaptor of a task
- Influenced by learning and cognitive information–processing theories regarding the therapeutic principle behind this approach
- *Not* being used to make a therapeutic change of underlying capabilities such as strength or memory

Using occupation as ends as an intervention serves as the goal to be learned or achieved. For example, Peter, who is undergoing inpatient rehabilitation after a spinal cord injury (SCI) left him paraplegic, may have a goal to independently transfer from his wheelchair to his car or to his bathtub. If you were to watch the therapist and Peter in action, they would be engaged in specifically chosen areas of occupation, and you may observe actual practice of these mobility skills: the therapist teaching Peter how to

BOX 30-1   EXAMPLES OF USING OCCUPATION AS ENDS

- Teaching a person who has just had a hip replacement adapt positions so that sexual activities can be engaged in safely
- Practicing of one-handed shoe tying after stroke or upper limb amputation
- Repetitive practice of components of meal preparation
- Teaching a child living with developmental delays to use an augmentative communication device
- Recommending magnifying devices so that a person living with macular degeneration can read the newspaper
- Recommending and training with vehicular hand controls so that a person who does not have use of his or her lower extremities after a spinal cord injury can drive again

- Teaching an adult living with schizophrenia a new leisure activity, such as photography
- Task-specific practice of handwriting, such as writing out a weekly grocery list
- Teaching a person who has survived a stroke how to propel a wheelchair using an arm and leg for functional mobility within the home
- Demonstrating and teaching the use of bilateral upper limb prostheses to eat a meal after upper limb amputations
- Demonstrating and teaching an adaptive swallowing technique to promote independent and safe self-feeding

use a sliding board to move from surface to surface; the therapist suggesting environmental modifications such as a tub bench and nonslip bath mats; and/or the therapist gradually decreasing the amount of physical, cognitive, and emotional support required to perform the task as the client becomes more independent. The occupations chosen are based on the occupations that the client wants to, needs to, or has to resume or continue in his or her various life roles. Using occupation as ends as an intervention approach makes the focus of OT quite clear, particularly when a collaborative approach to intervention planning is used (Box 30-1).

Occupation as Means as Intervention

Occupation as means refers to "the occupation acting as the therapeutic change agent to remediate impaired abilities or capacities" (Trombly, 1995, p. 964). Occupation as means as an intervention can be described as follows:

- Including a variety of interventions, such as arts and crafts, games, sports, and specifically chosen daily activities
- Requiring more constrained responses as compared to occupation as ends
- Chosen based on both client interest and potential to remediate an underlying impairment
- Providing a challenge that is slightly beyond what the client can easily achieve. This concept has also been described as finding "just the right challenge."

An assumption inherent in this intervention approach is "that acquisition or reacquisition of motor, cognitive, and psychological skills will ultimately result in successful performance of activities of daily living" (Weinstock-Zlotnick & Hinojosa, 2004, p. 594). Box 30-2 provides examples of using occupation as means as an intervention. Unlike occupation as ends, simply observing a client engaged in occupation as means may not provide the observer with a clear understanding of why the intervention was chosen. In many cases, this understanding emerges after a discussion with the OT practitioner as to the rationale for the choice of the intervention. Teaching someone a new board game may be considered occupation as ends if the client's goals include expanding their repertoire of leisure-based occupations. A board game may also be chosen as a therapeutic mechanism for a variety of reasons that may classify the intervention choice as occupation as means. Examples include using manipulation of game pieces to acquire or reacquire dexterity, placing game pieces out of reach to promote postural control, using the game to develop social skills such as turn taking, grading how long the client plays the game to improve sustained attention skills, and using the game to enhance self-efficacy or lessen anxiety. When this approach is used, the therapist *must* clearly link the potential change in underlying skills and client factors to improved occupational performance. Improved dexterity would not be considered the end product of OT. However, regaining the ability to manipulate fasteners to independently dress, independently finger feed, or be able to manipulate scissors while making holiday cards in school would all be considered examples of desired outcomes depending on client preference and the context of therapy.

When using occupation as means as the intervention, it is particularly important that the OT practitioner choose occupations that have meaning and that the rationale for the intervention is made explicit. Otherwise, clients may find it difficult to understand the focus of OT. It is important that clients do not leave a session simply thinking "we played cards in OT today."

BOX 30-2   EXAMPLES OF USING OCCUPATION AS MEANS

- Rolling out dough to strengthen an older adult's upper limbs so that he or she can regain independence in homemaking tasks such as washing dishes
- Engaging a child in a playground climbing activity to promote body awareness and motor planning so that he or she can engage in age-appropriate play such as bike riding
- Playing a game of Connect Four with game pieces placed on the left side to promote spatial awareness so that a person may be able to locate grooming items placed on the left side of the sink
- Using arts and crafts activities to improve self-esteem and/or lessen anxiety so that a person feels more confident when socializing with others

- Leading a group of adults in a session of water aerobics to promote joint flexibility so that they can maintain independence in home activities such as putting away groceries
- Engaging in a gardening task to develop reach and coordination skills that may then be used during self-care activities
- Engaging a client in a challenging occupation such as money management to promote awareness of cognitive deficits. This improved awareness may then result in the client understanding that he or she requires adaptive cognitive strategies to manage at home.

Combining Occupation as Means and as Ends

It is possible to combine aspects of occupation as ends and occupation as means (Figure 30-1). Using this method, a collaborative approach is used to determine goals and to understand a client's interests. The OT practitioner then uses his or her skills of occupational analysis to determine which underlying performance skills and/or client factors may need to be challenged. In her discussion of combining occupation as ends and means, Gray (1998) states,

> Rather than completing an assessment and using problem areas (components) to decide which activities to use for

treatment (e.g., macramé is great for coordination, parquetry puzzles are assumed to help visual perceptual deficits), the occupational therapist has the added challenge of looking into the client's occupational history and selecting activities related to the client's occupations and interests that can be modified and structured to improve coordination and visual perception. Perhaps that particular client enjoyed waxing the car, making fried chicken, or playing with his or her nieces. The occupational therapist could, with a little creativity and ingenuity, tailor those occupations to treat the very same coordination or visual perceptual deficits. (p. 358).

To be successful, this approach requires that the OT practitioner has mastered the skill of occupational analysis. See Chapter 25 for detailed information on occupational

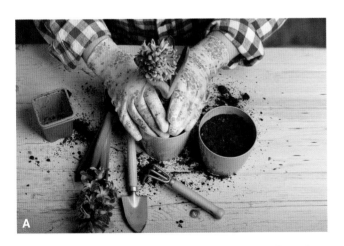
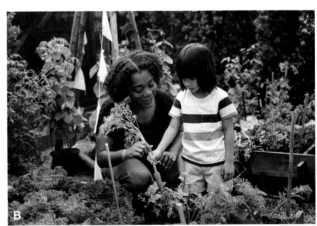

FIGURE 30-1 **A.** Gardening may be considered occupation as ends or means or both. If the client's goal is to resume leisure activities in his or her garden or work in a nursery, this would be considered occupation as ends. If the therapist chooses the enjoyable activity as garden as a way to improve endurance, balance, coordination, or organization skills, it would be considered occupation as means. Just by observing one can not tell. The therapist's rationale and client's goals must be investigated. **B.** For a child, gardening is most likely occupation as means.

TABLE 30-2	Combining Occupation as Means and Occupation as Ends
Goal: Independently Manage/Navigate a Subway System in order to Attend Alcoholics Anonymous Meetings	**Goal: Independent in Toileting**
Occupation as ends: Task-specific training of the occupation using graded physical and verbal cues for difficult aspects of the task such as interpreting a subway map. Helping the client perform parts of the task that are difficult (e.g., money management) so that the task can be completed. Adapting the task so that it can be completed (e.g., providing a prepaid fare card so that the client does not need to manage money).	*Occupation as ends*: Task-specific training of the occupation using graded physical and verbal cues for difficult aspects of the task such as maneuvering from a wheelchair to the commode. Helping the client perform parts of the task that are difficult (e.g., clothing management) so that the task can be completed. Adapting the task so that it can be completed (e.g., providing grab bars or a raised toilet seat).
Occupation as means: Managing and navigating the subway is used to challenge a variety of underlying skills and factors such as the following: • Manipulation of money • Way finding in new environments • Social skills development such as appropriately waiting in line for the attendant • Problem solving if there is a schedule or service change • Calculation of change after money exchange • Maintaining balance when the train is in motion • Endurance for ambulation, stair climbing, and standing tolerance	*Occupation as means*: Using aspects of toileting to challenge a variety of underlying skills and factors such as the following: • Postural control when transitioning from sitting to standing • Motor planning during manipulation of toilet paper • Sequencing the steps of the toileting task • Promoting safety awareness in reference to locking brakes and manipulating footplates out of the way • Challenging sitting balance • Manipulation skills when fastening pants • Awareness of body position in space when transitioning from chair to commode • Lower extremity strength and control to transition from sit to stand and stand to sit

analysis. In summary, occupation is always the ends and is the most frequent means with the addition of purposeful and preparatory methods as needed. See Table 30-2 for examples of combining occupation as ends and means. See Box 30-3 for further discussion regarding classifying interventions.

Specific Intervention Approaches

Occupational therapy practitioners address the interaction among client factors, performance skills, performance patterns, contexts and environments, and activity demands that influence occupational performance within those occupations

the person needs and wants to do. The intervention focus is on the following (AOTA, 2014, p. 313) (Table 30-3):

• Therapeutic use of occupations and activities
• Preparatory methods
• Education and training
• Advocacy (e.g., advocacy, self-advocacy)
• Group interventions

A variety of intervention approaches are available. In some cases, only one category of intervention is used to meet client goals. Other clinical situations require the use of several categories of intervention or a change in intervention choice based on a poor response, reimbursement issues, or a change in client status. Practitioners base their choice of interventions on a variety of factors including

BOX 30-3	INTERVENTIONS ARE NOT ALWAYS EASY TO CLASSIFY

It would be nice if we could neatly classify our OT interventions as occupation as means or occupation as ends. In reality, OT interventions are complex and often involve elements that address impairments, relate to caregivers, and involve both the client and the client's environment. This makes them difficult to name or fit into neat categories. For example, consider interventions focused on clinical challenges such as the following:

• Decreasing self-injurious behavior for people living with traumatic brain injury, dementia, autism, etc.
• Protecting caregivers from harm (e.g., biting) during activities of daily living assist

• Preventing wandering behaviors
• Preventing interaction with potentially dangerous substances such as household chemicals

These interventions may be categorized in a variety of ways beyond means and ends. Categories may include preparatory, education based, behavioral based, sensory based, or as a combination of categories. These interventions are clearly under our domain of concern as occupational therapists as they promote safe participation in occupation in the least restrictive environment.

TABLE 30-3	Types of Interventions Outlined in the AOTA Practice Framework
Type of Intervention	**Non-Inclusive Examples**
Occupations and activities Occupations (client-directed life activities that match participation goals)	Bathing a child Completing morning self-care Applying for job Building a Lego castle Participating on a bowling team Paying monthly bills Participating in a peaceful protest or rally Visiting parent in the hospital Attending and participating religious services
Activities (selected to improve or develop performance skills and patterns to improve occupational performance; components of occupation that hold meaning and relevance)	Practicing car transfers Shuffling cards Climbing a playground ladder Engaging in handwriting or keyboarding activities to type the alphabet Manipulating tools, locks, fasteners Writing out a medication schedule
Preparatory methods and tasks (prepares the client for occupational performance; used as *part of* a session; these methods are used in preparation for our concurrently with occupation and activities) (See Box 30-4.)	Thermal modalities Electrical modalities Edema massage Relaxation activities Splinting Experiencing a sensory room Strengthening via elastic bands or therapeutic putty
Education and training Education (imparting knowledge and information) (See Chapter 32.)	Teaching energy conservations skills to a group undergoing cancer treatments Educating a parent as to the best sleep position for their child with torticollis Educating a company who is planning expansion on universal design Developing a cumulative trauma prevention training course for a local factory
Training (training for the acquisition of everyday skills)	Instructing how to utilize a sip-and-puff wheelchair control Training a child to use a new prosthesis to self-feed Teaching a shelter dweller how to apply for housing or fill out a job application Teaching a person who has lost communication skills to access an augmentative communication device with an adapted switch
Advocacy and self-advocacy (efforts toward promoting occupational justice and empowering clients to obtain resources to participate in everyday life)	Collaborating with an employer to enact the Americans with Disability Act to make reasonable accommodations for your client with mental illness Becoming a board member of the local parks department to assure playgrounds are inclusive Connecting with local museums and arts initiative to promote sensory-friendly experiences A graduate student requests an accommodation for his attention deficit disorder via the university office of students with disabilities. A group of intensive care unit (ICU) nurses reach out to administration concerned over the recent increase in experienced back pain.
Group interventions (facilitate learning and skill acquisition through the dynamics of group and social interaction) (See Chapter 38.)	Running a group for recent widows and widowers to learn skills that were previously performed by their deceased spouses Engaging in a support/education group for those who have experienced a recent amputation Developing a group for children/adolescents with poor social skills to engage in social skills role-playing

From American Occupational Therapy Association. (2014). Occupational therapy practice framework: Domain and process (3rd ed.). *American Journal of Occupational Therapy, 68,* S1–S48.

client choice (see Chapter 37), interpretation of assessment findings (see Chapter 28), evidence (see Chapter 35), clinical experience and professional reasoning (see Chapter 34), knowledge of disease and disability, setting (see Chapter 62), length of stay, and reimbursement (see Chapter 74). The following paragraphs describe the specific approaches, give examples of evidence that support the approaches, and provide further examples in Table 30-4.

Preparatory Interventions

Preparatory interventions have been defined as "methods and tasks that prepare the client for occupational performance, used as *part of a treatment session* in preparation for or concurrently with occupations and activities or provided to a client as a home-based engagement to support daily occupational performance (AOTA, 2014, p. S29). Indeed, a

TABLE 30-4   Examples of Specific Intervention Approaches

Intervention Approach	Examples
Remediation or restoration of personal factors, performance skills, and/or performance patterns to improve occupational performance	• Therapeutic exercise to strengthen a muscle • Use of a video game to improve sustained attention • Goal-oriented reaching to improve upper limb function • Constraint-induced movement therapy to improve upper limb control • Mall walking program to improve endurance • Using homemaking tasks to challenge cognitive functions such as safety and judgment • Sensory integration techniques
Occupational skill acquisition	• Teaching meal preparation skills • Task-specific practice of handwriting • Mental practice of IADL • Teaching adaptive coping skills • Using motor learning principles such as random practice schedules to learn or relearn self-care skills • Teaching a recently widowed woman how to manage monthly bills (which her husband had previously taken care of) • Developing crawling ability in a nonambulatory child with developmental delays
Adaptation/compensation approach to improve occupational performance	• Using a wrist extension orthosis to allow keyboarding • Using a checklist system to perform assigned tasks in a supported employment program • Using a tub seat, handheld shower, and long-handled sponge to enable bathing • Using lightweight cookware during meal preparation • Using built-up handles on school supplies • Using a power scooter during grocery shopping • Using an augmentative communication device to interact with other students
Environmental modifications to improve occupational performance (See Chapter 33.)	• Performing a home visit and suggesting removing throw rugs, sliding shower doors, and unnecessary furniture to promote wheelchair access • Recommending appropriate playground equipment for children with varying skills • Recommending minimizing environmental stimuli (e.g., television on in the background, many people talking at once) for those who are easily distracted • Providing specific information regarding the gradient for a wheelchair ramp • Removing trip hazards in a home or work setting to decrease fall risks • Setting up a bathroom so that needed grooming and hygiene items are placed on the right for those who do not attend to the left • Assisting a family in developing a caretaker schedule for a loved one with a disability • Assisting parents in understanding the type and timing of verbal cues required for their child to focus on homework • Demonstrating how the ground floor of a two-story dwelling can be set up so that a nonambulatory person can live independently on one floor • Providing sensory input such as music to improve alertness during a therapy session
Educational approach to improve occupational performance (See Chapter 32.)	• Instructing caretakers on proper transfer techniques • Informing a person as to the signs and symptoms of emerging depression • Leading a stroke education group focused on community resources and leisure opportunities • Providing information about alternative community access after a driver's license is lost due to visual impairment • Instructing a client or caregiver on skin inspection techniques and the signs of skin breakdown
Prevention approach to maintain occupational performance	• Instructing a stock person in a retail store on proper lifting techniques • Instructing nursing staff on an appropriate in-bed turning schedule to prevent the development of decubitus ulcers • Educating a person who types most of the day on proper posture, rest breaks, and so forth to prevent carpal tunnel syndrome • Preventing social isolation by suggesting appropriate leisure-based after-work activities such as a bowling league, participation in a chorus, etc.
Palliative approaches	• Prescribing positioning equipment that allows more time out of bed • Engaging in reminiscence activities • Engage in activities related to leaving a legacy such as finally writing down and sharing a secret recipe, engagement in creative arts, scrapbooking, etc. • Physical agent modalities, positioning, edema management, and fabricating an orthosis to reduce pain • Teaching caregivers handling techniques for bed mobility assist as the client's physical status declines
Therapeutic use of self (See Chapter 37.)	• Developing rapport • Appropriate use of humor • Maintaining open communication • Being empathetic • Establishing trust • Being motivational • Maintaining a caring attitude • Active listening

IADL, instrumental activities of daily living.

BOX 30-4 **EXAMPLES OF PREPARATORY METHODS AND INTERVENTIONS USED IN CONJUNCTION WITH OR PREPARATION FOR ENGAGEMENT IN OCCUPATION**

- Applying a therapeutic hot pack to and stretching both shoulders prior to a remediation session that uses reaching into kitchen cabinets as a means to improve shoulder range of motion
- Teaching a person with an anxiety disorder to use deep breathing and guided imagery to promote relaxation prior to interviewing for a new job
- Teaching a morning flexibility program to be completed after a warm morning shower to prepare for a variety of morning activities such as making breakfast

- Having a hospitalized child who survived a burn interact with a therapy dog to decrease anxiety prior to a potentially painful therapy session
- Suggesting morning yoga as a method of promoting mental focus prior to facing the day
- Using biofeedback to manage increased muscle tone and maximize the use of an involved limb after traumatic brain injury
- Massaging edema out of a swollen hand to improve finger range of motion with the goal of enabling coin manipulation

recent systematic review (Amini, 2011) of OT for individuals with work-related injuries and illnesses as summarized by Arbesman, Lieberman, and Thomas (2011) documented

> the effectiveness of several preparatory activities such as exercise, the use of the thermal modality of heat, and early mobilization after fractures and acute trauma. Other preparatory methods have been found to be effective for specific clinical conditions, including splinting for osteoarthritis and carpal tunnel syndrome; scar massage to prevent hypertrophic scarring and promote extensibility; the use of sensory focusing, a cognitive pain control technique during burn dressing changes; and the use of pressure garment work gloves after burns. (p. 14)

These interventions are only used in preparation for or concurrently with occupation-based interventions (Box 30-4).

Remediation or Restoration of Client Factors, Performance Skills, and/or Performance Patterns to Improve Occupational Performance

The **remediation** or restoration approach is used to enhance client factors (body functions and body structures) such as range of motion, strength, endurance, thoughts, feelings, cognitive processing, etc., with the goal of improving occupational performance. The approach is also used to enhance performance skills and patterns in order to support occupational performance. It is imperative that clinicians link potential changes in underlying abilities to changes in occupational performance. For example, an objective improvement in strength on a manual muscle test or improved cognitive testing without a resultant change in performance

may reveal that this is the incorrect intervention approach for a client or that underlying impairment being treated was incorrectly chosen. Although some impairments are not amenable to remediation (e.g., severe memory loss, denervated muscles, endurance impairments that emerge during the end stages of disease), others are amenable but require substantial time, motivation, and commitment to achieve a positive outcome. These factors must be considered carefully when choosing this approach. See Figure 30-2 for an example of using pet therapy as part of an intervention designed to remediate coordination problems.

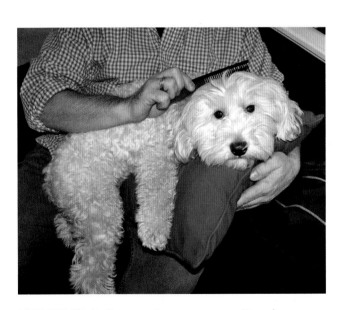

FIGURE 30-2 Occupation as means. Pet therapy can be used to increase range of motion, develop motor planning skills, improve coordination, or lessen anxiety. If the client was a pet owner with the goal of resuming care for his pet, this intervention may be considered occupation as ends.

Therapists working with a variety of shoulder conditions such as adhesive capsulitis, tears of the rotator cuff, and humeral fractures tend to adopt a remediation approach as part of an overall intervention plan. Marik and Roll (2017) evaluated the current evidence for interventions within the OT scope of practice that address pain reduction and increase participation in functional activities. Seventy-six studies were reviewed. Strong evidence was found that range of motion, strengthening exercises, and joint mobilizations can improve function and decrease pain.

A remediation approach called sensory integration may also be adopted when working with children who have varying abilities related to processing incoming sensory information (see Chapter 59). A recent systematic review addressed the question "What is the efficacy of occupational therapy using Ayres Sensory Integration® (ASI) to support functioning and participation?" The authors found that ASI intervention demonstrated positive outcomes for improving individually generated goals of functioning and participation as measured by Goal Attainment Scaling for children with autism. Moderate evidence supported improvements in impairment-level outcomes of improvement in autistic behaviors and skills-based outcomes of reduction in caregiver assistance with self-care activities. Child outcomes in play, sensory-motor, and language skills and reduced caregiver assistance with social skills had emerging but insufficient evidence (Schaaf, Dumont, Arbesman, & May-Benson, 2018).

Occupational Skill Acquisition (Development and Restoration of Occupational Performance)

Interventions that focus specifically on skill development (**occupational skill acquisition**) are frequently used in OT. "Skills for the job of living" is a phrase frequently associated with OT. Skills may include those that were previously developed and are now limited or lost. This situation may occur, for example, with an adolescent or adult who sustains a trauma. It is also an appropriate approach to develop skills for those with developmental delays such as a young adult with intellectual delay or a child with developmental coordination disorder. Lastly, it is appropriate for those who are required to learn new skills based on a change in their role. An example is that of a recent widow who depended on her husband for transportation because she had never learned to drive and is now required to learn to drive or use public transportation (Figure 30-3).

Social skills training is an example of this intervention, and evidence supports the use of this intervention for particular populations (see Chapter 61). A recent study compared the daily living skills of children with and

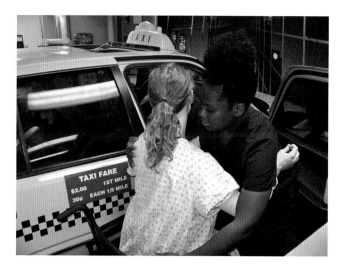

FIGURE 30-3 Occupation as ends. The therapist is using physical assist during a session focused on functional retraining of mobility using an adaptive transfer technique.

without attention-deficit/hyperactivity disorder (ADHD) and the influence of a social skills training group on these skills. Children in the group with ADHD were randomly selected to attend group treatment that focused on social skills training through meaningful occupations such as art, games, and cooking. The children were evaluated at the beginning of group treatment and after 10 sessions using the Assessment of Motor and Process Skills (AMPS). Ten children without ADHD were evaluated at similar intervals. Children with ADHD initially achieved significantly lower scores on the AMPS in all process skills and in the coordination motor subtest than children without ADHD. Children with ADHD significantly improved from the first to the second evaluation and no longer differed from the children without ADHD after treatment. The authors concluded that the results emphasize the need for a focus on occupation in assessment and treatment of children with ADHD (Gol & Jarus, 2005).

Community reintegration training also serves as an example of this intervention. A recent experiment was carried out to examine the effect of an OT intervention focused on improving community skills after a lower extremity major joint replacement. One hundred and seven subjects, status post total hip or total knee replacement, were examined pre- and post-community reintegration intervention involving practice of community skills in a natural environment. Skills included safely transferring out of the vehicle, managing outdoor obstacles such as uneven surfaces, ambulating throughout the destination, and appropriately transferring back into the car. Participants reported significantly higher scores postintervention on measures of satisfaction, performance, and confidence related to community living skills. Self-reported scores were significantly higher for individual community skills as well as the overall score (Gillen et al., 2007).

Adaptation/Compensation Approach to Improve Occupational Performance

The **adaptation** or compensation approach is used in a variety of situations. These include when a disability is considered permanent (e.g., after the amputation of a limb), underlying client factors or performance skills are not expected to improve (e.g., prolonged and severe short-term memory loss or severe and persistent lower limb weakness after an SCI), limited access to therapy prevents engagement in a remediation program, and/or clients and their families prefer this approach. This intervention is frequently combined with environmental modifications, which is described next. Many times, this approach is also used in conjunction with a remediation approach. A person who is recovering from the resection of a brain tumor may use adaptive activities of daily living (ADL) methods while they are undergoing motor control remediation interventions. Specific areas of occupation are the focus of this approach, with an emphasis on modifying the demands of the task and using adaptive equipment/assistive devices (Figure 30-4).

Gentry (2008) evaluated the effects of an OT training protocol using personal digital assistants (PDAs) as assistive technology for people with cognitive impairment related to multiple sclerosis. Following the training period, participants demonstrated the ability to learn how

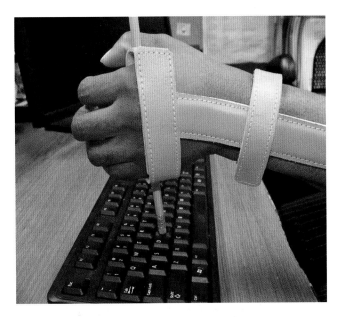

FIGURE 30-4 Adaptive device used to promote independence in typing, writing, feeding, and so forth for those with wrist and hand weakness.

to use basic PDA functions and retain learning for at least 8 weeks. Functional performance increased significantly with PDA use, and this gain was maintained at 8-week follow-up.

This approach can also be useful within the cognitive rehabilitation domain. Another example of evidence to support the use of this approach is a study that examined the effect of cognitive adaptation training (CAT) on a sample of people living with schizophrenia who had been in the community at least 3 months. Cognitive adaptation training is a series of adaptive supports and environmental modifications (see later) designed to compensate for deficits in cognitive functioning. Examples of supports include signs, alarms, labels, and organization of belongings to cue and sequence adaptive behavior in the client's home and work environments. Forty-five participants were randomly assigned to one of three conditions: (1) CAT, (2) a condition that controlled for therapist time and provided environmental changes unrelated to cognitive deficits or, (3) follow-up only. Results of repeated measures indicated that those participating in CAT had better adaptive function and quality of life and fewer positive symptoms than those in the two non-CAT conditions. The authors concluded that compensatory strategies may improve various outcomes in those living with schizophrenia (Velligan et al., 2002).

Environmental Modifications to Improve Occupational Performance

Modifying the environment (environmental modification) is also considered an adaptive approach as described earlier. It includes modifying both the physical environment that includes the natural (geographic terrain, sensory qualities of the environment, plants and animals) and built nonhuman environment (buildings, furniture, etc.) as well as the social environment (relationships and expectations of persons, organizations, populations) (AOTA, 2014). Physical environment modifications may include incorporating aspects of barrier-free and universal design into intervention plans. An example of social environment modifications would be teaching caregivers the most efficient cuing method to assure that the person living with dementia can continue to participate in family meals.

A variety of sources of evidence for the efficacy of environment-based interventions on the affect, behavior, and performance of people with Alzheimer disease and related dementias exists. Jensen and Padilla (2017) evaluated the effectiveness of environment-based interventions that address behavior, perception, and falls in the home and other settings for people with Alzheimer disease and related major neurocognitive disorders. The authors documented that strong evidence indicates that person-centered approaches can improve behavior. Moderate evidence supports noise regulation, environmental design, unobtrusive visual barriers, and environmental relocation strategies to reduce problematic behaviors. On the other hand, they found that evidence is insufficient for the effectiveness of mealtime ambient music, bright light, proprioceptive input, wander gardens, optical strategies, and sensory devices in improving behavior or reducing wandering and falls.

Another study examined the short-term effects of a home environmental intervention on self-efficacy and upset in caregivers and daily function of dementia patients. One hundred and seventy-one families were examined and were randomized to intervention or usual care control group. The intervention involved five 90-minute home visits by occupational therapists who provided education and physical and social environmental modifications. The intervention involved the following:

- Educating caregivers about the impact of the environment on dementia-related behaviors
- Helping caregivers simplify objects in the home (e.g., remove clutter), break down tasks (e.g., one- or two-step commands, lay out clothing in the order in which it is to be donned)
- Involving other members of the family network or formal supports in daily caregiving tasks

The authors demonstrated that, as compared with controls, intervention caregivers reported fewer declines in patients' IADL, less decline in self-care, and fewer behavior problems in patients. The intervention spouses reported reduced upset, women reported enhanced self-efficacy in managing behaviors, and women and minorities reported enhanced self-efficacy in managing functional dependency. The authors concluded that the environmental program appeared to have a modest effect on those with dementia IADL dependence as well as improve self-efficacy and reduce upset in specific areas of caregiving (Gitlin, Corcoran, Winter, Boyce, & Hauck, 2001).

Educational Approach to Improve Occupational Performance

Occupational therapy practitioners frequently take on the role of teacher and use an education-based approach when working with clients. Education approaches may be used in both individual and group settings. This approach may be aimed directly at the clients, their caregivers, significant others, employers, etc.

Teaching joint protection techniques would serve as an example of this approach. Researchers have assessed the effects on pain, disability, and health status of an educational joint protection program in a group of people with moderate-to-severe rheumatoid arthritis (RA). Eighty-five subjects were enrolled into the study and randomized into either an experimental group or a control group. The intervention consisted of four educational meetings. These included information on pathophysiology and evolution of RA, joint protection during ADL, suggestions on how to adapt the surrounding environment, and self-learning exercises to perform at home. The study showed that 8 months after attending an educational joint protection program, subjects with moderate-to-severe RA presented with less pain and disability and thus an enhanced health status (Masiero et al., 2007).

Teaching those with fatigue issues how to manage and conserve their energy throughout the day would also fall under this category of intervention. A recent study assessed the impact of a one-to-one fatigue management course on participants' fatigue, self-efficacy, quality of life, and energy conservation behaviors. Participants showed significant reductions in fatigue and significant increases in self-efficacy and quality of life at posttest. These beneficial effects were maintained at follow-up. The authors concluded that the one-to-one fatigue management course is a beneficial intervention for people with chronic conditions and fatigue (Van Heest, Mogush, & Mathiowetz, 2017).

Prevention Approach to Maintain Occupational Performance

The prevention intervention approach can be used for those living with or without a disability but who are at risk for developing limitations in occupational performance (AOTA, 2014). It can also be used to prevent secondary impairments that may limit occupational performance such as pain, contracture, skin breakdown, depression, etc.

The Lifestyle Redesign® for pressure ulcer prevention in SCI falls under this approach. The specific aim of this program is to develop a lifestyle intervention that promises to significantly reduce pressure ulcers in the population of adults with SCI. The intervention was developed based on the results of a qualitative investigation of lifestyle and ulcer risk among adults with SCI (Clark et al., 2006; University of Southern California, 2013).

Another example of a prevention approach is discussed in a systematic review explored the impact of fall prevention programs and home modifications on falls and the performance of community-dwelling older adults. The authors concluded that the strongest results were found for multifactorial programs that included home evaluations and home modifications, physical activity or exercise, education, vision and medication checks, or assistive technology to prevent falls. Positive outcomes included a decreased rate of functional decline, a decrease in fear of falling, and an increase in physical factors such as balance and strength. The strength of the evidence for physical activity and home modification programs provided individually was moderate (Chase, Mann, Wasek, & Arbesman, 2012).

Palliative Approaches

The **palliative** approach focuses on providing clients with relief from the symptoms, pain, and stress of a serious illness regardless of the diagnosis. The goal is to improve quality of life for both the client and their family. Unlike hospice care (end-of-life care), it can be carried out throughout the disease course and not just during the last months of life. Curative care interventions also may be considered under the umbrellas of the palliative approach; however, curative services are not provided when a client is receiving hospice care (AOTA, 2016). Palliative care is often part of end-of-life care.

The AOTA (2016) defines the roles and focus of the OT practitioner related to end-of-life care as the following:

- Occupational therapy practitioners' distinct value in end-of-life care is to facilitate quality of life for clients and their caregivers through engagement in occupations during the client's remaining days.
- The chosen occupations of a dying person or his or her caregiver may be familiar and routine, such as a goal of sharing a final family meal, or they may be dynamic and tied specifically to saying goodbye in a good way, such as resolving unfinished business or crafting a final gift for family members.
- Occupational therapy practitioners recognize the purpose of these occupations as twofold: (1) providing a means of self-expression and engagement while (2) serving as a vehicle by which the client finds peace with the dying process and prepares for death.
- Occupational therapy practitioners facilitate a good death experience for all involved in the dying process by enabling occupation.
- Practitioners consider environmental and contextual factors (e.g., accessibility of objects or places in the environment, caregiver training, social contacts available to prevent isolation) as well as personal factors (e.g., decreased endurance, increased anxiety) that may be limiting a client's abilities and satisfaction when performing desired occupations.
- Practitioners collaborate with the client and family members throughout the OT process to identify occupations that are especially meaningful and to incorporate strategies that support participation and quality of life rather than rehabilitation.

The AOTA (2016) further defines the roles and focus of the OT practitioner related to end-of-life care as it relates to caregivers as the following:

- Occupational therapy practitioners recognize the interdependent nature of relationships at end of life and caregivers' potential need for support in their caring role. At times, the needs of the caregiver may exceed the needs of the person who is dying yet be overshadowed by the immediate needs of the loved one.
- Occupational therapy practitioners extend services to caregivers in their own right.
- Practitioners are uniquely qualified to boost caregiver recognition and support by identifying people in caregiving roles and assessing their needs and preferences with regard to potential interventions.

Home-based OT is a typical context in which palliative care is delivered. A study examined OT for patients in the palliative stage of cancer care from the perspective of the patients and carers. This study defined the palliative stage of cancer care as the point from which the patient is no longer responsive to curative treatment until death. The study examined 30 clients and their primary informal carers via a structured interview. The results suggested that both patients and their carers valued the service provided and report high levels of satisfaction, although there were gaps identified in service provision. The authors concluded that there is a need to build on the good work being done by home-based occupational therapists in the area of palliative cancer care and increase education and resources to ensure that a client-centered, holistic approach to care is used, addressing both the needs of the patient and their carers (Kealey & McIntyre, 2005).

Therapeutic Use of Self

Therapeutic use of self, a component of the therapeutic relationship, should not be considered a separate intervention but should instead influence and inform all of the aforementioned intervention approaches. Although there is no consensus on a definition, therapeutic use of self has been defined as the "planned use of his or her personality, insights, perceptions, and judgments as part of the therapeutic process" (Punwar & Peloquin, 2000, p. 285). This term is also used to refer to therapists' conscious efforts to optimize their interactions with clients (Punwar & Peloquin, 2000).

Although this area of clinical practice can benefit from further research emphasis and attention in education programs (Taylor, Lee, Kielhofner, & Ketkar, 2009), it is a foundation of practice. A survey of 129 occupational therapists practicing in various areas found that therapists strongly emphasized empathy, rapport, and open communication as being important in the therapeutic relationship.

Participants also perceived the therapeutic relationship as critical to therapy outcomes (Cole & McLean, 2003).

Eklund and Hallberg (2001) reported the results from a survey investigating psychiatric occupational therapists' ($n = 292$) use of verbal interaction on a regular basis with their clients. Among predefined areas, verbal interaction, routine occupations, self-image, and ego-strengthening interventions were among the most frequently given alternatives. The content analysis indicated that the occupational therapists used verbal interaction to

- Enhance the therapeutic relationship. This was expressed as efforts to make contact, to stimulate motivation in the patient, or to enhance mutuality and make the patient participate actively.
- Give the patients opportunities to reflect on and articulate feelings and experiences (e.g., formulate feelings and opinions; make their own thoughts, feelings, and actions clear; have the patient reflect on his or her behavior in the OT sessions).
- Make assessments (i.e., to assess capacities, resources, functions, liabilities, problems, and motivation).
- Make treatment plans to arrive at an appropriate treatment plan together with the patient and set goals.
- Provide interventions in order to reach certain goals the intention of acting to remedy problems and give support in order to reach certain goals.
- Evaluate and follow up their practice.

See Table 30-4 for specific examples of interventions.

Case Vignettes

One may note that the aforementioned approaches are not mutually exclusive. As described earlier, you may use an *education*-based approach to *prevent* joint destruction and further decline in occupational performance for those living with arthritis. A therapist involved in *palliative* care with a client with a nonoperable brain tumor may use *adaptive* seating in a wheelchair to decrease back pain. In many cases, therapists use a variety of approaches with the same client, whereas in other cases may focus on one approach. The following case vignettes highlight this point. Cases include an occupational profile, relevant assessment findings, goals, and intervention choices (Case Studies 30-2 to 30-5).

Conclusion

Occupational therapy practitioners have a variety of intervention approaches available to choose from and combine. The correct choices of interventions are based on a variety of data including client choice, knowledge of disease/disability, assessment findings, clinical experience, and professional reasoning. No matter which approach is chosen, occupation is always the end and is the most frequent means with the addition of purposeful and preparatory methods as needed.

CASE STUDY 30-2   JAMES: A MARRIED BANKER WHO SURVIVED A STROKE

Occupational Profile

James is 62-year-old banker. He lives in a two-story house in a suburban town with his wife Carla, and Max, the family dog. James was in his usual state of health (hypertension and type 2 diabetes mellitus) when he woke up on the floor, unable to move his left limbs, drooling, and slurring his words when yelling for help. He was admitted to the neurology unit of the local hospital. After a 3-day stay, he was transferred to the inpatient rehabilitation unit. Upon initial meeting with his occupational therapist, Dan, the therapist learned that James has been looking forward to retiring soon to "spend time with my wife, fish in the lake, read classic novels, and get to know my children and grandchildren again." He reports that he is a workaholic and regrets "missing out" on key family functions. He states that he is "fiercely independent and mortified about the help he needs with basic hygiene." He also reports that he is "very left handed" and frustrated by the lack of motor output in his left limbs.

Assessment Findings

Dan first administered the Canadian Occupational Performance Measure (COPM), a self-report measure of occupational performance. James identified toileting, using his tablet computer to access work and personal e-mail, performing grooming using both hands, reading work documents, and holding his new grandchild as initial areas of focus. He rated his performance of these tasks as between 2 and 4 on a 1 to 10 scale. He rated his satisfaction with his performance as 2/10 for all five of the identified tasks. The Functional Independence Measure (FIM™) was used to objectively document his self-care and mobility skills. James required moderate assist for all aspects of self-care except that he was able to feed himself with minimal assist. James also required moderate assist for ambulation and all transfers. Based on behaviors noted during the FIM administration, Dan was concerned about the presence of left neglect. Left neglect is a neurologic phenomenon in which a client will overfocus on the right side of the environment and pay less attention to (i.e., neglect) the left side. Some behaviors that were noted included spending the majority of time brushing the right side of the mouth, leaving the left arm behind when rolling in bed, and multiple left-sided collisions when propelling his wheelchair. To document the impact of left neglect on daily function, the therapist administered the Catherine Bergego Scale (CBS). This scale is based on observation of ADL, mobility, and social interaction to objectify the quantity and quality of left-sided errors. James scored 17/30, with low scores indicating less impairment. Based on some statements James was making in therapy (e.g., "Why can't I read? It is my arm and leg that are weak. There is nothing wrong with my eyes!"), Dan decided to ask James to score himself on the client report version of the CBS. James scored himself as 5/30, indicating that James was overestimating his level of function and underestimating his level of impairment (i.e., the impact of the left neglect). Finally, James was quite concerned about using his limbs again. A manual muscle test revealed that his left limbs fell into the 1/5 to 2/5 range, with 5 indicating normal strength. Sensation was preserved.

Goals

Based on the occupational profile, the COPM results, and the analysis of occupational performance, James's initial short goals were set as (1) James will perform toilet transfers with minimal assistance, (2) James will perform grooming using both hands with minimal assist, and (3) James will read the daily weather report accurately with tactile and verbal cues four out of five times.

Interventions

Dan developed an intervention plan that combined *acquisition*, *adaptive*, *remediation*, and *environmental modification* approaches. As James stated multiple times that he was concerned and "embarrassed" about being helped with hygiene, Dan worked with James twice per day, and the morning session was focused on these tasks. Because of James's significant weakness, Dan first *modified the environment* by providing a raised toilet seat. Dan also checked that the already placed grab bars were secure. James was encouraged to use his left arm as a stabilizer on the grab bar (*remediation* of motor control). Dan also had to *adapt* the method in which James would perform the task. It was decided that James would use a stand-pivot technique to move from his wheelchair to the toilet. Once the method was decided, Dan worked with James to learn and *acquire* the skill. Dan used a variety of motor learning principles (see Chapter 57) to assist James in acquiring this skill. These included blocked practice at first followed by random practice, providing James with feedback about his performance, demonstrating the task for James, and decreasing the number of verbal and physical cues as

James's performance improved. Several of the cues that were provided were related to using his left limbs (*remediation*) as able ("push up with your left arm"; "straighten your left knee"). This session demonstrates the use of a combined *occupation as ends/means* approach. That is, the focus is toileting the "goal to be learned," and toileting is being used as a therapeutic change agent to remediate left-sided motor control and left-sided awareness.

In the grooming domain, both James's motor status and his left neglect limited his occupational performance. Dan first *modified the environment* by placing a colored piece of tape on the far left side of the sink and the left edge of the mirror. This "perceptual anchor" was used as an environmental cue to scan to the left (Gillen et al., 2015). Dan attempted to *remediate* his haphazard scanning ability. Prior to starting the task, Dan worked with James to find all of the objects required for the task by systematically scanning the workspace. He was taught to scan to the left until he saw the blue tape, scan back right, and so on. Although James is left handed, the therapist began to *remediate* James's left limb by showing him how to use his left hand as a nondominant assist. He was able to stabilize the toothpaste with the left hand and use his right hand to guide his left to control the faucets. Similar to the earlier discussion, a variety of cues and methods of feedback were used to help James *acquire* the skill of oral care. Again, using a combined *occupation as ends/means* approach, oral care is the goal to be learned, whereas grooming is also being used to improve scanning, left-sided attention, and left-sided motor control (Figure 30-5).

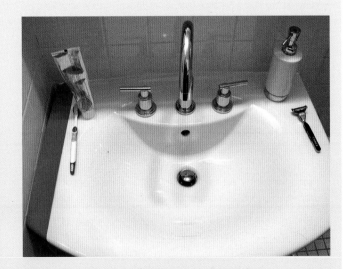

**FIGURE 30-5 Environmental modification.
A colored strip of tape on the sink used as a perceptual anchor to improve awareness to the left side of the environment.**

(continues)

CASE STUDY 30-2   JAMES: A MARRIED BANKER WHO SURVIVED A STROKE *(continued)*

In terms of reading, Dan was concerned that James was not aware of the reason that he could not read (i.e., his left neglect). Because reading was a critical aspect of both his work and planned leisure pursuits, Dan decided that starting with reading training proper would probably result in failure based on the assessment findings. Dan was concerned that failure may result in the possible development of anxiety/depression. Instead, Dan decided to use an *occupation as means* approach to begin with using activities on James's tablet computer as the therapeutic change agent. Dan first used the *adaptive* settings to enlarge the screen, and James was encouraged to hold the tablet vertically. It came up in casual conversation that James enjoyed playing solitaire. Dan decided to use this game as the method to begin to teach James, further scanning strategies (*remediation*), and begin introducing reading preparation (pre-skill *acquisition*). After the solitaire application loaded the cards, Dan asked James to read the initial seven cards dealt. James initially only read

the five cards biased toward the right. When this pointed out, James became concerned. Dan began to use this discussion as a way to *remediate* awareness regarding his neglect. It was pointed out that when he missed cards, they were always on the left. Dan made connections to the mistakes made during this game to other behaviors such as having difficulty finding objects on the left side of the sink, etc. Dan asked James to hold the tablet in both hands (*remediation* of motor function) and to use his left hand as the perceptual anchor (*adaptation*) to know when he has scanned far enough to the left. Dan then continued to use more complex games (e.g., word search) that required left to right scanning and reading skills. Dan continued these interventions until James became more proficient in using these skills and strategies. Dan then found Websites that had one to two line descriptors of the daily weather. Using the enlarged print command (*adaptation*) and the newly *acquired* scanning skills, James met his short-term goal.

CASE STUDY 30-3   SAHAR: AN 8-YEAR-OLD GIRL LIVING WITH CEREBRAL PALSY

Occupational Profile

Sahar is an 8-year-old girl who attends a mainstream school. Sahar receives occupational, physical, and speech therapy in school to manage her spastic cerebral palsy. She has an attendant with her at all times. Sahar enjoys art, pop music, playing with her dog, and, until recently, school. Until the recent past, she particularly enjoyed spelling and English classes. She recently started to make comments to her parents that she "does not fit in," is "tired of being teased," "does not want to feel different," and that she "is a bad friend." Her parents are concerned about her self-esteem and her new disinterest in school. They are getting reports from her teacher that she is "falling behind" and seems "disinterested."

Sahar recently started working with a new occupational therapist. Her assessment findings included the following:

- Environmental: Sahar's power wheelchair was ill fitting. Her seating system was not providing enough support, and she tended to lean to the left and sit with a flexed spine and neck. This position limited her eye contact, which resulted in difficulty seeing the teacher and information written on the blackboard. In addition, she

has recently started to drool occasionally because of her neck position. The wheelchair was too high to pull up to the desks and tables in the classroom so she was always positioned behind the class with her aide, which also added to her difficulty interacting with peers and seeing her teacher. Finally, due to her poor seated position, she was having trouble controlling the wheelchair, and her aide was now assisting her in navigating the school.

- Children's Assessment of Participation and Enjoyment (CAPE): The CAPE was used to measure Sahar's participation in activities outside of school. Sahar presented with overall low participation in activities. Specifically, she reported low participation in recreational, physical, and social activities. Many activities were engaged in alone and many were confined to her bedroom.

- School Function Assessment (SFA): Sahar scored 2 (participation in a few activities) for most items on the participation scale, 1 or 2 (moderate-to-extensive assistance and adaptions) for most items on the task supports scale, and 1 or 2 (does not perform or partial performance) for most items on the activity performance scale.

- Evaluation of Social Interaction (ESI): Sahar's score on the ESI was indicative of problematic social interactions severe enough to limit interactions with others (moderately to markedly ineffective and/or immature social interaction skills). Particular items that were difficult for Sahar included not approaching/starting interactions, physical difficulties not supporting interaction (looks, turns toward), not replying, and at times not taking turns.
- Vision: Sahar has worn glasses since she was 3 years old. The therapist found that Sahar's acuity was decreased (20/60) for far vision using a Snellen chart.

Goals

(1) Sahar will navigate her school in a power wheelchair with distant supervision. (2) Sahar will answer two questions per day during teaching lessons. (3) Sahar will improve her overall academic performance as indicated by her quarterly report card. (4) Sahar will initiate two conversations per day with peers during recess or other group activities.

Interventions

Sahar's new therapist took the lead in terms of managing this change in Sahar's function. He focused on maximizing her social and academic participation in school, making Sahar feel more comfortable about fitting in with peers, and improving her self-esteem. He used a variety of approaches including *environmental modifications* and *adaptive* and *acquisition* approaches. In addition, he referred Sahar to an eye care specialist to change the prescription in her glasses. Sahar's occupational therapist first collaborated with a wheelchair vendor to update the chair that she has outgrown and update her seating system. An *adapted* wheelchair frame that has the ability to tilt in space was ordered. A tilt system changed Sahar's orientation in space while maintaining fixed hip, knee, and ankle angles. This tilt helped to promote proper alignment including an extended spine. A headrest was provided to maintain Sahar's head in extension, expand her field of vision, and decrease the tendency to drool. Lateral supports were added to the system to further help maintain Sahar's posture. A removable lap tray was provided so that Sahar could use it as a work/play space when not at a table or desk. The occupational therapist ordered an *adapted* joystick with a "t-bar" to compensate for Sahar's poor hand function and promote independent mobility. The occupational therapist spent time with Sahar teaching her to *acquire* the skill of controlling the wheelchair both indoors and outdoors. Time was spent learning how to navigate doorways, ramps, and curb cuts. Particular attention was spent teaching Sahar how to safely navigate the playground and recess areas.

The occupational therapist collaborated with Sahar's teacher to *modify the environment*. Desks/tables were rearranged to assure that Sahar's chair could easily navigate the classroom. The therapist placed table risers on one table so that Sahar's wheelchair could fit underneath it. With these modifications, Sahar was able to navigate the classroom and sit with other students. This also served to facilitate her interactions with peers and her teacher during lesson plans.

Although these changes resulted in Sahar making statements that reflect improved esteem, the occupational therapist and Sahar's parents were concerned about her feeling socially isolated. The therapist then shifted back to an *acquisition* approach focused on social skills training. The therapist tapped into Sahar's love of art and collaborated with Sahar's teacher to integrate an arts and crafts lesson once a week. The focus of the lesson was for the students to make seasonal decorations for a bulletin board. The therapist provided *adaptive* art supplies such as a loop scissor mounted on the table and a paintbrush that was built up with foam. As Sahar's physical participation began to improve, the therapist used the arts and crafts sessions to encourage Sahar to initiate conversations, maintain eye contact, and answer appropriately when spoken to. Because Sahar had limited manipulation abilities, as her confidence grew, she took on the primary role of deciding the overall theme and design of the bulletin board while her peers took main responsibility for the implementation of the design. The interventions in total helped Sahar reach her goals.

CASE STUDY 30-4   LOIS: AN ADULT WITH SCHIZOPHRENIA LIVING AT HOME

Occupational Profile

Lois is a 32-year-old who is currently living with her parents in an apartment in a large city. Lois was diagnosed with schizophrenia in college when she began to develop delusions that her roommate was following her all over campus and that all the teachers "wanted me to fail." Her behavior became more erratic and disorganized, causing her to drop out of school. She was soon admitted to an inpatient unit for medical stabilization of her symptoms. Over the years, Lois has been inconsistent with her medications and has required at least two other hospitalizations. Her parents are concerned about her recent lack of structure secondary to quitting her job. They feel that when she lacks structure, her symptoms begin to worsen. They have noticed that she is not paying attention to personal hygiene and reports that she sits on the couch all day. Lois reports that she is just "busy." Her parents want her to contribute to household chores and make herself "useful."

Assessment Findings

An informal interview was conducted with Lois along with her parents. Lois agreed that it would be helpful if her parents were part of the therapy process. The occupational therapist, Nadia, inquired as to how Lois spent her days. Lois was able to describe her morning care routine and eating meals with her family but described little else in terms of active participation. Her parents corroborated that most of her day is spent watching television. Her parents then again articulated their concerns about Lois not contributing to the household management. Nadia asked Lois if she would be willing to take on household responsibilities. Reluctantly, Lois agreed to contribute to shopping and cooking simple meals such as lunch. Nadia first administered the Assessment of Motor and Process Skills (AMPS). The AMPS is an observational assessment that is used to measure the quality of a person's ADL. The quality of the person's ADL performance is assessed by rating the effort, efficiency, safety, and independence of 16 ADL motor and 20 ADL process skill items while the person is doing chosen, familiar, and life-relevant ADL tasks. Nadia observed three AMPS tasks including making canned soup, making a luncheon meat sandwich, and sweeping the floor. Skill items that were considered ineffective or markedly deficient included paces, chooses, search/locate, inquires, sequences, calibrates, benefits, adjusts, and accommodates. The Test of Grocery Shopping Skills (TOGSS) was also administered. The TOGSS is a performance-based assessment that measures how accurately and efficiently clients can locate items in a grocery store. Scales include accuracy (finding the correct item, correct size, and lowest price), time to locate the items, and redundancy (e.g., returning to the same aisle). Lois scored 17 out of a possible 30 on this measure.

Goals

Based on the interview with Lois and her parents as well as the standardized measures outlined earlier, two goals were set for Lois: (1) Lois will prepare grilled cheese safely and efficiently with distant supervision and verbal cues for sequencing and locating items and (2) Lois will successfully grocery shop for 10 items with 85% accuracy in less than 35 minutes.

Interventions

Acquisition, *adaptive*, *therapeutic use of self*, and *environmental modification* approaches were used to help Lois meet these goals. The intervention for teaching Lois grocery shopping skills was based on an evidence-based protocol (Brown, Rempfer, & Hamera, 2002). This intervention is designed to compensate (*adaptation*) for cognitive impairments by providing strategies that organize/simplify the task (*adaptation*) and environment (*environmental modifications*). During all sessions, Nadia used encouragement, positive feedback, and open communication to keep Lois motivated (*therapeutic use of self*). Based on the protocol, Nadia worked with Lois for nine sessions on *acquiring* this skill. The authors of the protocol integrated strategies from several learning theories to help clients acquire this skill. Examples of strategies that were used include repeated practice, structured feedback, motivational incentives, scripting of the process, situated cognitive approaches, and cuing (Brown et al., 2002). Training the skill was based on a script of three questions with corresponding strategies. These questions helped Lois sequence the task. The three aspects of training included "Where is it?" "Is this what I am looking for?" and "Is this the lowest price?" Examples of strategies for the "Where is it?" step include use overhead signs, know the store layout or use a map, and ask for help (Brown et al., 2002).

Based on the work of Duncombe (2004), Nadia assisted Lois in learning the skills of cooking using an *acquisition* approach. The first lesson emphasized the aspects of cooking required for a simple stovetop task (making pudding). Lois was given a guideline that listed 10 steps necessary for cooking simple foods (*adaptive*). The list included skills such as washing hands prior to cooking, clearing a space to work, gathering equipment and ingredients, safety, etc. Nadia hung these guidelines in Lois's kitchen. During the next two sessions, Nadia had Lois cook meals that were similar in the number of steps but differed in ingredients. The rationale was to help Lois begin to generalize and transfer the skills she was learning. During session 2, Lois made a sandwich, emphasizing 7 of the 10 cooking guidelines. During the next session, the task was upgraded to preparing soup during which all 10 of the guidelines were followed (Duncombe, 2004). The combined intervention approaches allowed Lois to meet her goals.

CASE STUDY 30-5   SHIRLEY: RECEIVING HOME HOSPICE WITH END-STAGE AMYOTROPHIC LATERAL SCLEROSIS

Occupational Profile

Shirley is a 60-year-old woman who was diagnosed with amyotrophic lateral sclerosis (ALS) 1 year ago. The occupational therapist on this case, Yin, first met Shirley when she was diagnosed and monitored her functional status during monthly clinic visits. Shirley is now homebound and receiving end-of-life care via home hospice. Shirley was a homemaker; and her pride and joy are her two children and, more recently, her three grandchildren, all younger than 3 years old. Occupational therapy was ordered for three to four home visits to implement *palliative* and *prevention* interventions and maximize the family's ability to care for her using both *adaptive* and *education* approaches, with an overarching theme of *therapeutic use of self* during this difficult time.

Assessment Findings

Prior to the home visit, Yin reviewed Shirley's medical record. Her last documented ALS Functional Rating Scale-Revised was 15. This tool estimates degree of functional impairment. The scores range from 0 to 48 (best). An informal interview indicated that the family was most concerned about keeping Shirley pain free as she recently started to wince when they were assisting her to move in bed, transfer, and dress. Shirley's husband, Tom, reported that he wanted to be very hands on with her care despite having the hospice team. He reported that his low back has been hurting him ever since Shirley developed a substantial loss of strength in her legs and trunk. Before this latest decline in status, Shirley had been typing letters to her three young grandchildren. Her plan was to give these letters to her children in a sealed envelope to be given to the grandchildren when they turned 16. Tom reported that Shirley was devastated that she would not see them grow up and she wanted to be remembered by them. Shirley was not able to talk despite being grossly cognitively intact. Yin established a yes/no system of responses using eye movements (one blink indicated "yes," two "no," and wide eyes indicated "pain"). Through this blinking system, Shirley was able to indicate that she was highly motivated to finish the letters and that it was painful in her low back, shoulders, and hips when she was being assisted with ADL/mobility. The Caregiver Burden Scale was administered to Tom. Findings suggested that Tom felt quite burdened in all five domains (general strain, isolation, disappointment, emotional involvement, and environment). In addition, Yin observed Tom assisting Shirley in and out of bed and from her bed to her wheelchair. Tom was noted to hold Shirley tightly under her arms during transfers and demonstrated poor body mechanics (twisting his back) during the transfer.

Goals

Based on Shirley and her family's concerns, the following goals were established: (1) Tom will demonstrate proper body mechanics and safe technique when transferring Shirley to her wheelchair with supervision; (2) Shirley will, with supervision, complete writing three letters with assistive devices; and (3) Tom will independently and safely position Shirley in bed.

Interventions

The first intervention was *education based* to *prevent* injury to Tom's back as well as to *prevent* Shirley from becoming injured during transfers and mobility. Yin demonstrated and discussed proper body mechanics and demonstrated proper transfer techniques. As Tom was still having difficulty, Yin further *adapted* the transfer method and showed Tom how to use a sliding board to assist Shirley from her bed to the wheelchair. Tom reported that he felt more secure with this technique. Continuing with an *education* approach, Yin demonstrated proper positioning in bed to keep Shirley's joints in neutral as to *prevent* contractures and pain. While Shirley was in bed, Yin additionally taught Tom to perform gentle passive range of motion following the application of heating pads on Shirley's shoulders and hips to help control pain (*palliative* approach). Yin told Tom that the heat could be used two to three times per day for 20 minutes to help control Shirley's pain.

At the next home-based session, Yin observed that Shirley was in a much better position in her bed. Yin asked to observe Tom transfer Shirley to her wheelchair. He transferred her safely and effectively. Yin borrowed three pieces of equipment from the ALS clinic to allow Shirley to complete her letters using an *adaptive* approach. Yin applied a static wrist orthosis to Shirley's right wrist for stability and applied a universal cuff to her right hand (refer back to Figure 30-4). The cuff is designed to give persons with limited grip or dexterity controlled use of items such as eating utensils and writing tools. A pencil was inserted into the universal cuff with the eraser side facing down. Next, Yin attached an overhead suspension sling to Shirley's wheelchair. Using this device, Shirley's arm was supported by a sling and suspended by an overhead rod. This device is used for people presenting with proximal weakness, with muscle grades in the 1/5 to 3/5 range. The sling acts to unweight Shirley's weak arm to allow her to use her remaining muscle strength to guide her hand to the proper letters on the keyboard. Using these adaptations, Shirley was able to complete her letters, albeit slowly.

Acknowledgments

The author would like to acknowledge the contributions of Anne E. Dickerson, PhD, OTR/L, FAOTA, and Elin Schold Davis, OTR/L, CDRS, for contributing the driving vignette. He would also like to acknowledge Emily Raphael-Greenfield, EdD, OTR/L, and Debra Tupé, PhD, OTR, for useful feedback. Thank you to Cathy Peirce, PhD, OTR/L, for thoughtful discussions on occupation.

 Visit thePoint to watch a video about OT for individuals.

REFERENCES

American Occupational Therapy Association. (2014). Occupational therapy practice framework: Domain and process (3rd ed.). *American Journal of Occupational Therapy, 68*, S1–S48.

American Occupational Therapy Association. (2016). The role of occupational therapy in end-of-life care. *American Journal of Occupational Therapy, 70*(Suppl. 2), 7012410075.

American Occupational Therapy Association. (2017). Philosophical base of occupational therapy. *American Journal of Occupational Therapy, 71*, 7112410045.

Amini, D. (2011). Occupational therapy interventions for work-related injuries and conditions of the forearm, wrist, and hand: A systematic review. *American Journal of Occupational Therapy, 65*, 29–36.

Arbesman, M., Lieberman, D., & Thomas, V. J. (2011). Methodology for the systematic reviews on occupational therapy for individuals with work-related injuries and illnesses. *American Journal of Occupational Therapy, 65*, 10–15.

Bennett, S., & Bennett, J. W. (2000). The process of evidence-based practice in occupational therapy: Informing clinical decisions. *Australian Occupational Therapy Journal, 47*, 171–180.

Bennett, S., Hoffmann, T., McCluskey, A., McKenna, K., Strong, J., & Tooth, L. (2003). Evidence-based practice forum. Introducing OTseeker (Occupational Therapy Systematic Evaluation of Evidence): A new evidence database for occupational therapists. *American Journal of Occupational Therapy, 57*, 635–638.

Brown, C., Rempfer, M., & Hamera, E. (2002). Teaching grocery shopping skills to people with schizophrenia. *Occupational Therapy Journal of Research, 22*, 90S–91S.

Chase, C. A., Mann, K., Wasek, S., & Arbesman, M. (2012). Systematic review of the effect of home modification and fall prevention programs on falls and the performance of community-dwelling older adults. *American Journal of Occupational Therapy, 66*, 284–291.

Clark, F. A., Jackson, J. M., Scott, M. D., Carlson, M. E., Atkins, M. S., Uhles-Tanaka, D., & Rubayi, S. (2006). Data-based models of how pressure ulcers develop in daily-living contexts of adults with spinal cord injury. *Archives of Physical Medicine and Rehabilitation, 87*, 1516–1525.

Cole, B., & McLean, V. (2003). Therapeutic relationships re-defined. *Occupational Therapy in Mental Health, 19*, 33–56.

Duncombe, L. W. (2004). Comparing learning of cooking in home and clinic for people with schizophrenia. *American Journal of Occupational Therapy, 58*, 272–278.

Eklund, M., & Hallberg, I. R. (2001). Psychiatric occupational therapists' verbal interaction with their clients. *Occupational Therapy International, 8*, 1–16.

Fisher, A. G. (1998). Uniting practice and theory in an occupational therapy framework, 1998 Eleanor Clarke Slagle lecture. *American Journal of Occupational Therapy, 52*, 509–522.

Gentry, T. (2008). PDAs as cognitive aids for people with multiple sclerosis. *American Journal of Occupational Therapy, 62*, 18–27.

Gillen, G., Berger, S., Lotia, S., Morreale, J., Siber, M., & Trudo, W. (2007). Improving community skills after lower extremity joint replacement. *Physical and Occupational Therapy in Geriatrics, 25*, 41–54.

Gillen, G., Nilsen, D. M., Attridge, J., Banakos, E., Morgan, M., Winterbottom, L., & York, W. (2015). Effectiveness of interventions to improve occupational performance of people with cognitive impairments after stroke: An evidence-based review. *American Journal of Occupational Therapy, 69*, 6901180040.

Gitlin, L. N., Corcoran, M., Winter, L., Boyce, A., & Hauck, W. W. (2001). A randomized, controlled trial of a home environmental intervention: Effect on efficacy and upset in caregivers and on daily function of persons with dementia. *The Gerontologist, 41*, 4–14.

Gol, D., & Jarus, T. (2005). Effect of a social skills training group on everyday activities of children with attention-deficit-hyperactivity disorder. *Developmental Medicine and Child Neurology, 47*, 539–545.

Gray, J. M. (1998). Putting occupation into practice: Occupation as ends, occupation as means. *American Journal of Occupational Therapy, 52*, 354–364.

Haynes, R. B., Devereaux, P. J., & Guyatt, G. H. (2002). Clinical expertise in the era of evidence-based medicine and patient choice. *ACP Journal Club, 136*, A11–A14.

Hemmingsson, H., & Jonsson, H. (2005). An occupational perspective on the concept of participation in the International Classification of Functioning, Disability and Health—Some critical remarks. *American Journal of Occupational Therapy, 59*, 569–576.

Jensen, L., & Padilla, R. (2017). Effectiveness of environment-based interventions that address behavior, perception, and falls in people with Alzheimer's disease and related major neurocognitive disorders: A systematic review. *American Journal of Occupational Therapy, 71*, 7105180030.

Kealey, P., & McIntyre, I. (2005). An evaluation of the domiciliary occupational therapy service in palliative cancer care in a community trust: A patient and carers perspective. *European Journal of Cancer Care, 14*, 232–243.

Law, M., Baptiste, S., & Mills, J. (1995). Client-centred practice: What does it mean and does it make a difference? *Canadian Journal of Occupational Therapy, 62*, 250–257.

Marik, T. L., & Roll, S. C. (2017). Effectiveness of occupational therapy interventions for musculoskeletal shoulder conditions: A systematic review. *American Journal of Occupational Therapy, 71*, 7101180020.

Masiero, S., Boniolo, A., Wassermann, L., Machiedo, H., Volante, D., & Punzi, L. (2007). Effects of an educational-behavioral joint protection program on people with moderate to severe rheumatoid arthritis: A randomized controlled trial. *Clinical Rheumatology, 26*, 2043–2050.

Owsley, C., & McGwin, G., Jr. (1999). Vision impairment and driving. *Survey Ophthalmology, 43*, 535–550.

Owsley, C., Sekuler, R., & Siemsen, D. (1983). Contrast sensitivity throughout adulthood. *Vision Research, 23*, 689–699.

Owsley, C., Stalvey, B. T., Wells, J., & Sloane, M. E. (1999). Older drivers and cataract: Driving habits and crash risk. *The Journals of Gerontology, 54*, M203–M211.

Punwar, J., & Peloquin, M. (2000). *Occupational therapy: Principles and practice* (3rd ed.). Philadelphia, PA: Lippincott Williams & Wilkins.

Sackett, D. L., Strauss, S. E., Richardson, W. S., Rosenberg, W., & Haynes, R. B. (2000). *Evidenced-based medicine: How to practice and teach.* Edinburgh, United Kingdom: Churchill Livingstone.

Schaaf, R. C., Dumont, R. L., Arbesman, M., & May-Benson, T. A. (2018). Efficacy of occupational therapy using Ayres Sensory Integration®: A systematic review. *American Journal of Occupational Therapy, 72*, 7201190010. doi:10.5014/ajot.2018.028431

Stutts, J., Martell, C., & Staplin, L. (2009). *Identifying behaviors and situations associated with increased crash risk for older drivers* (Report No. DOT HS 811 09). Washington, DC: National Highway Traffic Safety Administration.

Sumsion, T., & Law, M. (2006). A review of evidence on the conceptual elements informing client-centred practice. *Canadian Journal of Occupational Therapy, 73*, 153–162.

Taylor, R. R., Lee, S. W., Kielhofner, G., & Ketkar, M. (2009). Therapeutic use of self: A nationwide survey of practitioners' attitudes and experiences. *American Journal of Occupational Therapy, 63*, 198–207.

Trombly, C. A. (1995). Occupation: Purposefulness and meaningfulness as therapeutic mechanisms. 1995 Eleanor Clarke Slagle Lecture. *American Journal of Occupational Therapy, 49*, 960–972.

University of Southern California. (2013). *USC/Rancho Lifestyle Redesign® pressure ulcer prevention project.* Retrieved from http://www.usc.edu/programs/pups/

Van Heest, K. N. L., Mogush, A. R., & Mathiowetz, V. G. (2017). Effects of a one-to-one fatigue management course for people with chronic conditions and fatigue. *American Journal of Occupational Therapy, 71*, 7104100020.

Velligan, D. I., Prihoda, T. J., Ritch, J. L., Maples, N., Bow-Thomas, C. C., & Dassori, A. (2002). A randomized single-blind pilot study of compensatory strategies in schizophrenia outpatients. *Schizophrenia Bulletin, 28*, 283–292.

Weinstock-Zlotnick, G., & Hinojosa, J. (2004). Bottom-up or top-down evaluation: Is one better than the other? *American Journal of Occupational Therapy, 58*, 594–598.

World Health Organization. (1980). *International classification of impairments, disabilities and handicap (ICIDH)*. Geneva,Switzerland: Author.

World Health Organization. (2001). *International classification of functioning, disability and health (ICF)*. Geneva, Switzerland: Author.

World Health Organization. (2010). *International Classification of Diseases* (10th ed.). Geneva, Switzerland: Author. Retrieved from http://www.who.int/classifications/icd

World Health Organization. (n.d.a). *History of WHO*. Retrieved from http://www.who.int/about/history/en/

World Health Organization. (n.d.b). *WHO historical collection*. Retrieved from http://www.who.int/library/collections/historical/en/index1.html

World Health Organization. (n.d.c). *Disease classifications and nomenclature documents*. Retrieved from http://www.who.int/library/collections/historical/en/index1.html

thePoint® *For additional resources on the subjects discussed in this chapter, visit* **http://thePoint.lww.com/Willard-Spackman13e.** *See* **Appendix I, Resources and Evidence for Common Conditions Addressed in OT** *for more information about disease and disability.*

Occupational Therapy Interventions for Groups, Communities, and Populations

Marjorie E. Scaffa

LEARNING OBJECTIVES

After reading this chapter, you will be able to:

1. Identify client factors and performance patterns that apply to groups, communities, and populations.
2. Discuss the application of client-centered, evidence-based, and occupation-based interventions to groups, communities, and populations.
3. Describe potential outcomes of occupational therapy intervention for groups, communities, and populations.
4. Compare and contrast a variety of specific intervention approaches that are used for groups, communities, and populations receiving occupational therapy services.

Introduction

In many settings where occupational therapy (OT) is practiced, the term *client* refers to an individual who is receiving services. However, in the Occupational Therapy Practice Framework (Framework), *clients* are categorized as persons, groups, and populations (American Occupational Therapy Association [AOTA], 2014). *Persons* include individuals and their caregivers. *Groups* include collectives of individuals such as families, workers, students, and communities. *Populations* are collectives of groups living in the same geographic area or sharing similar characteristics or concerns (AOTA, 2014).

Green and Kreuter (1991) define a population as a group of "people identified by common values and mutual concern for the development and well-being of their group or geographical area" (p. 504). Examples of populations include homeless persons, veterans, refugees, and people with chronic mental and/or physical disabilities. The terms *communities* and *populations* are sometimes used interchangeably. However, typically, there may be a variety of populations within one community. For example, within my community, there are populations of students, professionals, persons who are homeless, veterans, and immigrants, among others.

Communities and populations, like individuals, may experience various challenges to engagement in occupations, including occupational delays, disparities, interruptions, and/or imbalances and therefore may benefit from OT intervention (Bass-Haugen, Henderson, Larson, & Matuska, 2005). Bass-Haugen (2009) identified several health disparities among children and adults across racial, ethnic, and socioeconomic groups that are appropriate for OT intervention. These include disparities in health behavior characteristics, activity profiles, home and work environments, and experiences and outcomes of health care services, which can ultimately impact occupational performance and participation. Although organizations are not considered clients in the Framework (AOTA, 2014), organizations often provide the context for the provision of OT services to persons, groups, and populations. Organization-based, community-based, and population-based services address the "needs of a group of individuals as a whole rather than the specific needs of an individual" (Moyers, 1999, p. 263).

Chapter 30 described OT interventions for individuals receiving services. This chapter focuses on interventions for groups, communities, and populations. The OT intervention process "consists of the skilled services provided by OT practitioners in collaboration with clients to facilitate engagement in occupation related to health, wellbeing, and participation" (AOTA, 2014, p. S14). Interventions addressing the needs of groups, communities, and populations are sometimes referred to as **programs**. Programs are "systematic efforts to achieve preplanned objectives such as changes in knowledge, attitudes, skills, and behaviors to maintain or improve function and/or health" (Brownson, 2001, p. 96).

According to Youngstrom and Brown (2005), OT interventions, whether designed for individuals, groups, communities, or populations, are client centered, context driven, occupation based, and evidence based.

The outcomes of OT intervention for groups, communities, and populations may include improved occupational performance, increased occupational participation, improved role competence, enhanced well-being and quality of life, prevention of occupational performance problems, and occupational justice for individuals and for the collective (AOTA, 2014).

Designing and implementing OT intervention for groups, communities, and populations require an understanding of the (1) people (lifestyles, health status, risk and resiliency factors, and performance patterns), (2) occupation and activity demands, and (3) environments in which these occupations occur (Watson & Wilson, 2003). The following sections describe client-centered, context-driven, evidence-based, and occupation-based approaches to intervention for groups, communities, and populations.

Client-Centered Approaches for Groups, Communities, and Populations

Regardless of whether the client is an individual, group, community, or population, OT practitioners provide client-centered care. This means ongoing collaboration and incorporation of the aggregate needs, priorities, and choices of the group, community, or population in the intervention. Client-centered intervention or program development for groups, communities, and populations is based

CENTENNIAL NOTES

Hull House

Hull House in Chicago was a settlement house for immigrants founded in 1889 by Jane Addams and Ellen Gates Starr (Figure 31-1). The primary purpose of Hull House was to provide social and educational opportunities for working class people. In addition, Hull House established the city's first public playground, gymnasium, and bathhouse (Bryan & Davis, 1991). In 1917, Eleanor Clarke Slagle (1870 to 1942) conducted training courses and provided OT services at Hull House (Pollock, 1942; Reed & Andersen, 2017). In essence, Hull House was the first community-based OT program.

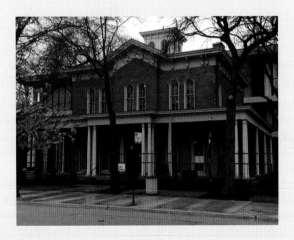

FIGURE 31-1 **Hull House.**

on two main principles: (1) the principle of relevance and (2) the principle of participation. The principle of relevance refers to starting "where the people are" and addressing the perceived needs of the program participants rather than those of the intervention planners. The principle of participation emphasizes the importance of involving clients in the intervention planning, implementation, and evaluation processes. Research has shown that participation in intervention planning itself is health enhancing and that clients meet their goals more effectively and efficiently when they are actively involved in the planning process (Baker & Brownson, 1998).

In order to be truly client centered, the intervention must address occupations the client finds meaningful and be focused on the client's interests, needs, and priorities. This is accomplished, in part, through the development of an occupational profile and the process of occupational performance analysis. An occupational profile includes the client's occupational history and experiences, patterns of daily living, roles, interests, values, and priorities (AOTA, 2014). Through an occupational performance analysis, the client's assets and problems or potential problems are identified including the degree of lifestyle and/or occupational balance. *Lifestyle balance* has been defined by Christiansen and Matuska (2006) as "a consistent pattern of occupations that results in reduced stress and improved health and well-being" (p. 50). Lifestyle imbalance can result in emotional disturbances, sleep deprivation, insufficient time for leisure and social participation, lack of need fulfillment, and inability to meet role demands. Lifestyle imbalance is not only a function of individual behavior but also of conditions in the organization or larger community (Christiansen & Matuska, 2006).

When the client is a group, community, or population, the occupational performance analysis involves profiling participation rates and barriers and facilitating factors for occupational performance and occupational participation. Occupational performance analysis focuses on client factors and occupational performance patterns. The characteristics of interest for groups, communities, and populations include the following:

• "Health indicators;
• The lifestyles of the community or cohort of people;
• Sociocultural values;
• Prevalence, incidence, and temporal trends in impairments, conditions, and risk behaviors, and
• Commitment to and preparedness for change." (Watson & Wilson, 2003, p. 30)

In addition, it is important to profile group, community, and/or population strengths and assets. **Assets** are the "inherent attributes and available resources of populations that might be used in attaining target outcomes" (Watson & Wilson, 2003, p. 37). Assets may be

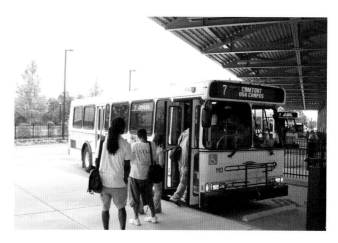

FIGURE 31-2 **Accessible transportation is a valuable community asset. (Photo courtesy of J. Schell.)**

economic, educational, environmental, religious, political, social, and/or cultural. An occupational therapist might ascertain community assets by gathering data on the number of options in the community for healthy leisure activity (parks, recreation centers, youth organizations, public swimming pools, etc.) and on the number and variety of healthy food outlets (grocery stores, fresh food markets, local produce, etc.) and public transportation to and from these venues (Figure 31-2).

Client Factors and Occupational Performance Patterns

Interventions for groups, communities, and populations may be designed to address client factors and/or performance patterns. *Client factors* are "specific capacities, characteristics, or beliefs" that "influence performance in occupations" (AOTA, 2014, p. S7). Client factors related to groups, communities, and populations include values and beliefs as evidenced by culture and religious traditions; functions such as economic, educational, political, and social; and structure, for example, similarities across individuals based on health-related conditions, genetics, and risk factors, among others. For example, group, community or population values may include honesty, commitment, equity, and tolerance. Beliefs may include the rights of individuals to self-determination, the importance of empowerment and independence, and the role of society in facilitating community inclusion for all regardless of age, gender, or ability.

Performance patterns are those routines, rituals, and roles that support or hinder occupational performance (AOTA, 2014). Clients may have the performance skills necessary for effective occupational participation; however, if performance patterns are lacking, the healthy enactment of occupations may be negatively affected. Routines in groups, communities and populations are "patterns of behavior that are observable, regular, and repetitive and that provide structure for daily life . . . and are embedded in cultural and ecological contexts" (AOTA, 2014, p. S27). Rituals in groups, communities, and populations are "shared social actions with traditional, emotional, purposive, and technological meaning contributing to the values and beliefs within the group or population" (AOTA, 2014, p. S27). Roles in groups, communities, and populations are "sets of behaviors by the group or population expected by society and shaped by culture and context" (AOTA, 2014, p. S27).

Performance patterns associated with groups, such as families and workers, may include the following:

* Rituals, such as birthdays, celebrations of accomplishment, retreats, among others
* Roles, for example, within families or of workers and departments at a worksite, and roles of a business in the community and in society
* Routines, such as regularly scheduled family meals and other activities, and worksite meetings and safety procedures

Performance patterns associated with communities and populations include the following:

* Rituals and cultural customs such as appropriate forms of greeting, and national, religious, and holiday celebrations
* Roles, for example, community leadership roles, roles of agencies within the community, and role of the community/population vis-à-vis other communities and populations
* Routines, such as regular health practices, annual community events, and seasonal work practices

Client-centered interventions address the unique client factors and occupational performance patterns of the group, community, or population served.

Context-Driven Approaches for Groups, Communities, and Populations

In addition to client factors and occupational performance patterns, occupational performance analysis requires identification of environmental and contextual factors that support or hinder occupational performance and participation. In the Framework, *environment* refers to the external physical and social setting or milieu within which occupations occur, and *context* refers to cultural, temporal, and virtual conditions in which the client is embedded (AOTA, 2014). Table 31-1 provides some examples of contexts and environments associated with groups, communities, and populations.

All interventions occur within a specific environment and context, which influences the design, implementation,

TABLE 31-1 **Examples of Environments and Contexts Associated with Groups, Communities, and Populations**

Environment or Context	Examples
Physical	
Group (family, workers, students)	Home, neighborhood, office, factory, school, hospital complex
Community/population	Public transportation system, city parks, natural resources
Social	
Group (family, workers, students)	Interaction with extended family, communication and social support among workers, appreciation from supervisors, positive feedback from teachers and peers
Community/population	Influence of city government, nonprofit agencies, and other community organizations on occupational performance and/or participation
Cultural	
Group (family, workers, students)	Interaction patterns and behavioral expectations within the group; for example, family prayer, dress down Fridays, professional behavior
Community/population	Cultural activities such as siestas, afternoon tea, Mardi Gras, etc.
Temporal	
Group (family, workers, students)	Birthdays, work schedule, semester breaks
Community/population	National and religious holiday celebrations, seasonal activities
Virtual	
Group (family, workers, students)	Videoconferencing, instant messaging, telephone conference calls
Community/population	Virtual community of gamers, Internet social networks

and effectiveness of the intervention. For example, the physical and social environments in which they are located would significantly impact the development and implementation of interventions for immigrant women and children. A program for homeless immigrant women and children living in temporary shelters would be much different than a church-based program for immigrant women and children hosted by foster families. Similarly, contextual factors also impact interventions for groups, communities, and populations. Cultural contexts, in particular, must be considered for population-based interventions to be effective. The incorporation of cultural values, beliefs, activity patterns, behavioral standards, and expectations in the intervention significantly enhance the likelihood of success.

The environment and/or context are often the primary features addressed in interventions for groups, communities, and populations (Youngstrom & Brown, 2005). Each environment or context provides unique barriers and supports for occupational performance. Therefore, modification of the environment and/or context can impact the occupational performance and participation of all members of a group, community, or population. Interventions focused on environmental factors are typically based on socioenvironmental and ecological models (ecological models are described in more detail in Chapter 43). For populations, interventions focus on the broad determinants of health through community-centered change. The World Health Organization (1986) has identified the fundamental conditions and resources for population health, which include food, shelter, education, income, a stable ecosystem, sustainable resources, peace, equity, and social justice. The lack of these resources for health produces stress, impairment, health problems, and occupational injustices that are amenable to OT intervention (Kronenberg & Pollard, 2006). See Chapter 45 for more details on occupational justice.

Evidence-Based Approaches for Groups, Communities, and Populations

As in all areas of practice, interventions provided to groups, communities, and populations should be based on the best available evidence. Although evidence on OT interventions for groups, communities, and populations specifically is not plentiful, some strong evidence exists in other disciplines that can guide the development of OT interventions (see "Commentary on the Evidence" box). Occupational therapy practice guidelines and official documents also

can be useful in this regard. Examples of useful documents relevant to providing interventions for groups, communities, and populations include, but are not limited to, the "Occupational Therapy Practice Framework: Domain and Process, (3rd edition)" (AOTA, 2014); "Occupational Therapy in the Promotion of Health and Wellbeing" (AOTA, 2013a); "AOTA's Societal Statement on Disaster Response and Risk Reduction" (AOTA, 2017); and "The Role of Occupational Therapy in Disaster Preparedness, Response, and Recovery: A Concept Paper" (AOTA, 2011).

Evidence in health education, health promotion, and public health suggests that interventions for groups, communities, and populations based on ecological models are most effective (Kok, Gottlieb, Commers, & Smerecnik, 2008; Sallis, Owen, & Fisher, 2008). Ecologically based interventions address multiple levels and include multiple approaches to achieve their goals and objectives. According to Brownson (2001), the levels addressed include the following:

- **Intrapersonal level**: characteristics of individuals within the organization or population that influence behavior and impact occupational performance, participation, and health
- **Interpersonal level**: relationships among family, friends, peers, and groups that provide support, identity, and role definition and facilitate or constrain occupational performance and/or participation and impact health
- **Organizational level**: rules, regulations, policies, procedures, programs, and resources within agencies and organizations that impact occupational performance and/or participation and impact health
- **Community level**: social networks, norms, trends, and standards that facilitate or constrain desired occupational performance and/or participation and impact health
- **Public policy/societal level**: local, state, and federal policies, laws, and programs that regulate, support, or constrain desired occupational performance and/or participation and impact health

In addition, effective interventions for groups, communities, and populations appear to adhere to certain core evidence-based principles (Davis, Schwartz, Wheeler, & Lancaster, 1998; Freudenberg et al., 1995). These interventions

- Are tailored to the expressed needs of a particular group, community, or population in a specific setting;
- Involve the participants in all phases of the intervention including planning, implementation, and evaluation;
- Incorporate intervention strategies at multiple levels;
- Improve client health, well-being, and quality of life by addressing various life concerns;
- Build on client strengths and cultural norms;

COMMENTARY ON THE EVIDENCE

Evidence to support OT interventions at the group, community, and population levels is limited at present. However, evidence from health education, health promotion, and public health can guide the design and evaluation of OT interventions. Evidence-based techniques vary depending on the desired outcomes and level of intervention. A few studies from OT and other disciplines providing evidence for the efficacy of interventions for groups, communities, and populations are briefly described in Table 31-2.

Occupational therapy interventions for individuals typically focus on the intrapersonal level and occasionally incorporate the interpersonal level. However, interventions for groups, communities, and populations require a broader focus and the incorporation of multiple levels of intervention. Obesity, particularly childhood obesity, is an example of a public health problem that has captured the attention of OT practitioners (AOTA, 2007; Kugel, 2010; Lau, 2011). It has become obvious that this epidemic must be addressed not only on the individual and family levels but also on the group, community, and population levels. Table 31-3 provides an example of addressing childhood obesity at several levels of intervention. Potential roles for OT are provided based on the Occupational Therapy Practice Framework: Domain and Process, third edition (AOTA, 2014). Although none of these roles is unique to OT, the pervasiveness of this public health problem invites the participation of occupational therapists and OT assistants.

TABLE 31-2 Selected Studies Providing Evidence of the Efficacy of Interventions for Organizations, Communities, and Populations

Authors	Findings
Coker-Bolt et al. (2017)	Demonstrates the effectiveness of a community-based program on women's personal hygiene through the use of health education and the distribution of sustainable personal hygiene supplies
Umeda et al. (2017)	Describes the provision of organization-level consultation to maximize community social participation of individuals with intellectual and developmental disabilities
Wenborn et al. (2016)	Discusses the importance of adapting complex community-based OT interventions to specific national contexts using an example of a program for persons with dementia and their family caregivers
Guoping, Yanchun, Yingjie, & Gongxiang (2010)	Describes a Tai Chi intervention for middle-aged and older adults that produced improved physical and mental health and quality of life. Muscle tone, body weight, balance, and flexibility were superior in the intervention group as compared to the control group.
Webb, Joseph, Yardley, & Michie (2010)	Investigates the characteristics of effective Internet-based health promotion interventions. The use of theory, multiple behavior change techniques, and various methods for interacting with participants were deemed to be significant factors.
Classen et al. (2007)	Identified 11 factors in three categories (behavioral, health, and environmental) related to safe driving for older adults that can be used as elements of a population-based health promotion intervention
Lamontagne, Keegel, Louie, Ostry, & Landsbergis (2007)	A systematic review indicated the efficacy of organizational-level primary prevention strategies addressing the causes and consequences of workplace stress in improving work productivity and decreasing job stress.
Maller, Townsend, Pryor, Brown, & St. Leger (2006)	Presents empirical and theoretical evidence of the importance contact with nature plays in human health and well-being and describes public health strategies to optimize the health-promoting effects of nature-based interventions
McClure et al. (2005)	An evidence-based review of the characteristics of effective population-based approaches to the prevention of falls among older people

TABLE 31-3 Addressing Childhood Obesity at Multiple Levels of Intervention

Level of Intervention	Potential Occupational Therapy Role[a]
Intrapersonal/individual	Facilitate regular physical activity through engagement in meaningful and enjoyable occupations (leisure participation, health management and maintenance)
Interpersonal	Teach children and their parents how to develop and implement healthy meal plans for the family (meal preparation)
Organizational	Consult with local agencies to provide developmentally appropriate after-school active play or leisure activities for children (play exploration and play participation) (see Figure 31-3)
Community	Advocate for accessible and safe walking and biking paths for persons of diverse abilities (safety and emergency maintenance, community mobility)
Public policy/government	Lobby for improvements in the nutritional value of school lunches and vending machine snacks (health management and maintenance)

[a]Terminology from Occupational Therapy Practice Framework (AOTA, 2014).

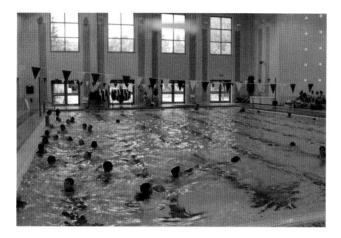

FIGURE 31-3 Practitioners can improve client health, well-being, and quality of life by addressing various life concerns using existing resources such as an open swim at a community pool. (Photo courtesy of J. Schell.)

- Use existing resources (see Figure 31-3);
- Advocate for needed policy and resource changes to achieve objectives; and
- Prepare clients to become effective self-managers and self-advocates.

Occupation-Based Approaches for Groups, Communities, and Populations

Occupation-based interventions are designed to enable the client to enact occupational performance effectively and to participate in desired occupations fully. As described in Chapter 30, occupational performance and occupational participation are the end goals and outcomes of OT for individuals and frequently the means or process of achieving those goals as well. These are also the end goals and outcomes of OT interventions for groups, communities, and populations.

Various intervention approaches may be used with groups, communities, and populations depending on the desired change and goals to be achieved. Some intervention approaches are designed to influence change in the client (restoration and skill acquisition training); others to modify the task, environment, or context (adaptation, compensation); and others to proffer the best client–environment fit (Youngstrom & Brown, 2005). Often, a combination of approaches produces the best results. The following paragraphs describe the specific approaches and their

application to groups, communities, and/or populations and provide further examples in Table 31-4. These categories of intervention approaches are not mutually exclusive. Some interventions may fit into multiple categories depending on the goal and level addressed.

Restoration approaches are designed to enhance performance capacities and/or reduce or eliminate performance constraints. Restoration interventions for populations may take the form of developing a program to enhance balance, endurance, and strength for residents of an assisted living facility in order to prevent falls or providing training in work simplification and energy conservation for a group of cancer survivors.

Occupational skill acquisition or training approaches are designed to develop or enhance an occupational performance skill or process. Occupational skill acquisition or training interventions for populations may take the form of developing and implementing an after-school anger management program for adolescents to enhance emotional regulation skills and reduce bullying or a parenting program to address the special needs of parents of children with disabilities.

Adaptation and compensation approaches are designed to diminish constraints by modifying contexts or activity demands in order to support occupational performance and occupational participation in natural contexts. Adaptation and compensation interventions for populations may take the form of adapting a task or providing special equipment in order to facilitate the participation of children with disabilities in a summer day camp or providing adaptive equipment and mobility devices in an emergency shelter to accommodate the needs of persons with disabilities.

The environmental modification approach is designed to reduce natural, built, and social environmental barriers to occupational performance and occupational participation. Environmental modification interventions for populations may take the form of designing accessible playgrounds based on universal design principles to enhance the development of children of all abilities or adapting the environment of senior housing to facilitate the safety of older adults with low vision.

Prevention and health promotion approaches are designed to avert the occurrence of illness, injury, and disability and enhance well-being and quality of life by reducing risk factors and enhancing protective and resiliency factors (Scaffa & Brownson, 2005). The World Health Organization (1986) defined *health promotion* as a "process of enabling people to increase control over and to improve their health" and the "science and art of helping people change their lifestyle to move toward a state of optimal health" and "enhance awareness, change behavior and create environments that support good health practices" (p. iii). The Well Elderly Study by Clark et al., a classic randomized controlled trial,

TABLE 31-4   Examples of Specific Intervention Approaches

Intervention Approach	Intervention Level	Examples
Remediation or restoration approach: using occupations and purposeful activities to improve occupational performance	Intrapersonal	Establishing a walking program at a local shopping mall for older adults to improve endurance
	Interpersonal	Providing social and occupation-based activities for young, single mothers to facilitate interpersonal support
	Organizational	Using a school facility after hours for a drop-in program for homeless adolescents focusing on healthy leisure occupations and assistance with school assignments
Skill acquisition or training approach: providing information, training, and practice to enhance a skill or process	Intrapersonal	Teaching occupation-based adaptive coping skills to clients in a substance abuse treatment program
	Interpersonal	Training adolescents in conflict resolution skills to improve relationships with parents, teachers, and peers and improve social participation
	Organizational	Incorporating regular training for police, firefighters, and emergency medical personnel regarding responding to the needs of persons with mental disorders
Adaptation or compensation approach: modifying tasks or using devices or equipment to enable occupational participation	Intrapersonal	Modifying home environments in order to facilitate aging in place
	Organizational	Adapting the policies and procedures of a worksite to address the needs of persons with mental disorders
	Community	Providing motorized scooters in public facilities for persons with mobility impairments
Environmental modifications approach: changing the physical and/or social environment and modifying contexts	Organizational	Providing specific information regarding the gradient for a wheelchair ramp to accommodate a newly hired employee
	Community	Addressing the stigma against mental disorders by modifying the social context through social media campaigns
	Public policy	Recommending the development and implementation of driver's license restrictions for older adults based on driving assessments
Prevention or health promotion approach: combining educational, social, and environmental intervention strategies to enhance health and prevent injury, disease, and disability	Intrapersonal	Providing occupation-based mental health services in a school following a traumatic event
	Organizational	Preventing compassion fatigue in health care workers by designing and creating a safe and comfortable space for emotional decompression and collegial support
	Community	Offering a chronic disease self-management program at a local church
Consultation approach: using the knowledge and skill of an expert to assist clients make better decisions or deal more effectively with situations	Organizational	Advising an organization that responds to disaster on how best to meet the needs of persons with disabilities in shelters
	Community	Advising local government officials regarding the integration of persons with mental disorders into the community after discharge from the state psychiatric hospital
	Public policy	Counseling state government agencies in establishing polices related to best practices for intervention for children with autism and their families
Advocacy approach: using the power of persuasion to alter opinions and mobilize resources	Organizational	Persuading management to modify the work environment to reduce the incidence of repetitive strain injuries
	Community	Advocating for the hiring of returning soldiers with disabilities to local businesses
	Public policy	Advocating for the establishment of policies that facilitate full participation of persons with disabilities in public recreational facilities

demonstrated the effectiveness of a population-based health promotion OT intervention for community-dwelling older adults (Clark et al., 2001; Clark et al., 1997). In comparison to subjects who participated in social activities and those who received no treatment, individuals who received OT services demonstrated improved vitality, physical and social functioning, life satisfaction, and general mental health. Other prevention and health promotion interventions for populations may take the form of teaching safe lifting techniques at a factory to avoid back injuries among workers or providing community-based programs on chronic disease self-management that have been shown to prevent the development of secondary conditions that limit occupational performance (Arbesman & Mosley, 2012).

Consultation is an indirect service provision approach designed to enable the client to solve occupation-related problems independently. Consultation involves establishing a collaborative relationship with the client in order to define the occupational concern to be addressed, identify potential solutions, and develop implementation strategies. However, the actual implementation of the intervention is the responsibility of the client. Consultation interventions for groups, communities, and populations may take the form of designing a wheelchair basketball program for a local boys and girls club or making recommendations for worksite compliance with the Americans with Disabilities Act of 1990.

Advocacy is another indirect service provision approach. It is designed to impact decision making within political, economic, and social systems and institutions to "promote occupational justice and empower clients to seek and obtain resources to fully participate in daily life occupations" (AOTA, 2014, p. S30). Advocacy interventions for populations may take the form of collaborating with community agencies to improve access to services for people with mental health disorders or serving on the board of a community nonprofit organization attempting to acquire funding for transition services for adolescents with disabilities.

Telehealth services have become a viable option for clients who live in remote or underserved areas. According to the AOTA (2013b), **telehealth** is "the application of evaluative, consultative, preventative, and therapeutic services delivered through telecommunication and information technologies" (p. S69). Telehealth service delivery can be synchronous, occurring in real time, through interactive technologies, or asynchronous relaying information that can be stored and accessed at the receiver's convenience. Telehealth increases access, removes barriers, and prevents unnecessary delays in receiving OT services. In addition, it allows outreach to communities and populations that may not otherwise receive our services (AOTA, 2013b).

Regardless of the intervention approach used, therapeutic use of self and establishing a therapeutic alliance with the client are critical to the success of any intervention with a group, community, or population. *Therapeutic use of self* is defined as an OT practitioner's "planned use of his or her personality, insights, perceptions, and judgments as part of the therapeutic process" (Punwar & Peloquin, 2000, p. 285). Developing rapport, communicating effectively, displaying empathy, establishing trust, providing motivation, listening actively, and maintaining a caring attitude are prerequisite to effectively interacting with any client.

Case Vignettes

The following case vignettes provide examples of OT interventions for a group, a community, and a population. As can be seen, multiple intervention approaches are incorporated in each scenario. Each case includes an occupational profile, occupational performance analysis findings, goals, and intervention approaches used.

Group-Based Case

An elementary school in Pensacola, Florida, has a significantly higher enrollment of children with parents on military deployment than other schools in the area. This is due in part to its location near multiple military bases. Approximately 40% of children attending the school have one or both parents deployed in the Middle East conflict zone. Many of these children are being cared for by grandparents or other relatives.

Over the past 6 months, teachers have noted increased absences, decreased classroom participation, reduced social interaction with peers, and falling grades among this group of children. The principal has asked Danielle, the school-based occupational therapist, to work with the school counselor to identify and address the needs of these children.

The school counselor administered a depression inventory and noted that approximately 70% of these children scored in the mild-to-moderate range for depressive symptoms. Teachers completed the Child Behavior Checklist (CBCL) (Achenbach, 2009). The scores on the CBCL indicated that the children had elevated scores on both the internalizing and externalizing scales. Internalizing behaviors include emotional reactivity, anxiety, depression, withdrawal, and somatic complaints. Externalizing behaviors include attention deficits and aggression.

The occupational therapist administered the Children's Assessment of Participation and Enjoyment (CAPE) (King et al., 2004), the Social Skills Rating System (SSRS) (Gresham & Elliott, 2007), and the School Function Assessment (SFA) (Coster, Deeney, Haltiwanger, & Haley, 1998) to children with deployed parents whom the teachers identified as at risk for academic failure. Results from the CAPE indicated a low level of social participation and a low level of enjoyment of activity participation among 65% of the children tested. The SSRS supported the results of the CBCL and indicated high levels of internalizing and externalizing behaviors including anxiety, sadness, and poor anger management. In addition, the SSRS indicated a high level of hyperactivity and impulsivity among a small number of the children.

The SFA (participation and activity performance sections only) data was collected by interviewing the classroom teachers. The children demonstrated low scores on playground/recess and social behaviors during transitions. They had few problems in physical tasks but demonstrated deficits in compliance with adult directives and school rules, task behavior/completion, positive interaction, and behavior regulation.

One of the strategies recommended (consultation) by the occupational therapist was to develop a mentoring program pairing a same gender high school student who has experienced parental deployments with an elementary school student with a currently deployed parent (interpersonal level). The program would be designed to increase play/leisure participation, improve academic performance, and enhance social participation. The pairs would meet once a week to play games, complete homework, take walks, and eat together.

In addition, the occupational therapist created an expressive arts program that teachers could incorporate into the regular classroom curriculum. These activities would provide an opportunity for children with deployed parents to have an outlet for nonverbal emotional expression and to socially interact with peers (interpersonal level). Danielle was careful to develop expressive art activities that were age appropriate for each grade level. Activities in the expressive arts program included, but were not limited to, arts and crafts, puppetry, drama, music activities, fairy tale enactments, dance and movement activities, and bibliotherapy (remediation or restoration approach). These activities were chosen based on research reported by Jackson and Arbesman (2005) that indicated the efficacy of creative art activities for emotional expression.

A program for parents and other caregivers was also developed by the occupational therapist and offered online via the school's Website (educational approach, organizational level). Topics included preparing children for a parent's deployment, identifying signs and responding to emotional distress, managing difficult behaviors, and preparing children for a parent's return (interpersonal level). Other topics to meet the parents' personal needs included stress management, occupational balance, routines and rituals, social support, and community resources.

Last, the occupational therapist and school counselor began researching and developing a grant proposal to establish an after-school program for children in military families regardless of deployment status. They also requested that the school board provide an additional school counselor and more hours of OT time for this particular school (advocacy approach).

Community-Based Case

Due to the closing of a state psychiatric facility, there has been a significant increase in the number of men with mental disorders who are homeless and wandering the streets. The local mental health services agency has an inadequate number of group homes to accommodate this sudden influx of persons needing housing. The executive director of the mental health agency has contacted the OT department at the local university and requested assistance in addressing the needs of persons with mental disorders who are homeless (consultation approach, organizational level).

In order to determine the needs and assets of the community, Michael, the occupational therapist, conducted a focus group consisting of five homeless men with mental health problems and key informant interviews with staff

of current group homes and members of the housing board. The staff of the group homes stated that a significant problem is the lack of life skills assessment of adults with mental disorders prior to placement in community housing. This leads to clients being placed in group homes who lack the basic skills for community living. As a result, these clients often "bounce back" to the inpatient psychiatric facilities or come to the hospital emergency room in psychiatric crisis. The members of the housing board were in consensus regarding the need for additional housing but stated that they did not have money to build housing or to provide support staff for the group homes.

After meeting with the stakeholders involved including the housing board, the mental health agency, the homeless coalition, and local elected officials, the occupational therapist facilitated a collaborative effort to address the problem (advocacy approach, public policy level). An old hotel that was no longer being used could be purchased and renovated by the housing board, the mental health agency would provide staffing, and the homeless coalition would provide basic furnishings. The local elected officials lobbied for funding from the State Department of Mental Health for support services and from the U.S. Department of Housing and Urban Development (HUD) for renovations to the site. Occupational therapy students at the university would be involved in administering screening and assessment tools and providing an independent living skills program (skill acquisition) for the residents based on an intervention developed by OT practitioners Helfrich, Chan, and Sabol (2011) and incorporating the evidence-based permanent supportive housing model (Substance Abuse and Mental Health Services Administration, 2010). Level I fieldwork students would assist mental health staff in the delivery of services.

Population-Based Case

A large hospital in a metropolitan area is designated as a transplant center. Individuals in need of transplants and their families often move from distant parts of the country to live near the transplant center. Currently, the hospital does not have services for families awaiting transplants or for those actively involved in the transplant process.

Courtney, an occupational therapist at a home care agency in the same city, has recently been receiving an influx of patients posttransplantation for evaluation and intervention. Many of the problems experienced by transplant recipients stem from physical deconditioning and emotional stress. The family members, especially the caregivers, also report high levels of fatigue and nervous tension.

The occupational therapist works with the transplant recipients to increase endurance and strength by working on activities of daily living. She is also teaching the patients energy conservation and work simplification techniques as well as providing assistive devices as needed. Initially, the occupational therapist included family members in the interventions so they could learn energy conservation and work simplification techniques themselves. In addition, the occupational therapist provided caregiver training that included the importance of good body mechanics and occupational balance in one's lifestyle (health promotion/prevention approach, intrapersonal and interpersonal levels).

After several months of working with these families, the occupational therapist approached the management of the home care agency about initiating a support group for families of persons awaiting transplantation and families of transplant recipients (advocacy approach, organizational level). Such a support group would assist family members in arranging, supervising, and providing care for their loved ones. The home care agency met with hospital staff, and the hospital agreed to provide the space and some funding for the support group. The occupational therapist and social worker began to collaboratively develop a 6-week group protocol to meet the needs of this population. The group would address psychosocial concerns especially stress management and provide practical occupation-based strategies for everyday living (educational approach, population level).

Conclusion

Occupational therapy practice is based on the premise that participation in meaningful occupations can improve occupational performance and overall health. If one agrees that occupation is a determinant of health, then it is not difficult to recognize the role of OT practitioners in developing, implementing, and evaluating occupation-based interventions for groups, communities, and populations. The profession of OT has unprecedented opportunity to respond to and help resolve various social problems that impact health and occupational participation including violence and abuse, homelessness, poverty, unintentional injury, joblessness, and social discrimination (Baum & Law, 1998). These social problems are best addressed through interventions designed to impact groups, communities, and populations. Collaboration with existing agencies and the development of funding streams will be vital to the successful participation of OT in these endeavors.

REFERENCES

Achenbach, T. M. (2009). *The Achenbach System of Empirically Based Assessment (ASEBA): Development, findings, theory, and applications.* Burlington, VT: University of Vermont Research Center for Children, Youth and Families. Retrieved from http://www.aseba.org/schoolage.html

American Occupational Therapy Association. (2007). Obesity and occupational therapy: Position paper. *American Journal of Occupational Therapy, 61,* 701–703.

American Occupational Therapy Association. (2011). The role of occupational therapy in disaster preparedness, response and recovery. *American Journal of Occupational Therapy, 65,* S11–S25.

American Occupational Therapy Association. (2013a). Occupational therapy in the promotion of health and wellbeing. *American Journal of Occupational Therapy, 67,* S47–S59.

American Occupational Therapy Association. (2013b). Telehealth. *American Journal of Occupational Therapy, 67,* S69–S90.

American Occupational Therapy Association. (2014). Occupational therapy practice framework: Domain and process (3rd ed.). *American Journal of Occupational Therapy, 68,* S1–S48.

American Occupational Therapy Association. (2017). AOTA's societal statement on disaster response and risk reduction. *American Journal of Occupational Therapy, 71,* 7112410060. doi:10.5014/ajot.2017.716S11

Americans With Disabilities Act of 1990, Pub. L. No. 101-336, 104 Stat. 328 (1991).

Arbesman, M., & Mosley, L. J. (2012). Systematic review of occupation- and activity-based health management and maintenance interventions for community-dwelling older adults. *American Journal of Occupational Therapy, 66,* 277–283.

Baker, E. A., & Brownson, C. A. (1998). Defining characteristics of community-based health promotion programs. *Journal of Public Health Management and Practice, 4,* 1–9.

Bass-Haugen, J. (2009). Health disparities: Examination of evidence relevant for occupational therapy. *American Journal of Occupational Therapy, 63,* 24–34.

Bass-Haugen, J., Henderson, M. L., Larson, B. A., & Matuska, K. (2005). Occupational issues of concern in populations. In C. H. Christiansen, C. M. Baum, & J. Bass-Haugen (Eds.), *Occupational therapy: Performance, participation, and well-being* (3rd ed., pp. 166–187). Thorofare, NJ: SLACK.

Baum, C., & Law, M. (1998). Community health: A responsibility, an opportunity, and a fit for occupational therapy. *American Journal of Occupational Therapy, 52,* 7–10.

Brownson, C. A. (2001). Program development for community health: Planning, implementation and evaluation strategies. In M. Scaffa (Ed.), *Occupational therapy in community-based practice settings* (pp. 95–118). Philadelphia, PA: F. A. Davis.

Bryan, M. L., & Davis, A. F. (1991). *One hundred years at hull house.* Bloomington, IN: Indiana University Press.

Christiansen, C. H., & Matuska, K. M. (2006). Lifestyle balance: A review of concepts and research. *Journal of Occupational Science, 13,* 49–61.

Clark, F., Azen, S. P., Carlson, M., Mandel, D., LaBree, L., Hay, J., . . . Lipson, L. (2001). Embedding health-promoting changes into the daily lives of independent-living older adults: Long-term follow-up of occupational therapy intervention. *Journal of Gerontology: Series A: Biological Sciences & Medical Sciences, 56,* 60–63.

Clark, F., Azen, S. P., Zemke, R., Jackson, J., Carlson, M., Mandel, D., . . . Lipson, L. (1997). Occupational therapy for independent-living older adults. A randomized controlled trial. *JAMA, 278,* 1321–1326.

Classen, S., Lopez, E., Winter, S., Awadzi, K. D., Ferree, N., & Garvan, C. W. (2007). Population-based health promotion perspective for older driver safety: Conceptual framework to intervention plan. *Clinical Interventions in Aging, 2,* 677–693.

Coker-Bolt, P., Jansson, A., Bigg, S., Hammon, E., Hudson, H., Hunkler, S., . . . Laurent, M. D. (2017). Menstrual education and personal hygiene supplies to empower young women in Haiti. *OTJR: Occupation, Participation, and Health, 37,* 210–217.

Coster, W., Deeney, T., Haltiwanger, J., & Haley, S. (1998). *School Function Assessment (SFA).* Retrieved from http://www.pearsonassessments.com/HAIWEB/Cultures/en-us/Productdetail.htm?Pid=076-1615-709&Mode=summary

Davis, J. R., Schwartz, R., Wheeler, F., & Lancaster, B. (1998). Intervention methods for chronic disease control. In R. C. Brownson, P. L. Remington, & J. R. Davis (Eds.), *Chronic disease epidemiology and control* (2nd ed., pp. 77–116). Washington, DC: American Public Health Association.

Freudenberg, N., Eng, E., Flay, B., Parcel, G., Rogers, T., & Wallerstein, N. (1995). Strengthening individual and community capacity to prevent disease and promote health: In search of relevant theories and principles. *Health Education Quarterly, 22,* 290–306.

Green, L. W., & Kreuter, M. W. (1991). *Health promotion planning: An educational and environmental approach* (2nd ed.). Mountainview, CA: Mayfield.

Gresham, F. M., & Elliott, S. N. (2007). *Social skills rating system.* Los Angeles, CA: Western Psychological Services.

Guoping, L., Yanchun, F., Yingjie, Z., & Gongxiang, D. (2010). *Effect of Tai Chi on physical and mental health of middle-aged and elderly population.* Retrieved from http://en.cnki.com.cn/Article_en/CJFDTOTAL-HLXZ201003003.htm

Helfrich, C. A., Chan, D. V., & Sabol, P. (2011). Cognitive predictors of life skill intervention outcomes for adults with mental illness at risk for homelessness. *American Journal of Occupational Therapy, 65,* 277–286.

Jackson, L. L., & Arbesman, M. (2005). *Occupational therapy practice guidelines for children with behavioral and psychosocial needs.* Bethesda, MD: AOTA Press.

King, G., Law, M., King, S., Hurley, P., Hanna, S., Kertoy, M., . . . Young, K. (2004). *Children's Assessment of Participation and Enjoyment (CAPE) and Preferences for Activities of Children (PAC).* San Antonio, TX: Harcourt Assessment.

Kok, G., Gottlieb, N. H., Commers, M., & Smerecnik, C. (2008). The ecological approach in health promotion programs: A decade later. *American Journal of Health Promotion, 22,* 437–442.

Kronenberg, F., & Pollard, N. (2006). Political dimensions of occupation and the role of occupational therapy. *American Journal of Occupational Therapy, 60,* 617–626.

Kugel, J. (2010). Combating childhood obesity through community practice. *OT Practice, 15*(15), 17–18.

Lamontagne, A. D., Keegel, T., Louie, A. M., Ostry, A., & Landsbergis, P. A. (2007). A systematic review of the job-stress intervention evaluation literature, 1990–2005. *International Journal of Occupational and Environmental Health, 13,* 268–280.

Lau, C. (2011). Food & fun for kids: Preventing childhood obesity through OT. *OT Practice, 16*(6), 11–17.

Maller, C., Townsend, M., Pryor, A., Brown, P., & St. Leger, L. (2006). Healthy nature healthy people: 'contact with nature' as an upstream health promotion intervention for populations. *Health Promotion International, 21,* 45–54.

McClure, R. J., Turner, C., Peel, N., Spinks, A., Eakin, E., & Hughes, K. (2005). Population-based interventions for the prevention of fall-related injuries in older people. *The Cochrane Database of Systematic Reviews,* (1), CD004441. doi:10.1002/14651858.CD004441.pub2

Moyers, P. A. (1999). Guide to occupational therapy practice. *American Journal of Occupational Therapy, 53,* 248–322.

Pollock, H. M. (1942). Eleanor Clarke Slagle. *The American Journal of Psychiatry, 99,* 472–474.

Punwar, J., & Peloquin, M. (2000). *Occupational therapy: Principles and practice.* Philadelphia, PA: Lippincott Williams & Wilkins.

Reed, K. L., & Andersen, L. T. (2017). Eleanor Clarke Slagle: Facts and myths. *Occupational Therapy in Health Care, 31,* 291–311. doi:10.1080/07380577.2017.1376365

Sallis, J. F., Owen, N., & Fisher, E. B. (2008). Ecological models of health behavior. In K. Glanz, B. K. Rimer, & K. Viswanath (Eds.), *Health behavior and health education: Theory, research, and practice* (4th ed., pp. 462–484). San Francisco, CA: Jossey-Bass.

Scaffa, M. E., & Brownson, C. A. (2005). Occupational therapy interventions: Community health approaches. In C. H. Christiansen, C. M. Baum, & J. Bass-Haugen (Eds.), *Occupational therapy: Performance, participation, and well-being* (3rd ed., pp. 476–493). Thorofare, NJ: SLACK.

Substance Abuse and Mental Health Services Administration. (2010). *Permanent supportive housing evidence-based practices kit.* Retrieved from http://store.samhsa.gov/product/Permanent-Supportive-Housing-Evidence-Based-Practices-EBP-KIT/SMA10-4510

Umeda, C. J., Fogelberg, D. J., Jirikowic, T., Pitonyak, J. S., Mroz, T. M., & Ideishi, R. I. (2017). Expanding the implementation of the Americans with Disabilities Act for populations with intellectual and developmental disabilities: The role of organization-level occupational therapy consultation. *American Journal of Occupational Therapy, 71,* 7104090010. doi:10.5014/ajot.2017.714001

Watson, D. E., & Wilson, S. A. (2003). *Task analysis: An individual and population approach* (2nd ed.). Bethesda, MD: AOTA Press.

Webb, T. L., Joseph, J., Yardley, L., & Michie, S. (2010). Using the Internet to promote health behavior change: A systematic review and meta-analysis on the impact of theoretical basis, use of behavior change techniques, and mode of delivery on efficacy. *Journal of Medical Internet Research, 12,* e4. doi:10.2196/jmir.1376

Wenborn, J., Hynes, S., Moniz-Cook, E., Mountain, G., Poland, F., King, M., . . . Orrell, M. (2016). Community occupational therapy for people with dementia and family carers (COTiD-UK) versus treatment as usual (Valuing Active Life in Dementia [VALID] programme): Study protocol for a randomised controlled trial. *Trials, 17,* 65.

World Health Organization. (1986). *The Ottawa charter for health promotion.* Retrieved from http://www.who.int/hpr/NPH/docs/ottawa_charter_hp.pdf

Youngstrom, M. J., & Brown, C. (2005). Categories and principles of interventions. In C. H. Christiansen, C. M. Baum, & J. Bass-Haugen (Eds.), *Occupational therapy: Performance, participation, and well-being* (3rd ed., pp. 396–419). Thorofare, NJ: SLACK.

the**Point** *For additional resources on the subjects discussed in this chapter, visit* http://thePoint.lww.com/Willard-Spackman13e.

Educating Clients

Sue Berger

"What we say doesn't matter as much as what patients understand, remember, and do. If their understanding is incorrect or incomplete, we did not find the right way to reach them."

—REGINA BENJAMIN

LEARNING OBJECTIVES

After reading this chapter, you will be able to:

1. Understand key factors that contribute to effective client education.
2. Understand the importance of health literacy throughout all types of client education.
3. State strategies to use to provide education to clients of varying abilities.
4. Choose and/or develop appropriate written client education materials.

Introduction

As health care professionals, occupational therapy (OT) practitioners are educators. We teach our clients the knowledge and skills they need to enhance their well-being and live as safely as possible (Figure 32-1). *Education and Training* is one of the five core categories of OT interventions as stated in our Practice Framework (American Occupational Therapy Association [AOTA], 2014). Not surprisingly, Sharry, McKenna, and Tooth (2002) found that client education was frequently used as a key intervention approach by occupational therapists. To be effective clinicians, we must know what specific strategies to teach our clients, and we need to know *how* to teach our clients. We need to know the various ways to stabilize a bowl for mixing when one has the use of only one arm, but we also need to know how to teach clients so they will remember the strategy, be successful with the strategy, and be able to generalize the strategy to all environments where they might cook. Therefore, this chapter focuses on specific education strategies and how to effectively use them. Chapter 48 provides additional theoretical background related to teaching and learning.

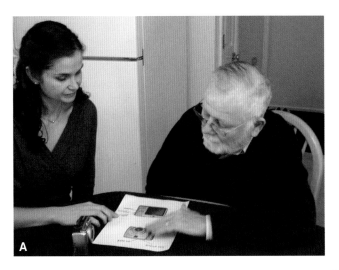
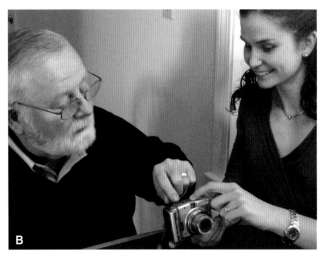

FIGURE 32-1 Reinforcing verbal directions in use of a digital camera, with a handout that includes a simple, clearly labeled photo.

Why Does the Information Need to Be Communicated?

Educating clients decreases anxiety, increases knowledge, improves satisfaction with services, and leads to better clinical outcomes (Berkman et al., 2011; Fredericks & Yau, 2017; Watson, Cosio, & Lin, 2014). Client education can shorten hospital stays and decrease costs of health care, especially for those living with chronic conditions (Dreeben, 2010). When individuals become ill, those who are educated about the illness and treatment stay motivated and adhere to recommendations (Drench, Noonan, Sharby, & Hallenborg, 2007). Client education maximizes an individual's ability to participate in daily activities. For all of this to occur, OT practitioners need to communicate information clearly, and more importantly, they need to ensure that clients understand the material conveyed.

Client education is more than telling someone what to do; rather, it is a complex yet important concept that includes careful consideration of teaching and learning strategies that ultimately will affect client outcomes in the clinic and at home (Dreeben, 2010). Effective client education is at the core of quality care.

Who Needs to Know the Information?

Just as the profession of OT uses the term *clients* to broadly refer to persons, groups, or populations who receive service (AOTA, 2014), the term *clients* in this chapter includes families, caregivers, teachers, employers, and relevant others. One must consider the unique learning needs of all clients that we work with. In addition, it is important to note that the learning needs of one client, for example, an individual living with a stroke, may be different than those of the partner, child, or other family member.

Along with communicating with clients, communicating clearly with other professionals is critical, both to support client outcomes and to clearly articulate OT practice (Brewer & Rosenwax, 2016; Lamb, 2015). Interprofessional practice is common practice in many settings but is only successful when professionals clearly share key information in a timely manner. Although the focus of this chapter is on client education, many of the principles discussed regarding the what, where, when, and how of client education relate to communicating and sharing information with other professionals as well. Occupational therapy practitioners must learn to effectively communicate with the different individuals and groups relevant to each situation.

As with all intervention, knowing the client and his or her strengths, limitations, culture, values, interests, age, primary language, and auditory ability is fundamental. Knowing the client's literacy skills is also important. Although the definition of literacy focuses on reading and writing, it also affects one's ability to comprehend oral information (Dreeben, 2010; van Servellen, 2009).

Literacy

Health literacy is defined as "the degree to which individuals have the capacity to obtain, process, and understand basic health information and services needed to make appropriate health decisions" (Institute of Medicine [IOM],

CENTENNIAL NOTES

Educating Clients

Patient education has been around for many years. For instance, in 1940, Pattee shared examples of prescribed "exercises" which were suggestions of activities one could do to strengthen specific areas of the body such as shown below:

Types of Exercises

If the hands are affected, the power of flexion and extension of the fingers may be increased by:	Washing dishes Polishing silver Polishing shoes Crumpling whole sheet of newspaper in one hand Dusting furniture Typewriting Playing the piano Shelling peas Squeezing a sponge, rubber ball, or water pistol
Power of flexion of fingers may be increased by:	Using a screw driver Using a plane (on soft wood first; hard wood later) Using a Dover egg beater (woman) Using a hand drill (man) Ironing
Power of extension of fingers may be increased by:	Playing crokinole or games which require the spinning of an arrow, such as Parcheesi and shooting marbles

The ways in which we educate the people we work with have changed dramatically since the beginning of our profession. Today, technology has enabled us to meet the many learning styles of our clients. Not only do we provide client education face-to-face and through written and video materials, but also we educate our clients virtually. For example, if the practice setting limits the ability to perform a home visit prior to discharge, family members can easily take a video of a bathroom set up and share it with the practitioner. If clients have questions between therapy appointments, they can e-mail the practitioner. We provide links for our clients for important resources.

When this chapter first appeared in *Willard & Spackman's Occupational Therapy* (11th edition), there was a small section on multimedia. The amount of information on technology and client education has doubled in just 10 years and for this edition could easily have been a chapter in and of itself. Who would have predicted the opportunities through telehealth when our profession just began in 1917? It is exciting to imagine the opportunities for educating our clients in the coming centuries.

2004, para. 1). Therefore, being health literate involves more than reading and writing; one also needs to have effective speaking and listening skills. Because technology has emerged as an important way to communicate and share information—especially health information—one also needs to be computer literate. Finally, motivation, cognitive ability, and social skills influence one's ability to gather, understand, and use health information. Health literacy includes the interaction between an individual's skills and the demands of the environment (U.S. Department of Health and Human Services, 2010), and this implies that an individual's health literacy changes depending on the clarity of the health-related materials. It is our responsibility as OT practitioners to assure that our clients are functioning at their highest literacy abilities by providing educational information in a way that they can effectively use (AOTA, 2011; Smith & Gutman, 2011).

Good observation skills can provide a great deal of information about reading level. When giving written material to a client, one should note whether the client states something similar to "I'll read this later so I can discuss it with my husband," "I left my glasses at home," or "I'll remember what you say—no need to write it down." Does the client appear to read something but then is unable to follow the instructions? Although there are standardized reading level assessments such as the Rapid Estimate of Adult Literacy in Medicine (REALM) (Davis et al., 1991) and the Test of Functional Health Literacy in Adults (TOFHLA) (Parker, Baker, Williams, & Nurss, 1995), they can be time-comsuming to administer and embarrassing for clients. Sometimes, a simple question such as "How confident are you in filling out medical forms?" can identify persons with limited health literacy as accurately (and quicker) than the TOFHLA (Sarkar, Schillinger, López, & Sudore, 2011).

Culture

Knowing the culture of an individual is critical to providing effective education. Terminology, topics, and ideas should all be relevant to the intended audience. When possible, communication should be in a person's primary language. Native speaker, professional interpreters are best to prevent miscommunication and ensure privacy (Centers for Disease Control and Prevention [CDC], 2009). At times, clients ask their family member to provide translation. Caution should be used in this situation, as family members' own opinions and reactions are often conveyed as well or instead of the client's (Brega et al., 2015).

Being culturally sensitive involves more than speaking in the client's primary language. One should consider the meaning of personal space and time within the client's culture, be careful about making judgments or interpretations without checking this out with the person, and use culturally relevant scenarios (Brega et al., 2015; van Servellen, 2009). For example, when addressing nutrition, discuss food and habits that are culturally appropriate for the client (e.g., soy sauce or ketchup; use of utensils or hands). Being cognizant of cultural differences and beliefs in health and wellness is the first step toward effective communication with individuals of cultures other than one's own. See Chapter 19 for more information on culture.

What Information Needs to Be Conveyed?

Several studies have found large discrepancies between what clients want to know and what health professionals believe is most important. For example, Murphy et al. (2015) found that many patients wanted to know about potential emotional issues related to their conditions but only a minority of people received this information. When clients don't receive the information from health care providers that they want to know, they seek out the information on their own, often through the Internet. However, with so much material available, clients struggle to know which information to trust (Kravitz & Bell, 2013). Collaborative goal setting can support OT practitioners in understanding what information is important to the client.

As OT practitioners, we teach our clients strategies to help them participate in daily life. We teach individuals strategies for using community transportation. We teach parents strategies to help their children participate in play activities. We teach mental health workers strategies to adapt the environment to best meet the needs of their patients. The list is endless. The key for all client education is to limit the objectives, focusing on information that clients want or need to know. Although something that is nice to know might seem valuable to include, more is often not better (Office of Disease Prevention and Health Promotion, 2016; Weiss, 2007). Remember to prioritize information by what is important to the client, not what you believe is important for the client to know.

Where Is the Best Place to Communicate the Information?

The environment in which client education occurs can influence comprehension and recall. Information should be shared in a shame-free environment (Osborne, 2011), a setting in which the client feels free to ask questions, admit lack of understanding, or ask for repetition. A quiet space with no distractions provides an environment where clients can focus on the topic being discussed. For example, ask for permission to turn off the television or radio or find a better time if a favorite show is playing. Find a private room or corner. If the client is reading material, be sure there is adequate lighting with little or no glare.

When Is the Best Time to Communicate the Information?

Internal distractions such as pain, anxiety, hunger, or need to use the bathroom affect one's ability to absorb and understand information. When possible, resolve these distractions prior to client education. Because some people are "morning people" and others are more alert and receptive to information in the evening, consider the timing of all client education. When working in schools, schedule evening hours to provide parent education. Parents who need to take time off from work to attend a meeting may arrive frustrated and angry and will be less open to hearing new information.

It is also important to consider timing of information over the course of care. For example, educational needs in the acute phase of health care differ from those during rehabilitation. Timing of client education needs to be considered related to both time of day and time in the recovery process.

How Is the Best Way to Communicate the Information?

Recall of information depends on how the information is presented. Organization of content helps clients understand and apply information. Although this is true for individuals with low literacy, all people—especially those who are in a new environment, are learning new information, are in pain, or are anxious—will benefit when material is presented clearly and in an organized manner. Therefore, plan the information to be conveyed before talking and remember to sequence your information logically (Centers for Medicare & Medicaid Services [CMS], 2017). For example, if you are working with a group of children to help them lighten their backpacks, begin by stating, "First, decide what needs to go in; second, put heavy books at the back of the pack; and third, put lighter objects in the front of the pack." When using numbers to represent quality, the higher number should always convey better quality (Berkman et al., 2011). Information that is given as a concrete suggestion is recalled more often than a general suggestion (CDC, 2009). For example, "Walk briskly for 30 minutes three times a week" would be recalled more often than "Exercise several times a week."

Using demonstrations, models, and pictures along with oral communication also helps people to understand information (Berkman et al., 2011; Weiss, 2007). When teaching clients about the importance of eliminating clutter for safety, show before and after pictures of a kitchen and point out safety hazards and ways they were resolved. When teaching use of adaptive equipment, explain and demonstrate. Use multiple teaching methods, especially when working with groups of individuals, because different people learn differently. Even when working with one client, multiple teaching methods help to emphasize key information and facilitate comprehension and memory.

Finally, one must verify understanding. The practitioner might believe that he or she was clear, organized, and consistent, but if the client did not understand the message, the practitioner was not successful. The individual who is passive or constantly nodding in agreement might not fully understand or adhere to the recommendations. Therefore, whenever possible, employ the "teach-back technique," having clients return demonstration, repeat in their own words, or explain a concept using a different example (Caplin & Saunders, 2015; Nouri & Rudd, 2015). This technique is effective in making sure that clients understand the information and, more importantly, in improving health outcomes. If appropriate, ask one client to demonstrate to or teach other clients. Clients are more likely to ask questions and admit lack of understanding with a peer than with a therapist.

In their extensive systematic review, Berkman et al. (2011) summarized key principles to consider for all forms of client education to improve health outcomes, including repetition, pilot testing of material, and emphasis on skill building. In general, there are three ways to communicate with clients: orally, in writing, and via technology.

Communicating Orally

Communicating with clients face-to-face is most effective because it provides the opportunity to use conversational style speaking, provides nonverbal cues for acknowledgement, and allows for interpretation of nonverbal cues to determine comprehension. Face-to-face communication is also often interactive because clients are able to demonstrate understanding through answering questions or performing the task. Oral communication also provides opportunity to develop rapport and trust, which ultimately can lead to better therapeutic outcomes (van Servellen, 2009).

In communicating verbally with someone with low literacy skills, it is helpful to be consistent with word choice. During a session on feeding skills, for example, the word *silverware* should be used throughout instead of alternating with *utensil*. Unusual or challenging words used in conversation should be defined, and acronyms should be explained (CDC, 2009). Words such as *assessment* or *intervention* should be defined, or more common words should be used. Acronyms such as *ROM* and *ADL* should be used only after they are fully explained; even then, be sure to verify comprehension. If you are unsure of word choice, ask the client what word he or she uses to describe an item, and use that word consistently. For example, you might ask your clients if they refer to shoes as *sneakers* or *tennis shoes*.

Communicating with clients who are hard of hearing poses other challenges. It is helpful to choose an environment that is quiet and free of distractions, get the client's attention before speaking, and position oneself directly in front of the client (Osborne, 2011). Often, a client hears better from one side than the other, so take the time to find this out and position oneself on the side which is better. If the person wears hearing aids, make sure they are in place and working. If hearing is severely impaired, use other methods of communication along with, or instead of, speaking.

Communicating in Writing

Most people forget much of what they are told during a patient–physician interaction, and what they believe they remember, they remember incorrectly (Sandberg, Sharma, & Sandberg, 2012). Reinforcing oral communication with print material can help recall and comprehension. Written forms of communication reinforce what is said, provide a record of what is said, and provide reminders of what is conveyed. The ability to understand verbal information differs from the ability to understand written information because the reader can control the pace of obtaining written information and can review it as often as needed (E. A. Wilson & Wolf, 2009). If it is worth the time to write down information, it is important to ensure that the reader can use the material. To effectively communicate in writing, one needs to consider the reading level and presentation of the material (CDC, 2009; National Institutes of Health, 2016).

Reading Level of the Material

Public information, such as newspapers, is often written at the 10th-grade level or higher, but many people read at a much lower level. Dignan and Hunter (2015) reviewed 97 documents used for patient education within a rehabilitation hospital and found the average reading level was about grade 16. In a study reviewing OT written educational materials, Griffin, McKenna, and Tooth (2006) found that the materials were written at a 9th- or 10th-grade level, whereas the clients mean reading ability was at a 7th- to 8th-grade level. Use of a low reading level in written materials meets the needs of a large number of people as all individuals appreciate receiving information in a clear and simple format (National Institutes of Health, 2016).

There are numerous assessments to determine the reading level of written material such as the Simplified Measure of Gobbledygook (SMOG) formula (McLaughlin, 1969; shown in Box 32-1) and the Gunning Fog index scale (Gunning & Kallan, 1994) along with computer-generated readability scores (Microsoft Office Online, 2017). In general, however, using short sentences and primarily one- or two-syllable words is a simple strategy that will keep the reading level low.

In addition to reading level, other factors influence the readability of printed material. For example, the use of all capital letters is more challenging to read than is a combination of uppercase and lowercase letters because readers use the shapes of words to help read (Harvard T.H. Chan School of Public Health, 2015; Weiss, 2007). For example,

---

BOX 32-1   SIMPLIFIED MEASURE OF GOBBLEDYGOOK READABILITY ACTIVITY

Try to determine the readability level of this chapter. Using the Simplified Measure of Gobbledygook formula, determine the number of words with three or more syllables in the following sentences: first 10 sentences of the chapter, last 10 sentences of the chapter, first 10 sentences of the section "Reading Level of the Material." Take that number, find the nearest perfect square (e.g., if there are 67 words with 3 or more syllables, the nearest perfect square is 64), take the square root of that (i.e., 8), and then add a constant of 3 (i.e., 11). This number equals the approximate grade/reading level of the material.

---

when typed in all capitals, *AND* looks like a rectangle and is visually very similar to *FOR*, *THE*, or any other three-letter word. If typed with lowercase letters, *and*, *for*, and *the*, all have different shapes, and it is therefore easier to quickly determine the word. Box 32-2 provides examples of easy and difficult to use layouts and fonts.

To make written information readable, use active rather than passive wording and use positive terminology (CDC, 2009). For example, write, "Put your right arm in first when getting dressed" instead of "Your right arm should be put in first when getting dressed," and state, "Raise your arm slowly" instead of "Do not raise your arm quickly."

Similar to oral communication, use of common words in writing makes reading easier (CDC, 2009; National

---

BOX 32-2   EXAMPLES OF EASY VERSUS DIFFICULT TO READ FONTS AND LAYOUT

1. It is easier to read material that is written using a combination of uppercase and lowercase letters THAN MATERIAL WRITTEN IN ALL CAPITALS.

2. It is easier to read basic fonts such as Arial, vs. *fancy fonts such as Informal Roman.*

3. It is easier to read material that uses a 12-point font than material that uses a 9-point font.

4. It is easier to read the material written above that is single-spaced than what you are reading right now, which is less than single space. Remember that spacing and allowing for white space are important.

Institutes of Health, 2016). Using the word *doctor* instead of *physician* is often appropriate. Most people understand the phrase *thinking skills* better than they do *cognition*. If it is important to use the term *cognition*, define it and use it consistently. Use of descriptions that are simple to visualize is another helpful strategy. In encouraging someone to lift only small items, the commonly used expression "no bigger than a bread box" is easier to understand than "no bigger than 2 ft by 1 ft by 1 ft."

Presentation of the Material

The overall presentation of all written communication is important. Presentation includes, but is not limited to, the type of paper used, the color of paper and print, font size and style, visuals, and organization. These factors affect one's ability to see the material, read the material, and understand the material as well as one's motivation to read the material.

Font and Paper.
To ensure that most people can see the written material, it should be typed in a font size of at least 12 points (National Institutes of Health, 2016). Font size of 14 or greater should be used for readers with low vision (Osborne, 2011) (see Box 32-2). Use of fancy fonts or italics should be avoided (National Institutes of Health, 2016). The use of san serif versus serif (the small lines at the end of characters) has been controversial. Whereas a study has found that people with aphasia understood significantly more information when written with a san serif font (L. Wilson & Read, 2016), another study found an increase in speed and comprehension of serif font by those with macular degeneration (Tarita-Nistor, Lam, Brent, Steinbach, & González, 2013). Centers for Disease Control and Prevention guidelines (2009) recommend serif font for information in the body of a text; however, they suggest using san serif for headings. Using san serif font for headings provides contrast to the font in the text and enables one to skim material by reading headings easily.

Matte paper should be used because glossy paper can cause glare and make reading difficult. Black print on white paper is often most effective for contrast (CMS, 2017; Osborne, 2011). Limit the use of color as it can be distracting and make material harder to read (CMS, 2017). If using color, do so in a way that supports comprehension (e.g., green for positive actions and red for negative actions).

Organization.
The organization of the material affects readability. Highlighting key information by making it bold or underlining it adds focus to important information. Headings are helpful to group information. Including white space, rather than filling up all the paper with words and pictures, facilitates self-efficacy (CDC, 2009; National Institutes of Health, 2016). Looking at a brochure that is unappealing and crammed with information will be discouraging for clients, regardless of the information in the brochure

(Figure 32-2). Include key information first or last because readers remember this information best (CDC, 2009).

Spacing is important for visual cues. Leave more space above headings and subheadings than below (CDC, 2009; National Institutes of Health, 2016). This ties information together at a quick visual glance. Consider using simple questions as headers, such as "What is energy conservation?" and "What are the key principles of energy conservation?" Chunking information into five or fewer categories facilitates recall. Information can be divided by rooms in a house (for a handout on environmental adaptations), by senses (for a handout on sensory processing), or according to any categorization that is appropriate for the topic.

When possible, the material should be personalized. This can be done simply by writing the user's name at the top of the material or by leaving blank space for adding individualized suggestions. Using terminology such as "your exercise program" rather than "the exercise program" has been shown to make a difference in both recall and satisfaction with the material (Wagner, Davis, & Handelsman, 1998).

Visuals.
The old saying "A picture is worth a thousand words" is true only if the picture is clear and relevant. Health literacy literature emphasizes the importance of visuals that are culturally appropriate, easy to understand, and used with simple captions (Agency for Healthcare Research and Quality [AHRQ], 2013; CDC, 2009). Use shapes with simple words that are universally recognized. For example, use a picture of a stop sign to reinforce the importance of stopping activity before pain occurs. Visuals, like words, should convey the positive. For example, include pictures of healthy foods rather than a picture of chips and cookies with a line through it. Some visuals can be confusing rather than helpful. For example, pictures with many arrows or bus schedules with small font and many columns are difficult to use. The purpose of using visuals is to facilitate comprehension. Pictures as decorations can detract from the message (CDC, 2009). All pictures that are included should convey an idea, enhancing the message in the text.

Assessing Print Material

The best way to develop effective printed material is to engage members of the intended audience in the development of the material, ask potential users for feedback of a draft, and revise accordingly (CMS, 2017; Harvard T.H. Chan School of Public Health, 2015). The Suitability Assessment of Materials (SAM) (Doak, Doak, & Root, 1996) and the Patient Education Materials Assessment Tool (PEMAT) (AHRQ, 2013) are two of several published assessments that can be used to ensure that written materials are developed well. The PEMAT also has a version that can be used to assess audio visual materials. Box 32-3 provides a quick checklist of items to consider in developing or choosing print material to use with clients.

Low Vision Tips

1. Improve the lighting
- Direct light onto the surface of reading or writing material.
- Bring light closer to surface.
- Turn on overhead light along with task light.
- Make sure all lights have working bulbs and be sure to turn them on.
- Keep on a nightlight or keep a flashlight by the bed.

2. Increase the contrast
- Consider painting walls "opposite" colors of the carpeting.
- Add high contrast throw pillows or afghan to chairs and couches.
- Use colored towels and floor mat to provide high contrast to bathroom walls.
- Use black marker on white paper.
- Choose hard covered books, which provide more contrast than paperbacks.

3. Decrease the glare
- Make sure the light bulb is fully covered by the shade.
- Wear baseball caps inside and outside.
- Wear wraparound filters when outside.
- Use low gloss or no gloss floor and table polish or use table cloths to cover shiny surfaces.

4. Increase the size
- Label items with large print, high contrast lettering.
- Borrow large print books from the library.
- Change the font on the computer to a

A

LOW VISION TIPS

IMPROVE THE LIGHTING

Direct light onto the surface of reading or writing material
Bring light closer to surface
Turn on overhead light along with task light
Make sure all lights have working bulbs and be sure to turn them on.
Keep on a nightlight or keep a flashlight by the bed.

INCREASE THE CONTRAST

Consider painting walls "opposite" colors of the carpeting.
Add high contrast throw pillows or afghan to chairs and couches.
Use colored towels and floor mat to provide high contrast to bathroom walls.
Use black marker on white paper.
Choose hard covered books, which provide more contrast than paperbacks

DECREASE THE GLARE

Make sure the light bulb is fully covered by the shade
Wear baseball caps inside and outside
Wear wraparound filters when outside
Use low gloss or no gloss floor and table polish or use table cloths to cover shiny surfaces

INCREASE THE SIZE

Label items with large print, high contrast lettering
Borrow large print books from the library
Change the font on the computer to a larger font
Purchase commercially available large print items (e.g., large print playing cards; large print wall clock, large print calendar)

USE YOUR OTHER SENSES

Mark items such as the stove and telephone with raised dots or bright colored stickers.
Purchase commercially available talking items (e.g., talking clock)
Smell certain items in refrigerator before eating to make sure they haven't gone bad.

B

FIGURE 32-2 **A.** Well-designed brochure that is easy to read. **B.** Poorly designed brochure (With the same content as part A) that would discourage the reader.

BOX 32-3   CHECKLIST OF THINGS TO CONSIDER IN DEVELOPING OR CHOOSING PRINTED MATERIALS

Characteristics of the User

___ Was the age of the user considered?
___ Was the education and/or reading level of the user considered?
___ Were the values, beliefs, and interests of the user considered?

Information Included

___ Is the information what the user might want to know?
___ Is the information what the user might need to know?
___ Is information limited to a few key objectives?

Reading Level of the Material

___ Is there a limited number of long and/or compound sentences?
___ Are there only a few three or more syllable words? Are the majority of these common, everyday words?
___ Are unusual words defined? Are all other words common, everyday words?
___ Is the same term used consistently?
___ Are common descriptions used to assist with visualization?
___ Is active terminology used?
___ Is terminology phrased in the positive?

Presentation of the Material

___ Is a font style that is clear and easy to read used?
___ Is the font size at least 12 points (greater for people with low vision)?
___ Is there a strong contrast between color of print and color of paper?
___ Is matte paper used?
___ Is bold or underlining used for emphasis?
___ Are headings and subheadings used to chunk information and for layout?
___ Is adequate white space used?
___ Is key information included first or last?
___ Is information personalized?

Visuals

___ Are visuals culturally appropriate?
___ Are simple captions included for each visual?
___ Are visuals conveyed in the positive?
___ Do the visuals convey information (not just for decoration)?

Cultural Relevance

___ Is the material relevant to the intended audience?
___ Is the terminology culturally appropriate?
___ Was the material reviewed with the intended audience prior to distribution?
___ Is the material available in the user's primary language?

Communicating through Technology

The explosion of technology has expanded the ways we educate clients. Beyond television and radio, computers, tablets, and smartphones provide many innovative ways to teach and reinforce important knowledge and skills through use of audio, video, and multimedia. Multimedia provide information in a consistent, repetitive manner and often in an environment with no time pressure and has been shown to be effective with clients of all levels of literacy (Bickmore et al., 2010; Kandula et al., 2009) and for those with a variety of health conditions (Jeste, Dunn, Folsom, & Zisook, 2008). Web-based technology has expanded multimedia options exponentially in recent years with innovation occurring daily. Interactive quizzes, slideshows, and games can be fun, motivating, and effective in conveying information.

Understanding someone's learning style is often the first step to effective client education (McNeill, 2012).

Some learn best by reading, others by listening, and others by seeing. For many, learning information in multiple forms reinforces the information and assists with recall.

Audio and Video

Audio and video options have been available for many years, but recently, the technology and options have advanced considerably. Podcasts are just one example of a relatively new audio tool useful for conveying health material. This format can be used for providing specific interventions (e.g., stress management relaxation podcasts) and for reinforcing content already discussed (e.g., complications from diabetes). Video technologies have advanced as well and are easy to use and accessible. Recommending a YouTube video about volunteering might encourage a client to consider this opportunity or developing a video of a home program that can be viewed on a tablet or smartphone can facilitate comprehension and support accurate follow-through.

In choosing or developing audio or video materials, similar considerations should be used as for written materials, keeping health literacy principles in mind (Weiss, 2007). Using plain language and limiting objectives are important no matter the media used to convey the information. Important information should be presented at the beginning of a video, although a review of the key information at the end is also needed (Frentsos, 2015). For audio, when possible, use voices of people like the intended audience, and for video, be sure that images are of people like the intended audience. When making a video for a specific client, take videos of the client doing the activity. When using audio or video, the text of the material should also be provided to increase accessibility for all (Office of Disease Prevention and Health Promotion, 2016).

Telehealth

Telehealth is a way of providing health care and education at a distance. It can be used throughout the scope of OT practice (Cason, 2012) and can be provided through four different modalities: "live" or synchronous, asynchronous, remote patient monitoring, and mobile health (Center for Connected Health Policy, 2017). Telehealth can incorporate all modes of communication including "face-to-face" communication over the Internet, video messages, written passages, interactive components, and e-mail communication. The benefits of telehealth are many including decreased travel time for both therapist and client, increased access to therapy and specialists, especially for clients in rural areas, and ability to understand occupational performance within the home context (AOTA, 2010; Serwe, Hersch, Pickens, & Pancheri, 2017). There are challenges to telehealth as well, including reimbursement, technology infrastructure, privacy concerns, and licensure issues (AOTA, 2010; Cason, 2012) along with logistical challenges such as background noise (Serwe et al., 2017).

Results of a survey, regarding patient perceptions of receiving electronic patient information, show that more than half of the people questioned prefer paper brochures; however, this did vary by age and gender (Hammar, Nilsson, & Hovstadius, 2016). Although there is evidence regarding the effectiveness of e-learning on clinician behavior, there are few studies that provide objective data regarding patient outcomes (Sinclair, Kable, Levett-Jones, & Booth, 2016). Clearly, there is still much information we don't know regarding the benefits and challenges of electronic forms of education.

Using Web-based materials requires both reading and computer literacy. Technology today, therefore, has increased the divide for those with low literacy skills and/or limited technology literacy (Mackert, Mabry-Flynn, Champlin, Donovan, & Pounders, 2016). If using computer technology for client education, be sure to consider the client's information technology knowledge, motivation and interest, the usability and functionality of the application, the costs of implementation and use, and the infrastructure and support (Ammenwerth, Iller, & Mahler, 2006). Health Literacy Online (Office of Disease Prevention and Health Promotion, 2016) is a wonderful resource to guide the development of Websites to make them accessible. This resource provides many simple strategies including putting the most important information first as often readers only read the first few words of a page or paragraph, limiting the number of links, and providing meaningful labels for buttons.

Keep in mind that 15% of Americans have no access to the Web except through their smartphone and more than half of people who own a smartphone have used it to find health information (Pew Research Center, 2015). Therefore, providing resources regarding health, appointments, or "homework" reminders through a mobile device is another way to reach individuals who may struggle accessing and interpreting other types of information.

Conclusion

No one method of client education is effective for all individuals (van Servellen, 2009). Some material is best suited for certain methods of teaching, and some individuals learn best via certain teaching strategies. "One size fits all" is not an effective motto for educating clients. Although more research is needed to determine the best ways to provide client education, considering multiple modes of communication and the specific needs of the individual or groups of individuals will help to convey valuable information to clients.

REFERENCES

Agency for Healthcare Research and Quality. (2013). *The Patient Education Materials Assessment Tool (PEMAT) and user's guide.* Retrieved from https://www.ahrq.gov/sites/default/files/publications/files/pemat_guide.pdf

American Occupational Therapy Association. (2010). Telerehabilitation. *American Journal of Occupational Therapy, 64,* S92–S102. doi:10.5014/ajot.2010.64S92

American Occupational Therapy Association. (2011). AOTA's societal statement on health literacy. *American Journal of Occupational Therapy, 65,* S78–S79. doi:10.5014/ajot.2011.65S78

American Occupational Therapy Association. (2014). Occupational therapy practice framework: Domain and process, 3rd edition. *American Journal of Occupational Therapy, 62,* 625–683. doi:10.5014/ajot.2014.682006

Ammenwerth, E., Iller, C., & Mahler, C. (2006). IT-adoption and the interaction of task, technology and individuals: A fit framework and a case study. *BMC Medical Informatics and Decision Making, 6,* 3. Retrieved from http://www.biomedcentral.com/content/pdf/1472-6947-6-3.pdf

Berkman, N. D., Sheridan, S. L., Donahue, K. E., Halpern, D. J., Viera, A., Crotty, K., . . . Viswanathan, M. (2011). *Health literacy interventions and outcomes: An updated systematic review* (Evidence Report/Technology Assessment, 199. AHRQ Pub. No. 11-E006). Rockville, MD: Agency for Healthcare Research and Quality.

Bickmore, T. W., Pfeifer, L. M., Byron, D., Forsythe, S., Henault, L. E., Jack, B. W., . . . Paasche-Orlow, M. K. (2010). Usability of conversational agents by patients with inadequate health literacy: Evidence from two clinical trials. *Journal of Health Communication, 15*(Suppl. 2), 197–210. doi:10.1080/10810730.2010.499991

Brega, A. G., Barnard, J., Mabachi, N. M., Weiss, B. D., DeWalt, D. A., Brach, C., . . . West, D. R. (2015). *AHRQ health literacy universal precautions toolkit* (2nd ed.). Rockville, MD: Agency for Healthcare Research and Quality.

Brewer, M. L., & Rosenwax, L. (2016). Can interprofessional practice solve the vexing question of 'What is occupational therapy'? *Australian Occupational Therapy Journal, 63,* 221–222.

Caplin, M., & Saunders, T. (2015). Utilizing teach-back to reinforce patient education: A step-by-step approach. *Orthopedic Nursing, 34,* 365–368.

Cason, J. (2012). Telehealth opportunities in occupational therapy through the Affordable Care Act. *American Journal of Occupational Therapy, 66,* 131–136.

Center for Connected Health Policy. (2017). *What is telehealth?* Retrieved from http://www.cchpca.org/what-is-telehealth

Centers for Disease Control and Prevention. (2009). *Simply put: A guide for creating easy-to-understand materials* (3rd ed.). Atlanta, GA: Author. Retrieved from https://www.cdc.gov/healthliteracy/pdf/simply_put.pdf

Centers for Medicare & Medicaid Services. (2017). *Toolkit for making written material clear and effective.* Retrieved from https://www.cms.gov/Outreach-and-Education/Outreach/WrittenMaterialsToolkit/index.html?redirect=/WrittenMaterialsToolkit

Davis, T. C., Crouch, M. A., Long, S. W., Jackson, R. H., Bates, P., George, R. B., & Bairnsfather, L. E. (1991). Rapid assessment of literacy levels of adult primary care patients. *Family Medicine, 23,* 433–435.

Dignan, M., & Hunter, E. (2015). Assessing and adapting patient educational materials: Addressing low health literacy in an inpatient rehabilitation setting. *American Journal of Occupational Therapy, 69,* 140–142. doi:10.5014/ajot.2015.69S1-RP204A

Doak, C. C., Doak, L. G., & Root, J. H. (1996). *Teaching patients with low literacy skills* (2nd ed.). Philadelphia, PA: J. B. Lippincott.

Dreeben, O. (2010). *Patient education in rehabilitation.* Boston, MA: Jones & Bartlett Learning.

Drench, M. E., Noonan, A. C., Sharby, N., & Hallenborg, V. S. (2007). *Psychosocial aspects of health care* (2nd ed.). Upper Saddle River, NJ: Pearson Education.

Fredericks, S., & Yau, T. (2017). Clinical effectiveness of individual patient education in heart surgery patients: A systematic review and meta-analysis. *International Journal of Nursing Studies, 65,* 44–53. doi:10.1016/j.ijnurstu.2016.11.001

Frentsos, J. M. (2015). Use of videos as supplemental education tools across the cancer trajectory. *Clinical Journal of Oncology Nursing, 19,* E126–E130.

Griffin, J., McKenna, K., & Tooth, L. (2006). Discrepancy between older clients' ability to read and comprehend and the reading level of written educational materials used by occupational therapists. *American Journal of Occupational Therapy, 60,* 70–80.

Gunning, R., & Kallan, R. (1994). *How to take the fog out of business writing.* Chicago, IL: Dartnell.

Hammar, T., Nilsson, A. L., & Hovstadius, B. (2016). Patients' views on electronic patient information leaflets. *Pharmacy Practice, 14,* 702. Retrieved from https://www.ncbi.nlm.nih.gov/pmc/articles/PMC4930857/pdf/pharmpract-14-702.pdf

Harvard T.H. Chan School of Public Health. (2015). *Health literacy studies web site.* Retrieved from https://www.hsph.harvard.edu/healthliteracy

Institute of Medicine. (2004). *Health literacy: A prescription to end confusion* (Report Brief). Washington, DC: The National Academies Press. Retrieved from http://www.iom.edu/Reports/2004/Health-Literacy-A-Prescription-to-End-Confusion.aspx

Jeste, D. V., Dunn, L. B., Folsom, D. P., & Zisook, D. (2008). Multimedia educational aids for improving consumer knowledge about illness management and treatment decisions: A review of randomized controlled trials. *Journal of Psychiatric Research, 42.* doi:10.1016/j.jpsychires.2006.10.004

Kandula, N. R., Nsiah-Kumi, P. A., Makoul, G., Sager, J., Zei, C. P., Glass, S., . . . Baker, D. W. (2009). The relationship between health literacy and knowledge improvement after a multimedia type 2 diabetes education program. *Patient Education and Counseling, 75,* 321–327. doi:10.1016/j.pec.2009.04.001

Kravitz, R. L., & Bell, R. A. (2013). Media, messages, and medication: Strategies to reconcile what patients hear, what they want, and what they need from medications. *BMC Medical Informatics and Decision Making, 13*(Suppl. 3). doi:10.1186/1472-6947-13-S3-S5

Lamb, G. (2015). Overview and summary: Care coordination: Benefits of interprofessional collaboration. *The Online Journal of Issues in Nursing, 20.* Retrieved from http://www.nursingworld.org/MainMenuCategories/ANAMarketplace/ANAPeriodicals/OJIN/TableofContents/Vol-20-2015/No3-Sept-2015/Overview-Summary-Care-Coordination.html

Mackert, M., Mabry-Flynn, A., Champlin, S., Donovan, E. E., & Pounders, K. (2016). Health literacy and health information technology adoption: The potential for a new digital divide. *Journal of Medical Internet Research, 18,* e264. doi:10.2196/jmir.6349

McLaughlin, G. H. (1969). SMOG grading—a new readability formula. *Journal of Reading, 12,* 639–646.

McNeill, B. E. (2012). You "teach" but does your patient really learn? Basic principles to promote safer outcomes. *Tar Heel Nurse, 74,* 9–16.

Microsoft Office Online. (2017). *Test your documents readability.* Retrieved from http://office.microsoft.com

Murphy, B. M., Higgins, R. O., Jackson, A. C., Edington, J., Jackson, A., & Worcester, M. U. (2015). Patients want to know about the 'cardiac blues.' *Australian Family Physicians, 44*(11), 826–832.

National Institutes of Health. (2016). *Clear and simple.* Retrieved from https://www.nih.gov/institutes-nih/nih-office-director/office-communications-public-liaison/clear-communication/clear-simple

Nouri, S. S., & Rudd, R. I. (2015). Health literacy in the "oral exchange": An important element of patient-provider communication. *Patient Education and Counseling, 98,* 565–571.

Office of Disease Prevention and Health Promotion. (2016). *Health literacy online.* Retrieved from https://health.gov/healthliteracyonline/

Osborne, H. (2011). *Health literacy from A to Z: Practical ways to communicate your health message* (2nd ed.). Burlington, MA: Jones & Bartlett Learning.

Parker, R. M., Baker, D. W., Williams, M. V., & Nurss, J. R. (1995). The test of functional health literacy in adults: A new instrument for measuring patients' literacy skills. *Journal of General Internal Medicine, 10,* 537–541.

Pattee, G. (1940). Prescribed exercise to be carried out at home. *Occupational Therapy and Rehabilitation, 19,* 169–175.

Pew Research Center. (2015). *The smartphone difference.* Retrieved from http://www.pewinternet.org/2015/04/01/us-smartphone-use-in-2015

Sandberg, E. H., Sharma, R., & Sandberg, W. S. (2012). Deficits in retention for verbally presented medical information. *Anesthesiology, 117,* 772–779. doi:10.1097/ALN.0b013e31826a4b02

Sarkar, U., Schillinger, D., López, A., & Sudore, R. (2011). Validation of self-reported health literacy questions among diverse English and Spanish-speaking populations. *Journal of General Internal Medicine, 26,* 265–271. doi:10.1007/s11606-010-1552-1

Serwe, K. M., Hersch, G. I., Pickens, N. D., & Pancheri, K. (2017). Caregiver perceptions of a telehealth wellness program. *American Journal of Occupational Therapy, 71,* 7104350010. doi:10.5014/ajot.2017.025619

Sharry, R., McKenna, K., & Tooth, L. (2002). Occupational therapists' use and perceptions of written client education materials. *American Journal of Occupational Therapy, 56,* 573–576.

Sinclair, P. M., Kable, A., Levett-Jones, T., & Booth, D. (2016). The effectiveness of internet-based e-learning on clinician behavior and patient outcomes: A systematic review. *International Journal of Nursing Studies, 57,* 70–81. doi:10.1016/j.ijnurstu.2016.01.011

Smith, D. L., & Gutman, S. A. (2011). Health literacy in occupational therapy practice and research. *American Journal of Occupational Therapy, 65,* 367–369. doi:10.5014/ajot.2011.002139

Tarita-Nistor, L., Lam, D., Brent, M. H., Steinbach, M. J., & González, E. G. (2013). Courier: A better font for reading with age-related macular degeneration. *Canadian Journal of Ophthalmology, 48,* 56–62. doi:10.1016/j.jcjo.2012.09.017

U.S. Department of Health and Human Services, Office of Disease Prevention and Health Promotion. (2010). *National Action Plan to Improve Health Literacy.* Washington, DC: Author.

van Servellen, G. (2009). *Communication skills for the health care professional: Concepts, practice, and evidence* (2nd ed.). Sudbury, MA: Jones & Bartlett Learning.

Wagner, L., Davis, S., & Handelsman, M. M. (1998). In search of the abominable consent form: The impact of readability and personalization. *Journal of Clinical Psychology, 54,* 115–120.

Watson, E. C., Cosio, D., & Lin, E. H. (2014). Mixed-method approach to veteran satisfaction with pain education. *Journal of Rehabilitation Research and Development, 51,* 503–514. doi:10.1682/JRRD.2013.10.0221

Weiss, B. D. (2007). *Health literacy and patient safety: Help patients understand* (2nd ed.). Chicago, IL: American Medical Association Foundation. Retrieved from http://www.ama-assn.org/ama1/pub/upload/mm/367/healthlitclinicians.pdf

Wilson, E. A., & Wolf, M. S. (2009). Working memory and the design of health materials: A cognitive factors perspective. *Patient Education and Counseling, 74,* 318–322. doi:10.1016/j.pec.2008.11.005

Wilson, L., & Read, J. (2016). Do particular design features assist people with aphasia to comprehend text? An exploratory study. *International Journal of Language & Communication Disorders, 51,* 346–354.

the**Point**®   *For additional resources on the subjects discussed in this chapter, visit* **http://thePoint.lww.com/Willard-Spackman13e**.

Modifying Performance Contexts

Patricia J. Rigby, Barry Trentham, Lori Letts

LEARNING OBJECTIVES

After reading this chapter, you will be able to:

1. Describe why occupational therapists view occupation in context.
2. Analyze how environmental factors contribute to performance context.
3. Describe interventions that can be applied in various contexts across the life course in clients' homes, workplaces, schools, and communities.
4. Critically reflect on how contextual factors may influence your practice as an occupational therapist.
5. Examine the evidence supporting specific environmental intervention approaches.

Introduction: The Role of Environment and Context in Occupational Therapy Practice

Each human lives in a life space that is built on a system of environments. Occupational therapists recognize that environmental factors have an important influence on their clients' engagement in and performance of occupations (American Occupational Therapy Association [AOTA], 2014; Townsend & Polatajko, 2013). The environment features prominently in numerous models of occupational behavior, performance, and engagement (e.g., Dunn, Brown, & McGuigan, 1994; Kielhofner, 2008; Law et al., 1996; Townsend & Polatajko, 2013). These models view environment broadly, and some emphasize the transactional person-environment-occupation (PEO) relationship. Conceptually, the outcome of a congruent PEO relationship or good PEO fit is optimal occupational performance and engagement (Law et al., 1996). When there is less congruence or a poor PEO fit, modifying the environment becomes an important strategy to improve fit and occupational performance and engagement.

Environments, as described in the *International Classification System for Functioning, Disability and Health* (ICF) (World Health Organization [WHO], 2001), can include physical elements (products and technology and natural environment and human-made changes to the environment); social elements (social support and relationships); attitudes (arising from

CENTENNIAL NOTES

Modifying Contexts

Early pioneers in occupational therapy (OT) carefully managed environments to provide patients with the opportunity to have their needs met, develop healthy habits, and endeavor to lead meaningful lives. Environments were seen as important to the therapeutic process (Friedland, 2011; Meyer, 1922). When OT began to "medicalize" from the 1920s to 1960s, the attention was more on the person's disorder than on the treatment context, although there was some attention to the creation of "healthy hospital environments" through the use of color, décor, and social activities to enhance "community spirit" (McColl, Law, & Stewart, 2015).

> One must assess the requirements of the environment, eliminate those impossible to meet, modify others as necessary and possible, and often devise new methods of assistance for the individual patient specifically tailored to him. This assessment of real disability and devising means of living normally again is developing into a specialty within the field of OT in many centers. It is a very important field and is the only one which can give a true picture of the patient-environment relationship by actual trial. (O'Reilly, 1954, p. 79)

In the return to an occupational paradigm in the late 1960s through the 1970s, the narrow focus of the medical model was questioned and the profession was influenced by the Independent Living Movement (McColl et al., 2015). Occupational therapy theorists began to describe how modifying environments can challenge, stimulate, and/or support clients in rehabilitation (e.g., Dunning, 1972; Parent, 1978). Occupational therapy departments in hospitals built replica apartments for assessment and training purposes, in order to prepare patients more realistically for their discharge. Movements to incorporate environment as a key factor in professional models was started in 1980s, continuing through the 1990s. A proliferation of models developed to guide OT practice such as the Model of Human Occupation (Kielhofner & Burke, 1980), followed by others that included the environment as central to assessment and intervention. These included the Ecology of Human Performance Model (Dunn et al., 1994), Person-Environment-Occupation Model (Law et al., 1996), Person-Environment-Occupation-Performance Model (Christiansen & Baum, 1991).

In the 2000s to the present, environmental applications continue to receive attention in the OT literature. Occupational therapists in various contexts have been involved in efforts to promote age-friendly cities, which take into account environmental factors, as a means to promote health and well-being.

---

customs, practices, ideologies, values, norms, and beliefs); and services, systems, and policies. These are described more fully in Box 33-1. The ICF also notes that **context** is the interconnection of personal factors such as gender, race, age, lifestyle, social background, education, occupation, and psychological characteristics with environmental factors (WHO, 2001).

The environment also plays an important role in shaping human experience and behavior over time. A person's values and beliefs are shaped by social and cultural elements of the environment. At the same time, people actively shape and influence the environments in which they live, work, and play. Occupations occur within a context that is unique to each person's circumstances. Consequently, the meaning attached to that occupation and to the place or environment in which the occupation takes place will influence a person's engagement in any given occupation, and this may vary across time. Thus, it is critical that we understand that our clients' occupational experiences cannot be separated from **contextual influences** (AOTA, 2014). In Chapter 22, the meaning of place and space was explored and explained. Those concepts and recommendations for OT practice are critically

important when considering interventions to modify the context for occupational performance and engagement.

Occupational therapists routinely modify environments and access environmental resources, such as assistive technologies (ATs), to support the health, well-being and occupational participation of their clients (AOTA, 2014). These modifications and supports can enhance performance and engagement in occupations, plus the safety and comfort of the client, caregivers, and others. Environmental modifications and resources may also affect others in a setting, not just our clients. Thus, we must consider what is most appropriate for all who use or could use the setting.

Environmental settings can afford people with possibilities for actions, which, depending on an individual's previous and current experiences, can be viewed as opportunities and resources or demands and barriers.

There is a growing body of evidence that demonstrates the efficacy of modifying context to enable occupational performance and engagement. For example, home modifications and ATs for the home, together with caregiver training and education, help improve clients' activities of daily living (ADL), prevent falls, and reduce injuries (Alguren, Lundgren-Nilsson, & Sunnerhagen, 2009; Niva & Skär, 2006;

BOX 33-1 ENVIRONMENT FACTORS OF THE INTERNATIONAL CLASSIFICATION SYSTEM FOR FUNCTIONING, DISABILITY AND HEALTH

1. **Products and technology:** the natural or human-made products or systems of products, equipment, and technology in an individual's immediate environment that are gathered, created, produced, or manufactured. Examples include wheelchairs and speech-generating devices.
2. **Natural environment and human-made changes to environment:** animate and inanimate elements of the natural or physical environment and components of that environment that have been modified by people as well as characteristics of the population in that environment. Examples include sound, temperature, and lighting.
3. **Support and relationships:** people or animals that provide practical physical or emotional support, nurturing, protection and assistance, and relationships to other persons in the home, place of work, school, at play, or in other aspects of their daily activities. Examples include family members, friends, and personal care workers.
4. **Attitudes:** Attitudes are the observable consequences of customs, practices, ideologies, values, norms, factual beliefs, and religious beliefs. The attitudes classified are those of people external to the person whose situation is being described, not of the person himself or herself. Examples include individual attitudes of family and professionals, societal attitudes, and social norms.
5. **Services, systems, and policies:** *Services* comprise structured programs, operations, and services—public, private, or voluntary—established at a local, community, regional, national, or international level by employers, associations, organizations, agencies, or government in order to meet the needs of individuals and includes the persons who provide these services. *Systems* and *policies*, respectively, comprise the administrative control and monitoring mechanisms and rules, regulations, and standards established by local, regional, national, and international government or other recognized authorities, which organize services, programs, and other infrastructural activities in various sectors of society. Examples include availability of and policies for accessible transportation and housing.

Sumathipala, Radcliffe, Sadler, Wolfe, & McKevitt, 2011). Participation in social- and community-based occupations is enabled when environmental barriers are removed (Lysack, Komanecky, Kabel, Cross, & Neufeld, 2007; Papageorgiou, Marquis, Dare, & Batten, 2016). Furthermore, occupational therapists agree that modifying performance contexts can be easier to achieve and have more immediate enabling effects than using interventions that try to "fix the person" (Anaby et al., 2014; Egilson & Traustadottir, 2009; Law, Di Rezze, & Bradley, 2010). Examples of evidence to support modifying specific contexts are provided throughout this chapter and in a special section at the end.

Terminology Use in This Chapter

Throughout this chapter, the term *client* may refer to individuals, groups, organizations, or communities regardless of their health or functional status. Although occupational therapists, for the most part, work with individual clients who live with physical or mental health conditions or disabilities, the authors of this chapter assume that clients may include anyone who experiences barriers to occupational performance or engagement. So, for example, people who are not disabled with respect to activity limitations may indeed still face barriers to occupational participation due to restrictive or discriminatory societal attitudes or life course

occupational transition difficulties and could therefore benefit from the expertise of an occupational therapist.

Human Rights and the Rights to an Inclusive and Accessible Environment

The Universal Declaration of Human Rights (U.S. Department of State, 2008) outlines the rights and freedoms to which all humans are entitled regardless of their status, including race, color, sex, social origins, or other status. In addition, the Convention on the Rights of Persons with Disabilities, the first comprehensive international human rights treaty, was adopted in 2006 (United Nations, 2016). From these, legislation has been developed across the world, bridging the gap from international treaties to state-level, municipal, or organizational policies. They all shape how social groups or individuals are included or not in the public domain.

Antidiscrimination laws have been developed in many jurisdictions to ensure **inclusion** of all minority groups, including peoples of minority ethnic, religious, or sexual identities. Many of these policies were hard-won achievements and, like the American Civil Rights Act of 1964, came at the expense of tremendous committed effort and even the lives of people dedicated to making the world a more socially inclusive place for all people. At an organizational level, companies and public institutions develop employment equity policies that ideally prevent discrimination. These laws and policies serve to ensure that all people have access to housing, work, education, and other publicly and privately funded opportunities. In essence, they enable or disable occupational engagement.

The rights of people with disabilities are typically protected in developed countries through human or civil rights laws. For example, the Americans with Disabilities Act (ADA, 1990) was designed to create equal opportunity and equal access to public environments, services, employment, accommodations, telecommunications, and transportation across the United States. The ADA Amendments Act of 2008 (ADA, 2016) provides a revised definition of "disability" to more broadly encompass impairments that substantially limit a major life activity, such as going to work. The ADA Standards for Accessible Design outline how both public and private sector services, programs, and facilities must comply with and implement accessibility requirements (U.S. Department of Justice, 2010). The focus of the ADA, and of similar legislation in many countries, is to enable people with disabilities to achieve social inclusion and independent living. Chapter 21 provides additional insight about these issues. Occupational therapists should become familiar with the policies and laws that influence marginalized populations and persons with disabilities because this knowledge will affect their practice.

These social policies undergo ongoing revision and development and provide a space for occupational therapists to promote equitable access to occupational engagement for all social groups. Indeed, many leaders in the field have called on occupational therapists as potential leaders themselves to become more involved in building healthy public policy (Kirsh, 2015; Scaffa & Bonder, 2009; Townsend & Polatajko, 2013) within whatever environmental contexts they potentially have influence. In short, to become leaders in society, occupational therapists must go beyond acting as gatekeepers and implementers of existing public policy to becoming active in the development and creation of inclusive social policy.

Framing Interventions to Modify Performance Contexts

Although the ICF is useful in rehabilitation because it classifies environmental factors and illustrates the complex relationship between disability, participation, and environment (WHO, 2001), the authors of this chapter feel it is also useful to view the environment from the perspective of Bronfenbrenner's (2005) Bioecological Model. His model describes the interrelationships between the various levels of environment. Although this model is primarily concerned with human development over time, the manner in which it conceptualizes the dynamic interplay of environmental systems is particularly relevant for OT's focus on occupational engagement and performance.

The model is composed of five systems: the *microsystem, mesosystem, exosystem, macrosystem,* and *chronosystem,* as shown in Figure 33-1. The nested systems interact and fuse with each other. The microsystem is where individuals have the most direct involvement and includes home, neighborhoods, places of worship, or schools. The mesosystem represents the interaction of various microsystems. For example, a child's family relationships in the home environment will impact how he or she performs within the school microsystem. The exosystem is a sphere that people have less involvement with but nevertheless impacts their occupational engagement. For example, government policies that define funding opportunities for ATs impact how an individual functions within any given microsystem. The macrosystem includes the cultural and social structures within which all people live. The values and traditions that guide how people interact with one another are examples of the contextual features of this system. One might consider how the values associated with the culturally dominant Western ways of thinking within a North American context shape shared understandings of the therapeutic process and how these interact with the many diverse cultural contexts within which therapists work. Finally, the chronosystem is concerned with the important element of time and history and how changing contexts over time impact on and interact with the life course transitions of individuals.

Importantly, Bonfrenbrenner's model recognizes that people engage within these environmental systems by taking on changing roles at different times throughout their lives. As well, as noted earlier, occupational therapists interact in different ways across these systems in order to enable the occupational performance of their clients. The case study of Gary Lau in this chapter illustrates how occupational therapists might engage with individuals within the home microsystem to improve physical access while **advocating** at the level of the exosystem for greater access to funding for home renovations and ATs. The case study also shows how both the client's and the therapist's cultural values interact at a macrosystem level, which influences the therapeutic relationship. Importantly, therapists need to be aware of how their own micro, meso, exo, macro, and chronological contexts shape their interactions with their clients. This requires a **reflexive** and critically self-aware stance.

CASE STUDY 33-1 GARY LAU READJUSTING TO HOME LIFE FOLLOWING AN ACQUIRED BRAIN INJURY

Gary Lau is a 52-year-old man who sustained a closed brain injury with diffuse axonal injury as the result of a motor vehicle accident. Before his brain injury, Gary worked full time as a mechanical engineer. He lives with his partner, Dan; they have no children. In the past, he enjoyed participating in social activities with family and friends, community volunteering, playing sports, and many outdoor activities. Gary perceives himself to be very independent, a risk taker, and stubborn at times.

The brain injury resulted in both cognitive and physical impairments. Following 5 months of intensive therapy, Gary was discharged home. Gary has left hemiplegia, decreased balance, and an unsteady gait; he uses a quad cane (a cane with four prongs) for walking. He has no voluntary spontaneous movement in his left hand and cannot grasp things with that hand. In addition to impairments to his short-term memory, he has limitations in his executive function, including difficulty initiating tasks, poor organization, and poor judgment and safety. He demonstrates decreased insight; although aware of his deficits, he does not fully appreciate how his deficits affect his occupational performance. Gary has made appreciable gains in recovery of cognition and physical abilities, and the rehabilitation team expressed confidence that he will recover more by returning to familiar occupations in familiar settings.

Currently, Gary requires assistance with some aspects of self-care. He is independent with dressing, toileting, and grooming (in a seated position). However, he has difficulty with bathtub transfers and needs help to wash his legs, feet, and back. He requires assistance with many housekeeping tasks, including laundry and meal preparation.

When Katya, who works as a home-care occupational therapist, first met Gary and Dan in their 1½ story bungalow home, she had misgivings about whether Gary could manage in a house with four steps at the entrance and a flight of stairs to the master bedroom suite. Her initial private thoughts were that Gary and Dan should move to a fully accessible home, such as a condominium. However, she soon learned that Gary and Dan loved their home and neighborhood and were eager to problem-solve with Katya to make Gary's return to his own home a success.

Katya interviewed Gary together with Dan using the Canadian Occupational Performance Measure (Law et al., 2014). From those results, they identified the following occupational performance goals for Gary: (1) to regain independent mobility within and into his home, (2) to become independent with bathing, (3) to be able to prepare a simple lunch for himself, and (4) to continue volunteering at a local community center.

The first priority for Gary and Dan was accessibility in the home. A ramp was installed at the side entrance to the house and a stair lift was installed to enable Gary to access the second floor. Katya helped access funding for these renovations through Gary's private health insurance.

Katya's initial assessment of the bathroom and the kitchen revealed numerous barriers. Katya then analyzed the accessibility of the bathroom in relation to Gary's occupational performance needs. This analysis led her to recommend several minor modifications using ATs, which included installing a bath transfer bench with a back, plus a clamp-on bar at the side of the tub and a vertical grab bar on the wall beside the tub. She also recommended he use a nonslip bath mat in the tub to reduce his chances of slipping and falling and a handheld shower, which will allow him to control the shower spray and provide him greater independence with bathing.

Gary presents with decreased safety and independence with meal preparation secondary to both cognitive and physical impairments. On assessing the kitchen environment, Katya could see that some physical features were not a good fit for Gary with his current functional limitations. The kitchen in Gary's home is very small and cluttered, and it has very limited counter space. Gary loved to do gourmet cooking and to make meals for his partner and their friends. He has many modern kitchen gadgets and heavy cast iron pots and pans. Katya was sensitive to the pride that Gary had for his cooking and for his kitchenware; thus, while they problem-solved through the occupation of making a meal, she gently educated Gary and Dan about Gary's functional challenges in relation to his safety and need to conserve energy (Table 33-1).

Katya discussed her recommendations for environmental modifications with Gary and Dan. Although Gary's condition might improve, some of the modifications were considered essential for safety. Gary and Dan followed through with the recommended environmental modifications. Katya met with Gary and Dan and trained them both in the safe use of all the modifications in the home. As a result of this environmentally based intervention, Gary has made several advancements in his occupational performance. Gary has greater independence and improved safety with bathing and can independently prepare a simple meal. He is less reliant on Dan to help him with these activities. Gary reports improved satisfaction and performance scores on the Canadian Occupational Performance Measure, although his personal abilities (cognition, strength, and range of motion) have not changed during this intervention. Gary and Dan are pleased with his increased independence and have expressed their appreciation for the extra time they now have to spend on leisure activities rather than on self-care.

CASE STUDY 33-1	GARY LAU READJUSTING TO HOME LIFE FOLLOWING AN ACQUIRED BRAIN INJURY *(continued)*

TABLE 33-1	Modifications to Gary Lau's Kitchen to Address the Occupational Performance Goal of Preparing a Simple Meal

Occupational Performance	Intervention Recommendations	Rationale for Intervention
Meal preparation • Mobility: Gary is ambulating around the kitchen with a quad cane, and he has impaired left hand function. He finds it difficult to transfer heavier items such as foods and plates.	• Recommend that Gary use a four-wheeled walker (rollator) with a tray/basket or a tea trolley. • Consider purchasing lightweight pots, pans, and plates.	• Enable him to independently and safely transfer items to and from counter, stove, and refrigerator to the table. • Enable him to safely lift and use items while conserving energy.
• Cupboards are installed high on walls, with dishes stored on the top shelves. Gary's ability to engage in overhead reaching is limited by poor balance and impaired fine and gross motor coordination.	• Lower the height of the cupboards. • Relocate items in the cupboards so the items that are most frequently used are in easy-to-reach places. • A long-handled reacher can be used for overhead reaching of light items.	• Allow Gary to have easy access and promote safe reaching. • Avoid unnecessary bending and reaching. • Reduce risk of falls due to overreaching (which can contribute to loss of balance).
• Deficits in short-term memory and executive function • Gary sometimes forgets and needs to be reminded to turn off the stove.	• Place written sign above stove that reads "TURN OFF STOVE." • Use a timer for reminder; when the timer sounds, that acts as a cue to turn off the stove. • When preparing a meal while home alone, prepare something that does not require use of the stove.	• Use compensatory strategies to enhance independence and safety.
• Deficits in short-term memory and executive function	• Group ingredients, tools, and items that Gary uses most frequently together in one area (in cupboard, in the refrigerator). • Label drawers and cupboards so that Gary knows exactly where to look to retrieve the cooking utensils and ingredients that he needs. • Gary and Dan could generate step-by-step instructions for commonly prepared items and place these in clear plastic jackets so that Gary can use an erasable marker to tick off steps as they are completed.	• Compensates for short-term memory deficits and increases independence

Interventions

When the assessment process is complete, interventions focusing on the client's identified targeted occupational goals are developed using a systematic approach such as the Occupational Therapy Practice Framework (AOTA, 2014) or the Canadian Practice Process Framework (Craik, Davis, & Polatajko, 2013). The goal of enabling occupational performance and engagement guides the development of the intervention plan.

In this section, we first present design approaches and technologies that support occupational performance and engagement and then describe various intervention strategies for the home, school, workplace, and community settings. Some interventions can be applied at the microsystem and

mesosystem level with individual clients, and others can be applied at the broader exosystem and macrosystem levels with groups and communities or at a societal level. Those interventions applied at the microsystem and mesosystem levels are typically client-centered and take into account the clients' specific needs and their situations, whereas interventions from the group or population perspective should be based on knowledge of the common and diverse challenges, expectations, and/or needs of that population (Iwarsson & Ståhl, 2003).

Interventions directed at modifying physical context involve making architectural changes to places and spaces and the provision of ATs. Modifying the social context can involve developing and mobilizing social resources, plus training and educating these resources about how best to support the occupational performance and engagement of

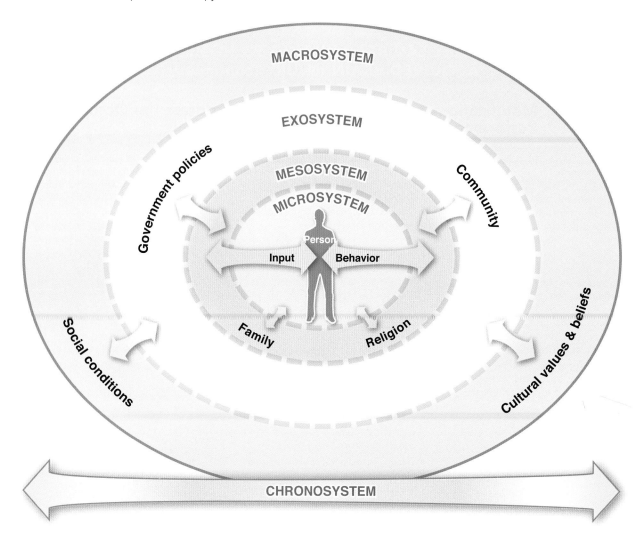

FIGURE 33-1 The dynamic interplay between levels of the environment as demonstrated by Bronfenbrenner's Bioecological Model.

our clients. Modifying social and cultural context can involve advocacy, consultation, education, and policy development at the mesosystem, macrosystem, and exosystem to broaden awareness, change attitudes and views, and support programs and services for our clients. Occupational therapists typically employ several of these strategies in concert. Throughout this chapter, examples from the case study of Gary Lau are used to illustrate various strategies for modifying the performance context, including those that use several strategies in concert.

Design Strategies and Technologies to Support Occupational Performance

Universal Design

Universal design (UD) is a way to create products and environments that are more usable by everyone, regardless of

age or ability (Steinfeld & Maisel, 2012). Universal design involves thinking about a range of human abilities before the environment is built. The seven principles of UD developed by the Center for Universal Design (2002) integrate accessibility and usability features in design. Today, UD is considered across most settings, including housing, office buildings, airports, restaurants, and parks. It recognizes human differences in shapes, sizes, ages, abilities, and cultures and promotes inclusion and ergonomic design for all people. For example, the level entrance and power sliding doors at the entrance to a grocery store makes the store accessible to everyone. In this case, the entrance design accommodates people who are pushing the grocery carts, those moving large objects on a cart as well as those using wheelchairs or mobility devices.

Accessible Design

Accessible design, also referred to as *barrier-free design*, adds accessibility to otherwise inaccessible buildings, products, and services to enable persons with disabilities to function independently (Iwarsson & Ståhl, 2003). For example, braille can be added to elevator keypads to enable persons with visual impairments to select the floor number they want. Often, accessible design responds to specific requirements and standards as laid out in legislation, such as the ADA and in building codes. It can be applied to make buildings, products, and services accessible to special populations. Accessible design can also be applied at the microsystem level with changes made to specific aspect of the environment in the home, school, or workplace to achieve PEO fit for individual clients. Occupational therapists routinely apply their knowledge about accessible design in their daily practice. The home modifications such as the ramp added to Gary's home in the case study exemplify accessible design.

Assistive Technologies

Assistive technologies are devices, adaptive equipment, or products that are designed to enable persons with disabilities to engage in daily occupations within their homes, schools, workplaces, and communities (Cook & Polgar, 2015). They fall into the products and technology category within the environmental factors domain of the ICF (WHO, 2001). As will be shown throughout this chapter, ATs are routinely prescribed by occupational therapists to address specific occupational performance goals of their clients, including those for ADL, mobility, and communication. These technologies range from simple devices such as grab bars and raised toilet seats to more complex devices such as powered wheelchairs and speech-generating devices (Figure 33-2).

Assistive technologies have undergone dramatic innovation over the past 30 years, and the availability and quality of the technologies have greatly improved (Cook & Polgar, 2015). Assistive technologies are widely used by persons with disabilities. There is growing evidence that ATs can improve occupational performance (e.g., Agree, 2014; Mitzner et al., 2010; Rigby, Ryan, & Campbell, 2009), enhance quality of life (e.g., Agree, 2014; Rigby, Ryan, & Campbell, 2011), and reduce caregiver burden (e.g., Marasinghe, 2016; Mortenson et al., 2012). In many jurisdictions, funding for ATs is provided by the state and/or charitable organizations. Occupational therapists assist their clients to obtain this funding.

Smart Technologies

Computers and smart technologies are transforming how people live and perform their daily occupations. Smartphones and mobile computers are rapidly developing and many have been developed using UD principles, making them very user-friendly and accessible. For example,

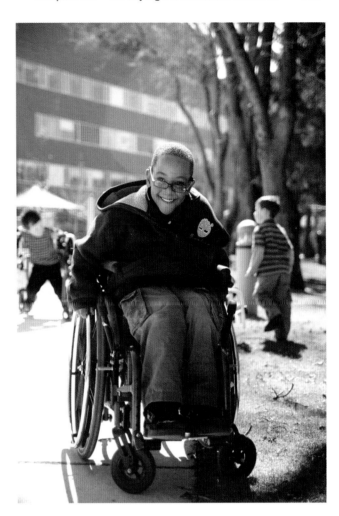

FIGURE 33-2 **Wheelchairs are a commonly used assistive technology for mobility and enable participation in daily life.**

many have easy to use and see LCD touch screens, enlarged keyboards, and menu-driven software. It is common to see many people, from children through older adults, using smartphones, computer tablets, and laptop computers in public spaces. Occupational therapists find many features and new applications made for these technologies helpful for enabling their clients' occupational performance. For example, persons with memory impairments can use the schedule reminder on their smartphone to organize their day, and persons with motor impairments can use voice commands to operate their phone.

Smart home technologies enable persons with physical, sensory, and/or cognitive disabilities to live in their own home, and older adults to age in place. They consist of electronic sensors and actuators used in the home to allow individuals to achieve greater independence and safety within their home and reduce the need for caregiver assistance. They can be used to monitor health wellness, emergency detection and response, and to prompt behaviors, such as steps to completing ADL. The development of this technology is rapidly evolving and there is growing evidence of its efficacy (Liu, Stroulia, Nikolaidis, Miguel-Cruz, & Rios Rincon, 2016).

Web-Based Technologies

Web-based technologies are rapidly changing and have changed the structure of communities (Figure 33-3). We are now a networked society in which we have multiple links to various work, community, and friendship networks. Social support, as experienced through online communities, has been shown to have correlates with ratings on mental health and well-being, life satisfaction, engagement in social activities, and sense of community (Aguilar, Boerema, & Harrison, 2010; Erickson & Johnson, 2011; Sum, Mathews, Pourghasem, & Hughes, 2009). Networked communities have been shown to support community development (CD) initiatives where neighborhood and interest group linkages have enabled groups to collectively advocate for shared interests and lobby companies or government officials for proposed changes (Hampton & Wellman, 2003).

Disabled and isolated persons stand to benefit in particular from online community engagement because they are no longer limited by physical access barriers, geographic distances, or perhaps discriminatory attitudes that disrupt information sharing. Enabling online participation is now an important consideration for occupational therapists. Much has been written about the potential barriers faced by people living with disabilities as well as the unique design features that should be considered when developing accessible Web spaces and online community formats (e.g., Trentham, Sokoloff, Tsang, & Neysmith, 2015).

Occupational therapists can play a vital role in assisting their clients to access and learn how to use these

various technologies in their daily lives. It is important that occupational therapists stay abreast of new developments and be open to their potential for enabling occupation.

Modifying the Home Environment

Home is the context for a broad range of occupations, from basic ADL like bathing to social events and celebrations with family. Home is a multidimensional concept, which includes a physical space within a geographic location but has emotional, cultural, and personal elements (Mitty & Flores, 2009). Home is frequently one of the most cherished environments in people's lives, and people make meaning out of their life events through their homes (Cristoforetti, Gennai, & Rodeschini, 2011). The home has been described as having three elements: physical, social, and personal (Tanner, Tilse, & de Jonge, 2008). The implications of modifications to a physical aspect of a home should be considered in light of these other elements. For example, what may be viewed as clutter to a therapist concerned about falls prevention could be seen as a threat to personal self-expression by an older adult with many important possessions. Similarly, bathroom modifications such as grab bars and a raised toilet seat to promote independent toileting for a client might be viewed negatively by the client if the bathroom is the main one that visitors would use. Chapter 22 provides more information on the meaning of place and space in daily life.

Often, the primary goal of clients in an inpatient setting is to go home; the goal of older adults with chronic conditions is to be able to stay home (American Association of Retired Persons, 2000). However, even if the living location needs to change when a person's health or social situation requires support in a congregate living environment, that new home can be given meaning with personal objects (Cipriani et al., 2009) and ideas associated with living in age-supportive environments that can be adjusted to adapt to need (Vasara, 2015).

Beyond considering the home as a physical space and the need for modifications of the physical environment within clients' homes, therapists need to be attentive to the nature of home as a social sphere, which might also be modified to support clients' return to or remaining home. **Social supports** at home can sometimes be implemented as an environmental intervention that can overcome physical barriers associated with the home environment. The elements of the social and personal meanings of home may help therapists and others understand the importance of home beyond its physical layout and features. This is illustrated in the case study of Gary Lau.

When dealing with clients' homes, several intervention strategies can be considered in the environment to maximize the person's ability to engage in his or her

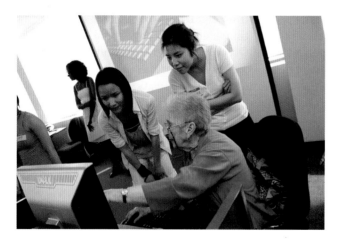

FIGURE 33-3 Occupational therapy students collaborating with an older adult on the use of Web-based, social media.

occupations. These can range from building a new home following a catastrophic injury to making minor changes to the living space like rearranging furniture. Modifications can also incorporate formal or informal supports, ranging from personal care workers to help with bathing to family assistance with meal preparations.

Occupational therapists should also keep in mind that any modifications to different types of homes, whether they are situated in suburban neighborhoods, urban apartments or condominiums, or within congregate living arrangements such as group homes or retirement homes, are contingent on different regulations and processes. Prior to making recommendations, therapists should inform themselves of the various policy and legal considerations and guidelines that apply to the various housing types. In addition, therapists must be aware of how home modifications will impact other residents. This is particularly an issue when working in congregate living settings.

Ideal Features of an Accessible Home

For people requiring accessible housing, ideal features vary depending on their needs. Most frequently, accessible housing is sought when people have issues related to mobility, requiring use of a mobility device such as a walker or manual or power wheelchair. Box 33-2 includes a number of the key features that can make a home accessible for someone with mobility impairments.

Assistive technologies can be incorporated to improve accessibility. For example, electronic aids to daily living, which enable a person to electronically control the physical environment, can be installed (e.g., for locking and unlocking entrances, opening and closing blinds, and manipulating home electronics such as the television). As smart home technologies have become more common, many of these ATs are broadly available.

Occupational therapists may provide consultation to clients if accessible housing is being sought or built. This may occur following an acquired disability resulting from an incident causing spinal cord injury or acquired brain injury. In these situations, it is important to work with the client and family to identify the most important accessibility features required.

Major Home Modifications

Not all clients are able to find accessible housing. Other clients are reluctant to move away from their family home. Both of these situations may result in a need to consider modifying the physical environment of the home in which the client is currently residing. The two most common areas of the home that require modifications are the entrance to the home and bathrooms.

Entrances are most frequently modified with the installation of either ramps or porch lifts. A major consideration in recommending these relates to the height from the ground level to the entrance. Because a ramp requires a minimum of 12 in of length for each inch of rise, there are occasions when a ramp is simply not feasible. When they are possible, a front or side door is typically designated for access.

In circumstances when the height from the ground to the entrance is too high to make a ramp feasible, the most common alternative used is a porch lift. In addition, some clients are unwilling to install a ramp because of concerns related to aesthetics, and they choose a lift because it can be more discreetly installed. Some considerations in the selection of lifts include back-up electrical or manual systems in case of power failures and a need to consider the climate in which the home is located. Ideally, there will be more than one entrance/exit accessible to the client so that in case of an emergency such as a fire, at least one exit is available. If there is only one accessible entrance, escape plans in case of emergencies are advised. In the case study of Gary Lau, the occupational therapist helped Gary and his partner consider the various options for making the entrance to his home accessible, and in his case, a ramp to the side entrance to his home was considered the best solution.

Bathrooms often require major modifications because they are typically small, making mobility within the space challenging. In addition, transferring to and from a toilet and bath/shower can present challenges. Although minor modifications such as grab bars and handheld showers might be adequate in some circumstances, other clients require major modifications in the bathroom. These can

---

BOX 33-2 PHYSICAL FEATURES OF AN ACCESSIBLE HOME

- Exterior walkway smooth and graded
- Level entrance
- Lever handles on all doors
- Inside doorway widths sufficient for mobility device
- Adequate turning space in bathrooms/entry
- Access to home systems (e.g., electrical panel, furnace)
- Ample lighting
- Cabinet heights in kitchen and bathroom allow seated access.
- Furniture arrangements allow mobility.
- Floor surface levels allow mobility.
- Structural supports for equipment such as ceiling tracks
- Access to environmental controls (e.g., light switches) and appliances
- Emergency exit available

range from moving or removing fixtures to installation of new fixtures such as roll-in shower stalls, higher toilets, and sink and tap fixtures that can be readily managed.

Because major modifications at the entrance and bathroom are costly, it is important for the therapist to work closely with the client and family to consider current as well as possible future needs.

Minor Home Modifications

Major modifications to the physical environment of a client's home are not always required. There are many times when minor modifications provide solutions to challenges experienced in the home. Assistive technologies such as a bath bench and handheld shower for someone who is unable to enter and stand for a shower is a common minor modification that occupational therapists provide. Therapists also recommend off-the-shelf products that support performance such as adding a handrail to the wall or stairs to the basement or an automatic shut-off kettle for someone with early cognitive decline.

Occupational therapists can also suggest that clients modify the way they use the physical environment. For example, they can teach individuals to make use of features of their existing environment in ways that make it safer or easier to perform daily activities. This may mean rearranging items in kitchen cupboards, organizing items in a basket to be carried up and down stairs, or programming the telephone to make use of autodial functions to make it easy for someone with memory issues to contact family.

Supports from others are often also important to consider. Sometimes, help from others can make it possible for someone to remain in his or her home environment. For example, having a neighbor collect mail from a community mailbox can not only overcome challenges with outdoor mobility but also provide a social connection for an older adult living alone. Having a personal support worker assist with bathing can be an alternative to installing assistive devices.

Considerations to Implementing Home Modifications

By focusing on the goals of the client, the therapist can generate several possible environmental strategies that can be implemented. There is often more than one environmental solution available to address an occupational issue. For example, in the case study for Gary Lau, modifications to the bathroom could be avoided if Gary were to receive personal assistance for transfers in and out of the bathtub and bathing (either from Gary's partner Dan or from a paid support worker). Another strategy would be to make major modifications to Gary and Dan's bathroom to replace the traditional tub and shower space with a walk-in shower with a modular seat. In the end, the occupational therapist, Gary, and Dan chose to use a combination of minor modifications (grab bars) and simple off-the-shelf products (bath mat, hand held shower). It is important to review with a client the range of environmental modifications that might address his or her goals and work together to consider current and future needs, the needs of others living in or using the home environment, costs, and complexity of each modification in order to support the client to choose the solution that is optimal.

Funding of home modifications is an important factor and can sometimes present a barrier to implementation of the optimal solution. Renovations can be expensive, and, depending on the client's circumstances, insurance companies may not provide financial supports. People often rely on personal resources or social service agencies to fund the modifications. Occupational therapists should be familiar with their local social service agencies that provide for such modifications and may need to work collaboratively with the client to apply for funding supports. Occupational therapists have an important duty to help justify the need for home modifications to payers (whether insurers, social service agencies, or other funding bodies). Although home renovations are costly, paid support workers are also expensive. Justification for modifications to the physical environment may in part be that the increased independence of the client will decrease costs associated with paid support workers.

A final consideration related to home modifications is the relationship between the various parties involved in any renovations. Although occupational therapists may recommend major or minor modifications to the physical environment, the implementation of any modifications is completed by others and should be overseen by the client or family. The AT vendor or a skilled family member can sometimes do minor modifications, such as installing grab bars. Major modifications or home renovations involve a complex team that might include an architect, contractor, trades people, AT vendors, or even builders in the case of a new home. However, occupational therapists can advise clients on strategies to consult and collaborate with all parties to oversee modifications to the home environment.

Modifying the School Context

Occupational therapists play a critical role in enabling students with various conditions and disabilities to succeed in school settings and to participate in classroom, playground, and extracurricular activities (Anaby et al., 2014; AOTA, 2011). Researchers describe how various environmental factors can help or hinder students' participation in school-based occupations and urge occupational therapists to modify school contexts to support students at school (Anaby et al., 2014; Egilson, 2014; Egilson & Traustadottir, 2009; Kennedy-Behr, Rodger, Graham, & Mickan, 2013). Examples provided subsequently demonstrate how therapists can modify the school context from the microsystem through exosystem levels. Further information about school-based practice is provided in Chapter 51.

Although it is now common to find legislation and policies that support the inclusion of students with *disabling* conditions in their local schools, inclusion can be challenging to achieve due to many environmental obstacles. Physical barriers, such as heavy doors, raised thresholds at doors, and absence of elevators in multilevel schools are still common. School culture and attitudes of teachers and classmates can also create barriers to inclusion. For example, a teacher may misunderstand the classroom behaviors and performance of a student with a learning disability and react in a manner that exacerbates the student's distress, and classmates might make fun of and exclude this same student. The participation and inclusion of students with disabilities cannot succeed until adequate resources and supports are put into place to address these barriers.

Modifying the performance context in schools can take many forms. The most common approach is to modify the physical environment by modifying and adapting furniture and educational materials, accessing ATs, and making architectural modifications to schools. Occupational therapists also use strategies to modify the social, cultural, and organizational environments of schools to support students' inclusion and participation. Examples include sensitivity education for school staff and students, advocating for social supports in the classroom (e.g., teaching assistants or peer mentors), collaborating with teachers to modify and adapt curricula to support students' learning, and coaching teachers to use specific teaching strategies tailored for individual students.

Modifications to the physical environment can happen at the microsystem level for individual students and at the exosystem level to make schools accessible for persons with disabilities. For example, therapists can consult about and advocate for architectural accessibility and the use of UD principles within schools. They can also consult with individual schools or school boards to prepare annual accessibility plans or to assist in the design and planning of new schools and planning for major renovations to make schools more accessible. Examples of specific modifications using ATs can include installing electronic door openers, lever-style taps at sinks, and grab bars in the toilet stall.

Classroom environments can have high levels of sensory stimuli in terms of noise, visual clutter, and the physical activity of a classroom full of students, which can have a disorganizing effect for children with sensory-processing problems. Occupational therapists assess the classroom environment to identify the sensory features that either facilitate or hinder students' ability to complete schoolwork and recommend modifying the space to better fit students' sensory-processing needs. For example, sound-absorbing partitions and low lighting can enable some students to focus their attention while working on individual assignments. The therapist might recommend setting up a quiet space in the classroom where a student with autism can use a rocking chair to seek calming sensory input and put on a headset to listen to music or a taped story.

The occupational therapist should become familiar with the conditions and terms for funding environmental modifications and special or adapted furniture and ATs for schools. Some environmental modifications can be made at little expense, whereas others will be costly and involve applying to the school board or a government agency for special funding.

Modifying the Workplace

For many people, the ability to work is a primary occupational goal. However, the workplace can contribute to illness and injury and can pose barriers to those with various chronic conditions and disabilities who wish to enter the workforce or return to work. The scope for OT in the workplace is broad; the focus can be on health promotion and wellness, injury prevention, or return to work. All of these areas involve making modifications to the work environment and can range from microsystem to exosystem levels and address physical, social, and attitudinal factors. The role of the occupational therapist in the workplace is explored in detail in Chapter 52. This chapter focuses on modifications to the workplace to enable individuals with occupational performance challenges to enter or return to work and successfully perform their jobs.

The ADA and similar human rights legislation in many countries support the individual's right to work by prohibiting discrimination against people with disabilities. In the United States, when people with disabilities can perform the essential functions of a job with accommodations, they are allowed to apply for and maintain a job. Under the ADA Section 101, an employer is responsible for providing the reasonable accommodations necessary for a qualified individual to perform the job. The ADA, in relation to work, is described more fully in Chapter 52.

When workplace accommodations are necessary, the occupational therapist can lead a team to identify the environmental resources and barriers that influence an employee's ability to work and help to access resources and/or remove these barriers. In addition to the occupational therapist, the team members typically include the employer, key employees, and the group that is responsible for implementing the environmental modifications. There is a growing body of evidence for the efficacy of workplace accommodations and modifications, but more research is needed to develop best practices (McDowell & Fossey, 2015; Nevala, Pehkonen, Koskela,

BOX 33-3   EXAMPLES OF JOB ACCOMMODATIONS FOR SPECIFIC WORK CHALLENGES

Work Performance Challenge: Gripping or Pinching Tools or Objects

People who have physical limitations that result in difficulty gripping or pinching objects. Accommodations may involve the office, industrial, service, and medical industries and can extend to personal needs. Options for the office include the following:

- Providing alternative telephone access: auto-dialers, gooseneck telephone holders, hands-free telephones, and computer-telephone integration
- Offering filing modifications such as modified filing trays, Lazy-Susan carousels, and automated filing systems
- Providing grip aids such as reachers and door knob grips
- Providing page turners and book holders

Work Performance Challenge: Working at Full Production

People may have physical limitations that result in difficulty working at full production levels. Accommodations may include the following:

- Reducing or eliminating physical exertion and workplace stress
- Scheduling periodic rest breaks away from the workstation
- Implementing ergonomic workstation design with ergonomic equipment (e.g., copy holders, electric hole punches, electric stapler, foot rests, forearm supports, headsets, etc.)
- Providing adjustable/ergonomic chairs or stand/lean stools
- Providing compact lifting devices
- Providing anti-fatigue matting and anti-vibration materials
- Providing a scooter or other mobility aid if walking cannot be reduced

Ruusuvuori, & Anttila, 2015; Padkapayeva et al., 2017). The Job Accommodation Network (n.d.) Website (see http://askjan.org/) provides an excellent resource for therapists, employers, and employees with disabilities to identify possible workplace modifications in relation to specific work performance challenges. Examples are provided in Box 33-3. Architectural changes to the environment, such as installing electronic door openers and modifying a bathroom, can make the workplace accessible for employees and others who use mobility aids such as a wheelchair. Assistive technologies are commonly prescribed, particularly for workers with motor weakness and/or impairments like Gary Lau in our case study. For example, because Gary has hemiplegia and is not able to use his left hand functionally, he can be enabled to use a computer with a one-handed keyboard with a reduced number of keys to depress when typing and/or speech recognition software that enters data to the computer via voice command. The social, cultural, and organizational aspects of the workplace can also be modified to support and enable workers to perform their job. For example, in order to accommodate Gary's cognitive impairments with organizational skills and short-term memory, his employer could assign him a peer mentor to assist Gary to break down daily tasks into achievable steps, create daily to-do lists, and provide him with daily guidance. His employer could also provide sensitivity training to coworkers.

Changing the physical environment can be expensive and complicated to implement. Under the ADA, workers are permitted "reasonable accommodations" as long

as these do not cause "undue hardship" to the employer. A small company that has a very small profit margin might not be required to pay for an elevator if it would cause the company bankruptcy, but the employer might be required to move the office of an employee with a mobility impairment to the first floor if space was available. The outcome of the job accommodation should be evaluated, and the continued success of the accommodations should be monitored over time to ensure the best worker-job-environment fit.

Modifying Community Contexts

The exosystem level of the environment contains spaces in which most people visit on a less frequent basis than the work or home environment. Examples include government agencies, cultural venues, shopping complexes, and stores. Although people often spend less time in these spaces, they serve as links between more private spaces such as work and home, and they contain critical goods and services necessary for successful participation in community life. Community contexts are important for socialization, recreation, and civic and social engagement. Socially exclusive environments with poor accessibility can negatively affect the community participation of people with disabilities and other marginalized groups.

Communities are important venues for social and physical change interventions. Communities can be fostered, developed, enabled, built, enhanced, created, or organized with the aim to enhance the wellness of their members. Scaffa and Bonder (2009) view wellness as distinct from health and use Gallup's (1999) definition of wellness as an individual's perception of physical and psychological well-being characterized by adequate physical capacity for accomplishment of desired activities, coupled with overall satisfaction with one's life situation. With this in mind, in the case example of Gary Lau, the

occupational therapist saw it as her role to influence both the *social structures* and physical access concerns of Gary's community center (see Case Study 33-2). The concepts of **community**, **community participation**, and **community development** are outlined subsequently and provide a basis from which therapists can bring about social and physical change.

CASE STUDY 33-2   GARY LAU AND COMMUNITY REINTEGRATION

Once the home-based physical accessibility issues were worked out, Katya met further with Gary to discuss his interest in reengaging with his local community. She spent time exploring his past leisure interests using the Occupational Performance History Interview-Second Version (OPHI-II) (Kielhofner et al., 2004), his values, culture, and spirituality. It became clear that volunteering is consistent with his past interests and the importance he and his partner place on being part of a community. Although neither Gary nor his partner identified with any religious community, it became clear that the values and traditions they now hold were influenced by their parents' Buddhist cultural roots (Gary is a third-generation American) as well as mainstream American values related to being neighborly and helping others out.

Once Gary and Katya identified a number of possible volunteering roles, she accompanied him to a local community center to assess any accessibility issues that he might experience. She suggested that Gary call the center prior to their visit to inquire about accessibility. They were assured that the center was fully accessible. Once there, an enthusiastic volunteer coordinator greeted them and quickly outlined the various volunteer opportunities available. Throughout the interview, the coordinator directed her comments and responses to Katya even when Gary asked the question. Katya noticed this and attempted on several occasions to redirect the coordinator's attention to Gary. At some point, Gary asked to use the toilet. Returning some time later, he pointed out to Katya that he had difficulty getting up from the toilet as there were no grab bars. Katya asked the coordinator if anything could be done to improve the accessibility of the bathrooms. The coordinator replied politely that she would check into it but that the center was not designed for crippled or mentally retarded people and that perhaps they should seek out other community programs.

Katya tactfully informed the coordinator that Gary did not label himself as crippled nor mentally retarded and that they were under the impression that public spaces such as this were to be fully accessible under the ADA guidelines. She asked if there was someone at the center whom she could talk to about accessibility and accommodation options. The coordinator gave her a name and number and encouraged her to call. Although it was clear that there were a number of opportunities available at the center that Gary was interested

in and could likely manage, both he and Katya were turned off by the polite brush-off that they felt from the coordinator.

Afterward, Katya discussed with Gary and his partner their interest in pursuing volunteer opportunities at this location. She offered to follow up with the contact given to her by the coordinator and to see what could be done regarding the center's approach to social inclusion of people with disabilities. They were both agreeable to this plan.

Katya was also aware of several other clients who lived in this area who could benefit from the opportunities available at this center. She was, however, reluctant to suggest this center given her experience. In keeping with Katya's knowledge and appreciation for the OT role in advocating for socially inclusive environments, Katya recognized the importance of doing something about the center's social barriers to people with disabilities. She considered how she might go about dealing with that at a broader level.

Fortunately, a component of Katya's position allowed her to work with community agencies on issues related to disability and inclusion. She set up a meeting with the community agency's executive director and identified her concerns about the attitudes conveyed by some of the staff regarding accessibility issues at the center. She informed the director that there were several people she worked with who, although living with some type of disability, would benefit from their participation in the community center if it were accessible not only in terms of the physical requirements but also the social attitudes conveyed by the staff. Katya offered her support to work with the center to develop this and suggested starting with an accessibility and social inclusion audit of the various programs at the center. Katya agreed also to provide education on relevant legislation and policies that organizations such as this one must adhere to. Katya had experience with working with design teams and running stakeholder focus groups for other community organizations. She emphasized the importance of including people living with disabilities on the design team and also as part of relevant focus groups. She suggested including several of her clients to assist in the development of education sessions aimed at informing the community center staff around issues of stigma and accessibility. Dilemmas faced by occupational therapists within the social environment are presented in the "Practice Dilemma" box.

Addressing Diversity Issues

Gary Lau's narrative presents several key dilemmas that occupational therapists may be faced with, particularly with respect to interventions aimed at the social environment.

As a social resource herself, Katya, the occupational therapist, can be considered a part of Gary's social environment. The ethnocultural values and social attitudes that she brings to Gary's situation can influence how she works with him and could determine how effective she will be in enabling his preferred occupations. The degree to which the therapist is aware of her own cultural values and attitudes and how they shape her therapeutic interactions will be of primary importance. Beyond her own self-awareness of the cross-cultural nature of this particular therapeutic relationship, her awareness of the social resources available to Gary and his partner will be crucial. Social attitudinal barriers and discrimination faced by many gay or lesbian people have been well documented (de Vries, 2015; Hammack & Cohler, 2009; Kirsh, Trentham, & Cole, 2006), and, as relevant for this case, the intersections between experiences of ageism and heterosexism impacts on their use of mainstream services. How open will Gary be to participating in any community organizations that might present such barriers? Similarly, a lack of knowledge about lesbian, gay, bisexual, and transgender (LGBT) culture, communities, and social and recreational resources limits the effectiveness of the therapist in supporting Gary's efforts to reintegrate into the community. A similar scenario can be imagined for any client who identifies with a culture, religion, or community that is different from that of the therapist. How well informed is the therapist to respond to these types of cross-cultural interactions?

Questions

1. Consider a situation where your cultural or religious values conflict with those of your client. How might you reconcile your need to enable the occupations of choice of your client while being true to your own values?
2. To what extent do you feel occupational therapists are obliged to become familiar with the cultural practices and health and social resources of their clients?
3. How might the therapist in this situation navigate the cross-cultural interaction?

The concept of community is often linked to ideas about human connection, social cohesiveness, or support. Less discussed are the less positive aspects of community that can also be associated with exclusivity as illustrated, for example, in the commonly used acronym NIMBYism (not in my backyard). As a result, communities can as often keep people out as to bring people together. Communities can offer opportunities for occupational engagement through the manner in which occupational roles are created, delegated, acknowledged, and made accessible. They can as likely create barriers to occupational engagement by creating inaccessible physical environments or by fostering discriminatory and stigmatizing social attitudes that alienate, segregate, and limit the participation of particular groups including people living with disabilities. At its most basic, however, community can refer to people living within a particular geographic area who share common services and/or to a group of people who simply share a common identity, for example, older people with disabilities.

In summary, despite the potential restrictive and constraining aspects of community, ideally, community can be a space where the unique value of each person can develop and through which individual needs for integration, participation, and relationship with others is realized. The view that communities serve as a forum for shared identity development, social occupational participation, and expression reflects a desire to understand community as a context for occupational role development and enablement. How then do occupational therapists enable community participation?

Enabling Community Participation

In this chapter, *participation* refers to active participation of individuals who both benefit and contribute to the community through their actions, ideas, knowledge, or skills. Community participation is about relating to others, to be in some sort of relationship with them. Communities or, at the very least, a sense of community can be fostered by the social spaces that occupational therapists work within, such as congregate living environments or neighborhoods. So, how then can communities be developed and how can occupational therapists be involved?

Community Development

Hoffman and Duponte (1992) state, "community development is about . . . helping people to develop the skills they need, and removing the structural barriers that prevent them from achieving their full potential as members of the community" (p. 21). Community development strategies aim to create supportive environments and strengthen the capacity of communities to respond to health problems (WHO, 1986).

Rothman and Tropman's (1987) classic taxonomy of three CD approaches can be helpful for occupational therapists considering this type of work. A *locality development* approach views the change process as involving many people, most often within one geographic community, in determining goals and action. Emphasis is placed on process components and on strengthening the connections among community members. Neighborhood safety committees use this approach. *Social planning* uses a top-down process where a governing body typically defines issues and solutions. Finally, *social action* demands a critical social analysis based on class, gender, ability, and race to create change and views problems as rooted within inequitable power structures (Alinsky, 1971); thus, efforts are directed at changing power structures. Building on Rothman and Tropman's taxonomy, occupational therapists Lauckner, Krupa, and Paterson (2011) further conceptualized the link between OT and community development. Their work emphasizes the role of the occupational therapist to enable "power sharing between sectors to create opportunities for meaningful engagement with(in) communities." (p. 267). Similarly, Leclair (2010) challenges occupational therapists to go beyond individualist assumptions within OT theory and to consider the notion of shared occupations as a helpful construct in work aimed at community change.

Social action approaches share many assumptions with what occupational therapists and occupational scientists referred to as *occupational justice*. Its growing discourse (Leclair, Ashcroft, Canning, & Lisowski, 2016; Stadnyk, Townsend, & Wilcock, 2010; Townsend & Polatajko, 2013) highlights the need for practitioners to become aware of the impacts of occupational injustice as experienced through occupational alienation, occupational marginalization, occupational imbalance (Stadnyk et al., 2010), or occupational deprivation (Whiteford, 2005). From this perspective, individuals and groups (e.g., cultural minorities) may be alienated from meaningful occupations and roles, prevented from access to decision making, may be over- or underemployed, or may be deprived of opportunities for meaningful occupational engagement. Chapter 45 is devoted to exploring occupational justice.

In one particularly illustrative example of CD strategies, occupational therapists working at a community health center in Canada articulated their role within an occupational approach (Trentham, Cockburn, & Shin, 2007). In response to a community needs survey that identified physical inaccessibility and social isolation of older adults, they invited older adults and others living with disabilities as members of an urban neighborhood to help create a more physically accessible and socially supportive neighborhood. Facilitated activities helped the participants envision the possibilities for a "senior-friendly" neighborhood.

The group began with achievable, less complex projects because the successful completion of smaller projects could help build the confidence of the working group while making meaningful change. The provision of optimal structure, group facilitation techniques, shared storytelling, active listening, and environmental adaptations helped to develop a more supportive and accessible community. Examples of the group's action outcomes included the creation of a grocery delivery guide for homebound seniors, an increased number of sidewalk curb cuts in the local area, and installation of street benches in strategic positions for seniors with less physical tolerance.

After working together for some time and gaining knowledge about advocacy approaches at the municipal level, the group became aware of the larger policy issues that impact on their lives. They shifted from using a locality development approach to a social action approach by focusing on broader level change directed at underlying inequities.

Such CD strategies provide a means to collaborate with clients to bring about both physical and social changes. Very often, however, the therapist may be working from a consultative framework rather than a facilitative approach and is charged with the task of providing recommendations to improve community accessibility. Knowledge of both the enabling and *disabling* aspects of both the physical and social environment is important and further discussed subsequently.

Enabling Community Participation— Modifying Physical Access in Public and Community Spaces

Public spaces are typically designed to meet the needs of average individuals and are based on general guidelines such as the ADA-Architectural Barriers Act (ABA) Accessibility Guidelines (U.S. Access Board, 2004). Greater accessibility can be achieved by working directly with clients, by working with community property owners or consultants, and by working as advocates in the community. For example, people with activity or participation restrictions may face barriers navigating public transportation systems, an important component of occupational performance. Iwarsson, Ståhl, and Carlsson (2003) described collaborative work between OT, traffic planning, and engineering in an initiative to understand the accessibility of transportation systems.

Barrier removal might not always be possible. In some cases, without regulatory incentives in place (e.g., mandatory accessibility guidelines), it might not be possible to make changes. It is the occupational therapist's role, however, to understand current legislation and minimum standards and to help clients advocate for change. It is also possible to identify barriers through the assessment process to help clients make decisions about how they could access and use spaces. In this case, understanding the physical environment is the goal, even though modification might not be possible.

Conclusions and Future Considerations

Physical, social, cultural, institutional, and technological aspects of environment can create barriers or provide resources and supports toward enabling optimal occupational performance and engagement. Occupational therapists

❝ COMMENTARY ON THE EVIDENCE

The Effectiveness of Environmental Modifications

Environmental modifications can be applied in many contexts and for a wide variety of purposes. The evidence for the effectiveness of modifying environments has grown exponentially. For this review, two common OT interventions are discussed: modifying the physical environment to prevent falls and modifying social and physical environments to support people with dementia and their caregivers.

Falls Prevention through Environmental Modifications

Falls prevention interventions for older adults can include many components that address physical performance of the person (e.g., through strengthening or balance exercises), medication reviews, group education, and assessment and modification of the home environment, often with a focus on home hazards. Sometimes, these are provided singly; in other work, a multicomponent intervention approach is used. Falls prevention research has included a large number of randomized controlled trials and subsequent systematic reviews and meta-analyses of the data from these studies (Law et al., 2010). Although not always provided as a single intervention, several reviews have examined the effectiveness of modifications of the physical environment as a strategy to prevent falls.

In 2016, Pighills, Ballinger, Pichering, and Chari compared two systematic reviews of the effectiveness of home assessment modifications for falls prevention in older adults. The two reviews both found that the home modification interventions were effective in preventing falls for people at high risk of falling, based on results from randomized controlled trials in which home modifications interventions could be isolated from other components of falls prevention strategies. Furthermore, the two reviews demonstrated that high-intensity interventions delivered by occupational therapists were most effective. Their conclusions are important, by emphasizing that environmental factors must be considered in the context of person- and activity-related factors, an approach to home modifications most commonly used by occupational therapists in practice.

Supporting People with Dementia and their Caregivers

Another area that has received attention in research is the value of home-based OT interventions designed to support caregivers and people with dementia living in their own homes. Typically, the interventions have included OT visits to identify goals, and the interventions focus on skills training for caregivers, introduction of simple home modifications, and activities modification for the person with dementia and their caregivers. Overall, the studies have identified significant improvements in the overall ADL (Gerner, 2013; Gitlin, Winter, Dennis, Hodgson, & Hauck, 2010; Graff et al., 2006) and quality of life for the person with dementia (Clare et al., 2010; Graff et al., 2007) and trends to decreased depression in their caregivers (Clare et al., 2010; Graff et al., 2007).

These interventions focus on caregivers managing their own actions (as part of the social environment of the person with dementia) as well as the physical environment to address challenges in managing people with dementia at home. Together, the results of these studies demonstrate that OT can result in positive effects for both the caregiver and the person with dementia by focusing on combinations of physical and social aspects of the environment.

have considerable experience and have demonstrated leadership and success with modifying home, school, work, and community contexts to support the participation of their clients in their daily pursuits. Today, more people who have previously been marginalized, excluded, or discriminated against are able to live with greater autonomy, go to school, return to work, and actively participate in their communities through efforts made by occupational therapists to reduce environmental barriers and harness environmental resources. To provide this leadership, it is critical that occupational therapists maintain a strong working knowledge about applicable policies and legislation, building codes, and accessibility guidelines that can improve the overall participation and empowerment of their clients. Beyond this awareness, however, as enablers of occupation, therapists can serve their clients by boldly participating in efforts to shape more inclusive social and public policies and to join the efforts of others, including their clients, in creating the spaces and opportunities that foster meaningful participation in life for all.

REFERENCES

Agree, E. M. (2014). The potential for technology to enhance independence for those aging with a disability. *Disability and Health Journal, 7*, S33–S39.

Aguilar, A., Boerema, C., & Harrison, J. (2010). Meanings attributed by older adults to computer use. *Journal of Occupational Science, 17*, 27–33.

Algurén, B., Lundgren-Nilsson, A., & Sunnerhagen, K. S. (2009). Facilitators and barriers of stroke survivors in the early post-stroke phase. *Disability and Rehabilitation, 31*, 1584–1591.

Alinsky, S. D. (1971). *Rules for radicals: A practical primer for realistic radicals.* New York, NY: Random House.

Amendment of Americans With Disabilities Act Title II and Title III Regulations to Implement ADA Amendments Act of 2008, 81 Fed. Reg. 53,204. (2016). Retrieved from https://www.gpo.gov/fdsys/pkg /FR-2016-08-11/pdf/2016-17417.pdf

American Association of Retired Persons. (2000). *Fixing to stay: A national survey on housing and home modification issues—executive summary.* Washington, DC: Author.

American Civil Rights Act of 1964, Pub. L. No. 88-352, § 78, Stat. 241 (1964). Retrieved from http://www.archives.gov/education/lessons /civil-rights-act/

American Occupational Therapy Association. (2011). Occupational therapy services in early childhood and school-based settings. *American Journal of Occupational Therapy, 65*(Suppl.), S46–S54.

American Occupational Therapy Association. (2014). Occupational therapy practice framework: Domain and process (3rd ed.). *American Journal of Occupational Therapy, 68*(Suppl. 1), S1–S48.

Americans with Disabilities Act of 1990, Pub. L. No. 101-336, 42 U.S.C. § 12101 (1990). Retrieved from http://www.ada.gov/

Anaby, D., Law, M., Coster, W., Bedell, G., Khetani, M., Avery, L., & Teplicky, R. (2014). The mediating role of the environment in explaining participation of children and youth with and without disabilities across home, school, and community. *Archives of Physical Medicine and Rehabilitation, 95,* 908–917.

Bronfenbrenner, U. (2005). *Making human beings human: Bioecological perspectives on human development.* Thousand Oaks, CA: Sage.

Center for Universal Design. (2002). *A blueprint for action: A resource for promoting home modifications.* Raleigh, NC: North Carolina State University. Retrieved from https://www.ncsu.edu/ncsu/design /cud/about_ud/udprinciples.htm (Original work published 1997)

Christiansen, C., & Baum, C. (Eds.). (1991). *Occupational therapy: Overcoming human performance deficits.* Thorofare, NJ: SLACK.

Cipriani, J., Kreider, M., Sapulak, K., Jacobson, M., Skrypski, M., & Sprau, K. (2009). Understanding object attachment and meaning for nursing home residents: An exploratory study, including implications for occupational therapy. *Physical and Occupational Therapy in Geriatrics, 27,* 405–422.

Clare, L., Linden, D. E., Woods, R. T., Whitaker, R., Evans, S. J., Parkinson, C. H., . . . Rugg, M. D. (2010). Goal-oriented cognitive rehabilitation for people with early-stage Alzheimer disease: A single-blind randomized controlled trial of clinical efficacy. *The American Journal of Geriatric Psychiatry, 18,* 928–939. doi:10.1097 /JGP.0b013e3181d5792a

Cook, A. M., & Polgar, J. M. (2015). *Cook and Hussey's assistive technologies: Principles and practice* (4th ed.). St. Louis, MO: Elsevier/Mosby.

Craik, J., Davis, J., & Polatajko, H. J. (2013). Introducing the Canadian Practice Process Framework (CPPF): Amplifying the context. In E. A. Townsend & H. J. Polatajko (Eds.), *Enabling Occupation II: Advancing an occupational therapy vision for health, well-being* (pp. 229–246). Ottawa, Canada: Canadian Association of Occupational Therapists.

Cristoforetti, A., Gennai, F., & Rodeschini, G. (2011). Home sweet home: The emotional construction of places. *Journal of Aging Studies, 25,* 225–232.

de Vries, B. (2015). Stigma and LGBT aging: Negative and positive marginality. In N. A. Orel & C. A. Fruhauf (Eds.), *The lives of LGBT older adults: Understanding challenges and resilience* (pp. 55–71). Washington, DC: American Psychological Association.

Dunn, W., Brown, C., & McGuigan, A. (1994). The ecology of human performance: A framework for considering the effect of context. *American Journal of Occupational Therapy, 48,* 595–607.

Dunning, H. (1972). Environmental occupational therapy. *American Journal of Occupational Therapy, 26,* 292–298.

Egilson, S. T. (2014). School experiences of pupils with physical impairments over time. *Disability and Society, 29,* 1076–1089.

Egilson, S. T., & Traustadottir, R. (2009). Participation of students with physical disabilities in the school environment. *American Journal of Occupational Therapy, 63,* 264–272.

Erickson, J., & Johnson, G. (2011). Internet use and psychological wellness during late adulthood. *Canadian Journal on Aging, 30,* 197–209.

Friedland, J. (2011). *Restoring the spirit: The beginnings of occupational therapy in Canada, 1890-1930.* Montreal, Canada: McGill-Queen's University Press.

Gallup, J. W. (1999). *Wellness centers: A guide for the design professional.* New York, NY: Wiley.

Gerner, A. (2013). *Effectiveness of an individualized home occupational therapy for persons with dementia—a randomized controlled trial* (Unpublished doctoral dissertation). Dresden University of Technology, Dresden, Germany.

Gitlin, L., Winter, L., Dennis, M., Hodgson, N., & Hauck, W. W. (2010). A biobehavioral home-based intervention and the well-being of patients with dementia and their caregivers: The COPE randomized trial. *JAMA, 304,* 983–991.

Graff, M. J. L., Vernooij-Dassen, M. J. M., Thijssen, M., Dekker, J., Hoefnagels, W. H. L., & Olderikkert, M. G. (2007). Effects of community occupational therapy on quality of life, mood, and health status in dementia patients and their caregivers: A randomized controlled trial. *The Journals of Gerontology, 62,* 1002–1009.

Graff, M. J. L., Vernooij-Dassen, M. J. M., Thijssen, M., Dekker, J., Hoefnagels, W. H. L., & Rikkert, M. G. M. (2006). Community based occupational therapy for patients with dementia and their care givers: Randomised controlled trial. *BMJ, 333,* 1196.

Hammack, P. L., & Cohler, B. J. (Eds.). (2009). *The story of sexual identity: Narrative perspectives on the gay and lesbian life course.* New York, NY: Oxford University Press.

Hampton, K., & Wellman, B. (2003). Neighboring in Netville: How the internet supports community and social capital in a wired suburb. *City & Community, 2,* 277–311.

Hoffman, K., & Duponte, J. (1992). *Community health centres and community development.* Ottawa, Canada: Health and Welfare Canada.

Iwarsson, S., & Ståhl, A. (2003). Accessibility, usability and universal design—positioning and definition of concepts describing person-environment relationships. *Disability and Rehabilitation, 25,* 57–66.

Iwarsson, S., Ståhl, A., & Carlsson, G. (2003). Accessible transportation: Novel occupational therapy perspectives. In L. Letts, P. Rigby, & D. Stewart (Eds.), *Using environments to enable occupational performance* (pp. 235–251). Thorofare, NJ: SLACK.

Job Accommodation Network. (n.d.). *SOAR: Searchable online accommodation resource.* Retrieved from http://askjan.org/soar/

Kennedy-Behr, A., Rodger, S., Graham, F., & Mickan, S. (2013). Creating enabling environments at preschool for children with developmental coordination disorder. *Journal of Occupational Therapy, Schools & Early Intervention, 6,* 301–313.

Kielhofner, G. (2008). *Model of human occupation: Theory and application* (4th ed.). Philadelphia, PA: Lippincott Wilkins & Williams.

Kielhofner, G., & Burke, J. P. (1980). A model of human occupation, part 1. Conceptual framework and content. *American Journal of Occupational Therapy, 34,* 572–581.

Kielhofner, G., Mallinson, T., Crawford, C., Nowak, M., Rigby, M., Henry, A., & Walens, D. (2004). *Occupational Performance History Interview II (OPHI-II) Version 2.1.* Chicago, IL: MOHO Clearinghouse.

Kirsh, B. (2015). Transforming values into action: Advocacy as a professional imperative. *Canadian Journal of Occupational Therapy, 82,* 212–223.

Kirsh, B., Trentham, B., & Cole, S. (2006). Diversity in occupational therapy: Experiences of consumers who identify themselves as minority group members. *Australian Occupational Therapy Journal, 53,* 302–313.

Lauckner, H., Krupa, T., & Paterson, M. (2011). Conceptualizing community development: Occupational therapy practice at the intersection of health services and community. *Canadian Journal of Occupational Therapy, 78*, 260–268.

Law, M., Baptiste, S., Carswell, A., McColl, M., Polatajko, H., & Pollock, N. (2014). *Canadian Occupational Performance Measure* (5th ed.). Ottawa, Canada: Canadian Association of Occupational Therapists.

Law, M., Cooper, B., Strong, S., Stewart, D., Rigby, P., & Letts, L. (1996). The person-environment-occupation model: A transactive approach to occupational performance. *Canadian Journal of Occupational Therapy, 63*, 9–23.

Law, M., Di Rezze, B., & Bradley, L. (2010). Environmental change to improve outcomes. In M. Law & M. A. McColl (Eds.), *Interventions, effects, and outcomes in occupational therapy: Adults and older adults* (pp. 155–182). Thorofare, NJ: SLACK.

Leclair, L. (2010). Re-examining concepts of occupation and occupation-based models: Occupational therapy and community development. *Canadian Journal of Occupational Therapy, 77*, 15–21.

Leclair, L., Ashcroft, M., Canning, T., & Lisowski, M. (2016). Preparing for community development practice: A Delphi study of Canadian occupational therapists. *Canadian Journal of Occupational Therapy, 83*, 226–236.

Liu, L., Stroulia, E., Nikolaidis, I., Miguel-Cruz, A., & Rios Rincon, A. (2016). Smart homes and home health monitoring technologies for older adults: A systematic review. *International Journal of Medical Informatics, 91*, 44–59.

Lysack, C., Komanecky, M., Kabel, A., Cross, K., & Neufeld, S. (2007). Environmental factors and their role in community integration after spinal cord injury. *Canadian Journal of Occupational Therapy, 74*, 243–254.

Marasinghe, K. M. (2016). Assistive technologies in reducing caregiver burden among informal caregivers of older adults: A systematic review. *Disability and Rehabilitation, 11*, 353–360.

McColl, M. A., Law, M. C., & Stewart, D. (2015). *Theoretical basis of occupational therapy* (3rd ed.). Thorofare, NJ: SLACK.

McDowell, C., & Fossey, E. (2015). Workplace accommodations for people with mental illness: A scoping review. *Journal of Occupational Rehabilitation, 25*, 197–206.

Meyer, A. (1922). The philosophy of occupational therapy. *Archives of Occupational Therapy, 1*, 1–10.

Mitty, E., & Flores, S. (2009). There's no place like home. *Geriatric Nursing, 30*, 126–129.

Mitzner, T. L., Boron, J. B., Fausset, C. B., Adams, A. E., Charness, N., Czaja, S. J., . . . Sharit, J. (2010). Older adults talk technology: Technology usage and attitudes. *Computers in Human Behaviour, 26*, 1710–1721.

Mortenson, W. B., Demers, L., Fuhrer, M., Jutai, J., Lenker, J., & DeRuyter, F. (2012). How assistive technology use by individuals with disabilities impacts their caregivers: A systematic review of the research evidence. *American Journal of Physical Medicine & Rehabilitation, 91*, 984–998

Nevala, N., Pehkonen, I., Koskela, I., Ruusuvuori, J., & Anttila, H. (2015). Workplace accommodation among persons with disabilities: A systematic review of its effectiveness and barriers or facilitators. *Journal of Occupational Rehabilitation, 25*, 432–448.

Niva, B., & Skär, L. (2006). A pilot study of the activity patterns of five elderly persons after a housing adaptation. *Occupational Therapy International, 13*, 21–34.

O'Reilly, J. A. (1954). Occupational therapy in the management of traumatic disabilities. *Canadian Journal of Occupational Therapy, 21*, 75–80.

Padkapayeva, K., Posen, A., Yazdani, A., Buettgen, A., Mahood, Q., & Tompa, E. (2017). Workplace accommodations for persons with physical disabilities: Evidence synthesis of the peer-reviewed literature. *Disability and Rehabilitation, 39*(21), 2134–2147 doi:10.1080/09638288.2016.1224276

Papageorgiou, N., Marquis, R., Dare, J., & Batten, R. (2016). Occupational therapy and occupational participation in community dwelling older adults: A review of the evidence. *Physical & Occupational Therapy in Geriatrics, 34*, 21–42.

Parent, L. (1978). Effects of a low-stimulus environment on behavior. *American Journal of Occupational Therapy, 32*, 19–25.

Pighills, A., Ballinger, C., Pickering, R., & Chari, S. (2016). A critical review of the effectiveness of environmental assessment and modification in the prevention of falls amongst community dwelling older people. *British Journal of Occupational Therapy, 79*, 133–143.

Rigby, P., Ryan, S. E., & Campbell, K. A. (2009). Effect of adaptive seating devices on the activity performance of children with cerebral palsy. *Archives of Physical Medicine and Rehabilitation, 90*, 1389–1395.

Rigby, P., Ryan, S. E., & Campbell, K. A. (2011). Electronic aids to daily living and quality of life for persons with tetraplegia. *Disability and Rehabilitation. Assistive Technology, 6*, 260–267.

Rothman, J., & Tropman, J. E. (1987). Models of community organization and macro practice perspectives: Their mixing and phasing. In F. M. Cox, J. L. Erlich, J. Rothman, & J. E. Tropman (Eds.), *Strategies of community organization: Macro practice* (4th ed., pp. 26–63). Itasca, IL: Peacock.

Scaffa, M., & Bonder, B. (2009). Health promotion and wellness. In B. Bonder & V. Dal Bello-Haas (Eds.), *Functional performance in older adults* (3rd ed., pp. 449–467). Philadelphia, PA: F. A. Davis.

Stadnyk, R., Townsend, E., & Wilcock, A. (2010). Occupational justice. In C. H. Christiansen & E. A. Townsend (Eds.), *Introduction to occupation: The art and science of living* (2nd ed., pp. 329–353). Upper Saddle River, NJ: Pearson.

Steinfeld, E., & Maisel, J. (2012). *Universal design: Creating inclusive environments*. Hoboken, NJ: Wiley.

Sum, S., Mathews, R. M., Pourghasem, M., & Hughes, I. (2009). Internet use as a predictor of sense of community in older people. *Cyberpsychology & Behavior, 12*, 235–239.

Sumathipala, K., Radcliffe, E., Sadler, E., Wolfe, C. D. A., & McKevitt, C. (2011). Identifying the long-term needs of stroke survivors using the International Classification of Functioning, Disability and Health. *Chronic Illness, 8*, 31–44.

Tanner, B., Tilse, C., & de Jonge, D. (2008). Restoring and sustaining home: The impact of home modifications on the meaning of home for older people. *Journal of Housing for the Elderly, 22*, 195–215.

Townsend, E. A., & Polatajko, H. J. (2013). *Enabling occupation II: Advancing an occupational therapy vision for health, well-being, & justice through occupation* (2nd ed.). Ottawa, Canada: Canadian Association of Occupational Therapists.

Trentham, B., Cockburn, L., & Shin, J. (2007). Health promotion and community development: An application of occupational therapy in primary health care. *Canadian Journal of Community Mental Health, 26*, 53–70.

Trentham, B., Sokoloff, S., Tsang, A., & Neysmith, S. (2015). Social media and senior citizen advocacy: An inclusive tool to resist ageism? *Politics, Groups & Identities, 3*, 558–571.

United Nations. (2016). *Convention on the Rights of Persons with Disabilities (CRPD)*. Retrieved from https://www.un.org/development/desa/disabilities/convention-on-the-rights-of-persons-with-disabilities.html

U.S. Access Board. (2004). *ADA and ABA accessibility guidelines*. Retrieved from http://www.access-board.gov/ada-aba/final.pdf

U.S. Department of Justice. (2010). *ADA standards for accessible design*. Retrieved from http://www.ada.gov/2010ADAstandards_index.htm

U.S. Department of State. (2008). *Appendix A: Universal declaration of human rights*. Retrieved from http://www.state.gov/g/drl/rls/irf/2008/108544.htm

Vasara, P. (2015). Not ageing in place: Negotiating meanings of residency in age-related housing. *Journal of Aging Studies, 35*, 55–64.

Whiteford, G. (2005). Understanding the occupational deprivation of refugees: A case study from Kosovo. *Canadian Journal of Occupational Therapy, 72*, 78–88.

World Health Organization. (1986). Ottawa charter for health promotion. *Health Promotions, 1*, iii–v.

World Health Organization. (2001). *International classification of functioning, disability and health*. Geneva, Switzerland: Author. Retrieved from http://www.who.int/classification/icf/

Resources

American Printing House for the Blind (provides materials, alternative media, tools, and resources for individuals who are blind or visually impaired): http://www.aph.org/

Americans with Disabilities Act: http://www.ada.gov/

Center for Inclusive Design and Environmental Access (IDeA): http://www.ap.buffalo.edu/idea/Home/index.asp

Center for Universal Design at North Carolina State University: https://www.ncsu.edu/ncsu/design/cud/

Centre for Accessible Environments, United Kingdom: http://www.cae.org.uk/

Home Modification Information Clearing House in Australia: https://www.homemods.info/

Job Accommodation Network (JAN): http://askjan.org/

National Centre on Accessibility (promotes access for people with disabilities in recreation): http://www.ncaonline.org

Services for People with Disabilities from Services Canada: http://www.faslink.org/Disability_Guide_ENG.pdf

U.S. Access Board (a federal agency committed to accessible design): https://www.access-board.gov/

U.S. Equal Employment Opportunity Commission: http://www.eeoc.gov/

thePoint® *For additional resources on the subjects discussed in this chapter, visit* **http://thePoint.lww.com/Willard-Spackman13e.** *See* **Appendix I, Resources and Evidence for Common Conditions Addressed in OT** *for more information on traumatic brain injury.*

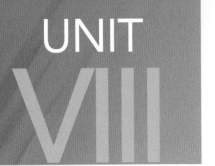

UNIT VIII

Core Concepts and Skills

"You treat a disease: you win, you lose. You treat a person; I guarantee you win—no matter what the outcome."

—Patch Adams

CHAPTER 34

Professional Reasoning in Practice

Barbara A. Boyt Schell

LEARNING OBJECTIVES

After reading this chapter, you will be able to:

1. Analyze important aspects of reasoning in occupational therapy practice.
2. Discuss how the reasoning process is embedded in the transactions that occur among the practitioner, the client, and the practice context.
3. Identify the different facets of professional reasoning based on personal reflection, practitioners' descriptions, and case studies.
4. Describe the process of developing expertise and discuss characteristic reasoning processes along a continuum of expertise.

Introduction

Professional reasoning is the process that practitioners use to plan, direct, perform, and reflect on client care. It is typically performed quickly because the practitioner has to act on that reasoning right away. It is a complex and multifaceted process, and it has been called by several different names. In the past, many authors referred to it as **clinical reasoning** (Mattingly & Fleming, 1994; Rogers, 1983; Schell & Cervero, 1993), but terms such as *professional reasoning* (Schell & Schell, 2018) and **therapeutic reasoning** (Kielhofner & Forsyth, 2002) have surfaced in an attempt to find a word that is not so closely aligned with medicine because occupational therapy (OT) practices not only in medical settings but also in many educational and community settings. When using these labels, authors are talking about how therapists *actually think* when they are engaged in practice. This requires metacognitive analysis or, in simple terms, *thinking about thinking*. This is important because newcomers to the field might incorrectly understand professional reasoning as something that practitioners "choose to do" or confuse it with the many OT intervention theories. It is neither of those things. Whenever you are thinking about or doing OT for an identified individual or group, you are engaged in professional reasoning. It is not a question of whether you are doing it, only a question of how well. Furthermore, many practice theories are discussed throughout this text that will inform your reasoning and help you to think about your clients. However, the research and theories about reasoning that are discussed in

CENTENNIAL NOTES

Clinical Reasoning

Clinical reasoning is a term that first gained prominence among American occupational therapists in the 1980s, when Joan Rogers made clinical reasoning the subject of her 1983 American Occupational Therapy Association (AOTA) Eleanor Clark Slagle Lecture (Rogers, 1983). In this speech, she shared research from professions such as medicine designed to understand how decisions were made in clinical practice. Rogers advocated for occupational therapists to examine the reasoning processes underlying their therapy actions. She felt it is important for OT reasoning to be described, both to figure out the most effective reasoning approaches and also to make it easier to teach students how to reason as occupational therapists. Her lecture stimulated research designed to explore what therapists *actually* thought when they engaged in therapy.

The next chapter in this story for OT came about in the late 1980s when a group of theorists and researchers met with Donald Schön to discuss how to "investigate clinical knowledge and expertise within the profession" (Mattingly & Fleming, 1994a, p. ix). Schön, a philosopher and a professor in urban planning, was already well known for his book, *The Reflective Practitioner* (Schön, 1983), in which he described commonalities in the thinking of a variety of professionals as they engaged in their work. Cheryl Mattingly, an anthropologist, and Schön's graduate student, teamed up with Maureen Fleming, an experienced OT faculty member at Tufts University, in Boston, to do an extensive study of occupational therapists at a large medical center in a major U.S. city (Mattingly & Fleming, 1994). This landmark study produced findings suggesting that occupational therapist used not just one clinical reasoning process, but several. This work had tremendous influence on the study of clinical reasoning in OT. Their subsequent publications in an *American Journal of Occupational Therapy* (AJOT) Special Issue on Clinical Reasoning (Cohn, 1991) and later in their book *Clinical Reasoning: Forms of Inquiry in a Therapeutic Practice* (Mattingly & Fleming, 1994) along with Roger's 1983 Slagle Lecture formed the basis of this a large body of research in the profession.

From that beginning until today, at least 140 studies have been reported in the OT literature on clinical and professional reasoning (Unsworth & Baker, 2016), and many more articles, studies, and book chapters have been published across many countries (Schell & Schell, 2018).

this chapter are focused on you as an OT practitioner and how you are likely to think as you engage in therapy. Thus, the focus is on the therapist, not on the client, although obviously, therapists do this thinking in the service of client care. Keep in mind these important distinctions as you become mindful of your own reasoning processes.

This chapter examines professional reasoning from several perspectives. To help you see real examples of the material discussed, the following Case Study 34-1, which is adapted with name changes from an actual situation, provides an example of an encounter between an occupational therapist Terry and her client Mrs. Munro. Read this case study before continuing with the text, paying special attention to the different kinds of issues and problems that the OT practitioner has to address. Then, keep referring back to it as you read about the nature of professional reasoning.

Reasoning in Practice: Using the Whole Self

With the case study in mind, let's explore the nature of reasoning during practice. Perhaps one of the first things to note is that professional reasoning is an **embodied** process involving the therapist's whole self as well as the context in which therapy occurs. That is one reason why it is a different experience to read a case study than to be the practitioner in the situation. Some professional reasoning involves straightforward thinking processes that the practitioner can easily describe. Examples include assessing occupational performance, such as daily living skills and work behaviors. Occupational therapy practitioners use their observations and theoretical knowledge to identify relevant client factors that contribute to occupational performance problems. Practitioners also attend to the contextual factors that affect performance. For instance, Terry was able to describe her concerns about Mrs. Munro's safety in returning home. In particular, Terry was addressing self-care and homemaking activities. She had analyzed relevant contextual factors about the home setting and Mrs. Munro's social and financial situation. Terry had identified some impairments in cognition and motor control that were affecting her client's occupational performance skills. This was all information that Terry could readily share with Barb. However, there was more knowledge from the therapy session that Terry either did not or could not put into words.

Part of Terry's professional reasoning involved knowledge that she gained from her senses. For instance, Terry

CASE STUDY 34-1 TERRY AND MRS. MUNRO: DETERMINING APPROPRIATE RECOMMENDATIONS

Terry, an occupational therapist, goes up to a client's room in the neurology unit of a regional medical center. Along the way, she shares her thoughts with Barb, a researcher who is observing Terry's practice. Terry fills Barb in on the client they are about to see. The client, Mrs. Munro, is a widow who lives alone in a house in town. A couple of days earlier, she had a stroke—a right cerebrovascular accident—and was brought by a neighbor to the hospital. Mrs. Munro has made a rapid recovery and demonstrates good return of her motor skills. She still has some left-sided weakness and incoordination, along with some cognitive problems. She is a delightful, pleasant older woman and is anxious to return home.

Terry is seeing this client for the third time, and her primary concern is to assess whether Mrs. Munro has any residual cognitive effects from her stroke that would put her at serious risk if she returned home alone. Terry plans to do some more in-depth activities of daily living with Mrs. Munro to see how well she demonstrates safety awareness. Terry thinks that she will probably have Mrs. Munro get out of bed, obtain her clothing and hygiene supplies, perform her morning hygiene routines at the sink, and then get dressed. Terry wants to see the degree to which Mrs. Munro is spontaneously able to manage these tasks as well as how good her judgment appears to be. Terry's thought is that if she can engage Mrs. Munro in several multistep activities that also require her to perform in different positions, Terry should be able to detect any cognitive and motor problems that pose a serious safety threat.

When Terry arrives at the room, she greets Mrs. Munro who says, "I am so excited. The doctor says I can go home today."

Terry turns to Barb and raises her eyebrows as if to say, "I told you so." On the way to the room, Terry had told Barb that she was worried that the physician who was managing Mrs. Munro's case tended to think that as soon as clients could physically get up, they should go home. Terry went on to defend the physician by saying that in today's cost-conscious environment, doctors were under a lot of pressure not to keep clients in the hospital.

As Terry converses with Mrs. Munro about generalities, she notices that Mrs. Munro is already dressed in her housecoat. When she talks to Mrs. Munro about doing some self-care activities, it becomes apparent that Mrs. Munro has already completed her bathing and dressing routines, with help from a nurse. When Terry suggests that she perhaps brush her teeth and comb her hair, Mrs. Munro is happy to get up out of bed but notes that her neighbor never did bring in her dentures. Mrs. Munro sits on the edge of the bed and, after a reminder from Terry, puts on her slippers. She then stands and walks to the nearby sink, finds her comb, and

combs her hair. While she is doing this, Terry looks around for some other ideas about what to do because Mrs. Munro has already completed the self-care tasks Terry had planned to do with her.

Terry's eyes light on some wilted flowers by the bed. She suggests to Mrs. Munro that she might want to dispose of the flowers and clean the vase so that it will be ready to pack when it is time to go home. Mrs. Munro agrees and proceeds to walk somewhat unsteadily over to the vase. Picking it up, she carries it to the sink, where she pulls out the dead flowers. Terry follows her, staying slightly behind and within reach of Mrs. Munro. When Mrs. Munro stops after removing the flowers, Terry suggests that she rinse out the vase, which she does. She then dries it and returns the vase to the bedside table. Terry reminds her to throw out the dead flowers. While Mrs. Munro does this, they talk some more about her plans to return home.

Mrs. Munro tells Terry that she has lived in her home for 40 years, and even though her husband died more than 10 years ago, she still feels his presence there. He used to love her cooking, and she still cooks three meals a day for herself. Mrs. Munro starts to cry when they talk about cooking but then cheers up. Terry tells her that it might be safer if she had someone around the house for a few weeks until she recovers a bit more from her stroke. Mrs. Munro thinks that she can get some help from her neighbor. Terry says she is also going to suggest some home care therapy, just to make sure Mrs. Munro is safe in the kitchen, bathroom, and so on, noting, "We sure don't want to see you have a bad fall just when you are doing so well after your stroke."

After reviewing some coordination activities for Mrs. Munro's left hand, Terry says good-bye. Terry and Barb leave the room. Terry stops at the nurses' station to note in the chart that Mrs. Munro demonstrated good safety awareness in familiar tasks at her bedside but did require cueing to complete multistep tasks. Terry also notes some motor instability in task performance during ambulation. Terry recommends a referral to a home health OT practitioner "to assess safety and equipment needs during bathroom activities, meal preparation, and routine homemaking tasks." Terry comments to Barb, as they walk off the unit, that she thinks Mrs. Munro did pretty well, but Terry remains concerned about the risks once Mrs. Munro goes home, particularly when she is tired. Terry wants someone to monitor Mrs. Munro in a familiar setting to see whether she handles her daily routines adequately. Terry would really like to see Mrs. Munro start to consider a more supported living environment, but the client doesn't have either long-term care insurance or the personal finances to support that. Terry believes that she might at least be

CASE STUDY 34-1   TERRY AND MRS. MUNRO: DETERMINING APPROPRIATE RECOMMENDATIONS *(continued)*

able to get one home care visit to evaluate home safety, particularly fall prevention. Staying in her own home seems to be Mrs. Munro's major goal, and Terry is going to do what she can to try to help her attain that goal. Terry will catch up with the social worker later to discuss the need for Mrs. Munro to have good support from any neighbors, friends, or relatives.

Questions and Exercises

1. How did Terry develop her concerns about Mrs. Munro?
2. How did Terry know what to do when her initial plans did not work out?
3. What factors seem to guide Terry's recommendations at the end?

used her sense of touch to feel the muscle tension (or lack of tension) in Mrs. Munro's affected arm when she was doing an activity. During her evaluation, Terry did some quick stretches to Mrs. Munro's elbow and wrist to determine whether she could feel evidence of spasticity, an abnormal reflex response that is commonly found in individuals who are recovering from a stroke. When Mrs. Munro stood up, Terry gauged the distance she stood from Mrs. Munro because Mrs. Munro was at some risk of falling. Terry was careful to stand not so close that she crowded or overprotected Mrs. Munro but close enough to protect her should she lose her balance. While close to Mrs. Munro, Terry could smell her, gaining a quick sense of possible hygiene or continence problems. Terry used her voice quality to display encouragement and support. Terry watched and listened carefully for clues about the nature of Mrs. Munro's emotional state. In particular, she watched facial expressions and listened for evidence of fear or insecurity during Mrs. Munro's performance of activities. All of these sensations contributed to an image of Mrs. Munro that influenced Terry's practice.

There are other aspects of reasoning during therapy that are even harder to describe. Fleming (1994c) described this as "knowing more than we can tell" (p. 24). She explained that much of the profession's knowledge is practical knowledge, which is "seldom discussed and rarely described" (Fleming, 1994c, p. 25). This tacit knowledge, combined with the rich sensory aspects of actual practice, helps to explain why reading about therapy and doing therapy are such different experiences. Kinsella summarizes this deeper understanding of reasoning when she notes "the mind can be revealed in the embodied *doings* of a person, mind is revealed in *practices*" (Kinsella, 2018, p. 111). Hooper (1997, 2018) has also noted the importance of how our own values, beliefs, and assumptions underpin each practitioner's grasp of the therapy process. So keep in mind that therapy always happens in the real world with real people, and you will see variations because each therapist is different.

Theory and Practice

There has been a long-standing discussion in many professions about the role of theory in professional practice (Kessels & Korthagen, 1996). Theories help practitioners to make decisions, although Cohn (1989) noted that the problems of practice rarely present themselves in the straightforward manner described in textbook theories. Professional reasoning involves the naming and framing of problems on the basis of a personal understanding of the client's situation (Schön, 1983). In problem identification and problem solution, practitioners blend theories with their own personal and practice experiences to guide their actions. Theoretical knowledge helps the practitioner to avoid unjustified assumptions or the use of ineffective therapy techniques and to reflect on how his or her own experiences in therapy are similar to or different from theoretical understandings (Parham, 1987). In Chapter 41, you will find more information about how theories inform practice as well as how our underlying assumptions shape our therapy actions. The point here is that, although practice can (and should) be informed by theories, it is ultimately a result of how each therapist interprets each therapy situation and then acts on that understanding.

Cognitive Processes Underlying Professional Reasoning

In the case study, Terry had to remember, obtain, and manage a great deal of information quickly to provide effective and efficient intervention. How did she do it? Research findings from the field of cognitive psychology and medical clinical reasoning help to explain how practitioners process information and how experience combined with reflection fosters increasing expertise. Individuals receive, store, and organize information in *frames* or *scripts*, which are complex representations or simulations representing perceptions gained from our experiences (Bruning, Schraw, & Ronning, 1999; Carr & Shotwell, 2018; Norman, 2005). This process involves both working memory and long-term memory. Working memory is where the thinking occurs, and it can hold very few thoughts at a time. That is one reason that one sometimes has to look at the directions two or three times in order to correctly assemble something unfamiliar, such as a new toy or piece of furniture. Similarly, students and new practitioners find it challenging to try to keep all the important considerations in mind when dealing with a client or attempting a new assessment or intervention procedure. Practitioners with extensive experience have this information organized and stored in their long-term memories and thus do not have to actively juggle all the details. Norman's research with physicians suggests the practitioner create exemplars in their minds which serve to guide analysis of new cases (Norman, 2005). For example, in school, Terry probably learned many of the common problems associated with someone who has had a stroke. She also has seen perhaps 100 people with strokes over the past several years. She has built up a general representation in her mind of what to expect when she receives a referral for someone who has had a stroke. She anticipates that many of these individuals will have extensive medical charts because they almost always have prior medical problems, such as diabetes and high blood pressure. She will not be surprised if the person is overweight. She expects to see impairments in cognition that often affect the person's ability to do everyday tasks, such as dressing, cooking, and driving. As part of her frame, Terry has built-in mental rules that help her to categorize and detect differences. For instance, although she knows that many people who have strokes have movement impairments, she knows that not all do. Furthermore, when movement is impaired, she expects individuals with a left cerebrovascular accident (CVA) to have right-sided weakness and those with a right CVA to have left-sided weakness. Additionally, she knows that a person's social support system is critical for promoting an adaptive response to disability. She may use certain cues, such as the presence or absence of frequent family visits, to prompt her to categorize a family as supportive or nonsupportive.

In addition to framing or "chunking" information, Terry also creates and uses scripts or procedural rules that guide her thinking (Bruning et al., 1999; Carr & Shotwell, 2018). Just as her mental frames help her to organize and retrieve her knowledge about common aspects of stroke, scripts help her to organize common occurrences or events. For instance, she understands that her role involves responding to the referral by seeing the client, writing her findings on the correct form, providing interventions, communicating verbally with the other team members,

and developing discharge plans. Terry likely has scripts about the implications for clients with supportive families and those without. In her experience, a supportive family cares for its family member at home regardless of the family's financial resources. Alternatively, clients with little family support are more likely to face institutional care. Again, these scripts are formed by Terry's observations and experiences over time and serve the purpose of helping her to anticipate likely events.

The mind appears to use frames, scripts, and exemplars to support effective processing of information by providing efficient mental frameworks for handling complex information (Carr & Shotwell, 2018; Norman, 2005). Each person individually constructs them. It is no surprise that students and new practitioners often struggle to retain and effectively use their therapy knowledge. It takes time and repetition of experiences to develop effective reasoning based on efficient storage in long-term memory allowing for targeted use of short-term memory as therapy happens. Important aspects of the process are as follows (Roberts, 1996):

- *Cue acquisition:* searching for the helpful and targeted information through observation and questioning
- *Pattern recognition:* noticing similarities and differences among situations
- *Limiting the problem space:* using patterns to help focus cue acquisition and knowledge application on the most fruitful areas
- *Problem formulation:* developing an explanation of what is going on, why it is going on, and what a better situation or outcome might be
- *Problem solution:* identifying courses of action based on the problem formulation

These cognitive processes are interactive and rarely occur in a linear fashion. Rather, the mind jumps around between the information at hand and that which has been stored up from prior learning while attempting to make sense of the situation. Now that we have a better understanding of the basic systems our mind uses to support our professional reasoning, we turn our attention to research on the different aspects of professional reasoning that have surfaced from research on occupational therapists.

Aspects of Professional Reasoning

Although there appear to be common processes underlying reasoning in practice, the focus of that mental activity appears to vary with the demands of the problems to be addressed. Fleming (1991) was the first within OT to describe how occupational therapists seemed to use different thinking approaches depending on the nature of the clinical problem they were addressing. She referred to this process as the "therapist with the three-track mind" (p. 1007). Since that time, others have examined the different aspects of OT professional reasoning. Most of this research has been done with occupational therapists, although at least one case study (Lyons & Crepeau, 2001) suggests there is some application for OT assistants as well. The most commonly agreed on aspects of professional reasoning are listed in Table 34-1, along with the typical focus clues for recognizing when that sort of reasoning is occurring. Note that other authors may name and characterize these somewhat differently, but all agree that there are multiple aspects that surface in research about professional reasoning (Sinclair, 2007; Unsworth, 2012).

Scientific Reasoning

Scientific reasoning is used to understand the condition that is affecting an individual and to decide on interventions that are in the client's best interest. It is a logical process that parallels scientific inquiry. Forms of scientific reasoning that are described in OT are diagnostic reasoning (Rogers & Holm, 1991) and procedural reasoning (Fleming, 1991, 1994b) in addition to the general use of hypothetical-deductive reasoning (Tomlin, 2018). Scientific reasoning is also referred to as *treatment planning* (Pelland, 1987) in which the therapist uses selected theories both to identify problems and to guide decision making.

Diagnostic reasoning is concerned with clinical problem sensing and problem definition. The process starts in advance of seeing a client. Occupational therapy practitioners, because of their domains of concern, look primarily for occupational performance problems. Furthermore, the nature of the problems they expect to find is influenced by the information in the requests for services. Some of Terry's diagnostic reasonings, described earlier, included information about the typical symptoms associated with having a stroke.

Procedural reasoning occurs when practitioners are "thinking about the disease or disability and deciding which intervention activities (procedures) they might employ to remediate the person's functional performance problems" (Fleming, 1991, p. 1008). This may involve an interview, an observation of the person engaged in a task, or formal evaluations using standardized measures. Although one hopes that procedural reasoning is science-based, Tomlin makes the important observation that procedural reasoning can become an unquestioned implementation of therapy protocols, in which case it becomes less scientific in nature (Tomlin, 2008). That is why there is such an emphasis on evidence-based practice, which challenges the practitioner to routinely evaluate customary

therapy approaches based on of the best information currently available (Holm, 2000; Law & MacDermid, 2008; Tickle-Degnen, 2000). In more recent work related to science-informed thinking (Dougherty, Toth-Cohen, & Tomlin, 2016; Tomlin, 2018), researchers suggest the scientific reasoning is part of an evidence-informed versus evidence-based process. Chapter 35 speaks on the importance of evidence-informed practice, and all of the chapters in this text, along with many other OT texts, include evidence that can help guide practice.

In the case study, Terry used a combination of interview and observation, both of which were guided by her working hypothesis that Mrs. Munro had cognitive problems that might affect her safe performance at home. She was likely operating on the basis of her understanding of cognitive theories (such as those described in Chapter 58) as well as her own experience with similar clients. As intervention begins, more data are collected, and the OT practitioner gains a sharper clinical image. This clinical image is the result of the interplay between what the OT practitioner expects to see (such as the usual course of the disease) and the client's actual performance. In the case study, there was congruence between Mrs. Munro's abilities and problems in performing activities of daily living and Terry's expectations of someone making a good recovery from a stroke.

Mattingly (1994b) made the point that occupational therapists have a "two-body practice" (p. 37). By that, she meant that OT practitioners view a person in two ways: the body as a machine, in which parts may be broken, and the person as a life, filled with personal meanings and hopes. Much of the procedural reasoning in OT addresses issues related to the body as machine, although current theories in the field do place much more emphasis on the need to understand the client as an open system, responsive to and acting on the environment. The next form of reasoning, narrative reasoning, provides the OT practitioner with a way to understand a person's illness experience.

Narrative Reasoning

Understanding the meaning that a disease, illness, or disability has to an individual is a task that goes beyond the scientific understanding of disease processes and organ systems. Rather, it requires that practitioners find a way to understand the meaning of this experience from the client's perspective. Mattingly (1994c) suggested that practitioners do this through a form of reasoning called narrative reasoning. Narrative reasoning is so named because it involves thinking in story form. It is not uncommon for an OT practitioner who is preparing to substitute for another with a client to ask the other practitioner, "So what is the client's story?"

TABLE 34-1   Aspects of Reasoning in Occupational Therapy

Reasoning Aspect	Clues for Recognizing in Therapist Discussions	Examples of the Therapy Problems or Questions which Draw Out This Reasoning
Scientific		
Reasoning involving the use of applied logical and scientific methods, such as hypothesis testing, pattern recognition, theory-based decision making, and statistical evidence	Impersonal, focused on the diagnosis, condition, guiding theory, evidence from research, or what "typically" happens with clients like the one being considered	What is the nature of the illness, injury, or development problem? What are the common impairments or disabilities resulting from this condition? What are the typical contextual factors that affect performance? What theories and research are available to guide assessment and intervention?
Diagnostic		
Investigative reasoning and analysis of cause or nature of conditions requiring OT intervention can be considered one component of scientific reasoning	Uses both personal and impersonal information. Therapists attempt to explain why client is experiencing problems using a blend of science- and client-based information.	What are the occupational performance problems this client has or may have in the future? What are the factors contributing to this problem (impairments, performance context)? How are these problems manifest (skills, habits, routines, occupational roles)?
Procedural		
Reasoning in which therapist considers and uses intervention routines for identified conditions; may be science-based or may reflect the habits and culture of the intervention setting	Characterized by therapist using therapy regimes or routines thought to be effective with problems identified and that are typically used with clients in that setting	What evaluation and intervention protocols are applicable to this person's situation? How are clients like this usually handled in my setting?
Narrative		
Reasoning process used to make sense of people's particular circumstances; prospectively imagine the effect of illness, disability, or occupational performance problems on their daily lives; and create a collaborative story that is enacted with clients and families through intervention	Personal, focused on the client, including past, present, and anticipated future. Involves an appreciation of client culture as the basis for understanding client narrative; relates to the "so what" of the condition for the person's life	What is this person's life story? What is the nature of this person as an occupational being? How has the health condition affected the person's life story or ability to continue his or her life story? What occupational activities are most important to this person? What occupational activities are both meaningful to this person and useful for meeting therapy goals?
Pragmatic		
Practical reasoning that is used to fit therapy possibilities into the current realities of service delivery, such as scheduling options, payment for services, equipment availability, therapists' skills, management directives, and the personal situation of the therapist	Generally not focused on client or client's condition but rather on all the physical and social "stuff" that surrounds the therapy encounter as well as the therapist's internal sense of what he or she is capable of and has the time and energy to complete	Who referred this person, and why? Who is paying for services, and what are their rules? What family or caregiver resources are there to support intervention? What are the expectations of my supervisor and workplace? How much time do I have to see this person? What therapy space and equipment are available? What are my practice competencies?
Ethical		
Reasoning directed toward analyzing an ethical dilemma, generating alternative solutions, and determining actions to be taken; systematic approach to moral conflict	Tension is often evident as therapist attempts to determine what is the "right" thing to do particularly when faced with dilemmas in therapy competing principles, risks, and benefits.	Are the benefits of therapy worth the cost? Are the risks of therapy worth the benefits? How should I prioritize my caseload? What are the limits of how I change my documentation to maximize payment? What should I do when other members of the treatment team are operating in ways that I feel conflict with the goals of the person receiving services?

TABLE 34-1	Aspects of Reasoning in Occupational Therapy *(continued)*	
Reasoning Aspect	**Clues for Recognizing in Therapist Discussions**	**Examples of the Therapy Problems or Questions which Draw Out This Reasoning**
Interactive		
Thinking directed toward building positive interpersonal relationships with clients, permitting collaborative problem identification and problem solving	Therapist is concerned with what client likes or does not like; use of praise, empathetic comments, and nonverbal behaviors to encourage and support client's cooperation	How can I best relate to this person? How can I put this person at ease? What is the best way for me to encourage this person? What nonverbal strategies should I use in this situation? Where should I place myself relative to this person so that I support him or her but do not "invade" the person? What cultural factors do I need to consider as I engage with the person?
Conditional		
A blending of all forms of reasoning for the purposes of flexibly responding to changing conditions or predicting possible client futures	Typically found with more experienced therapists who can "see" multiple futures based on the therapist's past experiences and current information	Where is this person going? How will the various therapy options play out, given this person's health condition, social situation, economic status, and culture? Given these future possible trajectories, what is the best action I can take now?

For more additional summaries of these aspects, refer to Carrier, Levasseur, Bédard, and Desrosiers (2010); Schell and Schell (2018); and Unsworth (2011).

In the case study, part of Terry's reasoning was concerned with making decisions in light of what was important to Mrs. Munro. This process of collaboration and empathy has been described as "building a communal horizon of understanding" (Clark, Ennevor, & Richardson, 1996, p. 376). Terry gained understanding by listening attentively to Mrs. Munro's stories about her husband and how he loved her cooking. It is apparent from this session that Mrs. Munro's home is more than just a house. It is the place in which she lived with her husband, where he died, and where she still felt his presence. Part of Mrs. Munro's story is that going home is going back to her husband. If this stroke were to prevent that, Mrs. Munro would lose more than her independence; she would lose symbolic connections to her husband. Although a logical case might be made that Mrs. Munro should start considering a more supportive living environment, Terry understands that for Mrs. Munro, this would not be an acceptable ending. Consequently, Terry worked hard to obtain the support systems that would be necessary for Mrs. Munro to function in her chosen environment, where she will continue her life story.

Often, OT practitioners work with individuals whose life stories are so severely disrupted that they cannot imagine what their future will look like. Mattingly (1994b) believed that in these situations, skillful practitioners help their clients to invent new life stories. This has been referred to as helping clients "recraft" their "occupational narratives" (Auzmendia, de las Heras, Kielhofner, & Miranda, 2008, p. 313). To some degree, these stories become visible as the OT practitioner and the client

develop goals together. The use of life stories is also apparent when activities are selected for both their healing potential and their particular significance to the person. To do this, one must first solicit occupational stories from the individual (Clark et al., 1996; Hamilton, 2018). With an understanding of clients' past occupational stories, practitioners can help individuals to create new stories and new futures for themselves. If Mrs. Munro's symptoms were more severe and she was in a more extended therapy process, Terry might explore Mrs. Munro's interest in cooking as an activity that she liked and that would offer many therapeutic opportunities. Furthermore, Mrs. Munro might find that she could express her pleasure in cooking for others by making special treats, first for other clients and then perhaps for neighbors in exchange for their help with chores. During this process, Mrs. Munro would not only be regaining coordination and dexterity but also her sense of self as a productive person. This narrative aspect of clinical reasoning, which ultimately focuses on the person as an occupational being, provides a link between the founding values of the profession and current practice demands (Gray, 1998).

Pragmatic Reasoning

Pragmatic reasoning is yet another strand of reasoning that goes beyond the practitioner–client relationship and addresses the world in which therapy occurs (Schell, 2018b; Schell & Cervero, 1993). This world is considered from two perspectives: the practice context and the personal context. Because reasoning during therapy is a practical activity, a number of everyday issues have been identified over the years that affect the therapy process. These include resources for intervention, organizational culture, power relationships among team members, reimbursement practices, and practice trends in the profession (Barris, 1987; Howard, 1991; Neuhaus, 1988; Rogers & Holm, 1991). Studies examining clinical reasoning have confirmed that OT practitioners both actively consider and are influenced by their practice contexts (Copley, Nelson, Turpin, Underwood & Flanigan, 2008; Creighton, Dijkers, Bennett, & Brown, 1995; Holmqvist, Kamwendo, & Ivarsson, 2009; Schell, 1994; Strong, Gilbert, Cassidy, & Bennett, 1995; Unsworth, 2005). An example of pragmatic reasoning in the case study was Terry's use of immediate resources (the flower vase) in Mrs. Munro's room as a therapy tool. Although Terry had thought of appropriate activities related to self-care, she had to identify practical alternatives quickly when it turned out that Mrs. Munro was already dressed. Practical constraints for Terry included (1) the time it would take to move Mrs. Munro to the clinic, where there might be more resources; (2) the need to get the required information on that day because Mrs. Munro was going home; and (3) the physical constraints of what was available within the room. Terry's invention of a feasible alternative was a product of both her therapeutic imagination and the cues that were provided within her practice setting.

Terry's attention to the influence of team members demonstrates pragmatic reasoning directed to interpersonal and group issues. She knew that the physician had the power to make discharge decisions. She was aware of the pressures on the physician by third-party payers to discharge clients as quickly as possible. Practice requires that practitioners' reason about negotiating their clients' interests within the practice culture.

The practitioner's personal situation also is part of the pragmatic reasoning process. Although less readily identified in research, Unsworth (2005) surfaced some examples in her research in which therapists "weighed their own therapy skills against the therapeutic needs of the clients" (p. 36) in order to decide whether to refer to others with more expertise. A person's clinical competencies, preferences, commitment to the profession, and life role demands outside of work all affect the therapy choices that are considered and thus enter into the reasoning process. For instance, if a practitioner does not feel safe helping a client stand or transfer to a bed, the therapist is more likely to use tabletop activities in which the client can participate from a wheelchair. Another OT practitioner might feel uncomfortable interacting with individuals who have depression and, therefore, might be quick to suggest that such clients are not motivated for therapy. A practitioner who has a young family to go home to might opt not to schedule clients late in the day so as to

get home as early as possible. These simple personal issues result in clinical decisions that affect the scope and timing of therapy services. Hooper (1997, 2018) suggested that fundamental issues, such as a practitioner's values and general worldview, strongly affect the way in which an individual constructs his or her reasoning. Such worldviews play an important role in the next kind of reasoning: ethical reasoning.

Ethical Reasoning

All of the forms of reasoning that have been described so far help the practitioner to respond to the following questions: What is this person's current occupational situation? What can be done to enhance the person's situation? Ethical reasoning goes one step further and asks: What should be done? Rogers (1983) framed these three questions (here paraphrased) in her Eleanor Clark Slagle Lecture and went on to state, "The clinical reasoning process terminates in an ethical decision, rather than a scientific one, and the ethical nature of the goal of clinical reasoning projects itself over the entire sequence" (p. 602). In the case study, Terry's ethical dilemma is to understand Mrs. Munro's personal wishes and to honor them when developing a therapy plan that realistically addresses Mrs. Munro's limitations. This can be particularly challenging when the pressures of financial realities (such as Mrs. Munro's limited income and the lack of insurance for supported living) come up against concerns for safety or similar therapy concerns. Several OT authors have addressed the ethical aspect of professional reasoning (Fondiller, Rosage, & Neuhaus, 1990; Howard, 1991; Neuhaus, 1988; Peloquin, 1993), and Chapter 36 of this text is devoted to the issue of the ethics of the profession. The purpose here is to introduce ethical reasoning as yet another of the components of professional reasoning in OT.

Interactive Reasoning

The provision of therapy is inherently a communicative process (Schwartzberg, 2002). In OT, practitioners must gain the trust of their clients and of people who are important in the clients' world. This is because OT involves "doing with" as opposed to "doing to" clients (Mattingly & Fleming, 1994, p. 178). A therapist gains this trust by entering the client's life world (Crepeau, 1991) and by using several interpersonal strategies that are designed to motivate clients. These include advocating, collaborating, empathizing, encouraging, instructing, and problem solving (Taylor, Lee, & Kielhofner, 2011), each of which is discussed more in Chapter 37. Once they are in the client's life world, OT practitioners can better understand how to help the individuals resolve performance problems. This form of therapist reasoning is referred to as *interactive reasoning* and is considered important to the OT process (Copley, Turpin, Brosnan, & Nelson, 2008).

It is likely that some reasoning focused on interaction is conscious, as when a practitioner remembers that "I need to be sure to praise the client often because he gets discouraged so easily." Other interpersonal acts might be quite automatic, such as when a therapist touches a person's arm to convey sympathy. It is sometimes easiest to detect the importance of effective interactive reasoning when the therapist makes a mistake or gets an unexpected reaction and is forced to regroup and rebuild the therapy relationship.

A Process of Synthesis in Shared Activity

The preceding section described commonly accepted aspects of professional reasoning separately to illustrate the different parts of the process. Table 34-1 includes examples of the kinds of questions that practitioners seek to answer with the different aspects of professional reasoning. As you read these, keep in mind that you can't characterize these by watching someone. You have to ask practitioners what they were thinking, as one person may perceive something as a purely technical problem requiring a "scientific solution" and thus responds with scientific reasoning, whereas another may frame it as one requiring attention to therapist–client collaboration and focus more on interactive reasoning.

Furthermore, these facets of reasoning are not separate or parallel processes; rather, the opposite appears to be the case. Virtually all the research about reasoning in practice suggest that these different forms interact and overlap with each other (Carrier et al., 2010; Mitchell & Unsworth, 2005). Furthermore, Toth-Cohen (2008) makes the point that the "shared activity" that occurs during the therapy process is an "integral part" of the reasoning process (p. 82).

Reasoning to Solve Problems

Scientific, narrative, pragmatic, ethical, and interactive reasoning processes are intertwined throughout the therapy process. Indeed, each perspective informs the other. In the case study, Terry's understanding of medical science helped her to know what might be the potential impairments and performance problems, but her narrative reasoning helped her to understand the importance to Mrs. Munro of returning home. Put together, these two forms of reasoning help Terry to reach an unspoken understanding that there would be a high risk for depression (which could worsen her client's medical condition) if Mrs. Munro did

not return to her home, which means so much to her. Furthermore, the practical constraints associated with the setting and Mrs. Munro's reimbursement prompted Terry to reason about the ethics of suggesting that she return home alone (where she might not be safe), consider more alternative supported living (which she may not want and probably can't afford), and finally of recommending that she return home with the support of home health care and neighbors.

Conditional Process

Not only must practitioners blend different aspects of reasoning in order to interact effectively with their clients but also they must flexibly modify interventions in response to changing conditions and to the context in which the therapy is occurring. Terry showed her flexibility by inventing an activity with the flower vase when her plan to work with Mrs. Munro on bathing and dressing did not pan out. Creighton and colleagues (1995) noticed that OT practitioners preplanned interventions in a hierarchical manner. They observed that practitioners typically brought several sets of supplies to an intervention session. One set would be directed to the expected level of performance, and the others to a stage higher and a stage lower than the expected performance. As an example, one practitioner, in preparation for a writing activity with a client who had a spinal cord injury, brought a short writing splint and unlined paper. This practitioner also brought a longer splint to provide wrist support (in case the client's hand control was worse than expected) and lined paper, which required more precision (in case the hand control was better than expected). This practitioner blended scientific and pragmatic concerns in a way that anticipated several possible situations that might occur.

On a larger scale, Fleming (1994a) described the ability of skilled OT practitioners to "form an image of future life possibilities for the person" (p. 234). The ability to form these images (or schemata, to use a cognitive terms) seems to require a blend of all the forms of clinical reasoning, along with sufficient clinical experience to have seen various different outcomes with former clients. These images help practitioners to select therapeutic activities on a day-to-day basis. For instance, the writing activity for the client who had a spinal cord injury not only is a good activity for increasing coordination but also presages occupations that will enable the client to regain control of his life through writing his own checks, signing his name on legal documents, and using various forms of technology for work and play. If this client were an accountant, these would be powerful images. Conversely, if the client were a professional athlete, the OT practitioner might have to create different activities to allow the client to develop a vision of himself as a future coach or teacher. The activities that are used in OT can help to meet specific short-term goals and shape long-term expectations. It is in this way that practitioners help individuals to reengage in their lives through the use of meaningful occupations.

Ecological View of Professional Reasoning

Units I, II, IV, and V contain many chapters which discuss how occupational performance is the result of complex transactions among a person's inherent capacities, the person's prior experiences, and the demands of the performance context. Similarly, the professional reasoning process and the resulting therapy actions represent transactions that occur among the practitioner, the client, the therapy context, and the actual therapy activity (Toth-Cohen, 2008; Unsworth & Schell, 2006). Schell (2018a) synthesized these many factors associated with professional reasoning into the Ecological Model of Professional Reasoning (Schell, 2018a) which is described here. Key assumptions of the model are shown in Box 34-1.

The practitioner's reasoning is shaped by both personal and professional perspectives as shown in Figure 34-1.

BOX 34-1   KEY ASSUMPTION OF SCHELL'S ECOLOGICAL MODEL OF PROFESSIONAL REASONING

The overarching assumption is that *professional reasoning is an ecological process that involves multiple therapist, client, and context factors.* Additional assumptions include the following:

1. Occupational therapy is a co-constructed process between the therapist and the client.
2. What actually happens in therapy is the result of a transaction among the therapist, the client, and the practice context.
3. There are a number of personal and practice context factors that influence professional reasoning, the client, and the therapy process. Some of these factors are known to the participants and some are tacit or unknown.
4. Therapy outcomes are affected by this nexus of factors, along with the nature of the occupational performance/participation problem, and the client's therapy-related actions outside of therapy.

Each practitioner brings to the therapy situation knowledge and skills that are grounded in life experiences, including personal characteristics such as physical capacities, personality, values, and beliefs that comprise their personal gestalt. These form a *personal* self that consist of the person's embodied characteristics along with their interpretation of the experiences or worldview. These personal factors shape each person's perception and interpretation of all life activities, and thus act as a *personal lens* through which each practitioner views all life events. Layered over or entwined with this personal self is the *professional self*, which includes the therapist's professional knowledge from education, experiences from prior clients, and beliefs about what is important to do in therapy along with knowledge of specific technical skills and therapy routines. Thus, a therapist views therapy situations through both a personal and *professional lens*, which over time likely merge into the therapist's customary ways of viewing the therapy process. The personal and professional selves act in concert to respond to various problems of practice.

Just as with the therapist, the client (also depicted in Figure 34-1) comes to therapy with his or her own life experiences and personal characteristics, life situation, and performance problems that prompted the need for therapy. The client may also come with his or her own theories about what is causing the performance problems, past experiences with therapy and health care, along with what to expect from the therapy process. The therapist and the client come together in a practice context to engage in therapy, as shown in Figure 34-2.

Because this therapy is happening in a finite time and place, it is inherently a process that is imbedded in the setting in which it occurs, called here the *practice context*. The practice context includes both physical and sociocultural aspects that influence therapy options. Examples might include outpatient medical setting, a client's home, or a student's classroom. Each of these settings shapes the therapy tools available as well as the rules or social and organizational expectations about what should occur. Other factors in the practice context include time, physical resources, social environment, caseload size and characteristics, and payment and discharge options.

The therapist and the client engage in therapy activities together within the practice context. These specific actors, working in the specific context, shape the nature, scope, and trajectory of the therapy process. Thus, professional reasoning is not just what occurs in the therapist's body–mind; it is an ecological process that comes together in a therapy activity that represents the transaction among the therapist, the client, and the therapy setting (Carrier et al., 2010; Schell, 2018a; Toth-Cohen, 2008; Unsworth, 2011). At different times, different aspects of this system will have greater influence on what will occur. Reflective therapists are encouraged

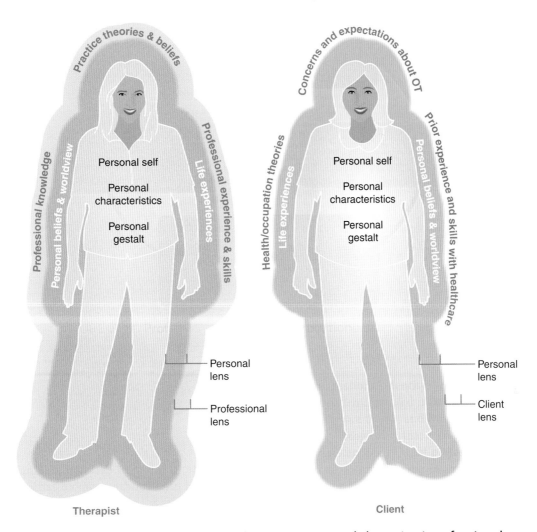

FIGURE 34-1 **Personal and professional lenses shape occupational therapists' professional reasoning.**

to be mindful of all these factors and their influence on their reasoning and associated therapy actions and therapy outcomes.

Developing and Improving Professional Reasoning

Understanding the complexity of professional reasoning helps students and practitioners alike to appreciate why it takes so long to truly become an excellent practitioner. Research shows that it typically takes a minimum of 10 years for individuals to gain expertise within a given field (Boshuizen & Schmidt, 2000), although some studies in OT show differing expertise levels showing up as early as 5 years (Rassafiani, Ziviani, Rodger, & Dalgleish, 2009). Although experience is necessary, experience alone is not sufficient to ensure advancement in clinical reasoning skills. Therapists must reflect on that experience in order to gain expertise.

Reflection in Practice

Schön (1983) proffered the term *reflective practitioner* to describe how experts think critically about their own experience. Reflection happens in two ways. First, practitioners "reflect in action" (Schön, 1983, p. 49). This involves the practitioners' ability to think in the midst of action and adapt to meet the demands of the situation. Reflection in action most often occurs when the usual approaches are not working. "Reflection on action" (Schön, 1983, p. 61) is the term Schön uses for critical thinking that occurs after the fact. Reflection about practice, identifying what worked and what did not, and being open to alternative conceptions are necessary to support the learning associated with advancing expertise. As described in Chapters 35 and 41, the use of research evidence to inform practice and the

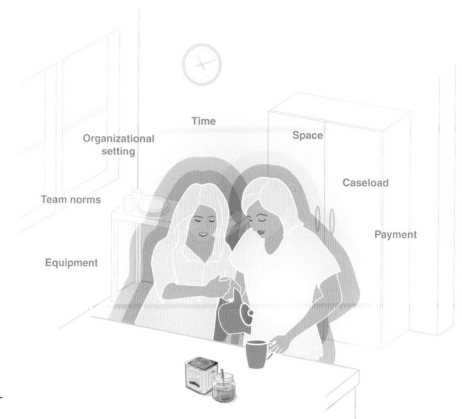

FIGURE 34-2 Schell's Ecological Model of Professional Reasoning. Professional reasoning is an ecological process in which the therapist and the client engage in therapy activities in a specific setting. All of these components transact to shape therapist reasoning, resulting actions with the client, and ultimately, therapy outcomes.

application of formal theories along with systematic observation and data collection are important to reflection and, thus, to expert professional reasoning.

Expertise Continuum

There is a slowly growing body of evidence about the nature of professional reasoning in OT. Dreyfus and Dreyfus's (1986) conceptualization of professional expertise has been applied to OT (Slater & Cohn, 1991) and elaborated on over time by several researchers, although often, the research dichotomizes beginners or novices from experts. Table 34-2 summarizes changes that have surfaced in research about the reasoning of occupational therapists as they develop expertise. Although the changes that are listed in Table 34-2 are associated with typical years of experience, it is important to recognize that development is dynamic and influenced by many factors beyond just the years of experience. One important consideration is the familiarity of the task and the context. Expertise is a function of how consistently a person is effective within a given context (Benner, 1984; Rassafiani et al., 2009; Toth-Cohen, 2008). Someone who demonstrates expertise at providing services in a school setting might be just minimally competent in a nursing home setting. Additionally, active reflection about one's experiences is critical to becoming an expert (Benner, 1984; Gambrill, 2012; Slater & Cohn, 1991). Recent research also suggests that the use

of systematic training in decision making relevant to a given type of problem can promote earlier acquisition of expertise (Harries & Tomlinson, 2012). Refer to Chapter 70 for more discussion about professional development, continuing competence, and expertise.

Conclusion

Professional reasoning is the process that practitioners use to plan, direct, perform, and reflect on client care. It is an embodied multisensory process that requires complex cognitive activity. Practitioners develop cognitive frames and scripts as they gain experience, forming the basis of professional knowledge and action. Professional reasoning is multifaceted and enables practitioners to understand client issues from different perspectives. Practitioners use the logical processes associated with scientific reasoning to understand the client's impairments, disabilities, and performance contexts and to predict the impact these have on occupational performance. Narrative reasoning helps practitioners to appreciate the meaning of occupational performance limitations to the client, thus supporting client-centered care. Practitioners use pragmatic reasoning when they address the practical realities associated with service delivery. All of these forms of reasoning lead to an ethical reasoning process by which practitioners select the best therapy action to respond to the client's occupational performance needs.

TABLE 34-2	Professional Reasoning Continuum and Characteristics	
Category and Reflective Experience	**Characteristics**
Novice (no experience in practice area)	• No experience in situation of practice; depends on theory to guide practice • Uses rule-based procedural reasoning to guide actions but does not recognize contextual cues; not skillful in adapting rules to fit situation • Narrative reasoning is used to establish social relationships but does not significantly inform practice. • Pragmatic reasoning is stressed in terms of job survival skills. • Recognizes overt ethical issues
Advanced beginner (<1 yr)	• Begins to incorporate contextual information into rule-based thinking • Recognizes differences between theoretical expectations and presenting problems • Limited experience impedes recognition of patterns and salient cues; does not prioritize well • Relies on external guides so as forms to guide reasoning • Gaining skill in pragmatic and narrative reasoning • Begins to recognize more subtle ethical issues
Competent (1–3 yr)	• Automatically performs more therapeutic skills and attends to more issues • Is able to develop communal horizon with people receiving service • Is able to sort relevant data and prioritize intervention goals related to desired outcomes • Planning is deliberate, efficient, and responsive to contextual issues. • Uses conditional reasoning to modify intervention but lacks flexibility • Recognizes ethical dilemmas posed by practice setting
Proficient (3–5 yr)	• Perceives situations as wholes • Reflects on expanded range of experiences, permitting more focused evaluation and more flexibility in intervention • Creatively combines different diagnostic and procedural approaches • More attentive to occupational stories and relevance for intervention • More skillful in negotiating resources to meet patient/client needs • Increased sophistication in recognizing situational nature of ethical reasoning
Expert (5–10 yr)	• Clinical reasoning becomes a quick intuitive process • Procedural and pragmatic reasoning more detailed • Able to flow conversation and action smoothly • Uses understanding of client and client's perspective to determine intervention • Relies on internal guides or images to support actions

From Benner (1984); Clark et al. (1996); Creighton et al. (1995); Dreyfus and Dreyfus (1986); Mattingly and Fleming (1994); Rassafiani et al. (2009); Slater and Cohn (1991); Strong et al. (1995); Unsworth (2001); and Mitchell and Unsworth (2005).

The process of professional reasoning involves a transaction among the practitioner's personal and professional perspectives, the client's perspectives, and the demands of the practice context that unfolds in therapy activities. Expertise develops as the practitioner gains experience and reflects on that experience for deeper understanding.

Acknowledgment

Selected portions of this chapter are from B. A. Schell & J. W. Schell (Eds.) *Clinical and professional reasoning in occupational therapy* (2nd ed., pp. 3–12). Philadelphia, PA: Lippincott Williams & Wilkins.

REFERENCES

Auzmendia, A. L., de las Heras, C. G., Kielhofner, G., & Miranda, C. (2008). Recrafting occupational narratives. In G. Kielhofner (Ed.), *Model of human occupation* (4th ed., pp. 313–336). Baltimore, MD: Lippincott Williams & Wilkins.

Barris, R. (1987). Clinical reasoning in psychosocial occupational therapy: The evaluation process. *Occupational Therapy Journal of Research, 7*, 147–162.

Benner, P. (1984). *From novice to expert*. Menlo Park, CA: Addison-Wesley.

Boshuizen, H. P. A., & Schmidt, H. G. (2000). The development of clinical reasoning expertise. In J. Higgs & M. Jones (Eds.), *Clinical reasoning in the health professions* (2nd ed., pp. 15–22). Boston, MA: Butterworth Heinemann.

Bruning, R. H., Schraw, G. J., & Ronning, R. R. (1999). *Cognitive psychology and instruction* (3rd ed.). Upper Saddle River, NJ: Merrill.

Carr, M., & Shotwell, M. (2018). Information processing theory and professional reasoning. In B. A. B. Schell & J. W. Schell (Eds.), *Clinical and professional reasoning in occupational therapy* (2nd ed., pp. 73–104). Philadelphia, PA: Wolters Kluwer.

Carrier, A., Levasseur, M., Bédard, D., & Desrosiers, J. (2010). Community occupational therapists' clinical reasoning: Identifying tacit knowledge. *Australian Occupational Therapy Journal, 57*, 356–365.

Clark, F., Ennevor, B. L., & Richardson, P. L. (1996). A grounded theory of techniques for occupational storytelling and occupational story making. In R. Zemke & F. Clark (Eds.), *Occupational science: The evolving discipline* (pp. 373–392). Philadelphia, PA: F. A. Davis.

Cohn, E. S. (1989). Fieldwork education: Shaping a foundation for clinical reasoning. *American Journal of Occupational Therapy, 43*, 240–244.

Cohn, E. S. (1991). Explicating complexity. *American Journal of Occupational Therapy, 45*, 969–971.

Copley, J., Nelson, A., Turpin, M., Underwood, K., & Flanigan, K. (2008). Factors influencing therapists' interventions for children with learning difficulties. *Canadian Journal of Occupational Therapy, 75*, 105–113.

Copley, J., Turpin, M., Brosnan, J., & Nelson, A. (2008). Understanding and negotiating: Reasoning processes used by an occupational therapist to individualize intervention decisions for people with upper limb hypertonicity. *Disability and Rehabilitation, 30*, 1486–1498.

Creighton, C., Dijkers, M., Bennett, N., & Brown, K. (1995). Reasoning and the art of therapy for spinal cord injury. *American Journal of Occupational Therapy, 49*, 311–317.

Crepeau, E. B. (1991). Achieving intersubjective understanding: Examples from an occupational therapy treatment session. *American Journal of Occupational Therapy, 45*, 1016–1025.

Dougherty, D. A., Toth-Cohen, S. E., & Tomlin, G. S. (2016). Beyond research literature: Occupational therapists' perspectives on and uses of "evidence" in everyday practice. *Canadian Journal of Occupational Therapy, 83*, 288–296.

Dreyfus, H. L., & Dreyfus, S. E. (1986). *Mind over machine: The power of human intuition and expertise in the era of the computer.* New York, NY: Free Press.

Fleming, M. H. (1991). The therapist with the three-track mind. *American Journal of Occupational Therapy, 45*, 1007–1014.

Fleming, M. H. (1994a). Conditional reasoning: Creating meaningful experiences. In C. Mattingly & M. H. Fleming (Eds.), *Clinical reasoning: Forms of inquiry in a therapeutic practice* (pp. 197–235). Philadelphia, PA: F. A. Davis.

Fleming, M. H. (1994b). Procedural reasoning: Addressing functional limitations. In C. Mattingly & M. H. Fleming (Eds.), *Clinical reasoning: Forms of inquiry in a therapeutic practice* (pp. 137–177). Philadelphia, PA: F. A. Davis.

Fleming, M. H. (1994c). The search for tacit knowledge. In C. Mattingly & M. H. Fleming (Eds.), *Clinical reasoning: Forms of inquiry in a therapeutic practice* (pp. 22–33). Philadelphia, PA: F. A. Davis.

Fondiller, E. D., Rosage, L. J., & Neuhaus, B. E. (1990). Values influencing clinical reasoning in occupational therapy: An exploratory study. *Occupational Therapy Journal of Research, 10*, 41–55.

Gambrill, E. (2012). *Critical thinking in clinical practice: Improving the quality of judgments and decisions* (3rd ed.). San Francisco, CA: Jossey-Bass.

Gray, J. M. (1998). Putting occupation into practice: Occupation as ends, occupation as means. *American Journal of Occupational Therapy, 52*, 354–364.

Hamilton, T. B. (2018). Narrative reasoning. In B. A. B. Schell & J. W. Schell (Eds.), *Clinical and professional reasoning in occupational therapy* (2nd ed., pp. 171–202). Philadelphia, PA: Wolters Kluwer.

Harries, P. A., & Tomlinson, C. (2012). Teaching young dogs new tricks: Improving occupational therapists' referral prioritization capacity with a web-based decision-training aid. *Scandinavian Journal of Occupational therapy, 19*, 542–546. doi:10.3109/11038128.2012.693945

Holm, M. B. (2000). The 2000 Eleanor Clarke Slagle Lecture. Our mandate for the new millennium: Evidence-based practice. *American Journal of Occupational Therapy, 54*, 575–585.

Holmqvist, K., Kamwendo, K., & Ivarsson, A. B. (2009). Occupational therapists' descriptions of their work with persons suffering from cognitive impairment following acquired brain injury. *Scandinavian Journal of Occupational Therapy, 16*, 12–24.

Hooper, B. (1997). The relationship between pretheoretical assumptions and clinical reasoning. *American Journal of Occupational Therapy, 51*, 328–338.

Hooper, B. (2018). Therapists' assumptions as a dimension of professional reasoning. In B. A. B. Schell & J. W. Schell (Eds.), *Clinical and professional reasoning in occupational therapy* (2nd ed., pp. 51–72). Philadelphia, PA: Wolters Kluwer.

Howard, B. S. (1991). How high do we jump? The effect of reimbursement on occupational therapy. *American Journal of Occupational Therapy, 45*, 875–881.

Kessels, J. P. A. M., & Korthagen, F. A. (1996). The relationship between theory and practice: Back to the classics. *Educational Researcher, 25*, 17–22.

Kielhofner, G., & Forsyth, K. (2002). Thinking with theory: A framework for therapeutic reasoning. In G. Kielhofner (Ed.), *A model of human occupation: Theory and application* (3rd ed., pp. 162–178). Baltimore, MD: Lippincott Williams & Wilkins.

Kinsella, E. A. (2018). Embodied reasoning in professional practice. In B. A. B. Schell & J. W. Schell (Eds.), *Clinical and professional reasoning in occupational therapy* (2nd ed., pp. 105–124). Philadelphia, PA: Wolters Kluwer.

Law, M., & MacDermid, J. (Eds.). (2008). *Evidence based rehabilitation: A guide to practice* (2nd ed.). Thorofare, NJ: SLACK.

Lyons, K. D., & Crepeau, E. B. (2001). The clinical reasoning of an occupational therapy assistant. *American Journal of Occupational Therapy, 55*, 577–581.

Mattingly, C. (1994a). Acknowledgments. In C. Mattingly & M. H. Fleming (Eds.), *Clinical reasoning: Forms of inquiry in a therapeutic practice* (pp. ix–xii). Philadelphia, PA: F. A. Davis.

Mattingly, C. (1994b). Occupational therapy as a two-body practice: The body as machine. In C. Mattingly & M. H. Fleming (Eds.), *Clinical reasoning: Forms of inquiry in a therapeutic practice* (pp. 37–63). Philadelphia, PA: F. A. Davis.

Mattingly, C. (1994c). The narrative nature of clinical reasoning. In C. Mattingly & M. H. Fleming (Eds.), *Clinical reasoning: Forms of inquiry in a therapeutic practice* (pp. 239–269). Philadelphia, PA: F. A. Davis.

Mattingly, C., & Fleming, M. H. (1994). Interactive reasoning: Collaborating with the person. In C. Mattingly & M. H. Fleming (Eds.), *Clinical reasoning: Forms of inquiry in a therapeutic practice* (pp. 178–196). Philadelphia, PA: F. A. Davis.

Mitchell, R., & Unsworth, C. A. (2005). Clinical reasoning during community health home visits: Expert and novice differences. *British Journal of Occupational Therapy, 68*, 215–223.

Neuhaus, B. E. (1988). Ethical considerations in clinical reasoning: The impact of technology and cost containment. *American Journal of Occupational Therapy, 42*, 288–294.

Norman, G. (2005). Research in clinical reasoning: Past history and current trends. *Medical Education, 39*, 418–427.

Parham, D. (1987). Toward professionalism: The reflective therapist. *American Journal of Occupational Therapy, 41*, 555–561.

Pelland, M. J. (1987). A conceptual model for the instruction and supervision of treatment planning. *American Journal of Occupational Therapy, 41*, 351–359.

Peloquin, S. M. (1993). The depersonalization of patients: A profile gleaned from narratives. *American Journal of Occupational Therapy, 47*, 830–837.

Rassafiani, M., Ziviani, J., Rodger, S., & Dalgleish, L. (2009). Identification of occupational therapy clinical expertise: Decision-making characteristics. *Australian Occupational Therapy Journal, 56*, 156–166.

Roberts, A. E. (1996). Clinical reasoning in occupational therapy: Idiosyncrasies in content and process. *British Journal of Occupational Therapy, 59*, 372–376.

Rogers, J. C. (1983). Eleanor Clarke Slagle Lectureship—1983; clinical reasoning: The ethics, science, and art. *American Journal of Occupational Therapy, 37,* 601–616.

Rogers, J. C., & Holm, M. B. (1991). Occupational therapy diagnostic reasoning: A component of clinical reasoning. *American Journal of Occupational Therapy, 45,* 1045–1053.

Schell, B. A. B. (1994). *The effect of practice context on occupational therapy practitioner's clinical reasoning* (Doctoral dissertation, University of Georgia, 1994). Dissertation Abstracts International, AAT 9507243.

Schell, B. A. B. (2018a). An ecological model of professional reasoning. In B. A. B. Schell & J. W. Schell (Eds.), *Clinical and professional reasoning in occupational therapy* (2nd ed., pp. 23–49). Philadelphia, PA: Wolters Kluwer.

Schell, B. A. B. (2018b). Pragmatic reasoning. In B. A. B. Schell & J. W. Schell (Eds.), *Clinical and professional reasoning in occupational therapy* (2nd ed., pp. 203–223). Philadelphia, PA: Wolters Kluwer.

Schell, B. A. B., & Cervero, R. M. (1993). Clinical reasoning in occupational therapy: An integrative review. *American Journal of Occupational Therapy, 47,* 605–610.

Schell, B. A. B., & Schell, J. W. (2018). *Clinical and professional reasoning in occupational therapy* (2nd ed.). Philadelphia, PA: Wolters Kluwer.

Schön, D. A. (1983). *The reflective practitioner: How professionals think in action.* New York, NY: Basic Books.

Schwartzberg, S. (2002). *Interactive reasoning in the practice of occupational therapy.* Upper Saddle River, NJ: Prentice Hall.

Sinclair, K. (2007). Exploring facets of clinical reasoning. In J. Creek & A. Lawson-Porter (Eds.), *Contemporary issues in occupational therapy: Reasoning and reflection* (pp. 143–160). Chichester, United Kingdom: Wiley.

Slater, D. Y., & Cohn, E. S. (1991). Staff development through analysis of practice. *American Journal of Occupational Therapy, 45,* 1038–1044.

Strong, J., Gilbert, J., Cassidy, S., & Bennett, S. (1995). Expert clinicians' and students' views on clinical reasoning in occupational therapy. *British Journal of Occupational Therapy, 58,* 119–123.

Taylor, R., Lee, S. W., & Kielhofner, G. (2011). Practitioners' use of interpersonal modes within the therapeutic relationship: Results from a nationwide study. *OTJR: Occupation, Participation and Health, 31,* 6–14. doi:10.3928/15394492-20100521-02

Tickle-Degnen, L. (2000). Evidence-based practice forum: Gathering current research evidence to enhance clinical reasoning. *American Journal of Occupational Therapy, 54,* 102–105.

Tomlin, G. (2008). Scientific reasoning. In B. A. B. Schell & J. W. Schell (Eds.), *Clinical and professional reasoning in occupational therapy.* Baltimore, MD: Lippincott Williams & Wilkins.

Tomlin, G. (2018). Scientific reasoning. In B. A. B. Schell & J. W. Schell (Eds.), *Clinical and professional reasoning in occupational therapy* (2nd ed., pp. 145–169). Philadelphia, PA: Wolters Kluwer.

Toth-Cohen, S. (2008). Using cultural-historical activity theory to study clinical reasoning in context. *Scandinavian Journal of Occupational Therapy, 15,* 82–94.

Unsworth, C. A. (2001). The clinical reasoning of novice and expert occupational therapists. *Scandinavian Journal of Occupational Therapy, 8,* 163–173.

Unsworth, C. A. (2005). Using a head-mounted video camera to explore current conceptualizations of clinical reasoning in occupational therapy. *American Journal of Occupational Therapy, 59,* 31–40.

Unsworth, C. A. (2011). The evolving theory of clinical reasoning. In E. A. S. Duncan (Ed.), *Foundations for practice in occupational therapy* (5th ed., pp. 209–231). New York, NY: Elsevier.

Unsworth, C. A. (2012). The evolving theory of clinical reasoning. In E. A. S. Duncan (Ed.), *Foundations for practice in occupational therapy* (5th ed., pp. 209–231). Edinburgh, United Kingdom: Churchill Livingstone Elsevier.

Unsworth, C. A., & Baker, A. (2016). A systematic review of professional reasoning literature in occupational therapy. *British Journal of Occupational Therapy, 79,* 5–16.

Unsworth, C. A., & Schell, B. A. (2006, July). *Clinical reasoning: Development of a theory-in-use.* Proceedings of the 14th International Congress of the World Federation of Occupational Therapists, Sydney, Australia.

*the***Point**°   *For additional resources on the subjects discussed in this chapter, visit* http://thePoint.lww.com /Willard-Spackman13e.

Evidence-Based Practice

Integrating Evidence to Inform Practice

Nancy Baker, Linda Tickle-Degnen

LEARNING OBJECTIVES

After reading this chapter, you will be able to:

1. Define evidence-based practice and how it is integrated into clinical practice.
2. Describe how to organize evidence around clinical tasks.
3. Name the basic steps of evidence-based practice.
4. Write answerable questions for different clinical tasks.
5. Identify key methods for searching research literature effectively.
6. Describe how to appraise the clinical relevance and trustworthiness of a research report.
7. Describe how to interpret the results of a study for generalizability and clinical importance.
8. Describe qualities of effective communication about evidence.

Introduction

Let's imagine a hypothetical occupational therapy (OT) student, Rhonda. Rhonda has been assigned Judy, who has rheumatoid arthritis (RA). Judy is not only a new client to Rhonda but also her first client, and one with an unfamiliar diagnosis. Rhonda discusses Judy with her supervisor to receive expert guidance and then looks over Judy's chart to orient herself to Judy's medical problem and current interventions. Judy has had RA for 2 years; she has recently experienced a decline in function and increase in hand pain. Rhonda completes a biomechanical assessment of Judy's impairments and talks with her about her goals. She identifies that Judy has mild structural deformities of the hand that limit occupational tasks requiring intensive hand use such as typing and housework. Judy has decreased hand strength and reports that pain is increasingly problematic. Rhonda identifies goals related to reducing pain, increasing hand strength, and improving activities of daily living (ADL) performance. She initiates a strengthening and pain management program but feels frustrated about identifying methods to teach techniques that will enable Judy and others like her to continue progressing at home. None of her colleagues have any suggestions of an educational program that may be effective post therapy.

NOTES

Evidence-Based Practice in Occupational Therapy

The concept of evidence-based practice (EBP) as the best method to inform practice is relatively new. Most medical practice prior to EBP, including OT, was eminence-based practice: experts, usually senior personnel, determined practice parameters. The term *evidence-based medicine* was first used in 1991 by Sackett and his colleagues at McMaster University in Canada (Sur & Dahm, 2011). Throughout the 1990s, this term grew to mean the critical appraisal of the literature as well as methods of incorporating evidence into everyday decision making. One of the earliest discussions of EBP in OT was in 1997 when the *British Journal of Occupational Therapy* published an issue on EBP. The *Canadian Journal of Occupational Therapy* followed shortly with its own issue about EBP in 1998. Both issues discussed the need for and ramifications of EBP in OT. The *American Journal of Occupational Therapy* started publishing articles describing methods of EBP in 1998 (Tickle-Degnen, 1998). Holm (2000) further reinforced the need for EBP when she identified EBP as a necessary and ethical requirement of OT practice in her 2000 Slagle lecture. Willard & Spackman was not far behind in its promotion of EBP to OT students. The first chapter discussing EBP was published in 2003 (Bailey, 2003). Although EBP in OT is only about 20 years old, it has fundamentally changed the face of OT.

This chapter demonstrates how **evidence-based practice** might create a different scenario for working with a client like Judy (Shin, Randolph, & Rauch, 2010). Rhonda recognized that she needed information or evidence to guide her provision of OT services to Judy. The forms of evidence that she used to inform her work with Judy were expert opinion, medical records about tests and interventions conducted with Judy, information from Judy herself, and direct observation of Judy's wrist function. Rhonda did not seek out or use evidence from research studies to inform her practice with Judy, the type of evidence meant in the term *evidence-based practice*. This chapter describes how evidence from research studies can be put into practice consistently and in a manner that enriches the contributions of OT and the outcomes of clients.

The Evidence-Based Practitioner

Implementing evidence-based practice is a priority within OT practice (Lin, Murphy, & Robinson, 2010). Because evidence-based practice has been associated with better outcomes (Shin et al., 2010), it has already started to affect daily practice, reimbursement, and policy. The shift to evidence-based practice started in the early 1990s. Health care practitioners realized that traditional information sources used in practice (textbooks, experts, and continuing education) were often out of date, ineffective, or just plain wrong (Straus, Glasziou, Richardson, & Haynes, 2011). In its earliest years, evidence-based practice focused on finding experimental studies and analyzing them to determine their credibility based on the validity of the study design and scientific rigor. If the experimental evidence was credible, "best evidence," it was used to determine practice. Practitioners placed little emphasis on clinical decision making (Shin et al., 2010). This original definition was predicated on the idea that the evidence was undeniably applicable to a medical situation, so that the translation from the evidence to the real world of the clinic was relatively straightforward. However, as clinicians have struggled with using evidence to make appropriate decisions for individual patients, a more pragmatic definition of evidence-based practice has emerged (Shin et al., 2010). This pragmatic approach uses evidence as part of a clinical decision-making process that also takes into consideration the relevance of the evidence to the treatment environment and the individual clients' values and circumstances (Mayer, 2010). These latter two areas are as important as the evidence in the decision-making process. Although evidence may support a treatment, if the environment lacks resources for the therapist and client to engage in that treatment, the treatment remains nonviable. In a like manner, even if the evidence supports a treatment but does not match a client's values and circumstances, it will not constitute client-centered practice—a cornerstone of OT. Thus, evidence-based practice is composed of three equal core components: (1) the current best evidence, (2) the treatment environment, and (3) each client's values and circumstances (Shin et al., 2010), which, in combination with a clinician's expertise, aid in clinical decision making. Figure 35-1 provides a schematic of the interaction between client, clinician, evidence, and environment representative of the current thinking about evidence-based

Organizing Evidence around Central Clinical Tasks

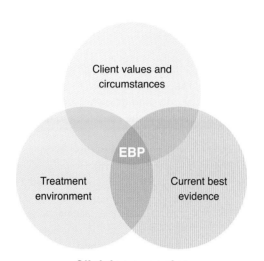

Client values and circumstances

EBP

Treatment environment

Current best evidence

Clinician expertise

FIGURE 35-1 Interaction between the elements of clinical decision making in evidence-based practice.

practice (Mayer, 2010; Shin et al., 2010). Although it is generally understood that occupational therapists are skilled in providing clinical expertise, understanding their clinical environment, and identifying client values and circumstances, their skill is more likely to be deficient in identifying "current best evidence."

Imagine yourself just about to meet the Judy of Rhonda's clinical experience. As an evidence-based practitioner, you would use scientific reasoning along with the current best evidence from research studies to support central clinical tasks, such as the selection of appropriate and valid assessment procedures, interventions, and procedures for monitoring clinical progress (Law & MacDermid, 2014; Straus et al., 2011). In evidence-based practice, research evidence does not replace reasoning that is informed by clinical experience, theory, core values of practice, and ethics. Nor does the use of research evidence replace the clinical use of information derived from observing clients and talking with their family members or from consulting with experts and peers. Evidence-based clinical reasoning involves the use of all forms of evidence in the pursuit of optimal client outcomes. It is the integration of scientific reasoning with reasoning that has been matured by clinical experience, validated practice theory, and client-centered values and ethics (Lee & Miller, 2003; Rappolt, 2003).

Table 35-1 shows how, you, the evidence-based practitioner, could organize the search for and interpret evidence around central clinical tasks, in general, and, specifically, with respect to Judy. One of the first clinical tasks that the practitioner faces in working with a client is *getting*

TABLE 35-1   Organizing Evidence around Clinical Tasks with Judy

Central Clinical Task	Research Evidence	Relevant Research Designs	Use of Evidence for Judy's Case
I. Get to know a client *a. Background*	Typical occupational experiences and needs of clients from populations who can be compared to Judy	Descriptive and exploratory research 1. Qualitative studies 2. Case series 3. Cohort studies 4. Cross-sectional studies	Generate a discussion with Judy about her own occupational experiences and needs in comparison with the research samples.
b. Diagnosis	Quality (e.g., reliability, validity, trustworthiness, usefulness) of occupational assessment procedures	Exploratory research that evaluate assessment tools 1. Cross-sectional studies 2. Case-control studies	Select the best assessment method to identify Judy's unique occupational experiences and needs.
II. Choose an effective treatment *Intervention*	Relative effectiveness of different types of treatments designed for this population	Experimental and exploratory research 1. Randomized clinical trials 2. Quasi-experimental studies 3. *N* of 1 studies 4. Cohort studies	Select, ideally in collaboration with Judy, potentially beneficial interventions.
III. Estimate the probable outcomes *Prognosis*	Based on factors such as comorbidities, previous and present circumstances identify the outcomes most commonly occurring for these populations	Exploratory and descriptive research 1. Cohort studies 2. Case-control studies 3. Case series	Assist with planning for discharge, training, and support services necessary for Judy.

to know the client. One aspect of getting to know a client is obtaining *background knowledge* about the client's disorder. Background knowledge provides basic information on the clinical nature of a disease (Mayer, 2010). It is often long-standing knowledge, and therefore, "current best evidence" may be readily available in textbooks or on credible Websites. The task of getting to know a client also involves gathering evidence that is descriptive of the experiences and needs of clients with the disorder in general (e.g., clients who have been research participants in published studies). Expert clinicians who have treated many people with a specific diagnosis may choose to forgo obtaining specific background information because their clinical expertise will already include pertinent information, but a novice clinician, such as Rhonda, should obtain background information before seeing a client. Research designs that would be relevant to this aspect of getting to know the client are **descriptive research**, such as **qualitative studies** and **case series**, and **exploratory research**, such as **cross-sectional studies** and **cohort studies**.

Background knowledge provides the foundation from which to develop treatment strategies, but it must be tempered with information coming from the specific client. **Diagnosis**, assessing the presence and degree of disorders and their effect on a client's current status with respect to occupational needs and status, is an important part of getting to know a client (Fritz & Wainner, 2001; Straus et al., 2011). Research on diagnostic studies tests the quality of assessment procedures for determining an individual client's unique experiences and needs. High-quality evidence on diagnostic tools ensures that services are relevant and beneficial, specifically for that person. Research designs that would be relevant to this task are exploratory research, such as cross-sectional studies and **case-control studies** (Oxford Centre for Evidence-Based Medicine Levels of Evidence Working Group, 2011).

With respect to Judy, descriptions of the occupational lives of women with RA or similar disorders that can affect the structural integrity of the hands could enhance your understanding of possible issues that Judy might face in her own life and could generate a discussion with Judy about her own life. Such a discussion might identify what specific types of in-depth information about Judy you want to learn in the assessment procedures. After targeting key areas to assess, you could go back to the research literature to find evidence about the **reliability** and **validity** of methods to select the most valuable methods for assessing those areas.

Another central clinical task is that of *choosing an effective treatment* approach and procedure for addressing the client's specific needs and goals. The research evidence that would be relevant to this task includes findings about the relative effectiveness of different types of interventions designed for individuals with a particular type of personal characteristic or health care condition. The task of choosing an effective intervention for a client involves gathering evidence that evaluates the **effectiveness** or **efficacy** of a type of intervention in comparison to alternative interventions or no intervention at all. Effectiveness evidence is published in studies that use an intervention or treatment research design or procedure. The most relevant research designs are **experimental research**, such as **randomized clinical trials (RCTs)**, **quasi-experimental studies**, and *N* **of 1 studies**, or exploratory research such as cohort studies (Oxford Centre for Evidence-Based Medicine Levels of Evidence Working Group, 2011). With respect to Judy, you could use **effectiveness evidence** about interventions designed for individuals with RA and similar disorders to select an appropriate intervention. In a client-centered approach, this selection would involve collaboration with Judy (Tickle-Degnen, 2002a).

A third central clinical task is *estimating the probable outcomes* based on variables such as the client age, history, comorbidities, symptoms, and response to treatment, often referred to as **prognosis** (Moons, Royston, Vergouwe, Grobbee, & Altman, 2009). This task assists the occupational therapist and patient to engage in long-range treatment planning as well as discharge planning, including additional therapies, home programs, education and training, and accessing resources. Relevant evidence tracks people over time and looks for relationships between baseline and long-term outcomes. The most relevant research designs are exploratory research, such as cohort studies and case-control studies, or descriptive research, such as case series (Oxford Centre for Evidence-Based Medicine Levels of Evidence Working Group, 2011).

For Judy, it would be important to identify the general prognosis of clients with RA. Prognosis in RA has actually changed in the last 10 years. Current prognostic evidence suggests that people with RA treated aggressively with disease-modifying antirheumatic drugs (DMARDs) and the appropriate biologic therapies, such as etanercept or adalimumab, are much less likely to experience the severe fixed deformities and significant joint degeneration experienced by previous generations of people with RA (Diffin et al., 2014). This shift in outcome makes it even more imperative that recent literature rather than textbooks or clinical experience be used to estimate prognosis.

The Steps of Evidence-Based Practice

Evidence-based practitioners systematically integrate research evidence into practice by carrying out a series of steps (Lin et al., 2010; Mayer, 2010; Straus et al., 2011; Taylor, 2017).

1. Writing an answerable clinical question
2. Gathering current published evidence that might answer the question

3. Appraising the gathered evidence to determine what is the "best" evidence for answering the question
4. Using the evidence to guide practice for individual clients by collaboratively communicating the results to patients

Step 1: Writing an Answerable Clinical Question

The first systematic step, writing an answerable question, helps the practitioner to focus on the specific type of evidence that would help a clinical task. The question must be written by using key words and terminology that tap into a general body of research literature that may hold an answer to the question and that locates evidence that is relevant to performing a particular clinical task with a specific client. There are two types of questions: **background questions** and **foreground questions** (Mayer, 2010; Straus et al., 2011; Taylor, 2017).

Background questions identify descriptive research that is used to better understand the nature of the problem.

There are two elements to a background question: a question's root (e.g., who, what, when, where) combined with a verb and a disorder, problem, or some aspect of patient care (Mayer, 2010; Straus et al., 2011). A background question for Judy is provided in Table 35-2.

Foreground questions are about current knowledge on the best practice treatment of a specific patient. They focus on recent interventions, diagnostic tests, potential patient outcomes, and theories about causation (Mayer, 2010). There are three to four elements to a foreground intervention research question (Lou & Durando, 2008; Mayer, 2010; Straus et al., 2011):

● The *patient, population, or problem* (P). The element identifies features of the client population of interest, such as the client's clinical condition or diagnosis, gender, ethnicity, age group, and socioeconomic status. Defining the patient, population, or problems establishes the acceptable characteristics of the sample of any research study. Important features are those that identify populations or subpopulations of which the client is a member, ensuring that retrieved evidence will be relevant to the client.

| TABLE 35-2 | **Examples of Answerable Questions for Each Type of Clinical Task** |

	Get to Know a Client		Choose an Effective Treatment	Estimate the Probable Outcomes
	Background	Diagnosis	Intervention	Prognosis
Example: Answerable questions	Root: How common Verb and problem: are hand structural deformities in RA?	P: 44-year-old woman with RA I: Reliable and valid test to evaluate hand dysfunction O: Identify changes in hand function.	P: 44-year-old woman with RA I: Behavioral-based joint protection program C: Standard education program O: Increase occupational performance and grip strength and reduce pain.	P: 44-year-old woman with RA I: On methotrexate and adalimumab O: Remain employed for 10 years following diagnosis
	How common are hand structural deformities in RA?	What is a valid and reliable test to identify changes in hand function in a middle-aged woman with RA?	Will a behaviorally based joint protection program cause greater increases in occupational performance and grip strength and greater reductions in pain than a standard education program for a middle-aged woman with RA?	How likely is it for a middle-aged woman with RA on methotrexate and adalimumab to remain employed for 10 years after diagnosis?
Example: Key terms (*MeSH* terms)	RA (*arthritis; rheumatic diseases; autoimmune diseases*) Hand structural deformities (*hand deformities, acquired*)	RA (*arthritis; rheumatic diseases; autoimmune diseases*) Test (*evaluation*) Hand function reliable or valid (*psychometrics*)	RA (*arthritis; rheumatic diseases; autoimmune diseases*) Joint protection program (*educational program; self-management program; health education; patient education*) Occupational performance (*Activities of daily living, work, participation*) Pain (*discomfort*) Grip (*grasp*)	RA (*arthritis; rheumatic diseases; autoimmune diseases*) Employment (*work; occupation*) Methotrexate or adalimumab (*biologics; TNF-inhibitors*)

C, comparison; I, intervention; MeSH, Medical Subject Headings; O, outcome; P, patient, population, or problem; RA, rheumatoid arthritis; TNF, tumor necrosis factor.

- The *intervention* of interest (I). This can be a specific technique or a general type of treatment.
- The *comparison* treatment (C). The best intervention studies are experimental and examine the effectiveness of one treatment in comparison to some other treatment. The "some other treatment" does not necessarily have to be specified in the answerable question, particularly if the clinician is not particularly interested if one treatment is better than another, only if the treatment works. Therefore, the comparison treatment may be omitted.
- The desired *outcomes* (O). These should be results that are directly applicable to occupational performance. Variables of interest are attributes of clients that are addressed in OT, such as their physical or psychosocial functioning, occupational performance, or satisfaction with outcomes. Models and theories of occupation and OT, such as the Person-Environment-Occupation Model (Law et al., 1996), as well as more general models of health that encompass an OT perspective, such as the International Classification of Functioning, Disability, and Health (World Health Organization, 2013), provide the language needed to identify occupational variables.

The foreground question is often referred to as a *PICO* question (the acronym of the first letters of each element). The PICO-type question has to be modified when looking for diagnostic or prognostic evidence. For diagnostic/assessment questions, the *intervention* will become a diagnostic tool, whereas the **outcome** will be the ability of the tool to accurately identify the degree of the problem, distinguish a diagnosis, or the psychometrics of the tool. Prognosis, too, requires modifications in the standard PICO question with the intervention becoming **predictor variables** that are expected to alter outcomes and the outcomes tending to focus on long-term participation, health and wellness, and quality of life. Table 35-2 provides examples of answerable questions for each type of clinical task.

Step 2: Gathering Current Published Evidence

Once a clinical question has been written, the practitioner draws on the elements of the question to search for and gather evidence to answer the question. Relevant research is published in various fields: OT, medicine, nursing, physical therapy, education, psychology, sociology, anthropology, and so on. Consequently, search strategies should tap into the research literature of different disciplines.

Each element of an answerable clinical question contains one or more *key terms* for searching the literature. A whole body of literature can be excluded inadvertently simply because the key terms that are used in the search do not match terminology used by the researchers or the cataloguers of the research literature. Some of the important terms that OT practitioners use to identify clinical conditions (e.g., sensory integrative disorder) or occupational variables (e.g., occupational performance) are not the most typical terms used to describe or catalogue research studies in the broader literature. Therefore, it is important to generate a list of synonyms for each key term in each element of the question before beginning the search.

One list of terms that is used by the national databases PubMed and Medline to structure the citations of over 5,400 of the leading biomedical journals is the U.S. National Medical Libraries *Medical Subject Headings* (*MeSH*) terminology (U.S. National Library of Medicine, 2017). Medical Subject Headings is a controlled vocabulary thesaurus, arranged in a 12-level hierarchy with broader, more encompassing terms connected to progressively more specific terms. Medical Subject Headings is designed to link multiple terms to its overall hierarchy and provides a good starting point for identifying common terminology. Freely accessible literature search services such as PubMed (National Center for Biotechnology Information, 2017) provide online tutorials so that evidence-based practitioners can learn how to more effectively search the literature with MeSH terms.

Table 35-2 shows examples of questions that you could write with respect to Judy for each of the clinical tasks. Possible key terms and alternatives that are synonyms and terms that are broader or more specific are listed. For diagnosis ("What is a valid and reliable test to document and identify changes in hand function in a middle-aged woman with RA?"), a combination of *hand function, rheumatoid arthritis, reliable*, and *test* yield six citations of various hand function tests using PubMed, suggesting that this search strategy is effective.

There are numerous free search engines available online for searching the literature as well as clearinghouses for summaries, systematic reviews, and other useful sources of evidence (Lin et al., 2010). One source available to all practitioners is Google Scholar (http://scholar.google.com/), which provides links to full text articles if they are available.

Step 3: Appraising the Evidence

The term *best evidence* is often used in relationship to evidence-based practice. Practitioners are encouraged to use the best evidence to guide practice. As should be apparent, the best evidence is not one type of study design or one type of source; it is dependent on the type of question being asked as well as the access to that evidence. Even after a research study has been identified and acquired, it must be appraised to determine if the study is best evidence for the clinical problem on hand. Evidence that is clinically useful and valuable (1) is relevant to the

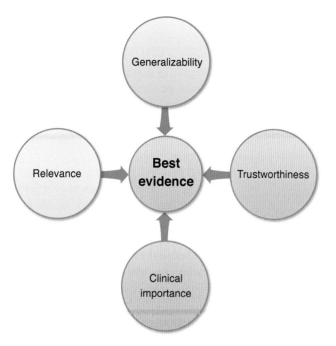

FIGURE 35-2 Elements of best evidence.

clinical task, (2) is trustworthy, (3) has **generalizability**, and (4) has clinically important results (Carter, Lubinsky, & Domholdt, 2011) (Figure 35-2). There are many excellent resources for guiding the appraisal of research evidence (e.g., Law & MacDermid, 2014; Straus et al., 2011).

Appraising the Relevance of a Research Study

The **relevance** of a research study is determined by the degree to which it answers the clinical question and how well its methods fit within the constraints and resources of the practitioner's context of practice (Tickle-Degnen, 2001, 2002b). Rarely will the search for evidence locate a study or set of studies that directly answers the clinical question. Studies are designed to answer the authors' research questions, not your clinical question. The most relevant research study is one that (1) investigates a variable that is the occupational variable of interest or one highly related to that variable, (2) includes research participants who are members of your client's population, and (3) offers clinical methods that are suitable to your context of practice.

To illustrate the process of examining relevance, we return to the citation retrieved in response to the intervention question in Table 35-2, "Will a behaviorally based joint protection program cause greater increases in occupational performance and grip strength and greater reductions in pain than a standard education program for a middle-aged woman with RA?" One citation was for a paper by Hammond and Freeman (2001), which can be retrieved from *Rheumatology*. This paper also has a companion piece

which examines the long-term outcomes of a joint protection program (Hammond & Freeman, 2004). Further examination of the literature finds that this article has been included in a systematic review of OT interventions for people with RA (Siegel, Tencza, Apodaca, & Poole, 2017).

Table 35-3 provides the aim and general methods of Hammond and Freeman's (2001) research study as applied to determining best evidence. The study tested the efficacy of a group focused on acquiring joint protection behaviors through behavioral training methods to reduce pain, impairment, and dysfunction at 1 year in comparison to a group focused on general, didactic education about managing RA. The researchers addressed pain, impairment, and functional outcomes, which are similar to the goals identified by Judy. The subjects are people with RA within Judy's age range, length of disease, and severity of disease. The group format is already used within your clinic, although the behavioral techniques described in the study do not match the current educational methods. They are feasible for your clinic because they do not require special equipment or knowledge. Overall, the article is relevant to your purposes, and you should continue with your appraisal of the trustworthiness of the findings of the study.

Appraising the Trustworthiness of a Research Study

The relevance of a research study is assessed primarily as a degree of fit between your clinical need, as represented in the clinical question, and the methods of the study. The trustworthiness of a research study is assessed primarily as a degree of fit between the researcher's research question, or purpose, and the methods of the study. A trustworthy study is one for which the conclusions are defensible with respect to the methods of the study, and there are few, if any, alternative plausible explanations—scientific explanations for the findings beyond the conclusions drawn from the study and its researchers (Carter et al., 2011). Trustworthiness is enhanced when the researcher carefully and rigorously maintains standards of discovery, description, and explanation (Carpenter & Hammell, 2000).

The most trustworthy research study is one that (1) uses a study design that will achieve the stated purpose and (2) provides methods to enhance trustworthiness with respect to standards of science. The evidence-based practitioner attempts to evaluate the degree to which a descriptive study provides a defensible description of a client or clinical population; the degree to which an assessment study provides a strong test of the reliability, validity, or usefulness of an assessment procedure; or the degree to which an intervention effectiveness study supports the conclusion that client outcomes were caused by the intervention and not by other factors.

The first area to assess to determine the trustworthiness of a study is that the best design was used to answer

| TABLE 35-3 | Evaluation of Hammond and Freeman (2001) as "Best Evidence" |

	Criteria	Hammond and Freeman (2001)
Aim of study		"To evaluate whether joint protection can reduce pain and local inflammation and maintain the integrity of joint structures and functional ability of people with RA 1 year after attending an educational-behavioral joint protection program." (p. 1045)
Relevance	Investigates an occupational variable of interest	Outcome variables included adherence with joint protection techniques (Joint Protection Behavior Assessment), ADL performance (Arthritis Impact Measurement Scale for ADL), hand pain experienced during moderate activity (100 mm VAS) and grip strength (kg).
	Study participants are members of your client's population	Inclusion criteria: diagnosed with RA within the last 5 years (mean disease duration ~19.4 months); age 18–65 years (mean age ~51 years); both genders; hand pain on activity; no other medical conditions affecting hand function; history of wrist and/or metacarpophalangeal (MCP) joint pain/inflammation; mild to severe disease rating
	Clinical methods suitable to your context of practice	Educational-behavioral joint protection program (intervention): Educators used multiple methods (educational, behavioral, motor learning, and self-efficacy enhancing strategies) to educate and practice joint protection techniques. Subjects developed goals for home implementation of joint protection techniques and problem solved as a group. Subjects also received education on RA and drug therapy. Group size: 3–6 people with RA and partners standard education program (control). Short talks from health professionals on RA, drug treatments, alternate therapies, diet, exercise, rest, energy conservation, joint protection, assistive devices, splinting, pain, and relaxation. Some practice time was included for topics such as joint protection. Group size was 6–10 people with RA and partners. Duration for both groups: 8 hours (four 2-hour sessions)
Trustworthiness	Type of design that will achieve the stated purpose	Randomized control study—considered to be the strongest evidence for an intervention study.
	Methods to enhance trustworthiness (Table 3)	Random assignment—Yes Concealed random allocation—Yes (allocation sequence preloaded in envelopes) Similar groups at study baseline—Yes (Table 1) Follow-up of subjects sufficiently long and complete—Yes (1 year) Subjects results analyzed in the groups to which they were allocated—Yes (Table 2) Subjects/study personnel blinded—Yes (independent assessor of outcome measures) Groups treated equally apart from the experimental intervention—Yes Attrition less than 20%—Yes (2%; Table 2)
Generalizability	p value $< .05$ (significance)	Statistical tests: unpaired t tests, Mann-Whitney U test, and chi-square tests. Significant between group differences at 1 year favoring the treatment group for using joint protection behaviors during activities ($p = .001$), hand pain ($p = .02$), and ADL ($p = .04$). Nonsignificant differences between groups at 1 year favoring the treatment group for grip strength ($p = .83$).
Clinical importance	Effect size	**Between Treatment and Control Groups** Joint Protection Behavior Assessment = large effect (Cohen's $d = 0.79$) Hand pain = small effect (Cohen's $d = -0.33$) ADL = negligible effect (Cohen's $d = -0.13$) Grip strength = negligible effect (Cohen's $d = 0.18$) / **Within Treatment Group (Baseline to 1 Year)** Joint Protection Behavior Assessment = large effect (Cohen's $d = 0.93$) Hand pain = small effect (Cohen's $d = -0.21$) ADL = negligible effect (Cohen's $d = -0.15$) Grip strength = small effect (Cohen's $d = 0.27$)
	MCID	VAS hand pain MCID is 2. The difference between 1 year VAS and baseline VAS was 0.56

ADL, activities of daily living; MCID, minimal clinically important difference; RA, rheumatoid arthritis; VAS, visual analogue scale.

TABLE 35-4	Common Research Study Designs

Study Design	Definition
Experimental (Test Hypotheses, Identify Cause and Effect)	
Randomized controlled trials (RCT)	An intervention study in which subjects are randomly assigned to the experimental treatment group or the control group.
Quasi-experimental	An intervention study in which subjects are non–randomly assigned to the experimental treatment group or the control group.
N of 1	An intervention study in which a **single subject** is the total population. This subject receives several treatment periods; one period involves the experimental treatment, and the others, alternative or placebo treatments. Usually, the subject receives multiple baseline measurements and multiple outcome measurements to determine if the intervention causes change.
Associative (Identify Risk Factors or Possible Causes; Hypothesis Generating)	
Cohort	A study in which subjects who represent a particular population are measured on suspected risk factors or predictors of outcome(s) of interest and are followed over time to determine (1) the incidence or natural history of the outcome and (2) the relationship between the predictors and the outcome(s).
Case-control	A retrospective study in which subjects with the outcome of interest (cases) are selected and matched to subjects without the outcome of interest (controls). The presence of risk factors or predictors is determined through self-report or chart review, and the relationship between these retrospective predictors and the outcome of interest is determined.
Cross-sectional	A study in which subjects who represent a particular population are measured simultaneously for suspected risk factors or predictors and outcome(s) of interest to determine (1) the prevalence of the outcome and (2) the relationship between the predictors and the outcome(s).
Descriptive (Describe Problem)	
Qualitative	A research paradigm based on the assumption that there are multiple constructed realities and that the purpose of research is to describe and analyze these realities to facilitate the understanding of the phenomena.
Case series (case study)	A study that tracks several patients over the course of a disease. The results are not aggregated and detailed information on the diagnosis, treatment, and outcomes is provided for each individual patient (a case study tracks a single patient in a like manner).

the research question. Over many decades, a set of basic study designs have evolved. Table 35-4 provides the most common types of study designs and their trustworthiness for different clinical tasks. Each type of study is best used for different types of questions; for example, RCTs and other experimental research are the strongest design for answering intervention questions because they are most suited to determining cause and effect. Cross-sectional studies are the strongest design for diagnosis because they capture subjects at a single point of time in the diagnostic continuum, allowing for an accurate determination if the instrument can accurately identify a problem or disease. Hierarchies of evidence have been developed to rank the trustworthiness of different study designs. Table 35-5

TABLE 35-5	Hierarchy of Trustworthiness of Study Designs

Diagnosis	Intervention	Prognosis
I. SR of cross-sectional studies with consistently applied **reference standards** and **blinding**.	I. SR of RCT or *N* of 1 studies	I. SR of inception cohort studies
II. Cross-sectional study with consistently applied reference standards and blinding.	II. RCT or **observational study** with dramatic effect	II. **Inception cohort study**
III. **Nonconsecutive** cross-sectional study or studies without consistently applied reference standards	III. Non–randomized controlled cohort study	III. Cohort study or **control arm** of RCT
IV. Case-control study	IV. Case-series, case-control study, or **historically controlled study**	IV. Case-series, case-control study, or poor quality prognostic cohort study
V. **Mechanism-based reasoning**	V. Mechanism-based reasoning	V. n/a

Hierarchy is represented by the Roman numerals from I (*strongest design*) to V (*weakest design*).

RCT, randomized controlled trial; SR, systematic review.

Adapted with permission from the Oxford Centre for Evidence-Based Medicine Levels of Evidence Working Group. (2011). *The Oxford Centre for evidence-based medicine 2011 levels of evidence.* Retrieved from http://www.cebm.net/index.aspx?o=5653

TABLE 35-6	Criteria for Determining Trustworthiness	
Diagnosis	**Intervention**	**Prognosis**
1. Independent, blind comparison of the new diagnostic test to a reference standard 2. Evaluation of the new diagnostic test on a full spectrum of patients 3. Both reference standard and new diagnostic test obtained on all study subjects	1. Random assignment 2. **Concealed random** allocation 3. Similar groups at study baseline 4. Follow-up of subjects sufficiently long and complete 5. Subjects results analyzed in the groups to which they were allocated 6. Subjects/study personnel blinded 7. Groups treated equally apart from the experimental intervention 8. **Attrition** less than 20%	1. Baseline data obtained on a defined, representative sample at a common point in their treatment 2. Follow-up of subjects sufficiently long and complete 3. Objective outcome measures applied at follow-up by blinded assessors 4. Adjustments for important prognostic **covariates** for subgroups with different prognostic outcomes 5. **Validation study** completed

Data from Straus, S. E., Glasziou, P., Richardson, W. S., & Haynes, R. B. (2011). *Evidence-based medicine* (4th ed.). New York, NY: Churchill Livingstone.

provides a hierarchy of evidence for the categories of diagnostic, intervention effectiveness, and prognosis evidence.

The second area to assess to determine the trustworthiness of a study is the use of methods to reduce bias and enhance validity. All studies have some form of bias (see Hartman, Forsen, Wallace, & Neely, 2002, for an excellent discussion of bias); nonetheless, some studies provide stronger evidence with respect to trustworthiness than others because they have attempted to carefully and rigorously address these and other potential limitations (Carter et al., 2011). There are numerous scales to assess trustworthiness (e.g., Hempel et al., 2011; Higgins & Green, 2011; Jadad et al., 1996; Maher, Sherrington, Herbert, Mosely, & Elkins, 2003). Table 35-6 provides one set of assessment criteria (Straus et al., 2011) that can identify studies that have the minimum controls to ensure truthful outcomes.

With respect to the study done by Hammond and Freeman (2001), the type of design is an RCT. The clinical task is one of identifying intervention effectiveness, and an RCT is the best choice for determining cause and effect (see Table 35-4). A review of the study using the eight criteria proposed for an intervention study in Table 35-6 suggests that this study has excellent general validity, and therefore, the results are probably trustworthy (see Table 35-4).

Interpreting the Results of a Study: Generalizability and Clinical Importance

Now that you have completed a basic evaluation of the relevance and trustworthiness of the evidence from the study, it is time to examine the results in terms of whether they can help answer the clinical question. First, the results must be generalizable from the sample to the population, and second, they must be clinically important (see Figure 35-2).

A hallmark of research and the scientific method is to understand general, population-centered truths rather than individual outcomes (Taylor, 2017). However, clinical research cannot be completed on a population because it is not feasible to access every person with the characteristics of interest. Therefore, research is performed on a sample of people who are assumed to be representative of the whole population. Research studies describe the characteristics of the sample (inclusion/exclusion criteria and demographics) so that readers can determine how well the sample of a study matches a population and how well their clients match the sample. All data generated from a study, therefore, is sample specific and represents the sample participants but may or may not represent the larger population. If the study is trustworthy, the results are considered to provide a good representation of a population. How do we know that these trustworthy, sample-specific results can translate to the population?

Inferential statistics determine how confident we should be that sample results can be generalized to the client population. The statistic that is commonly used to estimate the confidence that sample results can be generalized is the **p value**. By an arbitrary convention, the threshold to distinguish between statistically significant results that inspire higher confidence about generalizability versus nonsignificant results that inspire lower confidence is generally set at $p \leq .05$. Essentially, a $p \leq .05$ states "the probability that the results in this study are due to chance is less than 1 in 20, and based on this low probability, we feel somewhat confident that we can generalize the results to the population." Many methodologists have suggested that **confidence intervals** replace or augment the use of the p value statistic for interpretation of study results (Cohen, 1990; Cummings & Finch, 2005). Whereas the p value provides a probability value related to chance findings, the confidence interval indicates the range of possible results that are likely to be found in the larger population. The p value and confidence interval are statistically related to one another in that the higher the p value, the larger the confidence interval around the average finding; that is, the larger the range of possible results in the population.

Inferential statistics are applied to all evidence, yet for purposes of demonstrating the meaning of p values and confidence intervals, we provide an example of an intervention effectiveness study. A study found that participants in OT interventions scored an average of five points higher on a postintervention function test than participants in the control condition. The difference was statistically significant at $p < .05$. The confidence interval around the average difference ranged from 1 to 9 points. This finding suggests that in the population as a whole, we would be somewhat confident that the average postintervention function score would be 1 to 9 points higher in individuals receiving the intervention, and that there was a low probability that the average difference between the two conditions was due to chance.

An intervention study finding in which a p value is statistically nonsignificant (e.g., $p > .05$) indicates that we should not feel as confident in generalizing the sample results to the population and that the range of possible responses to the intervention is large. This nonsignificant finding does not tell us that the intervention is ineffective. Rather, it tells us that we cannot be sure that the intervention would or would not be effective. We must use caution in generalizing nonsignificant results to the population and to our client.

Note that inferential statistics, whether they yield statistically significant or nonsignificant results, tell us only about general tendencies in the population and not about our particular client's responses. However, the results of inferential statistics aid us in our clinical reasoning as we work with the client. We are more likely to feel confident in applying statistically significant results to our client's situation than nonsignificant results.

The results of Hammond and Freeman's (2001) study indicated that people in the **treatment group** did statistically significantly better than people in the control group at 1 year for joint protection behaviors, hand pain, and ADL performance. Grip strength, however, was not statistically significant (see Table 35-3). The authors reported p values but no confidence intervals. The p values associated with the results suggest that improvements in joint protection behaviors, hand pain, and ADL performance would also be seen on the average in the population, and therefore, we might expect Judy to show improvement with this type of intervention.

Separate from statistical significance is the concept of clinical importance. Statistical significance focuses on the ability to generalize the results from the sample to the population, regardless of how effective those results are. Statistical significance is strongly tied to sample size because it examines the probability that the results represent a true effect. Thus, with a large enough sample, *any* result can be statistically significant and represent a true effect, as long as the study was highly controlled and used

trustworthy, reliable, and valid assessment procedures. However, this true effect may not be large enough to affect clients in any meaningful way. Just providing whether or not a result is significant may not ultimately be useful for clinical practice. Recent best practice guidelines for reporting research results have identified the inclusion of effect sizes as a key aspect (Moher et al., 2010). It is important to know that small sample sizes that produce a nonsignificant result may actually have produced an effect that would generalize to the population if the study were to be replicated with a larger sample size. The study's sample size might be too small to detect that the effect would generalize to the population (i.e., it does not provide us with enough confidence in the generalizability of the findings).

An **effect size** describes the magnitude of the difference between two treatment effects or the magnitude of the relationship between two variables using some form of a standardized score (Ferguson, 2009). The standardized score eliminates the scale of the original instrument used to measure the variable, which allows effects sizes to be compared between instruments or between studies. There are many different forms of effect sizes, and the most appropriate type depends on the type of data being evaluated and the statistical analyses performed (Table 35-7). Often, the numerical effect size is translated into a verbal interpretation, such as "small," "moderate," or "large," to assist clinicians in estimating the magnitude of the effect on treatment (Ferguson, 2009; Portney & Watkins, 2009; Tickle-Degnen, 2001).

Another way to determine clinical effectiveness is the **minimal clinically important difference (MCID)**. The MCID is the smallest change in an outcome that will lead to some perceived clinically beneficial improvement. For example, Salaffi, Stancati, Silvestri, Ciapetti, and Grassi (2004) identified the MCID for pain for people with chronic musculoskeletal pain due to arthritis after a 3-month period using a numerical rating scale (NRS). A mean change of two corresponded with "much better" improvement. Thus, a study that reported a change of two on an NRS would suggest that the intervention had a clinically important effect on pain for the average client. More and more studies are examining the percentage of subjects who achieve an MCID during the study as one measure of outcome. The biggest barrier to using MCID in clinical practice is that clinicians must know the MCID for different outcome measures, and these are not always readily available. Clinicians should collect MCID for outcomes that are important to them to facilitate interpreting the clinical importance of different studies.

The effect sizes calculated for the Hammond and Freeman's (2001) study suggest that although the educational program had a large effect in altering joint protection behaviors (see Table 35-3) in the treatment group, these changes in behaviors only had a small corresponding

TABLE 35-7 Effect Sizes

Effect Size	Clinical Task	Definition	Citations
Sensitivity	Diagnosis	Proportion of people with the target disorder who have a positive result on the diagnostic test.	Fritz & Wainner (2001) Portney & Watkins (2009, pp. 619–634) Straus et al. (2011, pp. 73–77)
Specificity	Diagnosis	Proportion of people without the target disorder who have a negative result on the diagnostic test.	
Positive predictive value	Diagnosis	Proportion of people with a positive diagnostic test who have the target disorder.	
Negative predictive value	Diagnosis	Proportion of people with a negative diagnostic test who do not have the target disorder.	
Likelihood ratios	Diagnosis	The likelihood that a specific test result would be seen in a person with the target disorder.	
Kappa	Diagnosis	A reliability coefficient that identifies the degree of agreement between two measure made by two observers measuring the same item while controlling for chance agreement.	Portney & Watkins (2009, pp. 598–605)
Intraclass correlation coefficients (ICC)	Diagnosis	A reliability coefficient that evaluates the consistency of two measures made by observers measuring the same item.	Portney & Watkins (2009, pp. 588–598)
Cohen's d, Hedge's g, Glass's Δ	Intervention	Measures the magnitude of the difference between two means in standard deviation units (each cited measure uses a different variation of standard deviation units).	Lipsey & Wilson (2001, pp. 34–71) Tickle-Degnen (2001)
r	Intervention	The degree of shared variance between two measures.	
Number needed to treat (NNT)	Intervention	The number of patients who would need to receive treatment to produce a positive outcome in one patient who otherwise would have had a negative outcome.	Dalton & Keating (2000) Straus et al. (2011, pp. 73–77)
Odds ratio; risk ratio	Intervention; prognosis	Estimate of the difference in the risk for a particular outcome between two or more groups.	Portney & Watkins (2009, pp. 667–670)

effect on impairment and function. Overall, people in the treatment group had only small improvements in function in comparison to the control group, and even when the effect within the treatment group alone was evaluated from baseline to posttest at 1 year, the results remained negligible to small. The MCID for hand pain also suggests that the changes were not enough to affect clinical performance. Therefore, although the results are generalizable from the sample to the population (significance), they are not necessarily clinically important.

The small effect sizes from this study require the use of clinical reasoning to understand their implications for Judy and other similar clients. On one hand, the results suggest minimal benefit. However, these results are 1-year postintervention on a disease process that routinely causes continued deterioration of abilities. The fact that the participants in this study not only did not get worse but also improved in comparison to a group of similar individuals suggests that this treatment may be more beneficial than the effect sizes indicate. We do not know how Judy

would respond herself to this type of intervention. This clinical conundrum demonstrates the importance of clinician expertise and client input into the decision-making process.

Thus, best evidence is a combination of the relevance of the results to the clinician's practice, the trustworthiness of the research design in obtaining "true" sample results for the study sample, the ability to generalize the results from the sample to the population, and results that are not only "significant" but clinically important as well. Finally, best evidence should demonstrate replication; numerous studies should show similar results related to treatment, diagnoses, or prognoses. **Systematic reviews** are frequently cited as the best "best evidence" because they synthesize the results from multiple studies (Lin et al., 2010; Oxford Centre for Evidence-Based Medicine Levels of Evidence Working Group, 2011). A meta-analysis, a form of systematic review that includes statistical techniques to combine the results of multiple studies into a single effect size, provides one of the best overall reviews of evidence. The

Cochrane Collaboration is one group that has provided numerous high-quality systematic reviews on various topics (Cochrane Collaboration, 2017) including OT for RA (Steultjens et al., 2004), problems in ADL after stroke (Hoffmann, Bennett, Koh, & McKenna, 2010), and multiple sclerosis (Steultjens et al., 2003). Although systematic reviews provide overall evidence of the efficacy of a treatment, it may be limited in its use for individual clients. Often, the summaries address a heterogeneous group of subjects or broad treatment plans which reduce their relevance to day-to-day practice. Systematic reviews are best when a topic is well established. They are less effective for new and emerging practices where they may underestimate the effect due to small sample sizes or unreliable assessment procedures or overestimate it due to poorly controlled studies with biased assessment procedures. Systematic reviews are excellent sources of articles that deal with a specific sample or treatment topic; evidence-based practitioners can use the reviews to identify and obtain more specific articles for treatments that show an overall effectiveness.

There is one other consideration regarding best evidence. The best evidence is the best that can be found and not best in the sense of meeting all of the standards. The possible answer this best evidence delivers may be one about which you can feel a high, moderate, or low degree of confidence. You might not have enough time to gather and evaluate enough evidence to form a confident opinion, which is very likely, given, in this scenario, how busy you are as a practitioner in an outpatient clinic. Even with little research evidence about which you feel a modicum of confidence, you may go to the next step of evidence-based practice: communication about the evidence with the client, in this case, Judy, and other individuals who are important to the client.

Step 4: Using the Evidence to Guide Practice

By appraising the relevance of the evidence, you will have identified that a study can potentially be applied to your client; it matches his or her general characteristics and it is feasible within your clinical setting. You will also know from your appraisal that the study results are generally trustworthy and demonstrate potentially generalizable and important results. This study can now be used as a tool to help develop and implement treatment. However, before you decide to use the results of a study, you must determine if they truly match the values and circumstances of your client (see Figure 35-1). This is done by communicating the evidence to the client to inform the process of decision making about treatment.

As has been put forward in this chapter, evidence-based practice emerges from the core values and ethics of OT (American Occupational Therapy Association, 2010; Holm, 2000). Evidence-based practice occurs in a respectful, truthful, and collaborative relationship with the client and with those acting on the client's behalf. Clients are viewed as active contributors to the therapy process rather than as passive recipients of information or services (Law, Baptiste, & Mills, 1995). To be active rather than passive, that is, to act with as much autonomy as possible and the least amount of dependency, clients and those acting on their behalf must be informed rather than uninformed or misinformed. To be an informed client means to know the meaning of one's occupational status in relationship to one's quality of life, to know the nature and quality of possible OT assessments to be undertaken, to know the quality and probable outcomes of relevant interventions, and to have the means to assess one's own progress toward meaningful outcomes. Once informed, clients and those acting on their behalf can reason and act with the degree of autonomy of which they are capable.

The main goal of communicating about evidence is to inform decision making (Tickle-Degnen, 2000, 2002b). Wise decisions are ones that are likely to benefit the client and family members and are embraced by client, family members, you (the OT practitioner), and others of importance to the client, such as other practitioners. Communication that achieves these types of decisions (1) has content that accurately represents the research evidence, including its strengths and weaknesses related to relevance and trustworthiness; (2) involves language that is mutually understandable to all participants; and (3) encourages an open and mutual discussion of information and ideas rather than a closed-ended or unidirectional delivery of information from one individual to another. Even a small amount of evidence in which you have a small degree of confidence can be helpful in decision making if it is presented with these qualities in mind.

Communication with Judy about the joint protection program might be as follows: "Generally, clients' hand pain improves with behavioral joint protection programs. However, some improve more than others. Would you be interested in participating in a joint protection group?" In this communication, the findings are accurately portrayed in the past rather than present tense, and the pertinent relevance issue is addressed, enabling Judy to assess the evidence herself.

One implication of autonomous reasoning and action is that clients can choose to participate or not participate in OT assessments and interventions. Likewise, family members or other health practitioners may decide to encourage or discourage client participation. Evidence-based practice is not about the imposition of the will of one individual on the will of the other but rather is a mutual search for and discussion about information that will aid informed, wise decision making. The practitioner's responsibility is to provide information in such a manner that reasoned decision making is maximized.

Summary

Evidence-based practice has become an integral part of OT practice. In combination with the treatment environment and client values and circumstances, evidence forms a strong base to achieve best practice clinical decision making. To best inform the process of decision making, evidence can be clustered into three types of clinical tasks: getting to know the client, or diagnosis; choosing an effective treatment, or intervention; and estimating probable outcomes, or prognosis. Occupational therapists must develop the skills to identify answerable clinical questions, find and critically appraise research to identify the best evidence for each of the clinical tasks, use their clinical expertise to integrate this best evidence with their clients' values and needs, and implement it within their treatment environment. Critically appraising the evidence involves identifying the relevance, trustworthiness, generalizability, and clinical importance of research. Once best evidence is determined, occupational therapists must be able to communicate the evidence to clients to ensure collaborative and informed treatment decisions. Without skills in evidence-based practice, an occupational therapist will not be competitive in today's health care system. Evidence-based practice takes time and energy; the skills needed are acquired through active learning and practice. Throughout your career as an occupational therapist, you will refine and improve your skills and ensure that you use the best evidence to provide the best treatment for all of your clients.

REFERENCES

American Occupational Therapy Association. (2010). Occupational therapy code of ethics and ethics standards. *American Journal of Occupational Therapy, 64*, 151–160. Retrieved from http://www.aota.org/Pubs/AJOT_1.aspx

Bailey, D. (2003). Evidence-based practice: The link between research and practice. In E. B. Crepeau, E. S. Cohn, & B. A, B. Schell (Eds.), *Willard & Spackman's occupational therapy* (10th ed., pp. 972–974). Philadelphia, PA: Lippincott Williams & Wilkins.

Carpenter, C., & Hammell, K. (2000). Evaluating qualitative research. In K. W. Hammell, C. Carpenter, & I. Dyck (Eds.), *Using qualitative research: A practical introduction for occupational and physical therapists*. Edinburgh, United Kingdom: Churchill Livingstone.

Carter, R. E., Lubinsky, J., & Domholdt, E. (2011). *Rehabilitation research: Principles and applications* (4th ed.). St. Louis, MO: Elsevier Saunders.

Cochrane Collaboration. (2017). *The Cochrane collaboration.* Retrieved from http://www.cochrane.org/

Cohen, J. (1990). Things I have learned (so far). *American Psychologist, 45*, 1304–1312. Retrieved from http://www.apa.org/pubs/-journals/amp/index.aspx

Cumming, G., & Finch, S. (2005). Inference by eye: Confidence intervals and how to read pictures of data. *American Psychologist, 60*, 170–180. doi:10.1037/0003-066X.60.2.170

Dalton, G. W., & Keating, J. L. (2000). Number needed to treat: A statistic relevant for physical therapists. *Physical Therapy, 80*, 1214–1219. Retrieved from http://ptjournal.apta.org/content/80/12/1214.long

Diffin, J. G., Lunt, M., Marshall, T., Chipping, J. R., Symmons, D. P., & Verstappen, S. M. (2014). Has the severity of rheumatoid arthritis at presentation diminished over time? *The Journal of Rheumatology, 41*, 1590–1599. doi:10.3899/jrheum.131136

Ferguson, C. J. (2009). An effect size primer: A guide for clinicians and researchers. *Professional Psychology: Research and Practice, 40*, 532–538. doi:10.1037/a0015808

Fritz, J. M., & Wainner, R. S. (2001). Examining diagnostic tests: An evidence-based perspective. *Physical Therapy, 81*, 1546–1564. Retrieved from http://ptjournal.apta.org/

Hammond, A., & Freeman, K. (2001). One-year outcomes of a randomized controlled trial of an educational-behavioural joint protection programme for people with rheumatoid arthritis. *Rheumatology, 40*, 1044–1051. doi:10.1093/rheumatology/40.9.1044

Hammond, A., & Freeman, K. (2004). The long-term outcomes from a randomized controlled trial of an educational-behavioural joint protection programme for people with rheumatoid arthritis. *Clinical Rehabilitation, 18*, 520–528. doi:10.1191/0269215504cr766oa

Hartman, J. M., Forsen, J. W., Jr., Wallace, M. S., & Neely, J. G. (2002). Tutorials in clinical research: Part IV. Recognizing and controlling bias. *The Laryngoscope, 112*, 23–31. doi:10.1097/00005537-200201000-00005

Hempel, S., Suttorp, M. J., Miles, J. N. V., Wang, Z., Maglione, M., Morton, S., . . . Shekelle, P. G. (2011). *Empirical evidence of associations between trial quality and effect sizes.* Rockville, MD: Agency for Healthcare Research and Quality.

Higgins, J. P. T., & Green, S. (Eds.). (2011). *Cochrane handbook for systematic reviews of interventions version 5.1.0* [updated March 2011]. The Cochrane Collaboration, 2011. Retrieved from http://www.cochrane-handbook.org

Hoffmann, T., Bennett, S., Koh, C. L., & McKenna, K. T. (2010). Occupational therapy for cognitive impairment in stroke patients. *The Cochrane Database of Systematic Reviews*, CD006430. doi:10.1002/14651858.CD006430.pub2

Holm, M. (2000). The 2000 Eleanor Clarke Slagle Lecture. Our mandate for the new millennium: Evidence-based practice. *American Journal of Occupational Therapy, 54*, 575–585. doi:10.5014/ajot.54.6.575

Jadad, A. R., Moore, R. A., Carroll, D., Jenkinson, C., Reynolds, D. J. M., Gavaghan, D. J., & McQuay, H. J. (1996). Assessing the quality of reports of randomized clinical trials: Is blinding necessary? *Controlled Clinical Trials, 17*, 1–12. Retrieved from http://www.sciencedirect.com/science/journal/01972456

Law, M., Baptiste, S., & Mills, J. (1995). Client-centered practice: What does it mean and does it make a difference? *Canadian Journal of Occupational Therapy, 62*, 250–257. Retrieved from http://www.cmaj.ca/

Law, M., Cooper, B., Strong, S., Stewart, D., Rigby, P., & Letts, L. (1996). The person-environment-occupation model: A transactive approach to occupational performance. *Canadian Journal of Occupational Therapy, 63*, 9–23. Retrieved from http://www.cmaj.ca/

Law, M., & MacDermid, J. (Eds.). (2014). *Evidence-based rehabilitation: A guide to practice* (3rd ed.). Thorofare, NJ: SLACK.

Lee, C. J., & Miller, L. T. (2003). The process of evidence-based clinical decision making in occupational therapy. *American Journal of Occupational Therapy, 57*, 473–477. Retrieved from http://www.aota.org/Pubs/AJOT_1.aspx

Lin, S. H., Murphy, S. L., & Robinson, J. C. (2010). Facilitating evidence-based practice: Process, strategies, and resources. *American Journal of Occupational Therapy, 64*, 164–171. Retrieved from http://www.aota.org/Pubs/AJOT_1.aspx

Lipsey, M. W., & Wilson, D. B. (2001). *Practical meta-analysis.* Thousand Oaks, CA: Sage.

Lou, J. Q., & Durando, P. (2008). Asking clinical questions and searching for the evidence. In M. Law & J. MacDermid (Eds.), *Evidence-based rehabilitation* (2nd ed., pp. 95–117). Thorofare, NJ: SLACK.

Maher, C. G., Sherrington, C., Herbert, R. D., Mosely, A. M., & Elkins, M. (2003). Reliability of the PEDro scale for rating quality of randomized controlled trials. *Physical Therapy, 83*, 713–721. Retrieved from http://ptjournal.apta.org/

Mayer, D. (2010). *Essential evidence-based medicine* (2nd ed.). New York, NY: Cambridge University Press.

Moher, D., Hopewell, S., Schulz, K. F., Montori, V., Gøtzsche, P. C., Devereaux, P. J., . . . Altman, D. G. (2010). CONSORT 2010 explanation and elaboration: Updated guidelines for reporting parallel group randomised trials. *Journal of Clinical Epidemiology, 63*, e1–e37. doi:10.1016/j.jclinepi.2010.03.004

Moons, K. G. M., Royston, P., Vergouwe, Y., Grobbee, D., & Altman, D. G. (2009). Prognosis and prognostic research: What, why, and how. *BMJ, 338*, 1317–1320. doi:10.1136/bmj.b375

National Center for Biotechnology Information. (2017). *PubMed.* Retrieved from http://www.ncbi.nlm.nih.gov/pubmed/

Oxford Centre for Evidence-Based Medicine Levels of Evidence Working Group. (2011). *The Oxford Centre for evidence-based medicine 2011 levels of evidence.* Retrieved from http://www.cebm .net/index.aspx?o=5653

Portney, L. G., & Watkins, M. P. (2009). *Foundations of clinical research: Applications to practice* (3rd ed.). Upper Saddle River, NJ: Pearson Education.

Rappolt, S. (2003). The role of professional expertise in evidence-based occupational therapy. *American Journal of Occupational Therapy, 57*, 589–593. Retrieved from http://www.aota.org/Pubs/AJOT_1.aspx

Salaffi, F., Stancati, A., Silvestri, C. A., Ciapetti, A., & Grassi, W. (2004). Minimal clinically important changes in chronic musculoskeletal pain intensity measured on a numerical rating scale. *European Journal of Pain, 8*, 283–291. doi:10.1016/j.ejpain.2003.09.004

Shin, J., Randolph, G. W., & Rauch, S. D. (2010). Evidence-based medicine in otolaryngology, part 1: The multiple faces of evidence-based medicine. *Otolaryngology—Head and Neck Surgery, 142*, 637–646. doi:10.1016/j.otohns.2010.01.018

Siegel, P., Tencza, M., Apodaca, B., & Poole, J. L. (2017). Effectiveness of occupational therapy interventions for adults with rheumatoid arthritis: A systematic review. *American Journal of Occupational Therapy, 71*, 1–11. doi:10.5014/ajot.2017.023176

Steultjens, E. E. M. J., Dekker, J. J., Bouter, L. M., Cardol, M. M., Van de Nes, J., & Van den Ende, E. C. H. M. (2003). Occupational therapy for multiple sclerosis. *Cochrane Database of Systematic Reviews*, CD003608. doi:10.1002/14651858.CD003608

Steultjens, E. E. M. J., Dekker, J. J., Bouter, L. M., van Schaardenburg, D. D., Kuyk, M. A. M. A. H., & Van den Ende, E. C. H. M. (2004). Occupational therapy for rheumatoid arthritis. *Cochrane Database of Systematic Reviews*, CD003114. doi:10.1002/14651858.CD003114.pub2

Straus, S. E., Glasziou, P., Richardson, W. S., & Haynes, R. B. (2011). *Evidence-based medicine* (4th ed.). New York, NY: Churchill Livingstone.

Sur, R. L., & Dahm, P. (2011). History of evidence-based medicine. *Indian Journal of Urology, 27*, 487–489. doi:10.4103/0970-1591.91438

Taylor, R. R. (2017). *Kielhofner's research in occupational therapy* (2nd ed.). Philadelphia, PA: F. A. Davis.

Tickle-Degnen, L. (1998). Communicating with clients about treatment outcomes: The use of meta-analytic evidence in collaborative treatment planning. *American Journal Occupational Therapy, 52*, 526–530.

Tickle-Degnen, L. (2000). Communicating with clients, family members, and colleagues about research evidence. *American Journal of Occupational Therapy, 54*, 341–343. Retrieved from http://www.aota .org/Pubs/AJOT_1.aspx

Tickle-Degnen, L. (2001). From the general to the specific: Using meta-analytic reports in clinical decision making. *Evaluation & The Health Professions, 24*, 308–326. doi:10.1177/01632780122034939

Tickle-Degnen, L. (2002a). Client-centered practice, therapeutic relationship, and the use of research evidence. *American Journal of Occupational Therapy, 56*, 470–473. Retrieved from http://www.aota .org/Pubs/AJOT_1.aspx

Tickle-Degnen, L. (2002b). Communicating evidence to clients, managers, and funders. In M. Law (Ed.), *Evidence-based rehabilitation: A guide to practice* (pp. 221–254). Thorofare, NJ: SLACK.

U.S. National Library of Medicine. (2017). *Medical Subject Headings (MeSH).* Retrieved from http://www.nlm.nih.gov/mesh/meshhome.html

World Health Organization. (2015). *International classification of functioning, disability, and health.* Retrieved from http://www.who.int /classifications/drafticfpracticalmanual2.pdf?ua=1

Additional Resources

American Occupational Therapy Association's Evidence-Based Practice Resources: https://www.aota.org/Practice/Researchers.aspx
https://www.aota.org/-/media/Corporate/Files/Practice/Researcher /EBP%20Resources.ashx

the**Point**®   *For additional resources on the subjects discussed in this chapter, visit* **http://thePoint.lww.com /Willard-Spackman13e.** *See* **Appendix I, Resources and Evidence for Common Conditions Addressed in OT** *for more information on arthritis.*

Ethical Practice

Regina F. Doherty

"Practitioners must be grounded not only by a moral conscience to do what is right, but also by the courage to proceed and ensure the best interests of the patient."

—BRANDT & HOMENKO (2016)

LEARNING OBJECTIVES

After reading this chapter, you will be able to:

1. Recognize the ethical issues that occupational therapy practitioners encounter in professional practice.
2. Identify the virtues of health professionals.
3. Understand basic ethics problems, ethical theories, and approaches to ethics.
4. Understand and apply an ethical decision-making guide for case analysis.
5. Understand and apply ethical reasoning as a construct within the decision-making process.
6. Identify and know how to access ethics resources.
7. Understand effective communication strategies for difficult conversations.

Why Ethics?

Ask yourself the following questions:

- What would I say to a patient who asked me if I could be his "Facebook friend" while he was undergoing active treatment on the unit where I practice?
- What would I say to a colleague who asked me to change my documentation to indicate that a client is worse than he really is so that the client would qualify for additional services?
- How would I feel if the family of a client with autism told me they were discontinuing his occupational therapy (OT) services because they had no means to pay for his continued care?

Ethical questions like these often arise for OT practitioners in their day-to-day practice. They require practitioners to recognize ethical situations and have both the capacity and the willingness to address these situations systematically. In this chapter, ethical issues that arise in OT practice are discussed. This serves as a foundation to aid the reader in understanding, recognizing, and reasoning through ethical aspects of professional practice.

Occupational therapy practitioners in all professional roles will encounter ethical problems. Ethics is about reflecting, thinking, critically reasoning, justifying, acting on, and evaluating moral decisions. Ethical problems are often dynamic and complex, requiring additional knowledge, communication with interprofessional colleagues, and consultation with various resources. Consequently, knowledge and understanding of ethical reasoning and ethical decision making are essential for competent OT practice.

Ethics, Morality, and Moral Reasoning

The terms *ethical* and *moral* are often used interchangeably in professional practice, and although related, they have slightly different meanings. The term *ethics* stems from the Greek word *ethos*, meaning "character." Ethics is a branch of philosophy that involves systemic study and reflection providing language, methods, and guidelines to study and reflect on morality (Doherty & Purtilo, 2016). In contrast, the term *morality* refers to social conventions about right and wrong human conduct and sets the stage for ethical behavior. Values, duty, and moral character guide reasoning and inform ethical decisions (Beauchamp & Childress, 2013). Values are the beliefs or objects a person holds dear (e.g., life). Duties describe an action that is required (e.g., provide food and shelter to care for one's family). Moral character describes traits or dispositions that facilitate trust and human flourishing (e.g., compassion, honesty) (Doherty & Purtilo, 2016).

There are three types of morality: personal or individual, group or organizational, and societal (Glaser, 2005). Personal morality includes individual beliefs and values. Acting in accordance with these values preserves one's integrity. Group morality is the morality of the profession or organization to which an individual belongs. A professional organization, such as the American Occupational Therapy Association (AOTA), maintains collective values that guide group decisions. For occupational therapists, this might be the emphasis on collaborative practice and occupation. Societal morality is the morality of society as a whole. Societal values change over time, and different communities may fight for the protection of different values and rights. Tension often exists between these three realms of morality. It is important to reflect on how these different moralities interrelate because in a pluralistic society, no single vision of morality prevails, making ethical decision-making challenging.

Moral reasoning is a term used to describe the process of reflecting on ethical issues. Moral reasoning is about norms and values, ideas of right and wrong, and how practitioners make decisions in professional work (Barnitt, 1993; Doherty & Purtilo, 2016). Moral reasoning

is a reflective process that leads to ethically supported actions. It is a manifestation of moral character and mindful reflection (Slater, 2016). We use our moral reasoning to think critically about the meaning and values of a variety of situations including, but not limited to, the therapeutic relationship; the context of practice situations; and the institutional, cultural, and societal influences on the provision of health care (Delany, Edwards, Jensen, & Skinner, 2010). Consequently, effective moral reasoning and ethical decision making are closely linked to effective practice (Bebeau, 2002; Hartwell, 1995; Sisola, 2000; Unsworth & Baker, 2016).

Ethical Implications of Trends in Health Care and Occupational Therapy Practice

Health care systems are increasingly complex. Health care policy, as well as demographic and epidemiologic forces, will continue to change the delivery of health care services. New technologies, including those used in intensive care, life-sustaining treatment, reproductive medicine, organ/tissue transplantation, robotics, genetics, and genomics, have created ethical questions for health professionals, increasing the likelihood of encountering moral distress. **Moral distress** is an ethical problem that occurs when practitioners know the right thing to do but cannot achieve it because of external barriers or uncertainty about the outcome (Doherty & Purtilo, 2016). Common ethical concerns that OT practitioners encounter in practice are highlighted in Box 36-1. Issues that cause moral distress in OT practice with high frequency include

---

BOX 36-1   COMMON CAUSES OF MORAL DISTRESS

Common causes of moral distress in OT practice include the following:

- Reimbursement constraints
- Pressures surrounding billing and productivity
- Issues related to client decision-making capacity and safety
- Resource allocation and systematic issues
- Cultural, religious, and family considerations
- Confidentiality and disclosure
- Vulnerable patient populations
- Upholding professional standards and values
- Balancing benefits and burdens in care
- Difficult client behaviors
- Practice management
- Conflicting values surrounding goals of care

those surrounding billing and reimbursement, resource allocation, goals of care, client safety, and upholding professional standards and values (Bushby, Chan, Druif, Ho, & Kinsella, 2015; Doherty, Dellinger, Gately, Pullo, & Sullivan, 2012; Foye, Kirschner, Wagner, Stocking, & Siegler, 2002; Slater & Brandt, 2016).

Virtues of Health Professionals

Health professionals hold a unique societal role because the public expects them to uphold particular virtues. These include the virtues of integrity, benevolence, competence, kindness, trustworthiness, fairness, conscientiousness, caring, and compassion (Beauchamp & Childress, 2013; Devettere, 2009; Doherty & Purtilo, 2016; Gawande, 2002; Pellegrino, 1995, 2002; Purtilo, 2004). First and foremost, OT practitioners (occupational therapists and OT assistants) must be benevolent and focus on what is best for the client. Second, the practitioner must be competent. All practitioners are responsible for achieving and maintaining competence in their area of OT practice. They must use evidence to guide practice decisions and participate in continuing education. Third, practitioners must be caring. Care enhances comfort and recovery and is an essential feature of professional practice (Doherty & Purtilo, 2016; Fry & Veatch, 2000). Although most practitioners recognize that caring is inherent in the health professional's role, there are times when professionals interact with challenging clients or families. There may be lack of reciprocity and mutuality caused by the condition itself, such as combativeness resulting from a head injury, which can erode the caring relationship. Finally, practitioners must be compassionate. Compassion is "the recognition, empathic understanding of and emotional resonance with the concerns, pain, distress or suffering of others coupled with motivation and relational action to ameliorate these conditions" (Lown & McIntosh, 2015, p. 3). Compassion serves as a foundation for collaborative, client- and family-centered care. It informs shared decision making and contributes to positive outcomes for clients, practitioners, and organizations.

Distinguishing among Clinical, Legal, and Ethical Problems in Practice

Practitioners must learn to distinguish ethical questions from other questions that they encounter in the care of clients. Many times, what might appear to be an ethical issue is in fact something else, such as a miscommunication or a clinical

or legal issue. For example, a clinical question would be "Can clients with severe dysphagia due to end-stage amyotrophic lateral sclerosis (ALS) eat?" This is a clinical question because there is a diagnostic answer to it. Clients who pass a bedside swallowing evaluation and modified barium swallow (MBS) test are clinically able to eat. If they fail this test but want to continue eating orally, an ethical question could arise. The ethical question would be "Should clients with end-stage ALS who fail an MBS test eat?" This is an ethical question because it raises questions relative to quality of life and the risks and benefits of eating with diminished swallowing capacity.

Legal questions may also arise in patient care decision making. Law and ethics are related fields; however, they have different goals and sanctions. Both rely on analytical processes and ground rules for good decision making; however, laws are legislated and are legally enforceable (Horner, 2003). Laws prescribe what we cannot do. What may be permitted legally might not be justified ethically and vice versa. In the case of clients with ALS, a legal question would be "Do competent clients have the right to refuse medical advice and continue eating orally despite the recommendation of the team?" This example highlights the importance of distinguishing and interpreting the type of question to more critically reason through the problem. Interpretation is a critical step in professional reasoning because how the practitioner or team understands the situation has great influence on how they will respond to it (Sullivan & Rosin, 2008).

Reflection and Ethical Practice

Recognizing the morally significant features of a situation is one of the first steps in ethical reflection. **Reflection** is a form of self-assessment used to improve practice. Developing reflective capacity is a critical element in professional development and competence (Wald, Borkan, Taylor, Anthony, & Reis, 2012). When reflecting on ethical aspects of practice, practitioners must consider their own values and how those values might influence their work. A value is a belief or an ideal to which an individual is committed (Kanny, 1993). Practitioners, who are aware of their own value positions, critically examine their assumptions, and acknowledge judgment and biases have a better appreciation of the complexity of moral decisions (McAuliffe, 2014). For a values clarification exercise, see Exercise 36.A on thePoint.

Another form of reflection is mindfulness. Mindfulness is a way of tuning in to what is happening in and around us (Schoeberlein & Sheth, 2009). Mindful practice enables practitioners to be present, listen more attentively to clients' distress, recognize their own errors, refine their technical skills, make evidence-based decisions, and recognize the values necessary to act with compassion, competence, presence, and insight (Epstein, 1999; Olson & Kemper, 2014). Mindfulness is an effective way to foster reflective capacity, build resilience, and infuse ethical reasoning into professional practice.

CENTENNIAL NOTES

Ethical Core of the Profession

The field of OT has long upheld a strong commitment to professionalism and ethical practice. Decades before the official code of ethics, Mrs. Marjorie B. Greene, dean of the Boston School of Occupational Therapy, wrote to Thomas Kidner, president of the Occupational Therapy Board of Managers, expressing the desire to adopt a "Pledge and Creed for Occupational Therapists" (Figure 36-1). This pledge, which had been adopted by students at the school,

pledge and creed for occupational + therapists +

Reverently and earnestly do I pledge my whole-hearted service in aiding those crippled in mind and body.

To this end that my work for the sick may be successful, I will ever strive for greater knowledge, skill and understanding in the discharge of my duties in whatsoever position I may find myself.

I solemnly declare that I will hold and keep inviolate whatever I may learn of the lives of the sick.

I acknowledge the dignity of the cure of disease and the safeguarding of health in which no act is menial or inglorious.

I will walk in upright faithfulness and obedience to those under whose guidance I am to work and I pray for patience, kindliness and strength in the holy ministry to broken minds and bodies.

FIGURE 36-1 Pledge and Creed for Occupational Therapists. Reprinted with permission from the Tufts University Digital Collections and Archives and The Archives of the American Occupational Therapy Association.

was presented to the full board at its September 26, 1926 meeting in Atlantic City, New Jersey. The motion passed unanimously, and the Pledge and Creed was adopted by the Association as a whole (Board of Management, 1926). The values of altruism, fidelity, dignity, and lifelong learning can be gleaned from this early pledge and creed.

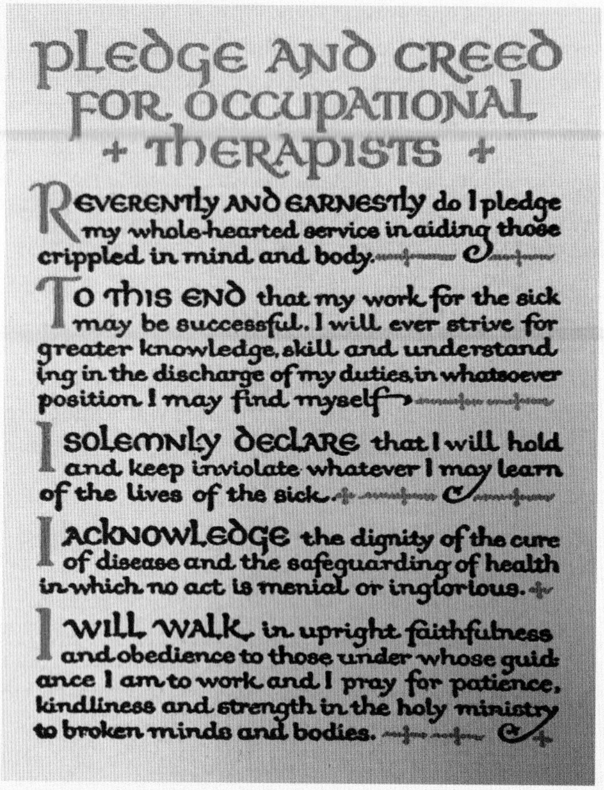

In the late 1960s and early 1970s, rapid advances in medicine and biology and abuses in experimental research introduced a wide range of ethical problems that led to an expansion of field of bioethics in the United States and abroad. In 1975, the first AOTA Ethics Commission was established, and in 1977, the Representative Assembly approved the first Principles of Occupational Therapy Ethics (AOTA, 1977), a full 50 years after adoption of the Pledge and Creed. These 12 principles were first published in the fifth edition of *Willard & Spackman's Occupational Therapy*. The code has been revised six times and went from 30 subprinciples in 2000, to 38 in 2005, and to 69 in 2015 (Howard & Kennell, 2017). Because the Code of Ethics is a living document, it changes as the profession, technology, and society change. As the global body of the profession, The World Federation of Occupational Therapists (WFOT) also publishes a Code of Ethics (WFOT, 2016). This code serves as an overarching guide to professional practice. It is based on tasks of the profession, responsibilities toward recipients of services, professional collaborators/employers, and society on a local and global level.

As the fields of science, public policy, medicine, and technology advance and intersect on a local and global level, the complexity of questions regarding what is best for the patient, the health care system, and society will continue to evolve. The moral imperative of acting in the best interest of clients will demand that health professionals collaborate to think critically and reflect on what it means for human beings and society to flourish. May we channel the words of our founders so that "whatsoever position" we may find ourselves in, we may "ever strive for greater knowledge, skill, and understanding in the discharge of our duties" (Tufts University Digital Collections and Archives, 1959, p. 2).

Identifying Different Types of Ethical Problems

When reflecting on ethical dimensions of practice, it is important to distinguish among the different types of ethical problems. An **ethical problem** is a situation that is believed to have negative implications regarding cherished moral values and duties *and* that will pose an

extremely difficult choice to an individual or group of individuals (Doherty & Purtilo, 2016). It may be manifested by an emotional reaction such as discomfort, anxiety, or anger and is often captured when the practitioner says, "This just doesn't feel right." This "not right" feeling is an emotional response that serves as a trigger to initiate ethical reflection. Being aware of ethical tension or sensing a threat to integrity often drives the need to

CASE STUDY 36-1   CONSIDERING VIRTUES

Victoria is an OT student completing her second Level II fieldwork affiliation in an inpatient rehabilitation setting. She is 8 weeks into her placement and has been enjoying the increased independence and confidence that comes with practice experience and mentorship. Victoria has been primarily assigned to the neurology unit but is working with Tara this week, a covering clinical instructor who practices on the orthopedic unit. She has enjoyed the change of pace and exposure to new diagnoses while working on this unit. Tara and Victoria receive a referral for a newly admitted client named Joe. Joe was injured in a motor vehicle crash 10 days prior to his admission to the rehab facility. His injuries include open ulna and radius fractures, status post open reduction and internal fixation with skin grafting to cover a soft tissue deficit, a tibia fracture, and a mild concussion.

Tara is excited to treat Joe. The surgical team told her about his upper extremity reconstruction in rounds this morning, requesting a splint to immobilize his forearm. Tara and Victoria go in together to meet Joe. He is sedated and very groggy. Tara introduces herself to Joe and tells him that she needs to make him a splint to protect his forearm where the surgery took place. Joe replies, "I'm too tired." Tara knows that Joe must have this fitted today so that the graft is protected, and so he can begin daily dressing changes to advance his soft tissue healing. Tara communicates the need for the procedure to happen today and tells Joe he can just "chill out" and she and Victoria will do all the work. Joe agrees to the session stating, "Ok I trust you ladies, just get it done and try not to hurt me."

Tara and Victoria begin the splint fabrication, and Victoria is so pleased that she is the student assisting in this intervention session. She has not seen any grafts on her fieldwork experiences so far and finds them a fascinating way to achieve soft tissue closure. Joe tolerates the session surprisingly well, with very little pain or discomfort at the operative site. When Joe's dressing is removed, Tara turns to Victoria and says, "Wow this is the best graft I have seen! Hold his arm up Victoria, I want to take a picture of it on my phone. It's perfect for my blog." Victoria holds Joe's arm but is immediately uncomfortable with this as Joe is sedated and not aware that the photo is being taken. She feels her uneasiness rise as Tara goes on to take several photos of Joe without his knowledge. She knows that she has a responsibility to do something but is unsure what to do. She broaches the subject by saying, "I know on the neurology unit, we have to get written consent for all photos we take of our clients. Don't you guys have the same policy on this unit?" Tara responds by saying, "Yeah, but he's out of it. No harm done. I'll ask him another time. I'm sure he won't mind. Now can you rotate his arm a little? I want to get a few more images." Victoria is frustrated, and her mind is awhirl thinking of what she should do next.

The case of Victoria highlights the need to call on both character and conduct in professional practice. It also highlights how quickly demands are placed on our reasoning in the practice environment, necessitating us to use our skills of discernment and moral reasoning.

- What are the virtues that should guide Victoria in this situation?
- Victoria is no doubt feeling vulnerable and is at a power differential with Tara. What are the consequences of speaking up versus staying silent in this scenario?
- How can Victoria best advocate for Joe and uphold the virtue of professional integrity?

take moral action and activates the cognitive processes for moral reasoning (Opacich, 2003; Rushton, Kaszniak, & Halifax, 2013).

Moral Distress

Moral distress (as defined earlier) results from the conflict of knowing the right thing to do but not being able to achieve it. This cognitive discomfort helps the practitioner realize the potential threat to ethical integrity. Often, multiple stakeholders are involved in the care of the client (e.g., the primary care physician, consulting specialists, rehabilitation practitioners, the organizational administrator, the private insurer, the family). Moral distress can occur when stakeholders hold different opinions regarding the goals of care, leaving practitioners with no clear course of action.

When conflict arises in the care of patients, the paramount goal should always be patient's welfare. Moral distress must be worked through so that this goal can be achieved. An example of moral distress can be found in the case of Etta Jorani.

Ethical Dilemma

An ethical dilemma is slightly different from a moral distress. A dilemma exists when the individual has obligations to do both X and Y but cannot do both (Horner, 2003). In a true dilemma, there is a strong persuasive argument both for and against a "right" course of action. Each choice, or course of action presented to the moral agent, is morally acceptable in some respects and morally unacceptable in others (Beauchamp & Childress, 2013). In other words, each choice has an element of right and wrong posing a moral conflict. Ethical dilemmas are more complex problems as they often pit values and cherished moral principles against each other (Wells, 2003).

CASE STUDY 36-2   EXPERIENCING MORAL DISTRESS

Etta is a 72-year-old woman who was visiting her daughter in New York City from her home in the Philippines. During her visit, Etta suffered a left middle cerebral artery (MCA) cerebrovascular accident (CVA) with severe right-sided hemiplegia.

Etta requires moderate assistance with all activities of daily living (ADL) and is motivated to work with OT despite her limited English skills. The neurologist caring for Etta lets the team know that she is medically ready for discharge. The occupational therapist, physical therapist (PT), and speech-language pathologist (SLP) all recommend inpatient rehabilitation; however, because Etta is not a U.S. citizen, she is not covered by insurance for this level of care in the United States. The case manager who coordinates the discharge services lets Etta know that she will not be eligible for rehabilitation care in the United States. Etta is visibly upset and says, "What do you mean? Where am I supposed to go? My daughter works and takes care of her own kids in a one-bedroom apartment. I can't stay with her and there is no way I can get back to the Philippines like this. I don't understand; you saved me only to leave me alone and helpless." The OT and the interprofessional team caring for Etta feel terrible. They do not want Etta to mistake the limitations in her resources as noncaring on the part of the providers. They are experiencing moral distress. They know the right thing to do (transfer Etta to an inpatient rehabilitation hospital for continued intense treatment), but a barrier (the lack of insurance) stands in the way. They all want the best outcome for Etta but are limited by the context and the constraints of her situation. They must work together to problem-solve through this moral distress so Etta and her family achieve the best outcome.

The case of Victoria presented earlier in this chapter is an ethical dilemma. As you will recall, Victoria is the student working with Joe, the client status post upper extremity reconstruction who was being photographed by Tara, his primary therapist, without his knowledge or consent. It is easy to see that Victoria is experiencing moral distress; however, she also has an ethical dilemma.

Victoria has dual obligations. She has a loyalty to her supervising therapist (and the organization) under whom she is practicing. Tara is a well-respected clinician and has been a resource to Victoria throughout her student affiliation. Victoria wants to honor the student–mentor relationship they have developed. At the same time, she questions whether honoring this relationship is supported because it would disregard the promise she made on entering the OT profession—to above all respect the rights of individuals and refrain from any actions that cause harm (AOTA, 2015a). Victoria knows that she also has an obligation to treat her supervisor with respect and discretion. Tara states that she will obtain consent from Joe later. Victoria wonders—does this meet the intent of consent and adequately protect Joe from harm? Can she trust this will happen? Victoria may also be thinking—I am just a student so technically I could just let this go. After all, what if there were repercussions for continuing to insist that Tara not take photos (and delete the ones she has already taken)? Upon reflection, Victoria also realizes that by holding Joe's arm she was an active participant in the session and may be responsible for any consequences of this action. She wonders if she could lose her student affiliation for this. She is feeling angry, anxious, and vulnerable.

Victoria weighs possible courses of action. One option would be to continue to trust Tara's supervisory guidance, allowing her to take the photos and obtain consent from Joe once he is more alert. Perhaps Tara is right; Joe won't mind (and may even be flattered) knowing the photos will be used to educate other therapists. Victoria justifies this action thinking—that would be a "good outcome"—no harm would be done and perhaps even some good would come out of it. By not objecting and deferring to Tara's judgment, Victoria avoids conflict and does not place her student affiliation at risk by bringing the incident to the attention of others.

Victoria then reasons through another option. In this option, she continues to advocate for Joe and insists that Tara not photograph Joe without his consent. In this way, Victoria upholds her professional responsibility by being both responsive (to the patient's well-being) and by sharing what she knows with her supervisor who is accountable for the action. This action takes both character and courage on Victoria's part as it may cause conflict within the student–mentor relationship. Tara may be upset. She may dismiss Victoria from the case, or Tara may be pleased and she may commend Victoria for her advocacy skills. Either way, if Victoria refrains from further participation in the session, she highlights for Tara that taking photographs without consent is a wrong act (both ethically and legally). This option ensures safety for the client, but it runs the risk of eroding the mentoring relationship, something Victoria greatly values. It also has potential professional repercussions for both Victoria and Tara. The fact is that Victoria cannot choose both options. She must act on one or the other. She has an ethical dilemma.

Moral Theories and Ethical Principles That Apply to Occupational Therapy Practice

Moral theories and ethical principles provide a language for diagnosing, communicating, analyzing, and reflecting on ethical questions. Moral theories are well-developed, systematic frameworks of rules and principles (Nash, 2002). They provide reasons and ideals for ethical standards. The most commonly used ethical approaches in health care are principle-based approaches, virtue- and character-based ethics, utilitarianism, and deontology.

Principle-Based Approach

A principle-based approach to ethics relies on ordinary shared moral beliefs as theoretical content. Principles are duties, rights, or other moral guidelines that provide a logical approach to analyzing ethical issues for a given situation. In case analysis, principles are identified, applied, and compared to weigh one principle against another in deciding a course of action. The following principles are commonly used in health care:

- **Autonomy.** Autonomy is the ability to act freely and independently on one's own decisions (Beauchamp & Childress, 2013). It is often called the principle of self-determination.
- **Beneficence.** Beneficence refers to actions done on or for the benefit of others.
- **Nonmaleficence.** Nonmaleficence is the duty not to harm others.
- **Fidelity.** Fidelity means being faithful to one's promises or commitments.
- **Justice.** Justice refers to equal treatment. It deals with the proper distribution of benefits, burdens, and resources. Procedural justice is often used to reflect impartial decision-making procedures. Distributive justice refers to the equitable allocation of societal resources such as health care (Horner, 2003).
- **Veracity.** Veracity refers to telling the truth.

Virtue and Character-Based Ethics

Virtues are dispositions of character and conduct that motivate and enable practitioners to provide good care (Fletcher, Miller, & Spencer, 1997). Virtue ethics, derived from Aristotle and Thomas Aquinas, focuses on moral agents and their good character. Using this approach, moral goodness is achieved when behaviors are chosen for the sake of virtue (caring and kindness) rather than obligation.

Utilitarianism

Utilitarianism, derived from the work of Jeremy Bentham and John Stuart Mill, is concerned with actions that maximize good consequences and minimize bad consequences. From this perspective, morally right acts produce the best overall results; that is, the ends justify the means. The ethical action is one whose outcome brings about the most good or the least harm overall (Doherty & Purtilo, 2016). Utilitarianism is often used in public policy development.

Deontology

Deontology is a duty-based moral theory that is based primarily on the work of Immanuel Kant. In this theory, moral rules are universal and never to be broken; consequently, doing one's duty is considered primary, regardless of the consequences. For example, truthfulness is an unconditional Kantian duty. A practitioner would never keep the truth from a client even if the truth would harm the client in some way. From a Kantian perspective, respect for people is a moral imperative; therefore, withholding the truth disrespects the client's right to know.

The Ethical Decision-Making Process

Ethical decision making is a key component of professional reasoning. The ethical decision-making process provides a structured and systematic way for practitioners to give due consideration to issues, reflect on them, formulate possible alternatives, and make thoughtful choices. It guides client-centered care with an emphasis on moral conduct (Doherty & Purtilo, 2016). There are various ethical decision-making models available to practitioners. Common aspects of all ethical decision-making models are the need for the practitioners to do the following (Bailey & Schwartzberg, 2003; Doherty & Purtilo, 2016; Gervais, 2005; Hansen & Kyler-Hutchison, 1989; Hunt & Ells, 2013; Scanlon & Glover, 1995; Swisher, Arslanian, & Davis, 2005):

1. Recognize and define the ethical question.
2. Gather the relevant data.
3. Formulate a moral diagnosis and analyze the problem using ethics theory/principles.
4. Problem-solve practical alternatives, weight options, and decide on an action.
5. Act on a morally acceptable choice.
6. Evaluate and reflect on the process/action/results.

Ethical Resources and Jurisdiction

Resources

Practitioners who face ethical issues must be knowledgeable about the resources that exist to support them in this dimension of their clinical reasoning. Resources are crucial for dealing with the uncertainties related to ethical issues that practitioners encounter at all levels of practice.

Ethics Committees

Ethics committees support practitioners who need assistance in reasoning about ethical dimensions of care. The three primary roles of ethics committees are consultation, education, and policy review and development. Accrediting agencies, such as The Joint Commission, require that all health care organizations have a process to address ethical issues involving patient care and organizational ethics. Ethics committees provide an environment for safe and open discussion of basic moral questions, ease the feelings of staff, provide knowledgeable resources, and empower practitioners and families to make morally justified decisions.

Effective ethics committees are interprofessional in makeup and have strong institutional support. They analyze cases from many different perspectives to ensure the best outcome for clients. Occupational therapy practitioners who are either interested novices or experts in ethics should serve as members of ethics committees because they can bring broad perspectives to ethics discussions, are resources for topics related to values clarification and quality of life, and are skilled in group facilitation. Practitioners in settings without ethics committees should seek counsel in a timely manner from mentors, managers, administrative supports, and professional organizations for appropriate assistance with ethical issues. Other organizational resources such as the office of patient care advocacy (also known as the ombudsman), office of social work, chaplaincy service, and office of legal counsel can also provide guidance with ethical issues.

Institutional Review Boards

Increased impetus for research and attention to evidence-based practice have resulted in an increase in the number of OT practitioners involved in research. All practitioners who are involved in research activity have a moral obligation to familiarize themselves with the rules, regulations, and ethical obligations of conducting responsible research. There are many ethical considerations in research (e.g., data integrity, conflict of interest, authorship), but the most compelling pertains to human subjects as research participants.

To ensure an objective review of ethical issues related to human subject research, any institution that receives federal funding is required to have an **institutional review board (IRB)**. An IRB is a panel of diverse individuals, including organization staff and at least one community member, who are responsible for reviewing all research proposals and grants to ensure that adequate protections for research participants are in place. These protections include informed consent, research design and methodology, recruitment, the balance of risks and benefits, and confidentiality. The three fundamental principles that guide the ethical conduct of research involving human participants are respect for persons (autonomy), beneficence, and justice (National Commission for the Protection of Human Subjects of Biomedical and Behavioral Research, 1979). Occupational therapy practitioners should refer to their organization's specific policies and regulations regarding oversight and training in the ethical conduct of research.

Codes of Ethics

Codes of ethics are written documents produced by professional associations, organizations, or regulatory bodies that state the commitment to a service ideal, core purpose, or standard of conduct. Ethical codes ensure public trust and safeguard the reputation of a profession. Codes of ethics are often aspirational, educational, and regulatory in nature (Banks, 2004). The values articulated in the ethical code serve to guide professional practice.

The "Occupational Therapy Code of Ethics" (AOTA, 2015a) serves as a guide for professional conduct. Along with the "Standards of Practice for Occupational Therapy" (AOTA, 2015b), this document serves as resource to all OT practitioners, educators, students, and researchers encouraging them to attain the highest level of professional behavior. The primary purpose of the "Occupational Therapy Code of Ethics" (AOTA, 2015a) is to

1. Provide aspirational Core Values that guide members toward ethical courses of action in professional and volunteer roles and
2. Delineate enforceable Principles and Standards of Conduct that apply to AOTA members.

It also serves to educate the general public and members regarding established principles and standards of conduct to which OT personnel are accountable and can guide OT personnel in recognition and resolution of ethical dilemmas (AOTA, 2015a, p. 1). In addition to the Code of Ethics, the profession is grounded in seven long-standing "Core Values." These values are altruism, equality, freedom, justice, dignity, truth, and prudence (AOTA, 2015a). When practitioners find themselves facing ethical challenges, they should return to these foundational values to guide

CASE STUDY 36-3 APPLYING THE ETHICAL DECISION-MAKING PROCESS

Nicole is an occupational therapist working in an early intervention (EI) setting. She has been working with an interprofessional team of practitioners treating the Suarez family. Their client, Gabriella Suarez, is a 2-and-a-half-year-old female status post embolic CVA.

Gabriella spent more than 3 months in the acute rehabilitation setting because she had lost her ability to perform all occupations including her ability to speak, eat, and play. The loss of these previously achieved developmental milestones was traumatic to the family, who surrounded this outgoing and loving toddler with support and encouragement throughout her rehabilitation. After weeks of OT and speech therapy, it was determined that Gabriella was ready to be transitioned back to taking food by mouth (since her stroke, she had been receiving nourishment through a gastric tube because she was unable to swallow without aspirating). She was awaiting an MBS test as the final step in this transition.

One afternoon, Nicole arrived to find Gabriella's mother feeding her daughter a cookie. Her initial reaction of joy at the fact that the child was able to enjoy a cookie for the first time in months was quickly overwhelmed by her sobering realization that she had not yet been cleared to eat solid foods. Over the last month, Nicole had become very close to both the child and her mother who were thrilled with this victory. Gabriella smiled, an expression of emotion that Nicole had never seen her exhibit before. This gave the mother great hope, something she had been without for many weeks. Nicole then realized that she was in a tough place when the mother then asked her to "please, please not tell anyone" that she had given her daughter the cookie.

To ensure a professional and caring response to this situation, Nicole must analyze the situation using an ethical decision-making process. This will help guide her thinking and her actions.

Identify the Ethical Question

First, Nicole must identify and reflect on the ethical questions that emerged in the case. This often begins with the question, "What should I do?" In the case of Gabriella and her mother, some questions would be the following: Should Nicole tell the team that the client's mother fed her the cookie? Should she honor the mother's request not to report the action, knowing that this may cause harm to the child? How can Nicole balance her obligations to the child, the mother, and the EI agency?

Gather the Relevant Data

The next step in ethical analysis is to gather the relevant data, identifying the known facts and beliefs about the case. It is important to distinguish between the two. Facts are needed to make judicious decisions. Facts regarding medical information

and factors such as family context, client preferences, social and cultural considerations, institutional factors, and provider considerations should be confirmed for accuracy. Additional information should be sought if needed. Take a moment and think about the facts and beliefs in this case.

Formulate a Moral Diagnosis and Apply Ethics Principles/Theory to the Case

Once the information has been gathered, a moral diagnosis must be formulated by identifying the type of ethical problem and the ethical principles that apply to the case. If there is more than one problem, they should be ranked in order of importance.

Having considered the ethical questions in the case of Gabriella, Nicole must decide whether the ethical problem is moral distress or ethical dilemma. She decides that she is facing moral distress. Nicole knows the correct course of action requires her to tell the team that the mother has fed the child prior to medical clearance. The relationship that she had with the child and her mother and the mother's emotional plea for her not to tell was a barrier to that disclosure. She was torn with how to best care for Gabriella and show care and concern to the mother. Key ethical principles that relate to this moral distress are beneficence and nonmaleficence. There are other principles and theories that apply; think about which ones as you continue to reason through the case.

Problem-Solve Practical Alternatives and Decide on a Course of Action

Now Nicole must begin to identify practical alternatives and decide what do. She must ask herself, "What is the good or right thing to do?" She would be wise to seek out resources in her facility and to ask her mentors for guidance in this ethical analysis. She might consult with various stakeholders, such as the interprofessional team, to identify strategies to best educate the family and ensure Gabriella's safety. She also could refer to the AOTA "Occupational Therapy Code of Ethics" (AOTA, 2015a) and "Standards of Practice for Occupational Therapy" (AOTA, 2015b). Generating a list of alternatives enables evaluation of the positive and negative consequences. Once the alternatives have been identified, ethical theory should be applied to support and justify the proposed action.

Nicole brainstormed a list of possible alternatives:

- Ask the mother why she gave Gabriella the cookie and why she does not want other members of the EI team to know. This is an important piece of information to explore. What were the motivating factors behind the mother's decision to give Gabriella the cookie? Did she want to be the first person to reintroduce food to her child? What are the cultural expectations and the meaning of food for the Suarez family?

(continues)

CASE STUDY 36-3   APPLYING THE ETHICAL DECISION-MAKING PROCESS *(continued)*

- Offer support to the mother. She may fear judgment of others or may feel that if the information is revealed, her daughter may suffer consequences of her action causing a delay in her progress.
- Deny the mother's request and inform the team.
- Say nothing to the mother but document the observation in the record. (It is important to note that this alternative is not one that has moral grounding, as it has the potential to cause more harm to all parties involved. It fractures the therapeutic relationship with the family, and although it may alleviate Nicole's anxiety, will only do so temporarily, creating possible future distress).
- Talk with the mother about the concerns Nicole has related to Gabriella's safety. In a supportive way, this allows the mother to gain better insight into the potential outcomes of her actions and participate in shared decision making. This conversation may even lead to a joint discussion with other members of the interprofessional care team regarding the mother's understanding of the process for transitioning back to oral feeding. Choice talk and option talk can enhance collaborative goal setting in the best interests of the client and family.
- Describe the situation with the EI nurse without identifying which family was involved.
- Tell the mother that she will not tell the team as long as the mother agrees to not give Gabriella any more food by mouth until medically cleared.

Nicole will need to reason through the alternatives, apply ethical theory to support her actions, and come to a judgment on the best approach. Having virtue, sensitivity to ethical issues, and a process for analyzing ethical questions are important elements in ethical decision making. If you were Nicole, which alternative would you choose?

Act on a Morally Acceptable Choice

Now that Nicole has decided on the course of action, she must act on the decision, bridging the gap between knowing what she ought to do and actually doing it. This is where the Aristotelian notion of practical wisdom and moral argument

join together with clinical judgment for action. Often, this is the most difficult step because it requires calling on moral courage to take positions that are unpopular or contrary to the interest of others (Aulisio, Arnold, & Younger, 2000). Moral courage is a skill. It involves facing and overcoming fear to uphold an ultimate good.

Nicole will need courage to talk with Gabriella's mother. She will need to be attentive to the interests and emotions of the mother and remember the ultimate goal, which is to ensure compassionate, quality care for Gabriella.

Evaluate and Reflect on the Process/Action/Results

Finally, Nicole must evaluate the results of her action. Evaluation includes both current and retrospective analysis. This reflection can guide future action by either avoiding or preventing a similar situation or knowing how to act should a similar situation arise in the future. Questions Nicole might ask are as follows:

- What was the most challenging aspect of this situation?
- What have I learned from this case to help improve future patient care?
- What did I learn from the family/team regarding my course of action?
- What have I learned that will contribute to my own moral life and to my virtues as a practitioner?
- How has this case affected me as a care provider? What would I do differently if faced with the same situation again?

Evaluation of the decision-making process in cases such as this one has the potential to change practice, policies, education, or service delivery systems. Evaluation provides the opportunity for personal and professional reflection that can lead to further professional development and greater confidence to respond to future moral distress. Nicole could also work with her colleagues and the EI agency to propose policies and staff education so that similar confusion does not occur in the future. Nicole should also consider how those she consulted with contributed to the case and should critique her own decision-making process to improve her future practice.

ethical practice. Additional information about the code and related documents and the AOTA Ethics Commission can be found at http://www.aota.org.

Regulatory Agencies

Three organizations provide oversight for OT practice: the AOTA, the National Board for Certification in Occupational Therapy (NBCOT), and state regulatory boards (SRBs).

Each has distinct concerns, sanctions, and jurisdiction, but one commonality is their concern for ethical practice.

The American Occupational Therapy Association

The AOTA, the professional association for OT, is the primary vehicle for influencing, promoting, and developing the profession's services to society (Doherty & Peterson, 2016). The AOTA develops standards of practice for all OT practitioners. These standards are an essential resource for practitioners, students, educators, and researchers.

Within AOTA, the Ethics Commission reviews the AOTA Occupational Therapy Code of Ethics every 5 years. Its primary responsibility is to recommend the ethics standards for the profession. It also educates members and consumers regarding ethics standards. Ethics Commission members and staff of the AOTA Ethics Program are resources for students, practitioners, educators, and consumers. They provide assistance with the interpretation of relevant ethical principles via advisory opinions, consultation, articles, and presentations. Finally, the Ethics Commission is responsible for the process of developing and implementing the enforcement procedures for the code. Disciplinary actions apply to members of AOTA and include reprimand, censure, probation, suspension, and permanent revocation of membership.

National Board for Certification in Occupational Therapy

The NBCOT is a credentialing agency that provides certification for the OT profession. Its mission is to "serve the public interest by advancing client care and professional practice through evidence-based certification standards and the validation of knowledge essential for effective practice in occupational therapy" (NBCOT, 2017). The NBCOT establishes minimum standards for certification to enter practice and ongoing recertification standards, including continuing competency through professional development. The NBCOT Certificant Code of Conduct (NBCOT, 2016) outlines professional responsibilities for certified OT practitioners. As in many organizational codes of conduct, the NBCOT Certificant Code of Conduct includes ethics-related principles such as integrity, responsibility, honesty, fairness, and technical competence. Violation of this code of conduct is grounds for sanction, which may entail reprimand, probation, or suspension or revocation of certification.

The NBCOT Qualifications and Compliance Review Committee oversees certification violation issues such as breaches of ethics and unprofessional practice. The NBCOT notifies SRBs and the public of any complaints it receives and the disciplinary action it takes in response to these complaints. Additional information about NBCOT and the NBCOT Certificant Code of Conduct can be found at http://www.nbcot.org.

State Regulatory Boards

State regulatory boards or licensing boards safeguard and promote the public welfare by ensuring that qualifications and standards for professional practice are properly evaluated, applied, and enforced (Doherty & Peterson, 2016). They ensure the health and safety of citizens in their respective states. Occupational therapy is regulated in all 50 states and in three U.S. territories. The level of regulation varies; therefore, all OT practitioners must be aware of the specific provisions and statutes for the state in which they work. Most states use professional licensure to regulate practice, but several states have certification, registration, or title protection. Licensure is a means of defining a lawful scope of practice. It ensures patient protections and legally articulates the domain of practice for the profession. Licensure also prevents nonqualified individuals from practicing OT or using the title "occupational therapist" or "occupational therapy assistant." Many states include codes of ethics statements (most adopt the AOTA code and ethics standards) in their licensure law or regulations. State regulatory boards have the authority by state law to discipline OT practitioners who violate regulations, including the state's code of conduct. Practitioners have the responsibility to understand the regulations under which they work and the procedure for processing a complaint.

Difficult Conversations

Communication is a fundamental aspect of respectful interactions, therapeutic relationships, and client-centered care (Haddad, Doherty, & Purtilo, 2018). The cases of Etta, Victoria, and Gabriella highlight how difficult conversations are a part of everyday interactions in health care. Some of these are with clients, some with families, and some with interprofessional colleagues. Although difficult conversations may be uncomfortable and awkward, practitioners can develop the skill and confidence to improve the quality and outcomes of their communications.

Open communication and empathetic listening are key components to the delivery of compassionate care. The following are suggestions for effective communication:

1. **Be present.** Always respect others. Try to minimize interruptions and ensure that the environment is as free of distractions as possible. Choose an appropriate communication style for the situation. Establish rapport by making good eye contact and show interest, care, warmth, and responsiveness. These factors are predictive of effective client communication (Levetown, 2008).

2. **Use open-ended communication and listen quietly.** Health care practitioners often say too much, which does not allow time for the other person to speak. Talk less and listen more. Phrases such as "go on" can encourage the person to examine issues at a deeper level (Cameron, 2004).

3. **Remain focused on the person and the goals of intervention.** Strive to understand the client's story. What are the connections between the circumstances, beliefs, values, and resources in the client narrative? Ask open-ended questions such as "What is your understanding of the situation?" or "What are your fears?" and "What are your hopes?" This helps you understand another's

perspective and can assist both practitioner and client in setting appropriate goals for care (Gawande, 2014; Hinkle, Fettig, Carlos, & Bosslet, 2017; Quill, 2000).

4. **Be contrite and humble.** If you do not know the answer to a question, say so and assure the person that you will find the answer. Then find the answer and follow up with the person. Share your uncertainty about the case or prognosis.

5. **Legitimize the losses that the person is experiencing.** It is important to acknowledge the person's experience. Many clients are not prepared to cope with their newly diagnosed condition. They never expected to be in a compromised state, and their family might not be able to cope with the personal or financial implications of this change. Denial, depression, and anger are common responses to disease and disability. Practitioners need to acknowledge these emotions openly by stating "What I am hearing you say is that you are angry that you can no longer live alone" or "Let me see if I can summarize what your daughter is trying to say . . . Is that correct?"

6. **Ensure shared decision making.** Questions surrounding new disability, quality-of-life, and end-of-life issues can be especially complex. Clients experience biographical disruption when confronted with illness challenging their fundamental values and autonomy (Mars, Kempen, Widdershoven, Janssen, & van Eijk, 2008). Occupational therapy practitioners are obligated to engage clients in shared decision making and to fully inform clients of the likelihood of the success or failure of therapeutic interventions. Shared decision making is a process in which information is exchanged *between* the professional and the client (Doherty & Purtilo, 2016).

7. **Make a team effort.** In today's complex health care environments, the interprofessional care team has a moral obligation to work collaboratively to deliver the best care possible. Ethical approaches must focus on interprofessional teamwork because it is unreasonable to expect that individuals can resolve complex situations and moral distress alone (Carpenter, 2010). Collective perspectives are foundational to collaborative care delivery. Effective interprofessional teams listen attentively, use understandable communication, provide feedback to others, respond to feedback from others, and address interprofessional conflict (Interprofessional Education Collaborative, 2016).

Conclusion

Ethical issues are ever present in professional practice and will continue to challenge OT practitioners as the fields of medicine, technology, and health care delivery evolve. Occupational therapy practitioners must recognize,

critically reason, act, and reflect on ethical issues that arise in their professional roles. Occupational therapy practitioners who are reflective and knowledgeable in ethical decision-making processes are best prepared to successfully address ethical aspects of practice. Ethical behavior is the responsibility of all OT professionals.

"The tools of ethical decision making include developing 'habits of thought' for reflection on complex, changing situations that are part of everyday practice."

—Jensen (2005)

REFERENCES

American Occupational Therapy Association. (1977). Representative Assembly—Resolution A, Principles of occupational therapy ethics. *American Journal of Occupational Therapy, 69,* 6913410057.

American Occupational Therapy Association. (2015a). Occupational therapy code of ethics (2015). *American Journal of Occupational Therapy, 69,* 6913410030.

American Occupational Therapy Association. (2015b). Standards of practice for occupational therapy. *American Journal of Occupational Therapy, 31,* 594.

Aulisio, M. P., Arnold, R. M., & Younger, S. J. (2000). Health care ethics consultation: Nature, goals, and competencies: A position paper from the Society for Health and Human Values-Society for Bioethics Consultation Task Force on Standards for Bioethics Consultation. *Annals of Internal Medicine, 133,* 59–69.

Bailey, D. M., & Schwartzberg, S. L. (Eds.). (2003). *Ethical and legal dilemmas in occupational therapy* (2nd ed.). Philadelphia, PA: F. A. Davis.

Banks, S. (2004). *Ethics, accountability, and the social professions.* New York, NY: Palgrave Macmillan.

Barnitt, R. E. (1993). Deeply troubling questions: The teaching of ethics in undergraduate courses. *British Journal of Occupational Therapy, 56,* 401–406.

Beauchamp, T. L., & Childress, J. F. (2013). *Principles of biomedical ethics* (7th ed.). New York, NY: Oxford University Press.

Bebeau, M. J. (2002). The defining issues test and the four component model: Contributions to professional education. *Journal of Moral Education, 31,* 271–293.

Board of Management. (1926, September 26). *Pledge and Creed. Minutes of the meeting of Board of Managers.* Archives of the American Occupational Therapy Association (Series 3, Box 13, Folder 81), Bethesda, MD.

Brandt, L. C., & Homenko, D. F. (2016). Balancing patient rights and practitioner values. In D. Y. Slater (Ed.), *Reference guide to the occupational therapy code of ethics and ethics standards* (2015 ed., pp. 151–153). Bethesda, MD: AOTA Press.

Bushby, K., Chan, J., Druif, S., Ho, K., & Kinsella, E. A. (2015). Ethical tensions in occupational therapy practice: A scoping review. *British Journal of Occupational Therapy, 78,* 212–221.

Cameron, M. (2004). Ethical listening as therapy. *Journal of Professional Nursing, 20,* 141–142.

Carpenter, C. (2010). Moral distress in physical therapy practice. *Physiotherapy Theory and Practice, 26,* 69–78.

Delany, C. M., Edwards, I., Jensen, G. M., & Skinner, E. (2010). Closing the gap between ethics knowledge and practice through active engagement: An applied model of physical therapy ethics. *Physical Therapy, 90*, 1068–1078.

Devettere, R. J. (2009). *Practical decision making in health care ethics: Cases and concepts* (3rd ed.). Washington, DC: Georgetown University Press.

Doherty, R., Dellinger, A., Gately, M., Pullo, R., & Sullivan, S. (2012, April). *Ethical issues in occupational therapy: A survey of practitioners.* Paper presented at the American Occupational Therapy Association 2012 Annual Conference, Indianapolis, IN.

Doherty, R. F., & Peterson, E. W. (2016). Responsible participation in a profession: Fostering professionalism and leading for moral action. In B. Braveman (Ed.), *Leading and managing occupational therapy services: An evidence-based approach* (2nd ed.). Philadelphia, PA: F. A. Davis.

Doherty, R. F., & Purtilo, R. B. (2016). *Ethical dimensions in the health professions* (6th ed.). St. Louis, MO: Elsevier Saunders.

Epstein, R. M. (1999). Mindful practice. *JAMA, 282*, 833–839.

Fletcher, J. C., Miller, F. G., & Spencer, E. M. (1997). Clinical ethics: History, content, and resources. In J. C. Fletcher, P. A. Lombardo, M. F. Marshall, & F. G. Miller (Eds.), *Introduction to clinical ethics* (2nd ed., pp. 3–20). Hagerstown, MD: University Publishing Group.

Foye, S. J., Kirschner, K. L., Wagner, L. C. B., Stocking, C., & Siegler, M. (2002). Ethics in practice: Ethical issues in rehabilitation: A qualitative analysis of dilemmas identified by occupational therapists. *Topics in Stroke Rehabilitation, 9*, 89–101.

Fry, S. T., & Veatch, R. M. (2000). *Case studies in nursing ethics.* Sudbury, MA: Jones & Bartlett Learning.

Gawande, A. (2002). *Complications: A surgeon's notes on an imperfect science.* New York, NY: Picador.

Gawande, A. (2014). *Being mortal: Medicine and what matters in the end.* New York, NY: Metropolitan Books.

Gervais, K. G. (2005). A model for ethical decision making to inform the ethics education of future professionals. In R. Purtilo, G. M. Jensen, & C. B. Royeen (Eds.), *Educating for moral action: A sourcebook in health and rehabilitation ethics* (pp. 185–190). Philadelphia, PA: F. A. Davis.

Glaser, J. W. (2005). Three realms of ethics: An integrating map of ethics for the future. In R. Purtilo, G. M. Jensen, & C. B. Royeen (Eds.), *Educating for moral action: A sourcebook in health and rehabilitation ethics* (pp. 169–184). Philadelphia, PA: F. A. Davis.

Haddad, A., Doherty, R., & Purtilo, R. (2018). *Health professional and patient interaction* (9th ed). St. Louis, MO: Elsevier Saunders.

Hansen, R., & Kyler-Hutchison, P. (1989, April). *Light at the end of the tunnel.* Workshop presented at the annual conference of the American Occupational Therapy Association, Baltimore, MD.

Hartwell, S. (1995). Promoting moral development through experiential teaching. *Clinical Law Review, 1*, 505–539.

Hinkle, L. J., Fettig, L. P., Carlos, W. G., & Bosslet, G. (2017). Twelve tips for just in time teaching of communication skills for difficult conversations in the clinical setting. *Medical Teacher, 39*, 920–925.

Horner, J. (2003). Morality, ethics, and law: Introductory concepts. *Seminars in Speech and Language, 24*, 263–274.

Howard, B., & Kennell, B. (2017, April). *Celebrating the history of occupational therapy ethics in the USA.* Paper presented at the American Occupational Therapy Association 2017 Annual Conference, Pennsylvania, PA.

Hunt, M. R., & Ells, C. (2013). A patient-centered care ethics analysis model for rehabilitation. *American Journal of Physical Medicine & Rehabilitation, 92*, 818–827.

Interprofessional Education Collaborative. (2016). *Core competencies for interprofessional collaborative practice: 2016 update.* Washington, DC: Interprofessional Education Collaborative.

Jensen, G. M. (2005). Mindfulness: Applications for teaching and learning in ethics education. In R. Purtilo, G. M. Jensen, & C. B.

Royeen (Eds.), *Educating for moral action: A sourcebook in health and rehabilitation ethics* (pp. 191–202). Philadelphia, PA: F. A. Davis.

Kanny, E. (1993). Core values and attitudes of occupational therapy practice. *American Journal of Occupational Therapy, 47*, 1085–1086.

Levetown, M. (2008). Communicating with children and families: From everyday interactions to skill in conveying distressing information. *Pediatrics, 121*, 1441–1460.

Lown, B. A., & McIntosh, S. (2015). *Recommendations from a conference on advancing compassionate, person- and family-centered care through interprofessional education for collaborative practice.* Retrieved from http://humanism-in-medicine.org/wp-content/uploads/2015/03/TripleCConferenceRecommendations.pdf

Mars, G. M. J., Kempen, G., Widdershoven, G., Janssen, P., & van Eijk, J. (2008). Conceptualizing autonomy in the context of chronic physical illness: Relating philosophical theories to social scientific perspectives. *Health, 12*, 333–348.

McAuliffe, D. (2014). *Interprofessional ethics: Collaboration in the social, health, and human services.* Port Melbourne, Australia: Cambridge University Press.

Nash, R. J. (2002). *Real world ethics: Frameworks for educators and human service professionals* (2nd ed.). New York, NY: Teachers College Press.

National Board for Certification of Occupational Therapy. (2016). *Code of conduct.* Retrieved from https://www.nbcot.org/-/media/NBCOT/PDFs/Code_of_Conduct.ashx?la=en

National Board for Certification of Occupational Therapy. (2017). *Home page.* Retrieved from https://www.nbcot.org

National Commission for the Protection of Human Subjects of Biomedical and Behavioral Research. (1979). *The Belmont report.* Retrieved from http://www.hhs.gov/ohrp/humansubjects/guidance/belmont.htm

Olson, K., & Kemper, K. J. (2014). Factors associated with well-being and confidence in providing compassionate care. *Journal of Evidence-Based Complementary & Alternative Medicine, 19*, 292–296.

Opacich, K. J. (2003). Ethical dimensions of occupational therapy management. In G. L. McCormack, E. G. Jaffe, & M. Goodman-Lavey (Eds.), *The occupational therapy manager* (pp. 491–512.). Rockville, MD: American Occupational Therapy Association.

Pellegrino, E. D. (1995). Toward a virtue-based normative ethics for the health professions. *Kennedy Institute of Ethics Journal, 5*, 253–277.

Pellegrino, E. D. (2002). Professionalism, profession and the virtues of the good physician. *The Mount Sinai Journal of Medicine, 69*, 378–384.

Purtilo, R. (2004). Professional–patient relationship: III. Ethical issues. In S. G. Post (Ed.), *Encyclopedia of bioethics* (3rd ed., pp. 2150–2158). New York, NY: Macmillan.

Quill, T. E. (2000). Perspectives on care at the close of life. Initiating end-of-life discussions with seriously ill patients: Addressing the "elephant in the room." *JAMA, 284*, 2502–2507.

Rushton, C. H., Kaszniak, A. W., & Halifax, J. S. (2013). A framework for understanding moral distress among palliative care clinicians. *Journal of Palliative Medicine, 16*, 1074–1079.

Scanlon, C., & Glover, J. (1995). A professional code of ethics: Providing a moral compass for turbulent times. *Oncology Nursing Forum, 22*, 1515–1521.

Schoeberlein, D., & Sheth, S. (2009). *Mindful teaching and teaching mindfulness: A guide for anyone who teaches anything.* Boston, MA: Wisdom.

Sisola, S. W. (2000). Moral reasoning as a predictor of clinical practice: The development of physical therapy students across the professional curriculum. *Journal of Physical Therapy Education, 14*, 26–34.

Slater, D. Y. (2016). *Reference guide to the occupational therapy code of ethic and ethics standards* (2nd ed.). Bethesda, MD: AOTA Press.

Slater, D. Y., & Brandt, L. C. (2016). Combating moral distress. In D. Y. Slater (Ed.), *Reference guide to the occupational therapy code of ethics and ethics standards* (2015 ed., pp. 117–123). Bethesda, MD: AOTA Press.

Sullivan, W. M., & Rosin, M. S. (2008). *A new agenda for higher education: Shaping a life of the mind for practice.* San Francisco, CA: Jossey-Bass.

Swisher, L., Arslanian, L. E., & Davis, C. M. (2005). The Realm-Individual-Process-Situation (RIPS) model of ethical decision making. *HPA Resource, 5,* 3–18.

Tufts University Digital Collections and Archives. (1959). *Pledge and creed for occupational therapists*, BSOT Student's Handbook 1959–1960, p.2, UA032.011.111.00006. Boston, MA: Tufts University.

Unsworth, C., & Baker, A. (2016). A systematic review of professional reasoning literature in occupational therapy. *British Journal of Occupational Therapy, 79,* 5–16.

Wald, H. S., Borkan, J. M., Taylor, J. S., Anthony, D., & Reis, S. P. (2012). Fostering and evaluating reflective capacity in medical education: Developing the REFLECT rubric for assessing reflective writing. *Academic Medicine, 87,* 41–50.

Wells, B. G. (2003). Leadership for ethical decision making. *American Journal of Pharmaceutical Education, 67,* 5–8.

World Federation of Occupational Therapists. (2016). *The World Federation of Occupational Therapists (WFOT) code of ethics.* Retrieved from http://www.wfot.org/ResourceCentre/tabid/132/did/780/Default.aspx

the**Point**®   *For additional resources on the subjects discussed in this chapter, visit* **http://thePoint.lww.com /Willard-Spackman13e.** *See* **Appendix I, Resources and Evidence for Common Conditions Addressed in OT** *for more information about fractures, traumatic brain injury, and cerebrovascular accident/stroke.*

CHAPTER 37

Therapeutic Relationship and Client Collaboration

Applying the Intentional Relationship Model

Renée R. Taylor

LEARNING OBJECTIVES

After reading this chapter, you will be able to:

1. Outline the evidence supporting therapeutic use of self in occupational therapy.
2. Describe the components of the Intentional Relationship Model.
3. Define and give examples of interpersonal events that can occur during the therapy process.
4. Compare the strengths and weaknesses of each of the six interpersonal modes.
5. Apply the interpersonal reasoning process, including the six modes to clinical scenarios and case examples.

Introduction: The Nature of the Therapeutic Relationship in Occupational Therapy

Occupational therapists carry the privilege and responsibility to maintain the trust that clients and interprofessional colleagues place in our ability to accompany people through their most difficult periods of rehabilitation. This is demonstrated by the growing evidence base from which we practice (Dirette, Rozich, & Viau, 2009; Marr, 2017). The Occupational Therapy Practice Framework (American Occupational Therapy Association, 2014, p. 52) emphasizes therapeutic use of self as "integral to the practice of occupational therapy [and] used in all interactions with clients." As defined by R.R. Taylor (2008), the therapeutic use of self is the application of empathy and intentionality to an interpersonal knowledge base and corresponding set of communication skills that are applied thoughtfully to resolve evocative interpersonal events in practice. An effective therapeutic use of self requires the therapist to strive toward a fundamental understanding of clients as human beings, at an interpersonal level.

During rehabilitation, clients are faced with fatigue, pain, economic expense, loss, and uncertainty about the future. These experiences can lead to feelings of disorientation or confusion, helplessness, isolation, abandonment, stigma, despair, and anxiety even in the highest functioning individuals (Johnson & Webster, 2002; Moorey & Greer, 2002). When problems arise, there is often an immediate need to focus on functional impairments and environmental barriers. Without an equivalent (or sometimes stronger) focus on the internal psychological and interpersonal aspects of a person's experience, the therapy process may be experienced as impersonal or dehumanizing.

To address these problems, some therapists apply personal intuition, past experience, or other theoretical or popular psychology strategies. Although some of these strategies may work in the short term, they are insufficient in the face of more complex and intractable interpersonal dynamics. Many therapists tend to view higher level complexities that may emerge during the therapeutic relationship as being outside of their roles, expertise, and scope of practice as occupational therapists. The *Intentional Relationship Model (IRM)* seeks to address all of these challenges in order to guide this understudied yet important area of practice. The IRM provides an evidence-based explanation of the client–therapist relationship, an interpersonal reasoning processes, and a set of concrete communication skills to be used in response to a client's evolving interpersonal characteristics and the inevitable interpersonal events of therapy.

Biopsychosocial Issues and Psychiatric Overlay

Beyond the usual range of negative emotions that clients experience lies a level of interpersonal complexity that is introduced by those with psychiatric overlay or coexisting mental health diagnoses. It has been estimated that roughly 15% to 39% of individuals with chronic illness or impairments also have clinically significant psychiatric overlay (Guthrie, 1996). Depending on the diagnosis, psychiatric overlay can introduce a host of challenges to the therapeutic relationship, ranging from behaviors that are often labeled as "noncompliance" or "resistance" to manipulative behaviors or excessive demands on the therapist's time and energy. An individual's personality and premorbid psychological history can play significant roles in adjustment to impairment because the impairment itself inevitably functions as an additional source of stress (S. E. Taylor & Aspinwall, 1990). Those with prior histories of trauma and psychopathology may be more vulnerable to developing an exaggerated emotional response to the impairment or to engaging in maladaptive health behaviors (White, 2001).

One study found that therapists reported remarkably high rates of difficult client emotions, behaviors, and interpersonal problems in a predominantly nonpsychiatric sample of occupational therapy (OT) clients (R. R. Taylor, Lee, Kielhofner, & Ketkar, 2009). Therapists from a wide range of practice settings and disciplines, treating clients ranging in age from neonates to older adults, found that between 20% and 30% of their clients frequently exhibited behaviors characterized as manipulative, demanding, or dependent. A further 10% to 16% described their clients as frequently hostile, oppositional, resistive, passive, self-denigrating, and unrealistic about treatment or in denial about their impairments. Surprisingly, between 2% and 9% of therapists described their clients as frequently exhibiting hostility, questioning their knowledge or criticizing their approach, uninvested in therapy, resisting feedback and suggestions, and having difficulties with rapport and trust.

From a psychological perspective, it can be argued that all of these behaviors can be attenuated or exacerbated within the therapeutic relationship depending on the experience and skill level of the therapist. Importantly, the way these behaviors are managed (or ignored) within the relationship has lasting consequences for OT outcomes—both immediately and in the long term.

Whereas some therapists feel comfortable addressing the challenging client attitudes and behaviors that sometimes manifest within the relationship, many wish they had more information and training. In a survey by R. R. Taylor and colleagues (2009), less than 5% of therapists reported having taken a course solely dedicated to developing skills to enhance the therapeutic relationship during their training to become an occupational therapist. Fewer than 30% felt there was sufficient knowledge about this area in the field of OT, and only 51% reported feeling adequately trained upon graduating from OT school (R. R. Taylor et al., 2009).

Background and Evidence Base

As a well-established health care discipline, OT traditionally emphasizes the value and importance of therapists' interactions with their clients. One of the most common terms used to refer to therapist–client interactions is the **therapeutic relationship** (Anderson & Hinojosa, 1984; Cole & McLean, 2003; Eklund, 1996; Rosa & Hasselkus, 1996). Literature and dialogue about the therapeutic relationship commonly address topics such as rapport building, communication, conflict resolution, emotional sharing, collaboration, and partnership between therapists and clients. *Therapeutic use of self* is a popular term used in OT to refer to the therapists' deliberate efforts to enhance their interactions with clients (Cole & McLean, 2003; Punwar, 2000).

Therapeutic Use of Self and Collaboration

Collaboration is a critical element in client-centered care. Collaboration refers to the process of mutual participation on the part of client and therapist (Jenkins, Mallett, O'Neill, McFadden, & Baird, 1994). It also

CENTENNIAL NOTES

Therapeutic Use of Self: Historical Perspectives

The importance of therapist demeanor and relationships with clients was recognized early in the profession. Throughout the history of OT, there have been varied definitions and emphases on how therapists are expected to optimize their interactions with clients. In addition to the current definition of therapeutic use of self that is presented in this chapter, the following definitions have been used.

- Ann Mosey discussed the importance of the conscious awareness of oneself. According to Mosey (1981, 1986), a conscious use of self represents an ability to deliberately use one's own responses to clients as a part of the therapeutic process. In order to determine how best to respond to a client, the therapist had to possess self-awareness, empathy, flexibility, humor, honesty, compassion, and humility.
- Denton (1987) emphasized respect and acceptance, with the ultimate purpose of restoring self-esteem.
- Similarly, Schwartzberg (2002) focused on understanding, empathy, and caring. The therapist was to remain neutral but engaged, accepting the client as he or she is, being tolerant and interested in the client's painful emotions, and being able to interpret the client's expectations of therapy accurately.
- Hagedorn (1995) defined therapeutic use of self as the artful, selective, or intuitive use of personal attributes to enhance therapy. The notion of an artful

use of self should not be confused with behaving in artificial or deceitful ways toward clients. Artfulness referred to selecting aspects of one's own personality, attitudes, values, or responses which were predicted to be relevant or helpful in a given situation. In turn, therapists were expected to control or suppress those aspects of self that were not appropriate for the situation. According to Hagedorn, therapists were not expected to be perfect, but instead, they were expected to be aware of their strengths and limitations, sensitive, honest, and genuine with clients. Therapists were also expected to manage stress effectively and to have personal integrity.
- Cara and MacRae (2005) called for therapists to develop an individual style that promotes change and growth in clients and helps to furnish them with a corrective emotional experience. A corrective emotional experience was described as one in which a therapist's behavior toward a client during therapy contradicts the way others have behaved toward the client in the past and demonstrates to the client that he or she is worthy of caring and empathy.
- Punwar and Peloquin (2000) defined therapeutic use of self as a "practitioner's planned use of his or her personality, insights, perceptions and judgments as part of the therapeutic process" (p. 285).

Taken together, all of these definitions influenced the current definition of therapeutic use of self presented in this chapter.

---

includes providing choice, involving clients in decision making, and encouraging clients to actively contribute and to set their own goals for therapy (Kielhofner, 2009; Palmadottir, 2006). Theoretically, all of this should occur within the context of an egalitarian relationship (Norrby & Bellner, 1995). One of the primary approaches to collaboration involves educating clients about all aspects of the treatment process and providing them with information about the purpose and relevance of any procedure or treatment approach. Providing a rationale at each session increases the likelihood of client involvement in therapy (Peloquin, 1988).

Relative to the vast conceptual literature on this topic, a smaller number of empirical studies have focused on examining the role of the therapeutic relationship, collaboration, or aspects of therapeutic use of self in OT. One study specifically examined the interpersonal strategies that occupational therapists use to respond to clients'

interpersonal needs and characteristics (R. R. Taylor, Lee, & Kielhofner, 2011). Findings from 563 practitioners revealed that therapists most preferred to encourage their clients by reminding them of their strengths, providing positive reinforcement, and by instilling hope and confidence. The second most preferred approach involved collaborating with clients by encouraging them to make more decisions during the therapy process, by supporting their perspectives, by gathering feedback from the client before selecting or recommending an activity, and by asking the client to recommend his or her own goals for therapy. Other approaches involving problem solving, empathizing, and instructing clients were less frequently used. Interestingly, these findings did not differ based on the age group of the clients being treated.

In a Swedish study, Eklund and Hallberg (2001) investigated the extent of use of verbal communication during OT in a psychiatric setting. In a sample of 292 occupational therapists, verbal interaction was used during assessment, intervention, treatment planning, and posttreatment evaluation. Verbal communication was deemed a significant component of the therapeutic relationship. Findings emphasized the need to study and develop the verbal as well as the doing aspect of OT.

Cole and McLean (2003) conducted another survey study that focused on approaches to communication among 129 practicing occupational therapists from various practice areas. They found that therapists strongly emphasized rapport, open communication, and empathy as important roles in the therapist–patient relationship. They also found that therapists perceived the therapeutic relationship as critical to therapy outcomes.

In a qualitative study that used focus groups as the main data source, Allison and Strong (1994) examined the use of verbal interaction among 23 occupational therapists in an adult general rehabilitation setting. They concluded that good clinical communicators accommodated their interactions to clients' needs. Similarly, Jenkins and colleagues (1994) systematically observed the communication patterns of eight practitioners in a geriatric setting. Therapists with more experience achieved more mutual participation in the therapy process than those with less experience.

Palmadottir's (2006) qualitative study explored adult clients' perceptions of the therapy relationship in a rehabilitation setting. Based on interviews with 20 adult clients, she recommended the following: Therapists needed to pay more attention to their clients' occupational issues and needs, involve them more in a goal-directed therapy process, and have more awareness of how their own attitudes are communicated and acted out in therapy.

Rosa and Hasselkaus (1996) interviewed 83 occupational therapists who were practicing nationwide. Their qualitative analysis concluded that therapists' personal identities seemed to be merged with their professional identities. They concluded that it is important to have a sense of "connecting" with clients in terms of helping and caring.

Guidetti and Tham (2002) interviewed 12 OT practitioners who worked on self-care training with clients with either stroke or spinal cord injury. Their study identified interpersonal strategies used by practitioners. They included relationship building, trust, motivating clients, and providing an enabling occupational experience.

Eklund (1996) investigated whether the therapeutic relationship was related to outcomes in mental health practice. In an observational study of 20 patients and 5 occupational therapists, she found that both therapists and clients perceived their working relationship as good. Although, no consistent relationships with outcomes were found using a measure of the quality of the working relationship, both clients' and therapists' perceptions of the extent of client participation in the treatment process were related to outcomes.

These studies form a beginning knowledge base concerning current attitudes and behaviors that comprise the therapeutic relationship in OT. They provide preliminary evidence to suggest that a wide range of interpersonal skills are necessary to sustain a productive therapeutic relationship. There is a clear need for increased self-awareness, empathy, and power sharing within the therapeutic relationship. Moreover, confidence, self-awareness, and an orientation toward the client's interpersonal needs may lead to improved therapeutic outcomes.

The Intentional Relationship Model

Today's practice environment requires a therapist to skillfully navigate a client's interpersonal challenges while simultaneously facilitating occupational engagement (R. R. Taylor, 2008). The IRM provides a practical skill set and an interpersonal reasoning approach that presents different approaches to communication that are necessary to sustain a positive working relationship with a client. According to IRM, it is the therapist's responsibility to work to develop a predictable and trusting relationship with the client irrespective of any interpersonal difficulties or misgivings that the client may bring into the therapy process (R. R. Taylor, 2008). This does not assume that the therapist will always be successful at building such a relationship. However, it does assume the therapist recognizes it is his or her responsibility to establish and maintain this relationship.

The IRM focuses on four main components of the therapist–client relationship. These include the client, the interpersonal events that occur during therapy, the therapist's use of self, and the occupation. The IRM asks therapists to observe and understand their clients from an interpersonal perspective, to be prepared to respond therapeutically to rifts and other significant interpersonal events, and to communicate within a **mode** that matches the client's interpersonal needs of the moment (R. R. Taylor, 2008). This model, which is diagrammed in Figure 37-1, provides a theoretical framework for attempting to understand the meaning of the communication and interpersonal behavior that occurs during therapy. It also provides guidance about how to therapeutically respond in a manner that best serves the client. Each of the central components of the model will be described in the following pages, and more extensive information is presented in R. R. Taylor (2008).

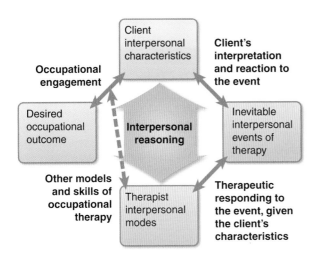

FIGURE 37-1 A Model of the Intentional Relationship in Occupational Therapy.

Client Interpersonal Characteristics

Individuals react to chronic conditions with tremendous variability. Recognizing and responding appropriately to psychological heterogeneity within and between clients is vital to a successful therapy outcome. Fear, anxiety, sadness, hopelessness, anger, and rage are inevitable emotions that any client with a chronic condition faces during the course of his or her experience. However, the duration and degree to which these emotions become entrenched and affect overall psychological, interpersonal, occupational, and health-related behavior and functioning vary considerably within and between individuals. For example, studies have shown that individuals with the same chronic condition can vary widely in terms of psychological response (Bombardier, D'Amico, & Jordan, 1990; Lacroix, Martin, Avendano, & Goldstein, 1991). Beck (1996) has acknowledged that there is a significant diversity in terms of the intensity of individuals' reactions to specific life circumstances over time, and there is also variation in terms of individuals' nonpathological psychological reactions to life events.

For these reasons, the IRM emphasizes the need for every therapist to gain an understanding of each client's interpersonal characteristics. This is typically accomplished by maintaining a mental (or written, if first beginning) list of features of a client's personality that represent strengths and weaknesses. For example, if a client has a heightened need for control, this will become clear the moment he or she asks what seems to be an unnecessary question for the third time. A client's reluctance to engage in an activity may become apparent when he or she appears not to have heard a given instruction. One quickly learns of a client's limited

capacity to assert his or her needs when he or she is found lying on a mat without a means to get up, not having asked anyone for help. Although these are common characteristics of clients in everyday practice, they are not traditionally discussed as fundamental aspects of OT care plans or documented in a client's chart notes. Understanding the more challenging aspects of a client's interpersonal characteristics from an objective but empathic perspective will assist a therapist to act in a way that is intentional and facilitating of occupational engagement.

Intentional Relationship Model defines the essential interpersonal characteristics of a client in terms of 12 categories, presented in Table 37-1.

Communication style refers to a client's ability to communicate in a clear, well-paced, and detailed yet succinct manner that is appropriate to his or her developmental level and cognitive ability. Reticence to communicate or, by contrast, excessive loquaciousness, will undoubtedly affect the therapeutic dynamic and the quality of occupational engagement that might otherwise be possible to achieve. Therefore, the IRM calls for therapists to consider communication difficulties such as these in building the therapeutic alliance, selecting an approach to communication, and, ultimately, in establishing the OT care plan. The same approach applies to the remaining categories of client characteristics. *Capacity for trust* refers to a client's ability to trust that the therapist has his or her best interests in mind and that every effort will be made to ensure his or her physical safety and emotional well-being.

Need for control is defined as the degree to which a client takes an active versus passive role within the relationship and in determining the course of therapy. *Capacity to assert needs* defines a client's approach to expressing his or her wishes and needs for support, information, resources, or other requests within the therapeutic relationship. *Response to change and challenge* refers to a client's ability to adapt to changes in the therapy plan or environment and his or her approach to OT tasks and situations that are new or challenging. *Affect* is defined as a client's general emotional expression during therapy, ranging from appropriately buoyant for the situation (flexible) to flat (absence of expression) to heightened (intensely emotional) to labile (fluctuating anywhere between elation, anger, angst, and despair). *Predisposition to giving feedback* involves a client's ability to provide the therapist with appropriate negative or positive comments about his or her reactions to the therapist and experience of therapy as either helpful or unhelpful. *Capacity to receive feedback* describes a client's ability to maintain perspective when receiving praise from the therapist or when receiving correction during performance, limits on behavior, or information about his or her strengths and weaknesses.

| TABLE 37-1 | Client Interpersonal Characteristics |

Interpersonal Characteristic	Practice Example
Communication style	Ana is a reluctant communicator. She tends to be quiet during therapy and only provides information when responding to a question. This makes it difficult for the therapist to read and understand her needs, and it limits the spontaneity of the interaction. This style causes the therapist to over function by asking Ana more questions than she would otherwise ask a client during therapy. This style was present from the first moment of therapy and has not changed.
Capacity for trust	Ana has a low capacity for trust. She demonstrates hesitancy in attempting new activities despite encouragement. She recoils from eye contact and does not look at the therapist often. She is guarded and will not share her thoughts, feelings, and reactions with the therapist.
Need for control	Ana is highly passive during therapy and has a low need for control. She is cooperative, but the therapist is unable to read what activities are more or less important and enjoyable for her. She appears to respond to every activity, particularly new ones, in the same hesitant but compliant manner.
Capacity to assert needs	Ana lacks the capacity to assert her needs in therapy. On one occasion, she wore her splint for a longer period than necessary because a fieldwork student had forgotten to have her take it off. Ana did not seem to care or react, despite any inconvenience or discomfort associated with wearing the splint.
Response to change and challenge	Unable to locate a regularly used paring knife for a baking activity, Ana gives up early and waits for the therapist to take control. When prompted to come up with an alternative solution, Ana remains puzzled and frozen.
Affect	Ana's affect vacillates between being flat and showing a slightly sad facial expression. In response to praise, she is either indifferent or displays a weak and almost pleading type of smile.
Predisposition to giving feedback	Ana never provides the therapist with unsolicited feedback about her experience in therapy. When the therapist asks for feedback, she frequently responds that everything is "fine" or weakly says, "I'm good."
Capacity to receive feedback	Ana responds well, almost robotically, to corrective feedback. She occasionally offers a weak smile but is generally indifferent to praise or reinforcement.
Response to human diversity	Ana does seem to show slightly more interest and enthusiasm when working with the physical therapist who is a male. Her occupational therapist is a female. It is not clear why this is the case.
Orientation toward relating	Ana shows a need to remain safely distant from the therapist and all others on the unit. She is unwilling to disclose information, including even superficial thoughts, feelings, and reactions in the moment. She appears indifferent to any personal disclosures or expressions of empathy made by the therapist and recoils from eye contact.
Preference for touch	Ana never initiates touch but does not flinch when the therapist does. At this time, it is unclear what Ana's preference for touch is, so the therapist tends to limit touch to that which is necessary to complete the more impairment-focused tasks of therapy.
Capacity for reciprocity	Ana does not appear interested in the therapist as a person and does not show any appreciation of therapy or expressions of gratitude. This appears consistent with her reactions to other providers on the unit.

Response to human diversity is defined by a client's reaction to ways in which he or she may be the same or different from the therapist in terms of observable sociodemographic characteristics (e.g., race, ethnicity, gender, age) and other interpretations of outward appearance or perceived worldview. Some clients have more difficulty than others relating to a therapist whom they perceive as differing from them in fundamental ways. *Orientation toward relating* defines a client's need for interpersonal closeness versus professional distance within the therapeutic relationship. Difficulties may occur when the client's expectations about the relationship differ from those of the therapist.

Preference for touch involves a client's observed comfort or discomfort with or expressed reaction to any type of physical touch, whether it be a necessary part of treatment or an expression of caring. *Capacity for reciprocity* refers to a client's ability to engage fully in the therapy process and/or show appreciation toward the therapist as a separate but connected partner within the therapy process. Some clients may be so focused on their own situations that they may lack this capacity, whereas others may function in an active and mutual way within the relationship. Regardless of the outcome, a client's capacity for reciprocity is always felt by the therapist and must be managed accordingly.

In summary, understanding client's interpersonal characteristics is fundamental to planning how to respond during therapeutic interactions. This becomes particularly important when clients present with more difficult or challenging interpersonal characteristics or when a therapist has a negative or apprehensive feeling about a client's personality. An extensive discussion of client characteristics may be found in R. R. Taylor (2008).

The Inevitable Interpersonal Events of Therapy

Similar to client characteristics, uncomfortable or emotionally laden situations that occur during therapy are a normal part of everyday practice for the experienced therapist. However, knowing how to anticipate and respond to them in a deliberate and therapeutic way is not necessarily an assumed, universal skill. According to IRM, an interpersonal event is a naturally occurring communication, reaction, process, task, or general circumstance that occurs during therapy and that has the potential to fortify or weaken the therapeutic relationship depending on how it is handled (R. R. Taylor, 2008). The 11 categories of interpersonal events, their definitions, and practice examples are presented in Table 37-2.

When interpersonal events occur, their interpretation by the client is a product of the client's unique set of interpersonal characteristics and mood. Sometimes, the event may have a significant effect on the client, and other times, a client will be unaffected or minimally affected. When such events occur, it is important that the therapist be aware that the event has occurred and takes responsibility for assessing the client's response and responding appropriately. According to R. R. Taylor (2008), interpersonal events are inevitable during the course of therapy and ripe with both threat and opportunity. Similar to our everyday relationships with coworkers, friends, and loved ones, when something significant happens, how we respond to that event typically has a lasting impact on that relationship. Interpersonal events are part of the constant give and take that occurs during therapy. If these events go unnoticed, are deliberately ignored, or are responded to without intentionality, these events can threaten both the therapeutic relationship and the client's occupational engagement. When optimally responded to, these events can provide opportunities for positive client learning or change and for solidifying the therapeutic relationship. Because they are unavoidable in any therapeutic interaction, one of the primary tasks of a therapist is to respond to these inevitable events in a way that leads to repair and strengthening of the therapeutic relationship (R. R. Taylor, 2008).

The Therapist's Use of Self: The Six Modes

According to IRM, effective use of self requires therapists to recognize and cultivate strengths within their personalities and develop less used aspects of their personalities through honest appraisal of the effects of their behavior on clients (R. R. Taylor, 2008). The first step in accomplishing this is through an understanding of the six therapist interpersonal modes. A **therapeutic mode** is a specific way of relating to a client. The IRM identifies six therapeutic modes:

1. **Advocating**
2. **Collaborating**
3. **Empathizing**
4. **Encouraging**
5. **Instructing**
6. **Problem solving**

A brief definition of each mode and an example of its use in a therapy situation is provided in Table 37-3.

Therapists naturally use therapeutic modes that are consistent with their fundamental personality characteristics. For example, a person who feels most confident and comfortable with others when teaching and sharing information with them would likely use instructing as a primary therapeutic mode in therapy. Therapists vary widely in terms of the range and flexibility with which they use modes in relating to clients. Some therapists relate to clients in one or two primary ways, whereas others draw on multiple therapeutic modes depending on the interpersonal characteristics of the client and the situation, or inevitable interpersonal events, at hand. One of the goals in using IRM is to become increasingly comfortable using any of six of the modes flexibly and interchangeably depending on the client's needs. A therapeutic mode or set of modes define a therapist's general **interpersonal style** when interacting with a client. Therapists able to use all six of the modes flexibly and comfortably and match those modes to the client and the situation are described as having a **multimodal** interpersonal style.

According to the IRM, a therapist's choice and application of a particular therapeutic mode or set of modes should depend largely on the interpersonal characteristics of the client and his or her reaction to any interpersonal events that may be occurring. Although a client may prefer that the therapist use one or two central modes, certain interpersonal events in therapy may call for a mode shift. A **mode shift** is a conscious change in one's way of relating to a client.

For example, if a client perceives a therapist's attempts at problem solving to be insensitive or off the mark, a therapist would be wise to switch from the **problem solving mode** to an *empathizing mode* so that he or she can get a better understanding of the client's reaction and the root of the dilemma. An **interpersonal reasoning** process,

TABLE 37-2	The Inevitable Interpersonal Events of Occupational Therapy	
Interpersonal Event	**Definition**	**Practice Example**
Expression of strong emotion	Observable manifestations of internal feelings that occur with a higher-than-usual level of intensity given a client's cultural context and norms; can be positive or negative expressions	Carl, a client in the neurosurgical intensive care unit, is justifiably angry because he is uncomfortable and the nursing staff is not responding to his calls. He proceeds to rip the vital sign monitors off his body so that a distress signal will be emitted and he will receive care.
Intimate self-disclosures	Statements or stories that reveal something personal or sensitive about the person making a disclosure. These can be stories about oneself or about close others.	During inpatient rehabilitation, Carl confides in the therapist that he intends to continue smoking when he returns home despite what his wife will think or do about it.
Power dilemmas	Feelings of stress or conflict that emerge when the client and therapist disagree about something. Power dilemmas can manifest overtly or covertly during therapy. They are more likely to occur when clients feel a lack or loss of control over their lives (which is a common feeling when undergoing rehabilitation).	Carl decides that he does not want to clean up the sawdust and woodworking tools after a therapy activity. Instead, he stands and watches while the therapist does it. The same behavior repeats itself during the following session. When the therapist says something about it, Carl tells her that he is the one paying her bill.
Nonverbal cues	Communications that do not involve the use of formal language. Some examples of these are facial expressions, movement patterns, body posture, and eye contact.	Carl stares at the therapist with anger in his eyes when he feels that a therapy task is pointless or undesirable.
Crisis points	Unanticipated, stressful events that cause clients to become absent or distracted from therapy. Examples include major weather disasters, a change in the client's health status, or an emergency involving a client's family member.	Carl collapses and experiences an unanticipated grand mal seizure while attempting to walk to the therapy room with the therapist.
Resistance and reluctance	Resistance is a client's passive or active refusal to participate in some or all aspects of therapy for reasons linked to the therapeutic relationship (e.g., unexpressed anger toward the therapist or situation). Reluctance is disinclination toward some aspect of therapy for reasons outside the therapeutic relationship, such as client anxiety about task difficulty or other concerns about performance.	Carl ignores the therapist's directions when he does not want to engage in a task or activity.
Boundary testing	A client behavior that violates or asks the therapist to disclose something or act in ways that the therapist is not comfortable with or that are outside the definition of a professional relationship	At the beginning of therapy, Carl asks the therapist a series of questions about her educational and employment history as well as what her qualifications are to treat him. Although these questions are within the parameters of the therapeutic relationship, they cause the therapist to feel that Carl has prejudices about her competence as a professional.
Empathic breaks	Any action initiated by the therapist, or something a therapist fails to notice or acknowledge, that results in a client feeling disappointed, disillusioned, insignificant, or emotionally injured	Carl asks the therapist to compare his progress with others with the same diagnosis, and the therapist tells him that she feels his progress would improve if he exerted more effort during sessions. Carl's facial expression appears deflated.
Emotionally charged therapy tasks and situations	Activities or circumstances that the client feels strongly about due to a past experience, a high level of value for the activity, or due to something embarrassing about the activity	During a physically challenging activity, Carl experiences increased oral secretions that he is unable to control. He immediately discontinues the activity with a shameful look on his face.
Limitations of therapy	Restrictions on the available or possible services, time, resources, or nature of the desired relationship with the therapist	Close to the time of discharge, Carl and the therapist review his accomplishments in therapy and his goals for the future. Carl asks the therapist if he could pay her out-of-pocket to continue home visits with him. The therapist informs Carl that she already works a 60-hour workweek and that she does not have the time to honor his request.
Contextual inconsistencies	Any aspect of a client's interpersonal or physical environment that changes during the course of therapy	When Carl is moved from intensive care into the step-down neurorehabilitation unit, he is initially nervous because of the decreased intensity of services provided.

TABLE 37-3 **The Six Therapeutic Modes**

Mode	Definition	Practice Example
1. Advocating	Ensuring that the client's rights are enforced and resources are secured; may require the therapist to serve as a mediator, facilitator, negotiator, enforcer, or other type of advocate with external persons and agencies	Upon discharge, the occupational therapist discusses with Carl's wife the possibilities of continuing to work on established goals for therapy and educates her on how she can support and encourage his continued efforts toward those goals.
2. Collaborating	Expecting the client to be an active and equal participant in therapy; ensuring choice, freedom, and autonomy to the greatest extent possible	The therapist shows respect and value for Carl's knowledge about his own medical condition and often asks him to provide his perspective regarding the objectives and tasks of therapy.
3. Empathizing	Ongoing striving to understand the client's thoughts, feelings, and behaviors while suspending any judgment; ensuring that the client verifies and experiences the therapist's understanding as truthful and validating	When Carl shares how he ripped the leads off his chest to attract the attention of the nursing staff when in pain during the night, the therapist summarizes and validates his feelings of desperation and anger in attempting to communicate and express his needs to staff.
4. Encouraging	Seizing the opportunity to instill hope in a client. Celebrating a client's thinking or behavior through positive reinforcement; conveying an attitude of joyfulness, playfulness, and confidence	When working in the kitchen, the therapist often jokes with Carl that he can cook better than she does. Carl appears to enjoy this banter.
5. Instructing	Carefully structuring therapy activities and being explicit with clients about the plan, sequence, and events of therapy. Providing clear instruction and feedback about performance; setting limits on a client's requests or behavior	The therapist typically prepares on certain evenings before sessions with Carl if she knows that they will be discussing some of his questions about assistive technologies or his functioning at work. During therapy, the therapist often cites empirical evidence and provides information about these technologies.
6. Problem solving	Facilitating pragmatic thinking and solving dilemmas by outlining choices, posing strategic questions, and providing opportunities for comparative or analytical thinking	When Carl presents the therapist with complex questions for which there are no right or wrong answers, the therapist often responds by asking him for his opinion or by helping him create a list of options and weigh pros and cons.

described in the following section, can be used to guide the therapist in deciding when a mode shift might be required and determining which alternative mode to select. Because the interpersonal aspects of OT practice are complex and require a therapist to possess a highly adaptive therapeutic personality, the IRM recommends that therapists learn to draw on all six of the therapeutic modes in a flexible manner according to the different interpersonal needs of each client and the unique demands of each clinical situation. See Case Study 37-1 for an example of how the interpersonal reasoning process and the six modes may be used during OT.

Interpersonal Reasoning

According to IRM, an important competency to develop as a therapist is the capacity to engage in an ongoing interpersonal reasoning process during therapy. This is particularly important when an interpersonal dilemma presents itself in therapy. Interpersonal reasoning is a step wise process by which a therapist decides what to say, do, or express in reaction to a client's interpersonal characteristics or behavior. It includes developing a mental vigilance toward the interpersonal aspects of therapy in anticipation that a dilemma might occur and a means of reviewing and

evaluating options for responding. The six steps of interpersonal reasoning and their definitions are presented in Table 37-4. An extensive description and discussion of these steps can be found in R. R. Taylor (2008). The following case study is a partially fictionalized extraction from an actual consultation provided to an occupational therapist by the author. Demographic information of the client has been changed to protect the client's anonymity.

Conclusion

In this chapter, we reviewed evidence that supports therapeutic use of self in OT. We learned about the field's emphasis on collaboration and about how the IRM can support that emphasis. The IRM is a conceptual practice model that explains how therapists can apply an interpersonal reasoning process to understand and respond supportively to clients in difficult or awkward moments. The model requires therapists to take responsibility for the emotional well-being of their clients during the therapy interaction by understanding the client's unique interpersonal characteristics and adjusting their therapeutic personalities accordingly. The model articulates six therapist

CASE STUDY 37-1 CYNTHIA: A WOMAN WITH A ROTATOR CUFF INJURY AND COMORBID POSTTRAUMATIC STRESS DISORDER

Cynthia is a 26-year-old woman who recently graduated with an associate degree to become a small-animal veterinary technician. She moved to Chicago, Illinois, from Madison, Wisconsin, where she had grown up and attended school. She is new to the large, fast-paced, and sometimes dangerous lifestyle of urban Chicago. On the way to take her certification exam for licensure, she was physically assaulted by an adolescent male on a metro platform in return for her wallet, ID card holder, and cell phone. In an attempt to keep her items, she engaged in a physical battle with the assailant and experienced facial abrasions, tooth breakage, and a complete rotator cuff injury requiring surgical repair. She presented to OT in the outpatient rehabilitation unit to address her shoulder issues. A review of her records revealed the presence of psychiatric overlay involving symptoms of posttraumatic stress disorder (PTSD).

Applying principles of Intentional Relationship Model (IRM) (R. R. Taylor, 2008), the treating occupational therapist immediately began the process of interpersonal reasoning before meeting with the client. Applying her knowledge of PTSD from a prior fieldwork experience, she reviewed its primary symptoms by referencing the *Diagnostic and Statistical Manual of Mental Disorders* and discussed typical features of the diagnosis during a brief consultation with a psychiatry resident in the cafeteria. Knowing that Cynthia is new to Chicago, likes animals, and engaged physically with her assailant gave her some preliminary data to anticipate the interpersonal events that might occur during therapy and some of the client interpersonal characteristics that might become important to watch in Cynthia's case.

In terms of client characteristics, the therapist prepared herself to assess Cynthia's need for control because she may have feelings of lost control due to the assault. For example, Cynthia may feel out of control when experiencing PTSD symptoms such as flashbacks and visceral reexperiencing of sights, sounds, smells, and sensations that trigger memories of the trauma. She may react to these feelings by exhibiting an abnormally high or abnormally low need for control during the therapy process. A second important characteristic to watch would be Cynthia's affect and how it may change in response to the different demands and activities of therapy, particularly when certain practices might induce pain or discomfort. A third important characteristic to watch for would be Cynthia's preference for touch because individuals with PTSD tend to be hypervigilant and have an exaggerated startle response if approached unexpectedly.

With respect to inevitable interpersonal events, it would be important to look for power dilemmas to occur, particularly if Cynthia exhibits a high need for control during therapy. Additionally, it would be important to watch for nonverbal cues signaling her discomfort with aspects of the therapy process. Finally, it would be important to anticipate therapy tasks or recommendations that might be emotionally charged for Cynthia, such as those involving using public transportation within the city of Chicago or those involving work with or care for animals, because animals appear to be important in her life.

During her consultation with Cynthia, many of the therapist's hypotheses about the interpersonal characteristics and events were confirmed. The therapist experienced Cynthia as a self-assured but traumatized young woman who had a fair amount of medical knowledge and a high need to express her knowledge and make decisions during therapy. The therapist deliberately avoided potential power dilemmas with Cynthia by selecting the *collaborating mode* as her primary mode, followed by the instructing mode when Cynthia's affect appeared anxious. The problem-solving mode was used when other nonverbal cues indicated that she was irritable and insecure.

The therapist was very careful to forewarn Cynthia each time she needed to help her partially disrobe and touch her shoulder. Each time, she was careful to use the instructing mode to explain the nature of the touch and why it was required to range, manipulate, or otherwise touch her shoulder in that particular way. When Cynthia's nonverbal cues and affect indicated that she was anticipating or experiencing discomfort, the therapist relied on the empathizing mode to validate Cynthia's reactions. Using the instructing mode, the therapist also mentioned to Cynthia that sometimes, touch can trigger symptoms of PTSD, and if that was the case, to be sure to let her know so that she can stop and be of support to her.

Although brief, what could have been an uncomfortable therapy process was optimized by the therapist's application of the interpersonal reasoning process to anticipate, select, and shift modes according to Cynthia's needs.

Now that you have read the case study and basic overview of the IRM, review the Practice Dilemma and questions. Can you see differences between the way the therapist managed the interpersonal dynamics with Cynthia versus the way she managed them with George? (See the Practice Dilemma.)

TABLE 37-4   The Six Steps of the Interpersonal Reasoning Process

Step of Interpersonal Reasoning	Definition
1. Anticipate	Based on your observations, information from others who have had experience with the client, and any experience you have had with the client, anticipate the likely interpersonal events that may occur during therapy and the modes that might work best. If you have met the client previously, be certain to incorporate your knowledge of the client's interpersonal characteristics in predicting events that might occur and modes that might work best.
2. Identify and cope	Use Intentional Relationship Model language to label a difficult client characteristic or interpersonal event when it occurs. Do what it takes to collect yourself and get emotional perspective on the situation. Remind yourself not to take it personally.
3. Determine if a mode shift is required	Ask yourself the following questions to determine whether a mode shift is required: What mode am I currently using with this client, if any? What are the effects of the mode on the client? Would another mode better serve the interpersonal needs of this client at this moment?
4. Choose a response mode or mode sequence	Interact within the mode or modes that you think the client prefers/needs at this moment. Think about a sequence of modes that you might use to accommodate changes in what the client might need from moment to moment.
5. Draw on any relevant interpersonal skills associated with the mode(s)	Think about other communication, rapport building, and/or conflict resolution skills that you might draw upon in association with your mode use.
6. Gather feedback	Gather nonverbal or verbal feedback from the client as to whether or not he or she feels comfortable with the way you approached the event or difficulty.

interpersonal modes that represent different facets of the therapeutic personality. Learning how to change those modes depending on each individual client's needs is a dynamic, lifelong process. Occupational therapists should strive to understand each client interpersonally, putting one's personal and emotional reactions to clients to productive use without prejudice or judgment.

🧍 PRACTICE DILEMMA

Gayle and George

George is a 54-year-old biomedical engineer who endured a mild traumatic brain injury and several bone fractures from a motor scooter accident. Following surgery on his pelvis, he was referred to Gayle, a newly licensed occupational therapist working in the inpatient rehabilitation unit of a major metropolitan teaching hospital. In passing, a nurse from the acute care unit informed Gayle that George has been causing a lot of disruption on the unit. He had made a series of complaints to the head of nursing about the lack of timeliness and intensity of his nursing care. Additionally, he had made excessive demands for incidental items such as specific newspapers and brand name toiletries that the hospital does not routinely provide.

Having graduated from an OT school with a high grade point average and an award for her outstanding performance in fieldwork, Gayle was not deterred by this information. Instead, she was determined to do everything she could to ensure that George was satisfied with the quality of care that she would provide him in therapy. Because she knew that George was highly educated and of high income, she decided to begin

therapy by giving her best explanation of what OT is and by asking him what his goals were. In her mind, she thought she was taking a client-centered approach. She was immediately disillusioned by his condescending tone of voice and sarcastic response: "My goal is to make sure my Vespa is salvageable and to be back on the road as soon as possible."

In an equally sarcastic tone, she immediately reacted by asking him if he planned to wear a helmet this time. She thought maybe he would find the comment humorous and that it might break the ice. Instead, the remainder of the session was occupied with an air of tension. Gayle initiated passive range of motion exercises and made numerous futile attempts to make conversation by asking George about his job and hobbies.

Following the session, George contacted the director of services at the hospital to file a complaint about Gayle. He reported that her attitude was arrogant and unprofessional during the session and that he felt she did not have the experience or maturity required to be of any help to him. He requested to be seen by a different therapist in the future. Upon hearing this news from her supervisor, Gayle was devastated and could figure out what she could have done differently with this challenging client.

Questions

1. After introducing herself and describing OT, which of the six modes did Gayle use to begin the session? Was this mode successful with George? Why or why not?
2. Did an empathic break occur during the session?
3. Is there anything that Gayle could have done differently during the session to prevent the complaint that George made about her?

REFERENCES

Allison, H., & Strong, J. (1994). Verbal strategies used by occupational therapists in direct client encounters. *OTJR: Occupation, Participation and Health, 14*, 112–129.

American Occupational Therapy Association. (2014). Occupational therapy practice framework: Domain and process, 3rd edition. *American Journal of Occupational Therapy, 68*, S1–S48.

Anderson, J., & Hinojosa, J. (1984). Parents and therapists in a professional partnership. *American Journal of Occupational Therapy, 38*, 452–461.

Beck, A. T. (1996). Beyond belief: A theory of modes, personality, and psychopathology. In P. M. Salkovskis (Ed.), *Frontiers of cognitive therapy* (pp. 1–25). New York, NY: Guilford Press.

Bombardier, C. H., D'Amico, C., & Jordan, J. S. (1990). The relationship of appraisal and coping to chronic illness adjustment. *Behaviour Research and Therapy, 28*, 297–304.

Cara, E., & MacRae, A. (2005). *Psychosocial occupational therapy: A clinical practice* (2nd ed.). Albany, NY: Delmar.

Cole, M. B., & McLean, V. (2003). Therapeutic relationships re-defined. *Occupational Therapy in Mental Health, 19*, 33–56.

Denton, P. L. (1987). *Psychiatric occupational therapy: A workbook of practical skills*. Boston, MA: Little, Brown and Company.

Dirette, D., Rozich, A., & Viau, S. (2009). Is there enough evidence for evidence-based practice in occupational therapy? *American Journal of Occupational Therapy, 63*, 782–786.

Eklund, M. (1996). Working relationship, participation and outcome in a psychiatric day care unit based on occupational therapy. *Scandinavian Journal of Occupational Therapy, 3*, 106–113.

Eklund, M., & Hallberg, I. R. (2001). Psychiatric occupational therapists' verbal interaction with their clients. *Occupational Therapy International, 8*, 1–16.

Guidetti, S., & Tham, K. (2002). Therapeutic strategies used by occupational therapists in self-care training: A qualitative study. *Occupational Therapy International, 9*, 257–276.

Guthrie, E. (1996). Emotional disorder in chronic illness: Psychotherapeutic interventions. *The British Journal of Psychiatry, 168*, 265–273.

Hagedorn, R. (1995). *Occupational therapy: Perspectives and processes*. Edinburgh, United Kingdom: Churchill Livingstone.

Jenkins, M., Mallett, J., O'Neill, C., McFadden, M., & Baird, H. (1994). Insights into "practice" communication: An interactional approach. *British Journal of Occupational Therapy, 57*, 297–302.

Johnson, C., & Webster, D. (2002). *Recrafting a life: Solutions for chronic pain and illness*. New York, NY: Psychology Press.

Kielhofner, G. (2009). *Conceptual foundations of occupational therapy* (4th ed.). Philadelphia, PA: F. A. Davis.

Lacroix, J. M., Martin, B., Avendano, M., & Goldstein, R. (1991). Symptom schemata in chronic respiratory patients. *Health Psychology, 10*, 268–273.

Marr, D. (2017). Fostering full implementation of evidence-based practice. *American Journal of Occupational Therapy, 71*, 7101100050p1–7101100050p5. doi:10.5014/ajot.2017.019661

Moorey, S., & Greer, S. (2002). *Cognitive behaviour therapy for people with cancer*. Oxford, United Kingdom: Oxford University Press.

Mosey, A. C. (1981). *Occupational therapy: Configuration of a profession*. New York, NY: Raven Press.

Mosey, A. C. (1986). *Psychosocial components of occupational therapy*. New York, NY: Raven Press.

Norrby, E., & Bellner, A. L. (1995). The helping encounter–occupational therapists' perception of therapeutic relationships. *Scandinavian Journal of Caring Sciences, 9*, 41–46.

Palmadottir, G. (2006). Client-therapist relationships: Experiences of occupational therapy clients in rehabilitation. *British Journal of Occupational Therapy, 69*, 394–401.

Peloquin, S. M. (1988). Linking purpose to procedure during interactions with patients. *American Journal of Occupational Therapy, 42*, 775–781.

Punwar, A. J. (2000). The art and science of practice. In A. J. Punwar & S. Peloquin (Eds.), *Occupational therapy: Principles and practice* (3rd ed.). Philadelphia, PA: Lippincott Williams & Wilkins.

Punwar, A. J., & Peloquin, S. M. (2000). *Occupational therapy: Principles and practice* (3rd ed.). Philadelphia, PA: Lippincott Williams & Wilkins.

Rosa, S. A., & Hasselkus, B. R. (1996). Connecting with patients: The personal experience of professional helping. *Occupational Therapy Journal of Research, 16*, 245–260.

Schwartzberg, S. L. (2002). *Interactive reasoning in the process of occupational therapy*. Upper Saddle River, NJ: Pearson Education.

Taylor, R. R. (2008). *The intentional relationship: Occupational therapy and use of self*. Philadelphia, PA: F. A. Davis.

Taylor, R. R., Lee, S. W., & Kielhofner, G. (2011). Practitioners' use of interpersonal modes within the therapeutic relationship: Results from a nationwide study. *OTJR: Occupation, Participation and Health, 31*, 6–14.

Taylor, R. R., Lee, S. W., Kielhofner, G., & Ketkar, M. (2009). Therapeutic use of self: A nationwide survey of practitioners' attitudes and experiences. *American Journal of Occupational Therapy, 63*, 198–207.

Taylor, S. E., & Aspinwall, L. G. (1990). Psychosocial aspects of chronic illness. In P. T. Costa & G. R. Vanden Bos (Eds.), *Psychological aspects of serious illness: Chronic conditions, fatal diseases, and clinical care* (pp. 3–60). Washington, DC: American Psychological Association.

White, C. A. (2001). *Cognitive behaviour therapy for chronic medical problems: A guide to assessment and treatment in practice*. West Sussex, United Kingdom: John Wiley & Sons.

the**Point**® *For additional resources on the subjects discussed in this chapter, visit* http://thePoint.lww.com /Willard-Spackman13e.

CHAPTER 38

Group Process and Group Intervention

Marjorie E. Scaffa

LEARNING OBJECTIVES

After reading this chapter, you will be able to:

1. Appreciate the complexity and value of small groups in occupational therapy.
2. Understand factors influencing group process dynamics.
3. Discuss the characteristics of effective group leadership.
4. Describe various types of occupational therapy intervention groups.
5. Identify the basic components of a group intervention protocol.
6. Outline group members' behaviors that indicate occupational performance deficits.

Introduction

According to the Occupational Therapy Practice Framework: Domain and Process, third edition (American Occupational Therapy Association [AOTA], 2014), the term *client* refers to persons, groups, or populations receiving occupational therapy (OT) services. A **group** is an aggregate of people who share a common purpose that can only be achieved through collaboration. Groups are organized systems of interrelated, interactive, and interdependent individuals. Occupational therapists provide intervention to groups in various settings, including schools, hospitals, skilled nursing facilities, psychiatric services, day care programs, independent living centers, and community social service agencies, to name a few. The age range of members of these groups is very broad, from children to older adults. In addition to a group being a client, a group may also be a method of service delivery (AOTA, 2014). Group interventions are described in The Framework as the "use of distinct knowledge and leadership techniques to facilitate learning and skill acquisition across the life span through the dynamics of group and social interaction" (AOTA, 2014, p. S31). In a survey of OT practitioners, 50% indicated they used group interventions in their practice. Physical activity, such as exercise and yoga, was the most common group intervention used. Task groups and sensory modulation groups were other frequently used modalities (Higgins, Schwartzberg, Bedell, & Duncombe, 2015).

Group interventions in OT provide opportunities to develop task skills and interpersonal interaction skills (Mosey, 1973) that would be difficult to develop through interventions directed at the individual. Change

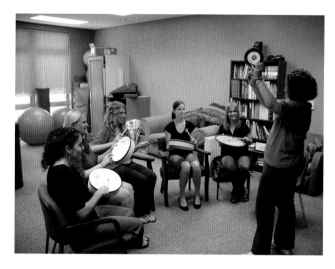

FIGURE 38-1 Occupational therapy often occurs within a group format. (Photo courtesy of Elizabeth Alford, MS, OTR).

occurs in individuals and in the group as a whole as a result of the interactions and feedback among group members (Figure 38-1). Yalom (1995) describes the benefits of an adaptive cycle whereby a growth-enhancing change in an individual creates improvements in his or her interpersonal environment, which precipitates additional personal change. Group interventions can occur in a variety of settings including inpatient units, outpatient clinics, skilled nursing facilities, schools, worksites, and in the community.

A group is a therapeutic social system and an agent of change. Although group work can be quite challenging, there are many benefits to be derived from developing and implementing group interventions. Based on years of research, Yalom (1995) developed a classification of "curative factors" or therapeutic factors that make group interventions particularly effective (Box 38-1). A therapeutic factor is "an element occurring in group therapy that contributes to improvement in a patient's condition and is a function of the actions of a group therapist, the patient, or fellow group members" (Bloch, 1986, p. 679). Some of the therapeutic factors are preconditions for change (e.g., group cohesiveness), others refer to what a participant learns (e.g., universality) by being in a therapy group, whereas others refer to changes in behavior (e.g., altruism). The relative importance of each of the therapeutic factors varies by the type of group and the stage of group development. Therapeutic factors "are interdependent and neither occur nor function separately" (Yalom, 1995, p. 2).

Groups used in OT intervention typically fall into four categories: functional groups, activity groups, task groups, and social groups (AOTA, 2014). Groups are planned based on the purpose or goal of the group and include, for example, energy conservation groups, psychoeducational groups, social skills groups, activities of daily living groups, reminiscence groups, leisure groups, and sensorimotor groups, among others (Table 38-1).

Group interventions provide a variety and multitude of benefits. Groups "allow clients to explore and develop skills for participation, including basic social interaction skills, tools for self-regulation, goal setting, and positive choice making" (AOTA, 2014, p. S31). Group interventions are cost effective and versatile, build social relationships, provide a context for vicarious learning and problem solving, and can be designed to achieve multiple goals simultaneously (Cole, 2012).

BOX 38-1   YALOM'S PRIMARY THERAPEUTIC FACTORS OF GROUPS

- Altruism: sharing with others, reaching out to others, giving of oneself to help others
- Catharsis: sharing feelings and experiences, expressing and releasing emotions
- Cohesiveness: sense of belonging, developing relationships based on trust, support, and caring
- Imitative behavior: observing the behaviors of others and then experimenting and applying positive behaviors modeled by other group members and the group leader to one's own life
- Imparting information: learning about one's health, illness, or disability through discussion with other group members

- Instillation of hope: receiving reassurance, experiencing optimism and positive expectations based on observation of improvement in others
- Interpersonal learning: learning about and from others in the group, developing an awareness of others, correcting past misinterpretations about others
- Self-understanding: discovering and accepting previously unknown aspects of the self, developing insight
- Socializing techniques: learning, practicing, and developing social skills
- Universality: recognizing shared feelings, developing an awareness that one is not alone and that others have similar problems and experiences

From Yalom, I. D. (1995). *The theory and practice of group psychotherapy* (4th ed.). New York, NY: Basic Books; and Yalom, I. D., & Leszcz, M. (2005). *The theory and practice of group psychotherapy* (5th ed.). New York, NY: Basic Books.

| TABLE 38-1 | Examples of Occupational Therapy Intervention Groups |

Occupational Therapy Intervention Group Type and Purpose	Occupational Therapy Practice Example
Psychoeducational Group	
Educates clients regarding health concerns that impact occupational performance, participation, and well-being; enhances the client's capacity for health management and maintenance Psychoeducational groups typically have a cognitive behavioral element embedded in the intervention.	A group of soldiers who are recovering from posttraumatic stress disorder (PTSD) attend OT sessions one night per week at an outpatient mental health facility to learn stress management strategies and how to incorporate them during their daily occupations.
Social Skills Group	
Provides opportunities for the development, establishment, and remediation of skills needed for social participation Creates a situation where group members are socially connected which allows members to develop social interaction skills and learn from one another	In an outpatient program for substance dependence, an occupational therapist provides group sessions that incorporate role-playing various social situations, which are generated based on concerns clients have expressed. The members help each other gain insight regarding how they are perceived by others and provide/receive social support.
Activities of Daily Living (ADL) Group	
Designed to establish, remediate, or restore ADL and instrumental ADL (IADL) skills. Group members gain awareness, knowledge, and skills necessary for mastery of occupational performance. Improved functional outcomes are realized through intervention focused on skill development and adaptations.	An occupational therapist facilitates an ADL group for persons with low vision at the local senior center. The members explore the strategies and adaptations suggested by the occupational therapist and by individuals who are successfully participating in home-management and self-care activities.
Reminiscence Group	
The goal is to support, maintain, protect, or preserve a person's current occupational interests and abilities by participating in meaningful activities from their past.	An OT assistant leads a recreation group for persons in the middle stages of dementia, who like to play cards. She plays a matching game using picture cards placed face up on the table. This parallel activity requires only simple recognition, which enhances the client's potential for success.
Leisure Group	
Provides opportunities to explore and participate in various leisure activities in order to achieve and maintain occupational balance	An occupational therapist is hired to develop community reintegration plans with members of a clubhouse program that incorporate activities offered by the local parks and recreation department.
Sensorimotor Group	
Designed to facilitate adaptation; activities are generally dependent on the developmental level of the group. It is common for sensorimotor groups to address neurological or cognitive dysfunction in a thematic format.	At a recreational group for adolescents with mild traumatic brain injury, an occupational therapist uses a parachute activity to help the members move to various types of music and rhythms.
Fall Prevention Group	
Group members participate in activities that focus on health promotion to reduce the incidence of a disease or disorder or to prevent secondary conditions in cases of progressive or degenerative diseases.	An occupational therapist at a continuing care retirement community (CCRC) develops a group to teach the principles of fall prevention to seniors and to help them incorporate these strategies into their daily occupational routines.

In this chapter, basic group processes are described, including various characteristics of intervention groups, and stages of group development. In addition, types of OT group interventions are discussed, and the development and implementation of OT group interventions are explored.

Group Process

The components of group OT are content and process. *Content* refers to the occupational activity in which the group engages. It is the information shared and the products produced by the group. The interrelationships and interactions between members, leaders, and the group as a whole are called group process. **Group process** "is the here-and-now experience in the group that describes how the group is functioning, the quality of relationships between and among group members and with the leader, the emotional experiences and reactions of the group, and the group's strongest desires and fears" (Brown, 2003, p. 228). Taylor (2008) advocates for a balance between a focus on activity and attention to interpersonal interactions.

CENTENNIAL NOTES

Fern Cramer-Azima

Dr. Fern Cramer-Azima was one of the first occupational therapists to conduct research on the effectiveness of group interventions (Figure 38-2). Her research on analytic group art therapy, in collaboration with her husband (H. Azima, MD) and a colleague (E. D. Wittkower, MD), was published in the *International Journal of Psychotherapy* in 1957 (Azima, Cramer-Azima, & Wittkower, 1957). The study was conducted at the Allan Memorial Institute of Psychiatry/Royal Victoria Hospital where Dr. Azima was the director of the child and adolescent service. As a pioneer in OT and an associate professor at McGill University in Montreal, Canada, Dr. Azima created the Azima Diagnostic Battery based on psychodynamic theory.

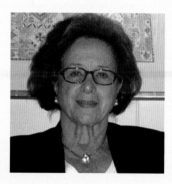

FIGURE 38-2 **Dr. Fern Cramer-Azima (1928–2013).**

The moment-to-moment interaction between leaders and members makes up the here-and-now process of a group. At a minimum, as an interdependent system, interaction operates simultaneously in six ways:

1. Member to member
2. Leader to member and member to leader
3. Subgroups
4. Group as a whole
5. Engagement in occupation
6. The culture or environment

There are sets of constantly changing dynamics that operate in small groups regardless of setting. In a system-centered model, the group is viewed as an organized body of mutually dependent interacting parts. "It is the interactive system that changes through the developmental stages, not the individual group members" (Howe & Schwartzberg, 2001, p. 22).

Characteristics of Groups

Intervention groups have the following characteristics:

- Group context and climate
- Boundaries/membership
- Roles
- Group cohesiveness
- Group norms
- Group goals

Groups are systems that exist within larger systems and occur within historical, social, and environmental contexts. These contexts impact the internal functioning of the group and its relationships with other systems. According to Schwartzberg, Howe, and Barnes (2008), "group climate refers to the physical and interpersonal or emotional environment affecting the group" (p. 8). An inviting physical environment and a safe, accepting interpersonal climate enhances group function.

Group boundaries may be flexible, rigid, or have variable degrees of permeability. Typically, intervention groups have inclusion and exclusion criteria for membership. Groups can be closed, with no new members added, or open with changing membership. Members can be selected to be similar to one another or heterogeneous. Small groups can range in size from 3 members to 10 or even 12 members. Group size influences group methods, leader strategies, and outcomes (Howe & Schwartzberg, 2001).

People take on various roles in intervention groups. A **role** is a set of socially agreed on behavioral expectations, rights, and responsibilities for a specific position or status in a group or in society. Roles may be related to task accomplishment or to the social/emotional needs of group members, both of which are critical to the effective functioning of the group. A list of task and social-emotional roles is provided in Box 38-2 (Benne & Sheats, 1978). The performance of roles within a group mirrors role expectations in all areas of life and provides an opportunity for the development of role competence. There may be a mismatch between the roles members take on and the demands of a situation. If everyone offers emotional support and no one carries out actions such as offering suggestions, the group falters. Conversely, if the group focuses only on getting the job done, the members will feel emotionally dissatisfied and isolated. Group cohesion results when the member roles are congruent with the task.

Group cohesiveness refers to the degree of understanding, acceptance, and feelings of closeness group members have toward each other and the value they place on the group. It is the group members' sense of liking, their trust and desire to work together, a feeling of togetherness, and sense of security. Group cohesiveness is both a therapeutic factor in its own right and a necessary precondition for the optimal functioning of other therapeutic factors.

BOX 38-2	TASK AND SOCIAL-EMOTIONAL ROLES IN INTERVENTION GROUPS

Task Roles

- Initiator/contributor
- Information seeker/information giver
- Opinion seeker/opinion giver
- Elaborator
- Coordinator
- Orienter
- Evaluator/critic
- Energizer (prods group to action)
- Procedural technician (performs routine tasks)

Social-Emotional Roles

- Encourager
- Harmonizer (mediates differences among group members)
- Compromiser (changes own behavior to maintain group harmony)
- Gatekeeper
- Standard setter
- Group observer (provides feedback on group process)
- Follower

In contrast to a noncohesive group, members of a cohesive group are more likely to participate willingly in group activities, be open to influence by other members, and experience a greater sense of security which allows them to experiment and try out new behaviors in a safe environment (Yalom, 1995). Group cohesiveness can be enhanced through frequent group meetings, emphasizing similarities among group members, competition against other groups, and consensus regarding the group's norms and goals.

Group norms reflect the value system of the group what members believe are appropriate ways of thinking, feeling, and behaving. Norms provide clear expectations of the individual and the group. Some norms are prescriptive and indicate what group members should do, whereas other norms are proscriptive and indicate behaviors that are unacceptable. Not all group norms facilitate the therapeutic process. Desirable norms include, but are not limited to, active involvement in the group, nonjudgmental acceptance of other group members, desire for self-awareness, and readiness for change. Group norms, once established, can be difficult to change. The leader helps to create a therapeutic group culture by modeling desirable behavior in a deliberate manner (Yalom, 1995). Norms can be explicit or implicit and change over time as the group develops and matures. Some groups have specific written rules or contracts that govern attendance, expectations, roles, and interpersonal interactions (Schwartzberg et al., 2008).

Occupational therapy groups typically focus on the performance of occupations, for example, instrumental activities of daily living, work, leisure, and social participation. **Group goals** are a future state toward which most group members' efforts are directed. Goals determine the group's focus and may be explicit or implicit. Goals give the group identity and provide meaning; goals are the standards by which the individual's and group's activities may be judged. Groups function best when members are clear about and invest in the group's purpose and goals (Schwartzberg et al., 2008). Group goals are stated in more general terms than individual goals. However, a variety of individual goals can be addressed effectively in occupation-based groups. The following are a few examples of group goals:

- Develop meal planning, preparation, and cleanup skills for independent living.
- Enhance social skills to facilitate social participation in a variety of settings.
- Explore adapted leisure activities available in the community.
- Acquire job-seeking and acquisition skills in order to obtain paid employment.

Group Leadership

Leadership implies a relationship between an individual and a group built around some common interest. A *leader* is "a person who can influence others to be more effective in working to achieve their mutual goals and maintain effective working relationships among members" (Johnson & Johnson, 2006, p. 168). The basic attitude of the leader/therapist in relationship to the group participants must be one of concern, acceptance, empathy, and genuineness. This therapeutic use of self takes precedence over everything else. Leadership styles include directive, facilitative, and advisory (see Box 38-3 for descriptions). There are advantages and disadvantages of each leadership style. Therefore, it is best to use the approach that is most appropriate for a given situation, level of client functioning, and stage of group development. For example, directive leadership is necessary for lower functioning clients who may not have adequate safety awareness and therefore may be at risk for injury during activity. The facilitative leadership style is most likely to lead to group cohesiveness, and the advisory leadership style is most appropriate for working with caregivers, families, and community organizations in a consultative role. For this reason, effective leaders have all three styles as part of their repertoire (Cole, 2012).

BOX 38-3   LEADERSHIP STYLES

- **Directive:** Leader defines the group, selects activities, and structures the group for therapeutic purposes.
- **Facilitative:** Facilitator earns the support of the members, members make decisions with leader's guidance, and the therapist serves as a resource person and educator.
- **Advisory:** Leader offers expertise as needed or requested but does not provide structure or goals; motivation comes from within the group.

Data from Cole, M. B. (2012). *Group dynamics in occupational therapy: The theoretical basis and practice application of group intervention* (4th ed.). Thorofare, NJ: SLACK.

A leader "helps members learn new behaviors that will increase their ability to balance the task and social-emotional aspects of the group" and "members learn to effectively and appropriately meet other members' needs while achieving group goals" (Schwartzberg et al., 2008, p. 59). In order to effectively facilitate this learning process, the leader employs the skills of interactive reasoning, including establishing rapport through empathic listening, building alliances, giving and receiving information and feedback, validating success, sharing personal stories, and reflective responding (Mattingly & Fleming, 1994).

Research indicates that there are four functions of leadership that are important to group members (Yalom & Leszcz, 2005):

- Emotional activation (eliciting feelings, facilitating emotional expression, challenging, and confronting as necessary)
- Caring (offering support, concern, acceptance, etc.)
- Meaning attribution (providing clarification, explanation, interpretation, etc.)
- Executive function (managing time, setting limits, recommending strategies and procedures)

Kouzes and Posner (2007) describe five practices of exemplary leadership. These include modeling the way, inspiring a shared vision, challenging the process, enabling others to act, and encouraging the heart. Modeling the way involves setting an example by clarifying, affirming, and acting on values shared by the group. Inspiring a shared vision based on collective aspirations builds commitment to action among group members. Challenging the process promotes initiative, creativity, and innovation among group members. Enabling others to act fosters relationship building, collaboration based on trust, and the development of individual and group competence. Encouraging the heart demonstrates appreciation for group members' contributions and creates a spirit of community in the group.

Group Development

Intervention groups can be short term (crisis intervention) or long term (recovery). Whether they are short term or long term, groups change over time. Various interpersonal concerns emerge as groups evolve. The phases of group development provide a conceptual model of the evolution of group issues. Tuckman (1965) identified four stages of group development: (1) forming (uncertainty of one's role in the group, purpose, and procedures of group), (2) storming (conflict and rebellion in group because members resist group influence), (3) norming (group discovers ways to work together, set norms to enable cohesiveness), and (4) performing (group is flexible in ways of working together to achieve aims). Gazda (1989) provided an updated description (Box 38-4). The phases or stages of group development often do not occur in a predictable, linear sequence but rather in a fluctuating, cyclical pattern. Groups may plateau or revert to earlier stages during times of stress and renegotiate norms, goals, and strategies in order to grow in a more positive direction.

Using Groups to Evaluate Client Function

Occupational performance is the product of the interaction between the client, the occupation, and the environment. As a result, groups can be a useful context for evaluating certain client factors, performance skills, and performance patterns. Although various client factors can be assessed during group activities, specific and global mental functions that are readily apparent in group situations include attention, memory, perception, thought, temperament and personality, energy, and drive.

Performance skills, particularly cognitive, emotional regulation, and social interaction kills, are easily assessed during group activities. Cognitive process skills such as judging, selecting, organizing, sequencing, prioritizing, and problem solving are evident when a client is planning and managing the performance of an occupation or activity in the group context and while interacting with other group members. Observing clients during craft activities, such as those included in the *Allen Diagnostic Module*, may be useful to evaluate cognitive skills during group task sessions. The Comprehensive Occupational Therapy Evaluation (COTE) can also be used to assess task-related behaviors and skills.

Emotional regulation skills are those "actions or behaviors a client uses to identify, manage, and express feelings while engaging in activities or interacting with others" (AOTA, 2008, p. 640). These behaviors include managing frustration and anger, empathizing and responding to the feelings of others, displaying emotions appropriately, and coping with stressful situations. Dialectical Behavioral

BOX 38-4   GAZDA'S (1989) STAGES OF GROUP DEVELOPMENT

Exploratory Stage

- Set ground rules/norms for the group.
- Clarify goals.
- Inform participants of their responsibilities.
- Leader centered
- Getting acquainted
- Establishing roles/functions in the group

Transition Stage

- Conflict and polarization
- Resistance to group influence
- Emotional responses
- Insecurity
- Defensiveness and frustration
- Problems seem insurmountable.
- Group survival is in question.

Action Stage

- Work/task focus
- Resistance is overcome.
- Trust and cohesiveness is developed.
- Increased self-disclosure
- Increased spontaneity
- Decreased reliance on the leader
- Problems are easily resolved.

Termination Stage

- Usually short duration
- Decreased self-disclosure
- Attempts at closure
- Need to say good-bye and move on

Therapy (DBT) diary cards are useful for clients to monitor their emotional reactions and their use of emotional regulation skills. By tracking emotions and behaviors on a daily basis, problematic patterns become apparent and can be addressed. An electronic version of the DBT diary card is available as an iPhone application (DBT iPhone App, 2012).

Communication and interpersonal skills are necessary for effective and satisfying relationships and social participation in the community. Social interaction skills are nearly impossible to evaluate outside of the group context. The skills that can be observed during group interaction include maintaining eye contact, initiating conversations, responding to questions, taking turns, sharing limited supplies, respecting the perspectives and beliefs of others, and using appropriate interpersonal distance. There are many useful OT assessments for communication and social skills, including the Assessment of Communication and Interaction Skills (ACIS) based on the Model of Human Occupation, the Social Interaction Scale (SIS) of the Bay Area Functional Performance Evaluation (BaFPE), and the COTE.

Intervention Groups in Occupational Therapy

Schwartzberg et al. (2008) provide several important reasons why OT practitioners should incorporate group interventions in their practice, including the following:

- "Groups provide an occupation-based experience that is reality-oriented and that promotes adaptation."
- "Groups are a natural environment that can provide feedback and support for individual and social needs."

- "Through participating in group activities that promote growth and change, members can learn and practice skills to master and achieve competence in activities required for daily life."
- "When groups provide an opportunity for dealing with real-life issues and objects, people can maintain, improve or enhance their occupational nature to fulfill social demand" (p. 39).

Occupational therapy intervention groups may take many forms, for example, client-centered groups, developmental groups, task groups, activity groups, and functional groups. Each of these is described briefly. However, it is important to realize that these forms of group intervention frequently overlap, combined into hybrid forms, and rarely used singularly.

Client-Centered Groups

A client-centered approach has become one of the major foundational underpinnings of OT practice and applies to planning and implementing group interventions as well as individual interventions. Client-centered practice is based primarily on the humanistic approach to mental health care. The client-centered intervention approach is based on the following principles that are incorporated into the group process:

- Clients know what they want from therapy and what they need to reach their optimum level of occupational performance.
- The only relevant frame of reference or vantage point for therapy is that of the client.
- The therapist cannot actually promote change; he or she can only create an environment that facilitates change.

- Respect for clients and their families and the choices they make is central to therapist–client interactions.
- Clients and families have the ultimate responsibility for decisions about daily occupations and OT services.
- Client participation is to be facilitated in all aspects of OT service.
- Occupational therapy service delivery should be flexible and individualized to the client's needs.
- The goal is to enable and empower clients to address their occupational performance issues.
- Intervention has a focus on the person-environment-occupation relationship (Law, 1998).

Client-centered groups facilitate client self-expression, identification of strengths and weaknesses, prioritization of problem areas, identification of goals, awareness of options and choice, and exploration of the impact of context on occupational performance and participation (Cole, 2012). Incorporating client-centered practice principles into group interventions can take many forms, including values-clarification exercises, group and individual goal setting and action planning, information seeking and sharing, role-playing, and occupational exploration. However, the primary client-centered intervention is the development of a therapeutic relationship with the clients in the group through therapeutic use of self.

Developmental Groups

Mosey (1970) was the first occupational therapist to describe the nature of developmental groups and postulated that group interaction skills develop in a specific sequence from parallel group participation, through project group, egocentric cooperative group, to cooperative group, and, finally, to mature group participation. This represents a continuum from leader-dependent to member-driven groups. Mature, adaptive group interaction skills are required to effectively function in various groups. Effective group functioning is satisfying to oneself and to other group members and meets the demands of the social environment.

Developmental groups are not age specific but rather a reflection of the group's level of functioning. Group experiences and activities are graded to facilitate the client's development of appropriate group interaction skills. Developmental groups represent simulations of groups typically encountered in the normal developmental process and are used in intervention as modalities for planned change. A few of the strategies that can be implemented to facilitate the development of group interaction skills include the following:

1. Encouraging clients to imitate the behaviors of the therapist or other group members
2. Encouraging clients to experiment with various behavioral responses within the safety of the group

3. Providing encouragement and positive feedback for engaging in productive group interactions
4. Discussing and role-playing possible behavioral options to various social situations (Mosey, 1970)

Donohue (2010) updated Mosey's work on developmental groups and described five levels of social participation (Box 38-5). In addition, Cole and Donohue (2011) developed and validated the Social Profile, an assessment designed to measure three categories of social participation: group membership, group interaction, and group activity behavior. Results from the Social Profile can be used to guide the planning and implementation of therapeutic group interventions.

Task Groups

Task groups provide an opportunity for active involvement in occupation in natural contexts. A *task* is defined as any activity or process that produces an end product or provides service for the group as a whole or for persons not in the group (Fidler, 1969). The group members work together to accomplish a task. In this way, task groups resemble demands persons encounter in community living.

Mosey (1981) believed that task group interventions facilitate the development of adaptive skills, including sensory integration skills, cognitive skills, dyadic interaction skills, group interaction skills, self-identity skills, and sexual identity skills. Task-oriented group interventions provide a shared work experience that facilitates the integration of thinking, feeling, and behavior and provides structure for interaction as well as opportunities for problem solving and skill development (Fidler, 1969). Task groups require collaboration, clear communication, interdependence, and shared decision making in real-life scenarios, thus enhancing the learning needed for functioning in home, school, work, and community contexts. Various task skills can be learned in a group setting (Box 38-6).

Choosing an appropriate task for the group requires the occupational therapist to analyze the level and types of skills required to successfully complete the task. Tasks chosen should provide the "just right challenge" for group members; tasks that are too easy or too difficult will not provide an experience conducive to skill development.

Activity Groups

Activity groups are similar to task groups. However, task groups focus on the group collaboratively completing a task, whereas activity groups focus on the process of engaging in meaningful activity with others. Activity groups are frequently designed to build a positive self-concept, manage and express emotions constructively, and improve communication skills among group members (DeCarlo & Mann, 1985). A study comparing the outcomes of an OT activity group with a verbal therapy group indicated that

BOX 38-5   DONOHUE'S (2010) FIVE LEVELS OF SOCIAL PARTICIPATION

Parallel Participation

- Carrying out activities in the presence of others in a supportive manner
- Working side by side
- Members show awareness of others.
- With minimal verbal or nonverbal interaction between group members

Associative Participation

- Brief verbal and nonverbal interactions, for example, greetings, short conversations
- Evidence of some beginning cooperation and competition
- Focus is on the task, minimal interaction outside the task.
- Can give and receive minimal assistance with the task

Basic Cooperative Participation

- Joint tasks carried out over time, emphasis is on completion of the project
- Members jointly select, implement, and execute activity.
- Members begin to express ideas and try to meet the needs of others.

- Mutual interest in the task, activity, or goal
- Members respect others' rights and follow group rules.

Supportive Cooperative Participation

- Emphasizes camaraderie and emotional sharing around a task
- Members of the group are typically homogeneous.
- Aim to fulfill each other's needs and derive mutual satisfaction from the activity
- Task is considered secondary to emotional support.
- Feelings are frequently expressed; members grow in personal and interpersonal insight.

Mature Participation

- Combines the skills of the basic and supportive cooperative participation levels
- Group members are often heterogeneous.
- Members take turns in various complementary roles teaching, learning, experimenting, and mentoring.
- Goal is to complete the activity harmoniously and efficiently while enjoying the process.
- Members balance task accomplishment with meeting social-emotional needs of group members.

---

the activity group produced higher levels of interpersonal communication skills as measured by the Interpersonal Communication Inventory (DeCarlo & Mann, 1985).

Expressive arts, crafts, music, dance, role-play scenarios, and games are typical modalities in activity groups. Participation in creative activity groups by persons with mental disorders has been shown to positively correlate with improved mental health. Reductions in self-reported

BOX 38-6   TASK SKILLS THAT CAN BE LEARNED IN A GROUP SETTING

- A fairly normal rate of performance
- Appropriate use of tools and materials
- Willingness to engage in doing tasks
- Sustained interest in a task
- Ability to follow demonstrated, oral, and written directions
- An acceptable level of neatness
- Appropriate attention to detail
- The ability to solve problems that arise in performing a task
- Ability to organize tasks in a logical manner

and clinician-rated symptoms were also evident (Caddy, Crawford, & Page, 2012). Haltiwanger, Rojo, and Funk (2011) describe a group intervention for women with cancer that is a combination of an expressive art activity group and a peer support group. Through the creative arts, participants can express their feelings as well as reestablish self-confidence. Through the peer support of others who have similar concerns, participants can learn adaptive behaviors and coping skills and the social isolation often associated with a cancer diagnosis is reduced.

Functional Groups

The goal of a **functional group** is to promote adaptation and health through group action and engagement in occupation (Schwartzberg et al., 2008). *Adaptation* refers to the process by which a person adjusts to his or her environment and life circumstances. The four types of actions that are characteristic of a functional group include (1) purposeful action, (2) **self-initiated action**, (3) **spontaneous action** or here-and-now action, and (4) **group-centered action** (Box 38-7). According to Schwartzberg et al. (2008), "it is through the dynamic interaction of these four types of action . . . that the group matures and members develop their ability to function" (p. 95).

Functional groups are experiential in nature; they are designed to motivate group members to meaningful action

BOX 38-7 **HOWE AND SCHWARTZBERG'S (2001) FUNCTIONAL GROUP ACTIONS**

- **Purposeful action:** meaningful for individuals and group as a whole
- **Self-initiated action:** Member takes initiative verbally or nonverbally.
- **Spontaneous action:** Action occurs in the here and now.
- **Group-centered action:** Member actions are interdependent.

in order to facilitate independent or interdependent function. Functional groups are occupation based and make use of the human and nonhuman environments for therapeutic purposes. In functional groups, "objects guide action" and "talking is used to clarify doing." The goal is not the product of the activity but rather the learning that occurs through group participation.

Occupations chosen for use in functional groups may be school, work, play, leisure, or social in nature. In selecting occupations to use for intervention, Schwartzberg et al. (2008) recommend considering the following:

- The occupational goals should be meaningful to the clients.
- Clients should have input in the choice of occupations.
- The demands of the occupation should be congruent with the clients' ability to participate.
- Clients should be able to interact with the environment at a subcortical level.
- Occupations should be chosen that are compatible with the clients' ages, skills, and performance levels (Case Study 38-1).

Implementing Intervention Groups in Occupational Therapy

Regardless of whether the group is client centered, developmental, task oriented, or functional in nature, the OT intervention group format is significantly different from verbal psychotherapy groups conducted by other mental health professionals. Cole (2012) has provided an excellent framework for implementing OT intervention groups that consists of a seven-step process (Box 38-8). A description of this process follows.

Step 1: Introduction

The introduction step is always included regardless of frame of reference or type of group. It is important for group members to learn each other's names and the name of the group leader. The warm-up exercise is designed to capture the group's attention, relax group members, and prepare them to participate in the activity. The warm-up exercise should be challenging but not beyond the group members' capabilities and can be formal or informal in nature. Examples of warm-up exercises include a feelings check-in, review of a previous session, or team-building activity. It is important during the introduction step to set the mood for the group session using the environment and verbal and nonverbal communication. The group leader communicates what is expected of group members and serves as a role model. The purpose of the group should be explained clearly; understanding leads to increased motivation and participation. The group leader describes the structure and processes to be used in the session, including how long the activity will last, what will be done after the activity, and who will keep any products of the activity.

Step 2: Activity

It is critical that the group leader is adequately prepared to lead the group, understands the therapeutic goals, and is aware of the physical and mental capabilities of the group members. The group leader must be knowledgeable in conducting the group activity and skilled in modifying and adapting the activity to meet client needs and goals. Instructions for the activity can be presented verbally, as written directions and/or through demonstration. It is important to get feedback from group members to be sure they understand the directions. This can be accomplished simply by asking group members to repeat the instructions back to you in their own words. It is a good idea to have the materials and supplies for the activity ready but out of view. This will help to decrease distractions while providing instructions.

Step 3: Sharing

The sharing step is designed to facilitate interpersonal learning as group members share their work or experience with the group. It is best to ask for a volunteer and not force anyone to share who is reticent. Role modeling how you want group members to share their activity experience facilitates the learning process. Make sure each group member has the opportunity to share and acknowledge each person's contribution to the group, either verbally ("thank you for sharing") or nonverbally (nodding and making eye contact).

CASE STUDY 38-1   MARCUS

Marcus is a 32-year-old sergeant in the U.S. Army. He is serving in his third deployment with the Airborne Ranger sniper team and is the current leader of his reconnaissance platoon. During his first deployment, Marcus sustained a blast injury to his right side in combat, which required extensive OT rehabilitation intervention. During this combat, he also witnessed the death of two members of his platoon. Although the death of his colleagues could not have been prevented, his injury had prevented him from employing a rescue attempt. For this, he suffered frequent nightmares and flashbacks. His right upper extremity, although functional, continued to be weak. The weakness of his dominant right upper extremity led to a repetitive use injury in his left shoulder that required him to be on pain medication.

The mission commander referred Marcus to the Combat and Operational Stress Control (COSC) unit because of growing concern that he was consuming an excessive amount of pain medication and potentially becoming drug dependent. It was also noted by his superiors, as well as his subordinates, that he was making critical decisions too quickly, reacting impulsively and sometimes explosively during mission planning and debriefing meetings. The sergeant was in danger of losing his position as the platoon leader.

The COSC prevention team, consisting of a U.S. Army occupational therapist, a physician extender, and a psychiatrist, performed a mental health evaluation. The evaluation revealed a history of substance and alcohol abuse, chronic pain related to an injury sustained in an automobile accident as a child, and posttraumatic stress disorder (PTSD) and major depressive disorder that had not been formerly diagnosed or treated. Marcus's treatment plan consisted of a planned reduction of pain medication dependence through incorporation of an individualized physical fitness program to include daily stretching and strengthening exercises.

A cognitive behavioral program was designed for Marcus to address his frequent expressions of distorted thinking,

impulsivity, and verbally explosive outbursts to his supervisor and his subordinates. The cognitive behavioral module was delivered through group therapy. The format of the group allowed soldiers to come together and discuss traumatic events. The U.S. Army occupational therapist, who led the group as a facilitator, gave the soldiers new opportunities to discuss events with a group of peers who had experienced similar traumas. The group leader used projective art techniques, leisure activities, pet therapy, stress reduction, and anger management strategies.

The group sessions were often saturated with strong emotions like anger, resentment, guilt, and grief. During a final session, Marcus shared an insight.

> Sometimes I just get so angry, and I don't even know what the anger is about. Jonathon, our group leader, asked me a question about something I said in our group and I got mad at him, really laid into him. The other members just stared at me. I told him that I didn't have to explain anything to him. But I realize now, it wasn't about his question or even about the group. What I learned is that I didn't want to answer questions because I was afraid I'd get it wrong and fail like I failed my soldiers when I didn't rescue them.

The occupational therapist used a facilitative approach and provided a format for progressive relaxation, diaphragmatic breathing, and mindfulness meditation at the close of each group session. The short-term goal and outcome for the group was to provide a sense of relief and closure that would facilitate gradual behavioral changes resulting in improved mental health. The long-term goal was to normalize traumatic events that are unfortunately associated with combat, to teach coping skills, and to educate soldiers about warning signs of posttraumatic stress. Perhaps the most important advantage for use of a therapeutic group in this case was the unmistakable peer support shown for one another. Peer support is a protective factor for mental health and facilitates resiliency in the face of danger and the physical and psychosocial effects of traumatic events.

Source: Case Study courtesy of Courtney Sase, MS, OTR, used with permission.

Step 4: Processing

The processing step is designed to facilitate emotional learning as group members share their feelings (about each other, about the experience, about the leader) with the group. In this step, as in the sharing phase, it is best to ask for volunteers, model appropriate responses, provide an opportunity for all who desire to share, and acknowledge each person's contribution. During the processing step, the group leader may discuss nonverbal aspects of the group,

for example, struggles for power and control, scapegoating, conflict, attraction, and avoidance. This is done in order to help the group understand its own processes.

Step 5: Generalizing

The generalizing step is designed to facilitate cognitive learning. Cognitive learning is facilitated when the group leader sums up the group experience in a few general principles. These principles are derived directly from the

BOX 38-8   COLE'S (2012) SEVEN-STEP GROUP PROCESS

Step 1: Introduction

- Introduce self (name, title, name of the group).
- Have group members introduce themselves.
- Warm-up exercise
- Communicate expectations of group members.
- Explain purpose of the group clearly.
- Brief outline of the session/structure of the group

Step 2: Activity

- Timing not more than one-third of group session, simple, short activity
- Consider the therapeutic goals to be accomplished by the activity.
- Consider the physical and mental capabilities of the group members.
- Modify/adapt to suit client needs and goals.
- Present instructions clearly, provide example or demonstration as appropriate.
- Get feedback from group members to be sure they understand the directions.
- Have materials and supplies ready but out of view.
- After activity, collect supplies.

Step 3: Sharing

- Members share their work or experience with the group.
- Role model sharing for group members
- Make sure each group member has an opportunity to share.
- Acknowledge each person's contribution verbally or nonverbally.

Step 4: Processing

- Members share their feelings (about each other, about the experience, about the leader) with the group.
- Role model sharing for group members
- Make sure each group member has an opportunity to share.
- Acknowledge each person's contribution verbally or nonverbally.

Step 5: Generalizing

- Sum up the group experience in a few general principles.
- Point out like or similar responses.
- Point out contrasts or differences.
- State one or two principles learned from the experience.

Step 6: Application

- Verbalize the meaning or significance of the experience.
- Discuss how principles learned in the group can be applied to everyday life.
- Relate the experience to issues/problems of members.
- Use concrete examples.

Step 7: Summary

- Emphasize the most important aspects of the group.
- Review goals, content, and process of the group.
- Verbally reinforce group's learning (interpersonal, emotional, and cognitive).
- Thank members for their participation.
- End group on time.

lived experience of the group members and are not pre-planned. These principles should relate to the group goals whenever possible. One way to derive these general principles from the group experience is to look for patterns in responses (similarities, differences). Another way is to observe group energy levels (what energized the group, what subdued the group) and present these observations as general principles to be learned by the group experience.

Step 6: Application

The application step is designed to facilitate the application of the principles learned in the group to everyday life. This is accomplished when the group leader and group members verbalize the meaning or significance of the experience to their problems and personal lives. This may take the form of group problem solving. The best examples of application are simple, concrete, and specific. The group leader may provide examples of how they use the principles in their personal and professional life.

Step 7: Summary

The summary step is designed to reinforce the group's interpersonal, emotional, and cognitive learning. The group leader emphasizes the most important aspects of the group; reviews the goals, content, and process of the group, and thanks group members for their participation. Ending the group on time demonstrates respect for group members' time and other obligations.

Developing Group Protocols

Occupational therapy group interventions involve the processes of observation, evaluation, planning, analyzing, responding, and documenting. Group protocols are one method for coordinating this process. Evaluating client needs is the first step in developing a group intervention.

THEORIES COMMONLY USED IN THE DEVELOPMENT OF GROUP INTERVENTIONS

- **Cognitive disabilities:** focuses on cognitive processes, functional behavior, and problem solving; incorporates cueing, environmental adaptation, and task modification
- **Cognitive behavioral:** focuses on social learning, cognitive distortions, and self-regulation; incorporates cognitive restructuring, role modeling, and behavioral techniques
- **Psychodynamic:** focuses on self-identity, interpersonal relationships, and spirituality; incorporates the symbolic and metaphorical meanings of activity
- **Model of Human Occupation (MOHO):** focuses on occupational performance, participation and adaptation, performance patterns, and skills; incorporates systems theory; contextual factors; and occupational choice, exploration, and mastery
- **Developmental:** focuses on normal developmental tasks, performance patterns, and life transitions; incorporates developmentally appropriate activities and emphasizes the application of learning to everyday life
- **Sensorimotor:** focuses on sensory, motor, and perceptual processes and the learning or relearning of motor skills; incorporates sensory stimulation, purposeful movement, and real-life tasks

Data from Cole, M. B. (2012). *Group dynamics in occupational therapy: The theoretical basis and practice application of group intervention* (4th ed.). Thorofare, NJ: SLACK.

The identification of clients' specific occupational concerns and priorities guides the selection of group goals, activities, structure, and process. The basic process of developing and implementing a group intervention involves the following:

1. Identifying and evaluating the client population
2. Selecting a model or theory or frame of reference to use in the design of the group intervention
3. Determining a focus area or problem for intervention
4. Searching for evidence that can be applied to the group intervention
5. Writing a group intervention outline
6. Developing individual group sessions
7. Implementing the group intervention
8. Evaluating the effectiveness of the group intervention

A **group protocol** is basically an intervention plan for a specific client population. Most groups consist of several sessions and the group protocol outlines the overall goals of the group and the objectives for each session. Each session is outlined in detail including the following:

- Group membership and size
- Session format
- Areas of occupation, performance patterns, or performance skills addressed
- Intervention approach
- Time and place
- A step-by-step description of the therapeutic activity to be used
- The role of the group leader
- Supplies and costs
- Environmental setup
- Potential safety issues
- Grading and adapting the activity
- Evaluation strategies (Cole, 2012)

Group protocols should be theory based and use the best available evidence on group interventions. Common theories used in developing group interventions are briefly described in Box 38-9.

Managing Disruptive Behaviors in Groups

Group dynamics can be productive and growth enhancing, or destructive and maladaptive. All interpersonal behaviors serve a specific need or purpose for at least one individual in the group. However, maladaptive dynamics are usually ineffective and result in negative feelings or outcomes. Examples of maladaptive dynamics include enmeshment, disengagement, competitiveness, manipulation, and scapegoating (O'Brien & Solomon, 2013).

According to the Intentional Relationship Model, clients possess certain interpersonal characteristics. These include the following:

- Communication style
- Capacity for trust
- Need for control
- Response to change and challenge
- Affect
- Predisposition to giving feedback
- Capacity to receive feedback
- Response to human diversity
- Orientation toward relating
- Preference for touch
- Capacity for reciprocity (Taylor, 2008)

These characteristics are often exhibited in groups, sometimes producing positive results and other times

TABLE 38-2	Managing Disruptive Behaviors in Groups	
Problem Behavior	Possible Therapeutic Modes to Employ	Example
Hallucinations and delusions	Instructing	Provide reality-based orientation; keep activity structured.
Akathisia	Empathizing and problem solving	Allow freedom of movement if needed, plan for movement-oriented breaks, select gross motor activities, or adapt fine motor activities.
Storming out of the group	Collaborating and problem solving	Determine the reason for the behavior and collaborate in addressing the client's concerns.
Demonstrating inappropriate sexual behavior	Instructing and empathizing	Explain in clear terms that the behavior is inappropriate and unacceptable. Help the person find appropriate ways to show affection or request attention.
Interrupting other members, excessive talking, or monopolizing discussions and leader's time	Instructing	Design structured activities. Ask questions that require answers from all members of the group. Teach and model methods of taking turns in a conversation, redirect the client's attention to group goals, activities, or discussions.
Using offensive language Displaying escalating or aggressive behavior	Instructing and problem solving	Actively listen, use a calm tone of voice, address problem behavior immediately, and adhere to boundaries, referring often to established group rules.
Excessive or inappropriate approval seeking	Collaborating	Ensure choice and autonomy, expect client to be an active participant and decision maker.
Lack of participation in group activity and/or interactions	Encouraging	Provide positive reinforcement for participation, celebrate accomplishments, and instill hopefulness.

negative outcomes. One of the challenges of facilitating effective intervention groups is managing the disruptive and difficult behaviors of group members. These behaviors may indicate anxiety, frustration, boredom, fear, or symptom exacerbation on the part of the client. Disruptive behaviors may be the client's way of alerting the occupational therapist that he or she needs or wants more structure, guidance, or reassurance. Interpersonal events may occur in the context of group therapy and can be precipitated by client resistance, therapist behavior, difficult circumstances within the group, and the display of strong emotions, among other causes. When difficult situations, or interpersonal events that arise during group interventions are handled effectively, client learning and growth is facilitated, and the therapeutic alliance with the therapist is enhanced. If handled poorly, these events can undermine the efficacy of the group intervention and harm relationships within the group.

Understanding the underlying cause or motivation for the behavior will help the occupational therapist determine the best response or therapeutic mode to employ. Therapeutic modes are described in more detail in Chapter 37 and include advocating, collaborating, empathizing, encouraging, instructing, and problem solving (Taylor, 2008). Some common problem behaviors and therapeutic management strategies or modes are outlined in Table 38-2.

PRACTICE DILEMMA 38-1

Just One of Those Days . . .

In a busy urban hospital outpatient behavioral health unit, an occupational therapist and a certified OT assistant (COTA) are responsible for the provision of a social skills group for clients recovering from traumatic brain injuries (TBIs). The group has five members not including the leaders. Martin is a 55-year-old former high school basketball coach who was involved in a serious car accident 5 months ago. He has frequent emotional outbursts and a tendency toward disruptive behaviors that escalate. Joanna is a 36-year-old mother of two children. She was involved in an accident at her job with the power company. She fell from a bucket truck while on the job, which resulted in a TBI. Joanna frequently displays manic behaviors and at times is sexually inappropriate toward other group members.

Louis is a 60-year-old street musician who was hit by an oncoming car when the driver lost control and ran up onto the sidewalk of a busy city square. Louis is quiet and mild mannered but often withdraws from the group activity or refuses to participate. He also experiences hallucinations. Marcella and Elaine are 22-year-old twins who were diagnosed with juvenile onset Huntington disease. Their frequent jerky movements and limited cognitive abilities are often complained about by other group members.

In order to develop and practice communication and social skills, the group is working on completion of a group collage requiring collaborative decision making and planning. Within the first 15 minutes of the session, the occupational therapist notes that Louis begins to have active hallucinations. About this time, a nurse, who had arrived to deliver medication, hurried through the door to the OT room, creating a draft that blew all of the magazine pictures to be used for the collage onto the floor. Martin, with his voice raised, shouted at the nurse, calling her stupid for knocking over all of the pictures.

Although this was a difficult project for Elaine and Marcella because of their decreased fine motor abilities, the occupational therapist had constructed larger, foam board pictures of various foods for the twins to use to contribute to the collage. Even with this adaptation, the clients were expressing frustration by talking loudly and abandoning the group activity. Joanna's akathisia and inappropriate sexual behavior seemed to be disrupting task completion and social interaction among group members.

The occupational therapist and the COTA discussed the group session later while preparing the documentation, analyzing the tremendous impact clients' problem behaviors had had on their group in a 1-hour session on a single day. The occupational therapist looked at the COTA and concluded, "Oh, well, I guess it is all in a day's work, and it was just one of THOSE days!"

Questions

1. Which of the disruptive behaviors in the practice dilemma would be the most difficult for you to address? Why?
2. What strategies or therapeutic modes might you employ in the practice scenario to manage each client's disruptive behaviors?
3. How might you have prevented these problems from occurring beforehand?

Special Considerations

Working with groups has many challenges and specific ethical and legal issues to be considered. Group leaders/therapists have a "dual responsibility (a) to protect the welfare of each individual group member and (b) to ensure that the group, as a whole, functions in a way that benefits everyone involved" (Herlihy & Flowers, 2010, p. 191). All of the ethical concerns related to OT services for individuals also apply to group work. In addition, due to the differences in the treatment approaches, there are some special considerations that must be addressed when providing group interventions. Confidentiality, managing boundaries, transference, and documentation issues briefly described here.

Confidentiality concerns are multiplied when providing group interventions because participants disclose personal information not only to the therapist but also to the group as a whole. It is incumbent on the group leader to emphasize the importance of confidentiality to group members. The leader must address violations of confidentiality or trust will be diminished and the boundaries of the group will be weakened.

Managing group boundaries is another challenge. This means not only the professional boundaries between therapist and client but also the boundaries among group members and boundaries between group members and nonmembers. Social relationships outside of the clinical setting between therapist and group members are discouraged. The boundaries between group members and nonmembers must be clear enough to prevent outside intrusion and to provide a sense of security for group members (Herlihy & Flowers, 2010).

Another concern relates to transference and countertransference in group situations. Transference occurs when clients transfer feelings, expectations, and impressions about a person in their past onto the therapist or other group members. For example, the therapist (or other group member) may remind a client of his or her parent or spouse and the client may interact in a way that recreates that former relationship (Haley & Carrier, 2010). Countertransference, where the therapist experiences transference with the client, is also possible. For example, when the group leader has positive or negative feelings toward a specific group member, it may be because the therapist is recreating a relationship with someone in his or her past.

Documentation of group interventions must conform to third-party payors, state, and federal requirements. In order for group interventions to be billable, the therapist must be an active participant in the process, and most of the group session should involve interaction between the participants and the therapist. Typically, each client's progress is documented following each group session, and notes are kept on the group's function as a whole. In addition, outcome measures may be used to determine the effectiveness of the group intervention in meeting client goals.

Conclusion

Occupational therapy intervention groups have the potential to incorporate many, if not all, of Yalom's (1995) therapeutic factors. One study indicated that psychiatric clients in four OT intervention groups most valued

of cohesiveness, instillation of
l learning (Falk-Kessler, Momich,
pation-based groups may be par-
promoting hopefulness because oc-
ion facilitates the development of
chievement. Hopefulness and a sense
key affective motivators for learning,
cha... ...wth. Falk-Kessler et al. (1991) propose,
"activities c... ...e used to facilitate the development of

helpful therapeutic factors and therapeutic factors can be used to maximize the inherent or prescribed therapeutic effect of the activities" (p. 65). The "Commentary on the Evidence" box outlines additional evidence of the efficacy of group interventions. It is therefore important to incorporate these therapeutic factors in the design and implementation of occupation-based group interventions regardless of the population served or the setting in which the intervention occurs.

COMMENTARY ON THE EVIDENCE

Evidence to support the use of group interventions comes from various disciplines, including counseling, psychology, social work, and OT. Research suggests that OT-related intervention in groups is effective in addressing outcomes in body function (e.g., mental functions) and occupational performance areas and skills such as social participation and communication/interaction skills (Howe & Schwartzberg, 2001). Evidence-based techniques vary depending on the desired outcomes and client problem. Intervention for performance areas and skills conducted in a group setting may result in greater client satisfaction and compliance with intervention regimes (Howe & Schwartzberg, 2001). Because the range of skills addressed is so varied, it is best to examine the literature specific to the client factor and outcome in question. There is a need to expand the evidence in all areas of OT intervention in which group process is applied to specific client problems.

A few studies providing evidence for the efficacy of group work are briefly described here.

Authors	Findings
Rosenberg, Maeir, Yochman, Dahan, & Hirsch (2015)	Preschoolers with attention-deficit/hyperactivity disorder and their parents attended a cognitive-functional OT group intervention and demonstrated increases in functional performance as measured by the Canadian Occupational Performance Measure (COPM) and goal attainment scaling.
Haltiwanger (2012)	A culturally tailored peer-led support group for Mexican-American older adults with type 2 diabetes demonstrated increases in self-efficacy and improved glycosylated hemoglobin test results.
Hewlett et al. (2011)	A cognitive behavioral group intervention was found to be effective in reducing the impact of fatigue, coping and perceived severity, and well-being for persons with rheumatoid arthritis.
Castle et al. (2010)	Participants in a manualized group-based intervention were less likely than those treated individually to have a relapse of their bipolar disorder and spent less time unwell.
Lamb et al. (2010)	A group cognitive behavioral intervention in a primary care setting was found to be efficacious and cost effective in enhancing quality of life and reducing disability associated with subacute and chronic low back pain.
Capasso, Gorman, & Blick (2010)	A study of persons with cerebrovascular accident and resultant hemiparesis demonstrated improved upper extremity function as a result of participation in a social breakfast group intervention as an alternative to repetitive exercise.
Starino et al. (2010)	An illness self-management group intervention for persons with severe mental disorders demonstrated increases in hope and recovery-related attitudes. Participants showed improvement in symptoms, but the change was not statistically significant.
Boisvert (2004)	A client-centered OT group (based on the Model of Human Occupation) for persons with substance dependence demonstrated significant improvement in participants' self-esteem.
Peterson (2003)	A randomized controlled trial designed to evaluate the efficacy of an eight-session, group-based fall prevention program for older adults demonstrated increased social participation and improved community mobility.
Bober, McLellan, McBee, & Westreich, 2002	An art-based activity group for persons with Alzheimer disease was effective in improving participants' ability to identify emotions and socialize with other group members.

REFERENCES

American Occupational Therapy Association. (2008). Occupational therapy practice framework: Domain and process, 2nd edition. *American Journal of Occupational Therapy, 62*, 625–683. doi:10.5014/ajot.62.6.625

American Occupational Therapy Association. (2014). Occupational therapy practice framework: Domain and process, 3rd edition. *American Journal of Occupational Therapy, 68*, S1–S48.

Azima, H., Cramer-Azima, F., & Wittkower, E. D. (1957). Analytic group art therapy. *International Journal of Psychotherapy, 7*, 243–260.

Benne, K. D., & Sheats, P. (1978). Functional roles of group members. In L. P. Bradford (Ed.), *Group development* (2nd ed., pp. 52–61). LaJolla, CA: University Associates.

Bloch, S. (1986). Therapeutic factors in group psychotherapy. In A. J. Frances & R. E. Hales (Eds.), *Annual review* (Vol. 5, pp. 678–698). Washington, DC: American Psychiatric Press.

Bober, S. J., McLellan, E., McBee, L., & Westreich, L. (2002). The feelings art group: A vehicle for personal expression in skilled nursing home residents with dementia. *Journal of Social Work in Long Term Care, 1*, 73–86.

Boisvert, R. A. (2004). Enhancing substance dependence intervention. *OT Practice, 9*(10), 11–16.

Brown, N. W. (2003). Conceptualizing process. *International Journal of Group Psychotherapy, 53*, 225–244.

Caddy, L., Crawford, F., & Page, A. C. (2012). "Painting a path to wellness": Correlations between participating in a creative activity group and improved measured mental health outcome. *Journal of Psychiatric and Mental Health Nursing, 19*, 327–333. doi:10.1111/j.1365-2850.2011.01785.x

Capasso, N., Gorman, A., & Blick, C. (2010). Breakfast group in an acute rehabilitation setting: A restorative program for incorporating client's hemiparetic upper extremities for function. *OT Practice, 5*(8), 14–18.

Castle, D., White, C., Chamberlain, J., Berk, M., Berk, L., Lauder, S., . . . Gilbert, M. (2010). Group-based psychosocial intervention for bipolar disorder: Randomised controlled trial. *The British Journal of Psychiatry, 196*, 383–388. doi:10.1192/bjp.bp.108.058263

Cole, M. B. (2012). *Group dynamics in occupational therapy: The theoretical basis and practice application of group intervention* (4th ed.). Thorofare, NJ: SLACK.

Cole, M. B., & Donohue, M. (2011). *Social participation in occupational contexts: In schools, clinics, and communities.* Thorofare, NJ: SLACK.

DBT iPhone App. (2012). *DBT diary card and skills coach.* Retrieved from http://www.diarycard.net/

DeCarlo, J. J., & Mann, W. C. (1985). The effectiveness of verbal versus activity groups in improving self-perceptions of interpersonal communication skills. *American Journal of Occupational Therapy, 39*, 20–27.

Donohue, M. (2010). *Five levels of social participation.* Retrieved from http://www.social-profile.com/social_levels.html

Falk-Kessler, J., Momich, C., & Perel, S. (1991). Therapeutic factors in occupational therapy groups. *American Journal of Occupational Therapy, 45*, 59–66.

Fidler, G. S. (1969). The task-oriented group as a context for treatment. *American Journal of Occupational Therapy, 23*, 43–48.

Gazda, G. M. (1989). *Group counseling: A developmental approach* (4th ed.). Boston, MA: Allyn & Bacon.

Haley, M., & Carrier, J. W. (2010). Psychotherapy groups. In D. Capuzzi, D. R. Gross, & M. D. Stauffer (Eds.), *Introduction to group work* (5th ed., pp. 295–320). Denver, CO: Love.

Haltiwanger, E. P. (2012). Effect of a group adherence intervention for Mexican-American older adults with type 2 diabetes. *American Journal of Occupational Therapy, 66*, 447–454.

Haltiwanger, E., Rojo, R., & Funk, K. (2011). Living with cancer: Impact of expressive arts. *Occupational Therapy in Mental Health, 27*, 65–86.

Herlihy, B. R., & Flowers, L. (2010). Group work: Ethical and legal considerations. In D. Capuzzi, D. R. Gross, & M. D. Stauffer (Eds.), *Introduction to group work* (5th ed., pp. 191–217). Denver, CO: Love.

Hewlett, S., Ambler, N., Almeida, C., Cliss, A., Hammond, A., Kitchen, K., . . . Pollock, J. (2011). Self-management of fatigue in rheumatoid arthritis: A randomised controlled trial of group cognitive-behavioural therapy. *Annals of the Rheumatic Diseases, 70*, 1060–1067.

Higgins, S., Schwartzberg, S., Bedell, G., & Duncombe, L. (2015). Current practice and perceptions of group work in occupational therapy. *American Journal of Occupational Therapy, 69*, 6911510223p1. doi:10.5014/ajot.2015.69S1-PO7096

Howe, M. C., & Schwartzberg, S. L. (2001). *A functional approach to group work in occupational therapy* (3rd ed.). Philadelphia, PA: Lippincott Williams & Wilkins.

Johnson, D. W., & Johnson, F. P. (2006). *Joining together: Group theory and group skills* (9th ed.). Boston, MA: Pearson.

Kouzes, J., & Posner, B. (2007). *The leadership challenge* (4th ed.). San Francisco, CA: Jossey-Bass Learning.

Lamb, S. E., Hansen, Z., Lall, R., Castelnuovo, E., Withers, E. J., Nichols, V., . . . Underwood, M. R. (2010). Group cognitive behavioural treatment for low-back pain in primary care. A randomised controlled trial and cost-effectiveness analysis. *Lancet, 375*, 916–923.

Law, M. (1998). *Client-centered occupational therapy.* Thorofare, NJ: SLACK.

Mattingly, C., & Fleming, M. H. (1994). *Clinical reasoning: Forms of inquiry in a therapeutic practice.* Philadelphia, PA: F. A. Davis.

Mosey, A. C. (1970). The concept and use of developmental groups. *American Journal of Occupational Therapy, 24*, 272–275.

Mosey, A. C. (1973). *Activities therapy.* New York, NY: Raven Press.

Mosey, A. C. (1981). *Occupational therapy: Configuration of a profession.* New York, NY: Raven Press.

O'Brien, J. C., & Solomon, J. W. (2013). *Occupational analysis and group process.* St. Louis, MO: Elsevier/Mosby.

Peterson, E. W. (2003). Evidence-based practice: A matter of balance. *OT Practice, 8*(3), 12–14.

Rosenberg, L., Maeir, A., Yochman, A., Dahan, I., & Hirsch, I. (2015). Effectiveness of a cognitive-functional group intervention among preschoolers with attention deficit hyperactivity disorder: A pilot study. *American Journal of Occupational Therapy, 69*, 6903220040p1–6903220040p8.

Schwartzberg, S. L., Howe, M., & Barnes, M. (2008). *Groups: Applying the functional group model.* Philadelphia, PA: F. A. Davis.

Starino, V. R., Mariscal, S., Holter, M. C., Davidson, L. J., Cooke, K. S., Fukui, S., & Rapp, C. A. (2010). Outcomes of an illness self-management group using wellness recovery action planning. *Psychiatric Rehabilitation Journal, 34*, 57–60.

Taylor, R. (2008). *The intentional relationship: Occupational therapy and use of self.* Philadelphia, PA: F. A. Davis.

Tuckman, B. W. (1965). Developmental sequence in small groups. *Psychological Bulletin, 63*, 384–399.

Yalom, I. D. (1995). *The theory and practice of group psychotherapy* (4th ed.). New York, NY: Basic Books.

Yalom, I. D., & Leszcz, M. (2005). *The theory and practice of group psychotherapy* (5th ed.). New York, NY: Basic Books.

the**Point** *For additional resources on the subjects discussed in this chapter, visit* http://thePoint.lww.com/Willard-Spackman13e. *See* **Appendix I, Resources and Evidence for Common Conditions Addressed in OT** *for more information on posttraumatic stress disorder, depression (included with mood disorders), and substance use disorders.*

CHAPTER 39

Professionalism, Communication, and Teamwork

Janet Falk-Kessler

LEARNING OBJECTIVES

After reading this chapter, you will be able to:

1. Understand what it means to be a professional.
2. Understand what types of behaviors are viewed as professional and as unprofessional, and why.
3. Understand the value of teamwork.
4. Be able to distinguish between different types of teams and how they function.
5. Be able to describe the "do's and don'ts" of social media participation.

Introduction

The purpose of this chapter is to review professionalism and collaborative behavior. In this chapter, professionalism encompasses how one presents oneself as a professional and the individual's responsibilities and obligations as a professional and to one's profession.

Professionalism is a concept that has many attributes. It includes behaviors that are on public display; knowledge and skill-based competencies that are continually sought and demonstrated; and overall responsibilities to one's clients, colleagues, profession, and society (Monrouxe, Rees, & Hu, 2011). Becoming a professional is a process—one that begins by learning what a professional is and does, enacting the professional role by meeting expectations, and eventually embodying and internalizing professional qualities. Implicit and explicit guidelines, rules, and expectations within social contexts contribute to professional development (Monrouxe et al., 2011).

Professionalism reflects the person as well as one's profession. Within medically related professions, professionalism at its core is a belief system that embraces a social contract on health care delivery that asserts competency and ethical standards (Wynia, Papadakis, Sullivan, & Hafferty, 2014). These characteristics echo how professionalism in occupational therapy (OT) has been described (Glennon & Van Oss, 2010; Hordichuk, Robinson, & Sullivan, 2015) and served as the foundation for one's behaviors, commitments, collaboration, and teamwork. As one's professionalism develops, one's role as a contributing member of the health care team and

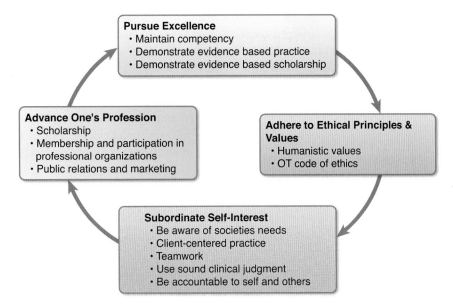

FIGURE 39-1 Professionalism and OT practitioners.

the OT profession is strengthened. This chapter reviews professionalism as it relates to each of these areas.

Professionalism has been garnering a vast amount of attention in both the public and professional media. Demonstrating professionalism has become a focus within many academic settings, with the emergence of professionalism assessments (Wang et al., 2017; Yuen, Azuero, Lackey, Brown, & Shrestha, 2016; Ziring et al., 2015). The development of values, attitudes, and behaviors that mirror one's profession is a process that continually evolves throughout one's career and is in part reflective of a contract between one's discipline and society in general (Cruess & Cruess, 2009; Hordichuk et al., 2015). Maintaining standards of practice, which include maintaining competency, demonstrating **evidence-based practice**, using appropriate judgment, and abiding by our profession's ethical code, is a professional responsibility (American Occupational Therapy Association [AOTA], 2015a, 2015b).

Participating in local, state, and national organizations that work to market OT services to various stakeholders—including consumers, third-party payers, and policymakers—and that sponsor continuing education opportunities, provide members with a range of literature, and inform members of legislation as well as other concerns of interest is part of one's professional responsibility. This is further articulated through the core tenets of Vision 2025 (AOTA, 2017b), which demands the highest standards of professionalism.

Historically, the transmission of professionalism relied on immersion in a professional environment. Distinct from professional identity, professionalism is defined by behaviors demonstrated in various contexts: with clients, on health care teams, and through all modes of communication. Recognizing that each generation brings a different understanding of what professionalism is, many have argued that simply being in professional environments may not be enough to learn the behaviors; instead, it is to be taught within academic and clinical programs (Cruess & Cruess, 2009; Lindheim, Nouri, Rabah, & Yaklic, 2016; Monrouxe et al., 2011; Ziring et al., 2015). These obligations and responsibilities are depicted in Figure 39-1.

Workplace Professionalism and Behavior

In the last few decades, many medical professionals have emphasized and embraced their long-held, traditional values. The "Occupational Therapy Practice Framework" (AOTA, 2014), with its emphasis on occupational engagement, similarly reminds therapists of the roots of professional practice and the professional responsibility to use terminology that reflects these values (Youngstrom, 2002) and affirms one's identity (Fawcett, 2013). The context for using terminology, however, is critical in one's communication; overly technical terminology with clients, for example, may actually result in a diminished professional presentation (Berman et al., 2016).

Regardless of situation or interaction (e.g., a professor, supervisor, client and/or the client's family, a team meeting, or conference presentation), professionalism is expected. Professional behavior has become so important that it is included in academic accreditation standards for all levels of OT education (Accreditation Council for Occupational Therapy Education, 2010) and is an integral part of the competencies expected in both level I (AOTA, 2017a) and level II (AOTA, 2002) fieldwork experiences.

Among the many characteristics that shape professionals are values about work, roles, and service recipients. Many believe that values, especially those that revolve around work ethic, cause conflict in academic and employment environments. In recent decades, attention has been paid to differences in work values and expectation that is generationally linked (Lyons & Kuron, 2014; Wiedmer, 2015). How one behaves is rooted in the cultural and societal norms and expectations in which one was raised. Today's society, which serves as the context of the health care culture, may have contributed to the unraveling of professionalism (Glennon & Van Oss, 2010).

When considering the characteristics of the different generations, one should not assume that all traits are exhibited by all within one generational cohort or are exhibited consistently regardless of the environment. Some traits, such as ease with technology, might not translate to professional settings (Hills et al., 2016), and one's identity within a generation, rather than one's birth date, may inform behavior (Campbell, Twenge, & Campbell, 2017; Lyons & Kuron, 2014). But it is nonetheless important to recognize that differences that distinguish cohorts impact both communication and one's perception of professionalism and work ethic (Kick, Contacos-Sawyer, & Thomas, 2015), along with one's expectation of the work environment (Anselmo-Witzel, Orshan, Heitner, & Bachand, 2017; Ozkan, & Solmaz, 2015; Wiedmer, 2015).

Understanding and respecting generational differences, however, is important for two overarching reasons: as a treating professional, when one considers the habits, values, and perceptions of the different generations, one is better prepared for client-centered care. Understanding how an older client might perceive a behavior demonstrated by a young therapist is critical to the client–therapist interaction.

The second consideration regarding generational differences involves one's role as a team member. Because there may be varying perspectives on what constitutes professional and unprofessional behavior, interpersonal conflict between professionals can arise (Johnston, 2006). Furthermore, one may acknowledge what is considered unprofessional behavior but rationalize this behavior as not unprofessional when they themselves display it (Aurora, Wayne, Anderson, Didwania, & Humphrey, 2008). This individual has no idea that he or she is perceived as

inappropriate, unreasonable, and even disrespectful. It has been suggested that these behaviors reflect how individuals perceive and understand rules and their expectations of and for themselves (Lake, 2009). As an example, those individuals of the more recent generations grew up within home, school, and societal environments that promoted self-esteem, emphasized individualism, and placed little emphasis on social rules. This can result in the expectation of entitlements (Twenge, 2006; Ventriglio & Bhugra, 2016). The previous generations grew up with a respect for authority and the notion that achievement is based on what one has actually accomplished. Table 39-1 presents the comparison of generations, using Pew Research Center information (Dimock, 2018) and recent consensus (Twenge, 2017) for cohort dates.

Differences in how one perceives work/career values and rewards can also lead to conflict (Lipscomb, 2010). When one considers that professionalism within academia and health care is typically defined by those from the Silent or Baby Boomer generations, it is not surprising that those from the more recent generations are unaware that their attitudes and behaviors are viewed as unprofessional. These attitudes and behaviors may be at the root of fieldwork and workplace difficulties rather than knowledge (Langenfeld, Cook, Sudbeck, Luers, & Schenarts, 2014). Student scenarios provided by academic and clinical colleagues across the country are presented in Table 39-2. Each example demonstrates behavior that has been considered unprofessional.

What is the underlying issue portrayed in the case study? Individuals from two different generations perceive behaviors in very different ways. These perceptions come from experiences specific to their "generational culture." Being from different generational cultures is not an excuse to maintain behaviors and expectations that are viewed by many as unprofessional, nor to hold on to behaviors and expectations that might no longer be appropriate. Although the supervisor in this case example is concerned by what he sees as a combination of laziness and unprofessional behaviors, the younger therapist believes in efficiency and flexibility while being dependent on his supervisor for knowledge. Both are coming from their own generational context. In practice settings, however, one must remember that the client's needs come first and that most likely, there are generational differences between therapist and client as well. Therefore, those joining the workforce will succeed if they are aware of how they are perceived and learn to demonstrate all aspects of professionalism that will garner them respect from the multigenerational contexts. Their supervisors will similarly have more satisfying relationships with those they oversee if they, too, understand how to adapt their supervisory styles in order to help the new therapists adapt and to not blame their supervisees for behaviors shaped by their culture.

CASE STUDY 39-1   JOHN ON FIELDWORK

John Dimet is a graduate student in OT and has just started his first level 2 fieldwork experience. He has completed all of his coursework. He is 26 years old, having spent the time between undergraduate and graduate school completing his prerequisites and engaging in volunteer work.

Prior to the start of his fieldwork, he sent his supervisor, who he had not yet met, the following e-mail: *Hey Fred, looking forward to starting on Monday. What time should I arrive, and is there a dress code? JD*

John met his supervisor on Monday at 8 a.m. as instructed, and they immediately went to morning rounds. His university's fieldwork coordinator had told him that there would be days he would need to arrive at 7 a.m. so that he could participate in activities of daily living (ADL) sessions with clients. The site was an inpatient rehabilitation setting with an average length of stay of 4 to 6 weeks.

During the first week, John participated in orientation along with three other OT students and shadowed his supervisor, Fred Hill. Fred had 20 years of OT experience plus several specialty certifications. He gave John a schedule of when he was to arrive at 7 a.m.

During their weekly supervision session of the second week, Fred asked John questions about the clinical conditions and functional challenges of the clients seen and pressed him to identify long-term goals for one of the clients. John had very superficial knowledge of the clinical conditions, and when asked about this limitation, John reported that his academic program did not go into depth on every condition. This surprised Fred, as he was knowledgeable about the academic program's curriculum. John also stated that he hadn't thought about goals for the clients seen, as he thought Fred would let him know what they were. In addition, Fred pointed out to John that during the shadowing time, he heard John's smartphone vibrate and saw John check its screen. He reminded John that all smartphones are to be off during work hours, but he can use it during his lunch break.

During the third week, John arrived late on 2 days, completely missing morning rounds 1 day and arriving late to rounds on the second day. He told Fred that he could get the information missed from one of the other students, and that if necessary, he can make up the time at the end of the day. He also asked if he really needed to attend rounds every morning, as not much changed from day to day. He suggested that because students have to be at the site at 7 a.m. twice a week, and on those days, each would attend rounds, whichever student attended rounds can easily text or e-mail the information to those not present. This would make the workday easier on everyone. John added that commute was close to an hour each way, and a flexible schedule would be very helpful to everyone.

Fred was troubled with John's professionalism and devoted their next supervision session to review what his concerns were. Fred and John had very different views on each of the behaviors:

- Being prepared:
  - Fred expected students to come to fieldwork prepared, which includes doing research on their own time in any area they had limited knowledge of. They are expected to be ready to discuss OT's role in promoting functional performance and participation, and to examine how one might apply evidence-based practice. By not putting in the time to learn, Fred believes that his student is either unmotivated or simply lazy.
  - John assumed it was his supervisor's responsibility to provide him with information about clinical conditions, be told by his supervisor what he needed to do, and if he needed to do anything "extra," he would be given time during the workday to do it. After all, isn't his supervisor a teacher, and as such shouldn't he be giving him the knowledge he needs to have?
- Electronic devices:
  - Fred views smartphone use as not just a distraction to patient care but also a demonstration of disrespect to those he needs to interact with.
  - John believes he has the ability to multitask; by keeping his smartphone on vibrate is actually showing respect, and he needs to check it just in case something important is shared. In addition, he does not wear a watch so this is how he knows the time.
- Interprofessional collaboration:
  - Fred believes in collaborative teamwork and participating in morning rounds not only keeps everyone up to date on any changes or progress made by patients but also provides an opportunity to engage with others around patient care. In addition, schedules and their related responsibilities are to be adhered to and not ignored as a matter of convenience.
  - John doesn't understand why attendance is required because there are more efficient ways of gathering the information. He also doesn't understand why making up the time later in the day isn't an option.
- Patient privacy:
  - Finally, Fred is very concerned that John would suggest texting information about patients, as this can easily result in Health Insurance Portability and Accountability Act (HIPAA) violations.
  - John views electronic communication as efficient and assures Fred that it will be shared only with students at the site.

TABLE 39-1   Generational Comparisons

	Silent Generation	Baby Boomers	Generation X	Generation Y	Generation Z
Also known as . . .	Traditionalists veterans	Sandwich generation	Slacker generation Me generation Latchkey kids	Millennials Nexters Trophy kids Echo boomers	Digital natives iGeneration Net Gen
Birth years	1928–1945	1946–1964	1965–1980	1981–1995	1996–2010 (some identify the mid-nineties as the start of this generation)
Descriptors	Loyal, formal	Optimistic, tactful	Skeptical, blunt	Pragmatic, polite	Socially and environmentally aware Self-confident Service-oriented
Learning styles	Process-oriented	Personal experiences Caring environment Handouts Note-taking	Efficient Only study what is personally useful Own pace, own time Detailed review and study guides Like technology	Collaborative Technology is necessary Experiential Immediate feedback Want it right the first time	Prefer digital access to information but do not assess the sources Expect instant feedback Prefer "customized" learning over lectures Experiential learners Teamwork
Career goals and rewards	To "build a legacy" Feel a personal responsibility for their organization Doing a good job is personally satisfying	"Build a stellar career" Achievement, recognition, financial remuneration	"Build a portable career" (career security vs. job security) Freedom	"Build parallel careers" Multitask at work; multiple careers in life Seek personally meaningful work	Flexible work environments Work–life balance Multitaskers Achievement- and reward-focused Want to make a difference
Workplace values and ethics	Loyalty, dedication, and sacrifice Hard work Respect for authority Respect for hierarchy, elders Adhere to rules Duty first Conformity Responds to directive leadership	Dedication Respect authority Want "face time" Team-oriented Personal growth and gratification Uncomfortable with conflict Can be overly sensitive to feedback Can be judgmental Responds to directive leadership	Work–life balance Want autonomy, flexibility, and informality Accept diversity Pragmatic/practical Self-reliant Reject rules Mistrust institutions Use technology Multitaskers	Need feedback and recognition Nurtured Seek fulfillment and fun Celebrate diversity Optimistic Self-inventive Rewrite rules Institutions are irrelevant Not awed by hierarchy, elders Expect technology Multitask fast Have difficulty dealing with "difficult people" issues	Need constant feedback and recognition Control their own work time and environments Expect clear goals Self-reliant Entrepreneurial Informal communication style Personal satisfaction is important Job change is expected Confident in authority

Information compiled from the following sources: Berkup (2014); Fogg (2008); Mohr, Moreno-Walton, Mills, Brunett, & Promes (2011); Tulgan (2009); Wiedmer (2015); and Zemke, Raines, & Filipczak (2013).

TABLE 39-2	Student Behaviors
Generational Factor (Lake, 2009)	**Behavior**
Rules "Have trouble understanding rules as guides for their behavior, unless particularized to them"	A student refused to go to her fieldwork assignment because ADL sessions started at 7:30 a.m., and she isn't "a morning person."
	A student is ½ hour late for an exam and asks for extra time to finish it.
	A student did not attend a Monday class because it interfered with her long weekend plans. She asked the professor to go over what she missed.
Rewards "Have grown up constantly rewarded, not punished"	A student earned a 94 on a case study. She made an appointment with her professor to complain because she felt she deserved a higher grade.
	A student complained to the administration that faculty won't let them redo assignments for a better grade.
	A student complained that he didn't get a higher grade in the course. After all, he attended all of the classes.
Avoidance "When confronted with rules . . . instinctively respond with avoidance behaviors . . . or find a way around it "	A student was absent from a fieldwork assignment and asked a friend to inform her supervisor.
	A professor asked a student to make an appointment with him. The student never followed through.
	After doing a literature search, many of the references that emerged were not available online but were available in the school's library. The student only used what he accessed online.
Decision makers "Often make their decisions in close connection with family members and friends."	A student's parents advised him to change his level 2 fieldwork placement because he had no intention of seeking a job with the client population to which he was assigned.
	A student expressed concern over a requirement she didn't know existed. She never visited the school or spoke with anyone from the school prior to attending. She relied on information she received from a friend who graduated 4 years earlier.

ADL, activities of daily living.

To further illustrate differences in how individuals from different generations perceive professionalism, consider Case Study 39-1.

Professionalism and Teamwork

Interprofessional teamwork is ubiquitous. Thus, an important feature of professionalism is one's ability to be an effective team member. **Teamwork** as applied in the health care environment is, simply put, "the ability to recognize and respect the expertise of others and work with them in the patient's best interest" (Cruess, Cruess, &

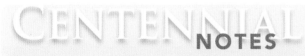

NOTES

Important Members of the Health Team

One of the earliest mention of occupational therapists as vital team members is from *Syllabus for Training of Nurses in Occupational Therapy* by Eleanor Clarke Slagle and Harriet A. Robeson, published in 1933:

> "She became one of the most important members of the health team, for today no doctor can successfully practice as an individualist. To aid him he has the nurse, the laboratory technician, the X-ray technician, the dietitian, the physiotherapist, the dentist, and now, no less important than the other members of the health team, the occupational therapist."

Steinert, 2009, p. 286). Interprofessional teams in particular enhance client safety and care and are based on the premise that no one person has all the skills and knowledge to meet the client's goals. As a result, competencies have been developed along with health care academic programs' accreditation standards to ensure collaborative practice (Interprofessional Education Collaborative [IPEC], 2016).

Effective teamwork is linked with improved client outcomes and improved client safety (Brock, et al., 2013; Ndoro, 2014; Zwarenstein, Goldman, & Reeves, 2009), including outcomes in rehabilitation settings (Sinclair, Lingard, & Mohabeer, 2009). Failures related to the environment's culture and to interpersonal communication can result in treatment errors (Deering, Johnston, & Colacchio, 2011). Improving health care is a direct result of improving communication and collaboration (Zwarenstein et al., 2009).

Teams are an outgrowth of the knowledge that an individual who functions alone is not as helpful to the client as a team that works well together. The reasoning process, when done in a group, is more effective than when done in isolation (Mercier & Sperber, 2011). This reduces the risk of ignoring information that does not fit within one's belief system and increases access to information from others, which helps decision making. Being a member of a team does not automatically result in collaboration (Thistlethwaite, 2012), however, and one must be aware that teams can be undermined by power relationships (Baker, Egan-Lee, Martimianakis, & Reeves, 2011). Facilitating interprofessional teamwork in clinical sites

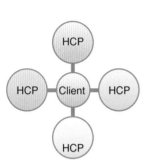

Multidisciplinary Team

Each works within their own silo, although they regularly meet to share information regarding the client's progress toward their respective discipline's goals.

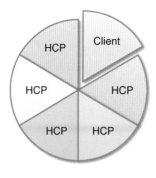

Interdisciplinary Team

They work together to determine goals and how each team member will contribute to their collaborative plan. Client is often involved in the decision making process.

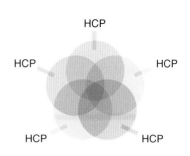

Transdisciplinary Team

Each team member brings one's own set of knowledge and skills to the team. When working with clients, there are overlapping responsibilities and reduced professional boundaries. Role blurring is common.

FIGURE 39-2 Interprofessional collaboration of health care practitioners (HCP).

is critical (Poston, Haney, Kott, & Rutledge, 2017), but providing educational opportunities during ones professional education is equally important (Anderson, Smith, & Hammick, 2016; Boet, Bould, Layat Burn, & Reeves, 2014; Brennan, Olds, Dolansky, Estrada, & Patrician, 2014; Brock, 2013; House, Sun, Sullivan, & Ross, 2016; Ndoro, 2014). Furthermore, interprofessional education must be competency-based (IPEC, 2016).

Effective teams, whether they be made up by two individuals such as an occupational therapist and an OT assistant or representing a group of health care professionals from varying disciplines, are all characterized by communication and collaboration, formal and informal learning opportunities, and, above all, trust (Cartmill, Soklaridis, & Cassidy, 2011; Jones & Jones, 2011; Kalisch, Lee, & Rochman, 2010). These attributes are developed through group cohesion, shared mental models, and objective leadership and often result in increased job satisfaction (Kalisch et al., 2010). Effective teams are characterized by individuals who collaborate and coordinate their work, share their knowledge and resources, learn about each other's roles, and share responsibilities when appropriate (Sims, Hewitt, & Harris, 2015). In addition, the explicit importance of team meetings, the role of shared objectives in conflict management, and the value of autonomy within the team (Jones & Jones, 2011) are further examples of effective interprofessional teams.

There are three categories of interprofessional teams that exist in health care: multidisciplinary, interdisciplinary, and transdisciplinary (Figure 39-2). Each is composed of individuals from various professional backgrounds, and each is focused on a common client. It is helpful to consider these teams as a continuum of interprofessional cooperation. Multidisciplinary teams emerged first, with other forms of teams developing as team objectives changed (Figure 39-3).

Multidisciplinary Teams

Coordination of care is essential if a patient is to benefit from multiple health care services provided by various health care professionals (Zwarenstein et al., 2009). The **multidisciplinary team**, like all interprofessional teams, is composed of individuals representing professional disciplines that serve the client. In the multidisciplinary team, each professional is responsible for identifying and carrying out one's own discipline-related evaluation and intervention. Multidisciplinary teams generally have access to each other's written record, as each typically contributes to chart notes, etc. If they meet as a group, which is often the case, they share information about their client's progress relative to the discipline-specific goals, and they may coordinate their efforts. For example, they may arrange intervention sessions to be on the same day. Multidisciplinary teams can also provide an opportunity for its members to

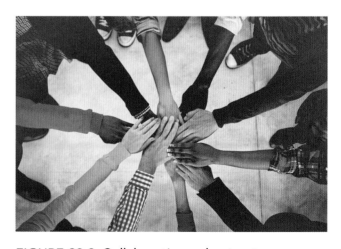

FIGURE 39-3 Collaboration = best outcomes.

learn from each other. The objective, however, is coordination and cooperation, not necessarily to share goals with a common outcome. Although the expectation is that knowledge of the expertise of other team members will promote cooperation and communication that ultimately benefits the client, each team member functions in a parallel fashion and maintains professional autonomy (Jessup, 2007).

The multidisciplinary team can be seen in various settings, from inpatient and community settings to global crisis intervention and management. Consider the intervention plan for an individual with vision loss secondary to diabetes. The internist oversees medical care. The ophthalmologist and optometrist monitor and manage diabetic retinopathy. The occupational therapist addresses the individual's functional ability and safety in light of vision loss and peripheral neuropathy (see AOTA, 2011, for the specific role and function of an occupational therapist in diabetes management). The nurse addresses wound care, blood glucose monitoring, and prevention of complications, and the nutritionist monitors and educates about diet. Although each of these professionals has a focused role, the client benefits because these professionals share their knowledge and progress with each other.

Interdisciplinary Teams

The **interdisciplinary team** is distinct from the multidisciplinary team. Although similarly composed of members representing and using knowledge and skills of their respective discipline, the team members identify goals and plan intervention collaboratively. They also discuss with each other how their intervention plans will be implemented. Although their skills may complement each other, team members become interdependent as they work toward improving health outcomes for their clients. It is common for interdisciplinary teams to meet as a group with the client, the client's family, etc. This type of team is further distinguished from the multidisciplinary team in that some interventions may be jointly carried out, and the client is often involved in the decision-making process (Cartmill et al., 2011; Jessup, 2007).

The benefits of interdisciplinary teams are many (Jessup, 2007; Zwarenstein et al., 2009). It is client-centered, giving the client a role in his or her care. Team members share their knowledge, which leads to respecting the roles and functions of each other. Because team members share a great deal with each other about how they implement intervention, a synergy develops in how different disciplines address common and complementary goals. Intervention plans for clients are developed holistically and cost-effectively. Job satisfaction is increased. Ultimately, client care and outcomes are enhanced.

There are several potential problems that can also emerge in the functioning of an interdisciplinary team. An overly assertive team member can dominate the meetings, thereby pushing an agenda that was not collaboratively agreed on. A silent or unassertive team member can easily be ignored, assuming his or her silence means compliance. A hierarchy may develop or a particular team member may assume he or she is the team's leader simply because of his or her profession. This can negatively affect decision making (Jessup, 2007) and promote feelings of being undervalued and disrespected (Baker et al., 2011). The important attributes of trust and mutual respect are keys in ensuring effective teamwork.

Interdisciplinary teams are seen in many settings. In fact, settings have designed specific models of interdisciplinary teams that are deemed effective (Deering et al., 2011; Medlock, McKee, Feinstein, Bell, & Tracy, 2011). Consider, as an example, a day hospital setting serving those with major mental illnesses. An interdisciplinary team may decide that for a particular client with schizophrenia, the goal is to have him be able to live in a group home, participate in chores, and be able to attend a sheltered workshop that prepares packages for shipment. Team members also are aware that he can become noncompliant with medication, has sensory processing issues, has difficulty with following instructions and making decisions, and complains about not seeing his brother often enough. In this team, different professionals address the same objectives and goals collaboratively but through their own profession's lens. For example, the psychiatrist and nurse monitor his medication, whereas the occupational therapist is able to observe if any medication side effects are interfering with function. The occupational therapist is addressing sensory and cognitive impairment while having the recreational therapist monitor changes in leisure function. The social worker is addressing family issues, with the occupational therapist and the nurse attending to activities of daily living (ADL) issues raised by the brother.

Transdisciplinary Teams

The **transdisciplinary team** is one that functions without discipline-centered boundaries. Members in these types of teams appear to have blurred roles because many of their role-related functions become interchangeable. As distinguished from interdisciplinary teams, the expertise related to discipline-specific tasks is shared and results in the taking on of each other's responsibilities (Cartmill et al., 2011). This type of team is most efficient and may be cost-effective because in some examples, fewer professionals interact with a specific client (King, Tucker, Desserud, & Shillington, 2009).

It has been suggested that there are three key elements for successful and responsible transdisciplinary teamwork. The first is overall assessment conducted by one professional but observed by all. This type of arena assessment allows each to provide information based on their unique base of knowledge and skill. Next is ongoing interaction between team members so that each can continuously contribute their knowledge to the plan of care. Perhaps most critical is the third element, which is role release. This allows interprofessional intervention to be carried out by one individual. Ideally and responsibly, this should be done under the direction of and continuous consultation from those responsible for what is being implemented (King et al., 2009).

The transdisciplinary team can be highly effective if used with the right population and in the right manner. A noncompetitive and nonhierarchical environment is important in order to allow for effective intervention. These teams are especially helpful in situations where interprofessional intervention is required, yet it is in the best interest of the client to have only one individual interact. A very good example of effective transdisciplinary teamwork can be seen in a report of a home-visiting program for infants in which the family benefits from the expertise of many professionals but interacts with only one (King et al., 2009). As described by these authors, a home-visiting program for infants with developmental disabilities is established, with the objectives of promoting child development along a series of domains. Rather than overwhelm the caregiver with various visiting professionals, one individual is assigned to each family. Team members learn theories and techniques from each other in order to provide service that spans disciplinary boundaries. The team is responsible for continually appraising and providing input to the professional who visits.

The transdisciplinary team approach is also useful in settings that can benefit from a system-wide approach, in settings with limited resources that do not have access to different professionals, in remote settings where access is limited, or following a crisis or natural disaster. The use of technology can support the functioning of transdisciplinary teams, ensuring a high level of competency.

Paramount for the success of transdisciplinary teams are the same elements identified for interdisciplinary teams: trust, communication, and respect. A major concern of transdisciplinary teamwork can arise when the "agent" for the team is not as skilled or knowledgeable as the team members being represented, resulting in diminished effectiveness of the intervention. Furthermore, if an individual professional providing intervention ceases to obtain ongoing input from fellow team members, the client is at risk for adverse events.

Transdisciplinary approaches have additional ethical and legal concerns. If, on a transdisciplinary team, members assume responsibilities of other professionals, regulatory violations and scope of practice concerns emerge. A team member should never perform the actions of which they are not educated for and approved for under their state regulations. This is not the case when there is overlap in assessment and intervention modalities or techniques. Each team member has a responsibility to provide service within his or her scope of practice and request the provision of direct service from another team member when it is necessary to provide service outside of one's scope of practice.

Research Teams

Although much of this section has focused on interprofessional teams in practice settings, there are two important arenas in which interprofessional teams are critical for their success. The first that warrants mention is the research team.

In medically related research, discipline-specific investigators focusing primarily on basic science have carried out investigations. In some circumstances, this is not only appropriate but also necessary. However, having one discipline central to a study can result in outcomes that isolate professions, perpetuate knowledge gaps, and limit information advancement (Bindler, Richardson, Daratha, & Wordell, 2012). The advantages of interprofessional research include being able to better address the complex issues involved in research, allow for innovative, including more technologically based, approaches (Bindler et al., 2012), and translate results into effective interventions that are functionally and clinically relevant. Like patient-oriented teams, multidisciplinary, interdisciplinary, and transdisciplinary research teams function in distinct ways, with research questions reflecting the nature of the team (Fawcett, 2013). The federal government has placed increased emphasis on interprofessional collaborative research and has set up structures to support the translation and application of basic research to practice-related outcomes (Bindler et al., 2012), although barriers continue to exist that impede translating interprofessional research into clinical practice (Fletcher, Whiting, Boaz, & Reeves, 2017).

⚕ PRACTICE DILEMMA

You are an occupational therapist with 2 years of experience. You have been educated and trained in the use of physical agent modalities and have used these in your practice as part of preparatory procedures to enhance occupational performance. You have recently moved to another state that restricts your use of physical agent modalities. Your new place of employment uses transdisciplinary teams. You are the "lead" on your team with a particular client for whom the team determined the use of deep thermal modalities. It is expected by the team that you provide this service because they are aware of your abilities in this area.

Question

1. As a new employee skilled in the use of such modalities, what do you do?

Health Care Policy Teams

Another area that warrants mention is health care policy development. Just as research and intervention addresses complex needs, health care policy deals with issues that are also multifaceted. From setting health care agendas to outlining their implementation in order to improve health service delivery, policymakers need to collaborate on teams to be effective. To ensure this, an interprofessional approach to policy development, just as with clinical care and with research, allows for access to varied sources of information and promotes perspectives that represents different areas of expertise. It has also been suggested that interprofessional team-based learning opportunities facilitate collaboration and enhances the development of effective health care policy (Rider, Brashers, & Costanza, 2008).

Scholarship: Presentations and Publications

Nearly two decades ago, Margo B. Holm (2000), in her Eleanor Clarke Slagle Lecture, called for occupational therapists to acquire evidence to support OT services and to practice based on that evidence (see Table 39-3 for steps to become an evidence-based practitioner). Evidence-based practice must undergird our clinical decisions and as such is embedded in our Vision 2025 (AOTA, 2017b) and in our practice standards (AOTA, 2015a). Using evidence in practice, however, is challenging for practitioners because of time constraints along with the process used when keeping up to date with the literature (Marr, 2017). Despite this, it is critical for professionals to use as well as generate outcome

---

TABLE 39-3   Steps for Being an Evidence-Based Practitioner

Six Steps for Evidence-Based Practice
1. Identify the clinical question.
2. Search for evidence.
3. Evaluate the evidence for validity and utility.
4. Incorporate your assessment of the evidence with your clinical experience and expertise and from a client-centered perspective.
5. After implementing a change based on the evidence, think about its effectiveness and ease of putting into practice.
6. Share what you have learned.

Source: Lin, S. H., Murphy, S. L., & Robinson, J. (2010). Facilitating evidence-based practice: Process, strategies, and resources. *American Journal of Occupational Therapy, 64,* 164–171. doi:10.5014/ajot.64.1.164

---

studies that have met standards of scientific rigor in order to justify OT interventions.

Two of the many reasons to be an evidence-based practitioner are competency and currency. As scientific knowledge continues to amass in an ever-changing health care environment, practitioners and educators alike need to embrace and be proficient in interventions proven to be efficacious and cost-effective. Learning from those with a proven scholarly record, such as individuals whose work has appeared in peer-reviewed journals or who are presenting research at conferences or workshops under organizations and/or companies that have met requirements for continuing education, such as AOTA's Approved Provider of Continuing Education, is important. The information learned must be reliable, accurate, and evidence-based. It is also incumbent on researchers to address questions pertinent to the practice of OT so that the services provided can be both efficacious and cost-effective. Thus, it is the responsibility of all OT practitioners to participate in learning opportunities based on the most recent knowledge that can be applied to practice.

Presenting and publishing is part of the professional role and provides another venue for sharing information (Table 39-4). When one has an opportunity to present or to publish, it is similarly important to consider the context in which one chooses to present and publish. Again, presenting under the auspices of an approved provider of continuing education enhances credibility.

Presentations take many forms. Within clinical settings, one presents in a team meeting, at a grand rounds, and at in-service training. Some of these settings may appear informal, but the presenter must remember that his or her style of presenting will reflect his or her integrity and professionalism. In conference type settings, one might present a poster or platform presentation in which key points along with graphics are printed on a poster that is usually mounted to a bulletin board. A poster session, which has varying lengths, allows the presenter to discuss points of interest to those who review the poster. A paper presentation, which can be anywhere from 20 minutes to 2 hours, is a formal presentation to an audience and typically includes audiovisual technology. Workshop presentations, which are somewhat modeled after a classroom setting, also include audiovisual technology and can be in a half-day format or as long as a 5-day format. Panel presentations consist of several experts on a single topic in which brief presentations are made to facilitate discussion with the audience. Although each of these types of presentations allow for the dissemination of information, it is equally important to be sure that one's manner of presenting is professional. There are many guidelines available electronically and in libraries that one can refer to on *how* to present (e.g., Eggleston, n.d.), guidelines that remind one to be articulate, focus on the question at hand,

TABLE 39-4   A Sample of Venues for Disseminating Knowledge

Presentations		Publications	
Professional Venues	Consumer Venues	Peer-Reviewed	Non–Peer-Reviewed
Team meeting	Community event	Practice-oriented periodicals [a]	Trade magazines
In-service presentation	Consumer organization	Journals	Practice-oriented periodicals [a]
Grand rounds		Book chapters [a]	Newsletters
Poster session		Websites [a]	News periodicals
Panel discussion			Book chapters [a]
Platform sessions			Self-published books
Workshops			Blogs
Courses			Websites [a]

[a] These venues may or may not be peer-reviewed.

and engage the audience, no matter how big or how small. These guidelines also include attention to eye contact; avoiding the use of filler words such as "um," "you know," and "like"; and maintenance of proper posture.

Similarly, there are various types of publication venues, from traditional, subscription-based journals to digital publications which might not be subscription-based. Each venue targets different audiences, has varying levels of review and rigor, along with perceived value. A publication's value is typically based on the review process used by a journal, along with a journal's quality, reputation, and impact factor. This applies to traditional and digital publications. Digital publications, which are becoming more prevalent, may be through open access (OA) publishing venues, such as an institutional OA repository where an author may upload ones work or work in progress, without any review; and OA journals which may or may not be peer-reviewed and often carry a fee charged to the author (Rowley, Johnson, Sbaffi, Frass, & Devine, 2017).

Understanding which media an author publishes in is important to both the writer and to the reader, as it may inform the content's trustworthiness. The **peer review** process, valued in the scholarly literature, simply refers to a procedure in which a manuscript, once submitted for publication, is reviewed by experts in the field who provide feedback and contribute to the decision of whether or not the manuscript meets the criteria for publication. Peer review provides a layer of critical evaluation to the publishing process, is often a more challenging route of publication for the writer, but gives the reader a level of trust in the information (Nicholas et al., 2015). Peer-reviewed articles are typically in scientific journals (Farrell, Magida Farrell, & Farrell, 2017) and may or may not be reviewed anonymously (Nobarany & Booth, 2017).

Non-peer review refers to manuscripts that are submitted or invited to be published in books, periodicals, or trade magazines and might be reviewed by an editor rather than go through a longer, more critical process (Jacobs, 2009). Non–peer-reviewed articles are in news or practice-oriented periodicals and trade publications. Non–peer

review also includes self-publication, such as blogs and personal Websites as well as self-published books. As indicated earlier, publishing in peer-reviewed or non–peer-reviewed media carries different perceived value as a result of the review process. Finally, papers in OA journals, which speed up the time between a paper's acceptance to its publication, may or may not be peer-reviewed.

Professionalism and Social Media: Opportunities and Pitfalls

There is a great deal of dependency on and use of social media. Whether used as a way to network professionally or personally, **social media** is becoming a tool that enables one to communicate quickly and to a very wide audience. As more and more consumers use Internet sites, including social media sites, to gain and share information about health care (Massey, 2016), a responsibility exists to ensure that this information is factual and evidence-based.

⚖ ETHICAL DILEMMA

You decided to attend a continuing education workshop on treating cognitive deficits because the location and timing of this was convenient. Although the program was not being offered by an approved provider of continuing education, you knew that you could tally the hours spent and record these as professional development units. At the workshop, you received copies of the slideshow but no reference list. During the presentation, you realized that you had seen some of these slides at another workshop taught by a reputable scholar in the field. There was no mention of this scholar's name during the presentation. In addition, many of the examples given were anecdotal, with little or no evidence to support it. Finally, the only places you could find references to some of the facts that were given were in an online discussion board and in a therapist's blog.

Questions

1. Have any ethics been violated, and if so, which one(s)?
2. What degree of scholarship was demonstrated by the presenter?
3. What responsibility do you have to the other attendees or potential attendees?
4. How might you handle your concerns without violating your ethical principles?

Reasons for using such sites include obtaining information and seeking social connectedness. The use of social media is also on the rise for hospitals and professional practices, which are turning to this technology in order to provide information related to medical updates and health information to their patients and the general public (Ficarra, 2011). Consumers actively use social media sites as a way to assess the quality of their health care provider (Rozenblum & Bates, 2013).

Relationships and communication are often nurtured through social networks (Bahk, Sheil, Rohm, & Lin, 2010), yet behavior on these networks has come under scrutiny. Indeed, attention is being paid to how social media and other forms of electronic communication are and have been used in a variety of academic and work contexts (Chretien, Greysen, Chretien, & Kind, 2009; Gerlich, Browning, & Westermann, 2010). The prevailing concern revolves around the individual's right to privacy and one's commitment to his or her professional environment.

Professionalism in the use of social media is important. Professionalism in part stems from a contract between one's discipline and society, and therefore, how one behaves is a reflection of his or her professionalism. Even accessing social media sites while at work (Piscotty, Martindell, & Karim, 2016) can be unprofessional. Because social media has such a widespread audience and that behavior on social media sites can reflect negatively on one's place of work and on one's profession, policies and guidelines are being developed (DeCamp, 2012; Greysen, Kind, & Chretien, 2010; Spector & Kappel, 2012).

Many have claimed that what one does on one's own time is an issue of individual rights and of privacy. Yet, by virtue of being on an Internet site, posted information and photos can be publically viewed (Langenfeld et al., 2014) and, if of a client, can potentially violate patient privacy (Hader & Brown, 2010). The Internet has not only allowed for efficient communication but has also widened the net with whom one communicates. As a result, professionals have an obligation to understand that their postings on any site can be viewed by unlimited numbers of individuals without restriction. Once information is posted, one can no longer control its intended audience no matter what privacy settings are used.

There continues to be evidence of the misuse of social media sites by professionals, including health care students and professionals. This includes posting disrespectful comments about their colleagues, clients, and place of work; photos and videos of work-related activities and people; and photos and videos of themselves or their friends engaged in compromising activities. Many of these types of postings have resulted in a wide range of disciplinary actions (Chretien et al., 2009; Greysen et al., 2010; Lagu, Kaufman, Asch, & Armstrong, 2008; Langenfeld et al., 2014; Thompson et al., 2008) with a call for guidelines of professionalism when on the Internet (DeCamp, 2012; Spector & Kappel, 2012). In addition to potential violations of Health Insurance Portability and Accountability Act (HIPAA) and Family and Educational Rights and Privacy Act (FERPA), legislative and ethical concerns have been raised. "Friending" patients and clients on Facebook, for example, may impact the therapeutic relationship (Guseh, Brendel, & Brendel, 2009). As stated earlier, inappropriate behaviors, even if subjectively inappropriate, can negatively impact the professional expectations held by the public.

Social media, however, can be an important tool in promoting one's profession. Just as it can be used to enhance learning opportunities at the college level (Gerlich et al., 2010), social media has and can be used to share relevant information with peers and to provide learning opportunities about health and wellness to the public (Greysen et al., 2010; McNab, 2009). Possible uses of social media include using blogs to teach persons with multiple sclerosis about energy conservation or fall prevention strategies to the elderly and providing tips on identifying cognitive impairment in daily activities or ways to identify the beginning signs of driving impairment. Using a Facebook site to promote a professional practice, share videos on sites such as YouTube that demonstrate an assessment or intervention technique, tweet about opportunities for community participation, and connecting with professionals to promote evidence-based research collaboration on a specific topic are also possible uses of social media.

When producing content electronically, it is helpful to remember the "do's and don't's." Table 39-5 provides a checklist for proper online content and conduct.

Summary

The professional role carries with it a great deal of responsibility. Professionals, whose responsibilities are to one's clients, to one's profession, and to society, are ambassadors

TABLE 39-5 Social Media and E-mail Checklist for the Professional

YES	NO	For social media sites, such as Facebook, LinkedIn, and Twitter as well as personal Websites and blogs; for e-mails and texts.
❏	❏	Did you target the correct audience for your posts?
❏	❏	Is the information you posted factual and backed up by evidence?
❏	❏	Are you in compliance with HIPAA and/or FERPA regulations?
❏	❏	Are you in compliance with your workplace's policies?
❏	❏	Are your remarks (and/or status updates) respectful (i.e., Did you avoid making comments that someone might find offensive or hurtful?)?
❏	❏	Did you use proper spelling, grammar, and punctuation in your professional postings? Did you avoid using "text" abbreviations, such as "u" or "r," on sites not limited in character number?
❏	❏	Did you avoid posting photographs or videos of yourself or others that can be considered improper, even if these photographs were taken and posted in non–work-related venues (i.e., Would you want your family, your professors, your boss, or your clients to see these)?
❏	❏	If you posted a photo or video, does it comply with HIPAA, FERPA, and/or additional workplace policies?
❏	❏	Did you send a communication to a colleague that is grammatically and structurally correct?
❏	❏	Did you remember to sign your name on all e-mails so that the recipient can identify you?
❏	❏	Did you remember that whatever you post will be accessible forever, in spite of privacy assurances from Websites?
❏	❏	Did you avoid overuse of punctuation marks, all capital letters, and boldface in your e-mail? These may cause the reader to misinterpret your intent or make it difficult to read.
❏	❏	Does your e-mail reflect the appropriate level of formality? For example, did you avoid using the greeting "Hey" in a message to a colleague?

HIPAA, Health Insurance Portability and Accountability Act; FERPA, Family Educational Rights and Privacy Act.

for their field. Whether or not one is at work, with friends, or in the virtual world, how one is perceived as a person may be a reflection of who one is as a professional.

The world of OT is an exciting one. Our science is growing, our practice areas are expanding, and our presence is ubiquitous. As an OT professional, you have an opportunity to not only participate in this wonderful profession but also to contribute to its development.

⚖ ETHICAL DILEMMA

You are working in a mental health setting. A member of your interdisciplinary team, who often takes client groups to events in your community, has "friended" you on Facebook. You also socialize with this colleague after work hours.

You check your Facebook newsfeed and see that your coworker/friend has posted a photograph of the backs of a few of the clients under the marquee of a show they are about to see. The status update with this photo is "fun at work." You also see a photo posted of her at a bar, holding up two beer bottles. The status update on this photo is "just getting started."

Questions

1. What action do you take after seeing these posts?
2. Do both posts warrant a response, as one was work-related and one was not?
3. What responsibility, if any, do you have to your employer?

REFERENCES

Accreditation Council for Occupational Therapy Education. (2010). *Accreditation Council for Occupational Therapy Education (ACOTE) standards and interpretive guidelines.* Bethesda, MD: American Occupational Therapy Association.

American Occupational Therapy Association. (2002). *Fieldwork performance evaluation for the occupational therapy student.* Bethesda, MD: Author.

American Occupational Therapy Association. (2011). *Occupational therapy's role in diabetes self-management.* Retrieved from http://www.aota .org/Practitioners/PracticeAreas/Aging/Tools/Diabetes.aspx?FT=.pdf

American Occupational Therapy Association. (2014). Occupational therapy practice framework: Domain and process, 3rd edition. *American Journal of Occupational Therapy, 68,* S1–S48. doi:10.5014 /ajot.2014.682006

American Occupational Therapy Association. (2015a). Occupational Therapy Code of Ethics (2015). *American Journal of Occupational Therapy, 69,* 6913410030p1–6913410030p8. doi:10.5014/ajot .2015.696S03

American Occupational Therapy Association. (2015b). Standards of practice for occupational therapy. *American Journal of Occupational Therapy, 69,* 6913410057p1–6913410057p6. doi:10.5014/ajot .2015.696S06

American Occupational Therapy Association. (2017a). *Level I fieldwork competency evaluation for OT and OTA students.* Retrieved from https://www.aota.org/~/media/Corporate/Files /EducationCareers/Educators/Fieldwork/LevelI/Level-I-Fieldwork -Competency-Evaluation-for-ot-and-ota-students.pdf

American Occupational Therapy Association. (2017b). Vision 2025. *American Journal of Occupational Therapy, 71,* 7103420010p1. doi:10.5014/ajot.2017.713002

Anderson, E., Smith, R., & Hammick, M. (2016). Evaluating an interprofessional education curriculum: A theory-informed approach. *Medical Teacher, 39,* 385–394.

Anselmo-Witzel, S., Orshan, S. A., Heitner, K. L., & Bachand, J. (2017). Are generation Y nurses satisfied on the job? Understanding their lived experiences. *The Journal of Nursing Administration, 47,* 232–237.

Aurora, V., Wayne, D., Anderson, R., Didwania, A., & Humphrey, H. (2008). Participation in and perceptions of unprofessional behaviors among incoming internal medicine interns. *JAMA, 300,* 1132–1134.

Bahk, C. M., Sheil, A., Rohm, C. E., & Lin, F. (2010). Digital media dependency, relational orientation and social networking among college students. *Communications of the IIMA, 10,* 69–78.

Baker, L., Egan-Lee, E., Martimianakis, M. A., & Reeves, S. (2011). Relationships of power: Implications for interprofessional education. *Journal of Interprofessional Care, 25,* 98–104.

Berkup, S. (2014). Working with generations X and Y in generation Z period: Management of different generations in business life. *Mediterranean Journal of Social Sciences, 5*(19), 218. Retrieved from http://www.mcser.org/journal/index.php/mjss/article/view/4247/4153

Berman, J. R., Aizer, J., Bass, A. R., Blanco, I., Davidson, A., Dwyer, E., . . . Pillinger, M. H. (2016). Fellow use of medical jargon correlates inversely with patient and observer perceptions of professionalism: Results of a rheumatology OSCE (ROSCE) using challenging patient scenarios. *Clinical Rheumatology, 35,* 2093–2099. doi:10.1007/s10067-015-3113-9

Bindler, B., Richardson, K., Daratha, D., & Wordell, D. (2012). Interdisciplinary health science research collaboration: Strengths, challenges, and case example. *Applied Nursing Research, 25,* 95–100.

Boet, S., Bould, M. D., Layat Burn, C., & Reeves, S. (2014). Twelve tips for a successful interprofessional team-based high-fidelity simulation education session. *Medical Teacher, 36,* 853–857. doi:10.3109/0142159X.2014.923558

Brennan, C. W., Olds, D. M., Dolansky, M., Estrada, C. A., & Patrician, P. A. (2014). Learning by doing: Observing an interprofessional process as an interprofessional team. *Journal of Interprofessional Care, 28,* 249–251. doi:10.3109/13561820.2013.839750

Brock, D., Abu-Rish, E., Chiu, C., Hammer, D., Wilson, S., Vorvick, L., . . . Zierler, B. (2013). Interprofessional education in team communication: Working together to improve patient safety. *BMJ Quality & Safety, 22,* 414–423.

Campbell, S. M., Twenge, J. M., & Campbell, W. K. (2017). Fuzzy but useful constructs: Making sense of the differences between generations. *Work, Aging and Retirement, 3,* 130–139.

Cartmill, C., Soklaridis, S., & Cassidy, J. D. (2011). Transdisciplinary teamwork: The experience of clinicians at a functional restoration program. *Journal of Occupational Rehabilitation, 21,* 1–8.

Chretien, K. C., Greysen, S. R., Chretien, J., & Kind, T. (2009). Online posting of unprofessional content by medical students. *JAMA, 302,* 1309–1315.

Cruess, R., & Cruess, S. (2009). Cognitive base of professionalism. In R. Cruess, S. Cruess, & Y. Steinert (Eds.), *Teaching medical professionalism* (pp. 7–30). New York, NY: Cambridge University Press.

Cruess, R., Cruess, S., & Steinert, Y. (2009). Core attributes of professionalism. In R. Cruess, S. Cruess, & Y. Steinert (Eds.), *Teaching medical professionalism* (pp. 285–286). New York, NY: Cambridge University Press.

DeCamp, M. (2012). Social media and medical professionalism: Toward an expanded program. *Archives of Internal Medicine, 172*(18), 1418–1419.

Deering, S. J., Johnston, L. C., & Colacchio, K. (2011). Multidisciplinary teamwork and communication training. *Seminars in Perinatology, 35,* 89–96.

Dimock, M. (2018). *Defining generations: Where millennials end and post-millennials begin.* Retrieved from http://www.pewresearch.org/fact-tank/2018/03/01/defining-generations-where-millennials-end-and-post-millennials-begin

Eggleston, S. (n.d.). *Key steps to an effective presentation.* Retrieved from http://www.theegglestongroup.com/writing/keystep1.php

Farrell, P. R., Magida Farrell, L., & Farrell, M. K. (2017). Ancient texts to PubMed: A brief history of the peer-review process. *Journal of Perinatology, 37,* 13–15. doi:10.1038/jp.2016.209

Fawcett, J. (2013). Thoughts about multidisciplinary, interdisciplinary, and transdisciplinary research. *Nursing Science Quarterly, 26,* 376–379.

Ficarra, B. (2011). *Social media: Medical social networking—part 2.* Retrieved from http://healthin30.com/2011/03/social-media-medical-social-networking-part-2/

Fletcher, S., Whiting, C., Boaz, A., & Reeves, S. (2017). Exploring factors related to the translation of collaborative research learning experiences into clinical practice: Opportunities and tensions, *Journal of Interprofessional Care, 31,* 543–545. doi:10.1080/13561820.2017.1303464

Fogg, P. (2008, July 18). When generations collide. *The Chronicle of Higher Education, 54*(45), p. B18.

Gerlich, R. N., Browning, L., & Westermann, L. (2010). The social media affinity scale: Implications for education. *Contemporary Issues in Education Research, 3,* 35–41.

Glennon, T., & Van Oss, T. (2010). Identifying and promoting professional behavior: Best practices for establishing, maintaining, and improving professional behavior by occupational therapy practitioners. *Occupational Therapy Practice, 15,* 13–16.

Greysen, S. R., Kind, T., & Chretien, K. C. (2010). Online professionalism and the mirror of social media. *Journal of General Internal Medicine, 25,* 1227–1229.

Guseh, J. S., II., Brendel, R., & Brendel, D. H. (2009). Medical professionalism in the age of online social networking. *Journal of Medical Ethics, 35,* 584–586.

Hader, A. L., & Brown, E. D. (2010). Patient privacy and social media. *AANA Journal, 78,* 270–274.

Hills, C., Ryan, S., Smith, D. R., Warren-Forward, H., Levett-Jones, T., & Lapkin, S. (2016). Occupational therapy students' technological skills: Are 'generation Y' ready for 21st century practice? *Australian Occupational Therapy Journal, 63,* 391–398. doi:10.1111/1440-1630.12308

Holm, M. B. (2000). The 2000 Eleanor Clarke Slagle lecture. Our mandate for the new millennium: Evidence-based practice. *American Journal of Occupational Therapy, 54,* 575–585.

Hordichuk, C. J., Robinson, A. J., & Sullivan, T. M. (2015). Conceptualising professionalism in occupational therapy through a western lens. *Australian Occupational Therapy Journal, 62,* 150–159. doi:10.1111/1440-1630.12204

House, J. B., Sun, J. K., Sullivan, A., & Ross, P. (2016). Introduction to interprofessional education using health professionals. *Medical Education, 50,* 579–580.

Interprofessional Education Collaborative. (2016). *Core competencies for interprofessional collaborative practice: 2016 Update.* Washington, DC: Author.

Jacobs, K. (2009). Professional presentations and publications. In E. B. Crepeau, E. S. Cohn, & B. A. Schell (Eds.), *Willard & Spackman's occupational therapy* (11th ed., pp. 411–417). Philadelphia, PA: Lippincott Williams & Wilkins.

Jessup, R. L. (2007). Interdisciplinary versus multidisciplinary care teams: Do we understand the difference? *Australian Health Review, 31,* 330–331. Retrieved from http://ezproxy.cul.columbia.edu/login?url=https://search.proquest.com/docview/231778493?accountid=10226

Johnston, S. (2006). See one, do one, teach one: Developing professionalism across the generations. *Clinical Orthopaedics and Related Research, 449,* 186–192.

Jones, A., & Jones, D. (2011). Improving teamwork, trust and safety: An ethnographic study of an interprofessional initiative. *Journal of Interprofessional Care, 25,* 175–181.

Kalisch, B. J., Lee, H., & Rochman, M. (2010). Nursing staff teamwork and job satisfaction. *Journal of Nursing Management, 18,* 938–947.

Kick, A. L., Contacos-Sawyer, J., & Thomas, B. (2015). How generation Z's reliance on digital communication can affect future workplace relationships. *Competition Forum, 13*(2), 214–222. Retrieved from http://ezproxy.cul.columbia.edu/login?url=https://search.proquest.com/docview/1755486105?accountid=10226

King, G., Tucker, M., Desserud, S., & Shillington, M. (2009). The application of a transdisciplinary model for early intervention services. *Infants & Young Children, 22,* 211–223.

Lagu, T., Kaufman, E. J., Asch, D. A., & Armstrong, K. (2008). Content of weblogs written by health professionals. *Journal of General Internal Medicine, 23,* 1642–1646.

Lake, P. (2009, April 17). Student discipline: The case against legalistic approaches. *The Chronicle of Higher Education, 55*(32), pp. A31, A32.

Langenfeld, S. J., Cook, G., Sudbeck, C., Luers, T., & Schenarts, P. J. (2014). An assessment of unprofessional behavior among surgical residents on Facebook: A warning of the dangers of social media. *Journal of Surgical Education, 71,* 028–032.

Lin, S. H., Murphy, S. L., & Robinson, J. (2010). Facilitating evidence-based practice: Process, strategies, and resources. *American Journal of Occupational Therapy, 64,* 164–171. doi:10.5014/ajot.64.1.164

Lindheim, S. R., Nouri, P., Rabah, K. A., & Yaklic, J. L. (2016). Medical professionalism and enculturation of the millennial physician: Meeting of the minds. *Fertility and Sterility, 106,* 1615–1616.

Lipscomb, V. (2010). Intergenerational issues in nursing: Learning from each generation. *Clinical Journal of Oncology Nursing, 14,* 267–269. doi:10.1188/10.CJON.267-269

Lyons, S., & Kuron, L. (2014). Generational differences in the workplace: A review of the evidence and directions for future research. *Journal of Organizational Behavior, 35,* S139–S157.

Marr, D. (2017). Fostering full implementation of evidence-based practice. *American Journal of Occupational Therapy, 71,* 7101100050p1–7101100050p5. doi:10.5014/ajot.2017.019661

Massey, P. M. (2016). Where do U.S. adults who do not use the internet get health information? Examining digital health information disparities from 2008 to 2013. *Journal of Health Communication, 21,* 118–124.

McNab, C. (2009). What social media offers to health professionals and citizens. *Bulletin of the World Health Organization, 87,* 566.

Medlock, A., McKee, E., Feinstein, J., Bell, S. H., & Tracy, C. S. (2011). Applying an innovative model of interprofessional team practice: The view from occupational therapy. *Occupational Therapy Now, 13,* 7–9.

Mercier, H., & Sperber, D. (2011). Why do humans reason? Arguments for an argumentative theory. *The Behavioral and Brain Sciences, 34,* 57–111. doi:10.1017/S0140525X10000968

Mohr, N., Moreno-Walton, L., Mills, A. M., Brunett, P. H., & Promes, S. B. (2011). Generational influences in academic emergency medicine: Teaching and learning, mentoring, and technology (Part I). *Academic Emergency Medicine, 18,* 190–199.

Monrouxe, L., Rees, C. E., & Hu, W. (2011). Differences in medical students' explicit discourses of professionalism: acting, representing, becoming. *Medical Education, 45,* 585–602.

Ndoro, S. (2014). Effective multidisciplinary working: The key to high-quality care. *British Journal of Nursing, 23,* 724–727. doi:10.12968/bjon.2014.23.13.724

Nicholas, D., Watkinson, A., Jamali, H. R., Herman, E., Tenopir, C., Volentine, R., . . . Levine, K. (2015). Peer review: Still king in the digital age. *Learned Publishing, 28,* 15–21. doi:10.1087/20150104

Nobarany, S., & Booth, K. S. (2017). Understanding and supporting anonymity policies in peer review. *Journal of the Association for Information Science and Technology, 68*(4), 957–971.

Ozkan, M., & Solmaz, B. (2015). The changing face of the employees—generation Z and their perceptions of work (a study applied to university students). *Procedia Economics and Finance, 26,* 476–483.

Piscotty, R., Martindell, E., & Karim, M. (2016). Nurses' self-reported social media and mobile device use in the work setting. *Online Journal of Nursing Informatics (OJNI), 20*(1). Retrieved from http://www.himss.org/ojni

Poston, R., Haney, T., Kott, K., & Rutledge, C. (2017). Interprofessional team performance, optimized. *Nursing Management, 48,* 36–43. doi:10.1097/01.NUMA.0000520722.55679.7c

Rider, E. A., Brashers, V. L., & Costanza, M. E. (2008). Using interprofessional team-based learning to develop health care policy. *Medical Education, 42,* 519–520.

Rozenblum, R., & Bates, D. W. (2013). Patient-centred healthcare, social media and the internet: The perfect storm? *BMJ Quality & Safety, 22,* 183–186.

Rowley, J., Johnson, F., Sbaffi, L., Frass, W., & Devine, E. (2017). Academics' behaviors and attitudes towards open access publishing in scholarly journals. *Journal of the Association for Information Science and Technology, 68,* 1201–1211. doi:10.1002/asi.23710

Sims, S., Hewitt, G., & Harris, R. (2015). Evidence of collaboration, pooling of resources, learning and role blurring in interprofessional healthcare teams: A realist synthesis. *Journal of Interprofessional Care, 29,* 20–25.

Sinclair, L. B., Lingard, L. A., & Mohabeer, R. N. (2009). What's so great about rehabilitation teams? An ethnographic study of interprofessional collaboration in a rehabilitation unit. *Archives of Physical Medicine and Rehabilitation, 90,* 1196–1201.

Slagle, E. C., & Robeson, H. A. (1933). *Syllabus for training of nurses in occupational therapy* (2nd ed.). Utica, NY: State Hospitals Press.

Spector, N., & Kappel, D. M. (2012). Guidelines for using electronic and social media: The regulatory perspective. *Online Journal of Issues in Nursing, 17*(3), 1–11. doi:10.3912/OJIN

Thistlethwaite, J. (2012). Interprofessional education: A review of context, learning and the research agenda. *Medical Education, 46,* 58–70.

Thompson, L. A., Dawson, K., Ferdig, R., Black, E. W., Boyer, J., Coutts, J., & Black, N. P. (2008). The intersection of online social networking with medical professionalism. *Journal of General Internal Medicine, 23,* 954–957.

Tulgan, B. (2009). *Not everyone gets a trophy.* San Francisco, CA: Jossey-Bass.

Twenge, J. M. (2006). *Generation me: Why today's young Americans are more confident, assertive, entitled—and more miserable than ever before.* New York, NY: Free Press.

Twenge, J. M. (2017, April 12). Here comes the iGen—and businesses can rejoice. *Psychology Today Online.* Retrieved from https://www.psychologytoday.com/blog/our-changing-culture/201704/here-comes-the-igen-and-businesses-can-rejoice

Ventriglio, A., & Bhugra, D. (2016). Age of entitlement and the young: Implications for social psychiatry. *The International Journal of Social Psychiatry, 62,* 107–109.

Wang, J., He, B., Miao, X., Huang, X., Lu, Y., & Chen, J. (2017). The reliability and validity of a new professionalism assessment scale for young health care workers. *Medicine, 96,* e7058.

Wiedmer, T. (2015). Generations do differ: Best practices in leading traditionalists, boomers, and generations X, Y, and Z. *Delta Kappa Gamma Bulletin, 82,* 51–58.

Wynia, M. K., Papadakis, M. A., Sullivan, W. M., & Hafferty, F. W. (2014). More than a list of values and desired behaviors: A foundational understanding of medical professionalism. *Academic Medicine, 89,* 712–714.

Youngstrom, M. (2002). The occupational therapy practice framework: The evolution of our professional language. *American Journal of Occupational Therapy, 56,* 607–608.

Yuen, H. K., Azuero, A., Lackey, K. W., Brown, N. S., & Shrestha, S. (2016). Construct validity test of evaluation tool for professional behaviors of entry-level occupational therapy students in the United States. *Journal of Educational Evaluation for Health Professions, 13,* 22.

Zemke, R., Raines, C., & Filipczak, B. (2013). *Generations at work: Managing the clash boomers, gen Xers, and gen Yers in the workplace* (2nd ed.). New York, NY: AMACOM.

Ziring, D., Danoff, D., Grosseman, S., Langer, D., Esposito, A., Jan, M. K., . . . Novack, D. (2015). How do medical schools identify and remediate professionalism lapses in medical students? A study of U.S. and Canadian medical schools. *Academic Medicine, 90,* 913–920.

Zwarenstein, M., Goldman, J., & Reeves, S. (2009). Interprofessional collaboration: Effects of practice-based interventions on professional practice and healthcare outcomes. *Cochrane Database of Systematic Reviews,* CD000072. doi:10.1002/14651858.CD000072 .pub2

the**Point**® *For additional resources on the subjects discussed in this chapter, visit* **http://thePoint.lww.com /Willard-Spackman13e.**

Documentation in Practice

Karen M. Sames

"I thought primarily of occupation therapy, of getting the patient to do things, and getting things going which did not work but which could work with proper straightening out."

—ADOLF MEYER, 1893

LEARNING OBJECTIVES

After reading this chapter, you will be able to:

1. Identify the primary reasons for documentation of occupational therapy services.
2. Describe the types of clinical, educational, and administrative documentation used in occupational therapy practice.
3. Compare and contrast the key features of occupational therapy documentation in clinical and educational settings.
4. Identify the components of well-written goals.
5. Write a SOAP note.
6. Discuss ethical issues in documentation.

Introduction

Occupational therapy (OT) practitioners communicate with many different types of people on a daily basis. They provide instructions for home programs to clients and their caregivers. They inform other professionals on the care team about the client's progress in OT. They write letters to foundations seeking funding for new programs. This chapter addresses the various audiences and types of documentation that OT practitioners may use at some point during their careers.

Audience

How one documents depends greatly on who will read it—one's audience. How a letter to an insurance company is worded might be very different from the way a letter to a parent or physician is worded. Documentation that is read by members of the clinical care team might use more precise anatomical and technical words than would an Individualized Family Service Plan (IFSP) that is shared with the parents of a 2-year-old. Knowing who

NOTES

Adolf Meyer Hits the Right Note

Adolf Meyer is well known for being the first to articulate the philosophy of OT (Meyer, 1922). Additional key achievements include his innovations in the field of psychiatry and his influence on the modern medical record. Born in Switzerland and trained as a physician, Meyer immigrated to the United States in 1882 (Christiansen, 2007; Lief, 1948; Scull & Schulkin, 2009). While a pathologist at the Illinois Eastern Hospital for the Insane at Kankakee, he was tasked to study the connection between brain lesions in deceased patients and their psychiatric diagnoses (Christiansen, 2007; Scull & Schulkin, 2009). He found that the lack of accurate records of the patient's symptoms during the hospitalization made his efforts pointless (Scull & Schulkin, 2009). Meyer tried to develop a more systematic way of recording information about patients' histories and symptoms, but he was met with resistance (Lief, 1948). He soon moved on to the State Lunatic Hospital in Worcester, Massachusetts, where he had more success in implementing a practical documentation system that recorded concise case histories which included the following:

1. A sizing up of the situation
2. The somatic material of adaptation (a physical exam)

3. The mental status
   a. General demeanor and adaptation to the environment (discrete observations)
   b. The patient's spontaneous utterances
   c. Special features such as moods, emotional traits, ruminations, and delusions and/or hallucinations
   d. Grasp of the past and present; orientation to person, place, and time
   e. Patient's insight into situation and disease
   f. Evolution of the symptoms (Meyer & Kirby, 1908, as published in Lief, 1948, pp. 207–209)

Meyer believed the record should list more than statistics about the patient and include information to help the staff handling the patient (Meyer, 1911, as cited in Lief, 1948). In this way, he set the standard for medical records today, a delicate balance between providing adequate information to support best care while not spending so much time documenting that there is little time left to spend with the client. His initial push for standardization of the medical record has evolved to the electronic health record we use every day. If he were alive today, he would be admonishing us to use the record as more than a series of check boxes and dropdown menus but rather including the unique course of the patient's development or recovery.

will read what is being communicated is an important aspect of effective documentation.

The potential audiences for OT documentation include the following:

- Medical professionals (e.g., doctors, nurses, psychologists, physical therapists, speech-language pathologists, social workers)
- Education professionals (teachers, principals, etc.)
- Lawyers, judges, and juries
- Accreditation agencies (The Joint Commission, Commission on Accreditation of Rehabilitation Facilities [CARF], Department of Education, etc.)
- Payers (e.g., managed care companies, Medicare contractors, Medicaid reviewers)
- The client or the client's guardian

Each audience reads documentation through a different lens, depending on practice setting, educational level, motivation, and cultural background (Sames, 2015).

Communicating with medical professionals requires the writer to be very precise. Nurses need to know more than that the patient needs assistance with dressing; they need to know how much assistance and the nature of

the assistance. The physical therapist needs to know how long the client was standing at the sink while working on grooming and hygiene.

When one is communicating in a school setting, there is a need to focus on the educationally relevant information. The entire team working with the child might not understand medical jargon, so educational terms are more appropriate.

Occupational therapy practitioners need to communicate with each other and with other professionals. The word choices and the tone of the writing or speech used in professional, or formal, communication are very different from those used in informal communication between friends. Professional communication requires a level of respect and formality that is not found in informal communication (Sames, 2015).

Professional communication uses complete sentences and avoids slang or emotionally charged words. Professional writing uses active voice and is free from bias. When writing appeal letters, official memos, or progress notes, the writer might or might not know the person on the receiving end of the communication. This is where first impressions count and more formal writing is called for.

| BOX 40-1 | DOCUMENTATION TIPS |

- Use correct
  - Grammar
  - Spelling
  - Syntax
  - Word choice
  - Literacy level for the reader(s)
- Read spell-checker and grammar checker recommendations carefully; sometimes, it is better to click "Ignore" than to use what they recommend.
- Follow directions carefully.
- Have a dictionary and a writing manual handy.
- Write legibly.
- Proofread, proofread, and proofread again (Sames, 2015).

Formal documentation often requires compliance with specific standards. For example, the Individuals with Disabilities Education Act (IDEA) requires that specific items be included on the Individualized Education Program (IEP), and Medicare requires specific documentation elements for outpatient therapy reimbursement. The Joint Commission requires that certain abbreviations be avoided to minimize the likelihood of medical errors due to abbreviations that are remarkably close in appearance (The Joint Commission, 2017). In addition, employers might have policies or procedures that further direct the method (electronic or paper and pen), timing, placement, and word choices of the documentation. Box 40-1 contains some documentation tips that apply to all documentation.

Two important considerations for all documentation are the following:

1. People form an impression of your professionalism and intelligence by reading what you write.
2. What you write can be used as evidence in a court proceeding, whether you are on trial or not (Sames, 2015).

Legal and Ethical Considerations

Health records are legal documents. Health records can be entered as evidence in any type of legal proceeding involving **malpractice**, **fraud**, **negligence**, or **incompetence**. Occupational therapy documentation can be called into court, with or without the occupational therapist being there to explain the documentation, even years after the

services were provided. What was written at or near the actual time the event or events in question occurred is stronger evidence than what a person can recall months or years after the event. To remain mindful that all documentation is legal evidence, some people mentally preface their documentation by saying to themselves "Ladies and gentlemen of the jury . . ." before putting pen to paper (Sames, 2015).

Medicare and other payers can review clinical documentation and client billing records at any time to determine whether fraud has been committed. If documentation is not adequate to support the charges, they can refuse to pay for the services. The OT practitioner responsible for documenting the services in question could face both civil and criminal penalties (e.g., fines) as well as loss of certification and licensure (Centers for Medicare & Medicaid Services [CMS], 2012; Fremgen, 2012; Kornblau & Burkhardt, 2012).

In addition to legal issues of documentation, there are ethical concerns. The American Occupational Therapy Association (AOTA) Code of Ethics (2015) states in Principle 3.H that OT practitioners shall "maintain the confidentiality of all verbal, written, electronic, augmentative, and nonverbal communications . . . " (6913410030p4). Principle 4.O affirms that OT documentation complies with relevant laws and regulations. Principle 5.B states that OT practitioners should not be involved in writing anything that contains false or misleading information. Thus, the key ethical issues in documentation include confidentiality, accuracy, and compliance.

Documentation in Clinical Settings

In hospitals, rehabilitation facilities, primary care clinics, outpatient clinics, long-term care, mental health centers, home health, and related settings, similar types of documentation are used, although the frequency of documentation may vary. Clinical documentation generally involves reporting and interpreting the clients' responses on assessments and to interventions in a clinical record. Clinical documentation is important for the following reasons:

- Continuity of care within the department
- Communication across shifts, disciplines, departments
- Chronological record of care
- Legal record
- Reimbursement requirements (Sames, 2015)

It is critical that the objective information reported in the documentation be clearly differentiated from the subjective information or interpretations. Both are important. If a practitioner states that a client appeared depressed, that is an interpretation. It is a conclusion drawn from the practitioner's observations. To make an objective statement, the practitioner should describe what was seen or heard that would logically lead to the conclusion that the client appeared depressed. For example, the practitioner could say, "Client stared at the floor for the entire session. She slouched forward in her chair, responded to questions with one syllable words, and did not initiate any conversations with peers."

⚖️ ETHICAL DILEMMA

Documentation Standards

You work for a company that provides on-call OT personnel to hospitals and long-term care facilities in a large metropolitan area. You have been asked to work at a large, long-term care facility that normally has a part-time occupational therapist and a full-time OT assistant (OTA). The occupational therapist went into labor early, so she is not there to orient you. You have never worked in this facility before, but you have worked in other long-term care facilities and are familiar with the documentation requirements for Medicare and Medicaid.

On your first day there, you open the file for your patients and see that a few patients should have had 90-day intervention plans (renewals) written last week, but you can find no evidence that this was done. You ask the OTA whether the documentation could be somewhere else, and he says no. You find some progress notes on these patients, but they are irregular and inconsistent. Mostly, they just list some activities the patients worked on and say that the patients continue to progress toward their goals. Ten minutes later, you get a call from the medical records director saying that there are five patients for whom she cannot find a discontinuation summary and that the discontinuation summaries are needed for reimbursement. She asks you to write them, even though you have never seen the patients and the patients were discharged from the facility over a week ago. You know that the documentation must be done in order for the facility to get paid, but you feel uncomfortable documenting the care of patients you have never seen. The OTA says that he cannot help you because he is too busy with his own patients and he did not pay a lot of attention to the patients the occupational therapist was working with. What do you do?

All clinical documentation must be done in compliance with the standards of the setting and the payers as well as standards set by the profession. For example, every entry in the clinical record must be dated (AOTA, 2013). With electronic documentation, the date and time are automatically recorded by the system. If the documentation is handwritten, the date must be put either at the top of the documentation or at the bottom, by the signature, whichever is the standard at the facility. The essential features of all clinical documentation are as follows (items with an * are automatic in an electronic health record):

- *Date of completion of report
- *Full signature and **credentials**
- *Type of document
- *Client name and case number
- Acceptable abbreviations as determined by the facility
- Acceptable terminology as determined by the facility
- Record storage and disposal that complies with federal and state laws and facility procedures
- Protections of confidentiality (AOTA, 2013; Sames, 2015)

The OT practitioner's rationale—the reasons behind the intervention—should be made clear in the documentation. For example, clients with mental health challenges might have problems in living that are not as visible as physical challenges. Whereas people who use wheelchairs might have difficulty with grocery shopping because they cannot reach all the shelves or push the cart while seated in a wheelchair, people with bipolar disorder might have difficulty shopping because of an inability to control impulses to buy everything and talk to everyone in the store. Simply saying a client is working on shopping is not sufficient; the rationale for working on this occupation must be made clear.

Documentation of the Initiation of Occupational Therapy Services

The first type of clinical documentation reflects the first steps in the clinician–client interaction. In some settings, such as in a long-term care facility, the first step is a **screening** of all new admissions to the facility. A screening is used to determine whether or not the person would benefit from an OT evaluation. In other settings, the first step might be an introduction, or it might be the beginning of the evaluation process.

If the client is seen for a screening or introduction prior to an **evaluation**, a short note is usually written in the health record summarizing the conversation and/or results of the screening. The occupational therapist or OT assistant writes a short summary and indicates the next step in the intervention process.

Evaluation reports are written by occupational therapists to document the starting point of OT intervention. Occupational therapy assistants may contribute to the evaluation, but the responsibility for writing the evaluation report rests with the occupational therapist (AOTA, 2015). Evaluation reports contain factual data collected during the evaluation process and an interpretation of the evaluation findings. The report must show the distinct value of OT by documenting which occupations are limited or at risk of being limited. Often, there will be an initial **plan of care** (also called care plan, treatment plan, or intervention plan) embedded in the evaluation report. This plan includes measurable, functional, and time-limited goals for the client (Gateley & Borcherding, 2012; Sames, 2015).

The AOTA (2013) guidelines for documentation identify content needed for an evaluation. The evaluation report content is based on the Occupational Therapy Practice Framework: Domain and Process, third edition (AOTA, 2014). In an acute care setting, especially for short-stay clients, a complete evaluation might not be conducted. Although AOTA recommends that a complete evaluation be conducted and documented for each client, the time constraints of certain settings might require that the occupational therapist abbreviate the evaluation process.

Typically, the evaluation report contains the following:

- Identifying and background information (e.g., client's name, age, diagnoses or conditions, date of referral, date of report, **precautions**, and **contraindications)**
- Referral information (date, time, who referred the client and why)
- Evaluation procedures and/or tests used
- **Occupational profile**
- Findings or results of the evaluation process (**occupational analysis)**
- An interpretation of the meaning of the findings or results that reflects the occupational needs of the client
- A plan, including goals, frequency, duration, and location of intervention
- Signature and credentials of the occupational therapist (AOTA, 2013; Sames, 2015)

The occupational profile (AOTA, 2013) is critical for demonstrating the distinct value of OT services. It summarizes the client's "occupational history and experiences, patterns of daily living, interests, values, and needs" (p. S33). This information is gathered primarily through interviewing the client (or client's surrogate). It will help the occupational therapist understand the client's needs, concerns, and goals and be useful in selecting outcome measures. The AOTA offers a template that every OT practitioner can use to document the occupational profile (AOTA, 2017). The occupational profile is now a requirement when billing for an OT evaluation using Current Procedural Terminology (CPT) evaluation codes (AOTA, 2017).

The occupational analysis is the process of selecting and administering appropriate assessment tools, and then using this information, along with the information gathered from the occupational profile, to develop a hypothesis about what is going on with the client and set goals to help the client achieve desired outcomes (AOTA, 2014).

The initial plan of care is based on the occupational profile and occupational analysis. The initial plan of care sets long- (outcome) and short-term goals and describes the types of interventions that will be used to help the client achieve his or her goals.

The occupational therapist, with input from the OT assistant, and in collaboration with the client, sets short- and long-term goals. Long-term goals describe what the client will do by the time of discharge from OT—the outcome of OT interventions. Short-term goals describe what the client will do in the next 1 to 30 days. If the client will receive OT services for just a couple days, for example, during a short stay in the acute care hospital before moving on to a transitional care setting, only one set of goals may be developed rather than separate long- and short-term goals. All goals must address performance in areas of occupation, describe observable behavior, be measureable, and be time limited (state target date for when the goal will be met) (Sames, 2015). See Table 40-1 for examples of poorly written goals and how to improve them.

The goals and interventions will help the client create or promote health, establish (habilitate) or restore (rehabilitate or remediate) function, maintain or preserve occupational performance, modify (compensate or adapt) the task or the environment to enable occupational participation, or prevent barriers to performance (AOTA, 2014).

Documentation of Continuing Occupational Therapy Services

In clinical settings, there are two types of notes written to show the client's progress in OT: daily (session) notes and progress reports. The documentation of progress should include more than a list of the activities the client engaged in during the session; it must also show how the client's performance has changed since the last intervention session, any functional improvements, adaptive equipment provided, and client or caregiver understanding of any instructions (Sames, 2015).

Daily (contact) notes are usually written at the end of or after each intervention session. The OT practitioner who provided the service writes the daily note. Although Medicare does not require that notes written by an OT assistant be cosigned by the occupational therapist, state licensure laws may dictate whether or not a note needs to be cosigned (CMS, 2017; Sames, 2015). These daily notes and progress reports may be written in narrative, SOAP, or flow sheet formats.

TABLE 40-1 Examples of Poorly Written Goals and Improved Goals

Examples of Poorly Written Goals	Examples of Improved Goals	Why the Improved Goal Is Better
Increase elbow range of motion	By June 1, 2017, Maria will use elbow flexion and extension to fold three t-shirts.	It specifies by when the goal will be met and describes performance in an area of occupation.
Jamal will dress himself independently.	Jamal will consistently dress himself, including shoes and socks, independently by discharge.	It is more specific about what is included in "dressing himself" and specifies by when the goal will be achieved.
Tsoyushi will use an adapted pencil to write legibly by the end of the year.	By June 15, 2017, Tsoyushi will write two complete, legible sentences within 5 minutes.	It is more specific about the length of the goal and includes a measurement (two legible sentences within 5 minutes).
By September 13, 2017, Agnes will make toast and tea.	By September 13, 2017, Agnes will prepare toast and tea with no more than one verbal cue.	It includes a measurement.
Jenny will put six golf tees in each bag, completing each bag in 2 minutes or less, with 90% accuracy on 75% of trials on 3 consecutive days within 2 weeks.	By December 8, 2017, Jenny will package golf tees accurately on 75% of trials.	It is clearer—the original goal had too many measurements, and providing an end date for the goal is clearer than saying within 2 weeks.

Progress reports summarize OT interventions at regular intervals between updated plans of care. Medicare requires that the occupational therapist write a progress note at least once every 30 days or 10 treatment days, whichever is less (CMS, 2017; Sames, 2015).

One of the most common forms of documenting the client's progress is called a **SOAP note**. This note-writing format is used by many medical disciplines, a practice that strengthens communication among professionals. Dr. Lawrence Weed developed the SOAP note format in the 1960s as part of a problem-oriented medical record (Gateley & Borcherding, 2012; Sames, 2015). Each letter of the word SOAP represents a different component of the note (Gateley & Borcherding, 2012; Sames, 2015):

Subjective: the subjective experience of the client, what the client says

Objective: the clinician's objective observations and measurements

Assessment: the clinician's interpretation of the meaning of the "O" section

Plan: description of what will happen next (frequency, duration, location)

The most difficult part of writing a SOAP note is separating the objective information from the interpretation of it (assessment). Every statement in the "A" section needs to be supported with evidence in the "S" and the "O" sections (Sames, 2015). Box 40-2 shows an example of a SOAP note.

An updated plan of care is written in settings in which clients are seen for an extended period of time (up to 90 calendar days, depending on the setting). This documents the progress that has occurred since the last plan of care was written (or an explanation for lack of progress); updates the short-term goals and sets new ones; and verifies the frequency, duration, and location of continued intervention (AOTA, 2013). The long-term goal, the outcome goal, usually remains the same.

BOX 40-2   SOAP NOTE

S: "It hurts to reach items on the second shelf. No way could I reach the top shelf. I can't even put my hair in a ponytail."

O: Client reached items on the second shelf of the kitchen cabinet with her right hand, expressing discomfort throughout the range. Client did not attempt to reach items on the top shelf. Client pointed to the anterior aspect of the glenoid fossa when asked where it hurt. Scapular elevation and trunk rotation substituted for part of shoulder flexion and abduction; she never raised her arm above 80°. Client used internal rotation to place items retrieved from the shelf on the counter with no complaints. Client did not use external rotation in replacing objects on shelf, reporting severe pain using that kind of motion. She rated her pain a 9 on a 0–10 point scale.

A: Right shoulder range of motion is severely limited and very painful. Limited range of motion interferes with household tasks, dressing, hygiene, and grooming.

P: Occupational therapy 2 times per week, for 30 minutes outpatient sessions to instruct client in use of reacher, discuss environmental adaptation principles related to placement of objects within comfort zone, and develop a home program to facilitate regaining pain-free range of motion.

Documentation of Termination of Occupational Therapy Services

Once clients have met their long- and short-term goals or other circumstances require that OT services end, a **discontinuation summary** (discharge summary) is written (AOTA, 2013; Sames 2015). This summary includes the following:

• Client identification and background information
• Summary of the client's functional status at the initiation of OT services
• Summary of change in functional status at the close of OT services
• Results of outcome measures
• Recommendations for follow-up
• Signature, credentials, and date

According to AOTA (2014), outcomes of OT intervention can include occupational performance, prevention, health and wellness, quality of life, participation, role competence, well-being, and occupational justice. Outcomes are reflected in subjective and objective data gathered at the end of OT interventions. Subjective data would be based on client reports, and objective data would come from standardized or nonstandardized testing (AOTA, 2013).

Electronic Health Records

Electronic health records have replaced paper charts in most practice settings. Electronic health records require health care providers to enter clinical data into a computerized system. These systems may use desktop, laptop, or tablet computers; smartphones; or other handheld devices (Figure 40-1). Because these systems are electronic, special precautions need to be taken to assure the security and confidentiality of each client's health record. These systems allow members of the client's health care team nearly instant access to updated information about the client's health care, test results, medications, and consultation reports.

Occupational therapy practitioners (and all other health care providers) need to log in and log out of the system even if they are going to be away from their computer (or other device) for only a minute or two. No computer can be left unattended while a client's health record is open. When you are logged in, every client record you access, every note you write, and every error you make and correct, is recorded under your "signature."

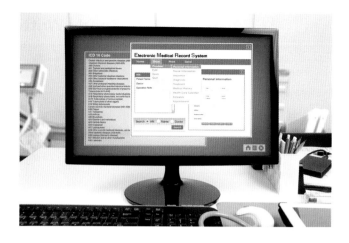

FIGURE 40-1 Electronic health records require health care providers to enter clinical data into a computerized system.

Access to any client's health record has to be limited to those who have a need to know what is in that record. Thirty-two employees of a health system in Minnesota were fired because they looked at the health records of people involved in a highly publicized case (several teens overdosed at a party) when they were not involved in the care of any of the teens. They were caught because of routine audits that check to see who has viewed selected health records (Lauritsen, 2011).

Documentation of Telehealth

When a client is being treated by an OT practitioner using telehealth technology, documentation is completed in the same way as it would be if the session was conducted in person. One addition to the daily notes would be to indicate that the session was conducted using approved telehealth technology. Individual payers may have additional requirements for documenting and billing for services provided via telehealth.

Documentation in School Settings

Documentation in educational settings can be very different from clinical documentation, but the same documentation principles apply. Documentation in school systems includes documentation of notice and consent as well as specific documentation depending on the age of the student (Sames, 2015). See Chapter 51 for more detail related to OT in education settings.

Documentation of Notice and Consent

According to the IDEA, notice and consent forms are required to communicate with parents or guardians of children being served by the school district. Documents may include notices of team meetings, notice and consent for evaluation or reevaluation, referral for an initial evaluation, procedural safeguards, and a report of an IFSP or IEP meeting (Sames, 2015).

Documentation of Services from Birth through Age 2 Years

Services for infants and toddlers are described in Part C of IDEA (Clark & Handley-More, 2017). Individualized Family Service Plans are written to address these services. Each state designates a lead agency (education, health, or human services) to serve the needs of infants and toddlers with special needs to help ready them for school. The lead agency (e.g., school district, health department, or contracted agency) is responsible for creating an IFSP for each child served that is tailored to the specific needs of the child and the child's family. An IFSP includes the following:

- A summary of the child's present level of performance (physical, cognitive, communicative, social or emotional, and adaptive development)
- Identification of the family's concerns, priorities, and resources
- A summary of expected outcomes (measurable goals)
- Identification of early intervention services needed, including frequency, intensity, and service delivery method
- Identification of the child's natural environment (where services will be delivered)
- Date services will start and the anticipated length of services
- Identification of a service coordinator for the child
- Identification of the steps that will be taken to help the toddler transition to the preschool setting (IDEA, 2004).

Documentation of Services from Age 3 to 21 Years

The IEP is the document that guides services for a child with disabilities between the ages of 3 and 21 years (Clark & Handley-More, 2017). The requirements for IEPs are described in Part B of IDEA. Individualized Education Program services may include both **special education** and **related services**. For the purposes of the IEP, OT services are considered related services. As a related service

provider, the occupational therapist would contribute to the process of writing and revising the IEP. The IEP is written every year and reviewed at least every 6 months (Sames, 2015).

An IEP must contain the following elements:

- Present level of educational performance
- Annual goals
- Special education and related services
- Participation with nondisabled children
- Participation in statewide and districtwide tests
- Starting date and location of services
- Transition services (for children aged 14 years and older transitioning to adult programs or work settings)
- Measurement of progress (IDEA, 2004)

The fundamental difference between the IFSP and the IEP is that the IFSP is more family-centered; the IEP is more education focused (Clark & Handley-More, 2017). An IEP must be educationally related. Each state or each school district within a state may establish its own forms for these documents; the federal regulations do not require use of specific forms. The federal regulations mandate the timetables for completing the documents and the content of the documents (Clark & Handley-More, 2017; Sames, 2015).

Documentation in Emerging Practice Settings

Occupational therapy practitioners are now working in community-based programs such as homeless shelters, prisons, sheltered workshops, home hospice, and summer camps. The clinical approach to documentation might not be appropriate, especially if there is no health record in which to enter OT documentation. It is advisable that the occupational therapist develop evaluation, intervention plan, progress, and discontinuation reports that are consistent with the AOTA documentation guidelines (2013) to the greatest extent possible. However, if the OT practitioners are providing services at a community or population level, they may simply provide the agency with periodic consultation reports with a less structured format. Most consultation reports are narrative descriptions of the needs assessment, plan, implementation, and/or outcomes of the OT program.

Because OT practitioners in emerging practice settings are demonstrating the distinct value of OT in new ways, they may use their documentation as a mechanism to demonstrate successful outcomes and benefits of OT services.

Tatiana is a 16-month-old girl. Three weeks ago, while under the care of her mother's boyfriend, she was allegedly shaken violently.

Excerpt from Evaluation Report

Tatiana did not focus on or visually track any objects in any direction. She did not reach for any toys that were quietly placed in front of her, but she did turn her head to localize sounds and flailed her hands in reaction to sound. Her fingers closed around a rattle placed in the palm of her hand. Passive range of motion was within normal limits in all extremities. Muscle tone was low. When placed on her stomach, she rolled her head from side to side but did not lift her head. When placed in a sitting position, she was unable to hold her head up or maintain sitting unassisted. She is fed through a nasogastric tube; therefore, chewing and swallowing were not evaluated at this time. She cried and made other noises but did not form any words. Tatiana will need adaptive seating with head support and OT

intervention to maximize her abilities to actively interact with people and her environment.

Excerpt from Prior Authorization Letter

This 16-month-old girl was diagnosed with shaken baby syndrome resulting in severe head trauma. She has low muscle tone and cannot assume or maintain a seated position unassisted. This child will need adaptive seating and positioning devices to ensure proper positioning of her trunk and limbs and to prevent deformities. Proper positioning is also important for her cognitive, social, and physical development. She is functionally blind. In a seated position, she will better be able to localize sound, use her arms and hands, and begin to engage in social interactions. Please refer to the attached list of recommended adaptive positioning devices and their respective costs. In addition, I recommend OT intervention twice a week for 3 months (24 visits) to work on developing the movement, social, and cognitive skills needed to enable participation in daily life activities of typical toddlers.

Administrative Documentation

Occupational therapists in any setting may have to write an incident report, a letter of appeal to a payer source, a grant proposal, or **policies** and **procedures**. These types of documentation are administrative because they are necessary for the ongoing administration of OT services. For example, to be paid for delivering OT services, OT practitioners may need to write letters to request funding or to respond to a denial of a payment. Policies and procedures must be written clearly so that all employees of the department understand and follow the departmental standards, ensuring that the department functions well. To effectively do their jobs, aides—who may be high school graduates with some on-the-job training—as well as professional staff must understand policies and procedures.

Administrative documentation requires the use of terminology that anyone can understand; people who have limited understanding of OT jargon or medical terms may read these documents. Often, the first person who reads an appeal letter will be someone who is trained to interpret insurance company standards but who might not have a medical background.

Box 40-3 shows an example of a section of an evaluation report written for a medical record and how it might be translated in a letter to an insurance company requesting authorization for services.

Conclusion

Individual agencies may opt to develop or purchase their own documentation formats. However, it is critical that whatever documentation formats are chosen conform to federal and state laws; OT documentation, practice, and ethical standards; and the requirements of reimbursement sources. It is the OT practitioner's responsibility to be aware of and comply with all documentation requirements.

REFERENCES

American Occupational Therapy Association. (2013). Guidelines for documentation of occupational therapy. *American Journal of Occupational Therapy*, 67, S32–S38. doi:10.5014/ajot.2013.67S32

American Occupational Therapy Association. (2014). Occupational therapy practice framework: Domain and process, 3rd edition. *American Journal of Occupational Therapy*, 62, S1–S48. doi:10.5014/ajot.2014.682006

American Occupational Therapy Association. (2015). Occupational therapy code of ethics (2015). *American Journal of Occupational Therapy*, 69, 6913410030p1–6913410030p8. doi:10.5014/ajot.2015.696S03

American Occupational Therapy Association. (2017). *AOTA Occupational profile template.* Retrieved from https://www.aota.org/~/media/Corporate/Files/Practice/Manage/Documentation/AOTA-Occupational-Profile-Template.pdf

Centers for Medicare & Medicaid Services. (2012). *Medicare fraud and abuse: Detection, prevention, and reporting.* Retrieved from http://www.jointcommission.org/topics/patient_safety.aspx

Centers for Medicare & Medicaid Services. (2017). *Medicare benefit policy manual: Chapter 15—covered medical and other health*

services. Retrieved from https://www.cms.gov/Regulations-and
-Guidance/Guidance/Manuals/downloads/bp102c15.pdf

Christiansen, C. H. (2007). Adolf Meyer revisited: Connections
between lifestyle, resilience and illness. *Journal of Occupational
Science, 14,* 63–76.

Clark, G. F., & Handley-More, D. (2017). *Best practices for documenting
occupational therapy services in schools.* Bethesda, MD: American
Occupational Therapy Association.

Fremgen, B. F. (2012). *Medical law and ethics (5th ed.).* Upper Saddle
River, NJ: Prentice Hall.

Gateley, C. A., & Borcherding, S. (2012). *Documentation manual for
occupational therapy: Writing SOAP notes.* Thorofare, NJ: SLACK.

Individuals with Disabilities Education Act of 2004, 20 U.S.C. § 1414
(2004). Retrieved from http://www.gpo.gov/fdsys/pkg/PLAW
-108publ446/html/PLAW-108publ446.htm

Kornblau, B. L., & Burkhardt, A. (2012). *Ethics in rehabilitation: A clinical perspective.* Thorofare, NJ: SLACK.

Lauritsen, J. (2011). *Allina fires 32 employees for snooping at patient
records.* Retrieved from http://minnesota.cbslocal.com/2011/05/06
/allina-fires-32-employees-for-snooping-at-patient-records/

Lief, A. (1948). *The commonsense psychiatry of Dr. Adolf Meyer: Fifty-
two selected papers edited, with biographical narrative.* New York,
NY: McGraw-Hill.

Meyer, A. (1922). The philosophy of occupation therapy. *Archives of
Occupational Therapy, 1,* 1–10.

Sames, K. M. (2015). *Documenting occupational therapy practice
(3rd ed.).* Upper Saddle River, NJ: Pearson Prentice Hall.

Scull, A., & Schulkin, J. (2009). Psychobiology, psychiatry, and psychoanalysis: The intersecting careers of Adolf Meyer, Phyllis
Greenacre, and Curt Richter. *Medical History, 53,* 5–36. doi:10.1017
/s002572730000329x

The Joint Commission. (2017). *Facts about the official "Do Not Use" list
of abbreviations.* Retrieved from http://www.jointcommission.org
/topics/patient_safety.aspxhttps://www.jointcommission.org/facts
_about_do_not_use_list/

thePoint® *For additional resources on the subjects
discussed in this chapter, visit* http://thePoint.lww.com
/Willard-Spackman13e.

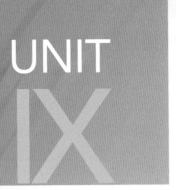

UNIT IX

Occupational Performance Theories of Practice

"I long to accomplish a great and noble task;
but it is my chief duty to accomplish small tasks as if
they were great and noble."

— Helen Keller

Examining How Theory Guides Practice

Theory and Practice in Occupational Therapy

Ellen S. Cohn, Wendy J. Coster

"In theory there is no difference between theory and practice. In practice there is."

—YOGI BERRA

LEARNING OBJECTIVES

After reading this chapter, you will be able to:

1. Compare and contrast the personal and formal theories.
2. Analyze the distinction between tacit and explicit knowledge.
3. Assess assumptions and propositions guiding practice.
4. Critically examine assumptions and propositions of a theory.

When occupational therapy (OT) practitioners meet a client[1] for the first time, they must quickly figure out why the client has come for intervention, what is important to the client, what might be helping or interfering with his or her desired occupations, and what might be the best possible intervention to enable the client to achieve his or her goals. Figuring out what to do requires complex professional reasoning processes that involve ongoing analysis and reflection on the OT practitioner's knowledge, observations, and understanding of the lives of clients and what matters to them.

In order to enable clients to achieve their occupational performance goals, OT practitioners must decide which interventions are most likely to achieve these goals. When we propose an intervention that involves particular actions or steps, our reasoning about what to do is guided by our ideas of how change might occur. These ideas include theoretical assumptions and propositions that guide us in what to observe and how to describe, explain, or predict outcomes from the interventions we might use. That is, in addition to client priorities, our experience, and available research evidence, we are guided by theories. The theories that guide professional reasoning are both personal and formal and both tacit and explicit. Whatever their form, theories help practitioners reason about what to assess, how

---

[1] "The person or persons (including those involved in the care of the client), group (collective of individuals, e.g., families, workers, students, or community members), or population (collective of groups of individuals living in a similar locale—e.g., city, state or country—or sharing the same or like concerns)" (American Occupational Therapy Association, 2014, p. S41)

to understand occupational performance problems, how to intervene, and what to expect from the intervention. Often, we need to articulate our reasoning process to others (clients, other professionals, peers, supervisors, third party payers, etc.) to communicate what they may expect from OT intervention.

The purpose of this chapter is to provide a structure to help OT practitioners "unpack" or critically examine the theories they use to understand the problems clients present and to guide intervention. Our goal is to help practitioners clarify and evaluate the assumptions and propositions that guide their practice. This analysis is important for several reasons. First, it helps us to determine whether our professional reasoning is sound. Then, based on whether we conclude that it is sound or not, we may need to modify our reasoning and potentially the services we provide. Finally, examining our thinking helps us to articulate our professional reasoning to others so we can explain why we are using the assessments we have chosen, how the intervention we are providing works, and what outcomes we expect. The scenario in Case Study 41-1 illustrates a common challenge many OT students confront during their fieldwork experience.

Propositions and Assumptions

To begin our discussion, we make a distinction between two types of ideas that are part of most theories: propositions and assumptions. **Propositions** are formal statements about causes and effects or the nature of relationships among features of the world. Their distinguishing feature is that it is possible (hypothetically at least) to test them and therefore to prove them false—a characteristic that is referred to in philosophy of science as "falsifiability" (Popper, 1959). Sometimes, it is possible to test a proposition directly, for example, to test the proposition that a virus causes a particular illness. Other times, evidence accumulates from various sources and that eventually makes clear that the "old" ideas about the world do not fit with the data as, for example, when scientists challenged the proposition that the sun revolved around the earth. Modern science is built around the posing and testing of hypotheses, which are propositions about how the world "works." In order to make the proposed relationships among the factors explicit, it can be helpful to formulate

---

CASE STUDY 41-1　ALEX

Alex, a 9-year-old child, has been referred to you, an OT student completing your Level II fieldwork experience in an outpatient private practice for children. Alex is reluctant to try new activities, is beginning to have difficulty keeping up with his peers in school, wanders around the periphery of the playground during recess, and refuses to participate in gym class. The other children have begun to tease Alex, and he has not developed friendships. After observing Alex struggle to complete a variety of fine and gross motor activities, you conduct formal assessments and document delays in both fine and gross motor development. You also complete the Perceived Efficacy and Goal Setting System (PEGS) with Alex to gain insight into his perspectives and concerns. The PEGS is a standardized system designed to enable young children with disabilities to self-report their perceived competence in everyday activities and to set goals for intervention. Alex wants to be able to play baseball, shuffle playing cards, and type on the computer. You are now clear about the outcomes Alex hopes to achieve but need to determine how to best intervene to help Alex achieve his goals in an effective and efficient manner. Your supervisor asks you to explain the "theoretical rationale" of the intervention you propose for Alex. Your supervisor wants to know what you think the "mechanisms of action" are for the intervention.

Before reading further, take a moment to think about and write down your ideas about the following:

1. Why might Alex have trouble developing friendships?
2. Why might Alex be reluctant to try new activities?

Go back and review your explanations for why Alex might have trouble developing friendships and be reluctant to try new activities.

3. Which ideas are testable (i.e., are propositions)?
4. How might you test the propositions?
5. Which are more like assumptions?
6. Can you identify the sources of some of your assumptions?

Before reading further, take another moment to think about this question:

Are your ideas about Alex's challenges with friendships and new activities based on personal theories or some formal theories that you may have learned in your studies to date?

7. Identify in writing the personal theories that guided your reasoning about Alex.
8. Identify in writing the formal theories (either broad or discrete) that guided your reasoning about Alex.

TABLE 41-1	Examples of Propositions with If/Then Statements	
Proposition	**If/Then Statement**	**How It Would Be Tested**
Practice of a skill in the context in which it will typically be applied leads to more effective long-term mastery.	If a person practices a skill in the natural context in which it is typically performed, then he or she will achieve more effective long-term mastery than if the skill is practiced in a contrived context.	A controlled comparison of the transfer of a skill learned under two different conditions: in typical context and in a laboratory or contrived context
Organization of movement is different when reaching toward a desired object (i.e., a goal) than when simply reaching into space.	If a person reaches toward a goal, then his or her movement is organized differently than when he or she reaches into space without a goal.	Kinematic analysis of specific characteristics of reaching movements by the same person under the two different conditions
Sensory defensiveness is a defining characteristic of children with autism.	If a child has autism, then he or she will display sensory defensiveness.	Use of a structured protocol to examine responses to sensory stimuli in a large sample of children with autism. Calculate prevalence of sensory defensiveness and compare this rate to that of a sample with a different diagnosis.

propositions as "if/then" statements. Table 41-1 presents some examples of propositions, their corresponding if/then statements, and how they might be tested.

In contrast, **assumptions** are ideas we "believe to be true." This term is used a little differently in everyday language and in the language of science. In everyday language, we use the term to refer to a wide variety of situations where we have drawn a conclusion without having definite evidence. For example, we might tell our friend we "assume" that Mary took her book because she was the last person we saw reading it. In this situation, although we don't have the evidence on hand to prove our statement, we could readily gather evidence by asking Mary if she has the book. In other words, our conclusion is "falsifiable" and thus more like a proposition. In the language of science, the term *assumption* is applied much more specifically to ideas that really cannot be definitively proven true or false, for example, the idea that people have an inherent drive for mastery of their environment. Evidence can be judged to be more or less consistent with a particular assumption like this, but there is no way to obtain definitive proof.

Because assumptions are so completely accepted, it can be hard at first to recognize when a particular idea is an assumption rather than a proposition that is well supported by evidence. Our assumptions may derive from different sources. Some may have been learned during formal education, for example, from study of the theories of an academic discipline. Others reflect our personal theories and our assumptions derived from our culture and individual life experience. (See Chapter 34 for a more thorough discussion of personal theories.) The distinction between personal and "academic" assumptions is not always clearcut; often, our preference for a particular formal theory is based on its compatibility with our personal assumptions. For example, we may find it easier to accept theories that

emphasize personal control over outcomes because we have a personal assumption that "people are in control of their fates." Table 41-2 gives some examples of how personal and theory-based assumptions might be expressed in the literature or in a person's statements regarding his or her observations.

Our assumptions about the nature of human behavior and corresponding views of reality may shape what we attend to when planning the evaluation process and developing intervention strategies with clients. Our day-to-day practices are rooted in both assumptions and propositions (Hooper, 1997). Often, propositions and assumptions are confounded, viewed as the same things, or confused with each other. Making a distinction between them helps us to identify them more easily, to reflect on how they may influence our reasoning about evaluation and intervention, and to evaluate whether they make sense. If we distinguish our propositions and assumptions, we can then search for relevant evidence to evaluate the propositions, evaluate whether our assumptions are logical and consistent with current knowledge, and reflect on how both the assumptions and propositions are influencing our reasoning and expectations for intervention outcomes.

Note that some of the examples in Table 41-2 have elements that could be tested or checked for their consistency with the evidence. However, the *broader* assumptions would be hard to prove or disprove. For example, how would one *prove* that all people want to be as independent as possible? This is one reason why it is important to evaluate the evidence supporting your ideas about how to intervene with a client. If you cannot find any evidence, that is one clue that you may be basing your approach on assumptions.

It is important to keep in mind that we all make assumptions; they provide answers to important

TABLE 41-2 **Examples of How Personal and Theory-Based Assumptions Might Be Expressed**

Types of Assumptions	Examples of Assumptions	How the Assumption Might Be Expressed in a Formal Theory	How the Assumption Might Be Expressed in a Personal Theory
Assumptions about causes	Behavior is largely controlled by external social influences.	A theory proposes that negative social influences (e.g., unsafe neighborhood, low socioeconomic status) explain poor outcomes among youth.	"You can't blame him, given the kind of neighborhood he grew up in."
	Behavior is largely controlled by unconscious motives and conflicts.	A theory proposes that unconscious conflicts stemming from early experiences explain a person's current behavior.	"She's doing that because she's in denial about what happened."
Assumptions about the nature of the person	People are largely aware of and can report accurately on the reasons for their behavior.	A theory proposes that information gained through self-report on motives and goals accurately reflects the real causes of their behavior.	"Once we have talked with her, we should have a much better idea of what caused her to do that."
	People are largely in control of their own behavior.	A theory proposes that behavior is directed by commitment to personal goals.	"If she really wanted to, she would put in the effort" to change that bad habit.
	People have an inherent drive to experience sensory stimulation.	A theory proposes that the experiences derived from sensory input are highly rewarding.	"Providing rich sensory experiences for their child is one of the most important things a parent can do."
	People have an inherent drive to make sense of their experience.	A theory proposes that people automatically formulate explanations of their experience without being taught to do so.	"There must be a reason why this happened to me."
	People are inherently rational.	A theory proposes that given adequate information, people will choose their actions based on an accurate weighing of the pros and cons of various options.	"I don't get it: I explained the importance of doing this, but he's still resisting!"
	All people desire to be independent as much as possible.	A theory proposes that being able to do things without the support of others is the greatest indication of success.	"Even though he says he likes living in the group home, I'm sure he really wants to live on his own."
Assumptions about human development	There is a universal, optimal sequence to developing competence.	A theory proposes that failure to follow a standard sequence for mastering skills will result in less optimal functioning.	"If we don't focus on fine motor skills first, he will never be able to write well."
	There is a timetable of experiences required for optimal development that is universal across cultures.	A theory proposes that if a child does not have certain experiences at a particular time, he or she will not achieve the same skills as his or her peers.	"It is important to make sure you talk to your baby to develop his attention and listening skills for school."
Assumptions about knowledge and learning	The essence of learning is acquiring more information.	A theory proposes that lack of accurate or sufficiently detailed information explains why people act ineffectively.	"We have a lot of parents who aren't providing the right kind of experiences for their child. We should offer a presentation about typical motor development."
	The essence of learning is changing the way we think about something.	A theory proposes that people must integrate new information into their existing personal system of knowledge before they can organize new ways to act.	"An interactive teaching session observing how their child solves movement 'problems' will help parents change their approach to supporting their child."

fundamental questions such as "What is the nature of the person?" or "Am I in control of my fate?" It is not really possible to construct theories without them. However, because assumptions cannot be fully disproved, we need to be cautious in applying them as guides for practice. The propositions of a theory, on the other hand, can be tested so that we can determine whether or not they are accurate guides for achieving desired changes. This systematic testing is what leads to new discoveries and therefore more effective practice.

Tacit and Explicit

Sometimes our reasoning is **tacit**; that is, implicit or based on information or experiences that we cannot easily put into language. Experienced practitioners have an implicit or tacit understanding of what they do in practice and will make adjustments to the intervention to address the subtle and complex cues observed in the process of intervention. For example, through experience, a therapist might determine that the strength of a muscle "just doesn't seem right" and the therapist then automatically adjusts the activity to compensate for the person's limited strength. Another therapist might instinctively sing a calming, gentle song to soothe a young child who is screaming and agitated. The philosopher Polanyi (1966/2009, p. 4) eloquently summarized this process when he noted, "We can know more than we can tell." Tacit reasoning is important to our practice because it allows us to work quickly and effectively in the moment. However, in order to evaluate whether the approach was effective (and if we should continue to use it), we need to be able to translate our tacit or implicit reasoning into clear *explicit* propositions about what we think promoted the desired change for the client. In order to evaluate whether our model of change is logical and is supported by evidence, we need to describe the exact mechanism that we think caused the change. For example, on reflection, we may realize that we asked a client to repeat the same movement numerous times as we increased the task demands because we hypothesized, based on motor learning theory, that "repetition under condition of ever-increasing task demands" will promote change in the movement (Plautz, Milliken, & Nudo, 2000). Then, we could review whether the evidence supports this theoretical proposition.

Theories Vary in Specificity

In OT, authors have used many different terms to define similar concepts (theory, conceptual foundation, frame of reference, paradigm, practice model). Different authors may provide very different definitions of the same terms, which can be confusing. Rather than try to clarify the subtle distinctions across these definitions, this chapter takes a different approach. We suggest that theories can be located along a continuum that reflects their degree of specificity.

Broad

One definition of a theory (2010) is "a plausible or scientifically acceptable general principle or body of principles offered to explain phenomena." This definition is broad, global, and explanatory. A broad theory serves as an "overarching model that helps to explain a large set of findings or observations" (Whyte, 2006, p. 100). A broad or global theory provides a way of organizing or systematizing the elements of the phenomenon being observed and helps us focus our observations and decide what cues to attend to. A **broad theory** specifies how concepts or factors are related and gives a name to a set of elements that share something in common. However, propositions about change are not specified in precise detail in broad theories. For example, ecological theory tells us to pay attention to the person–environment interaction, but it does not tell us how to intervene to enable the client to participate more satisfactorily in desired occupations. Therefore, broad theories do not provide precise information on how we can intervene to enable change.

In OT, we often use ecological and systems theories,[2] which propose a transactional relation between the mind, the body, and the environment. We consider the context or environment in its broadest sense (including culture and social aspects) and assume that humans have an innate drive to explore and be competent in their environments. Some broad ecological theories explain the influence of the environment in greater detail than others. These broad theories commonly suggest that in order to explore and be competent in our environments, people need skills and abilities, and we judge our competence by the feedback we receive from the environment. Consequently, in this example, the broad theories help us focus our initial observations of human behavior on the complex transactions among mind, body, and environment.

Several ecological theorists in the field of human development have offered explanations of the transactional relationship between person and environment. Bronfenbrenner (1979), a social scientist, proposed an ecological theory to explain how a person's biology and interactions among ever-changing and multilevel environments are key to human development. Bronfenbrenner proposed that social factors such as families, friends, communities,

---

[2]For a thorough description of these theories, see primary sources.

BOX 41-1   CHARACTERISTICS OF BROAD AND DISCRETE THEORIES

Broad ➡ **Discrete**

Broad	Discrete
• Global	• Testable specific postulates about causal relationships
• Explanatory: help explain a large set of findings or observations	• Specify how to behave in intervention, what to say or do, under what conditions changes will occur
• Map out the elements of phenomena being observed	• Explanatory: help explain how intervention works
• Specify what is related to what and gives a name to a set of elements that share something in common	• Predictive: specify what might happen or what to expect as a result of intervention
• Help us focus our initial observations (i.e., what is important to attend to rather than what to do)	• Each particular proposition of the theory is supported by evidence and specified so you can anticipate what the outcome is likely to be.

or institutions can enhance or inhibit development. Gibson's (1979) concept of affordances describes the idea that people's perception of the relationship between objects in the environment and their own personal capabilities enables action. Lawton (1986) proposed the concept of press to explain the idea that the demands of the environment or task impact human performance and suggested that "goodness of fit" between a person's abilities and the demands of the task influences human performance. Numerous theories proposed by occupational therapists (Ecology of Human Performance [Dunn, Brown, & McGuian, 1994], Person-Environment-Occupation [Law et al., 1996], Person-Environment-Occupation Performance [Baum & Christiansen, 2005], and Model of Human Occupation [Kielhofner, 2008; Kielhofner & Burke, 1980]) are based on these ecological principles. When observing occupational performance, ideas drawn from these ecological theories direct the occupational therapist to focus his or her observations on the person, the environment, and the occupation and how these elements influence each other.

Discrete

Another definition of a theory (2010) is a "hypothesis assumed for the sake of argument or investigation." This definition describes a **discrete theory**. Discrete theories often draw on the ideas of broad theories and describe specific causal relationships. These theories may be efforts to identify the specific causes of a problem or may propose how an aspect of intervention leads to therapeutic change. Because discrete theories identify ways in which a phenomenon can be changed or controlled, they help us determine what to do or say in providing interventions and they inform our treatment or intervention theories. A treatment

theory helps to narrow the scope of possibilities for change and states how a specific intervention is believed to act. By clearly specifying the **mechanisms of action**,[3] that is, how specific intervention strategies lead to particular outcomes, treatment theories explicate how change proceeds and the particular conditions under which an intervention achieves the desired results. Consequently, treatment or intervention theories also help us determine what types of clients might benefit from the intervention, how the intervention is best delivered, and what outcomes we might expect.

Broad and discrete theories both make claims about hypothesized relationships. However, these theories are on a continuum in terms of the degree of development and specificity regarding how to intervene, clarity about the essential features, or element of the intervention and evidence to support their propositions. One way to determine where a theory may be on the broad to discrete continuum is to examine the degree to which each causal relationship proposed in the theory is supported by sound evidence. Theories with more developed propositions include clear assertions of the effects of an intervention, the mechanism through which the intervention is believed to exert these effects, and identification of the components of the intervention that are most responsible for the effects. Because research is conducted to test the hypothesized relationships, theories become more refined and we gain greater clarity about the effectiveness of the various components of an intervention. Box 41-1 provides a simple schematic of the continuum from broad to discrete theories.

---

[3] You may also see the term "mechanism of change" used in the literature to describe ideas about how change happens during intervention. These terms are essentially equivalent.

Where Do Theories Come From?

What prompts someone to propose a new or a revised theory? Recall that theories are an effort to *explain* a particular phenomenon or process and to *organize* information about that phenomenon. Thus, theories, particularly clinical or practice theories, are often developed in response to an observation or experience that the person cannot adequately account for using existing explanations. For example, when Jean Ayres (1972) was working with children in the 1970s, she found that the accepted theories about learning difficulties did not adequately account for the full range of difficulties that she saw in the children she worked with and didn't offer useful guidance for how to intervene. Eventually, this experience led her to develop sensory integration theory and develop a new approach to intervention based on this theory. Sometimes, theory or research in a related field suggests new ways to understand or intervene with clinical problems. For example, Taub, Uswatte, and Pidikiti (1999) developed constraint-induced movement therapy for people with stroke after observing what they termed "learned non-use" in monkeys who had central nervous system (CNS) damage.

Clinical theories are based on the knowledge available at the time they are first developed. Over time, more evidence will become available about whether or not the propositions of the theory are correct or whether they need to be modified. For example, evidence may show that a specific feature of the intervention is particularly effective in achieving the desired change and that other features of the intervention may not be necessary. Therefore, it is important for practitioners to remain current in the research related to the theories they are applying in practice.

Cognitive Orientation to Daily Occupational Performance

After a thorough review of interventions to address the needs of children with motor coordination challenges, we discover the Cognitive Orientation to Daily Occupational Performance (CO-OP Approach™) intervention developed by occupational therapists Polatajko et al. (2001). The CO-OP Approach™ was developed because various intervention approaches offered to children with mild-to-moderate movement difficulties were primarily impairment-oriented, focusing on remediating underlying impairments thought to interfere with functional performance (Mandich, Polatajko, Macnab, & Miller, 2001).

Scratching a Clinical Itch: The CO-OP Approach™ Model

The CO-OP Approach™ was originally introduced into the OT literature in 2001 in response to an identified "clinical itch." That is, there was a need for effective interventions to help children diagnosed with developmental coordination disorder (DCD) meet their occupational performance goals in real-world contexts. A series of studies documented that CO-OP Approach™ was an effective alternative to bottom-up neurodevelopment interventions that were prominent in clinical practice at the time. Since 2001, there have been 27 studies conducted to examine the efficacy or effectiveness, application, and adaptations of CO-OP Approach™ with eight different populations including children with autism spectrum disorder, Asperger syndrome, or acquired brain injury. Within the adult population, CO-OP Approach™ has been studied with people 6 months poststroke, with acute stroke, and with traumatic brain injury (TBI). All of the studies documented positive improvements in occupational performance (Scammel, Bates, Houldin & Polatajko, 2016). Continued clinical trials to examine the CO-OP Approach™ will help us further understand who is mostly likely to benefit from the use of CO-OP Approach™. For example, we have learned from prior studies that the client must have occupational performance goals and sufficient language ability to participate in the goal-plan-do-check and problem-solving processes with the therapist. Although the CO-OP Approach™ has evolved into an evidence-based and theoretically based intervention model with demonstrated positive outcomes for people with certain conditions, the boundaries of the intervention in relation to physical and cognitive abilities, the nature of the injury or impairment, the length of time since onset, dosage, and specificity of intervention format are still being tested.

Dissatisfied with the lack of generalization to skilled action, occupational therapists Helene Polatajko and Angela Mandich turned to literature about growing understanding of motor control and skill learning to develop a highly individualized metacognitive approach to help children master motor skills for real world performance. The CO-OP Approach™ is an occupation-based, client-centered, metacognitive, performance-based, and evidence-based intervention that combines motor learning principles with other theories that emphasize the role of cognitive processes and goal setting in developing movement skills.

The CO-OP Approach™ is an example of a theory-based intervention informed by multiple theoretical perspectives from a range of disciplines, including behavioral and cognitive psychology, education, human movement science, and OT. The original purpose of the intervention was to teach children to use cognitive strategies that support skill acquisition through a process of guided discovery.

The CO-OP Approach™ might be an effective intervention to help Alex achieve his goals to play baseball, shuffle playing cards, and type on the computer. The overarching broad assumption of the CO-OP Approach™ is that successful participation in everyday occupation is essential to health and well-being. Figure 41-1 provides a general overview of the key theoretical propositions and essential and structural elements of the CO-OP Approach™. The approach is composed of seven key features: client-chosen goals, dynamic performance analysis, cognitive strategy use, guided discovery, enabling principles, significant other involvement, and intervention format. Table 41-3 presents the if/then statements for the key theoretical propositions.

Based on principles of motor learning and goal setting, the therapist would help Alex to identify goals and discover the relevant aspects of the task, examine how he is currently performing the task, identify where he is getting "stuck," and generate alternative solutions. Bandura (1997) noted that children's actual experiences performing an activity contribute to their self-perceptions and that when children set their own goals, they feel more empowered to work toward achieving their goals. A global strategy is used to provide a consistent framework to help Alex discover task-specific strategies. This structure was based on the problem-solving structure first described by Luria (1976), who drew from Vygotsky's (1967) observation of problem-solving attempts of children, and then further developed by Meichenbaum (1977), a psychologist now known as the founder of cognitive behavioral modification therapy. Meichenbaum adopted a rubric, known as "goal-plan-do-check," originally developed by educators Camp and Bash (1982) for helping aggressive boys to use problem-solving techniques in social situations. In addition to the global problem-solving strategy proposed by Meichenbaum, occupational therapist Angela Mandich (Mandich, Polatajko, Missiuna, & Miller, 2001), who was a graduate student at the time Polatajko and her colleagues were developing the CO-OP Approach™, identified eight domain-specific strategies directly related to specific task performance problems. Mandich proposed that task knowledge and cognitive strategies specific to the performance challenges were necessary "mechanisms of action" to support children's competence in their desired occupations. Informed by principles of mediated learning described by educators Feuerstein, Hoffman, Jensen, Tzuriel, and Hoffman (1986)

and Haywood (1988), the OT structures the environment by asking probing questions to facilitate Alex's awareness and reflection on his performance. Once Alex identifies a helpful strategy, the therapist uses questions to help Alex think about how he might apply or generalize the strategy to other situations.

Figure 41-2 provides a conceptual mapping of what the practitioner actually does to implement the CO-OP Approach™ in a way that reflects the theoretical propositions. We could actually test the propositions of the theory by observing the therapist's actions and Alex's responses. For example, to test the proposition related to goal setting, we could observe the therapist asking Alex to identity three skills that he needs, wants, or is expected to do at school, home, or when playing. We could determine whether Alex increases his efforts to catch a small ball after setting a goal focused on ball catching.

The intervention process is dynamic and continuously changes over time as we learn more and reflect on our initial propositions. As we continue to work with Alex to achieve his goals, we are constantly reflecting on and examining our intervention approaches to determine if they are effective. If the approach is not effective, we must be open to changing or adapting the approach. We might discover that, for Alex, verbalizing the strategies to prompt the motor movement is only effective when there are no other distracters in the immediate context. Based on this ongoing examination of the intervention, we might modify the context as distracting stimuli emerged as an important element influencing Alex's performance. We might also discover the CO-OP Approach™ works well with Alex, but that does not mean that we stop reflecting on the propositions because the research evidence is constantly evolving and our understanding of the causal relationships may also change. For example, Batte and Polatajko (2006) analyzed videotapes of children during the CO-OP Approach™ and other intervention approaches to determine the role of practice in skill acquisition. Because the CO-OP Approach™ is a cognitive-based intervention, the children who received the CO-OP Approach™ spent more intervention time discussing performance. The children who received other interventions had more practice time than the children receiving the CO-OP Approach™. Yet, the children who received the CO-OP Approach™ showed significantly greater gains in performance, illustrating that strategy use, in addition to practice, is an important "mechanism of action" in the CO-OP Approach™. Such research evidence helps us clarify what to do in the intervention process. As the research evolves, the theoretical propositions also evolve (Miller, Polatajko, Missiuna, Mandich, & Macnab, 2001). Therefore, the question we must always ask is "Is there a basis to what I'm doing in the intervention that is supported by theory and evidence?"

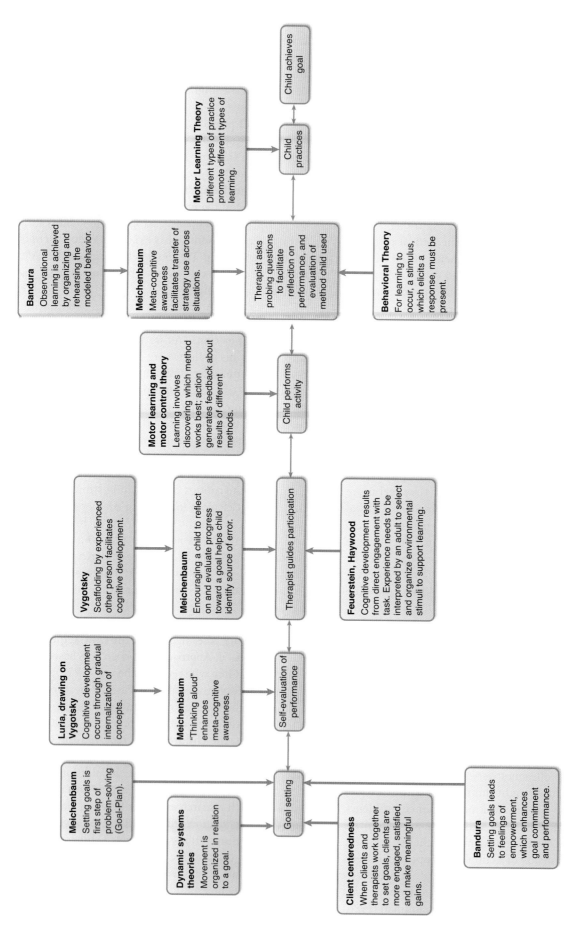

FIGURE 41-1 Theoretical propositions and key features of the Cognitive Orientation to Daily Occupational Performance (CO-OP Approach™).

| TABLE 41-3 | Theoretical Propositions and If/Then Statements of the CO-OP Approach™ |

Intervention Feature	If/Then Statements from Key Theories
Essential Elements: Key Elements to Be Considered in the CO-OP Approach™	
Goal setting: client-chosen, occupation-based goals	If a movement is directed toward a goal, then that movement will be organized uniquely in relation to that goal.
	If the person is collaboratively engaged in setting a goal, then his or her problem-solving process in relation to that goal will be facilitated.
	If the person is collaboratively engaged in setting a goal, then he or she will experience increased self-efficacy.
	If the person's self-efficacy is increased, then his or her motivation and commitment to the goal will be enhanced.
Dynamic performance analysis: dynamic (on-going), analytical process of identifying performance problems that engages both the practitioner and the client; initially led by therapist and then becomes collaborative	If a person can identify performance problems and where the performance is breaking down, then this information can be used to guide the person to discover, learn, and apply strategies to support performance.
Cognitive strategy use: goal-directed and consciously controlled cognitive processes that facilitate or support performance and skill acquisition. Strategies may be global (general) or domain (task) specific.	If a person engages in talking aloud while attempting to solve a problem (cognitive scaffolding), then awareness of his or her performance will be enhanced.
	If a person develops strategies to address the challenges/sources of error, then using the strategies will develop competence in the desired activity.
	If a person engages in talking aloud while attempting to solve a problem, then the problem-solving process will be facilitated.
	If a person engages in self-evaluation of performance, he or she will develop a structure for self-monitoring (check) and evaluating performance.
Guided discovery: Practitioner asks logical and sequential questions that guide client to discover a concept, rule, principle, or action to support performance that was not previously known.	If a more experienced person guides and supports (scaffolds) a learner who is attempting to solve a problem, then the learner's problem-solving capacity (cognitive development) will be enhanced.
	If the therapist asks appropriate questions, then the child's ability to identify effective strategies will be enhanced.
	If an adult models the thinking process to be mastered and if the child repeats the steps of that process aloud, then the child's learning of the process will be enhanced.
Enabling principles based on learning and motor behavior: instructional and feedback methods that promote learning, facilitate goal attainment, promote generalization and transfer	If the child performs an activity, then he or she will receive meaningful feedback about the results of a particular approach to the activity.
	If the therapist engages the child in "thinking out loud" about his or her performance, then the child's ability to evaluate the effectiveness of his or her strategies will be enhanced.
Structural Elements: Key Elements That Are Preferred or Suggested, May Be Altered to Meet Specific Needs of Person, Practice Setting, or Other Factors	
Parent or support person involvement: Important people in the client's life are aware of and use guided discovery and enabling principles outside the intervention environment.	If people important to the client's real-world performance can use guided discovery and enabling principles in a range of environments, then the client will continue skill development beyond the intervention environment.
Intervention format: Setting, number of intervention sessions, and sequence of sessions may vary. Sessions may be group or individual, delivered in person or by telerehabilitation.	If the intervention includes the essential elements specified by the CO-OP Approach™, then the number and sequence of sessions may vary to meet client needs.

Sources: Based on Polatajko, H., McEwen, S., Dawson, D. R., & Skidmore, E. R. (2017). Cognitive orientation to daily occupational performance. In M. Curtin, M. Egan, & J. Adams (Eds.), *Occupational therapy for people experiencing illness, injury or impairment: Promoting occupation and participation* (7th ed., pp. 636–647). Toronto, Canada: Elsevier; and Skidmore, E., McEwen, S., Green, D., van den Houten, J., Dawson, D., & Polatajko, H. (in press). Essential elements and key features of the CO-OP Approach™. In D. Dawson, S. McEwen, & H. Polatajko (Eds.), *Enabling participation across the lifespan: Advancements, adaptations and extensions of the CO-OP Approach*. Bethesda, MD: AOTA Press.

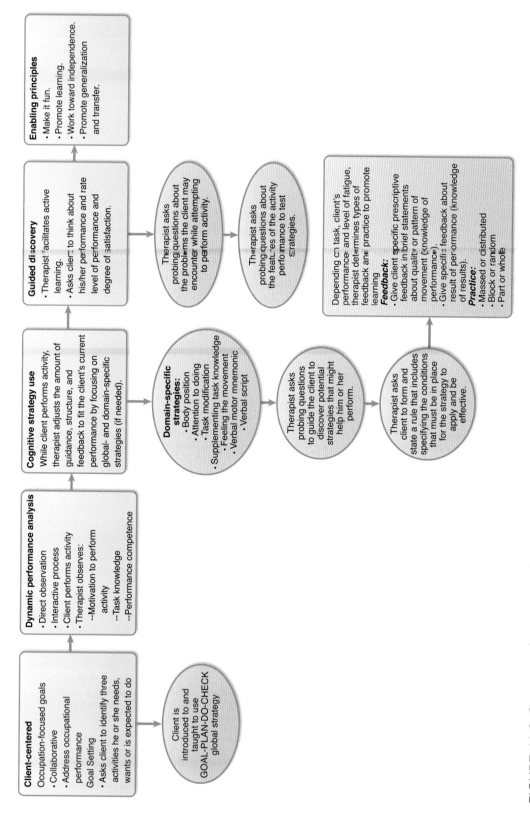

FIGURE 41-2 Conceptual mapping of practitioner's actions.

Occupational Therapy Task-Oriented Approach

Let's consider another scenario and another theoretical approach, the Occupational Therapy Task-Oriented Approach for people who have had stroke, developed by occupational therapists Virgil Mathiowetz and Julie Bass-Haugen (1994). The Occupational Therapy Task-Oriented Approach is another example of a theory and evidence-based intervention informed by multiple theoretical perspectives from a range of disciplines. During the early 1990s, many researchers began to question the assumptions and propositions of theories of motor development (Thelen & Ulrich, 1991) and motor behavior change (Jongbloed, Stacey, & Brighton, 1989; Sabari, 1991). Therapists were using interventions based on assumptions such as (1) the CNS is hierarchically organized, (2) normal movement can be facilitated by providing specific patterns of sensory input, and (3) recovery from brain damage follows a predictable sequence. Clients were not making desired changes, and practitioners were searching for a better understanding of the challenges clients presented. Therapists and clients were particularly dissatisfied that retraining of normal movement patterns did not result in carryover to functional daily living skills.

The Occupational Therapy Task-Oriented Approach includes assumptions and propositions from broad OT theories, a systems model of motor control, an ecological approach to perception and action, and dynamic systems theory. This multidisciplinary approach represents understanding of motor control and learning from the neuropsychological, biomechanical, and behavioral sciences. An overarching assumption of the Occupational Therapy Task-Oriented Approach is that movement is organized around a goal and influenced by the environment. Movement emerges as an interaction among many systems, each contributing to motor control.

The term *task-oriented approach* was first proposed by a physical therapist at a professional conference focused on contemporary management of motor control problems (Horak, 1991). Occupational therapists revised the task-oriented approach to consider task performance in relation to a person's valued life roles. The inclusion of role performance in the Occupational Therapy Task-Oriented Approach is based on Trombly's (1995) proposition that to engage satisfactorily in a life role, a person must be able to do the activities and tasks that, in the person's opinion, make up that role. As research and theories have evolved, the Occupational Therapy Task-Oriented Approach continues to evolve and become more discrete as new research helps us refine the specific mechanisms of action (Bass-Haugen, Mathiowetz, & Flinn, 2008; Mathiowetz, 2011; Preissner, 2010).

As we examine the Occupational Therapy Task-Oriented Approach, consider Case Study 41-2 and how a

CASE STUDY 41-2   PABLO

Pablo, a 52-year-old successful businessman, had a right middle cerebral artery stroke with resulting left-sided weakness and decreased balance 3 weeks ago. He lives with his wife and two sons, ages 11 and 13 years. Pablo loves to cook food from his Ecuadorian homeland for his family. He is eager to regain function so he can return to his job as a financial consultant. His family enjoys sledding with his children in the winter and camping in the summer—activities he hopes to continue. How will the occupational therapist use theory to guide his or her reasoning about the best possible intervention for Pablo?

The occupational therapist begins the evaluation by focusing on Pablo's roles and then proceeds to identify his priorities and goals for intervention. First, the therapist administers the Role Checklist (Oakley, Kielhofner, Barris, & Reichler, 1986), a self-report measure to assess roles significant to Pablo and his motivation to engage in tasks or activities necessary to fulfill valued roles. The practitioner may discuss with Pablo and his wife which roles Pablo had before his stroke and which roles he wants or must do in the future. Together, Pablo, his wife, and the practitioner identify goals for OT intervention. The initial emphasis on role performance

is congruent with Trombly's (1995) theoretical propositions that to satisfactorily engage in a life role, a person must be able to do the activities and tasks that, in the person's opinion, make up that role and that clients who are actively engaged in their treatment achieve self-identified goals and better outcomes. These initial evaluation and goal-setting processes are also supported by propositions from client-centered perspectives: When clients and therapist work together to achieve goals, clients are more engaged, are satisfied, and make meaningful gains.

After discussing Pablo's important life roles and his goals for OT, Pablo and the occupational therapist decide to try making a fruit drink in the OT department kitchen in the rehabilitation hospital. As Pablo cuts a papaya, the occupational therapist notices that Pablo places his left arm on the table to stabilize the bowl as he puts the cut-up pieces of papaya in the bowl. When cued to use his left hand, he tries to pick up a mango, but the mango drops to the floor because Pablo's grasp is too weak to hold the mango. The therapist then completes performance-based assessments to determine if Pablo has the necessary performance skills to complete desired tasks.

practitioner working with Pablo following a stroke might adopt the Occupational Therapy Task-Oriented Approach to inform his or her reasoning related to evaluation and intervention.

The OT practitioner also uses the Occupational Therapy Task-Oriented Approach to guide Pablo's intervention. The emphasis of intervention is on enabling clients to successfully engage in tasks and activities associated with the roles and occupations clients are expected to, need to, or want to fulfill; purposeful and meaningful tasks are the primary intervention modality. The practitioner believes that the Occupational Therapy Task-Oriented Approach might be an effective intervention to help Pablo achieve his goals to cook, return to work, and enjoy outdoor activities with his family. The overarching assumptions of the Occupational Therapy Task-Oriented Approach are presented in Box 41-2.

Figure 41-3 provides a general overview of the key theoretical propositions and features of the Occupational Therapy Task-Oriented Approach. Table 41-4 presents if/then statements for the key theoretical propositions outlined in Figure 41-3.

Following an assessment of Pablo's performance in relation to desired tasks and activities, the therapist and Pablo will consider whether to develop compensatory approaches for challenging tasks or attempt to remediate skills necessary for successful task completion. Based on dynamical systems theory, the therapist continuously analyzes the critical control parameters—personal and environmental variables—that may have potential to impact task performance. A review of available evidence will support the practitioner's reasoning regarding the probability of changing a control parameter to support performance. The dynamic systems perspective that proposes that movement is organized in relation to a goal echoes the propositions informed by other theoretical perspectives. Together, these theoretical perspectives inform the practitioner's actions with Pablo. It is possible to test these propositions, and numerous researchers have conducted studies to demonstrate support for these propositions (for one example, see Trombly, Radomski, & Davis, 1998).

At first glance, the CO-OP Approach™ and the Occupational Therapy Task-Oriented Approach appear quite similar because both approaches are based on the proposition that if a person is engaged in the process of setting goals for intervention based on his or her values and preferences, he or she will engage in more effective problem solving and be more motivated to engage in the intervention activities. Guided practice with specific feedback is another common feature of the two approaches. Yet, the CO-OP Approach™ is informed by metacognitive theories, whereas the Occupational Therapy Task-Oriented Approach is derived from motor learning and behavioral control theories; thus, the discrete propositions are different; intervention strategies, the resulting therapist actions, and expected outcomes might differ. Baking cookies and a cake provide a useful metaphor for capturing this distinction. We might use the ingredients of flour, sugar, and butter in preparing both cake and cookies. Yet, in order to achieve our goal or desired outcome, we need to use the appropriate amount or dose of ingredients, perhaps select among different forms of the ingredients, add other unique ingredients, and introduce the ingredients in a particular order or sequence. In contrast to baking, OT is a complex and dynamic process, and the outcome being sought is unique to each client. This complexity requires a unique approach for each client that is constructed and continually revised through application of the therapist's professional reasoning. In order to ensure that one's intervention is optimally suited to the client's capacities and effective to achieve the client's goals, the therapist must continually articulate and examine the assumptions and propositions underlying his or her actions and be prepared to revise his or her approach when desired outcomes are not achieved or the evidence does not support the reasoning.

BOX 41-2 **ASSUMPTIONS OF OCCUPATIONAL THERAPY TASK-ORIENTED APPROACH**

- Personal and environmental systems, including the CNS, are heterarchically organized.
- Functional tasks help organize behavior.
- Occupational performance emerges from the interaction of persons and their environment.
- Experimentation with various strategies leads to optimal solutions to motor problems.
- Recovery is variable because patient factors and environmental contexts are unique.
- Behavioral changes reflect attempt to compensate to achieve task performance.

CNS, central nervous system.

Conclusion

Within OT, some of our interventions and treatment theories are more developed than others. As we develop a more refined understanding of the causal relationships represented in our intervention theories and deconstruct how the intervention works, we can be more precise in our intervention. We can also articulate the basis of what

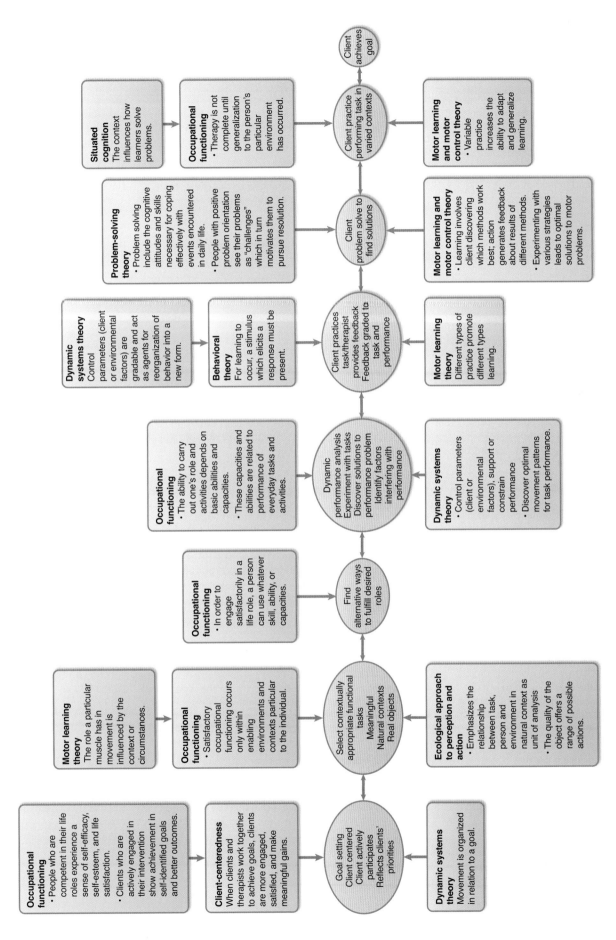

FIGURE 41-3 General overview of Occupational Therapy Task-Oriented Approach.

TABLE 41-4 Theoretical Propositions and If/Then Statements of the Occupational Therapy Task-Oriented Approach

Intervention Feature	If/Then Statements from Key Theories	Evidence to Support Proposition
Goal setting: client guides selection of tasks for intervention • Client-centered • Intervention reflects client's priorities. • Elicit active participation of client	If the client sets goals for intervention, then he or she will be more engaged in intervention and achieve desired outcomes.	Law, Babtiste, and Mills (1995) Law and Mills (1998) Siegert and Taylor (2004) Trombly (1995)
Functional and meaningful tasks	If the task is functional and meaningful to the client, then quality of movement during execution of the task will be better.	Lin, Wu, Tickle-Degnen, and Coster (1997) Wu, Wong, Lin, and Chen (2001)
Natural context (if rehabilitation setting, should simulate real-life setting as much as possible)	If the intervention is provided in a natural context, then clients will develop more flexible movement patterns for the task and context.	Bernstein (1967) Burgess (1989) Gillen and Wasserman (2004)
Real objects	If a person uses real objects, rather than rote exercise without objects, then quality of movement will be better.	Mathiowetz and Wade (1995) Nelson et al. (1996) Wu, Trombly, Lin, and Tickle-Degnen (2000)
Help clients adjust to role and task performance limitations	If clients can find alternative ways to fulfill roles or perform associated tasks, then they will be able to continue desired roles.	Trombly (1995)
Dynamic performance analysis • Experiment with functional tasks to discover efficient strategies for optimal solutions to performance problems. • Identify salient client or environmental factors interfering with effective and efficient task performance	If the client experiments with functional activities, then he or she will discover the most effective and efficient way to perform task. If a client factor (e.g., strength, sensation) is critical to occupational performance of desired task and there is potential to change that factor, then remedial techniques should be used. If a client, after a stroke, has active wrist and finger extension in the involved extremity, then the client is likely to benefit from constraint-induced movement therapy (CIMT). • If a client has active extension of the wrist >10° starting at neutral, some active abduction of the carpometacarpal (CMC) joint of thumb and 10° of active extension in elbow flexion, then the client is likely to benefit from modified constraint-induced therapy (mCIT). If remediation is unlikely, then adaptive and compensatory approaches should be used.	Bonaiuti, Rebasti, and Sioli (2007) Flinn (1995) Gillen (2002) Van Peppen et al. (2004)
Adapt task to promote optimal performance	Changing task and environmental characteristics can elicit changes in the client's movement forms and patterns.	Davis and Burton (1991)
Client practices task and therapist provides feedback to facilitate learning. • Feedback graded to task and performance	If the therapist provides graded feedback for the type of task and client performance, then the client will learn the task. If the feedback is gradually tapered, then the client will learn how to use his or her own feedback mechanisms to monitor and evaluate his or her own performance.	Crutchfield and Barnes (1993)
Problem-solve with client	If the client can break down the task and problem-solve on his or her own, then he or she will be more likely to generate solutions in other contexts and environments.	D'Zurilla & Nezu (2007) Elliott (1999)
Practice performing tasks outside of therapy context • Follow-up	If the client uses abilities discovered in therapy in varied contexts, then abilities will become more automatic.	Gillen and Wasserman (2004) Trombly (1995)

we are doing more clearly to others. Thus, for example, we can explain to Pablo how the activities he is engaging in during an intervention session relate to achieving the goal he has set for himself or explain to the supervisor why we expect CO-OP Approach™ to be more effective for Alex than simple practice of desired skills with feedback. It is our professional responsibility to continually examine the assumptions and theoretical propositions guiding our intervention approaches so that we can improve practice and achieve desired outcomes for clients.

REFERENCES

American Occupational Therapy Association. (2014). Occupational therapy practice framework: Domain and process (3rd edition). *American Journal of Occupational Therapy, 68*(Suppl. 1), S1–S48. doi:10.5014/ajot.2014.682006

Ayres, A. J. (1972). *Sensory integration and learning disorders.* Los Angeles, CA: Western Psychological Services.

Bandura, A. (1997). *Self-efficacy: The exercise of control.* New York, NY: W. H. Freeman.

Bass-Haugen, J., Mathiowetz, V., & Flinn, N. (2008). Optimizing motor behavior using the occupational therapy task-oriented approach. In M. V. Radomski & C. A. T. Latham (Eds.), *Occupational therapy for physical dysfunction* (6th ed., pp. 598–617). Philadelphia, PA: Lippincott Williams & Wilkins.

Batte, M., & Polatajko, H. J. (2006). *CO-OP vs. practice for children with developmental coordination disorder: A question of strategy* (Unpublished dissertation). University of Toronto, Canada.

Baum, C. M., & Christiansen, C. H. (2005). Person-environment-occupation-performance: An occupation-based framework for practice. In C. H. Christiansen, C. M. Baum, & J. Bass-Haugen (Eds.), *Occupational therapy: Performance, participation, and well-being* (pp. 242–266). Thorofare, NJ: SLACK.

Bernstein, N. (1967). *The coordination and regulation of movements.* Elmsford, NY: Pergamon Press.

Bonaiuti, D., Rebasti, L., & Sioli, P. (2007). The constraint induced movement therapy: A systematic review of randomized controlled trials on the adult stroke patients. *Europa Medicophysica, 43,* 139–146.

Bronfenbrenner, U. (1979). *The ecology of human development: Experiments by nature and design.* Cambridge, MA: Harvard University Press.

Burgess, M. K. (1989). Motor control and the role of occupational therapy: Past, present, and future. *American Journal of Occupational Therapy, 43,* 345–348.

Camp, B. W., & Bash, M. S. (1982). *Think aloud: Increasing social and cognitive skills—a problem solving program for children: Primary level.* Champaign, IL: Research Press.

Crutchfield, C. A., & Barnes, M. R. (1993). *Motor control and motor learning in rehabilitation.* Atlanta, GA: Stokesville.

Davis, W. E., & Burton, A. W. (1991). Ecological task analysis: Behavior theory into practice. *Adapted Physical Activity Quarterly, 8,* 154–177.

Dunn, W., Brown, C., & McGuian, M. (1994). The ecology of human performance: A framework for considering the effect of context. *American Journal of Occupational Therapy, 48,* 595–607.

D'Zurilla, T., & Nezu, A. (2007). *Problem-solving therapy: A positive approach to clinical intervention* (3rd ed.). New York, NY: Springer.

Elliott, T. R. (1999). Social problem-solving abilities and adjustment to recent-onset spinal cord injury. *Rehabilitation Psychology, 44,* 315–332.

Feuerstein, R., Hoffman, M., Jensen, M., Tzuriel, D., & Hoffman, D. (1986). Learning to learn: Mediated learning experiences and instrumental enrichment. *Special Services in Schools, 3,* 48–82.

Flinn, N. (1995). A task-oriented approach to the treatment of a client with hemiplegia. *American Journal of Occupational Therapy, 49,* 560–569.

Gibson, J. J. (1979). *The ecological approach to visual perception.* Boston, MA: Houghton Mifflin.

Gillen, G. (2002). Improving mobility and community access in an adult with ataxia. *American Journal of Occupational Therapy, 56,* 462–466.

Gillen, G., & Wasserman, M. (2004). Mobility: Examining the impact of environment on transfer performance. *Physical and Occupational Therapy in Geriatrics, 22,* 21–29.

Haywood, H. C. (1988). Bridging: A special technique of mediation. *The Thinking Teacher, 4,* 4–5.

Hooper, B. (1997). The relationship between pretheoretical assumptions and clinical reasoning. *American Journal of Occupational Therapy, 51,* 328–338.

Horak, F. B. (1991). Assumptions underlying motor control for neurologic rehabilitation. In M. J. Lister (Ed.), *Contemporary management of motor control problems: Proceeding of the II STEP conference* (pp. 11–27). Alexandria, VA: Foundation for Physical Therapy.

Jongbloed, L., Stacey, S., & Brighton, C. (1989). Stroke rehabilitation: Sensorimotor integrative treatment versus functional treatment. *American Journal of Occupational Therapy, 43,* 391–397.

Kielhofner, G. (2008). *The model of human occupation: Theory and application* (4th ed.). Philadelphia, PA: Lippincott Williams & Wilkins.

Kielhofner, G., & Burke, J. P. (1980). A model of human occupation, part 1. Conceptual framework and content. *American Journal of Occupational Therapy, 54,* 572–581.

Law, M., Babtiste, S., & Mills, J. (1995). Client-centered practice: What does it mean and does it make a difference? *Canadian Journal of Occupational Therapy, 62,* 250–257.

Law, M., Cooper, B., Strong, S., Stewart, D., Rigby, P., & Letts, L. (1996). The person-environment-occupational model: A transactive approach to occupational performance. *Canadian Journal of Occupational Therapy, 63,* 9–23.

Law, M., & Mills, J. (1998). Client-centered occupational therapy. In M. Law (Ed.), *Client-centered occupational therapy* (pp. 1–18). Thorofare, NJ: SLACK.

Lawton, M. P. (1986). *Environment and aging* (2nd ed.). Albany, NY: Plenum Press.

Lin, K., Wu, C., Tickle-Degnen, L., & Coster, W. (1997). Enhancing occupational performance through occupationally embedded exercise: A meta-analytic review. *Occupational Therapy Journal of Research, 17,* 25–47.

Luria, A. R. (1976). *Cognitive development: Its cultural and social foundations.* Cambridge, MA: Harvard University Press.

Mandich, A., Polatajko, H. J., Macnab, J. J., & Miller, L. T. (2001). Treatment of children with developmental coordination disorder: What is the evidence? *Physical and Occupational Therapy in Pediatrics, 20,* 51–68.

Mandich, A. D., Polatajko, H. J., Missiuna, C., & Miller, L. T. (2001). Cognitive strategies and motor performance in children with developmental coordination disorder. *Physical and Occupational Therapy in Pediatrics, 20*(2–3), 125–143.

Mathiowetz, V. (2011). Task-oriented approach to stroke rehabilitation. In G. Gillen (Ed.), *Stroke rehabilitation* (pp. 80–99). St. Louis, MO: Elsevier Mosby.

Mathiowetz, V., & Bass-Haugen, J. (1994). Motor behavior research: Implications for therapeutic approaches to CND dysfunction. *American Journal of Occupational Therapy, 48,* 733–745.

Mathiowetz, V. G., & Wade, M. (1995). Task constraints and functional motor performance of individuals with and without multiple sclerosis. *Ecological Psychology, 7*, 99–123.

Meichenbaum, D. (1977). *Cognitive behaviour modification*. New York, NY: Plenum Press.

Miller, L. T., Polatajko, H. J., Missiuna, C., Mandich, A. D., & Macnab, J. J. (2001). A pilot trial of a cognitive treatment for children with developmental coordination disorder. *Human Movement Science, 20*, 183–210.

Nelson, D. L., Konosky, K., Fleharty, K., Webb, R., Newer, K., Hazboun, V. P., . . . Licht, B. C. (1996). The effects of an occupationally embedded exercise on bilaterally assisted supination in persons with hemiplegia. *American Journal of Occupational Therapy, 50*, 639–646.

Oakley, F., Kielhofner, G., Barris, R., & Reichler, R. (1986). The Role Checklist: Development and empirical assessment of reliability. *Occupational Therapy Journal of Research, 6*, 157–170.

Plautz, E. J., Milliken, G. W., & Nudo, R. J. (2000). Effects of repetitive motor training on movement representations in adult squirrel monkeys: Role of use versus learning. *Neurobiology of Learning and Memory, 74*, 27–55.

Polanyi, M. (2009). *The tacit dimension*. Chicago, IL: University of Chicago Press. (Original work published 1966)

Polatajko, H. J., Mandich, A. D., Missiuna, C., Miller, L. T., Macnab, J. J., Malloy-Miller, T., & Kinsella, E. A. (2001). Cognitive orientation to daily occupational performance (CO-OP): Part III—the protocol in brief. In C. Missiuna (Ed.), *Children with developmental coordination disorder: Strategies for success* (pp. 107–123). New York, NY: Haworth Press.

Polatajko, H., McEwen, S., Dawson, D. R., & Skidmore, E. R. (2017). Cognitive orientation to daily occupational performance. In M. Curtin, M. Egan, & J. Adams (Eds.), *Occupational therapy for people experiencing illness, injury or impairment: Promoting occupation and participation* (7th ed., pp. 636–647). Toronto, Canada: Elsevier.

Popper, K. (1959). *The logic of scientific discovery*. Oxford, United Kingdom: Basic Books.

Preissner, K. (2010). Use of the occupational therapy task-oriented approach to optimize the motor performance of a client with cognitive limitations. *American Journal of Occupational Therapy, 64*, 727–734. doi:10.5014/ajot.2010.08026

Sabari, J. S. (1991). Motor learning concepts applied to activity-based intervention with adults with hemiplegia. *American Journal of Occupational Therapy, 45*, 523–530.

Scammel, E. M., Bates, S. V., Houldin, A., & Polatajko, H. J. (2016). The Cognitive Orientation to Daily Occupational Performance (CO-OP): A scoping review. *Canadian Journal of Occupational Therapy, 83*, 216–225. doi:10.1177/0008417416651277

Siegert, R. J., & Taylor, W. J. (2004). Theoretical aspects of goal-setting and motivation in rehabilitation. *Disability and Rehabilitation, 26*, 1–8.

Skidmore, E., McEwen, S., Green, D., van den Houten, J., Dawson, D., & Polatajko, H. (in press). Essential elements and key features of the CO-OP Approach™. In D. Dawson, S. McEwen, & H. Polatajko (Eds.), *Enabling participation across the lifespan: Advancements, adaptations and extensions of the CO-OP Approach*. Bethesda, MD: AOTA Press.

Taub, E., Uswatte, G., & Pidikiti, R. (1999). Constraint-induced movement therapy: A new family of techniques with broad application to physical rehabilitation. *Journal of Rehabilitation Research and Development, 6*, 237–251.

Thelen, E., & Ulrich, B. D. (1991). Hidden skills. *Monographs of the Society for Research in Child Development, 56*, 1–98.

Theory. (2010). In *Merriam-Webster Online Dictionary*. Retrieved from http://www.merriam-webster.com/dictionary/theory

Trombly, C. A. (1995). Occupation: Purposefulness and meaningfulness as therapeutic mechanisms. *American Journal of Occupational Therapy, 49*, 960–972.

Trombly, C., Radomski, M. V., & Davis, E. S. (1998). Achievement of self-identified goals by adults with traumatic brain injury: Phase I. *American Journal of Occupational Therapy, 52*, 810–818.

Van Peppen, R. P., Kwakkel, G., Wood-Dauphinee, S., Hendriks, H. J., Van der Wees, P. J., & Dekker, J. (2004). The impact of physical therapy on functional outcomes after stroke: What's the evidence? *Clinical Rehabilitation, 18*, 833–862.

Vygotsky, L. S. (1967). Play and its role in the mental development of the child. *Soviet Psychology, 5*, 6–18.

Whyte, J. (2006). Using treatment theories to refine the designs of brain injury rehabilitation treatment effectiveness studies. *Journal of Head Trauma Rehabilitation, 21*, 99–106.

Wu, C., Trombly, C. A., Lin, K., & Tickle-Degnen, L. (2000). A kinematic study of contextual effects on reaching performance in persons with and without stroke: Influences of object availability. *Archives of Physical Medicine and Rehabilitation, 81*, 95–101.

Wu, C., Wong, M., Lin, K., & Chen, H. (2001). Effects of task goal and personal preference on seated reaching kinematics after stroke. *Stroke, 32*, 70–76.

The Model of Human Occupation

Kirsty Forsyth, Renée R. Taylor, Jessica M. Kramer, Susan Prior, Lynn Ritchie, Jane Melton

LEARNING OBJECTIVES

After reading this chapter, you will be able to:

1. Describe the personal factors addressed by the Model of Human Occupation and articulate how each concept affects occupational life.
2. Explain the environmental factors that are addressed by the Model of Human Occupation and articulate how each concept affects occupational life.
3. Identify dimensions of doing that the Model of Human Occupation uses to describe and examine a person's engagement in occupations.
4. Outline the steps of therapeutic reasoning in the Model of Human Occupation.
5. Articulate how change occurs in occupational therapy and identify client actions and therapeutic strategies that lead to change.
6. Analyze how the Model of Human Occupation can be applied to clients with various diagnoses across the life course in different practice contexts.

Stephen is a man in his mid-30s who was diagnosed with schizophrenia in his final year of university. Due to fluctuating mental health, he became socially withdrawn and, throughout his adulthood, was unable to secure paid employment. Stephen's mental health improved recently, and he is keen to obtain an employment. He self-referred to occupational therapy (OT) vocational rehabilitation program with the goal of returning to paid employment.

John is a 7-year-old boy who wants to be a computer engineer like his dad when he grows up. He lives at home with his parents and his brother. His family describes him as a lovable, endearing boy. However, John's schoolteacher raised concerns about his awkward movement within classroom, distractibility, and laborious handwriting. The concern was raised that if these issues are not resolved, John will not be able to keep up with his class peers in terms of academic performance. As a result, it was decided that John would benefit from a specialist OT assessment.

Each of these clients' OT practitioners chose to use the Model of Human Occupation (MOHO) to guide their intervention. In the course of this chapter, these cases are used to illustrate the theory and application of this model.

CENTENNIAL NOTES

Where Did Model of Human Occupation Come From?

The earliest debt of the Model of Human Occupation (MOHO) is owed to Mary Reilly and her graduate students who, over many years, developed the Occupational Behaviour Tradition in which MOHO has its roots. Gary Kielhofner was a latecomer to this community and inherited a rich tradition in which important themes and concepts were already identified. The MOHO was developed to transform Occupational Behaviour into concepts useful to OT *practice* inclusive of how to use the concepts within assessment and interventions. The MOHO first took shape in a rudimentary form in the process of Gary Kielhofner writing his master's thesis during which Linda Florey, Nancy Takata, and Phillip Shannon were important influences. Uncounted hours of conversation and debate between Gary Kielhofner, Janice Burke, numerous colleagues, and students resulted in shaping MOHO as it was originally published in *American Journal of Occupational Therapy* in 1980; Kielhofner, 1980a, 1980b; Kielhofner & Burke, 1980; Kielhofner & Igi, 1980). Janice's original work on spelling out the dimensions of personal causation became exemplary for elaborating other concepts in the model. Roann Barris had an important role in first extending the models view of the environment and later

collaborating to extend many other concepts. The MOHO was truly a community of effort from its origins with numerous authors bringing the first edition of the text to life in 1985 (Kielhofner, 1985), inclusive of Janice Burke, Gloria Furst, Marion Kavanagh, Fran Oakley, Jayne Shephard, Florence Clark, Sally Jackson, Jana Green, Betty Herlong Harlan, Kathy Kaplan, Ellen Koldner, Sue Hirsch Knox, Ruth Ellen Schlemm, Mike Lyons, Jeanne Madigan, Zoe Mailloux, Carole Lee McLellan, Peggy Neville, Joan Owens, Lillian Hoyle Parent, Joan Rogers, Charlotte Brasic Royeen, Cheryl Salz, Teena Snow, Cynthia Stabenow, and Janet Hawkins Watt.

Where Is Model of Human Occupation Now?

Evidence indicates that MOHO is now the most widely used occupation-based model in practice worldwide; 76% of occupational therapists make use of MOHO in their practice (Haglund, Ekbladh, Thorell, & Hallberg, 2000; Law & McColl, 1989; Lee, Taylor, Kielhofner, & Fisher, 2008; National Board for Certification in Occupational Therapy, 2004; Wilkeby, Pierre, & Archenholtz, 2006). Therapists report that MOHO allows them to have an occupation-focused practice, a clearer professional identity, provides a holistic view of clients, supports client-centered practice, and provides a useful structure for intervention planning (Lee et al., 2008).

Introduction

The MOHO (Kielhofner, 2008; Taylor, 2017) is an approach to OT practice that is occupation-focused (Pedretti & Early, 2001), theory-driven (Elenko, Hinojosa, Blount, & Blount, 2000), client-centered (Law, 1998), and evidence-based (Law et al., 1997). The MOHO was introduced 30 years ago by three practitioners seeking to articulate an approach to occupation-based intervention. They described MOHO as a theory to guide thinking about clients and the therapy process (Kielhofner, 1980a, 1980b; Kielhofner & Burke, 1980; Kielhofner, Burke, & Heard, 1980). Evidence indicates that MOHO is now the most widely used occupation-based model in practice worldwide (Haglund et al., 2000; Law & McColl, 1989; National Board for Certification in Occupational Therapy, 2004; Wilkeby et al., 2006). A national study of occupational therapists in the United States (Lee et al., 2008) indicated that 75.7% of therapists make use of MOHO in their practice. These therapists reported that MOHO allows them to have an occupation-focused practice and a clearer professional identity. They also reported that MOHO provides a holistic view of clients, supports

client-centered practice, and provides a useful structure for intervention planning (Lee et al., 2008).

The MOHO has been developed through the efforts of an international community of practitioners and scholars. It is supported by a substantial evidence base of well over 400 articles and chapters that present theoretical, applied, or research aspects of the model. This chapter provides a brief overview of this model's focus, theory, and resources for application in practice.

Why the Model of Human Occupation Is Needed?

The MOHO emerged at a time when the field was just beginning to rediscover the importance of occupation as an outcome and means of intervention. In the 1970s, when MOHO was being formulated as an approach to practice, most OT theory and practice focused on understanding and reducing impairment. The impetus for developing MOHO was the recognition that many factors beyond motor, cognitive, and sensory impairments contribute to difficulties in everyday occupation. These include occupational barriers posed by the physical and social environment, difficulties in choosing and finding meaning in occupations, and the challenge of maintaining positive involvement in life roles and routines. The MOHO was developed to address these factors.

Consequently, the MOHO concepts address (1) the motivation for occupation, (2) the routine patterning of occupations, (3) the nature of skilled performance, and (4) the influence of environment on occupation. These concepts serve as a framework for gathering data about a client's situation, enable therapists to identify the client's occupational strengths and limitations, and help therapists and clients plan and implement a course of OT. The MOHO is appropriate for clients with a wide range of impairments (physical, mental, cognitive, and sensory) throughout the life course.

The Model of Human Occupation Concepts

The MOHO explains how occupations are chosen, patterned, and performed (Kielhofner, 2008). The MOHO is concerned with how people participate in daily occupations and achieve a sense of competence and identity (Figure 42-1). The model begins with the idea that a person's characteristics and his or her environment are linked together when someone is engaged in an occupation. Moreover, the model asserts that motives, patterns of performance, and skills are maintained and changed through

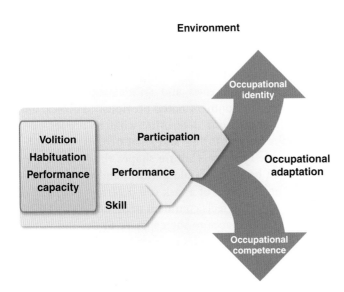

FIGURE 42-1 Model of Human Occupation concepts.

engagement in occupations. The MOHO understands OT as a process in which practitioners support client engagement in occupations in order to shape the clients' choices, their routine ways of doing things, and their skills.

Model of Human Occupation Concepts Related to the Person

To explain how occupations are chosen, patterned, and performed, MOHO conceptualizes people as composed of three interacting elements: volition, habituation, and performance capacity. The sections that follow discuss these elements.

Volition

Volition refers to the process by which people are motivated toward and choose what activities they do. The concept of volition asserts that all humans have a desire to engage in occupations and that this desire is shaped by previous experiences. Volition occurs in a cycle of anticipating possibilities for doing, choosing what to do, experiencing what one does, and subsequent interpretation of the experience. These thoughts and feelings are influenced by underlying personal factors, for example, how capable and effective one feels (called *personal causation*), what one holds as important (called *values*), and what one finds enjoyable and satisfying (called *interests*).

Personal causation refers to thoughts and feelings about one's abilities and effectiveness as he or she does everyday activities. These include, for example, recognizing one's strengths and weaknesses, feeling confident or anxious when faced with an occupation, and reflecting on how well one did after doing something.

Values are beliefs and commitments about what is good, right, and important to do. They include thoughts and feelings about activities that are worth doing, beliefs about the proper way to complete those activities, and the meanings that are ascribed to the things one does. Values specify what is worth doing, how to perform, and what goals or aspirations deserve commitment.

Interests develop through the experience of pleasure and satisfaction derived from occupational engagement (Matsutsuyu, 1969). Therefore, the development of interests depends on available opportunities to engage in occupations.

Volition has a pervasive influence on occupational life. Volition guides choices of what to do and determines the experience of doing. It shapes how people make sense of what they have done. Volition is also central to the OT process. All therapy requires that clients make choices to do things; therefore, it *must* engage clients' volition. Moreover, how clients experience what they do in therapy (a function of volition) to a large extent determines therapy outcomes.

Habituation

Habituation refers to a process whereby people organize their actions into patterns and routines. Through repeated action within specific contexts, people establish habituated patterns of doing. These patterns of action are governed by habits and roles, which shape how people go about the routine aspects of their lives.

Habits involve learned ways of doing things that unfold automatically. Habits operate in cooperation with context, using and incorporating the environment as a resource for doing familiar things. They influence how people perform routine activities, use time, and behave. For instance, habits shape how people intuitively go about self-care each morning, organize the weekly routine, and complete a familiar task.

Roles provide a cultural script for one's identity and provide a set of responsibilities and obligations that are associated with that identity. People see themselves as students, workers, and parents and recognize that they should behave in certain ways to fulfill these roles. Much of what people do is done as a spouse, parent, worker, or student. People learn how to acquire each of these roles successfully through the expectations that others have for a role and the social environment in which each role is located. Thus, through interaction with others, people internalize an identity and a way of behaving that is associated with each role they have internalized.

Habits and roles make up how people routinely interact with their physical and social environments. When habituation is challenged by impairments and/or environmental circumstances, people can lose a great deal of what has given life familiarity and consistency. One of the major tasks of therapy may be to reconstruct habits and roles so that the person can more routinely participate in life occupations within the everyday environment.

Performance Capacity

Performance capacity refers to a person's underlying mental and physical abilities and how those abilities are used and experienced in occupational performance. The capacity for performance is affected by the status of musculoskeletal, neurological, cardiopulmonary, and other bodily systems that are called on when a person does things. Biomechanical, motor control, cognitive, and sensory integration approaches to practice address these aspects of performance capacity that can be observed, measured, and modified (Ayres, 1979; Trombly & Radomski, 2001).

The MOHO recognizes the importance of approaches that address physical and mental capacities for occupational performance, and it is typically used in conjunction with such models. The MOHO stresses the importance of also paying attention to how people experience impairments. This includes paying attention to how people's bodies feel to them and how they perceive the world when they have impairments.

Model of Human Occupation Concepts Concerning the Environment

The MOHO stresses that all occupation results from an interaction of the person (volition, habituation, and performance capacity) with the characteristics of the physical and social environment. The **environment** can be defined as the particular physical, social, cultural, economic, and political features within a person's context that influence the motivation, organization, and performance of occupation. There are several dimensions of the environment that may have an impact on an individual's occupational life. For example, people encounter different physical spaces, objects, and people as well as expectations and opportunities for doing things. At the same time, the larger culture, economic conditions, and political factors also exert an influence. Accordingly, the environment includes the following dimensions:

- The objects that people use when they do things
- The spaces within which people do things
- The tasks that are available, expected, and/or required of people in a given context and that provide a set of social norms and conventions for engaging in recognizable occupations (such as "studying," "cleaning the house," or "playing cards")
- The social groups (e.g., family, friends, coworkers, neighbors) that make up the context and the expectations those social groups hold
- The surrounding culture, political, and economic forces

Objects and spaces together comprise the **physical environment**. The **social environment** includes both tasks and social groups.

The things that people do and how they think and feel about these things reflect a complex interplay of motives, habits and roles, and abilities with the dimensions of the environment noted previously. Political and economic conditions determine what resources people have for doing things and what occupational roles are available to them. Culture shapes the formation of ideas about how one should perform and what is worth doing. The demands of a task can determine the extent to which a person feels confident or anxious. The match of objects and spaces to the capacity of the individual influences how the person performs. In these and a myriad of other ways, the environment has an impact on what people do and how they think and feel about their doing. In turn, people also choose and modify their environments. For instance, people select environments that match and allow them to realize their values and interests.

Dimensions of Doing

As Figure 42-1 shows, MOHO identifies three levels at which we can examine a person's engagement in occupations: occupational participation, occupational performance, and occupational skill.

Occupational participation refers to engaging in work, play, or activities of daily living (ADL) that are part of one's sociocultural context and that are desired and/or necessary to one's well-being. This is the highest "level" of conceptualizing engagement in occupations. Examples of occupational participation are volunteering for an organization, working in a full- or part-time job, regularly getting together with friends, doing self-care, maintaining one's living space, and attending school. Each area of occupational participation involves a cluster of related tasks that one does. For example, participating to maintain one's living space may include paying the rent, doing repairs, and cleaning. Doing a task related to participation in a major life area is referred to as **occupational performance**.

During occupational performance, we carry out discrete purposeful actions. For example, making tea is a culturally recognizable task in many cultures. To do so, one *gathers* together tea, kettle, and a cup; *handles* these materials and objects; and *sequences* the steps necessary to brew and pour the tea. These actions that make up occupational performance of a task are referred to as skills. Skills are goal-directed actions that a person uses while performing (Forsyth, Salamy, Simon, & Kielhofner, 1998). In contrast to *performance capacity*, which refers to underlying ability (e.g., range of motion and strength), **skill** refers to the actions *within* an occupational performance such as reaching or sequencing. There are three types of skills: motor skills, process skills, and communication and interaction skills. Detailed taxonomies of each of the three types of skills have been developed (Bernspang & Fisher, 1995; Doble, 1991; A. Fisher & Kielhofner, 1995; Forsyth, Lai, & Kielhofner, 1999; Forsyth et al., 1998). See Chapter 26 for more detail on performance skills.

Occupational Identity, Competence, and Adaptation

Over time, what people do creates their **occupational identity**. This identity, generated from experience, is the cumulative sense of who people are and who they wish to become as occupational beings. The degree to which people are able to sustain a pattern of doing that enacts their occupational identity is referred to as **occupational competence**. These two essential elements of **occupational adaptation** entail the creation of an occupational identity and the ability to enact this identity in various circumstances.

The Process of Change and Therapy

A basic premise of MOHO is that all change in OT is driven by clients' occupational engagement. The term **occupational engagement** refers to clients' doing, thinking, and feeling under certain environmental conditions in the midst of therapy or as a planned consequence of therapy.

When clients engage in tasks in therapy or as a result of therapy, volition, habituation, and performance capacity are all involved in some way. For example, a client may be (1) drawing on performance capacity to exercise skill in occupational performance, (2) evoking old habits that shape how the occupational performance is done, (3) enacting or working toward acquiring a role, (4) experiencing a level of satisfaction and enjoyment (or dissatisfaction) with occupational performance, (5) assigning meaning and significance to what is done (i.e., what this means for the client's life), or (6) feeling able (or unable) when doing an occupation.

Each of these aspects of what the client does, thinks, and feels shapes the change process. For this reason, practitioners using MOHO are mindful of their clients' volition, habituation, performance capacity, and environmental conditions in the midst of therapy and how these elements are interacting as the therapy unfolds. To help practitioners think about the process of occupational engagement, MOHO identifies the nine dimensions of occupational engagement shown in Table 42-1. These nine dimensions provide a basic structure for thinking about how clients achieve change and for planning how therapy goals will be achieved. This process is discussed in the next section.

Using Model of Human Occupation in Practice: Steps of Therapeutic Reasoning

Using MOHO in practice involves thinking with its concepts—a process referred to as *therapeutic reasoning*. Therapeutic reasoning refers specifically to the use of MOHO concepts in thinking about clients' needs throughout the OT process (American Occupational Therapy Association, 2014). The therapeutic reasoning process has six steps:

1. Generating questions about the client
2. Gathering information on and with the client
3. Using the information gathered to create a theory-based explanation of the client's situation

TABLE 42-1   **Dimensions of Client Occupational Engagement**

Dimensions of Occupational Engagement	Definition
Choose/decide	Anticipate and select from alternatives for action.
Commit	Decide to undertake a course of action to accomplish a goal or personal project, fulfill a role, or establish a new habit.
Explore	Investigate new objects, spaces, social groups, and/or occupational forms/tasks; do things with altered performance capacity; try out new ways of doing things; and examine possibilities for occupational participation in one's context.
Identify	Locate novel information, alternatives for action, and new feelings that provide solutions for and/or give meaning to occupational performance and participation.
Negotiate	Engage in a give-and-take with others that creates mutually agreed-on perspectives and/or finds a middle ground between different expectations, plans, or desires.
Plan	Establish an action agenda for performance or participation.
Practice	Repeat a certain performance or consistently participate in an occupation with the intent of increasing skill, ease, and effectiveness of performance.
Reexamine	Critically appraise and consider alternatives to previously held beliefs, attitudes, feelings, habits, or roles.
Sustain	Persist in occupational performance or participation despite uncertainty or difficulty.

4. Generating goals and strategies for therapy
5. Implementing and monitoring therapy
6. Determining outcomes of therapy

Practitioners generally move back and forth between these steps over the course of therapy. Each step is briefly discussed below.

Generating Questions

Practitioners must come to understand their clients in order to plan and implement therapy. This understanding begins with asking questions about their clients (Table 42-2). The MOHO concepts allow a practitioner to generate these questions systematically. That is, the major concepts of the theory (environmental impact, volition, habituation, performance capacity, participation, performance, skills, occupational identity, and occupational competence) orient the practitioner to be concerned about certain things when learning about a client. For example, practitioners using MOHO would ask what their clients' thoughts and feelings are in relation to personal causation, values, and interests. Moreover, they would ask about their clients' roles and habits and how these affect the clients' routines. These questions would, of course, be tailored to the clients' circumstances.

Gathering Information

To answer the questions generated in the first step, practitioners must gather information on and with the client. Practitioners may take advantage of naturally occurring opportunities to gather information. For example, a practitioner might learn about a client's personal causation by observing the client's emotional reaction when attempting to learn a challenging new task. Practitioners may also use structured MOHO assessments. Some MOHO assessments will capture comprehensive information on several aspects of the person and the environment. Some MOHO assessments attempt to capture more in-depth information on one aspect of MOHO, such as assessments that focus on volition. A wide range of MOHO-based assessments has been developed; they are summarized in Table 42-3. Thus, practitioners using MOHO have a range of choices when they decide which assessment(s) to use. Some OT services have developed assessment protocols to indicate service response to assessment needs.

Creating a Theory-Based Understanding of the Client

The information that the practitioner gathers to answer questions about a client is used to create a theory-based understanding of that client. In this step, the practitioner uses MOHO theory as a framework for creating an explanation of that particular client's situation. As will be demonstrated in the cases of Stephen and John, the therapists use MOHO to create an explanation of each of these client's occupational circumstances to guide the next step of generating goals and strategies for therapy.

As part of creating an explanation of clients' circumstances, practitioners identify problems or challenges that need to be addressed in therapy as well as strengths that

TABLE 42-2 **Model of Human Occupation (MOHO)-Based Therapeutic Reasoning Questions**

MOHO Concept	Questions
Occupational identity	• What is the person's sense of who he or she has been, is, and wishes to become in relation to family life, school, friendships, hobbies, and interests? • What is the family's sense of who this person has been, is, and what do they wish him or her to become? How does this affect the person's occupational identity?
Occupational competence	• To what extent has this person sustained a pattern of satisfying occupational participation over time? • Does this person feel that he or she can do the things he or she needs to do in school, with friends, and in the community? • To what extent has this person's life sustained patterns of occupational participation over time that reflect his or her occupational identity?
Participation	• Does the person currently engage in work, play, and ADL that are part of his or her sociocultural context and that are desired and/or necessary for his or her well-being?
Performance	• Can this person do the occupations that are part of the work, play, and ADL that make up, or should make up, his or her life? • Can the person do the occupations that are expected of his or her roles?
Skill	• Does the person exhibit the necessary communication/interaction, motor, and process skills to perform what he or she needs and wants to do?
Environment	• Does the family support the person in developing the necessary volition, habituation and communication/interaction, motor, and process skills needed for participation? • What impact do the opportunities, resources, constraints, and demands (or lack of demands) of the environment have on how this person thinks, feels, and acts? • How do the opportunities, resources, constraints, or demands provided by spaces, objects, occupations/tasks, and social groups affect the person's skill, performance, and participation?
Volition	• What is this person's view of his or her personal capacity and effectiveness? • What does this person think is important? • What are this person's interests? What does this person enjoy doing?
Habituation	• What routines does this person participate in, and how do routines influence what he or she does? • What are the roles with which this person identifies with, and how do they influence what he or she routinely does?

ADL, activities of daily living.

can be drawn on in therapy. Problems and challenges may be a function of volition, habituation, performance capacity, or the environment.

Generating Measurable Goals and Strategies

This step involves creating therapy goals (i.e., identifying what will change as a result of therapy), deciding what kinds of occupational engagement will enable the client to change, and determining what kind of therapeutic strategies will be needed to support the client to change.

Goals (Table 42-4) indicate the kinds of changes that therapy will aim to achieve. Change is required when the client's characteristics and/or environment are contributing to occupational problems or challenges. For instance, if a client feels ineffective, therapy would seek to enable the client to feel more effective, or if a client has too few roles development of new roles would become the focus

of therapy. In this way, identifying challenges or problems in the third step allows one to select the goals in the fourth step.

The next element in this step is to identify how the goals will be achieved. This involves indicating what occupational engagement on the part of the client will contribute to achieving these goals and how the practitioner will support the client. The previous section on change offered nine dimensions of occupational engagement, and these serve as a framework for thinking in this step. The MOHO also identifies key therapeutic strategies that practitioners will use; these are listed in Box 42-1.

The fifth edition of *Kielhofner's Model of Human Occupation: Theory and Application* (Taylor, 2017) provides a comprehensive resource, the Therapeutic Reasoning Table, for this component of the therapeutic reasoning process. It identifies a wide range of problems and challenges that correspond to the concepts of MOHO along with types of changes that would be warranted. The table also indicates what types of occupational engagement

TABLE 42-3 **Model of Human Occupation (MOHO) Assessments Summary**

MOHO Assessment	Method of Administration	Description
Active in Children Health Integrating Evidence Valuing Experience (ACHIEVE) assessment (Forsyth, Whitehead, Owen, & Gorska, 2012)	Questionnaire, interview or observation	The assessment can be administered by mail or over the telephone and is completed by the child's teacher with a separate rating scale for the parent or guardian. It affords an opportunity for teachers or parents to share their view of how the child is participating in everyday activities. It asks for information on the frequency of their child's engagement in home, community, and school activity and then asks MOHO orientated questions as to why this engagement is positive or negative.
Assessment of Communication and Interaction Skills (ACIS) (Forsyth et al., 1998)	Observation	Gathers information about the communication and interaction skills that a person displays while engaged in an occupation across the domains of physicality, information exchange, and relations. Used to generate goals for therapy related to communication/interaction skills and to assess outcomes/changes in skill.
Assessment of Motor and Process Skills (AMPS) (A. G. Fisher, 2003)	Observation	Gathers information about the motor and process skills that a person displays while engaged in an occupation. Used to generate goals for therapy related to motor and process skills and to assess outcomes/changes in skill.
Assessment of Occupational Functioning-Collaborative Version (AOF-CV) (Watts, Hinson, Madigan, McGuigan, & Newman, 1999)	Interview and/or client self-report	Yields qualitative information and a quantitative profile of the impact of a client's personal causation, values, roles, habits, and skills on occupational participation. Used to inform intervention.
Child Occupational Self Assessment (COSA) (Keller, Kafkes, Basu, Federico, & Kielhofner, 2005)	Client self-report	Children and youths rate their occupational competence for engaging in 25 everyday activities in the home, school, and community and the importance of those activities. Used to generate goals and assess outcomes/change in competence and values.
Interest Checklist (Matsutsuyu, 1969)	Client self-report	Checklist that indicates strength of interest and past, present, and future engagement in 68 activities. Used to inform intervention.
Model of Human Occupational Screening Tool (MOHOST) (Parkinson, Forsyth, & Kielhofner, 2006)	Observation, interview(s), and/or chart review	Information gathered assesses impact of volition, habituation, skills, and environment on client's occupational participation. Used to generate goals and assess outcomes or changes in participation.
National Institutes of Health Activity Record (Frust, Gerber, Smith, Fisher, & Shulman, 1987; Gerber & Frust, 1992)	Client self-report	Self-report "log" records information in half-hour intervals throughout the day on perceptions of competence, value, enjoyment, difficulty, and pain experienced when engaging in various occupations in that time period. Used to inform intervention and assess outcomes or change in participation.
Occupational Circumstances Assessment Interview and Rating Scale (OCAIRS) (Forsyth et al., 2005)	Interview	Interview yields information to assess values, goals, personal causation, interests, habits, roles, skills, readiness for change, and environmental impact on participation. Used to generate goals and assess outcomes or changes in participation.
Occupational Performance History Interview-II (OPHI-II) (Kielhofner et al., 2004)	Interview	Detailed life history interview that yields (1) scales measuring competence, identity, and environmental impact and (2) a narrative representation/analysis of the life history. Used as an in-depth, comprehensive assessment to generate goals, inform intervention, and build the therapeutic relationship.
Occupational Therapy Psychosocial Assessment of Learning (OT PAL) (Townsend et al., 1999)	Observation or interview	This assessment evaluates a student's volition (the ability to make choices), habituation (roles and routines), and environmental fit within the classroom setting. The manual includes reproducible assessment and data summary forms.
Occupational Questionnaire (OQ) (Smith, Kielhofner, & Watts, 1986)	Client self-report	Self-report "log" records information in half-hour intervals throughout the day on perceptions of competence, value, and enjoyment experienced when engaging in various occupations in that time period. Used to inform intervention and assess outcomes or change in participation.
Occupational Self Assessment (OSA) (Baron, Kielhofner, Iyenger, Goldhammer, & Wolenski, 2006)	Client self-report	Clients rate their occupational competence for engaging in 21 everyday activities and the importance of those activities. Allows clients to set priorities for change. Used to generate goals and assess outcomes or change in competence and values.
Pediatric Interest Profiles (PIP) (Henry, 2000)	Client self-report	Assessment includes three age-appropriate scales (some with line drawings) for children and adolescents to indicate participation, interest, and perceived competence in various play and leisure activities. Used to generate goals and assess outcomes or changes in participation.
Pediatric Volitional Questionnaire (PVQ) (Basu, Kafkes, Geist, & Kielhofner, 2002)	Observation	Guides a systematic observation of a child across multiple environments to assess volition and the impact of the environment on volition. Used as an in-depth assessment of volition to generate goals and assess outcomes or change in volition.

TABLE 42-3 **Model of Human Occupation (MOHO) Assessments Summary (*continued*)**

MOHO Assessment	Method of Administration	Description
Residential Environment Impact Survey (REIS) (G. Fisher, Arriaga, Less, Lee, & Ashpole, 2008)	Observation or interview	Assesses how well the home environment is meeting the needs of the residents as a whole. Ratings in 24 areas provide a summary of the data and a structure for generating recommendations to enhance the qualities of the environment. The intent of this assessment tool is to not only assess the residential environment but also to determine the impact of the environment on the residents and to make recommendations to improve the quality of life for the residents and the work life of the staff.
Role Checklist (Oakley, Kielhofner, & Barris, 1985)	Client self-report	Checklist provides information on past, present, and future role participation and the perceived value of those roles. Used to inform intervention and assess outcomes or changes in role performance.
Short Child Occupational Profile (SCOPE) (Bowyer, Ross, Schwartz, Kielhofner, & Kramer, 2006)	Observation, interview(s), and/or chart review	Information gathered assesses impact of volition, habituation, skills, and environment on child's or adolescent's occupational participation. Used to generate goals and assess outcomes or changes in participation.
School Setting Interview (SSI) (Hemmingson, Egilson, Hoffman, & Kielhofner, 2005)	Interview	Interview works with students to gather information on student-environment fit and identify need for accommodations. Used to generate goals, inform intervention, and assess outcomes or changes in student-environment fit.
Volitional Questionnaire (VQ) (de las Heras, Lierena, & Kielhofner, 2003)	Observation	Guides a systematic observation of a client across multiple environments to assess volition and the impact of the environment on volition. Used as an in-depth assessment of volition to generate goals and assess outcomes or change in volition.
Worker Role Interview (WRI) (Braveman et al., 2005)	Interview	Interview yields information to rate the impact that volition, habitation, and perceptions of the environment have on psychosocial readiness for the worker role or return to work. Used to generate goals and assess outcomes or changes in psychosocial readiness for work.
Work Environment Impact Scale (WEIS) (Moore-Corner, Kielhofner, & Olson, 1998)	Interview	Interview works with client to assess environmental impact on participation in the worker role and to identify needed accommodations. Used to generate goals and inform intervention.

TABLE 42-4 **Model of Human Occupation (MOHO)-Based Therapy Goals: Examples**

MOHO Concept	Measurable Goal
Volition	Within [time frame], [client] will be *able to identify* (number of) occupations that are significant to his or her occupational life (or roles) and are consistent with his or her current skills and abilities [action] within [setting] independently [degree] Within [timeframe], [client] will *make the choice* to engage in (name occupation) having *identified* this as significant to his or her (successful performance of/or as a step in the progress toward) his or her performance as a (name role) [action] within [setting] with minimal support [degree]
Habituation	Within [time frame], [client] will be able to *identify* the responsibilities for roles that are valuable and meaningful to the person [action]; this will be achieved with minimal support [degree] within [setting] Within [time frame], [client] will be able to *practice* and develop a habit pattern that will support achievement of a single occupation [action]; this will be achieved with minimal support [degree] within [setting]
Skill	Within [time frame], [client] will be able to perform within (name the occupation) using (name skills) [action] within [setting], independently [degree] Within [time frame], [client] will be able to perform in (name the occupation) using adapted techniques to support lack of skill [action] within [setting], independently [degree]
Performance capacity	Within [time frame], [client] will be able to incorporate damaged or estranged parts of the body into completion of occupations [action], within [setting] independently [degree] Within [time frame], [client] will be able to manage symptoms while engaged in (name the occupations) [action] within [setting] independently [degree]
Environment	Within [time frame], [client] will be able to *perform* in (name the occupation) [action] within his or her physical and social home environment [setting], independently [degree] Within [time frame], [client] will be able to *perform* in the occupation using adapted objects or new objects [action] within [setting], independently [degree]

Adapted from Kielhofner, G. (2007). *A model of human occupation: Theory and application* (4th ed.). Baltimore, MD: Lippincott Williams & Wilkins.

BOX 42-1	THERAPEUTIC STRATEGIES IDENTIFIED BY MODEL OF HUMAN OCCUPATION

- **Validating:** Attending to and acknowledging the client's experience
- **Identifying:** Locating and sharing a range of personal, procedural, and/or environmental factors that can facilitate occupational performance
- **Giving feedback:** Sharing your understanding of the client's situation or ongoing action
- **Advising:** Recommending intervention goals/strategies
- **Negotiating:** Engaging in a give-and-take with the client

- **Structuring:** Establishing parameters for choice and performance by offering client alternatives, setting limits, establishing ground rules
- **Coaching:** Instructing, demonstrating, guiding, verbally and/or physically prompting
- **Encouraging:** Providing emotional support and reassurance in relation to engagement in an occupation
- **Providing physical support:** Using one's body to provide support for a client to complete an occupational form/task

could contribute to achieving those changes and what type of support from the practitioner could facilitate change. Table 42-5 shows one small section from this Therapeutic Reasoning Table related to personal causation.

Implementing and Monitoring Therapy

To implement therapy means not only following the plan of action that was set out in the previous step but also monitoring how the therapy process unfolds. This monitoring process might confirm the practitioner's understanding of the client's situation or require the practitioner to reformulate the client's situation. The monitoring process also can confirm the usefulness of therapy and whether a change to the goals and/or plan is required. When things do not turn out as expected, the practitioner returns to earlier steps of

generating questions, selecting methods to gather information, formulating the client's situation, setting goals, and establishing plans.

Collecting Information to Assess Outcomes

Determining therapy outcomes is an important final step in the therapy process. Typically, therapy outcomes are documented by examining the extent to which goals have been achieved and readministering structured assessments that were administered initially. Both of these approaches are valuable in documenting outcomes. Assessing outcomes by examining goal attainment is helpful in reflecting on the extent to which the therapeutic reasoning process resulted in good decisions for therapy. Using structured MOHO assessments also allows one to compare change

TABLE 42-5	Excerpt from the Therapeutic Reasoning Table Showing a Problem/Challenge Related to Personal Causation and Corresponding Intervention Goals and Strategies

Problem/Challenge	Goal	Client Occupational Engagement	Therapeutic Strategies to Support the Client
• Feelings of lack of control over occupational performance leading to anxiety (fear of failure) within occupations	• Reduce client's anxiety and fear of failure in occupational performance (e.g., "The client will complete a simple 3-step meal in 20 minutes without verbalizing anxiety or concern."). • Build up confidence to face occupational performance demands (e.g., "The client will identify and participate in 3 new leisure activities with minimal support in 1 week.").	• *Reexamine* anxieties and fears in the light of new performance experiences. • *Choose* to do relevant and meaningful things that are within performance capacity. • *Sustain* performance in occupational forms tasks despite anxiety.	• *Validate* how difficult it can be to do things that provoke anxiety. • *Identify* client's strengths and weaknesses in occupational performance. • Give *feedback* to client about match/mismatch between choice of occupational forms/tasks and performance capacity. • Give *feedback* to support a positive reinterpretation of his or her experience of engaging in an occupation. • *Advise* client to do relevant and meaningful things that match performance capacity.

From Kielhofner, G. (2008). *A model of human occupation: Theory and application* (4th ed.). Baltimore, MD: Lippincott Williams & Wilkins.

across different clients or when different strategies are used. In this way, they can contribute to evidence-based therapy.

Case Studies

Collecting Information and Creating a Theory-Based Understanding of Stephen

Who Is Stephen?

Stephen is in his mid-30s and lives with his parents. He is very close to his supportive parents and younger brother who lives in the same city. He described himself as a helpful son, supportive brother, loyal friend, and devoted dog owner. He enjoys the outdoors and sports, and he is currently unemployed.

Background

Stephen did well academically at school but became unwell and was diagnosed with schizophrenia in his final year of university. He left without completing his degree. Throughout this period, Stephen worked part-time in various jobs: retail, hospitality, and caregiving. He also volunteered in local day center for the elderly. Throughout his 20s, Stephen's mental health was poor with regular long admissions to hospital. He became socially withdrawn, only spending time with family members and health professionals; he rarely participated in swimming and running, which had previously been daily occupations. During this period, Stephen's family helped him find several temporary jobs in retail and catering, all of which he left due to deterioration in his mental health.

Recently, Stephen's mental health has improved, which he attributes to an improved medication regime. He is engaging in sporting activities and is keen to return to employment. In the past, he attended an OT prevocational training project where he participated in office administration tasks. His goal was to return to employment. He gradually built confidence and on discharge from the project and went on to a college course. He attained a vocational qualification in office administration but had been unable to secure employment.

The OT service provides an evidence-based vocational MOHO rehabilitation program, based on supported employment, where service users are supported to find a job quickly and rehabilitation is focused on maintaining the job ("place then train") as opposed to prevocational training ("train then place"). More information about the service is contained in *The WORKS: Occupational Therapy and Evidence Based Vocational Rehabilitation* (Prior, Forsyth, &

Ritchie, 2011). The service operates a self-referral system, and Stephen contacted the service with the goal of returning to paid employment.

Generating Questions

The occupational therapist was initially interested to explore Stephen's perceptions of his past, present, and future worker roles, including the following:

- What work activities does Stephen enjoy and value and how able does he feel doing these activities (volition)?
- How are his present roles and routines impacting on his engagement in work or impacting on work (habituation)?
- What level of support is offered in social and physical work environment?
- Stephen had not reported any specific challenges in motor, process, or communication and interaction skills, and therefore, early reflection on questions did not relate to these areas.

Gathering Information

The occupational therapist used the following assessment strategy to answer the previous questions:
    Initial assessment

- Worker Role Interview (WRI) (Braveman et al., 2005)—The assessment was administered during the initial meeting between the occupational therapist and Stephen (Figure 42-2).
- Work Environment Impact Scale (Moore-Corner et al., 1998)—The assessment was selected by the occupational therapist to complement information gathered through the WRI to better understand the impact that previous work environments have had on Stephen's participation in his worker role (Figure 42-3).

Creating a Theory-Based Understanding of the Client

The following occupational formulation was created from the assessment findings.

- *What is Stephen's occupational identity?* Stephen is a son, brother, friend, and dog owner. He is a regular runner and swimmer. Stephen recognizes himself as an unemployed person who is seeking work.
- *What is Stephen's occupational competence?* Stephen enjoys and feels competent in all roles he is currently pursuing. He reported a tendency to underestimate his abilities; the standards he applies to his own work performance usually exceed those of his colleagues and managers. This has interfered with Stephen's personal causation in relation to work and has led him to doubt his competence in previous work roles. However, given improvements in mental health and his strong work ethic, he is confident that he will succeed in a worker role.

Initial Assessment

Personal causation			Values		Interests		Roles		Habits			Environment			
Assesses Abilities & Limitations	Expectation of Success in Work	Takes Responsibility	Commitment to Work	Work Related Goals	Enjoys Work	Pursues Interests	Appraises Work Expectations	Influence of Others Roles	Work Habits	Daily Routines	Adapts Routine to Minimize Difficulties	Perception of Physical Work Setting	Perception of Family and Peers	Perception of Boss and/or Company	Perception of Co-workers
SS	**SS**	SS	**SS**	SS	**SS**	SS	**SS**	**SS**	SS	SS	SS	**SS**	**SS**	SS	SS
S	S	**S**	S	S	S	S	S	S	S	S	S	S	S	S	S
I	I	I	I	**I**	I	**I**	I	I	**I**	**I**	**I**	I	I	**I**	**I**
SI	SI	SI	SI	SI	SI	SI	SI	SI	SI	SI	SI	SI	SI	SI	SI
N/A	N/A	N/A	N/A	N/A	N/A	N/A	N/A	N/A	N/A	N/A	N/A	N/A	N/A	N/A	N/A

Outcome Assessment

Personal causation			Values		Interests		Roles		Habits			Environment			
Assesses Abilities & Limitations	Expectation of Success in Work	Takes Responsibility	Commitment to Work	Work Related Goals	Enjoys Work	Pursues Interests	Appraises Work Expectations	Influence of Others Roles	Work Habits	Daily Routines	Adapts Routine to Minimize Difficulties	Perception of Physical Work Setting	Perception of Family and Peers	Perception of Boss and/or Company	Perception of Co-workers
SS	**SS**	SS	**SS**	**SS**	**SS**	**SS**	**SS**	**SS**	SS	SS	SS	**SS**	**SS**	SS	SS
S	S	**S**	S	S	S	S	S	S	**S**	**S**	**S**	S	S	**S**	S
I	I	I	I	I	I	I	I	I	I	I	I	I	I	I	**I**
SI	SI	SI	SI	SI	SI	SI	SI	SI	SI	SI	SI	SI	SI	SI	SI
N/A	N/A	N/A	N/A	N/A	N/A	N/A	N/A	N/A	N/A	N/A	N/A	N/A	N/A	N/A	N/A

Rating Scale:	**SS** Strongly Supports	**S** Supports	**I** Interferes	**SI** Strongly Interferes	**N/A** Not Applicable

WRI (Version 10.0), (Braveman et al., 2005)
Addresses psychosocial and environmental factors that impact return to work. Complimenting other work/physical capacity assessments to ensure a well rounded picture of the client and their needs that should be addressed to ensure return to work.

FIGURE 42-2 Stephen—Worker Role Interview (Version 10.0) ratings. (From Braveman, B., Robson, M., Velozo, C., Kielhofner, G., Fisher, G., Forsyth, K., & Kerschbaum, J. [2005]. *The Worker Role Interview* [WRI; Version 10.0]. Chicago, IL: Model of Human Occupation Clearinghouse.)

• *What are the occupational issues Stephen is having difficulty with?* Stephen reported frustration in his lack of success in applying for work. Previous worker roles had all been in entry-level jobs, and he had no aspirations for career development beyond attaining a paid job. Stephen described a lack of enjoyment of previous worker roles in hospitality and retail; in particular, he found the fluctuating demands of the role difficult to manage with high levels of noise and stress at busy times contrasting with lack of routine tasks in quiet periods. There was limited opportunity for Stephen to work with any autonomy in organizing his tasks. All the positions he had previously held were temporary, low paid entry-level jobs and had offered little reward. Stephen has previously had poor relationships with colleagues and managers and has felt stigmatized due to his mental health condition. Stephen's life at the time of assessment lacked structure and routines; his roles as family member, friend, and dog owner were important but demanded little time.

Initial Assessment

Time demands	Task demands	Appeal of work tasks	Work schedule	Co-worker interaction	Work group membership	Supervisor interaction	Work role standards	Work role style	Interaction with others	Rewards	Sensory Qualities	Architecture / arrangement	Ambience / mood	Properties of objects	Physical amenities	Meaning of objects
4	4	4	4	4	4	4	4	4	4	4	4	4	4	4	4	4
3	3	3	3	3	3	3	3	3	3	3	3	3	3	3	3	3
2	2	2	2	2	2	2	2	2	2	2	2	2	2	2	2	2
1	1	1	1	1	1	1	1	1	1	1	1	1	1	1	1	1
N/A	N/A	N/A	N/A	N/A	N/A	N/A	N/A	N/A	N/A	N/A	N/A	N/A	N/A	N/A	N/A	N/A

Outcome Assessment

Time demands	Task demands	Appeal of work tasks	Work schedule	Co-worker interaction	Work group membership	Supervisor interaction	Work role standards	Work role style	Interaction with others	Rewards	Sensory Qualities	Architecture / arrangement	Ambience / mood	Properties of objects	Physical amenities	Meaning of objects
4	4	4	4	4	4	4	4	4	4	4	4	4	4	4	4	4
3	3	3	3	3	3	3	3	3	3	3	3	3	3	3	3	3
2	2	2	2	2	2	2	2	2	2	2	2	2	2	2	2	2
1	1	1	1	1	1	1	1	1	1	1	1	1	1	1	1	1
N/A	N/A	N/A	N/A	N/A	N/A	N/A	N/A	N/A	N/A	N/A	N/A	N/A	N/A	N/A	N/A	N/A

Rating Scale: 4 Strongly Supports   3 Supports   2 Interferes   1 Strongly Interferes   N/A Not Applicable

WEIS (Version 2.0) (Moore-Corner et al., 1998)
Identifies environmental characteristics that facilitate successful employment experiences. Factors that inhibit worker performance and satisfaction and which may require accommodation are also addressed in order to maximize the "fit" of the worker and their skills to the job environment

FIGURE 42-3 Stephen—Work Environment Impact Scale (Version 2.0) ratings. (From Moore-Corner, R. A., Kielhofner, G., & Olson, L. [1998]. *A user's guide to work environment impact scale.* Chicago, IL: Model of Human Occupation Clearinghouse.)

- *What are the positive occupational issues for Stephen?* Stephen has a strong commitment to being in paid employment. He has a clear understanding of the expectations of work roles he has held in the past. He has a strong supportive network of family and friends. They are very encouraging and had in the past used contacts to secure employment on his behalf.
- *Why is Stephen unable to work or having challenges engaging in work?* Previous worker roles Stephen has held were mainly in retail and hospitality and were a poor fit with his interest in office administration. His current methods for seeking employment have been unsuccessful, and he has been unable to adjust his strategies. His current routine lacks routine due to the absence of a worker role, and Stephen is concerned that he will find adjusting to the greater demands of a worker role challenging. Stephen has experienced difficulty in unsupportive relationships with coworkers and managers in past worker roles and is concerned this may occur in the future.

Generating Therapy Goals and Strategies

The following goals were jointly generated:

- Within 2 weeks, Stephen (with the support of the occupational therapist) will identify jobs that match his interests and preferred working style using online and paper-based career planning material at the therapy clinic.
- Within 4 weeks, Stephen's (with the support of the occupational therapist) assistant will develop a résumé and begin applying for jobs in his local library.
- Within 6 weeks, Stephen will independently spend time daily identifying, researching, and applying for jobs at home, in the job center, and in the library.

- Within 6 weeks, Stephen and the occupational therapist will investigate potential opportunities for unpaid internship in positions relevant to preferred worker role.

The therapist used the format featured in Table 42-4 to create a clear goal structure for Stephen. For example, the first goal indicates the following:

- The time frame as "2 weeks"
- The degree (or amount of assistance) as "with the support of the occupational therapist"
- The action as "identify jobs which match his interests and preferred working style using online and paper-based career planning materials"
- The setting as "the therapy clinic"

The goals also include examples of occupational engagement that will help Stephen achieve the change necessary to obtain these goals. For example, the occupational engagement in the first goal is "identify."

Implementing and Monitoring Therapy

The intervention plan includes the therapeutic strategies (in italics) that will support Stephen's achievement of his goals.

- Stephen and the occupational therapist worked together, and exploring a range of employment options and *negotiating* which types of worker roles offered the best fit with his interests and working styles.
- The occupational therapist *coached* Stephen in how to use career-planning material and *encouraged* him to discuss his future worker roles with his natural social support network of family and friends.
- The OT assistant *coached* Stephen and assisted in *structuring* how to build a résumé and complete application forms.
- The therapist regularly met with Stephen to review his increasing work routine; during these sessions, the occupational therapist offered *advice* and *encouragement* and *gave feedback*.
- Initially, the occupational therapist *identified* opportunities and barriers for establishing a work routine for Stephen and offered support by *structuring* increasing participation. As he became more confident and independent, the occupational therapist offered *encouragement*.
- The occupational therapist with Stephen identified a relevant unpaid internship opportunity; they then met with the manager of the workplace to *negotiate* and *structure* a placement of gradually increasing demand.
- The occupational therapist and Stephen discussed the social environment of the work placement in advance of commencing the internship. Stephen was anxious about establishing new relationships with coworkers. The therapist listened to Stephen's concerns based on previous

negative experience and demonstrated respect by *validating* his perspective. The therapist *coached* Stephen in strategies for meeting and conversing with new people at work. Stephen chose not to disclose his mental health condition to coworkers and so role-playing allowed Stephen to practice tricky conversations.

- The therapist offered advice to Stephen and his manager about managing mental health and well-being in the workplace.
- The therapist regularly communicated with Stephen's wider mental health team to share information, feedback progress, and ensure compatibility of care plans and objectives.

Collecting Information to Assess Outcomes

After 3 months, Stephen was established in his internship—working 2.5 days per week, totaling 16 hours. He was also regularly applying for similar paid roles and had secured two interviews. The occupational therapist chose to assess outcomes to date (Figures 42-2 and 42-3). The assessment strategy was

Goal attainment (i.e., review of initial goals)

- Stephen and the occupational therapist worked together, establishing that Stephen had gained the greatest levels of satisfaction in administrative roles; this had been his chosen course of study at college.
- Stephen has a résumé that he tailors and shares with local employers, and he regularly applies for relevant available jobs, recently securing two interviews.
- Stephen has established a work routine of activities related to applying for employment.
- The occupational therapist secured an unpaid internship at a local leisure center where Stephen gradually built up his routine from 3 half days per week to 2 full days and 1 half day. The manager of the leisure center is very positive about Stephen as a worker and has provided an excellent reference. The manager would be willing to appoint Stephen if a post was available.

Collecting Information and Creating a Theory-Based Understanding of John

Who Is John?

John is a 7-year-old boy who is a third grader in elementary school, a son, a grandson, a brother, a friend, a swimmer, and a bike rider. He wants to be a computer engineer like his dad when he grows up. He is described by his family as a lovable, endearing boy and by his schoolteacher as chaotic, disorganized, and worried.

Background

John lives at home with his two parents and his brother. John has been referred for a specialist assessment by his elementary schoolteacher who was concerned about his awkward movement within the classroom, distractibility, and laborious handwriting. These issues have been long standing; the strategies tried within the school have not been helpful and the challenges persist. The teachers within John's school had already tried some of the strategies from *Inclusive Learning and Collaborative Working: Teachers Ideas in Practice* (CIRCLE Collaboration, 2009b). This is a resource based on what teachers have found helpful when supporting children with additional support needs. They had identified supports and strategies from the motor skill section, namely, task breakdown, hand-over-hand support, modeling, and additional verbal instructions. There is a concern that if the issues are not resolved, John will not be able to keep up with his class peers in terms of academic performance. Following discussion between John's class teacher and the headmaster, it was decided that it would be appropriate to refer John for an OT assessment.

Generating Questions

The occupational therapist started with an intention to understand what was important to John, his teacher, and his family. The therapist wanted to use MOHO as a framework for understanding how the issues raised on the referral affected John's engagement and participation in everyday occupations. Therefore, the therapist asked the following questions:

- What is important to John (his values) and what motivates him to participate in occupations at school?
- How do John's distractibility and awkward movement impact his ability to fulfill his responsibilities, maintain his routines, interact with others, and organize activities?
- What is John's view of his abilities and his limitations?
- How does John's occupational performance vary in different environments (home and school)?

Gathering Information

When John was referred into a local therapy facility, the therapists chose an assessment pattern that would provide information for the previous questions.

Prior to Attendance at the Therapy Clinic

- Active in Children Health Integrating Evidence Valuing Experience (ACHIEVE) Assessment (Forsyth et al., 2012)—This assessment was administered by mail and was completed by John's mother and by John's teacher. It affords an opportunity for John's mother/teacher to share their view of how their child is participating in everyday activities (Figure 42-4).

- As the teacher indicated on the referral form that John's movement was awkward, the ACHIEVE Assessment also included a Developmental Coordination Disorder Questionnaire (DCDQ) (Wilson, Kaplan, Crawford, Campbell, & Dewey, 2000), which is a brief questionnaire designed to screen for coordination disorders in children aged 5 to 15 years.

During Therapy Clinic

- Review and verification of the findings of the ACHIEVE Assessment (Forsyth et al., 2012) with parent
- Movement Assessment Battery for Children (ABC) (Henderson & Sugden, 1992)—This assessment identifies, describes, and guides the treatment of motor impairment. It is used to assess children's motor skills disabilities and determine intervention strategies (Table 42-6).
- Standardized assessment of handwriting, *The Handwriting File* (Alston & Taylor, 1988), was completed to understand if John's writing skill was significantly slower that would be expected of a child his age (Table 42-7).

After the Therapy Clinic

- Short Child Occupational Profile (SCOPE) (Bowyer et al., 2006)—This is an assessment that is completed by the therapist using information gathered in various ways.
- The therapist rated the SCOPE using information gathered from the other assessments as well as during an observation of John's participation within the classroom (Figure 42-5). This allowed for "triangulation" between the parents' view, the teacher's view, and the therapist's view on how different personal and environment factors impacted John's participation. This provides a range of views to build a comprehensive understanding of John.

Creating a Theory-Based Understanding of the Client

The following occupational formulation was created from the assessment findings.

- *What was important to John, his family, and his teacher?* John stated, "Writing is not my thing," and wanted to be able to keep up with his friends and not feel his cheeks getting hot and feeling panicky about being the last to complete writing tasks. John's mother wanted him to be able to write better and not find it so difficult to do this. John's teacher wants John to be less clumsy, less distractible, and for his writing to be less laborious.
- *What is John good at and what does he enjoy?* Comparing teacher and parent assessments, John performs more consistently in activities at home than at school. John has many areas of strength including home and community activities; for example, able to get dressed/undressed, able to ride a bike, able to take part in social events. John's teacher reports that John enjoys math and physical education.

SUMMARY SCORES - Baseline

Name: ...John..Date of Birth: ....

Age: ...7.........Yrs....................................Months   CHI Number: ....

Clinician(s) Scoring: ....

PARENT QUESTIONNAIRE

PARENTAL OBSERVATIONS OF ACTIVITY FREQUENCY - WHAT

		None of the time	Some of the time	Most of the time	All of the time
Home Activities	a. Able to dry after bath/shower	1	2	3	4
	b. Able to clean after toileting	1	2	3	4
	c. Able to get un/dressed	1	2	3	4
	d. Able to make a simple snack	1	2	3	4
	e. Able to use a knife and fork	1	2	3	4
	f. Able to get ready in the morning	1	2	3	4
School Activities	a. Able to use learning materials	1	2	3	4
	b. Able to make effective shapes/letters/writing	1	2	3	4
	c. Able to engage in sports/leisure	1	2	3	4
	d. Able to engage in curriculum	1	2	3	4
	e. Able to clean after toilet at school	1	2	3	4
	f. Able to get dressed after P.E./gym	1	2	3	4
Community Activities	a. Able to ride bike/rollerblade etc	1	2	3	4
	b. Able to play with friends in activities	1	2	3	4
	c. Able to take part in out of school clubs	1	2	3	4
	d. Able to take part in social events	1	2	3	4
	e. Able to take part with family in leisure activity	1	2	3	4
	f. Able to manage clothes before/after activities	1	2	3	4

PARENTAL OBSERVATIONS OF CHARACTERISTICS OF CHILD - WHY

		None of the time	Some of the time	Most of the time	All of the time
Routine	a. Understands sequence/structure of routine	1	2	3	4
	b. Organises routines	1	2	3	4
	c. Copes with change in routine	1	2	3	4
	d. Copes with change in how activity's done	1	2	3	4
	e. Copes with a variety of activities	1	2	3	4
Responsibility	a. Understands their responsibilities	1	2	3	4
	b. Accepts their responsibilities	1	2	3	4
	c. Manages multiple responsibilities	1	2	3	4
	d. Understands rules associated with activities	1	2	3	4
	e. Accepts leadership roles at home	1	2	3	4
Confidence	a. Confident in their abilities	1	2	3	4
	b. Enjoys daily activities	1	2	3	4
	c. Satisfied with performance in activities	1	2	3	4
	d. Identifies what he/she wants to get better at	1	2	3	4
	e. Keeps trying despite challenges	1	2	3	4
Social Skills	a. Plays well with others	1	2	3	4
	b. Chatty/sociable and talks with friends	1	2	3	4
	c. Speaks clearly when with others	1	2	3	4
	d. Understands other's feelings	1	2	3	4
	e. Can ask for the support he/she needs	1	2	3	4
Organisational Skills	a. Organises and uses objects for activities	1	2	3	4
	b. Maintains concentration throughout activities	1	2	3	4
	c. Works out problems if stuck on a task	1	2	3	4
	d. Follows through instructions for activities	1	2	3	4
	e. Does the steps of an activity in the right order	1	2	3	4
Environment	a. Can navigate around physical environment	1	2	3	4
	b. Community environment has opportunities	1	2	3	4
	c. Access to the things to help them take part	1	2	3	4
	d. Family members are available for support	1	2	3	4
	e. School environment supports school activities	1	2	3	4
	f. Does activities in usual/accepted way	1	2	3	4

PARENTAL OBSERVATIONS OF MOTOR SKILLS (DCD Q) - WHY

		Not at all like	A bit like	Mod. like	Quite like	Extremely like
Control During Movement	1. Throws ball	1	2	3	4	5
	2. Catches ball	1	2	3	4	5
	3. Hits ball/birdie	1	2	3	4	5
	4. Jumps over	1	2	3	4	5
	5. Runs	1	2	3	4	5
	6. Plans activity	1	2	3	4	5
	TOTAL				20/30	
Fine Motor/ Handwriting	1. Writing fast	1	2	3	4	5
	2. Writing legibly	1	2	3	4	5
	3. Effort and pressure	1	2	3	4	5
	4. Cuts	1	2	3	4	5
	TOTAL				8/20	
General Coordination	1. Likes sport	1	2	3	4	5
	2. Learning new skills	1	2	3	4	5
	3. Quick and competent	1	2	3	4	5
	4. "Bull in shop"	1	2	3	4	5
	5. Does not fatigue	1	2	3	4	5
	TOTAL				16/25	
	OVERALL TOTAL				44/75	

Children aged 5 years 0 months to 7 years 11 months (tick as appropriate)
15-46: Indication of DCD or suspect DCD ☑
47-75: Probably not DCD ☐

Children aged 8 years 0 months to 9 years 11 months (tick as appropriate)
15-55: Indication of DCD or suspect DCD ☐
56-75: Probably not DCD ☐

Children aged 10 years 0 months to 15 years (tick as appropriate)
15-57: Indication of DCD or suspect DCD ☐
58-75: Probably not DCD ☐

SCHOOL QUESTIONNAIRE

TEACHER OBSERVATIONS OF ACTIVITY FREQUENCY - WHAT

		None of the time	Some of the time	Most of the time	All of the time
Home Activities that relate to School	a. Able to clean after toileting	1	2	3	4
	b. Able to get dressed in morning	1	2	3	4
	c. Able to use a knife and fork	1	2	3	4
	d. Able to make a simple snack	1	2	3	4
	e. Able to prepare for school in the morning	1	2	3	4
	f. Able to prepare for school activities	1	2	3	4
School Activities	a. Able to use learning materials	1	2	3	4
	b. Able to make effective shapes/letters/writing	1	2	3	4
	c. Able to engage in sports/leisure	1	2	3	4
	d. Able to engage in curriculum	1	2	3	4
	e. Able to organise themselves	1	2	3	4
	f. Able to get dressed after P.E./gym	1	2	3	4
Community Activities	a. Able to ride bike/rollerblade etc	1	2	3	4
	b. Able to play with peers in activities	1	2	3	4
	c. Able to take part in after school clubs	1	2	3	4
	d. Able to take part in social events	1	2	3	4
	e. Able to take part with family in leisure activity	1	2	3	4
	f. Able to manage clothes before/after activities	1	2	3	4

TEACHER OBSERVATIONS OF CHARACTERISTICS OF CHILD - WHY

		None of the time	Some of the time	Most of the time	All of the time
Routine	a. Understands sequence/structure of routine	1	2	3	4
	b. Organises routines	1	2	3	4
	c. Copes with change in routine	1	2	3	4
	d. Copes with change in how activity's done	1	2	3	4
	e. Copes with a variety of activities	1	2	3	4
Responsibility	a. Understands their responsibilities	1	2	3	4
	b. Accepts their responsibilities	1	2	3	4
	c. Manages multiple responsibilities	1	2	3	4
	d. Understands rules associated with activities	1	2	3	4
	e. Accepts leadership roles at school	1	2	3	4
Confidence	a. Confident in their abilities	1	2	3	4
	b. Enjoys school activities	1	2	3	4
	c. Satisfied with performance in activities	1	2	3	4
	d. Identifies what he/she wants to get better at	1	2	3	4
	e. Keeps trying despite challenges	1	2	3	4
Social Skills	a. Plays well with others	1	2	3	4
	b. Chatty/sociable and talks with friends	1	2	3	4
	c. Speaks clearly when with others	1	2	3	4
	d. Understands other's feelings	1	2	3	4
	e. Can ask for the support he/she needs	1	2	3	4
Organisational Skills	a. Organises and uses objects for activities	1	2	3	4
	b. Maintains concentration throughout activities	1	2	3	4
	c. Works out problems if stuck on a task	1	2	3	4
	d. Follows through instructions for activities	1	2	3	4
	e. Does the steps of an activity in the right order	1	2	3	4
Environment	a. Can navigate around physical environment	1	2	3	4
	b. Community environment has opportunities	1	2	3	4
	c. Access to the things to help them take part	1	2	3	4
	d. School staff are available for support	1	2	3	4
	e. School environment supports school activities	1	2	3	4
	f. Does activities in usual/accepted way	1	2	3	4

TEACHER OBSERVATIONS OF MOTOR SKILLS (DCD Q) - WHY

		Not at all like	A bit like	Mod. like	Quite like	Extremely like
Control During Movement	1. Throws ball	1	2	3	4	5
	2. Catches ball	1	2	3	4	5
	3. Hits ball/birdie	1	2	3	4	5
	4. Jumps over	1	2	3	4	5
	5. Runs	1	2	3	4	5
	6. Plans activity	1	2	3	4	5
	TOTAL				15/30	
Fine Motor/ Handwriting	1. Writing fast	1	2	3	4	5
	2. Writing legibly	1	2	3	4	5
	3. Effort and pressure	1	2	3	4	5
	4. Cuts	1	2	3	4	5
	TOTAL				8/20	
General Coordination	1. Likes sport	1	2	3	4	5
	2. Learning new skills	1	2	3	4	5
	3. Quick and competent	1	2	3	4	5
	4. "Bull in shop"	1	2	3	4	5
	5. Does not fatigue	1	2	3	4	5
	TOTAL				9/25	
	OVERALL TOTAL				32/75	

Children aged 5 years 0 months to 7 years 11 months (tick as appropriate)
15-46: Indication of DCD or suspect DCD ☑
47-75: Probably not DCD ☐

Children aged 8 years 0 months to 9 years 11 months (tick as appropriate)
15-55: Indication of DCD or suspect DCD ☐
56-75: Probably not DCD ☐

Children aged 10 years 0 months to 15 years (tick as appropriate)
15-57: Indication of DCD or suspect DCD ☐
58-75: Probably not DCD ☐

FIGURE 42-4 John—Active in Children Health Integrating Evidence Valuing Experience (ACHIEVE) Assessment scores: baseline and reassessment.

SUMMARY SCORES – Re-assessment

Name: ...John...Date of Birth: ....

Age: ..7.........Yrs...................................Months   CHI Number: ....

Clinician(s) Scoring: ....

PARENT QUESTIONNAIRE

PARENTAL OBSERVATIONS OF ACTIVITY FREQUENCY - WHAT

	Item	None of the time	Some of the time	Most of the time	All of the time
Home Activities	a. Able to dry after bath/shower	1	2	3	4
	b. Able to clean after toileting	1	2	3	4
	c. Able to get un/dressed	1	2	3	4
	d. Able to make a simple snack	1	2	3	4
	e. Able to use a knife and fork	1	2	3	4
	f. Able to get ready in the morning	1	2	3	4
School Activities	a. Able to use learning materials	1	2	3	4
	b. Able to make effective shapes/letters/writing	1	2	3	4
	c. Able to engage in sports/leisure	1	2	3	4
	d. Able to engage in curriculum	1	2	3	4
	e. Able to clean after toilet at school	1	2	3	4
	f. Able to get dressed after P.E./gym	1	2	3	4
Community Activities	a. Able to ride bike/rollerblade etc	1	2	3	4
	b. Able to play with friends in activities	1	2	3	4
	c. Able to take part in out of school clubs	1	2	3	4
	d. Able to take part in social events	1	2	3	4
	e. Able to take part with family in leisure activity	1	2	3	4
	f. Able to manage clothes before/after activities	1	2	3	4

PARENTAL OBSERVATIONS OF CHARACTERISTICS OF CHILD - WHY

	Item	None of the time	Some of the time	Most of the time	All of the time
Routine	a. Understands sequence/structure of routine	1	2	3	4
	b. Organises routines	1	2	3	4
	c. Copes with change in routine	1	2	3	4
	d. Copes with change in how activity's done	1	2	3	4
	e. Copes with a variety of activities	1	2	3	4
Responsibility	a. Understands their responsibilities	1	2	3	4
	b. Accepts their responsibilities	1	2	3	4
	c. Manages multiple responsibilities	1	2	3	4
	d. Understands rules associated with activities	1	2	3	4
	e. Accepts leadership roles at home	1	2	3	4
Confidence	a. Confident in their abilities	1	2	3	4
	b. Enjoys daily activities	1	2	3	4
	c. Satisfied with performance in activities	1	2	3	4
	d. Identifies what he/she wants to get better at	1	2	3	4
	e. Keeps trying despite challenges	1	2	3	4
Social Skills	a. Plays well with others	1	2	3	4
	b. Chatty/sociable and talks with friends	1	2	3	4
	c. Speaks clearly when with others	1	2	3	4
	d. Understands other's feelings	1	2	3	4
	e. Can ask for the support he/she needs	1	2	3	4
Organisational Skills	a. Organises and uses objects for activities	1	2	3	4
	b. Maintains concentration throughout activities	1	2	3	4
	c. Works out problems if stuck on a task	1	2	3	4
	d. Follows through instructions for activities	1	2	3	4
	e. Does the steps of an activity in the right order	1	2	3	4
Environment	a. Can navigate around physical environment	1	2	3	4
	b. Community environment has opportunities	1	2	3	4
	c. Access to the things to help them take part	1	2	3	4
	d. Family members are available for support	1	2	3	4
	e. School environment supports school activities	1	2	3	4
	f. Does activities in usual/accepted way	1	2	3	4

PARENTAL OBSERVATIONS OF MOTOR SKILLS (DCD Q) - WHY

	Item	Not at all like	A bit like	Mod. like	Quite like	Extremely like
Control During Movement	1. Throws ball	1	2	3	4	5
	2. Catches ball	1	2	3	4	5
	3. Hits ball/birdie	1	2	3	4	5
	4. Jumps over	1	2	3	4	5
	5. Runs	1	2	3	4	5
	6. Plans activity	1	2	3	4	5
	TOTAL					20/30
Fine Motor/ Handwriting	1. Writing fast	1	2	3	4	5
	2. Writing legibly	1	2	3	4	5
	3. Effort and pressure	1	2	3	4	5
	4. Cuts	1	2	3	4	5
	TOTAL					8/20
General Coordination	1. Likes sport	1	2	3	4	5
	2. Learning new skills	1	2	3	4	5
	3. Quick and competent	1	2	3	4	5
	4. "Bull in shop"	1	2	3	4	5
	5. Does not fatigue	1	2	3	4	5
	TOTAL					16/25
	OVERALL TOTAL					44/75

Children aged 5 years 0 months to 7 years 11 months (tick as appropriate)
15-46: Indication of DCD or suspect DCD ☑
47-75: Probably not DCD ☐

Children aged 8 years 0 months to 9 years 11 months (tick as appropriate)
15-55: Indication of DCD or suspect DCD ☐
56-75: Probably not DCD ☐

Children aged 10 years 0 months to 15 years (tick as appropriate)
15-57: Indication of DCD or suspect DCD ☐
58-75: Probably not DCD ☐

SCHOOL QUESTIONNAIRE

TEACHER OBSERVATIONS OF ACTIVITY FREQUENCY - WHAT

	Item	None of the time	Some of the time	Most of the time	All of the time
Home Activities that relate to School	a. Able to clean after toileting	1	2	3	4
	b. Able to get dressed in morning	1	2	3	4
	c. Able to use a knife and fork	1	2	3	4
	d. Able to make a simple snack	1	2	3	4
	e. Able to prepare for school in the morning	1	2	3	4
	f. Able to prepare for school activities	1	2	3	4
School Activities	a. Able to use learning materials	1	2	3	4
	b. Able to make effective shapes/letters/writing	1	2	3	4
	c. Able to engage in sports/leisure	1	2	3	4
	d. Able to engage in curriculum	1	2	3	4
	e. Able to organise themselves	1	2	3	4
	f. Able to get dressed after P.E./gym	1	2	3	4
Community Activities	a. Able to ride bike/rollerblade etc	1	2	3	4
	b. Able to play with peers in activities	1	2	3	4
	c. Able to take part in after school clubs	1	2	3	4
	d. Able to take part in social events	1	2	3	4
	e. Able to take part with family in leisure activity	1	2	3	4
	f. Able to manage clothes before/after activities	1	2	3	4

TEACHER OBSERVATIONS OF CHARACTERISTICS OF CHILD - WHY

	Item	None of the time	Some of the time	Most of the time	All of the time
Routine	a. Understands sequence/structure of routine	1	2	3	4
	b. Organises routines	1	2	3	4
	c. Copes with change in routine	1	2	3	4
	d. Copes with change in how activity's done	1	2	3	4
	e. Copes with a variety of activities	1	2	3	4
Responsibility	a. Understands their responsibilities	1	2	3	4
	b. Accepts their responsibilities	1	2	3	4
	c. Manages multiple responsibilities	1	2	3	4
	e. Accepts leadership roles at school	1	2	3	4
Confidence	a. Confident in their abilities	1	2	3	4
	b. Enjoys school activities	1	2	3	4
	c. Satisfied with performance in activities	1	2	3	4
	d. Identifies what he/she wants to get better at	1	2	3	4
	e. Keeps trying despite challenges	1	2	3	4
Social Skills	a. Plays well with others	1	2	3	4
	b. Chatty/sociable and talks with friends	1	2	3	4
	c. Speaks clearly when with others	1	2	3	4
	d. Understands other's feelings	1	2	3	4
	e. Can ask for the support he/she needs	1	2	3	4
Organisational Skills	a. Organises and uses objects for activities	1	2	3	4
	b. Maintains concentration throughout activities	1	2	3	4
	c. Works out problems if stuck on a task	1	2	3	4
	d. Follows through instructions for activities	1	2	3	4
	e. Does the steps of an activity in the right order	1	2	3	4
Environment	a. Can navigate around physical environment	1	2	3	4
	b. Community environment has opportunities	1	2	3	4
	c. Access to the things to help them take part	1	2	3	4
	d. School staff are available for support	1	2	3	4
	e. School environment supports school activities	1	2	3	4
	f. Does activities in usual/accepted way	1	2	3	4

TEACHER OBSERVATIONS OF MOTOR SKILLS (DCD Q) - WHY

	Item	Not at all like	A bit like	Mod. like	Quite like	Extremely like
Control During Movement	1. Throws ball	1	2	3	4	5
	2. Catches ball	1	2	3	4	5
	3. Hits ball/birdie	1	2	3	4	5
	4. Jumps over	1	2	3	4	5
	5. Runs	1	2	3	4	5
	6. Plans activity	1	2	3	4	5
	TOTAL					15/30
Fine Motor/ Handwriting	1. Writing fast	1	2	3	4	5
	2. Writing legibly	1	2	3	4	5
	3. Effort and pressure	1	2	3	4	5
	4. Cuts	1	2	3	4	5
	TOTAL					8/20
General Coordination	1. Likes sport	1	2	3	4	5
	2. Learning new skills	1	2	3	4	5
	3. Quick and competent	1	2	3	4	5
	4. "Bull in shop"	1	2	3	4	5
	5. Does not fatigue	1	2	3	4	5
	TOTAL					9/25
	OVERALL TOTAL					32/75

Children aged 5 years 0 months to 7 years 11 months (tick as appropriate)
15-46: Indication of DCD or suspect DCD ☑
47-75: Probably not DCD ☐

Children aged 8 years 0 months to 9 years 11 months (tick as appropriate)
15-55: Indication of DCD or suspect DCD ☐
56-75: Probably not DCD ☐

Children aged 10 years 0 months to 15 years (tick as appropriate)
15-57: Indication of DCD or suspect DCD ☐
58-75: Probably not DCD ☐

FIGURE 42-4 (*Continued*)

TABLE 42-6	John—Movement Assessment Battery for Children-2 (ABC2) Scores
Movement ABC2 Scores	Manual dexterity: 9th percentile, which is suggestive of being at risk of movement difficulties Aiming and catching: 75th percentile, no movement difficulties detected Balance: 9th percentile, which is suggestive of being at risk of movement difficulties
Overall Percentile	9th percentile, which is suggestive of being at risk of movement difficulties

The Movement ABC2 assesses a child's fine motor ability, for example, pencils and scissors skills, performance with ball skills, and balance. The test scores provide information about how your child's motor performance compares to his or her peers and can provide an indication of the severity of the motor difficulties. Below 5th percentile: significant movement difficulties; 5th–15th percentile: suggestive of being at risk of movement difficulties; above 15th percentile: no movement difficulties detected.

From Henderson, E., & Sugden, D. (1992). *The movement assessment battery for children*. London, United Kingdom: Psychological Corporation.

- *Why does John have these strengths?* Despite concerns, John can achieve 26 letters per minute (normative performance is 28 letters per minute for a 7-year-old) *when focused*. John's mother, teacher, and therapists identified that John has structured routines at both home and school. His mother, teacher, and therapists agree that John mostly understands responsibilities, has appropriate social skills, and has a supportive school and home environment matched to his abilities and skills.

- *What does John find challenging?* John doesn't have any areas of challenge at home. John was, however, observed in the classroom to have challenges using learning materials effectively (e.g., pens, pencils, crayons, rules, glue sticks, scissors) and being able to make effective shapes or letters and writing within a school context.

- *Why does John have these challenges?* Parents were concerned about John's motor skill development; however, from their point of view, there are no other health concerns. Indeed, John's teacher reported he has challenges navigating around his physical school environment. Although the DCDQ indicates challenges in fine motor or handwriting and general coordination within school and the Movement ABC was within the 9th percentile (which is suggestive of being at risk of movement difficulties with manual dexterity and balance), it is likely that these scores have been significantly impacted by John's distractibility or lack of attention. John was observed to be *highly* distractible during both the therapy clinic and classroom. This is further supported by John's handwriting being normative for his age group when formally tested—when he was focused in a quiet

TABLE 42-7	John—The Handwriting File Scores
Test	Handwriting file
Performance indicator	Letters per minute
Score	26 letters per minute (7-year-old normally able to manage 28 letters per minute)

From Alston, J., & Taylor, J. (1988). *The handwriting file* (2nd ed.). Wisbech, United Kingdom: LDA.

environment. Moreover, John's teacher reports that John has significant challenges in the area of organizational ability in school (i.e., extremely poor concentration throughout written tasks, lack of effort in writing tasks, following through on instructions), which was consistent with the therapist's observation. The impact on John's confidence in school was noticeable in the classroom (i.e., having confidence in abilities, enjoyment or having satisfaction in school activities, and not trying despite challenges). This was consistent with John giving up easily within the therapy clinic, although he was competitive when performing against a timer.

Generating Therapy Goals and Strategies

Although the initial referral from the teacher was framed as challenges in movement and coordination, the assessment process identified that the main areas of occupational change to target in therapy was

- Improvement in use of learning materials through developing organizational skills and increase confidence for tasks completed within the classroom

The joint measurable goal shared between therapy and education was therefore

- Within 4 weeks, John will be able to confidently use learning materials (such as books, writing utensils) through organizing objects and maintaining concentration within his classroom independently.

A meeting was arranged between the therapist, the parent, and the teacher to exchange strategies that worked for John at home and resulted in John performing better within the home environment (i.e., routine praise for completing activities regardless of outcome or speed), making eye contact with John before sharing instructions, and creating an environment with limited distractions when completing homework. The parent, teacher, and occupational therapists therefore identified strategies—from *Intervention Descriptions: Occupational Therapy* (CIRCLE Collaboration, 2009c)—of (1) modifying the school environment, (2) recreating volition, and (3) process skill building.

Baseline

Volition	1	2	3	4		Habituation	1	2	3	4
Exploration	**1**	2	3	4		Daily activities	1	2	3	**4**
Expressions of enjoyment	**1**	2	3	4		Response to transitions	1	2	3	**4**
Preferences & choices	**1**	2	3	4		Routine	1	2	3	**4**
Response to challenge	**1**	2	3	4		Roles	1	2	3	**4**

Communication & Interaction skills	1	2	3	4		Process Skills	1	2	3	4
Non verbal	1	2	**3**	4		Understands/uses objects	**1**	2	3	4
Verbal expression	1	2	3	**4**		Orientation to environment	**1**	2	3	4
Conversation	1	2	**3**	4		Plan/make decisions	**1**	2	3	4
Relationships	1	2	**3**	4		Problem solving	**1**	2	3	4

Motor skills	1	2	3	4		Environment	1	2	3	4
Posture/mobility	1	**2**	3	4		Physical space	1	**2**	3	4
Coordination	1	**2**	3	4		Physical resources	1	**2**	3	4
Strength	1	2	3	**4**		Social groups	1		**3**	4
Energy/Endurance	1	**2**	3	4		Activity demands	1	**2**	3	4

Re-assessment

Volition	1	2	3	4		Habituation	1	2	3	4
Exploration	1	2	3	**4**		Daily activities	1	2	3	**4**
Expressions of enjoyment	1	2	3	**4**		Response to transitions	1	2	3	**4**
Preferences & choices	1	2	3	**4**		Routine	1	2	3	**4**
Response to challenge	1	2	3	**4**		Roles	1	2	3	**4**

Communication & Interaction skills	1	2	3	4		Process Skills	1	2	3	4
Non verbal	1	2	**3**	4		Understands/uses objects	1	2	3	**4**
Verbal expression	1	2	3	**4**		Orientation to environment	1	2	3	**4**
Conversation	1	2	**3**	4		Plan/make decisions	1	2	3	**4**
Relationships	1	2	**3**	4		Problem solving	1	2	3	**4**

Motor skills	1	2	3	4		Environment	1	2	3	4
Posture/mobility	1	2	**3**	4		Physical space	1	2	3	**4**
Coordination	1	2	**3**	4		Physical resources	1	2	3	**4**
Strength	1	2	3	**4**		Social groups	1	2	**3**	4
Energy/Endurance	1	2	**3**	4		Activity demands	1	2	3	**4**

Scale: 1 = Facilitates participation in occupation
2 = Allows participation in occupation
3 = Inhibits participation in occupation
4 = Restricts participation in occupation

FIGURE 42-5 John—Short Child Occupational Profile (SCOPE) scores: baseline and reassessment. (From Bowyer, P., Ross, M., Schwartz, O., Kielhofner, G., & Kramer, J. [2006]. *The Short Child Occupational Profile* [SCOPE; Version 2.1]. Chicago, IL: Model of Human Occupation Clearinghouse.)

Implementing and Monitoring Therapy

The philosophy of the school therapist was to empower those around a child to provide therapeutic supports to allow for a more consistent approach to supporting a child's occupational participation. The understanding of John was shared with the teacher through the use of the *Collaborative Communication Chart* (CIRCLE Collaboration, 2009a) and *Therapy Manual: Occupational Therapy* (CIRCLE Collaboration, 2009d). This chart was created by therapists and teachers as a structured set of language to support consistent communication.

This provided a common language for the therapist and teacher to discuss strategies that John could use to improve his organizational skills and concentration in the classroom.

The following was agreed as the intervention package:

- John was given a pencil grip.
- John's desk was moved to a front corner of the classroom from his current position in the center of the class to reduce distractions. He was also provided with a bigger desk that would have adequate space for work materials and support materials.

- John was provided with a range of objects that provide sensory feedback during writing (i.e., rubber grips, weighted pencils, weighted wristbands).
- John's teacher provided praise on completion of activities and displayed work alongside others to show its equal value.
- John's teacher created writing tasks where John could write about strong interests.
- John's teacher made him more aware of when he was feeling enjoyment during writing tasks.
- Teacher facilitated positive feedback on his writing by his friends in the classroom.
- Teacher was positive about any perceived failure to support task perseverance despite challenges.
- Teacher was more aware of John disengaging from his writing task; and when she noticed disengagement, she supported John to use his concentration strategies to ensure continued focus.
- John's teacher made eye contact with John before providing instruction on writing task.
- Integrate into John's strong routines setting up and clearing away his workstation space on daily basis.
- John was provided with a timer and taught how to use it to work in 10-minute increments.
- The therapist and John collaborated to make a checklist for materials and for checking task completion that John could then reference independently at the beginning and end of each class work period.

The teacher was encouraged to contact the therapist if there were any concerns or insurmountable challenges during the intervention period. Otherwise, the intervention was provided solely by the teacher.

Collecting Information to Assess Outcomes

The expected therapeutic change in John's occupational participation was within school. A reassessment after 4 weeks was arranged and the following review was completed.

- Goal attainment (i.e., review of joint therapy or educational goal)
- ACHIEVE Assessment (Forsyth et al., 2012) (see Figure 42-4)
- SCOPE (Bowyer et al., 2006) (see Figure 42-5)

John reached his 4-week goal of being able to perform within the classroom more confidently. This was supported by his teacher reporting (see Figure 42-4) improved confidence and organizational skills. He was observed to use his self-monitored strategies. She also reflected that John was "calmer" and more "focused" within the classroom and less disruptive. Classroom observations using the SCOPE also revealed improved scores for confidence and organizational ability (see Figure 42-5). Most importantly, John stated that he felt less panicked

when writing tasks were assigned, and his posture and demeanor were more relaxed. He proudly showed his workstation to the therapists as his space.

Conclusion

This chapter provided an overview of the concepts and practice resources of MOHO. Two cases were used to demonstrate how MOHO concepts are used to guide the process of therapeutic reasoning. As the cases illustrate, therapists can use MOHO to support a client-centered and occupationally focused practice. This chapter was able to demonstrate only a small fraction of the theoretical, empirical, and practical resources that are available under this model. Anyone who wishes to use MOHO is encouraged to take advantage of those resources.

REFERENCES

Alston, J., & Taylor, J. (1988). *The handwriting file* (2nd ed.). Wisbech, United Kingdom: LDA.

American Occupational Therapy Association. (2014). Occupational therapy practice framework: Domain and process. *American Journal of Occupational Therapy, 68*, S1–S48.

Ayres, A. J. (1979). *Sensory integration and the child.* Los Angeles, CA: Western Psychological Services.

Baron, K., Kielhofner, G., Iyenger, A., Goldhammer, V., & Wolenski, J. (2006). *The Occupational Self Assessment* (OSA; Version 2.2). Chicago, IL: Model of Human Occupation Clearinghouse.

Basu, S., Kafkes, A., Geist, R., & Kielhofner, G. (2002). *The Pediatric Volitional Questionnaire* (PVQ; Version 2.0). Chicago, IL: Model of Human Occupation Clearinghouse.

Bernspang, B., & Fisher, A. (1995). Differences between persons with a right or left cerebral vascular accident on the assessment of motor and process skills. *Archives of Physical Medicine and Rehabilitation, 75,* 1144–1151.

Bowyer, P., Ross, M., Schwartz, O., Kielhofner, G., & Kramer, J. (2006). *The Short Child Occupational Profile* (SCOPE; Version 2.1). Chicago, IL: Model of Human Occupation Clearinghouse.

Braveman, B., Robson, M., Velozo, C., Kielhofner, G., Fisher, G., Forsyth, K., & Kerschbaum, J. (2005). *The Worker Role Interview* (WRI; Version 10.0). Chicago, IL: Model of Human Occupation Clearinghouse.

CIRCLE Collaboration. (2009a). *Collaborative communication chart.* Edinburgh, United Kingdom: City of Edinburgh Council, Queen Margaret University, and NHS Lothian.

CIRCLE Collaboration. (2009b). *Inclusive learning and collaborative working: Teachers' ideas in practice.* Edinburgh, United Kingdom: City of Edinburgh Council, Queen Margaret University, and NHS Lothian.

CIRCLE Collaboration. (2009c). *Intervention descriptions: Occupational therapy.* Edinburgh, United Kingdom: City of Edinburgh Council, Queen Margaret University, and NHS Lothian.

CIRCLE Collaboration. (2009d). *Therapy manual: Occupational therapy.* Edinburgh, United Kingdom: City of Edinburgh Council, Queen Margaret University, and NHS Lothian.

de las Heras, C. G., Lierena, V., & Kielhofner, G. (2003). *Remotivation process: Progressive intervention for individuals with severe volitional challenges* (Version 1.0). Chicago, IL: Department of Occupational Therapy, University of Illinois at Chicago.

Doble, S. (1991). Test-retest and interrater reliability of a process skills assessment. *Occupational Therapy Journal of Research, 11,* 8–23.

Elenko, B. K., Hinojosa, J., Blount, M.-L., & Blount, W. (2000). Perspectives. In J. Hinojosa & M.-L. Blount (Eds.), *The texture of life: Purposeful activities in occupational therapy* (pp. 16–35). Bethesda, MD: American Occupational Therapy Association.

Fisher, A. G. (2003). *Assessment of Motor and Process Skills* (5th ed.). Fort Collins, CO: Three Star.

Fisher, A., & Kielhofner, G. (1995). Skill in occupational performance. In G. Kielhofner (Ed.), *A model of human occupation: Theory and application* (2nd ed., pp. 113–137). Baltimore, MD: Lippincott Williams & Wilkins.

Fisher, G., Arriaga, P., Less, C., Lee, J., & Ashpole, E. (2008). *The Residential Environment Impact Survey* (REIS; Version 2.0). Chicago, IL: Model of Human Occupation Clearinghouse.

Forsyth, K., Deshpande, S., Kielhofner, G., Henriksson, C., Haglund, L., Olson, L., . . . Kulkarni, S. (2005). *The Occupational Circumstances Assessment Interview and Rating Scale* (OCAIRS; Version 4.0). Chicago, IL: Model of Human Occupation Clearinghouse.

Forsyth, K., Lai, J., & Kielhofner, G. (1999). The assessment of communication and interaction skills (ACIS): Measurement properties. *British Journal of Occupational Therapy, 62*, 69–74.

Forsyth, K., Salamy, M., Simon, S., & Kielhofner, G. (1998). *Assessment of communication and interaction skills* (Version 4.0). Chicago, IL: Model of Human Occupation Clearinghouse.

Forsyth, K., Whitehead, J., Owen, C., & Gorska, S. (2012). *A users guide to the Active in Children Health Integrating Evidence Valuing Experience (ACHIEVE) Assessment*. Edinburgh, United Kingdom: Queen Margaret University.

Frust, G., Gerber, L., Smith, C., Fisher, S., & Shulman, B. (1987). A program for improving energy conservation behaviors in adults with rheumatoid arthritis. *American Journal of Occupational Therapy, 41*, 102–111.

Gerber, L., & Frust, G. (1992). Scoring methods and application of the activity record (ACTRE) for patients with musculoskeletal disorders. *Arthritis Care and Research, 5*, 151–156.

Haglund, L., Ekbladh, E., Thorell, L., & Hallberg, I. R. (2000). Practice models in Swedish psychiatric occupational therapy. *Scandinavian Journal of Occupational Therapy, 7*, 107–113.

Hemmingson, H., Egilson, S., Hoffman, O., & Kielhofner, G. (2005). *School Setting Interview* (SSI; Version 3.0). Nacka, Sweden: Swedish Association of Occupational Therapists.

Henderson, E., & Sugden, D. (1992). *The movement assessment battery for children*. London, United Kingdom: Psychological Corporation.

Henry, A. D. (2000). *The pediatric interest profiles: Surveys of play for children and adolescents*. Unpublished manuscript, Model of Human Occupation Clearinghouse, Department of Occupational Therapy, University of Illinois, Chicago, IL.

Keller, J., Kafkes, A., Basu, S., Federico, J., & Kielhofner, G. (2005). *A user's guide to Child Occupational Self Assessment* (COSA; Version 2.1). Chicago, IL: University of Illinois, Chicago.

Kielhofner, G. (1980a). A model of human occupation: 2. Ontogenesis from the perspective of temporal adaptation. *American Journal of Occupational Therapy, 34*, 657–663.

Kielhofner, G. (1980b). A model of human occupation: 3. Benign and vicious cycles. *American Journal of Occupational Therapy, 34*, 731–737.

Kielhofner, G. (1985). *A model of human occupation: Theory and application*. Baltimore, MD: Lippincott Williams & Wilkins.

Kielhofner, G. (2008). *A model of human occupation: Theory and application* (4th ed.). Baltimore, MD: Lippincott Williams & Wilkins.

Kielhofner, G., & Burke, J. (1980). A model of human occupation: 1. Conceptual framework and content. *American Journal of Occupational Therapy, 34*, 572–581.

Kielhofner, G., Burke, J., & Heard, I. C. (1980). A model of human occupation: 4. Assessment and intervention. *American Journal of Occupational Therapy, 34*, 777–788.

Kielhofner, G., & Igi, C. H. (1980). A model of human occupation: 4. Assessment and intervention. *American Journal of Occupational Therapy, 34*, 777–788.

Kielhofner, G., Mallison, T., Crawford, C., Nowak, M., Rigby, M., Henry, A., & Walens, D. (2004). *Occupational Performance History Interview-II* (OPHI-II; Version 2.1). Chicago, IL: Model of Human Occupation Clearinghouse.

Law, M. (1998). *Client-centered occupational therapy*. Thorofare, NJ: SLACK.

Law, M., Cooper, B. A., Strong, S., Stewart, D., Rigby, P., & Letts, L. (1997). Theoretical contexts for the practice of occupational therapy. In C. Christiansen & C. Baum (Eds.), *Occupational therapy: Enabling function and well-being* (2nd ed., pp. 73–102). Thorofare, NJ: SLACK.

Law, M., & McColl, M. A. (1989). Knowledge and use of theory among occupational therapists: A Canadian survey. *Canadian Journal of Occupational Therapy, 56*, 198–204.

Lee, S. W., Taylor, R., Kielhofner, G., & Fisher, G. (2008). Theory use in practice: A national survey of therapists who use the model of human occupation. *American Journal of Occupational Therapy, 62*, 106–117.

Matsutsuyu, J. (1969). The interest checklist. *American Journal of Occupational Therapy, 23*, 323–328.

Moore-Corner, R. A., Kielhofner, G., & Olson, L. (1998). *A user's guide to Work Environment Impact Scale*. Chicago, IL: Model of Human Occupation Clearinghouse.

National Board for Certification in Occupational Therapy. (2004). A practice analysis study of entry-level occupational therapists registered and certifies occupational therapy assistant practice. *OTJR: Occupation, Participation and Health, 24*, S1–S31.

Oakley, F., Kielhofner, G., & Barris, R. (1985). An occupational therapy approach to assessing psychiatric patients' adaptive functioning. *American Journal of Occupational Therapy, 39*, 147–154.

Parkinson, S., Forsyth, K., & Kielhofner, G. (2006). *A user's manual for the model of human occupation screening tool* (MOHOST; Version 2.0). Chicago, IL: University of Illinois, Chicago.

Pedretti, L. W., & Early, M. B. (Eds.). (2001). Occupational performance and models of practice for physical dysfunction. In *Occupational therapy: Practice skills for physical dysfunction* (5th ed.). St. Louis, MO: Mosby.

Prior, S., Forsyth, K., & Ritchie, L. (2011). *ActiVate collaboration: Occupational therapy & evidence based vocational rehabilitation*. Edinburgh, United Kingdom: Queen Margaret University, NHS Lothian.

Smith, N. R., Kielhofner, G., & Watts, J. (1986). The relationship between volition, activity pattern, and life satisfaction in the elderly. *American Journal of Occupational Therapy, 40*, 278–283.

Taylor, R. T. (2017). *Kielhofner's model of human occupation: Theory and application* (5th ed.). Baltimore, MD: Lippincott Williams & Wilkins.

Townsend, S., Carey, P. D., Hollins, N. L., Helfrich, C., Blondis, M., Hoffman, A., . . . Blackwell, A. (1999). *The Occupational Therapy Psychosocial Assessment of Learning* (OT PAL; Version 2.0). Chicago, IL: Model of Human Occupation Clearinghouse.

Trombly, C. A., & Radomski, M. V. (2001). *Occupational therapy for physical dysfunction* (5th ed.). Philadelphia, PA: Lippincott Williams & Wilkins.

Watts, J. H., Hinson, R., Madigan, M. J., McGuigan, P. M., & Newman, S. M. (1999). The assessment of occupational functioning—Collaborative version. In B. J. Hempill-Pearson (Ed.), *Assessments in occupational therapy in mental health*. Thorofare, NJ: SLACK.

Wilkeby, M., Pierre, B. L., & Archenholtz, B. (2006). Occupational therapists' reflection on practice within psychiatric care: A Delphi study. *Scandinavian Journal of Occupational Therapy, 13*, 151–159.

Wilson, B. N., Kaplan, B. J., Crawford, S. G., Campbell, A., & Dewey, D. (2000). Reliability and validity of a parent questionnaire on childhood motor skills. *American Journal of Occupational Therapy, 54*, 484–493.

Ecological Models in Occupational Therapy

Catana E. Brown

LEARNING OBJECTIVES

After reading this chapter, you will be able to:

1. Outline the historical foundations of ecological models and how these concepts contributed to the development of occupational therapy ecological models.
2. Evaluate the role of the environment in understanding occupational performance.
3. Compare and contrast the similarities and differences among the four ecological models described in the chapter (Ecology of Human Performance, Person-Environment-Occupation, and Person-Environment-Occupational-Performance, Canadian Model of Occupational Performance and Engagement).
4. Analyze and apply the ecological models (Ecology of Human Performance, Person-Environment-Occupation, Person-Environment-Occupational-Performance, Canadian Model of Occupational Performance and Engagement) and their concepts to occupational therapy practice.
5. Distinguish the five intervention strategies: establish/restore, adapt/modify, alter, prevent, and create.

Introduction

Models provide occupational therapy (OT) practitioners with a representation along with language to help the practitioner understand and explain practice. Occupational therapy practitioners are ultimately concerned with what the person wants or needs to do, in other words, occupational performance. Before intervention begins, the OT practitioner must first identify barriers and facilitators to performance. This is where the ecological models are helpful. These models provide the profession with a greater appreciation for the role of the environment.

In the 1990s, different groups of occupational therapists working independently created four separate models that emphasized the importance of considering the environment in OT practice. The four models, the Ecology of Human Performance (EHP) model (Dunn, Brown, & McGuigan, 1994), the Person-Environment-Occupational-Performance (PEOP) model (Christiansen & Baum, 1997), the Person-Environment-Occupation (PEO) model (Law et al., 1996) and the Canadian Model of Occupational

CENTENNIAL NOTES

Occupational therapy: The *Doing* Profession

From our beginnings, OT could be distinguished from other disciplines because of our emphasis on doing and not talking. Because occupational therapists engage clients in occupational performance, we need to use "things" in our therapy. Therefore, one component of the environment that has always been a part of OT involves the objects used in practice. In the early years of OT, the objects used in therapy were heavily focused on arts and crafts (Marshall, Myers, & Pierce, 2017).

When the profession had yet to be established, two individuals used pottery work as both a means and an end of therapy. Herbert Hall, identified as a near founder and later a president of American Occupational Therapy Association established a workshop at a sanatorium in Marblehead, Massachusetts, for young people with neurasthenia (Peloquin, 1991). Although several types of arts and crafts were used, pottery was at the forefront.

Philip King Brown was inspired by Hall and founded the Arequipa Sanatorium where pottery was also used and in this case for young women with tuberculosis (Harley & Schwartz, 2013).

In both instances, Hall and Brown used pottery as a way to address the illness (means) as well as social inequality (end). Pottery had the physical benefits of getting people out of bed and moving. The wet nature of the clay made it less problematic for those with breathing issues. Psychological benefits included the provision of a sense of purpose and a connection with others.

Pottery work also served as an end because it provided employment. Both Hall and Brown emphasized the importance of the patients receiving remuneration for their work, and because pottery was a highly desirable product, their work was marketable. This legacy continues today as Marblehead pottery is displayed at the Marblehead Museum (http://www.marbleheadmuseum.org/archives/marblehead-pottery/) and continues to be sold in galleries.

Performance (CMOP) (Canadian Association of Occupational Therapists, 1997) share many similarities and a few distinctions. The four dynamic models consider occupational (task) performance as a primary outcome of interest to occupational therapists. In 2013, the CMOP model became the CMOP-E model to indicate OT extends beyond occupational performance to include occupational engagement (Townsend & Polatajko, 2013).

In addition, all of the models indicate that occupational performance is determined by the person, environment (context), and occupation (task). However, of the constructs of person, environment, and occupation, there was a concern by the developers of the models that the environment was the construct not receiving adequate attention. There is a tendency to focus on person factors and neglect the influence of the environment on occupational performance. Therefore, the ecological models were developed so that along with consideration for the person and occupation, OT practice includes assessments and interventions that focus on the environment. The differences in these models lie primarily in the definitions, components, and structures of the models.

Intellectual Heritage

The ecological models were built on social science theory, earlier OT models, and the disability movement. Each of the ecological models draws heavily on social science theories that describe person–environment interactions (Bronfenbrenner, 1979; Gibson, 1979; Lawton, 1986; Csikszentmihalyi, 1990) as well as earlier models of OT such as the Model of Human Occupation (Kielhofner, 2004) and Occupational Adaptation (Schkade & Schultz, 1992).

Perhaps most importantly, the ecological models in OT were influenced by the disability civil rights movement. Health care practice is dominated by a focus on impairment in the person and interventions that are designed to fix that impairment. Individuals with disabilities have challenged this perspective. People in the independent living movement pointed out that environmental barriers are typically the greatest impediment to a successful and satisfying life (DeJong, 1979; Shapiro, 1994). Furthermore, individuals with psychiatric disabilities revealed that the power of stigma and subsequent discrimination interfere with full participation in community life (Chamberlin, 1990; Deegan, 1993).

The disability movements advocated for civil rights for individuals with disabilities and promoted self-determination and empowerment. The ecological models embrace the values of the disability movement. This is reflected in both the emphasis on the environment as a significant barrier and facilitator of occupational performance and the adoption of principles of client-centered practice.

Definitions

Person

The EHP, PEO, PEOP, and CMOP-E models have similar definitions of the *person*. The holistic view of the person acknowledges the mind, body, and spirit. Variables associated with the person include values and interests, skills and abilities, and life experiences. Values and interests help to determine what is important, meaningful, and enjoyable to the person. Skills and abilities include cognitive, social, emotional, and sensorimotor skills as well as abilities such as reading and knowing how to balance a checkbook. Life experiences form the person's history and personal narrative. In CMOP-E, spirituality is emphasized as the essence of the person and is the place where determination and meaning happen.

The person influences and is influenced by the environment. For example, a person's family and friends contribute to the development of particular values and interests. A child might develop a love of reading because of the availability of books in the home and parents who read to the child, whereas having a child in the home might cause the parents to be more concerned about having healthy foods at home and creating a safe physical environment.

Environment

The environment is also described similarly across the four models. The environment is where occupational performance takes place and consists of physical, cultural, and social components. The EHP model also includes the temporal environment, and the CMOP-E model includes the institutional environment. The physical environment is the most tangible. It includes built and natural features, large elements such as the terrain or buildings, and small objects such as tools. The cultural environment is based on shared experiences that determine values, beliefs, and customs. The cultural environment includes, but is not limited to, ethnicity, religion, and national identity. For example, individuals may also adopt values and beliefs from the culture of their family, profession, organizations or clubs, and peer group.

The social environment is made up of many layers. It includes close interpersonal relationships such as family and friends. Another layer includes work groups or social organizations to which the individual belongs. A larger layer consists of political and economic systems, which can have a profound effect on the daily life of people with disabilities. These systems make decisions related to the rights of people with disabilities, availability of services, and financial benefits, such as social security disability and health insurance. This larger layer of the social

environment is comparable to the institutional environment in CMOP-E. The temporal environment is made up of time-oriented factors associated with the person (developmental and life stage) and the task (when it takes place, how often, and for how long).

Occupational performance cannot be understood outside of the context or environment. The environment can both create barriers to performance and enhance occupational performance. For example, a well-organized and familiar grocery store that provides foods that are culturally familiar and consistent with the person's likes might be described as an adaptive environment. Conversely, the grocery store might be a barrier if the person is overwhelmed by many choices, cannot find the items he or she is looking for, and is anxious when there are too many people around.

Occupation or Task

One difference in the four models is found in the concepts related to occupations or *tasks*. The PEO, PEOP, and CMOP-E use the term *occupation*, whereas EHP uses *task*. The developers of EHP were intentional about the selection of the term *task* because a primary purpose of the model was to facilitate interdisciplinary collaboration. It was felt that the term *task* would be more accessible to other disciplines. Tasks are defined as objective representations of all possible activities available in the universe. Although this was not explicitly expressed in the early writings of EHP, occupations exist when the person and context factors come together to give meaning to tasks (Dunn, McClain, Brown, & Youngstrom, 2003). In CMOP-E, occupation is the link between the person and the environment.

The PEO and PEOP models describe a series of nested concepts that make up occupations. In PEO, activities are the basic units of tasks. Tasks are purposeful activities, and occupations are self-directed tasks that a person engages in over the life course. The PEOP model involves actions, which are observable behaviors; tasks, which are combinations of actions with a common purpose; and occupations, which are goal-directed, meaningful pursuits that typically extend over time. For example, chopping vegetables might be the observable behavior or activity, embedded within the task of preparing soup, which falls under the larger occupation of cooking dinner for the family.

Occupational Performance

Occupational performance is the outcome that is associated with the confluence of the person, environment, and occupation factors. The degree to which occupational performance is possible depends on the goodness of fit of

PEO model

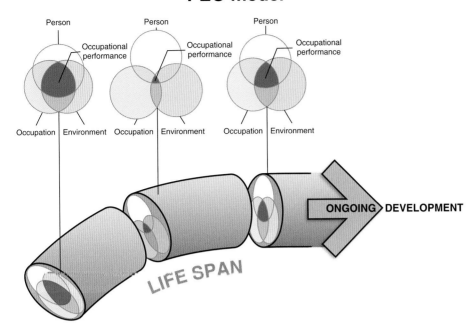

FIGURE 43-1 Person-Environment-Occupation Model. (Reprinted with permission from Law, M., Cooper, B., Strong, S., Stewart, D., Rigby, P., & Letts, L. [1996]. The person-environment-occupation model: A transactive approach to occupational performance. *Canadian Journal of Occupational Therapy, 63,* 9–23.)

these factors. The structures of the models are depicted in slightly different ways. In PEO, a Venn diagram is used to illustrate the meeting of person, environment, and occupation variables (Figure 43-1). The space in which the three circles come together is occupational performance. The PEOP is similar; however, there are four circles instead of three (Figure 43-2). Person and environment touch but do not overlap. Occupation and performance are two separate circles that overlay person and environment. These circles come together to form occupational performance and

participation. In EHP, the person is embedded inside the context, with tasks floating all around (Figure 43-3). The performance range includes the tasks that are available to the person because of the existing environment supports and his or her own skills, abilities, and experiences. In COMP-E, occupation connects the person and environment with occupation as our core domain of interest (Figure 43-4).

In all of the models, the performance range or occupational performance area is constantly changing as the

PEOP model

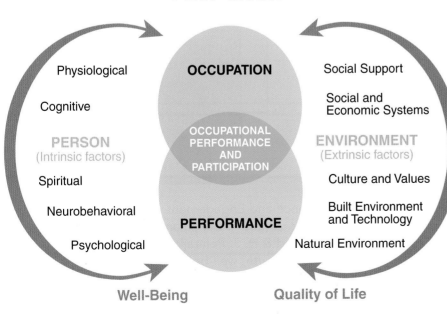

FIGURE 43-2 Person-Environment-Occupational-Performance model. (Reprinted with permission from Christiansen, C., Baum, C., & Bass-Haugen, J., [Eds.]. [2005]. *Occupational therapy: Performance, participation, and well-being* [3rd ed.]. Thorofare, NJ: SLACK.)

EHP model

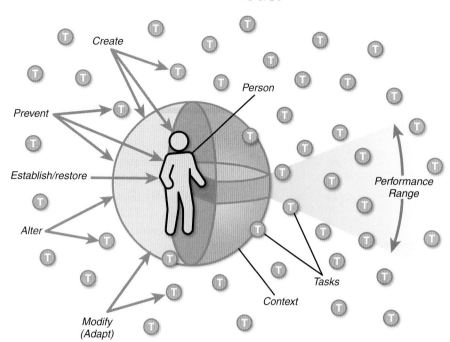

FIGURE 43-3 Ecology of Human Performance model. (Reprinted with permission from Dunn, W., McClain, L. H., Brown, C., & Youngstrom, M. J. [2003]. The ecology of human performance. In E. B. Crepeau, E. S. Cohn, & B. A. B. Schell [Eds.], *Willard & Spackman's occupational therapy* [10th ed., pp. 223–226]. Philadelphia, PA: Lippincott William & Wilkins.)

CMOP-E model

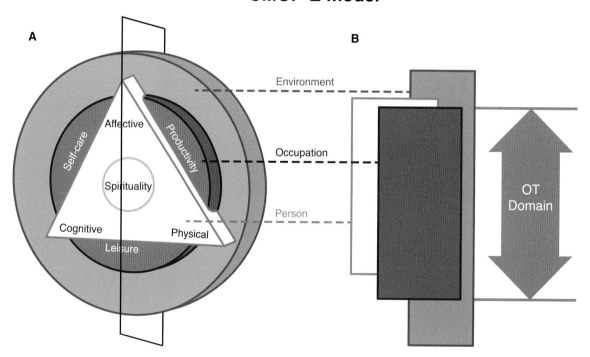

FIGURE 43-4 Canadian Model of Occupational Performance and Engagement. (Reprinted with permission from Polatajko, H. J., Townsend, E. A., & Craik. J. [2007]. Canadian Model of Occupational Performance and Engagement [CMOP-E]. In E. A. Townsend & H. J. Polatajko (Eds.), *Enabling occupation II: Advancing an occupational therapy vision of health, well-being, & justice through occupation* (p. 23). Ontario, Canada: Canada Association of Occupational Therapists.

other variables change. The area of occupational performance increases or the performance range expands when the person acquires new skills. Likewise, expansion occurs when stigma is decreased, physical barriers are removed, additional social supports are acquired, or schedules are accommodating. Unfortunately, people with disabilities are often faced with limited personal capacities and multiple environmental barriers. The role of the occupational therapist is to change this dynamic so that more occupations are available to the person.

Intervention Strategies

Additional terms that are included in the EHP model are five different intervention strategies: (1) *establish/restore*, (2) *adapt/modify*, (3) *alter*, (4) *prevent*, and (5) *create*. These interventions were spelled out so that occupational therapists would consider the full range of options. In particular, the enumeration of intervention choices was designed to encourage occupational therapists to use more interventions directed at the environment.

- **Establish/restore interventions** target the person and are aimed at developing and improving skills and abilities so that the person can perform tasks (occupations) in context. Increasing range of motion so that an individual can better manage self-care tasks and teaching someone how to use a microwave oven for meal preparation involve establish/restore strategies.
- **Adapt/modify interventions** change the environment or task to increase the individual's performance range. Using assistive devices such as an adapted car for driving or a built-up handled spoon for eating are interventions that change the typical environment. Changes to the physical environments are most common in OT; however, it is important to consider interventions that target the social and cultural environment as well. Adapt/modify strategies can include providing education about disabilities to students in an elementary school classroom so that the child with special needs will be more accepted. This is an adapt/modify strategy because the social environment is being changed.
- **Alter interventions** do not change the person, task, or environment but are designed to make a better fit. Occupational therapists may overlook alter interventions because it does not appear that they are "doing" anything. However, alter interventions can be very effective because they take advantage of what is already naturally occurring. Making a good match requires that the occupational therapist have strong skills in activity analysis and environmental assessment. Moving from a two-story house with stairs to a ranch home would for someone with limited endurance and matching the person's skills with a particular job are examples of alter interventions.

- **Prevent interventions** are implemented to change the course of events when a negative outcome is predicted. Prevention can use interventions that change the person (establish/restore), change the environment (adapt/modify), or make a better match (alter), but these occur before the problem develops. Teaching at-risk parents skills in facilitating developmentally appropriate play is an example of a prevent strategy, as is using a special cushion in a wheelchair to prevent pressure ulcers.
- **Create interventions** do not assume that a problem has occurred or will occur but are designed to promote and enrich performance in context. Like the prevent strategies, create interventions can use establish/restore, adapt, or alter approaches. Setting up a study space within a quiet area with adequate lighting is an example of a create intervention.

Assumptions of the Ecological Models

- The relationships between people, environments, and occupations are dynamic and unique. They interact continually and across time and space. Therefore, occupational therapists should approach each situation as ever changing and distinct.
- The environment is a major factor in the prediction of successful and satisfying occupational performance. Environments can either facilitate or inhibit occupational performance. All aspects of the environment (physical, social, cultural, and temporal) should be evaluated to determine relevant environmental influences.
- Rather than exclusively using interventions that change the person, it is often more efficient and effective to change the environment or find a person–environment match.
- Occupational performance is determined by the confluence of person, environment, and occupation factors. People, environments, and occupations are constantly changing, and as these factors change, so does occupational performance.
- Occupational therapy practice begins by identifying what occupations the person wants or needs to perform. Using a top–down approach, the targeted area of occupational performance is identified first by the client or family. This is followed by an assessment of barriers and facilitators within the person, environment, and occupation that affect occupational performance.
- Occupational therapy practice involves promoting self-determination and the inclusion of people with disabilities in all environments. The person or system that is the service recipient is the primary decision maker in the OT process. Occupational therapists should act as advocates for people with disabilities and should support their clients in self-advocacy.

Application to Practice

The ecological models provide a framework for thinking about OT practice but do not delineate specific assessments or techniques. Using an ecological model requires an intentional effort on the part of the occupational therapist to consider the environment as extensively as he or she considers the person. An overarching value of the ecological models is a client-centered approach to practice. The person and occupational therapist collaborate throughout all stages of the OT process, and the process begins by identifying what the person wants or needs to do in his or her life (Box 43-1). Consequently, the stage is set so that assessment and intervention are not driven by the therapist but are framed in terms of what is most important to the person. The person is not viewed in isolation but instead is considered in terms of the environment in which occupational performance takes place. The dynamic interrelationships of person, environment, and occupation compel the therapist to appreciate the uniqueness of each situation. This means that practice is not an unyielding protocol applied to everyone with the same diagnosis but a thoughtful, reasoned, and collaborative process of evaluation and intervention tailored to each individual.

Once the person identifies the relevant area(s) of occupational performance, the evaluation process determines what features of the person, environment, and occupation support or interfere with occupational performance. Therefore, OT assessment must be comprehensive

---

BOX 43-1 CLINICAL QUESTIONS RELATED TO CONSTRUCTS OF THE ECOLOGICAL MODELS

Person

Skills (cognitive, social, psychological, sensory, motor)
- What are the person's inherent strengths?
- What are potential areas of cognitive, social, or sensorimotor impairment?

Life skills
- What life skills has the person learned and what skills has the person not learned?
- What life skills has the person mastered and what skills are problematic?

Interests
- What does the person like to do?

Experiences
- What are the life experiences that contribute to or interfere with occupational performance?
- What are the major life events for the person?
- What are themes in the person's life story?

Environment/Context

Culture
- What cultural groups does the person identify with?
- What values does the person derive from these cultural groups?
- Are the beliefs and expectations of these cultural groups accepting of the person?

Social
- Are friends and family available to provide support?
- What providers are involved?
- How does public policy influence the person's ability to engage in tasks or occupations?

Physical
- What cultural groups does the person identify with?
- What values does the person derive from these cultural groups?
- Are the beliefs and expectations of these cultural groups accepting of the person?

Temporal
- Is the person able to engage in occupations that are consistent with the person's developmental or life phases?
- Does the person have too much time or not enough time to perform important tasks or occupations?

Occupation or Tasks
- What does the person want or need to do?
- What occupations or tasks come together to create roles or identity for the person?
- What occupations or tasks give meaning to the person's life?

Performance or Performance Range
- Which tasks or occupations fall inside or outside of the performance range?
- Are there factors related to the person, environment/context, or occupation that interfere with performance?

Therapeutic Intervention
- What intervention approach would be the most efficient and have the most desirable outcomes?
- Is there evidence to support the intervention approach?
- Which intervention approach does the service recipient want?

and include measures that consider the person, environment, and occupation. Assessments that are conducted in the natural environment or specifically measure the impact of the environment on occupational performance and engagement are consistent with the ecological models.

Ecological models provide a framework for practice but do not provide specific guidelines or theory about intervention techniques. However, the selection of practice models should be faithful to the values of the ecological models. Mostly, this means that the practice models that are used to guide intervention cannot be limited to person and occupational factors but must address the environment as well. The dynamic nature of the ecological models acknowledges that situations are constantly changing, indicating that regular reevaluation should occur.

The five intervention options proposed by the EHP model require occupational therapists to use a wide range of intervention approaches. Intervention can take many directions, and those interventions that target the environment should always be considered as one option. The association of ecological models with disability rights means that occupational therapists should also be involved at the systems level, supporting policy that promotes full participation in all aspects of community life. The case study (Case Study 43-1) on The Asbury Café demonstrates the ecological model in practice.

Evidence Supporting the Ecological Models

The ecological models are large conceptual frameworks, making them difficult to study in their entirety. However, research indicating a relationship between environment and occupational performance, studies of environmental assessments and efficacy studies of environmental interventions, provides support for the ecological models. This section provides examples of both types of research.

Research examining the relationship between the environment and occupational performance has implications for rehabilitation. For example,

- Neighborhood characteristics affect social participation for older adults such that greater population density was associated with more attendance in sports and social clubs and greater social cohesion was associated with greater attendance of nonreligious organizations (Hand & Howrey, 2017).
- Environmental features affect participation for individuals with mobility impairments. Negative attitudes, physical barriers and inadequacy of systems, services and policies affect participation in multiple areas such participation in education, employment and health care (Wong et al., 2017).

- A qualitative study found that the sensory environment could interfere with participation for children with autism. If the occupation was deemed essential, then additional efforts or strategies were often required. However, if the occupation was nonessential, it was often avoided (Pfeiffer et al., 2017).

Other research that is useful to occupational therapists examines environmental assessments.

- One study supported the validity of the Young Children's Participation and Environment Measure which assesses several aspects of the environment in terms of its impact on children's participation (Khetani, 2015).
- Construct validity of the Environmental Factors Item Banks, which measures four aspects of the environment for people with disabilities, was supported in a study correlating the measure with seven existing measures (Heinemann et al., 2016).
- An assessment that identifies environmental barriers to performance of daily caregiving activities, the I-HOPE Assist was found to have good interrater reliability, internal consistency and convergent validity (Keglovits, Somerville, & Stark, 2015.

There are several examples of research that support the efficacy of OT intervention with an ecological basis.

- One study established the feasibility and satisfaction of a sensory-adapted dental environment for children with autism (Cermak et al., 2015).
- The Community Aging in Place—Advancing Better Living for Elders (CAPABLE) intervention using an occupational therapist, nurse, and handyman successfully addressed personal and environmental risk factors to reduce activities of daily living (ADL) disability in older adults living at home (Szanton et al., 2015).
- A weight loss intervention that included targeted changes to the obesogenic environment of people with serious mental illness was effective in reducing waist circumference and cardiometabolic risk (Looijmans et al., 2017).

The research here provides just a few examples of this rapidly growing body of research. The research evidence suggests occupational therapists are now more informed about the role of the environment as it relates to occupational performance and better prepared to provide relevant and useful assessments and interventions using an ecological approach.

Conclusion

Occupational therapy practice is aimed at promoting occupational performance. Ecological models provide a framework for understanding the multiplicity of factors

CASE STUDY 43-1   THE ASBURY CAFÉ

The Asbury Café is an employment program developed by the author. The Asbury Café operates every Wednesday night at a local church. Five individuals with serious mental illness are employees of the café. A meal is served at a reasonable cost for church members, neighbors, and friends. An occupational therapist oversees the running of the café, assisted by volunteers and college students. It is an example of a program that uses the principles of the ecological models to promote work performance for people with psychiatric disabilities. However, that is just one of the aims of the program, which on a larger scale aspires to make changes in social and cultural environments to reduce the stigma associated with serious mental illness. People with serious mental illness are frequently depicted in the media as dangerous, peculiar, and in need of care and protection. Although serious mental illness is not uncommon, many people do not disclose their diagnosis because of the associated stigma. The Asbury Café provides an opportunity for people with and without mental illness to come together and interact in a positive environment (Figure 43-5).

The first aim of the program is to provide employment to individuals with psychiatric disabilities. Individuals who are referred by the vocational team to this worksite are typically individuals who have less work experience, have

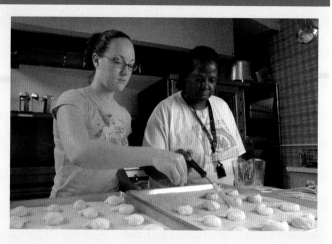

FIGURE 43-5 Jess and Janet at the Asbury Café. (Photo courtesy of C. Brown.)

more overt symptomatology, and need more extensive adaptations to the work environment. No formal assessments are completed; however, extensive skilled observation and task analysis are used to match employees with tasks and to make adaptations to the task and environment.

Target Area of Occupational Performance: Work

Ecological Model Components	Interventions
Person Factors	
Individuals with serious mental illness often have cognitive impairments that slow information processing and interfere with learning of the job tasks.	Establish/restore: Provide simple instructions with demonstration, models, and regular feedback. Alter: Match worker with café task that best meets the person's interests and abilities. Adapt: Pair workers so that one with stronger skills can model, help focus, and provide feedback to the worker with developing skills.
Psychiatric symptoms such as anxiety and auditory hallucinations can make it more challenging to focus on work tasks.	Establish/restore: Teach the worker individual strategies to use when feeling anxious (e.g., deep breathing) or experiencing hallucinations (e.g., talk aloud to others). Adapt: Allow for frequent breaks, set up an environment of acceptance and support, use the environment to create distractions from hallucinations or worries.
Environmental Factors	
Fewer job opportunities are available to the employees of the café in the neighborhoods where they live, and typical worksites do not offer the limited schedule needed and desired by current employees.	Adapt: The full Asbury Café program is an adapt strategy. Supervisors and volunteers have experience in mental health services. Employees at the café are individuals who need more extensive supports for successful work performance.
Employees at the café do not have cars, and no public transportation is available to the work location.	Adapt: Although this is not ideal, the mental health center provides transportation.
Occupation	
The major occupation is work in the area of meal preparation, serving, and cleanup. Each task has many subcomponents.	Alter: Over time, the best matches become known, and individual workers assume responsibility for their tasks. They are able to perform these tasks without assistance or oversight. Adapt: The tasks are often adapted so that there are fewer steps or one task is done by two or three people so that the full task is not too difficult for an individual.

CASE STUDY 43-1   THE ASBURY CAFÉ (continued)

The second purpose of the Asbury Café is to reduce the stigma associated with serious mental illness by promoting positive social interactions between people with and without mental illness.

The Asbury Café demonstrates how OT can have an impact outside of a traditional service setting. The café is true to the values of the ecological models, which emphasize

client-centered practice and full participation in community life. The program enhances occupational performance in the areas of work and social interaction by providing interventions targeting the person, environment, and occupation. The program itself is designed to change the stigmatizing social and cultural environment that is currently so pervasive for people with serious mental illness.

Target Area of Occupational Performance: Social Interaction

Ecological Model Components	Interventions
Person Factors	
Many of the customers at the café have limited exposure to individuals with serious mental illness.	Alter: Employees with mental illness are assigned work tasks so that they have opportunities to interact directly with the café customers (taking money, serving meals). Employees with mental illness are also assigned work tasks that require regular contact with church staff. This provides an opportunity for real work relationships to develop.
Environmental Factors	
Our culture tends to portray individuals with serious mental illness as dangerous, unpredictable, and in need of protection. Yet, the church is an environment that is open to accepting diverse individuals and welcomes the program.	Establish/restore: Educational opportunities are provided through the church in the form of lectures, articles in the newsletter, and presentations by consumers of the mental health center to provide accurate information to potential café customers about serious mental illness. Adapt: The program director and volunteers create an environment that models positive interactions with individuals with serious mental illness (e.g., avoiding distinguishing between those who do and do not have mental illness; in addition to working alongside one another, also socializing together during breaks).
Occupation	
Eating together socially.	Alter: The Asbury Café provides a naturally occurring opportunity for people to socialize in a natural setting. The café workers, supervisor, and volunteers eat during the time when the customers are eating so that there are more times for interaction.

that must be taken into account in assessing and providing interventions to enhance occupational performance. These models require that the occupational therapist use a client-centered approach and always consider the importance of the environment in the OT process.

REFERENCES

Bronfenbrenner, U. (1979). *The ecology of human development: Experiments by nature and design.* Cambridge, MA: Harvard University Press.

Canadian Association of Occupational Therapists. (1997). *Enabling occupation: An occupational therapy perspective.* Ontario, Canada: Author.

Cermak, S. A., Stein Duker, L. I., Williams, M. E., Dawson, M. E., Lane, C. J., & Polido, J. C. (2015). Sensory adapted dental environments to enhance oral care for children with autism spectrum disorders: A randomized controlled pilot study. *Journal of Autism and Developmental Disorders, 45,* 2876–2888.

Chamberlin, J. (1990). The ex-patients' movement: Where we've been and where we're going. *Journal of Mind and Behavior, 11,* 323–336.

Christiansen, C., & Baum, C. (Eds.). (1997). *Occupational therapy: Enabling function and well-being* (2nd ed.). Thorofare, NJ: SLACK.

Christiansen, C., Baum, C., & Bass-Haugen, J. (Eds.). (2005). *Occupational therapy: Performance, participation, and well-being* (3rd ed.). Thorofare, NJ: SLACK.

Csikszentmihalyi, M. (1990). *Flow: The psychology of optimal experience.* New York, NY: Harper & Row.

Deegan, P. E. (1993). Recovering our sense of value after being labeled mentally ill. *Journal of Psychosocial Nursing and Mental Health Services, 31*(4), 7–11.

DeJong, G. (1979). Independent living: From social movement to analytic paradigm. *Archives of Physical Medicine and Rehabilitation, 60,* 435–446.

Dunn, W., Brown, C., & McGuigan, A. (1994). The ecology of human performance: A framework for considering the effect of context. *American Journal of Occupational Therapy, 48,* 595–607.

Dunn, W., McClain, L. H., Brown, C., & Youngstrom, M. J. (2003). The ecology of human performance. In E. B. Crepeau, E. S. Cohn, & B. A. B. Schell (Eds.), *Willard & Spackman's occupational therapy* (10th ed., pp. 223–226). Philadelphia, PA: Lippincott William & Wilkins.

Gibson, J. J. (1979). *The ecological approach to visual perception.* Boston, MA: Houghton Mifflin.

Hand, C. L., & Howrey, B. T. (2017). Associations among neighborhood characteristics, mobility limitation, and social participation in late life. *Journals of Gerontology, Series B: Psychological Sciences.* Advance online publication. doi:10.1093/geronb/gbw215

Harley, L., & Schwartz, K. B. (2013). Philip King Brown and Arequipa Sanatorium: Early occupational therapy as medical and social experiment. *American Journal of Occupational Therapy, 67*, e11–e17.

Heinemann, A. W., Miskovic, A., Semik, P., Wong, A., Dashner, J., Baum, C., . . . Gray, D. B. (2016). Measuring environmental factors: Unique and overlapping international classification of functioning, disability and health coverage of 5 instruments. *Archives of Physical Medicine and Rehabilitation, 97*, 2113–2122.

Keglovits, M., Somerville, E., & Stark, S. (2015). In-Home Occupational Performance Evaluation for Providing Assistance (I-HOPE Assist): An assessment for informal caregivers. *American Journal of Occupational Therapy, 69*, 6905290010.

Khetani, M. A. (2015). Validation of environmental content in the Young Children's Participation and Environment Measure. *Archives of Physical Medicine and Rehabilitation, 96*, 317–322.

Kielhofner, G. (2004). *Conceptual foundations of occupational therapy* (3rd ed.). Philadelphia, PA: F. A. Davis.

Law, M., Cooper, B., Strong, S., Stewart, D., Rigby, P., & Letts, L. (1996). The person-environment-occupation model: A transactive approach to occupational performance. *Canadian Journal of Occupational Therapy, 63*, 9–23.

Lawton, M. P. (1986). *Environment and aging* (2nd ed.). Albany, NY: Plenum Press.

Looijmans, A., Stiekema, A. P. M., Bruggeman, R., van der Meer, L., Stolk, R. P., Schoevers, R. A., . . . Corpeleijn, E. (2017). Changing the obesogenic environment to improve cardiometabolic health in residential patients with a severe mental illness: Cluster randomised controlled trial. *British Journal of Psychiatry, 211*, 296–303.

Marshall, A., Myers, C., & Pierce, D. (2017). A century of therapeutic use of the physical environment. *American Journal of Occupational Therapy, 71*, 7101100030p1–7101100030p10.

Peloquin, S. M. (1991). Occupational therapy service: Individual and collective understandings of the founders, part 2. *American Journal of Occupational Therapy, 45*, 733–744.

Pfeiffer, B., Coster, W., Snethen, G., Derstine, M., Piller, A., & Tucker, C. (2017). Caregivers' perspectives on the sensory environment and participation in daily activities of children with autism spectrum disorder. *American Journal of Occupational Therapy, 71*, 7104220020p1–7104220028p9.

Polatajko, H. J., Townsend, E. A., & Craik, J. (2007). Canadian Model of Occupational Performance and Engagement (CMOP-E). In E. A. Townsend & H. J. Polatajko (Eds), *Enabling occupation II: Advancing an occupational therapy vision of health, well-being, & justice through occupation* (pp. 22–36). Ontario, Canada: CAOT Publications.

Schkade, J. K., & Schultz, S. (1992). Occupational adaptation: Toward a holistic approach for contemporary practice, part 1. *American Journal of Occupational Therapy, 46*, 829–837.

Shapiro, J. P. (1994). *No pity: People with disabilities forging a new civil rights movement.* New York, NY: Three Rivers Press.

Szanton, S. L., Wolff, J. L., Leff, B., Roberts, L., Thorpe, R. J., Tanner, E. K., . . . Gitlin, L. N. (2015). Preliminary data from community aging in place, advancing better living for elders, a patient-directed, team-based intervention to improve physical function and decrease nursing home utilization: The first 100 individuals to complete a Centers for Medicare & Medicaid Services innovation project. *Journal of the American Geriatrics Society, 63*, 371–374.

Townsend, E. A., & Polatajko, H. J. (2013). *Enabling occupation II: Advancing an occupational therapy vision for health, well-being, and justice through occupation* (2nd ed.). Ontario, Canada: Author.

Wong, A. W. K., Ng, S., Dashner, J., Baum, M. C., Hammel, J., Magasi, S. . . . Heinemann, A. W. (2017). Relationships between environmental factors and participation in adults with traumatic brain injury, stroke, and spinal cord injury: A cross-sectional multi-center study. *Quality of Life Research, 26*, 2633–2645.

the**Point**® *For additional resources on the subjects discussed in this chapter, visit* http://thePoint.lww.com /Willard-Spackman13e.

CHAPTER 44

Theory of Occupational Adaptation

Lenin C. Grajo

LEARNING OBJECTIVES

After reading this chapter, you will be able to:

1. Articulate occupational adaptation as an internal, normative human process that results from the transaction of the person and the occupational environment.
2. Evaluate the four core constructs of occupational adaptation: person, occupational environment, press for mastery, and occupational participation.
3. Apply the five essential elements of occupational adaptation as an intervention model.
4. Analyze ways in which the construct and theory of occupational adaptation can be used in daily clinical practice and research.

The Reconceptualization of Schkade and Schultz's Occupational Adaptation Theory

This chapter presents a reconceptualization of Schkade and Schultz's (1992) theory presented from two previous works (Grajo, 2017; Grajo, 2018). The reconceptualization aims to facilitate easier understanding and use of the theory in daily practice, education, and research. Occupational adaptation (OA) theory can be summarized in two core, interrelated principles (Figure 44-1):

1. Occupational adaptation is a normative, internal human process.
2. Occupational adaptation is an intervention process that can guide an occupational therapist's critical thinking and clinical reasoning within the therapeutic process and relationship.

A major disruption in the normative process in humans (principle 1) as a result of illness, disease, or disability; a major life transition; or an alteration of typical human development may be a basis for seeking occupational therapy (OT) intervention (principle 2). The goal of OT intervention (principle 2) is to facilitate the OA process in the person (principle 1).

NOTES

Development of the Theory of Occupational Adaptation

In 1987, Drs. Janette Schkade, Sally Schultz, and several faculty members began the development of the Theory of Occupational Adaptation (OA) as a theoretical framework to guide the doctor of philosophy in OT program at Texas Woman's University. Drawing from two foundational constructs—occupation and adaptation—Schkade and Schultz were influenced by the rich historical literature in OT (Schultz, 2014). Some of the historical underpinnings of the theory (Grajo, 2017, p. 288) included use of occupation to facilitate adaptation (Meyer, 1922/1977); man's need to master the environment (Reilly, 1962); occupation as a way to achieve competency, mastery, and motivation (Florey, 1969; Llorens, 1970; White, 1959); the importance of self-initiated occupation (Yerxa, 1967); and different perspectives and definitions of adaptation, competence, and resilience as a result of doing, active involvement, and choice (Fidler, 1981; Fidler & Fidler, 1978; Fine, 1991; Kielhofner, 1977; King, 1978; Kleinman & Bulkley, 1982; Nelson, 1988).

The theory of OA was first introduced as a two-part publication in the *American Journal of Occupational Therapy* (Schkade & Schultz, 1992; Schultz & Schkade, 1992). It was first published in *Willard & Spackman's Occupational Therapy* in the 8th edition of the text (1988). OA has been referred to in Willard and Spackman's book as a frame of reference (8th and 9th editions, 1988 and 1998, respectively); a theory derived from occupational behavior perspectives (9th and 10th editions, 1998 and 2003, respectively); as a conceptual basis for practice (11th edition, 2009); and as an occupational performance theory of practice (12th edition, 2014).

Between 1993 and 2015, the OA theory has been cited at least 74 times in published research articles as a primary influence in the understanding of the process of adaptation in humans, both in quantitative and qualitative studies (Grajo, Boisselle, & DaLomba, 2018) and more body of work using the theory continue to emerge.

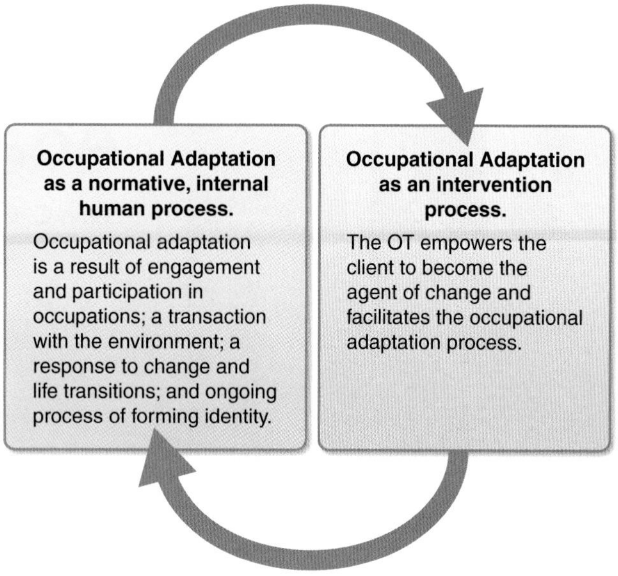

FIGURE 44-1 Summarizing the principles of the theory of occupational adaptation.

in occupations; a transaction with the environment; a manner of responding to change, altered situations, and life transitions; and a manner of forming identity. Figure 44-2 illustrates a summary of these definitions of OA as a normative process.

Four main constructs (also termed as *constants*; Schkade & Schultz, 2003) are essential in understanding this normative process

Person

The person is an occupational being with an inherent **desire to master** occupations through transactions with the environment (Grajo, 2017). Three person systems, in typical human development, enable the person to perform and participate in occupations: cognitive (i.e., neurological and processing abilities), sensorimotor (i.e., integrated sensory, perceptual, and motor capacities), and psychosocial systems (i.e., emotional, social, behavior-related abilities) (Schkade & Schultz, 1992).

Core Principle 1: Occupational Adaptation as an Internal Normative Process

A scoping study of literature (Grajo et al., 2018) identified four themes to define the construct of OA. **Occupational adaptation** is a product of engagement and participation

Occupational Environment

The occupational environment includes settings and contexts that influence occupational performance and participation. The occupational environment includes the physical and social environments and the temporal, virtual, and cultural contexts (American Occupational Therapy Association [AOTA], 2014). The occupational environment asserts a *demand for mastery* from the person. Circumstances (e.g., limited time, norms, and cultural expectations) as well as aspects of the built environment

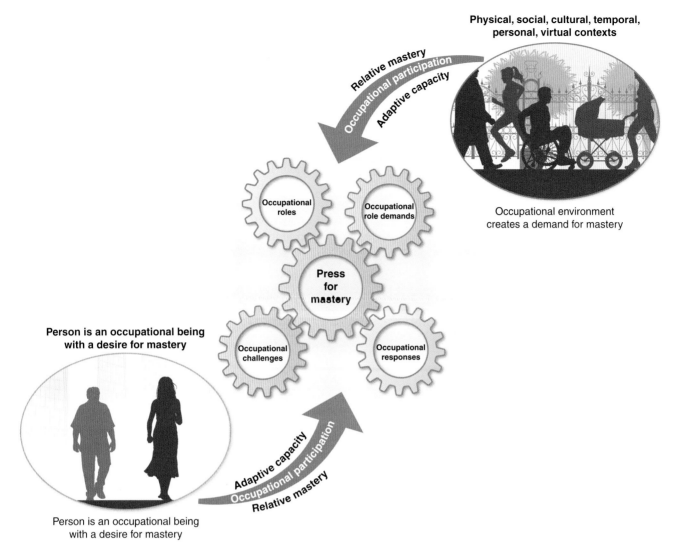

Physical, social, cultural, temporal, personal, virtual contexts

Occupational environment creates a demand for mastery

Person is an occupational being with a desire for mastery

FIGURE 44-2 A reconceptualization of Schkade and Schultz's occupational adaptation process illustration. (Reprinted with permission from Grajo, L. [2017]. Occupational adaptation. In J. Hinojosa, P. Kramer, & C. Royeen [Eds.], *Perspectives in occupation* [2nd ed., pp. 287–311]. Philadelphia, PA: F. A. Davis.)

and expectations by society may all create various forms and levels of demand for mastery from the person to behave, perform, and participate in life in ways that may facilitate or hinder the OA process.

Occupational Participation

A revision to the "Philosophical Base of Occupational Therapy" states the influence of occupational participation in a person's adaptation process: "Participation in meaningful occupation is a determinant of health and leads to adaptation" (AOTA, 2017, p. 1). Occupational participation is the mechanism for OA as an internal, normative process to manifest. Occupational participation leads to increased adaptation. Increased adaptation leads to improved occupational participation. Occupations have three important

properties: (1) They require active engagement, (2) they have meaning to the individual, and (3) they are goal oriented (i.e., they produce a tangible or intangible product as a result of participation) (Grajo, 2017; Schkade & Schultz, 1992).

Press for Mastery

When the person and the occupational environment transact during occupational participation, the press for mastery is manifested. The situational element of the press for mastery is observed when the person perceives the level of demand for mastery (asserted by the occupational environment), analyzes the skill demands of the occupation (cognitive, sensorimotor, and psychosocial demands), and assesses his or her desire for mastery of the occupation.

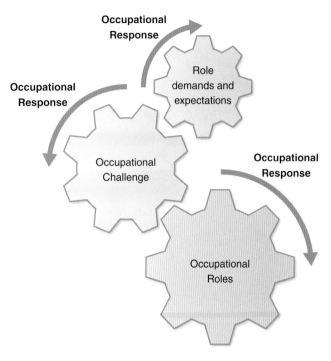

FIGURE 44-3 **Press for mastery.**

The press for mastery manifests as a series of simultaneously or concurrently occurring processes, dependent on the features of the occupation, and factors within the person and the occupational environment (Figure 44-3). These processes include the following:

a. Occupational roles. These are person-defined sets of behaviors based on expectations of society and are heavily influenced by culture and context (AOTA, 2014, p. S27).

b. Occupational challenges. Based on the person's current abilities, desire for mastery of the occupation and the environment, and assessment of the level of demand for mastery from the environment, certain occupational challenges may surface. Some occupational challenges may be easy to overcome, whereas some occupational challenges may hinder the OA process and cause a temporary or persistent level of **occupational dysadaptation**.

c. Role demands or expectations. Occupational roles assert a combination of internal and/or external role demands. Internal role demands are those perceived by the person (e.g., a single father perceives the need to work two jobs to provide for the family). External role demands are asserted by the occupational environment (e.g., some cultures may dictate that mothers need to spend more time with children than at work).

d. Occupational responses. During transaction with the environment and participation in occupations,

the person evaluates the level of occupational challenge, roles expected by society or assumed by the person, and role demands. The person then identifies a way to respond to these challenges, roles, and role demands or expectations. This configuration of a response involves creating an **adaptation gestalt**. The adaptation gestalt allows the person to assess how to respond and what responses to produce to achieve mastery and competence in occupational participation. The person may choose an old response that previously worked for him or her, develop a new response, or modify old responses to create new responses that may overcome the occupational challenge based on cognitive, sensorimotor, and psychosocial abilities.

The Adaptation Gestalt

The adaptation gestalt is an assessment of the amount and level of cognitive, sensorimotor, and psychosocial capacities needed to respond to occupational challenges, roles, and role demands and perform an occupation with a level of mastery and competence (Schkade & Schultz, 1992). Occupations require different levels of skills and demands from the person systems. Some occupations may have higher cognitive demands (e.g., studying for a final exam), higher psychosocial skills demands (e.g., making new friends), or higher demands from sensory and motor abilities (e.g., completing a 60-minute upper body workout). A pie chart (Figure 44-4) can be used to visually configure the adaptation gestalt (Schultz & Schkade, 1997). The person system that is required more to perform an occupation takes a bigger piece of the pie. The pie chart configuration also helps determine the person's skill strengths and challenges. Experiences by the person

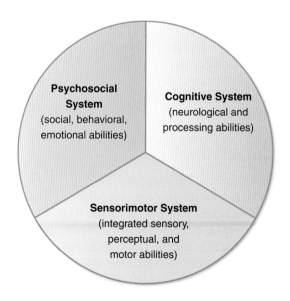

FIGURE 44-4 **The adaptation gestalt.**

CASE STUDY 44-1   RACHEL

Rachel is a retired nurse who was diagnosed with breast cancer and had a mastectomy. She is a single mother to a teenage daughter with intellectual disabilities. She completed six rounds of chemotherapy but had to discontinue chemotherapy due to enlargement of the heart as a result of the strong drugs. She has low physical endurance to do many basic activities of daily living, some weakness and limited range of motion on her right upper extremity (due to mastectomy), and always feels fatigued and often confused when performing activities that require multiple steps. Her daughter relies on her for daily routines and basic activities such as preparing meals, driving to school and therapies, and helping with completing school work.

Let us try to understand Rachel's occupational adaptation process: *Rachel is undergoing significant changes in life as a result of her breast cancer diagnosis and treatments.*

- Desire for mastery: Rachel (person) wants to be able to perform basic daily activities for herself and for her daughter.
- Demand for mastery: Rachel's daughter (social environment) expects that she will continue to support her with her many daily life needs.

- Press for mastery:
  a. Important occupational role: mother
  b. Role expectations/demands: Continue participating in occupations to fulfill the mother role such as helping with the daily needs of her daughter with intellectual disabilities (drive to school and therapies, assist with homework, prepare meals).
  c. Occupational challenges: difficulties with various, multistep tasks (e.g., driving, preparing daily meals) due to low endurance, upper extremity weakness, easy fatigability; impacted cognitive abilities
  d. Positive (adaptive) occupational responses: She may seek assistance of friends and family members with driving daughter; she can potentially identify ways to do tasks in smaller chunks and steps.
  e. Negative (dysadaptive) occupational responses: She may experience depression and feelings of inadequacy and helplessness; feelings of guilt because of her inability to support daughter's needs.

- Potential need for OT programming guided by occupational adaptation: OT can facilitate Rachel's adaptive functioning to allow her to fulfill important occupational roles, participate in occupations, and master the occupational environment.

---

based on occupations performed and challenges encountered form variations of adaptation gestalts. The person, when transacting with the occupational environment, identifies a configuration of the gestalt that will enable him or her to participate in occupations with mastery and competence.

The case of Rachel provides an overview of how to apply the four core constants of the OA theory (Case Study 44-1).

Adaptive and Dysadaptive Responses

Schkade and Schultz (2003) described complex and layered **adaptive response subprocesses**. The adaptive response subprocesses can be understood as an iterative process of identifying, producing, evaluating, and modifying occupational responses to various occupational challenges to allow the person to participate in occupations with mastery and competence. Experience heavily influences this iterative adaptive response subprocesses. Occupational responses may be described as **adaptive**. Adaptive responses overcome or help manage the occupational challenge and promote mastery and competence in the occupation. Other occupational responses maybe described as *dysadaptive* (a term coined in the original

Schkade and Schultz [1992] publication). Dysadaptive responses do not overcome the occupational challenge and may make the person feel "stuck" and unable to perform occupations and transact with the occupational environment with mastery and competence. Throughout the person's growth and development, he or she will produce, evaluate the effectiveness of, and modify a variety of adaptive and dysadaptive responses to enable him or her to participate in daily occupations.

Relative Mastery and Adaptive Capacity: Assessing Occupational Adaptation

Two terms have been used in the OA theory to describe how to evaluate the normative process of OA and when a state of occupational adaptiveness is achieved are *relative mastery* and *adaptive capacity*.

Relative Mastery. Relative mastery has three components (Grajo, 2017; Schkade & McClung, 2001):

- Effective participation in occupations is assessed based on how well people achieve their set goals of occupational engagement and participation.

- Efficiency is a person's good and appropriate use of available personal resources and resources in the occupational environment (e.g., time, energy, task objects and materials, social supports).
- Satisfaction is the extent to which people are content with their occupational performance and the congruence between occupational participation and performance expectations. Satisfaction is measured based on self and satisfaction of important others.

Adaptive Capacity. Adaptive capacity can be understood using a "tools in a toolbox" analogy (Grajo, 2017). Adaptive capacity can be defined as the person's ability to perceive the need to change, modify, or refine a variety of responses to occupational challenges in the environment (Schkade & Schultz, 2003). When faced with difficulties in life and when participating in occupations that may pose challenges, does the person have enough tools in his or her toolbox to solve the challenge? Is the person able to develop new tools or modify old tools to overcome the occupational challenge?

A major life transition, or the experience of illness or disability may impact a person's relative mastery and adaptive capacity and, therefore, the OA process. When the life event makes the person unable to resume important roles, unable to perform occupations due to major life transitions, feel overwhelmed by role demands and responsibilities, or unable to use appropriate tools or strategies to overcome occupational or task performance breakdown, a persistent state of **occupational dysadaptation** may occur (Grajo, 2018). In these cases, an occupational therapist may need to support and assist the person (the client) to reestablish important roles, resume participation in meaningful occupations, and facilitate the OA process.

Core Principle 2: Occupational Adaptation as an Intervention Process

The occupational therapist may use the OA theory to guide him or her in the therapeutic process and relationship with the client. The OA-guided intervention is not a protocol, collection of techniques, or a series of action steps to do or to take (Schkade & Schultz, 2003). The OA-guided intervention is a manner of using critical and clinical reasoning skills to assist the therapist in assessment and intervention. Establishing a meaningful therapeutic relationship is critical in OA-guided intervention. OA-guided intervention has five essential elements, as shown in Figure 44-5 (adapted from Grajo, 2017, Grajo, 2018; Schultz, 2014):

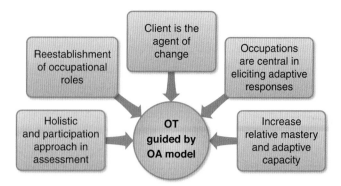

FIGURE 44-5 Essential elements of occupational adaptation (OA)-guided intervention. OT, occupational therapist. (Adapted and used with permission from Grajo, L. [2018]. Occupational adaptation as a normative and intervention process—new perspectives on Schkade and Schultz's professional legacy. In L. C. Grajo & A. K. Boisselle [Eds.], *Adaptation through occupation: Multidimensional perspectives.* Thorofare, NJ: SLACK.)

Element 1: A Holistic Approach and Participation Approach to Assessment

Based on the OA theory, assessments should not only measure static outcomes but also assess the impact of the intervention on the client's engagement and personally meaningful life roles (Schultz, 2014). An OA-guided occupational therapist will use a combination of standardized and nonstandardized assessments to create a holistic picture of the client. The occupational therapist will assist the client in creating an *occupational profile* to identify strengths and weaknesses and meaningful occupational roles. Norm-referenced tools can be used in combination with patient report–type tools, tools that assess perceptions of roles, and participation in occupations, and observational assessments of occupational performance and participation (Grajo, 2018). The OA-guided occupational therapist must evaluate the client's effectiveness, efficiency, and satisfaction in performing occupations (relative mastery) and the client's ability to assess and use a variety of tools and responses to overcome challenges (adaptive capacity).

Element 2: Reestablish Important Occupational Roles

Life roles provide the context for expressing our competence in occupational functioning (Schkade & McClung,

2001). Critical in OA-guided intervention is a focus on reestablishing roles rather than developing performance skills (Schkade & Schultz, 2003). When intervention focuses on improving a client's occupational adaptiveness based on important roles, the client is better able to participate in occupations and use and improve performance skills (Grajo, 2018; Schultz, 2014). Fulfillment of roles provides meaning and satisfaction in life.

Element 3: The Client Is the Agent of Change

The OA-guided intervention focuses on making the client the agent of change in the therapeutic process. The occupational therapist must use the therapeutic relationship to help facilitate the OA process within the client. This can be done in a variety of ways:

- Learning when to push and when to hold back: The occupational therapist must assume the role of a facilitator rather than an instructor. Instead of telling the client what to do, how to do, and what strategies to use to perform tasks and participate in occupations, the occupational therapist can use a series of facilitated questions and probing statements. The occupational therapist must also learn how to provide clients with opportunities to problem-solve, experience difficulties, and support the client to identify ways to solve occupational challenges instead of always providing insights for the client.
- Facilitating the use of occupations: The occupational therapist must allow the client to self-initiate and choose occupations that they want to work on rather than the prescribing of or identifying goals and tasks that the client needs to complete. When using occupations to facilitate the OA process, the occupational therapist must also make the client in charge of setting the levels of difficulty (grading or modifying the task difficulty) to make occupations less or more challenging.
- Facilitating the occupational environment: The occupational therapist must also involve the client in identifying ways in which the occupational environment can support masterful and competent occupational participation. The occupational therapist must be skillful in identifying contextual and environmental factors that may facilitate or hinder the OA process. The transaction with the occupational environment (as manifested in the press for mastery) is situation dependent. Aldrich and Heatwole-Shank (2018) asserted that the OA process can be seen as occurring within the person–environment relationship where both individual and social factors play a role in shaping possible solutions to a problematic situation.

Whereas Aldrich and Heatwole-Shank believe that OA cannot be an intervention outcome, Schkade and Schultz (2003) asserted that facilitated and self-initiated transactions with the occupational environment can provide mechanisms for the internal OA process to improve.

The occupational therapist must also be cognizant of a tendency to become a "fixer" for the client. Innate in occupational therapists is the willingness to help the client in all aspects of living. By focusing on the client as the agent of change, the therapist must creatively learn how to navigate the therapeutic relationship to avoid assuming a "fixer" role.

Element 4: Occupations Are Central in Eliciting Adaptive Responses

When a client feels "stuck" and in a constant or intermittent state of occupational dysadaptation, the OT can use occupations to facilitate the client to "unstick" him- or herself (Grajo, in press). Occupations can be used in two ways to elicit adaptive responses (Schkade & Schultz, 1992): *occupational readiness and occupational activities*. **Occupational readiness** are preparatory activities or performance skill-building approaches. Body function limitations may need to be addressed to prepare the client for occupations. This may include reducing spasticity or edema and addressing strength limitations or cognitive deficits. However, the occupational therapist must not only rely on occupational readiness methods alone but should also move right away to facilitating client's participation in actual occupations (originally termed **occupational activities**). The OT guided by OA must try to move away from occupational readiness and use of simulated tasks as quickly as possible and encourage use of materials, tools, and environments from where natural occupational participation occurs (Grajo, 2018).

Element 5: Increase Relative Mastery and Adaptive Capacity

The OA-guided therapist consistently assesses the client's relative mastery and adaptive capacity during the therapeutic process. Successful OT intervention empowers the normative process of OA in the client and an increase in relative mastery and adaptive capacity. Successful OA-guided OT intervention also facilitates transfer and generalization of skills. When the client is able to use adaptive responses to overcome occupational challenges in similar situations and/or when the client is able to develop new or modified occupational responses when presented with new challenges or situations, then we know that the client has increased relative mastery and adaptive capacity.

⚖️ ETHICAL DILEMMA

During a weekly case discussion with the OT staff and clinic manager, an occupational therapist reported that the pediatric client he has been treating for the past 6 months has shown remarkable improvements in all areas of concern (e.g., handwriting difficulties, impulsive behaviors that impact school performance) and has achieved documented goals. However, during the most recent reevaluation using a standardized test, the client still exhibits low average ability to modulate sensory stimuli. The occupational therapist believes this might be the client's optimal level of sensory functioning at this point and has demonstrated ways to manage challenges with sensory functioning on his own or with prompting from a parent or teacher. The occupational therapist is recommending discharge. The pediatric clinic manager, however, recommended keeping the client for OT services for another 2 to 3 months to continue addressing the sensory issues until the client scores within normal range of sensory modulation skills. The clinic manager suggested ways on how to document this finding so that the referring physician and the insurance company will find this recommendation a medical necessity.

The OA-guided therapist believes that his or her role is not to fix everything for the client and to facilitate the client's OA process to allow him or her to overcome difficulties and challenges in life. Using clinical reasoning and critical thinking skills and principles of OA theory, how should the occupational therapist respond to the recommendation of the clinic manager? What potential issues with the code of ethics of OT practice might arise with the clinic manager's recommendations?

Summary

Schkade and Schultz's theory of OA presents a manner of understanding mechanisms of occupational participation and the person–environment relationship. The theory of OA presents a guide to OT assessment and intervention. As an internal human process, with constructs grounded and supported by theoretical underpinnings in the history of OT, it is important to understand the factors and mechanisms that may facilitate or disrupt this normative process. As an intervention model, the OA theory is not a manner of doing OT but rather a manner of thinking that can guide specific actions and steps that the occupational therapist can take to support the client. The OA theory can be used with frames of reference or specific intervention approaches (e.g., cognitive models, motor learning theories, sensory processing approaches, specific rehabilitation techniques, cognitive-behavioral approaches) to develop a holistic intervention approach.

❝ COMMENTARY ON THE EVIDENCE

The theory of occupational adaptation has been used as a guide in understanding the lived experiences of disability, life transition, and altered life situations that disrupt the normative occupational adaptation process. Although this is not an exhaustive list, some contemporary examples include understanding the occupational adaptation process in adults with multiple sclerosis (Lexell, Iwarsson, & Lund, 2011), older adults with stroke (Williams & Murray, 2013), adults with posttraumatic stress disorder (Lopez, 2011), adults with acquired brain injuries (Parsons & Stanley, 2008), traumatic brain injuries (Hoogerdijk, Runge, & Haugboelle, 2011), normative changes as a result of the aging process (Moyers & Coleman, 2004), and women who immigrated to a foreign country (Nayar & Stanley, 2015).

The OA theory has also been used to guide intervention across different populations and settings. Some applications include adolescents with limb deficiencies (Pasek & Schkade, 1996), adults with stroke (Dolecheck & Schkade, 1999; Gibson & Schkade, 1997; Johnson & Schkade, 2001), adults with hip fracture (Buddenberg & Schkade, 1998; Jackson & Schkade, 2001), community-dwelling older adults (Spencer, Hersch, Eschenfelder, Fournet, & Murray-Gerzik, 1999), older adults with various physical disabilities (Bontje, Kinébanian, Josephsson, & Tamura, 2004), adults with psychiatric illness (Adami & Evetts, 2012; Whisner, Stelter, & Schultz, 2014), and children with reading difficulties (Grajo & Candler, 2016) and in settings like schools (Orr & Schkade, 1997) and prison systems (Stelter & Whisner, 2007).

Despite emerging and increasing evidence in the use of the OA theory, Grajo et al. (2018) suggested that there is a need to produce more rigorous studies on the effectiveness of the OA-guided intervention using randomized controlled trials and to develop more assessments that are explicitly based on the constructs of the OA theory.

REFERENCES

Adami, A. M., & Evetts, C. (2012). A natural approach in mental health practice: Occupational adaptation revealed. *Occupational Therapy in Mental Health, 28*, 170–179. doi:10.1080/0164212X.2012.679589

Aldrich, R., & Heatwole-Shank, K. (2018). An occupational science perspective on occupation, adaptation, and participation. In L. C. Grajo & A. K. Boisselle (Eds.). *Adaptation through occupation: Multidimensional perspectives.* Thorofare, NJ: SLACK.

American Occupational Therapy Association. (2014). Occupational therapy practice framework: Domain and process (3rd edition). *American Journal of Occupational Therapy, 68*, S1–S48. doi:10.5014/ajot.2014.682006

American Occupational Therapy Association. (2017). Philosophical base of occupational therapy. *American Journal of Occupational Therapy, 71*, 7112410045p1. doi:10.5014/ajot.2017.716S06

Bontje, P., Kinébanian, A., Josephsson, S., & Tamura, Y. (2004). Occupational adaptation: The experiences of older persons with physical disabilities. *American Journal of Occupational Therapy, 58*, 140–149. doi:10.5014/ajot.58.2.140

Buddenberg, L. A., & Schkade, J. K. (1998). A comparison of occupational therapy intervention approaches for older patients after hip fracture. *Topics in Geriatric Rehabilitation, 13*, 52–68.

Dolecheck, J. R., & Schkade, J. K. (1999). Effects on dynamic standing endurance when persons with CVA perform personally meaningful versus non-meaningful tasks. *OTJR: Occupation, Participation and Health, 19*, 40–54.

Fidler, G. (1981). From crafts to competence. *American Journal of Occupational Therapy, 35*, 567–573. doi:10.5014/ajot.35.9.567

Fidler, G., & Fidler, J. (1978). Doing and becoming: Purposeful action and self-actualization. *American Journal of Occupational Therapy, 32*, 305–310. doi:10.5014/ajot.64.1.142

Fine, S. (1991). Resilience and human adaptability: Who rises above adversity? *American Journal of Occupational Therapy, 45*, 493–503. doi:10.5014/ajot.45.6.493

Florey, L. (1969). Intrinsic motivation: The dynamics of occupational therapy theory. *American Journal of Occupational Therapy, 23*, 319–322.

Gibson, J., & Schkade, J. (1997). Occupational adaptation intervention with patients with cerebrovascular accident: A clinical study. *American Journal of Occupational Therapy, 51*, 523–529. doi:10.5014/ajot.51.7.523

Grajo, L. (2017). Occupational adaptation. In J. Hinojosa, P. Kramer, & C. Royeen (Eds.), *Perspectives on human occupation: Theories underlying practice* (2nd ed., pp. 287–311). Philadelphia, PA: F. A. Davis.

Grajo, L. (2018). Occupational adaptation as a normative and intervention process—new perspectives on Schkade and Schultz's professional legacy. In L. C. Grajo & A. K. Boisselle (Eds.), *Adaptation through occupation: Multidimensional perspectives.* Thorofare, NJ: SLACK.

Grajo, L., Boisselle, A., & DaLomba, E. (2018). Occupational adaptation as a construct: A scoping review of literature. *The Open Journal of Occupational Therapy, 6*(1), 2. doi:10.15453/2168-6408.1400

Grajo, L., & Candler, C. (2016). An occupation and participation approach to reading intervention (OPARI) part II: Pilot clinical application. *Journal of Occupational Therapy, Schools and Early Intervention, 9*, 86–98. doi:10.1080/19411243.2016.1141083

Hoogerdijk, B., Runge, U., & Haugboelle, J. (2011). The adaptation process after traumatic brain injury: An individual and ongoing occupational struggle to gain a new identity. *Scandinavian Journal of Occupational Therapy, 18*, 122–132. doi:10.3109/11038121003645985

Jackson, J., & Schkade, J. (2001). Occupational adaptation model versus biomechanical-rehabilitation model in the treatment of patients with hip fractures. *American Journal of Occupational Therapy, 55*, 531–537. doi:10.5014/ajot.55.5.531

Johnson, J., & Schkade, J. (2001). Effects of an occupation-based intervention on mobility problems following a cerebral vascular accident. *Journal of Applied Gerontology, 20*, 91–110.

Kielhofner, G. (1977). Temporal adaptation: A conceptual framework for occupational therapy. *American Journal of Occupational Therapy, 31*, 235–242.

King, L. J. (1978). 1978 Eleanor Clarke Slagle Lecture: Toward a science of adaptive responses. *American Journal of Occupational Therapy, 32*, 429–437.

Kleinman, B., & Bulkley, B. (1982). Some implications of a science of adaptive responses. *American Journal of Occupational Therapy, 36*, 16–19. doi:10.5014/ajot.36.1.15

Lexell, E. M., Iwarsson, S., & Lund, M. L. (2011). Occupational adaptation in people with multiple sclerosis. *OTJR: Occupation, Participation and Health, 31*, 127–134. doi:10.3928/15394492-20101025-01

Llorens, L. (1970). Facilitating growth and development: The promise of occupational therapy. *American Journal of Occupational Therapy, 24*, 93–101.

Lopez, A. (2011). Posttraumatic stress disorder and occupational performance: Building resilience and fostering occupational adaptation. *Work, 38*, 33–38. doi:10.3233/WOR-2011-1102

Meyer, A. (1977). The philosophy of occupation therapy. *American Journal of Occupational Therapy, 31*, 639–642. (Original work published 1922)

Moyers, P. A., & Coleman, S. D. (2004). Adaptation of the older workers to occupational challenges. *Work, 22*, 71–78.

Nayar, S., & Stanley, M. (2015). Occupational adaptation as a social process in everyday life. *Journal of Occupational Science, 22*, 26–38. doi:10.1080/14427591.2014.882251

Nelson, D. (1988). Occupation: Form and performance. *American Journal of Occupational Therapy, 42*, 633–641.

Orr, C., & Schkade, J. (1997). The impact of classroom environment on defining function in school-based practice. *American Journal of Occupational Therapy, 51*, 64–69. doi:10.5014/ajot.51.1.64

Parsons, L., & Stanley, M. (2008). The lived experiences of occupational adaptation following acquired brain injury for people living in a rural area. *Australian Occupational Therapy Journal, 55*, 231–238. doi:10.1111/j.1440-1630.2008.00753.x

Pasek, P. B., & Schkade, J. K. (1996). Effects of a skiing experience on adolescents with limb deficiencies: An occupational adaptation perspective. *American Journal of Occupational Therapy, 50*, 24–31. doi:10.5014/ajot.50.1.24

Reilly, M. (1962). Occupational therapy can be one of the greatest ideas of 20th century medicine (1961 Slagle Lecture). *American Journal of Occupational Therapy, 16*, 1–9.

Schkade, J. K., & McClung, M. (2001). *Occupational adaptation in practice: Concepts and cases.* Thorofare, NJ: SLACK.

Schkade, J. K., & Schultz, S. (1992). Occupational adaptation: Toward a holistic approach for contemporary practice, part 1. *American Journal of Occupational Therapy, 46*, 829–837. doi:10.5014/ajot.46.9.829

Schkade, J. K., & Schultz, S. (2003). Occupational adaptation. In P. Kramer, J. Hinojosa, & C. B. Royeen (Eds.), *Perspectives in human occupation: Participation in life* (pp. 181–221). Baltimore, MD: Lippincott Williams & Wilkins.

Schultz, S. (2014). Theory of occupational adaptation. In B. A. B. Schell, G. Gillen, & M. E. Scaffa (Eds.), *Willard & Spackman's occupational therapy* (12th ed., pp. 527–540). Philadelphia , PA: Lippincott Williams & Wilkins.

Schultz, S., & Schkade, J. K. (1992). Occupational adaptation: Toward a holistic approach for contemporary practice, part 2. *American Journal of Occupational Therapy, 46*, 917–925.

Schultz, S., & Schkade, J. K. (1997). Adaptation. In C. Christiansen & C. Baum (Eds.), *Occupational therapy: Enabling function and wellbeing* (2nd ed., pp. 458–481). Thorofare, NJ: SLACK.

Spencer, J., Hersch, G., Eschenfelder, V., Fournet, J., & Murray-Gerzik, M. (1999). Outcomes of protocol-based and adaptation-based occupational therapy interventions for low-income elders on a transitional unit. *American Journal of Occupational Therapy, 53,* 159–170. doi:10.5014/ajot.53.2.159

Stelter, L., & Whisner, S. (2007). Building responsibility for self through meaningful roles: Occupational adaptation theory applied in forensic psychiatry. *Occupational Therapy in Mental Health, 23,* 69–84.

Whisner, S. M., Stelter, L. D., & Schultz, S. (2014). Influence of three interventions on group participation in an acute psychiatric facility. *Occupational Therapy in Mental Health, 30,* 26–42. doi:10.1080/0164212X.2014.878527

White, R. (1959). Motivation reconsidered: The concept of competence. *Psychological Review, 66,* 297–333.

Williams, S., & Murray, C. (2013). The lived experiences of older adults' occupational adaptation following a stroke. *Australian Occupational Therapy Journal, 60,* 39–47. doi:10.1111/1440-1630.12004

Yerxa, E. (1967). Authentic occupational therapy (1966 Slagle Lecture). *American Journal of Occupational Therapy, 21,* 1–9.

the**Point**® *For additional resources on the subjects discussed in this chapter, visit* http://thePoint.lww.com/Willard-Spackman13e.

Occupational Justice

Ann A. Wilcock, Elizabeth A. Townsend

LEARNING OBJECTIVES

After reading this chapter, you will be able to:

1. Analyze occupational justice in relation to the absence of illness, social, mental, physical, and population health.
2. Appreciate, synthesize, and apply occupational justice within occupational therapy.
3. Plan and evaluate approaches to advance occupational rights and reduce injustices at both individual and population levels.

Introduction

This chapter outlines the emergence and growth of occupational justice in conceptual terms and discusses how the health of all people is potentially subject to injustices. Occupational therapists are encouraged to consider the centrality of occupation to peoples' survival, health, and well-being as a human rights issue and to incorporate action to address occupational injustices and health outcomes experienced by populations, communities, and individuals. Advancing the concept is complex, calling occupational therapists to take up assessments and interventions that may be unfamiliar to them in line with the directives of the United Nations (UN), World Health Organization (WHO), and World Federation of Occupational Therapists (WFOT).

"Occupational justice" is an idea that seems to prompt strong reactions. It challenges the long-term individual medically founded practices of occupational therapy (OT) by requiring consideration of the occupational needs of people in terms of communal equity, fairness, and opportunity. Some are energized by the language, ideas, and practice possibilities that validate justice-oriented work and open new doors within OT. Those who are skeptical, however, may not recognize a role for OT in addressing social illness or changing sociopolitical will and funding sources to cover justice-oriented work.

Looking back now in 2017, the first occupational justice workshop in 2000 in Australia attracted those who wanted to talk about doing occupational justice as well as those who expressed concern that such a topic may not belong in OT. Participants in this and later workshops as well as readers of chapters and articles on occupational justice by many writers have engaged the occupational science and OT communities in lively

CENTENNIAL NOTES

Occupation Finds Justice

At a lively lunch in Adelaide, Australia, in 1998, Ann Wilcock and Elizabeth (Liz) Townsend discussed "justice" in relation to "occupation" and together decided to advance the idea of "occupational justice." In December 2016, Hiromi Yoshikawa dramatized this exciting meeting of minds using Playback Theatre with actors portraying "occupation" and "justice" at a session within the 20th Occupational Science conference in Nagoya, Japan.

With a critical lens on society, occupational justice builds on the 1917 foundation objectives of the American Society to "study of the effect of occupation upon the human being" (Certificate of Incorporation of the National Society for the Promotion of Occupational Therapy, Inc., 1917). It also reflects the World Federation of Occupational Therapists (WFOT) position that "abuses of the right to occupation may take the form of economic, social, or physical exclusion, through attitudinal or physical barriers,

or through control of access to necessary knowledge, skills, resources, or venues where occupation takes place" (WFOT, 2006).

Occupational justice challenges but does not negate medically determined individual OT. Rather, it suggests a widening of practice to address occupational inequities arising from "societal conditions in which people are born, grow, live, work and age" (World Health Organization, 2011a, 2011b) that impact on the health of populations. From the first workshop in 2000 to the present, lively debates have addressed how occupational justice can advance long-standing, well-known efforts in many fields to theorize, write, and act on social injustice; to encourage the development of places, structures, and policies that enable equitable and diverse participation in personal, collective, and civic occupations; and to create disability-friendly, age-friendly, and mental health–friendly places to do, be, belong, and become (Wilcock & Hocking, 2015).

conversations. Some conversations have been highly practical such as "Does advocacy for community ramps constitute occupational justice work?" Not surprisingly, some people have said yes, whereas others have said no. Most people who have encountered the language, ideas, and practice possibilities that are potentially aligned with occupational justice have confirmed that advocating for one ramp is well worth doing. However, with a critical lens on society, many people have called for occupational therapists to consider not only individualized approaches but the needs of communities and populations as well. In a sense, doing occupational justice requires consideration of collectives of people and collective occupations and subsequent action. For example, occupational therapists could address occupational injustice by advocating collectively with an array of others to create disability-friendly, age-friendly, and mental health–friendly places to live and work; that is, to say places where the structures and policies of society enable equitable, diverse participation in personal, collective, and civic occupations.

Many ask how occupational justice advances long-standing, well-known efforts in many fields to theorize, write, and act on social injustice and justice. Certainly, one of the ongoing conversations for the future is how to distinguish what is the additive force beyond social justice of naming issues of justice as occupational. In this centennial edition of *Willard & Spackman's Occupational Therapy*, we (Ann and Liz) see each chapter and article on occupational injustice or occupational justice as opening new insights. For particular populations, changing situations can

influence and/or alter physical, mental, or social health in ways that extend beyond typical societal concerns for social justice. Maybe the growth of occupational science and OT "literacy" over the next 100 years will provide knowledge and skills to think, talk, write, speak, and organize occupations so that justice ensues as an integral part of the human search for health-giving, purposeful, and meaningful occupations, and occupational injustice is reduced.

Occupational Justice as an Idea and a Need

From the genesis of humankind, individuals and the communities in which they live have needed occupation to survive healthily, or, indeed, to survive at all. They have had to balance activity and rest, find food, make shelter, and nurture their young as future occupational beings and their old as the custodians of accumulated occupational lore and wisdom. In these fundamental terms, occupationally just situations are essential. A societal system that is occupationally just would be one in which each person and community could meet their own and others' survival, physical, mental, and social health needs through occupations that recognize and encourage individual and communal strengths and respect the environment to meet the needs of future generations. An occupationally unjust situation occurs when the reverse is the case. Common examples well known to occupational therapists are scarcity or absence of suitable or supportive employment; inadequate support for youth, adults, and seniors who lack the resources or opportunities to live and sustain their mental, physical, social, and spiritual health; limited recreational opportunities; and absent, unsuitable, or insufficient housing or shelter. When accepting unjust conditions of this kind, occupational therapists are part of the "system" that perpetuates injustice. Although finding strategies to change existing injustices can be complex and daunting, the WFOT advocates that its members engage in occupationally just practices based on individual and population occupational rights (WFOT, 2006, 2014, 2016).

Despite an apparent need for occupational justice throughout human time, it was not named as such until the mid-1990s. Naming arose from two directions of study in different parts of the globe. One of these directions made the discovery that many societal and practice determinants "overruled" occupational therapists' "good intentions" of enabling justice with clients who could be populations, organizations, communities, groups, families, or individuals (Townsend, 1993, 1996, 1998, 2003a, 2003b, 2007). The other direction of study concerned with understanding the relationship between occupation and health made the discovery that beneficial or negative health outcomes of the relationship were often dependent on sociopolitical and cultural determinants which could be framed in social justice terms (Wilcock, 1993, 1995, 1998, 2001, 2002, 2006; Wilcock & Hocking, 2015) and led to the first published definition of occupational justice as:

> The promotion of social and economic change to increase individual, community, and political awareness; resources and equitable opportunities for diverse occupational opportunities that enable people to meet their potential and experience well-being. (Wilcock, 1998, p. 257)

Both study directions generated occupational terminology and new insights on justice including considerations about whether or not social justice sufficiently addresses the rights of people, individually or collectively, to participate in what they define as meaningful occupations (Wilcock & Townsend, 2000). With this common focus, Townsend and Wilcock have explored together what they describe as occupational justice (Stadnyk, Townsend, & Wilcock, 2010; Townsend & Wilcock, 2004).

The following explanations outline the meanings the authors ascribe to occupation, social justice, and occupational justice.

Occupation

Occupation is viewed broadly as referring to all the things that people want, need, or have to do whether of a physical, mental, social, sexual, political, or spiritual nature and is inclusive of sleep and rest. It refers to all aspects of actual human doing, being, belonging, and becoming at individual or population levels. The practical, everyday medium of self-expression or of making or experiencing meaning, occupation is the activist element of human existence whether occupations are contemplative, restful, reflective and meditative, or action-based. Occupation is also a unit of economy shaped by time, place, and social conditions. It is a fundamental means of achieving implicit or explicit goals, so power relations are central to possibilities and limitations in pursuing goals: The power to participate in occupations may be controlled through physical force, or invisibly through regulation; the media; technology; and sociocultural, spiritual, or familial expectations. Those forces can suppress or foster physical activity, the self, being, belief, spirit, autonomy, and individual, group, or population identity and can therefore be health-threatening as well as health-enhancing. Humans require occupation not only to thrive but also to survive. Like air, water, and food, humans cannot survive without occupation.

Social Justice

Social justice is a central concern in growing numbers of postmodern societies. It can be described as just and nondiscriminatory relationships between individuals, groups, and the society in which they live. It is applied to the ethical distribution and sharing of resources, rights, and responsibilities between people recognizing their equal worth, "their equal right to be able to meet basic needs, the need to spread opportunities and life chances as widely as possible", and "reduce and where possible eliminate unjustified inequalities" (UN Commission on Social Justice, 1994, p. 1). It is assessed for differences according to wealth and social privilege, racial and gender equality, and opportunity for personal and population activity including for those with social, mental, or physical disability and those who are environmentally displaced. Theories of social justice grew, in part, from the vision of reformers such as Robert Owen (Owen, 1813/1995). They emerged gradually in the wake of the industrial revolution and the parallel development of socialist doctrine with the ideology of fair and compassionate distribution of economic growth (UN, 2006). Social justice was the central ideology of the Arts and Crafts movement that influenced the beginnings of OT in both the United States and England (Wilcock, 2001, 2002).

Occupational Justice

Occupational justice and **occupational rights** are concerned with ethical, moral, and civic issues such as equity and fairness for individuals and collectives, specific to engagement in diverse and meaningful occupation that

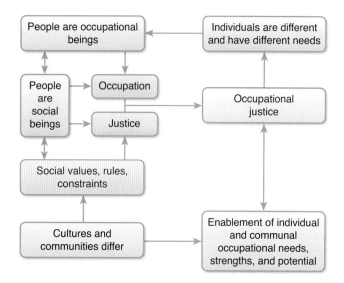

FIGURE 45-1 An exploratory theory of occupational justice: intersecting ideas. (©2016 CH Christiansen & EA Townsend, used with permission.)

is inclusive of "doing, being, belonging and becoming" (Wilcock & Hocking, 2015). In their exploratory theory of occupational justice, Townsend and Wilcock (2004) proposed that occupation highlights the reality of justice in the occupations of daily life (Figure 45-1). It exposes the everyday individual, group, and population experiences within broad social conditions and structures that shape options for and against justice in the lives of people in different cultures around the world. Their theory accepts that occupation is central to human existence. The theory recognizes that people are occupational beings, they participate in occupations as autonomous beings and as members of particular communities, participation in occupation is interdependent and contextual, and the context for occupational engagement is a determinant of health and well-being or the cause of illness and ill-being. Occupations are subject to societal pressures and governance so there are options or limits for choice in doing, being, belonging, and becoming that can affect health and well-being. The theory puts forward the principles that human **empowerment** is achieved or not through occupation, that empowerment is highly dependent on the power relations that shape the context for occupational engagement, that a broad view of occupation demands a more inclusive occupational classification beyond paid or volunteer work, that occupations have both economic and social value, and that societies are responsible for the individual and collective enablement of the diverse occupational potential of each occupational being individually and as members of populations. The exploratory theory with these principles states that, for justice

to prevail, there must be an ethical distribution and sharing of resources, rights, and responsibilities regarding what both population groups and individuals want, need, or are obliged to do within their socioeconomic milieu.

The naming of occupational justice may be recent and visionary, but respected scholars, over millennia, have considered the notion that what people do, and their actions toward being, belonging, and becoming are largely socially determined and not a matter of individual choice. Some have deplored the occupational injustices and illnesses caused by biased expectations, assumptions, rules, protocols, and political expediencies. Ruskin (1865), for example, asked, "Which of us . . . is to do the hard and dirty work for the rest, and for what pay? Who is to do the pleasant and clean work, and for what pay?"(p. 107). Similar concerns about occupational justice in the present day can be linked without much effort to the politics of economic growth and the growing disparity of wealth and power (Hocking, 2017; Werner, 1998). The disparity is pronounced between agrarian, industrializing, industrialized, and postindustrial countries, but in the first two of these, many people are unable to provide the necessities of life that are a prerequisite to health, and in all of them, some people face ill-health or are unable to achieve positive well-being through what they do. Indeed, occupational illness, deprivation, imbalance, and alienation are recognized consequences of financially limited lifestyles for people everywhere (Wilcock, 1998, 2006; Wilcock & Hocking, 2015). Those who live in poverty are the most likely to suffer the direct effects of such injustices, but in advanced economies, too, many flounder, unable to realize their talents or achieve their aspirations and are conditioned to particular occupations and ways of life that may not meet their needs or that may lead to illness. It is perhaps a lack of understanding as well as systemic forces that undermine the occupational rights of populations, communities, and individuals across the globe. Occupational injustice can mean that many people are unable to meet even basic needs, or have unequal opportunities to reach their occupational potential. Throughout the world, many individuals and population groups are constrained, deprived, marginalized, oppressed, or alienated from occupational engagement that could provide them with personal, family, and/or community necessities, or satisfaction, meaning, personal growth, life balance, well-being, and health (Townsend, 2003a; Wilcock, 1998, 2006; Wilcock & Hocking, 2015).

Social and occupational justice share two powerful social requirements:

1. The creation of families, groups, and communities as structures in which people can define what they can and want to do, who they will be and become, and how they belong or not in particular social and populations contexts

2. The organization of economic and human resources in which people are enabled to participate according to their potential, experience well-being, reduce illness, and thrive (Stadnyk, 2007; Stadnyk et al. 2010; Whiteford & Townsend, 2011; Wilcock & Hocking, 2015)

These social requirements point to the primary purpose for developing a theory of occupational justice including principles that define possibilities and limits for occupational justice to prevail.

Occupational Justice and Health

The WHO is, arguably, the ultimate global authority on health issues, so its relevant directives are woven through this section about occupational justice and health. From its inception in 1946, the WHO recognized that health encompasses not only the absence of illness but also the presence of mental, physical, and social well-being. In 1986, the WHO built on that initial concept with the definitive call for action to improve health throughout the world that is found within the 1986 WHO Ottawa Charter for Health Promotion (OCHP). With the understanding that health is a fundamental right of all human beings without distinction of race, religion, political belief, or economic or social condition, the Charter called for "enablement," "mediation," and "advocacy" (WHO, 1986) to reduce health inequities between and within countries where inequities are unfair and unacceptable. Key strategies in the Charter are the building of healthy public policy, the creation of environments that are supportive of health, the strengthening of community action for health, the development of personal skills, and the reorientation of health services. A world was envisaged in which all people are able to satisfy needs, cope with the environment, and realize aspirations by "reducing differences . . . and ensuring equal opportunities and resources to enable all people to achieve their fullest health potential" (WHO, 1986, p. 1). The interaction of those strategies with occupation—with what people are actually doing in their lives—cannot be disputed. But the interaction is so complex that the relationship has largely been considered from other viewpoints and political expediencies. A holistic approach that considers, fosters, strengthens, and reorients the health building occupational needs and natures of all people has yet to be fully understood and developed. From an occupational justice perspective, health-giving occupations to meet biological, mental health, social, and economic needs should be regarded as a fundamental right for all human beings. The Charter remains current having been reaffirmed many times over the ensuing years in subsequent worldwide

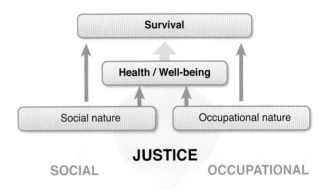

FIGURE 45-2 Occupational justice and social justice enabling survival through the meeting of biological needs and providing the means to health.

health promotion conferences to the present time (WHO, 1988, 1991, 1997, 2005, 2009, 2013, 2016) (Figure 45-2).

Occupational Justice and the Absence of Illness

The simplest definition of health—equated with the absence of disease—would lead to a definition of the promotion of health as an effort to remove diseases and diminish the numbers of individuals who suffer from them. (Sartorius, 2006, p. 662)

Most people experience illness at some time. Following medical prescription, treatment, and regimes to be free of illness appears to be what many, including governments, describe as health care. Doctors of medicine are acknowledged as the experts in exploring and managing recovery, and numerous occupational therapists work in this sphere. Illness is a matter of importance including financial and ethical concerns, and in affluent nations, the need for more and more sophisticated medical treatment appears paramount and increasingly dominant in the allocation of health-related resources. Consideration of ways to reduce the incidence of illness is seldom financed sufficiently by those with the power to make a significant difference.

Illness is disproportionately concentrated among those who are poor. This is especially true for women and children with a child dying from poverty-related conditions every 3.5 seconds (World Bank, 2014). In the developing world, many are vulnerable to political and economic oppression, often lacking information about available services and appropriate practices. Many lack access to education, work, or recreational opportunities and adequate shelter or nutrition as well as quality health care. In countries with more developed health services, its poorer members remain the least advantaged, in part because of "the potentially catastrophic effects of out-of-pocket health care costs" (World Bank, 2014, p. 1).

A variety of occupations are necessary for people to avoid illness, injury, or violent assault, to be free of extreme fear or anxiety or of dying prematurely (Nussbaum, 2011). In any community, health may be affected by restriction to participation in occupations of choice or variety. The causes of limitations or restrictions may be invisible, but causes could be regulations; the media; changing technology; and sociocultural, spiritual, or familial expectations or physical force. The Commission on Social Determinants of Health talks of the "causes of the causes" explaining them as "the fundamental structures of social hierarchy and the socially determined conditions these create in which people grow, live, work, and age" (Marmot, 2007, p. 1153). The causes of causes can marginalize or exploit. They can disempower, restrict, alienate, and inflict physical, psychological, and spiritual harm on people who have too little or too much to do (Whiteford & Townsend, 2011). Indeed, the personal and population consequences of insufficient, beneficial occupations are not discrete. They are the foundations of life and death, illness, or health for individuals, groups, communities, and countries wherever people live.

Occupational Justice, Social Health, and Well-Being

The *Universal Declaration of Human Rights* (UN, 1948) advocates for all people to have a standard of living adequate for health and well-being; equal rights to participate in the cultural life of a community; meaningful work with free choice for employment; and rest, leisure, and holidays. Included are rights to take part in the arts and in national governments and access education directed to the full development of the human personality. Subsequent publications call for the promotion and protection of societal and individual rights and fundamental freedoms and equality of opportunities as well as the amendment of social injustices that separate people from different sociocultural backgrounds and environments (Brown, 2016; UN, 1998, 2006). The WHO and many others have acknowledged the interaction between population, social, and individual health that in turn is dependent on people meeting the biological needs to do and to belong through the fair and just structure of social groups (Argyle, 1987; Blaxter, 1990; Cohen et al., 1982; Isaksson, 1990; Warr, 1990; Wilcock, 1998; Wilcock & Hocking, 2015; WHO, 1986, 2011a). Rights, freedoms, and tensions in power relations provide directions for debate and action in relation to occupational empowerment, and debate and action to ensure choice and opportunity are central to social health and to what people need or hope to do. The tension between justice for the common good and for individuals underpins debate and action on occupational rights and **social health**.

Social injustices for particular population groups have been embedded in occupations over the centuries. Women, for example, have had and can still have their occupations restricted. A Nigerian study recommended "public enlightenment and mass education" about women's right to paid work to ensure their empowerment and emancipation, after the study revealed women's "relative deprivation, male dominance, and subordination" (Bassey, Ojua, Archibong, & Bassey, 2012, p. 238). Many have also questioned the fairness of differing occupational opportunities for those who are institutionally confined. A study of asylum seekers in detention found increased levels of distress and decreased levels of health and well-being associated with occupational deprivation (Morville, 2014). Similarly, immigrants, refugees, people in war-torn regions or homeless, and communities where people live in poverty experience limited engagement in meaningful occupations (Watson & Swartz, 2004). Globally, the numbers of homeless people in situations of occupational poverty and disadvantage are rising alarmingly. The UN Refugee Agency estimated that 45.2 million people were forcibly displaced in 2012 due to conflict and persecution, with most of those seeking asylum originating from Afghanistan, Somalia, Iraq, Syria, and Sudan.

Despite deplorable situations around the globe, understanding about the negative or positive consequences of occupation as a social health issue is frequently overlooked. This is despite recognition in the OCHP that "changing patterns of life, work and leisure have a significant impact on health," indeed, that communities as well as individuals "must be able to identify and realize aspirations, to satisfy needs and to change or cope with the environment" as "a source of health" (WHO, 1986, p. 3). Accepting that the fundamental conditions and resources for health are peace, shelter, education, food, income, a stable ecosystem, sustainable resources, social justice, and equity, the WHO OCHP (1986) called for the development of personal skills and the strengthening of community action for health as well as the building of healthy public policy, the creation of environments that are supportive of health, and the reorientation of health services as key strategies. Those conditions and resources relate directly or indirectly to what people do, with millions around the world unable to meet such primary needs. The OCHP and its authoritative recognition of the complex and wide ranging requirements for health stimulated the growth of the New Public Health during the 1980s. This called for intervention beyond the provision of conventional medical and health services because "the struggle for health is essentially a struggle for equity and compassion" in "all sectors and aspects of life" (Werner, 1998, p. 2). "If health is ever to be construed as a human right . . . disparities of outcome in and between countries" is a major challenge (Farmer, Furin, & Katz, 2004, p. 1832). In the 1990s, the development of "active societies" and "enabling states" began to be addressed within international organizations (Gilbert, 1995; Kalisch, 1991; Organization for Economic Cooperation and Development, 1989). Sir John Elvidge (2017), a permanent secretary to the Scottish Government, for example, argued the enabling state as a new model of government "supporting individuals and communities to take a more active role in maximizing their own wellbeing" (p. 1). In the United States, the Clinton Administration encouraged a "blueprint for a new America" in which an "enabling state be organized around the goals of work and individual empowerment" and "the poor as the prime agents of their own development, rather than as passive clients of the welfare system" (Marshall & Schram, 1993, p. 228).

It is easy to ignore that many people are channelled into both vocational and avocational occupations by where they live; their gender, social, religious, and family expectations; class systems; necessity; and financial circumstances. Commonly, children and adolescents in more affluent countries, for example, are pressured to put aside particular interests and talents to excel within a limited range of occupations to follow the current rage or family or community traditions or be financially successful as adults. Such pressure may be a contributing factor to young people experiencing increased unhappiness in life as evidenced by the growing numbers of suicides. In Australia, for example, suicide among those aged 15 to 24 years was the leading cause of premature death in 2010 to 2012 (Australian Institute of Health and Welfare, 2017). Occupational therapists working in schools, universities, or with community organizations might have a role assisting in the practical exploration of present lifestyles and future occupational options to reduce suicide. Population and individual perspectives interact, so appreciating and improving both needs to be the norm in any intervention.

Another common problem is the pressure put on older people to change their interests and decrease levels of activity at a given chronological age whatever they feel about it themselves or whatever their health status (Nilsson & Townsend, 2010). The right of seniors to participate in meaningful occupations to maintain and enhance health requires facilities for active living in communities that encourage and value their opinions and expertise, are fully accessible, and increasingly provide assistance to keep abreast of everyday technology and evolving communication systems (Nilsson & Townsend, 2010; Townsend, 2007; Townsend & Wilcock, 2004). Decreasing activity increases the likelihood of illness and early death. A 13-year study of 2,761 older Americans found that doing social and productive occupations carried as much weight in terms of lowering the risk of all causes of death as doing exercise (Glass, de Leon, Marottoli, & Berkman, 1999). Later studies after Glass et al. (1999) support this finding (Agahi & Parker, 2008; Lennartsson & Silverstein, 2001; Mendes de

Leon, 2005; Wang, Karp, Winblad, & Fratiglioni, 2002). Occupational therapists should seek opportunities to be involved in developing occupationally just solutions toward "ageing in place" other than in institutions (Trentham & Cockburn, 2011).

Paul-Ward (2009) argues, "As the social justice movement builds momentum . . . occupational therapy is ideally situated to work with marginalized groups to achieve full participation" (p. 1). In the United Kingdom, occupational inequities have been identified resulting from sociopolitical, economic, and environmental factors (Hocking & Hammell, 2017; Pollard & Sakellariou, 2007; Sakellariou & Pollard, 2016). That is probably the case in most countries, supporting the call for updated systems to reflect occupational justice issues (Hammell, 2015; Pizzi, Reitz, & Scaffa, 2010). Interventions will often require consultation and interactive practices with other disciplines because the complexity of opportunities for participation by diverse people and populations are unequally distributed and may be the result of unexpected or unanticipated factors beyond a single discipline's expertise. When action is required, care must be taken to avoid unintentionally worsening or causing injustice (Thibeault, 2013). "Those who intervene must critique their own worldview to avoid imposing their ways of being onto others" because "situations of injustice are complex manifestations of local and global forces operating through social, cultural, political, economic and historical institutions" (Bailliard, 2016, p. 3).

The World Federation of Occupational Therapists (2006; 2014) recognizes social health issues and occupational justice as occupational therapists' human rights responsibilities, deploring global conditions such as poverty, social discrimination, displacement, disease, disasters, and armed conflict that threaten the right to occupational engagement and choice. It recommends that occupational therapists become "partners in world changing initiatives related to regions dealing with the aftermath of war, social upheaval and revolution" working "in partnership with others to ensure clean water, safe housing, education and meaningful community engagement." The WFOT *Minimum Standards for the Education of Occupational Therapists* have been updated to go "beyond education on bodily dysfunction" and to include health and wellness to "advance human rights" (WFOT, 2016, p. 11) as core principles across all areas of practice. These latest *Minimum Standards* call for social inclusion and participation to be advanced globally, with the application of practical understanding of the social determinants of health and occupational justice. Meeting the new *Minimum Standards* for enabling social as well as individual health requires major changes away from medically organized OT curricula. Practitioners will need to think differently about their roles and practices, and they will need an understanding that a focus on human rights and justice is "something that already intersects with practice, not something that practitioners must choose whether to take up" (Aldrich, Boston, & Daaleman, 2017, p. 1). Occupational therapists must recognize the contributions they can provide if they are to keep informed and actively pursue the holistic vision that WFOT subscribes.

Occupational Justice, Mental Health, and Well-Being

Occupational justice is an essential component of mental health and well-being—with issues of justice long recognized especially by those working with people in prisons (Howard, 1789). Mental health is a state in which people realize their own abilities; cope with the normal stresses of life; work productively and fruitfully; seek response to their spiritual quest for meaning, purpose, and belonging; and make contributions to their community. Justice in promoting mental health can be enhanced by attending to multiple and interacting social, psychological, and biological factors using assessments and interventions that respect and protect basic rights (Herrman, Shekhars, & Moodie, 2005, p. XIX). Mental health promotion is a fairly recent branch of public health associated with the WHO OCHP (1986). Around much of the world, promotion of mental health is integral to the empowerment of people individually and at a population level, having the potential to enable and activate governments to design interventions aimed at early disorders of children and youth in disadvantaged populations and the empowerment of women and to fund appropriate supports for ageing populations as well as vulnerable groups such as indigenous peoples, migrants, refugees, and victims of disasters (Herrman et al., 2005).

In order to eradicate "attitudes that perpetuate stigma and discrimination that have isolated people" with mental illness since ancient times, the WHO 66th World Health Assembly embedded the idea of mental health as an international human right separate from mental illness, defining it as

> A state of well-being in which every individual realizes his or her own potential, can cope with the normal stresses of life, can work productively and fruitfully, and is able to make a contribution to her or his community. (WHO, 2014, p. 1)

As a result of this Assembly, the WHO through the Calouste Gulbenkian Foundation (2014) recommended a multi-layered and multi-sectoral "health in all policies" approach to promote the mental health of populations and to reduce the risk of mental disorders throughout life. World Health Organization has called for action to improve the circumstances in which people are born, grow, live, work, and age; address disparities in the social determinants of mental health; and include interventions at environmental, structural, local, community, and national levels when

necessary. Focusing solely on the most disadvantaged people will not adequately reduce health inequalities for overall benefit. Approaches must be universal, span societies as a whole, and protect mental health at several different levels. Given that mental health promotion is about enhancing mental well-being and improving quality of life (WHO, 2016), occupational therapists could be proactive in instigating programs that assist the acquisition and empowerment of life skills as a matter of occupational justice for those who need to achieve a greater sense of control and improve quality of life and health potential. A multi-layered and intersectoral approach provides an avenue for occupational justice initiatives (Blair, Hume, & Creek, 2008).

Despite a long and varied history, the treatment of mental illness is now largely medicalized. There were times when therapeutic milieus included ridicule, neglect, mental and physical abuse, and other times when the opposite was true and religion, peace, and tranquility were the order of the day. In the mid-nineteenth century, programs to meet individual needs for justice, benevolence, and occupation like the one described by Browne (1837) were the forerunner of twentieth century OT. Browne's ideas still have value if they combine personal interests and growth with enabling opportunities for social interaction and necessary *change at population levels*. That is especially true because of the apparent increase of disorders such as child, gender, and substance abuse; violence; depression; and anxiety. Such disorders are more problematic where there is low income, high unemployment, stressful work conditions, limited education, gender discrimination, human rights violations, and unhealthy lifestyles. Poorer members of societies around the world are especially vulnerable to stressful, difficult, or hazardous living conditions and exploitation that can increase the risk of mental disorders and decrease access to treatment (WHO, 2001). The "vicious circle of poverty and mental health disorders" (WHO, 2001, p. 1) is rarely broken. As well as poverty, in both the developed and developing world, the risk of mental illness appears to be associated with rapid social change such as multiculturalism or when displaced people seek asylum in new countries where they experience insecurity and hopelessness, the risks of violence, and physical ill-health (Patel & Kleinman, 2003). However, within the constraints of "painful, distressing, or debilitating symptoms," those who live with ongoing mental illness can attain effective well-being; experience "a satisfying, meaningful, contributing life"; and attain effective well-being (WHO, 2014, p. 12). In that regard, occupation-based programs have much to offer.

Individual occupation-based programs for people with mental illness have decreased with economic rationalism, the dominance of medication-focused programs, and changes from institutional to home-based services. Advocacy to address the current scarcity of OT interventions and raise community and government awareness about occupational imbalance, occupational deprivation, and occupational alienation that compound mental health problems is long overdue (Wilcock & Hocking, 2015). Gruhl (2014) argues that occupational therapists across the globe need to ensure that vulnerable people and particularly those with serious mental illness have access to participation in therapeutic regimes that address occupational justice and injustices they and their family members face. Families from all backgrounds and communities need to be involved. Occupation-based programs must enable people to cope with the normal stresses of life and provide purpose (doing), meaning (being), community involvement (belonging), and the means for people to strive toward their potential (becoming). The guideline of "doing, being, belonging, and becoming" is useful to bear in mind as it integrates active, passive, reflective, familial, social, communal, world citizenship, and personal growth (Wilcock, 1998; Wilcock & Hocking 2015). Such initiatives must respect, protect, and advance basic civil, political, economic, social, cultural, and occupational rights, even if therapists are required to challenge institutional or public policy (Townsend & Wilcock, 2004; Whiteford & Pereira, 2012; Whiteford & Townsend, 2011). A dilemma that can face occupational therapists in establishing population-based programs is lack of information and experience outside the prevalent education and practice focus on individual function and dysfunction. The newest *Minimum Standards* (WFOT, 2016) require entry-level OT education programs worldwide to include theories and practice experiences that will prepare practitioners with an adequate understanding and methods to address human rights issues and collective occupational injustices at population levels. The implication is that all OT entry-level education programs in the world will now be required to include *population health*.

Occupational Justice, Physical Health, and Well-Being

Occupational justice is an essential component of physical health and well-being. Too much, too little, or ill-chosen occupation can lead directly to illness or death. Bernadino Ramazzini (1705), a pioneer figure of occupational health, raised very practical concerns about the early death and disorders suffered by workers in many types of basic and necessary employment in the eighteenth century. His extensive research is a testament to the occupational injustices of that time and resonates with what still happens in many poor communities around the world in agrarian, industrializing, and industrialized countries. Currently, opportunities to inform and assist people to prevent physical illness are haphazard even though prevention is emphasized as a

priority of the WHO. So, too, opportunities to assist recovery through occupation are random, limited, and in short supply especially in the most disadvantaged countries. This may be a matter of priorities, funding, or available expertise (Curtin, Egan, & Adams, 2017). It may be because those who finance or prescribe services have an incomplete understanding of the relationship between health, justice, human rights, and what people do, or it may be a reticence to change existing medical regimes. In any case, occupational therapists and occupational scientists need to advance their own and public literacy on occupation for thinking, talking, writing, and speaking publicly and professionally in the "right places" about the strength of the relationship between occupation, health, human rights, and justice (Townsend, 2015). Whatever the cause, absent, limited, or random assessment and programming targeted on meaningful occupation as part of health care is a global injustice, especially as physical inactivity has now been identified as the fourth leading risk factor in global mortality: Inactivity is one of only a few largely preventable risk factors that account for the majority of illness throughout the world (WHO, 2004, 2010, 2011a, 2013, 2017a).

Arguing that increasing industrialization, urbanization, economic development, and food market globalization have led to a significant decrease in physical activity, the WHO prescribes regular, moderate engagement in activity to reduce the risk of a range of common disorders such as cardiovascular diseases, diabetes, hip and vertebral fractures, disorders of weight, some cancers, and depression (WHO, 2017b). In low- and middle-income countries, the relationship between occupation and such diseases is a little realized cause of poverty that hinders economic development and is the cause of 80% of deaths (WHO, 2011a). In 2013, the WHO published a global action plan for the prevention and control of noncommunicable diseases (NCD) (Chestnov, 2013). This plan recognizes that health and quality of life are influenced by lifestyles and the conditions in which people live and work recommending physical activity for the 1 in 4 adults and more than 80% of adolescents who are not sufficiently active. The WHO action plan describes physical activity as

> Any bodily movement produced by skeletal muscles that requires energy expenditure—including activities undertaken while working, playing, carrying out household chores, travelling, and engaging in recreational pursuits. (WHO, 2013, p. 1)

Activity to improve physical dysfunction needs to engage individuals or communities in whatever they need, want, or are required to do and be in line with human rights, the social determinants of health, prevailing societal beliefs about disability or disfigurement, and the risk of contagion (Hocking & Hammell, 2017; Mandelstam, 2003).

The UN High Commissioner for Human Rights and the WHO (2008) recognized the relationships between health, poverty, and discrimination, urging governments to give priority to improving the health of vulnerable and marginalized groups through efforts that directly address the social determinants of health. Only improvement in human rights can lead to improvements in health and disability (Hocking & Hammell, 2017; Wilcock & Hocking, 2015). Multisectoral action is required to reduce the global threat of NCD that accounts for some of the disadvantage, discrimination, and disempowerment experienced by physically ill people. Even in countries with advanced economies, those with a disability are among the most poor, excluded, and disenfranchised, as poverty can be a cause or consequence of impairment and disability and can adversely affect neurological development (Canadian Medical Association, 2013).

Well-chosen occupations can aid in the repair of illness and be a source of health for individuals, communities, and populations. Widely recognized at the start of the twentieth century, this idea, value, and philosophy lead to the advent of OT as a formal discipline. However, occupation-based remedial programs have decreased in regular health care facilities for people experiencing physical illness except perhaps for those aimed at improving independence in personal care. The decrease can be blamed on increased medical costs and priorities, shortened stays within health facilities, downgrading ideas about activity as a personal rather than a societal responsibility, and a reluctance to accept that what people do in their everyday lives (apart from visits to the gym, perhaps) can affect physical health and well-being. Reliance on medication and surgery has become the norm. Dilemmas for occupational therapists include how to increase community understanding of the physical health benefits of meeting wide-ranging occupational needs, how to continue occupation-based rehabilitation programs beyond shortened institutional stays, and how to assist compensatory cases to improve their fitness whilst under the restrictive jurisdiction of insurers.

Occupational Justice within Occupational Therapy

Many occupational therapists contend that since the formal birth of OT in the United States early in the last century, social justice has been an implicit aspect of this profession. Early efforts to use occupation as therapy drew on ideas championed by women like Florence Nightingale with Victorian interests in education and helping the poor (Burstyn, 2016; West, 2011; Woodham-Smith, 1952). Perhaps that is why interest in occupational justice

has grown so rapidly in various parts of the world since evolving in Australasia and Canada in 1998. At the 2003 conference of the European Network of Occupational Therapists in Higher Education (ENOTHE), Townsend (2003a) asked, "Why would occupational therapist be concerned with occupational justice?" She explained how injustices experienced when people are barred, trapped, confined, segregated, restricted, prohibited, unable to develop, disrupted, alienated, imbalanced, deprived, or marginalized can exclude them from participating optimally in the occupations they need and want to do to sustain health throughout the life course. By 2005, Wood, Hooper, and Womack were discussing the place of occupational justice within OT education, and about the same time Kronenberg, Algado, and Pollard (2005) challenged occupational therapists to work in places and situations where people are occupationally marginalized and exploited. Arguing that occupational justice is a professional responsibility and an ethical issue of global citizenship for occupational therapists, the notion of occupational apartheid was introduced to raise critical awareness of the political nature of occupation (Pollard, Sakellariou, & Kronenberg, 2009). Publications began to appear in which occupational therapists were encouraged to work in underresourced communities and countries to help overcome occupational injustices and to achieve occupationally just goals in community development (Hocking & Townsend, 2015; Hocking et al., 2015; Pollard et al., 2009). Occupational therapists are now emphasizing the necessity of learning to integrate justice with practice (Sakellariou & Pollard, 2016). This demands greater than traditional understanding of sociopolitical issues and other systemic injustices such as homelessness, poverty, disaster relief, displacement, torture, human trafficking, or ineffective anti-discriminatory legislation (Hocking & Hammell, 2017; Newton & Fuller, 2005; Pollard et al., 2009; Townsend, 1998, 2003b; Wilcock & Hocking, 2015). For actually enabling occupational justice (Townsend & Marval, 2013), occupational therapists need consciousness raising experiences and support to reduce potential professional isolation and technical competency expectations that minimize the complex work of enabling occupational justice.

Occupational therapists face major challenges until social health is recognized as a legitimate field of work in the profession (Malfitano, Lopes, Magalhães, & Townsend, 2014). A social health focus means accepting the professional responsibility of raising awareness of occupational injustices within communities and developing occupation-based programs that address injustices such as occupational deprivation, imbalance, and alienation (Trentham & Cockburn, 2011; Wilcock, 1993, 2006). Possibly, a greater challenge for many is coming to terms with a population approach to illness and becoming active in addressing social/occupational injustice at that level. Although, as Scott & Reitz (2013) recognize, social justice has always been part of the tradition of OT practice, it is individual rather than population interventions around injustice that have been at the forefront of practice for a century, and only a minority of therapists have seriously challenged the accepted medical order (American Occupational Therapy Association [AOTA], 2017). Individual "therapy" is so embedded in OT thought, speech, education, and literature, and the shift to population-based practice is extremely difficult. The language of population health is different and much more political than that of mainstream OT, and trying to think and write in that genre can be challenging and take time to achieve. Although regarding as imperative that occupational therapists reconsider initiatives and goals from an occupational justice and social health perspective, such initiatives are different than previous OT interventions that rarely touched social phenomena such as homelessness, sexual abuse, or domestic violence (Wilcock & Hocking, 2015).

The concept of occupational justice is influencing the governance, planning and policies of OT's national professional organizations such as AOTA (2006, 2017). The UN Universal Declaration of Human Rights was endorsed by the WFOT when the latter published a Position Statement that includes its stand on human rights and occupational justice as a right and condemns the global conditions that threaten that right including "poverty, disease, social discrimination, displacement, natural and man-made disasters and armed conflict" (WFOT, 2006, p. 1). The Statement called for occupational therapists to identify and support individuals, groups, communities, and societies experiencing occupational injustices and to work with them to enhance participation in occupation. This position was expanded in the 2016 WFOT *Minimum Standards.*

Although the first initiatives recognizing occupational justice came from the West, occupational therapists throughout the world are now exploring the idea with attention to cultural variations. Exploration is a regular feature in textbooks and journals, with discussions covering diverse practice, individual, community, and population health initiatives with increasingly explicit reference to addressing injustice (Bailliard, 2016; Durocher, Gibson, & Rappolt, 2014; Frank, 2012; Sakellariou & Pollard, 2016; Sakellariou & Simó Algado, 2006; Smith & Hilton, 2008; Trentham & Cockburn, 2011; Wilcock, 2006; Windley, 2011). Some see occupational justice and the related issues of occupational rights as the profession's core purpose, expanding its focus from individual to community and societal outcomes and guiding practice according to new ways for viewing the world (Hammell, 2008; Molineux & Baptiste, 2011, p. 3; Paul-Ward, 2009; White, 2009). The future practice of OT—in truth, the future existence

of this profession—may rest on the profession's success in putting occupational justice explicitly on the public agenda and showing what an occupation-based, justice-driven, socially responsive profession can accomplish.

Reducing Occupational Injustices and Advancing Occupational Rights

Occupational therapy is founded on the belief that participation in occupation is central to health. If the move toward an occupationally just and healthy world is not achieved, occupational injustice will remain a problem. For the authors of this chapter, the lack of understanding about the just distribution of occupational opportunities and resources is the major societal health problem that occupational therapists need to address. The task of reducing occupational injustices and advancing occupational rights demands a committed effort. For some, a focus on justice can be integrated within formal education or understood by practitioners as "something that already intersects with practice" (Aldrich et al., 2017, p. 1). For others, it is actually about changing the world. This may sound both grandiose and overwhelming, yet Margaret Mead (1901–1978) reminded us:

> Never doubt that a small group of thoughtful, committed citizens can change the world. Indeed, it is the only thing that ever has.

A questionnaire is provided as a checklist and guideline to document injustices and encourage action. Occupational therapists can start their commitment where they work, linking their individual, local actions to a global vision of an occupationally just world. Some occupational therapists may find like-minded colleagues to form a local group or to network nationally and internationally. For occupational therapists with a passion to influence global change, there are collective options to work through the WFOT and national OT organizations, nongovernmental organizations (NGOs), media and consumer-based programs, local political networks, or through individual efforts to generate collective action.

Because occupational justice requires proactive initiatives that explore, inform, and inspire changes to basic community structures and organizational health strategies, the three cases summarized in the following section suggest what therapists could do in various spheres of work. Figure 45-3 illustrates the cases as a visual tool for action not as literal examples rather to stimulate ideas and dialogue, take action, and evaluate progress toward occupational justice and occupational rights. The figure shows how local, group, and collective actions are linked.

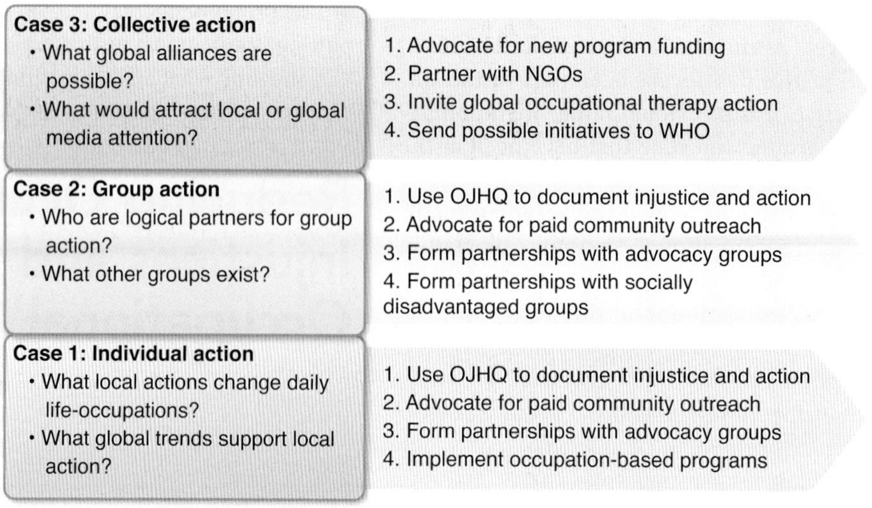

Case 3: Collective action
- What global alliances are possible?
- What would attract local or global media attention?

1. Advocate for new program funding
2. Partner with NGOs
3. Invite global occupational therapy action
4. Send possible initiatives to WHO

Case 2: Group action
- Who are logical partners for group action?
- What other groups exist?

1. Use OJHQ to document injustice and action
2. Advocate for paid community outreach
3. Form partnerships with advocacy groups
4. Form partnerships with socially disadvantaged groups

Case 1: Individual action
- What local actions change daily life-occupations?
- What global trends support local action?

1. Use OJHQ to document injustice and action
2. Advocate for paid community outreach
3. Form partnerships with advocacy groups
4. Implement occupation-based programs

FIGURE 45-3 Linking individual, group, and collective action for local and global change. *OJHQ,* Occupational Justice and Health Questionnaire; *NGOs,* nongovernmental organizations; *WHO,* World Health Organization.

The opening questions in this figure emphasize the importance of partnerships, media attention, documentation, and daily life occupation as important media for change. The arrows suggest actions that are targeted for individual, group, or collective action or for all of these because they are interrelated. An individual may start actions that attract others to engage in collective action; conversely, collective action, such as collaborating with a justice-based NGO, could stimulate ideas and dialogue for individual or group action in particular directions or situations. Evaluation of individual, group, and collective action can be facilitated by setting objectives that can be measured, narrated, or otherwise documented for review in a stated time frame and place, for funders, managers, the public, insurers, or other interested audiences.

The first case relates to rehabilitation practices in health facilities where occupational therapists work primarily with individuals who have physical, mental, cognitive, and other bodily challenges. In enabling occupational justice, rehabilitation practitioners would watch for individuals who have experienced long-term discrimination on the basis of disability or old age. The question is often raised whether occupational therapists in these traditional places of work should focus on enabling occupational justice where work to change the environment or address client rights is not funded or recognized as necessary by those in charge. However, not to find opportunities for enabling occupational justice demonstrates a failure to further the profession's philosophical foundations. Each therapist is an agent with the power to shape future health care and other sectors in society from housing to education and transportation. Occupational therapists can change the profession—that is, if advocates of change work

with professional leaders, and the evaluation of practice actions is documented in reports that can be distributed to health and other hierarchies, the media, or interested parties. An action by occupational therapists could be to develop occupational injustice checklists suited to particular situations, such as the two offered as samples in this chapter: *Occupational Justice and Health Questionnaire* (OJHQ) (Table 45-1) and *Occupational Injustice and Seniors Checklist* (Box 45-1).

The second case in Figure 45-3 addresses occupational injustice relating to the promotion of mental health. It suggests action with a group of interested colleagues. There are advantages in the strength and support of numbers and in brainstorming opportunities to discover innovative, feasible group action about occupational injustice in communities and health services. Whether in face-to-face, e-mail, teleconference, or other means, occupational therapists can access colleagues working in the geographical area or belonging to the same interest groups. The challenge to a group is to be daring and innovative in using OT knowledge, occupational injustice checklists, and questionnaires. With such tools and using data from multiple occupational therapists to record occupational justice issues, group action could start by raising awareness of injustices and progress made to enlist community action toward changing them.

The third case in Figure 45-3 suggests collective action through raising questions capable of generating debate and innovation to change an occupationally unjust world. Action could take many forms such as innovative programming and media arousal, perhaps through presenting at rallies and meetings; publicizing stories about occupationally unjust situations and actions; presenting statistics

TABLE 45-1	Occupational Justice and Health Questionnaire

Instructions: Tick column 2 if client or community is able to meet the right listed in column 1.
Tick one or more of columns 3–6 if client or community is unable according to the reason(s) stated.

Client: Individual, Community, or Population: _____   **Date:** _____

DETERMINANTS	ABLE	UNABLE Health	UNABLE Political	UNABLE Social	UNABLE Economic	COMMENT
Basic Needs World Health Organization [WHO]						
Peace						
Shelter						
Education						
Food						
Income						
Sustainable resources						
Social equity						
Social, Physical, and Mental Well-Being (WHO)						
Life pattern = well-being						
Work = well-being						
Leisure = well-being						
Can realize aspirations						
Can satisfy specific needs						
Has regular physical activity						
Change/cope with environment						
Validate personal uniqueness						
United Nations Rights—Living Standard Adequate for Health and Well-Being. Free Choice to:						
Employment						
Rest						
Leisure						
Holidays						
Community cultural life						
The arts						
Scientific advancement						
Participate in government						
Education toward full development of personality						
World Federation of Occupational Therapists (WFOT) Rights 5 As above plus free choice to participate in:						
Cultural beliefs and customs						
Local events						
SUMMARY: Instructions: Tick one or more if occupational injustice results from the community issues listed below.						
WHO and WFOT—The right to health and well-being through occupation is decreased because of:						

Poverty	Low incomes
High unemployment	Stressful work conditions
Gender discrimination	Social discrimination
Limited education	Occupational discrimination
Unhealthy lifestyles	Displacement
Lack of health facilities	Political unrest
Lack of recreational opportunities	Human rights violations
Natural/man-made disasters	Armed conflict

RECOMMENDATIONS/ACTION

BOX 45-1   **OCCUPATIONAL INJUSTICE AND SENIORS CHECKLIST**

Check all that apply.

- ❏ Not attended to when they talk about what they have done in their lives
- ❏ Not asked for advice or listened to if they give it
- ❏ Given no chance to help others
- ❏ Taken for outings in which they have no interest
- ❏ Are told they can't do something they would enjoy "for their own good"
- ❏ Insufficient advice, practical assistance, equipment, or support to remain in their own environment if they wish to do so
- ❏ Prevented from doing what they want in the name of risk management

- ❏ Placement in sheltered accommodation away from their own people, pets, interests, and environment
- ❏ Sitting alone in nursing homes or other confined settings with nothing to do except watch others in the same situation or a television that shows program after program they did not choose
- ❏ Lack of resources, helpers, services, or support to enable satisfying occupations to match their interests
- ❏ Social contact restricted to paid service providers who bring food, help with personal care, and change beds
- ❏ Restricted, deprived, or alienated by the policies of people in authority or by legislation

of concern and using population data to monitor change; creating and critiquing visual images of occupational injustices and actions; and consultation, cooperation, and contributions to national and international organizations such as the WFOT and WHO. The use of occupational justice language to pinpoint the issues is an example of using occupational literacy for writing and speaking about occupation (Townsend, 2015) as a powerful skill for this case.

Initiatives following suggestions in this third case are congruent with the tradition of collective action that was central to the emergence of OT in the early twentieth century and to the profession's growth around the world (West, 2011). Early occupational therapists, despite minuscule numbers, stimulated the profession's rapid growth because of their belief in the effectiveness of occupation as therapy and their commitment to it demonstrated through collective action. Since then, the profession's leaders have negotiated positions driven in diverse situations by client need, workplace agreements, professional regulation, and other structures, sometimes without attention to occupational justice. Ideally, present and future actions will be designed to advance occupational justice with strategies that meet people's occupational needs and contribute to society while also developing the profession and a more occupationally just world.

Conclusion

Proactivity toward an occupationally just world is the next challenge in the occupation for health journey in all corners of the world. Advancing the concept is complex. It demands a different mindset and focus than the profession's current emphasis on individual, bodily health aligned with medical priorities. It also requires the development of

unfamiliar, proactive interventions on personal, community, national, and world stages. Meeting these demands would place the development of OT practice clearly in line with the directives of the UN, WHO, and occupational justice principles.

REFERENCES

Agahi, N. I., & Parker, M. G. (2008). Leisure activities and mortality: Does gender matter? *Journal of Aging and Health, 20,* 855–871.

Aldrich, R. M., Boston, T. L., & Daaleman, C. E. (2017). Justice and U.S. occupational therapy practice: A relationship 100 years in the making. *American Journal of Occupational Therapy, 71,* 1.

American Occupational Therapy Association. (2006). The role of occupational therapy in disaster preparedness, response, and recovery. *American Journal of Occupational Therapy, 60,* 642–649.

American Occupational Therapy Association. (2017). *Congressional affairs.* Retrieved from https://www.aota.org/Advocacy-Policy/Congressional-Affairs.aspx

Argyle, M. (1987). *The psychology of happiness.* New York, NY: Methuen and Co.

Australian Institute of Health and Welfare. (2017). *Authoritative information and statistics to promote better health and wellbeing.* Bruce, Australia: National Mortality Database.

Bailliard, A. (2016). Justice, difference and the capability to function. *Journal of Occupational Science, 23,* 3–16.

Bassey, A. O., Ojua, T. A., Archibong, E. P., & Bassey, U. A. (2012). Nigeria gender and occupation in traditional African setting: A study of Ikot Effanga Mkpa Community, Nigeria. *American International Journal of Contemporary Research, 2,* 238–245.

Blair, E. E., Hume, C. A., & Creek, J. (2008). Occupational perspectives on mental health and well-being. In W. Bryant, J. Fieldhouse, & K. Bannigan (Eds.), *Creek's occupational therapy and mental health* (4th ed., pp. 17–27). Churchill Livingstone.

Blaxter, M. (1990). *Health and lifestyles.* London, United Kingdom: Tavistock/Routledge.

Brown, G. (Ed.). (2016). *The universal declaration of human rights in the 21st century: A living document in a changing world.* Cambridge, United Kingdom: Open Book.

Browne, W. A. F. (1837). *What asylums were, are, and ought to be.* Edinburgh, United Kingdom: Adam and Charles Black.

Burstyn, J. N. (2016). *Victorian education and the ideal of womanhood. Routledge Library Editions: Education 1800–1926*. London, United Kingdom: Routledge.

Canadian Medical Association. (2013). *Health care in Canada. What makes us sick?* Ontario, Canada: Author.

Certificate of Incorporation of the National Society for the Promotion of Occupational Therapy, Inc. (1917). *Then and now: 1917–1976*. Rockville, MD: American Occupational Therapy Association.

Chestnov, O. (2013). *Introduction to the WHO 2013. Global action plan for the prevention and control of NCDs*. Geneva, Switzerland: World Health Organization.

Cohen, P., Struening, E. L., Muhlin, G. L., Genevie, L. E., Kaplan, S. R., & Peck, H. B. (1982). Community stressors, mediating conditions and wellbeing in urban neighborhoods. *Journal of Community Psychology, 10*, 377–390.

Curtin, M., Egan M., & Adams, J. (Eds.). (2017). *Occupational therapy for people experiencing illness, injury or impairment: Promoting occupation and participation* (7th ed.). Edinburgh, United Kingdom: Elsevier.

Durocher, E., Gibson, B., & Rappolt, S. (2014). Occupational justice: A conceptual review. *Journal of Occupational Science, 21*, 418–430.

Elvidge, J. (2017). *Alliance magazine for philanthropy and social investment worldwide*. Retrieved from alliancemagazine.org/blog/from-welfare-state-to-enabling-state-what-role-for-foundations/

Farmer, P. E., Furin, J. J., & Katz, J. T. (2004). Global health equity. *Lancet, 363*, 1832.

Frank, G. (2012). Occupational therapy/occupational science/occupational justice: Moral commitments and global assemblages. *Journal of Occupational Science, 19*, 25–35.

Gilbert, N. (1995). *Welfare justice: Restoring social equity*. London, United Kingdom: Yale University Press.

Glass, T. A., de Leon, C. M., Marottoli, R. A., & Berkman, L. F. (1999). Population based study of social and productive activities as predictors of survival among elderly Americans. *BMJ, 319*, 478–483.

Gruhl, K. L. R. (2014). Strengths and challenges to practice, in advancing occupational therapy in mental health practice. In E. A. McKay, C. Craik, K. H. Lim, & G. Richards (Eds.), *Advancing occupational therapy in mental health practice*. Chichester, United Kingdom: John Wiley & Sons.

Hammell, K. W. (2008). Reflections on . . . well-being and occupational rights. *Canadian Journal of Occupational Therapy, 75*, 61–64.

Hammell, K. W. (2015). Occupational rights and critical occupational therapy: Rising to the challenge. *Australian Occupational Therapy Journal, 62*, 449–451.

Herrman, H., Shekhars, S., & Moodie, R. (Eds.). (2005). *Promoting mental health. Concepts, emerging evidence*. Geneva, Switzerland: World Health Organization.

Hocking, C. (2017). Occupational justice as social justice: The moral claim for inclusion. *Journal of Occupational Science, 24*, 1.

Hocking, C., & Hammell, K. W. (2017). Process of assessment and evaluation. In M. Curtin, M. Egan, & J. Adams (Eds.), *Occupational therapy for people experiencing illness, injury or impairment: Promoting occupation and participation* (7th ed., pp. 171–184). Edinburgh, United Kingdom: Elsevier.

Hocking, C., & Townsend, E. A. (2015). Driving social change: occupational therapists' contributions to occupational justice. *World Federation of Occupational Therapists Bulletin, 71*(2), 68–71. doi:10.1179/2056607715Y.0000000002

Hocking, C., Townsend, E. A., Gerlach, A., Huot, S., Rudman, D. L., & van Bruggen, H. (2015). "Doing" human rights in diverse occupational therapy practices. *Occupational Therapy Now, 17*, 18–20.

Howard, J. (1789). *An account of the Principal Lazarettos in Europe*. Warrington, United Kingdom: William Eyres.

Isaksson, K. (1990). A longitudinal study of the relationship between frequent job change and psychological well-being. *Journal of Occupational Psychology, 63*, 297–308.

Kalisch, D. (1991, August). The active society. *Social Security Journal*, 3–9.

Kronenberg, F., Algado, S. S., & Pollard, N. (Eds.). (2005). *Occupational therapy without borders: Learning from the spirit of survivors*. Edinburgh, United Kingdom: Elsevier/Churchill Livingstone.

Lennartsson, C., & Silverstein, M. (2001). Does engagement with life enhance survival of elderly people in Sweden? The role of social and leisure activities. *The Journals of Gerontology, 56*, S335–S342.

Malfitano, A. P., Lopes, R. E., Magalhães, L., & Townsend, E. A. (2014). Social occupational therapy: Conversations about a Brazilian experience. *Canadian Journal of Occupational Therapy, 81*, 298–307. doi:10.1177/0008417414536712

Mandelstam, M. (2003). Disabled people, manual handling, and human rights. *British Journal of Occupational Therapy, 66*, 528–530.

Marmot, M. (2007). Achieving health equity: From root causes to fair outcomes. *Lancet, 370*, 1153–1163.

Marshall, W., & Schram, M. (Eds.). (1993). *Mandate for change*. New York, NY: Berkley.

Mead, M. (1901–1978). *Laura Moncur's motivational quotations*. Retrieved from http://www.quotationspage.com/quote/33522.html

Mendes de Leon, C. F. (2005). Social engagement and successful aging. *European Journal of Ageing, 2*, 64–66.

Molineux, M., & Baptiste, S. (2011). Emerging occupational therapy practice: Building on the foundations and seizing the opportunities. In M. Thew, M. Edwards, S. Baptiste, & M. Molineux (Eds.), *Role emerging occupational therapy: Maximising occupation-focused practice* (pp. 3–14). Oxford, United Kingdom: Wiley-Blackwell.

Morville, A-L. (2014). *Daily occupations among asylum seekers: Experience, performance and perception*. Lund, Sweden: Department of Health Sciences, Lund University.

Newton, E., & Fuller, B. (2005). The occupational therapy international outreach network: Supporting occupational therapists working without borders. In F. Kronenberg, N. Pollard, & D. Sakellariou (Eds.), *Occupational therapy without borders: Towards an ecology of occupation-based practices* (pp. 361–373). Edinburgh, United Kingdom: Elsevier/Churchill Livingstone.

Nilsson, I., & Townsend, E. A. (2010). Occupational justice—Bridging theory and practice. *Scandinavian Journal of Occupational Therapy, 17*, 57—63.

Nussbaum, M. (2011). *Creating capabilities: The human development approach*. Cambridge, United Kingdom: The Belknap Press.

Organization for Economic Cooperation and Development. (1989, July). The path to full employment: Structural adjustment for an active society [Editorial]. *Employment Outlook*, 7–12.

Owen, R. (1995). *A new view of society and other writings*. London, United Kingdom: Penguin Classics, Mass Market Paperback. (Original work published 1813)

Patel, V., & Kleinman, A. (2003). Poverty and common mental disorders in developing countries. *Bulletin of the World Health Organization, 81*, 609–615.

Paul-Ward, A. (2009). Social and occupational justice barriers in the transition from foster care to independent adulthood. *American Journal of Occupational Therapy, 63*, 1.

Pizzi, M. A., Reitz, M., & Scaffa, M. E. (2010). Assessments for health promotion practice. In M. E. Scaffa, S. M. Reitz, & M. A. Pizzi (Eds.), *Occupational therapy in the promotion of health and wellness* (pp. 173–194). Philadelphia, PA: F. A. Davis.

Pollard, N., & Sakellariou, D. (2007). Occupation, education and community-based rehabilitation. *British Journal of Occupational Therapy, 70*, 171–174.

Pollard, N., Sakellariou, D., & Kronenberg, F. (Eds.). (2009). *A political practice of occupational therapy*. Edinburgh, United Kingdom: Elsevier/Churchill Livingstone.

Ramazzini, B. (1705). *A treatise of the diseases of tradesmen, Shewing the various influence of particular trades upon the state of health.* London, United Kingdom: Andrew Bell.

Ruskin, J. (1865). *Sesame and lilies.* Orpington, United Kingdom: George Allen.

Sakellariou, D., & Pollard, N. (2016). *Occupational therapies without borders: Integrating justice with practice* (2nd ed.) Edinburgh, United Kingdom: Elsevier/Churchill Livingstone.

Sakellariou, D., & Simó Algado, S. (2006). Sexuality and disability: A case of occupational injustice. *British Journal of Occupational Therapy, 69,* 69–76.

Sartorius, N. (2006). The meanings of health and its promotion. *Croatian Medical Journal, 47,* 662–664.

Scott, J. B., & Reitz, S. M. (Eds.). (2013). *Practical applications for the occupational therapy code of ethics and ethics standards.* Bethesda, MD: American Occupational Therapy Association.

Smith, D. L., & Hilton, C. L. (2008). An occupational justice perspective of domestic violence against women with disabilities. *Journal of Occupational Science, 15,* 166–172.

Stadnyk, R. (2007). Occupational justice and injustice. In S. Coppola, S. Elliott, P. Toto, & E. Varela-Burstein (Eds.), *Strategies to advance gerontology excellence.* Bethesda, MD: American Occupational Therapy Association.

Stadnyk, R., Townsend, E. A., & Wilcock, A. A. (2010). Occupational justice. In C. Christiansen & E. A. Townsend (Eds.). *Introduction to occupation: The art and science of living* (2nd ed., pp. 329–358). Thorofare, NJ: Prentice Hall.

Thibeault, R. (2013). Occupational justice's intents and impacts: From personal choices to community consequences. In M. P. Cutchin & V. A. Dickie (Eds.), *Transactional perspectives on occupation* (pp. 245–256). Dordrecht, NL: Springer.

Townsend, E. A. (1993). Muriel driver memorial lecture: Occupational therapy's social vision. *Canadian Journal of Occupational Therapy, 60,* 174–184.

Townsend, E. (1996). Enabling empowerment: Using simulations versus real occupations. *Canadian Journal of Occupational Therapy, 63,* 113–128.

Townsend, E. A. (1998). *Good intentions overruled: A critique of empowerment in the routine organization of mental health services.* Ontario, Canada: University of Toronto Press.

Townsend, E. A. (2003a). *Occupational justice: Ethical, moral and civic principles for an inclusive world.* Prague, Czech Republic: European Network of Occupational Therapy Educators. Retrieved from http://www.enothe.hva.nl/meet/ac03/acc03-text03.doc

Townsend, E. A. (2003b). Power and justice in enabling occupation. *Canadian Journal of Occupational Therapy, 70,* 74–87.

Townsend, E. A. (2007). Justice and habits: A synthesis of habits III. *OTJR: Occupation, Participation and Health, 27,* 69S–78S.

Townsend, E. A. (2015). The 2014 Ruth Zemke Lectureship in Occupational Science. Critical occupational literacy: Thinking about occupational justice, ecological sustainability, and aging in everyday life. *Journal of Occupational Science, 22,* 389–402. doi:10.1080/14427591.2015.1071691

Townsend, E. A., & Marval, B. (2013). Can professionals enable occupational justice? *Occupational Therapy Journal, 21,* 215–228 (English; Portuguese: pp. 229–242).

Townsend, E. A., & Wilcock, A. A. (2004). Occupational justice and client-centred practice: A dialogue in progress. *Canadian Journal of Occupational Therapy, 71,* 75–87.

Trentham, B., & Cockburn, L. (2011). Promoting occupational therapy in a community health centre. In M. Thew, & M. Edwards, S. Baptiste, & M. Molineux (Eds.), *Role emerging occupational therapy: Maximising occupation-focused practice* (pp. 97–110). West Sussex, United Kingdom: Blackwell.

United Nations. (1948). *Universal declaration of human rights.* Geneva, Switzerland: United Nations General Assembly.

United Nations. (1998). *Declaration on human rights defenders.* Geneva, Switzerland: United Nations General Assembly.

United Nations. (2006). *The International Forum for Social Development. Social justice in an open world: The role of the United Nations.* The International Forum for Social Development. New York, NY: Author.

United Nations Commission on Social Justice. (1994). *Social Justice: Strategies for national renewal. The report of the Commission on Social Justice.* London, United Kingdom: Vintage.

United Nations High Commissioner for Human Rights, & World Health Organisation. (2008). *The Right to health, a fact sheet.* Geneva, Switzerland: United Nations General Assembly.

Wang, H., Karp, A., Winblad, B., & Fratiglioni, L. (2002). Late-life engagement in social and leisure activities is associated with a decreased risk of dementia: A longitudinal study from the Kungsholmen project. *American Journal of Epidemiology, 155,* 1081–1087.

Warr, P. (1990). The measurement of well-being and other aspects of mental health. *Journal of Occupational Psychology, 63,* 193–210.

Watson, R., & Swartz, L. (2004). *Transformation through occupation: Human occupation in context.* London, United Kingdom: Wiley.

Werner, D. (1998, November). *Health and equity: Need for a people's perspective in the quest for world health.* Paper presented at the "PHC21—Everybody's Business" Conference, Almaty, Kazakhstan.

West, T. (2011). *The curious Mr Howard: Legendary prison reformer.* Hampshire, United Kingdom: Waterside Press.

White, J. A. (2009). Questions for occupational therapy. In E. B. Crepeau, E. S. Cohn, & B. Schell (Eds.), *Willard & Spackman's occupational therapy* (11th ed., pp. 262–272). Philadelphia, PA: Lippincott Williams & Wilkins.

Whiteford, G., & Pereira, R. (2012). Occupation, inclusion and participation. In G. Whiteford, & C. Hocking (Eds.), *Occupational science, inclusion, participation* (pp. 187–208). West Sussex, United Kingdom: Wiley-Blackwell.

Whiteford, G., & Townsend, E. (2011). Participatory occupational justice framework: Enabling occupational participation and inclusion. In N. Kronenberg, D. Pollard, & D. Sakellariou (Eds.), *Occupational therapy without borders: Towards an ecology of occupation-based practices* (2nd ed., pp. 65–84). Edinburgh, United Kingdom: Elsevier/Churchill Livingstone.

Wilcock, A. A. (1993). A theory of the human need for occupation. *Journal of Occupational Science: Australia, 1,* 17–24.

Wilcock, A. A. (1995). The occupational brain: A theory of human nature. *Journal of Occupational Science: Australia, 2,* 68–73.

Wilcock, A. A. (1998). *An occupational perspective of health.* Thorofare, NJ: SLACK.

Wilcock, A. A. (2001). *Occupation for Health: Vol. 1. A journey from self-health to prescription.* London, United Kingdom: College of Occupational Therapy.

Wilcock, A. A. (2002). *Occupation for Health: Vol. 2. A journey from prescription to self-health.* London, United Kingdom: College of Occupational Therapy.

Wilcock, A. A. (2006). *An occupational perspective of health* (2nd ed.). Thorofare, NJ: SLACK.

Wilcock, A., & Hocking, C. (2015). *An occupational perspective of health* (3rd ed.). Thorofare, NJ: SLACK.

Wilcock, A. A., & Townsend, E. A. (2000). Occupational terminology interactive dialogue: Occupational justice. *Journal of Occupational Science, 7,* 84–86.

Windley, D. (2011). Community development. In M. Thew, M. Edwards, S. Baptiste, & M. Molineux (Eds.), *Role emerging occupational therapy: Maximising occupation-focused practice* (pp. 123–134). Blackwell.

Wood, W., Hooper, B., & Womack, J. (2005). Reflections on occupational justice as a subtext of occupation-centred education. In F. Kronenberg, S. S. Algado, & N. Pollard (Eds.), *Occupational therapy without borders: Learning from the spirit of survivors* (pp. 378–389). Edinburgh, United Kingdom: Elsevier/Churchill Livingstone.

Woodham-Smith, C. (1952). *Florence Nightingale* (2nd ed., p. 71). London, United Kingdom: The Reprint Society.

World Bank. (2014, August). *Poverty-health*. Retrieved from www .worldbank.org/en/topic/health/brief/poverty-health

World Federation of Occupational Therapists. (2006). *Position statement on human rights*. Retrieved from wfot.org/office_files /Human%20Rights%20Position%20Statement%20Final%

World Federation of Occupational Therapists. (2014). *Position statement on global-health informing occupational therapy practice*. Retrieved from http://www.wfot.cm2014_Japan_PS

World Federation of Occupational Therapists. (2016). *Minimum standards for the education of occupational therapists*. London, United Kingdom: World Federation of Occupational Therapists.

World Health Organization. (1946). *Constitution of the World Health Organization*. Geneva, Switzerland: Author.

World Health Organization. (1986). *Ottawa charter for health promotion*. Ontario, Canada: Author.

World Health Organization. (1988). *Second international conference on health promotion*. Adelaide, South Australia: Author.

World Health Organization. (1991). *Third international conference on health promotion*. Sundsvall, Sweden: Author.

World Health Organization. (1997). *Jakarta declaration on leading health promotion into the 21st century. Fourth international conference on health promotion*. Jakarta, Indonesia: Author.

World Health Organization. (2001). *Mental disorders affect one in four people*. Geneva, Switzerland: Author.

World Health Organization. (2004). *Global strategy on diet, physical activity and health*. Geneva, Switzerland: Author. Retrieved from http://www.who.int/mediacentre/factsheets/fs385/en/

World Health Organization. (2005). *Bangkok Charter for health promotion in a globalized world*. 6th Global Conference on health promotion. Geneva, Switzerland: Author.

World Health Organization. (2009). *7th Global Conference on health promotion*. Nairobi, Kenya: Author.

World Health Organization. (2010). *Global recommendations on physical activity for health*. Geneva, Switzerland: Author.

World Health Organization. (2011a). *Global strategy on diet, physical activity and health*. Geneva, Switzerland: Author. Retrieved from http://www.who.int/mediacentre/factsheets/fs385/en/

World Health Organization. (2011b). *Rio political declaration on social determinants of health*. Geneva, Switzerland: Author.

World Health Organization. (2013). *Global action plan for the prevention and control of NCDs 2013–2020*. Geneva, Switzerland: Author.

World Health Organization. (2014). *Mental health: A state of well-being. The 66th World Health Assembly*. Retrieved from http://www .who.int/dg/speeches/2013/launch_mental_health_action_plan/en/

World Health Organization. (2016). *9th Global Conference on Health Promotion*. Shanghai, China: Author.

World Health Organization. (2017a) *Global strategy on diet, physical activity and health*. Geneva, Switzerland: Author. Retrieved from http://www.who.int/mediacentre/factsheets/fs385/en/

World Health Organization. (2017b). *Physical activity. WHO Fact sheet. Updated February*. Geneva, Switzerland: Author.

World Health Organization, & Calouste Gulbenkian Foundation. (2014). *Social determinants of mental health*. Geneva, Switzerland: Author.

the**Point**® *For additional resources on the subjects discussed in this chapter, visit* **http://thePoint.lww.com /Willard-Spackman13e.**

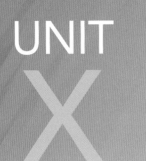

UNIT X

Broad Theories Informing Practice

"In order to understand anything well, you need at least three good theories."

—Laurent Daloz (1986)

From *Effective teaching and mentoring: Realizing the transformational power of adult learning experiences*, page 43. London: Jossey-Bass

Recovery Model

Skye Barbic, Terry Krupa

LEARNING OBJECTIVES

After reading this chapter, you will be able to:

1. Describe contemporary perspectives on recovery in the mental health field.
2. Identify elements or components of the recovery process.
3. Integrate various frameworks or models of the recovery process.
4. Summarize approaches to measure recovery systematically in practice.
5. Apply recovery-oriented principles in occupational therapy practice.

Introduction

The concept of recovery is rooted in the simple and yet profound realization that people who have been diagnosed with mental illness are human beings. . . . The goal is to become the unique, awesome, never to be repeated human being that we are called to be. Those of us who have been labeled with mental illness are not de facto excused from this fundamental task of becoming human. In fact, because many of us have experienced our lives and dreams shattered in the wake of mental illness, one of the most essential challenges that face us is to ask who can I become and why should I say yes to life. (Deegan, 1996, p. 92)

This opening quote is by Patricia Deegan (1996), who is widely credited with coining the term "recovery" to describe the phenomena whereby people come to live rich and meaningful lives despite experiencing mental illness. As a person with lived experience of mental illness, Deegan provides a powerful real-life example of how recovery can unfold within a life situation characterized by despair, isolation, and deprivation. Deegan has poignantly described how mental health service providers have the power to be either insensitive and hardened or enabling and supportive of the struggles that people with mental illness experience in determining "who to become" and in "saying yes to life." Indeed, becoming familiar with the range of Deegan's writings and speeches might be considered foundational knowledge for occupational therapists learning about recovery (see for example, Deegan, 1988, 1990, 1996, 2001).

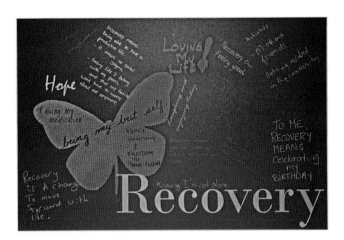

FIGURE 46-1 Recovery-oriented services create a vision of recovery that includes the voices of people served.

In this chapter, the reader is introduced to recovery as it is evolving in the mental health field. Multiple perspectives on recovery are presented, but particular emphasis is placed on the perspectives of people with lived experience of mental illness (Figure 46-1). The recovery construct is not free of debate in the mental health field. Understanding the controversy surrounding recovery can position occupational therapists to better evaluate their own practice and to contribute to the ongoing evolution of the recovery vision and emerging science. This chapter begins with the definitions of recovery. Conceptual frameworks and models of recovery are then presented. These are followed by a discussion of recovery in practice that reviews recovery intervention programs and issues related to evaluation. In the final section of this chapter, the relationship between recovery and occupational therapy (OT) are discussed.

Defining Recovery

Recovery as a Personal Life Journey

In this chapter, **recovery** is defined as a process experienced by people with mental illness whereby they come to a life that is defined less by illness and pathology and defined more by a personal sense of purpose, agency and control, and active participation in valued and meaningful activities (Noordsy et al., 2002). The understanding of recovery as a *process* is important; it denotes an ongoing personal life journey, rather than

an endpoint, or some final outcome. As with everyone's life journey, it suggests that there will be ups and downs, high points and low points, and successes and failures. Yet the overarching expectation is that the journey of recovery will provide opportunities for greater well-being, positive growth, and community participation.

This definition of recovery also highlights that the process of recovery belongs to and is the personal responsibility of people with mental illness themselves. It is consistent with what Slade (2009) has referred to as *personal recovery*. Deegan stresses that service providers are not responsible for making people recover, but they can play an important role by creating conditions that will invite people to engage in the recovery journey and to negotiate the struggles that will inevitably present (Deegan, 1988, 1996). Recovery-based training for service providers is increasingly available in a variety of countries with a broad range of cultures. Common to most training courses is how to communicate with a person about his or her personal recovery journey. This includes contextualizing how to negotiate one's illness or symptoms within the context of the needs and priorities of the person in recovery. The U.S. Substance Abuse and Mental Health Services Administration (SAMHSA) describes four dimensions that support a life in recovery:

1. *Health*—overcoming or managing one's disease(s) or symptoms—for example, abstaining from use of alcohol, illicit drugs, and nonprescribed medications if one has an addiction problem—and, for everyone in recovery, making informed, healthy choices that support physical and emotional well-being
2. *Home*—having a stable and safe place to live
3. *Purpose*—conducting meaningful daily activities, such as a job, school volunteerism, family caretaking, or creative endeavors, and the independence, income, and resources to participate in society
4. *Community*—having relationships and social networks that provide support, friendship, love, and hope

The dimensions resonate clearly with OT, where health is understood within the context of what is important and meaningful to a person. As well, these dimensions highlight that recovery is a continual process and requires ongoing evaluation of how personal, environmental, and occupational factors influence the recovery trajectory of a person. Finally, perhaps the most important point for consideration is that these dimensions are relevant to most people, regardless if diagnosed with a mental illness or not. Del Vecchio (2012) describes the journey of recovery as highly personal, may occur via many pathways, and is characterized by continual growth and improvement in one's health and wellness.

Conflicting Perspectives on Recovery

Recovery has gained international prominence as a guiding vision for the development of mental health services and systems. Yet, despite its influence, confusion persists, and there is no guarantee that discussions about recovery in mental health will start from a shared agreement about its meaning. Practice Dilemma 46-1 illustrates divergent views on the meaning of recovery and expectations regarding participation in occupations for persons with mental illness.

⚓ PRACTICE DILEMMA 46-1

Shandra, an occupational therapist, works for a community mental health program that is focused on helping people with serious mental illness to live successfully in the community. At their annual retreat, the agency set aside time to discuss practices related to employment and other vocational or productive activities. Shandra examined the employment and productivity participation of the people receiving services and informed the team that fewer than 15% of the 90 people served identified any regular involvement in productivity activities such as work, school, or volunteering. During the ensuing discussion, team members made comments such as "the people we serve are too sick to work," "we don't have the time or resources to focus on work—that isn't our job," "no one I work with has said they want to work," and "work will make their symptoms flare up." The team encouraged Shandra to follow up on her interest in employment and productivity but left the discussions without any firm plans for follow-up.

Questions

1. Evaluate the service response to the issue of employment and productivity with respect to contemporary perspectives on recovery.
2. Shandra decides to give some thought to how she might respond to this discussion, so that she can facilitate a shift to more recovery-oriented services. What might she say to challenge the idea that addressing employment and productivity is not within the scope of the service?
3. The practice dilemma does not reflect the voices of people with mental illness. How might Shandra engage their involvement in this discussion about employment and productivity?

Clinical versus Personal Perspectives on Recovery

Definitions of recovery that have emerged from mental health professionals have tended to focus on the amelioration of the mental illness, evidenced by symptom remission and the reduction in the need for intensive treatment services. Slade (2009) refers to this as a definition of "recovery as cure" and distinguishes it as a clinical perspective on recovery rather than the personal perspective of recovery that emerges from people with lived experience. Davidson and Roe (2007) suggest that *clinical interpretations* are perhaps best described as "recovery from mental illness," whereas *personal interpretations* are best described as "being in recovery." The ongoing confusion between personal and clinical definitions of recovery has historical roots. It is occurring within a mental health system that has long been dominated by biomedical perspectives on illness.

The assumption underlying the clinical perspective is that illness management is central to recovery and occurs in the context of treatments—treatments that are largely developed and offered by mental health professionals who have expertise. The assumptions underlying personal recovery—that people with mental illness can be largely in control of managing their illnesses, that effective illness management strategies exist outside the realm of the authority of mental health professionals, and that people with mental illness can enjoy a life of inclusion in their communities—have been largely overlooked and, at worst, depreciated. Davidson, Rakfeldt, and Strauss (2010), in their study of the historical roots of the recovery movement, pointed out that although other branches of health care have largely accepted that people who experience chronic forms of disease or significant disability should not "put their lives on hold until the illness resolves" (p. 4), this notion has not received the same broad acceptance in the mental health service arena.

Recovery as a Citizenship Movement

Another perspective on recovery, although perhaps less prevalent, is the argument that definitions of recovery have been highly individualistic and ultimately unable to integrate the influence of exceptional levels of disadvantage and marginalization that characterize the social position of people with mental illness. From this perspective, it is argued that people with mental illness in their recovery process encounter injustices embedded within social structures, such as discrimination, oppressive public policies, and social segregation. Social perspectives on recovery highlight the extent to which the daily lives of people with serious mental illness are characterized by conditions of social and economic poverty, marginalization, and stigma. There is evidence to support that these social and financial strains will have a negative impact on the recovery process (Mattsson, Topor, Cullberg, & Forsell, 2008; Pelletier et al., 2015). From this social perspective, recovery is conceptualized as a civil rights movement focused on securing full citizenship rights and responsibilities for people with mental illness.

The Definition Matters

More than a play of words, the definition of recovery does matter—a great deal. With recovery being adapted as a guiding vision for mental health services in many jurisdictions, the definition selected will ultimately influence how human and material resources are distributed, how success in the system will be evaluated, and what kinds of service activities and supports will be expected. The choice of definition is the foundation from which communication can take place.

The perspective of personal recovery offers an important opportunity for a fundamental transformation in the mental health service arena toward an integrated system that is able to address illness, health, well-being, and citizenship in a synergistic fashion. In response to this challenge, efforts have been directed to describing how the concepts and ideals of personal recovery can be translated to reform service delivery and service systems, avoiding the very real risk that conflicting perspectives on recovery will lead to the conclusion that only small tweaks are required or, worse, that recovery-oriented practices are already in place. For example, Tondora and Davidson (2006) and Davidson et al., (2007) have advanced practice guidelines to direct the development of recovery-oriented services and to identify what people in recovery should expect from the mental health service system. As well, Barbic (2016) has advanced practice by working with people with lived experience to conceptualize recovery as a linear continuum and map the types of evidence-based services that a person could consider.

> ### 👤 PRACTICE DILEMMA 46-2
>
> Samantha, an occupational therapist, works for an assertive community treatment (ACT) team that focus on helping people with serious mental illness to live successfully in the community. In preparation for their staff meeting, her manager asks her to present to her team about the types of services OT can provide for a person in recovery.

Questions

1. In preparation for this presentation, Samantha decides to meet with some of her clients to ask them what their recovery journey looks like. If recovery can be mapped as a continuum from low to high, what might that Samantha's clients say to describe what high (optimal) recovery looks like? What might low levels of recovery look like?
2. What types of OT assessments are available to evaluate her clients as they move along their recovery journey from low to high?
3. What types of evidence-based OT interventions exist to support her clients along the recovery journey?
4. What can Samantha tell her team about the value of OT services to support individuals receiving ACT services?

Recovery Frameworks or Models

To date, no single theory or conceptual model of recovery has been developed and accepted, but the mental health field is replete with systematic efforts to capture critical elements of an overarching framework for recovery.

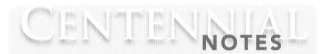

Determining What "Matters" to Clients in Mental Health Practice

In the last 100 years, systematic approaches to defining client priorities in OT for mental health have not been developed. However, OT is not alone in that status. In a recent editorial published in the *British Medical Journal*, Coulter (2017) notes that the behavior of measuring what matters to patients is "surprisingly rare" in medicine, with a mere 11% of patient-reported outcome measures actually asking patients which outcomes are worth measuring (Coulter, 2017).

With our profession's long-standing history of client-centered practice, occupational therapists are naturally suited to lead initiatives over the next century to ensure that assessments, treatments, policies, and funding are aligned with our clients' needs and priorities. The natural intersection between recovery and client-centered practice in the field of mental health has potential to drastically improve health care, limit costs, and foster excellence in person-centered care and innovation.

Empirically constructed conceptualizations of the personal recovery process incorporate a common understanding of the components or elements of the recovery process and the phases and tasks central to the process.

Elements of the Recovery Process

Based on an analysis of published qualitative accounts of recovery, Davidson (2005) identified and described elements that appear common to the experience of the recovery process, including

- Renewing hope and commitment,
- Redefining self,
- Incorporating illness,
- Being involved in meaningful activities,
- Overcoming stigma,
- Assuming control,
- Becoming empowered,
- Exercising citizenship,
- Managing symptoms, and
- Being supported by others.

The elements provide an understanding of the nature of the personal transformations that are experienced in the recovery process. The renewal of hope provides the individual with a growing sense that the future holds possibilities. The individual develops a growing sense that the illness need not be the defining feature of one's identity; there are other stories about the self that are waiting to be explored and developed. A transition from passive acceptance of circumstances to a growing sense of control and personal agency occurs. The illness experience is not ignored but becomes integrated into this broader view of the self and the self in the world. The sense of personal agency, or self-determination, is extended to developing a personal understanding of the illness that supports these processes of growth and change and the development of strategies to manage the illness experience. The critical elements include actions that connect the individual to living a full life in the broader community.

The 10 components of recovery identified in the *National Consensus Statement on Mental Health Recovery* by the SAMHSA (2006) have similarities to those proposed by Davidson (2005) but are written more from a perspective that guides mental health service delivery and the design of service systems (Box 46-1). The components highlight important elements of the mental health service system, such as peer support. At its core, the recovery process reflects a release of strengths and a growth of abilities, capacities, and possibilities that should be valued and nurtured by others. All of the components are interdependent and act synergistically toward the goal

of recovery (Figure 46-2). The consensus statement concludes with a very powerful statement that recovery benefits not only the individual in recovery but also society.

Stage and Task Models of Recovery

There have been several efforts to understand how the recovery process unfolds and how the various defined elements of the process are related to each other over time. These have led to the development of several stage models of the process, largely developed empirically from persons in recovery (see Andresen, Oades, & Caputi, 2003, for an integrated review of several stage models).

One such model was developed by people with lived experience of mental illness who are considered leaders across the United States in their roles as members of a Recovery Advisory Group (Ralph, 2005). They described a six-stage model of the recovery process: (1) anguish, described as an experience of despair related to the accepted label of "mentally ill"; (2) awakening, reflecting the beginning sense that things can change; (3) insight, or the growing understanding and personalization of possibilities of change; (4) action planning, reflecting the increase in doing toward well-being and meaning; (5) determined commitment to become well, describing the growing resolution for action and self-determination; and (6) well-being and empowerment, an experience of belief in the self to help the self and others. A particularly helpful feature of the model is the inclusion of specific domains of change—four internal (occurring within the self) and four external (responses or actions)—and descriptions of changes that occur in these domains across the six stages.

Another example of a linear model of recovery is that developed from the Personal Recovery Outcome Measurement study led by Barbic (2016). In this model, a set of indicators are hypothesized to reflect a person's journey of recovery from low to high. The model summarizes a hierarchy of items that describe basic requirements for recovery (such as safety, resources, hope), moderate needs (energy, goals, purpose), and high needs (contribution to the community, intimacy, peace of mind). The model has also been use to guide the development of a 30-item measure of personal recovery called the Personal Recovery Outcome Measure (PROM).

Although stage models advance our understanding and provide empirical support for the recovery process, they are inherently problematic. If we are to conceptualize recovery as an individual and nonlinear process, then how can defining moments of the recovery process be ordered in any sort of generalizable way? The field will need to evaluate how stage models capture the range of expressions of recovery.

BOX 46-1 NATIONAL CONSENSUS STATEMENT ON MENTAL HEALTH RECOVERY: THE 10 FUNDAMENTAL COMPONENTS OF RECOVERY

Self-direction: Consumers lead, control, exercise choice over, and determine their own path of recovery by optimizing autonomy, independence, and control of resources to achieve a self-determined life. By definition, the recovery process must be self-directed by the individual, who defines his or her own life goals and designs a unique path toward those goals.

Individualized and person-centered: There are multiple pathways to recovery based on an individual's unique strengths and resiliencies as well as his or her needs, preferences, experiences (including past trauma), and cultural background in all of its diverse representations. Individuals also identify recovery as being an ongoing journey and an end result as well as an overall paradigm for achieving wellness and optimal mental health.

Empowerment: Consumers have the authority to choose from a range of options and to participate in all decisions—including the allocation of resources—that will affect their lives, and are educated and supported in so doing. They have the ability to join with other consumers to collectively and effectively speak for themselves about their needs, wants, desires, and aspirations. Through empowerment, an individual gains control of his or her own destiny and influences the organizational and societal structures in his or her life.

Holistic: Recovery encompasses an individual's whole life, including mind, body, spirit, and community. Recovery embraces all aspects of life, including housing, employment, education, mental health and health care treatment and services, complementary and alternative health services, addictions treatment, spirituality, creativity, social networks, community participation, and family supports as determined by the person. Families, providers, organizations, systems, communities, and society play crucial roles in creating and maintaining meaningful opportunities for consumer access to these supports.

Nonlinear: Recovery is not a step-by-step process but one based on continual growth, occasional setbacks, and learning from experience. Recovery begins with an initial stage of awareness in which a person recognizes that positive change is possible. This awareness enables the consumer to move on to fully engage in the work of recovery.

Strengths-based: Recovery focuses on valuing and building on the multiple capacities, resiliencies, talents, coping abilities, and inherent worth of individuals. By building on these strengths, consumers leave stymied life roles behind and engage in new life roles (e.g., partner, caregiver, friend, student, employee). The process of recovery moves forward through interaction with others in supportive, trust-based relationships.

Peer support: Mutual support—including the sharing of experiential knowledge and skills and social learning—plays an invaluable role in recovery. Consumers encourage and engage other consumers in recovery and provide each other with a sense of belonging, supportive relationships, valued roles, and community.

Respect: Community, systems, and societal acceptance and appreciation of consumers—including protecting their rights and eliminating discrimination and stigma—are crucial in achieving recovery. Self-acceptance and regaining belief in one's self are particularly vital. Respect ensures the inclusion and full participation of consumers in all aspects of their lives.

Responsibility: Consumers have a personal responsibility for their own self-care and journeys of recovery. Taking steps toward their goals may require great courage. Consumers must strive to understand and give meaning to their experiences and identify coping strategies and healing processes to promote their own wellness.

Hope: Recovery provides the essential and motivating message of a better future—that people can and do overcome the barriers and obstacles that confront them. Hope is internalized but can be fostered by peers, families, friends, providers, and others. Hope is the catalyst of the recovery process. Mental health recovery not only benefits individuals with mental health disabilities by focusing on their abilities to live, work, learn, and fully participate in our society but also enriches the texture of American community life. America reaps the benefits of the contributions individuals with mental disabilities can make, ultimately becoming a stronger and healthier nation.

In contrast to stage models, Slade (2009) proposed a model of recovery based on the tasks that people are engaged in over the course of the recovery process. The tasks are highly consistent with empirically derived elements of recovery, account for recovery as both an internal process and a process that is positioned within a larger social environment, and are only loosely ordered, acknowledging considerable individual variability.

The four tasks include (1) developing a positive identity, (2) framing the mental illness, (3) self-managing the illness, and (4) developing valued social roles. As shown in Table 46-1, each of these tasks requires personal work ranging from changing one's own self-perception to the development of expertise and supports needed to manage the mental illness within the broader context of one's life.

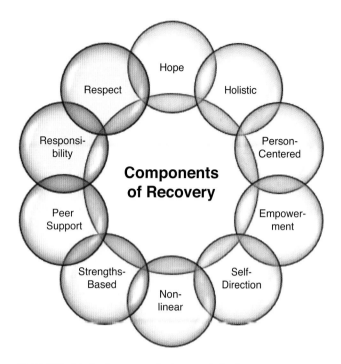

FIGURE 46-2 A synergistic model of recovery.

Recovery in Practice

Evaluating Recovery

The complexity of the recovery process extends to design and methodological issues related to research and evaluation. If, for example, recovery is an ongoing process, how can any meaningful outcome associated with recovery be conceptualized and evaluated? How can we reconcile the notion of recovery as a process experienced and owned by people with mental illness within a health care system (and research funding system) that highly values controlled trials, researcher objectivity, and quantified results?

TABLE 46-1	Slade's Task Model of Recovery

Task	Personal Work Involved
Developing a positive identity	Developing a multifaceted view of a valued sense of self
Framing the mental illness	Making sense of the illness experience as an important challenge to be negotiated within the context of important broader life experiences
Self-managing the illness	Developing expertise in controlling the experience of mental illness
Developing valued social roles	Connecting to others and the broader world through personally and socially valued activities

People with mental illness have long been concerned that innovations in practice and advances in research have largely occurred without their input and voice. The popular slogan "Nothing about us without us" became a sort of rallying call against a mental health system that did not, in any meaningful way, include the voices of the people it served. The understanding of recovery as a personal journey experienced and owned by people with mental illness has advanced this movement because it has relied on first-person narratives of the lived experience. This has led to a greater understanding of the value of the experiential knowledge of people who live with mental illness and has subsequently contributed to the growth of valued, formal peer support services in the mental health system and the development of research relationships with people in recovery that engage them to a varying extent—from seeking their perspectives to involving them as partners in research (Figure 46-3).

Advances in the conceptual development of recovery are providing a good foundation for advancing evaluation. A wide array of measures to evaluate individual recovery have now been developed and been subject to psychometric testing. Most measures are self-report measures, such as the Recovery Process Inventory (Jerrell, Cousins, & Roberts, 2006) which asks people with mental illness to rate themselves on six dimensions (anguish, connection to others, confidence or purpose, others care or help, living situation, and hopeful). Many of these measurement tools are available electronically on the Web and are not subject to restrictive copyright rules (see, for example, Barbic, 2016; Campbell-Orde, Chamberlin, Carpenter, & Leff, 2005).

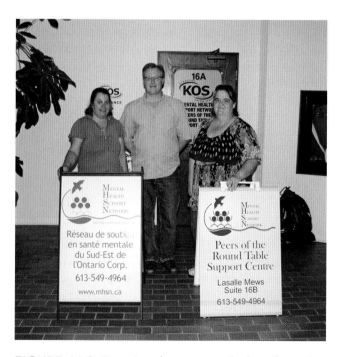

FIGURE 46-3 Peer involvement including formal peer support services is a critical element of a recovery-oriented service system.

In addition to generic measures of recovery such as the Recovery Assessment Scale (Corrigan, Salzer, Ralph, Sangster, & Keck, 2004) and the newly developed Recovery Quality of Life Scale (Keetharuth, Brazier, Connell, Carlton, Taylor Buck, Ricketts, & Barkham, 2017) evaluation can be designed to focus on particular elements of the recovery process. For example, it is widely accepted that a fundamental shift in agency occurs in the recovery process whereby individuals with mental illness move from attitudes and behaviors that reflect passivity, internalized stigma, the absence of expectations, and helplessness to positions of control and a growing sense of expectations for the self in the larger world. With this in mind, evaluators may choose to focus on the changing sense of empowerment within the recovery process and use established measures such as the Empowerment Scale (Rogers, Chamberlin, Ellison, & Crean, 1997)—a self-report scale developed by individuals with mental illness, which operationalizes the many dimensions of empowerment in 28 items reflecting five factors of self-efficacy and self-esteem, power and powerlessness, community activism, righteous anger, and optimism toward the future.

Another recently discussed outcome important to personal recovery is time use. The Illness Management Recovery (IMR) scale (Salyers, Godfrey, Mueser, & Labriola, 2007) has a specific item that asks people about time use. As well, occupational therapists are familiar with many other time-use assessments including diaries and time logs. Targeting time use is an outcome of important consideration for occupational therapists working in mental health (Eklund, Leufstadius, & Bejerholm, 2009). "Time" has a common unit that most people clearly understand, and how people spend their time meaningfully to achieve health and well-being has been developed by occupational therapists as a concern for public health (Gewurtz et al., 2016). Depending on the chosen definition of recovery, meaningful time use is an important target for OT treatment.

Remembering that the personal journey of recovery occurs within a larger mental health care context, recovery-related evaluation has also been directed to operationalizing and measuring the shifts expected within this context. Clear descriptions of how programs and services are structured and administered within a recovery-oriented system have contributed to the ability to evaluate system change. For example, the Recovery Self-Assessment (RSA) tool has been used to engage services in adopting a recovery orientation (O'Connell, Tondora, Croog, Evans, & Davidson, 2005). Similarly, shifts in service provider knowledge and practice are expected, and this has included the clear articulation of recovery competencies or the attitudes, knowledge, and behaviors expected from providers in a recovery-oriented system. In New Zealand and Canada, for example, a set of recovery competencies was developed for all mental health service providers to inform the development of standards in care (Mental Health Commission of Canada, 2015; Mental Health Commission of New Zealand, 2001). In addition, there have been efforts to develop recovery competencies to meet the needs of specific contexts, where the principles and values of recovery are compromised by restrictive contexts. For example, occupational therapists Chen, Krupa, Lysaght, McCay, and Piat (2013, 2014) developed a recovery competency framework for the inpatient mental health context and developed and evaluated an accompanying recovery education program for interdisciplinary inpatient mental health service providers. With the development of evaluation tools such as the Recovery Knowledge Inventory (RKI) (Bedregal, O'Connell, & Davidson, 2006), changes in provider attitudes and knowledge about recovery can be evaluated over time.

Threats to recovery-oriented care have been documented recently by Parker and colleagues (2017). These include staff burnout and external pressure to accept clients who are "not ready" for recovery. Parker and colleagues recommend active vigilance to maintain a focus on recovery and rehabilitation and that leadership focus on adapting services to the emergent needs of people receiving mental health services.

Recovery Approaches and Strategies

Various intervention approaches and strategies have been developed in response to the growing understanding of the recovery process. Evidence demonstrating the effectiveness of these strategies is emerging. Generally, these intervention approaches attempt to operationalize key elements of recovery-oriented practice. The *Recovery Workbook* (Spaniol, Koehler, & Hutchinson, 1994) takes individuals with mental illness through a series of activities meant to increase their awareness of recovery, increase their knowledge about and control of psychiatric conditions, understand the importance of stress, build a meaningful and enjoyable life and personal supports, and begin to develop sustained plans of action. A pilot research study, using a randomized controlled trial design, evaluated the effectiveness of a modified version of the workbook that shortened the 30 weekly sessions to 12 sessions. Findings suggested that participants experienced positive changes in perceived levels of hope, empowerment, and general measures of recovery (Barbic, Krupa, & Armstrong, 2009). The well-known *Wellness Recovery Action Plan* (Copeland, 1997) engages people with mental illness in activities designed to identify and implement personalized wellness strategies and raise awareness of benefits of peer support. A large-scale study using randomized controlled trials demonstrated positive changes in experiences of psychiatric symptoms, increased levels of hopefulness, and enhanced quality of life (Cook et al., 2012). As well, the Illness Management and Recovery intervention program uses a series of activities based on five practices for teaching illness self-management, including psychoeducation, behavioral training focused on integrating medications into daily routines, relapse prevention planning, coping skills training, and social skills training to enhance social support (Gingerich & Mueser, 2005). A randomized controlled trial of the intervention program suggested that participants experienced improvements in illness self-management, as evaluated by both self and clinician ratings (Levitt et al., 2009). Finally, new evidence exists to support an OT-based intervention called "Action Over Inertia" (Krupa et al., 2010) which aims to allow individuals with mental illness to increase their activity engagement and community participation. To date, the authors have shown evidence for the intervention based on how peoples' time use patterns have changed to be more reflective of patterns associated with health and well-being (Edgelow & Krupa, 2011).

Recovery and Occupational Therapy

Recovery-oriented practice is not considered the domain of any one discipline or professional group. Rather, efforts to instill a recovery-oriented vision in our mental health systems have depended on all providers to consider their own practice with respect to the evolving understanding of recovery processes. The relationship between recovery and OT is reciprocal. Occupational therapy can contribute to the growing knowledge and evidence base of recovery, and recovery concepts can inform OT practice.

Many occupational therapists have actively contributed to efforts to realize the vision of recovery in the mental health services sector. They have served as study investigators on research advancing our understanding of recovery. Occupational therapists have been hired to serve as recovery facilitators to assist mental health organizations in achieving the difficult transformation to recovery-oriented care. Occupational therapists have worked in close collaboration with groups of individuals with lived experience to advocate for and implement structures that ensure their meaningful involvement in creating recovery-oriented practices, services, and systems.

Of particular interest in this chapter, however, is the consideration of how the distinct knowledge and practice base of the OT profession might contribute to the ongoing evolution of recovery. From this perspective, the question engages occupational therapists in

considering how their particular focus on their domain of concern—occupation—can advance recovery knowledge and practice. The connection between occupation and recovery is explicit, given that participation in personally and socially meaningful activities and roles has been considered a critical element of the recovery process. Davidson and colleagues (2010) in their history of the roots of the recovery movement express that participation in the everyday but meaningful activities of daily life is not the outcome of recovery but rather the foundation of recovery. Consistent with OT theory and practice, the authors contend that the recovery process can be positively influenced by the actual doing of activities, particularly when supported by others in their engagement in occupations. Lamenting the loss of attention to activity-based approaches within the mental health service system with the closure of psychiatric hospitals, they suggest, "There currently are glimmers of hope that the recovery movement may bring about a bit of renaissance of OT and science within psychiatry" and state they would "heartily welcome such a development, and suggest that the recovery movement would have much to learn from this discipline" (Davidson et al., 2010, p. 237). The remainder of this section describes how occupational therapists have or could advance their expertise in the area of occupation to further the vision of recovery.

Although goal identification and planning has been an integral element of several recovery interventions, the Canadian Occupational Performance Measure (COPM) (Law et al., 1990) is a client-centered tool that engages individuals with mental illness in collaboration with service providers in the identification of priority occupations and the evaluation of both performance and satisfaction with these occupations over time. In their review of the relevance of the COPM to recovery-oriented practice, Kirsh and Cockburn (2009) point out that consistent with recovery, "the COPM enables clients and service providers to work in partnership and direct their gaze towards the roles and activities that compromise people's identity, enhancing opportunities for self-actualization" (p. 174). The authors raise several possible points of contention surrounding the COPM, including concerns about its sensitivity to diversity and culturally specific occupations, as well as the susceptibility of clients to the perspectives of clinicians even in the context of interactions that are meant to be collaborative. These are not concerns exclusive to the COPM but rather reflect healthy, critical discourse that should underlie all recovery practice.

Contextualizing care planning in a person's goals is increasingly becoming best practice on most community mental health teams. Increased research has focused on the importance of recovery plans to be strengths focused. Xie (2013) highlights that strengths-based approaches to recovery planning move the focus away from deficits of people with mental illnesses (consumers) and focuses on the strengths and resources of the person receiving services. The implications for this approach have been shown to improve outcomes such as client engagement, functioning, satisfaction with care, and quality of life (Lyons, Uziel-Miller, Reyes, & Sokol, 2000; Rapp & Goscha, 2012; Rust, Diessner, & Reade, 2009).

An important systematic review of other occupation- or activity-based interventions examines the extent to which these interventions lead to positive changes in areas of community integration and normative life roles for adults with serious mental illness (Gibson, D'Amico, Jaffe, & Arbesman, 2011). The study considered a range of interventions from training in social skills to instrumental activities of daily living (IADL) and life skills training and role development. Not all interventions were developed specifically by occupational therapists (e.g., supported employment and education and neurocognitive training), but all interventions were considered within the OT scope of practice. The review suggested that the evidence for social skills training was strong, whereas the evidence supporting the effectiveness of neurocognitive training paired with skills training across domains of occupational performance and training in life skills and IADL was only moderate. The review provides a valuable summary of evidence-based, occupation-focused interventions and perhaps offers a prototype for how a range of seemingly disparate interventions might be organized conceptually within the framework of recovery.

People with mental illness frequently experience profound disruptions in both their performance of important occupations and in their experience of these occupations. Descriptions of the nature of these disruptions are being advanced by the profession with a view to connecting the experience of occupations closely with intervention and support approaches. For example, an individual whose occupational patterns are characterized by an exceptional lack of involvement might best be characterized as disengagement or difficulties associated with emotional detachment, or it might be more characterized by deprivation or exceptional levels of disadvantage with respect to opportunities (Krupa, Fossey, Anthony, Brown, & Pitts, 2009). In the former case, the individual in recovery and the therapist might work together to identify and build sources of meaning in occupation, whereas in the latter, they might assertively organize opportunities and resources of occupation. Developing ways to talk directly about occupation is important for the evolution of recovery as a guiding vision for mental health service delivery. It can, for example, provide a way to talk about people who experience mental illness as social and community beings rather than focusing on illness and pathology. Rebeiro Gruhl (2008) suggests that the occupational issues facing

people with serious mental illness needs to be conceptualized as an issue of occupational injustice, highlighting that social and structural issues constrain and restrict their occupational lives and that this needs to be reconciled if the recovery vision in mental health is to be realized. These highlight the importance of advocacy as a fundamental element of OT practice within a recovery framework.

Consistent with recovery, occupational therapists have advanced the development of a range of approaches to collaboratively develop occupational lives that are characterized by health and well-being. Assessment tools, such as the Occupational Performance History Interview, have been developed to engage individuals in telling their occupational stories in a way that can build on the individual's lived experiences and reveal strengths and potential opportunities (Ennals & Fossey, 2009). Similarly, assessment tools that measure time use help to capture the actual occupational patterns of people with mental illness to facilitate collaborative planning (Eklund et al., 2009). Other tools such as the Profile of Occupational Engagement (Bejerholm, Hansson, & Eklund, 2006) can help with the interpretation of occupational patterns by considering how elements of well-being and health are being experienced through occupation. For example, occupational patterns might be explored with respect to the extent to which they provide the individual with structure and routine, provide a good level of satisfaction, and provide opportunities for social interactions and access to a range of community environments. Occupational therapists have used the evidence-based practice of psychoeducation to explicitly inform people with mental illness and their support networks about the link between activity, occupation, and recovery. Figure 46-4 provides an example of a handout used in one such initiative, Action Over Inertia, which addresses the activity health needs of people with serious mental illness. Initial testing of Action Over Inertia has suggested that it may be effective in enabling people to make meaningful changes in their occupational patterns (Edgelow & Krupa, 2011; Krupa et al., 2010). However, it should be noted that the role of OT in recovery has rarely been explicitly tested in recovery interventions. Although the guiding principles of recovery are much in line with OT's values and scope, future evidence is needed to support the unique evidence-based role of the profession practicing in this new model of care.

Conclusion

The core values, assumptions, and philosophy of OT are remarkably consistent with those espoused within contemporary perspectives on personal recovery. It is important to remember, however, that occupational

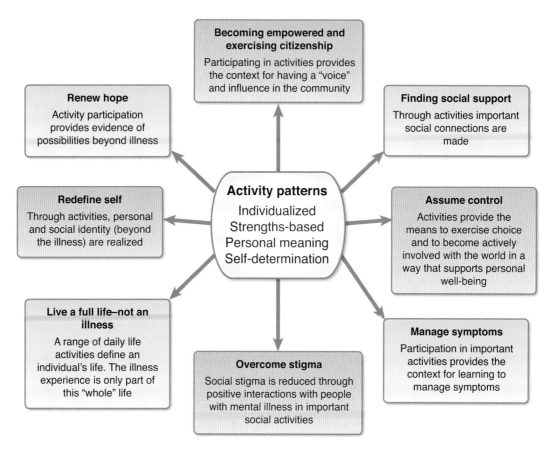

FIGURE 46-4 The recovery benefits of activity participation. (Adapted from Krupa, T., Edgelow, D., Radloff-Gabriel, D., Perry, A., Mieras, C., Bransfield, M., . . . Almas, A. [2010]. *Action over inertia: Addressing the activity-health needs of individuals with serious mental illness.* Ottawa, Canada: Canadian Association of Occupational Therapists. Reprinted with permission.)

therapists have and do practice within a health service delivery system where there have been major challenges and obstacles to implementing a recovery-oriented vision. It would be unreasonable to think that occupational therapists have somehow not been influenced by these obstacles and that their practice has always been recovery-oriented within a larger system that has had such difficulty with this transformation. For example, Davidson, O'Connell, Tondora, Styron, and Kangas (2006) identified several concerns about recovery that emerged during efforts to transform a state mental health system. These concerns include such difficulties as practicing from the assumption that recovery is possible for only a selection of people with mental illness; difficulties with orienting professional expertise to practice that is assertively supportive of self-determination, personal agency, and control; and difficulties with refining practice to actively develop evidence-based approaches and interventions that will enable recovery.

Occupational therapists need to stay sensitive to the fact that recovery-oriented practice cannot reflect "business as usual" in the mental health field. It will necessitate continual reflection related to assumptions underlying practice, the development of new forms of partnership with the people they serve as individuals and as a group, engaging actively with the broader community to create real opportunities for participation and citizenship, and innovation in service delivery. Of critical importance to the profession is evaluating these innovations and explicitly documenting the contributions of OT knowledge and expertise. Such evidence will provide much needed strength and leadership to advocate for the rights of people with mental illness to experience personally and socially meaningful occupational lives.

REFERENCES

Andresen, R., Oades, L., & Caputi, P. (2003). The experience of recovery from schizophrenia: Towards an empirically validated stage model. *Australian and New Zealand Journal of Psychiatry, 37,* 586–594.

Barbic, S. (2016, April). *Development and testing of the Personal Recovery Outcome Measure (PROM) for people with mental illness.* Paper presented at the Canadian Association of Occupational Therapists, Banff, Canada.

Barbic, S., Krupa, T., & Armstrong, I. (2009). A randomized controlled trial of the effectiveness of a modified recovery workbook program: Preliminary findings. *Psychiatric Services, 60,* 491–497.

Bedregal, L. E., O'Connell, M., & Davidson, L. (2006). The Recovery Knowledge Inventory: Assessment of mental health staff knowledge and attitudes about recovery. *Psychiatric Rehabilitation Journal, 30,* 96–103.

Bejerholm, U., Hansson, L., & Eklund, M. (2006). Profiles of occupational engagement in people with schizophrenia (POES): The development of a new instrument based on time-use diaries. *British Journal of Occupational Therapy, 69,* 58–69.

Campbell-Orde, T., Chamberlin, J., Carpenter, J., & Leff, H. S. (2005). *Measuring the promise: A compendium of recovery measures* (Vol. 2). Retrieved from http://www.power2u.org/downloads/pn-55.pdf

Chen, S., Krupa, T., Lysaght, R., McCay, E., & Piat, M. (2013). The development of recovery competencies for in-patient mental health providers working with people with serious mental illness. *Administration and Policy in Mental Health, 40,* 96–116.

Chen, S. P., Krupa, T., Lysaght, R., McCay, E., & Piat, M. (2014). Development of a recovery education program for inpatient mental health providers. *Psychiatric Rehabilitation Journal, 37,* 329–332.

Cook, J. A., Copeland, M. E., Jonikas, J. A., Hamilton, M. M., Razzano, L. A., Grey, D. D., . . . Boyd, S. (2012). Results of a randomized controlled trial of mental illness self-management using wellness recovery action planning. *Schizophrenia Bulletin, 38,* 881–891.

Copeland, M. E. (1997). *Wellness recovery action plan.* Brattleboro, VT: Peach Press.

Corrigan, P. W., Salzer, M., Ralph, R. O., Sangster, Y., & Keck, L. (2004). Examining the factor structure of the recovery assessment scale. *Schizophrenia Bulletin, 30,* 1035–1041.

Coulter, A. (2017). Measuring what matters to patients. *BMJ, 356,* j816.

Davidson, L. (2005). Recovery in serious mental illness: Paradigm shift or shibboleth. In L. Davidson, C. Harding, & L. Spaniol (Eds.), *Recovery from severe mental illnesses: Research evidence and implications for practice* (pp. 5–26). Boston, MA: Centre for Psychiatric Rehabilitation, Boston University.

Davidson, L., O'Connell, M., Tondora, J., Styron, T., & Kangas, K. (2006). The top ten concerns about recovery encountered in mental health system transformation. *Psychiatric Services, 57,* 640–645.

Davidson, L., Rakfeldt, J., & Strauss, J. (2010). *The roots of the recovery movement in psychiatry: Lessons learned.* West Sussex, United Kingdom: Wiley-Blackwell.

Davidson, L., & Roe, D. (2007). Recovery from versus recovery in serious mental illness: One strategy for lessening confusion plaguing recovery. *Journal of Mental Health, 16,* 459–470.

Davidson, L., Tondora, J., O'Connell, M., Kirk, T., Jr., Rockholz, P., & Evans, A. (2007). Creating a recovery-oriented system of behavioral health care: Moving from concept to reality. *Psychiatric Rehabilitation Journal, 31,* 23–31.

Deegan, P. (1988). Recovery: The lived experience of rehabilitation. *Psychosocial Rehabilitation Journal, 11*(4), 11–19.

Deegan, P. (1990). Spirit breaking: When the helping professions hurt. *The Humanistic Psychologist, 18,* 301–313.

Deegan, P. (1996). Recovery as a journey of the heart. *Psychiatric Rehabilitation Journal, 19,* 91–97.

Deegan, P. (2001). Recovery as a self-directed process of healing and transformation. *Occupational Therapy in Mental Health, 17,* 5–21.

del Vecchio, P. (2012). *SAMHSA working definition of recovery updated.* Rockville, MD: Substance Abuse and Mental Health Services Administration. Retrieved from https://blog.samhsa.gov/2012/03/23/defintion-of-recovery-updated/#.Wa3l07pFwrE

Edgelow, M., & Krupa, T. (2011). Randomized controlled pilot study of an occupational time-use intervention for people with serious mental illness. *American Journal of Occupational Therapy, 65,* 267–276.

Eklund, M., Leufstadius, C., & Bejerholm, U. (2009). Time use among people with psychiatric disabilities: Implications for practice. *Psychiatric Rehabilitation Journal, 32,* 177–191.

Ennals, P., & Fossey, E. (2009). Using the OPHI-II to support people with mental illness in their recovery. *Occupational Therapy in Mental Health, 25,* 138–150.

Gewurtz, R., Moll, S., Letts, L., Larivière, N., Levasseur, M., & Krupa, T. (2016). What you do every day matters: A new direction for health promotion. *Canadian Journal of Public Health, 107,* e205–e208.

Gibson, R. W., D'Amico, M., Jaffe, L., & Arbesman, M. (2011). Occupational therapy interventions for recovery in the areas of community integration and normative life roles for adults with serious mental illness: A systematic review. *American Journal of Occupational Therapy, 65,* 247–256.

Gingerich, S., & Mueser, K. T. (2005). Illness management and recovery. In R. E. Drake, M. R. Merrens, & D. W. Lynde (Eds.), *Evidence-based mental health practice: A textbook* (pp. 395–424). New York, NY: Norton.

Jerrell, J. M., Cousins, V. C., & Roberts, K. M. (2006). Psychometrics of the Recovery Process Inventory. *The Journal of Behavioral Health Services and Research, 33,* 464–473.

Keetharuth, A., Brazier, J., Connell, J., Carlton, J., Taylor Buck, E., Ricketts, T., & Barkham, M. (2017). *Development and validation of the Recovering Quality of Life (ReQoL) Outcome Measures.* Retrieved from http://www.eepru.org.uk/article/development-and-validation-of-the-recovering-quality-of-life-reqol-outcome-measure/

Kirsh, B., & Cockburn, L. (2009). The Canadian Occupational Performance Measure: A tool for recovery-based practice. *Psychiatric Rehabilitation Journal, 32,* 171–176.

Krupa, T., Edgelow, D., Radloff-Gabriel, D., Perry, A., Mieras, C., Bransfield, M., . . . Almas, A. (2010). *Action over inertia: Addressing the activity-health needs of individuals with serious mental illness.* Ottawa, Canada: Canadian Association of Occupational Therapists.

Krupa, T., Fossey, E., Anthony, W. A., Brown, C., & Pitts, D. (2009). Doing daily life: How occupational therapy can inform psychiatric rehabilitation practice. *Psychiatric Rehabilitation Journal, 32,* 155–161.

Law, M., Baptiste, S., McColl, M. A., Opzoomer, A., Polatajko, H., & Pollock, N. (1990). The Canadian Occupational Performance Measure: An outcome measure for occupational therapy. *Canadian Journal of Occupational Therapy, 57,* 82–87.

Levitt, A. J., Mueser, K. T., DeGenova, J., Lorenzo, J., Bradford-Watt, D., Barbosa, A., . . . Chernick, M. (2009). Randomized controlled trial of illness management and recovery in multiple-unit supportive housing. *Psychiatric Services, 60,* 1629–1636.

Lyons, J. S., Uziel-Miller, N. S., Reyes, F., & Sokol, P. T. (2000). Strengths of children and adolescents in residential settings: prevalence and associations with psychopathology and discharge placement. *Journal of the American Academy of Child and Adolescent Psychiatry, 39,* 176–81.

Mattsson, M., Topor, A., Cullberg, J., & Forsell, Y. (2008). Association between financial strain, social network and five-year recovery from first episode psychosis. *Social Psychiatry and Psychiatric Epidemiology, 43,* 947–952.

Mental Health Commission of Canada. (2015). *Recovery guidelines.* Ontario, Canada. Retrieved from https://mentalhealthcommission.ca/sites/default/files/MHCC_RecoveryGuidelines_ENG_0.pdf

Mental Health Commission of New Zealand. (2001). *Recovery competencies for New Zealand mental health workers.* Retrieved from http://www.maryohagan.com/resources/Text_Files/Recovery%20Cometencies%20O%27Hagan.pdf

Noordsy, D., Torrey, W., Mueser, K., Mead, S., O'Keefe, C., & Fox, L. (2002). Recovery from severe mental illness: An intrapersonal and functional outcome definition. *International Review of Psychiatry, 14,* 318–326.

O'Connell, M. J., Tondora, J., Croog, G., Evans, A. C., & Davidson, L. (2005). From rhetoric to routine: Assessing perceptions of recovery-oriented practices in a state mental health and addiction system. *Psychiatric Rehabilitation Journal, 28*, 378–386.

Parker, S., Dark, F., Newman, E., Korman, N., Rasmussen, Z., & Meurk, C. (2017). Reality of working in a community-based, recovery-oriented mental health rehabilitation unit: A pragmatic grounded theory analysis. *International Journal of Mental Health Nursing, 26*, 355–365. doi:10.1111/inm.12251

Pelletier, J. F., Corbière, M., Lecomte, T., Briand, C., Corrigan, P., Davidson, L., & Rowe, M. (2015). Citizenship and recovery: Two intertwined concepts for civic-recovery. *BMC Psychiatry, 15*, 37.

Ralph, R. (2005). Verbal definitions and visual models of recovery: Focus on the recovery model. In R. O. Ralph & P. W. Corrigan (Eds.), *Recovery in mental illness: Broadening our understanding of wellness* (pp. 131–145). Washington, DC: American Psychological Association.

Rapp, C., & Goscha, R. (2012). *The strengths model: A recovery-oriented approach to mental health services* (3rd ed.). New York, NY: Oxford University Press.

Rebeiro Gruhl, K. (2008). Strengths and challenges to practice: Reconciling occupational justice issues as a prerequisite to mental health recovery. In E. A. McKay, C. Craik, K. H. Lim, & G. Richards (Eds.), *Advancing occupational therapy in mental health practice* (pp. 103–117). Malden, MA: Blackwell.

Rogers, E. S., Chamberlin, J., Ellison, M. L., & Crean, T. (1997). A consumer-constructed scale to measure empowerment among users of mental health services. *Psychiatric Services, 48*, 1042–1047.

Rust, T., Diessner, R., & Reade, L. (2009). Strengths only or strengths and relative weaknesses? A preliminary study. *The Journal of Psychology, 143*, 465–476.

Salyers, M. P., Godfrey, J. L., Mueser, K. T., & Labriola, S. (2007). Measuring illness management outcomes: A psychometric study of clinician and consumer rating scales for illness self-management and recovery. *Community Mental Health Journal, 43*, 459–480.

Slade, M. (2009). *Personal recovery and mental illness: A guide for mental health professionals.* Cambridge, United Kingdom: Cambridge University Press.

Spaniol, L., Koehler, M., & Hutchinson, D. (1994). *Recovery workbook: Practical coping and empowerment strategies for people with psychiatric disability.* Boston, MA: Centre for Psychiatric Rehabilitation, Boston University.

Substance Abuse and Mental Health Services Administration. (2006). *National consensus statement on mental health recovery.* Rockville, MD: U.S. Department of Health and Human Services. Retrieved from http://store.samhsa.gov/shin/content//SMA05-4129/SMA05-4129.pdf

Tondora, J., & Davidson, L. (2006). *Practice guidelines for recovery-oriented behavioural health care.* Hartford, CT: Connecticut Department of Mental Health and Addiction Services.

Xie, H. (2013). Strengths-based approach for mental health recovery. *Iran Journal of Psychiatry and Behavioral Sciences, 7*(2), 5–10.

the**Point**® *For additional resources on the subjects discussed in this chapter, visit* http://thePoint.lww.com /Willard-Spackman13e. *See* **Appendix I, Resources and Evidence for Common Conditions Addressed in OT** *for more information on various mental health disorders such as anxiety disorders, eating disorders, mood disorders, posttraumatic stress disorder, personality disorders, schizophrenia, and substance use disorders.*

CHAPTER 47

Health Promotion Theories

S. Maggie Reitz, Kay Graham

LEARNING OBJECTIVES

After reading this chapter, you will be able to:

1. Outline occupational therapy's role in promoting health, well-being, and quality of life.
2. Apply an understanding of health determinants and health disparities to occupational therapy practice.
3. Differentiate theories of health behavior and health promotion that can be used to inform occupational therapy practice.
4. Examine considerations in combining occupational therapy theories with health behavior theories.
5. Apply theory to the development of occupation-based occupational therapy health promotion interventions in interdisciplinary health promotion practice.
6. Examine the evidence available related to occupational therapy health promotion and health behavior health promotion interventions.
7. Demonstrate how health promotion can and should be used throughout occupational therapy practice to maximize health, well-being, and quality of life in individuals, groups, and populations.

Introduction

Health promotion activities have long been engaged in by a small portion of occupational therapy (OT) practitioners (American Occupational Therapy Association [AOTA], 2010a; Reitz, 1992) and seen as an appropriate role for the profession (Brunyate, 1967; Finn, 1972; Jaffe, 1986; Johnson, 1986; Kaplan & Burch-Minakan, 1986; West, 1967, 1969; Wiemer, 1972). Health and wellness was identified as one of the major practice areas in the AOTA's Centennial Vision (Baum, 2006). In addition, health promotion is an important part of the remaining five identified practice areas, which include children and youth; productive aging; mental health; rehabilitation, disability, and participation; and work and industry (Baum, 2006). Health and wellness as well as quality of life (QOL) were identified as possible outcomes of OT intervention in the AOTA (2008) "Occupational Therapy Practice Framework," hereafter referred to as the *Framework*. More recently, well-being was added as a potential outcome of OT services in the most recent edition of the Framework (AOTA, 2014). The term *well-being* also has a prominent place in the new Vision 2025—"occupational therapy maximizes health, well-being, and QOL for all people, populations, and communities through effective solutions that facilitate participation in everyday living" (AOTA, 2017b, p. 1).

Within this chapter, OT's potential to enhance the health of clients through the use of health promotion interventions will be detailed in the hope of encouraging greater involvement in this important area of practice. Clients can be individuals, families, communities, or populations (AOTA, 2008, 2014). This information will be provided through a lens of theory-driven practice, based on the assumption that ethical OT practice is theory-based, occupation-based, and evidence-driven (AOTA, 2008, 2010b, 2010c, 2014). The objective is to demonstrate how theory can be used to support and strengthen OT's role in health promotion thereby maximizing the health and well-being of the society we serve.

Definitions of Health, Health Promotion, Well-Being, and Quality of Life

Definitions of health promotion and the focus of health promotion interventions vary across the many disciplines that engage in this type of practice; however, the definition of health is generally agreed on. The following definition of health from the World Health Organization (WHO) is probably the most frequently cited. **Health** is "the complete state of physical, mental and social well-being and not just the absence of disease or infirmity" (WHO, 1947, p. 29). **Health promotion** is the use of discipline-specific techniques to assist people in achieving their health-related goals. *Occupational therapy–directed health promotion* is the client-centered use of occupations, adaptations to context, or alteration of context to maximize individuals', families', communities', and groups' pursuit of health and QOL. Health promotion is a process that can vary in length, intensity, and audience. For example, it can include providing a specific short-term standardized intervention such as a fall prevention program or a more complex, community-wide initiative such as developing a community garden in an urban food desert. A food desert is a geographic area where inhabitants "lack access to affordable fruits, vegetables, whole grains, low-fat milk, and other foods that make up the full range of a healthy diet" (Centers for Disease Control and Prevention [CDC], 2017, para. 2).

Health promotion is a process of maximizing health through structured interventions, whereas **wellness** is the outcome of health promotion and ultimately is the responsibility of the individual, family, community, or society (Reitz & Scaffa, 2010). The Framework, using Hettler's (1984) definition, delineates wellness as an active process where clients "become aware of and make choices toward a more successful existence" (AOTA, 2014, p. S34), whereas well-being is defined as being content with one's life including physical, mental, and social aspects (AOTA, 2014).

In recent years, especially within the field of gerontology, there has been an increased focus on well-being and QOL. Quality of life is the self-appraisal of the client's life satisfaction, hope, sense of self, health, function, and socioeconomic status (SES) (AOTA, 2014). Health-related quality of life (HRQOL) is a more specific type of QOL that considers "an individual's or group's perceived physical and mental health over time" (CDC, 2016, para. 1). Although OT practitioners conceptually link participation in occupations to health and QOL, little direct evidence exists; therefore, the profession should strive to "evaluate and document health and QOL from the client's perspective" (Pizzi & Richard, 2017, p. 2).

Determinants of Health

In a U.S. national government report entitled Healthy People 2020, determinants of health are described within five broad categories: biology and genetics, individual behavior, social environment, physical environment, and health services (U.S. Department of Health and Human Services [USDHHS], 2017a). These five determinants are shown in Figure 47-1 together with the mission of Healthy People 2020 and the overarching goals for the next decade for improving health of the nation. Healthy People 2020 is a framework available for usage by federal, state, and local governments, nonprofits, and businesses to address and assess outcomes of programs and policies that aim to improve the health and QOL of populations living in the United States (USDHHS, 2017a). If a community or population has not already identified a health need, then a review of the objectives identified in this report may be of assistance to start the conversation.

The process to develop Healthy People 2030 is underway (USDHHS, 2017b). The guiding principles for this work include those in the following list, items appears verbatim, including bold text.

- Health and well-being of the population and communities are essential to a **fully functioning, equitable society**.
- Achieving the full potential for health and well-being for all provides **valuable benefits to society**, including lower health care costs and more prosperous and engaged individuals and communities.

Healthy People 2020
A society in which all people live long, healthy lives

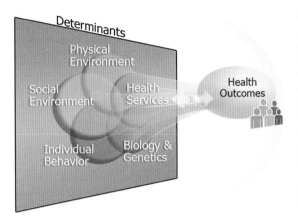

Overarching Goals:

• Attain high quality, longer lives free of preventable disease, disability, injury, and premature death.

• Achieve health equity, eliminate disparities, and improve the health of all groups.

• Create social and physical environments that promote good health for all.

• Promote quality of life, healthy development and healthy behaviors across all life stages.

FIGURE 47-1 Graphic model of Healthy People 2020. (From U.S. Department of Health and Human Services. [2017a]. *Healthy people 2020: Framework* [p. 3]. Retrieved from http://healthypeople .gov/2020/consortium /HP2020Framework.pdf)

- Achieving health and well-being requires **eliminating health disparities, achieving health equity**, and **attaining health literacy**.
- **Healthy physical, social and economic environments** strengthen the potential to achieve health and well-being.
- Promoting and achieving the nation's health and well-being is a **shared responsibility** that is distributed among all stakeholders at the national, state, and local levels, including the public, profit, and not-for-profit sectors.
- Working to attain the full potential for health and well-being of the population is a component of **decision-making and policy formulation** across all sectors.
- Investing to maximize health and well-being for the nation is a critical and efficient use of resources.

It is interesting to note that these guiding principles are consistent with AOTA's Occupational Therapy Code of Ethics (AOTA, 2015b).

World Health Organization, through a document entitled *Ottawa Charter for Health Promotion* published in 1986, identified eight prerequisites for health. These prerequisites include the following (WHO, 1986, p. 1):

1. Education
2. Food
3. Income
4. Peace
5. Shelter
6. Social justice and equity
7. Stable ecosystem
8. Sustainable resources

A comparison of the determinants of health identified by the USDHHS to the prerequisites for health developed by WHO shows the WHO places less emphasis on the individual and health services and a greater emphasis on access to basic human needs that are required to live a healthy life. Successful health promotion programs should address both those prerequisites and determinants of health that are applicable to the population, based on the population's self-determination, which will be influenced by geopolitics, geographical location, and other contextual features. Occupational therapy practitioners also should consider the impact of health determinants on their clients when conducting occupational profiles with their clients. For example, the occupational therapist can ask the individual, family, or group, "What keeps you from participating in your favorite activities?"

Access to occupations, or occupational enrichment (Molineux & Whiteford, 2011), is an important contributor to health mediated through health determinants and prerequisites for health. Lack of access to occupation can result in occupational deprivation, which in turn can have a significant negative impact on the health of individuals, families, and communities. **Occupational deprivation**, which is the lack of access to engagement in an array of self-selected occupations that have meaning to the individual, family, or community, can result in ill health (Wilcock, 2006) and cascading occupational injustice. The divergent paths for those who experience occupational enrichment, and thus the prerequisites for health, from those who experience occupational deprivation are displayed in Figure 47-2. Examples of the potential relationships between occupational deprivation and health determinants are depicted in Table 47-1.

From a health promotion perspective, occupational deprivation is one of the unfortunate results of health disparities. Hallmarks of health disparity are inequality, discrimination, or limitations placed on a group of people which then create negative effects on health of persons in that group (Box 47-1).

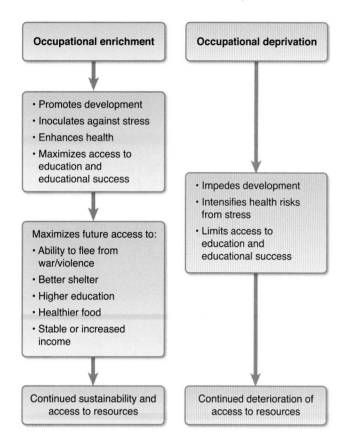

FIGURE 47-2 Divergent health paths based on access to occupation. (Adapted from U.S. Department of Health and Human Services. [2017a]. *Healthy people 2020: Framework* [p. 3]. Retrieved from http://healthypeople.gov/2020 /consortium/HP2020Framework.pdf)

| | TABLE 47-1 | Occupational Deprivation and Health Impacts |

Occupational Deprivation	Relationship to Health Determinants
Children with congenital sensory and motor challenges who do not have opportunities to play with peers on adaptive playgrounds	• Biology and genetics • Social environment • Physical environment
Rural teenagers with limited opportunities to access various positive group occupations with peers turn to unhealthy habits to cope with boredom and isolation	• Individual behavior • Social environment • Physical environment
Working parents' limited access to health care and/or educational services due to lack of proof of citizenship	• Health services • Social environment
Older adults who cannot negotiate exit from house become imprisoned in own home	• Social environment • Physical environment

Persistent health disparities exist, for example, in terms of life expectancy (i.e., years of life one is expected to live) due to geographic location, race, SES, or educational level. For example, in a 10-mile area in Atlanta, Georgia, there is a 10- to 12-year discrepancy in life expectancy (Virginia Commonwealth University Center on Society and Health, 2017). This geographic disparity also follows racial and SES divisions as well. Such factors must be considered in program or intervention planning. Because many of the areas in Atlanta with lower life expectancy also are areas lacking healthy options for food (i.e., food deserts), plans for the group or client to address the high rates of obesity or heart disease in these areas must consider the barriers within the environmental context in addition to specific client factors. The AOTA's Societal Statement on Health Disparities stresses that OT practitioners should intervene when clients (both individuals and communities) face limitations to participation due to inequalities by advocating for access to services (AOTA, 2013a).

Each of the examples in Table 47-1 can be the beginning of a negatively reinforcing relationship leading to additional threats to health as occupational deprivation increases. For example, the rural teenager with limited access to age-appropriate group occupations can move from using tobacco and abusing alcohol alone near home to driving long distances after drinking or exploration of controlled substances. Either of these in turn could lead to a driving under the influence (DUI) conviction, a manslaughter charge, or the use of illegal drugs, any of which could result in a period of incarceration, which then can result in decreased access to various self-chosen occupations and an acceleration of health problems. An adaption of a well-known Ben Franklin quote summarizes the

| BOX 47-1 | HEALTH DISPARITIES DEFINED |

Health disparity is a particular type of health difference that is closely linked with social, economic, and/or environmental disadvantage. Health disparities adversely affect groups of people who have systematically experienced greater obstacles to health based on their racial or ethnic group; religion; socioeconomic status; gender; age; mental health; cognitive, sensory, or physical disability; sexual orientation or gender identity; geographic location; or other characteristics historically linked to discrimination or exclusion. (USDHHS, Office of Disease Prevention and Health Promotion, 2008, p. 28).

potential benefit of occupation-based interventions on health determinants:

> **An ounce of occupation can prevent the need for pounds and dollars of cure.**

Health Promotion and Occupational Therapy

The development of noteworthy documents has helped to support and communicate the profession's contribution to health promotion. A sample of these documents is listed in Box 47-2. The AOTA, through the statement "Occupational Therapy in the Promotion of Health and Well-Being" (AOTA, 2013b), describes the role of OT in health promotion for not only individuals but also for families, communities, and populations. The philosophical link and match of occupational values to national and international policies on health promotion are reviewed to provide the context for a series of examples of potential assessments, interventions, and strategies. Examples and case studies are provided for each of the three levels of prevention (i.e., primary, secondary, and tertiary) and with various clients (i.e., individuals, groups, and populations). These are excellent sources of ideas for potential interventions at the person and policy levels.

The AOTA, World Federation of Occupational Therapists (WFOT), and other national OT associations, through publication of documents, also advocate for access to prerequisites for health, including access to meaningful occupations in the community. For example, the document entitled "AOTA's Societal Statement on Livable Communities" (AOTA, 2016b) informs the public, students, and new practitioners about the profession's support for access to services, establishment of policies, and implementation of design features that will allow both older adults to age in place and individuals with disabilities to fully engage in the community and reach their full occupational potential. The WFOT (2004), through the *Position Paper on Community Based Rehabilitation*, also advocates for equal access to the right of occupational engagement of individuals with disabilities and their families. Lack of such access or occupational deprivation leads to cascading health problems and further injustices as was depicted earlier in Figure 47-2.

Health Literacy

Health literacy is an essential aspect of ensuring clients' abilities to participate in their own health management. Health literacy has been defined as the "the degree to which individuals have the capacity to obtain, process, and understand basic health information and services needed to make appropriate health decisions" (USDHHS, *Office of Disease and Prevention* 2010, p. iii). Thus, health literacy includes reading literacy but also considers numeracy abilities such as calculating sliding scale dosage for diabetes or interpreting risk of disease as well as ability to advocate for self by discussing health with health care providers. The AOTA's Societal Statement on Health Literacy states that

CENTENNIAL NOTES

Why Should Occupational Therapy Practitioners Be Involved in Health Promotion?

The question of why the profession should be involved in health promotion can be answered by reflecting on the early history of the profession as well as more recent events. Founders and early leaders in the profession studied and used the health-promoting properties as well as the healing properties of occupation (Reitz, 2010). Supporters also articulated the value of occupation to health. For example, as early as the 1930s, Dr. Losada, a physician, noted that OT had the potential not only to do more than quicken the rate of recovery from injury or disease but to also "be an agent for positive health" (Losada, 1936, p. 285).

Historically, OT practitioners have engaged in health promotion activities primarily through instructing clients in basic preventive strategies such as energy conservation or the use of ergonomic principles. Fewer engage in community- or population-based health promotion activities. Data from AOTA membership surveys indicate that from 1970 to 2010, few OT practitioners taking part in the surveys practiced primarily with the well population, in health promotion, or at the population level (AOTA, 1982, 1987, 1991, 2001, 2006, 2010a, 2015a; Jantzen, 1979).

There are many barriers that have limited OT practitioners' engagement in community- or population-based health promotion practice. Besides difficulty in seeking and receiving reimbursement, minimal education and exposure to health promotion, a shortage of mentors and evidence, and confusion about role delineation also can be contributing factors.

BOX 47-2   SAMPLING OF OCCUPATIONAL THERAPY DOCUMENTS RELATED TO HEALTH PROMOTION

- "The AOTA's Societal Statement on Disaster Response and Risk Reduction" (AOTA, 2017a)
- "AOTA's Societal Statement on Health Disparities" (AOTA, 2013a)
- "AOTA's Societal Statement on Health Literacy" (AOTA, 2016a)
- "AOTA's Societal Statement on Livable Communities" (AOTA, 2016b)
- "Occupational therapy in the promotion of health and well-being" (AOTA, 2013b)

- "Health Promotion in Occupational Therapy" (British Association of Occupational Therapists and College of Occupational Therapists, 2008)
- "World Federation of Occupational Therapists' (WFOT) Position Paper on Community Based Rehabilitation" (WFOT, 2004)
- "World Federation of Occupational Therapists' Position Paper on Disaster Risk Reduction" (WFOT, 2016)

OT practitioners have a responsibility to promote health by developing programs and associated materials that are "understandable, accessible, and usable by the full spectrum of consumers" and tailored to person factors and context (AOTA, 2017c, p. 1-2). Attention to health literacy can help facilitate self-management skills associated with enhanced participation in the instrumental activity of daily living of health management and maintenance.

Addressing and promoting health literacy is critical due to the poor health outcomes such as higher mortality, longer hospital stays, and increased visits to emergency room associated with lower health literacy (Heijmans, Waverijn, Rademakers, van der Vaart, & Rijken, 2015). Only 12% of Americans surveyed in 2003 had proficient health literacy (e.g., were able to use a table to calculate employee share of health insurance costs) and 35% had basic or below basic health literacy levels (e.g., read instructions and determine what they can and cannot drink prior to a medical test). Race/ethnicity, older age, lower SES, and low education levels were associated with lower health literacy levels (USDHHS, Office of Disease Prevention and Health Promotion, 2008).

Promoting health literacy is a common goal shared across public health and health care professionals. In fact, the Agency for Healthcare Research and Quality (AHRQ) has developed the Health Literacy Universal Precautions online resource to encourage all professionals working in health care to assume that all patients might have difficulty understanding and accessing health information and services. There are multiple resources available to assess health literacy levels of clients. These include screenings such as the Vital Signs and the Rapid Estimate of Adult Literacy in Medicine (REALM), organizational assessments, intervention recommendations, and training resources available at their website (AHRQ, 2017). Practitioners can ensure adequate client understanding by using techniques such as teach back, show me, verbal rehearsal, and providing clear, concise materials at

appropriate reading levels. Refer to Chapter 32 for examples of effective educational methods for use with clients.

Program Planning and Implementation: Needs Assessment, Intervention, and Evaluation

The process of developing appropriate interventions and programs to address aspects of prevention and to promote health should follow several basic steps. Occupational therapy practitioners must (1) understand the role of OT in health promotion and prevention and the potential to assist in making meaningful change, (2) identify the clients' needs and wants, (3) select an appropriate theory to guide reasoning and joint decision making, (4) develop an intervention based on available evidence, (5) ethically implement the intervention, and (6) evaluate the program for effectiveness during and after the program is completed.

This process mirrors the evaluation and intervention process outlined in the AOTA Practice Framework. The individual or community needs assessment is equivalent to the occupational profile. For health promotion, the target individuals, group, or population should share enough in common so that program will address their common needs. Part of this initial needs assessment should include client or key informant priorities, a review of statistics and health disparities to assist with prioritization of key areas, identification of deficits in occupational performance or participation, and assets. An appropriate theory should guide interventions to address identified problems and assets. Occupational therapy models and theories and health promotion theories

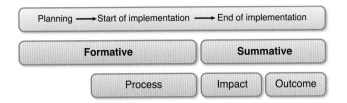

FIGURE 47-3 Processes of evaluation.

can be used together to enhance the preventative aspects of health and well-being programming and care.

It is helpful to note the meaning of common terms in the public health arena that are related to assessment of effectiveness. In OT, the term *evaluation* is typically used to denote the initial analysis of occupational performance (based on a variety of assessments), and the term *reevaluation* is typically used for subsequent checks during the course of care, culmination in the evaluation of outcomes achieved (AOTA, 2014). In public health and other health disciplines, the first process is referred to as a *needs assessment*. Then, the term *evaluation* is used for methods to assess program or intervention effectiveness at several different time points, including in the midst of a program (i.e., formative/process evaluation), immediately following the program (i.e., impact evaluation), and finally toward evaluation of whether the program met broader goals geared to QOL and well-being over time (i.e., outcome evaluation). See Figure 47-3 for clarification of these terms and their timing in the process.

PRECEDE-PROCEED: A Framework for Planning Health Promotion Programs

The acronym PRECEDE-PROCEED is a shorthand way of referring to a model designed to support program planning. PRECEDE refers to Predisposing, Reinforcing, and Enabling Constructs in Educational/Environmental Diagnosis and Evaluation. PROCEED refers to Policy, Regulatory, and Organizational Constructs in Educational and Environmental Development. The PRECEDE-PROCEED model is not a theory but rather a planning framework comprising eight phases. These phases are helpful to guide ethical health promotion interventions at the community or population level (Green & Kreuter, 2005; National Cancer Institute [NCI], 2005). The originators clearly share OT's value of client-centered care by communicating the importance of the community or population as decision makers. Community engagement starts immediately in the PRECEDE portion of the

framework in which the community guides the health promotion experts in the selection of the priority health concern that is to be addressed. In the next group of steps called the PROCEED section, models such as the ones describe earlier are used to guide the specific details of the chosen intervention. The PROCEED portion of the framework also details the evaluation process of the intervention. The phases of the PRECEDE-PROCEED framework (Green & Kreuter, 2005; NCI, 2005) and potential actions for each phase are described in Table 47-2. This is an introductory table; additional reading on the framework would be required before using it to plan or evaluate a health promotion program.

The PRECEDE-PROCEED framework has the potential to work well with the AOTA Practice Framework (AOTA, 2014) as well as a number of OT theories in order to develop occupation-based health promotion programs. To illustrate, refer to Case Study 47-1 which describes the development of a dating etiquette program designed to decrease dating and partner violence among adolescents and young adults.

Health Promotion Theories

Health promotion interventions beyond those typically offered to individual clients or families are most often conducted by interdisciplinary teams or in close consultation with other disciplines. Thus, an understanding of theories commonly used in health promotion is important in enhancing communication and understanding. Three health behavior theories will be briefly introduced—the Health Belief Model (HBM), the Stages of Change Model, and Social Cognitive Theory (SCT). These theories and framework were selected from many possibilities due to either past experience combining them with OT theories or easily seen commonalities for future blending. An additional potential model is the Social Ecological Model, which is described elsewhere (Reitz, Scaffa, Campbell, & Rhynders, 2010). Prior to using any of these theories or framework, additional knowledge should be sought through reading, mentoring, continuing education, or working toward a specialized doctoral degree.

Health Belief Model

The HBM is one of the first and most widely used models to explore and facilitate health behavior change. It was originated by public health social psychologists in the 1950s (NCI, 2005). Occupational therapy practitioners frequently recommend that their clients change occupational behaviors. This model explores the way people examine and balance competing factors when deciding to adopt or

TABLE 47-2 PRECEDE-PROCEED Planning Framework

Phase	Description	Potential Change Strategies
PRECEDE		
1. Social assessment and situational analysis	Engaging the community in identifying current social problems and their vision of an improved quality of life	• Review available data on the status of the prerequisites of health in the community • Share data at meetings with community stakeholders; focus groups with community members to elicit their decision as to priorities for interventions and assets and community capacities that can be tapped • Formalize relations with a community-identified group or institute a community board
2. Epidemiological assessment	Reviewing health and health-related data that is linked to the social health concerns identified in Phase 1	• Review summary of data and data sources with community board • Identify need for additional data or sources for data
3. Educational and ecological assessment	Identifying the predisposing factors, enabling factors, and reinforcing factors linked to the identified social problem	• Review summary of data and data sources with community board and government leaders if none are on the board • Identify need for additional data or sources for data
4. Administrative and policy assessment and intervention alignment	Identifying potential policy and resource barriers to initiate and maintain program; developing and securing needed policy changes and additional resources	• Review findings with community board and local government leaders
PROCEED		
5. Implementation	Launching and conducting the program	• Facilitate a culturally relevant kickoff for the program with the community board
6. Process evaluation	Evaluating success of continued community involvement and utilization of community resources	• Review program implementation as it is occurring and solicit feedback from community board, stakeholders, and participants
7. Impact evaluation	Evaluating short-term progress toward goals of program such as access to resources and gaining of skills and knowledge	• Collect data from participants through previously planned strategy (e.g., post portion of a pretest posttest plan, focus group)
8. Outcome evaluation	Evaluating long-term achievement of goals of program related to quality of life and health indicators	• Continue to collect data from participants through previously planned strategy (e.g., post portion of a pretest posttest plan, focus group) • Review and share with community board the current social and epidemiological data to determine if there were changes in desired quality of life and health indicators

Adapted from National Cancer Institute. (2005). *Theory at a glance* (2nd ed., p. 42, Table 10). Bethesda, MD: National Institutes of Health. Retrieved from http://www.cancer.gov/theory.pdf

not to adopt health recommendations. The constructs of the model are described together with strategies to promote behavior change related to each specific construct in Table 47-3. Various health promotion programs can be designed using these constructs.

The basis of this model is the balancing of threats (i.e., perceived susceptibility and perceived severity) with barriers (e.g., time, financial cost) of taking the recommended action (e.g., time, financial cost) and the potential benefits. When the individual, family, or community believes the threat outweighs the cost of action, then change will occur (NCI, 2005). Other components of the model include **self-efficacy** and cues to action. A cue to action can be an artifact such as the "save the ta-tas" bumper stickers that can serve as a reminder to perform breast self-examinations. The bumper sticker cue to action will be

more likely to result in a woman performing a breast self-exam if the woman feels confident in her ability to perform the exam (e.g., self-efficacy).

The impact and relationship of these constructs can be shown through a description of the potential roles of a health educator and an OT practitioner on an interdisciplinary smoking cessation program development team. Health educators have the background knowledge and expertise to ensure the perceived severity (e.g., ill health, death, decreased life course) and susceptibility are appropriately represented in the program without causing undue fear. Although both health educators and occupational therapists can be familiar with barriers to behavior change, occupational therapists can add a perspective in terms of establishing new habits to support health decisions while unhealthy habits are extinguished through an

CASE STUDY 47-1   USING PRECEDE-PROCEED TO REDUCE DATING AND PARTNER VIOLENCE ON CAMPUS

The need for programs to reduce dating/partner violence is important, especially for high school– and college-age students. Most intimate partner violence (IPV) happens in adolescence and young adulthood. Approximately one-quarter of women and 14% of men have experienced severe IPV (Smith et al., 2017). Based on this knowledge, an OT student and a health education student approached the student government association (SGA) with a request for funds to develop a program to increase awareness of IPV. They shared that fellow students were concerned about campus safety and had approached their respective student organizations to take the lead in developing a solution (Phase 1). The two were identified by the groups to represent them and their plan to take action. The pair also shared with the SGA data that showed the incidence of IPV both on their campus and other campuses as well as reports from the literature of health impacts of such violence that had been gathered and vetted by the leadership of both student groups (Phases 2 and 3). Meeting with the SGA, requesting funds, and meetings with the vice president of student affairs, which preceded the request for funds, were parts of Phase 4. An evaluation plan

for the program was shared with the SGA, which included process, impact, and outcome evaluation (Phases 6, 7, 8).

The program was developed to meet the needs of the specific student group using recommendations from the CDC Division of Violence Prevention (Niolon et al., 2017). During implementation, process measures assessed if the program was being administered according to protocol. Impact assessments immediately following the educational program included a pre/post-knowledge/awareness survey results from attendees as well as the number of total attendees reached by the program. Outcome evaluation at 1 year had an increase in IPV reported to campus security. This was expected because the program goal was to increase awareness of IPV; an increase in reported IPV did not necessarily mean that IPV incidence had increased but could have been due to increased reporting. The second year outcome report showed that reported IPV levels had decreased from the first year post-program levels. The program was considered as one of the factors that had resulted in this decrease, thus funding to sustain the program was earmarked in the student affairs budget.

occupation lens. For example, an OT practitioner may suggest to highlight additional negative aspects of smoking related to social consequences that health educators may not as readily identify but could increase the level of perceived seriousness (e.g., social ostracization due to tobacco odor, marginalization of smokers due to smoking bans).

In order to strengthen the likelihood of a person taking a positive health action and decreasing the negative consequences of smoking, an occupational therapist may suggest implementing a peer buddy occupation-based strategy. In order to successfully stop smoking, a change in social occupations and friends often is needed to prevent relapse.

TABLE 47-3   Health Belief Model

Concept	Definition	Potential Change Strategies
Perceived susceptibility	Beliefs about the chances of getting a condition	• Define what population(s) are at risk and their levels of risk • Tailor risk information based on an individual's characteristics or behaviors • Help the individual develop an accurate perception of his or her own risk
Perceived severity	Beliefs about the seriousness of a condition and its consequences	• Specify the consequences of a condition and recommended action
Perceived benefits	Beliefs about the effectiveness of taking action to reduce risk or seriousness	• Explain how, where, and when to take action and what the potential positive results will be
Perceived barriers	Beliefs about the material and psychological costs of taking action	• Offer reassurance, incentives, and assistance; correct misinformation
Cues to action	Factors that activate "readiness to change"	• Provide "how to" information, promote awareness, and employ reminder systems
Self-efficacy	Confidence in one's ability to take action	• Provide training and guidance in performing action • Use progressive goal setting • Give verbal reinforcement • Demonstrate desired behaviors

Reprinted from National Cancer Institute. (2005). *Theory at a glance* (2nd ed., p. 14). Bethesda, MD: National Institutes of Health. Retrieved from http://www.cancer.gov/theory.pdf

When first stopping smoking, for example, it is best to avoid social and physical contexts that reinforce smoking such as happy hours at an outside bar that permits smoking (e.g., barrier). The buddy strategy pairs successful ex-smokers (e.g., a cue to action) with individuals desiring to stop smoking. Through the use of an instrument such as the activity checklist, alternate activities and identification of a new peer group of nonsmokers could be identified. Engagement in one of more of these occupations with the buddy can increase the likelihood of success while broadening a person's occupational repertoire and social supports. Thus, instead of losing an identity and pleasurable occupation, they gain a friend, a new identity as an ex-smoker, and one or more new pleasurable occupations.

The HBM has been used to help explain the poor results from the use of a curriculum for parents of children with sickle cell disease (Drazen, Abel, Lindsey, & King, 2014). In this program, parents were not following the recommendations for caring for their children, which was explained as possibly due to lack of perception of serious risk for the children rather than disinterest in the program. In another example of HBM theory in research, a multidisciplinary research team investigated factors associated with older adult decisions to discuss their fall risks with health professionals using HBM to guide development of the survey questions (Lee et al., 2013). Other OT researchers have used it to explore occupation-based health behaviors such as eating habits (Deshpande, Basil, & Basil, 2009), physical activity engagement (Juniper, Oman, Hamm, & Kerby, 2004), and weight management (James, Pobee, Oxidine, Brown, & Joshi, 2012).

Transtheoretical Model of Change/Stages of Change Model

The originators of this model first investigated why some people were better able to quit smoking than others (Prochaska & DiClemente, 1982, 1983). Their work led to the development of a model that can be used to study people's readiness for change—ceasing a poor health habit such as smoking or starting a good health habit such as exercise. Literature regarding the model refers to it as either the *transtheoretical model of change* or the *stages of change model*. According to the proponents of the model, there are potentially five stages that an individual goes through as he or she changes a health-related behavior. These stages include precontemplation, contemplation, decision, action, and maintenance (NCI, 2005). The components of this model are presented in Table 47-4 and discussed in greater detail in other sources (NCI, 2005; Reitz et al., 2010) and in a table later in this chapter.

There are two aspects of the model that are particularly helpful to OT health promotion practice. One is the belief that relapse can be part of the normal cycle of behavior change. Therefore, neither the OT practitioner nor the client should give up hope. The second is the belief that specific strategies can be matched to each of the stages. For example, *consciousness raising* is a process that is well matched for moving someone from the precontemplation to the contemplation stage. Occupational therapy practitioners can be helpful in moving someone closer to smoking cessation through consciousness raising. For example, if a smoker reports concerns about walking to the corner store for milk, the OT practitioner, besides offering energy conservation strategies, also can suggest that they may be less out of breath walking if they stopped or decreased the number of cigars smoked.

Contingency management can help people be successful once they take action and to then maintain their new behavior. Following the earlier smoking cessation example, if a new ex-smoker was invited to a work event where people may be smoking, he or she may want to have a contingency plan such as inviting their antismoke buddy for support and suggestions on how to negotiate the experience. This model has contributed to the design and success of various health behaviors at the individual and group levels. For example, a program for children with

TABLE 47-4	Stages of Change Model	
Stage	**Definition**	**Potential Change Strategies**
Precontemplation	Has no intention of taking action within the next six months	Increase awareness of need for change; personalize information about risks and benefits
Contemplation	Intends to take action within the next six months	Motivate; encourage making specific plans
Preparation	Intends to take action within the next thirty days and has taken some behavioral steps in this direction	Assist with developing and implementing concrete action plans; help set gradual goals
Action	Has changed behavior for less than six months	Assist with feedback, problem solving, social support, and reinforcement
Maintenance	Has changed behavior for more than six months	Assist with coping, reminders, finding alternatives, avoiding slips/relapses (as applicable)

Reprinted from National Cancer Institute. (2005). *Theory at a glance* (2nd ed., p. 15). Bethesda, MD: National Institutes of Health. Retrieved from http://www.cancer.gov/theory.pdf

fibromyalgia used a pain outcome measure based on the stages of change model that measured adolescents' motivation to change and accept responsibility for pain control by engaging in an intensive program of physical therapy, OT, and psychotherapy rather than medication (Sherry et al., 2015). Another example is a faith-based community weight loss program (Kim et al., 2008) named WORD (wholeness, oneness, righteousness, deliverance).

Social Cognitive Theory

Social Cognitive Theory is a model that is a good fit for OT health promotion program development and evaluation due to its emphasis on "how" to change behavior, the importance placed on self-efficacy, and mastery gained through doing (Cook, 2004). According to Bandura (2004), the developer of SCT, this type of approach promotes "effective self-management of health habits that keep people healthy through their lifespan" (p. 144). The primary construct of the model is self-efficacy. Additional constructs include knowledge, a prerequisite for behavior change; outcome expectations, including physical, social, and self-evaluative; health goals; and sociostructural factors, including facilitators and impediments. The constructs of the model are described in Table 47-5 together with strategies to promote behavior change (Bandura, 2004; Cook, 2004) specific to each construct.

Returning to the earlier smoking cessation example, the SCT could be used to support both health educator and OT contributions to the smoking cessation program. Prior to instituting the antismoking buddy intervention, the health educators would again be responsible for ensuring the participants had sufficient knowledge regarding the relationship of smoking to ill health. In this example,

the buddy intervention is supported by the SCT because it serves to maximize self-efficacy through the use of social supports to achieve client-selected goals. A good resource for using this model in OT is Cook (2004) who used the SCT to develop an OT health promotion program for older adults. Others have used SCT for various populations, participation in a SCT program heavily based in promoting self-efficacy and self-management was found to increase activity participation in adults with multiple chronic conditions (Garvey, Connolly, Boland, & Smith, 2015).

Selecting and Blending Theories

Weighing possible theories for the best fit should take place throughout the health promotion process but at a minimum should be a part of decision making when determining the occupation and health need to be addressed and how. There are a variety of factors to consider in the selection of a health promotion theory; first and foremost must be the ease with which the theory and its constructs can be translated into lay language or the language of the cultural group requesting the intervention or assistance. Second is whether there is evidence that this theory has been useful in developing programs or evaluating health promotion interventions.

There are various health behavior theories as well as OT theories available to guide health promotion interventions as well as research that can inform interdisciplinary health promotion efforts. Health behavior theories generally lack an essential occupation perspective, whereas OT theories often can be strengthened through the application

TABLE 47-5 Social Cognitive Theory

Concept	Definition	Potential Change Strategies
Knowledge	Information related to health practices and their benefits and risks	• Provide tailored information connected to people's values, cultural, contextual, and educational level
Self-efficacy	Confidence in the ability to implement a health behavior change(s)	• Provide authentic positive feedback from a respected source at each stage of health behavior change • Build on effective behavior change strategies previously used
Outcome expectations	Determination whether the effort of the person or group to overcome the perceived barriers is worth the potential benefits of taking action	• Assist client or group in weighing of potential cost and benefits through a listing or section activity
Goals	Concrete, measurable goals and action steps to achieving goals	• Facilitate development of a system such as a blog, diary, or computerized reminder system to review progress toward steps and goal(s) on a predetermined schedule
Perceived facilitators	Social and physical supports for change	• Develop an artifact that symbolically represents assets for change
Perceived impediments	Social and physical barriers to change	• Develop an artifact that symbolically represents barriers to change, which can be either physically removed or erased and crossed out when barrier is no longer a threat

Adapted from National Cancer Institute. (2005). *Theory at a glance* (2nd ed., p. 20, Table 5). Bethesda, MD: National Institutes of Health. Retrieved from http://www.cancer.gov/theory.pdf

TABLE 47-6	Comparison of Theories to Support Health Promotion	
Theory	**Focus**	**Key Constructs**
Ecology of Human Performance (Dunn, Brown, & McGuigan, 1994)	How performance range can be maximized through skill, habit, or role development and/or modification of the environment	Establish or restore Adapt Alter Prevent Create
Health Belief Model (National Cancer Institute [NCI], 2005)	How individuals or communities balance the threat posed by a health problem with the benefits of avoiding the threat, the cost to avoid the threat, and other factors that influence the decision to act	Perceived susceptibility Perceived severity Perceived benefits Perceived barriers Cues to action Self-efficacy
Occupational Adaptation (Schultz, 2009)	How the ability to use adaptive capacities to solve problems, experience relative mastery, and enhance occupational performance can be enhanced	Adaptive capacity Adaptation energy Adaptive response Relative mastery
Model of Human Occupation (Kielhofner, 2009)	How individuals and communities develop performance capacity to perform habitual occupations to support participation and occupational adaption	Volition Habituation Performance capacity Occupational adaptation Occupational competency Occupational identity
Stages of Change Model (Prochaska & DiClemente, 1982, 1983)	Identification of when individuals or communities are ready to change a problem behavior, their current stage of change, and the optimal matching of intervention to current stage of change	Precontemplation Contemplation Decision Action Maintenance Relapse

Adapted from National Cancer Institute. (2005, p. 45, Table 11). *Theory at a glance* (2nd ed.). Bethesda, MD: National Institutes of Health. Retrieved from http://www.cancer.gov/theory.pdf

of constructs from one or more health behavior theories. Pyatak, Carandang, and Davis (2015) used SCT, the transtheoretical model, and the social ecological theory combined with Lifestyle Redesign® principles regarding meaningful occupation to help inform the theoretical framework for a manualized intervention for diabetes called REAL (Resilient, Empowered, Active Living with Diabetes).

A selection of the available theories to use in health promotion intervention and research that were introduced earlier is described in Table 47-6 together with a selection of OT theories. This was done in order to identify potential natural pairings between complementary OT theories and health behavior theories (Box 47-3). Table 47-7 provides an example of the use of a blended theory approach to developing a healthy weight program for high school girl students. This is discussed further in the Practice Dilemma box. Although pragmatic blending of theories can strengthen health programs, this work should be extended beyond simple evaluation of program outcomes in order to facilitate the creation of new, more powerful theories from the initial constituent theories, thus leading to broader benefit.

BOX 47-3 POTENTIAL OCCUPATIONAL THERAPY AND HEALTH PROMOTION THEORY PAIRINGS

- Health Belief Model and Ecology of Human Performance
- Health Belief Model and Model of Human Occupation
- Stages of Change and Occupational Adaptation
- Stages of Change and Model of Human Occupation
- Stages of Change and Person-Environment-Occupation

🧍 PRACTICE DILEMMA

At the request of a high school, you, together with a health educator, have successfully developed a weight management program for female high school students based on the theories shown in Table 47-7. The program includes occupation-based activities such as complicated line or group dances; healthy cooking classes, which emphasize portion control; a dress for success for all body

| TABLE 47-7 | Use of Multiple Frameworks and Theories in a Health Promotion Intervention to Reduce Obesity |

Step	Models to Partially Apply	Objective	Healthy Weight Example
1	PRECEDE portion of PRECEDE-PROCEED	Apply structure to work with community to identify occupation and health needs	Parents and school officials raise concerns regarding an increase in obesity rates among high school students
2	Health Belief Model	Determine level of threat (i.e., perceived seriousness and susceptibility weighed against benefits), relevant cues to action, and self-efficacy	Conduct separate groups prior to program development with parents, school employees, students, and local pediatricians to discuss culturally relevant cues to actions and approaches
	Stages of Change	Determine readiness for change	Develop mechanisms to identify and recruit students in the precontemplation, contemplation, and preparation stages
	Ecology of Human Performance	Determine which skills need to be established or restored through appropriate occupation-based intervention, which context or tasks be adapted or context altered to prevent harm; determine what programs or initiatives warrant being created	Assess environmental supports by identifying what foods are available for meals and snacks; observe meal and snack time behaviors of students; conduct formative or process evaluations with student participants to modify program as needed to ensure needed skills and knowledge are being obtained
3	PROCEED portion of PRECEDE-PROCEED	Plan and implement program evaluation to include process, impact, and outcomes evaluations	Involve student leaders, parents, and school officials in program evaluation planning

types lecture series; and a culminating fashion show. Each of these activities focused on establishing skills (Ecology of Human Performance [EHP] construct) and self-efficacy (HBM and SCT construct) as well as social support to live a healthy life. A series of outings also were taken to local healthy fast-food restaurants to sample healthier alternatives to fried food and red meat with the goal of permanently altering locations (EHP construct) of after-school meals to foster continued healthy food choices. The use of nondieting strategies were incorporated into the education portion of the program based on the work of Cole and Horacek (2009) who used the PRECEDE-PROCEED framework to develop an intuitive eating approach to weight management. More recently, the PROCEED portion of the framework was used to develop a weight management program for young adults from disadvantaged backgrounds (Walsh, White, & Kattelmann, 2014).

Based on your success, you have been asked to replicate your program with middle school boys and girls. The health educator you developed the program with has retired and is no longer available to assist you.

1. Given the retirement of the health educator, do you have the knowledge and skills to deliver an effective adaption of the current program to the new population? Explain your answer.
2. What are the implications to the use of the currently chosen theories with the new population?
3. Is there a place for developmental theory or other theory to guide you in adaptations to the programs for the new populations?

In addition to incorporating theory, OT health promotion interventions should be based on evidence. An example of evidence is provided in the "Commentary on the Evidence" box. Several systematic reviews also are available in a special issue of the *American Journal of Occupational Therapy* that directly relate to the impact of health promotion on the health and well-being of older adults (AOTA, 2012). Although randomized trials are seen by many as the most important level of evidence, by their nature, they require tight control over all aspects of the program development and evaluation. Generally, to be effective at a community level, programs must also go through translation studies in order to evaluate if programs will still produce results in "real-world" settings. Other programs may begin from an even stronger client-centered perspective by using a participatory action research approach that arises from community needs and champions and incorporates the researcher as a mentor for the community team.

Examples of Occupational Therapy Health Promotion in Action

Although there are many examples of OT health promotion activities, the link of the program development to theory is not always explicit. A small sampling of initiatives is provided here to show the potential for OT's role in the

Evidence-Based Practice

The Well Elderly Study (Clark et al., 2001; Clark et al., 1997) and falls prevention initiatives (e.g., Clemson et al., 2004) are examples of interventions that have been evaluated through randomized controlled trials. The Well Elderly Study in California demonstrated through a randomized clinical trial design that a preventive OT intervention (i.e., Lifestyle Redesign®) resulted in measurable benefits in health, function, and QOL (Clark et al., 1997), and these results were sustained after a 6-month follow up (Clark et al., 2001). The Well Elderly Trial 2 was conducted over a 5-year period for the purpose of replicating and assessing the effectiveness and cost-effectiveness of Lifestyle Redesign® among a more ethnically and economically diverse group of elders from a great number of sites around Los Angeles than in the first well-elderly trial. "The primary goal of the intervention was to enable the elders to develop a sustainable and customized healthy lifestyle in their daily context" (Clark & Jackson, 2010, para. 2). Results indicated that the intervention had a greater impact on measures of mental well-being (e.g., vitality, social function, life satisfaction) at statistically significant levels than on physical, health, and well-being measures (Clark et al., 2012). Lifestyle Redesign® was found to be a cost-effective intervention for use in ethnically diverse urban communities (Clark & Jackson, 2010; Clark et al., 2012). Recently, the Lifestyle Redesign® program was successfully used with 45 patients with chronic pain to improve patient function, self-efficacy, and QOL (Simon & Collins, 2017).

A mixed methods study continued research on the *Let's Go* community mobility program using the Person-Environment-Occupation-Performance (PEOP) model's fit between intrinsic (personal) and extrinsic (environmental) factors using group and individual sessions in a 4-week period (Mulry, Papetti, De Martinis, & Ravinsky, 2017). Content included participants identifying desired occupations and supports as well as barriers for community mobility. Significant improvement in participation, confidence, and community mobility was found at both 4 weeks and 6 months postprogram. This program addressed the needs of marginalized older adults to promote wellness, participation, and quality of life. Although the authors referenced only PEOP, it is easy to see an application with the HBM from the language used to describe the study (i.e., benefits, barriers, and self-efficacy).

Persch, Lamb, Metzler, and Fristad (2015) discussed multiple research-based interventions that support healthy habits for children in the areas of sleep, physical activity, and nutrition. They advocated that OT practitioners are well-situated via their expertise in activity analysis to apply healthy habit interventions within a variety of school settings. Suarez-Balcazar and colleagues (2016) researched a 16-week program on healthy habits for Latino families who had at least one child with a disability. They partnered with a local community organization for the program which included goal setting and action planning around, physical activity, and identification of barriers in community using concepts associated with the social ecological theory and Model of Human Occupation (MOHO). Although only 28% of the family goals were met at the conclusion of the study, researchers noted that all 17 families achieved at least 1 of the average 3 goals they had set. In addition, all families in the study reported they were planning to continue to address their other unmet goals.

promotion of health via research, program development, and program evaluation. These examples primarily fall into two categories: school-age children and older adults. Each initiative is linked to a potentially supporting health promotion theory, either identified by the developer of the program or suggested by the authors.

AOTA's National School Backpack Awareness Day

One initiative for children and youth is the AOTA's National School Backpack Awareness Day (Jacobs, Wuest, Markowitz, & Hellman, 2011). The AOTA's National School Backpack Awareness Day happens annually in September with the express goal of having students wear their backpack over both shoulders and to monitor the weight they carry. The programs can use a combination of fun activities to ensure that the students understand their potential susceptibility for an injury and the potential seriousness of an injury (two constructs from the HBM) as well as the proper techniques. Self-efficacy also can be promoted by students performing the correct techniques, which provide feedback about their ability to perform the task (SCT and HBM constructs) as well as to feel firsthand the benefits (HBM construct).

Powerful Tools for Caregivers via Telehealth

In recent years, technology has improved to allow virtual face-to-face meetings and as a result, telehealth has become an increasing popular option, especially for those with limited access to services (AOTA, 2013c). An existing caregiver program offered at many Area Agencies on

Aging, Powerful Tools for Caregivers, was piloted using a synchronous, face-to-face telehealth approach (Serwe, Hersch, Pickens, & Pancheri, 2017). Qualitative data collected via focus group following the program reflected positive participant experiences with attending the program this way; however, learning to use the technology was challenging for some participants. This study exemplifies how OT practitioners working in the field of health promotion can effectively use their skills to advance use and research of existing evidence-based programs.

CarFit

Stav (2010) has linked CarFit, a program developed jointly by AOTA, AARP (formerly the American Association of Retired Persons), and the American Automobile Association (AAA), to assess the fit between older drivers and their vehicles to theoretical constructs from the HBM and the Person-Environment-Occupation (PEO) Model (Law et al., 1996). CarFit sessions are offered in the community often in between rush hours when older adults are more typically running errands. The evaluations are scheduled in 30-minute increments to ensure that the 12-step checklist can be completed without rushing.

The primary purpose of the program is for older adults to gain information about the fit between their body and their car while sitting in their car (PEO constructs). Needed mirror, steering wheel, and seat adjustments can be made immediately, and other recommendations for additional adaptations when indicated are provided. Participants are educated about the findings that proper seating and alignment of mirrors decreases risk for a crash (HBM construct) due to increased visibility. At the end, participants walk around the car and reenter and can reassess the increased visibility leading to self-efficacy (HBM and SCT construct). The social atmosphere and encouragement in a group of peers acts as a sociostructural facilitator (SCT construct).

Conclusion

Occupation can be prescribed to promote health and well-being of individuals, families, and communities. However, this prescription must be unique and designed to be culturally relevant, client-centered, and based on theory and the most current evidence available. Using a blend of theories drawn from health behavior and OT has the potential to strengthen OT health promotion program design and success. The prescription or intervention then must be evaluated to determine if outcomes are achieved, whether the prescription or program needs to be modified, and whether the theoretical foundation needs to evolve.

CENTENNIAL NOTES

The Future of Health Promotion

Although the potential contributions of health promotion to social participation and the health of society have been and are currently a focus of the profession's leadership, they also are a current focus of U.S. governmental efforts to enhance the nation's health while controlling costs (USDDHS, Office of Disease Prevention and Health Promotion, 2010). One of these efforts has been the development of a framework by the Institute for Health care Improvement (IHI), coined the Triple Aim, to guide future efforts to maximize the outcomes of healthy systems. The Triple Aim seeks to influence the development of new health systems and approaches by focusing on three dimensions (IHI, 2017):

- Improving the patient experience of care (including quality and satisfaction)
- Improving the health of populations
- Reducing the per capita cost of health care

A policy document from the CDC further details how the triple aim can help frame efforts to support the development of and payment for sustainable population health initiatives (Hester, Stange, Seeff, Davis, & Craft, 2015). Occupational therapy practitioners can contribute to efforts to reduce costs while improving QOL and overall well-being through health promotion initiatives crafted with clients and built on evidence and theory.

REFERENCES

Agency for Healthcare Research and Quality. (2017). *AHRQ health literacy universal precautions toolkit* (2nd ed.) Retrieved from https://www.ahrq.gov/professionals/quality-patient-safety/quality-resources/tools/literacy-toolkit/index.html

American Occupational Therapy Association. (1982). *1982 Member data survey*. Rockville, MD: Author.

American Occupational Therapy Association. (1987). *1986 Member data survey: Interim report #1*. Rockville, MD: Author.

American Occupational Therapy Association. (1991). *1990 Member data survey: Summary report*. Rockville, MD: Author.

American Occupational Therapy Association. (2001). *AOTA 2000 member compensation survey*. Rockville, MD: Author.

American Occupational Therapy Association. (2006). *AOTA 2006 Workforce and compensation report*. Rockville, MD: Author.

American Occupational Therapy Association. (2008). Occupational therapy practice framework: Domain and process, 2nd edition. *American Journal of Occupational Therapy, 62*, 625–683.

American Occupational Therapy Association. (2010a). *2010 Occupational therapy compensation and workforce study*. Bethesda, MD: Author.

American Occupational Therapy Association. (2010b). Occupational therapy code of ethics and ethics standards (2010). *American Journal of Occupational Therapy, 64*, S17–S26. doi:10:5014/ajot2010.62S17-64S26

American Occupational Therapy Association. (2010c). Standards of practice for occupational therapy. *American Journal of Occupational Therapy, 64,* S10–S11. doi:10.5014/ajot.2010.64 S106–64S111

American Occupational Therapy Association. (2012). Special issue on productive aging: Evidence and opportunities for occupational therapy practitioners. *American Journal of Occupational Therapy, 66,* 263–265.

American Occupational Therapy Association. (2013a). AOTA's societal statement on health disparities. *American Journal of Occupational Therapy, 67,* S7–S8.

American Occupational Therapy Association. (2013b). Occupational therapy in the promotion of health and well-being. *American Journal of Occupational Therapy, 67,* S47–S59.

American Occupational Therapy Association. (2013c). Telehealth [Position paper]. *American Journal of Occupational Therapy, 67,* S69–S90.

American Occupational Therapy Association. (2014). Occupational therapy practice framework: Domain and process, 3rd edition. *American Journal of Occupational Therapy, 68,* S1–S48.

American Occupational Therapy Association. (2015a). *2015 AOTA salary and workforce survey.* Bethesda, MD: Author.

American Occupational Therapy Association. (2015b). Occupational therapy code of ethics (2015). *American Journal of Occupational Therapy, 64,* S17–S26.

American Occupational Therapy Association. (2016a). AOTA's societal statement on health literacy. *American Journal of Occupational Therapy, 70,* 7012410010p1–7012410010p2. doi:10.5014/ajot.2016.706S2OffDoc

American Occupational Therapy Association. (2016b). AOTA's societal statement on livable communities. *American Journal of Occupational Therapy, 70,* S1–S2.

American Occupational Therapy Association. (2017a). AOTA's Societal Statement on Disaster Response and Risk Reduction. *American Journal of Occupational Therapy, 71,* 7112410060. doi:10.5014/ajot.2017.716S11

American Occupational Therapy Association. (2017b). Vision 2025. *American Journal of Occupational Therapy, 71,* 1.

American Occupational Therapy Association. (2017c). AOTA's societal statement on health literacy. *American Journal of Occupational Therapy, 71,* 7112410065p1–7112410065p2. doi:10.5014/ajot.2017.716S14

Bandura, A. (2004). Health promotion by social cognitive means. *Health Education & Behavior, 31,* 143–164.

Baum, M. C. (2006). Presidential address, 2006: Centennial challenges, millennium opportunities. *American Journal of Occupational Therapy, 60,* 609–616.

British Association of Occupational Therapists and College of Occupational Therapists. (2008). *Health promotion in occupational therapy.* London, United Kingdom: College of Occupational Therapists.

Brunyate, R. W. (1967). From the president: After fifty years, what stature do we hold? *American Journal of Occupational Therapy, 21,* 262–267.

Centers for Disease Control and Prevention. (2016). *Health related quality of life (HRQOL).* Retrieved from https://www.cdc.gov/hrqol/

Centers for Disease Control and Prevention. (2017). *Food deserts.* Retrieved from http://www.cdc.gov/Features/FoodDeserts/

Clark, F., Azen, S. P., Carlson, M., Mandel, D., LaBree, L. Hay, J., . . . Lipson, L. (2001). Embedding health-promoting changes into the daily lives of independent-living older adults: Long-term follow-up of occupational therapy intervention. *The Journal of Gerontology, 56B,* P60–P63.

Clark, F., Azen, S. P., Zemke, R., Jackson, J., Carlson, M., Mandel, D., . . . Lipson, L. (1997). Occupational therapy for independent-living older adults: A randomized controlled trial. *Journal of the American Medical Association, 278,* 1321–1326.

Clark, F, & Jackson, J. (2010). *Well Elderly II clinical trial results: Effectiveness and cost-effectiveness of the Lifestyle Redesign intervention in community settings.* Retrieved from http://www.wfot.org/wfot2010/program/pdf/1457.pdf

Clark, F., Jackson, J., Carlson, M., Chou, C., Cherry, B. J., Jordan-Marsh, M., . . . Azen, S. P. (2012). Effectiveness of a lifestyle intervention in promoting the well-being of independently living older people: Results of the well elderly 2 randomised controlled trial. *Journal of Epidemiology and Community Health, 66,* 782–790. doi:10.1136/jech.2009.099754

Clemson, L., Cumming, R. G., Kendig, H., Swann, M., Heard, R., & Taylor, K. (2004). The effectiveness of a community-based program for reducing the incidence of falls in the elderly: A randomized trial. *Journal of the American Geriatrics Society, 52,* 1487–1494.

Cole, R. E., & Horacek, T. (2009). Applying PRECEDE-PROCEED to develop an intuitive eating nondieting approach to weight management pilot program. *Journal of Nutrition Education and Behavior, 41,* 120–126.

Cook, A. (2004). Health education programming for older adults based on social cognitive theory. *American Occupational Therapy Association Gerontology Special Interest Section Quarterly, 27*(1), 1–4.

Deshpande, S., Basil, M. D., & Basil, D. Z. (2009). Factors influencing healthy eating habits among college students: An application of the health belief model. *Health Marketing Quarterly, 26,* 145–164.

Drazen, C. H., Abel, R., Lindsey, T., & King, A. A. (2014). Development and feasibility of a home-based education model for families of children with sickle cell disease. *BMC Public Health, 14,* 116.

Dunn, W., Brown, C., & McGuigan, A. (1994). The ecology of human performance: A framework for considering the effect of context. *American Journal of Occupational Therapy, 48,* 595–607.

Finn, G. (1972). The occupational therapist in prevention programs. *American Journal of Occupational Therapy, 26,* 59–66.

Garvey, J., Connolly, D., Boland, F., & Smith, S. M. (2015). OPTIMAL, an occupational therapy led self-management support programme for people with multimorbidity in primary care: a randomized controlled trial. *BMC Family Practice, 16,* 59.

Green, L. W., & Kreuter, M. W. (2005). *Health promotion planning: An educational and ecological approach* (4th ed.). New York, NY: McGraw Hill.

Heijmans, M., Waverijn, G., Rademakers, J., van der Vaart, R., & Rijken, M. (2015). Functional, communicative and critical health literacy of chronic disease patients and their importance for self-management. *Patient Education and Counseling, 98,* 41–48. doi:10.1016/j.pec.2014.10.006

Hester, J. A, Stange, P. V., Seeff, L. C., Davis, J. B., & Craft, C. A. (2015). *Toward sustainable improvements in population health: Overview of community integration structures and emerging innovations in financing.* Atlanta, GA: Centers for Disease Control and Prevention. Retrieved from https://www.cdc.gov/policy/docs/financepaper.pdf

Hettler, W. (1984). Wellness—The lifetime goal of a university experience. In J. D. Matarazzo, S. M. Weiss, J. A. Herd, N. E. Miller, & S. M. Weiss (Eds.), *Behavioral health: A handbook of health enhancement and disease prevention* (pp. 1117–1124). New York, NY: Wiley.

Institute for Healthcare Improvement. (2017). *Triple aim initiative.* Retrieved from http://www.ihi.org/Engage/Initiatives/ TripleAim/Pages/default.aspx

Jacobs, K., Wuest, E., Markowitz, J., & Hellman, M. (2011). Get packing: Planning your own National School Backpack Awareness Day event. *OT Practice, 16*(13), 11–14.

Jaffe, E. (1986). Nationally speaking—The role of occupational therapy in the disease prevention and health promotion. *American Journal of Occupational Therapy, 40,* 749–752.

James, D. C. S., Pobee, J. W., Oxidine, D., Brown, L., & Joshi, G. (2012). Using the health belief model to develop culturally appropriate weight-management materials for African-American women. *Journal of the Academy of Nutrition and Dietetics, 112,* 664–670.

Jantzen, A. (1979). The current profile of occupational therapy and the future—Professional or vocational. In American Occupational Therapy Association (Ed.), *Occupational therapy: 2001* (pp. 71–75). Rockville, MD: American Occupational Therapy Association.

Johnson, J. A. (1986). *Wellness: A context for living.* Thorofare, NJ: Slack.

Juniper, K. C., Oman, R. F., Hamm, R. M., & Kerby, D. S. (2004). The relationships among construct in the health belief model and the transtheoretical model among African-American college women for physical activity. *American Journal of Health Promotion, 18,* 354–357.

Kaplan, L. H., & Burch-Minakan, L. (1986). Reach out for health: A corporation's approach to health promotion. *American Journal of Occupational Therapy, 40,* 777–780.

Kielhofner, G. (2009). *Conceptual foundations of occupational therapy* (4th ed.). Philadelphia, PA: F. A. Davis.

Kim, K. H., Linnan, L., Campbell, M. K., Brooks, C., Koenig, H. G., & Wiesen, C. (2008). The WORD (wholeness, oneness, righteousness, deliverance): A faith-based weight-loss program utilizing a community-based participatory action research approach. *Health Education & Behavior, 35,* 634–650.

Law, M., Cooper, B., Strong, S., Stewart, D., Rigby, P., & Letts, L. (1996). The person-environment-occupation model: A transactive approach to occupational performance. *Canadian Journal of Occupational Therapy, 63,* 9–23.

Lee, D. C. A., Day, L., Hill, K., Clemson, L., McDermott, F., & Haines, T. P. (2015). What factors influence older adults to discuss falls with their health care providers? *Health Expectations, 18,* 1593–1609.

Losada, C. A. (1936). Some values in occupational therapy. *Occupational Therapy and Rehabilitation, 15,* 285–289.

Molineux, M. L., & Whiteford, G. E. (2011). Prisons: From occupational deprivation to occupational enrichment. *Journal of Occupational Science, 6,* 124–130. doi:10.1080/14427591.1999.9686457

Mulry, C. M., Papetti, C., De Martinis, J. D., & Ravinsky, M. (2017). Facilitating wellness in urban-dwelling, low-income older adults through community mobility: A mixed methods study. *American Journal of Occupational Therapy, 71,* 7104190030p1–7104190030p7. doi:10.5014/ajot.2017.025494

National Cancer Institute. (2005). *Theory at a glance* (2nd ed.). Bethesda, MD: National Institutes of Health. Retrieved from http://www.cancer.gov/theory.pdf

Niolon, P. H., Kearns, M., Dills, J., Ramo, K., Irving, S., Armstead, T., & Gilbert, L. (2017). *Preventing intimate partner violence across the lifespan: A technical package of programs, policies, and practices.* Atlanta, GA: National Center for Injury Prevention and Control, Centers for Disease Control and Prevention.

Persch, A. C., Lamb, A. J., Metzler, C. A., & Fristad, M. A. (2015). Healthy habits for children: Leveraging existing evidence to demonstrate value. *American Journal of Occupational Therapy, 69,* 6904900010p1.

Pizzi, M. A., & Richards, L. G. (2017). Promoting health, well-being, and quality of life in occupational therapy: A commitment to a paradigm shift for the next 100 years. *American Journal of Occupational Therapy, 71,* 7104170010p2. doi:10.5014/ajot.2017.028456

Prochaska, J. O., & DiClemente, C. C. (1982). Transtheoretical therapy: Toward a more integrative model of change. *Psychotherapy: Theory, Research and Practice, 19,* 276–288.

Prochaska, J. O., & DiClemente, C. C. (1983). Stages and processes of self-change of smoking: Toward an integrative model of change. *Journal of Counseling and Clinical Psychology, 51,* 390–395.

Pyatak, E. A., Carandang, K., & Davis, S. (2015). Developing a manualized occupational therapy diabetes management intervention: Resilient, empowered, active living with diabetes. *OTJR: Occupation, Participation and Health, 35,* 187–194. doi:10.1177/1539449215584310

Reitz, S. M. (1992). A historical review of occupational therapy's role in preventive health and wellness. *American Journal of Occupational Therapy, 46,* 50–55.

Reitz, S. M. (2010). Historical and philosophical perspectives of occupational therapy's role in health promotion. In M. E. Scaffa, S. M. Reitz, & M. A. Pizzi (Eds.), *Occupational therapy in the promotion of health and wellness* (pp. 1–21). Philadelphia, PA: F. A. Davis.

Reitz, S. M., & Scaffa, M. E. (2010). Public health principles, approaches, and initiatives. In M. E. Scaffa, S. M. Reitz, & M. A. Pizzi (Eds.), *Occupational therapy in the promotion of health and wellness* (pp. 70–95). Philadelphia, PA: F. A. Davis.

Reitz, S. M., Scaffa, M. E., Campbell, R. M., & Rhynders, P. A. (2010). Health behavior frameworks for health promotion practice. In M. E. Scaffa, S. M. Reitz, & M. A. Pizzi (Eds.), *Occupational therapy in the promotion of health and wellness* (pp. 46–69). Philadelphia, PA: F. A. Davis.

Schultz, S. (2009). Occupational adaptation. In E. B. Crepeau, E. S. Cohn, & B. A. B. Schell (Eds.), *Willard & Spackman's occupational therapy* (11th ed., pp. 462–475). Philadelphia, PA: Lippincott Williams & Wilkins.

Serwe, K. M., Hersch, G. I., Pickens, N. D., & Pancheri, K. (2017). Caregiver perceptions of a telehealth wellness program. *American Journal of Occupational Therapy, 71,* 7104350010p1. doi:10.5014/ajot.2017.025619

Sherry, D. D., Brake, L., Tress, J. L., Sherker, J., Fash, K., Ferry, K., & Weiss, P. F. (2015). The treatment of juvenile fibromyalgia with an intensive physical and psychosocial program. *The Journal of Pediatrics, 167,* 731–737.

Simon, A. U., & Collins, C. R. (2017). Lifestyle Redesign® for chronic pain management: A retrospective clinical efficacy study. *American Journal of Occupational Therapy, 71,* 7104190040.

Smith, S. G., Chen, J., Basile, K. C., Gilbert, L. K., Merrick, M. T., Patel, N., . . . Jain, A. (2017). *The National Intimate Partner and Sexual Violence Survey (NISVS): 2010–2012 State Report.* Atlanta, GA: National Center for Injury Prevention and Control, Centers for Disease Control and Prevention. Retrieved from https://www.cdc.gov/violenceprevention/pdf/ipv-technicalpackages.pdf

Stav, W. (2010). CarFit: An evaluation of behavior change and impact. *British Journal of Occupational Therapy, 73,* 589–597.

Suarez-Balcazar, Y., Hoisington, M., Orozco, A. A., Arias, D., Garcia, C., Smith, K., & Bonner, B. (2016). Benefits of a culturally tailored health promotion program for Latino youth with disabilities and their families. *American Journal of Occupational Therapy, 70,* 7005180080p1. doi:10.5014/ajot.2016.021949

U.S. Department of Health and Human Services. (2017a). *Healthy people 2020: Framework.* Retrieved from http://healthypeople.gov/2020/consortium/HP2020Framework.pdf

U.S. Department of Health and Human Services. (2017b). *The Secretary's Advisory Committee Report on Approaches to Healthy People 2030.* Retrieved from https://www.healthypeople.gov/sites/default/files/Full%20Committee%20Report%20to%20Secretary%205-9-2017_0.pdf

U.S. Department of Health and Human Services, Office of Disease Prevention and Health Promotion. (2008). *America's health literacy: Why we need accessible health information.* Retrieved from https://health.gov/communication/literacy/issuebrief/

U.S. Department of Health and Human Services, Office of Disease Prevention and Health Promotion. (2010). *National action plan to improve health literacy.* Washington, DC: Author. Retrieved from https://health.gov/communication/hlactionplan/pdf/Health_Literacy_Action_Plan.pdf

Virginia Commonwealth University Center on Society and Health. (2017). *Mapping life expectancy.* Retrieved from http://www.societyhealth.vcu.edu/work/the-projects/mapsatlanta.html

Walsh, J. R., White, A. A., & Kattelmann, K. K. (2014). Using PRECEDE to develop a weight management program for disadvantaged young adults. *Journal of Nutrition Education and Behavior, 46,* 1–9.

West, W. (1967). The occupational therapist's changing responsibility to the community. *American Journal of Occupational Therapy, 21,* 312–316.

West, W. (1969). The growing importance of prevention. *American Journal of Occupational Therapy, 23,* 226–231.

Wiemer, R. (1972). Some concepts of prevention as an aspect of community health. *American Journal of Occupational Therapy, 26,* 1–9.

Wilcock, A. A. (2006). *An occupational perspective of health* (2nd ed.). Thorofare, NJ: Slack.

World Health Organization. (1947). Constitution of the World Health Organization. *Chronicle of the World Health Organization, 1*(1), 29–40. Available at http://apps.who.int/gb/bd/PDF/bd47/EN /constitution-en.pdf?ua=1

World Health Organization. (1986). *The Ottawa charter for health promotion.* Retrieved from http://www.who.int/hpr/NPH/docs /ottawa_charter_hp.pdf

World Federation of Occupational Therapists. (2004). *WFOT position paper on community based rehabilitation.* Retrieved from http:// www.wfot.org/ResourceCentre.aspx

World Federation of Occupational Therapists. (2016). *WFOT position paper on disaster risk reduction.* Retrieved from http://www.wfot .org/ResourceCentre.aspx

the**Point**® *For additional resources on the subjects discussed in this chapter, visit* **http://thePoint.lww.com /Willard-Spackman13e.**

CHAPTER 48

Principles of Learning and Behavior Change

Christine A. Helfrich

LEARNING OBJECTIVES

After reading this chapter, you will be able to:

1. Identify and describe five theories of learning: behaviorist, social cognitive, constructivist, self-efficacy, and motivational.
2. Compare the essential elements and assumptions of each theory of learning.
3. Explain how different theories of learning contribute to occupational therapy intervention.
4. Analyze a learning need and synthesize information to select the most appropriate strategy.

Introduction

Think of the many things you may have taught different people. Perhaps you taught a younger sibling how to share toys, a friend how to navigate a bus or subway system, grandparents how to keep track of their medicines, a classmate how to organize information and prepare for an important test, a son or daughter how to overcome a fear or anxiety, and yourself a new leisure activity or how to use a new cell phone. How did you decide *how* to teach the person? Why did you teach the skill or behavior *in a particular way*? What *strategies* did you use? *What beliefs about how people learn guided you in your selection of strategies*? In your efforts to teach others, you have likely developed a beginning set of beliefs about how people learn best. Hopefully, you have also begun to notice that different strategies work best for different people and/or different situations.

This chapter presents an overview of selected *theories of learning*. In general, "learning theories" explain a perspective on what is "knowing" and how a person "comes to know" (Fosnot, 2005, p. ix). Learning theories have provided the foundation for many occupational therapy (OT) theories and frames of reference such as Cognitive Disabilities and the Model of Human Occupation. It is important to understand the basic concepts of learning when using theoretical approaches considered unique to OT. Five different overall ways of thinking about and conceptualizing theories of learning are reviewed in this chapter: behaviorist, social cognitive, constructivist, self-efficacy, and motivational.

CENTENNIAL NOTES

Teachers of Occupation

Lori T. Andersen

Elizabeth Greene Upham (later Davis), a pioneer occupational therapist, wrote a report entitled *Training of Teachers for Occupational Therapy for the Rehabilitation of Disabled Soldiers and Sailors* (1918) for the Federal Board for Vocational Education. This report offered a plan for the rehabilitation of disabled soldiers and sailors. In World War I, the military emphasized the importance of the teaching role for reconstruction aides in OT, requiring " . . . good teachers; knowledge and skill in the particular occupation to be taught, attractive, and forceful personality, teaching ability, sympathy, tact, judgment, industry" (M. E. Haggerty, 1918, p. 29). Recognizing that some reconstruction aides were ill prepared to work with soldiers with disabilities, hospital training was also required starting June 1918 (McDaniel, 1968, p. 72).

In the 1920s, the National Society for the Promotion of Occupational Therapy (NSPOT) had lively discussions on whether specially trained nurses or experts in crafts should provide OT. The leaders of NSPOT believed that craft teachers without appropriate medical training to work with people with various disabilities were detrimental to the new profession. In a Round Table discussion, Eleanor Clarke Slagle declared " . . . he [doctor] depends on her not only to teach the crafts and handle the patient, but very generally to choose what the patient shall do and what is best for the patient, and unless the therapist has a broad vision and good understanding, not only of human nature but of human ills, there is great danger of much harm being done" (Round Table on Training Courses, 1923, p. 129). Susan E. Tracy, a nurse, promoted nurses by virtue of their medical training. Susan Cox Johnson, an arts and crafts teacher, suggested that nurses had neither the time for this specialized education nor time to develop OT programs for patients. Johnson proposed that a new field was emerging, one that combined knowledge of occupations and knowledge of medicine for therapeutic purposes.

Occupational therapists emerged as a new classification of worker, and training standards were developed to differentiate these new workers from craft teachers. Today, understanding of learning processes and teaching methods remains an important part of OT practice (Giles, in press).

Why Should Occupational Therapists Study Theories of Learning?

Svinicki (2004) identified several reasons to study theories of learning. Many of these are relevant to occupational therapists. Box 48-1 summarizes six important reasons for OT practitioners to study theories of learning as well as theory in general.

- Theory provides an overall *foundation for assessment and treatment* in all areas of practice. People often come to OT because they want to learn new ways of doing what is important to them, and OT practitioners help people to change behaviors so that they can engage in meaningful occupations. Theory provides the basis for designing specific interventions to address client issues.
- Theory *guides* and *informs* practice. Theory provides us with a conceptual framework related to observations of human behavior. Theories offer guidance about what to observe and answer questions about how best to facilitate behavior change.
- Theory presents an organizing framework of ideas about how people learn that leads to questions that can be

tested in practice—in other words, *research*. Asking and answering questions about OT practice through research is a core responsibility for all OT practitioners.

- The primary goal of OT is to help people function in their daily occupations. Interventions may be designed, suggested, and implemented in many different ways. Practitioners who understand different perspectives on how people learn are likely to be more *effective* at presenting a range of interventions that match their clients' learning needs and learning styles. And when problems do arise, it is important to be able to analyze why the intervention may not be working. Understanding

---

BOX 48-1   REASONS TO STUDY THEORIES OF LEARNING

1. Provides a foundation for practice
2. Guides and informs practice
3. Leads to researchable questions
4. Enhances practitioners' effectiveness and ability to solve problems
5. Promotes individualized and creative interventions
6. Core professional responsibility

theories of learning will help you to *solve problems* that emerge during intervention and generate new approaches with your client when an intervention strategy is not effective.

- Each client with whom you work will have different values, interests, needs, abilities, and preferred ways of learning. Understanding theories of learning will help you to design *individualized* and *creative* interventions that respond to each client's unique strengths and limitations.
- Occupational therapy practice should always be moving forward; it is not static. Neither is theory. Ongoing exploration of theory and theory development is a *professional responsibility* of all OT practitioners.

In addition to the reasons to study theories of learning listed in Box 48-1, theories of learning serve several other purposes as well. At perhaps the most basic level, they provide us with a way to organize vast amounts of knowledge that are used in practice. Theory helps us to put our knowledge together, to organize otherwise random knowledge into a cohesive set of ideas that explains some phenomenon—in this case, learning. Theories of learning enable us to see how interesting and complex even the most seemingly simple things can be. This does not mean that theory makes things more *complicated*. Rather, theory helps you to see that there is usually more to any teaching–learning situation than meets the eye. Theories of learning reflect beliefs about how people think and how they store and use information (Svinicki, 2004). According to Hergenhahn (1976),

> since most human behavior is learned, investigating the principles of learning will help us understand why we behave as we do. An awareness of the learning process will not only allow greater understanding of normal and adaptive behavior, but will also allow greater understanding of the circumstances that produce maladaptive and abnormal behavior. (p. 12)

Therefore, in any intervention situation, practitioners need to understand the reason or reasons that contribute to problematic behavior.

Where to Begin?

What is learning? How do we know when someone is learning? Under what conditions does learning occur? Why does learning occur? What does the learner do to cause the learning? What are the outcomes of learning? The answer to all of these questions is "it depends." It depends because different learning theories attribute different causes, reasons, actions, and circumstances to learning. And because the therapist is treating an individual who is unique, the challenge may be to determine the most appropriate theory to treat that person.

Behaviorist Theory

Behaviorist theory focuses on how observable, tangible behaviors are learned in response to some environmental stimulation (Martin & Pear, 2015). Behaviorist theorists focus on observable events rather than on mental processes. For example, how does a child learn to take turns while playing a game with friends, how might a person with a developmental disability learn to respond appropriately in a conversation, and how would a person learn to propel and navigate a wheelchair in an urban community? In these examples, the observable events are the child waiting for and taking his or her turn during a game of kickball, a person waiting for a conversation partner to finish speaking before providing new information, and a person successfully navigating curbs and crowds in a wheelchair. The overall emphasis in behavioral theories of learning is on the relationship between an environmental stimulus and a behavioral response and on how learning is indicated by an observed change in behavior.

Essential Elements and Assumptions of Behaviorist Learning Theory

Behaviorists use the term *conditioning* to explain changes in behavior rather than learning because behaviorist theory asserts that a person's behavior is conditioned by events in the environment. A behavior is gradually shaped, changed, and molded as it reflects the environment's response to the behavior. There are several key terms that you will notice in most types of behavioral theory: **conditioning** (a behavior modification process that increases or decreases the likelihood of a behavior being performed), **stimulus** (verbal, sensory, or environmental input that prompts a behavior), **response** (the reaction to the stimulus), **fading** and **shaping** (strategies to develop closer and closer approximations of a behavior), **chaining** (a stepwise process for teaching a multistep task), **reinforcement** (a stimulus that causes a behavior to be strengthened and performed again [positive or negative reinforcement]), **punishment** (an aversive stimulus that causes a behavior to decrease in frequency), and **extinction** (the process of reducing the frequency of a behavior by withholding reinforcement). Each of these terms is further defined and discussed in more detail.

Behavioral Theorists

Many well-known theorists have contributed to the development of the behavioral perspective, such as Ivan Pavlov (1849–1936), Edward Thorndike (1874–1949),

John Watson (1878–1958), and Burrhus Frederic (B. F.) Skinner (1904–1990). Although their theories are slightly different from each other, they do share common assumptions about the nature of learning—chiefly the need to focus on external, observable events as evidence of learning (Ormrod, 2015).

Ivan Pavlov developed the theory of *classical conditioning*, which resulted from his initial studies of a dog's salivation response to a neutral stimulus paired with an *unconditioned stimulus* (*food*), which caused an *unconditioned response* (*salivation*). After many pairings, the *neutral stimulus* (*bell*) became a *conditioned stimulus*, which then caused a *conditioned response* (*salivation*). As a result of his experiments and observations, Pavlov concluded that changes in behavior (learning) are due to *experience*.

Edward Thorndike's perspective is known as *connectionism*, whereby learning is seen as a process of making connections between things, understanding the relationship of a stimulus to a response. This concept may also be referred to as the *Law of Effect* (Driscoll, 2005). Thorndike studied how people established those connections and therefore how people developed and maintained behaviors. He emphasized the role of practice and experience in strengthening or weakening the connections between a stimulus and a response. Through a series of experiments, Thorndike concluded that behavior is learned via the consequences of the behavior. So responses to a behavior that were followed by a satisfying experience would be rewarded, thus strengthening the connection, the neural bond between the stimulus and the response, and increasing the likelihood that the behavior would be produced again.

John Watson introduced the term *behaviorism*. He emphasized the importance of focusing on observable behaviors. Watson was greatly influenced by the work of Pavlov. As he expanded on Pavlov's work, Watson proposed two "laws" that explained the relationship between stimulus and response and ultimately how behavior is learned. The *Law of Frequency* proposes that "the more frequently a stimulus and response occur in association with each other, the stronger that stimulus-response habit will become" (Ormrod, 2015, p. 20). The *Law of Recency* proposes that "the response that has most recently occurred after a particular stimulus is the response most likely to be associated with that stimulus" (Ormrod, 2015, p. 20).

B. F. Skinner was influenced by both Pavlov and Watson. He coined the term **operant conditioning**. Skinner's basic principle was that a response followed by some reinforcement is likely to be strengthened. And because a response is a change in behavior, then from a behaviorist perspective, this indicates learning. Any behavior, positive or negative, can be reinforced. Skinner used the term *reinforcement* rather than *reward* for two reasons.

First, he believed that the term *reward* implies something pleasant or desirable, but sometimes people intentionally do things to produce an unpleasant consequence (e.g., Katelyn might wear her sister's clothes just to annoy her because Katelyn enjoys watching her sister get angry). Second, the terms *reward*, *pleasant*, and *desirable* are highly subjective terms.

There are three important factors in operant conditioning. First, the reinforcement must follow, not precede the response. Second, the reinforcement should immediately follow the behavior in order to have the greatest effect. Third, the reinforcement must be contingent on the response; it should not be given for an unintended or unrelated response.

How is operant conditioning different from classical conditioning? In classical conditioning, there is an unconditioned stimulus and a conditioned stimulus. The conditioned stimulus brings about the conditioned response. The response is *automatic and involuntary*. In operant conditioning, a response is *followed by* a reinforcing stimulus. The response is *voluntary*. The organism has control over whether it emits the response. For example, consider John, a 77-year-old man attending a community behavioral health center senior. An example of *classical conditioning* would be if the living center was playing old songs (stimulus) that reminded John of past experiences with friends. This could make John feel comfortable and pleasant (response) and cause John to want to attend the center more often. *Operant conditioning* would occur if after John went to the community behavioral health center (response), he received praise and enthusiasm (reinforcing stimulus) and then attended the center more regularly as a result.

Behavioral Intervention Approaches: Positive and Negative Reinforcement, Punishment, and Extinction

There are several different types of interventions that are designed to strengthen or increase behavior, whereas others decrease or eliminate behavior.

- *Positive reinforcement* is the presentation of a reinforcer (stimulus) immediately following a behavior that causes the behavior to be more likely to reoccur. Different types of reinforcement may include consumable (i.e., food), manipulative (i.e., toy to play with), social (i.e., positive feedback or attention), activity (i.e., swinging or bouncing on lap or watching television), and possession (i.e., money or tokens). The reinforcer must be appealing to the individual for it to be effective.

- *Negative reinforcement* occurs when the removal of a stimulus immediately after a response causes the response to be strengthened or to increase in frequency (Martin & Pear, 2015). For example, if Anna gets in her car and begins pulling out of her driveway, a seatbelt alarm will sound until Anna fastens her seatbelt. In this case, removal of the aversive stimulus of the alarm causes the seatbelt-wearing response to be strengthened.
- **Punishment** is the presentation of an aversive stimulus contingent on a response that reduces the rate of that response. Such an approach is common in parenting, as for example, the practice of putting a child who misbehaves into "time-out" each time the misbehavior occurs.
- **Extinction** is the process of reducing the frequency of a behavior by withholding reinforcement. Extinction can be challenging to enact because it may be difficult to know which reinforcer is the one actually reinforcing the undesirable behavior. For example, a child who hits other children and is given a time-out for that behavior may actually be receiving positive reinforcement (in the form of social contact) for that behavior from the adult giving the time-out. When trying to extinguish a behavior, you may also see an extinction burst or spontaneous recovery. An **extinction burst** occurs when the behavior being extinguished gets worse before it gets better. For example, an individual who is diagnosed with diabetes and told she must eliminate all sweets from her diet goes out to a dessert buffet every night for a week before starting her new diet. *Spontaneous recovery* occurs when the behavior being extinguished reappears after a delay, even though typically it is not as severe. An example of this is a child who has stopped taking other's toys and then begins to do so again, seemingly for no reason. Often, spontaneous recovery can be linked to a stressful or anxiety-producing event for the individual. Reimplementing the behavioral strategies that extinguished the behavior initially can usually be done quite quickly and successfully.

Reinforcement Schedule, Differential Reinforcement, Stimulus Discrimination, and Generalization

Each type of reinforcement used to change a behavior is delivered on a schedule. A **reinforcement schedule** indicates which instances of behavior, if any, will be reinforced. There are two main types of reinforcement schedules. **Continuous reinforcement** reinforces every instance of the behavior and is most often used at the beginning of treatment. **Intermittent reinforcement** only reinforces certain demonstrations of the behavior

and is more effective at maintaining the desired response. **Intermittent reinforcement** can be delivered using one of the following four types of reinforcement schedules: (1) *ratio schedules*: reinforcement is based on the number of behaviors required, (2) *interval schedules*: reinforcement is based on the passage of time between behaviors occurring, (3) *fixed schedules*: the requirements for reinforcement are always the same, and (4) *variable schedules*: the requirements for reinforcement change randomly. It is easiest for someone to change his or her behavior initially when he or she knows when he or she will receive his or her next reinforcement; however, variable reinforcement is more effective at maintaining behavior change. For example, if the goal is for Gavin to get to school on time every day, you would begin by giving him positive reinforcement *each* day he arrived on time (*continuous*). Once he was arriving on time consistently, you might only reward him each time he arrived 3 days in a row (*ratio*) or every fourth day (*interval*) he arrived on time. Once either or both of these patterns were achieved, you would provide random reinforcement (*variable schedule*) for his on-time arrival to school.

Differential reinforcement teaches individuals to discriminate between *desired* and *undesired* behavior and can be used to *increase* or *decrease* behavior. There are four types of differential reinforcement. *Differential reinforcement at low rates* (DRL) and *differential reinforcement of zero responding* (DRO) involve the simple decrease or absence of behavior (i.e., decreases or stops talking out in class) (DRL or DRO). *Differential reinforcement of incompatible responding* (DRI) and *differential reinforcement of alternative behavior* (DRA) involve adding an incompatible or alternative behavior to replace the original behavior (i.e., eating a lollipop instead of sucking one's thumb [DRI], rolling cigarettes instead of spending food money on expensive cigarettes [DRA]). Note: Harm reduction programs use forms of differential reinforcement by reinforcing less harmful behaviors that replace more harmful behaviors (e.g., going to a needle exchange program instead of sharing needles to use heroin [DRA], taking Antabuse to decrease alcohol use [DRI]).

Stimulus discrimination learning is the procedure by which an individual can learn to emit a behavior under certain conditions instead of others. For example, children learn to raise their hands to be called on in the classroom if they wish to speak, whereas at the family dinner table, they wait for a pause in the conversation to speak (without raising their hands). In contrast, **stimulus generalization** occurs when a behavior becomes more probable in the presence of one stimulus as a result of being reinforced in the presence of another similar stimulus. For example, a child who has been abused by his father may *generalize his response* to being fearful of all men and demonstrate this fear by avoiding males in general.

Behavioral Techniques: Fading, Shaping, and Chaining

Whereas different types of reinforcement are used to *increase* or *decrease* specific behaviors, *fading*, *shaping*, and *chaining* are behavioral methods used to teach skills that involve *more than one step*.

- **Fading** occurs when prompts or cues that guide the performance of a complex behavior are gradually withdrawn. A *prompt* is a stimulus (physical, verbal, or visual) introduced to control the desired behavior during the early part of a learning program. For example, when Mariana is learning how to swing a golf club, the instructor will first provide hand-over-hand guidance to show Mariana how to hold and swing the club, then will move to using only verbal cues, and next will use fewer and fewer verbal cues until eventually Mariana is swinging the club on her own.
- **Shaping** occurs by reinforcing successively closer approximations to the target behavior while extinguishing preceding approximations of the behavior. For example, when baby Jennifer is learning how to talk and says "Je" when first attempting to say her own name, her parents reinforce her behavior with smiles and verbal praise. With practice, Jennifer next refers to herself as "Jen," then "Jen-fer," and finally as "Jennifer." As Jennifer's pronunciation improves, her parents provide smiles and verbal praise for each improved pronunciation while no longer reinforcing previous versions. For example, once Jennifer learns to say "Jen-fer," she is no longer praised for referring to herself as "Je."

Both fading and shaping involve a gradual change. Fading involves a gradual change in stimulus while the response stays the same. Shaping uses the same stimulus to establish a gradual change in the response.

- **Chaining** is used to teach a complex behavior by reinforcing the performance of each part of the behavior separately, but in order, until the individual can complete the entire sequence.

There are three types of chaining: (1) *Forward chaining* begins with reinforcing the first step and then adding sequential steps while fading the prompts/reinforcers for previous steps as they are learned. Forward chaining is the natural way that you would teach yourself a task that you had to read directions for, such as setting up a new computer system. (2) *Backwards chaining* begins with reinforcing the final step of the complex behavior and then the second-to-last step, and so on, until the behavior is learned. For example, Raisa recently had a cerebrovascular accident (CVA) and needs to learn to feed herself again. You would prepare her food, cut it into pieces, and place her fork correctly in her hand, and then she would complete the

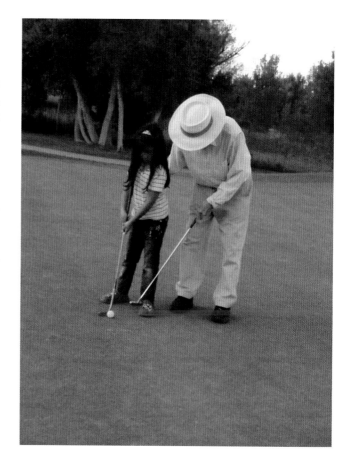

FIGURE 48-1 A great uncle uses backwards chaining to teach his young niece to golf by first reinforcing the final step of putting the golf ball into the hole.

last step: placing the food in her mouth—a natural reinforcement. The advantage of backwards chaining is that it is a natural reinforcer because the task is already completed and sometimes there is less frustration (Figure 48-1). (3) *Total task training* occurs when the individual is asked to attempt to do all the steps from the beginning to the end. Prompting may be provided along the way, and reinforcement is provided following the last step. This method often instills confidence when an individual is relearning a previously learned skill or learning a skill he or she may consider insulting to be taught yet may be necessary for safety or independence evaluations (i.e., dressing, cooking).

Behavior Modification: Assessment and Treatment

There are four phases of a successful behavioral modification program: (1) screening, (2) baseline, (3) treatment, (4) follow-up. Behavioral assessment can be carried out throughout the whole behavioral modification program or during each phase of the program.

Three sources of getting information for the baseline assessment include indirect assessment, direct assessment, and functional assessment. Indirect assessment includes interviews, questionnaires, role-playing, consulting with other professionals, and client self-monitoring.

Direct assessment records the *characteristics* of behaviors that are observed, including (1) *topography*: form of a particular response, (2) *amount*: frequency and duration of the behavior, (3) *intensity* (*force* or *magnitude*), (4) *stimulus control*: a certain behavior occurs in the presence of certain stimuli, (5) *latency*: the time between the occurrence of a stimulus and the beginning of a response, and (6) *quality of behavior*.

Functional assessment is used to identify the *cause* of a problem behavior. There are several approaches to completing a functional assessment including (1) questionnaires, (2) observations: observe and describe the antecedents and immediate consequences of the behavior in natural settings, and (3) functional analysis: directly assesses the effects of controlling variables on the problem behavior. In functional analysis, environmental events are systematically manipulated to test their roles as antecedents or as consequences in controlling and maintaining specific behaviors.

Occupational Therapy and Behaviorist Theory

Occupational therapy practitioners using behaviorist theory to understand human learning and guide their intervention would analyze a complex behavior that needs to be learned (e.g., a child's need to take turns when she plays) and sequence that behavior from simple to complex. Sometimes the process of *learning* a new behavior also involves *extinguishing* a problem behavior. Intervention would consists of opportunities for the person to participate in increasingly complex behaviors, using behaviorist principles such as reinforcement, shaping, and chaining. Progress would be measured by clients' observed occupational performance and their ability to complete increasingly complex behaviors necessary for occupational performance.

Occupational therapy practitioners have used the behavioral theory of learning in several ways to guide their interventions with clients. For example, Giles and Wilson (1988) and Giles, Ridley, Dill, and Frye (1997) described programs to help retrain people who had sustained severe brain injuries. The clients had severe physical and cognitive impairments and needed help with washing and dressing: basic self-care behaviors. The practitioners designed and implemented a program that consisted of individualized plans to break down each larger activity (getting dressed) into its smaller elements. Practitioners used a specific set of instructions to gradually add skills to each

person's repertoire (shaping) and eventually teach the entire behavior.

Katzmann and Mix (1994) presented a case report of a 34-year-old woman with viral encephalitis. The woman had difficulty processing written and verbal information and had great difficulty with various complex self-care tasks. The practitioners' intervention was influenced by behavioral theories, using such techniques as prompting with step-by-step instructions, shaping, and verbal or physical cues. The practitioners identified and sequenced all of the steps required for the woman to complete her washing, dressing, and grooming routine, which began with getting out of bed and ended with going to breakfast in the rehabilitation facility. A series of step-by-step instructions, gradual and consistent shaping of behavior, verbal cues, and physical assistance helped the woman to improve her overall activities of daily living (ADL) functioning. The practitioners used forward chaining by cueing the woman with directions or providing physical assistance for a step that needed to be completed and gradually removed the cues as she initiated and completed the task independently.

Behaviorist theories emphasize observable behavior, rewarding and reinforcing desirable behavior, and reducing problematic behaviors. Clients who might benefit from intervention approaches that are grounded in behaviorist theories of learning include people who have difficulty planning and organizing activities, those who have problems with memory and/or attention, those who have deficits in sequencing activities, and those who demonstrate inappropriate social behaviors. For instance, some strategies that could help a young girl to develop sharing and turn-taking skill include praising appropriate behavior (to provide positive reinforcement for sharing), not giving attention every time she takes toys from others (to decrease the negative reinforcement for the undesired behavior), using a sticker chart to document sharing (to gradually shape appropriate behavior), and providing rewards for good sharing, such as letting her stand first in line to go to the playground.

Social Learning and Social Cognitive Theory

The social learning and social cognitive theory of learning are an outgrowth of behaviorist theories. Theorists such as Piaget (1970) and Bandura (1977b) were dissatisfied with the limits of behaviorist theory because they believed that there was more to learning than just the interaction of a person with the environment. They developed theories of learning that integrated *social* and *cognitive* processes with behavioral processes. Although there are individual variations and areas of focus, in general, social cognitive theory explains learning as occurring in a social context, that is, the "where, what, when, with whom, how often, and under what circumstances" aspects of our lives. Humans learn by observing others, cognitively processing observations, storing those observations and thoughts, and then using them sometimes at a much later time. This is an important contrast with behavioral theorists, who view learning as an observable change in behavior at a specific point in time. Social learning/social cognitive theorists disagree and say that *learning can occur even in the absence of an observable change in behavior* (Ormrod, 2014). Social and cognitive processes such as observation, storing observations in memory, self-assessment, and self-appraisal promote learning. The *interactions* between a person, behavior, and the environment are emphasized.

Five major assumptions are inherent to social learning/social cognitive theory (Ormrod, 2014).

1. *People can learn by observing others.* For example, a college freshman, new to living and eating in a dormitory, may be unfamiliar with a waffle maker available to her in the breakfast line. She might casually watch others make waffles until she feels confident that she knows the process well enough to try it herself.

2. *Learning is an internal process* that may or may not lead to an observable change in behavior. For example, people might observe various social skills, such as how to introduce themselves to someone they meet, how to end a conversation politely, and how to maintain an appropriate social distance during a conversation. These skills might be stored in memory for future use and not be immediately demonstrated.

3. *People are generally motivated to achieve goals for themselves*, and their behavior is typically directed toward those goals.

4. *Learning occurs as people regulate and adjust their own behavior* instead of learning being a direct response to and dependent on environmental stimuli. This means that people would observe others, determine their own individual standards, and then work to behave according to those standards.

5. *Feedback via reinforcement and punishment affect learning and behavior indirectly* (not directly, as behaviorists believe). This means that people can adjust their behavior on the basis of *anticipated* (positive or negative) consequences. Or, people might observe the outcomes of a behavior demonstrated by others and adjust their behaviors on the basis of that observation (Ormrod, 2014). Box 48-2 summarizes these major assumptions.

It is important for a person to observe skills and behaviors via models and to note the reinforcement that models receive for behaviors. Models can be *live* (a person with whom the learner has actual contact) or *symbolic*

> **BOX 48-2   MAJOR ASSUMPTIONS OF SOCIAL COGNITIVE THEORY OF LEARNING**
>
> - People can learn by observing others.
> - Learning is an internal process.
> - People are motivated to achieve goals.
> - People regulate and adjust their own behavior.
> - Reinforcement and punishment may have an indirect effect on behavior.

(a pictorial or abstract representation of behavior, such as through television or other media). Whatever the source, the modeled behavior serves as information for the observer/learner. A person can also learn *vicariously*, increasing or decreasing a given behavior on the basis of the reinforcement that the person observes someone else is receiving (also an indirect form of modeling because the reinforcement is being modeled). For example, if a model's behavior is positively reinforced, the observer might increase that behavior. Other determining factors include how much attention gets paid to the model, how credible or prestigious the model is, and how the model is rewarded (Ormrod, 2014).

Because people can learn by observing others, *attention* to the behavior is a very important factor. A learner is more likely to remember information when the learner consciously attends to the behavior, rehearses it in his or her own mind, and develops personal verbal or visual ways to represent the information (Ormrod, 2015). A person should be able to describe the behavior or have a picture of that behavior in his or her mind, stored for future use.

People develop expectations about what they think will happen as a result of different behaviors. Thus, *incentive* is an important consideration. Incentive is the anticipation that something will happen (reinforcement) if a particular behavior is performed or not performed. This is another difference from behaviorist theory. According to operant conditioning theory, the reinforcement must come after the behavior has been performed. According to social cognitive theory, an anticipated outcome might precede the behavior being performed (or not performed).

Occupational Therapy and Social Learning/Social Cognitive Theory

An OT practitioner working with Jake, a 14-year-old who is having difficulty at school, might have Jake *identify* specific problem situations (e.g., being distracted in class, using minimal effort to complete projects, or becoming bored in class) and then identify specific strategies to address these difficulties (e.g., sitting at the front of the classroom, setting "effort goals" for himself, identifying at least one interesting aspect of any project), *set* manageable and measurable goals, and then *develop* a mechanism to determine how well he has achieved his goals. The OT practitioner might also encourage Jake's teacher to pair him with classmates who demonstrate good study habits and who are highly motivated for learning. Or, the practitioner might role-play conversations that Jake is likely to have with his parents or teachers about his feelings and attitudes toward schoolwork. The role-play conversations could help Jake to articulate his concerns and then work to support his learning.

Kramer and colleagues studied transition age youth with intellectual and developmental disabilities (I/DD) who completed e-mentoring, with a peer mentor with I/DD, during *Project TEAM* (Kramer, Hwang, Helfrich, Samuel, & Carrella, 2018). Peer mentors guided youth through the problem-solving process and shared examples from their own lives in which they identified and resolved physical, social, or sensory environmental barriers. The peer-mentored participants experienced sustained changes in self-determined behavior and had significantly higher goal attainment in comparison to a goal setting intervention that did not include peer mentoring.

Helfrich, Chan, and Sabol (2011) described a life skills intervention in the community for individuals who were homeless using *situated learning*. Situated learning theory, which is derived from social learning theory (Lave & Wenger, 2003), posits that behavior results from interaction between the person and the situation. The learner is placed in contexts that allow for simulated and actual application to everyday situations, whereas peers enhance the learning experience with feedback. In social situations, individuals gain motivational support from others and access both expertise and collaborative thinking, increasing opportunities to acquire and apply new knowledge. This approach allowed group participants functioning at a variety of levels to benefit from others' experiences with the life skills being taught.

Most of these programs emphasize the importance of learning in a social context, providing numerous opportunities for clients to develop or relearn essential skills for living, and employ activities such as role-play, observation, problem solving, and practice in real-life situations.

Constructivist Theory

Suppose you are an OT practitioner working in a community behavioral health center. Your clients are typically recovering from substance abuse or might have chronic mental illness. Part of your intervention includes a series of life skills sessions that are designed to help people learn or relearn different instrumental ADL. A new session will begin next week with five new clients. One segment of your program focuses on time use and leisure planning. Will all five clients come to the course with the same life experiences? Will all five people have the same outlook on life? How might you understand the teaching-learning process, given these individual differences and experiences?

A constructivist would assert that individual differences are to be expected, that "everyone's construction of the world is unique even though we share a great many concepts" (Svinicki, 2004, p. 14). Although there are several "traditional" methods of providing information, such as through imparting information or finding information in books or on the Internet, this does not necessarily indicate or result in learning, according to constructivism. For constructivists, the learner must *access* information, use this information to *alter* or modify existing knowledge and understanding, and *integrate* the new information with previous information to *create* a new understanding that is relevant to himself or herself (Marlowe & Page, 1998). For the life skills challenge posed earlier, a constructivist would embrace the members' different perspectives and perceive them as essential to individual learning. Although this approach may sound very similar to situated learning as described previously, *constructivism* speaks more to the role of the client as an individual learner, responsible for his or her own learning. Situated learning places the role of learning more in the context of an apprenticeship or mentoring model.

There are some basic assumptions about the teaching-learning process that are common to constructivism. First, learners must be *active participants* in their learning. Second, the learner is capable of *creating* his or her own *knowledge* through interaction with the human and nonhuman environment. Third, when learners participate in this type of learning environment, they develop the *ability to think critically* to solve problems. Fourth, when actively engaged in constructing their own knowledge, people *gather information and develop strategies* at the same time (Marlowe & Page, 1998).

Bruner (1961) has had a major influence in the development of constructivism or "discovery" learning. According to Bruner, a constructivist approach fosters *intellectual potency*, meaning that when people seek and find information for themselves, that information is more meaningful, relevant, and powerful for them. Furthermore, people organize information they find for themselves so that it is more efficiently and effectively retrieved for future use. Constructivists call this a *conservation of memory*. Second, because the learners "own" the information, this approach fosters *intrinsic motivation*. Rather than settling into a pattern in which learners conform to what the instructor wants them to learn, learners *discover* for themselves.

BOX 48-3 MAJOR ASSUMPTIONS OF CONSTRUCTIVIST THEORY OF LEARNING

- Learners must be active participants in their learning.
- Learners are capable of discovering and creating their own knowledge.
- Active participation in the learning environment enhances critical thinking and problem-solving abilities.
- In learning, people gather information and develop problem-solving strategies simultaneously.
- Active participation in the learning environment enhances the meaning and relevance of the learning experience and motivation for learning.

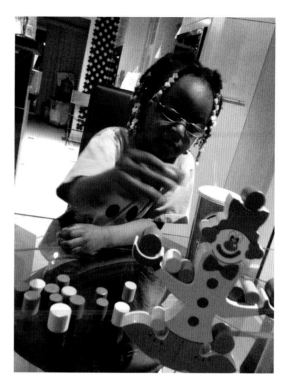

FIGURE 48-2 A young girl actively participates in her own learning by exploring principles of balance through play with blocks of different sizes and weights.

This promotes motivation to learn. Third, the only way to improve one's ability to think, question, and discover is to do it actively and repeatedly—to engage in the process. Constructivism fosters people's learning the *process of discovery*. Box 48-3 summarizes the major assumptions of constructivism.

A practitioner who uses a constructivist approach in the teaching-learning process emphasizes skills and activities such as asking questions, independent exploration, identifying problems, brainstorming, and gene-rating individual solutions to problems. The practitioner emphasizes the *client's essential role in the process* and sees his or her own role as facilitating client's progress. The practitioner views the therapy process as recognizing, embracing, respecting, and encouraging people to develop individual meanings to promote and enhance the client's knowledge and skill.

In this perspective, clients are expected to actively direct what needs to be learned and how the learning will occur. Clients help to determine the resources that will enhance their learning. Independent thinking, collaborative problem solving, and using past experience to reframe and revise new learning are all important. The practitioner's knowledge and expertise are still very essential; however, in this perspective, the practitioner uses his or her knowledge and expertise as a point of reference. In many ways, the practitioner takes a "back seat" as the client pursues learning; the practitioner's role is to address problems that arise. The practitioner facilitates the process, using himself or herself to promote the client's ability to identify, address, and solve problems. The OT practitioner does not provide "the intervention" but instead works to facilitate the person developing his or her own strategies to deal with his or her own issues. The practitioner is alert to major issues but is neither prescriptive nor directive (Lederer, 2001) (Figure 48-2).

PRACTICE DILEMMA 48-1

Constructivist Perspective on Learning

If each person constructs his or her own learning and therefore there is no "objective reality," what challenges does that present to an OT practitioner who advocates a constructivist perspective on learning? What opportunities does it provide to the practitioner and/or to the person with whom the practitioner is working? What are some strategies that you could implement to address clients' time use and leisure skill development in the life skills program described earlier? How would you address this individual's goals in a group setting?

Self-Efficacy Theory

The self-efficacy theory of learning focuses on a person's individual beliefs about how effective he or she is or will be at learning or completing a new skill or behavior. Albert Bandura (1977a) first articulated a theory of self-efficacy. His perspective on how behaviors are learned and changed involved behavioral *and* cognitive processes. His central thesis is that a person's **efficacy expectations**, the person's beliefs about how successful or unsuccessful he or she will be at performing a skill or occupation, will greatly influence his or her execution of that skill or occupation. The emphasis here is on the *person's beliefs* and *how those beliefs influence his or her performance*. For example, a person might believe that a particular action performed or executed by a person *in general* will produce a certain outcome. However, this is different from the person's belief that he or she has the ability to perform the action and that it will result in a successful outcome. A person's efficacy expectations also influence the person's *persistence* with different occupations. "Efficacy expectations determine how much effort people will expend and how long they will persist in the face of obstacles and aversive experiences. The stronger the perceived self-efficacy, the more active the efforts" (Bandura, 1977a, p. 194).

Efficacy expectations have three important dimensions: magnitude, generality, and strength (Bandura, 1977a). *Magnitude* involves the level of difficulty for a task—for example, making a sandwich versus making an elaborate dinner. *Generality* involves the degree to which a person's perceived self-efficacy for one task transfers to another—for example, maneuvering a wheelchair around the OT clinic versus maneuvering a wheelchair in a busy urban community. *Strength* refers to the degree to which people believe they can be successful—for example, being very confident about one's success versus being only slightly confident.

Typically, a person's self-efficacy is developed over time and through four sources of information: outcomes that were generated by the person's own *personal accomplishments*; through *vicarious experience*, that is, seeing others perform a skill and through that vicarious experience believing that "if the other person can accomplish the skill, so can I"; by being *persuaded* by others that the person can be successful; and by *feeling calm and relaxed* when performing a skill (Bandura, 1977a). Given these information sources, the person's *own cognitive appraisal* of how successful or unsuccessful he or she will be has the greatest impact on the person's efficacy expectation.

Although perceived self-efficacy and self-esteem are related, the two concepts are not the same. Perceived self-efficacy is what you believe you can do with your skill. *Self-esteem* refers to a person's negative or positive sense of self. So a person might feel that he or she is competent and successful in completing a variety of occupations but might have an overall negative feeling about himself or herself. Certainly, perceived self-efficacy might contribute to a person's self-esteem, but they are two separate concepts (Gage & Polatajko, 1994).

According to Bandura (1977b), self-efficacy relates to behavior change very directly. If a person has only weak expectations for his or her success, it is likely that unsuccessful experiences will quickly result in the person's not performing the skill or behavior. If the person's beliefs about his or her success are strong, then it is likely that the

person will persist, even through negative or unsuccessful experiences.

Motivational Theory

Motivational theories view change as coming from within the person and his or her motivation to make a change. The most common and well-developed theory is the Transtheoretical Model (TTM) of intentional change, which assesses individuals' readiness to change and measure progress toward goals over the course of an intervention (Brady et al., 1996; Finnell, 2003; J. O. Prochaska, Redding, & Evers, 1997). The theory, developed from the disciplines of psychology and psychotherapy, proposes that a person may progress through five stages of behavior change: precontemplation, contemplation, preparation, action, and maintenance (J. O. Prochaska, 2001; J. O. Prochaska & DiClemente, 1983). The TTM proposes that effective interventions address an individual's present stage of change and cautions that without intervention, individuals may not progress (Finnell, 2003; L. A. Haggerty & Goodman, 2003). The transtheoretical stages of change model has been applied to a variety of health behaviors and systems issues, such as smoking cessation (J. O. Prochaska & DiClemente, 1983), addressing health risk behaviors (Nigg et al., 1999), arthritis self-management (Keefe et al., 2000), organizational change (J. M. Prochaska, Prochaska, & Levesque, 2001), and weight control (Plotnikoff et al., 2009; Sarkin, Johnson, Prochaska, & Prochaska, 2001) (see Chapter 47 for detailed examples). This model has two essential elements: the five integrated stages of change and the various processes that can facilitate a person's moving from one stage to the next.

The stages of change begin with *precontemplation*. Here, a person demonstrates a behavior that is perceived by others as needing to be changed. These behaviors are often harmful or destructive (e.g., a substance use or addiction, poorly controlled anger or stress, or general health and wellness issues). The person might be unaware or minimally aware of his or her problem, or the person might be aware of the problem but resistant to fully acknowledge or address it. In the second stage, *contemplation*, the person is likely to be aware of his or her problem and is thinking about overcoming it but is not quite ready to take action. In the third stage, *preparation*, the person begins to make some small changes in his or her behavior. In the fourth stage, *action*, the person is committed to making the change and is involved in change behaviors on a regular basis. The person is putting forth great energy to modify behaviors, the environment, or his or her experiences to effect serious change. In the fifth stage, *maintenance*, the person struggles to maintain the change, working to sustain accomplishments and prevent relapse (J. O. Prochaska, DiClemente, & Norcross, 1992).

These stages might appear to be linear, occurring in a step-by-step progression from one stage to the next.

However, J. O. Prochaska et al. (1992) explain change as occurring in a spiral fashion because most people experience relapses or other setbacks as they work to change behaviors. In fact, relapse is expected. Relapse can occur back to *any* stage; however, the subsequent progress usually is easier for the individual. Think about a time that you or a friend set out to change a certain behavior and achieved stage 3 (preparation) or stage 4 (action) only to experience some setback and spiral back down to an earlier stage. According to the TTM, this is common and to be expected.

The processes of change explain how to promote the shifts. Because individuals may lack self-efficacy regarding their ability to change, it may be critical to increase the skills needed for change and to allow opportunities to practice change behaviors. According to J. O. Prochaska et al. (1992), people who have reached the contemplation stage are ready to understand the processes that can contribute to behavioral change. Their research indicates that people who are in the precontemplation stage lack the awareness to engage in or benefit from the processes of change. Others (Helfrich, Chan, Simpson, & Sabol, 2012) have disputed this assumption. Their research has demonstrated that people in the precontemplation stage of change may move to the contemplation stage, or yet a higher stage, through the process of being exposed to treatment interventions. The process of introducing the possibility of change may allow an individual to risk changing. People who have progressed to the contemplation stage may benefit from *consciousness-raising* strategies that help them to get information about their problem and themselves, by being encouraged to express their feelings about their problems through various *dramatic relief* strategies such as role-playing, and by *environmental reevaluation* to assess how their behavior affects their physical and social surroundings (e.g., perhaps a person's smoking deters family or friends from visiting or there are stains and cigarette burns on the person's furnishings). Strategies such as values clarification exercises to enhance *self-reevaluation*, or how one thinks and feels about himself or herself, can be helpful as one moves to the preparation stage. Making a real commitment to change, believing in one's ability to change, and using techniques such as personal goal setting to enhance *self-liberation* or will power can be helpful during the action stage. Several processes are important in the maintenance stage, such as fostering *helping relationships* and social supports that encourage the person to be open and honest about his or her problems; avoiding things that elicit the problem behavior and substituting alternatives (*stimulus control* and *counterconditioning*); and *reinforcement management*, rewarding oneself for making changes. *Social liberation* helps to promote change across various stages through advocacy, empowerment, and social change mechanisms (J. O. Prochaska et al., 1992). See Case Study 48-1 for a practice example.

Motivational interviewing (MI) is another clinical process (technique) that encourages people to consider and implement change. "Motivational interviewing is a collaborative conversation style for strengthening a person's own motivation and commitment for change" (Miller & Rollnick, 2013, p. 12). The spirit of MI includes (1) partnership, (2) acceptance, (3) compassion and (4) evocation. The processes used during MI which are both sequential and recursive include (1) engaging, (2) focusing, (3) evoking, and (4) planning (Miller & Rollnick, 2013). Box 48-4 summarizes the processes of MI.

There are five key communication skills that are suggested to implement these principles of MI: (1) asking open questions, (2) affirming, (3) reflective, (4) summarizing, and (5) providing information and advice with permission. In addition, the therapist should always be listening for *change talk* and to elicit the possibility of change talk during conversation with the client. Box 48-5 describes the six themes of change talk.

The key to success for this model is the careful, systematic, and close fit between the person, the stage, and the process. According to J. O. Prochaska et al. (1992), "efficient self-change depends on doing the right things (processes) at the right time (stages)" (p. 1110). Table 48-1 summarizes the stages and processes of change as outlined by J. O. Prochaska et al. (1992).

Occupational Therapy, Self-Efficacy Theory, and Motivational Theory

Both self-efficacy theories and motivational theories have great relevance for OT. Often, a person's self-perceptions and beliefs about his or her ability to be successful with an occupation influence the person's decision about whether to participate in that occupation. For example, a person who believes that he or she has good interview skills will be more likely to respond to a job advertisement even though he or she might not have direct experience with the type of work that needs to be done. A person who did not have that sense of effectiveness might be less likely to pursue the job. Intervention strategies to promote a person's perceived self-efficacy in the job interview situation described here would include determining with the person that he or she had all the requisite skills to be successful, using peer role models so that the person could practice or "try on" the essential skills and behaviors, having the person practice interview skills, providing feedback on specific successes, and encouraging the person to evaluate his or her skills in a personal way rather than comparing these skills to someone else's. These theories all emphasize the importance of an individual's participation in *meaningful* occupations as both the foundation and result of motivation and self-efficacy (Figure 48-3).

CASE STUDY 48-1   OLIVIA: BEHAVIOR CHANGE

Olivia, a 55-year-old woman, has always been severely overweight. Over the years, she has tried many different diets and has joined (and quit) numerous exercise programs and groups. After a recent episode of chest pain, Olivia's health care provider strongly recommended that she participate in organized nutrition, exercise, and overall health-promotion activities.

- How might you help Olivia to understand and reflect on her challenges with health and wellness issues over the years through the transtheoretical perspective?
- What stage might she be at currently?
- How might you help her move from one stage to the next?
- How might you work to minimize any setbacks to the process and remedy those setbacks when they occur?
- How would each theory of learning presented in this chapter be helpful with this case?

Strategies might include the following:

- The OT practitioner would first work with Olivia to help her understand the processes of change. Their work together would include helping Olivia to understand how change occurs, the spiraling nature of change, and the natural, to-be-expected gains and setbacks that occur. The OT practitioner would use counseling and discussion to encourage Olivia's conscious reflection on her behavior and recognition of the different stages of change. Olivia's current stage could be seen as preparation.
- Olivia would be presented with the behaviors she has demonstrated that have contributed to her weight gain and interfered with her weight loss. She would also be presented with the health consequences of those

behaviors. With support, as needed, from the therapist, Olivia would go to the health library and identify the long-term results of not addressing these concerns.

- A variety of intervention strategies, such as personal goal setting, developing social supports, creating a self-reward system for positive change or progress, and evaluation and reevaluation of progress, could be introduced using motivational interviewing techniques. As Olivia applied and practiced these strategies in her life, she could come back to the occupational therapist to problem-solve and revise those that did not work as well as update her self-reward system for those that were successful.
- The OT practitioner would recommend that Olivia participate in a group based on social learning principles so that she could benefit from hearing others' strategies. This type of group would also help to build her self-esteem as she shared her own accomplishments and strategies with others as well. After the group sessions, Olivia would meet individually with the OT practitioner to identify one or two new strategies that she heard to try each week. Olivia would develop a plan, with coaching, as needed from the occupational therapist, to go out and try the new strategy.
- Olivia would also be encouraged to view earlier obstacles or setbacks to change as typical and predictable. When setbacks do occur, the OT practitioner would reinforce the importance of conscious understanding of the spiraling nature of progress, the success of identifying setbacks when they occur, the opportunity to prevent any setback from spiraling too far down, and a return to strategies that were successful in the past or continuing to develop new strategies. The OT practitioner would reinforce the ongoing nature of change and progress.

BOX 48-4   PROCESSES OF MOTIVATIONAL INTERVIEWING

1. *Engaging* involves both establishing a helpful connection and a working relationship. Engaging with the client is essential before change can take place.
2. *Focusing* is the process of developing and maintaining specific direction in the conversation about change. Guiding the client back to the difficult topic of change facilitates progress.
3. *Evoking* involves eliciting the client's own motivation for change. Client's respond better to their own words and reasons for making a change.
4. *Planning* which encompasses both developing commitment to change and formulating a concrete plan of action. The therapist listens for the client to begin identifying solutions and strategies for change and then collaborates with them to develop a concrete plan.

BOX 48-5 SIX THEMES OF CHANGE TALK

1. **Desire:** Verbs include *want*, *like*, and *wish*. These tell you something that the person wants. (i.e., I *wish* I could lose some weight.)
2. **Ability:** The prototypical verb is *can* (*could*). These show you what the person perceives as within his or her ability. (i.e., I *could* probably cut down a bit.)
3. **Reasons:** There are no particular verbs here, but words used always express specific reason for a certain change. (i.e., This pain keeps me from playing the guitar!)
4. **Need:** Marker verbs include *need*, *have to*, *got to*, *should*, *ought*, and *must*. These tell you some necessity. (i.e., I *must* quit smoking.)
5. **Commitment:** Most used verbs are *will*, *intend to*, and *going to*. These can be presented with strong or lower level of commitment. (i.e., I *will* go to Alcoholics Anonymous [AA] group once a month.)
6. **Taking steps:** Reporting recent specific action (step) towards change. (i.e., I quit drinking for a couple of weeks but then started again.)

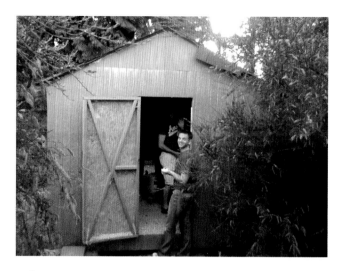

FIGURE 48-3 Two men who work in finance and value sustainability successfully build their own chicken coop to raise chickens and sell eggs, demonstrating self-efficacy and Prochaska's "action" stage of change.

PRACTICE DILEMMA 48-2

Promoting Self-Efficacy

If you are asked to evaluate a man who presents with severe problems with activities of daily living and he self-rates himself as not having a problem (not needing to change his behavior), what do you do? How would you discuss the problem behavior with the individual? Which theories of learning would be most helpful in working with this individual? Would you start with one theory and then shift to another theory at a different point in treatment? How might your approach be different for different diagnoses?

Conclusion

Behaviorist, social cognitive, constructivist, self-efficacy, and motivational theories of learning have great relevance and use for OT practitioners. Table 48-2 summarizes the five different theories of learning that were presented in this chapter and highlights their relevance to OT practice. The information presented in this chapter can be used to influence how you think about the learning needs of patients and clients, to reinforce the importance of designing optimal learning environments, to contribute to your ongoing professional development, and to promote your clients' abilities to achieve their goals.

TABLE 48-1   Stages and Processes of Change

Stage	Process (How to Promote Change)
Precontemplation	Strategies are not effective because the person lacks awareness to engage in or benefit from change.
Contemplation	Consciousness-raising strategies to learn about problem, role-play strategies to express feelings, assessment of how behavior affects physical and social environment
Preparation	Values clarification exercises to promote reevaluation of feelings or self-perception
Action	Goal-setting strategies and techniques
Maintenance	Development of social supports, substitution of alternatives to problem behavior, avoidance of experiences that elicit the problem behavior, rewarding oneself for making changes

TABLE 48-2 Summary Table

Theory	Major Emphases	Application to Occupational Therapy Practice
Behaviorist	• Learned behavior as an observable event (not a mental process) • Behavior is conditioned by the environment. • Environmental response alters subsequent behaviors.	• Analyze and sequence behaviors from simple to complex. • Measure progress as the person completes increasingly complex behaviors. • Use strategies including reinforcement, shaping, and rewards.
Social learning/ social cognitive	• Integrates behavior, social, and cognitive processes • Learning occurs in a social context. • Learning may occur without observable behavior change. • Person regulates and adjusts his or her own behavior.	• Emphasize client learning essential skills for living. • Use role-play, peer observation, role modeling, problem solving, and real-life practice activities to promote learning. • Encourage the client to identify the problem, set goals, develop a plan, evaluate outcomes.
Constructivist	• Learner is an active participant in his or her own learning. • Learner creates/constructs knowledge through past experience and interaction with the environment. • Self-constructed knowledge has great meaning and relevance for the learner. • Self-constructed knowledge promotes the learner's motivation for learning.	• Client actively directs what is to be learned and how learning will occur. • Use strategies including brainstorming, individual problem solving, independent exploration, asking questions. • Occupational therapist facilitates but does not direct the learning process.
Self-efficacy	• Emphasize a person's beliefs about how effective he or she is or will be. • Efficacy expectations influence a person's persistence with an activity. • Efficacy expectations are influenced by the difficulty of the task, how well completing a task transfers to other situations, and the degree to which a person believes that he or she will be successful. • Self-efficacy is developed over time and through experience.	• Personal accomplishment has the greatest effect. • Self-evaluation and personal appraisal are important. • Tasks should be challenging but not overwhelming, should be transferable to other situations. • Vicarious, observation experiences and/or persuasion to enhance the person's beliefs that he or she can be successful are less effective
Motivational	• Learning and change occurs in a spiral fashion. It is not linear. • A person's readiness (desire) for change will influence the outcomes. • Relapses are common and to be expected.	• Intervention processes must match behavior stage. • Intervention processes become increasingly active, self-directed, self-motivated, and self-monitored.

Acknowledgment

We would like to acknowledge Perri Stern for her contributions to the previous edition of this chapter.

REFERENCES

Bandura, A. (1977a). Self-efficacy: Toward a unifying theory of behavioral change. *Psychological Review, 84,* 191–215.

Bandura, A. (1977b). *Social learning theory.* Englewood Cliffs, NJ: Prentice-Hall.

Brady, S., Hiam, C. M., Saemann, R., Humbert, R., Fleming, M. Z., & Dawkins-Brickhouse, K. (1996). Dual diagnosis: A treatment model for substance abuse and major mental illness. *Community Mental Health Journal, 32,* 573–578.

Bruner, J. S. (1961). The act of discovery. *Harvard Educational Review, 31,* 21–32.

Driscoll, M. P. (Ed.). (2005). *Psychology of learning for instruction* (3rd ed.). Boston, MA: Allyn & Bacon.

Finnell, D. S. (2003). Addictions services: Use of the transtheoretical model for individuals with co-occurring disorders. *Community Mental Health Journal, 39,* 3–15.

Fosnot, C. T. (Ed.). (2005). *Constructivism: Theory, perspectives, and practice* (2nd ed.). New York, NY: Teachers College Press.

Gage, M., & Polatajko, H. J. (1994). Enhancing occupational performance through an understanding of perceived self-efficacy. *American Journal of Occupational Therapy, 48,* 452–461.

Giles, G. M. (in press). *2018 Eleanor Clarke Slagle Lecture: Neurocognitive rehabilitation: Skills or strategies?* Manuscript submitted for publication.

Giles, G. M., Ridley, J. E., Dill, A., & Frye, S. C. (1997). A consecutive series of adults with brain injury treated with a washing and dressing retraining program. *American Journal of Occupational Therapy, 51,* 256–266.

Giles, G. M., & Wilson, J. C. (1988). The use of behavioral techniques in functional skills training after severe brain injury. *American Journal of Occupational Therapy, 42,* 658–665.

Haggerty, L. A., & Goodman, L. A. (2003). Stages of change-based nursing interventions for victims of interpersonal violence. *Journal of Obstetric, Gynecologic, and Neonatal Nursing, 32,* 68–75.

Haggerty, M. E. (1918). Where can a woman serve? A big field is open for reconstruction aides. *Carry On, 1*(3), 26–29.

Helfrich, C. A., Chan, D. V., & Sabol, P. (2011). Cognitive predictors of life skill intervention outcomes for adults with mental illness at risk for homelessness. *American Journal of Occupational Therapy,* 65, 277–286. doi:10.5014/ajot.2011.001321

Helfrich, C. A., Chan, D. V., Simpson, E., & Sabol, P. (2012). Readiness-to-change cluster profiles among adults with mental illness who were homeless participating in a life skills intervention. *Community Mental Health Journal,* 48, 673–681. doi:10.1007/s10597-011-9383-z

Hergenhahn, B. R. (1976). *An introduction to theories of learning.* Englewood Cliffs, NJ: Prentice Hall.

Katzmann, S., & Mix, C. (1994). Improving functional independence in a patient with encephalitis through behavior modification shaping techniques. *American Journal of Occupational Therapy,* 48, 259–262.

Keefe, F. J., Lefebvre, J. C., Kerns, R. D., Rosenberg, R., Beaupre, P., Prochaska, J., . . . Caldwell, D. S. (2000). Understanding the adoption of arthritis self-management: Stages of change profiles among arthritis patients. *Pain,* 87, 303–313.

Kramer, J., Hwang, I., Helfrich, C., Samuel, P., & Carrellas, A. (2018). Evaluating the social validity of Project TEAM: A problem-solving intervention to teach transition age youth with developmental disabilities to resolve environmental barriers. *International Journal of Disability, Development and Education,* 65, 57–75.

Lave, J., & Wenger, E. (2003). *Situated learning: Legitimate peripheral participation.* Cambridge, United Kingdom: Cambridge University Press.

Lederer, J. M. (2001). The application of constructivism to concepts of occupation using a group process approach. *Occupational Therapy in Health Care,* 13, 81–93.

Marlowe, B. A., & Page, M. L. (1998). *Creating and sustaining the constructivist classroom.* Thousand Oaks, CA: Corwin Press/Sage.

Martin, G., & Pear, J. (2015). *Behavior modification: What it is and how to do it* (10th ed.). New York, NY: Routledge.

McDaniel, M. L. (1968). Occupational therapists before World War II (1917–1940). In R. S. Anderson, H. S. Lee, & M. L. McDaniel (Eds.), *Army Medical Specialist Corps* (pp. 69–97). Washington, DC: Office of the Surgeon General, Department of the Army.

Miller, W. R., & Rollnick, S. (Eds.). (2013). *Motivational interviewing: Helping people change* (3rd ed.) New York, NY: Guilford Press.

Nigg, C. R., Burbank, P. M., Padula, C., Dufresne, R., Rossi, J. S., Velicer, W. F., . . . Prochaska, J. O. (1999). Stages of change across ten health risk behaviors for older adults. *Gerontologist,* 39, 473–482.

Ormrod, J. E. (2014). *Educational psychology: Developing learners* (8th ed.). Upper Saddle River, NJ: Prentice Hall.

Ormrod, J. E. (2015). *Human learning: Principles, theories and educational applications* (7th ed.). New York, NY: Macmillan.

Piaget, J. (1970). Piaget's theory. In P. H. Mussen (Ed.), *Carmichael's manual of child psychology* (3rd ed., 703–732). New York, NY: Wiley.

Plotnikoff, R. C., Hotz, S. B., Johnson, S. T., Hansen, J. S., Birkett, N. J., Leonard, L. E., & Flaman, L. M. (2009). Readiness to shop for low-fat foods: A population study. *Journal of the American Dietetic Association,* 109, 1392–1397.

Prochaska, J. M., Prochaska, J. O., & Levesque, D. A. (2001). A transtheoretical approach to changing organizations. *Administration and Policy in Mental Health,* 28, 247–261.

Prochaska, J. O. (2001). Treating entire populations for behavior risks for cancer. *Cancer Journal,* 7, 360–368.

Prochaska, J. O., & DiClemente, C. C. (1983). Stages and processes of self-change of smoking: Toward an integrative model of change. *Journal of Consulting and Clinical Psychology,* 51, 390–395.

Prochaska, J. O., DiClemente, C. C., & Norcross, J. C. (1992). In search of how people change. Applications to addictive behaviors. *American Psychologist,* 47, 1102–1114.

Prochaska, J. O., Redding, C. A., & Evers, K. E. (1997). The transtheoretical model and stages of change. In K. Glanz, F. M. Lewis, & B. K. Rimer (Eds.), *Health behavior and health education: Theory, research, and practice* (2nd ed., pp. 60–80). San Francisco, CA: Jossey-Bass.

Round Table on Training Courses. (1923). Round table on training courses. *Archives of Occupational Therapy,* 2(2), 119–132.

Sarkin, J. A., Johnson, S. S., Prochaska, J. O., & Prochaska, J. M. (2001). Applying the transtheoretical model to regular moderate exercise in an overweight population: Validation of a stages of change measure. *Preventive Medicine,* 33, 462–469.

Svinicki, M. D. (2004). *Learning and motivation in the postsecondary classroom.* Bolton, MA: Anker.

Upham, E. G. (1918). *Training of teachers for occupational therapy for the rehabilitation of disabled soldiers and sailors.* Washington, DC: Government Printing Office.

thePoint® *For additional resources on the subjects discussed in this chapter, visit* http://thePoint.lww.com/Willard-Spackman13e.

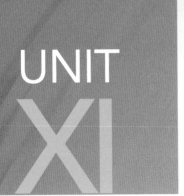

UNIT XI

Evaluation, Intervention, and Outcomes for Occupations

The Question

I walk into the room, say hello with a smile.

The patient is weak. She's been sick for a while.

She squints at my nametag. I give her my name.

I tell her my title. Her question's the same.

What is "Occupation"? Why is it therapy?

How will it help me get well . . . like I want to be?

I say: Occupation is life, the essence of you.

You become who you are by what you consistently do.

The tasks that you do, we call occupation.

They differ with age and your life's situation.

Occupations are work, self-care, and play.

The tasks that you do that fill up each day.

The tasks that you do, your routines and roles:

They define who you are. They help accomplish your goals.

Occupations bring meaning, control, sense of self,

Things you can't find on a pharmacy shelf.

Good health can't be purchased by buying a pill.

Health is built day by day with your hands, mind, and will.

If you want to get well and become a new you,

Wellness is earned by what you consistently do.

No matter your age or your life's situation,

Engage and live fully.

Life is occupation.

—Randy Hollman, MS, OTR/L

Reprinted with permission from
OT Reflections from the heart: The question.
OT Practice, August 7, 2017, p. 32

Introduction to Evaluation, Intervention, and Outcomes for Occupations

Glen Gillen, Barbara A. Boyt Schell

LEARNING OBJECTIVES

After reading this chapter, you will be able to:

1. Understand classification systems used to discuss areas of occupation.
2. Appreciate the complexity of occupation and the potential difficulties in applying these classification systems.

Categories of Occupation

As occupational therapists, we consider the many types of occupations in which clients engage across the course of the day. These occupations fall under the category of **activities** and **participation** in the World Health Organization's (WHO, 2001) *International Classification of Functioning, Disability, and Health* (ICF). The WHO (2001) defines *activity* as "the execution of a task or action by an individual" and participation as "involvement in a life situation" (p. 123). Furthermore, they define the term **activity limitations** as "difficulties an individual may have in executing activities" and **participation restrictions** as "problems an individual may experience in involvement in life situations" (WHO, 2001, p. 123). Within the ICF, the domains for the Activities and Participation component are presented as a single list that covers the full range of life areas. Examples of included areas are mobility, self-care, domestic life, interpersonal interactions, major life areas (e.g., education, work, economic life), communication, etc.

Occupational therapy (OT) classification systems typically sort the broad ranges of activities or occupations into categories called **areas of occupation**. There is no standardized classification system, and these areas of occupation have been categorized and classified in a variety of ways. For example, the Canadian Occupational Performance Measure (Law et al., 2014), which is a standardized measure of occupational performance, uses a three-category system of self-care, productivity, and leisure. On the other hand, the American Occupational Therapy Association (AOTA, 2014) categorizes these areas of occupation as eight kinds of life activities in which people, populations, or organizations engage. Because the AOTA categories for the areas of occupation are used as the basis for the major chapters in this unit, they are briefly described here, using the AOTA Practice Framework (AOTA, 2014) as the primary source. Readers are referred to the chapters themselves for more in-depth definitions and discussions about each category of occupations.

Activities of Daily Living

Activities of daily living (ADL) are activities that focus on caring for one's body and which are directed toward basic survival. Examples include bathing, grooming, dressing, swallowing/eating, feeding, functional mobility, sexual activity, personal device care, etc.

Instrumental Activities of Daily Living

Instrumental activities of daily living (IADL) are grouping of activities that also are necessary for daily life but which go beyond basic bodily care and survival. They typically involve a broader context, including family and community. A variety of activities are categorized as IADL including child rearing, pet care, financial management, religious and spiritual activities, meal preparation, shopping, and home management.

Education

Educational occupations are focused on formal and informal learning. Examples include formal educational participation (academic, nonacademic, extracurricular, and vocational participation), informal personal educational needs or interest explorations, and informal personal education participation.

Work

The category of work includes productive activities such as work and volunteer activities. It includes employment interests and pursuits, employment seeking and acquisition, job performance, retirement preparation and adjustment, volunteer exploration, and volunteer participation.

Play and Leisure

Play and leisure are activities that are characterized by enjoyment or diversion, and which typically arise out of interests and motivation of the person, as opposed to social obligation or survival requirements. This grouping encompasses play exploration and play participation, and it includes both leisure exploration and participation.

Rest and Sleep

The activities associated with rest and sleep are more recently included in the AOTA Practice Framework, in recognition of the role they play in supporting all other occupational functioning. Beyond rest and sleep, this area of occupation also includes sleep preparation and sleep participation. Examples include bedtime routines, ability to manage cues for waking such as the use of wake-up signals, as well as the management of the physical environment for comfort and safety. Occupations in this category may include negotiating the needs and requirements of others within the social environment such as sleep partners and children.

Social Participation

Social participation refers to the interweaving of occupations to support desired engagement in community and family activities as well as those involving peers and friends.

Cautions about Categorization

Personal Perspectives

An important consideration when using any classification system to guide evaluation and intervention is to fully understand the way that the person engaging in the occupation perceives the particular activity. For instance, making a meal may be considered work to a busy parent who sees it as part of his or her "job" as a parent to feed the family. Individuals who live by themselves or who take responsibility for this occupation as a part of family chores may consider meal preparation an IADL. Others may classify meal preparation as a leisure activity because it may help them to relax or decrease their stress levels. A chef in a restaurant is most likely to classify meal preparation as work. Finally, meal preparation may be considered under the heading of Social Participation. Examples include participating in a weekly neighborhood soup kitchen to serve meals to the homeless or being part of a group of friends or family engaged in making a holiday feast. Care of pets is another of many other examples that to consider. Depending on one's perspective, this may be considered as an IADL, as part of leisure/play, or as work for someone employed as a part-time dog walker (Figure 49-1).

Occupational Blends versus Categories

Some occupational scientists suggest that rather than trying to classify occupations into discrete categories, it might be more helpful to consider the relative mix within a particular activity. For example, someone who loves his or her job may have parts of the job that really feel like work, parts that are fun and feel like play, and parts that

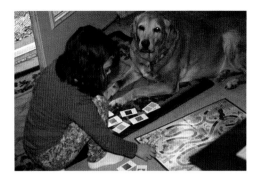

FIGURE 49-1 In this picture, the child is hard at work playing . . . but is the dog resting or playing? Or both? Or perhaps engaged in child care?

feel like IADL, such as using a calendar to coordinate work and home life. Indeed, in her paper "Work and Leisure: Transcending the Dichotomy," Primeau (1996) cites the work of Csikszentmihalyi (1975) who was an early challenger of the work versus leisure dichotomy: "One way to reconcile this split is to realize that work is not necessarily more important than play and play is not necessarily more enjoyable than work" (p. 202). Thus, client-centered care relies in part on the practitioner seeking to understand clients' particular perspective on their daily occupations in order to avoid incorrect assumptions.

Attention to Scope and Detail

In her discussion of using broad categories to classify occupations, Hasselkus (2006) expressed concern that we as OT practitioners " . . . risk losing sight of the unique contexts and individual small behaviors of everyday life and everyday occupation that make up those sweeping categories" (p. 629). However, a positive aspect of having a variety of classification systems is that it serves as a reminder to OT practitioners to inquire and evaluate a person's occupational engagement as a whole. Too often, OT may be overfocused on an occupation of particular interest in that setting. For instance, in medical rehabilitation, there is a strong focus on self-care retraining. We need to always reflect that our scope is much greater and holistic. As far back as 1995, Radomski reminded us that "there is more to life than putting on your pants" (p. 487). Likewise, in school-based practice, the need in the United States to justify services to be educationally related does not preclude the importance of appreciating that a child engages in a range of occupations during a school day and goes home to even more with his or her family.

Client Values and Choice

It is of critical importance to understand the value that our clients place on chosen occupations. Although self-care

may be important and valued by many clients, exclusive focus on this area of occupation may not serve our clients well in terms of giving them the ability to engage in occupations that are considered quality-of-life changers. For one client, this may be focused on regaining the ability to drive, for another to be able to interact with grandchildren, for another to access e-mail via the Internet, and for another to feed himself or herself independently. The OT profession has discussed the importance of client-centered care and client-centered assessment for more than two decades. A continued emphasis on this aspect of care will assure that we are truly collaborating with our clients and placing our therapy focus on meaningful client-chosen occupations regardless of how they might be classified.

Orchestrating Life

Finally, practitioners must not only consider specific occupations and engagement in occupations but also understand how clients orchestrate their engagement over time and within various environments (Molineux, 2007). Many of our clients are required to engage in multiple occupations at the same time, alternate back and forth between occupations based on changing priorities. They must organize and sequence occupations into a routine, which is satisfactory to themselves and those important to them. This may require that they balance participation in an array of occupations in a variety of familiar and unfamiliar contexts.

No Simple Hierarchies

The chapters that follow in this unit place specific focus on evaluating and intervening to maximize participation in specific categories of areas of occupation. Readers are cautioned that the order of presentation of these topics does not represent a hierarchy. New practitioners may wrongly assume that basic ADL are foundational skills and that clients must gain competence in these before tackling other areas. However, both clinical experience and current research suggests that other activities such as making a hot beverage or hand washing dishes may be much easier as compared to upper body grooming and total body dressing, depending on the patterns of performance skill abilities and limitations that a client presents with (Fisher & Jones, 2012).

Conclusion

In summary, the domain of OT is best described as "achieving health, well-being, and participation in life through engagement in occupation" (AOTA, 2014, p. S4). Knowledge gained from this unit should give the readers a range of therapy options to help our clients engage in their chosen occupations, maximize our clients' ability to participate fully, and assure satisfaction with the care we provide.

 Visit thePoint to watch a video about evaluation and interventions.

REFERENCES

American Occupational Therapy Association. (2014). Occupational therapy practice framework: Domain and process (3rd ed.). *American Journal of Occupational Therapy, 68,* S1–S48.

Csikszentmihalyi, M. (1975). *Beyond boredom and anxiety: Experiencing flow in work and play.* San Francisco, CA: Jossey-Bass.

Fisher, A. G., & Jones, K. B. (2012). *Assessment of motor and process skills: Development, standardization, and administration manual* (7th ed., Rev ed.). Fort Collins, CO: Three Star Press.

Hasselkus, B. R. (2006). The world of everyday occupation: Real people, real lives. *American Journal of Occupational Therapy, 60,* 627–640.

Law, M., Baptiste, S., Carswell, A., McColl, M. A., Polatajko, H., & Pollock, N. (2014). *Canadian Occupational Performance Measure* (5th ed.). Ottawa, Canada: Canadian Association of Occupational Therapists.

Molineux, M. (2007). The occupational careers of men living with HIV infection in the United Kingdom: Insights into engaging in and orchestrating occupations. *Australian Occupational Therapy Journal, 54,* 85.

Primeau, L. A. (1996). Work and leisure: Transcending the dichotomy. *American Journal of Occupational Therapy, 50,* 569–577.

Radomski, M. V. (1995). There is more to life than putting on your pants. *American Journal of Occupational Therapy, 49,* 487–490.

World Health Organization. (2001). *International classification of functioning, disability, and health.* Geneva, Switzerland: Author.

thePoint® *For additional resources on the subjects discussed in this chapter, visit* **http://thePoint.lww.com** **/Willard-Spackman13e.**

CHAPTER 50

Activities of Daily Living and Instrumental Activities of Daily Living

Anne Birge James, Jennifer S. Pitonyak

LEARNING OBJECTIVES

After reading this chapter, you will be able to:

1. Describe the purposes of an occupational therapy activities of daily living (ADL) and instrumental activities of daily living (IADL) evaluation.
2. Given a case, identify client and contextual factors that would influence the evaluation plan.
3. Develop client-centered goals that will drive the intervention process.
4. Describe contextual considerations that influence goal development.
5. Explain the most common approaches to ADL and IADL intervention.
6. Describe the role of client and caregiver education in intervention of ADL and IADL impairments.
7. Grade intervention activities to progress clients toward increased participation in ADL and IADL.

Introduction

This chapter focuses on the occupational therapy (OT) process for occupations that are classified as activities of daily living (ADL) and instrumental activities of daily living (IADL) in the Occupational Therapy Practice Framework: Domain and Process, 3rd edition (OTPF) (American Occupational Therapy Association [AOTA], 2014). Dysfunctions in ADL and IADL are termed *activity limitations* in the *International Classification of Functioning, Disability, and Health* (ICF) framework (World Health Organization, 2002). Evaluation and intervention of ADL and IADL dysfunction are central to individuals' participation in meaningful occupation. Individuals may value ADL and IADL as meaningful in and of themselves and as prerequisite tasks to meaningful engagement in education, work, play, leisure, and social participation.

Definition of Activities of Daily Living and Instrumental Activities of Daily Living

Conceptually, the term **activities of daily living** could apply to all activities that individuals perform routinely. In the OTPF, however, ADL are defined more narrowly as "activities oriented toward taking care of one's own body" (AOTA, 2014, p. S41), which include nine activity categories: bathing/showering, toileting and toilet hygiene, dressing, swallowing/eating, feeding, functional mobility, personal device care, personal hygiene and grooming, and sexual activity. **Instrumental activities of daily living** are defined as "activities that support daily life within the home and community and that often require more complex interactions than those used in ADL" (AOTA, 2014, p. S43). The IADL include 12 activity categories: care of others, care of pets, child rearing, communication management, driving and community mobility, financial management, health management and maintenance, home establishment and management, meal preparation and cleanup, religious and spiritual activities and expression, safety and emergency maintenance, and shopping.

The OTPF's (AOTA, 2014) definitions of ADL and IADL are consistent with those of the National Center for Health Statistics (2009); however, other health care practitioners or occupational therapists outside the United States might use other terms to refer to these same ADL and IADL concepts or use the same terms but define them differently. For example, some define ADL more broadly, referring to activities performed in daily life (e.g., Archenholtz & Dellhag, 2008). Other terms that are used to refer specifically to functional mobility and personal care are *basic ADL* and *personal ADL* (AOTA, 2014). The term *instrumental activities of daily living* appears outside the OT literature in a less consistent way. Measures of IADL vary considerably according to the activities that are included in the scales (Chong, 1995); for example, the Nottingham Extended ADL Scale includes leisure activities, tasks that fall outside the OTPF definition of IADL (das Nair, Moreton, & Lincoln, 2011). The crucial point is to understand that terms that refer to daily activities are used in variable ways, so it is important to look for operational definitions of terms used by authors and to find out the conventional language used by practitioners.

This chapter focuses on the evaluation and intervention of occupational performance limitations specifically related to ADL and IADL as defined by the OTPF. It is essential to have a fundamental understanding of the OT process before reading this chapter; the process is described in Chapter 27. The reader should be aware that ADL and IADL, although often a primary focus of OT practice, do not typically represent the full complement of occupational performance tasks needed for satisfying and meaningful participation in individual and societal roles. Evaluation and intervention should always begin with a comprehensive occupational profile (AOTA, 2014). Intervention should address all of the client's priorities, which will typically extend beyond ADL and IADL, although the rest of this chapter focuses exclusively on ADL and IADL.

Evaluation of Activities of Daily Living and Instrumental Activities of Daily Living

Evaluation refers to the overall process of gathering and interpreting data needed to plan intervention, including developing an evaluation plan, implementing the data collection, interpreting the data, and documenting the evaluation results (AOTA, 2015). **Assessment** refers to the specific method or tools that are used to collect data, which is one component of the evaluation process (AOTA, 2015). Standardized assessment methods are referred to as *assessment tools* or *instruments*. The evaluation is carried out by an occupational therapist. An OT assistant may participate in administering selected assessments under the supervision of an occupational therapist who is responsible for interpreting assessment data for use in intervention planning.

The ADL/IADL evaluation is discussed in two stages in this chapter: (1) planning the evaluation, which includes selecting specific assessment methods, and (2) implementing the evaluation, which includes gathering assessment data, making critical observations, generating hypotheses, and performing ongoing revision of the evaluation plan until adequate data have been collected. Keep in mind that ADL and IADL evaluation is only one part of a more comprehensive OT evaluation.

Evaluation Planning: Selecting the Appropriate Activities of Daily Living and Instrumental Activities of Daily Living Assessments

Occupational therapists can choose from various ADL and IADL assessments designed to meet the varied needs of clients and intervention settings. Selecting an appropriate assessment will facilitate optimal intervention planning and can be initiated by following these steps:

1. Identify the overall purpose(s) of the evaluation.
2. Have clients identify their needs, interests, and perceived difficulties with ADL and/or IADL as part of the occupational profile.
3. Further explore the client's relevant activities so that the activities are operationally defined.
4. Estimate client factors that affect occupational performance and/or the assessment process.
5. Identify contextual features that affect assessment.
6. Consider features of assessment tools.
7. Integrate the information from steps 1 to 6 to select optimal ADL and IADL assessments.

Although these steps appear to follow a linear progression, in practice, the steps become integrated because the occupational therapist continually blends knowledge and experience with information from and about the client.

Step 1: Identify the Purpose of the ADL/IADL Evaluation

The ADL and IADL may be evaluated for different purposes. At the level of individual client care, evaluation may be done to assess activity limitations to plan OT intervention or to facilitate decision making concerning discharge environment, competency, conservatorship, and/or involuntary commitment. At the programmatic level, evaluation may be done to document the need for program development and to appraise outcomes. The occupational therapist must determine how the information will be used so that appropriate and sufficient data are obtained.

Evaluation to Plan and Monitor Occupational Therapy Interventions.
When an evaluation is conducted to plan OT intervention, certain types of data are needed to establish a client's baseline performance (Dunn, 2017). First, occupational performance deficits need to be identified so that intervention can focus on tasks that are dysfunctional while simultaneously maintaining and enhancing those that are functional. Second, data are needed about the cause or causes of the activity limitation. For example, a limitation in cooking might be caused by low vision, a kitchen that is not wheelchair accessible, or poor motivation to cook. Occupational therapy intervention to increase independence in cooking is different for each of these causes. To understand the etiology of an activity limitation in ADL or IADL, data about occupational performance needs to be supplemented with data about the client's performance patterns and skills, client factors, activity demands, and contexts (Dunn, 2017). Third, the OT evaluation should provide practitioners with

possibilities for modifying the client's activity performance. Information about the activity demands and context should include consideration of which aspects might be modifiable to support performance and which features cannot be changed. The potential to change performance patterns and skills or client factors must also be assessed. Interventions that involve skill acquisition are feasible for some clients, depending on the cause of the problem. For example, a child with impaired balance secondary to cerebral palsy may have the potential to increase balance to support participation across several ADL and IADL, whereas a person with similar deficits from Parkinson disease might not because the disorder is progressive. All three types of data (performance deficit, underlying causes, and potential for change) are needed to devise adequate intervention plans.

Evaluation to Facilitate Decision Making about Eligibility or Discharge Environment.
Clients may also be referred for evaluation of ADL and IADL to facilitate decision making about eligibility or discharge environment. The ability to care for oneself and one's home can make the difference between independent and supported or assisted living. Supported living represents a continuum of options that includes in-home services (e.g., chore services), assisted living centers, group homes, supervised apartments, long-term care facilities, and more. Varied levels of support are offered within these settings to maintain or enhance daily living skills. When ADL and IADL are evaluated to inform eligibility or discharge decisions, the evaluation may be less comprehensive than those for planning individual interventions. The primary question to be answered is "Does the client meet the functional criteria for the discharge environment?"

A somewhat similar evaluation objective occurs when OT practitioners are asked to make recommendations regarding legal competence for independent living. This usually involves competence in caring for oneself or managing one's property. **Guardianship** is a legal association in which a protected individual's personal affairs are managed by one or more people or an agency. **Conservatorship** is a legal relationship, like guardianship, but is limited to managing the protected individual's financial affairs and property (Moye, 2005). Evaluation may also be requested in conjunction with involuntary commitments to psychiatric facilities to appraise the influence of psychiatric status on daily living. When competence is used in the legal sense, the capacity to make judicious or responsible decisions usually takes precedence over the capacity to perform activities. Individuals who have the ability to procure services and supervise caregivers in managing their personal care and living situation are viewed as competent, even though they might not be able to perform these activities themselves. Thus, OT evaluations that are conducted with guardianship, conservatorship, or involuntary commitment in mind must take into account the decisional capacities and supervisory skills needed by clients.

Evaluation for Programmatic Uses. Although this chapter emphasizes evaluation for individual client care, it is important to recognize that data gathered about clients may be aggregated for programmatic purposes (Law & MacDermid, 2017). For example, data about the ADL and IADL characteristics of clients who are served in an OT clinic can be used to document the extent of particular activity limitations and to support the development of new or expanded programs to manage them. In the current health care climate of cost-effectiveness and cost containment, health professionals must provide evidence for the effectiveness of their programs (Radia-George, Imms, & Taylor, 2014). Occupational therapy practitioners are often expected to measure and document ADL and IADL data consistently across clients so that they can be used effectively for program evaluation, such as the Uniform Data System for Medical Rehabilitation that is used by 70% of rehabilitation facilities in the United States (Galloway et al., 2013).

Step 2: Have Clients Identify Their Needs, Interests, and Perceived Difficulties with ADL/IADL

Once the purpose of the ADL/IADL evaluation has been determined, the occupational therapist must identify the specific activities to be evaluated. This is *one* component of the occupational profile, which will also encompass other aspects of occupational performance, including education, play, leisure, work, and social participation (AOTA, 2014). Developing the client's occupational profile is a crucial step in a client-centered evaluation by discovering the ADL and IADL problems of concern to the *client* (Law & Baum, 2017). Practitioners can expect the priorities to vary significantly for a 10-year-old elementary school student, a 29-year-old homemaker with young children, and a 49-year-old business executive; the client evaluations need to be tailored to take clients' lifestyle differences into account. It is easy to make assumptions about a client's priorities based on both clinical and personal experience and values; however, it is important to remember that unique circumstances may affect clients' ADL or IADL priorities for intervention. Clients' perception of their ADL and IADL problems, needs, and goals can be gathered through a semistructured interview process or through a more formal assessment, such as the Canadian Occupational Performance Measure (COPM) (Law et al., 2014), Occupational Performance History Interview II (Kielhofner et al., 2004), or Perceived Efficacy and Goal Setting System (Vroland-Nordstrand, Eliasson, Jacobsson, Johansson, & Krumlinde-Sundholm, 2015).

Step 3: Further Explore Clients' Relevant Activities So That the Activities Are Operationally Defined

The nature of the tasks that make up selected ADL and IADL can vary in relevance and meaning among individuals. For example, negotiating social services (affordable housing, accessible transportation, etc.) is a part of the daily routine for some persons with disabilities that is not encompassed in usual definitions of ADL and IADL activities (Magasi, 2012). In order to understand the process of negotiating social services and what activities this entails, the practitioner may need to engage in interprofessional collaboration with a case manager, social worker, or others who support clients in this process. Therefore, before activities can be evaluated, they must have an operational definition; that is, the OT practitioner and client must be clear on the precise nature of each task. For example, meal preparation for a middle school student might consist of making cereal for breakfast and packing a lunch, whereas meal preparation for a homemaker feeding a family of five involves many food preparation tasks and a very different set of skills. Assessment tools may define activities differently, so it is important to select an instrument that is congruent with activities as defined by the client. For example, in assessing feeding, clients are rated "independent" on the Barthel Index if they can feed themselves, which includes cutting up food and spreading butter on bread (Mahoney & Barthel, 1965). Clients are rated as "needing assistance" if they can get food from the plate to the mouth but need help cutting food into bite-sized pieces. The Katz Index of ADL, however, does not include preparation of food on the plate (e.g., cutting and spreading butter on bread) in the operational definition of feeding, so clients are rated independent if they can get food from the plate to the mouth, even if they cannot cut food or butter bread (Katz, Ford, Moskowitz, Jackson, & Jaffe, 1963). Many adolescents and adults would be dissatisfied with their feeding performance if their food had to be cut or their bread buttered by another person, so the Katz Index of ADL would not be an appropriate measure for these individuals.

Occupational therapy practitioners also need to consider relevant performance parameters when planning an evaluation. Performance parameters include independence, safety, and adequacy. Operational definitions of acceptable ADL and IADL performance should include attention to all relevant parameters in order to establish appropriate baseline data and intervention outcomes.

Level of Independence. Although clients often wish to be independent in ADL and IADL, practitioners should not make this assumption because some level of assistance, either verbal or physical, might be acceptable. For example, many clients who undergo total hip replacements must follow movement precautions for 2 months that make it impossible to don shoes and socks independently without adaptive equipment. A person who lives with others might prefer to have temporary assistance rather than purchasing and using adaptive equipment. As long they have someone who is willing and able to assist, a goal for assisted lower extremity dressing is perfectly appropriate, and intervention may focus on making sure that the client and caregiver can complete the task together while adhering to total hip precautions. Independence is the performance parameter that is the focus of most assessment tools, so occupational therapists can select from various assessment tools that measure independence.

Safety. Many assessment tools address safety indirectly by specifying that performance be completed in a safe manner in order to be rated as independent (e.g., the Functional Independence Measure [FIM™]; Centers for Medicare & Medicaid Services, 2018). Some tools do not address safety directly (e.g., the Katz Index of ADL; Katz et al., 1963), and a few rate safety separately from independence (e.g., the Performance Assessment of Self-Care Skills; Chisholm, Toto, Raina, Holm, & Rogers, 2014). When safety is a particular concern, for example, with clients who have cognitive deficits that impair judgment, a separate measure of safety can be more effective for documenting progress toward goals and making it clear in the OT documentation that safety has been addressed.

Adequacy. Clients may have criteria regarding the efficiency of task performance and the acceptability of the outcome of the performance, and these should be considered in selecting assessment tools. For example, a client might be safe and independent in lower body dressing but deem her performance inefficient because it takes her an hour to complete the task and she ends up too exhausted to work, or a client might be independent and safe in feeding himself but finds his performance outcome unacceptable because he drops food onto his clothing at each meal and does not wish to wear a bib, especially when eating with others. An assessment tool that measures only independence and safety makes it hard to justify intervention in either of these examples because both clients were safe and independent. There are, however, occupational performance problems that warrant intervention; that is, decreasing the time needed to complete lower body dressing or eliminating food spilled on clothing during eating. Adequacy parameters to consider in ADL and IADL performance include perceived difficulty, pain, fatigue, dyspnea (shortness of breath), societal standards, satisfaction, aberrant behaviors, and past experience with the activity. Practitioners must keep in mind that independence might not be the only important performance parameter to assess in the OT evaluation.

Step 4: Estimate the Client Factors That Affect ADL/IADL and the Assessment Process

One purpose of the ADL/IADL evaluation is to provide insight into the problems underlying occupational performance deficits. However, some estimate of these deficits prior to the assessment can help the occupational therapist to select the assessment tools that will be most effective in identifying and documenting occupational performance problems and the underlying deficits. Occupational therapists use their knowledge of pathology and how it affects occupational performance when selecting assessment tools. For example, some instruments rely on self-report, which is a very efficient way to gather information about a wide range of activities. However, self-reported measures could be inaccurate if the client has cognitive deficits (e.g., a person with Alzheimer disease), distorted thought functions (e.g., a person with schizophrenia), or little experience with the disorder (e.g., a teenager who sustained a spinal cord injury with tetraplegia just 5 days earlier). Additionally, insight into clients' underlying problems will be enhanced by actually seeing the client attempt to perform tasks rather than relying on a description of the problem. For example, a client who has had a stroke might report that he or she is unable to reach items stored above chest height with his or her affected hand, but the OT practitioner gains valuable information for intervention planning by observing the client reaching into cabinets and using skilled observation to see if the movement problem is due to limitations in movement of the scapula, glenohumeral joint, or elbow or some combination of the three.

Knowledge of underlying pathology and anticipated impairments also enables occupational therapists to select appropriate assessment tools that are designed for specific diagnostic groups, focusing on activities that are more commonly problematic for that population. For example, the Arthritis Impact Measurement Scale was developed for adults with rheumatic diseases and includes not only measures of ADL and IADL performance but also symptoms that are commonly experienced by people with arthritis during or following activities, such as pain and fatigue (Meenan, Mason, Anderson, Guccione, & Kazis, 1992).

Step 5: Identify Contextual Features That Affect Assessment

In this step, the occupational therapist considers the intervention context and its impact on the evaluation of ADL and IADL. These include physical context, social context, safety, the client's experience, time constraints, the practitioner's training and experience, availability of resources, and mandates from facilities or **third-party payers**.

Physical Context. Practitioners may observe clients performing occupational tasks under natural or clinical conditions. Natural conditions, which can often be met in long-term care settings and home-based care, provide the most accurate assessment of clients' performance (Rogers et al., 2003). Although the therapy setting will dictate where an assessment takes place, the influence of the physical context on activity performance should be considered so that valid conclusions about performance can be drawn (Bottari, Dutil, Dassa, & Rainville, 2006). Occupational therapy clinics are designed to promote function with adaptive features, which may make it easier for clients to perform activities in the clinic than in their own homes (Holm & Rogers, 2017). Conversely, performance might be more difficult for some tasks because clients are unfamiliar with the clinic setting. Research in this area is limited but demonstrates the variable impact of context on performance. For example, Brown, Moore, Hemman, and Yunek (1996) found that clients with mental illness performed similarly on a simulated purchasing task in the clinic and an actual purchasing task in a store, whereas Provencher, Demers, Gélinas, and Giroux (2013) found that older adults' process skills during IADL were typically higher in their homes than in clinic settings. Provencher, Demers, and Gélinas (2009) did a systematic review examining the impact of setting on IADL performance in adults and found varied results for studies of mixed-aged populations and some evidence that performance in home settings was better for older adults. The home advantage seemed to be more evident in activities that require interaction with the environment and not just task objects (e.g., cooking vs. managing finances).

Social Context. The OT evaluation also occurs in a social context. Practitioners must oversee activity performance during assessment, and their very presence can affect the manner and adequacy of the activities performed. The practitioner's presence especially affects the client's ability to initiate participation in ADL or IADL because the structure of the assessment process itself prompts clients to engage in the tasks. If initiation of task performance is impaired, the practitioner must supplement performance measures from a structured therapy session. For example, the Independent Living Scale includes a subscale for initiation (Ashley, Persel, & Clark, 2001). Alternatively, family members might be asked, for example, to keep track of the number of days the client completed pet care responsibilities without being asked. Clients' occupational performance might be impacted by the differences in social context between clinic and natural environments. For example, a client with a spinal cord injury who must be skilled in directing a personal care attendant during ADL might give directions effectively to a rehabilitation aide who is familiar with caring for people with similar needs

but might not give detailed enough instructions for an employee in the home who has less experience. Conversely, a client who requires setup to feed himself or herself will be more independent at home than in the clinic if he or she lives in a family where meals are routinely set up for the entire family by a caregiver who does all the cooking.

Safety. Occupational therapists must assess risks associated with ADL or IADL that have been identified as priorities by clients and might need to defer assessment of a task that they believe could be unsafe. Identifying the potential risk of a given assessment is based on occupational therapists' expertise in determining activity demands combined with their estimate of client problems, outlined in step 4 earlier. Occupational therapists may opt to defer or modify an assessment that they deem is unsafe. For example, a client who experienced a recent stroke resulting in very poor sitting balance might identify showering as an important goal; however, getting the client onto a shower chair in a wet environment might be unsafe, given the level of assistance she needs for maintaining balance. Instead, the occupational therapist might suggest an assessment of bathing skills completed at bedside and defer a shower assessment until sitting balance is improved. Simulating an occupational performance task may also be a way to minimize risk during an evaluation. For example, driving is an IADL with a critical safety component, and although on-road assessments are considered to be the most accurate, driving simulators offer a safe alternative for gathering data to determine whether or not the client is appropriate to assess on city streets (Bédard, Parkkari, Weaver, Riendeau, & Dahlquist, 2010).

The Client's Experience. Clients will come with varied experience with ADL and IADL based on personal context. Typically, ADL practice begins in childhood, and the societal expectation is that adolescents and adults have a wide range of experience with these activities and can perform them adequately. However, a similar expectation does not hold for IADL, where people have more options. Clients may not have developed proficiency in all IADL activities. Some might have no experience in planning and preparing meals, doing the laundry, or managing finances. Children with developmental disabilities often experience delays in the acquisition of ADL and IADL skills and might lack experience that a typically developing child would have at a given age. Clients' activity performance history is essential for understanding their current performance level. An activity limitation is interpreted differently for a client who has had no or little prior experience performing the activity than for one who had been doing it effectively prior to OT intervention.

Time Constraints. The time that is available for OT assessment and intervention is often limited by several factors, including reimbursement policies, so the evaluation must be done efficiently. For clients with a long list of ADL and IADL goals, selecting key activities is necessary so that the intervention to enhance occupational performance can be initiated in a timely manner. As goals are met, additional assessments may be initiated to document baseline performance of other ADL or IADL and to justify additional OT goals and intervention.

The Occupational Therapy Practitioner's Training and Experience.
An OT practitioner's experience can also affect the selection of assessment tools. Familiarity with an instrument increases efficiency of use and ability to accurately interpret assessment results. Some assessment tools require specialized training, so are not options for therapists who lack the training. For example, the Assessment of Motor and Process Skills (AMPS) (Fisher & Jones, 2011) relies on software that can be accessed only by practitioners who have completed the training course and calibration process (Holm & Rogers, 2017).

Availability of Resources.
The materials that are required for ADL and IADL assessments vary, and the OT practitioner must make sure that the necessary materials are readily available. A cooking assessment using a client's favorite cookie recipe might be an excellent choice for examining the client's performance, but the logistics and cost of procuring the ingredients for this activity make it impractical for an OT practitioner in a hospital setting. However, a client who is being seen in home-based therapy might have the required resources for making cookies readily available. Some assessments require special test kits, which can be costly, and facilities might have only a few such tools available for use.

Mandates from Facilities or Third-Party Payers.
Many facilities or third-party payers have assessment forms or procedures that must be completed for all clients. For example, rehabilitation facilities must use the Inpatient Rehabilitation Facility-Patient Assessment Instrument (IRF-PAI), which includes the FIM™ for measuring ADL (Centers for Medicare & Medicaid Services, 2016). If a client's description of a selected ADL differs from that of the FIM™ or if the client would like to address adequacy parameters in addition to independence and safety, then the occupational therapist must use a supplemental assessment because documentation of the FIM™ scores is required.

Step 6: Consider Features of Assessment Tools

The occupational therapist must be familiar with available assessments and consider what tasks are included in the assessment, how tasks are defined, the psychometric properties, the type of data to be collected, and the method of data collection.

Tasks Assessed.
Tasks that are included in an ADL or IADL assessment should be consistent with clients' priorities, and the operational definition of effective performance should fit clients' needs and address all parameters of importance. For example, many assessment instruments measure independence, but if clients would also like to complete tasks independently without experiencing shortness of breath or pain, occupational therapists might want to use a dyspnea or pain scale in conjunction with the independence measure.

Types of Assessments and Data.
Some assessments are not standardized; that is, the individual therapist designs the assessment and decides the type of information to gather. Results of nonstandardized assessments are often reported using qualitative data; that is, the salient characteristics of clients' activity performance are observed or obtained through client or caregiver descriptions. Clients' status is documented by simply describing their performance. Nonstandardized assessments lack testing of psychometric properties, such as reliability, validity, or sensitivity to change in a client's status (Dunn, 2017). **Standardized assessments** rely on a well-described, uniform approach, which makes the assessment more reliable when it is used for reassessment or by multiple therapists. For example, the term *moderate assistance* could be interpreted in several ways, but if it is operationally defined as "the patient requires more help than touching, or expends between 50% and 74% of the effort" (UB Foundation Activities, 2002, p. III-7), agreement among therapists using the instrument is likely to be higher. There is variability in the extent to which the psychometric properties of standardized assessments have been established. Some assessments have been extensively studied and include a wide range of psychometric statistics to support the reliability and validity of the tool. When possible, it is best to use an assessment with established psychometric properties (Dunn, 2017). Standardized measures that reduce observed behavior to a number also make it efficient for reporting data in documentation. However, loss of qualitative data can make it difficult for the reader to get a clear understanding of the client's limitations. Often, documentation includes quantitative assessment data accompanied by some qualitative data to provide a more comprehensive picture of client performance. A brief case, presented in Table 50-1, compares descriptive and quantitative data from two cases. See Chapter 29 for more information on types of assessments.

It is possible to rely entirely on qualitative data to document a client's baseline status, which is needed to

TABLE 50-1	Comparison of Descriptive and Quantitative Data from a Dressing Assessment of Two Children

Aiden	Brody
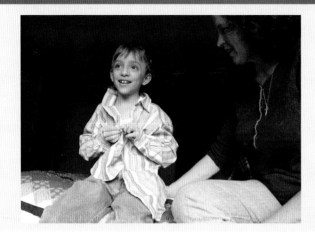	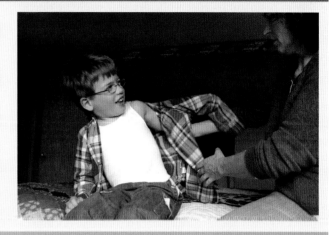

Client Description

Aiden is a 7-year-old child who sustained a traumatic brain injury. Before his injury, he was a typically developing child who dressed himself independently.	Brody is a 7-year-old child with cerebral palsy affecting the right side of his body. His mother has been helping him dress prior to this assessment.

Descriptive Data from Observing Dressing

• Well-coordinated and smooth movements of both upper extremities (UEs) when manipulating clothing • Maintenance of appropriate posture, sitting unsupported on the bed • Reached all areas of his body (behind, overhead, feet) without loss of balance • Frequently stopped midtask to verbalize thoughts, which were disjointed and difficult to follow • Made repeated (total of five) attempts to get his left arm in a sleeve turned inside out; did not attempt to self-correct or respond to verbal directions to turn the sleeve right side out. The practitioner turned the sleeve right side out after giving three verbal cues and gesturing toward the sleeve. • Aiden left the dressing task to look out the window when he heard a plane and continued to talk about the plane when asked to return to the dressing task. • Aiden returned to the task when the practitioner physically guided him to the bed and placed one of his arms in the sleeve. He then completed putting the shirt on his other arm on his own. • When asked to button his shirt, he completed two of six buttons, which were misaligned. When asked how well his shirt was buttoned, he looked down at himself and said, "It's perfect" and then skipped out of the room saying that he wanted to watch TV.	• Started to put left (stronger) UE in his shirtsleeve first; responded immediately to verbal cue to dress the right side of the body first • Wavering of trunk when using both UEs to position the shirt. Practitioner steadied Brody's trunk to prevent him from falling forward when he pulled the shirt across his back. He could not get the shirt far enough around to reach the sleeve. The practitioner moved the shirt so he could reach it with the left arm. • Left UE movements were smooth and well coordinated. • Right UE movement was minimal, and he could not use his hand for fine tasks, such as buttoning. Several attempts were required to complete the bottom three buttons with the left hand, and the practitioner had to complete the top three. • Putting on his shirt took 15 minutes. Brody reported he felt "pretty tired" at the end. He was focused during the task, even when his little brother ran into and out of the room. • Brody followed instructions consistently and made five attempts to help solve problems encountered along the way, for example, suggesting he wear pullover shirts that do not have buttons. • When asked which arm he will dress first when he tries the task tomorrow, Brody responded, "My right arm."

Quantitative Data Based on the WeeFIM™

Upper Body Dressing = 4	Upper Body Dressing = 4

determine whether or not progress is made in OT; however, this can be difficult and time-consuming. For example, if Aiden's and Brody's occupational therapists had to document the status of *all* ADL and IADL as presented in Table 50-1, the evaluation report would take a great deal of time to write and to read. Additionally, the OT practitioner

who is documenting qualitative data should be very careful to distinguish between *observations* and *clinical judgments* (subjective interpretations about the observations). The statements listed in Table 50-1 are observations. A statement of clinical judgment is interpretive, and several plausible interpretations could be made from the more objective observations. For example, the OT practitioner could conclude that Brody has weak trunk muscles that interfere with balance. This conclusion should be presented as a hypothesis, not as an observation, because Brody's inability to maintain balance while dressing could be due to other factors, such as impaired vestibular and proprioceptive input that interferes with his ability to detect when he is starting to fall to one side.

A quantitative assessment measure is a more efficient way to document progress, although it might not provide the reader with complete information. For example, although Aiden and Brody have the same quantitative score on the WeeFIM™, the qualitative information enables readers to see that there are very different underlying problems. Occupational therapists can document key qualitative data to support their evaluation and intervention plan, but most observations are simply used by therapists for planning intervention, whereas quantitative data are recorded in documentation (Gateley & Borcherding, 2017). Many standardized, quantitative ADL scales are available; however, it can be difficult for OT practitioners to find standardized assessments for some IADL. Therefore, using a nonstandardized approach provides a reasonable option for the assessment of selected tasks for which no standardized measure exists.

Data about ADL and IADL performance can be gathered by report or through direct observation. Reported data about the client's abilities and limitations in performance can be gathered from the client, the caregiver, and/or another health professional. The OT practitioner poses questions about ADL and IADL performance in oral or written format, using interviews or questionnaires, respectively. Although the questioning is frequently done face to face, either format can be done without physical interaction. Interviews may be conducted over the telephone. Questionnaires may be completed while the client is waiting for an appointment or can be mailed out in advance of a session. Gathering data via report can be done informally; that is, the practitioner develops the questions to be asked or through the use of a standardized protocol such as the COPM (Law et al., 2014), the Occupational Self Assessment (Baron, Kielhofner, Iyenger, Goldhammer, & Wolenski, 2006), or the Child Occupational Self Assessment (Keller, Kafkes, Basu, Federico, & Kielhofner, 2005). Although self-report is an efficient way to measure ADL and IADL, it is not always consistent with actual performance (Brown & Finlayson, 2013; Goverover, Chiaravalloti, Gaudino-Goering, Moore, & DeLuca, 2009; Rogers et al., 2003), and the occupational therapist should select performance-based assessments when the client's accuracy is in question. Additionally, gathering data about selected ADL or IADL through both self-report and performance-based measures can provide the occupational therapist with valuable insight into the accuracy of the client's self-awareness regarding the impact of his or her disability.

In some situations, clients might be unable to respond on their own behalf, so caregivers or other proxies can be queried on behalf of clients. The usefulness of information from caregivers or proxies depends on their familiarity with the client's ADL and IADL. For example, if the proxy has not observed a client bathing recently, the information might be based more on opinion than on concrete knowledge of bathing performance. In addition, there are known biases in the reporting tendencies of caregivers and proxies. Cohen-Mansfield and Jensen (2007) examined accuracy of spouses' perceptions of each other's self-care practices and found spouses agreed "exactly" 58% of the time and had "close/partial agreement" 75% of the time. Caregivers and proxies can readily observe evaluation parameters such as independence, safety, and aberrant activity behaviors. Some evaluation parameters, however, are subjective, so clients are the only appropriate respondents (e.g., values, satisfaction with performance, and activity-related pain).

Assessments that rely on self-report or caregiver's report are particularly useful for screening for activity limitations because a large number of activities can be queried in a short amount of time. Questioning is also the data-gathering method of choice when information is needed about daily living *habits*—that is, about what clients usually do on a daily basis—or to learn about clients' ADL and IADL experience. However, reporting is less useful in evaluating limitations for the purposes of intervention because clients might not be able to describe their limitations in sufficient detail to target the components of activities that are problematic.

Assessment data can also be gathered through direct observation of ADL and IADL, which gives the practitioner more information about how the client performs a task. Observation of performance, however, requires more time and material resources and is therefore more costly. Direct observation of performance can also be done in a nonstandardized way or through use of a standardized assessment. The constraints of practice settings, often imposed by third-party payers or limited funding, can place restrictions on the time an occupational therapist has available for evaluation. Occupational therapists must be strategic in selecting ADL and IADL assessments that will provide information relevant to the client and can be generalized to other tasks so that the practitioner does not have to observe all meaningful ADL and IADL that may be addressed in OT. For example, if a client requires assistance with cooking because of an inability to transport food and cooking equipment safely while using a walker, the occupational therapist can reasonably project, without having to observe performance, that the same client will require assistance in doing laundry because laundry also requires the transportation of task objects.

Selected standardized ADL and IADL assessments are listed in Table 50-2. The assessments that are included in Table 50-2 are readily available and either are commonly

TABLE 50-2	**Summary of Selected Activities of Daily Living (ADL) and Instrumental Activities of Daily Living (IADL) Instruments**			
Title	**Areas Addressed**	**Population**	**Method**	**Learning to Use the Assessment**
ADL-focused Occupation-based Neurobehavioral Evaluation (A-ONE)	Feeding, dressing, grooming and hygiene, transfers and mobility, and communication	16 years and older with central nervous system dysfunction	Observation of ADL	Training required to rate reliably (Árnadóttir, 1990, 2011)
Assessment of Motor and Process Skills (AMPS)	125 calibrated ADL and IADL activities; client and therapist select two or three for assessment	Children (age >2 years) and adults	Identify two to three ADL or IADL tasks for observation.	Training required. Software for scoring and required rater calibration available only through course. Course information and extensive reference list are available from the Center for Innovative OT Solutions Website: https://www.innovativeotsolutions.com/tools/amps
Barthel Index	10 ADL skills	Adults	Based on "best evidence," observation, self- or proxy-report	Test items and guidelines for administering can be found at http://www.strokecenter.org/wp-content/uploads/2011/08/barthel.pdf
Canadian Occupational Performance Measure (COPM)	Measures performance and satisfaction in self-care (ADL and some IADL), productivity (some IADL and work), and leisure	Children and adults	Self-report using a semistructured interview; five most important problems rated for performance and satisfaction	Training and purchase information (paper manual, electronic PDF, and the COPM App) is available at: http://www.thecopm.ca/
Functional Independence Measure (FIM™)	18 activities, 13 ADL tasks, and 5 communication and social cognition skills (no IADL)	Adolescents and adults	Observation of ADL	Training is recommended for interrater reliability. Training often provided by employer. Also available from the Uniform Data System for Medical Rehabilitation: http://www.udsmr.org
Goal-Oriented Assessment of Lifeskills (GOAL)	Assesses functional motor abilities needed for daily living using seven common occupational tasks	Children ages 7 to 17 years	Observation of intervention targets	Available for purchase at Pearson Assessments: http://www.pearsonassessments.com
Independent Living Scale (ILS)	Assesses information/performance and comprehension on 68 items in five areas: memory and orientation, managing money, managing home and transportation, health and safety, and social adjustment	Adolescents and adults with cognitive impairment	Observation of functional activities	Available for purchase at Pearson Assessments: http://www.pearsonassessments.com
Instrumental Activities of Daily Living (IADL) Scale	Eight IADL tasks	Adults	Self- or proxy-report	The instrument is available at http://www.strokecenter.org/wp-content/uploads/2011/08/lawton_IADL_Scale.pdf

(continues)

| TABLE 50-2 | Summary of Selected Activities of Daily Living (ADL) and Instrumental Activities of Daily Living (IADL) Instruments *(continued)* |

Title	Areas Addressed	Population	Method	Learning to Use the Assessment
Kohlman Evaluation of Living Skills (KELS)	13 living skills in five areas: self-care, safety and health, money management, community mobility and telephone, and employment and leisure	Adults with cognitive impairments	Observation and self-report of task performance	Manual included in test kit describes testing procedures. The KELS can be purchased from the AOTA: https://myaota.aota.org /shop_aota/search.aspx#q=KELS &sort=relevancy
Long-Term Care Facility Resident Assessment Instrument—Section G: Functional Status Scale	10 ADL tasks activities	Residents in long-term care	Observation and/or self- or proxy-report	The Centers for Medicare & Medicaid has training resources at https://downloads.cms.gov /files/1-MDS-30-RAI-Manual -v115R-October-1-2017-R.pdf
Outcome and Assessment Information Set (OASIS)	18 ADL and IADL tasks	Clients in home care	Observation and/or self- or proxy-report	The Centers for Medicare & Medicaid has training resources at https://www.cms.gov/Medicare /Quality-Initiatives-Patient -Assessment-Instruments /HomeHealthQualityInits /Downloads/OASIS-C2-Guidance -Manual-Effective_1_1_18.pdf
Pediatric Evaluation of Disability Inventory (PEDI)	Measures functional abilities in self-care, mobility, and social function. The PEDI is a normed test.	Children 6 months to 7+ years	Report of parent, clinician, or educator	Manual includes detailed instructions and cases to practice scoring the PEDI. Available for purchase at Pearson Assessments: http://www.pearsonassessments .com
Performance Assessment of Self-Care Skills (PASS)	26 tasks, including ADL and home management IADL tasks; different protocols for both client's home- and clinic-based.	Adults	Observation of independence, safety, and adequacy	Validity, reliability, and standardized procedures are described in the manual. The PASS is available through: http://www.shrs.pitt .edu/ot/about/performance -assessment-self-care-skills-pass
WeeFIM™ II	Measures 18 items in self-care, mobility, and cognition	Children from 6 months to 7 years	Observation, interview, or both	Training information at https://www .udsmr.org/WebModules/WeeFIM /Wee_About.aspx

used in practice (e.g., the FIM™) or research (e.g., the Barthel Index) or provide a unique approach to assessment. For example, the Independent Living Scale measures task initiation (Ashley et al., 2001). Resources with more information about the assessments, including learning to use them, are also provided. The IADL instruments that were selected include a range of activities.

Step 7: Integrate the Information from Steps 1 to 6 to Select the Optimal Activities of ADL/IADL Assessment Tools

After establishing the purpose of the evaluation and the client's priorities and gathering some preliminary information about the client and relevant contextual features, assessment instruments can be selected that are client centered, yield appropriate data, are reliable and valid, and are feasible to administer. Occupational therapists should engage in best practice by considering the evidence regarding the selection and use of assessments, for example, the reliability of instruments and the validity for a given clinical situation. Additional considerations for evidence-based evaluation are discussed in the "Commentary on the Evidence" box on putting evidence into practice through the use of standardized assessments. Perhaps the best data-gathering strategy is to use a combination of methods and sources, relying on the convergence of data for the best profile of clients' activity abilities and limitations.

COMMENTARY ON THE EVIDENCE

Standardized Assessments

Putting Evidence into Practice through the Use of Standardized Assessments

Best practice in OT indicates that standardized activities of daily living (ADL) and instrumental activities of daily living (IADL) assessments should be used because they provide objective measures that are both reliable and valid, accurately reflecting changes in clients' performance (Dunn, 2017; Fasoli, 2014). Third-party payers also prefer documentation that describes clients' status and progress toward goals with standardized assessments. In spite of this, many clinicians continue to rely on nonstandardized assessments in clinical practice, often citing barriers, including beliefs that standardized outcome measures are not clinically relevant or are too time-consuming to be practical, or they lack the necessary skills to administer assessments (Colquhoun, Letts, Law, MacDermid, & Edwards, 2010).

Many of these barriers may be relatively easy to overcome. Some standardized ADL and IADL assessments do not require much, if any, additional time or effort to conduct once practitioners are familiar with assessment protocols. For example, clinicians begin their assessment with an interview to establish an occupational profile and clients' priorities (Egan & Dubouloz, 2014; Stewart, 2010). The Canadian Occupational Performance Measure (COPM) not only gathers descriptive data, as an informal interview does, but also includes reliable and valid quantitative measures of clients' self-reported performance ability and satisfaction on client-selected occupational performance tasks (Law et al., 2014). Clients' initial COPM scores serve as an objective baseline measure, and reassessment of clients' perceived progress can be quickly done by asking clients to rerate their performance and satisfaction on previously rated tasks. Practitioners who volunteered to begin using the COPM as part of a research study did not find that it required additional evaluation time and reported that the information gained enhanced their ability to plan and carry out intervention (Colquhoun et al., 2010).

Standardized tests that do not require extensive additional time can also be selected when practitioners need to observe clients' actual performance. For example,

the Performance Assessment of Self-care Skills (PASS) uses a standardized approach in assessing several ADL and IADL, often by structuring observations of key elements of a task, such as sweeping up cereal placed on the floor by the therapist rather than having to observe the client sweep the entire kitchen (Chisholm et al., 2014). The assessment yields measures of three different parameters: independence, safety, and adequacy. Any or all of these performance parameters can be tracked and reported to document clients' progress toward goals. At first glance, the PASS administration and scoring procedures may seem complicated, but the assessment is very user friendly once practitioners become familiarized with the instrument.

Many standardized assessments are available for measuring ADL performance (Dunn, 2017), but many practitioners continue to use informal ADL assessments in clinical practice. Klein, Barlow, and Hollis (2008) conducted an action research design to identify ADL measures that were most reflective of the principles of OT practice and identified six instruments, including the ADL Profile, Assessment of Motor and Process Skills (AMPS), Functional Performance Measure, Rivermead ADL Assessment, Edmans ADL Index, and the Melville-Nelson Self-Care Assessment.

Appropriate assessment tools for IADL are more difficult to find. Standardized assessment of IADL is more challenging because of the variability and complexity of IADL tasks. One potential limitation in using standardized assessments for IADL is that many IADL assessments that examine a range of IADL tasks (rather than a single skill, such as cooking) rely on self-report or proxy report; examples are the Extended ADL (Nouri & Lincoln, 1987), COPM (Law et al., 2014), Assessment of Living Skills and Resources (Williams et al., 1991), and some parts of the *Kohlman Evaluation of Living Skills* (Kohlman Thomson & Robnett, 2016). The limitations of using reported performance were addressed earlier in this chapter. The development of reliable and valid IADL assessments that enable OT practitioners to objectively measure observed performance across many IADL tasks would increase their ability to engage in evidence-based evaluation.

It is often most effective to begin the evaluation with a questioning approach to provide an overall profile of the client's abilities and limitations, to understand clients' priorities, and to target activities that require in-depth evaluation. Questioning is then followed by observational assessments. If observational assessments raise additional

questions about the client's activity performance abilities, the evaluation plan can be modified to gather more or different data.

Planning an effective ADL and IADL evaluation is best illustrated by Case Study 50-1, which follows the seven steps for selecting an ADL/IADL assessment tool.

CASE STUDY 50-1   EVALUATION OF A CLIENT WITH MORBID OBESITY AND RESPIRATORY FAILURE

Mrs. Howard is a 59-year-old woman with a history of morbid obesity (5 ft tall and 376 lb). She was admitted to a hospital with difficulty breathing secondary to an allergic reaction. She went into respiratory arrest and required a tracheostomy and mechanical ventilation for 3 weeks. After 1 month in acute care, Mrs. Howard was transferred to a rehabilitation hospital where she participated in OT for activities of daily living (ADL) and instrumental activities of daily living (IADL) training and physical therapy (PT) for mobility training. She was dependent in all areas of ADL and IADL on admission and made considerable gains in function before her discharge home 3 months after her initial hospitalization. At discharge, she was ambulating short distances (up to 50 ft) independently with a rolling walker. She had an extra wide wheelchair for limited community outings (e.g., doctor's appointments), but the chair did not fit in her home. She continued to require supplemental oxygen. Mrs. Howard was referred for home-based services, including skilled nursing, nutritional counseling, home health aide (3 days a week, 2 hours each day), PT, and OT.

Occupational Profile

Mrs. Howard lives with her husband of 30 years. He works full time but is physically able and willing to assist his wife when he is home. Mr. and Mrs. Howard have two grown children and two school-age grandchildren who live in the area. Before hospitalization, Mrs. Howard was independent in ADL and IADL. She had primary responsibility for cooking, light housekeeping, and laundry. She worked 20 hours a week at the public library. Mrs. Howard had several close friends she enjoyed meeting for lunch or shopping, especially bargain hunting at flea markets. She and her husband also frequently attended their grandchildren's sports events in a nearby town. The following considerations were used to select appropriate ADL and IADL assessments for Mrs. Howard:

1. **Identify the overall purpose(s) of the evaluation.** The purpose is to plan and monitor OT intervention, so baseline data needs be effective for determining progress toward goals.
2. **Have clients identify their needs, interests, and perceived difficulties with ADL and/or IADL.** Mrs. Howard's primary goal is to regain her independence in ADL, IADL, and leisure. She identified ADL and IADL, including driving, as priorities because she is concerned about being a burden on her husband. She reported that her biggest difficulties are with lower body ADL (unable to reach) and with all IADL (fatigue, shortness of breath, limited reach, and mobility). She has frequent medical appointments and lives in a rural area, and she hates relying on others for getting to and from appointments.

3. **Further explore the client's relevant activities so that the activities are operationally defined.** The "problem activities" that Mrs. Howard identified were briefly discussed for more detail. The ADL were completed in the typical fashion. She reported that sexual activity is not currently a priority, but she would like to address it later, once she had sufficient energy for and independence in other ADL/IADL. Priorities for Mrs. Howard include the following:
   - Transporting laundry from bedroom to kitchen (top-loading washer) and out to the clothesline (no dryer)
   - Cooking complete dinners, including accessing the refrigerator, oven, stovetop, cooking utensils, dishwasher, and sink. A sample dinner would include fish, baked potatoes, steamed green beans, and a salad.
   - Driving and riding in her minivan
   - Accessing all areas of her one-story home except the basement, including home office for doing finances and using the computer, linen closets, and so forth

   Additionally, Mrs. Howard reported adequacy parameters, including the ability to complete ADL and IADL in a timely manner and regain the ability to sustain activity without fatigue or shortness of breath.

4. **Estimate the client factors that affect occupational performance and/or the assessment process.** Mrs. Howard's primary occupational performance problems are caused by her obesity, which limits her reach and ability to move and causes fatigue and dyspnea. Cognition and perception do not appear to be factors that interfere with function on review of her rehabilitation records and the initial interview.

5. **Identify contextual features that affect assessment.** Contextual features that support the evaluation process include the following:
   - The assessment will occur in Mrs. Howard's home, her natural environment.
   - There is a ramp into the home, providing access to the yard and driveway.
   - Mrs. Howard has years of experience with all of the tasks she wished to return to.

   Contextual features that are barriers to the evaluation process include the following:
   - Clutter in the home that presents a safety issue, restricting mobility and access
   - Use of supplemental oxygen, with the unit in the bedroom and a very long tube that she has to manage as she moves around the house

- The evaluation will occur midweek. The therapist is alone with the client whose weight presents a safety concern to the therapist when guarding her during new tasks.
- Mrs. Howard has private insurance, which requires that the OT evaluation be completed in one visit.

6. **Consider features of assessment tools.** This step is included in the discussion of step 7.

7. **Integrate the information from steps 1 to 6 to select the optimal ADL and IADL assessment tools.** The time limit of one visit (approximately 60 to 75 minutes) has a significant impact on which assessments are selected. The occupational therapist decided to start with the Canadian Occupational Performance Measure (COPM) based on the following considerations:

- The COPM has well-established psychometric properties and assesses both ADL and IADL and leisure (Law et al., 2014).
- The COPM relies on self-report; however, Mrs. Howard is cognitively intact and has been learning to live with her disability for the past 3 months. One advantage of self-report is that it does not pose safety hazards. For example, the occupational therapist gets a baseline performance and satisfaction rating on driving her car (including getting in and out) without having to attempt the task with Mrs. Howard.
- Mrs. Howard felt stress about burdening her husband. The COPM will help the occupational therapist prioritize ADL and IADL to reduce caregiver burden.
- The COPM included a satisfaction measure, which reflects some of the adequacy parameters that Mrs. Howard identified (e.g., if she can dress independently but it takes her 45 minutes, she would give that a low satisfaction score).
- The COPM can be completed in about 20 minutes.

After the COPM, the occupational therapist selects the Functional Independence Measure (FIM™) subtests of transfers, lower body dressing, and grooming. Other FIM™ tasks are not observed because Mrs. Howard reported no difficulty with them (including feeding, toileting, and upper body dressing) or because of time constraints (e.g., bathing). The FIM™ is an appropriate measure because of the following reasons:

- Mrs. Howard reports that she requires physical assistance for lower body dressing and getting out of bed (included in FIM™ transfer subtest), and the scale is believed to have adequate sensitivity in levels of physical assistance to document progress.
- The occupational therapist has discharge FIM™ scores from the rehabilitation center, so performance in the clinic and at home can be compared using the same tool to examine the impact of the home context on performance and aid in problem solving for intervention.
- These tasks can all be completed in 25 minutes.

Two additional parameter measures are used to supplement the FIM™. Lower body dressing and grooming are timed, which requires no additional assessment time. Dyspnea will be measured after each of the three subtasks, using a 100-mm visual analogue scale where 0 = "no shortness of breath," 50 mm = "moderate shortness of breath," and 100 mm = "severe shortness of breath" (Lansing, Moosavi, & Banzett, 2003). Completion of the dyspnea scales requires little additional time, fitting into the 25 minutes allowed for the FIM™.

At this point, Mrs. Howard needs a rest, although the occupational therapist wants to include some observation of IADL in the evaluation. While Mrs. Howard rests, the therapist uses the walker to do an informal accessibility assessment for several key areas in the home (e.g., dresser, closet, personal computer, kitchen appliances, and cabinets). Although standardized home assessments are available, the occupational therapist uses a nonstandardized approach because Mrs. Howard's walker requires additional room for accessibility and the therapist needs to focus on a few key areas because time is limited. The occupational therapist also begins some intervention by making a list of suggestions to make Mrs. Howard's environment more accessible and reviewing them with Mrs. Howard so she can enlist a friend or family member in modifying the context to enhance performance. The informal assessment of context and review with Mrs. Howard is completed in 15 minutes.

At this point, Mrs. Howard and her occupational therapist are about 1 hour into the initial evaluation. The therapist would like to observe Mrs. Howard complete a simple cooking task and also assess her potential to return to driving by having her get in and out of her car, including folding and storing the walker. However, Mrs. Howard is fatigued, and 15 minutes is not enough time for both. Mrs. Howard has a minivan that requires a significant step up. Given her level of fatigue with lighter activities and concerns about safely guarding someone of her size, the occupational therapist opts to have Mrs. Howard make a cup of tea, deferring the car assessment to another session. The kettle is placed in a low cabinet to assess her ability to retrieve it. The tea is in an over-counter cabinet. The therapist gathers qualitative data, times the task, and uses the visual analogue scale to measure dyspnea on completion. The task takes less than 10 minutes. After the assessment, Mrs. Howard settles into her favorite chair to enjoy her cup of tea.

Implementing the Evaluation: Gathering Data, Critical Observation, and Hypothesis Generation

Gathering Data and Critical Observation

Once occupational therapists develop an evaluation plan, they must carry it out. The thoughtful and deliberate selection of appropriate assessments described previously is key in making the data gathering run smoothly. A few additional considerations about the actual implementation of the evaluation warrant discussion. The OT practitioner who is doing an assessment should do the following:

- *Collect all equipment and supplies* needed for carrying out the evaluation plans, making sure test kits are complete and organized and that necessary equipment and supplies are available, including clients' personal items (e.g., clothing from home).
- *Schedule assessment sessions in the best environment available and the most appropriate time of day.* For example, a client in an inpatient rehabilitation center would find it more comfortable to dress in his or her room than in a curtained-off area in a busy clinic and may find it more meaningful and motivating to dress early in the day.
- *Be sensitive to individual needs for modesty,* which can vary greatly among clients. Many ADL are personal tasks that are typically done alone, including dressing, bathing, and toileting. Assessment for potential impairment in sexual activity should be included in ADL assessments but must be handled with sensitivity.
- *Structure the optimal social context.* For example, the practitioner might wish to have family members present during an interview to gain their perspectives about a client's abilities or needs, whereas having several family members observing a performance-based assessment of cooking might be distracting to the client and interfere with the evaluation process.
- *Bring appropriate tools to record data.* A well-planned evaluation session will reveal a lot of information about a client. Standardized tests often come with forms for recording data. The practitioner might also want to jot down relevant observations, for example, noting that a client complained of shoulder pain when putting a shirt on overhead or that a client's grocery list included primarily nonnutritious foods. If possible, practitioners should record directly into the client's health record to reduce time needed for completing the evaluation report.

During the evaluation, the practitioner should engage in critical observation, which can be framed by questions the practitioners ask themselves throughout the process, such as the following:

- *What are some of the possible underlying causes of the occupational performance deficits that are being observed or reported?* For example, various different factors may limit a client's ability to reach the clothes in her closet, including upper extremity weakness, impaired passive range of motion (ROM), poor coordination, diminished standing balance, or a clothes rod that is out of reach for the client's height. Observations made as the client tries to get clothes from the closet can provide clues to the underlying causes that will aid the occupational therapist in making sound intervention decisions, as shown in Figure 50-1.
- *What changes might need to be made in the initial evaluation plan based on the data from the first assessments?* For example, a cooking assessment might reveal mild cognitive deficits that were not apparent during initial interactions with a client, so the occupational therapist may add a cognitive assessment to the evaluation plan.
- *Are there discrepancies in the evaluation data that were collected?* Discrepancies need to be clarified and reconciled and can provide valuable insight into the nature of the client's ADL and IADL limitations. For example, a practitioner might observe during performance testing that a client can execute bed-to-wheelchair transfers, yet the client might insist that he cannot. The inconsistency might arise because, although the client performs the transfer independently with the practitioner present, he feels insecure about his abilities and will not transfer on his own. In this example, the use of different data sources identified a performance discrepancy between skill and habit that would not have been apparent from the use of one source alone.

Hypothesis Generation

The evaluation data that are obtained through questioning, observing, and testing methods must be analyzed, synthesized, and integrated into a cohesive problem statement (Gateley & Borcherding, 2017). This integration of data is accomplished through diagnostic or scientific reasoning, a component of clinical reasoning (Tomlin, 2018) that occurs as a kind of internal dialogue about the interpretation of the data. Evidence supporting one interpretation is weighed against evidence rejecting that interpretation, and the interpretation that has the most compelling evidence is selected. If the evidence fails to sufficiently support one interpretation over another, more evaluative data are collected to supplement the reasoning process. This process is best illustrated through an example based on the cases presented in Table 50-1. Aiden and Brody had

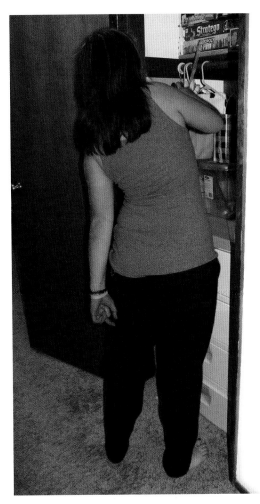

FIGURE 50-1 Observations made during reach: Lateral flexion of the trunk suggests that the client is compensating for an inability to raise the arm, which could be from limited passive range of motion or decreased strength. The height of the closet rod relative to the client's size should require only about 50% of typical shoulder flexion. Balance does not appear to be an issue because the client appears stable even while shifting her center of gravity toward the left as she reaches.

- What are their strengths, that is, what skills support each one's dressing performance?
- What observed behaviors led to your conclusions about each boy's strengths and limitations?

For Aiden, limited attention, impaired awareness of occupational performance deficits, and inconsistent response to feedback seemed to be underlying problems that limited his ability to dress independently. This is a hypothesis or clinical judgment rather than an objective observation because constructs such as attention and awareness of deficits cannot be directly observed and must be inferred from specific behaviors. At the same time, Aiden's physical capabilities seemed to be an asset and supported performance in many ways. Compare the observations and clinical judgments made by the occupational therapist about Aiden to those made about Brody. In both cases, the children required verbal cueing and occasional physical assistance; however, descriptive data led the occupational therapist to a very different hypothesis about Brody's dressing limitations. The underlying problems for Brody were physical impairments, for example, impaired sitting balance, incoordination of the right upper extremity, and decreased endurance. Behaviors that supported performance included attention to task, follow-through with feedback, the ability to recall adaptive strategies, and engagement in active problem solving. Generating hypotheses about the nature of the occupational performance deficit is crucial for selecting effective intervention, which must address the underlying problem. For example, adaptive equipment could be provided to help Brody reach his feet independently or to compensate for limited right hand function during buttoning; however, this equipment would be of no help to Aiden and would likely impede performance by distracting him from the task.

Through this process, the occupational therapist arrives at a cohesive understanding of the ADL and IADL performance of the client, factors that are interfering with performance, and appropriate therapeutic actions given the nature of the client's deficits. This understanding is presented to clients or their proxies for verification and collaborative decision making concerning the therapeutic action to be implemented.

the same dressing scores on the FIM™, a quantitative ADL assessment, but the occupational therapist's clinical interpretation of the descriptive data will lead to very different assumptions about the problems that are causing dressing impairments for the two children. Before reading on, take a minute to reflect on the different observations reported in Table 50-1 and consider the following for both Aiden and Brody:

- What are the underlying factors that interfere with each boy's ability to dress independently?

Establishing Clients' Goals: The Bridge between Evaluation and Intervention

The OTPF includes the establishment of clients' goals as the final step in the evaluation process and as the first component of the intervention plan (AOTA, 2014), so this important step really serves as a transition from evaluation to intervention. Synthesizing evaluation results into an effective intervention plan is a complex cognitive task and can be overwhelming for the student or new OT practitioner. The process of planning and implementing interventions is much easier for practitioners who have reasonable, attainable, and measurable goals or outcomes. The following section is designed to guide novice practitioners in the clinical reasoning used for establishing effective client goals.

Establishing goals requires analysis of the evaluation results in conjunction with additional factors that influence outcomes, such as the client's self-awareness and ability to learn, prognosis, time allocated for intervention, discharge disposition, and ability to follow through with new routines or techniques. The next section focuses on using performance parameters to establish meaningful goals for clients that have a clearly identified behavior; that is, what the client is expected to *do*. The behavior must be observable and include an appropriate *assist level*; that is, a characteristic of the behavior that is measurable, for example, "independently" or "without pain" (Gateley & Borcherding, 2017).

Identifying Appropriate Goal Behaviors

A comprehensive evaluation examines ADL and IADL performance across relevant performance parameters. Four of these performance parameters—value, level of difficulty, safety, and fatigue and dyspnea—are particularly relevant to consider in order to identify goals for intervention that target realistic and appropriate client behaviors.

Value

Occupational therapists should select goal behaviors (i.e., ADL and IADL tasks) that reflect the values defined by the client during the evaluation. The value that clients place on given activities influences their motivation for participation in any intervention aimed at improving performance for that activity (Doig, Fleming, Cornwell, & Kuipers, 2009; Jack & Estes, 2010). Because many OT interventions require the acquisition of new skills through practice, motivation can greatly influence the ultimate functional outcome. Clients who put little value on the activity that is being addressed during an intervention might appear uncooperative and are unlikely to follow through with programs outside of direct intervention that are necessary for improving skill in that activity.

Clients' self-awareness of ADL and IADL performance deficits can have an impact on identifying goals and their relative value. Clients with cognitive deficits and poor self-awareness may not value ADL or IADL goals if

they perceive they are already independent, efficient, and effective in their performance of those tasks. Doig et al. (2009) found that the process of collaborative goal setting with clients with traumatic brain injury and their significant others actually facilitated clients' self-awareness and increased their participation in OT. Occupational therapy practitioners who work with children may also face challenges in collaborative goal setting, although young school-age children with neurodevelopmental disabilities were able to engage effectively in setting goals with support of an assessment instrument that measured their perceived competence in various physical tasks (Vroland-Nordstrand et al., 2015). Clients with good insight into their occupational performance challenges may be more easily engaged in collaborative goal setting, but OT practitioners must carefully attend to the complex issues that can impact clients' priorities.

ADL and IADL are often highly valued by both children and adults because of the dependency on others that accompanies role dysfunction (Vroland-Nordstrand et al., 2015). However, OT practitioners should be careful not to assume that ADL and IADL are immediate priorities. Some people, especially those with severe activity limitations, might need or want to accept assistance from others in ADL so that they can focus on improving other areas of occupational performance. This was the case with Mr. Fritz, a 32-year-old man with a recently sustained spinal cord injury resulting in C6 tetraplegia. He was married, had three small children, and was self-employed as a tax accountant, and the family depended on Mr. Fritz's income. The ADL outcomes were initially established for Mr. Fritz, but self-care retraining was met with resistance and frustration. Further discussion of the intervention outcomes revealed that Mr. Fritz was anxious to return to work and wanted to focus on computer skills. Although he did want to be independent in self-care eventually, he felt it was best for him to return to work to minimize the financial burden on his family. His wife was able and willing to help him, and they both felt that self-care retraining could be delayed until the family business was again operational. With intervention outcomes refocused on activities most valued by Mr. Fritz—namely, computer access and home mobility—he became highly motivated to participate in therapy.

Clients' values should drive long-term goals, but OT practitioners may need to help clients focus on ADL initially when they have identified priorities for more complex occupational performance areas (e.g., IADL, work, or leisure) that may be difficult to treat effectively early in the intervention process (Cipriani et al., 2000). Self-care training often helps clients develop capacities and problem-solving skills that can later be applied to activities that are more complex, particularly when dealing with severe disorders of sudden onset (e.g., stroke and traumatic injuries). For example, suppose Mr. Fritz could not work from a home office and wanted to focus on driving to get to work—a realistic long-term goal for someone with C6 tetraplegia. Initiating intervention with driver training, however, would be impractical because Mr. Fritz lacked the prerequisite functional mobility skills early in his rehabilitation. The ADL training—involving bathing, dressing, transferring, and wheelchair mobility—can facilitate the development of functional mobility skills. Such training, therefore, would logically precede driver training. If Mr. Fritz had been in this situation, his needs may have been met through a referral to social services for assistance with financial planning to help the family manage until he could return to work. The OT practitioner would have also needed to educate Mr. Fritz about the commonalities among skills needed for both self-care and driving. This plan would simultaneously recognize Mr. Fritz's valued roles and progress him to the desired outcome in the most efficient way possible.

When the most valued activities and roles are beyond the client's potential skill level, the OT practitioner helps the client refocus priorities so goals are realistic and achievable. If Mr. Fritz were the owner and cook of a small restaurant, for example, it is unlikely that he would meet the essential job requirements of a short-order cook even if the kitchen were adapted for wheelchair accessibility because the activities require bilateral hand function and must be done quickly. It is possible, however, that he could perform the activities of restaurant owner, including managing personnel and finances, operating the cash register, and seating customers. In this and similar situations, OT practitioners use their expertise in activity analysis and functional adaptation to assist clients in creating a realistic yet meaningful life for themselves and help them establish achievable goals to progress them to that vision (Doig et al., 2009; Liddle & McKenna, 2000).

Difficulty

The perceived ease with which a client completes an activity and the projected difficulty that will remain after intervention are important considerations in selecting goal behaviors (Thornsson & Grimby, 2001). The OT practitioner, who is skilled in activity analysis and has knowledge of pathology and impairment, must determine the prognosis for functional difficulty. This prognosis must then be communicated to clients so that decisions about acceptable levels of difficulty can be made collaboratively. Clients set intervention priorities, in part, by weighing the projected level of difficulty within the context of value—that is, how much difficulty they are willing to tolerate to be independent in an activity. The frequency with which an activity is performed should also be considered in establishing goals for ADL and IADL that are likely to remain difficult for a client to perform. In general, a higher level of proficiency is needed for activities that need to be done routinely, whereas a lower level of proficiency may be acceptable for activities that are done only occasionally.

For example, James is a 7-year-old boy with spina bifida, resulting in paralysis from the waist down. He has a neurogenic bladder and requires regular intermittent catheterization. He identified self-catheterization as a critical task for fulfilling his role as a student because he does not want to have help with this personal task from school personnel. James will need to be able to self-catheterize independently and efficiently for this task to fit into his school day. The occupational therapist believes that James will be capable of achieving independence with little difficulty after a period of practice. The goal is agreed on, and intervention begins. Another client, Amy, also has spina bifida, but it affects her upper extremities as well as her trunk and lower extremities. Unlike James, the spinal cord damage is incomplete, so she can usually empty her bladder without self-catheterization. On occasion, however, she has episodes of urinary retention, requiring catheterization within about 1 hour of experiencing symptoms. Amy would also like to be independent in self-catheterizing at school, so she does not need help from school personnel. The occupational therapist thinks that independent self-catheterization using safe and clean technique is a reasonable goal for Amy, but it will always be difficult because of her impaired hand function and difficulty positioning herself so that she can see and reach to insert the catheter. Amy will need to go to the nurse's office to transfer to a bed. Despite the difficulty, Amy opts to work on this goal. Because she has to catheterize herself so infrequently, she believes that her skill level will be adequate for meeting her needs.

Safety

The degree of risk inherent in the person-task-environment transaction must also be considered when establishing client goals. The IADL tasks tend to pose more safety risks, for example, working with sharp or hot objects while cooking, driving, or operating snow blowers or lawn mowers for home maintenance. However, some ADL can also pose safety risks for people, such as bathing, managing medications, or using safe-sex practices during sexual activity. Oftentimes, intervention is effective in reducing safety risks to an acceptable level; however, if the occupational therapist believes that performance cannot be effectively modified to meet safety standards, then those tasks may not be appropriate goals.

Safe driving has received increasing attention in the health care literature as the number of older drivers, many with health-related impairments, continues to increase. Occupational therapists are often the health professionals who evaluate and treat this important IADL (Korner-Bitensky, Menon, von Zweck, & Van Benthem, 2010).

Because of the potentially grave consequences of unsafe driving, occupational therapists must develop the skills to identify when it is appropriate to pursue driving goals and when safety precludes a return to driving and intervention should focus on driving cessation and goals that address alternative transportation methods, such as using public transportation (Kartje, 2006).

Understanding and implementing "safe-sex" practices to prevent sexually transmitted diseases may be an important safety-related goal for clients that is often not addressed by OT practitioners. Clients with cognitive deficits that may impair decision making (e.g., developmental disability, traumatic brain injury, or mental health disorders) may benefit from education about the potential health threats associated with unprotected sex. Clients with physical disabilities may require adaptations for safe-sex tasks, such as applying condoms.

Fatigue and Dyspnea

Fatigue, the sensation of tiredness that is experienced during or following an activity, and dyspnea, difficult or labored breathing, can interfere with activity performance (Seo, Roberts, LaFramboise, Yates, & Yurkovich, 2011; Van Heest, Mogush, & Mathiowetz, 2017) and both are likely to be exacerbated by activity performance. The occupational therapist uses activity analysis to take into account the effort required to perform a task and its typical duration. In addition, the client's entire daily routine must be examined so that the energy demands of one activity can be weighed in relation to the client's other activities (Mathiowetz, Matuska, & Murphy, 2001). Assisting clients to examine the physical demands of their preferred activities can help them to prioritize activities so that appropriate goals can be established. Similar to budgeting money, clients must be encouraged to look at their "energy dollars" and decide how they wish to spend them. The OT practitioner contributes to this decision-making process by bringing valuable information about options for activity adaptation that can reduce the energy demands of activities, thereby saving clients' energy for other tasks.

For example, Mrs. Hernandez lived alone in an apartment in a retirement community. Her sister and brother-in-law also resided in the community as well as many close friends. She has had multiple sclerosis for many years, with some weakness and spasticity, but she remained independent in her ADL until a recent exacerbation required hospitalization.

Increased fatigue and decreased strength resulted in the need for physical assistance with dressing and bathing and the use of a wheelchair for mobility. The retirement community required residents to manage their own ADL and prepare breakfast and a light evening snack. A hot meal was provided at midday. The OT practitioner explained to Mrs. Hernandez that although independence in

ADL and simple meal preparation were reasonable goals, completing her ADL would likely be time-consuming and fatiguing, leaving her limited energy for other activities. Mrs. Hernandez was enthusiastic about beginning therapy, indicating that she was willing to engage in fewer IADL and leisure activities in order to be independent in tasks that would enable her to remain in the retirement community with family and friends.

A different scenario played out with Mrs. McKay, who also had multiple sclerosis. Like Mrs. Hernandez, she had a recent exacerbation that caused a functional decline, and achieving independence in ADL was likely to expend much of her daily energy. Mrs. McKay had been working full time as a programmer for a local radio station and was the mother of two young children. She perceived her role as a self-carer to be important, along with those of worker and mother. However, when it became apparent that independence in ADL would leave her with little energy for performing work and parenting roles, she decided not to establish goals for independence in ADL, opting instead to hire a personal care attendant for assistance so she could focus on work and parenting goals.

Identifying an Appropriate Degree of Performance

Occupational therapy goals must include a measurable outcome that indicates how well or at what level the identified behavior will be done, sometimes referred to as the *degree of performance* (Kettenbach, 2009). Independence is the most common degree of performance; however, several performance parameters can also provide effective goals, especially when the client is independent, but occupational performance deficits remain that warrant intervention. For example, this would be the case when a client can open jars independently, but it is painful and results in deforming forces to the hand joints.

Independence

Independence is the performance parameter most commonly focused on in OT interventions (Bonikowsky, Musto, Suteu, MacKenzie, & Dennis, 2012), and it becomes the level of assist, the measurable part of the goal (Gateley & Borcherding, 2017). Across all ages and disabilities, the goal is generally to increase the level of independence (Clarke et al., 2009; Eyres & Unsworth, 2005; Legg, Drummond, & Langhorne, 2006; Pillastrini et al., 2008). Independence in activity performance includes three phases: initiation of a task, continuation of a task, and completion of a task. The most common OT goals focus on the completion of the task, which implies that initiation and continuation of the task occurred; for example, a goal might be "Client will be independent in feeding her cats 3/3 meals a day by December 12, 2018" or "Client will require moderate assistance for bed to/from wheelchair transfers in 1 week."

Initiation is an aspect of activity performance that is frequently overlooked when goals are established, in part because it is difficult to evaluate and treat. The very presence of the OT practitioner may be a cue to initiate a task. Adults are typically expected to initiate ADL and IADL independently. Expectations for children also exist, depending on the children's ages and skills and the division of task responsibilities among family members. Impairments in activity initiation may occur as a result of many diseases and disorders, such as attention-deficit disorder, dementia, depression, schizophrenia, brain injury from trauma or stroke, multiple sclerosis, and Parkinson disease. Family members generally find it frustrating to have to cue ("constantly nag") a client with impaired initiation for each aspect of a daily routine. The occupational therapist may write an independence goal that includes initiation, such as "Client will initiate and complete bathing independently three to seven times a week by November 30, 2018." In this example, measuring progress toward the goal would require the client or a proxy to record the number of times in a week that the client initiated bathing without cueing or assistance from another person.

Safety

Although some goals may not be feasible at all because of safety concerns, other times, it is possible to improve a person's safe performance of ADL/IADL, so safety becomes a part of the goal. Because safety is a quality of the person-task-environment transaction, it cannot be observed or treated in isolation from independence (Chui & Oliver, 2006; Russell, Fitzgerald, Williamson, Manor, & Whybrow, 2002). Goals related to safety are typically linked to independence outcomes; that is, independent performance is assumed to be safe (Bonikowsky et al., 2012; Tamaru, McColl, & Yamasaki, 2007) because an occupational therapist could not ethically create a goal for independent performance that was not deemed to be safe. Although OT practitioners agree that safety is an intervention priority, there is less consensus about specific activity behaviors that are safe or unsafe. Many behaviors fall into a questionable zone, where some would rate them as safe, whereas others perceive them as unsafe, for example, standing to pull-up pants during dressing. In determining acceptable risk for setting independence goals, it is useful to consider clients' comfort level with risk; their ability to analyze the risks associated with a particular activity and devise a plan for managing them; and, most important, their ability to implement the plan expeditiously despite impairments. At times, the goal for level of independence in activity performance might need to be sacrificed for safety. A comparison of two clients with bilateral lower

extremity fractures sustained in car accidents who are learning independent transfers illustrates this point.

Ted and Ryan were both recently injured, are non–weight bearing on both lower extremities, and are learning to transfer with a transfer board. Ted demonstrates good judgment and a realistic perception of his skills. The occupational therapist has determined that the following goal is realistic: "Client will be independent in transfers with a transfer board from wheelchair to/from bed within three therapy sessions." Through training, Ted learns to execute a safe transfer with the transfer board while keeping weight off his fractured legs. After a couple of sessions, his goal of independence in transferring from wheelchair to bed and back is met. Ryan's injuries are similar to Ted's, but he also incurred a mild brain injury. Although Ryan's motor skills are comparable to Ted's, Ryan has difficulty recalling the steps for a safe transfer and forgets to keep weight off his lower extremities, which could interfere with fracture healing. The occupational therapist considers safety when setting a goal for Ryan by aiming for a lower level of independence, for example, "Client will require supervision and verbal cues for transfers from wheelchair to/from bed using a transfer board while adhering to weight-bearing precautions within six therapy sessions." The degree of independence and the time frame in Ryan's goal were adjusted to reflect his capacity for safe transfer performance.

In some situations, it may be better to establish client goals in which the goal behavior is directly related to safety rather than being assumed in the degree of independence indicated. Goals can be aimed at the occupational performance level, that is, the IADL "safety and emergency maintenance" (AOTA, 2014); for example, the goal might be "Client will verbally describe correct responses to a minimum of 10 potential home emergencies with 100% accuracy within 3 weeks." Safety goals may also be aimed at developing safe habits; for example, "Client will pause when entering a room and scan for obstacles on the floor 100% of the time to reduce fall risk during functional mobility by December 1, 2018."

Adequacy

Several aspects of activity performance contribute to the adequacy or quality of the behavior stated in the goal, which can also be reflected in the goal as the degree to which the behavior is expected to be done. In addition to independence, these performance parameters may be crucial components of meaningful goals, especially for clients who are independent and safe with their performance but who feel dissatisfied with the process or some other aspect of the outcome. Goals with measurable adequacy parameters can be used to justify OT even if clients are independent in tasks. Six adequacy parameters can be used as measurable outcomes: pain, fatigue and dyspnea, duration, societal standards, satisfaction, and aberrant task behaviors. Some of these parameters may be interdependent within a single client. For instance, pain might lead to changes in duration of activity performance (e.g., the activity takes longer) as well as the ability to meet normative standards and personal satisfaction. A goal should include only one measurable parameter so that it is clear what has changed in documenting progress toward goals.

Pain. Pain, either during or following an activity, can negatively influence engagement in ADL or IADL even if the activity is completed independently (Covinsky, Lindquist, Dunlop, & Yelin, 2009; Dudgeon, Tyler, Rhodes, & Jensen, 2006; Liedberg & Vrethem, 2009). The source of pain and the prognosis for it must be carefully considered in establishing goals and selecting an intervention approach. Both the evaluation and goals must include an index of pain so that intervention remains focused on achieving the projected level of independence while simultaneously reducing the presence of pain. For example, the goal might be "Client will prepare a simple meal (soup, sandwich, and beverage) independently with a maximum pain level of 2 cm on a 10-cm visual analogue scale 4/5 times within 2 weeks."

Fatigue and Dyspnea. Fatigue and dyspnea can influence the actual task behaviors that are selected for client goals, as was described earlier in this section, but when fatigue or dyspnea can be reduced through task adaptation or conditioning, goals can be established that use these performance parameters as performance criteria outcomes. The initial evaluation should include baseline data for comparison. For example, a goal might be "Client will complete morning care routine (shower, grooming, dressing) with a maximum score of 12 on the Borg Rate of Perceived Exertion Scale 75% of the time by November 28, 2018." As long as the Borg Scale (Centers for Disease Control and Prevention, 2015) was used during the initial evaluation, a lower number (meaning less exertion) can be used in a goal to indicate progress toward becoming less fatigued during ADL or IADL tasks. Dyspnea can be monitored in a similar way, using a visual analogue scale or numerical rating scale (Gift & Narsavage, 1998). Diagnosis is important to consider when goals are formulated relative to fatigue and dyspnea. Overexertion can exacerbate symptoms or even the disease process itself for conditions such as cardiac disease and multiple sclerosis. Prognosis is another important consideration in setting goals that measure fatigue or dyspnea. Clients with chronic obstructive pulmonary disease are likely to become worse; therefore, goals must be reasonable to achieve through activity adaptations and might need to accommodate a decline in function. A client with paraplegia secondary to spinal cord injury, by contrast, experiences fatigue from having to use the smaller muscles of the upper extremity for wheelchair mobility to compensate for the larger lower extremity muscles previously used for walking. Endurance is likely to improve significantly as upper extremity strength and muscle endurance increases with use, and more ambitious goals for reducing fatigue could be appropriate.

Duration. The length of time that is required to complete activities is typically thought of as a reflection of efficiency, which may be affected by many types of impairments, including poor endurance, impaired coordination, and cognitive deficits such as reduced attention for tasks. Although measuring performance time may be relatively simple, interpreting time data in a meaningful way is often difficult. The duration of ADL/IADL depends highly on the nature of the activity and the task objects that people choose to use in performing the activity. Most of us spend more time dressing when we are going out to dine in an elegant restaurant than we do when we are going to a fast-food establishment. Therefore, it is difficult to establish meaningful time norms for ADL and IADL, but duration is often a parameter that clients wish to incorporate into their OT goals when they are frustrated by slow performance.

Establishing acceptable time frames for ADL goals must be done collaboratively with clients and their significant others. Occupational therapists also should consider safety and independence parameters when establishing goals with time frames. Clients may be at increased risk when they rush through activities or even when they attempt them at a typical pace. For example, clients with swallowing deficits might need to eat more slowly than people without such deficits to avoid choking. People with poor fine motor coordination or sensory deficits might need to slow down when using sharp knives to improve control of the knives and prevent injury. In these examples, setting goals to decrease the duration of performance would be inappropriate because it could result in unsafe performance.

Societal and cultural standards also need to be taken into consideration in establishing outcomes for activity duration. In the United States, timeliness is highly valued, and efficient performance in community skills is expected. Shoppers might become irritated when they are standing in a checkout line behind a customer who takes 5 minutes to identify and count currency, even though in other cultures, this delay might go unnoticed. A person living in America who has cognitive or visual impairments that interfere with the ability to count currency might wish to decrease the time required for this activity to reduce embarrassment when shopping. The goal, then, needs to include an efficiency measure to reflect this performance parameter, for example, "Client will independently complete a simple cash transaction (select appropriate currency and count change) in less than 1 minute within 3 weeks to support participation in shopping."

Societal Standards. Performance standards, determined by the society and culture in which the client lives, are likely to exist in terms of both the end result and the process through which it is achieved. The line between acceptable and unacceptable performance is likely to be wide rather than narrow and may vary considerably, depending on characteristics such as age, gender, and cohort (generation) membership.

Societal standards exist for neatness, for example. A client might dress safely and independently, but if clients select clothing with clashing colors or their appearance is disheveled (the end product), then dressing might not meet societal standards. If the client is a teenager, such an appearance might be considered acceptable. However, if the client is a public relations manager going to work, it could well put the client's job in jeopardy. Identifying societal standards might seem subjective and difficult, but the use of measurable indicators of societal standards is critical for effective goals and can justify intervention. A goal for a client who eats rapidly, putting food in his mouth when it is still full, might include a measure of societal standard, such as "When eating during a social event, the client will demonstrate appropriate pacing as evidenced by completing a meal in no less than 15 minutes and swallowing each bite before putting additional food in his mouth by December 10, 2018."

Satisfaction. In addition to societal standards, clients have their own standards of acceptable performance, which also need to be incorporated into goals (Eklund & Gunnarsson, 2008). Setting goals with satisfaction measures requires collaboration with clients because personal standards will vary greatly from person to person. Mr. Balouris, for example, is always losing things. He never seems to know where his wallet and keys are, and he is always searching for something. Nonetheless, items seem to turn up, and he sees no reason to go to the trouble of organizing his apartment better to help him keep track of his belongings. Mr. Johnson, however, has always been meticulously neat and could put his hands on items the minute he wanted them. Recently, he sought medical attention for memory problems. He complained that he needed to search for items because he failed to put them in their usual places. He was particularly concerned about his memory problem because of a family history of Alzheimer disease. He was referred to OT to learn strategies to help him remember where items are placed. Objectively, Mr. Johnson's performance is similar to Mr. Balouris; however, Mr. Johnson is dissatisfied with his performance, which he views as impaired.

Client satisfaction can be measured quickly and easily with a visual analog scale or numerical scale, such as the 10-point scale that is used in the COPM (Law et al., 2014) that can be easily incorporated into goals to reflect specific conditions for performance, for example, "Client will be independent in locating items needed for ADL and IADL in the home with a satisfaction rating of at least 8/10 within 3 weeks to support participation in ADL and IADL."

Aberrant Task Behaviors. Goals and interventions may also address any aberrant task behaviors that interfere with activity performance (Ashley et al., 2001). Aberrant task behaviors vary widely and include unwanted motor behavior such as athetoid or ballistic movements and behavioral problems such as self-stimulation or hitting caregivers. Exploration of the underlying cause of the aberrant task behavior facilitates the establishment of realistic goals and the selection of effective intervention strategies. Goals are aimed at eliminating or diminishing aberrant task behavior typically by replacing it with more functional behaviors in the context of ADL and IADL tasks, for example, for a client with tongue thrusting during eating, a goal might be "Client will use tongue lateralization to form a bolus during eating, within 2 months, in order to support safe and adequate oral intake." Tongue lateralization is incompatible with tongue thrust and would indicate a reduction of that behavior. Goals focused on performance inconsistent with aberrant behaviors are preferable than those that simply reflect a reduction in those behaviors.

Additional Considerations for Setting Realistic Client Goals

The occupational therapist uses performance parameters to identify goal behaviors and degrees of performance, but several additional factors that can affect goal achievement must also be considered. The process of setting goals is complex and must be based not only on clients' hopes but also what changes are realistic (Wade, 2009). Several contextual factors must be considered, such as physical and social environment, financial resources, time available for intervention, and the client's past experience and learning ability. The prognosis for recovery, given the client's disability, can also affect goal achievement.

Prognosis for Impairments

The client's potential for improvement of performance skills and patterns and client factors must be examined within the context of any existing disease or disorder and resulting impairments (Egan & Dubouloz, 2014). First, the practitioner must consider precautions or contraindications pursuant to the diagnosis that could preclude the use of certain intervention strategies. For example, compare two clients whose endurance significantly limits their performance. Mrs. Tanaka has chronic fatigue syndrome, a disorder that may worsen if she becomes overfatigued. An aggressive program to increase endurance is contraindicated for her, so alternative intervention strategies should be explored, and goals for increasing endurance for ADL must be reasonable, given Mrs. Tanaka's potential for exacerbation of her disease. Conversely, Mr. Krull is deconditioned from inactivity resulting from major depressive illness and would like to increase his endurance to support participation in heavy home maintenance tasks, such as mowing the lawn and finishing an addition on his house. A rigorous activity program to increase endurance is not contraindicated and would help to increase Mr. Krull's participation in IADL.

Second, the prognosis for improvement of impairments, given the client's diagnosis, must be considered. Increasing impairment is expected in progressive disorders, such as muscular dystrophy and Alzheimer disease. Goals must be established with potential declines in mind so that the goals are realistic.

Occupational therapy practitioners must consider various impairments separately, however, because progressive diseases might affect bodily structures and functions differently. For example, Jorge, a teenager who has muscular dystrophy, has significant muscle weakness in the trunk and all four extremities with limitations in pelvic and ankle passive ROM that preclude maintaining an optimal position for functioning from his wheelchair. His muscle strength is expected to decline, even with intervention. His passive ROM restrictions are secondary to the muscle weakness and not a direct result of the disease process. Gains can be expected in passive ROM with intervention, despite the overall prognosis. In turn, increased passive ROM can enhance function by improving Jorge's position in the wheelchair.

Stable or diminishing impairments may be anticipated in many disorders and after injury. Pharmacological intervention, for example, may improve impairments associated with depression so that OT intervention can be focused on transferring gains made in mental and psychological capacities into ADL and IADL performance.

Typically, clients of any age with brain injuries from trauma or stroke can expect some spontaneous return of body functions in the early stages of recovery. Projected intervention goals should take into account the typical improvements for this diagnosis. Predicting "typical improvements" takes time and experience to develop, and the novice practitioner might find it helpful to consult with more experienced clinicians to facilitate the ability to set realistic goals.

Experience

Information gathered in the evaluation about a client's past and recent experience with an activity is important to consider when setting goals. Recent experience may facilitate progress in reestablishing independence in an activity because the client is learning a new way to do the activity rather than developing a new skill. For example, Mrs. McCarthy needs to relearn cooking skills following a stroke. She uses a wheelchair for mobility and has minimal use of her right (dominant) hand. Her cognitive skills are intact, and she can easily follow a recipe. Furthermore, she demonstrates good problem-solving skills in adapting cooking activities to improve her performance. Miranda, a 19-year-old with spastic hemiplegia secondary to cerebral palsy, like Mrs. McCarthy, has limited use of one hand and uses a wheelchair for mobility.

Miranda wants to cook simple meals and bake cookies. Her intervention will require more time and guidance than Mrs. McCarthy's intervention because Miranda has to learn basic cooking skills along with the activity adaptations to compensate for her impairments.

Many clients are faced with learning new activities, particularly skills needed to manage new impairments, such as performing self-catheterization, donning pressure garments, or learning to operate assistive technology. Whenever a skill is unfamiliar to a client, additional intervention time and education will be needed for basic skill acquisition and should be incorporated into the goal and the intervention plan.

Client's Capacity for Learning and Openness to Alternative Methods

The client's capacity for learning and openness to using alternative methods for task completion must be evaluated because intervention often requires learning new methods of completing activities (Flinn, 2014). Clients with limited learning capacity due to cognitive or affective impairments can still learn new skills if appropriate teaching approaches are used and the duration of the intervention is adequate (Davis, 2005). Some clients might resist intervention that incorporates adaptive equipment if they do not want to use a special device to do a task that most people do without a device (Lund & Nygård, 2003). Clients with a good capacity for learning and openness to alternative methods may be able to address more task deficits because of increased intervention options and the reduced time required for learning. It is important to view capacity for learning on a continuum; clients can fall between the extremes, and capacity might be better for some tasks than for others.

Clients' capacity for learning may also change as they progress through the rehabilitation process, particularly for clients with a new disability. The focus of learning should progress from more directive, therapist-initiated learning to client-initiated learning, where the client is more autonomous in identifying goals and directing his or her own learning (Greber, Ziviani, & Rodger, 2007; Jack & Estes, 2010). Autonomous learning strategies enable clients to solve problems long after therapy has ended and enables them to develop their own adaptive strategies. The ability to be an independent problem solver can be learned, so occupational therapists should structure intervention activities that promote self-directed learning whenever possible (Greber et al., 2007).

Projected Follow-through with Program Outside of Direct Intervention

Efforts to contain health care costs have led to increasingly shorter lengths of stay in hospitals and rehabilitation centers and a reduction in outpatient and home health visits. Clients are expected to take an active role in their therapy programs and to supplement formal interventions with home programs (Novak, Cusick, & Lannin, 2009). Goals therefore need to be established with some estimate of the client's capacity to follow through with a self-directed program because this may influence the success of an intervention (Radomski, 2011).

Several of the performance parameters that were previously described can give the OT practitioner guidance in this area. Clients have more motivation for programs aimed at activities that they highly value than at those that they do not value, making a client-centered approach critical for success (Doig et al., 2009). In addition, performance parameters such as difficulty, fatigue, pain, and satisfaction must be considered so that self-directed programs are manageable for the client. Manageability of the program must be determined by clients in consultation with the OT practitioner and should take into consideration clients' daily activities and responsibilities, tolerance for frustration, and perseverance.

Many clients require some assistance to practice activities, and the OT practitioner must be sure that these resources are available, for example, someone to set up an activity or provide assistance. Impairments can affect a client's ability to initiate or persevere with activities, so assistance may be needed for initiation and follow-through in the home program. Occupational therapy practitioners need to interact with and educate caregivers about their critical role and home programs must accommodate caregiver needs.

Time for Intervention

The projected timeline for OT may be influenced by multiple factors, including the client's functional prognosis, motivation for improvement, and finances. Third-party payers vary in their reimbursement allowances for therapy visits, which can impact access to services and intervention outcomes (Arango-Lasprilla et al., 2010). Ongoing changes in Medicare impact services across settings, such outpatient rehabilitation (Simpson et al., 2015). Occupational therapy goals must be tailored to meet a client's needs as much as possible within the time allotted. Nonetheless, it must also be recognized that best practice takes into account *all* the client's needs. Occupational therapy practitioners need to

be aware of their professional responsibility to clients to request intervention extensions and to support these requests through detailed documentation and to appeal payment denials for needed services (Gateley & Borcherding, 2017). They must also establish intervention timelines that meet the needs of the client, rather than the needs of the facility, which may benefit from providing services that extend beyond the client's needs or tolerance level, as described in the "Ethical Dilemma" box.

⚖️ **ETHICAL DILEMMA**

Can Client-Centered Care Conflict with the Needs of an Organization?

Jessica is an occupational therapist working in a subacute rehabilitation unit in a skilled nursing facility. She completed an evaluation on Mrs. Cabrini, an 82-year-old woman with multiple medical problems, including a recent total hip replacement secondary to a fracture, cardiovascular disease, and rheumatoid arthritis.

Mrs. Cabrini would like to be independent in transfers, indoor mobility, and toileting, which would enable her to return to her home in an assisted living facility. She reported that she could get daily help with dressing and bathing and would prefer to do that because she fatigues quickly and wants to save her energy for the daily craft group. During the evaluation, Mrs. Cabrini tolerated about 30 minutes of therapy in the morning and 30 minutes in the afternoon, divided between OT and physical therapy (PT). Jessica established client-centered goals collaboratively with Mrs. Cabrini. The physical therapist agreed that the client could work productively for only two 30-minute sessions a day, and they opted to split the time, so Jessica documented that the intensity of OT would be 30 minutes daily, 7 days a week.

Jessica's supervisor approached Jessica and asked her to increase Mrs. Cabrini to 45 minutes a day so that Mrs. Cabrini would qualify for a higher Resource Utilization Group (RUG) under the Medicare prospective payment system. The supervisor told Jessica that if the facility cannot increase reimbursement rates by having more clients in higher RUGs, they might need to lay off staff, which would have an overall negative impact on client care. Jessica's supervisor also suggested that it would be easy to justify the increased therapy time if Jessica added more ADL goals, such as independence in dressing and bathing, to Mrs. Cabrini's care plan.

Questions

1. What should Jessica do in this situation?
2. How might client-centered care influence Jessica's actions?
3. How can Jessica balance the needs and wishes of her client with the needs of the facility?

Expected Discharge Context and Resources

Clients' expected discharge environments must be considered in establishing goals and selecting interventions that will be relevant to the environment in which clients will ultimately perform tasks (Law & Dunbar, 2007; Nakanishi, Sawamura, Sato, Setoya, & Anzai, 2010). The social context is critical for clients who require assistance from others after discharge; that is, it is important to determine whether there are people who are willing and able to provide needed assistance. Clients' needs vary broadly in terms of the type and duration of assistance required. Some clients need only supportive services, such as help with shopping or housecleaning. Those with significant activity limitations and intact cognition might require considerable physical assistance but can be left alone once ADL have been completed, they have eaten, and they are mobile in their wheelchairs. Clients with cognitive impairments do not always need physical assistance but might need verbal cueing to initiate or sustain activities or to perform them in a safe manner. This assistance might be specific to certain tasks (e.g., when cooking or interacting with small children) or it may need to be constant. Inadequate support in the client's expected environment may necessitate a change in the discharge plan. Some families or friends might be able to provide the level and type of assistance needed, whereas others may not.

The physical environment must also be considered in setting realistic goals (Gitlin, Corcoran, Winter, Boyce, & Hauck, 2001). For example, Mr. Feng has reached his goal of independence in bathing during his hospital-based rehabilitation. He requires a transfer tub seat, a hand-held shower hose, and a grab bar to bathe safely without help (Figure 50-2). The OT practitioner wants to order this equipment for him. However, Mr. Feng reports that he must shower in a 4 × 4 ft shower stall because the only bathtub is on the second floor and he cannot manage stairs. His shower will not accommodate the transfer tub bench that he requires for safe transfers and balance during showering. An alternative bathing goal should have been established at the beginning of intervention so that Mr. Feng's program focused on developing skills he could use at home, such as sponge bathing at the sink.

The adaptability of the discharge environment must also be explored before setting goals. A house that is high above the street on a small lot with 21 steps to the front door makes the installation of a properly graded ramp impossible. Wall grab bars cannot be installed on some fiberglass tub surrounds, making a safety rail placed on the side of the bathtub the only feasible option regardless of where the client really needs the most support.

Established functional goals must also be achievable within the client's available resources, including property

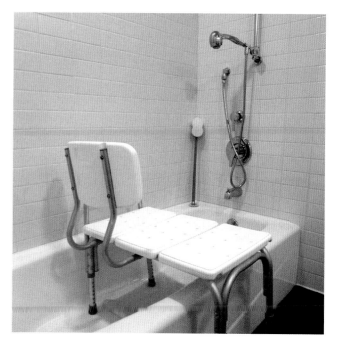

FIGURE 50-2 A transfer tub seat requires more space than Mr. Feng's small bathroom and shower can accommodate. Knowing the client's discharge environment can help practitioners determine interventions that will be successful after discharge.

and financial resources. For example, clients living in rental units might be unable to make structural alterations as desired because they do not own the unit. Some individuals may benefit from equipment or devices that they cannot afford and are not covered by their third-party payer. This situation can result in a practice dilemma for the occupational therapist, as described in the "Practice Dilemma" box.

PRACTICE DILEMMA

How Does One Provide Optimal Care with Limited Resources?

Jon is an occupational therapist in a large rehabilitation hospital in a major city. The OT department recently installed the latest **electronic aids to independent living (EADL)**, also known as **environmental control units**, in an on-site apartment that they use during therapy. Henry is a 16-year-old who has muscular dystrophy very limited use of his upper extremities. He operates a reclining power wheelchair independently with a head switch. Henry lives alone with his mother who works in a low-wage job. He receives Medicaid.

Henry's disease has progressed such that he is no longer able to get into and out of his home without assistance or operate common electronic devices, including the television, telephone, and lights. Because his mother works during the day, Henry must attend an after-school program that is primarily for small children. Henry said that his most important OT goal is to be independent in getting into and being home after school when no one is in the house. The occupational therapist is sure that this could be an achievable goal for Henry with an EADL system that would enable him to be independent in unlocking and opening the door, turning lights and electronic devices on and off, and using the telephone and computer. The therapist is also aware, however, that Medicaid will not pay for an EADL in his state.

Questions

1. How should Jon proceed? Should he train Henry in the use of the EADL, even if it will not be possible for him to purchase it?
2. What team members might the occupational therapist consult with to help progress Henry toward his goal?
3. Does the diagnosis of muscular dystrophy, a progressive disorder, affect the approach that Jon would take to solve this problem to help Henry achieve his goal?

Last, all of the various places in which a client expects to function after discharge must be explored if activities are likely to be performed in more than one place. Clients in a hospital-based setting may be focused primarily on returning home, but most people do not confine themselves to a single environment. Adaptations for toilets, such as raised toilet seats and toilet armrests, are commonly used for people with limited mobility. Home adaptations are easily made, but clients are often in environments that have not been adapted, such as public buildings, friends' homes, airplanes, hotels, and portable toilets at the local fair. If clients are likely to be in these environments, their goals should address their ability to perform tasks in varied settings.

Interventions for Activities of Daily Living and Instrumental Activities of Daily Living Impairments

Interventions for ADL and IADL problems are based on clients' goals and involve selecting intervention approaches and activities, carrying out the intervention, and reviewing the intervention to ensure that it is effective in progressing clients toward their goals.

Planning and Implementing Intervention

Five approaches to intervention are described in the OTPF: create/promote, establish/restore, maintain, modify, and prevent (AOTA, 2014). Although all of these approaches can be used to support or enhance ADL and IADL performance, modify and establish/restore are the most commonly used in practice and will be the focus of intervention discussed in this chapter. Both modify and establish/restore approaches need to be combined with client and/or caregiver education to ensure carryover of the program to function in everyday life (Flinn, 2014). Occupational therapy practitioners select specific intervention activities for clients that are guided by a range of theory-guided approaches, sometimes referred to as *frames of reference*. Specific OT approaches are beyond the scope of this chapter, but examples can be found in Unit IX. The following subsection focuses on broader intervention approaches and related strategies and includes a discussion of client and caregiver education and strategies for grading activities to progress clients to the established goals.

Selecting an Intervention Approach

The OT practitioner considers several variables when deciding whether it is more appropriate to focus on compensating for a client's deficits through adaptation or restoring underlying skills needed to reach goals or a combination of both (Buzaid, Dodge, Handmacher, & Kiltz, 2013). These considerations are addressed in the sections that follow.

Modify. Activity performance can be enhanced through modifications that compensate for limitations rather than restore previous capacities. This is often necessary when restoration is not an option. For example, a client with a complete C5 tetraplegia will not regain hand function regardless of the restorative approach used, so compensation is needed for successful participation in ADL and IADL. Even for clients for whom restoration is possible, a modify approach might be more appropriate if time limitations or client motivation would lead to less than optimal outcomes. Compensatory strategies may also be warranted when some, but not full, restoration of function is achieved. Generally, compensatory strategies require less intervention time for achieving functional outcomes compared with restorative strategies, although skilled intervention is warranted for selection and training in appropriate devices (Zanatta et al., 2017).

There are three general intervention strategies for compensation, which may be used alone or in combination: Modify the activity or task method, modify the task objects, or modify the environment. Examples of these three intervention strategies for selected ADL and IADL are included in Table 50-3.

• **Modify the Task Method.** The task objects and contexts are unchanged, but the method of performing the task

TABLE 50-3   Examples of the Three Approaches to Modifying Tasks to Compensate for Impairments

Task	Modify the Task Method	Modify the Task Objects	Modify the Task Environment
Bathing	Substitute washing at sink for someone unable to get in/out of the tub safely even with adaptive equipment.	Use a bath mitt and soap on a rope so that a person who cannot retrieve objects does not drop them.	Install grab bars and a transfer tub seat to enable a client to remain seated during bathing.
Grooming	Client stabilizes small containers with the ulnar digits and unscrews lids with the radial digits to compensate for loss of the use of one hand.	An extended handle is added to a razor so that a woman can shave her legs without bending forward.	A daily schedule is posted in the bathroom for a client with impaired attention to improve adherence to a daily grooming routine.
Toileting	Use an alarm watch to encourage regular emptying of the bladder.	Use a toilet aid to extend the range of reach for toilet hygiene.	Install a bidet to eliminate the need for manipulating toilet paper for hygiene.
Dressing	Learn to dress the affected side first to compensate for loss of use of one side of the body.	Use a sock aid to put socks on without having to reach the feet.	Lower clothing racks or replace a high dresser with a low one to increase access to clothes.
Feeding	Serve different food items (e.g., meat, starch, vegetable) in consistent places on the plate for someone who is blind.	Use a built-up handled utensil to compensate for diminished prehension in the hand.	Have a second grader with an attention disorder eat with a few friends in a small room rather than the loud and busy cafeteria.
Sexual activity	Identify alternate erogenous zones for a person without sensation in the genital area.	Use a vibrator for satisfying a female partner for a male partner with erectile dysfunction.	Provide bed rails or overhead trapeze to facilitate repositioning during sexual activity in bed.
Transfers	Sit first in the car seat before swinging the legs in rather than entering by leading with the leg.	Use a sliding board to eliminate the need for the lower extremities to support body weight.	Rearrange furniture to allow the wheelchair to be positioned near to the bed or a favorite chair.
Child care	Use safe lifting techniques when lifting a child out of a crib or onto a changing table.	Add a handle to a baby bottle to reduce finger grip needed to hold and position the bottle.	Install a wall-mounted changing table that allows for easy wheelchair access.
Caregiving for an adult	Change from showers to sponge baths to reduce the need for multiple transfers during morning care.	Use of a slip sheet to reduce friction when repositioning a person in bed.	Add high contrast stickers to the bottom of the tub to make the bottom visible and reduce fear of bathing for an adult with dementia.
Cooking	Sit at the kitchen table to chop vegetables to conserve energy.	Use a cutting board with aluminum nails to hold vegetables for cutting or peeling.	Install a mirror above the stove to enable a wheelchair user to see items cooking.
Driving	Enter the vehicle by sitting first then swinging the legs in.	Provide hand controls to compensate for paralysis of the legs.	Restrict driving to daylight or low-volume hours.
Shopping	Shift to online shopping to reduce the need for community mobility.	Purchase a walker basket for carrying items.	Request assistance from a grocery store employee to help reach items.

is altered to make the task feasible given the client's impairments. Many one-handed techniques for tasks that are normally done with two hands use this strategy, such as one-handed shoe tying (Figure 50-3) and one-handed typing techniques. Another example is minimizing tremors or **ataxia** by having a client stabilize her forearms on tabletops, armrests, or walls to improve hand coordination when performing a range of ADL (Gillen, 2000).

To master an altered task successfully, clients require the capacity to learn. The necessary level of learning capacity depends on the complexity of the method that is to be learned (Flinn, 2014). Occupational therapy practitioners should also attend to the level of automaticity clients may wish to achieve for specific ADL and IADL. People often rely on automatic processing for well-learned tasks, which means they require little direct attention. Automatic processing of routine tasks frees the individual for other things, such as planning one's workday while getting ready in the morning or chatting with a child during meal preparation. Practice is a necessary component of all learning and is especially crucial for clients

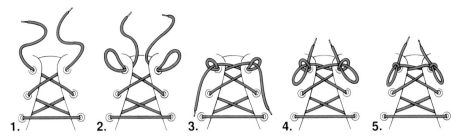

1. Lace laces in usual way.
2. Put both lace ends back through the holes they exited until the loops formed are small.
3. Put the lace ends through the opposite loops and pull to tighten loops, allowing just enough room to put the lace end back through the loop.
4. Put lace ends back through the loops, forming another loop.
5. Pull on these loops alternately to tighten.

FIGURE 50-3 **One-handed shoe-tying method.**

who wish to develop or return to automatic performance of ADL or IADL. Clients benefit from follow-through with a training program that includes the practice and repetition needed to meet adequacy parameters, such as reducing difficulty and duration of performance and increasing satisfaction.

- **Modify the Task Objects or Prescribe Assistive Devices.** The objects that are used for the task may be adapted to facilitate performance. For example, handles can be built up on utensils for clients with decreased active finger ROM or training in the use of memory aids (e.g., checklists, cue cards, and electronic devices) may help clients who have difficulty initiating tasks (Gillen, 2009; specifically Chapter 9). For some task adaptations, the task method does not change much, so the need for learning may be minimal. When this is the case, the need for practice is also reduced, and performance can improve quickly. Examples of simple adaptations include utensils with enlarged or extended handles, a cutting board with nails to stabilize food while cutting, and elastic shoelaces. Some adaptations, however, require more extensive training, for example, learning to drive with hand controls.

The prescription of assistive devices must take into account the client's capabilities and willingness to use the device as well as the features of the device. For example, a sock aid can help a client with poor sitting balance to reach her feet without leaning forward, which could throw her off balance. However, if the client's balance deficit is secondary to hemiplegia and she also has poor use of one hand, it will be very difficult or impossible for her to get the sock onto the sock aid, which typically requires both hands (Figure 50-4). Figure 50-5 depicts the number of decisions that an OT practitioner makes when

selecting an adapted spoon, a very simple type of adaptive equipment.

One disadvantage of adapting task objects is that the adapted item must be available to clients whenever or wherever they engage in the task. This may pose a problem, depending on the task and the adaptation. Clients who rely on phone alerts to remember appointments have their adaptation within a device they would normally have with them throughout the day. If a client requires built-up utensils for eating, however, and wishes to eat at a restaurant, the utensils must be taken along. This is cumbersome, and some clients find it embarrassing.

Finally, some clients find that the use of adaptive equipment reduces satisfaction with task performance. To enhance personal satisfaction with task performance, they might be willing to cope with the increased difficulty of doing a task without adapted tools. For example, a man with multiple sclerosis, who finds that using a wheelchair for outdoor mobility reduces fatigue, may opt to walk if his desire to be ambulatory in public outweighs his desire to save energy.

- **Modify the Task Environment.** Modification of the environment itself may facilitate task performance (Chard, Liu, & Mulholland, 2009; Padilla, 2011). Typically, when the environment is modified, the demand for learning and practice is less than that required for learning an alternative method or using adapted task objects. Environmental modifications are often fixed in place so that clients do not need to remember to bring along the necessary adaptations and the adaptations cannot be easily displaced (e.g., dropped out of reach). The task method is often unchanged, or only minimally changed, so that clients can rely on previous experience. Examples include installing a wheelchair ramp, increasing available light, labeling cupboard doors to compensate for

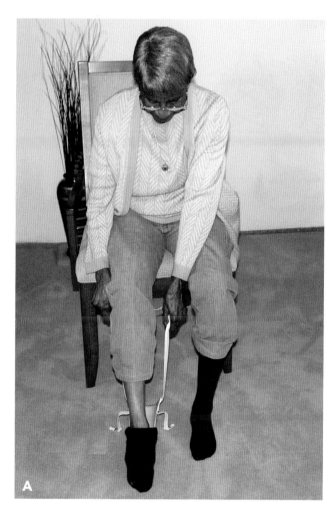

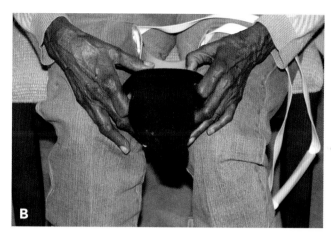

FIGURE 50-4 **A.** A sock aid is useful for people with limited reach, for example, from limited balance or range of motion. **B.** However, the client needs to have the use of both hands to get the sock onto the device, which could make it impractical for some clients.

cognitive deficits, and installing a toilet seat frame (Figure 50-6). Environmental control systems and now smart home technology are also environmental modifications that enable people to operate home electronics (e.g., computer, phone, lights, stereo, television) and even open doors by using an accessible switch, user display, and a processor (Brandt, Samuelsson, Töytäri, & Salminen, 2011).

The biggest drawback of environmental modifications is that clients might become limited in terms of performance context. They must do the task in the modified environment or in one that has been similarly modified because the modifications are not easily transportable and might be custom designed for a specific setting. However, interprofessional practice between OT providers and architects in the area of community mobility and universal design holds promise for expanding the accessibility of built environments (Hitch, Larkin, Watchorn, & Ang, 2012).

Establish/Restore. An establish or restorative approach typically focuses intervention at the impairment

level with the aim of restoring or establishing the capacities that are needed for functional tasks (AOTA, 2014), such as strength, endurance, ROM, short-term memory, visual scanning, and interests (Buzaid et al., 2013). More information about specific techniques can be found in the chapters in Unit XII. Regardless of the underlying theories or techniques used, one must always establish the link between the impairment and the resulting activity limitations. Careful documentation of the evaluation contributes to interprofessional collaboration by assisting other providers and third-party payers to understand the connection between the intervention and the established occupation-based outcomes (Gateley & Borcherding, 2017). Clients must be educated about the relationship between the capacities they are addressing in therapy and the occupations they support so that they understand how the intervention will ultimately lead to improved performance. Intervention must include opportunities to transfer new performance skills into everyday activities; for example, hanging laundry or pinning pictures on a bulletin board is a treatment activity that requires a client to use increased shoulder passive ROM in a functional

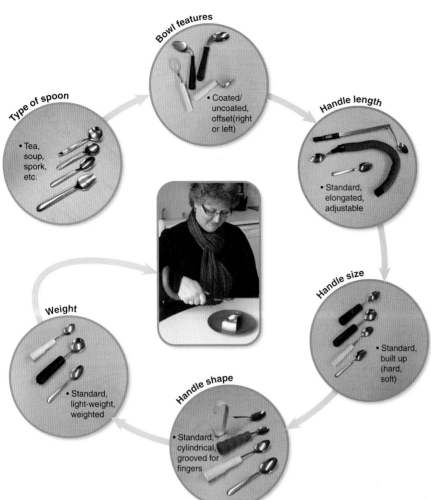

FIGURE 50-5 Potential decisions for prescribing an adapted spoon, a simple assistive device.

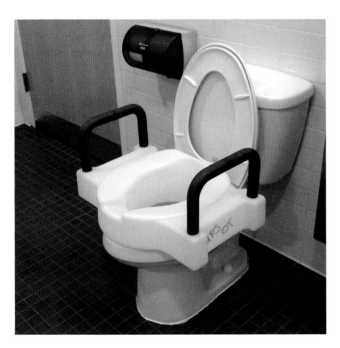

FIGURE 50-6 A toilet frame used to help the individual move between sitting and standing and to increase stability during transfers.

context (Figure 50-7). Table 50-4 includes additional examples.

Intervention that is aimed at establishing or restoring capacities is often most efficient for clients who have a few impairments that affect many tasks, and those impairments are expected to improve. For example, Mr. Stapinski had circumferential burns to both upper extremities.

The resulting bilateral restrictions in elbow flexion prevented him from completing most ADL because he could not reach his face, head, or trunk. Tasks could be easily adapted by using long-handled devices, but extended tools would have been needed for many ADL tasks (e.g., eating utensils, toothbrush, comb, brush, bath sponge). Because people with burns can usually regain passive ROM with stretching, scar management, and exercise, intervention aimed at increasing Mr. Stapinski's elbow flexion was most efficient. Adapting selected task objects improved his ADL performance in the short term; however, restoring Mr. Stapinski's capacity to flex his elbows enhanced function across many different tasks.

For clients with some types of impairments, carefully selected and graded intervention activities can restore or establish capacities while simultaneously permitting the

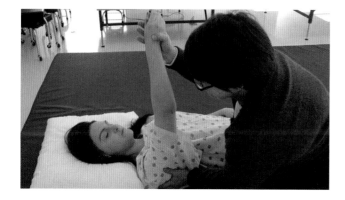

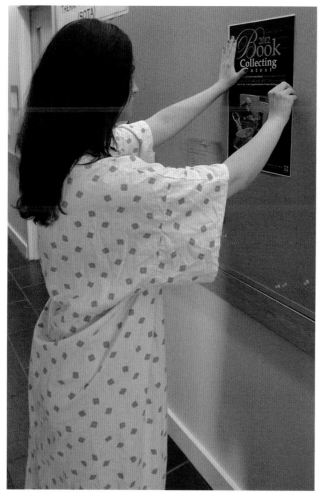

FIGURE 50-7 Stretching to restore passive range of motion (PROM) may be an effective treatment for improving reach **(A)**, but practitioners should be sure to incorporate PROM gains into occupation-based activities **(B)**.

practice of the meaningful occupations. Clients with limited endurance due to deconditioning could do aerobic exercise to increase cardiopulmonary endurance, shifting to meaningful activities when an adequate increase in cardiopulmonary capacity is achieved. Instead, an intervention that graded the intensity and duration of daily activities

could be as effective in increasing cardiovascular fitness while enabling the client to participate in desired tasks. Children and adults may engage more effectively in play or leisure activities that incorporate the necessary repetitive movements compared to a rote exercise (Melchert-McKearnan, Deitz, Engel, & White, 2000). Practice and participation in ADL and IADL programs also give clients with a new disability an opportunity to become familiar with their altered bodies (Guidetti, Asaba, & Tham, 2007) and may be more effective in overall outcomes, particularly in IADL (Orellano, Colón, & Arbesman, 2012).

Depending on the performance impairment, intervention time needed to establish or restore underlying skills may be longer than that required for compensatory approaches. This increased time must be considered, particularly for clients who have limited reimbursement for OT. In addition, clients must recognize that the rehabilitation period might be longer and that follow-through with a home program is vital if gains are to be made. Telehealth offers a possible means of follow-up with clients to support adherence with a home program and performance of health management and maintenance activities among persons with chronic conditions (Arif, El Emary, & Koutsouris, 2014).

Integrating Intervention for Impairments and Activity Limitations. A carefully crafted intervention plan may include both modify and establish/restore approaches to enable a client to be more functional through the use of compensatory strategies while at the same time working to restore underlying capacities (Buzaid et al., 2013). It is critical that the OT practitioner reduce the use of compensatory strategies as clients make gains in skill performance when using the two approaches.

For example, Mr. Stapinski, whose burns resulted in bilateral limitations in elbow flexion, might benefit from using utensils with extended handles to feed himself independently during the 2 to 3 weeks that it takes to increase his elbow flexion sufficiently for him to feed himself without these utensils. The extended handles should be fabricated to require him to flex fully within his available range and should be shortened as gains in passive ROM are made so that the new range is used whenever he feeds himself.

Whenever OT practitioners anticipate that task or environmental adaptations will be temporary, they must consider the cost in relationship to the anticipated time the adaptations will be needed and the potential benefit to clients. Thermoplastic extensions can be added to the handles of regular utensils rather than prescribing the more costly commercially available utensils with elongated handles. Safety concerns, of course, supersede cost considerations. Using a collapsible lawn chair in the shower would be an inexpensive alternative to a shower chair, but it would not provide adequate stability for most clients.

TABLE 50-4 Integrating Treatment Gains from an Establish or Restore Approach into Functional Tasks

Impairment	Preparatory Activity to Reduce Impairment	Task to Integrate Gains Made into ADL/IADL	Functional Outcomes
Impaired grip strength	Hand putty exercises	Cooking task with light resistance (e.g., stirring Jello) that progresses to more resistive tasks (e.g., brownies then cookies)	Increased ability to grasp task objects firmly (e.g., opening containers, doors, pulling up pants)
Decreased upper extremity muscle endurance	Using an arm ergometer	Wheelchair mobility, increasing time and difficulty (e.g., progress from flat surfaces to ramps)	Increased ability to engage in sustained upper extremity work (e.g., propelling a wheelchair, shampooing hair, washing windows)
Dyspnea	Practice diaphragmatic and pursed-lip breathing seated, doing nothing else.	Incorporate breathing techniques into seated ADL, progressing to standing and moving.	Ability to minimize dyspnea by improving oxygen intake during ADL and IADL
Hyperresponsiveness to tactile stimuli	Brushing skin	Progress from bathing in a tub to a shower, which provides a stronger stimulus.	Ability to tolerate tactile stimuli in everyday tasks, including dressing, brushing teeth, and interacting with others
Anxiety in new situations	Practice progressive relaxation in a quiet place to reduce anxiety.	Use progressive relaxation in community outings with the therapist.	Ability to function effectively in new situations without experiencing excessive anxiety (e.g., job interview, cultural events, travel)

ADL, activities of daily living; IADL, instrumental activities of daily living.

Education of the Client or Caregiver

Instructional Methods. Various instructional methods are available for client and caregiver education (Greber et al., 2007), and methods should be selected that best meet the person's needs. When a facility has a client population with similar goals, group instruction can be an efficient method for education that also provides learning through peer interaction and problem solving.

Individualized instruction is more appropriate for many clients and caregivers because the personal nature of many ADL are not conducive to group instruction. One-on-one client or caregiver education gives the OT practitioner immediate feedback from the person as the session progresses so the amount and focus of learning can be adjusted accordingly.

A vast array of media are available to facilitate the client's or caregiver's learning process. Written materials may be developed specifically for a client or caregiver, or published materials can be used if they meet the client's needs. Digital audio and visual recorders are usually available on the client's or caregiver's phone, and custom-made videos can be an effective teaching tools. The Internet contains a wealth of information about various disorders that is specifically geared toward clients and caregivers, or practitioners can develop and upload customized educational content to accessible sites, such as YouTube, as long as client confidentiality is maintained. Health care professionals, including occupational therapists, are using teleconferencing for educational purposes, for example, to engage in occupation-based coaching for parents of children with autism to increase children's participation in daily activities (Little, Pope, Wallisch, & Dunn, 2018).

Care must be taken to assess the match between client and caregiver skills and the educational content. For example, adults living in developed countries have mean reading skills that range from fifth to eighth grade, so written materials should be designed with these literacy levels in mind in order to improve clients' learning (McKenna & Scott, 2007). More information on client education can be found in the "Commentary on the Evidence" box.

Caregiver Training. Caregiver training may be implemented to maximize a client's functional outcome (Buzaid et al., 2013; Chard et al., 2009; DiZazzo-Miller, Winston, Winkler, & Donovan, 2017) while minimizing the efforts of the caregiver (Dooley & Hinojosa, 2004). For example, Mr. Ford had a stroke and required minimal physical assistance with verbal cues for wheelchair transfers. Mrs. Ford was physically fit but had no experience assisting a person with transfers. One day, she decided to help her husband move from his hospital bed to the chair. She had seen it done but did not know some of the important strategies, so they both fell onto the bed. No one was hurt but Mrs. Ford was distraught as she thought she could not care for her husband at home and he would have to go to a nursing home. She was open to transfer training from the OT practitioner and delighted to find that by using specific physical and verbal techniques, she could easily and safely assist

COMMENTARY ON THE EVIDENCE

Client Learning

Finding the Best Educational Strategies for Client Learning

As individual therapy time has been reduced by third-party reimbursement plans, client and caregiver education has played a more important role in intervention. Many studies have demonstrated the effectiveness of different and varied educational programs. For example, patient education programs have been effective in improving self-management and reducing pain and disability for people with rheumatoid arthritis (Siegel, Tencza, Apodaca, & Poole, 2017), reducing the impact of fatigue in people with chronic conditions (Van Heest et al., 2017), and increasing fall threats knowledge and fall prevention behaviors in older adults (Schepens, Panzer, & Goldberg, 2011). K. Eklund, Sonn, and Dahlin-Ivanoff (2004) compared a health education program for people who have visual impairment with traditional individualized intervention and reported that participants in the health education program had higher perceived security for several ADL and IADL. Researchers typically describe the educational programs used in their studies, and the educational methods reported vary significantly. Although there is ample research to support the efficacy of patient education

programs on client outcomes, few studies were found that compared varied educational approaches for clients to identify best practice in this area. For example, research on group intervention that includes active participation, collaborative problem solving, and learning tasks that relate to a current, relevant problem seem to be more effective in equipping clients with tools needed to meet challenges in the future (K. Eklund & Dahlin-Ivanoff, 2006). Learning is a complex process, and factors such as motivation and authenticity of training should be addressed in planning learning experiences (Schepens et al., 2011). Many educational programs are aimed at changing clients' habits, such as engaging in home exercise programs or incorporating energy conservation techniques into daily activities, which require behavioral approaches for supporting the development of new habits and follow-up studies to examine program effectiveness (Mathiowetz, Matuska, Finlayson, Luo, & Chen, 2007). Future research should also examine the impact of varied impairments on the effectiveness of education, for example, problems with initiation, attention, or executive function. Gathering additional evidence will enable practitioners to become even more effective in helping clients to reach their goals (see Chapters 32 and 48).

her husband. In this example, caregiver training increased the client's level of independence and the probability that he could go home at discharge.

Like clients, caregivers have varied learning styles, capacities, and experience. In many situations, the caregiver is a family member who is still coping with the emotional impact of having a family member with a disability, whether a new parent with a child with cerebral palsy or the spouse of someone who has had a stroke. Caregivers experiencing emotional stress have impaired learning and memory (Mackenzie, Wiprzycka, Hasher, & Goldstein, 2009) and often need more time and repetition to process information accurately. In other cases, caregivers have been providing care for years and bring a wealth of caring expertise to the OT session. The OT practitioner should work collaboratively with all caregivers but may move into a more consultative role with experienced caregivers who can articulate problems and engage actively in problem solving based on prior learning (Toth-Cohen, 2000). When caregivers must assist clients physically, their physical capacity for providing this assistance also warrants evaluation, and training must match their physical capacity.

When caregivers are helping to carry out an intervention program, the goals and general intervention strategies should be made clear to them (McKenna & Scott, 2007). Caregivers are often pivotal in motivating clients. Spurring clients on who have disorders that impact motivation, such

as depression, can be particularly challenging. Helping caregivers to understand that disinterest and lack of motivation are a part of the disorder, and providing concrete strategies for managing the "getting going" phase of the home program will foster its success (Resnick, 1998). For clients with behavior problems, such as the reactions that may accompany autism or Alzheimer disease, teaching caregivers behavior management strategies that prevent or defuse potentially volatile situations can be invaluable to their success as caregivers.

When caregivers need to provide physical assistance, they should be trained in using proper body mechanics, especially during transfers or bed mobility and for wheelchair positioning. Hinojosa and Rittman (2009) found that caregivers with greater educational needs were more likely to have sustained a physical injury, suggesting that caregiver education may reduce the risk of injury. Taking care of the caregiver is frequently overlooked in OT, but it is an essential component of the person-task-environment transaction, particularly when it is anticipated that the client will require assistance over a long period of time.

Grading the Intervention Program

It is important to progress the client continually toward established intervention goals and to set new goals as initial goals are met. The specific means of grading intervention when a restoration approach is being implemented

CENTENNIAL **NOTES**

Changes in Adaptations Over Time

Some adaptations have changed drastically over time, . . .

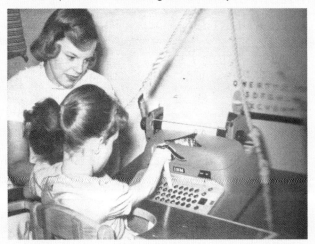

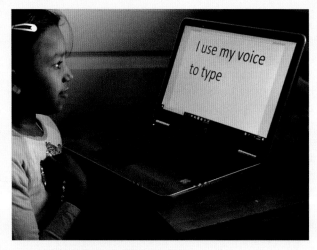

1963, 3rd edition
A child with cerebral palsy using a typewriter with keyboard shield tipped to the necessary position.

2018
A child typing by use of voice-to-text software.

. . . whereas others have remained the same.

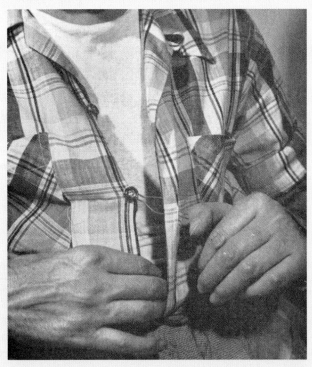

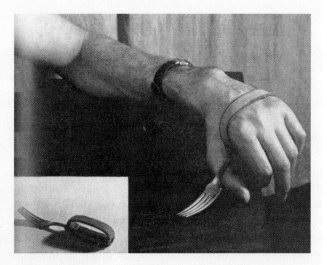

1954, 2nd edition
A simple adaptation that permits a disabled person to eat without assistance.

1954, 2nd edition
Use of adapted buttonhook for buttoning a shirt.

depends on the impairments and the intervention strategies that are being used (Piersol, 2014). If the intervention plan blends establish/restore and modify/adapt approaches, the program can be graded by reducing the amount of task and environmental adaptations as clients' capacities are restored.

Grading Task Progression from Easier to Harder. One means of grading an intervention program is to begin with easier ADL or IADL tasks and progress to more difficult ones. Task difficulty will be relative to a client's activity limitations and underlying impairments. For example, paying bills might be relatively easy for a client with tetraplegia to perform once the use of a writing tool is mastered, whereas lower extremity dressing is much more difficult. Conversely, a client with an acquired brain injury who has significant cognitive impairment but relatively preserved motor skills is likely to find lower extremity dressing to be relatively easy but money management extremely difficult.

Increasing Complexity within the Task. Rather than progressing only from easier to harder activities, intervention may also be graded by increasing the complexity within an activity or by progressing from simple to more complex ways of doing it. Cooking skills might extend from simple preparations such as cold sandwiches to more complex, multiple-course dinners. Even seemingly simple tasks can often be graded. A sock-donning intervention, for example, might be scaled from using looser ankle socks to tighter knee socks and finally to tight antiembolus hose.

Same Task in Varied Performance Environments. A critical part of a graded intervention program involves progression from the intervention environment to the real-life environment. This can involve transfer from a clinic to a home setting or the more subtle dynamics associated with the transfer of help from the OT practitioner to the natural caregiver. The client who is independent in donning a jacket while sitting on a mat table in the clinic might be unable to do so when sitting on a chair with a back or when standing. Providing practice in increasingly demanding performance environments can facilitate the generalization of skills, thereby enhancing the client's functional flexibility.

Therapist-Facilitated to Client-Facilitated Problem Solving. Clients with permanent disabilities or chronic diseases must develop problem-solving skills in order to meet new challenges in their lives after discharge from OT services. Initially, when facing a new task or becoming familiar with a changed body or mind, therapists may use explicit instruction or demonstration to help clients learn new approaches to ADL and IADL. Intervention can be graded by engaging the client in problem solving,

for example, by asking a client who is a new wheelchair user to come up with strategies for traveling after completing more direct training in community mobility in a familiar setting.

Intervention Review: Reevaluation to Monitor Effectiveness

The ADL and IADL are evaluated on entry to OT to provide a measure of the client's baseline performance status. Regardless of the extent and length of the intervention, reevaluation of ADL and IADL performance is needed to ascertain whether the intervention is resulting in improvement, whether the intervention should be continued or changed, or whether maximal benefit from OT has been achieved and activity performance has reached a plateau (AOTA, 2014). Occupational therapy practitioners routinely engage in informal review of interventions by observing clients' performance during intervention and considering the actual or potential impact of their performance on established goals.

Periodically, a more formal intervention reevaluation is needed to objectively measure clients' progress toward goals and to document progress in clinical records. The best strategy for reevaluation is to readminister the same assessments done in the initial evaluation, which enhances the possibility of detecting change in the client's performance attributable to intervention. If the reevaluation assessments vary from a prior evaluation, the potential for detecting change is reduced. For example, if ADL performance is assessed initially by self-report but is reassessed with a performance-based measure, differences in level of assistance may reflect an actual change in performance or simply differing views of the client and the therapist.

Conclusion

This chapter described the OT process for clients with ADL and IADL deficits. Performance parameters of value, independence, safety, and adequacy were reviewed, and their relevance to the selection of specific assessment tools was described. Occupational therapists should establish objective baseline measures through the use of standardized ADL and IADL assessments whenever possible; however, the realities of the intervention setting may also require the use of nonstandardized assessments. Developing objective goals that address all relevant performance parameters is a crucial first step in implementing intervention by providing a "road map" for guiding client care. General approaches that occupational therapists use to increase participation in ADL and IADL include modifying the task or environment, establishing or restoring underlying impairments, and providing client and caregiver education. Grading activities effectively will maximize clients' progress toward goals. Specific intervention activities vary significantly according to the clients' ages and disabilities and are beyond the scope of this chapter. Readers should use this chapter to guide them in the overall process of ADL and IADL intervention and refer to sources that focus on specific client populations and service delivery models when selecting specific intervention activities.

Acknowledgments

Anne Birge James thanks Dr. Margo B. Holm and Dr. Joan Rogers for inviting her to coauthor far earlier editions of the ADL/IADL chapters for *Willard & Spackman's Occupational Therapy*. Dr. Holm and Dr. Rogers conceptualize OT practice in ways both scholarly and practical, and their contributions are still evident in this chapter. We also thank clients, students, and colleagues who posed for photographs, especially Lucretia and Michael Berg, for their generous assistance taking and editing photos.

 Visit thePoint to watch a video about ADL and IADL.

REFERENCES

American Occupational Therapy Association. (2014). Occupational therapy practice framework: Domain and process (3rd ed.). *American Journal of Occupational Therapy, 68*, S1–S48. doi:10.5014/ajot.2014.682006

American Occupational Therapy Association. (2015). Standards of practice for occupational therapy. *American Journal of Occupational Therapy, 69*, 6913410057. doi:10.5014/ajot.2015.696S06

Arango-Lasprilla, J. C., Ketchum, J. M., Cifu, D., Hammond, F., Castillo, C., Nicholls, E., . . . Deng, X. (2010). Predictors of extended rehabilitation length of stay after traumatic brain injury. *Archives of Physical Medicine and Rehabilitation, 91*, 1495–1504. doi:10.1016/j.apmr.2010.07.010

Archenholtz, B., & Dellhag, B. (2008). Validity and reliability of the instrument Performance and Satisfaction in Activities of Daily Living (PS-ADL) and its clinical applicability to adults with rheumatoid arthritis. *Scandinavian Journal of Occupational Therapy, 15*, 13–22. doi:10.1080/11038120701223165

Arif, M. J., El Emary, I. M., & Koutsouris, D. D. (2014). A review on the technologies and services used in the self-management of health and independent living of elderly. *Technology and Health Care, 22*, 677–687. doi:10.3233/THC-140851

Árnadóttir, G. (1990). *The brain and behavior: Assessing cortical dysfunction through activities of daily living.* St. Louis, MO: Mosby Elsevier.

Árnadóttir, G. (2011). Impact of neurobehavioral deficits on activities of daily living. In G. Gillen (Ed.), *Stroke rehabilitation: A function-based approach* (3rd ed., pp. 456–500). St. Louis, MO: Mosby Elsevier.

Ashley, M. J., Persel, C. S., & Clark, M. C. (2001). Validation of an Independent Living Scale for post-acute rehabilitation applications. *Brain Injury, 15*, 435–442.

Baron, K., Kielhofner, G., Iyenger, A., Goldhammer, V., & Wolenski, J. (2006). *The Occupational Self-Assessment* (Version 2.2). Chicago, IL: University of Illinois at Chicago, College of Applied Health Sciences, Department of Occupational Therapy, Model of Human Occupation Clearinghouse.

Bédard, M., Parkkari, M., Weaver, B., Riendeau, J., & Dahlquist, M. (2010). Brief report—Assessment of driving performance using a simulator protocol: Validity and reproducibility. *American Journal of Occupational Therapy, 64*, 336–340.

Bonikowsky, S., Musto, A., Suteu, K. A., MacKenzie, S., & Dennis, D. (2012). Independence: An analysis of a complex and core construct in occupational therapy. *British Journal of Occupational Therapy, 75*, 188–195. doi:10.4276/030802212X13336366278176

Bottari, C., Dutil, E., Dassa, C., & Rainville, C. (2006). Choosing the most appropriate environment to evaluate independence in everyday activities: Home or clinic? *Australian Occupational Therapy Journal, 53*, 98–106. doi:10.1111/j.1440-1630.2006.00547.x

Brandt, Å., Samuelsson, K., Töytäri, O., & Salminen, A.-L. (2011). Activity and participation, quality of life and user satisfaction outcomes of environmental control systems and smart home technology. A systematic review. *Disability and Rehabilitation: Assistive Technology, 6*, 189–206. doi:10.3109/17483107.2010.532286

Brown, C. L., & Finlayson, M. L. (2013). Performance measures rather than self-report measures of functional status predict home care use in community-dwelling older adults. *Canadian Journal of Occupational Therapy, 80*, 284–294. doi:10.1177/0008417413501467

Brown, C. L., Moore, W. P., Hemman, D., & Yunek, A. (1996). Influence of instrumental activities of daily living assessment method on judgments of independence. *American Journal of Occupational Therapy, 50*, 202–206.

Buzaid, A., Dodge, M. P., Handmacher, L., & Kiltz, P. J. (2013). Activities of daily living: Evaluation and treatment in persons with multiple sclerosis. *Physical Medicine and Rehabilitation Clinics of North America, 24*, 629–638. doi:10.1016/j.pmr.2013.06.008

Centers for Disease Control and Prevention. (2015). *Perceived exertion (Borg Rating of Perceived Exertion Scale).* Retrieved from https://www.cdc.gov/physicalactivity/basics/measuring/exertion.htm

Centers for Medicare & Medicaid Services. (2016). *Inpatient Rehabilitation Facility (IRF) Quality Reporting Program (QRP).* Retrieved from https://www.cms.gov/Medicare/Quality-Initiatives-Patient-Assessment-Instruments/IRF-Quality-Reporting/index.html

Centers for Medicare & Medicaid Services. (2018). *Inpatient Rehabilitation Facility-Patient Assessment Instrument* (OMB No. 0938-0842). Retrieved from https://www.cms.gov/Medicare/Medicare-Fee-for-Service-Payment/InpatientRehabFacPPS/IRFPAI.html

Chard, G., Liu, L., & Mulholland, S. (2009). Verbal cueing and environmental modifications: Strategies to improve engagement in occupations in persons with Alzheimer's disease. *Physical & Occupational Therapy in Geriatrics, 27*, 197–211. doi:10.1080/02703180802206280

Chisholm, D., Toto, P., Raina, K., Holm, M., & Rogers, J. (2014). Evaluating capacity to live independently and safely in the community: Performance Assessment of Self-care Skills. *British Journal of Occupational Therapy, 77*, 59–66. doi:10.4276/030802214X13916969447038

Chong, D. K. (1995). Measurement of instrumental activities of daily living in stroke. *Stroke, 26*, 1119–1122. Retrieved from http://stroke.ahajournals.org/cgi/content/full/26/6/1119

Chui, T., & Oliver, R. (2006). Factor analysis and construct validity of the SAFER-HOME. *OTJR: Occupation, Participation and Health, 26*, 132–142.

Cipriani, J., Hess, S., Higgins, H., Resavy, D., Sheon, S., Szychowski, M., & Holm, M. (2000). Collaboration in the therapeutic process: Older adults' perspectives. *Physical and Occupational Therapy in Geriatrics, 17*, 43–54.

Clarke, C. E., Furmston, A., Morgan, E., Patel, S., Sackley, C., Walker, M., . . . Wheatley, K. (2009). Pilot randomized controlled trial of occupational therapy to optimize independence in Parkinson's disease: The PD OT trial. *Journal of Neurology, Neurosurgery, & Psychiatry, 80,* 976–978. doi:10.1136/jnnp.2007.138586

Cohen-Mansfield, J., & Jensen, B. (2007). Adequacy of spouses as informants regarding older persons' self-care practices and their perceived importance. *Families, Systems, & Health, 25,* 53–67. doi:10.1037/1091-7527.25.1.53

Colquhoun, H., Letts, L., Law, M., MacDermid, J., & Edwards, M. (2010). Feasibility of the Canadian Occupational Performance Measure for routine use. *British Journal of Occupational Therapy, 73,* 48–54. doi:10.4276/030802210X12658062793726

Covinsky, K. E., Lindquist, K., Dunlop, D. D., & Yelin, E. (2009). Pain, functional limits, and aging. *Journal of the American Geriatric Society, 57,* 1556–1561. doi:10.1111/j.1532-5415.2009.02388.x

das Nair, R., Moreton, B. J., & Lincoln, N. B. (2011). Rasch analysis of the Nottingham Extended Activities of Daily Living Scale. *Journal of Rehabilitation Medicine, 43,* 944–950. doi:10.2340/16501977-0858

Davis, L. A. (2005). Educating individuals with dementia: Perspectives for rehabilitation professionals. *Topics in Geriatric Rehabilitation, 21,* 304–314.

DiZazzo-Miller, R., Winston, K., Winkler, S. L., & Donovan, M. L. (2017). Family Caregiver Training Program (FCTP): A randomized controlled trial. *American Journal of Occupational Therapy, 71,* 7105190010. doi:10.5014/ajot.2017.022459

Doig, E., Fleming, J., Cornwell, P. L., & Kuipers, P. (2009). Qualitative exploration of a client-centered, goal-directed approach to community-based occupational therapy for adults with traumatic brain injury. *American Journal of Occupational Therapy, 64,* 559–568.

Dooley, N. R., & Hinojosa, J. (2004). Improving quality of life for persons with Alzheimer's disease and their family caregivers: Brief occupational therapy intervention. *American Journal of Occupational Therapy, 58,* 561–569.

Dudgeon, B. J., Tyler, E. J., Rhodes, L. A., & Jensen, M. P. (2006). Managing usual and unexpected pain with physical disability: A qualitative analysis. *American Journal of Occupational Therapy, 60,* 92–103.

Dunn, W. (2017). Measurement concepts and practices. In M. Law, C. Baum, & W. Dunn (Eds.), *Measuring occupational performance: Supporting best practice in occupational therapy* (3rd ed., pp. 17–28). Thorofare, NJ: SLACK.

Egan, M., & Dubouloz, C.-J. (2014). Practical foundations: For practice: Planning, guiding, documenting and reflecting. In M. V. Radomski & C. A. Trombly Latham (Eds.), *Occupational therapy for physical dysfunction* (7th ed., pp. 24–49). Philadelphia, PA: Lippincott Williams & Wilkins.

Eklund, K., & Dahlin-Ivanoff, S. (2006). Health education for people with macular degeneration: Learning experiences and the effect on daily occupation. *Canadian Journal of Occupational Therapy, 73,* 272–280. doi:10.2182/cjot.06.004

Eklund, K., Sonn, U., & Dahlin-Ivanoff, S. (2004). Long-term evaluation of a health education programme for elderly persons with visual impairment. A randomized study. *Disability and Rehabilitation, 26,* 401–409.

Eklund, M., & Gunnarsson, A. B. (2008). Content validity, clinical utility, sensitivity to change and discriminant ability of the Swedish Satisfaction with Daily Occupations (SDO) instrument: A screening tool for people with mental disorders. *British Journal of Occupational Therapy, 71,* 487–495.

Eyres, L., & Unsworth, C. A. (2005). Occupational therapy in acute hospitals: The effectiveness of a pilot program to maintain occupational performance in older clients. *Australian Occupational Therapy Journal, 52,* 218–224. doi:10.1111/j.1440-1630.2005.00498.x

Fasoli, S. E. (2014). Assessing roles and competence. In M. V. Radomski & C. A. Trombly Latham (Eds.), *Occupational therapy for physical dysfunction* (7th ed., pp. 76–102). Philadelphia, PA: Lippincott Williams & Wilkins.

Fisher, A. G., & Jones, K. B. (2011). *Assessment of Motor and Process Skills: Development, standardization, and administration manual* (7th ed., Rev. ed.). Ft. Collins, CO: Three Star Press.

Flinn, N. A. (2014). Learning. In M. V. Radomski & C. A. Trombly Latham (Eds.), *Occupational therapy for physical dysfunction* (7th ed., pp. 394–411). Philadelphia, PA: Lippincott Williams & Wilkins.

Galloway, R. V., Granger, C. V., Karmarkar, A. M., Graham, J. E., Deutsch, A., Niewczyk, P., . . . Ottenbacher, K. J. (2013). The Uniform Data System for Medical Rehabilitation Report of Patients with Debility Discharged from Inpatient Rehabilitation Programs in 2000-2010. *American Journal of Physical Medicine & Rehabilitation, 92,* 14–27. doi:10.1097/PHM.0b013e31827441bc

Gateley, C., & Borcherding, S. (2017). *Documentation manual for writing SOAP notes in occupational therapy* (4th ed.). Thorofare, NJ: SLACK.

Gift, A. G., & Narsavage, G. (1998). Validity of the numeric rating scale as a measure of dyspnea. *American Journal of Critical Care, 7,* 200–204.

Gillen, G. (2000). Improving activities of daily living performance in an adult with ataxia. *American Journal of Occupational Therapy, 54,* 89–96.

Gillen, G. (2009). *Cognitive and perceptual rehabilitation: Optimizing function.* St. Louis, MO: Mosby Elsevier.

Gitlin, L. N., Corcoran, M., Winter, L., Boyce, A., & Hauck, W. W. (2001). A randomized, controlled trial of a home environmental intervention: Effect on efficacy and upset in caregivers and on daily function of persons with dementia. *Gerontologist, 41,* 4–14.

Goverover, Y., Chiaravalloti, N., Gaudino-Goering, E., Moore, N., & DeLuca, J. (2009). The relationship among performance of instrumental activities of daily living, self-report of quality of life, and self-awareness of functional status in individuals with multiple sclerosis. *Rehabilitation Psychology, 54,* 60–68. doi:10.1037/a0014556

Greber, C., Ziviani, J., & Rodger, S. (2007). The four-quadrant model of facilitated learning (Part 2): Strategies and applications. *Australian Occupational Therapy Journal, 54,* S40–S48. doi:10.1111/j.1440-1630.2007.00663.x

Guidetti, S., Asaba, E., & Tham, K. (2007). The lived experience of recapturing self-care. *American Journal of Occupational Therapy, 61,* 303–310.

Hinojosa, M. S., & Rittman, M. (2009). Association between health education needs and stroke caregiver injury. *Journal of Aging and Health, 21,* 1040–1058. doi:10.1177/0898264309344321

Hitch, D., Larkin, H., Watchorn, V., & Ang, S. (2012). Community mobility in the context of universal design: Inter-professional collaboration and education. *Australian Occupational Therapy Journal, 59,* 375–383. doi:10.1111/j.1440-1630.2011.00965.x

Holm, M. B., & Rogers, J. C. (2017). Measuring performance in instrumental activities of daily living. In M. Law, C. Baum, & W. Dunn (Eds.), *Measuring occupational performance: Supporting best practice in occupational therapy* (3rd ed., pp. 305–331). Thorofare, NJ: SLACK.

Jack, J., & Estes, R. I. (2010). Documenting progress: Hand therapy treatment shift from biomechanical to occupational adaptation. *American Journal of Occupational Therapy, 64,* 82–87.

Kartje, P. (2006, October). Approaching, evaluating, and counseling the older driver for successful community mobility. *OT Practice, 11*(19), 11–15.

Katz, S., Ford, A. B., Moskowitz, R. W., Jackson, B. A., & Jaffe, M. A. (1963). Studies of illness in the aged. The Index of ADL: A standardized measure of biological and psychosocial function. *Journal of the American Medical Association, 185,* 914–919.

Keller, J., Kafkes, A., Basu, S., Federico, J., & Kielhofner, G. (2005). *The Child Occupational Self Assessment* (Version 2.1). Chicago, IL: University of Illinois at Chicago, College of Applied Health Sciences, Department of Occupational Therapy, Model of Human Occupation Clearinghouse.

Kettenbach, G. (2009). *Writing patient/client notes: Ensuring accuracy in documentation* (4th ed.). Philadelphia, PA: F. A. Davis.

Kielhofner, G., Mallinson, T., Crawford, C., Nowak, M., Rigby, M., Henry, A., & Walens, D. (2004). *Occupational Performance History Interview II (OPHI-II)* (Version 2.1). Chicago, IL: University of Illinois at Chicago, College of Applied Health Sciences, Department of Occupational Therapy, Model of Human Occupation Clearinghouse.

Klein, S., Barlow, I., & Hollis, V. (2008). Evaluating ADL measure from an occupational therapy perspective. *Canadian Journal of Occupational Therapy, 75,* 69–81.

Kohlman Thomson, L., & Robnett, R. (2016). *Kohlman Evaluation of Living Skills* (4th ed.). Bethesda, MD: American Occupational Therapy Association.

Korner-Bitensky, N., Menon, A., von Zweck, C., & Van Benthem, K. (2010). Occupational therapists' capacity-building needs related to older driver screening, assessment, and intervention: A Canadawide survey. *American Journal of Occupational Therapy, 64,* 316–324.

Lansing, R. W., Moosavi, S. H., & Banzett, R. B. (2003). Measurement of dyspnea: Word labeled visual analog scale vs. verbal ordinal scale. *Respiratory Physiology & Neurobiology, 3,* 77–83.

Law, M., Baptiste, S., Carswell, A., McColl, M. A., Polatajko, H., & Pollock, N. (2014). *The Canadian Occupational Performance Measure* (5th ed.). Ontario, Canada: Canadian Association of Occupational Therapists.

Law, M., & Baum, C. (2017). Measurement in occupational therapy. In M. Law, C. Baum, & W. Dunn (Eds.), *Measuring occupational performance: Supporting best practice in occupational therapy* (3rd ed., pp. 1–16). Thorofare, NJ: SLACK.

Law, M., & Dunbar, S. B. (2007). Person-environment-occupation model. In S. B. Dunbar (Ed.), *Occupational therapy models for intervention with children and families* (pp. 27–49). Thorofare, NJ: SLACK.

Law, M., & MacDermid, J. (2017). Guiding therapist decisions for measuring outcomes in occupational therapy. In M. Law, C. Baum, & W. Dunn (Eds.), *Measuring occupational performance: Supporting best practice in occupational therapy* (3rd ed., pp. 43–56). Thorofare, NJ: SLACK.

Legg, L., Drummond, A., & Langhorne, P. (2006). Occupational therapy for patients with problems in activities of daily living after stroke. *Cochrane Database of Systematic Reviews,* (4), 1–47. doi:10.1002/14651858.CD003585.pub2

Liddle, J., & McKenna, K. (2000). Quality of life: An overview of issues for use in occupational therapy outcome measurement. *Australian Occupational Therapy Journal, 47,* 77–85.

Liedberg, G. M., & Vrethem, M. (2009). Polyneuropathy, with and without neurogenic pain, and its impact on daily life activities—A descriptive study. *Disability and Rehabilitation, 31,* 1402–1408. doi:10.1080/09638280802621382

Little, L. M., Pope, E., Wallisch, A., & Dunn, W. (2018). Occupation-based coaching by means of telehealth for families of young children with autism spectrum disorder. *American Journal of Occupational Therapy, 72,* 7202205020. doi:10.5014/ajot.2018.024786

Lund, M. L., & Nygård, L. (2003). Incorporating or resisting assistive devices: Different approaches to achieving a desired occupational self-image. *OTJR: Occupation, Participation and Health, 23,* 67–75.

Mackenzie, C., Wiprzycka, U., Hasher, L., & Goldstein, D. (2009). Associations between psychological distress, learning, and memory in spouse caregivers of older adults. *Journals of Gerontology Series B: Psychological Sciences & Social Sciences, 64B,* 742–746. doi:10.1093/geronb/gbp076

Magasi, S. (2012). Negotiating the social service systems: A vital yet frequently invisible occupation. *OTJR: Occupation, Participation and Health, 32,* S25–S33.

Mahoney, F. I., & Barthel, D. W. (1965). Functional evaluation: The Barthel Index. *Maryland State Medical Journal, 14,* 61–65.

Mathiowetz, V. G., Matuska, K. M., Finlayson, M. L., Luo, P., & Chen, H. Y. (2007). One-year follow-up to a randomized controlled trial of an energy conservation course for persons with multiple sclerosis. *International Journal of Rehabilitation Research, 30,* 305–313.

Mathiowetz, V., Matuska, K. M., & Murphy, M. E. (2001). Efficacy of an energy conservation course for persons with multiple sclerosis. *Archives of Physical Medicine and Rehabilitation, 82,* 449–456.

McKenna, K., & Scott, J. (2007). Do written education materials that use content and design principles improve older people's knowledge? *Australian Occupational Therapy Journal, 54,* 103–112. doi:10.1111/j.1440-1630.2006.00583.x

Meenan, R. F., Mason, J. H., Anderson, J. J., Guccione, A. A., & Kazis, L. E. (1992). AIMS2: The content and properties of a revised and expanded Arthritis Impact Measurement Scales Health Status Questionnaire. *Arthritis and Rheumatism, 35,* 1–10.

Melchert-McKearnan, K., Deitz, J., Engel, J. M., & White, O. (2000). Children with burn injuries: Purposeful versus rote exercise. *American Journal of Occupational Therapy, 54,* 381–390.

Moye, J. (2005). Guardianship and conservatorship. In T. Grisso (Ed.), *Evaluating competencies: Forensic assessments and instruments* (2nd ed., pp. 309–390). Retrieved from https://www.springer.com/gp/book/9780306473432

Nakanishi, M., Sawamura, K., Sato, S., Setoya, Y., & Anzai, N. (2010). Development of a clinical pathway for long-term inpatients with schizophrenia. *Psychiatry and Clinical Neurosciences, 64,* 99–103. doi:10.1111/j.1440-1819.2009.02040.x

National Center for Health Statistics. (2009). *Limitations in activities of daily living and instrumental activities of daily living, 2003-2007.* Retrieved from http://www.cdc.gov/nchs/health_policy/ADL_tables.htm

Nouri, F. M., & Lincoln, N. B. (1987). An Extended Activities of Daily Living Scale for stroke patients. *Clinical Rehabilitation, 1,* 301–305.

Novak, I., Cusick, A., & Lannin, N. (2009). Occupational therapy home programs for cerebral palsy: Double-blind, randomized, controlled trial. *Pediatrics, 124,* e606–e614. doi:10.1542/peds.2009-0288

Orellano, E., Colón, W. I., & Arbesman, M. (2012). Effect of occupation- and activity-based interventions on instrumental activities of daily living performance among community-dwelling older adults: A systematic review. *American Journal of Occupational Therapy, 66,* 292–300. doi:10.5014/ajot.2012.003053

Padilla, R. (2011). Effectiveness of interventions designed to modify the activity demands of the occupations of self-care and leisure for people with Alzheimer's disease and related dementias. *American Journal of Occupational Therapy, 65,* 523–531. doi:10.5014/ajot.2011.002618

Piersol, C. V. (2014). Occupation as therapy: Selection, gradation, analysis, and adaptation. In M. V. Radomski & C. A. Trombly Latham (Eds.), *Occupational therapy for physical dysfunction* (7th ed., pp. 360–393). Philadelphia, PA: Lippincott Williams & Wilkins.

Pillastrini, P., Mugnai, R., Bonfiglioli, R., Curti, S., Mattioli, S., Maioli, M. G., . . . Violante, F. S. (2008). Evaluation of an occupational therapy program for patients with spinal cord injury. *Spinal Cord, 46,* 78–81.

Provencher, V., Demers, L., & Gélinas, I. (2009). Home and clinical assessments of instrumental activities of daily living: What could explain the difference between settings in frail older adults, if any? *British Journal of Occupational Therapy, 72,* 339–348.

Provencher, V., Demers, L., Gélinas, I., & Giroux, F. (2013). Cooking task assessment in frail older adults: Who performed better at home and in the clinic. *Scandinavian Journal of Occupational Therapy, 20,* 374–385. doi:10.3109/11038128.2012.743586

Radia-George, C., Imms, C., & Taylor, N. F. (2014). Interrater reliability and clinical utility of the Personal Care Participation Assessment and Resource Tool (PC–PART) in an inpatient rehabilitation setting. *American Journal of Occupational Therapy, 68,* 334–343. doi:10.5014/ajot.2014.009878

Radomski, M. V. (2011). More than good intentions: Advancing adherence with therapy recommendations. *American Journal of Occupational Therapy, 65,* 471–477. doi:10.5014/ajot.2011.000885

Resnick, B. (1998). Motivating older adults to perform functional activities. *Journal of Gerontological Nursing, 24,* 23–30.

Rogers, J. C., Holm, M. B., Beach, S., Schulz, R., Cipriani, J., Fox, A., & Starz, T. W. (2003). Concordance of four methods of disability assessment using performance in the home as the criterion method. *Arthritis Care & Research, 49,* 640–647.

Russell, C., Fitzgerald, M. H., Williamson, P., Manor, D., & Whybrow, S. (2002). Independence as a practice issue in occupational therapy: The safety clause. *American Journal of Occupational Therapy, 56,* 369–379.

Schepens, S. L., Panzer, V., & Goldberg, A. (2011). Research Scholars Initiative—Randomized controlled trial comparing tailoring methods of multimedia-based fall prevention education for community-dwelling older adults. *American Journal of Occupational Therapy, 65,* 702–709. doi:10.5014/ajot.2011.001180

Seo, Y., Roberts, B. L., LaFramboise, L., Yates, B. C., & Yurkovich, J. M. (2011). Predictors of modifications in instrumental activities of daily living in persons with heart failure. *Journal of Cardiovascular Nursing, 26,* 89–98.

Siegel, P., Tencza, M., Apodaca, B., & Poole, J. L. (2017). Effectiveness of occupational therapy interventions for adults with rheumatoid arthritis: A systematic review. *American Journal of Occupational Therapy, 71,* 7101180050. doi:10.5014/ajot.2017.023176

Simpson, A. N., Bonilha, H. S., Kazley, A. S., Zoller, J. S., Simpson, K. N., & Ellis, C. (2015). Impact of outpatient rehabilitation Medicare reimbursement caps on utilization and cost of rehabilitation care after ischemic stroke: Do caps contain costs? *Archives of Physical Medicine and Rehabilitation, 96,* 1959–1965. doi:10.1016/j.apmr.2015.07.008

Stewart, K. B. (2010). Purposes, processes, and methods of evaluation. In J. Case-Smith & J. C. O'Brien (Eds.), *Occupational therapy for children* (6th ed., pp. 193–211). Maryland Heights, MO: Mosby Elsevier.

Tamaru, A., McColl, M. A., & Yamasaki, S. (2007). Understanding 'independence': Perspectives of occupational therapists. *Disability and Rehabilitation, 29,* 1021–1033. doi:10.1080/09638280600929110

Thornsson, A., & Grimby, G. (2001). Ability and perceived difficulty in daily activities in people with poliomyelitis sequelae. *Journal of Rehabilitation Medicine, 33,* 4–11.

Tomlin, G. (2018). Scientific reasoning and evidence in practice. In B. A. B. Schell & J. W. Schell (Eds.), *Clinical and professional reasoning in occupational therapy practice* (2nd ed., pp. 145–169). Philadelphia, PA: Lippincott Williams & Wilkins.

Toth-Cohen, S. (2000). Role perceptions of occupational therapists providing support and education for caregivers of persons with dementia. *American Journal of Occupational Therapy, 54,* 509–515.

UB Foundation Activities. (2002). *IRF-PAI training manual.* Retrieved from https://www.cms.gov/Medicare/Medicare-Fee-for-Service-Payment/InpatientRehabFacPPS/downloads/irfpai-manualint.pdf

Van Heest, K. N. L., Mogush, A. R., & Mathiowetz, V. G. (2017). Effects of a one-to-one fatigue management course for people with chronic conditions and fatigue. *American Journal of Occupational Therapy, 71,* 7104100020. doi:10.5014/ajot.2017.023440

Vroland-Nordstrand, K., Eliasson, A.-C., Jacobsson, H., Johansson, U., & Krumlinde-Sundholm, L. (2015). Can children identify and achieve goals for intervention? A randomized trial comparing two goal-setting approaches. *Developmental Medicine and Child Neurology, 58,* 589–596. doi:10.1111/dmcn.12925

Wade, D. T. (2009). Goal setting in rehabilitation: An overview of what, why, and how. *Clinical Rehabilitation, 23,* 291–295.

Williams, J. H., Drinka, T. J., Greenberg, J. R., Farrel-Holtan, J., Euhardy, R., & Schram, M. (1991). Development and testing of the Assessment of Living Skills and Resources (ALSAR) in elderly community-dwelling veterans. *Gerontologist, 31,* 84–91.

World Health Organization. (2002). *Towards a common language for functioning, disability, and health: ICF.* Retrieved from http://www.who.int/classifications/icf/training/icfbeginnersguide.pdf

Zanatta, E., Rodeghiero, F., Pigatto, E., Galozzi, P., Polito, P., Favaro, M., . . . Cozzi, F. (2017). Long-term improvement in activities of daily living in women with systemic sclerosis attending occupational therapy. *British Journal of Occupational Therapy, 80,* 417–422. doi:10.1177/0308022617698167

thePoint *For additional resources on the subjects discussed in this chapter, visit* **http://thePoint.lww.com/Willard-Spackman13e.** *See* **Appendix I, Resources and Evidence for Common Conditions Addressed in OT** *for more information about the disorders and impairments discussed in this chapter and* **Appendix II, Table of Assessments** *for more ADL and IADL assessments.*

CHAPTER 51

Education

Yvonne Swinth

LEARNING OBJECTIVES

After reading this chapter, you will be able to:

1. Identify different educational settings in which an occupational therapist may provide services.
2. Outline the occupational therapy process within an educational setting.
3. Explain key requirements of occupational therapy services under guiding legislation such as the Individuals with Disabilities Education Improvement Act.
4. Compare and contrast an Individualized Family Service Plan (IFSP), an Individualized Education Program (IEP), and an Individualized Transition Plan (ITP).
5. Describe how a disability may affect the occupation of student.
6. Identify new occupation-based initiatives impacting the professional reasoning of occupational therapists working in educational settings.

Occupational Therapy in Educational Settings

Occupational therapy (OT) practitioners work in a variety of educational settings. These may include public schools, charter schools, private schools, alternative schools, vocational schools, and university settings. Across these settings, practitioners work with children and adolescents, generally from birth to 21 years old in a variety of contexts. For example, an OT practitioner might work with infants and families in a 0 to 3 center, young children in a preschool on the playground, elementary school-age children in the classroom, or adolescents in an alternative high school at a worksite. Occupational therapists might also work with an older adult client who is returning to school to learn a new skill after an injury (e.g., work hardening, job retraining) or for personal enhancement (i.e., leisure activity). Approximately 24.5% of occupational therapists and 17.8% of OT assistants who are members of the American Occupational Therapy Association (AOTA) identify public school/early intervention as their primary work setting (AOTA, 2015). According to the Bureau of Labor Statistics, U.S. Department of Labor (2018), continued growth (24%) is expected for the profession of OT, including working in educational settings, early intervention, and transition to work environments. We are beginning to see a developing niche for occupational therapists working in other educational settings (e.g., colleges, universities, community colleges, and continuing education venues) as these children become young adults and desire to continue their education (Quinn, Gleeson, & Nolan, 2014).

The primary focus of this chapter is on occupational performance within early intervention and public schools because this is the most common educational setting that employs OT practitioners. However, the reader is encouraged to consider the wide variety of educational settings that may benefit from the skills and expertise of an occupational therapist. These types of OT services may be innovative and preventive and may increase the occupational performance of individuals in ways that historically have not been explored or considered. For example, OT practitioners might develop a health promotion program for an entire school system to increase students' engagement in physical activity or work in collaboration with other school staff to establish programs to support mental health across school contexts such as the *Comfortable Cafeteria* or *Refreshing Recess* programs of *Every Moment Counts* (Demirjian, Horvath, & Bazyk, 2014). Colleges or universities may benefit from an occupational therapist's expertise in addressing universal design, access to curricular materials for students with disabilities, and training/supporting university faculty when teaching students with disabilities or ergonomic needs of staff and students. For example, an occupational therapist may work with a disability counselor at a university to help a student on the autism spectrum successfully participate in his or her school day (Quinn et al., 2014).

Legislation Guiding Practice

The Centennial Notes feature gives a historical perspective of legislation and services in educational settings. Practice across educational settings is guided by federal legislation, with a focus on the occupation of education and the role of the student through a variety of legislative and funding sources. Although the Individuals with Disabilities Education Improvement Act (2004) specifically addresses services in early intervention and schools that receive public funds, every educational setting must meet the requirements of Section 504 of the Rehabilitation Act (1973) as well as the Americans with Disabilities Act (ADA) of 1990 (Pub. L. 101-336). Thus, OT services in settings such as private schools, universities, and continuing education

venues can be provided under Section 504 and the ADA. Section 504 supports reasonable accommodations for individuals with a disability, a history of a disability, or a perceived disability if accommodations are needed to allow the individual to participate in educational settings. The ADA is a civil rights act and provides protection to individuals with disabilities similar to those provided to individuals on the basis of race, color, sex, national origin, age, and religion. Furthermore, the ADA supports the right of individuals with disabilities to have equal opportunities to live, work, and play within society (including educational settings). See Table 51-1 for an overview of this legislation.

Since 1975, the key goals of the IDEA 2004 (originally the Education for All Handicapped Children Act [EHA]) have remained the same (Box 51-1), with an increasing shift from the old paradigm of "if we cannot fix them, we exclude them" to a new paradigm of "disability as a natural and normal part of the human experience" (Silverstein, 2000, p. 1761). Thus, the role of OT under the IDEA 2004 has shifted to include a focus on contextual factors such as access to the environment so that individuals with disabilities can participate in their environments rather than on "fixing" the disability of the child or adolescent.

The IDEA 2004 has four parts, A to D; however, this chapter primarily addresses parts B and C. (Part A addresses the general provisions of the IDEA, and Part D addresses research and training.) Under Part C of the IDEA 2004, OT can be a primary service for infants and toddlers from birth to 2 years of age who are eligible for early intervention services (AOTA, 2007). Part B of the IDEA 2004 identifies OT as a related service for children ages 3 to 21 years for whom the team determines the service is *necessary* in order for students to benefit from their special education program. Two key concepts of Part B of the IDEA 2004 are a **free appropriate public education (FAPE)** in the **least restrictive environment (LRE)** (see Box 51-2 for definition of key terms found within the IDEA 2004). The IDEA 2004 allows each state and local education agency some latitude in how the federal legislation will be implemented as long as the FAPE and LRE provisions are not compromised. Thus, there are differences across states and local programs regarding the specifics of how services are provided.

The purpose of the IDEA 2004 is "to ensure that all children with disabilities have available to them a FAPE that emphasizes special education and related services designed to meet their unique needs and prepare them for further education, employment and independent living" (§ 300.1). Occupational therapy practitioners in the public school setting provide services within this structure and are generally a related (supportive) service to the educational program (specially designed instruction). Students come to school to get an education, and in the schools, OT serves this priority.

TABLE 51-1 Occupational Therapy Services in Educational Settings

Legislation/Sources of Funding	Population Served	Role of Occupational Therapist
Individuals with Disabilities Education Improvement Act (IDEA) of 2004	Students who are eligible for special education and require the related service of occupational therapy in order to receive free appropriate public education (FAPE) in the least restrictive environment (LRE). (IDEA 2004 is applicable only for students [age 0 to 21 years] who receive special education services through their early intervention or public school setting.)	To collaborate with the Individualized Education Program (IEP) team to determine the student's needs and then to provide services as outlined in the IEP in order to support student performance relevant to the educational environment
Section 504 of the Rehabilitation Act	Students who have a disability, a history of a disability, or a perceived disability that affects their performance in school. (In the public schools, these are generally students who are not eligible for special education.) Students who meet the definition of "individual with a disability" are defined as those individuals who have a physical or mental impairment that substantially limits one or more major life activities.	To collaborate with the 504 team to provide the accommodations and adaptations that the student needs to access the school environment and services
Americans with Disabilities Act (ADA)	The ADA ensures equal opportunity for individuals with disabilities in employment, state and local government services, public accommodations, commercial facilities, and transportation. Thus, it is a civil rights legislation that supports participation in the educational setting by students who have a disability.	To provide support through consultation and monitoring to ensure that students with disabilities have access to and can participate in the educational setting. It often involves working with environmental adaptations, accommodations, and the use of assistive devices.
Other funding sources: • General education funds (for public schools) • Private insurance • Private agencies (e.g., United Cerebral Palsy) • State agencies (e.g., Division of Vocational Rehabilitation)	Any student who needs the support of an occupational therapy practitioner	To support student performance in occupations relevant to the educational environment

Adapted from Swinth, Y., Chandler, B., Hanft, B., Jackson, L., & Shepherd, J. (2003). *Personnel issues in school-based occupational therapy: Supply and demand, preparation, and certification and licensure.* Gainesville, FL: Center on Personnel Studies in Special Education. Retrieved from http://www.coe.ufl.edu/copsse

Occupational Therapy Process in Educational Settings

A variety of factors affect the OT process in educational environments. Services that are provided under the structure of the IDEA 2004 often are influenced by the educational team. Collaboration across stakeholders through effective teaming often results in positive outcomes for children and adolescents (Hanft & Shepherd, 2016). Regardless of the educational setting in which the practitioner works, a team of professionals typically influence the OT process.

Decision Making

Effective and efficient delivery of services in the school environment requires a systematic process for team decision making and problem solving that attends to the ethical

responsibilities of the school-based practitioner. There is a tendency by OT professionals to identify a need and immediately start proposing and implementing solutions without first identifying the necessary outcomes needed for the student to participate in the educational environment.

BOX 51-1   KEY ASSUMPTIONS OF THE INDIVIDUALS WITH DISABILITIES EDUCATION ACT

1. Equality of opportunity for all individuals
2. Full participation (empowerment)
3. Independent living
4. Economic self-sufficiency

Adapted from Silverstein, R. (2000). Emerging disability policy framework: A guidepost for analyzing public policy. *Iowa Law Review, 85,* 1757–1802.

CENTENNIAL NOTES

A Brief History of Occupational Therapy in Education

Ever since the birth of OT, practitioners around the world have considered education and learning as part of their intervention. They have supported the learning of children with disabilities in hospitals, clinics, specialized schools, and public schools (Brackett, 1928; Whittier, 1922) and the learning of adults in hospitals, clinics, outpatient centers, and formalized educational institutions (Kidner, 1910). For more than 75 years, OT practitioners can be found in formal educational settings increasingly around the world. The specific settings in which they work and how they work in these settings depends on the educational system of the country, state, or city of which the educational setting is a part of. Some countries have legislation specific to working in the schools, whereas in other countries, most children with disabilities are in specialized schools and occupational therapists work in these schools. True to the core of OT, practitioners who work in educational settings strive to ensure that they are addressing key skills, habits, and routines needed by children, youth, and adults to successfully participate. Thus, there has been an evolution from a more clinical approach in educational settings (e.g., training of specific client factors) to identifying strengths and challenges in order to maximize performance across the educational context (e.g., use of accommodations and adaptations, universal design for learning). Additionally, as needs of the students have evolved based on changes in society so has the focus of OT in educational settings to include addressing assistive technology, telehealth, and social participation.

A quick overview of the legislation in the United States framing OT practice illustrates the evolution of practice in schools as practitioners respond to the changes in understanding "disability" and the changes in occupational needs within society. Occupational therapists formally began working in the public schools more than 83 years ago under a special section of the Social Security Act (1935). Services were provided in **segregated settings** or special schools and primarily to children with orthopedic and neurological impairments. In 1975, the Education for

All Handicapped Children Act (EHA) (Pub. L. 94-142) was enacted that required the provision of services, including OT, to all eligible children ages 6 to 21 years. Amendments to the EHA in 1986, Pub. L. 99-457, added services for preschoolers (ages 3 to 5 years). In 1990, the EHA was renamed the Individuals with Disabilities Education Act (IDEA) (Pub. L. 101-476), and assistive technology devices and services, services for children from birth to 3 years old, transition services (to prepare them for life after school), and programs for children with emotional disturbances were added. These amendments encourage more **integration** and services in general education settings. Further amendments were made to the IDEA in 1997 (Pub. L. 105-117) emphasizing **access to and participation in the general education curriculum** for students with disabilities. This continued into the current 2004 amendments when the name was changed to the Individuals with Disabilities Education Improvement Act— IDEA 2004 (Pub. L. 108-446). This latest reauthorization also increased the emphasis on prereferral intervention or **early intervening services** (commonly referred to as *response to intervention* or RtI). The amendments also place an emphasis on the use of scientifically based (research-based, evidence-based) practices, high-quality preservice training and professional education, increased representation of minorities in fields such as teaching and OT, and the use and development of appropriate technology (including assistive technology).

What has this historically perspective meant for OT practitioners in the educational contexts? The movement from segregation to participation in educational settings for students with disabilities means that OT practitioners have gone from replicating a clinical model of practice in the schools to providing more embedded services across educational contexts. Students have the opportunity to practice and learn skills in the context(s) they will use the skills. It is expected that OT services in educational settings will continue to refine and more therapists will be seen working to provide systems supports and to facilitate student support across context through collaboration with other stakeholders.

Educational teams have access to a variety of tools that support a systematic process of decision making and team problem solving (e.g., McGill Action Planning System [MAPS], Choosing Outcomes and Accommodations for Children). Through working with educational teams, practitioners are better able to identify and address priority educational needs. Additionally, school-based practitioners may encounter ethical dilemmas unique to practicing in educational settings. This may include a mismatch between the Occupational Therapy Code of Ethics and special education law, non-OT practitioners writing the services on the Individualized Education Plan without collaborating with the occupational therapist and more (Reed & Polichino, 2013). School-based practitioners should be aware of when educational legislation and priorities may conflict with the Occupational Therapy Code of Ethics and then have a framework for decision making that can help negotiate any incongruences.

BOX 51-2   COMMON TERMS IN THE INDIVIDUALS WITH DISABILITIES EDUCATION ACT 2004

Early intervening services: academic and behavior support to succeed in general education but is not part of special education

Free appropriate public education (FAPE): special education and related services provided at public expense that meets the standards of the state education agency (SEA)

General education: the environment, curriculum, and activities that are available to all students

General education curriculum: the same curriculum as for nondisabled children

Individualized Education Program (IEP): a commitment of services that ensures that an appropriate program is developed that meets the unique educational needs of children ages 3 to 21 years

Individualized Family Services Plan (IFSP): a commitment of services that ensures that an appropriate program is developed that meets the unique developmental and preeducational needs of children 0 to 3 years old and their families

Least restrictive environment (LRE): the environment that provides maximum interaction with nondisabled peers and is consistent with the needs of the child/student

No Child Left Behind: Pub. L. 107-110, aimed at improving the educational performance of all students by increasing accountability for student achievement. It emphasizes standards-based education reform with the belief that high expectations will result in success for all students.

Related services: transportation and such developmental, corrective, and other supportive services (including speech-language, audiology, psychological, and physical and occupational therapy services) needed to help the child benefit from special education

Response to intervention (RtI): an integrated approach to service delivery that includes both general and special education and includes high-quality instruction, interventions matched to student need, frequent progress monitoring, and data-based decision making

Special education: specially designed instruction at no cost to parents to meet the unique needs of a child with a disability

Educational Teams

The concept of teaming, or collaborating as a team, to make decisions about the program and services to be provided has been a guiding principle of OT services in public schools since the inception of federal law (Hanft & Shepherd, 2016). Working collaboratively as part of an interprofessional team provides a framework to ensure that all strengths and needs specific to participation across educational settings are addressed. With the reauthorization in 1997, the IDEA became more explicit regarding the emphasis on teaming and collaboration among professionals and families to make effective decisions about student need(s). The IDEA 1997 clearly specified that whenever decisions are made about a student, the parents or caregivers must be involved. Two types of teams are involved in a student's program: the evaluation team and the Individualized Education Program (IEP) team (Individualized Family Service Plan [IFSP] for children 0 to 3 years and Individualized Transition Plan [ITP] for adolescents 16 years and older). Both teams must include qualified professionals who are knowledgeable about the student and his or her need(s). If a decision is being made about OT involvement in a student's program, then an occupational therapist must be involved in the teaming process. In the public schools, the specific composition of each team is driven by the student's needs and may include general and special education teachers, therapists (physical, occupational, and speech), psychologists, counselors, parents, the student, and different community members. The focus of the team decision-making process must be on student outcomes and performance with an emphasis on participation in the general education environment as appropriate. In other educational settings, although the IDEA 2004 requirement to have a "team of qualified professionals" is not mandated, it is consistent with best practice. In most other settings, the team will be smaller but seldom does an OT practitioner makes decisions in isolation.

Other Factors Affecting Decision Making

In addition to ethics and working with a team, other factors may impact the decision making of a school-based practitioner. Education initiatives across educational settings are constantly evolving. Whereas the IDEA 2004 is the key legislation guiding school-based OT services, the school-based practitioner needs to develop and maintain a knowledge base of educational history, educational philosophies, and other key general education and special educational initiatives that may impact programs, placements, and services. One such legislation is the Every Student Succeeds Act (ESSA, 2015). This act reemphasizes a long-standing commitment to equal opportunity for all students and provides a framework for the consideration of OT services to support students across educational contexts, including general education students. Each of these factors is part of the professional reasoning considerations as OT practitioners implement the OT process within educational settings.

Evaluation Requirements in the Schools

In the public schools, a team of qualified individuals, which may include an occupational therapist, school psychologist, special education and general education teachers, physical therapist, speech-language pathologist, and others, is responsible for conducting the evaluation. Ideally, the evaluation is a collaborative process across team members (Hanft & Shepherd, 2016). The purpose of the evaluation process is not only to determine the student's needs in order to have access to and participate in the educational environment to the maximum extent appropriate but also to determine the student's needs in order to perform within the school setting including identifying needed supports, accommodations, adaptations, and/or modifications. Additionally, the IDEA 2004 requires that the evaluation help to determine services that will support a student's ability to demonstrate outcomes with a focus on the general education curriculum. Therefore, the evaluation process is driven by contextual factors (the school environment) and student (client) needs (Bazyk & Case-Smith, 2010; Chapparo & Lowe, 2012). The emphasis of the evaluation is on the occupational performance area of *education*. As defined by IDEA 2004, education includes not only academics but also physical education, after-school activities, and preparation for life after schools. Thus, other areas of occupation such as activities of daily living (ADL), leisure participation, and social participation might need to be addressed if participation in these areas is affecting educational performance or is needed to successfully engage in life activities postgraduation. Several key requirements underlie the evaluation process in schools under the IDEA 2004 that OT practitioners may not have to address in other settings. These requirements are briefly discussed.

Referral

The process of referral within the school setting is different from that in a clinical setting. As with any procedures within special education, specific steps can vary from state to state or from setting to setting. However, in most public schools, if there is a concern about student performance, a team of professionals will discuss and implement different strategies within the general education classroom before referring the student for special education. Some school

districts have a more formal process for these prereferral interventions called response to intervention (RtI) or Multi-Tiered Systems of Support (MTSS). If these strategies are not successful, then the student is referred for a special education evaluation to determine eligibility for services. Occupational therapy may or may not be involved in this step of the process. However, increasingly educational settings are recognizing the key contributions that can be provided by OT practitioners early in the process.

If the prereferral supports are not successful, then the student is referred to special education. At this point, the team completes an initial evaluation. Often the occupational therapist is part of this team. However, if OT is not involved in the initial evaluation process, then the team may request an OT evaluation at any time after determining that the student is eligible for special education. If the occupational therapist is working in a state where the OT practice act requires a physician referral for services, then such a referral may be necessary before starting the evaluation. If a physician refers a student for an OT evaluation, this referral does not guarantee services in a school setting. The occupational therapist in the public school must first ensure that the student is eligible for special education and then determine if services are necessary for the student to benefit from the education program.

Not all special education evaluations result in eligibility for services. Sometimes it is determined that a student does not require specially designed instruction (special education) in order to receive FAPE in the LRE but may only require accommodations/adaptations in order to participate in the educational program. Such support is provided under Section 504 of the Rehabilitation Act and depending on the policy and procedures of a district, the OT practitioner may or may not be involved in providing these supports as part of the 504 team. Ideally, the occupational therapist should be involved throughout the decision-making process if the evaluation team feels that the student might require the services of an OT practitioner or that the student has needs that might require the expertise of an occupational therapist.

In other educational settings, the referral process may be less formal. For example, in some university settings, a referral might come through the center for disability access (e.g., a student access concern) or human resources (e.g., a staff ergonomic concern). Therapists who provide services in these types of settings might need to develop a referral system to ensure that the process meets the needs of the client(s). If a physician referral is required by a state practice act, then the occupational therapist must comply with this requirement regardless of the setting.

As with other OT practice areas, the evaluation process in the schools is dynamic and ongoing and often continues during intervention. According to the IDEA 2004, the evaluation determines whether a child has a disability and the nature and extent of the special education and related services that the child needs (§ 300.15). The IDEA 2004 does not require use of a specific type of assessment method or tool. Rather, it requires that a variety of tools and strategies be used to gather relevant "functional and developmental information" related to enabling the child to "be involved in and progress in the general education curriculum" (§ 300.304[1]). In addition, the evaluation should help to determine the child's educational needs and how the disability affects the child's participation across school contexts and activities.

A child does not "qualify" for OT on the basis of testing under the IDEA 2004. Instead, OT services should be recommended by the occupational therapist, based on the evaluation results, and provided for a child if necessary to "benefit from their special education program." Even though the evaluation process in the schools is guided by federal law, occupation remains the core of the OT practitioner's theoretical perspective. Within the educational setting, therapy practitioners draw on the appropriate frames of reference to guide the evaluation process (Frolek-Clark, Polichino, & Jackson, 2004).

The evaluation process should be individualized (student centered) and should use a top–down, occupation/participation-based approach (Chapparo & Lowe, 2012). This means that the OT evaluation should start by looking at student performance within context versus evaluating specific client factors out of context. As with any OT evaluation, a broad view of the student (client) must be considered. Thus, the emphasis is on the educational context, including physical, temporal, social, and cultural considerations. Within the educational setting, the focus of special education and related services is on student outcomes. If the educational staff and/or parents require services (e.g., specialized training) for the student to reach his or her outcomes, then the practitioner is responsible for addressing these needs as well as broader systems issues (e.g., curriculum, environmental adaptations) that might require OT input and support (Chapparo & Lowe, 2012; Frolek Clark & Chandler, 2013). Under the IDEA 2004, OT services are supportive in nature in order to help the child be successful in school as well as in after-school activities (Giangreco, 2001). Additionally, services can be provided "on behalf of" the child and "to the parents, teachers, and other staff" so that these individuals can better support the child's learning (Table 51-2).

When OT is involved in the evaluation process, the occupational therapist uses the "Occupational Therapy Practice Framework" (AOTA, 2014) as a guide to the process. The special education process closely parallels the OT process described in the framework. Following is a brief description of the OT evaluation process. The specific role of the occupational therapist during the evaluation process for any given student will depend on the expertise and skills of all the team members as well as the referral concerns. There may be overlap across professional disciplines regarding specific skills assessed (e.g., gross motor skills with physical therapy, feeding with speech therapy, or psychosocial issues with psychology or counseling), but the input of

TABLE 51-2	Clients to Consider during the Occupational Therapy Evaluation Process
Client	**Evaluation Consideration(s)**
Student	Gather data regarding the occupational profile and occupational performance.
Parents/educational staff	On the basis of the student's occupational profile and occupational performance, determine whether there is any need for specific training, support, and/or dissemination of information.
System	On the basis of the student's occupational profile and occupational performance, determine whether any system supports (e.g., environmental modifications, curriculum development) are needed.

an occupational therapist is needed because of the unique emphasis of OT on occupation and context/environmental factors that affect occupational performance.

The occupational therapist in the school setting focuses the evaluation on what is needed for the student to engage and participate in meaningful and purposeful school occupations. Based on the educational needs and program of the student, the OT evaluation addresses the student's areas of strengths and concerns in any area of occupation, including ADL, education/work, play/leisure, and social participation. In each of these areas, the performance skills and the student's physical, sensory, neurological, and cognitive/mental function are evaluated. As in all other settings in which OT practitioners work, the occupational therapist is responsible for the administration of the evaluation methods and measures, the interpretation and documentation of results, and the communication of evaluation results with other team members. However, if an OT assistant is part of the team, he or she may contribute to any part of the process under the direct supervision of the occupational therapist in alignment with a state's practice act. First, an occupational profile is developed in collaboration with the team, including the family and student, as appropriate. This profile is followed by an analysis of the student's occupational performance within the educational setting.

Occupational Profile

The occupational profile is developed by gathering data from the student, family, and educational staff (AOTA, 2014). The OT assistant, community providers, and others who know the student also may contribute to this process. Often, the development of the occupational profile occurs over time. Several assessments and procedures that have been designed for use in the educational setting may be used to develop the occupational profile. Table 51-3 and

TABLE 51-3 Common Evaluation Methods and Tools Used in Educational Settings

Assessment	Participation		Areas of Occupation					Client Factors	
	Characteristics	Contextual Factors	Activity			Experience		Performance Skills	Abilities
			Activity Interests	Activity Choices	Subjective Experience	Personal Meaning	Satisfaction		
Part I: Process-Oriented Assessment Tools: Support Gathering Data for the Occupational Profile and Analysis of Occupational Performance									
Assessment of Motor and Process Skills (School Version [AMPS])	♦	♦	♦	♦	♦	♦	♦	♦	♦
Children's Assessment of Participation and Enjoyment (CAPE)/Preferences for Activities of Children (PAC)	♦	♦	♦	♦	♦	♦	♦	♦	♦
Choosing Outcomes and Accommodations for Children (COACH)	♦	♦	♦	♦	♦	♦	♦	♦	♦
Canadian Occupational Performance Measure (COPM)	♦	♦	♦	♦	♦	♦	♦	♦	♦
Goal-Oriented Assessment of Lifeskills (GOAL)			♦	♦		♦	♦	♦	♦
Making Action Plans (MAPs)	♦	♦	♦	♦	♦	♦	♦	♦	♦
Miller Function & Participation Scales			♦	♦		♦	♦	♦	♦
Planning Alternative Tomorrows with Hope (PATH)	♦	♦	♦	♦	♦	♦	♦	♦	♦
Perceived Efficacy and Goal Setting Scale (PEGS)	♦	♦	♦	♦	♦	♦	♦	♦	♦
Interview with the student, educational staff, parents, and others	♦	♦	♦	♦	♦	♦	♦	♦	♦
School Function Assessment (SFA)	♦	♦			♦			♦	♦
Sensory Processing Measure	♦	♦			♦			♦	♦
Skilled observation	♦	♦	♦			♦	♦	♦	♦
Vermont Interdependent Services Team Approach (VISTA)	♦	♦	♦	♦	♦	♦	♦	♦	♦
Part II: Assessments of Client Factors: Supports Analysis of Occupational Performance with Specific Performance Skills, Patterns, and Tasks									
Beery Developmental Test of Visual-Motor Skills (Beery VMI)								♦	♦
Bruininks-Oseretsky Test of Motor Proficiency, Second Edition (BOT-2)								♦	♦
Children's Handwriting Evaluation Scale (CHES)								♦	♦
Development Test of Visual Perception (DTVP)								♦	♦
Evaluation Tool of Children's Handwriting (ETCH)								♦	♦
Gross Motor Function Measure (GMFM)	♦						♦	♦	
Knox Preschool Play Scale					♦			♦	
Interest Checklist			♦						
Leisure Diagnostic Battery	♦	♦			♦	♦			
Minnesota Handwriting Assessment								♦	♦
Motor-Free Visual Perception Test (MVPT)								♦	♦
Peabody Developmental Motor Scales, Second Edition (PDMs-2)								♦	♦

TABLE 51-3 Common Evaluation Methods and Tools Used in Educational Settings *(continued)*

Assessment	Participation — Characteristics	Participation — Contextual Factors	Areas of Occupation — Activity — Activity Interests	Areas of Occupation — Activity — Activity Choices	Areas of Occupation — Activity — Subjective Experience	Areas of Occupation — Experience — Personal Meaning	Areas of Occupation — Experience — Satisfaction	Client Factors — Performance Skills	Client Factors — Abilities
Pediatric Evaluation of Disability Inventory (PEDI)	◆	◆						◆	◆
Sensory Profile 2	◆							◆	◆
Social Skills Rating System	◆					◆	◆	◆	
Test of Handwriting Skills								◆	◆
Test of Visual Perceptual Skills (TVPS)								◆	◆
Test of Visual Motor Skills (TVMS)								◆	◆

This is not an inclusive list nor is it an endorsement of any one assessment.

Appendix II list some of the assessments and procedures that are used in educational settings.

Most of these assessments are process oriented and must be completed with input from all team members, including the student and family. Ideally, the assessments should have a problem-solving focus that addresses the student's strengths and concerns as well as contextual factors that may affect student performance and outcomes. The assessments also will help the OT practitioner to identify strengths and challenges specific to the student's performance patterns and activity demands. By completing one or more of these process-oriented assessments, the OT practitioner will have addressed most of the occupational profile questions that are outlined within the "Occupational Therapy Practice Framework" (Box 51-3).

For example, the MAPS consists of seven specific questions that support the planning process and identification of team-generated outcomes for students with disabilities (O'Brien, Forest, Snow, Pearpoint, & Hasbury, 1989). The questions include the following:

1. What is the student's history?
2. What are your dreams for the student?
3. What are your fears for the student?
4. Who is the student? (one-word statements that describe the student)
5. What are the student's strengths, gifts, and abilities?
6. What are the student's needs?
7. What would the student's ideal day at school look like and what must be done to make it happen?

A typical MAPS planning session can take 2 hours or more. The entire team (parents, students, therapists, and teachers) as well as other invited members (siblings, other family members, or community members) provide input in answer to each question. The questions provide a strong foundation from which to develop the student's program, including any OT services. The process focuses on the value of integrating the student in neighborhood schools and in general education classes in order to develop friendships and to ensure a high-quality education for the child. By the time the team members are addressing

BOX 51-3 OCCUPATIONAL PROFILE QUESTIONS FROM THE OCCUPATIONAL THERAPY PRACTICE FRAMEWORK (ADAPTED FOR THE EDUCATIONAL SETTING)

1. Who is the student?
2. Why was the student referred to special education and/or for an OT evaluation in the schools?
3. In what areas of educational occupations (activities of daily living, education, work, play/leisure, and/or social participation) is the student successful, and what areas are causing problems or risks?
4. What contexts support engagement in desired educational occupations, and what contexts are inhibiting engagement?
5. What is the student's occupational history?
6. What are the student's, family's, and educational staff's priorities and desired target outcomes?

question 6 ("What are the student's needs?"), they have the background to be able to establish both short- and long-term outcomes. These outcome goals are then used to guide a discussion regarding the student's ideal day and how to get there.

Analysis of Occupational Performance

Often concurrent with the development of the occupational profile, the occupational therapist works with the team to determine whether more specific assessments are needed to help further determine a student's needs. Within the educational setting, the occupational therapist addresses performance in all areas of occupation as it relates to the child's educational needs (Table 51-4). Often, the process-oriented tools not only help with the development of the occupational profile but also help the occupational therapist better understand contextual factors, potential "whole-school approaches," and curricular and extracurricular issues. These tools help the occupational therapist to communicate observations of the person-activity-environment fit as it relates to the student's occupational performance in school.

If it is determined that additional information about occupational performance related to physical, sensory, neurological, and/or mental functions of the student is needed, the occupational therapist may use standardized or nonstandardized assessments that focus on client factors (see Chapter 23). These assessments can help to determine specific information about occupational performance but should not be used without one or more of the process-oriented assessments. Additionally, the occupational therapist may use observation, parent or teacher interviews, and file review to support the analysis of a student's performance. Case Study 51-1 describes the process of developing an occupational profile for Kristi, a junior high school student with cerebral palsy, as well as other steps of the OT process. These findings and recommendations were included in the special education evaluation report, and the team used them to develop Kristi's special education program. Once her program was developed, the team discussed Kristi's need for OT support to meet her educational goals and objectives.

Intervention

Occupational therapy services address a student's performance based on the evaluation results in order to support the student's participation in the curriculum, access to the school contexts, and participation in extracurricular activities (Figures 51-1 and 51-2). Generally, services should only as specialized as necessary and should be provided within the context or environment the skill will be used and should emphasize maximizing the student's strengths.

Factors That Influence Occupational Therapy Interventions in Educational Environments

In addition to the setting and legislation, a variety of factors affect the planning and implementation of intervention by OT practitioners within educational environments. These include the unique characteristics of the system, the range of services provided, and the research evidence supporting intervention.

TABLE 51-4   **Occupational Performance Areas Addressed from the Occupational Therapy Practice Framework (Adapted for the Educational Setting)**

Occupational Performance Area	How Addressed in the Educational Setting
Activities of daily living (basic and instrumental)	Cares for basic self needs in school (e.g., eating, toileting, managing shoes and coats, dressing up and down for physical education [PE]); uses transportation system and uses communication devices to interact with others
Education	Participates and performs in the educational environment including academic (e.g., math, reading, writing), nonacademic (e.g., lunch, recess, after-school activities), prevocational, and vocational activities
Work	Develops interests, aptitudes, and skills necessary for engaging in work or volunteer activities for transition to community life on graduation from school
Play/leisure	Identifies and engages in age-appropriate toys, games, and leisure experiences; participates in art, music, sports, and after-school activities
Social participation	Interacts with peers, teachers, and other educational personnel during academic and nonacademic educational activities including extracurricular and preparation for work activities

Adapted from Swinth, Y., Chandler, B., Hanft, B., Jackson, L., & Shepherd, J. (2003). *Personnel issues in school-based occupational therapy: Supply and demand, preparation, and certification and licensure.* Gainesville, FL: Center on Personnel Studies in Special Education. Retrieved from http://www.coe.ufl.edu/copsse

CASE STUDY 51-1   PROCESS FOR DEVELOPING AN OCCUPATIONAL PROFILE FOR KRISTI, A 13-YEAR-OLD STUDENT WITH CEREBRAL PALSY

Background

Kristi is a 13-year-old student with tetraplegia cerebral palsy. She has received OT in the past in both clinical and school-based settings. Kristi and her family had recently moved, and the education team in her new school district decided to complete an evaluation to determine her educational needs.

Occupational Profile

The occupational therapist started gathering data for the occupational profile by talking to Kristi and her family and reviewing Kristi's past records. Through this process, the occupational therapist began to develop a summary of Kristi's occupational history and her strengths and concerns in the areas of occupation related to Kristi's educational program. The therapist then observed Kristi in her academic courses, physical education (PE) class, lunch, and transitional periods (e.g., on and off the bus, between classes). The team

also met with Kristi and her parents to complete a McGill Action Planning System.

Analysis of Occupational Performance

On the basis of the data that had been gathered, the occupational therapist summarized Kristi's occupational performance (strengths and concerns) related to most of Kristi's physical, sensory, neurological, and/or mental functions. Because Kristi had some difficulty with handwriting, the therapist also completed a Test of Visual Perceptual Skills and a Test of Visual Motor Skills to assess potential underlying client factors affecting Kristi's handwriting performance. The therapist also assessed both functional and passive strength and range of motion.

Summary

The occupational therapist summarized the following findings and recommendations to the educational team:

Occupational Performance Area	Strengths and Concerns
Activities of daily living (basic and instrumental)	Kristi is able to take care of her basic self-care needs within her school environment at this time. However, she has difficulty with some dressing activities that could affect her ability to participate in PE activities when she moves to the junior high and high school settings. Kristi and her mother also want Kristi to take a cooking class as soon as possible to determine Kristi's need for adaptive equipment for cooking. Kristi uses a school bus with a lift to get to and from school. She is able to communicate with her peers and teachers without any difficulty.
Education	Kristi is able to participate and complete assignments in her general education classes with accommodations and adaptations. She requires additional time to complete written assignments and uses a computer with word prediction for longer papers. She needs to develop the self-determination skills necessary to independently problem-solve and implement accommodations/adaptations.
Work	Kristi states that she would like to be a lawyer or special education teacher. At age 16 years, the team will collaborate with Kristi and her parents to begin to develop her transition plan. This plan will support the assessment and address her needs for future environments.
Play/leisure	Kristi rides horses, swims at the YMCA, and enjoys playing computer games and watching television.
Social participation	Kristi tends to keep to herself at school. Her mother states that Kristi is very social when at home with her family but that she has minimal interaction with other students her age. Kristi reports that she enjoys sports and that even though she cannot play, she would like to be involved by keeping scores or helping in some other way.

Unique Characteristics of the System

Each educational setting has unique characteristics that must be considered in planning and implementing intervention. Even within the same school district, different schools have unique strengths and barriers. Many occupational therapists working in educational settings are itinerant and work among three or more schools. Variability can make it challenging for therapists to keep

track of the uniqueness of different settings. Additionally, the different legislation (e.g., ADA, 1990; Section 504 of the Rehabilitation Act, 1973) and different emphasis (e.g., public schools, universities, continuing education, virtual classroom) also affect the uniqueness of the system. Therapists in educational settings need to attend to systemic issues, changes, and challenges as well as ethical considerations in order to provide the most effective services.

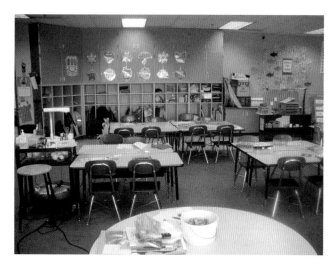

FIGURE 51-1 Occupational therapists may work with teachers to help engineer a classroom to support student participation.

Range of Services

Occupational therapy practitioners provide a range of services in educational settings. Intervention may include hands-on services (such as one-on-one or group activities) or team supports to identify and implement environmental adaptations and modifications to the physical layout of the school campus or the classroom. Finally, services may include system supports, which are activities such as working with the curriculum committee of a district to establish a handwriting curriculum or working with an elementary school principal to help design an accessible play area to be used during recess (Hanft & Shepherd, 2016) (see Table 51-5 for examples of the range of services in the schools). Regardless of how services are provided, practitioners working in public schools must be aware of curricular issues such as education reform, standards-based assessment, and the requirements of general education. The IDEA 2004 requires that students with disabilities be considered for and have access to the general education curriculum and contexts whenever possible and be included in education reform and statewide assessments. Therefore, OT services should consider and address the requirements of general education. For example, in some states, occupational therapists work collaboratively with an interprofessional team to address alternative assessments for students who have severe disabilities, or to make decisions about reasonable testing accommodations for students with learning disabilities or to set up access to a computer or tablet to use for testing for a student with a disability. To fully participate in these discussions and to support the implementation of the recommendations, the occupational therapist must have a basic understanding of the identified general educational outcomes and testing requirements.

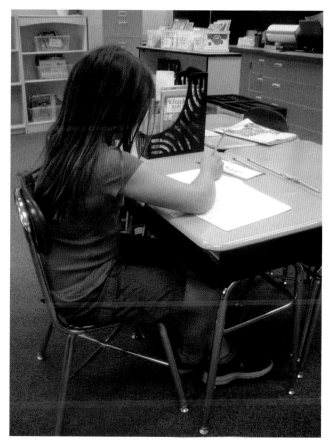

FIGURE 51-2 Occupational therapy works with classroom staff to support proper positioning in the classroom.

Additionally, occupational therapists need to understand the difference between accommodations and modifications and how these affect learning outcomes. Often, these terms are used interchangeably, but in educational settings, the same strategies may be used in both categories, yet they have very different outcomes. *Accommodations* are adaptations or strategies that support student learning but require the same learning outcome as other students. *Modifications* are adaptations or strategies that change the learning outcome by requiring the student to learn something different or to learn less (Nolet & McLaughlin, 2000). Table 51-6 provides some examples of accommodations and modifications to illustrate these differences. The goal is to use accommodations rather than modifications so students have the same learning outcome expectations as their peers.

Multi-Tiered Systems of Support

As mentioned earlier, MTSS are used by many but not all school districts (National Association of State Directors of Special Education [NASDSE], 2005). The MTSS are a research-based framework that targets struggling students in areas such as academics and

TABLE 51-5   Occupational Therapy Interventions in School Settings

Performance Skill	Student Interventions	Educational Staff Interventions	Systems Intervention
Process Skills			
• Energy • Knowledge • Temporal orientation • Organizing space and objects • Adaptation	• Learning about self-regulation/levels of arousal and attention • Use of sensory media during intervention • Sensory integrative techniques • Initiates activities and sustains attention to complete them • Organization of desk and other work areas • Accommodates/adapts to changes in the routine • Work on visual perceptual skills • Orientation to time and place • Problem solving • Self-determination • Behavior management • Teach calming techniques.	• Teach staff how to use sensory processing techniques in the classroom. • Provide in-services on programs such as the Alert Program (Williams & Shellenberger, 1996) to help students learn to recognize how alert they are feeling and to identify sensorimotor experiences that can be used to change the level of alertness. • Training and collaborative program development	• Participate on curriculum committees. • Educate the system about specific environmental factors that support self-regulation and arousal in the school. • Environmental modifications • Training about developmental trauma and impact on school performance • Embedded activities to support mental health
Motor Skills			
• Posture • Mobility • Coordination • Strength and effort • Energy	• Participation in physical education and recess activities • Participation in classroom activities such as written work • Posture/body alignment during school activities • Mobility within the school environment • Accessing assistive technology • Teach energy conservation techniques.	• Training on use of adaptive equipment and accommodations and modifications • Training on positioning, lifting, and transferring	• Work with the school system to adopt a handwriting curriculum. • Application of universal design to physical environment and the curriculum • Ordering appropriate adaptive equipment (e.g., lifts) for staff safety • Campaign for proper use of backpacks • Adapted equipment (e.g., weight training machines)
Communication/Interaction Skills			
• Physicality • Information exchange • Relations	• Social skill development • Psychosocial skill development • Peer interactions • Development of self-determination skills	• Training and collaborative program development	• Staff development activities • Participation on curriculum committees

This is not an inclusive list of interventions; rather, it is an outline of some possibilities. Specific needs of the student, staff, and system would help to define the specific interventions to be used.

TABLE 51-6   Examples of Accommodations and Modifications

Accommodations	Modifications
Alternative acquisition modes • Sign-language interpreters • Voice-output computers • Tape-recorded books	Teaching less content • Discriminating between animals and plants versus telling the distinguishing characteristics of animal and plant cells
Content enhancements • Advance organizers • Visual displays • Study guides • Peer-mediated instruction	Teaching different content • Identifying different animals versus learning the human anatomy
Alternative response modes • Scribe • Untimed response situations	

behavior and supports successful school participation through a tiered approach to intervention prior to referring a student for special education. The MTSS are implemented systematically as part of core instruction. The MTSS use differentiated instruction and universal design for learning (UDL) strategies. It is data driven and progress monitoring is key to support decision making. The MTSS include RtI, positive behavioral interventions and support (PBIS) and may also be referred to as Early Intervening Services or Positive School Climate.

Within the IDEA 2004, up to 15% of special education funds can be used for early intervening services (also known as *pre-referral interventions* or *whole-school approaches*). These are services that are provided for students, not in special education, who need "additional academic and behavioral support to succeed in a general education environment" (§ 300.226). Increasingly, research is suggesting that students need effective support when they first start having difficulty in school. Thus, IDEA 2004 has included early intervening services within the statutes. These services are for students "kindergarten through 12th grade (with particular emphasis on kindergarten through grade 3) who are not currently identified as needing special education or related services, but who need additional academic and behavioral support to succeed in a general education environment" (CFR, § 300.226[a]).

All MTSS are based on research evidence and student outcome data and are integrated approaches to service delivery that includes both general and special education that includes high-quality instruction, interventions matched to student need, frequent progress monitoring, and data-based decision making (NASDSE, 2005). It is a whole-school approach to services that are specifically directed at student need and based on a problem-solving model in which the team defines the problem, analyzes what is happening, develops a plan, and evaluates the effectiveness of the plan. In some cases, effective prereferral interventions, such as the use of a move-and-sit cushion for a fidgety student or the development and implementation of a handwriting curriculum, may successfully support the student within the educational environment and further intervention might not be needed.

This model generally uses a three-tiered approach to support (Figure 51-3). The first tier involves screening and group intervention; this approach will generally address about 80% of the problems. The second tier is targeted,

short-term interventions, addressing another 15% of the student needs. The final tier is intensive instruction, which is required by about 5% of the students. The role of OT at each tier varies across school districts. Some districts feel that the first tier should be addressed by the immediate team, whereas others include the occupational therapist early in the process. If the underlying concern is within the domain of OT, a therapist may be involved in the second or third tier of interventions. Case Study 51-2 provides an illustration of how OT may be involved in early intervening services. At this time, MTSS, although a promising practice, is not mandated in the IDEA 2004 and thus not all occupational therapists or schools provide early intervening services.

If the early intervening services are not effective, the student is then referred to a special education evaluation team and the process is followed as described earlier. The evaluation team determines whether the special education process, as outlined in the IDEA 2004, should be initiated or whether the student should be referred for some other type of support, such as a 504 plan.

In educational systems such as universities or continuing education settings, a range of OT services may be provided as well. However, at this time, most OT services in these settings tend to be more collaborative/consultative or focus on facilitating recommendations or accommodations rather than direct hands-on therapy services. For example, an occupational therapist might consult to a university computing center to recommend appropriate ergonomic arrangements or provide resources related to healthy computing. Or, the occupational therapists may

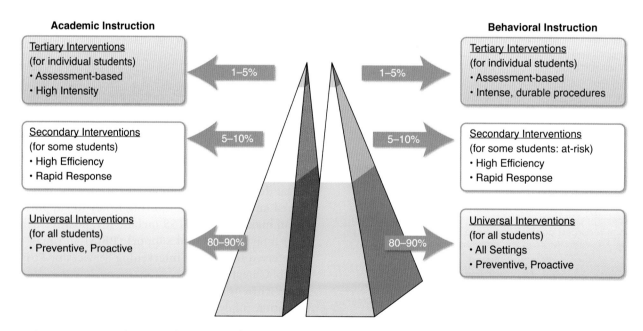

FIGURE 51-3 Multi-Tiered System of Support (MTSS): A schoolwide system for student success that includes both academic and behavioral instruction. (Used with permission from http://www.pbis.org/school/mtss.)

CASE STUDY 51-2   EARLY INTERVENING SERVICES TO SUPPORT DEVON'S EDUCATIONAL PROGRAM

Background

Devon is 7 years old and in first grade. He has been having difficulty with literacy activities in the classroom since the beginning of the school year and has been acting up or refusing to work. His kindergarten teacher reports that Devon struggled the previous year as well but always "just made it." His first grade teacher is concerned that if Devon continues to struggle, he will eventually fall too far behind his peers to catch up. The elementary school that he attends has just started implementing the Multi-Tiered Systems of Support (MTSS) model.

Tier One

Devon's student response team discusses his case with his first grade teacher. His teacher reports that he has difficulty copying and writing more than one or two words during any writing assignment. He often refuses to participate in reading activities as well. She reports that during literacy activities, Devon is fidgety and easily distracted and at times has behavioral outbursts. Using a problem-solving model, they determine that because it is November, they need to provide some proactive support to prevent future difficulties. The team decides to put Devon in a specialized literacy group that is explicitly designed to target first grade literacy outcomes. One team member used the *Calm Moment Cards* which were developed by a team of school-based OT practitioners from the Every Moment Counts Web site (http://www.everymomentcounts.org /view.php?nav_id=213) to help decrease stress and anxiety in her classroom and shared this resource with Devon's teacher. Although OT was not directly involved during this first meeting because the team did not feel that there were concerns about Devon's performance that required

the skills and expertise of an occupational therapist, the embedded strategies from the *Calm Moment Cards* used an OT framework. And, the occupational therapist provided some input as Devon's teacher started to implement the program in her classroom.

Tier Two

For 3 months, Devon participated in the specialized literacy group, the *Calm Moment Cards* were used by his classroom teacher, and data were systematically recorded to track the interventions that were used and Devon's progress. Devon's reading and writing skills improved, but he continued to be fidgety and easily distracted and to exhibit behavior problems during literacy activities even after using some of the strategies from the *Calm Moment Cards*. The team invited the occupational therapist to the second team meeting, wondering whether additional sensory strategies may support Devon's performance. The occupational therapist recommended strategies to the classroom teacher to support Devon's sensory processing (e.g., use of a move-and-sit cushion, allowing Devon to hold small objects in his hand to fidget, use of a water bottle) during literacy activities. Devon's parents also agree to try these strategies at home. The teacher introduced the strategies to the entire group and allowed anyone to use them. Data were recorded to help Devon and the team determine the best strategies for him. The combination of the targeted instruction by the teacher, use of the *Calm Moment Cards* as an embedded program, and specific sensory strategies recommended by the occupational therapist resulted in improved performance, and Devon did not need to receive Tier Three intervention. One year later, he was still doing well.

work with the disabilities services on a university campus to put together a resource on UDL that professors can use to support student participation in their university classrooms.

Development of the Individualized Family Service Plan, Individualized Education Program, or Individualized Transition Plan

Once the evaluation has been completed, the IFSP, IEP, or ITP team collaborates to design the child or student's

program (Giangreco, 2001). *IFSPs* are plans that include the child and family needs and are used in early intervention (age 0 to 3 years services) programs. *IEPs* are programs that address the needs of students in preschool through high school. *ITPs* are developed by the time a student turns 16 years and reflect the student's skills and aptitudes and guides teams to discuss and prepare the student for postschool programs (i.e., work, higher education, adult day health) (Figure 51-4). When developing the IFSP, IEP, or ITP, the team, which includes the parents and student (whenever appropriate), first reviews the evaluation results and writes a summary of the student's educational performance, called *present levels of academic achievement and functional performance*. The present levels describe the student's strengths and areas of concern in relation to the expectations of the general education

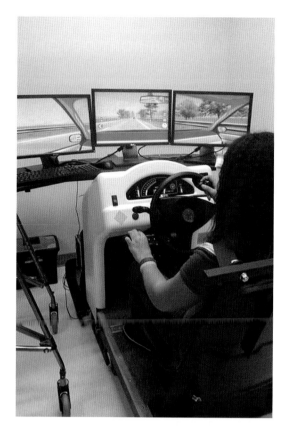

FIGURE 51-4 School-based therapists can support transition planning through activities such as adaptive driving.

curriculum. The team then develops the student's *goals and objectives* on the basis of the data summarized in the present levels and the agreed-on outcomes that the team has identified.

Different settings have different requirements for how goals and objectives are written. Under the IDEA 2004, the ideal is that goals and objectives are developed as a team. Thus, there might not be an "occupational therapy goal page." This is particularly common in some early intervention settings and is becoming increasingly common across all settings. Generally, it is expected that goals and objectives will identify a functional outcome, will state what the student will do and under what conditions the skill or behavior will be performed, and will include a timeline for completion (Park, 2012).

As discussed previously, collaborating with the team is an important aspect of OT service delivery in the schools. This collaboration sets the stage for focusing intervention strategies on specific student outcomes. Because parents (and older students) are involved in the team planning and decision-making process, their perspectives are well represented in the occupational profile that the occupational therapist develops. Throughout the collaborative process, the occupational therapist identifies where he or she may be able to support the student's occupational

performance in the educational environment. Case Study 51-3 provides an example of the goal-setting documentation for Shanna, a sixth grade middle school student with spina bifida.

After the goals and objectives have been developed, the team discusses which professional(s) should address particular goals (e.g., teacher and occupational therapist or maybe occupational therapist and speech-language pathologist), when they will be addressed (e.g., during physical education, during art, when walking in the hall), and where they will be addressed (e.g., in the general education classroom, in the cafeteria, on the playground). Each of these decisions is made on the basis of the student's need, not the personal preferences of professionals. Thus, if needed, the occupational therapist designs the OT intervention plan on the basis of the outcomes that the entire educational team has identified.

The Occupational Therapy Intervention Plan

Once the team has developed the program and determines that a student would benefit from receiving OT services, in order to reach anticipated outcomes, the OT practitioner develops a specific OT intervention plan. The intervention plan addresses the occupational performance areas as well as the performance skill or student factor(s) that are affecting the student's ability to fully participate in the educational environment. The IFSP, IEP, or ITP goals may be the goals on the intervention plan. However, if the goals were written collaboratively, then the OT intervention plan may have OT specific goals.

As in other settings, the OT practitioner considers student factors such as motor skills, process skills, and communication/interaction skills when determining student needs. Additionally, the practitioner considers performance patterns, such as habits and routines, the activity demands in the school setting, and the entire school context when determining student needs. With occupational performance as the core, a variety of conceptual frameworks for practice and frames of references guide OT interventions in educational settings. The primary perspectives may include occupational behavior, developmental, neurodevelopmental, learning, biomechanical, sensory integration, and coping perspectives (Kramer & Hinojosa, 2009). However, there are limited randomized controlled trials supporting or refuting specific OT interventions strategies in the schools. Thus, throughout OT intervention, the OT practitioner uses systematic data collection to inform intervention decisions, ensure the effectiveness of the intervention for the specific student, and help to support the best outcomes for the student (e.g., see Case Study 51-3 for information about Shanna's intervention plan).

CASE STUDY 51-3   GOAL-SETTING DOCUMENTATION FOR SHANNA

Shanna is in the sixth grade at the Norwood Middle School. She has spina bifida and some cognitive delays. The school psychologist, Shanna's teacher, the occupational therapist, the physical therapist, and the speech therapist each completed an individualized evaluation. The OT evaluation included an occupational profile and an analysis of Shanna's occupational performance in her educational setting. As a result of the individual assessments, an evaluation report was written, and the following are some of the strengths and concerns identified:

Strengths

- Able to independently move about the school in her wheelchair
- Social skills with peers
- Verbal expressive language
- Creativity

Concerns

- Easily distracted in the classroom
- Cannot transfer in and out of her wheelchair independently
- Receptive language
- Written language
- Fine and gross motor skills

(This is not an inclusive list of strengths and concerns.)

Excerpts from Shanna's Present Levels of Academic Achievement and Functional Performance

(Note: These excerpts and goal examples were developed and written as a team, not solely by the occupational therapist.)

Shanna currently participates in her general education classroom throughout her day. Her assignments are modified so that she can complete them in the same amount of time as her peers. Noise and visual stimuli can easily distract Shanna within her classroom environment. She goes to the resource room for assistance with math and written language when she cannot complete the assignment independently in her general education classroom. Fine and visual motor challenges impact her ability to complete written language assignments. She is unable to control a writing utensil for a sustained period (more than 5 minutes). Her difficulty with fine motor skills also affects her ability to complete art projects with her peers.

Shanna can move about her school environment without assistance using her manual wheelchair. In the classroom, she requires physical assistance to transfer from her wheelchair to desk chair and back. Her delays in gross motor skills affect her ability to participate in physical education and

recess activities. With accommodations, she is motivated to participate in PE and recess.

Shanna demonstrates good adaptive skills during social interactions with her peers. However, she is becoming increasingly aware of her disability and limitations. This awareness has caused some episodes of depression and has resulted in extended absences from school. Shanna demonstrates emerging self-determination skills in other areas as well. She can describe potential accommodations and adaptations that she would like to her parents and other familiar adults, but she does not advocate for herself during school.

Goal Examples

To address psychosocial skills: Shanna will demonstrate improved self-determination and self-advocacy by collaborating with her therapists and teachers to identify and implement any needed modifications and adaptations into her educational program from less than 50% of the time to 90% of the time as measured by therapist and teacher data by June.

To address written language: Shanna will use identified accommodations/adaptations and/or assistive technology (e.g., word processor, spell-checker, adapted writing utensil) in order to complete her classroom assignments within the general education setting within the same amount of time as her peers from 75% of the time to 100% of the time as measured by therapist and teacher data by June.

Using the team-identified goals and objectives as a guide, Shanna's occupational therapist developed an intervention plan. This plan included some direct therapy to identify and to teach Shanna how to implement any needed accommodations or adaptations and how to use any assistive technology. The occupational therapist also worked with Shanna to teach other school district personnel about her accommodations and adaptations and assistive technology. Ongoing consultation and monitoring were included to ensure that Shanna was able to participate within her educational environment, specifically during physical education (PE) and recess. Finally, because Shanna also received therapy from a community-based occupational therapist, the school therapist contacted the community therapist at least every 6 months to discuss Shanna's program. The therapist did not directly address written language or work on improving handwriting. This was part of the teacher's lesson plan. Rather, the occupational therapist collaborated with the teacher to address the underlying concerns affecting handwriting performance, including the implementation of accommodations and adaptations.

Service Delivery

Planning Intervention

When planning the intervention implementation, occupational therapists must consider the LRE requirement of the IDEA 2004: "to the maximum extent appropriate, children with disabilities are to be educated with children who are not disabled . . . removal of these children from the general educational environment occurs only when the nature or severity of the disability is such that education in regular classes with the use of supplementary aids and services cannot be achieved satisfactorily (Least Restrictive Environment)" (§ 300.114[a][2][i]). Thus, OT is provided and strategies are embedded in the student's typical environment to the extent possible. Such environments may include the classroom, lunchroom, bathroom, on/off the bus, transitions between settings, or playground.

Historical Background

With the start of EHA and through each reauthorization, service delivery by OT practitioners, in the schools, has been refined (see Centennial Notes). The three most commonly described models in the OT literature are direct services, consultation, and monitoring as first described by Dunn (1988). However, recently, there has been an increased recognition of the need for practitioners to work more deliberately within the general education environment to embed OT strategies within the day-to-day routine in order to support ongoing student engagement and participation. Additionally, occupational therapists are beginning to work more interdisciplinary at a systems level in order to impact the system as a whole. Newer publications (Hanft & Shepherd, 2016) are using terms such as *hands-on* (includes one-on-one, small group services, and the like in pullout or natural contexts), *team supports*, and *system supports* to describe services in the schools. Although terms to describe services in the schools continue to be refined, a variety of different terms, including *direct*, *consult*, and *monitoring*, continue to be used to describe OT services depending on the setting, state, or system in which the therapist works.

Service Delivery Models

Many different service delivery models are used within the educational setting. The IDEA 2004 defines four different categories for service delivery:

- Specially designed instruction
- Related services
- Supplemental aids and services
- Services on behalf of the child

In most educational settings, occupational therapists provide related services, supplemental aids and services, and services on behalf of the child. Depending on the rules and regulations in a particular state, an occupational therapist might provide the specially designed instruction, but this is rare. For example, a student with normal cognition but significant motor delays (e.g., muscular dystrophy, spina bifida, cerebral palsy) might require more support than just accommodations or adaptations in order to participate within his or her educational setting.

The rest of this section will use a model (Hollenbeck, 2012a) to contextualize services (Figure 51-5) that recognizes the unique skills and expertise of OT practitioners and represents current research and best practice trends in schools. Student need is the driving factor in deciding how services should be provided. As discussed previously, the need of a student represents the interaction among the client factors, performance skills and patterns, and program and placement (Giangreco, 2001). The IDEA 2004 mandates that services be provided in the LRE as much as possible. Thus, practitioners in the schools may provide systems supports (Frolek-Clark & Chandler, 2013; Hanft & Shepherd, 2016). At times, services provided at a systems level, such as playground redesigned to address universal access, has a greater impact on a larger number of children rather than working one-on-one with a student to learn to navigate a traditional climbing structure (Figure 51-6). Information sharing can be a powerful service delivery option in the schools. Occupational therapy practitioners in the schools can help other stakeholders in the schools better understand the unique needs of students in the schools. Key areas of information sharing can include AOTA initiatives such as backpack awareness (Figure 51-7), obesity prevention, and social skills. If the information sharing and training would result in the child receiving FAPE in the LRE, then a greater intensity of services (e.g., hands-on services in context) may not be needed. Service delivery may also include identifying, setting up, and training on the use of accommodations (as defined earlier in this chapter). The OT practitioners' skills in activity analysis enable them to be able to support the team in determining the best fit related to needed accommodations.

The need for increased collaboration in the schools, by all partners, has been receiving increased attention (Hanft & Shepherd, 2016; Hanft & Swinth, 2011) with positive results for students, families, and school staff (Henry & McClary, 2011; Shasby & Schneck, 2011). Collaboration reflects the interactive communication among team members (Friend & Cook, 2009; Snell & Janney, 2005) and collaborative consultation involves working closely with other team members to support student outcomes. For example, the practitioner may collaborate with the school counselor to integrate sensory processing strategies into a social skills curriculum used by the counselor or the practitioner may work with the classroom teacher on classroom redesign and dynamic seating options to help increase attention and engagement (Gochenour & Poskey, 2017).

Continuum of OT Service Delivery in the Schools

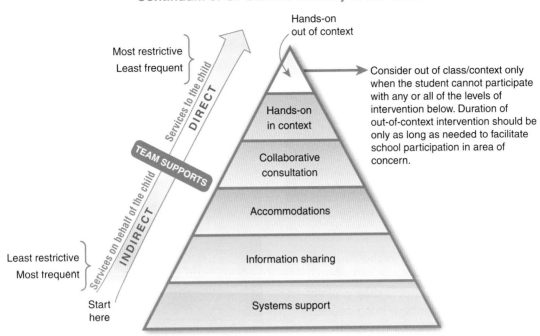

Hands-on
out of context

Most restrictive
Least frequent

Services to the child

DIRECT

TEAM SUPPORTS

Services on behalf of the child

INDIRECT

Hands-on
in context

Collaborative
consultation

Consider out of class/context only
when the student cannot participate
with any or all of the levels of
intervention below. Duration of
out-of-context intervention should be
only as long as needed to facilitate
school participation in area of
concern.

Accommodations

Least restrictive
Most frequent

Information sharing

Start
here

Systems support

FIGURE 51-5 Occupational therapy service delivery in the schools. (Adapted with permission from Hollenbeck, J. [2012b]. *Supporting students with SPD in school.* Retrieved from http://publicschoolot.com/currenttopics/sensory-integration/how-to -guides/115-supporting-students-with-spd-in-school.)

The previous examples of service delivery reflect *indirect services* or services where the occupational therapist is not working hands-on with the child. In the terms of IDEA, these can be included as a related service, but some districts document these services as supplemental aid and services (especially if provided in the general education setting) or services on behalf of the child when they are provided around a specific need of a specific student.

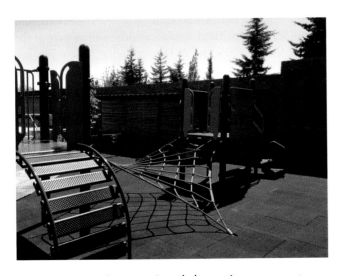

FIGURE 51-6 Occupational therapists support student participation on the playground and may be involved in playground design.

Some systems supports, information sharing, and accommodations may be provided not only as part of special education but also as part of programs such as MTSS or may not be specific to any student but benefit all students.

For some students, a greater intensity of services may be needed. These services are often referred to as *direct services* and may include hands-on services either in context or out of context. The goal is to provide services *in context* (e.g., in the classroom, lunchroom, during recess) whenever possible. Removing a student from the educational setting to go to a therapy room (or any other specialize space) should only be done if the skill cannot be addressed in context because this is a more restrictive environment. As soon as possible, an LRE option of service delivery should be implemented. Often, services are provided *out of context* for brief periods of time to help a child learn a new skill (e.g., a dressing technique). But once the skill is learned in a 1:1 setting, the student should practice and refine the skill as part of the natural school routine. Regardless of the type of service delivery provided by the practitioner, *team supports* should be considered (AOTA, 2007; Hanft & Shepherd, 2016). Table 51-7 provides a definition and additional examples of the different service delivery options.

Interagency Collaboration

Another important aspect of OT service delivery in educational settings includes collaboration between school

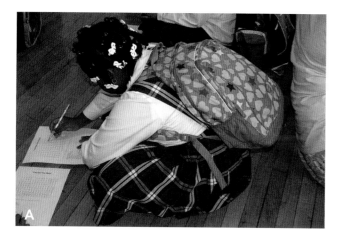

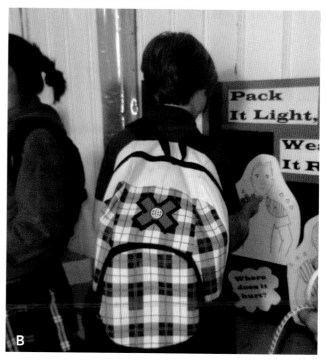

FIGURE 51-7 **A,B.** Participating in the American Occupational Therapy Association's (AOTA's) backpack campaign in the schools may prevent future injury for some students. (Photo courtesy of Karen Jacobs, EdD, OTR/L, CPE, FAOTA.)

personnel and staff from any clinic a child might be attending as well as collaboration with other agencies. Interagency collaboration is particularly necessary if the OT practitioner is providing services for students who use assistive technology or during transition planning for older students. Such collaboration is important for any other educational setting. For example, if a student with a disability who is attending university needs specialized adaptive equipment in order to fully participate, the Department of Vocational Rehabilitation might help with the procurement of such device. Or, if an occupational therapist is providing a continuing education course and one of the attendees is deaf, a sign-language interpreter might be needed.

Periodic Review

Inherent in service delivery in any setting is the documentation of services. Documentation serves as a communication tool to the students and families regarding the individualized program. Additionally, all decision making about OT intervention in the schools should be based on data, including research to the maximum extent possible. The IDEA 2004 requires that the IFSP, IEP, or ITP be reviewed at least annually, with regular updates to the family regarding the student's progress. These updates regarding student progress on IEPs/ITPs must be at least at the same intervals as general education report cards. However, the occupational therapist should consistently (more often than quarterly) reevaluate the intervention plan to ensure that the student is moving toward achieving targeted outcomes. If necessary, the OT intervention plan or even the IFSP, IEP, or ITP might need to be modified before the annual review.

Emerging Practice Considerations

Services in the schools continue to evolve based on the unique, changing, occupational needs of the students and system. Occupational therapy practitioners with their unique skills in activity analysis and their awareness of the interaction among the client, occupation and environment are well equipped to collaborate and partner with many other professionals in the schools in order to support participation and performance. Some practice considerations due to changing occupational needs in education include child mental health, social skills, obesity, telehealth, and school leadership. These areas are addressed as part of the AOTA Vision 2025, the AOTA evidence review project, and AOTA workgroups.

Child Mental Health

Occupational therapy has strong roots in mental health and addressing psychosocial needs of children and youth. There has been an increase emphasis on mental health and the link to learning and school participation in the educational community (AOTA, 2009, 2016b). Some of this increased awareness is being driven by the increasing numbers of students on the spectrum. Additionally, the increased awareness of developmental trauma and the impact on the student's behavior as well as ability to engage, learn, and/or interact with others increases the need for service providers in the schools who understand the unique needs of this

TABLE 51-7	Service Delivery Examples	
Type of Service	**Definition**	**Example**
Systems support	Working at a systems level (e.g., school, district) to meet the needs of all students, not just students with disabilities	Playground redesign
Schoolwide approaches to address sensory needs
Implementation of a handwriting curriculum
Support policies related to evacuation.
Positive behavioral supports
Address child mental health needs or psychosocial needs.
Implementation of embedded mental health activities
Information sharing	Reframing, educating, teaching, supporting, and other ways to share information regarding a student, disability, program, or need	Provide in-services.
Information sheets for teacher
Reframe a student behavior based on the disability.
Occupational therapy corner in school newsletter
Participate in teacher meetings.
Participate on curriculum committees.
Develop a program to support students with developmental trauma.
Accommodations (see Table 51-6 for additional information)	Support is provided without changing the content or outcome expectations.	Dynamic seating
Sensory tools
Assistive technology supports
Collaborative consultation	An interactive process that focuses teams and agencies on enhancing the functional performance, educational achievement, and participation of children and youth with disabilities in school, community, and home environments (Hanft & Shepherd, 2016)	Team meetings
Evaluate/observe collaboratively.
Collaborative e-mails
Feedback regarding collaborative goals
Hands-on in context	Contextual hands-on interventions designed to support student across settings, routines, and skills	Addressing needs:
In the classroom
On the playground
During extracurricular activities
On field trips
In the bathroom
During physical education
In the lunchroom
On the bus
In the community
Small social skills groups
Hands-on out of context	Hands-on interventions in settings that are not part of the naturally occurring school/classroom routines	Working in the therapy room
Working 1:1 in the gym
Each type of service delivery is important and valuable and should be viewed as integrated feature of an entire service delivery approach. In many cases, to meet a student's identified need(s), therapy practitioners working in the schools may use a variety of approaches concurrently (e.g., some hands-on, some information sharing, and some collaborative services).

This is not an inclusive list; rather, it represents examples of possibilities.

Adapted with permission from Hollenbeck, J. (2012a). *Service delivery.* Retrieved from http://publicschoolot.com/sped-process/service-delivery

population (Blodgett & Dorado, n.d.; Chafouleas, Koriakin, Roundfield, & Overstreet, 2018). Occupational therapists are well positioned to be able to support this need and help school teams address mental health and psychosocial needs. Therapy practitioners in the schools may collaborate with school counselors or school psychologists to run social groups. They may be part of preventative teams to address bullying or other such initiatives. Bazyk (2011) lays a foundation in her book, *Mental Health Promotion, Prevention, and Intervention with Children and Youth*, that can be used by OT practitioners to talk to other professionals about OT's contribution to this need.

Social Skills

With the emphasis on social participation in the "Occupational Therapy Practice Framework" (AOTA, 2014) and the necessity of appropriate social skills to be successful in postschool outcomes (AOTA, 2016a), OT practitioners may work as part of the team to support student engagement in this area of occupation. There is increasing awareness of the need to explicitly teach social skills and social thinking (Winner, 2007). Additionally, for some children, particularly those on the spectrum, sensory processing needs may impact social participation, and so the two issues may need to be addressed simultaneously (Baltazar-Mori & Piantanida, 2007; Kuypers, 2011). Again, the unique skills and expertise of the school-based practitioner is well served to work with the team to help address this area of need (see Chapter 61 for more details).

Obesity

Occupational therapy practitioners can play important roles in addressing childhood obesity in a variety of settings, including in schools and communities and at home. In each setting, intervention may focus on a number of areas, including culturally appropriate healthy food preparation and meals, enjoyable physical and social activities, and strategies for decreasing weight bias/stigma and bullying. Messages should focus on "health and a healthy lifestyle" rather than weight loss. Services can help children identify personal character strengths (e.g., creativity, humor, thoughtfulness) and build on them. Occupational therapy practitioners can play a critical role in working with school teachers, nutritionists, and other professionals to enhance healthy lifestyles in all children and youth (AOTA, 2012b).

With the Vision 2025 emphasis on Health and Wellness and the statistics regarding the increase in childhood obesity, there are many things school-based practitioners can consider as part of their intervention for students with special needs as well as within the school system as a whole. This area of intervention is one that is recently getting increased attention both within the field of OT and the American population as a whole.

Telehealth

Telehealth is a developing service delivery model for educational settings, specifically for rural settings or small school districts where there are only a few students who require services from a school-based practitioner (Criss, 2013). Zylstra (2013) completed an evidence review on the use of telehealth in pediatrics, including schools. She found that there was evidence to support the use of this service delivery approach due to satisfaction with the services. This service delivery approach can be more cost-effective for rural school districts by decreasing travel time as well as for smaller

school districts that have a limited need for OT services. Although some of the traditional hands-on services by an OT practitioner cannot be provided through telehealth, this model of service delivery can be very effective for collaborative services through consultation and facilitation of services which allows for the OT recommendations to be implemented throughout the school day. Additionally, telehealth may help address the shortage of school-based practitioners in some areas. As with any other OT services, school-based practitioners using telehealth need to attend to ethical considerations specific to this service delivery method.

School Leadership

In recent years, school-based practitioners are beginning to seek leadership positions in the schools. Although this can be difficult due to the different training of between occupational therapists and educators and the lack of a specific career track for OT practitioners to move into leadership positions, occupational therapists are well suited for this role in the schools. Many therapists take leadership positions over therapy teams, but other positions such as program coordinators and directors of special education are sought after and filled by a small group of therapists. The AOTA has a workgroup looking at this issue and how to support occupational therapists desiring school leadership positions.

Outcomes

Whether addressing traditional practice arenas or emerging practice trends in educational settings, outcomes are determined by increased ability of the client (child, student, other professional[s], family, etc.) to participate (or support participation) in the occupation of being a student (Figure 51-8). With the emphasis in today's educational

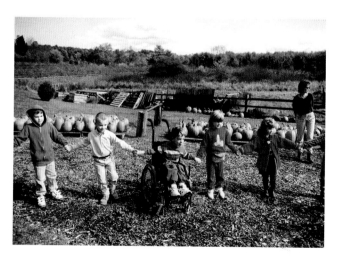

FIGURE 51.8 A functional outcome for a child in a preschool setting is participation with classmates during a field trip to pick pumpkins.

settings on evidence-based practices, it is important that occupational therapists working in these settings use strategies and techniques that are supported by research or effective or promising practices (Frolek-Clark & Chandler, 2013; Swinth, Spencer, & Jackson, 2007). The challenge for most therapists in these settings is that there is limited research and the research that exists tends to be descriptive. However, in the public schools, the federal government has recognized this dearth in research and therefore supports emerging and promising practices. Occupational therapy

practitioners working in educational settings can respond to this challenge by systematically collecting data when working with their clients and then using these data to support or change intervention. It is important that occupational therapists use professional reasoning that includes research, to the extent possible, to inform their practice but that they not allow the lack of more experimental research to limit the scope of their practice in education settings. See the "Commentary on the Evidence" box for an example.

COMMENTARY ON THE EVIDENCE

School-Based Practice

The Individuals with Disabilities Education Act (IDEA) 2004 requires that therapists use "scientifically based instructional practices, to the maximum extent possible" (§ 601[c][5][E]). This requirement is congruent with OT in any setting and is applicable to all professionals who provide services in public schools. Occupational therapy practitioners can use research evidence to examine the assumptions that guide their practice. For example, the value of consultation and education approaches and providing intervention within natural performance contexts is well documented in the research literature and serves as a guideline for best practice (Spencer, Turkett, Vaughan, & Koenig, 2006).

Although some research evidence is available, rigorous studies supporting effective practice in schools are still emerging. Swinth et al. (2007), in a paper developed for the Center on Personnel Studies in Special Education (COPSSE), summarized the current state of research supporting effective practices in the schools. (The reader is referred to the full report for specifics and in-depth information.) Because the mandate of IDEA is for services to be provided within the natural context as much as possible, Swinth and colleagues recommend that "occupational therapists working within the schools must consider outcomes within the context of the environment as well as the expectations in which their services are provided" (p. 8). Considering outcomes within the educational setting creates a challenge for therapy practitioners because some intervention strategies that have a strong research base in a clinical setting might not be as appropriate or as effective in educational settings. For example, rather than working on sensory processing in a one-on-one setting down the hall from the classroom in an environment that simulates a clinical setting, therapists in the schools might work with the teacher and student to implement sensory processing strategies in the classroom. The school-based therapist might work with the teacher to integrate tools such as move-and-sit cushions, a ball chair, and fidgets into the classroom routine (Gochenour & Poskey, 2017). Additionally, the therapist might work with the teacher to adjust the classroom environment, such as playing

low music, decreasing the lights or using natural lighting, or developing a "quiet corner" where students can go to decrease the amount of sensory input they are receiving.

The COPSSE review of the evidence specific to school-based practice revealed a lack of high-level research-based evidence due to the few randomized controlled trials or meta-analyses of such trials related to school-based OT services. Despite this finding, a growing body of descriptive research does exist. "Thus, currently occupational therapists must rely more on effective or promising practices, clinical expertise and client values as well as systematically collected data when delivering effective practices" (Swinth et al., 2007, p. 34). To increase the breadth and depth of the evidence, a culture of inquiry needs to be established among school-based practitioners. Within this culture of inquiry, a strong research agenda should be established to help inform and shape school-based practice. This research agenda should study current practice strategies (e.g., the use of sensory principles in the classroom, the best use of the skills and expertise of an occupational therapist to address handwriting) as well as the current assumptions of school-based OT service delivery (e.g., therapy in a therapy room versus in the classroom, the effectiveness of collaborative service delivery). Frolek-Clark and Chandler (2013) edited *Best Practices for Occupational Therapy in Schools*. This book provides the latest research for school-based practice specific to decision making, evaluation, intervention, and more. However, research continues to be needed across many areas of practice such as to help inform OT practitioners and others about how services can be provided effectively within natural contexts as well as how other approaches to service delivery (such as team supports or system supports) can be provided efficiently and effectively to improve student outcomes. Finally, high-level experimental and quasi-experimental studies that address the effectiveness of specific OT practices on students' educational access, participation, and performance (outcome measures) are needed.

Evidence reviews related to school-based practice are available from AOTA (AOTA, 2012a; Jackson & Arbesman, 2005). Although these reviews are not specific to OT services under the IDEA 2004, some of the summaries and data

(continues)

COMMENTARY ON THE EVIDENCE *(continued)*

that are contained in the reviews can help to inform OT services in the schools. Additionally, there are individual critical appraisals of papers (CAPS) available on AOTA's Web page that are specific to interventions in the schools, such as handwriting that can help inform practitioner decision making.

School-based OT practitioners must balance the current state of the research with the need to make the best decisions possible to support student outcomes. Ilott (2004) has noted that OT is a "research emergent" profession. At times, the profession, including practitioners working in the schools, lacks a sufficient evidence base to fully determine which practices and interventions are most effective.

> As a result, the competent school-based occupational therapist must think about "effective practice" and engage in systematic data collection related to desired student outcomes. At all times, the therapist must utilize student/client evaluation and intervention activities to collect and document student performance (outcomes) which justify on-going decisions [related to] OT service continuation, modification, or discontinuation. (Swinth et al., 2007, p. 35)

The following table provides an example of how school-based therapists can use research evidence to support their reasoning about intervention.

Conclusion

On the basis of the evidence review, the occupational therapist determined that a greater emphasis on team and system support might better support the handwriting needs of the students in his district. The therapist felt that intervention for each student who is referred to OT could be best served through collaboration with teachers to develop handwriting clubs, implement adaptations in the classroom (e.g., pencil grasps, writing templates, assistive technology), promote daily handwriting practice and activities within the natural context of the classroom, and implement a comprehensive handwriting curriculum across the district. Direct OT services through one-on-one or group intervention would be provided only if it was determined through an OT evaluation that a student had underlying client factors (e.g., biomechanical, visual-motor, fine motor) affecting handwriting performance that could be improved through such direct intervention and then for short periods of time. The therapist hypothesized that by providing services through a team or system support approach, more children would benefit from OT, albeit indirectly, and that the number of referrals to OT would decrease so that the therapist would be evaluating only those children with handwriting concerns that had underlying client factors.

Question	Evidence Reviewed	Implications for Intervention Outcomes
Should school-based occupational therapists provide hands-on direct services in a one-on-one setting to address the handwriting needs of students?	• Case-Smith (2000) • Case-Smith (2002) • Denton, Cope, & Moser (2006) • Cooley (2004) • Mackay, McCluskey, & Mayes (2010) • Ratzon, Efraim, & Bart (2007) • Santangelo & Graham (2016) • Wells, Sulak, Saxon, & Howell (2016)	Occupational therapy practitioners should consider the following when determining the type(s) of intervention provided to support a student's handwriting performance: • Although the research supports direct intervention to improve handwriting, it might not be the best use of the skills and expertise of an occupational therapist to address this need. • Use of a specific handwriting curriculum may support better outcomes. • The implementation of a sensorimotor aspect to handwriting instruction may not be as effective as therapeutic practice. • Use of play with younger children may support improved fine motor skills. • Occupational therapy may help to improve letter legibility but might not affect speed or numerical legibility. • The dynamic tripod grasp is not the only functional pencil grip used in handwriting activities. • Short periods of intervention in small groups may be an effective intervention strategy. • Use of an iPad is not as effective as traditional methods of handwriting instruction. • Motor instruction/activities were not as effective as direct handwriting instruction in improving legibility and fluency.

Summary

Occupational therapy intervention in the schools is guided by the IDEA 2004. Practitioners working in the schools collaborate with the educational team to determine student needs and targeted outcomes. Once these needs and outcomes have been defined in the educational plan and the team determines that OT services are needed, then the occupational therapist designs the specific OT intervention plan. Occupational therapy intervention in the schools focuses on the occupational performance of the student within the educational environment. Practitioners may also provide services that are directed to the needs of the educational staff, parents, or system. Specific intervention strategies and approaches should be based on research to the maximum extent possible. When research is not available but preliminary data indicate that a particular intervention or service delivery could be effective (promising), then the OT practitioner should use systematic data-based decision making to inform decisions about intervention for individual students.

 Visit thePoint to watch a video about interventions for school-age children.

REFERENCES

American Occupational Therapy Association. (2007). *Occupational therapy services for children and youth under IDEA* (3rd ed.). Bethesda, MD: Author.

American Occupational Therapy Association. (2009). *Occupational therapy and school mental health.* Bethesda, MD: Author.

American Occupational Therapy Association. (2012a). *AOTA Evidence briefs. School based interventions.* Retrieved from http://www.aota.org/Educate/Research/EB/School.aspx

American Occupational Therapy Association. (2012b). *Occupational therapy's role in mental health promotion, prevention, & intervention for children and youth: Childhood obesity.* Bethesda, MD: Author.

American Occupational Therapy Association. (2014). Occupational therapy practice framework: Domain and process, 3rd edition. *American Journal of Occupational Therapy, 68,* S1–S48.

American Occupational Therapy Association. (2015). *Salary and workforce survey: Executive summary.* Bethesda, MD: Author.

American Occupational Therapy Association. (2016a). *Mental health in children and youth: The benefit and role of occupational therapy.* Bethesda, MD: Author.

American Occupational Therapy Association. (2016b). *Occupational therapy in school settings.* Bethesda, MD: Author.

Americans with Disabilities Act of 1990, 42 U.S.C.A. § 12134 (1990).

Baltazar-Mori, A., & Piantanida, D. B. (2007). *Every child wants to play: Simple and effective strategies for teaching social skills.* Torrance, CA: Pediatric Therapy Network.

Bazyk, S. (2011). *Mental health promotion, prevention, and intervention with children and youth: A guiding framework for occupational therapy.* Bethesda, MD: AOTA Press.

Bazyk, S., & Case-Smith, J. (2010). School-based occupational therapy. In J. Case-Smith & J. O'Brien (Eds.), *Occupational therapy for children* (6th ed., pp. 713–743). Philadelphia, PA: Mosby.

Blodgett, C., & Dorado, J. (n.d.). *A selected review of trauma-informed school practice and alignment with educational practice.* Retrieved from http://extension.wsu.edu/cafru/wp-content/uploads/sites/62/2015/02/CLEAR-Trauma-Informed-Schools-White-Paper.pdf?x99454

Brackett, V. K. (1928). The organization and work of the industrial school for crippled and deformed children. *Occupational Therapy and Rehabilitation, 7,* 305–312.

Bureau of Labor Statistics, U.S. Department of Labor. (2018). *Occupational outlook handbook, occupational therapists.* Retrieved from https://www.bls.gov/ooh/healthcare/occupational-therapists.htm

Case-Smith, J. (2000). Effects of occupational therapy services on fine motor and functional performance in preschool children. *American Journal of Occupational Therapy, 54,* 372–380.

Case-Smith, J. (2002). Effectiveness of school-based occupational therapy intervention on handwriting. *American Journal of Occupational Therapy, 56,* 17–25.

Chafouleas, S. M., Koriakin, T. A., Roundfield, K. D., & Overstreet, S. (2018). Addressing childhood trauma in school settings: A framework for evidence-based practice. *School Mental Health.* Advance online publication. doi:10.1007/s12310-018-9256-5

Chapparo, C., & Lowe, S. (2012). School: Participating in more than just the classroom. In S. Lane & A. Bundy (Eds.), *Kids can be kids: A childhood occupations approach* (pp. 83–101). Philadelphia, PA: F. A. Davis.

Cooley, C. (2004). *Is the dynamic tripod grasp the most functional grip for handwriting? UPS evidence-based practice symposium.* Retrieved from https://www.region10.org/r10website/assets/File/tripod_grasp.pdf

Criss, M. J. (2013). School-based telerehabilitation in occupational therapy: Using telerehabilitation technologies to promote improvements in student performance. *International Journal of Telerehabilitation, 5,* 39–46.

Demirjian, L., Horvath, F., & Bazyk, S. (2014). *Creating a comfortable cafeteria program: A model program for every moment counts.* Washington, DC: U.S. Department of Education, Office of Special Education Programs.

Denton, P. L., Cope, S., & Moser, C. (2006). The effects of sensorimotor-based intervention versus therapeutic practice on improving handwriting performance in 6- to 11-year-old children. *American Journal of Occupational Therapy, 60,* 16–27.

Dunn, W. (1988). Models of occupational therapy service provision in the school system. *American Journal of Occupational Therapy, 42,* 718–723.

Education for All Handicapped Children Act of 1975, Pub. L. No. 94-142, 20 U.S.C., § 1401, Part H, § 677 (1975).

Education of the Handicapped Act Amendments of 1986, Pub. L. No. 99-457, 20 U.S.C. § 1400 (1986).

Every Student Succeeds Act of 2015, Pub. L. No. 114-95 § 114 Stat. 1177 (2015).

Friend, M., & Cook, L. (2009). *Interactions: Collaboration skills for school professionals* (6th ed.). Boston, MA: Allyn & Bacon.

Frolek-Clark, G., & Chandler, B. (Eds.). (2013). *Best practices for occupational therapy in schools.* Bethesda, MD: AOTA Press.

Frolek-Clark, G., Polichino, J., & Jackson, L. (2004). Occupational therapy services in early intervention and school-based programs (2004). *American Journal of Occupational Therapy, 58,* 681–685.

Giangreco, M. (2001). Interactions among program, placement, and services in educational planning for students with disabilities. *Mental Retardation, 39,* 341–350.

Gochenour, B., & Poskey, G. A. (2017). Determining the effectiveness of alternative seating systems for students with attention difficulties: A systematic review. *Journal of Occupational Therapy, Schools, & Early Intervention, 10,* 284–299. doi:10.1080/19411243.2017.1325817

Hanft, B., & Shepherd, J. (2016). *Collaboration and teamwork: Essential to school-based occupational therapy* (2nd ed.). Bethesda, MD: AOTA Press.

Hanft, B., & Swinth, Y. (2011). Commentary on collaboration. *Journal of Occupational Therapy, Schools, & Early Intervention, 4*, 2–7.

Henry, D. A., & McClary, M. (2011). The Sensory Processing Measure-Preschool (SPM-P)—Part two: Test–retest and collective collaborative empowerment, including a father's perspective. *Journal of Occupational Therapy, Schools, & Early Intervention, 4*, 53–70.

Hollenbeck, J. (2012a). *Service delivery.* Retrieved from http://public schoolot.com/sped-process/service-delivery

Hollenbeck, J. (2012b). *Supporting students with SPD in school.* Retrieved from http://publicschoolot.com/currenttopics/sensory-integration/how-to-guides/115-supporting-students-with-spd-in-school

Ilott, I. (2004). Evidence-based practice forum: Challenges and strategic solutions for a research emergent profession. *American Journal of Occupational Therapy, 58*, 347–352.

Individuals with Disabilities Education Act Amendments of 1990, Pub. L. No. 101-476, 20 U.S.C. §1400–1485, 104 Stat. 1142 (1990).

Individuals with Disabilities Education Act Amendments of 1997, Pub. L. No. 105-117, 20 U.S.C. 1400 *et se*, 111 Stat. 37 (1997).

Individuals with Disabilities Education Improvement Act of 2004, Pub. L. No. 108-446, 20 U.S.C. § 1400 *et seq*, 118 Stat. 2647 (2004).

Jackson, L., & Arbesman, M. (2005). *Occupational therapy practice guidelines for children with behavioral and psychosocial needs.* Bethesda, MD: AOTA Press.

Kidner, T. B. (1910). *Educational handwork.* Toronto, Canada: Educational Book.

Kramer, P., & Hinojosa, J. (2009). *Frames of reference for pediatric occupational therapy* (3rd ed.). Philadelphia, PA: Lippincott Williams & Wilkins.

Kuypers, L. (2011). *The zones of regulation: A curriculum designed to foster self-regulation and emotional control.* San Jose, CA: Think Social.

Mackay, N., McCluskey, A., & Mayes, R. (2010). The log handwriting program improved children's writing legibility: A pretest–posttest study. *American Journal of Occupational Therapy, 64*, 30–36.

National Association of State Directors of Special Education. (2005). *Response to intervention: Policy considerations and implementation.* Alexandria, VA: Author.

No Child Left Behind Act of 2001, Pub. L. No. 107-110, 115 Stat. 1425 (2002).

Nolet, V., & McLaughlin, M. J. (2000). *Accessing the general curriculum: Including students with disabilities in standards-based reform.* Thousand Oaks, CA: Corwin Press.

O'Brien, J., Forest, M., Snow, J., Pearpoint, J., & Hasbury, D. (1989). *Action for inclusion: How to improve schools by welcoming children with special needs into regular classrooms.* Toronto, Canada: Inclusion Press.

Park, S. (2012). Setting goals that express the possibilities: If we don't know where we are going, how will we know when we get there? In S. Lane & A. Bundy (Eds.), *Kids can be kids: A childhood occupations approach* (pp. 349–367). Philadelphia, PA: F. A. Davis.

Quinn, S., Gleeson, C. I., & Nolan, C. (2014). An occupational therapy support service for university students with Asperger's syndrome (AS). *Occupational Therapy in Mental Health, 30*, 109–125. doi:10.1080/0164212X.2014.910155

Ratzon, N. Z., Efraim, D., & Bart, O. (2007). A short-term graphomotor program for improving writing readiness skills of first-grade students. *American Journal of Occupational Therapy, 61*, 399–405.

Reed, K., & Polichino, J. (2013). Best practices in ethical decision making for school occupational therapy practitioners. In G. Frolek-Clark & B. Chandler (Eds.), *Best practice in the schools.* Bethesda, MD: AOTA Press.

Rehabilitation Act of 1973, 29 U.S.C. § 504 (1973).

Santangelo, T., & Graham, S. (2016). A comprehensive meta-analysis of handwriting instruction. *Journal Educational Psychology Review, 28*, 225–265. doi:10.1007/s10648-015-9335-1

Shasby, S., & Schneck, C. (2011). Commentary on collaboration in school-based practice: Positives and pitfalls. *Journal of Occupational Therapy, Schools, & Early Intervention, 4*, 22–33.

Silverstein, R. (2000). Emerging disability policy framework: A guidepost for analyzing public policy. *Iowa Law Review, 85*, 1757–1802.

Snell, M., & Janney, R. (2005). *Collaborative teaming* (2nd ed.). Baltimore, MD: Paul H. Brookes.

Social Security Act of 1935, Pub. L. No. 74-271, 49 Stat. 620 (1935).

Spencer, K. C., Turkett, A., Vaughan, R., & Koenig, S. (2006). School-based practice patterns: A survey of occupational therapists in Colorado. *American Journal of Occupational Therapy, 60*, 81–91.

Swinth, Y. L., Chandler, B., Hanft, B., Jackson, L., & Shepherd, J. (2003). *Personnel issues in school-based occupational therapy: Supply and demand, preparation, and certification and licensure.* Gainesville, FL: Center on Personnel Studies in Special Education. Retrieved from http://www.coe.ufl.edu/copsse

Swinth, Y. L., Spencer, K. C., & Jackson, L. (2007). *Occupational therapy: Effective school-based practices within a policy context.* Gainesville, FL: Center on Personnel Studies in Special Education.

Wells, K. E., Sulak, T. N., Saxon, T. F., & Howell, L. L. (2016). Traditional versus iPad-mediated handwriting instruction in early learners. *Journal of Occupational Therapy, Schools, & Early Intervention, 9*, 185–198.

Whittier, I. L. (1922). Occupation for children in hospitals. *Archives of Occupational Therapy, 1*(1), 41–47.

Williams, M. S., & Shellenberger, S. (1996). *How does your engine run? A leader's guide to the Alert Program for self-regulation.* Albuquerque, NM: TherapyWorks.

Winner, M. G. (2007). *Thinking about YOU thinking about ME* (2nd ed.). San Jose, CA: Think Social.

Zylstra, S. E. (2013). Evidence for the use of telehealth in pediatric occupational therapy. *Journal of Occupational Therapy, Schools, & Early Intervention, 6*, 326–355. doi:10.1080/19411243.2013.860765

the**Point**® *For additional resources on the subjects discussed in this chapter, visit* http://thePoint.lww.com/Willard-Spackman13e. *See* **Appendix I**, **Resources and Evidence for Common Conditions Addressed in OT** *for more details about cerebral palsy and obesity.*

Work

Julie Dorsey, Holly Ehrenfried, Denise Finch, Lisa A. Jaegers

LEARNING OBJECTIVES

After reading this chapter, you will be able to:

1. Define work in the context of occupational therapy (OT), including theoretical foundations, and discuss opportunities within the profession.
2. Describe work participation across the life course, including the varied meaning and value of work.
3. Articulate the distinct role of OT as part of the interprofessional team for work-related practice.
4. Identify common settings, reimbursement/payment systems, and legislation related to work participation.
5. Discuss various work-related evaluation and assessment methods including development of the occupational profile and job analysis.
6. Analyze client-centered, work-related intervention approaches and evidence for work and non–work-related injury, illness, and disease.

Introduction

> "What do you want to be when you grow up?"
>   "What's your major?"
>   "Where do you work?"

It is very likely that you have been asked these questions many times in your life, and that you often have asked these questions of others. Remember that you are reading this textbook as part of your work—as a student learning about occupational therapy (OT) or a practitioner expanding your knowledge.

Work as an occupation is defined in the Occupational Therapy Practice Framework (OTPF) as employment interests and pursuits, employment seeking and acquisition, job performance, and retirement preparation and adjustment (American Occupational Therapy Association [AOTA], 2014a). Participation in work contributes to an individual's sense of identity and development of meaning and purpose in life. It adds structure and routine to the day, provides valuable opportunities for making social connections and contributions to society, and allows us to seek financial security.

CENTENNIAL NOTES

Work: A Part of Occupational Therapy Since the Beginning

Work has been a part of OT since the beginning of the profession. In the 1800s and early 1900s, prior to the official designation of the profession in 1917, work was used for restorative functions (E. D. Bond, 1925), to increase self-esteem (Davis, 1945), and to meet unconscious needs (Medd, 1934). In the 1920s, OT workshops provided competitive, graded work with minimal compensation (Hanson & Walker, 1992). During the 1930s, industrial workshops, work evaluation services, and vocational rehabilitation programs thrived (Marshall, 1985).

During and after World War II, there was an increased demand to rehabilitate returning soldiers for return to work (Hanson & Walker, 1992; Johnson, 1971). In the 1950s, maintenance tasks were performed by psychiatric patients in mental hospitals (Ivany & Rothschild, 1951).

Research into the area of work began in the United States in 1960s with shared statistics on the working population, the effects and values of work ethics, information regarding new federal labor laws, and the relationship between work and leisure (Marshall, 1985), which helped to inform OT practice. The Occupational Safety and Health Act of 1970 required employers to provide work environments free from hazards that cause death or injury (Occupational

Safety and Health Administration [OSHA], n.d.b) which set the stage for a focus on injury prevention and work hardening programs (Hanson & Walker, 1992).

In the 1980s, occupational therapists began to perform work aptitude assessments, work hardening, job evaluations, job skill assessments, and industrial consultation (Reed & Peters, 2006), and in 1987, the AOTA created the *Work Programs Special Interest Section*— later known as *Work & Industry Special Interest Section* (WISIS). Opportunities for U.S. OT practitioners to assist workers expanded when the Americans with Disabilities Act of 1990 provided individuals with disabilities equal protection in employment (Americans with Disabilities Act of 1990).

Currently, OT practitioners aim to improve occupational performance and engagement through job and worker analysis (Braveman & Page, 2012) and serve as consultants to industry for wellness and prevention (Hanson & Walker, 1992).

Work practice continues to thrive and changes in response to societal trends, such as more people continuing to work well past retirement. The history of work within OT tells us that OT practitioners will continue to adapt and develop new strategies to keep work in the forefront of OT practice.

Occupational therapy practitioners work with individuals, groups, and populations across the life course and across settings to address the occupation of work (AOTA, 2014a). Work holds different meanings for different people and at different phases, stages, or times in their lives. Consider the following scenarios:

- A 17-year-old with Autism Spectrum Disorder is working with an OT practitioner to explore career interests.
- A 28-year-old is taking time away from paid work to work at home and raise a family.
- A 54-year-old who is the primary financial contributor in the family is injured at work.
- A 67-year-old who recently retired is looking for new ways to contribute to the community.

Although all of these situations are different in terms of what the OT process would involve, there are common issues related to occupational participation that are explored in this chapter. It is essential for OT practitioners to understand how individuals value work participation and to take these values into account throughout the OT process while also recognizing work within context of an employer and the broader culture in a region or country.

Within OT practice, work can be used as both a means and an ends. For example, an artist who experienced stroke and is being treated on an inpatient rehabilitation unit may enjoy painting at an easel to practice weight shifting and weight bearing, visual scanning, and impulse control. Returning to work may not directly be addressed within the OT plan of care, as the emphasis may be on safely returning home. Rather, work can be used as a meaningful occupation to engage the client in addressing underlying problem areas. However, that same artist may bring specific concerns about returning to work when seeking outpatient services.

In other situations, OT practitioners may address an individual's underlying skills needed for work participation, the work environment, and the work demands as part of a return to work treatment plan. Occupational therapy practitioners are responsible for addressing work as a means and/or ends across all practice settings and populations. Even if work participation is not the primary emphasis of a treatment plan, it is a meaningful occupation for clients and warrants specific attention.

Occupational therapy practitioners need to be responsive to the dynamic needs of their clients within the broader context of a changing society. In workplaces, there is a rise in workers with chronic physical, mental health, and other conditions that impact work participation and engagement, such as obesity, diabetes, opioid and other substance abuse, autism spectrum disorders, general aging, anxiety, cancer, and mild traumatic brain injury (mTBI). These populations present opportunities for OT practitioners to provide direct and indirect services in the form of preventing injuries, facilitating workplace health and well-being, advocating for clients' needs, recommending workplace accommodations, and other services. Population health interventions such as the National Institute for Occupational Safety and Health's (NIOSH) Total Worker Health® (Jaegers, 2015) and opportunities within primary care (AOTA, 2014b) can be valuable strategies for addressing the needs of these growing populations.

Additional considerations and trends in workplaces include the following:

- Increased use of technology (e.g., accessing more documents electronically, Web-conferencing programs to allow for virtual meetings and working from home or other remote locations, and home computer workstations)
- Shifts toward more active work environments (e.g., desk exercise programs, sit-stand stations, walking meetings)
- Increased acceptance and interest in workplace health and wellness initiatives by employers (e.g., safe patient handling initiatives, incentives for participating in fitness programs, onsite wellness programs)
- Trends in building design, such as "green" buildings through Leadership in Energy and Environmental Design (LEED) certification, which can impact the worker (e.g., large windows for passive solar and lighting benefits that result in excessive glare for workers)
- Focus on work in underserved populations (e.g., community reentry for incarcerated individuals, low-income individuals, migrant workers, and individuals who are homeless as well as services for veterans)

Theoretical Foundations and Models to Guide Practice

There is a broad spectrum of OT practice areas related to work. Work is an occupation that spans nearly all populations, practice settings, and social-ecological levels (e.g., individual, group, organization, community, and population). The primary goal of work-related OT practice is to promote participation and engagement in work activities. **Work participation** describes involvement in situations and activities that explore, support, or engage in work. **Work engagement** is performance of work participation occupations in which the activities are a "result of choice, motivation, and meaning within a supportive context

and environment" (AOTA, 2014a, p. S4). Lack of work or an overabundance of work can be detrimental to health. Individuals who are deprived of the opportunity to engage in occupations that they find meaningful have a reduced sense of well-being (Durocher, Gibson, & Rappolt, 2014). Conversely, individuals who are overworked may experience serious adverse health issues, and this situation can even result in death (Eguchi, Wada, & Smith, 2016). To address the occupation of work, a conceptual framework to guide practice, research, and knowledge acquisition was developed that highlights the broad scope of work, including preparation, accommodation, and adaptation; health promotion, wellness, and disease prevention; injury prevention and ergonomics; rehabilitation and return to work; and evaluation and practitioner education (Jaegers, Finch, Dorsey, & Ehrenfried, 2015). The importance of science-driven and practice-informed evidence (Hinojosa, 2013) is stressed throughout the framework for advancing knowledge and ensuring the use of efficacious interventions in work-based practice.

Although much of work-related OT practice focuses on individual and organizational level interventions, the health of human populations (e.g., the workforce, the population of unemployed individuals, and the aging population of workers) is also addressed. **Population health** is the outcome of efforts across the wide array of social determinants of health (Kindig, 2017), including health systems and services, employment, housing, transportation, education, social environment, public safety, and the physical environment (National Academies of Sciences, Engineering, and Medicine, 2017). Occupational therapy practitioners seek to improve health inequities that have consequences on health factors that affect a person's ability to participate in work-related activities and must be cognizant of health inequities surrounding their practice. It is also important to consider factors concerning occupational and social justice and underserved populations to be inclusive and provide a holistic approach.

Several models and theories can be used to guide the OT process in the area of work. *General systems theory* is useful in shaping our understanding of the complex interactions of the various parts within a system. Concepts from systems theory are the basis for multiple models within OT, including the following occupation-based models (see Chapters 42 and 43):

- Person-Environment-Occupation (PEO) (Law et al., 1996)
- Model of Human Occupation (Kielhofner, 2009)
- Person-Environment-Occupation-Performance (Baum, Christiansen, & Bass, 2015)

These models can provide a foundation for evaluation and interventions to address the occupation of work, as they provide practitioners with a holistic perspective from which to view the client. For example, a practitioner using the PEO model may structure an ergonomic assessment of an individual at their computer workstation by evaluating the person (e.g., posture, stress levels, height of person), the environment (e.g., height of desk, lighting, noise levels), and the occupation (e.g., specific work tasks, repetition and frequency of tasks). Once a mismatch is identified, an intervention plan can target the specific area(s) of the person, environment, and occupation.

There are also *health promotion models* that can guide the OT process in the area of work. Models related to individual behavior change such as the Transtheoretical Model and the Health Belief Model help practitioners identify and understand the various factors that can lead to behavior changes in the workplace. At the population level, theories and models such as Diffusion of Innovations Theory, Social Marketing approach, and the PRECEDE-PROCEED Model can guide practitioners on how to facilitate more widespread changes within a workplace, employment system, or community (Rimer & Glanz, 2005). Occupational therapy practitioners select a model/theory/framework based on what needs to be understood and addressed through the OT process.

Overview of Legislation Related to Work

There are many relevant pieces of legislation that influence OT practice in the area of work. Several pieces of key legislation are discussed in this section to provide context for the chapter.

Americans with Disabilities Act

The Americans with Disabilities Act (ADA) of 1990 was the first comprehensive civil rights law to address the needs of people with disabilities. Related to work, the ADA prohibits discrimination in employment and mandates **reasonable accommodations** in the workplace for people with disabilities who meet the prerequisite job requirements and who can perform the essential functions of the job with or without modification. The ADA was amended in 2008 (Americans with Disabilities Act Amendments Act—ADAAA) to clarify the definition of disability, to make it simpler for individuals seeking protection, and to shift the focus to discrimination versus the disability.

The ADAAA (2008) defines a person with a disability as follows:

1. "Has a physical or mental impairment that substantially limits one or more major life activities" (29 C.F.R. § 1630.2[g][1][i])
2. "A record of a physical or mental impairment that substantially limited a major life activity" (29 C.F.R. § 1630.2[g][1][ii])
3. "Is regarded as having a disability or substantially limiting impairment" (29 C.F.R. § 1630.2[g][1][iii])

Occupational therapy practitioners need to understand the provisions of the ADA when recommending job modifications and advocating for reasonable accommodations for people with disabilities who wish to remain in or enter the workforce. Job analyses can be used to help identify, describe, and measure essential job functions versus marginal or nonessential functions and examine opportunities for modifications to promote work participation.

Accommodations and modifications may be related to accessibility and/or task completion. Changes to the built environment, objects, tools, and/or routines at the workplace provide opportunities to improve the match between the workers' (individuals, groups, and populations) capacities and the job demands for successful engagement in work activities. The Job Accommodation Network (JAN) (https://askjan.org/) is a useful source for exploring accommodation options by diagnosis or type of accommodation.

Accommodation is a method for enabling individuals to access or perform work through technology and adjustments or modifications to a job or work environment. **Reasonable accommodations** are described in ADA as "any change or adjustment to a job or work environment that permits a qualified applicant or employee with a disability to participate in the job application process, to perform the essential functions or a job, or to enjoy benefits and privileges of employment equal to those enjoyed by employees without disabilities." These accommodations ensure individuals are able to perform the **essential functions** (i.e., the basic job duties an employee must be able to perform with or without reasonable accommodation) of a job while remaining feasible for the employer to support them (U.S. Equal Employment Opportunity Commission [EEOC], n.d.). Decisions regarding accommodations related to a person with disability require careful attention to company policies, local workers compensation laws (if applicable), and federal legislation such as the ADA (ADAAA, 2008). Reasonable accommodations must be considered carefully because each employer has a variety of resources available to them; what may be reasonable to one employer may not be to another employer.

Occupational therapy practitioners also can help employers assess job demands by creating **functional job descriptions** (FJDs). These reports identify essential job functions and critical demands; employers can use them in hiring, making return to work decisions, and determining necessary accommodation. The FJD is also beneficial to individuals with disabilities because the essential functions and specific critical demands of a job are identified and can be made available for review to help the individual make an informed decision about job selection.

ADA-compliant job descriptions should include employees during the data collection, information exchange, and review processes of FJD development (U.S. EEOC, 2005). The final determination of what is included as an essential function is the employer's decision, but the

EEOC (2005) provides a number of guidelines including (1) whether the reason the job exists is to perform that function, (2) the number of people available to complete the function, and (3) the degree of expertise required to perform the function.

Accessibility to work areas, meeting rooms, rest rooms, and other public spaces as well as communication opportunities within a company allow employees with disabilities to engage in activities related to work and meet social and personal needs in the workplace. The United States Access Board (USAB) is responsible for the development and updates of the design guidelines referred to as the Americans with Disabilities and Architectural Barriers Act Accessibility Guidelines (ADAAG) (USAB, n.d.). The ADAAG provides information regarding the design of and changes to the built environment necessary to accessibility for people with disabilities (USAB, 2004). The USAB (n.d.) states

> ADAAG, as issued under titles of the ADA (II and III) covering public access, makes a distinction between public or common use areas, which must be fully accessible, and areas used only by employees as work areas. Access is required to, not fully within, work areas in part because the ADA (title I) treats access for employees with disabilities as an accommodation made when the need arises. Employee spaces used for purposes other than job-related tasks (breakrooms, lounges, parking, shower and locker rooms, etc.) are considered "common use" and are required to be fully accessible. Work areas that also function as public use space, such as patient exam rooms, must be fully accessible for public access; fixtures and controls within used only by employees are not required to comply. Work areas must be accessible for "approach, entry, and exit," which means location on an accessible route so that people using wheelchairs can enter and back out of the space. This includes accessible entry doors or gates.

The U.S. Department of Justice more recently published the "2010 ADA Standards for Accessible Design" (ADA.gov, n.d.) which are the revised, enforceable accessibility standards for new construction and alterations to remove barriers as described under Title II: State and Local Government and Title III: Public Accommodations and Commercial Facilities sections of the ADA (1990). Occupational therapy practitioners can use these guidelines and standards to identify potential areas of change in the built environment.

Web accessibility is another area of concern for persons with disabilities. Access to electronic information such as human resources information, company e-mails/announcements, and other Web-based information via the computer is a critical factor at work. For example, if the employer posts a job application or promotion application in their Website in pdf format, a person with low vision using screen reader software designed to convert text to speech cannot read the document. The document needs to be available in HTML format for equal access to all employees. Additional information on Web accessibility for use of computers and Internet at work is provided in the online materials for this chapter.

Workers Compensation

Workers compensation insurance (WCI), worker safety, and employer/employee guidelines are regulated at the state level for most business entities including local government agencies. Workers compensation insurance is purchased by the employer and provides coverage for workers who have been injured on the job, including payment for medical services to treat the work injury and payment of lost wages if unable to resume work immediately after the injury as well as payment for permanent impairment such as loss of a limb. State labor boards regulate WCI carriers; each state has its own laws related to WCI.

Both state and federal programs provide guidelines and protections to the employee and the employer in the event of a workplace injury or illness. It is essential that OT practitioners treating injured workers and working with employers through workers compensation have a full understanding of the state laws or federal laws providing coverage for the work-related injuries. For example, in New Hampshire, employers with five or more employees are required to temporarily provide alternative work for workers who have sustained a work-related injury (New Hampshire Workers' Compensation Law, 2009). Therefore, the employee experiencing a work injury has the opportunity to remain engaged in work tasks within their capacity during the recovery period. Employers, insurance carriers, and practitioners then have a clear understanding of return to work/stay at work requirements. To facilitate work participation, an occupational therapy practitioner may provide treatment in the clinic to manage client factors and improve occupational performance and/or complete a job analysis to identify appropriate work tasks for modified work or investigate ergonomic risk factors. In some instances, therapy sessions occur at the work site and may include observing the worker completing tasks, providing cueing and training to modify set up or method of completing the task, and grading work activities to build work capacity.

Social Security Disability Insurance

Social Security Disability Income (SSDI) provides payments to individuals who cannot work due to medical conditions expected to last more than 1 year or that result in death (Social Security Administration [SSA], 2017). Eligibility and payments are determined by a number of factors including how long a person has worked and their age at time of disability. After receiving SSDI benefits for 2 years, people become eligible for health insurance through Medicare. In addition, Supplemental Security Income through the SSA is available to qualified persons with disabilities, older adults, and children who acquired a disability before age 22 years who are in need of supplemental income to pay for basic needs such as clothing, food, and shelter (SSA, 2017).

It can be difficult for people to transition off of SSDI and Supplemental Income Benefits through part-time or gradual return to work because benefits paid may be reduced due to income from temporary or part-time work, and/or their disability status may be challenged. To address this issue, the SSA also administers the "Ticket to Work" program. This is a free and voluntary program designed to help people receiving SSDI or Supplemental Income Benefits reenter the workforce and reduce reliance on disability benefits. Services are coordinated through eligible "employment networks" and vocational rehabilitation agencies and may include training, job placements, career counseling, and vocational rehabilitation (SSA, 2017).

The Occupational Therapy Process

The evaluation portion of the OT process includes the occupational profile and occupational performance analysis (AOTA, 2014a). Building rapport with the individual through interview and discussion leads to the answering of important questions related to why the individual is seeking services; concerns related to engagement in occupations; occupational history; performance in roles, routines, and habits; supports and barriers to occupational engagement; and priorities and preferred outcomes to target (AOTA, 2017). Job analysis is one of the main evaluation methods used by occupational therapists to address the occupational performance of work and is discussed in detail in the next section. Examples of formal work evaluation tools are available through AOTA at https://www.aota.org/wisis.

Service provision by OT practitioners includes direct and indirect services, consultation, advocacy, and education (AOTA, 2017). Work-related interventions commonly "address factors affecting work participation. The approaches fall into the following basic categories: create, promote, establish, restore, maintain, modify, compensate, adapt, or prevent" (AOTA, 2017, p. 4).

Understanding Work through Job Analysis

In OT, activity analysis is used to "analyze the demands of an activity or occupation" in order to "understand the specific body structures, body functions, performance skills, and performance patterns that are required and to determine the generic demands the activity or occupational makes on the client" (AOTA, 2014a, p. S12). **Job analysis** is a form of activity analysis that is specific to work tasks and includes the process of gathering and analyzing data related to job task requirements or demands, the environment, and human capacities needed to complete job functions.

Job analysis can be generic (i.e., related primarily to measuring and recording job activities and demands), problem or occupation based (i.e., addresses work activities and demands related to a specific person or population), or related to identification of ergonomic risk factors. For working adults with injuries, disability, or disease, as well as those who seek jobs or volunteer positions, job analysis can be an important part of the OT evaluation process, as it informs decision making related to interventions and outcomes to promote work participation. The scope and type of job analysis vary depending on the needs of the individual, group, or population as well as work environment factors, reimbursement or referral sources, and OT service settings.

Job analysis is a broad term used by a number of professionals including employers, vocational rehabilitation professionals, ergonomists, safety professionals, and OT practitioners. For OT practitioners, the most frequently used types of evaluations are the following:

- Occupation-based or problem-based job analysis
- Functional demands or functional job analysis
- Musculoskeletal disorder (MSD) ergonomic risk assessment

Each of these types of job analysis is described in Table 52-1.

Job analysis data is useful when planning interventions and outcomes for clients experiencing challenges with sustaining, returning to, or gaining work participation. Examples include injured workers; young adults with disabilities transitioning from school into the workforce; adults with mental illness; and adults with disease or disability such as a traumatic brain injury (TBI), low vision, and multiple sclerosis. Job analysis data can also be used to assist special populations such as older workers, prison personnel, farmers, volunteers, and those preparing for retirement to remain healthy at work or sustain participation.

For person-specific environmental interventions, careful attention to client factors such as strength, range of motion, and soft tissue status and pain as well as occupational performance as compared to job demands (e.g., work schedules, sequencing of tasks, cognitive and social demands, equipment used, equipment set up, body postures, and physical demands) help to identify mismatches and potential modifications.

TABLE 52-1 Types and Uses of Job Analyses

Type of Job Analysis	Purpose and Uses
Occupation-based or problem-based job analysis Evaluation and intervention related to a specific client for rehabilitation, accommodation, and/or modification	• Identify primary or essential physical, cognitive, and social demands in environment related to client's strengths and weaknesses • Measure specific physical demands (e.g., lifting weights, height range, and frequency) • Assess cognitive demands (e.g. complexity of processes and decision-making, attention) • Assess responsibilities and tasks related to social interaction and communication • Gather person- or group-specific information regarding client factors, roles, habits, routines, performance patterns, and performance skills
Functional analysis Measurement/evaluation of job requirements for hiring, job matching, or other evaluation (e.g., post-offer testing, ADA-related job accommodation and modification decisions, functional job descriptions)	• Gather and analyze information related to required job functions for job or job category rather than for a specific person • Assess required knowledge, background, and qualifications • Determine essential/marginal functions of job and time spent in those functions • Measure specific physical demands (e.g., lifting, moving, placing, holding, typing) related to job function • Assess environmental factors such as noise, lighting, temperature, number of people, tools, equipment, flooring/ground type, and exposure to weather • Determine cognitive demands • Determine responsibilities and tasks related to social interaction and communication • Formats vary and may be determined by employer or reimbursement source.
Musculoskeletal Disorder Risk Assessment (also called Ergonomic Risk Assessment and Risk Analysis) Injury prevention and health and wellness promotion	• Using risk assessment tools, measure risk factor exposures such as force, repetition, sustained postures, awkward postures, extreme temperatures, vibration, contact stress, and job stress • Gather additional data such as injury patterns in the worker and group or population health information • The results can help to identify effective interventions to resolve or reduce symptoms, vary work methods, modify the work environment or work organization, or redesign a job task or work area. A number of MSD risk assessments are available to evaluate jobs tasks (Table 52-2).

MSD, musculoskeletal disorder; ADA, Americans with Disabilities Act.

TABLE 52-2 Selected Musculoskeletal Disorder Risk Assessment Tools

Assessment Tool	Purpose and Application	Source
The Revised NIOSH Lifting Equation	Evaluates lifting loads to identify potential risk of back injury; uses a formula to identify the maximum acceptable load for a lifting task	https://www.cdc.gov/niosh/docs/94-110/pdfs/94-110.pdf
Rapid Upper Limb Assessment (RULA)	Used to evaluate upper extremity postures that are not highly repetitive or forceful	http://www.rula.co.uk/
WISHA Hazard Zone Checklist	Screens to review movements or postures that are a "regular and foreseeable part of the job" and identify related risk factors	http://www.lni.wa.gov/safety/SprainsStrains/evaltools/HazardZoneChecklist.PDF
Quick Exposure Checklist	Provides a risk factor score that considers exposures to multiple body parts, tasks performed, duration, work cycles, and worker perceptions	http://www.lni.wa.gov/Safety/SprainsStrains/pdfs/QECReferenceGuide.pdf
Computer Workstations eTool	This online checklist and evaluation resource provides information to evaluate computer workstations, related equipment setup and the work process. It also provides recommendations for improving ergonomics.	https://www.osha.gov/SLTC/etools/computerworkstations/
NIOSH Generic Stress Questionnaire	This 22-module subjective questionnaire gathers information from workers including their health, perceived demands and workload, conflict, and job satisfaction.	https://www.cdc.gov/niosh/topics/workorg/tools/pdfs/NIOSH%20Generic%20Job%20Stress%20Questionaire.pdf
Body picture pain diagram	Collects subjective symptom information; consists of an outline of a full body, anterior and posterior views. Clients are asked to mark the location of the pain or discomfort on the body chart and then describe the qualities of the pain.	https://www.cdc.gov/niosh/docs/97-117/pdfs/97-117.pdf
Observation-Based Posture Assessment: Review of Current Practice and Recommendations for Improvement	Describes observational approach for assessing work postures and provides related evidence	https://www.cdc.gov/niosh/docs/2014-131/

NIOSH, National Institute for Occupational Safety and Health; WISHA, Washington Industrial Safety and Health Act.

Job analysis services may be part of many OT service settings that provide work-related OT services including the following:

- Business and industrial environments
- Acute care and rehabilitation facilities
- Outpatient clinics
- Community-based settings such as mental health centers
- Sheltered or supported workshops
- Schools and universities
- Vocational programs
- U.S. Military Vocational Rehabilitation and Education Divisions (AOTA, 2017)

Requests for a job analysis may come from the employer, the medical or rehabilitation team, the vocational rehabilitation team, the WCI company, long-term disability insurance carrier, or the individual client. The source of the referral will often determine the payment source as well. Reimbursement sources include private pay by the employer or individual client, various insurance companies, or vocational rehabilitation.

Prior to scheduling the job analysis, it is helpful to determine the desired outcome in order to select the most appropriate analysis format (problem based, functional job demands, MSD risk assessment), to gather tools required to conduct the analysis, and to estimate the time needed. Regardless of the source, it is important to contact the referral source and employer's human resources representative to discuss and agree on the purpose of the analysis, the desired outcome, how the analysis will be conducted, and the data and report format.

A conversation with the individual about the job analysis and expected outcomes facilitates a client-centered approach that addresses the needs of multiple stakeholders including the employee, employer, the payer, and referring source. Employers may also require adherence to specific security, safety, and/or confidentiality procedures related to documentation, data collection, access to the worksite, and completion of the job analysis.

Preparation for a job analysis includes assembling the equipment needed to gather the desired data such as the following:

- Camera/video recorder
- Measuring tape
- Goniometer
- Push/pull force gauge
- Scale
- Pinch/grip gauge
- Light meter
- Pedometer or other device to measure walking distance
- Stopwatch
- Borg exertion scale (Borg, 1982)
- Forms (outline for data collection, risk assessment, task and tool measures, etc.)

Gathering Data

Occupational therapy practitioners can gather job analysis data in a number of ways to obtain comprehensive and accurate data regarding the job requirements and environment. Some methods of data collection include the following:

- On-site observation: This may be time intensive and requires ½ hour to 4 or more hours of observation depending on the type of job analysis required and complexity of the job. Typically, this includes talking to the supervisor and employee(s) to identify the individual tasks to be evaluated, observing completion of job tasks, measuring the work area and equipment, and recording the information.
- Videotape and photos obtained by the OT practitioner, the employer, or other stakeholders provide visual information that can depict or clarify job tasks and features of the job that may be difficult to describe. Video is particularly helpful when analyzing specific motion patterns or complicated jobs. Video and photos can also serve as a record of what components of a job were analyzed.
- Remote observation of the job site via synchronous, real-time electronic media such as robots, Facetime, Skype, etc.
- Production and job description information from the employer
- Generic job demands data for specific jobs and job categories are available through O*NET, an online job description database sponsored by the U.S. Department of Labor. It provides generic job descriptions for over 1,000 occupations in a wide variety of job categories (O*NET, 2017). Data from O*NET can be used to review job demands for a specific job category, assist with job searches, create plans for skill training, and structure more detailed job analyses.
- Self-report/daily task log by worker: The client describes the workday pattern including tasks, how long tasks take to complete, nonscheduled and scheduled breaks, and other factors that may influence tasks. For example, in some jobs, workload may increase around the holidays due to increased number of orders.
- Symptom log: The worker tracks work activities for several days with a focus on identifying patterns of activity that may influence symptoms such as pain, fatigue, and stress.
- Review of injury records: For MSD injury prevention programming, reviewing records, including the type and frequency of injury, provides useful information to target risk assessments and injury prevention programming.

Reporting formats vary widely and could include a combination of FJDs, physical demands analyses, and MSD ergonomic risk assessments. The ideal scenario is to complete a job analysis at the work setting, but when an on-site visit is not possible, job analysis may occur via simulation in the clinic using actual parts or tools from the worksite when available, through use of client and employer job descriptions, and via video/photographs. These methods may be sufficient for some individual level treatment planning and interventions. However, the use of remote technology or media to capture critical job information for detailed job analysis, in lieu of physical presence at the worksite, has not been studied extensively at this time. Table 52-3 provides examples of data that may be collected.

When conducting job analyses, it is essential to have an understanding of the various risk factors that can contribute to injuries and illnesses at work.

Physical Risk Factors

Musculoskeletal disorders can result from both work- and non–work-related tasks. With some exclusions, MSDs are considered work related if "an event or exposure in the work environment either caused or contributed to the resulting condition or significantly aggravated a preexisting injury or illness" (Bureau of Labor Statistics, 2016b, para. 1). The NIOSH (2017) further defines MSD type injuries as "Disorders of the muscles, nerves, tendons, ligaments, joints, cartilage or spinal discs that

- are caused by sudden or sustained physical exertion
- are not the result of any instantaneous non-exertion event (e.g., slips, trips, or falls)
- range in severity from mild/occasional to intense/chronic pain"

Musculoskeletal disorders include diagnoses such as low back pain, lateral epicondylitis, carpal tunnel syndrome (CTS), and neck pain (NIOSH, 2016b). The presence of risk factors does not mean that an injury will definitely occur, however, injury risk is associated with the intensity, duration, and frequency of exposure to risk factors, such as the following:

- Force (weight, grip, pinch, push/pull)
- Awkward postures (body positions that are potentially damaging such as working with the arms overhead, extreme wrist deviations, or twisting of the spine)

TABLE 52-3 Job Analysis Data Collection: Categories of Information and Examples

Data Category	Examples of Data
Job title and brief description	• Assembler I: assembles electronic components while seated at a workbench • Customer service representative: answers customer calls while seated at a computer; uses computer to search for solution and enters data to record interaction
Shift and breaks	• Full-time Monday through Friday 8:00 a.m. to 4:30 p.m. • Four 10-hour days with one 30-minute lunch and two 15-minute breaks
Number of people who complete the job	• One person completes this job per shift. • Eight people complete this task on first shift. • Four people work in a "cell" and rotate between tasks every 2 hours.
Tasks (brief description, frequency, and duration)	• Assembles parts 5.5 hours • Completes setup 15 minutes for every new part (two to four times per shift) • Uses phone while typing on computer 4 hours per shift • Computer work requires about 50% typing, 5% number pad use, and 45% mouse use.
Physical demands (postures, actions and motions)	• Lifts 30 lb two times per hour from floor to 50 in shelf • Reaches to the mouse with 45° shoulder flexion two per minute • Grips tool for 30 seconds every 2 minutes • Head tilted up to view computer screen
Physical environment (layout, tools, equipment, temperature, vibration, lighting, noise, stairs, heights, indoor/outdoor footing/flooring)	• Soldering tool, tweezers, workbench, adjustable tool, parts weighing <1 lb • Boxes of parts weighing 25 lb are 10 in high, 20 in wide, and 30 in long • Computer, computer screen, keyboard, mouse, phone, adjustable chair • Space is indoors and temperature controlled. • Overhead lighting or task lighting (light meter) • Environment is noisy.
Other physical skills (visual acuity, hearing acuity)	• Requires color vision to distinguish differences in wire colors • Machine for quality testing emits "beep" when part passes inspection.
Cognitive demands and social demands (decision making, multitasking, concentration, organizational skills, frequency of contact with other people, supervisory skills, communication)	• Work requires organization of materials in space, interpretation of blueprints, and completion of multistep process to build parts and meet quality guidelines. • Computer used to relay report data, instant message coworkers and alert customers regarding product orders, • Fifteen other people work in this area. • Interacts with coworker 4 times per hour to discuss progress.
Worker, group, or population demographics	• Number of male/female workers • Age range • Socioeconomic status • General health information of group or population of workers

- Static postures (defined by duration of sustained position)
- Repetition (variable definitions based on work cycle or actual number of movements during a period of time)
- Contact stress/compression (typically refers to external compression of the tissue from a sharp edge, tool handle or surface)
- Vibration
- Lack of rest and recovery time
- Extremes in temperature

Research conducted to understand the dose–response relationship between certain types of risk factors and the risk of developing an MSD is ongoing. Home activities and demands such as lifting children, computer use, woodworking, playing video games, and yard work may also expose clients to physical risk factors. Therefore, clinical decision making should be guided by careful analysis of evidence, understanding the job demands, consideration of nonwork tasks demands, and client factors. Assumptions such as "they do repetitive work so that must be why they have wrist pain" should be avoided. For example, Fan et al. (2015) found that hand force was strongly associated with the prevalence of CTS, whereas repetition as a single risk factor and wrist posture were not. This information can guide employers and employees to consider the use of forceful hand exertions and possible modifications to reduce the frequency, duration, and/or intensity of hand force during work and nonwork activities to reduce the intensity of or prevent CTS.

Work Organization and Psychosocial Risk Factors

Job stress is a concern relative to the overall health of workers, and stress occurs when the requirements of the job do not match the "capabilities, resources and needs of the worker" (NIOSH, n.d.). In the publication "Stress at Work", NIOSH (n.d.) reports that coping style and personality are personal factors that may influence how workers manage job stress; however, there are a number of workplace conditions that are believed to affect most people. To address work organization and psychosocial risk factors, risk assessments, surveys, and other tools that provide information regarding work organization and psychosocial conditions should include the following (NIOSH, n.d.):

- High physical, mental, or emotional demands
- Machine pacing or time pressure
- Shiftwork
- Low participation in decision making
- Badly designed, inadequate, or faulty equipment
- Poor communication
- Low social support
- Social/physical isolation
- Role ambiguity or role conflict
- Job insecurity

Data concerning work organization and psychosocial risk factors can inform interventions to promote health, wellness, and participation in the workplace.

Personal Risk Factors

Personal risk factors refer to individual characteristics such as age, body mass index (BMI), gender, smoking, and other medical conditions. The interactions between physical risk factors in job tasks, personal and psychosocial risk factors such as high workloads and tight deadlines, and the causal relationships to specific work injuries are not well understood due to the complexity of variables. The difficulty of identifying a single risk factor as the cause of an injury is apparent in a study conducted by Fan et al. (2015) wherein a sample of approximately 3,000 U.S. workers, CTS was associated with older than 35 years, female gender, obesity, prior upper extremity disorder, participating in recreational hand activities, and other medical conditions such as diabetes. In another study of 60 workers with low back pain, Govindu and Babski-Reeves (2014) reported that both direct and interactive effects of physical risk factors and psychosocial and personal risk factors influenced ratings of low back pain severity.

The findings from these studies suggest selecting intervention approaches that incorporate solutions to address potential contributions of personal and psychosocial as well as physical risk factors could help to reduce the severity or incidence of these types of MSD disorders. It is important to note, however, that the degree to which each type of factor contributes to the injury and the determination as to work relatedness is as much a legal matter managed by the workers' compensation laws as a medical diagnosis issue. Consideration of person factors, physical and social environments, and activities and tasks is an inherent part of OT practice.

Promoting Work Participation and Engagement

In a person's life course, there is an ebb and flow of occupational transitions related to work. An **occupational transition** is "a major change in the occupational repertoire of a person in which one or several occupations change, disappear, and/or are replaced by others" (Jonsson, 2010, p. 212). For example, life changes can occur as a result of a family change, such as a parent who chooses to place his or her career on hold in order to care for a child and then faces new preparations for returning to the paid workforce. Work participation may also be influenced by work or nonwork injury, disease, or disability. Individuals with a disability may need accommodations or adaptations to the physical and/or operational aspects of a job in order to fully engage in work activities. There can be obstacles to performing and accessing work that may lead to occupational imbalance, alienation, marginalization, and deprivation (Durocher, Gibson, & Rappolt, 2014).

Adaptation describes methods for adjusting equipment or physical aspects of work to improve access, usability, and ability to work. For instance, a person experiencing low vision may be recommended to adjust computer monitor display settings and lighting to improve visual contrast as adaptations to word processing tasks. Adaptions can also address workplace practices, for example, to facilitate an inclusive office culture and environment for individuals who are transitioning gender (Human Rights Campaign, 2017). These workplace changes may include policy and guidelines, everyday work practices, access to facilities, and employee education.

Occupational therapy practitioners provide services to promote work participation and engagement in the following areas:

- Health promotion and wellness
- Ergonomics, injury prevention, and workplace modifications
- Work-related injuries
- Work hardening and work conditioning
- Functional capacity evaluation
- Transitional work programs
- Non–work-related injury, illness, or disease
- Addressing work with individuals with disabilities

Health Promotion and Wellness

Health promotion is a process for enabling individuals to increase their control over and ultimately improve their health (Smith, Tang, & Nutbeam, 2006) and includes wellness and chronic disease prevention. Population health interventions such as the NIOSH Total Worker Health® (Jaegers, 2015; Schill, 2017) and opportunities within primary care (AOTA, 2014b) can be valuable strategies for addressing the needs of workers. Total Worker Health® is a holistic approach to workplace health protection and health promotion that encourages participatory methods for hazard assessment and mitigation. Occupational therapy practitioners seek health outcomes as a result of OT practices and utilize wellness participation and engagement as a means to achieve mental, physical, and social well-being (NIOSH, 2014). According to the OTPF (AOTA, 2017; Hettler, 1984), wellness is "an active process through which individuals [or groups or populations] become aware of and make choices toward a more successful existence." According to the WHO, there are two main focal concerns of wellness: (1) an individual's realization of their fullest physical, psychological, social, spiritual, and economic potential and (2) the fulfillment

of an individual's expectations in family, workplace, community, place of worship, and other settings (Smith, Tang, & Nutbeam, 2006). Wellness practices can be individual, but they are often practiced in workgroups or at the workplace level to address the needs of organizations. Chronic disease prevention practices address the health epidemic surrounding heart disease, stroke, and related conditions such as hypertension, diabetes, and obesity (Centers for Disease Control and Prevention [CDC], 2017). One example of a wellness intervention is the a Total Worker Health® initiative that spans company-wide participation for where a participatory team of employees identifies problems and solutions regarding the balance among work, leisure, and family life (group) (AOTA, 2017).

With the passage of the Affordable Care Act, improving the health of employees and promoting wellness have become increasingly important to employers as a way to reduce private health insurance costs and work-related injury claims and related costs. Poor worker health can be costly to employers. For example, workers who had a BMI in obesity class III (BMI $\geq$40) had an elevated rate of lost work time, lost workdays, and higher medical claim costs when compared with workers at their recommended weight (Ostbye, Dement, & Krause, 2007). Additionally, workers with anxiety, stress, and other related conditions had 50% more days away from work than workers with other injuries or illnesses (CDC, 2016).

The health and well-being of workers is of interest to OT practitioners as it influences engagement in occupations and in particular work participation. Occupational therapy practitioners view workers from a holistic perspective, and they can contribute significantly to the health and wellness of individuals, groups, and populations in work environments by working with employers and employees to identify areas of concern, determine possible strategies, and implement solutions to create a fully engaged and capable workforce. The OT practitioner may provide indirect services as part of a planning team as a consultant or manager or provide direct services. For example, to improve return to work program outcomes for individuals who have depression, employees and managers would need to have an understanding of mental health disorders and recovery to avoid stereotypes and bias in the workplace. Occupational therapy has been shown to increase long-term depression recovery and increase probability of long-term return to work (Hees, de Vries, Koeter, & Schene, 2013). Occupational therapy practitioners working in a mental health setting can address an employee's return to work, which can be very unsettling for individuals with mental illness. Occupational therapy practitioners are well prepared to discuss strategies to help such individuals address their mental health in both the acute and outpatient settings and can teach strategies to facilitate a successful return to work without sacrificing self-care and leisure occupations.

Aging workers are another group of focus for employers and OT practitioners. Increasing numbers of older workers are in the workplace as a result of longer life courses and improved health as well as a financial need to work past the traditional retirement age. The perception exists among some employers that older workers are more costly than younger workers because of higher absenteeism, higher wages, higher pensions, and increased use of health care and other benefits (Taskforce on the Aging of the American Workforce, 2008). This can negatively impact employability of older workers due to stereotypes and discrimination. In contrast, some employers report that older workers have greater knowledge of the job tasks they perform than their younger colleagues, willingly learn new tasks quickly, bring experience and resilience to work, and are able to keep up with the physical demands of their jobs (Munnell, Sass, & Soto, 2006; Vasconcelos, 2015).

Occupational therapy practitioners can serve the older adult demographic by educating and assisting employers in making the workplace more "friendly" to the aging worker and working directly with individuals to consider adaptive strategies, promote health, and prevent the risk of injury and illness. Interventions may include teaching adaptive strategies and improving work capacity, such as by addressing changes in physical strength, vision and hearing deficiencies, fall risk, and other age related changes. The OT can also advocate in the workplace for universal design and age-friendly procedures that are beneficial to the older adult and most employees of the organization.

⚖️ ETHICAL DILEMMA

You are consulting for a large corporate client who asks you to develop a post-offer test for their new hires so they can avoid hiring workers who may get injured. The human resources manager at the corporation asks you to make the test much harder than the actual job so they can make sure they "only hire strong people who won't get hurt." The corporation hires many new workers and could bring in an abundance of revenue for your hospital.

If you develop the screen and make it more difficult than the actual job as per the employer's request, you are violating the U.S. Equal Employment Opportunity Commission (EEOC) by developing a test that is not an actual reflection of the job demands. The result could potentially eliminate hiring people who could do the job because they are not capable of performing higher levels of physical exertion. If you do not develop the test as requested, the employer may take their business elsewhere and your hospital will lose revenue.

What is your responsibility in this matter? How do you handle this situation without violating your ethical principles and keep your corporate client happy?

Ergonomics, Injury Prevention, and Workplace Modifications

The problem of workplace injuries is significant with MSD injuries accounting for 31% of the total injury cases for all workers in 2015 (Bureau of Labor Statistics, 2016b). To reduce the risks for injuries and illness including MSDs and maximize work performance, employers look to **ergonomics** to improve the fit between the work and the worker (International Ergonomics Association [IEA], 2017). Based on this concept, ergonomics is often considered part of workplace safety. Workplace safety is the purview of the OSHA (n.d.b) through the U.S. Department of Labor, which guides safe work practices through standards, training, and outreach. Their work is informed by the NIOSH (2016a), which supports the transfer of research to occupational safety and health practices. Both the OSHA and NIOSH Websites provide excellent resources related to workplace safety, ergonomics, and injury prevention programming.

Although often associated with safety, the field of ergonomics is very broad and concepts are applied to both the design and redesign of tasks and environments. The field of ergonomics is compatible with OT and provides useful information regarding anthropometrics, human capacity, equipment design, space design, and organizational structure to consider when working with clients to improve occupational performance. The IEA defines ergonomics as follows:

> Ergonomics (or human factors) is the scientific discipline concerned with the understanding of interactions among humans and other elements of a system, and the profession that applies theory, principles, data and methods to design in order to optimize human well-being and overall system performance. Practitioners of ergonomics and ergonomists contribute to the design and evaluation of tasks, jobs, products, environments and systems in order to make them compatible with the needs, abilities and limitations of people. (IEA, 2017)

Occupational therapists are well suited to evaluate work tasks and environments including conducting ergonomic or MSD risk assessments with background in anatomy and physiology, psychology, client factors, environmental factors, and occupational performance. Job analysis in the form of MSD ergonomic risk assessments is used to identify injury risk factors related to a particular job or task, develop programs to prevent work injuries, or identify specific ergonomic problems and solutions for an individual worker.

Anthropometrics provides critical ergonomic information to assist in determining changes to improve the match between the work, worker, and the environment. **Anthropometry** is a field of science that studies and defines the physical measures of a person's size (e.g., overall height and weight, length of leg, elbow, height in sitting and standing, size of head) and functional capacities (e.g., range of motion, strength, and aerobic capacity). In the workplace, this information is used to design tasks, tools, machines, and personal protective equipment (PPE) to maximize the fit and usability of equipment to promote safety and injury prevention (NIOSH, 2018). Gathering data from a wide variety of populations is important as individual dimensions and capacities vary greatly depending on geographic location, personal factors, and gender. The NIOSH gathers data from specific populations, such as firefighters and emergency medical technicians (EMTs) to create profession-specific databases to use in the design of job-specific tools and work environments. Such anthropometric data informs ergonomics and is useful to OT practitioners when conducting ergonomic assessments, selecting work equipment such as chairs and tools, and working as part of an ergonomics team to design new or suggest modifications to existing work environments, tools, and tasks.

As OT practitioners, we may refer to environmental interventions as modifications, adaptations, or accommodations to the environment or adaptation on the part of the person. The language of ergonomic interventions refers to these types of changes as engineering controls, administrative/work practice controls, and personal protective equipment (PPE).

Engineering controls are changes to equipment or physical demands of the job that result in the reduction or removal of potential injury risk factors. For example, providing a tool with a small grip span for persons with smaller hands, providing a pneumatic lifting device to assist with lifting heavy boxes, or redesigning machinery to reduce the force necessary to turn a lever. These types of controls could also include simple changes such as adjusting the height of a computer screen to improve head position or reducing the reaching distance required to pick up a part. When possible, implementation of engineering controls that "design out" the potential risk factor are preferable over other types of controls.

Administrative and work practice controls refer to changes in task sequences or assignments in an effort to reduce exposure to strenuous or high demand job tasks. Job rotation, reducing the speed of work, or implementing more breaks may provide needed changes to alter exposure to or increase recovery time from highly repetitive or difficult tasks. These types of controls also include training workers to complete tasks in a particular way that may reduce stress to the body such as how to adjust a chair or set up a computer workstation properly.

Personal protective equipment controls refer to use of equipment that an employee wears such as safety glasses to prevent chemicals or metal shards from contacting the eye and earplugs to protect the ears from loud noises.

Examples of PPE controls include antivibration gloves, splints, or back belts issued to the worker to use during their job performance. It is important to note that the evidence to support use of these devices to prevent injuries is scant or mixed. For example, a rigid wrist splint may reduce bending at the wrist but increase stress to the wrist flexor and extensor muscles or shoulder if the person is pushing against the splint or adjusting their shoulder to compensate for the limited wrist movement. Therefore, the use and potential complications of using PPE devices need to be carefully reviewed prior to implementation.

Ergonomic interventions can be provided at the individual and group levels. Group level interventions can target job areas that are associated with higher rates of injury, turnover, and worker discomfort complaints with the focus on reducing injury rates, improving worker satisfaction, and preventing injury. The NIOSH (2017) provides resources to create and implement effective ergonomics programs to prevent or reduce the incidence of workplace injuries. An example of a group level intervention is the ergonomics program for lab workers conducted by Boynton and Darragh (2008). They created a worker-centered education and hands-on training programs focused on workstation redesign and body position changes to improve ergonomic fit. Records indicated that the year following the training, there were no work-related injuries reported. Although these types of programs often address cumulative type MSD injuries, workers may also experience acute injuries, such as TBI from a fall or blunt force incident. Occupational therapists have built evidence-based interventions to prevent falls and reduce injuries and deaths from falls from ladder and building surfaces (Kaskutas, Buckner-Petty, Dale, Gaal, & Evanoff, 2016).

At the individual level, multifaceted interventions can be helpful in addressing ergonomic concerns and return to work. For example, workplace modifications including ergonomics and graded return to work as part of coordinated care planning among health care professionals, including OT practitioners, were effective in reducing time out of work and improving functional status (Lambeek, van Mechelen, Knol, Loisel, & Anema, 2010). Similarly, in a review of factors affecting return to work following injury or illness, Cancelliere et al. (2016) found that stakeholder participation, work modification/accommodation, and return to work coordination were associated with positive return to work outcomes. Furthermore, in a systematic review conducted by Nevala, Pehkonen, Koskela, Ruusuvuori, and Anttila (2015), self-advocacy, changes in work schedules, work organization, and transportation availability promoted employment among people with disabilities. Interventions such as self-advocacy, ergonomic modification, work modification and accommodations, and graded return to work promote work participation and highlight the valuable contribution of OT in the area of ergonomics in the workplace.

TABLE 52-4 Work Posture Guidelines for Computer Users

Body Part	Work Posture Guidelines
Upper extremity	• Shoulders relaxed • Minimal shoulder abduction and flexion • Elbow bent midrange at about 90° • Wrist flexion and extension at <30°
Lower extremity	• Hip angle 90° or slightly more • Knee angle at 90° or slightly more • Feet on the floor or foot rest
Head and back	• Head aligned over shoulders • Natural curves of spine maintained

Equipment	Suggested Features/Placement
Keyboard/mouse platform—seated	• Adjustable between 22 and 28.5 in from the floor to the front edge of the platform • Place keyboard at about elbow height.
Keyboard/mouse platform—standing	• Adjustable between 37.4 and 46.5 in from floor to front edge of platform • Place keyboard at about elbow height.
Computer screen	• Place the computer screen at least 20 in from the eyes. • Position monitor so the top line of the screen falls below the horizontal gaze (eye level) of the user.
Chairs	• 4.5 in adjustment capacity within the recommended range of 15–22 in as measured from the floor to the top of the seat • Rounded front seat edge • Adjustable lumbar support

Computer Workstation Ergonomics

Many websites and handouts provide good basic information about ergonomic guidelines for computer workstations. For more detail, the American National Standards Institute/Human Factors and Ergonomics Society (ANSI/HFES) standard 100–2007: Human Factors Engineering of Computer Workstations (HFES, 2007) provides detailed workstation design standards related to seating, posture, computer equipment, workstations, and lighting. The standards serve as a resource for ergonomics for the office environment. Several guiding principles of interest can be found in Table 52-4. Opportunities to vary work postures throughout the day are also suggested. Healthy work postures for computer work can be seen in Figures 52-1 and 52-2.

The frequency of use, style or design, and location of keyboards, mouse input devices, computer screens, desks, and chairs influence the users' accessibility, work postures, and activity demands. There are a number of computer workstation assessment and screening tools available to assess the ergonomic factors of office workstations, such as the Rapid Office Strain Assessment (ROSA) (Sonne, Villalta, & Andrews, 2012) and the Computer Workstation eTool (OSHA, n.d.a) which is an online problem-solving tool that provides suggestions on how to select and arrange various workstation components.

Although ergonomic guidelines and screening tools serve as a general reference, person-specific evaluation of performance and selection of modifications to the computer workstation equipment or tasks may be necessary to accommodate individual needs. For example, an individual with right elbow pain that increases while holding the mouse with the wrist in extension may benefit from placing

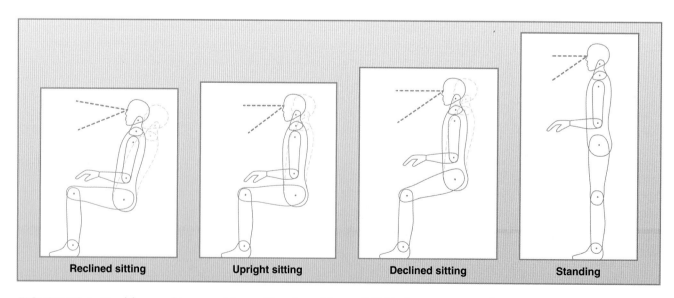

FIGURE 52-1 Healthy working positions. (Reprinted from OSHA Computer workstations eTool: Good working positions. Retrieved from https://www.osha.gov/SLTC/etools/computerworkstations/positions.html)

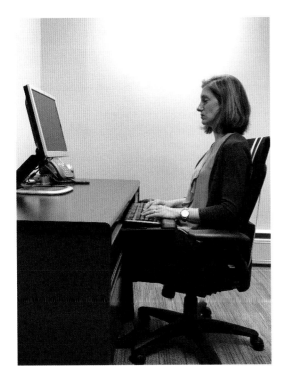

FIGURE 52-2 **Seated computer workstation position.** Person seated with arms relaxed and near side of body. Keyboard positioned at about elbow height. Top of screen is slightly below eye level. Back and feet supported.

the mouse at elbow height, to the left side of the keyboard, or using a different style input device (Figure 52-3).

Ergonomics in Non-Office Work Environments

People work in a wide array of environments, including general manufacturing of parts for cars, computers, and other equipment; laboratories that require use of microscopes and small hand tools; warehouses where workers lift and handle boxes or parts; food service settings such as cafeterias and restaurants; and health care facilities such as hospitals, nursing homes, and clinics. Each of these environments has unique workspaces, tools, equipment, and work demands.

The design of workplace tools and equipment has an impact on user comfort, postures, and the degree of effort required to complete a task. Poorly designed tools, workplaces, and tasks can expose workers' bodies to stresses and strains that contribute to musculoskeletal injury (NIOSH, 2016b). Worker-centered ergonomic programs, along with changes to tools, workplaces, tasks, and routines can help reduce musculoskeletal stressors and injuries. Ergonomic changes may address the underlying task, tool, equipment, or job design features (engineering controls) that create injury risk. Reducing risk exposures may also be controlled by changing work routines to limit high risk or problem tasks (administrative controls) or changing work methods such as altering lifting technique or using a stronger position such as gripping rather than pinching when holding a tool.

Back injuries are a significant concern, with 31% of all MSD cases in 2015 related to lifting exertions (Bureau of Labor Statistics, 2016a). Changes to the workplace, such as reducing the size and weight of a box, placing heavier items on middle shelves, and using a mechanical device to move objects are examples of changes that can help reduce injury risk exposure or modify a job for an individual with a back injury or limited capacity for lifting.

In the health care setting, careful analysis of patient lifting and transfers in emergency rooms, operating rooms, patient rooms, and therapy rooms can identify areas of concern related to body postures, unpredictable patient movements, and unanticipated events that put the person(s) involved in the transfer, including the patient, at risk of injury. Decision-making processes to help health care personnel identify when help (another person or device)

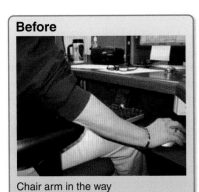

Before

Chair arm in the way

Shoulder rotated outward

Arm reaching forward

Wrist in severe extension

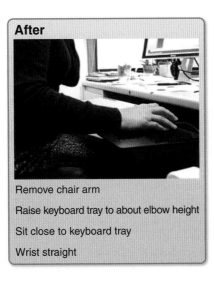

After

Remove chair arm

Raise keyboard tray to about elbow height

Sit close to keyboard tray

Wrist straight

FIGURE 52-3 **Before and after ergonomic solutions.** This individual experienced right elbow pain that increased when holding the mouse with the wrist in extension.

TABLE 52-5	Ergonomics and Injury Prevention Program Resources
Resources	**Content examples**
Ergonomic Guidelines for Manual Materials Handling (https://www.cdc.gov/niosh/docs/2007-131/pdfs/2007-131.pdf)	• Data gathering process • Assessment tools such as NIOSH lifting equation and materials handling checklist • Ergonomic suggestions • Guidelines for materials handling techniques
Safe Patient Handling and Mobility (SPHM) (https://www.cdc.gov/niosh/topics/safepatient/)	• Patient handling hazards • Patient handling ergonomics • Additional resources and tools
Guidelines for Nursing Homes: Ergonomics for the Prevention of Musculoskeletal Disorders (https://www.osha.gov/ergonomics/guidelines/nursinghome/final_nh_guidelines.pdf)	• Identifying management support • Decision-making trees for patient transfers and repositioning • Suggestions for assistive devices related to patient handling, housekeeping, kitchen tasks, and laundry
Guidelines for Retail Grocery Stores: Ergonomics for the Prevention of Musculoskeletal Disorders (https://www.osha.gov/Publications/osha3192.pdf)	• This resource reviews ergonomic hazards of work activities related to shelf stocking, stockrooms cashiering, bagging, produce handling, deli work, and baker work. • Suggestions include workstation design for cashiers and cake decorating stations, using sharp tools, and rearranging work routines for difficult tasks
A Guide to the Selection of Non-Powered Hand Tools (https://www.cdc.gov/niosh/docs/2004-164/)	• Ergonomic hazards related to hand tools • Ergonomics for hand tool design

NIOSH, National Institute for Occupational Safety and Health.

is needed when transferring or repositioning a client and selecting appropriate assistive devices are some solutions to reduce injury risk.

In manufacturing and construction environments, highly repetitive, forceful tasks using tools such as knives, screwdrivers, and other hand tools may place strain on wrist and forearm muscles, causing injury. Changing the tool handle size or shape, reducing vibration, and keeping tools sharp can help reduce risk factors exposures and strain on the arm. Ergonomic assessment tools as well as task- and industry-specific suggestions for ergonomic changes are available through a variety of OSHA and NIOSH publications. These resources and others can be found in Table 52-5.

Rehabilitation and Return to Work/Stay at Work

When a person experiences an injury, illness, or disease, the OT practitioner is a key provider of rehabilitation services to facilitate readiness for return to work. Rehabilitation after a hand injury such as tendon laceration involves treatment activities to address activities of daily living (ADL) such as self-care, scar remodeling, active range of motion, strengthening, and overall functional use of the hand for activity performance. For individuals who experienced a TBI, OT provides a holistic approach to motor skill retraining, executive function, coping skills, and a variety of related treatment approaches to assist with rehabilitation and work preparation.

Return to work focuses on multilevel aspects of work participation (e.g., individual preparation, workplace policy, and environmental adaptation) that are impacted by changes in work status due to a personal need such as taking care of a family member experiencing terminal cancer, being unemployed due to a job layoff, or being unable to work due to an injury or illness. Return to work also affects veterans moving from active duty to civilian work, wounded warriors, individuals incarcerated and transitioning to the community, and many others who experience a major change in their participation in work.

Work-Related Injuries

Interrupted or altered participation in work for individuals affected by work injuries across the United States is significant. In 2015, approximately 1.5 million workers in private industry experienced a work injury that required time out of work, a job transfer, or restriction of work activities (Bureau of Labor Statistics, 2016a). Occupational therapy practitioners involved in work programs may perform their duties in a variety of settings, such as outpatient clinics, hospitals, office settings, manufacturing environments, and warehouses. Occupational therapy practitioners need not confine their services to specially designed "occupational medicine" clinics to address work issues with their clients. Work should be addressed with all clients who want to work with the goal of improving the match between work demands and the worker's capacities for effective participation and engagement.

Acute Injury Management

When an individual is injured on the job and referred by a physician for OT, the occupational therapist performs an initial evaluation that includes an occupational profile. This portion of the evaluation includes identifying what the client needs and wants to do, barriers and facilitators related to occupational engagement including work, and occupational history.

Occupational performance analysis related to completion of work tasks, use of tools, and other activity demands is completed to identify factors related to effective participation. Depending on the specific diagnosis, the therapist evaluates client factors, such as muscle functions, movement-related functions, and sensory functions (e.g., pain or thermal awareness). For work participation issues, information about the job demands may be obtained from the client, job description or a job analysis, if available. Information of interest includes physical demands of the job, method of injury, length of time on the job, and current work status. An intervention plan is developed in conjunction with the client, keeping in mind the goal of returning to work. Interventions are selected to meet the targeted outcomes related to work, such as being able to lift, sustain grip on a tool, reach overhead, or working at a computer for 45-minute intervals.

As described in the OTPF (AOTA, 2014a), a variety of intervention types may be used, including occupations and activities, preparatory methods and tasks, education and training, and advocacy. Examples of these types of interventions include addressing hand coordination to improve keyboarding with an individual who has had a stroke and wants to return to work in an office environment, fabricating an orthotic device for a client who sustained a distal radius fracture, educating a client on proper positioning when lying down so back pain can be minimized, and advocating for a client to obtain reasonable light duty restrictions to avoid aggravation of symptoms while working on a light duty job. When the client's primary reason for attending therapy is beginning to resolve, the OT practitioner may need to consider work conditioning or work hardening as methods to return the client back to employment if the client physical abilities do not match the physical demands required to perform their job.

An accurate understanding of job demands provides key information when selecting and creating occupation-based interventions and recommending environmental modifications, such as ergonomic changes to reduce the impact of injury or facilitate resolution of the injury. Although a full job analysis may not be necessary, a focused review of symptom-aggravating tasks can yield useful information.

Work Hardening and Work Conditioning

Clients are typically ready to participate in a work conditioning or work hardening program when the client factors such as swelling, acute inflammation, or trauma that limit occupational performance in the acute OT intervention phase have resolved or are under control. **Work conditioning** is an approach to restore the performance of a worker recovering from an injury or illness; the focus is on restoring the musculoskeletal and cardiovascular systems and promoting safe work performance (AOTA, 2017). Work conditioning is typically performed using work simulation 3 to 5 days per week, 2 to 4 hours per day. **Work hardening** is similar to work conditioning; however, there are several key differences: work hardening is multidisciplinary and may include psychology, vocational rehabilitation, physical therapy, and OT. Work hardening strategies may include counseling, coaching, work simulation, cardiovascular conditioning, and ergonomic assessment. It is typically performed 5 days per week. Completing occupation-based activities is an important predictor of success in an occupational rehabilitation program (Hardison & Roll, 2017), and this is often achieved through the use of work simulation activities.

Typically, work hardening has been viewed as an intervention for individuals seeking to return to work who have physical limitations resulting from a musculoskeletal injury such as a back or shoulder injury. However, cognitive work hardening is a return to work intervention strategy for individuals with mental health problems, particularly depression. It is a recent arrival in the area of work rehabilitation and an appropriate area for OT practitioners to exercise their skills. **Cognitive work hardening** uses graded work tasks to simulate a person's actual work tasks and/or the cognitive demands of the person's job to develop the cognitive skills required for job performance (Wisenthal & Krupa, 2013). The tasks usually include concentration, memory, multitasking, and planning, which are often impaired as a result of illnesses such as depression. Cognitive work hardening is an excellent choice for a worker experiencing a mental health condition and whose job has high cognitive demands. The intervention strategies may address stress management, how to address interpersonal issues, following a work schedule, learning effective communication strategies, organizational skills, pacing, and focusing on mental stamina for returning to work. An example of this would be to have a client who has been diagnosed with depression begin a cognitive work hardening program by participating in an initial evaluation to determine the client's current status. The client is interviewed, and a collaborative treatment plan is established to return the client back to work. The emphasis of the program will be to arrive on time each day, participate in all activities, and discuss any issues that arise with the occupational therapy practitioner. The program will increase in intensity each day depending on how the client did the previous day. Activities will simulate the client's job and will either increase in length or difficulty each day. For example, if the worker assembles light switches, the occupational therapy practitioner may be able to get actual product from the employer to use in the clinic or could use another hand assembly task. The client

CASE STUDY 52-1   DELIA: ADDRESSING RIGHT ARM PAIN

Delia is a right hand–dominant 50-year-old woman with pain on the lateral part of her right elbow and forearm. She reports that she types all day long and feels her work is repetitive. She states she went to her family doctor and was told she had "tennis elbow" and her job was probably causing all of her pain. Her employer has asked for an assessment of her work area to determine if there are any areas of concern for development of this problem and to make recommendations for improvements. In addition, she has been referred for OT for treatment of this condition.

1. What should you consider during her occupational performance analysis?
2. How can you get information about her work requirements, work setup, and work techniques?
3. Why is it important to look at all tasks and not just work tasks?

When analyzing the work environment and occupational performance related to computer tasks, it is important to consider what may stress the injured tissue including work and nonwork activities. Ideally, you should visit the worker at the work location. By visiting, you can observe the worker in her environment and how she interacts with her office equipment as well as noting the location of supplies and office equipment in her office area. Steps to follow may include the following:

1. Speaking with the worker about her job and what she does, work hours, breaks, work routine, types of equipment she uses and how often she uses it, and a description of her discomfort. Discuss off work activity to determine if there are other activities aggravating or contributing to this condition.
2. Observation of the worker performing her job duties. You can take photos of the worker (with their permission) and then show her the photo so she can see her posture.
3. Take relevant measurements of the work area. Using tape measure, document the height of all relevant areas such as desk height, knee space, and reach distances. Also, note type of chair and its features and the monitor size as well as need for glasses/bifocals.
4. Review your recommendations with the worker and follow up with a written report to the employer.

After interviewing Delia, she verbalizes that she has had pain in her right elbow for several months and it becomes progressively worse throughout the day. She reports she works through her lunch each day and does not take her breaks. She takes her laptop home with her and works an additional 4 hours each night on her laptop using an external mouse. When asked about leisure participation, she states she just joined a scrapbooking group and has pain when she uses the scissors. Upon observation, it becomes evident that the client uses the mouse on an elevated surface with the right arm stretched forward. The wrist is extended and in ulnar deviation for 50% of the time during computer keyboard and mouse tasks both at work and at home. Her laptop external mouse is also used in a wrist extension position. The height of the work surface is 32 in, and she is 5 ft 5 in resulting in her reaching to use the mouse because it is too high for her. Her chair is adjustable, but she is not sure how to adjust it correctly or what all the adjustable features do on her chair. Photographs from the side and posterior reveal a rounded shoulder and forward head posture with the right shoulder being depressed and protracted. The neck is tilted to the right side.

A written report should be sent to the employer reviewing findings and recommendations for reduction of risk factors present in this job. The employer can then make any changes or obtain devices as needed in consultation with the OT. A clinical evaluation is conducted separately in the OT clinic to evaluate right upper extremity active range of motion (AROM), strength, and function. The methods used may include use of a goniometer to record range of motion, a grip and pinch dynamometer to record strength and pain provoking positions, and special testing to determine areas of pathology. Outcome measures such as the DASH (Disabilities of the Arm, Shoulder and Hand) can be used to determine perceived functional impairment. Occupational therapy will establish a clinical treatment plan to address limitations found in the evaluation.

Along with typical clinical interventions to reduce pain and regain strength, work simulation tasks can inform and provide opportunities to alter work methods, habits, and routines to alter wrist position. In addition, reducing the stress to the injured tissue may involve ergonomic changes such as changing the type of mouse based on wrist posture, positioning the mouse and keyboard at elbow height, or reducing the duration of right handed mouse use. Delia was also given instruction on alternate types of scissors that require less effort and less wrist extension to use with her scrapbooking hobby and advised to keep the scissors sharp to reduce strain on the wrist.

may assemble for 10 minutes one day and 20 minutes the next day depending on how the client is progressing. The occupational therapy practitioner will give positive feedback when it is relevant and will discuss ways of dealing with negative feedback with the client so the client can strategize for handling negative comments in the workplace.

Functional Capacity Evaluation

A **functional capacity evaluation** (FCE) is a clinical evaluation to determine an individual's capacity to perform work activities related to his or her participation in employment (Soer, van der Schans, Groothoff, Geertzen, & Reneman, 2008). An FCE can be performed by professionals other than OT practitioners, but OT practitioners are distinctly qualified to perform FCEs because of their ability to evaluate an individual's ability to perform activities, analyze activity (job analysis), and measure the environment using a wide variety of methods.

Functional capacity evaluations are usually performed in a clinic. They can be several hours in duration or extend up to 2 consecutive days. Functional capacity evaluations can be classified as either generic or job specific. A generic FCE assesses worker capacities compared to physical demands, as described by the U.S. Department of Labor (2014), and provides a complete view of all the client's physical abilities such as lifting, carrying, pushing, pulling, bending, sitting, crawling, kneeling, reaching, and grasping. Cognitive FCEs are a growing area and occupational therapists are well suited to conduct these detailed evaluations. Through cognitive FCE, OTs can evaluate cognitive capacities as related to job demands.

The generic FCE typically does not compare the client's abilities to the targeted job's physical or cognitive demands; rather, it documents the client's abilities as related to a list of general physical or cognitive demands. Thus, it typically does not determine if the client can return to a specific job. The information gleaned from a generic FCE can be utilized to make disability determinations for clients who are unable to work.

With job-specific FCEs, there is a targeted job for the client. An FJD should be obtained to identify specifics about the job such as weight capacities, distances, and frequencies of tasks. The FCE tests only those areas required for the job and determines if the client's abilities match the required job demands. The written report will give a recommendation as to whether or not the client can perform the job duties. Job-specific FCEs have been shown to have a high predictive validity in relation to recommendations to return to the previous job or change job in individuals with nonspecific low back pain (Cheng & Cheng, 2010) and with patients with a specific injury (e.g., distal radius fracture) than patients with a nonspecific injury (Cheng & Cheng, 2011).

At the conclusion of an FCE, a report is written to detail the results of the evaluation, including a review of the medical history; musculoskeletal or cognitive assessment; description of job duties; summary of strengths and limitations, any inconsistences in performance, and pain behaviors; and detailed results of the FCE including the maximum safe abilities to perform tasks. The report may also list suggested accommodations or modifications to increase the chances of a successful return to work process.

Post-Offer Pre-employment Testing

Employers want to hire individuals who are capable of performing the physical demands of the job. A *post-offer test* is one way an employer can identify if an applicant who has been offered the job is physically capable of performing the job. By hiring an employee who is physically capable of

performing the job, it is less likely the employee will sustain a work-related injury. The post-offer test can be developed based on the FJD and the physical demands identified; a job-specific test can be developed that simulates the most physically demanding job tasks. The test should be validated by having workers who perform the job take the test and give feedback regarding whether it adequately simulates the job demands. The test should be an accurate reflection of the job—not easier or more difficult than the actual job. Occupational therapy practitioners can develop a post-offer test utilizing their skills at analyzing activities.

Transitional Work Programs

Transitional work is a process performed at the client's actual job location and uses the client's job duties to assist in a safe gradual return to work process. The OT practitioner works closely with the client's employer, physician, and perhaps worker's compensation insurance representatives to arrange appointments at the client's job. After gaining a thorough understanding of the job by performing a job analysis, the OT practitioner selects job tasks with frequencies and durations the client can perform on the job and makes any recommendations for modifications in the job. The OT practitioner then obtains approval from the client's physician to initiate an adapted work program based on the information about the client's physical abilities, the physical demands of the job, and the employer's level of cooperation. After the client returns to work performing the modified job duties, they are closely monitored by the employer and OT practitioners. Work duties are graded up or down based on how the client is tolerating the job duties. The process is continued until the client achieves full, unrestricted duty; however, if this is not possible, the OT practitioner can make recommendations for accommodations or alternative job placement.

Non–Work-Related Injury, Illness, and Conditions

Injuries affecting a person's capacity to work are not always a cumulative type of musculoskeletal injury or sustained on the job. For example, individuals can fall at home and sustain a fracture while walking on ice or injure their back working in the garden; the end results are the same, and the client may or may not be able to return to work. The difference with a work-related injury is that an employer may be more willing to offer a light duty assignment to avoid any lost time away from the job (a cost factor for WCI), whereas modified work assignments may not be readily considered with a non–work-related injury, illness, or condition.

Illnesses and injuries such as cancer, stroke, and concussion as well as the normal aging process can affect an individual's ability to perform the physical, social, and/or cognitive demands of a job. Whether the occupation of work is disrupted by an acute injury (e.g., TBI, spinal cord injury), the side effects of disease or illness (e.g., cancer, depression), progressive disorders (e.g., amyotrophic lateral sclerosis, multiple sclerosis), or the normal aging process, it is important to consider the barriers and facilitators to work participation in conjunction with the person, their capacities and skills, required work tasks, and the work environment. Occupational therapy practitioners can address the factors that limit work participation at the level of the person through individualized interventions. To address environmental and task-oriented concerns, a job analysis can be particularly valuable. The data can be used to plan and select interventions, identify outcomes, and strategize for workplace accommodations.

The American Cancer Society (2017) estimates there will be nearly 1.7 million new cancer cases in 2017. A systematic review investigated the effects and characteristics of intervention studies on breast cancer survivors in which the goal was to return to work (Hoving, Broekhuizen, & Frings-Dresen, 2009). The results indicated that there were no methodologically sound intervention studies specific to breast cancer and return to work; the researchers suggested that evidence from general return to work interventions should be applied to breast cancer survivors, developed further, and evaluated. Issues that frequently occur among breast cancer patients were identified as fatigue, diminished physical work capacity and psychosocial functioning, cognitive limitations, difficult mobility, difficulty managing stress and anxiety, difficulty coping with new self-image, and changed attitude toward work (Hoving et al., 2009). Occupational therapy and return-to-work planning for the breast cancer survivor must be carefully considered and discussed with the patient and the physicians involved in the medical care. An example is as follows: a 42-year-old female patient status post right axillary radiation and chemotherapy for metastatic breast cancer has been referred to OT for strengthening and conditioning due to fatigue. The evaluation reveals not only fatigue limiting her performance of a full workday as an elementary school teacher but also peripheral neuropathy in her fingers as a side effect of the chemotherapy drugs. The neuropathy decreases her sensation in her hands limiting her ability to type on a computer, write with a pen, and write on a dry-erase board in class, and causes her drop objects. The fatigue is addressed through promotion of a walking program up to 20 minutes each day, journaling to keep track of fatigue patterns, and monitoring fatigue as it is related to medications. The neuropathy proves to be a very limiting factor in the return to work process, but the occupational therapist teaches her how to compensate by using her eyes to type, and use voice recognition software on her computer and smartphone. She uses a pop socket on her phone and a lanyard for her keys so she does not drop them. The patient made a successful return to work and utilized combination of adaptive strategies and accommodations provided by her employer.

Mild traumatic brain injury such as concussion and mild stroke can impact the ability to participate in work.

When individuals of working age sustain a concussion, return to work may be compromised due to impairment in a variety of cognitive, physical, and social interaction capacities. Assisting clients to engage in their chosen occupations and roles is a complex process, and helping them to engage in the role as a worker can be argued as the most complex (Wolf, 2010). Research has shown a relationship between executive functioning and employment outcomes in individuals with TBI (Hartmann, 2010; Ownsworth & McKenna, 2004). Executive functioning is often impaired in mTBI, including shifting, planning, and strategy use as well as emotional regulation, attention, and decision making. Even when awareness is intact, deficits in executive functioning can significantly impact daily life activities, including leisure, employment, and overall initiation (Erez, Rothschild, Katz, Tuchner, & Hartman-Maeir, 2009).

Project CAREER is an example of a program in which OT addresses TBI and concussions in college-aged students experiencing cognitive impairments that may lead to barriers in work participation and engagement (Jacobs et al., 2015). This program is active on three college campuses across the United States and uses cognitive support technology (e.g., iPads) to assist with career planning and vocational support including transitioning from college to a career.

The effects of mild stroke can produce similar executive function deficits as mTBI that may not be recognized when in the acute hospital setting. Wolf, Baum, and Connor (2009) reported that almost 50% of people having strokes are of working age with neurologically mild effects. They are typically independent in self-care, do not have motor impairment, have no speech issues, and are therefore discharged with little to no rehabilitation services. O'Brien and Wolf (2010) reported that these individuals may not have any outward signs of impairment, so it is often assumed that they can return to their prestroke activities including work. This study showed that, of the individuals who were working at the time of their stroke, close to 40% never returned to work, and another 15% were unemployed 6 months later.

Executive function deficits are commonly missed in the acute care environment, resulting in individuals being unable to successfully return to work. Occupational therapy in acute care is focused on rehabilitating functional ADL and home independence, which may deflect attention from performance skills that are necessary to successfully return to work. That is, although the emphasis on ADL is important to the overall functioning of the individual, it can fail to address how an injured or ill individual such as a stroke survivor will be able to complete activities within the complex social context of everyday life (Wolf et al., 2009). Wolf, Stift, Connor, and Baum (2010) conducted a study to determine if the Executive Function Performance Test (EFPT) could be used in the acute phase of stroke to detect executive function deficits. The results provided evidence that the EFPT is effective in the acute phase of stroke when compared with results of a previous study validating the EFPT

6 months poststroke. If executive function deficits are noted early in the acute phase of stroke, the deficits can be addressed and potentially prevented a failed return to work.

Executive function deficits can impair an individual's ability to perform their job when prior to the mTBI they had no job performance issues. For example, Rita is a 45-year-old woman who fell on the ice and hit her head resulting in a concussion. She is a waitress and prided herself in her ability to take multiple orders and customer requests and not have to write things down. After the concussion, she returned to work and realized she was unable to remember multiple meal orders and was confusing customer requests and making mistakes. Her employer was getting frustrated with her work and started disciplinary proceedings for her poor work skills. She recognized her problems and went to a physician and eventually was referred to OT where an evaluation revealed high-level executive function deficits in ability to memorize, multitask, and pay attention to details. She was able to educate her employer and participate in an OT program to eventually return to work at her previous level of function.

Addressing Work with Individuals with Disabilities

Occupational therapy practitioners play an important role in addressing work with individuals with disabilities such as intellectual disability, autism spectrum disorder, behavioral disorders, and other chronic physical and mental health illnesses. *Preparation* for work occurs under a variety of circumstances and at any point in time from childhood to adulthood. However, much of this work occurs in the school system for individuals up to age 21 years and within the community (college, trade schools, on-the-job training, sheltered workshops) for adults. It is imperative that the needs of this population are addressed, as there are poorer employment outcomes for adults with disabilities for all age groups and education levels. People with disabilities have lower rates of employment (Bureau of Labor Statistics, 2017) and often have lower mean annual wages compared with those without disabilities. Although 66% of people with serious mental illness indicate that they would like to be employed, less than 15% actually are (G. Bond et al., 2015). Occupational therapy practitioners are distinctly qualified to address the needs of adolescents and adults with disabilities as related to work participation and engagement.

School-to-Work Transition

Society values work performance and engagement, and work for individuals with disabilities is often considered the next step after secondary school completion, especially if postsecondary education is not a goal. Students covered under the Individuals with Disabilities Education Improvement Act of 2004 (IDEA; Pub. L. No. 108-446) have individualized education plans (IEPs) that address developmental, academic, and social challenges in the role of student. IDEA Part B mandates that transition from adolescence to adulthood must begin to be addressed by age 16 years, as related to training, education, employment, and independent living skills when appropriate (U.S. Department of Education, n.d.).

Occupational therapy practitioners may be part of the interdisciplinary transition team when students have an IEP that includes OT (see Chapter 51). This is an underserved area, however, as data from the National Longitudinal Transition Study-2 found that only 7.5% of eligible students with disabilities actually receive OT services during the transition years (Eismann et al., 2017). Occupational therapy practitioners need to advocate for their important role in transition in order to facilitate work participation and engagement for people with disabilities. Occupational therapy practitioners can use a person-centered approach to assist in the following:

- Identify appropriate and meaningful work opportunities through person-centered job matching that addresses interests, preferences, skills, and abilities.
- Evaluate motor, process, and communication and interaction skills as relevant to work participation.
- Build work-related skills (e.g., establish a timely morning routine specific to preparing for a workday—appropriate clothing, packing lunch).
- Modify or adapt work tasks to match the skills of the student (e.g., use assistive technology, flexible work schedule, on-the-job supports).
- Promote workplace communication skills, social behaviors, and social inclusion (e.g., ability to receive feedback from a supervisor, managing interactions with coworkers).
- Address environmental and social supports in the desired work environment as well as in the student's family and community.
- Promote self-determination and advocacy during the transition period.
- Address ADL and instrumental ADL skills that are important for work participation such as self-care, community mobility, laundry, shopping, medication management, and money management.
- Implement other direct, consultative, and/or advocacy-related interventions and approaches.

Career Interests, Job Exploration, and Job Matching

Adolescents and adults with disabilities may need support in identifying potential jobs that match their interests, skills, and abilities. Occupational therapy practitioners can assist with investigating career interests, performing job analysis based on the essential functions of the job, and recommending reasonable accommodations to promote job placement and success. Many career interest assessment tools are available, including the O*NET's Interest Profiler (National Center for O*NET Development, 2017), and such tools can be a valuable first step in client-centered job exploration.

"Job matching is the collaborative, data-based decision-making process used by transition teams to determine the best fit between an individual's abilities and preferences and the job's environmental and occupational demands" (Persch, Cleary, et al., 2015, p. 271). The Vocational Fit Assessment (VFA) was designed to "assess job demands, identify the pros and cons of each potential job match, and identify areas of need that are suitable for intervention" (Persch, Gugiu, Onate, & Cleary, 2015). This can be a useful tool for occupational therapists as it is based on job analysis for multiple subscales (e.g., cognitive abilities, communication skills, interpersonal skills, safety, self-determination) and can be used as an outcome measure.

Community-Based Work

Occupational therapy practitioners may work with people with disabilities through agencies that provide work opportunities and support within the community. This is often referred to as a *supported employment model* in which occupational therapy practitioners are part of an interdisciplinary team. The Workforce Innovation and Opportunity Act (Pub. L. No. 113-128) of 2014 (WIOA) defines **supported employment** as "competitive integrated employment, including customized employment, or employment in an integrated work setting in which individuals are working on a short-term basis toward competitive integrated employment, that is individualized and customized consistent with the strengths, abilities, interests, and informed choice of the individuals involved, for individuals with the most significant disabilities." Examples of supported employment opportunities include the following (Carrasco, Hermes, & Burgos, 2012):

- Sheltered workshops
- Individual placement—place and support
- Enclaves
- Mobile work crews
- Entrepreneurial business employment
- Transitional employment
- Supported jobs

As the first legislative reform in 15 years for the public workforce system, WIOA is designed to increase access to the employment, education, training, and support services necessary for employment success. Among other goals, WIOA aims to improve services to individuals with disabilities, and this presents many opportunities for occupational therapy practitioners.

"WIOA increases individuals with disabilities' access to high quality workforce services and prepares them for competitive integrated employment:

- American Job Centers will provide physical and programmatic accessibility to employment and training services for individuals with disabilities.

- Youth with disabilities will receive extensive pre-employment transition services so they can successfully obtain competitive integrated employment.
- State vocational rehabilitation agencies will set aside at least 15 percent of their funding to provide transition services to youth with disabilities.
- A committee will advise the Secretary of Labor on strategies to increase competitive integrated employment for individuals with disabilities.
- VR state grant programs will engage employers to improve participant employment outcomes" (https://www.doleta.gov/WIOA/Overview.cfm)

Other Work Transitions

Work transitions occur across the life course and with changes in life situations. The population of aging adults can benefit from work OT to explore interests and needs for transition from work to retirement, volunteer, and other work participation activities. Exploration of a current career and ideas for reinvention or encore are often of interest to individuals who seek to retire but want to continue using their skills in a new way (Arbesman, 2015). Transitions also occur with life changes such as after active military duty or postincarceration or losing a job. The process outlined earlier for individuals with disabilities seeking work transition opportunities is applicable to a variety of individuals and their life situations.

Interprofessional Teams and Relationships

Occupational therapy practitioners will interact with many other professionals who have similar goals in addressing work participation and engagement. These professionals work in variety of settings including schools, community agencies, therapy clinics, medical provider offices, vocational rehabilitation agencies, insurance companies, and employers. Understanding the complementary and distinct roles of other professionals is important to facilitate desired outcomes in any setting, as a team approach can strengthen these outcomes. For those roles that are not profession specific, OT practitioners are appropriate candidates, given their educational background, skills, and practice. An example of an occupational therapist working collaboratively with other professionals to return an injured worker back to their job might include the following scenario. An occupational health physician has referred a patient to OT for acute injury management of right lateral epicondylitis. The patient's symptoms have resolved after several weeks of treatment, but in direct communication with the physician, both agreed the patient may be at risk of reinjury due to possible musculoskeletal risk factors present during performance of the job. The certified case manager contacts the human resource manager at the patient's employer and requests the ability of the occupational therapist to assess the patient's work area to determine if there are potential areas of concern to compromise a successful return to work and to make recommendations to reduce exposure to the risk factor. The human resource manager is pleased with the suggestion, and the occupational therapist meets with the plant manager and the employee's direct supervisor to obtain information about

the job. It is determined there are several risk factors the employer should address prior to the worker returning to the job such as moving items closer to the worker, reducing the weight of certain boxes, and sharpening several tools. The interprofessional collaboration between all disciplines assured a successful return to work for the patient.

Table 52-6 summarizes common professionals with whom OT practitioners may encounter and highlights their distinct and complementary roles.

TABLE 52-6 Interprofessional Team Members

Profession	Description
Job coaches	Job coaches most commonly work with individuals with disabilities to learn and accurately carry out job duties.
Occupational and environmental medicine physician (https://www.acoem.org/WhatIsOEM.aspx)	The American College of Occupational and Environmental Medicine (ACOEM) is a board-certified specialty for physicians in preventive medicine that focuses on the diagnosis and treatment of work-related injuries and illnesses.
Physical therapist (https://www.apta.org/ScopeOfPractice/)	Physical therapy practitioners are licensed health care professionals who can help patients improve or restore mobility using treatment techniques to promote the ability to move, reduce pain, restore function, and prevent disability.
Occupational and environmental health nurses (OHN) (http://aaohn.org/page/what-is-occupational-and-environmental-health-nursing)	Occupational and environmental health nurses deliver health and safety programs to workers and worker populations to focus on promotion and restoration of health, prevention of illness and injury, and protection from work-related and environmental hazards.
Certified occupational health nurse (COHN) (https://www.abohn.org/employers)	This specialty designation for nurses focuses on case management and direct care services related to work injuries and employee health.
Certified Case Manager (CCM) (https://ccmcertification.org/sites/default/files/issue_brief_pdfs/changing_roles_and_functions.pdf)	Nurses, OT practitioners, and other professionals who meet the required qualifications can become CCM. Case managers may work for insurance companies, managed care groups, occupational health practices, or employers, and work with a wide variety of populations experiencing complex or challenging medical situations.
OT assistant	The OT assistant works under the supervision of and collaborates with the OT practitioner in the implementation of treatment plans to promote return to work. Supervision requirements for OT assistants are regulated by state practice acts and vary from state to state.
Human resource (HR) professionals (https://www.opm.gov/policy-data-oversight/hr-professionals/)	HR professionals act as a resource for supervisors and managers as they deal with employee performance or conduct related issues or concerns. They also hire, facilitate implementation of accommodations, and develop retention programs in the workplace.
Occupational health and safety professionals (http://www.asse.org/assets/1/7/ASSEFactSheet_1014.pdf)	Occupational health and safety professionals work in many industries, and they anticipate, identify, and evaluate a wide range of hazardous conditions and practices in order to prevent injury, illness, or death.
Physician/nurse practitioner—primary care providers (PCPs) at the worksite	The onsite PCP provides treatment to injured employees at the work site and may consult OT to address injured worker issues at the job.
Human factors/ergonomics (HFE) practitioners (referred to as ergonomists or human factors engineers) (IEA, 2017)	The HFE practitioners' goal is optimal well-being and performance of humans and effective systems using knowledge of a person's cognitive, physical capabilities, needs, and limitations.
Industrial hygienist (http://www.abih.org/content/ih-defined)	The science of industrial hygiene focuses on identifying, analyzing, and controlling the hazards that affect the health and safety of people at work and in their communities including chemical, physical, biological, and ergonomic stressors.
Labor union (https://www.unionplus.org/page/what-union)	A labor union is an organization of workers dedicated to protecting members' interests and improving working conditions.
Plant manager	The plant manager will be aware of current and pending activities/projects and how they will impact the workplace. The plant manager has an understanding of the financial aspects of the business and the impact safety and health hazards have on the financial well-being of the business.
Workplace personnel	Direct supervisors and team leads will know the workers and the work on an intimate level. These individuals are key to obtaining information about issues occurring within the workplace and reasons why injuries may be occurring.

Visit thePoint to watch a video about work adaptations.

REFERENCES

ADA Amendments Act of 2008, Pub. L. No. 110-325, 122 Stat. 3553 (2008).

ADA.gov. (n.d.). *ADA standards for accessible design.* Retrieved from https://www.ada.gov/2010ADAstandards_index.htm

American Cancer Society. (2017). *Cancer facts & figures 2017.* Atlanta, GA: American Cancer Society. Retrieved from https://www.cancer.org/research/cancer-facts-statistics/all-cancer-facts-figures/cancer-facts-figures-2017.html

American Occupational Therapy Association. (2014a). Occupational therapy practice framework: Domain and process, 3rd edition. *American Journal of Occupational Therapy, 68,* S1–S48. doi:10.5014/ajot.2014.682006

American Occupational Therapy Association. (2014b). The role of occupational therapy in primary care. *American Journal of Occupational Therapy, 68,* S25–S33. doi:10.5014/ajot.2014.686S06

American Occupational Therapy Association. (2017). Occupational therapy services in facilitating work participation and performance. *American Journal of Occupational Therapy, 71,* 7112410040p1–7112410040p13. Retrieved from https://www.aota.org/ñ/media/Corporate/Files/Secure/Practice/OfficialDocs/Statements/off

Americans with Disabilities Act of 1990, Pub. L. No. 101-336, 104 Stat. 328, 42 U.S.C. § 12101 (1990).

Arbesman, M. (2015). Finding new work and reinventing oneself. In L. A. Hunt & C. E. Wolverson (Eds.), *Work and the older person: Increasing longevity and well-being* (pp. 125–134). Thorofare, NJ: SLACK.

Baum, C. M., Christiansen, C. H., & Bass, J. D. (2015). The Person-Environment-Occupation-Performance Model. In C. H. Christiansen, C. M. Baum, & J. D. Bass (Eds.), *Occupational therapy: Performance, participation, and well-being* (4th ed., pp. 49–56). Thorofare, NJ: SLACK.

Bond, E. D. (1925). The development of occupational therapy in private hospitals for mental and nervous diseases. *Archives of Occupational Therapy, 2,* 83–100.

Bond, G., Kim, S. J., Becker, D. R., Swanson, S. J., Drake, R. E., Krzos, I. M., . . . Frounfelker, R. L. (2015). A controlled trial of supported employment for people with severe mental illness and justice involvement. *Psychiatric Services, 66,* 1027–1034. doi:10.1176/appi.ps.201400510

Borg, G. (1982). Psychophysical bases of perceived exertion. *Medicine and Science in Sports and Exercise, 14,* 377–381.

Boynton, T., & Darragh, A. R. (2008). Participatory ergonomics intervention in a sterile processing center: A case study. *Work, 31,* 95–99.

Braveman, B., & Page, J. J. (2012). *Work: Promoting participation & productivity through occupational therapy.* Philadelphia, PA: F. A. Davis.

Bureau of Labor Statistics. (2016a). *Nonfatal occupational injuries and illnesses requiring days away from work, 2015.* Retrieved from https://www.bls.gov/news.release/osh2.nr0.htm

Bureau of Labor Statistics. (2016b). *Occupational safety and health definitions.* Retrieved from https://www.bls.gov/iif/oshdef.htm

Bureau of Labor Statistics. (2017). *Persons with a disability: Labor force characteristics summary.* Retrieved from https://www.bls.gov/news.release/disabl.nr0.htm

Cancelliere, C., Donovan, J., Stochkendahl, M. J., Biscardi, M., Ammendolia, C., Myburgh, C., & Cassidy, J. D. (2016). Factors affecting return to work after injury or illness: Best evidence synthesis of systematic reviews. *Chiropractic & Manual Therapies, 24,* 32. doi:10.1186/s12998-016-0113-z

Carrasco, R. C., Hermes, S., & Burgos, B. B. (2012). Supported and alternative employment. In B. Braveman & J. J. Page (Eds.), *Work: Promoting participation and productivity through occupational therapy* (pp. 117–137). Philadelphia, PA: F. A. Davis.

Centers for Disease Control and Prevention. (2016). *Work organization and stress-related disorders program.* Retrieved from https://www.cdc.gov/niosh/docs/2016-150/default.html

Centers for Disease Control and Prevention. (2017). *Workplace health promotion.* Retrieved from https://www.cdc.gov/workplacehealthpromotion/index.html

Cheng, A. S. K., & Cheng, S. W. C. (2010). The predictive validity of job-specific functional capacity evaluation on the employment status of patients with nonspecific low back pain. *Journal of Occupational and Environment Medicine, 52,* 719–724. doi:10.1097/JOM.0b013e3181e48d47

Cheng, A. S. K., & Cheng, S. W. C. (2011). Use of job-specific functional capacity evaluation to predict the return to work of patients with a distal radius fracture. *American Journal of Occupational Therapy, 65,* 445–452. doi:10.5014/ajot.2011.001057

Davis, J. E. (1945). An introduction to the problems of rehabilitation. *Mental Hygiene, 29,* 217–230.

Durocher, E., Gibson, B. E., & Rappolt, S. (2014). Occupational justice: A conceptual review. *Journal of Occupational Science, 21,* 418–430. doi:10.1080/14427591.2013.775692

Eguchi, H., Wada, K., & Smith, D. R. (2016). Recognition, compensation, and prevention of karoshi, or death due to overwork. *Journal of Occupational and Environmental Medicine, 58,* e313–e314. doi:10.1097/jom.0000000000000797

Eismann, M. M., Weisshaar, R., Capretta, C., Cleary, D. S., Kirby, A. V., & Persch, A. C. (2017). Characteristics of students receiving occupational therapy services in transition and factors related to postsecondary success. *American Journal of Occupational Therapy, 71,* 7103100010p1–7103100010p8. doi:10.5014/ajot.2017.024927

Erez, A. B. H., Rothschild, E., Katz, N., Tuchner, M., & Hartman-Maeir, A. (2009). Executive functioning, awareness, and participation in daily life after mild traumatic brain injury: A preliminary study. *American Journal of Occupational Therapy, 63,* 634–640. doi:10.5014/ajot.63.5634

Fan, Z. J., Harris-Adamson, C., Gerr, F., Eisen, E. A., Hegmann, K. T., Bao, S., . . . Rempel, D. (2015). Associations between workplace factors and carpal tunnel syndrome: A multi-site cross sectional study. *American Journal of Industrial Medicine, 58,* 509–518. doi:10.1002/ajim.22443

Govindu, N. K., & Babski-Reeves, K. (2014). Effects of personal, psychosocial and occupational factors on low back pain severity in workers. *International Journal of Industrial Ergonomics, 44,* 335–341. doi:10.1016/j.ergon.2012.11.007

Hanson, C. S., & Walker, K. F. (1992). The history of work in physical dysfunction. *American Journal of Occupational Therapy, 46,* 56–62. doi:10.5014/ajot.46.1.56

Hardison, M. E., & Roll, S. C. (2017). Factors associated with success in an occupational rehabilitation program for work-related musculoskeletal disorders. *American Journal of Occupational Therapy, 71,* 7101190040p1–7101190040p8. doi:10.5014/ajot.2016.023200

Hartmann, K. (2010). Assistive technology: A compensatory strategy for work production post mild brain injury. *Work, 36,* 399–404. doi:10.3233/WOR-2010-1048

Hees, H. L., de Vries, G., Koeter, M. W., & Schene, A. H. (2013). Adjuvant occupational therapy improves long-term depression recovery and return-to-work in good health in sick-listed employees with major depression: Results of a randomised controlled trial. *Occupational and Environmental Medicine, 70,* 252–260. doi:10.1136/oemed-2012-100789

Hettler, W. (1984). Wellness—The lifetime goal of a university experience. In J. D. Matarazzo, J. A. Herd, N. E. Miller, & S. M. Weiss (Eds.),

Behavioral health: A handbook of health enhancement and disease prevention (pp. 1117–1124). New York, NY: Wiley.

Hinojosa, J. (2013). The evidence-based paradox. *American Journal of Occupational Therapy, 67*, e18–e23. doi:10.5014/ajot.2013.005587

Hoving, J. L., Broekhuizen, M. L., & Frings-Dresen, M. H. (2009). Return to work of breast cancer survivors: A systematic review of intervention studies. *BMC Cancer, 9*, 117. doi:10.1186/1471-2407-9-117

Human Factors and Ergonomics Society. (2007). *ANSI/HFES 100-2007: Human factors engineering of computer workstations*. Santa Monica, CA: Author.

Human Rights Campaign. (2017). *Transgender inclusion in the workplace: Recommended policies and practices*. Retrieved from https://www.hrc.org/resources/transgender-inclusion-in-the-workplace-recommended-policies-and-practices

Individuals with Disabilities Education Improvement Act of 2004, Pub. L. No. 108-446, 20 U.S.C. 1400 *et seq.* (2004).

International Ergonomics Association. (2017). *Definition and domains of ergonomics*. Retrieved from http://www.iea.cc/whats/

Ivany, E., & Rothschild, D. (1951). Relationship of the occupational therapy department to hospital industries. *American Journal of Occupational Therapy, 5*, 16–22.

Jacobs, K., Rumrill, P., Hendricks, D., Elias, E., Leopold, A., Sampson, E., . . . Stauffer, C. (2015). Project CAREER: Interprofessional support to transition college students with traumatic brain injuries to employment. *American Journal of Occupational Therapy, 69*, 6911510217p1. doi:10.5014/ajot.2015.69S1-PO6106

Jaegers, L. (2015). Total Worker Health™: An opportunity for integrated occupational therapy practice. *Work and Industry Special Interest Section Quarterly, 29*, 1–4.

Jaegers, L., Finch, D., Dorsey, J., & Ehrenfried, H. (2015). Supporting occupational therapy practice in work & industry: Hot topics. *Work & Industry Special Interest Section Quarterly, 29*, 1–4.

Johnson, J. A. (1971). Consideration of work as therapy in the rehabilitation process. *American Journal of Occupational Therapy, 25*, 303–308.

Jonsson, H. (2010). Occupational transitions: Work to retirement. In C. H. Christiansen & E. A. Townsend (Eds.), *Introduction to occupation: The art and science of living* (2nd ed., pp. 211–230). Upper Saddle River, NJ: Pearson Education.

Kaskutas, V., Buckner-Petty, S., Dale, A. M., Gaal, J., & Evanoff, B. A. (2016). Foremen's intervention to prevent falls and increase safety communication at residential construction sites. *American Journal of Industrial Medicine, 59*, 823–831. doi:10.1002/ajim.22597

Kielhofner, G. (2009). *Conceptual foundations of occupational therapy practice* (4th ed.). Philadelphia, PA: F. A. Davis.

Kindig, D. (2017). Population health equity: Rate and burden, race and class. *JAMA, 317*, 467–468. doi:10.1001/jama.2016.19435

Lambeek, L. C., van Mechelen, W., Knol, D. L., Loisel, P., & Anema, J. R. (2010). Randomised controlled trial of integrated care to reduce disability from chronic low back pain in working and private life. *BMJ, 340*, c1035. doi:10.1136/bmj.c1035

Law, M., Cooper, B., Strong, S., Stewart, D., Rigby, P., & Letts, L. (1996). The Person-Environment-Occupation Model: A transactive approach to occupational performance. *Canadian Journal of Occupational Therapy, 63*, 9–23.

Marshall, E. M. (1985). Looking back. *American Journal of Occupational Therapy, 39*, 297–300. doi:10.5014/ajot.39.5.297

Medd, M. R. (1934). Individualizing occupational therapy for the mental patient. *American Journal of Physical Medicine & Rehabilitation, 13*, 241–256.

Munnell, A. H., Sass, S. A., & Soto, M. (2006). *Employer attitudes towards older workers: Survey results*. Retrieved from https://ideas.repec.org/p/crr/crrwob/wob_3.html

National Academies of Sciences Engineering and Medicine. (2017). *Communities in action: Pathways to health equity*. Washington, DC: The National Academies Press. doi:10.17226/24624

National Center for O*NET Development. (2017). *O*NET interest profiler*. Retrieved from https://www.mynextmove.org/explore/ip

National Institute for Occupational Safety and Health. (2014). *National occupational research agenda. Proposed national Total Worker Health™ agenda for public comment*. Retrieved from http://www.cdc.gov/niosh/docket/review/docket275/pdfs/NationalTWHAgendaFinalDraft9_5_14.pdf

National Institute for Occupational Safety and Health. (2016a). *About NIOSH*. Retrieved from https://www.cdc.gov/niosh/about/default.html

National Institute for Occupational Safety and Health. (2016b). *Musculoskeletal disorders and ergonomics*. Retrieved from https://www.cdc.gov/workplacehealthpromotion/health-strategies/musculoskeletal-disorders/index.html

National Institute for Occupational Safety and Health. (2017). *Elements of ergonomics programs*. Retrieved from https://www.cdc.gov/niosh/topics/ergonomics/ergoprimer/default.html

National Institute for Occupational Safety and Health. (2018). *Anthropometry*. Retrieved from https://www.cdc.gov/niosh/topics/anthropometry/default.html

National Institute for Occupational Safety and Health. (n.d.). *Publication No. 99=101. Stress at work*. Retrieved from https://www.cdc.gov/niosh/docs/99-101/pdfs/99-101.pdf

Nevala, N., Pehkonen, I., Koskela, I., Ruusuvuori, J., & Anttila, H. (2015). Workplace accommodation among persons with disabilities: a systematic review of its effectiveness and barriers or facilitators. *Journal of Occupational Rehabilitation, 25*, 432–448. http://link.springer.com/article/10.1007/s10926-014-9548-z

New Hampshire Workers' Compensation Law, Title XXIII Labor Chapter 281-A § 281-A:23-b (2009).

O'Brien, A. N., & Wolf, T. J. (2010). Determining work outcomes in mild to moderate stroke survivors. *Work, 36*, 441–447.

Occupational Safety and Health Administration. (n.d.a). *Computer workstations eTool: Good working positions*. Retrieved from https://www.osha.gov/SLTC/etools/computerworkstations/positions.html

Occupational Safety and Health Administration. (n.d.b). *OSHA law & regulations*. Retrieved from https://www.osha.gov/law-regs.html

O*NET. (2017). *The O*NET resource center*. Retrieved from https://www.onetcenter.org/overview.html

Ostbye, T., Dement, J. M., & Krause, K. (2007). Obesity and workers' compensation: Results from the Duke Health and Safety Surveillance System. *Archives of Internal Medicine, 167*, 766–773. doi:10.1001/archinte.167.8.766

Ownsworth, T., & McKenna, K. (2004). Investigation of factors related to employment outcome following traumatic brain injury: A critical review and conceptual model. *Disability and Rehabilitation, 26*, 765–783.

Persch, A., Cleary, D., Rutkowski, S., Malone, H., Darragh, A., & Case-Smith, J. (2015). Current practices in job matching: A project SEARCH perspective on transition. *Journal of Vocational Rehabilitation, 43*, 259–273. doi:10.3233/JVR-150774

Persch, A. C., Gugiu, P. C., Onate, J. A., & Cleary, D. S. (2015). Development and psychometric evaluation of the Vocational Fit Assessment (VFA). *American Journal of Occupational Therapy, 69*, 6906180080p1–6906180080p8. doi:10.5014/ajot.2015.019455

Reed, K. L. & Peters, C. (2006, October 9). Occupational therapy values and beliefs, Part II: The great depression and war years: 1930–1949. *OT Practice,11*(18), 17–22.

Rimer, B. K., & Glanz, K. (2005). *Theory at a glance: A guide for health promotion practice* (2nd ed.). Bethesda, MD: U.S. Department of Health and Human Services, National Institutes of Health, National Cancer Institute.

Schill, A. L. (2017). Advancing well-being through Total Worker Health®. *Workplace Health & Safety, 65*, 158–163. doi:10.1177/2165079917701140

Smith, B. J., Tang, K. C., & Nutbeam, D. (2006). WHO health promotion glossary: New terms. *Health Promotion International, 21*, 340–345. doi:10.1093/heapro/dal033

Social Security Administration. (2017). *Disability benefits*. Retrieved from https://www.ssa.gov/pubs/EN-05-10029.pdf

Soer, R., van der Schans, C. P., Groothoff, J. W., Geertzen, J. H., & Reneman, M. F. (2008). Towards consensus in operational definitions in functional capacity evaluation: A Delphi survey. *Journal of Occupational Rehabilitation, 18*, 389–400.

Sonne, M., Villalta, D. L., & Andrews, D. M. (2012). Development and evaluation of an office ergonomic risk checklist: ROSA—Rapid Office Strain Assessment. *Applied Ergonomics, 43*, 98–108. doi:10.1016/j.apergo.2011.03.008

Taskforce on the Aging of the American Workforce. (2008). *Report of the Taskforce on the aging of the American workforce*. Retrieved from https://www.doleta.gov/reports/FINAL_Taskforce_Report _2_27_08.pdf

United States Access Board. (2004). *Americans with Disabilities Act and Architectural Barriers Act accessibility guidelines*. Retrieved from https://www.access-board.gov/attachments/article/412/ada -aba.pdf

United States Access Board. (n.d.). *About the ADA standards*. Retrieved from: https://www.access-board.gov/guidelines-and-standards /buildings-and-sites/about-the-ada-standards

U.S. Department of Education. (n.d.). *Building the legacy: IDEA 2004*. Retrieved from http://idea.ed.gov/explore/view.html

U.S. Department of Labor. (2014). *Work capacity evaluation musculoskeletal conditions*. Retrieved from http://www.dol.gov/owcp/dfec /regs/compliance/OWCP-5c.pdf

U.S. Equal Employment Opportunity Commission. (2005). *The ADA: Your employment rights as an individual with a disability*. Retrieved from www.eeoc.gov/facts/ada18.html

U.S. Equal Employment Opportunity Commission. (n.d.). *Procedures for providing reasonable accommodation for individuals with disabilities*. Retrieved from https://www.eeoc.gov/eeoc/internal /reasonable_accommodation.cfm#1

Vasconcelos, A. F. (2015). Older workers: Some critical societal and organizational challenges. *Journal of Management Development, 34*, 352–372. doi:10.1108/JMD-02-2013-0034

Wisenthal, A., & Krupa, T. (2013). Cognitive work hardening: A return-to-work intervention for people with depression. *Work, 45*, 423–430. doi:10.3233/WOR-131635

Wolf, T. J. (2010). Participation in work: The necessity of addressing executive function deficits. *Work, 36*, 459–463.

Wolf, T., Baum, C., & Connor, L. T. (2009). Changing face of stroke: Implications for occupational therapy practice. *American Journal of Occupational Therapy, 63*, 621–625.

Wolf, T. J., Stift, S., Connor, L. T., & Baum, C. (2010). Feasibility of using the EFPT to detect executive function deficits at the acute stage of stroke. *Work, 36*, 405–412.

the**Point**® *For additional resources on the subjects discussed in this chapter, visit* **http://thePoint.lww.com /Willard-Spackman13e.**

CHAPTER 53

Play and Leisure

Anita C. Bundy, Sanetta H. J. Du Toit

LEARNING OBJECTIVES

After reading this chapter, you will be able to

1. Compare and contrast play and leisure, describing the characteristics that distinguish them from each other and from other occupations.
2. Describe play and leisure as reflections of identity.
3. Evaluate existing assessments to determine which, if any, characteristics of play and leisure they reflect.
4. Distinguish between interventions in which play and leisure are means to meet other goals and those for which play and leisure are the targeted outcomes of intervention.
5. Use Hammell's (2009) categories (engagement in doing; belonging, connectedness, contribution; restoration; life continuity and hope) to evaluate the benefits associated with particular interventions promoting play and leisure.
6. Assess the environment and context for factors that promote, or detract from, play and leisure.
7. Synthesize the state of existing research demonstrating the effectiveness of interventions to promote play and leisure and that using play and leisure as means to meet other objectives.

Introduction

Occupational therapy (OT) practitioners have a long, if somewhat ambivalent, relationship with play and leisure (Parham, 2008). Founders of the profession believed that the "play spirit" was essential to a worthwhile life (E. B. Saunders, 1922; Slagle, 1922; Ziegler, 1924). However, even Slagle and Robeson (as cited in Kielhofner, 2009, p. 21) spoke of play as a means to an end. They wrote,

> Let our minds be engaged with the spirit of fun and competitive play and leave our muscles, nerves and organs to carry on their functions without conscious thought—then our physical exercise will be correspondingly more beneficial and we can readily picture the effect exerted on the mood of the sullen, morose patient by the genial glow which suffuses the body following active exercise.

As practitioners and theorists became increasingly concerned with the scientific and technical aspects of intervention, the value of play and leisure became viewed almost entirely as the means for meeting other goals rather than as occupation for its own sake. Speaking of OT for the treatment of physical disabilities, Ayres wrote,

> While the interest and pleasure of [crafts and games] are important [albeit not scientifically demonstrated], they do not provide the most fundamental and vital concept of occupational therapy. (as cited in Kielhofner, 2009, p. 31)

In time, occupational therapists came to believe that a "[mechanistic paradigm] would bring OT recognition as an efficacious medical service and increase its scientific respectability" (Kielhofner, 2009, p. 31). Thus, when they were considered at all, play and leisure were second-class occupations—relegated to **discretionary time**. Only people who could not engage in productive occupations—the very young, the elderly, and people in untoward circumstances—could claim discretionary time legitimately. But, as Hammell (2009) cautioned, "Placing occupations in a hierarchy easily justifies placing the doers of those occupations in a similar hierarchy" (p. 108).

A single voice in the wilderness, Reilly (1974) guided her students to explore play in OT in a scholarly way. They offered *Play as Exploratory Learning*, the first textbook on the subject in the field. Nonetheless, in this text, only Reilly explored play itself. In the Preface, she wrote,

> [*Play as Exploratory Learning*] is divided into two parts. Each part is an aspect of an heuristic approach to the phenomenon of play. Part One [Reilly's portion] searches for the most general questions about external and internal reality that play can answer; Part Two [student contributions] applies specific play questions to the behavior of disabled people. What the reader should realize is *that the theoretical approach of Part One is not applied in Part Two* [emphasis added]. . . . The heuristic

strategies, it needs also to be said, grew from the remedial setting in which occupational therapists use play. As an applied field, occupational therapy is not obliged to hold any allegiance to a specific science of theoretical methodology. The graduate student contributors in Part Two used play as a masters thesis theme . . . and drew upon their abundant clinical experiences acquired in rehabilitation clinics. Both the strengths and weaknesses of the contributors are that they were under no compulsion to make their data fit a particular scientific methodology or theoretical foundation (p. 10).

Prominent publications in OT, such as the *Willard and Spackman* text, largely ignored play and leisure for a long time. Up to the third edition of Willard and Spackman's *Occupational Therapy* textbook, there is no mention of play *or* children (Willard & Spackman, 1963). In the third edition, the word *leisure* is included in a table of aspects to consider when working in geriatrics. In the fifth edition, play is discussed as a treatment modality (i.e., medium), and reference is made to play behavior (Willard, Spackman, Hopkins, & Smith, 1978). The fifth edition does not mention leisure. However, it *does* include the word *recreation* in the index, referring readers to "play." Finally, for the first time in the eighth edition, Susan Knox contributed a seven-page chapter devoted to play and leisure (Willard, Spackman, Hopkins, & Smith, 1993).

Perhaps unsurprisingly, the majority of studies of play and leisure in OT, even now, describe the consequences of impairment to children or adults, often comparing their play or leisure with that of typically developing peers. See Table 53-1 for a listing of such studies.

Beginning in the early 1990s and growing steadily to the present, scholars in OT and occupational science have reclaimed play and leisure as significant domains of human

TABLE 53-1 Studies Describing Play and Leisure of Various Diagnostic Groups

Diagnostic Group	References
Acquired or traumatic brain injury	Bier, Dutil, & Couture (2009); Fleming et al. (2011); Law, Anaby, DeMatteo, & Hanna (2011); Mortenson & Harris (2006)
Amputation	Couture, Caron, & Desrosiers (2010)
Arthritis	Hackett (2003); Reinseth & Arild Espnes (2007)
Attention-deficit/hyperactivity disorder (ADHD)	Cordier, Bundy, Hocking, & Einfeld (2009, 2010a, 2010b, 2010c); Leipold & Bundy (2000); Shimoni, Engel-Yeger, & Tirosh (2010)
Autism spectrum disorder (ASD)	Desha, Ziviani, & Rodger (2003); Kuhaneck & Britner (2013); LaVesser & Berg (2011); Ziviani, Rodger, & Peters (2005)
Cerebral palsy and other congenital, physical, developmental, and communication impairments	Boucher, Dumas, Maltais, & Richards (2010); Hamm (2006); Imms (2008); Majnemer et al. (2008); Majnemer et al. (2010); Pfeifer, Pacciulio, Santos, Santos, & Stagnitti (2011); Raghavendra, Virgo, Olsson, Connell, & Lane (2011); Shikako-Thomas, Majnemer, Law, & Lach (2008); Specht, King, Brown, & Foris (2002)
Developmental coordination disorder (DCD)	Engel-Yeger & Hanna Kasis (2010); Kennedy-Behr, Rodger, & Mickan (2013)
Down syndrome	Oates, Bebbington, Bourke, Girdler, & Leonard (2011)
Mental illness	Pieris & Craik (2004)
Motor impairments	Kolehmainen et al. (2015)
Sensory processing disorder (SPD)	Cosbey, Johnston, Dunn, & Bauman (2012); Ismael, Lawson, & Cox (2015); Watts, Stagnitti, & Brown (2014)
Spinal cord injury	O'Brien, Renwick, & Yoshida (2008)
Stroke	McKenna, Liddle, Brown, Lee, & Gustafsson (2009); O'Sullivan & Chard (2010)
Vision loss	Berger (2010)

occupation (e.g., Bundy, 1993; Canadian Association of Occupational Therapy, 1996; Parham, 1996; Primeau, 1996; Suto, 1998). Researchers and theorists linked play and leisure as occupations to life satisfaction, quality of life and mental health for individuals of all ages, with and without disability (Goltz & Brown, 2014; Hess & Bundy, 2003; King, Law, Petrenchik, & Hurley, 2013; Parham, 2008; Pereira & Stagnitti, 2006; Rodríguez, Látková, & Sun, 2008). Importantly, some researchers (e.g., Wang et al., 2012) suggested that engaging in occupation leisure may provide a "buffer" against some forms of disability. Thus, play and leisure are important concerns of OT (e.g., Parham, 2008; Wilcock, 2007). In fact, Parham (2008) felt that play was so important that we should describe a rhetoric of "play as health."

Reflecting the regained status of play and leisure, occupational science researchers have recently applied a broader lens to these occupations. For example, Lynch, Hayes, and Ryan (2016) explored sociocultural influences on infant play in Irish homes. Graham, Truman, and Holgate (2014) studied the ways in which parents expanded the concept of play for their children with severe cerebral palsy. Gerlach, Browne, and Suto (2014) explored how indigenous children's play is shaped by historical, political, and economic structures. Ramugondo (2012) examined intergenerational play in one South African family, revealing both persistence and change.

Play and leisure have much in common; however, they are not synonymous. Neither does the age of participants distinguish them. That is, play is not an occupation solely of children and leisure of adults. Nonetheless, because play is an important contributor to development, it is often associated only, but incorrectly, with childhood. Similarly, the restorative and self-expressive outcomes of leisure mean that it is often, but equally incorrectly, considered only an adult occupation.

The Centennial Note highlights a historical perspective on leisure engagement and current challenges experienced in practice. We are now in an era where people are living well and longer and, therefore, have access to substantial "unobligated time," but we persist to focus primarily on functional independence in our practice.

CENTENNIAL NOTES

A Historical Perspective on Leisure and a Challenge to Practitioners

Leisure is an ancient idea. In primitive cultures, people engaged in celebrations and leisure activities when they had met their needs for food, security, and other basics. Early advanced cultures clearly differentiated between roles; "superior" members of the community were allowed leisure (Godbey, 1994; Jackson & Burton, 1999; Torkildsen, 1986, 1999). The Greeks, for example, associated work with the *toil of manual labor and with providing the necessities of life, while leisure was valued as those moments of life in which one contemplated the eternal truths, and participated in music or drama* (Torkildsen, 1986, p. 170).

In contrast, although the Romans enjoyed leisure as a way to promote fitness and prepare for war, up to the Middle Ages, they glorified work and perceived idleness as evil. However, class differences nonetheless prevailed (Torkildsen, 1986).

During the Renaissance, leisure pursuits became more readily available to the masses, but the Industrial Revolution had a profound impact on work and leisure patterns (Jackson & Burton, 1999; Torkildsen, 1986). People uprooted from small towns and villages to live in cities where cramped conditions meant little room to play and hardly any time to enjoy leisure. Leisure only became the right of the masses with the advent of Saturday half-day and a reduction in working hours. It took a long time for leisure pursuits to be enjoyed by people from all walks of life.

In contrast, too much unobligated time within nursing home facilities appears to be a modern-day problem. Rather than being occupied with personally meaningful activities, boredom and time killing activities negatively impact on well-being (Power, 2010; W. H. Thomas, 1996). Residents typically spend up to 69% of their day inactive (Causey-Upton, 2015; Cohen-Mansfield, 2005; Morgan-Brown, Ormerod, Newton, Manley, & Fitzpatrick, 2011). Despite active ageing, successful ageing, and healthy ageing agendas pushed by policy makers, health professionals, and academics, aged care organizations continue to provide repetitive activities that simply fill time (Dionigi, 2017; Raymore, Barber, Eccles, & Godbey, 1999).

The situation is even more complex for residents living with advanced dementia in institutional settings. Nursing home staff and health care workers, in general, expect that older adults with dementia will experience increased difficulty making decisions and retaining control of their lives resulting in what Swaffer (2015) termed Prescribed Disengagement™. Despite research indicating that engagement in leisure pursuits is the factor that most strongly impacts well-being within residential care (J. E. Thomas, O'Connell, & Gaskin, 2013), staff expectations of residents with dementia are low, and meaningful activity is lacking, leaving many residents trapped in a constant state of inactivity, isolation, and helplessness.

Causey-Upton (2015) has challenged occupational therapists to consider our responsibility as advocates for vulnerable client groups. Access to resources and prejudice associated with a diagnosis of dementia constitutes a form of social injustice. An occupational justice approach complements this view and focuses on individuals' right to engage in meaningful leisure. Therefore, it is paramount for occupational therapists to support the right to leisure for all clients, including those who are frail and disabled.

Play and Leisure: Characteristics That Define and Differentiate Them

Scholars have proposed multiple definitions of *play* and *leisure*. However, there is no consensus on either term (Hurd & Anderson, 2010). And, although single, precise, all-purpose definitions, responsive to the needs of the entire profession, may not be required (Hurd & Anderson, 2010; Parham, 2008), we argue that a lack of definitional clarity hampers practitioners' assessment and promotion of play and leisure.

Scholars commonly define play and leisure by the characteristics that separate them from each other and from other occupations. This is a particularly useful way for OT practitioners to define them because it allows clients to determine which activities they classify as their personal play or leisure. Although there is no consensus on the exact characteristics that define play or leisure, there is nonetheless marked similarity among scholars.

Expanding on Neumann's (1971) work, Bundy and colleagues proposed that three traits define play and separate it, along a continuum, from nonplay: internal control, intrinsic motivation, and suspension of reality (Bundy, 2012; Skard & Bundy, 2008). Neumann argued that, like play and nonplay, each trait comprises a continuum. A transaction would be play if a greater presence of some traits offset the lesser presence of others. (Figure 53-1). Skard and Bundy (2008) further argued intrinsic motivation, internal control, and suspension of reality were sufficient to capture most all of the traits that scholars commonly attribute to play (Table 53-2).

In further defining play, (Bundy, 2012; Skard & Bundy, 2008) placed a frame around the scale shown in Figure 53-1. Drawing from Bateson's (1972) work, the frame represents cues that, like a picture frame, separate play from "reality."

Play can therefore be defined as a transaction characterized by relative intrinsic motivation, relative internal control, and suspension of reality that is framed in such a way as to separate it from "real life."

Bundy, Du Toit, and Clemson (2018) similarly defined leisure by its traits. They applied a variation of Bundy's model, describing a continuum of engagement in leisure that ranged from "distracted" to "absorbed" (i.e., totally engaged).

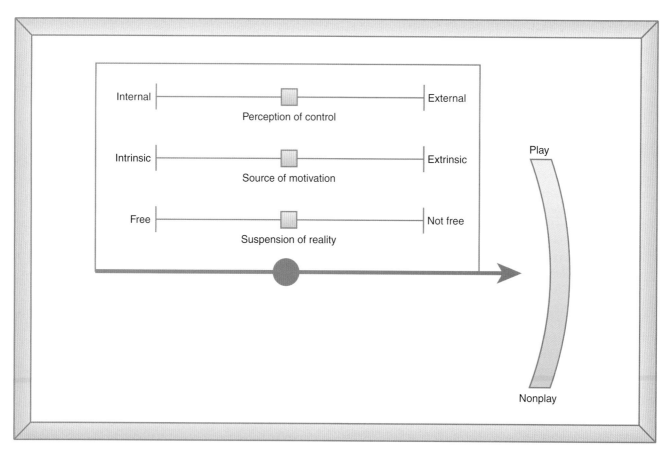

FIGURE 53-1 Elements of play.

Play Element	Play Trait	Theorist
Intrinsic motivation	Play is all absorbing.	Csikszentmihalyi (1975a, 1975b, 1990)
	Play involves more attention to the process than to the product.	Rubin, Fein, & Vandenberg (1983)
	Play is usually thought to be fun, although that perception may be clearer after the play has ended than while it is happening.	Csikszentmihalyi (1975a, 1975b)
	Play is more surprising than predictable.	Caillois (1979)
Internal control	Play is more safe than risky.	Caillois (1979)
	In play, the player reaches beyond himself or herself to meet a challenge.	Csikszentmihalyi (1975a, 1975b, 1990)
Internal control Suspension of reality	In play, the player makes things come out the way he or she wants or acts out his or her worst fears. The player can be whomever he or she desires. The player can control material things and make them do whatever his or her competence allows.	Connor, Seipp, & Williamson (1978)
Suspension of reality	In play, the usual meanings of objects no longer apply.	Rubin et al. (1983)
	"As if" serves the same function as rules. Rules create fiction. No activity in real life corresponds to games with rules.	Caillois (1979)

TABLE 53-2 Relationship of Commonly Cited Play Traits to the Three Primary Elements of Play

They proposed that control, motivation, and disengagement from unnecessary constraints of reality, collectively, determine whether or not a person becomes totally engaged in a leisure activity. They further associated total engagement with self-actualization.

Bundy et al. (2018) indicated that each element of leisure reflects a continuum; they were not all-or-none phenomena. The summative contributions of "control," "motivation," and "disengagement from the constraints of real life" to total engagement in leisure are illustrated in Figure 53-2. As with play, the elements of leisure are mutually influencing. That is, an individual engaging in an activity in which he or she feels little control is unlikely to be able to disengage from the constraints of real life. The converse also is likely true.

So, **leisure** can be defined as a transaction characterized by relative intrinsic or self-determined extrinsic motivation, relative internal control, and disengagement from reality that is framed in such a way as to separate it from "real life."

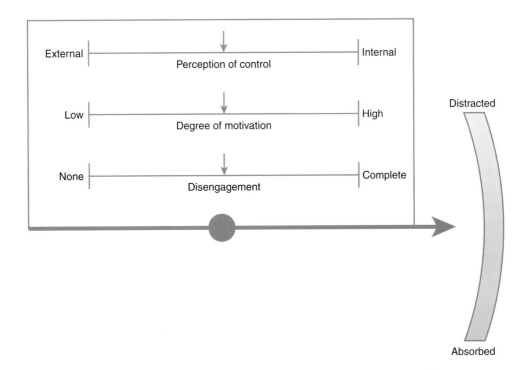

FIGURE 53-2 Summative contribution of the elements to total engagement in leisure.

Defining play and leisure by the characteristics that separate them from other occupations allows two individuals to consider the same activity as play or nonplay, leisure or nonleisure. For example, a highly skilled individual might consider soccer to be a cherished play or leisure activity, whereas an individual with developmental coordination disorder might find soccer the furthest thing from play or leisure. The highly skilled individual feels in control of her body and the ball and loves the feelings of engaging in the sport. She loves to win the game (an extrinsic motivator), but she enjoys playing even when her team loses. When she plays soccer, she is free, for a short time, from the everyday tasks she left behind (e.g., homework, cooking dinner). She becomes completely engaged in the game.

Because of the personalized nature of play and leisure experiences, the same activity can serve different purposes (Hammell, 2009; Jonsson, 2008). For example, some people enjoy reading for intellectual stimulation, whereas others seek relaxation and restoration. Understanding the motivation for a play or leisure activity is key to client-centered practice. For example, singing in a choir may be deemed involvement in a cultural activity, but it also could be performed primarily for socialization with choir members. Or, both socialization and the cultural aspects may be equally important. Understanding the motivations fulfilled by being a choir member facilitates replacement of that activity/role should that be necessary.

Distinguishing Play from Leisure

Earlier we said that play and leisure are not synonymous, although they share many of the same traits. We also said that, although age of a participant does not distinguish play from leisure, outcomes might. Development is commonly associated with play, whereas restoration and self-expression are associated with leisure. Some activities can be play *or* leisure.

When is an activity considered play but not leisure, or vice versa? Admittedly, this may be of more interest theoretically than practically but surely the way practitioners think about play and leisure influences the way we assess and promote them. We propose that aspects of motivation, suspension of reality, and framing distinguish play from leisure. Although each of these elements is equally important to both play and leisure, they can look quite different in one versus the other.

Motivation

Most theorists agree that **intrinsic motivation** is a defining feature of both play and leisure. Drawing from Rubin et al. (1983), Parham (2008) described the meaning of intrinsic motivation in play as "motivated by the experience of the

play itself, not by the promise of rewards that are external to the play" (p. 5). The sources of intrinsic motivation are individually determined and varied. They commonly include, for example, mastery (e.g., White, 1959), social interaction, sensation (e.g., Caillois, 1979), and the pleasure of being a cause (e.g., Sutton-Smith, 1997). Of course, play may also have extrinsic motivators (e.g., the desire to win or gain praise), but the driving force must be intrinsic for a transaction to be play.

In contrast, some authors found that intrinsic motivation and **self-determined extrinsic motivation** (i.e., activities performed for their own long-term gain or for another's benefit) are equally correlated with leisure satisfaction (Losier, Bourque, & Vallerand, 1993; Mannell, Zuzanek, & Larson, 1988). Although not specifically discussing leisure, Ryan and Deci (2017) described such activity as having integrated regulation (i.e., the goals of the activity, although extrinsic, are fully assimilated within the self). Although self-determined extrinsic motivators are undoubtedly powerful drivers for leisure, they seem less associated with play.

As occupations and identities evolve across the life course, individuals' motivations for engaging in play and leisure also change. For example, Passmore and French (2003) categorized leisure of adolescents according to whether activities met an intrinsic need for achievement, social interaction, or time-out. They associated achievement leisure with engagement in competitive and challenging pursuits, like team sports and music performances. But achievement leisure could also include creative activities like drawing. Achievement activities require regular commitment and organization. Social leisure activities (e.g., visiting friends, eating out, chatting/texting online) involve friends and social experiences and fulfill a need for belonging. Time-out leisure encompasses relaxing and calming experiences. Time-out leisure (e.g., listening to music, watching television, or keeping a diary) has low demand, can be undertaken alone, and includes time for reflection.

Suspension of Reality

Albeit by slightly different names, the bottom continua in the scales shown in Figures 53-1 and 53-2 refer to freedom from unnecessary constraints of reality. In defining play, we name that element **suspension of reality**, whereas in defining leisure, we refer to "disengagement" as a release from everyday reality. Neumann (1971) described suspension of reality by noting that a player is free to determine the degree to which a transaction resembles objective reality. A child swinging on a backyard swing could choose to "just swing"—the fun being in the sensation or from swinging as high as possible. Alternatively, the child could choose to "become a super hero": flying to save a "victim" from "sure death." The choice is the child's.

Pretending is a common form of suspending reality. A player can be whoever he or she chooses, pretend an object is something it is not, or pretend to be doing something he or she is not. Playful joking, teasing, mischief, and clowning are other ways of stepping outside of reality (Skard & Bundy, 2008).

We argue that, although both play and leisure depend on being free from unnecessary constraints of everyday life, the presence of pretend, playful joking, clowning, mischief, and teasing distinguishes play from leisure. Further, although pretending may be more common in children, adults also pretend. When taking a self-report version of the Test of Playfulness, many of the German adult participants in Weigl and Bundy's (2013) study revealed that they pretended in the context of everyday activities like choir practice. Glynn and Webster (1992) found that flights of playful joking and banter were not only common in the workplace but also contributed to productivity. And, more than one longstanding cartoon (e.g., *Rose Is Rose* by Pat Brady and *Foxtrot* by Bill Amend) depict adults and adolescents pretending. Cartoons are only funny because readers readily identify with the characters. See, for example, Box 53-1. "Zhipo" assumed an alter ego every day when he went off to work, pretending changed his entire outlook on life. We argue that playful clowning, joking, teasing, mischief, and

pretend are common in both adults and children and are characteristic of play but not of leisure.

Framing

Framing is the use of cues to separate play transactions from "real life." Cues reveal how a player wishes to be viewed and treated by others (Bateson, 1972). A child on all fours entering the kitchen barking gives a clear cue that he is a puppy and that his parents should interact with him accordingly. A father, exaggerating his motions, roaring and chasing after his child, likewise gives cues that he is a monster and his child should run away in mock fear. Of course, that father must alter his cues in response to the reactions of his child. Otherwise, the play may turn to nonplay. Importantly, overt cues do not accompany all pretending. Although Zipho (see Box 53-1) pretended overtly—changing his clothing to support a make believe role—many adults pretend more in their imaginations than in action.

Framing also happens outside of pretend play. The rules of a game, for example, are a frame that distinguishes what is allowed in the game and what is not (Caillois, 1979). Of course, players can renegotiate the rules. By changing what is allowed in the game, they change the frame.

The ability to frame play is critical to being a good playmate. Cordier et al. (2010a, 2010b) found that children with attention-deficit/hyperactivity disorder (ADHD) tended to have difficulty with framing. They suggested that responding to play cues is a reflection of empathy. Later, Wilkes-Gillan and colleagues developed an intervention in which they successfully taught cue-reading skills to children with ADHD (Wilkes, Cordier, Bundy, Docking, & Munro, 2011; Wilkes-Gillan, Bundy, Cordier, & Lincoln, 2014a, 2014b, 2016; Wilkes-Gillan, Bundy, Cordier, Lincoln, & Chen, 2016; Wilkes-Gillan, Bundy, Cordier, Lincoln, & Hancock, 2015; Wilkes-Gillan et al., 2017). Kent, Cordier, Joosten, Wilkes-Gillan, and Bundy (2018) have since extended their intervention to children with autism who also have issues giving and reading cues.

Framing is important to leisure as well as play. Caillois (1979; cited in Henricks, 2010, p. 180) wrote about indicators of collective affiliation where play becomes "a special world isolated from everyday affairs." These indicators are seen, for example, in the uniforms of sporting teams or other organized groups (e.g., scouting, cheerleading). Even solitary runners and bicyclists often don "uniform" clothing as a cue about how others should view them. Caillois (1979) described these indicators of group membership in reference to games and play, but we argue that such cues are more related to leisure (as we define it) than play. Adults assuming a theatrical role also give cues about how other cast members and the audience should interact with them. Arguably, however, those cues are about collective membership.

BOX 53-1   PRETENDING ENABLES ALTERNATE REALITIES

Suspending reality through pretend provides unique opportunities to take on roles and embrace identities not otherwise possible, especially for members of marginalized groups as demonstrated by the main character, Zipho, in The Script's music video *Superheroes* (https://www.youtube.com/watch?v=WIm1GgfRz6M). Zipho supports his daughter financially by working in a garbage dump. But every morning, Zipho leaves home dressed in a suit and tie. He travels to the dump, changes his clothing, works all day, changes back to his suit and tie, and returns home to his daughter. When Zipho and his daughter go out together in the evening, he wears his suit and tie. Dressing up allows Zipho to pretend to have a role he believes will make his daughter proud. When he can, Zipho rescues a discarded toy from the rubbish he sorts, cleans it, and presents it to his daughter. They share make-believing that his business is doing well, and he can afford to spoil her with gifts. One might ask, "Which is the real Zipho and which is the pretend Zipho?"

Play and Leisure as Statements of Identity

Because play and leisure activities are freely chosen, they make important statements about the identities of participants (Kelly, 1982; Neulinger, 1974; Scraton & Holland, 2006). In fact, Plato is credited with having said that you could learn more about a person in an hour of play than in a year of conversation. Theorists and researchers clearly link occupation and selfhood in general (Eakman, Atler, Rumble, & Gee, in press) and leisure and identity in particular. Families commonly decorate their homes with mementos of leisure experiences (Csikszentmihalyi & Halton, 1981; Rockwell-Dylla, 1992). Some of the most compelling photographs of children are taken while they play. Mementos make statements of accomplishments, selfhood, and things that bring great joy. When at risk of losing valued play or leisure unintentionally, individuals also risk losing important reflections of themselves.

Because of their importance and healing properties, play and leisure may counter the negative effects of adverse personal circumstances, preserving identity. Numerous individuals described the importance of play to children facing crises imposed by war (Figure 53-3), weather, and other untoward circumstances (e.g., Casey, Assi, Maharjan, Wirunrapan, & Gupta, 2017). Similarly, Pereira and Stagnitti (2006) indicated that older adults displaced by immigration found traditional leisure activities associated with their culture of origin to be very important. In Case Study 53-1 (adapted from Bundy et al., 2018), we relay an account of an OT assessment and intervention with leisure at the heart. This intervention went a long way to preserving identity.

The link between play and identity is not as well supported as the link between leisure and identity. Although play and identity are linked, both logically and theoretically, that link is largely undemonstrated in research (Sutton-Smith, 1997). Sutton-Smith (1997) indicated that research

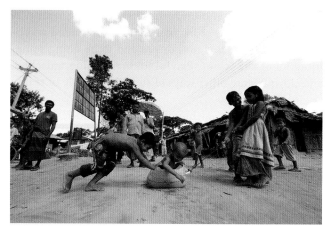

FIGURE 53-3 Rohingya children playing at a refugee camp in Bangladesh.

and theory about childhood play are driven, largely, by a rhetoric of progress (i.e., play promotes development). Although he also ascribed a rhetoric of power and identity to children's play, Sutton-Smith felt that the progress rhetoric was a way of adults maintaining power over children. Sutton-Smith posited that rhetorics of power and identity explain a lot about the substance of children's play and how children learn their place in a social hierarchy. Sutton-Smith described the research of Beresin (1993) and Hughes (1993a, 1993b) who, by studying children playing together, illustrated children's capacity for creating their own culture. About Hughes's study, Sutton-Smith said, "Playing games for the sake of games is always playing games for the sake of games *in a particular social context with its own particular social arrangements* [emphasis added]. There is no lasting social play without play culture" (p. 120). Finding one's place in a social hierarchy is surely about finding and expressing one's identity. As Henricks (2017, p. 13) wrote, play "asks us to confront the relationship between what is very basic in us and what is socially contrived."

CASE STUDY 53-1   SARAH: THE SAILING GRANDMOTHER

At age 74, following a stroke, Sarah was depressed not only because she had lost physical capability but also because her children wanted her to go into a retirement village to receive "the kind of care they felt she needed." Sarah chose instead to attend a Day Therapy Center where the occupational therapist completed an assessment of Sarah's leisure using an interest checklist supplemented by interview. The therapist, learning that, as a child, Sarah and her family had been avid sailors, developed an intervention plan that included an adapted sailing program called Sailability. Sarah flourished. She became

a "sailing grandmother," won a championship race, and was featured in a local newspaper. These achievements were turning points in her recovery. Sarah did not have the strength or movement to handle the sails, but she said, "I'm the captain. I choose who rolls the sails and tell them how to do it. You have to think or you might hit another boat." Sailing renewed her identity and self-confidence. Sailability kept her independent and mentally alert. She went every week. Clearly, leisure, for Sarah, not only reflected identity but also contributed to a renewed identity.

The Benefits of Play and Leisure

Hammell (2004b, 2009) indicated that all occupations (defined here as anything people do with their time) should be classified by the intrinsic needs they meet, in other words, by their benefits. Hammell categorized those intrinsic needs as (1) engagement in doing; (2) belonging, connecting, and contributing; (3) restoration; and (4) life continuity and hope for the future. Similarly, Pierce (2001a, 2003, 2014) labeled restoration, pleasure, and productivity as the motivations for engaging in occupations, including leisure. Productivity, pleasure, and restoration are interrelated and not categories unto themselves. Thus, horseback riding, needlepoint, playing with Barbies, and playing Nintendo are all occupations that foster an intrinsic need. Notably, the connection of pleasure with process, rather than outcome, is reminiscent of the definition of play. Categorizing occupations associated with play and leisure by benefits is appealing because occupational therapists often need a reminder of the enormous benefits of play and leisure.

Benefits of Engagement in Doing

Hammell (2009) cited her own earlier work (Hammell, 2004a, 2004b) and that of Laliberte-Rudman, Yu, Scott, and Pajouhandeh (2000); Nagle, Cook, and Polatajko (2002); and Ville, Ravaud, and Tetrafigap Group (2001), indicating that having something meaningful and purposeful to wake up and do contributed to self-perceptions of capability and value and to other indicators of well-being. Similarly, Atler (2014) indicated that the interrelated nature of productivity, pleasure, and restoration, and the understanding that pleasure is associated with process rather than the outcome of an experience, directs what individuals *do* every day in order to meet their needs.

Doing is certainly a hallmark of play. In fact, a cursory look at the major OT texts that describe play (i.e., Parham, 2008; Reilly, 1974) reveals that large portions of both describe doing associated with play. All of the assessments cited in *Play in Occupational Therapy for Children* (Parham, 2008) are about doing play, most notably the skills children use in play and the activities that children at various ages prefer. Similarly, the five chapters about play in practice in *Play as Exploratory Learning* (Reilly, 1974) describe doing and the assessment of doing in play.

Whether motivated intrinsically or by self-determined extrinsic sources (Ryan & Deci, 2017), doing is an important aspect of leisure. As with play, many assessments of leisure that occupational therapists use examine the activities people enjoy doing. Further, based on a longitudinal study of Swedish workers transitioning to retirement, Jonsson (2011) distinguished between free time as fully engaging and "killing time." In contrast to time-killing occupations, Johnsson viewed doing meaningful occupations as significant to enhancing personal well-being.

Benefits of Belonging, Connecting, and Contributing

Observation of play and leisure almost always reveals a social side (Figure 53-4). In their synthesis of qualitative research, Eakman et al. (in press) indicated that belonging and helping are two important aspects of the social meaning of occupation. Other authors (e.g., Ryan & Deci, 2017), although not writing specifically about play or leisure, made clear that feeling connected is necessary to intrinsic motivation. In turn, intrinsic motivation is a hallmark of play and of much of leisure.

Although social interaction is clearly an important motivator for play, most research and theory in OT related to social play deal primarily with the acquisition and relative competence of social skills in children, especially children with disabilities (see, for example, Parham, 2008). The recent works of occupational scientists are exceptions (Gerlach et al., 2014; Graham et al., 2014; Lynch et al., 2016; Powrie, Kolehmainen, Turpin, Ziviani, & Copley, 2015; Ramugondo, 2012). Based on a systematic review of qualitative research exploring the meaning of leisure (which also included play) for children and young people with physical disabilities, Powrie et al. (2015) argued persuasively that friendship is a universal trait, being more important than the activity itself. What is more, when young people played alone, they usually did not experience fun *or* leisure.

In addition to the importance of belonging, connecting, and contributing as benefits of play, we argue that occupational therapists and occupational scientists should give serious consideration to Sutton-Smith's (1997)

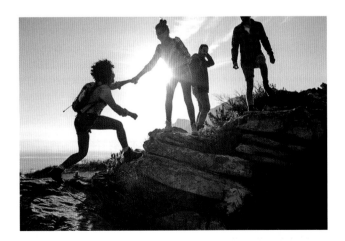

FIGURE 53-4 **Hiking can be a solo or group activity.**

rhetorics of power and identity in play. These rhetorics emphasize how children learn their place (i.e., connect with others) in a social hierarchy. This may be of particular relevance to children and young people with disabilities. Several authors wrote about the value of comparing oneself against similar others (Jessup, Bundy, & Cornell, 2013; Jessup, Cornell, & Bundy, 2010; Powrie et al., 2015).

Powrie et al. (2015) indicated that

Leisure in segregated settings, such as camps and sports teams, generally provided a sense of camaraderie and connectedness with others with disabilities. Participants could be themselves, and there was a sense of shared understanding and acceptance, without the negative interactions they experienced in other settings. (p. 1008)

Contributing to an OT perspective on connecting and contributing in leisure, Raber et al. identified that, even when older adults with dementia experience a decline in abilities, they continue to embrace opportunities for connectedness and belonging (Raber, Teitelman, Watts, & Kielhofner, 2010). When provided with freedom to engage as an observer, rather than join in physically, Raber's and colleagues' (2010) participants nonetheless contributed to activities by providing feedback and advice to others. Raber et al. further found that the adapted doing of older adults with dementia included relying on others, who also were engaged in the activity, to initiate and provide structure. In other words, doing in leisure, for these participants, required connectedness and co-occupation of two or more people (Pierce, 2009).

Benefits of Restoration

Restoration is an important benefit of leisure, although it is less readily associated with the busy doing of play. Pierce (2001a) described restoration as a subjective "experience that restores our energy levels and ability to continue to engage in our daily lives" (p. 253). She believed restoration was the most neglected and poorly understood dimension of occupation. Leisure can be highly restorative, especially for clients who are "very disorganized, depleted, or discouraged" (Pierce, 2011a, p. 254). Waking restoration is highly individualized and could include such quiet-focus leisure activities as reading, listening to music, knitting, viewing art (Figure 53-5); it might also include activities that yield solitude: being in nature, a solitary physical workout, or prayer and meditation (Pierce, 2001a).

Benefits of Life Continuity and Hope for the Future

Hammell (2009) indicated that continuity and hope for the future are especially important to people enduring life crises. Leisure that reflects hope for the future allows people to become who they want to be, despite changing circumstances and altered abilities (Hammell, 2007).

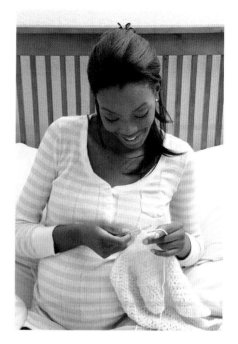

FIGURE 53-5 Crocheting a baby blanket is form of waking restoration for this expectant mother.

Researchers suggest that individuals maintain a core set of leisure activities across the life course (Atchley, 1989, 1993; Kelly, 1993). Some of these activities are learned early in life and derive their meaning from culture and the influence of significant others (Csikszentmihalyi & Kleiber, 1991; Iso-Ahola, Jackson, & Dunn, 1994; McGuire, Boyd, & Tedrick, 2004). For example, Pöllänen and Hirsimäki (2014) revealed that persons with dementia in residential care found pleasure in craft-related reminiscence, especially when they had enjoyed crafting earlier in life (Figure 53-6). Craft activities led to shared experiences and talking about crafts in general, promoting social interaction and higher quality reciprocal language.

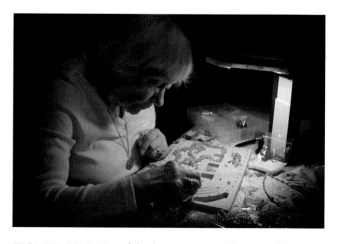

FIGURE 53-6 An elderly woman enjoys making beaded jewelry.

Numerous researchers promote life stories for identifying former interests and previously enjoyed activities of nursing home residents (Chung, 2004; Lape, 2009; Pöllänen & Hirsimäki, 2014; Warchol, 2006; Wood, Harris, Snider, & Patchel, 2005). In-depth examination of the benefits of previous leisure facilitates participation in new activities, when necessary, thereby promoting life continuity and hope for the future. Superficial acknowledgment of previous leisure pursuits cannot replace a thorough analysis. For example, although it might seem appropriate to offer a similar-themed Wii game as replacement for fishing, an individual who enjoyed fishing as an outdoor pursuit probably would not find Wii to be a good replacement.

Importantly, leisure may provide a "buffer" against some forms of age-related disability, such as dementia (Coleman & Iso-Ahola, 1993; Fabrigoule et al., 1995; Kleiber, Hutchinson, & Williams, 2002; Sorman, Sundström, Rönnlund, Adolfsson, & Nilsson, 2013; Wang et al., 2012). Therefore, leisure is an important concern of occupational therapists (Bevil, O'Connor, & Mattoon, 1994; Freysinger, 1993; Griffin & McKenna, 1999; Lau, Chi, & McKenna, 1998; Mishra, 1992; Pereira & Stagnitti, 2006; Tatham & McCree, 1993; Voelki, 1993; Wilcock, 2007). When Raber and colleagues (2010) applied the Volitional Questionnaire in a nursing home setting, they found that a lack of meaningful activity could be more disabling to older people with moderate dementia than the decrease in their abilities.

In their systematic review of qualitative research exploring the meaning of leisure, including play, for children and young people with physical disabilities, Powrie et al. (2015) provided evidence that the benefits of life continuity and hope for the future associated with leisure (and also with play) apply to children and young people as well as adults. Children and young people "described how leisure allowed them to experience fulfillment by proving their abilities, demonstrating their potential, countering assumptions about their abilities, and showing that there is more to their identity than being disabled" (Powrie et al., 2015, p. 1006).

Combining Benefits: Doing and Social

Opportunities for shared doing support reciprocity, the feeling that, overall, what people receive is similar to what they give (Goodman, 1984). Feeling as though one is giving to another is often the most important motivator for leisure for older individuals (K. R. Allen & Chin-Sang, 1990; Havighurst, 1979; Jacobson & Samdahl, 1998; Lawton, 1993). Without reciprocity, a state of indebtedness develops (Goodman, 1984). Indebtedness alters a relationship and prohibits the experiences of control, choice, comfort, and freedom characteristic of leisure.

Doing does not have to be with other *people*. At the turn of the century, people with AIDS experienced social isolation due to prejudice. In a small-scale study, J. M. Allen, Kellegrew, and Jaffe (2000) explored pet ownership, finding that not only were participants rewarded with unconditional love but they also engaged in daily walks and social events with other pet owners. Pet ownership offered both "normalized" experiences and a reason to care for themselves (i.e., hope for the future), as this quote illustrates: "He keeps me from giving up" (p. 276).

Context and the Environment

Context and environmental supportiveness are critical for promoting play and leisure. García-Martín et al. showed that the socially supportive context of small groups enhanced perceived control and self-efficacy for older adults engaging in self-determined, meaningful activity (García-Martín, Gómez-Jacinto, & Martimportugués-Goyenechea, 2004). Unfortunately, although centers and adult day programs may get participants "out of the house" and occupied, they often fail to create real leisure (Tse & Linsey, 2005). True leisure is reflected in the experience, not in activities.

Open spaces are important to many people's play and leisure, and lack of access to open spaces can impact negatively on health and well-being. Many adults enjoy walking, hiking, skiing, fishing, hunting, and other outdoor activities, experiencing the exhilaration of physical activity and the solace of nature. Children's outdoor play is associated with a variety of positive developmental, physical, and mental health outcomes (Figure 53-7) (Brussoni et al., 2015; Engelen et al., 2013; Sandseter & Kennair, 2011).

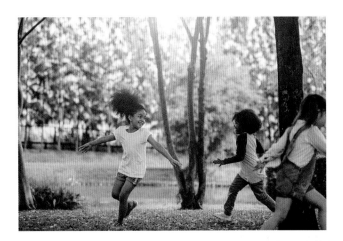

FIGURE 53-7 **Playing outdoors is associated with positive physical and mental outcomes.**

Despite this, parents', educators', and other caregivers' fears have resulted in unnecessary restrictions on children's outdoor play, which, in turn, may contribute to sedentary lifestyles and difficulties with coping and other aspects of mental health.

The context in which participation occurs includes a wide array of interrelated variables that affect performance (American Occupational Therapy Association [AOTA], 2014). Opportunities to experience control, choice, comfort, and freedom are fundamental to leisure. Relocating to a nursing home, for example, is often associated with loss of autonomy, control, roles, and privacy (Lee, Woo, & Mackenzie, 2002). The demands of group living and the regimentation of daily routines could lead to passive acceptance and perceived loss of control (Burack, Reinhardt, & Weiner, 2012; C. Thomas, du Toit, & van Heerden, 2014). Occupational therapists can enhance personal control in simple ways—by advocating for, and providing, *real* choice. For example, OT practitioners can provide the possibility of solitary pursuits indoors and outdoors as well as a range of group opportunities (Duncan-Myers & Huebner, 2000). If leisure opportunities do not address residents' needs and interests, declining participation may be the only way they have to exert control (Lee et al., 2002).

In 1953, Nash, a pioneer in understanding free time, unsurprisingly, found that free time is not always about leisure (Figure 53-8). Free time can be detrimental to well-being, resulting in risk to the self or society (e.g., drug taking, vandalism), as shown in Figure 53-9. Hence, context and the environment, including access to resources, are important factors ensuring that free time has positive outcomes.

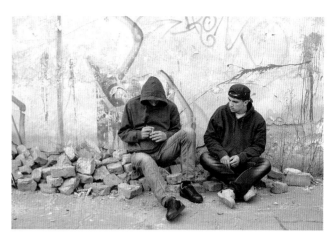

FIGURE 53-9 Teenagers with too much free time can cause injury to themselves or to society.

Evaluation of Play and Leisure

Best practice in OT means that evaluation begins with clients (often including family members and other caregivers) and practitioners collaboratively identifying what clients *want* to do (AOTA, 2014) and the extent to which they actually engage in desired activities (Coster, 1998). Broadly, evaluation of play and leisure addresses how context, environment, and client strengths facilitate or inhibit engagement. Further, best practice suggests that evaluation takes place in everyday life settings using a top–down approach (AOTA, 2014).

Logically, assessments of play and leisure would parallel their respective definitions. We defined play and leisure as the characteristics that separate them from other occupations. Nonetheless, although some assessments explicitly capture the characteristics of play, Hammell's (2009) occupational categories (i.e., doing, belonging, restoration, and life continuity) offer a somewhat more inclusive way of thinking about assessments of play and leisure.

Evaluation of Play

Play is a multifaceted and complex phenomenon. In practice, although play is a lifelong occupation, therapists are more likely to evaluate play in children than in adults. Hammell's (2009) category "engagement in doing" seems to capture the content of most existing play assessments for children. Although there are some relatively new assessments of adult playfulness (e.g., Shen, Chick, & Zinn, 2014a, 2014b; Waldman-Levi & Bundy, 2016), those that occupational therapists have developed (e.g., Waldman-Levi & Bundy, 2016) tend to be about how adults facilitate the play of children.

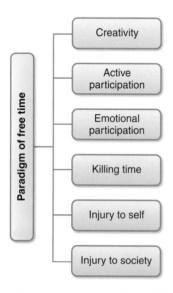

FIGURE 53-8 Free time as explained by Nash's (1953) model.

We argue that a complete OT assessment of play would comprise five aspects listed as follows. However, although play is multifaceted, generally, it is neither necessary nor practical to evaluate each aspect for any individual. Thus, practitioners must consider carefully which are most important in a given situation and choose assessments that reflect those aspects. Such choices require practitioners to carefully evaluate the items of an assessment.

Factors of a complete play assessment include the following:

1. The player's *capacity* to play (i.e., skills used in play)
2. *What* players do (i.e., play activities)
3. How players approach play (i.e., playfulness)
4. The relative supportiveness of the environment
5. The *motivations* for play (i.e., why players choose particular play activities)

Capacity to Play

Probably because of the importance attached to learning through play, most children's play assessments focus on skills. Assessments such as Knox's Revised Preschool Play Scale (Knox, 2008) and Linder's (2008) Transdisciplinary Play-Based Assessment provide reliable and valid data comparing the skills of a particular child with those of peers. Stagnitti (2007) developed an assessment of pretend play, the Child-Initiated Pretend Play Assessment (CHIPPA) that seems to fall into this category because examiners use it to determine level of pretend play, a reflection of cognitive development. All of these assessments can be useful for planning intervention to promote development, but they do not tell us much about play itself or how to promote it.

What Players Do

Assessments such as Henry's (2008) Pediatric Interest Profiles (PIP) and, to a lesser extent, the Children's Assessment of Participation and Enjoyment (CAPE) and the Preferences for Activities of Children (PAC) (King et al., 2004) offer reliable and valid ways of assessing *what* players do. All of these assessments concentrate on factors such as interest, intensity, enjoyment, and context. The various versions of the PIP (Kid Play Profile and Preteen Play Profile) focus exclusively on play activities, whereas the CAPE and PAC extend beyond play to include a range of activities children do outside of school. A version of the PIP, the Adolescent Leisure Interest Profile, includes activities that may be classified as play or leisure. Scores for the various versions of the PIP offer comparisons with preferences of peers, although this information may be somewhat outdated, and not all activities are relevant to all geographic locations or cultures. All of these assessments provide descriptive data about individual children that can be useful for planning interventions. However, it can be difficult to interpret the meaning of scores from any of these interest-checklist-type assessments. Is it better to have a lot of preferred activities or just a few in which one is intensely engaged? And, how important is it that preferred activities match a child's skills (Clifford & Bundy, 1989)?

The Approach to Play

So far as we know, there is only one OT assessment, the Test of Playfulness (ToP) that targets children's approach to play (Skard & Bundy, 2008). And although there are not many adult assessments of play (Waldman-Levi & Bundy, 2016; Shen et al., 2014a, 2014b), they seem to fit best under this category. The ToP is occasionally used with adults as a self-report measure (e.g., Weigl & Bundy, 2013).

In the ToP, Skard and Bundy (2008) applied operational definitions of the characteristics of play (i.e., intrinsic motivation, etc.) to players themselves, arguing that these traits also characterized playful people. They further argued that playfulness is relevant to many occupations—not only to play. The ToP scores offer a comparison of playfulness across children of a range of ages and abilities. And although Skard and Bundy offered a means to compare individual ToP scores with those of a large data set, the meaning of relative amounts of playfulness is not yet clear. Importantly, some researchers have linked playfulness to coping, which may provide insight in this area (Hess & Bundy, 2003; I. Saunders, Sayer, & Goodale, 1999).

Supportiveness of the Environment

Assessments such as the Test of Environmental Supportiveness (TOES) by Skard and Bundy (2008) and the Young Children's Participation and Environment Measure (YC-PEM) by Khetani et al. take very different approaches to evaluating aspects of environmental supportiveness (Khetani, Coster, Law, & Bedell, 2013; Khetani, Graham, Davies, Law, & Simeonsson, 2015). The TOES is set in the context of a player's motivations for play (i.e., what players seem to be seeking). In administering the TOES, practitioners determine the extent to which four environmental components (playmates, caregivers, play objects, and space) promote or detract from players' abilities to meet their motivations for play. The TOES is best used as a tool for consultation with adults seeking to promote play by optimizing the supportiveness of the play environment. The YC-PEM items allow practitioners to assess the effect of environmental features (e.g., physical layout, sensory qualities, adult supports, peer relationships) on participation of young children at home, in daycare/preschool, and in the community. Play is an important aspect of participation for young children in all of these settings.

Motivations for Play

Numerous researchers and theorists studied motivation and wrote about ways of capturing and understanding it (Csikszentmihalyi, 1975a, 1975b, 1990; Ryan & Deci, 2017; White, 1959; Ziviani, Poulsen, & Cuskelly, 2012). The work of these authors applies to play and beyond. As described, knowledge of the source of motivation for play forms the basis for the TOES. However, so far as we know, there are no formal assessments for determining a child's motivations for particular play activities. Practitioners must glean information about motivation through observation and interview. To do so, they seek answers to questions such as: What does the child get from particular play activities? What play activities bring the child great joy? In what kinds of activities does the child become totally immersed?

⚖ PRACTICE DILEMMA

You work in a private practice that sees children with learning and behavioral difficulties. Your practice highly values client-centered care, which the owner of the practice interprets as meaning you address the goals a family asks you to address. The mother of 6-year-old Casey is seeking services for her son. Casey is the youngest of four children; the three oldest are honor students. Casey's mother is particularly worried that Casey is not keeping up in school. She has heard that occupational therapists are experts at visual motor integration, and she thinks that is Casey's problem. As part of the evaluation, and with the parents' permission, you speak with Casey's teacher. His teacher says that Casey is performing in the middle of his class in all subjects. She does not see any problem with his academic performance. *However, she is worried* about Casey socially. She says he wanders the playground at recess and rarely joins with any other children. She also mentioned that two boys in the class had birthday parties recently, and Casey was not invited to either. You ask Casey's mother about the teacher's observations and suggest that you assess Casey's play. Casey's mother is not interested. She says that her priority is his school work. His brother and sisters are "A" students, and she expects the same from Casey. She came to OT so Casey would do better in school. She certainly is not going to waste her money on play.

Question

1. How should you handle this situation?

Evaluation of Leisure

As with play, we know of no assessments of leisure that parallel our definition (i.e., the characteristics that separate leisure from other occupations). To structure our discussion of assessment, we use Hammel's (2009) categories of the benefits of leisure: (1) engagement in doing; (2) belonging, connecting, and contributing; (3) restoration; and (4) life continuity and hope for the future. Importantly, Hammell warned against prescribing how clients *should* use their time to obtain a balance between self-care, leisure, and productive occupations. Clients are the only ones

who can determine a balance that ensures their priorities and needs are met.

A range of assessments is available to support leisure assessment. Honoring client-centered assessment, we recommend the following, much of which, in addition to (and occasionally instead of) standardized assessment, requires interviewing clients and sometimes caregivers:

- Collaborating to identify meaningful activities that clients consider leisure
- Examining motivations for/benefits sought in leisure
- Examining the degree of control participants can and want to experience and the form they want that control to take
- Gaining an understanding of personal, environmental, and contextual factors that impact leisure choices and participation

Many self-report checklists query clients' interest in activities commonly associated with leisure as well as factors such as intensity and enjoyment. Clients describe any that they engage in presently or have done previously and those that are potential future pursuits. These include the Modified Interest Checklist by Kielhofner and Neville (Taylor, 2017), the Occupational Performance History Interview–Second Version (OPHI-II) by Kielhofner et al. (Taylor, 2017), and the Activity Card Sort (ACS) (second edition) by Baum and Edwards (2001). However, because the lists are predetermined, unless supplemented by interview, they may provide limited insight. Further, *being physically able to do a particular leisure activity, even if it was once highly valued, does not ensure full engagement or feelings of belonging, hope, or restoration in the present.*

When clients cannot self-report on opportunities and experiences they find meaningful, the Assessment Tool for Social and Occupational Engagement (ATOSE) by Morgan-Brown and Chard (2014) can be useful. In addition, in institutional settings, tools such as the Residential Environmental Impact Scale (REIS) that employ observation and interview can guide assessment (Fisher et al., 2014).

Importantly, when leisure is the primary occupation, the focus of assessment should be on the process and not the outcome (Fenech & Collier, 2017). Identifying personal strengths, abilities, preferences, and resources is particularly important (Townsend & Polatajko, 2007; Townsend & Wilcock, 2004). Functional outcomes are secondary to creating moments of shared joy and the sense of belonging (Du Toit, Shen, & McGrath, 2018; Hitch, Pépin, & Stagnitti, 2014).

Play and Leisure in Intervention

Play and leisure are meaningful, lifelong occupations. Thus, improved play or leisure is an important outcome in its own right. However, perhaps because of cultural and remaining professional beliefs that play and leisure are not as important as other occupations, they rarely seem to be explicit goals of intervention. Not surprisingly, few rigorously designed studies in OT have tested the effectiveness of interventions for promoting play and leisure.

In contrast, many OT practitioners use play as a means to achieve performance-related intervention goals (Blanche, 2008; Munier, Myers, & Pierce, 2008). As Pierce (2001b) indicated, a careful blend of pleasure, productivity, and restoration is likely to increase clients' motivation to participate in intervention.

Play and Leisure as Outcomes

Only very recently have OT researchers used rigorous research designs to examine the effectiveness of interventions for increasing play and related skills in children. The research in leisure is even less well developed than that in play.

Play Interventions

Two basic types of OT interventions focusing on play have been the subject of rigorous research: (1) modeling and facilitated play and (2) loose parts intervention and risk reframing. Wilkes-Gillan and colleagues engaged children with ADHD and a familiar playmate in direct and indirect intervention to increase play and social skills (Barnes, Wilkes-Gillan, Bundy, & Cordier, 2017; Cantrill, Wilkes-Gillan, Bundy, Cordier, & Wilson, 2015; Wilkes-Gillan, Bundy, Cordier, & Lincoln, 2016; Wilkes-Gillan et al., 2015; Wilkes-Gillan et al., 2017; Wilkes-Gillan et al., 2011). Their approach was based on Cordier's earlier studies of the patterns of play deficit common in children with ADHD (Cordier et al., 2009, 2010a, 2010b, 2010c). The intervention, conducted as a randomized controlled trial, involved video and therapist modeling and engaged the children in facilitated play to help them respond appropriately to playmates' cues. Parents carried out a home program using a video story of an alien whose earthling friends helped him see that he would have more fun if his playmate was also having fun. The researchers demonstrated maintained effectiveness 18 months after the intervention concluded. Cordier and colleagues are currently extending this intervention to children with autism (Cordier et al., 2009, 2010a, 2010b, 2010c).

In two cluster trials, Bundy and colleagues placed loose parts of recycled materials with no obvious play value on school playgrounds for children to play with at recess (Bundy et al., 2017; Bundy, Naughton, et al., 2011; Bundy et al., 2015; Engelen et al., 2013). Simultaneously, Niehues and colleagues conducted small-group interventions with parents and school staff to help them reconsider the value of manageable risk taking in play (Niehues, Bundy, Broom, & Tranter, 2015, 2016; Niehues et al., 2013; Spencer et al., 2016). Participating children (who were typically developing) in the first trial had increased physical activity at recess. Time spent playing also increased, but the change was not statistically significant. Most recently, the team applied the same interventions to children with autism and intellectual disability, targeting coping and quality of play on the playground (Bundy et al., 2015).

Using less rigorous research designs, OT researchers have reported the results of five other interventions designed to influence play—with varying results. Sonday and Gretschel (2016) utilized qualitative methodology to examine the effects, which were marked, of powered wheelchairs on the play of two children with physical disabilities. Three studies utilized single group, pretest–posttest designs (Bundy, Naughton, et al., 2011; Keen, Rodger, Doussin, & Braithwaite, 2007; O'Connor & Stagnitti, 2011; Stagnitti, O'Connor, & Sheppard, 2012). Two additional studies employed a pretest–posttest design and compared child and parent outcomes at multiple points (Fabrizi & Hubbell, 2017; Fabrizi, Ito, & Winston, 2016). Notably, all but one (Bundy, Naughton, et al., 2011) occurred in a natural setting (i.e., home, school or community-based play group). Two (Bundy, Kolrosova, et al., 2011; Keen et al., 2007) were parent interventions: one with parents of children with varying disabilities and one with parents of children with autism. Two (Fabrizi & Hubbell, 2017; Fabrizi et al., 2016) focused on the children but included parents as part of the playgroup intervention.

Fabrizi and colleagues found increases in child playfulness across playgroup types (Fabrizi & Hubbell, 2017; Fabrizi et al., 2016). However, they did not find increases in parent outcomes (parent competence or participation). In a hospital-based group intervention, Bundy, Naughton, et al. (2011) failed to find increases in child playfulness, but parents reported positive changes in interactions among family members. Keen et al. (2007) employed a combined workshop and home-based format (Stronger Families). Although parents reported some changes in communication and symbolic behaviors, those were not supported by evaluator-scored observation. Both Keen et al. and Stagnitti and colleagues targeted symbolic play in young children with autism in a small-group, school-based direct intervention that involved adults modeling play scripts (Learn to Play) (Keen et al., 2007; O'Connor & Stagnitti, 2011; Stagnitti et al., 2012). They did not find increases in pretend play. However, they reported increased social interaction and language and decreased social disconnection; they also found relationships between language and pretend play.

> ⚖️ **ETHICAL DILEMMA**
>
> You have recently taken a position with an agency that promotes nontraditional OT interventions. During the summer, the agency plans to run a day camp with a "magic" theme for school-age children with hemiplegic cerebral palsy. Professional magicians teaching magic tricks are expected to be a big draw for participants.

Children will come every weekday, all day, for 2 weeks. They will spend at least an hour every day engaged with an occupational therapist, helping them master the magic tricks, which they are expected to perform using both hands. The children also will spend time daily in bilateral gross motor games that you organize. The plan is to have three occupational therapists at the camp because there are 12 children in each session. The agency wants to bill third-party payers for OT to recoup the costs of the camp. You know it is unlikely that third-party payers would see occupational therapist to master magic tricks or gross motor games as medically necessary. What should you do?

- The children and their parents could set bilateral activities of daily living (ADL) or instrumental activities of daily living (IADL) goals at the start of camp and structure time every day for OT to meet those goals. Those sessions are more likely to be billable.
- Before hiring the two additional therapists, you could be upfront with the agency director about your concerns for billing and suggest that you work with OT students who could provide the interventions under your supervision.

Leisure Interventions

Occupational therapy research exploring interventions to promote leisure is sketchy. Practitioners frequently use adapted procedures to enhance leisure. Among occupational therapists who reported using leisure assessments to plan their intervention, 11% focused on developing ways to adapt leisure activities to match clients' skills (Turner, Chapman, McSherry, Krishnagiri, & Watts, 2000). However, most support for effectiveness is anecdotal. We know of no research to support the effectiveness.

In a textbook focusing on OT interventions for the elderly, Bundy and Clemson (2009) described the intervention for an elderly woman who reported that cooking for her family that had once been her primary leisure was no longer satisfying after she had a stroke. The occupational therapist intervened by teaching adapted procedures that the client could use to compensate for the mild weakness and abnormal muscle tone in her affected arm (e.g., sliding pans onto and off the cooktop rather than lifting them). Instead of focusing intervention on performance skills and remediation of motor control, the practitioner used the client's preferred leisure activity of cooking as a means to enable her to regain the experience of leisure.

Use of electronic media as an outcome is an area in which occupational therapists could expand our scope of practice. Researchers from other disciplines have explored how virtual worlds contribute to opportunities for leisure participation of people with disabilities (e.g., Stendal, Balandin, & Molka-Danielsen, 2011; Vizenor, 2014).

Studies are needed to explore the role of technology as an OT intervention to promote play and leisure, considering the boundaries between health and electronic media usage.

Play and Leisure as a Means for Meeting Other Goals

Practitioners using play or leisure as a means for meeting other goals are likely doing so to engage their clients fully in therapy. People learn skills through practice, and clients are more likely to keep practicing when it is fun. Nonetheless, little is known about the effectiveness of this approach—and so far as we know, there are no rigorous studies of play or leisure as a medium.

Play as a Medium

In the Sydney Playground Project, Bundy and colleagues implemented loose parts and risk-reframing interventions to increase physical activity and coping skills (Bundy & Clemson, 2009; Bundy et al., 2017; Bundy, Naughton, et al., 2011; Engelen et al., 2013). Because improving play also was a target of this intervention, we described it in the section on play as an outcome.

In reasonably large-scale surveys of occupational therapists working with young children, Couch, Deitz, and Kanny (1998) and, more recently, Miller Kuhaneck et al. found that therapists regarded play primarily as a motivator to entice children to participate in interventions to meet performance goals (Miller Kuhaneck, Tanta, Coombs, & Pannone, 2013). Several correlational studies suggest that engaging in play may enhance developmental skill acquisition (Harris & Reid, 2005), school readiness (Long, Bergeron, Doyle, & Gordon, 2006), and coping (Hess & Bundy, 2003; I. Saunders et al., 1999).

Leisure as a Medium

In a review of eight primarily cross-sectional studies investigating the effect of engaging in leisure activities on depression or self-esteem in elder adults, Fine (2001) concluded that participation had a positive effect on mental health. However, only one of the three most rigorous studies revealed a statistically significant effect on mental health, and in that study, relaxation had a greater effect than participation in active leisure (Bensink, Godbey, Marshall, & Yarandi, 1992).

We often rely on traits associated with leisure to promote participation in intervention to help clients gain or regain movement, especially when they experience discomfort or pain on moving. Case Study 53-2 describes an intervention where leisure was the medium. The case demonstrates how interest, motivation, and creativity supported a marine in improving strength and range of motion in his injured hand.

CASE STUDY 53-2   LEISURE AS A MEANS OF MEETING OTHER GOALS

Arthur is a 26-year-old marine stationed at Fort Worth and attending outpatient rehabilitation services. He damaged his right (preferred) hand in a motor vehicle accident. He was in the back seat, resting his elbow on the window frame with his hand gripping the roof. As a result of the accident, he experienced an arthrodesis of the interphalangeal joints of his right hand. Hand function was the target of the OT intervention. Although range of motion had improved, Arthur still experienced challenges with grip and strength. He found sessions with Theraputty™ and hand-exercise equipment

distressing and painful. Thus, the occupational therapist suggested that they make a gift for Arthur's girlfriend using different colors of grated soap, course sea salt, and dried lavender to create bath salts. (Arthur had often mentioned that his girlfriend was angry with him for not making sure the driver had been sober on the night of the accident.) Grating different shapes and sizes of soap and cutting and drying lavender sprigs improved his grip strength and provided him with profound satisfaction when he presented his girlfriend with the end product.

Conclusion

In a class lecture in the 1990s, Jeanne Pretorius, a lecturer at the University of the Free State in South Africa, dubbed leisure as the "stepchild of occupational therapy." About the same time, Bundy (1993) published a paper in the *American Journal of Occupational Therapy* addressing the problem of play and leisure: Despite being primary, lifelong occupations, neither was important enough to devote resources to developing valid and reliable assessments on which to base interventions. Almost a decade later, Turner et al. (2000) surveyed 103 therapists: 75% reported using leisure assessments to plan interventions, and 35% said that they used leisure activity in intervention to promote their clients' future leisure participation. Nonetheless, we uncovered no rigorous research examining the effectiveness of such interventions.

Play has fared better—but only slightly. In 1998 and again in 2015, researchers (Couch et al., 1998; Miller Kuhaneck et al., 2013) surveyed occupational therapists working with preschool-age children. All respondents in both surveys regarded play primarily as a motivator to entice children to participate in intervention to elicit improvement in other areas. Nonetheless, so far as we know, there are no rigorous studies of play as a medium. There are a handful of rigorous studies done by two groups of researchers—Cordier and colleagues (Barnes et al., 2017; Cantrill et al., 2015; Wilkes-Gillan et al., 2016; Wilkes-Gillan et al., 2015; Wilkes-Gillan et al., 2017; Wilkes et al., 2011) and Bundy and colleagues (Bundy & Clemson, 2009; Bundy et al., 2017; Bundy, Naughton, et al., 2011; Engelen et al., 2013)—promoting play as an outcome. Several other groups have attempted to promote play using somewhat less rigorous research designs with varying results.

A quarter of a century later, we have made some, but not nearly enough, progress in promoting play and leisure as primary, lifelong occupations. As proponents of social and occupational justice, we have a duty to ensure access to non–income-generating ("non-productive") occupations

that support engagement in doing, belonging, connecting, and contributing; restoration; life continuity; and hope for the future.

 Visit thePoint to watch a video about therapeutic play.

REFERENCES

Allen, J. M., Kellegrew, D. H., & Jaffe, D. (2000). The experience of pet ownership as a meaningful occupation. *Canadian Journal of Occupational Therapy, 67,* 271–278.

Allen, K. R., & Chin-Sang, V. (1990). A lifetime of work: The context and meanings of leisure for aging black women. *The Gerontologist, 30,* 734–740.

American Occupational Therapy Association. (2014). Occupational therapy practice framework: Domain and process (3rd ed.). *American Journal of Occupational Therapy, 68,* S1–S48.

Atchley, R. C. (1989). A continuity theory of normal aging. *The Gerontologist, 29,* 183–190.

Atchley, R. C. (1993). Continuity theory and the evolution of activity in later adulthood. In J. R. Kelly (Ed.), *Activity and aging* (pp. 5–16). Newbury Park, CA: Sage.

Atler, K. (2014). The daily experiences of pleasure, productivity and restoration profile: A measure of subjective experiences. In D. Pierce (Ed.), *Occupational science for occupational therapy* (pp. 187–199). Thorofare, NJ: SLACK.

Barnes, G., Wilkes-Gillan, S., Bundy, A., & Cordier, R. (2017). The social play, social skills and parent–child relationships of children with ADHD 12 months following a RCT of a play-based intervention. *Australian Occupational Therapy Journal, 64,* 457–465.

Bateson, G. (1972). Toward a theory of play and phantasy. In G. Bateson (Ed.), *Steps to an ecology of the mind* (pp. 14–20). New York, NY: Bantam.

Baum, C. M., & Edwards, D. (2001). *ACS: Activity card sort.* St Louis, MO: Washington University School of Medicine.

Bensink, G. W., Godbey, K. L., Marshall, M. J., & Yarandi, H. N. (1992). Institutionalized elderly. Relaxation, locus of control, self-esteem. *Journal of Gerontological Nursing, 18,* 30–36.

Beresin, A. (1993). *The play of peer cultures in a city school yard: "reeling," "writhing," and "a rhythmic kick"* (Doctoral dissertation). University of Pennsylvania, PA.

Berger, S. (2010). The meaning of leisure for older adults living with vision loss. *OTJR: Occupation, Participation and Health, 31,* 193–199.

Bevil, C. A., O'Connor, P. C., & Mattoon, P. M. (1994). Leisure activity, life satisfaction, and perceived health status in older adults. *Gerontology & Geriatrics Education, 14,* 3–19.

Bier, N., Dutil, E., & Couture, M. (2009). Factors affecting leisure participation after a traumatic brain injury: An exploratory study. *The Journal of Head Trauma Rehabilitation, 24,* 187–194.

Blanche, E. I. (2008). Play in children with cerebral palsy: Doing with—Not doing to. In L. D. Parham & L. S. Fazio (Eds.), *Play in occupational therapy for children* (2nd ed., pp. 375–393). St. Louis, MO: Mosby.

Boucher, N., Dumas, F., Maltais, D. B., & Richards, C. L. (2010). The influence of selected personal and environmental factors on leisure activities in adults with cerebral palsy. *Disability and Rehabilitation, 32,* 1328–1338.

Brussoni, M., Gibbons, R., Gray, C., Ishikawa, T., Sandseter, E. B., Bienenstock, A., . . . Tremblay, M. (2015). What is the relationship between risky outdoor play and health in children? A systematic review. *International Journal of Environmental Research and Public Health, 12,* 6423–6454.

Bundy, A. C. (1993). Assessment of play and leisure: Delineation of the problem. *American Journal of Occupational Therapy, 47,* 217–222.

Bundy, A. C. (2012). Play: The primary occupation of childhood: Can I play too? In S. J. Lane & A. C. Bundy (Eds.), *Kids can be kids. A childhood occupations approach* (pp. 29–43). Philadelphia, PA: F. A. Davis.

Bundy, A. C., & Clemson, L. M. (2009). Leisure. In B. Bonder (Ed.), *Functional performance in older adults* (3rd ed., pp. 290–306). Philadelphia, PA: F. A. Davis.

Bundy, A., DuToit, S., & Clemson, L. (2018). Leisure. In B. Bonder & V. D. Bello-Haas (Eds.), *Functional performance in older adults* (4th ed., pp. 295–311). Philadelphia, PA: F. A. Davis.

Bundy, A., Engelen, L., Wyver, S., Tranter, P., Ragen, J., Bauman, A., . . . Naughton, G. (2017). Sydney playground project: A cluster-randomized trial to increase physical activity, play, and social skills. *The Journal of School Health, 87,* 751–759.

Bundy, A., Kolrosova, J., Paguinto, S.-G., Bray, P., Swain, B., Wallen, M., & Engelen, L. (2011). Comparing the effectiveness of a parent group intervention with child-based intervention for promoting playfulness in children with disabilities. *Israeli Journal of Occupational Therapy, 20,* e95–e113.

Bundy, A. C., Naughton, G., Tranter, P., Wyver, S., Baur, L., Schiller, W., . . . Brentnall, J. (2011). The Sydney playground project: Popping the bubblewrap—Unleashing the power of play: A cluster randomized controlled trial of a primary school playground-based intervention aiming to increase children's physical activity and social skills. *BMC Public Health, 11,* 680–688.

Bundy, A., Wyver, S., Beetham, K. S., Ragen, J., Naughton, G., Tranter, P., . . . Sterman, J. (2015). The Sydney playground project—Levelling the playing field: A cluster trial of a primary school-based intervention aiming to promote manageable risk-taking in children with disability. *BMC Public Health, 15,* 1125. doi:10.1186/s12889-015-2452-4

Burack, O. R., Reinhardt, J. P., & Weiner, A. S. (2012). Person-centered care and elder choice: A look at implementation and sustainability. *Clinical Gerontologist, 35,* 390–403.

Caillois, R. (1979). *Man, play and games.* New York, NY: Schocken Books.

Canadian Association of Occupational Therapy. (1996). Occupational therapy and children's play. *Canadian Journal of Occupational Therapy, 63,* 1–20.

Cantrill, A., Wilkes-Gillan, S., Bundy, A., Cordier, R., & Wilson, N. J. (2015). An eighteen-month follow-up of a pilot parent-delivered play-based intervention to improve the social play skills of children with attention deficit hyperactivity disorder and their playmates. *Australian Occupational Therapy Journal, 62,* 197–207.

Casey, T., Chatterjee, S., Assi, M., Maharjan, S., Wirunrapan, K., & Gupta, S. (2017, September). *Unleashing the power of play in situations of crisis.* Paper presented at the 20th International Play Association Triennial World Conference, Calgary, Alberta, Canada.

Causey-Upton, R. (2015). A model for quality of life: Occupational justice and leisure continuity for nursing home residents. *Physical & Occupational Therapy in Geriatrics, 33,* 175–188.

Chung, J. C. (2004). Activity participation and well-being of people with dementia in long-term—Care settings. *OTJR: Occupation, Participation and Health, 24,* 22–31.

Clifford, J. M., & Bundy, A. C. (1989). Play preference and play performance in normal boys and boys with sensory integrative dysfunction. *Occupational Therapy Journal of Research, 9,* 202–217.

Cohen-Mansfield, J. (2005). Nonpharmacological interventions for persons with dementia. *Alzheimer's Care Quarterly, 6,* 129.

Coleman, D., & Iso-Ahola, S. E. (1993). Leisure and health: The role of social support and self-determination. *Journal of Leisure Research, 25,* 111.

Connor, F. P., Siepp, J. M., & Williamson, G. G. (1978). *Program guide for infants and toddlers with neuromotor and other developmental disabilities.* New York, NY: Teachers College Press.

Cordier, R., Bundy, A., Hocking, C., & Einfeld, S. (2009). A model for play-based intervention for children with ADHD. *Australian Occupational Therapy Journal, 56,* 332–340.

Cordier, R., Bundy, A., Hocking, C., & Einfeld, S. (2010a). Comparison of the play of children with attention deficit hyperactivity disorder by subtypes. *Australian Occupational Therapy Journal, 57,* 137–145.

Cordier, R., Bundy, A., Hocking, C., & Einfeld, S. (2010b). Empathy in the play of children with attention deficit hyperactivity disorder. *OTJR: Occupation, Participation and Health, 30,* 122–132.

Cordier, R., Bundy, A., Hocking, C., & Einfeld, S. (2010c). Playing with a child with ADHD: A focus on the playmates. *Scandinavian Journal of Occupational Therapy, 17,* 191–199.

Cosbey, J., Johnston, S. S., Dunn, M. L., & Bauman, M. (2012). Playground behaviors of children with and without sensory processing disorders. *OTJR: Occupation, Participation and Health, 32,* 39–47.

Coster, W. (1998). Occupation-centered assessment of children. *American Journal of Occupational Therapy, 52,* 337–344.

Couch, K. J., Deitz, J. C., & Kanny, E. M. (1998). The role of play in pediatric occupational therapy. *American Journal of Occupational Therapy, 52,* 111–117.

Couture, M., Caron, C. D., & Desrosiers, J. (2010). Leisure activities following a lower limb amputation. *Disability and Rehabilitation, 32,* 57–64.

Csikszentmihalyi, M. (1975a). *Beyond boredom and anxiety: The experience of play in work and games.* San Francisco, CA: Jossey-Bass.

Csikszentmihalyi, M. (1975b). Play and intrinsic rewards. *Humanistic Psychology, 15*(3), 41–63.

Csikszentmihalyi, M. (1990). *Flow. The psychology of optimal experience.* New York, NY: HarperPerennial.

Csikszentmihalyi, M., & Halton, E. (1981). *The meaning of things: Domestic symbols and the self.* Cambridge, United Kingdom: Cambridge University Press.

Csikszentmihalyi, M., & Kleiber, D. A. (1991). Leisure and self-actualization. In B. L. Driver, P. J. Brown, & G. L. Peterson (Eds.), *Benefits of leisure* (pp. 91–102). State College, PA: Venture.

Desha, L., Ziviani, J., & Rodger, S. (2003). Play preferences and behavior of preschool children with autistic spectrum disorder in the clinical environment. *Physical & Occupational Therapy in Pediatrics, 23,* 21–42.

Dionigi, R. (2017). Leisure and recreation in the lives of older people. In M. Bernoth & D. Winkler (Eds.), *Healthy ageing and aged care* (pp. 204–220). Oxford, United Kingdom: Oxford University Press.

Duncan-Myers, A. M., & Huebner, R. A. (2000). Relationship between choice and quality of life among residents in long-term-care facilities. *American Journal of Occupational Therapy, 54,* 504–508.

Du Toit, S. H. J., Shen, X., & McGrath, M. (2018). Meaningful engagement and person-centered residential dementia care: A critical interpretive synthesis. *Scandinavian Journal of Occupational Therapy.* Advance online publication. doi:10.1080/11038128.2018.1441323

Eakman, A. M., Atler, K. M., Rumble, M., & Gee, B. M. (in press). A qualitative research synthesis of positive subjective experiences in occupation from the Journal of Occupational Science (1993–2010). *Journal of Occupational Science.*

Engelen, L., Bundy, A. C., Naughton, G., Simpson, J. M., Bauman, A., Ragen, J., . . . van der Ploeg, H. P. (2013). Increasing physical activity in young primary school children—It's child's play: A cluster randomised controlled trial. *Preventive Medicine, 56,* 319–325.

Engel-Yeger, B., & Hanna Kasis, A. (2010). The relationship between developmental co-ordination disorder, child's perceived self-efficacy and preference to participate in daily activities. *Child: Care, Health and Development, 36,* 670–677.

Fabrigoule, C., Letenneur, L., Dartigues, J. F., Zarrouk, M., Commenges, D., & Barberger-Gateau, P. (1995). Social and leisure activities and risk of dementia: A prospective longitudinal study. *Journal of the American Geriatrics Society, 43,* 485–490.

Fabrizi, S., & Hubbell, K. (2017). The role of occupational therapy in promoting playfulness, parent competence, and social participation in early childhood playgroups: A pretest posttest design. *Journal of Occupational Therapy, Schools and Early Intervention, 10,* 346–365.

Fabrizi, S. E., Ito, M. A., & Winston, K. (2016). Effect of occupational therapy–led playgroups in early intervention on child playfulness and caregiver responsiveness: A repeated-measures design. *American Journal of Occupational Therapy, 70,* 700220020p1–700220020p9.

Fenech, A., & Collier, L. (2017). Leisure as a route to social and occupational justice for individuals with profound levels of disability. In D. Sakellariou & Pollard, N. (Eds.), *Occupational therapies without borders: Integrating justice with practice* (2nd ed., pp. 126–133). Edinburgh, United Kingdom: Elsevier.

Fine, J. (2001). The effect of leisure activity on depression in the elderly: Implications for the field of occupational therapy. *Occupational Therapy in Health Care, 13,* 45–59.

Fisher, G., Forsyth, K., Harrison, M., Angarola, R., Kayhan, E., Noga, P., . . . Irvine, L. (2014). *Resident Environment Impact Scale (REIS) (Version 4.0 User's Manual).* Chicago, IL: University of IL at Chicago Department of Occupational Therapy, The MOHO Clearinghouse.

Fleming, J., Braithwaite, H., Gustafsson, L., Griffin, J., Collier, A. M., & Fletcher, S. (2011). Participation in leisure activities during brain injury rehabilitation. *Brain Injury, 25,* 806–818.

Freysinger, V. J. (1993). The community, programs, and opportunities: Population diversity. In J. R. Kelly (Ed.), *Activity and aging* (pp. 211–230). Newbury Park, CA: Sage.

García-Martín, M. Á., Gómez-Jacinto, L., & Martimportugués-Goyenechea, C. (2004). A structural model of the effects of organized leisure activities on the well-being of elder adults in Spain. *Activities, Adaptation & Aging, 28,* 19–34.

Gerlach, A., Browne, A., & Suto, M. (2014). A critical reframing of play in relation to indigenous children in Canada. *Journal of Occupational Science, 21,* 243–258.

Glynn, M. A., & Webster, J. (1992). The adult playfulness scale: An initial assessment. *Psychological Reports, 71,* 83–103.

Godbey, G. (1994). *Leisure in your life: An exploration* (4th ed.). State College, PA: Venture.

Goltz, H., & Brown, T. (2014). Are children's psychological self-concepts predictive of their self reported activity preferences and leisure participation? *Australian Occupational Therapy Journal, 61,* 177–186.

Goodman, C. C. (1984). Natural helping among older adults. *The Gerontologist, 24,* 138–143.

Graham, N., Truman, J., & Holgate, H. (2014). An exploratory study: Expanding the concept of play for children with severe cerebral palsy. *British Journal of Occupational Therapy, 77,* 358–365.

Griffin, J., & McKenna, K. (1999). Influences on leisure and life satisfaction of elderly people. *Physical & Occupational Therapy in Geriatrics, 15*(4), 1–16.

Hackett, J. (2003). Perceptions of play and leisure in junior school aged children with juvenile idiopathic arthritis: What are the implications for occupational therapy? *British Journal of Occupational Therapy, 66,* 303–310.

Hamm, E. M. (2006). Playfulness and the environmental support of play in children with and without developmental disabilities. *OTJR: Occupation, Participation and Health, 26,* 88–96.

Hammell, K. W. (2004a). Dimensions of meaning in the occupations of daily life. *Canadian Journal of Occupational Therapy, 71,* 296–305.

Hammell, K. W. (2004b). Quality of life among people with high spinal cord injury living in the community. *Spinal Cord, 42,* 607–620.

Hammell, K. W. (2007). Reflections on . . . a disability methodology for the client-centred practice of occupational therapy research. *Canadian Journal of Occupational Therapy, 74,* 365–369.

Hammell, K. W. (2009). Self-care, productivity, and leisure, or dimensions of occupational experience? Rethinking occupational "categories." *Canadian Journal of Occupational Therapy, 76,* 107–114.

Harris, K., & Reid, D. (2005). The influence of virtual reality play on children's motivation. *Canadian Journal of Occupational Therapy, 72,* 21–29.

Havighurst, R. J. (1979). The nature and values of meaningful free-time activity. In R. W. Kleemeier (Ed.), *Aging and leisure* (pp. 309–344). New York, NY: Arno Press.

Henricks, T. S. (2010). Caillois's "Man, Play, and Games": An appreciation and evaluation. *American Journal of Play, 3,* 157–185.

Henricks, T. (2017). Foreword. In C. L. Phillips, G. R. Adams, S. G. Eberle, & R. Hogan. (Eds.), *Play for life: Play theory and play as emotional survival.* Rochester, NY: The Strong.

Henry, A. (2008). Assessment of play and leisure in children and adolescents. In L. D. Parham & L. S. Fazio (Eds.), *Play in occupational therapy for children* (2nd ed., pp. 95–191). St. Louis, MO: Mosby.

Hess, L. M., & Bundy, A. C. (2003). The association between playfulness and coping in adolescents. *Physical & Occupational Therapy in Pediatrics, 23,* 5–17.

Hitch, D., Pépin, G., & Stagnitti, K. (2014). In the footsteps of Wilcock, part one: The evolution of doing, being, becoming, and belonging. *Occupational Therapy in Health Care, 28,* 231–246.

Hughes, L. (1993a). Children's games and gaming. In B. Sutton-Smith (Ed.), *Children's folklore: A sourcebook* (pp. 93–120). New York, NY: Garland.

Hughes, L. A. (1993b). "You have to do it with style": Girls' games and girls' gaming. In T. Hollis, L. Pershing, & M. J. Young (Eds.), *Feminist theory and the study of folklore* (pp. 130–148). Urbana, IL: University of Illinois Press.

Hurd, A. R., & Anderson, D. M. (2010). *The park and recreation professional's handbook.* Champaign, IL: Human Kinetics.

Imms, C. (2008). Children with cerebral palsy participate: A review of the literature. *Disability and Rehabilitation, 30,* 1867–1884.

Ismael, N. T., Lawson, L. M., & Cox, J. A. (2015). The relationship between children's sensory processing patterns and their leisure preferences and participation patterns. *Canadian Journal of Occupational Therapy, 82,* 316–324.

Iso-Ahola, S. E., Jackson, E. L., & Dunn, E. (1994). Starting, ceasing, and replacing leisure activities over the human life-span. *Journal of Leisure Research, 26,* 227–249.

Jackson, E. L., & Burton, T. L. (1999). *Leisure studies prospects for the twenty-first century.* State College, PA: Venture.

Jacobson, S., & Samdahl, D. M. (1998). Leisure in the lives of old lesbians: Experiences with and responses to discrimination. *Journal of Leisure Research, 30,* 233–255.

Jessup, G., Bundy, A. C., & Cornell, E. (2013). To be or to refuse to be? Exploring the concept of leisure as resistance for young people who are visually impaired. *Leisure Studies, 32,* 191–205.

Jessup, G., Cornell, E., & Bundy, A. C. (2010). The treasure in leisure activities: Fostering resilience in young people who are blind. *Journal of Visual Impairment & Blindness, 104,* 419–430.

Jonsson, H. (2008). A new direction in the conceptualization and categorization of occupation. *Journal of Occupational Science, 15,* 3–8.

Jonsson, H. (2011). The first steps into the third age: The retirement process from a Swedish perspective. *Occupational Therapy International, 18,* 32–38.

Keen, D., Rodger, S., Doussin, K., & Braithwaite, M. (2007). A pilot study of the effects of a social-pragmatic intervention on the communication and symbolic play of children with autism. *Autism, 11,* 63–71.

Kelly, J. R. (1982). Leisure in later life: Roles and identities. In N. J. Osgood (Ed.), *Life after work* (pp. 268–292). New York, NY: Praeger.

Kelly, J. R. (1993). Theory and issues. In J. R. Kelly (Ed.), *Activity and aging* (pp. 5–16). Newbury Park, CA: Sage.

Kennedy-Behr, A., Rodger, S., & Mickan, S. (2013). A comparison of the play skills of preschool children with and without developmental coordination disorder. *OTJR: Occupation, Participation and Health, 33,* 198–208.

Kent, C., Cordier, R., Joosten, A., Wilkes-Gillan, S., & Bundy, A. (2018). Peer-mediated intervention to improve play skills in children with autism spectrum disorder: A feasibility study. *Australian Occupational Therapy Journal.* doi:10.1111/1440-1630.12459

Khetani, M., Coster, W., Law, M., & Bedell, G. (2013). *Young children's participation and environment measure.* Ontario, Canada: CanChild.

Khetani, M. A., Graham, J. E., Davies, P. L., Law, M. C., & Simeonsson, R. J. (2015). Psychometric properties of the young children's participation and environment measure. *Archives of Physical Medicine and Rehabilitation, 96,* 307–316.

Kielhofner, G. (2009). *Conceptual foundations of occupational therapy practice* (4th ed.). Philadelphia, PA: F. A. Davis.

King, G., Law, M., King, S., Hurley, P., Hanna, S., Kertoy, M., . . . Young, N. (2004). *Children's Assessment of Participation and Enjoyment (CAPE) and Preferences for Activities of Children (PAC).* San Antonio, TX: Harcourt Assessment.

King, G., Law, M., Petrenchik, T., & Hurley, P. (2013). Psychosocial determinants of out of school activity participation for children with and without physical disabilities. *Physical & Occupational Therapy in Pediatrics, 33,* 384–404.

Kleiber, D. A., Hutchinson, S. L., & Williams, R. (2002). Leisure as a resource in transcending negative life events: Self-protection, self-restoration, and personal transformation. *Leisure Sciences, 24,* 219–235.

Knox, S. (2008). Development and current use of the revised Knox Preschool Play Scale. In L. D. Parham & L. S. Fazio (Eds.), *Play in occupational therapy for children* (2nd ed., pp. 55–70). St. Louis, MO: Mosby.

Kolehmainen, N., Ramsay, C., McKee, L., Missiuna, C., Owen, C., & Francis, J. (2015). Participation in physical play and leisure in children with motor impairments: Mixed-methods study to generate evidence for developing an intervention. *Physical Therapy, 95,* 1374–1386.

Kuhaneck, H. M., & Britner, P. A. (2013). A preliminary investigation of the relationship between sensory processing and social play in autism spectrum disorder. *OTJR: Occupation, Participation and Health, 33,* 159–167.

Laliberte-Rudman, D., Yu, B., Scott, E., & Pajouhandeh, P. (2000). Exploration of the perspectives of persons with schizophrenia regarding quality of life. *American Journal of Occupational Therapy, 54,* 137–147.

Lape, J. (2009). Using a multisensory environment to decrease negative behaviors in clients with dementia. *OT Practice, 14*(9), 9–13.

Lau, A., Chi, I., & McKenna, K. (1998). Self-perceived quality of life of Chinese elderly people in Hong Kong. *Occupational Therapy International, 5,* 118–139.

LaVesser, P., & Berg, C. (2011). Participation patterns in preschool children with an autism spectrum disorder. *OTJR: Occupation, Participation and Health, 31,* 33–39.

Law, M., Anaby, D., DeMatteo, C., & Hanna, S. (2011). Participation patterns of children with acquired brain injury. *Brain Injury, 25,* 587–595.

Lawton, M. P. (1993). Meanings of activity. In J. R. Kelly (Ed.), *Activity and aging* (pp. 25–41). Newbury Park, CA: Sage.

Lee, D. T., Woo, J., & Mackenzie, A. E. (2002). A review of older people's experiences with residential care placement. *Journal of Advanced Nursing, 37,* 19–27.

Leipold, E., & Bundy, A. C. (2000). Playfulness in children with attention deficit hyperactivity disorder. *Occupational Therapy Journal of Research, 20,* 61–82.

Linder, T. (2008). *Transdisciplinary play-based assessment* (2nd ed.). Baltimore, MD: Paul Brookes.

Long, D., Bergeron, J., Doyle, S. L., & Gordon, C. Y. (2006). The relationship between frequency of participation in play activities and kindergarten readiness. *Occupational Therapy in Health Care, 19,* 23–42.

Losier, G. F., Bourque, P. E., & Vallerand, R. J. (1993). A motivational model of leisure participation in the elderly. *The Journal of Psychology, 127,* 153–170.

Lynch, H., Hayes, N., & Ryan, S. (2016). Exploring socio-cultural influences on infant play occupations in Irish home environments. *Journal of Occupational Science, 23,* 352–369.

Majnemer, A., Shevell, M., Law, M., Birnbaum, R., Chilingaryan, G., Rosenbaum, P., & Poulin, C. (2008). Participation and enjoyment of leisure activities in school-aged children with cerebral palsy. *Developmental Medicine and Child Neurology, 50,* 751–758.

Majnemer, A., Shikako-Thomas, K., Chokron, N., Law, M., Shevell, M., Chilingaryan, G., . . . Rosenbaum, P. (2010). Leisure activity preferences for 6- to 12-year-old children with cerebral palsy. *Developmental Medicine and Child Neurology, 52,* 167–173.

Mannell, R. C., Zuzanek, J., & Larson, R. (1988). Leisure states and "flow" experiences: Testing perceived freedom and intrinsic motivation hypotheses. *Journal of Leisure Research, 20,* 289–304.

McGuire, F. A., Boyd, R., & Tedrick, R. T. (2004). *Leisure and aging: Ulyssean living in later life* (2nd ed.). Champaign, IL: Sagamore.

McKenna, K., Liddle, J., Brown, A., Lee, K., & Gustafsson, L. (2009). Comparison of time use, role participation and life satisfaction of older people after stroke with a sample without stroke. *Australian Occupational Therapy Journal, 56,* 177–188.

Miller Kuhaneck, H., Tanta, K. J., Coombs, A. K., & Pannone, H. (2013). A survey of pediatric occupational therapists' use of play. *Journal of Occupational Therapy, Schools and Early Intervention, 6,* 213–227.

Mishra, S. (1992). Leisure activities and life satisfaction in old age: A case study of retired government employees living in urban areas. *Activities, Adaptation & Aging, 16,* 7–26.

Morgan-Brown, M., & Chard, G. (2014). Comparing communal environments using the Assessment Tool for Occupation and Social Engagement: Using interactive occupation and social engagement as outcome measures. *British Journal of Occupational Therapy, 77,* 50–58.

Morgan-Brown, M., Ormerod, M., Newton, R., Manley, D., & Fitzpatrick, M. (2011). Social and occupational engagement of staff in two Irish nursing homes for people with dementia. *Irish Journal of Occupational Therapy, 39,* 11–17.

Mortenson, P. A., & Harris, S. R. (2006). Playfulness in children with traumatic brain injury: A preliminary study. *Physical and Occupational Therapy in Pediatrics, 26*(1–2), 181–198.

Munier, V., Myers, C. T., & Pierce, D. (2008). Power of object play for infants and toddlers. In L. D. Parham & L. S. Fazio (Eds.), *Play in occupational therapy for children* (2nd ed., pp. 219–249). St. Louis, MO: Mosby.

Nagle, S., Cook, J. V., & Polatajko, H. J. (2002). I'm doing as much as I can: Occupational choices of persons with a severe and persistent mental illness. *Journal of Occupational Science, 9,* 72–81.

Nash, J. B. (1953). *Philosophy of recreation and leisure.* Dubuque, IA: William C. Brown.

Neulinger, J. (1974). *The psychology of leisure: Research approaches to the study of leisure.* Springfield, IL: Charles C. Thomas.

Neumann, E. A. (1971). *The elements of play.* New York, NY: MSS Information.

Niehues, A. N., Bundy, A., Broom, A., & Tranter, P. (2015). Parents' perceptions of risk and the influence on children's everyday activities. *Journal of Child and Family Studies, 24,* 809–820.

Niehues, A. N., Bundy, A., Broom, A., & Tranter, P. (2016). Reframing healthy risk taking: Parents' dilemmas and strategies to promote children's well-being. *Journal of Occupational Science, 23,* 449–463.

Niehues, A. N., Bundy, A., Broom, A., Tranter, P., Ragen, J., & Engelen, L. (2013). Everyday uncertainties: reframing perceptions of risk in outdoor free play. *Journal of Adventure Education & Outdoor Learning, 13,* 223–237.

Oates, A., Bebbington, A., Bourke, J., Girdler, S., & Leonard, H. (2011). Leisure participation for school-aged children with Down syndrome. *Disability and Rehabilitation, 33,* 1880–1889.

O'Brien, A., Renwick, R., & Yoshida, K. (2008). Leisure participation for individuals living with acquired spinal cord injury. *International Journal of Rehabilitation Research, 31,* 225–230.

O'Connor, C., & Stagnitti, K. (2011). Play, behaviour, language and social skills: The comparison of a play and a non-play intervention within a specialist school setting. *Research in Developmental Disabilities, 32,* 1205–1211.

O'Sullivan, C., & Chard, G. (2010). An exploration of participation in leisure activities post-stroke. *Australian Occupational Therapy Journal, 57,* 159–166.

Parham, L. D. (1996). Perspectives on play. In R. Zemke & (Eds.), *Occupational science: The evolving discipline* (pp. 71–80). Philadelphia, PA: F. A. Davis.

Parham, L. D. (2008). Play and occupational therapy. In L. D. Parham & L. S. Fazio (Eds.), *Play in occupational therapy for children* (2nd ed., pp. 3–39). St. Louis, MO: Mosby.

Passmore, A., & French, D. (2003). The nature of leisure in adolescence: A focus group study. *British Journal of Occupational Therapy, 66,* 419–426.

Pereira, R. B., & Stagnitti, K. (2006, July). *The relationship between leisure experiences and health in an ageing Italian community in Australia.* Paper presented at the 14th World Federation of Occupational Therapists Congress, Sydney, Australia.

Pfeifer, L. I., Pacciulio, A. M., Santos, C. A., Santos, J. L., & Stagnitti, K. E. (2011). Pretend play of children with cerebral palsy. *Physical & Occupational Therapy in Pediatrics, 31,* 390–402.

Pierce, D. (2001a). Occupation by design: Dimensions, therapeutic power, and creative process. *American Journal of Occupational Therapy, 55,* 249–259.

Pierce, D. (2001b). Untangling occupation and activity. *American Journal of Occupational Therapy, 55,* 138–146.

Pierce, D. (2003). *Occupation by design: Building therapeutic power.* Philadelphia, PA: F. A. Davis.

Pierce, D. (2009). Co-occupation: The challenges of defining concepts original to occupational science. *Journal of Occupational Science, 16,* 203–207.

Pierce, D. (2014). *Occupational science for occupational therapy.* Thorofare, NJ: SLACK.

Pieris, Y., & Craik, C. (2004). Factors enabling and hindering participation in leisure for people with mental health problems. *British Journal of Occupational Therapy, 67,* 240–247.

Pöllänen, S. H., & Hirsimäki, R. M. (2014). Crafts as memory triggers in reminiscence: A case study of older women with dementia. *Occupational Therapy in Health Care, 28,* 410–430.

Power, G. A. (2010). *Dementia beyond drugs: Changing the culture of care.* Baltimore, MD: Health Professions Press.

Powrie, B., Kolehmainen, N., Turpin, M., Ziviani, J., & Copley, J. (2015). The meaning of leisure for children and young people with physical disabilities: A systematic evidence synthesis. *Developmental Medicine and Child Neurology, 57,* 993–1010.

Pretorius, J. (1993). *Recreation, the stepchild of occupational therapy. Recreation lecture* (ABT114). University of the Free State, South Africa.

Primeau, L. A. (1996). Work and leisure: Transcending the dichotomy. *American Journal of Occupational Therapy, 50,* 569–577.

Raber, C., Teitelman, J., Watts, J., & Kielhofner, G. (2010). A phenomenological study of volition in everyday occupations of older people with dementia. *British Journal of Occupational Therapy, 73,* 498–506.

Raghavendra, P., Virgo, R., Olsson, C., Connell, T., & Lane, A. E. (2011). Activity participation of children with complex communication needs, physical disabilities and typically-developing peers. *Developmental Neurorehabilitation, 14,* 145–155.

Ramugondo, E. L. (2012). Intergenerational play within family: The case for occupational consciousness. *Journal of Occupational Science, 19,* 326–340.

Raymore, L. A., Barber, B. L., Eccles, J. S., & Godbey, G. C. (1999). Leisure behavior pattern stability during the transition from adolescence to young adulthood. *Journal of Youth and Adolescence, 28,* 79–103.

Reilly, M. (1974). An explanation of play. In M. Reilly (Ed.), *Play as exploratory learning: Studies of curiosity behavior* (pp. 117–149). Beverly Hills, CA: Sage.

Reinseth, L., & Arild Espnes, G. (2007). Women with rheumatoid arthritis: Non-vocational activities and quality of life. *Scandinavian Journal of Occupational Therapy, 14,* 108–115.

Rockwell-Dylla, L. A. (1992). *Older adults' meaning of environment: Hospital and home.* Chicago, IL: University of Illinois at Chicago.

Rodríguez, A., Látková, P., & Sun, Y.-Y. (2008). The relationship between leisure and life satisfaction: Application of activity and need theory. *Social Indicators Research, 86,* 163–175.

Rubin, K., Fein, G., & Vandenberg, B. (1983). Play. In P. H. Mussen (Ed.), *Handbook of child psychology: Socialization, personality and social development* (Vol. 4, pp. 693–774). New York, NY: Wiley.

Ryan, R. M., & Deci, E. L. (2017). *Self-determination theory: Basic psychological needs in motivation, development, and wellness.* New York, NY: Guilford Press.

Sandseter, E. B. H., & Kennair, L. E. O. (2011). Children's risky play from an evolutionary perspective: The anti-phobic effects of thrilling experiences. *Evolutionary Psychology, 9,* 257–284.

Saunders, E. B. (1922). Psychiatry and occupational therapy. *Archives of Occupational Therapy, 1,* 99–114.

Saunders, I., Sayer, M., & Goodale, A. (1999). The relationship between playfulness and coping in preschool children: A pilot study. *American Journal of Occupational Therapy, 53,* 221–226.

Scraton, S., & Holland, S. (2006). Grandfatherhood and leisure. *Leisure Studies, 25,* 233–250.

Shen, X. S., Chick, G., & Zinn, H. (2014a). Playfulness in adulthood as a personality trait: A reconceptualization and a new measurement. *Journal of Leisure Research, 46,* 58–83.

Shen, X. S., Chick, G., & Zinn, H. (2014b). Validating the Adult Playfulness Trait Scale (APTS): An examination of personality, behavior, attitude, and perception in the nomological network of playfulness. *American Journal of Play, 6,* 345–369.

Shikako-Thomas, K., Majnemer, A., Law, M., & Lach, L. (2008). Determinants of participation in leisure activities in children and youth with cerebral palsy: Systematic review. *Physical & Occupational Therapy in Pediatrics, 28,* 155–169.

Shimoni, M. A., Engel-Yeger, B., & Tirosh, E. (2010). Participation in leisure activities among boys with attention deficit hyperactivity disorder. *Research in Developmental Disabilities, 31,* 1234–1239.

Skard, G., & Bundy, A. C. (2008). Test of playfulness. In L. D. Parham & L. S. Fazio (Eds.), *Play in occupational therapy for children* (2nd ed., pp. 71–94). St. Louis, MO: Mosby.

Slagle, E. C. (1922). Training aides for mental patients. *Archives of Occupational Therapy, 1*, 11–19.

Sonday, A., & Gretschel, P. (2016). Empowered to play: A case study describing the impact of powered mobility on the exploratory play of disabled children. *Occupational Therapy International, 23*, 11–18.

Sörman, D. E., Sundström, A., Rönnlund, M., Adolfsson, R., & Nilsson, L.-G. (2013). Leisure activity in old age and risk of dementia: A 15-year prospective study. *The Journals of Gerontology, 69*, 493–501.

Specht, J., King, G., Brown, E., & Foris, C. (2002). The importance of leisure in the lives of persons with congenital physical disabilities. *American Journal of Occupational Therapy, 56*, 436–445.

Spencer, G., Bundy, A., Wyver, S., Villeneuve, M., Tranter, P., Beetham, K., ... Naughton, G. (2016). Uncertainty in the school playground: Shifting rationalities and teachers' sense-making in the management of risks for children with disabilities. *Health, Risk & Society, 18*, 301–317.

Stagnitti, K. (2007). *The child initiated pretend play assessment.* West Brunswick, Victoria: Co-ordinates Publications.

Stagnitti, K., O'Connor, C., & Sheppard, L. (2012). Impact of the Learn to Play program on play, social competence and language for children aged 5–8 years who attend a specialist school. *Australian Occupational Therapy Journal, 59*, 302–311.

Stendal, K., Balandin, S., & Molka-Danielsen, J. (2011). Virtual worlds: A new opportunity for people with lifelong disability? *Journal of Intellectual & Developmental Disability, 36*, 80–83.

Suto, M. (1998). Leisure in occupational therapy. *Canadian Journal of Occupational Therapy, 65*, 271–278.

Sutton-Smith, B. (1997). *The ambiguity of play.* Cambridge, MA: Harvard University Press.

Swaffer, K. (2015). Dementia and Prescribed Disengagement™. *Dementia, 14*, 3–6.

Tatham, M. G., & McCree, S. (1993). Leisure facilitator: The role of the occupational therapist in senior housing. *Journal of Housing for the Elderly, 10*, 125–138.

Taylor, R. R. (2017). *Kielhofner's model of human occupation: Theory and application.* Philadelphia, PA: Wolters Kluwer Health.

Thomas, C., du Toit, S. H. J., & van Heerden, S. M. (2014). Leadership: The key to person-centred care. *South African Journal of Occupational Therapy, 44*, 34–39.

Thomas, J. E., O'Connell, B., & Gaskin, C. J. (2013). Residents' perceptions and experiences of social interaction and participation in leisure activities in residential aged care. *Contemporary Nurse, 45*, 244–254.

Thomas, W. H. (1996). *Life worth living: How someone you love can still enjoy life in a nursing home: The Eden alternative in action.* St. Louis, MO: VanderWyk & Burnham.

Torkildsen, G. (1986). *Leisure and recreation management* (2nd ed.). London, United Kingdom: Spon Press.

Torkildsen, G. (1999). *Leisure and recreation management* (4th ed.). London, United Kingdom: Spon Press.

Townsend, E. A., & Polatajko, H. J. (2007). *Advancing an occupational therapy vision for health, well-being, and justice through occupation.* Ontario, Canada: Canadian Association of Occupational Therapists.

Townsend, E., & Wilcock, A. (2004). Occupational justice and client-centred practice: A dialogue in progress. *Canadian Journal of Occupational Therapy, 71*, 75–87.

Tse, T., & Linsey, H. (2005). Adult day groups: Addressing older people's needs for activity and companionship. *Australasian Journal on Ageing, 24*, 134–140.

Turner, H., Chapman, S., McSherry, A., Krishnagiri, S., & Watts, J. (2000). Leisure assessment in occupational therapy: An exploratory study. *Occupational Therapy in Health Care, 12*, 73–85.

Ville, I., Ravaud, J.-F., & Tetrafigap Group (2001). Subjective well-being and severe motor impairments: The Tetrafigap survey on the long-term outcome of tetraplegic spinal cord injured persons. *Social Science & Medicine, 52*, 369–384.

Vizenor, K. V. (2014). *Binary lives: Digital citizenship and disability participation in a user content created virtual world.* Buffalo, NY: State University of New York at Buffalo.

Voelki, J. E. (1993). Activity and aging. In J. R. Kelly (Ed.), *Activity and aging* (pp. 380–389). Newbury Park, CA: Sage.

Waldman-Levi, A., & Bundy, A. (2016). A glimpse into co-occupations: Parent/caregiver's support of young children's playfulness scale. *Occupational Therapy in Mental Health, 32*, 217–227.

Wang, H.-X., Jin, Y., Hendrie, H. C., Liang, C., Yang, L., Cheng, Y., ... Gao, S. (2012). Late life leisure activities and risk of cognitive decline. *The Journals of Gerontology, 68*, 205–213.

Warchol, K. (2006). Facilitating functional and quality-of-life potential: Strength-based assessment and treatment for all stages of dementia. *Topics in Geriatric Rehabilitation, 22*, 213–227.

Watts, T., Stagnitti, K., & Brown, T. (2014). Relationship between play and sensory processing: A systematic review. *American Journal of Occupational Therapy, 68*, e37–e46.

Weigl, R., & Bundy, A. (2013). Die spielerische Herangehensweise (Playfulness) Erwachsener an ihre Freizeitaktivitäten. The Experience of Leisure Scale (TELS) mit deutsch-sprachigen Erwachsenen [The playful approach of adults to their leisure time activities with German-speaking adults]. *Ergoscience, 8*, 11–21.

White, R. W. (1959). Motivation reconsidered: The concept of competence. *Psychological Review, 66*, 297–323.

Wilcock, A. A. (2007). Active ageing: Dream or reality. *New Zealand Journal of Occupational Therapy, 54*, 15–20.

Wilkes, S., Cordier, R., Bundy, A., Docking, K., & Munro, N. (2011). A play-based intervention for children with ADHD: A pilot study. *Australian Occupational Therapy Journal, 58*, 231–240.

Wilkes-Gillan, S., Bundy, A., Cordier, R., & Lincoln, M. (2014a). Evaluation of a pilot parent-delivered play-based intervention for children with attention deficit hyperactivity disorder. *American Journal of Occupational Therapy, 68*, 700–709.

Wilkes-Gillan, S., Bundy, A., Cordier, R., & Lincoln, M. (2014b). Eighteen-month follow-up of a play-based intervention to improve the social play skills of children with attention deficit hyperactivity disorder. *Australian Occupational Therapy Journal, 61*, 299–307.

Wilkes-Gillan, S., Bundy, A., Cordier, R., & Lincoln, M. (2016). Child outcomes of a pilot parent-delivered intervention for improving the social play skills of children with ADHD and their playmates. *Developmental Neurorehabilitation, 19*, 238–245.

Wilkes-Gillan, S., Bundy, A., Cordier, R., Lincoln, M., & Chen, Y.-W. (2016). A randomised controlled trial of a play-based intervention to improve the social play skills of children with attention deficit hyperactivity disorder (ADHD). *PLoS One, 11*(8), 1–22.

Wilkes-Gillan, S., Bundy, A., Cordier, R., Lincoln, M., & Hancock, N. (2015). Parents' perspectives on the appropriateness of a parent-delivered intervention for improving the social play skills of children with ADHD. *British Journal of Occupational Therapy, 78*, 644–652.

Wilkes-Gillan, S., Cantrill, A., Cordier, R., Barnes, G., Hancock, N., & Bundy, A. (2017). The use of video-modelling as a method for improving the social play skills of children with attention deficit hyperactivity disorder (ADHD) and their playmates. *British Journal of Occupational Therapy, 80*, 196–207.

Willard, H. S., & Spackman, C. S. (1963). *Occupational therapy* (3rd ed.). Philadelphia, PA: Lippincott Williams & Wilkins.

Willard, H. S., Spackman, C. S., Hopkins, H. L., & Smith, H. D. (1978). *Willard & Spackman's occupational therapy* (5th ed.). Philadelphia, PA: Lippincott Williams & Wilkins.

Willard, H. S., Spackman, C. S., Hopkins, H. L., & Smith, H. D. (1993). *Willard & Spackman's occupational therapy* (8th ed.). Philadelphia, PA: Lippincott Williams & Wilkins.

Wood, W., Harris, S., Snider, M., & Patchel, S. A. (2005). Activity situations on an Alzheimer's disease special care unit and resident environmental interaction, time use, and affect. *American Journal of Alzheimer's Disease and Other Dementias, 20,* 105–118.

Ziegler, L. H. (1924). Some observations on recreations. *Archives of Occupational Therapy, 3,* 255–265.

Ziviani, J., Poulsen, A., & Cuskelly, M. (2012). *The art and science of motivation: A therapist's guide to working with children.* London, United Kingdom: Jessica Kingsley.

Ziviani, J., Rodger, S., & Peters, S. (2005). The play behaviour of children with and without autistic disorder in a clinical environment. *New Zealand Journal of Occupational Therapy, 52,* 22–30.

thePoint® *For additional resources on the subjects discussed in this chapter, visit* http://thePoint.lww.com /Willard-Spackman13e. *See* **Appendix I, Resources and Evidence for Common Conditions Addressed in OT** *for more information about cerebrovascular disease (stroke) and dementia.*

Sleep and Rest

Jo M. Solet

LEARNING OBJECTIVES

After reading this chapter, you will be able to:

1. Understand the elements of sleep architecture and sleep changes through the life cycle.
2. Develop an epidemiological perspective on sleep deficiency.
3. Relate sufficient sleep to individual health outcomes, memory, cognition, and occupational performance.
4. Describe multiple factors that may influence sleep.
5. Recognize common medical and psychiatric diagnoses treated by occupational therapists in which sleep may be implicated.
6. Organize client options for sleep hygiene, including sleep habits and environments; relate these to self-care and occupational balance.
7. Describe common primary sleep disorders.
8. Provide basic client sleep education and screening assessment and anticipate need for specialized referrals and occupational therapy participation on the treatment team.

Why Learn About Sleep?

We spend one-third of our lives asleep. Once thought of as a period of simple repose enforced by limited daylight, we now know sleep is a complex, dynamic state critical to growth and development. Many common medical and psychiatric disorders treated by occupational therapists affect client sleep or carry sleep-related signs and symptoms (Zee & Turek, 2006). Disordered sleep is a major public health concern affecting both genders, all races, and socioeconomic levels (Choi et al., 2006; Hale, 2005; Kim & Young, 2005) that increases with age (Ancoli-Israel & Cooke, 2005; Basner et al., 2007; Hale, 2005; Hale & Do, 2007; Patel et al., 2004). Sleep has documented impacts on health and safety, psychological well-being, learning and memory, and cognitive and occupational performance (Classen et al., 2011; Connor et al., 2002; Dorrian, Sweeney, & Dawson, 2011; Drake et al., 2010; Pizza et al., 2010; Poe, Walsh, & Bjorness, 2010; Smith & Phillips, 2011; Van Dongen, Maislin, Mullington, & Dinges, 2003). Inadequate sleep has been implicated in performance deficits and can place individuals and those they are responsible for at risk. Excessive sleepiness has contributed to environmental disasters such as oil spills, air traffic control failures, medical errors,

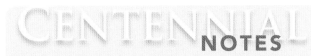

Sleep and Bedtime Routines

One hundred years ago when the profession of occupational therapy (OT) was beginning, the electroencephalogram (EEG) had yet to be invented. No one understood how active the brain really is during sleep or that sleep was composed of cycles of differing brainwave frequencies. However, early advocates of occupation therapy (also called moral treatment, labor, or employment) did recognize the importance of sleep, focusing the need for "employment . . . to *procure rest*, give strength, promote appetite, and facilitate recovery" (Dunton, 1917, p. 381, attributed to Dr. Samuel B. Woodward, Worcester Hospital). Additionally, Slagle's habit training schedules included bedtime and retiring as components (Slagle, 1934).

and auto and truck accidents. Sleep medicine is a dynamic, evolving field; research is underway at multiple levels, from genetic through epidemiological (Hobson, 2011; Shepard et al., 2005). New insights with clinical significance can be expected on a continuing basis. The 2008 "Occupational Therapy Practice Framework" (American Occupational Therapy Association, 2008) categorizes sleep as an occupation. This chapter provides a sleep foundation in this emerging area of practice for occupational therapists.

Now, as our technology continues to evolve, we have developed the ability to monitor sleep outside the laboratory and even to detect some disorders through our personal devices. These same devices can now also deliver personalized sleep health behavior support through artificial intelligence (AI) counseling for problems such as insomnia. Already under development are techniques for enhancing learning and memory through sleep stage, wave-specific subliminal stimulation.

The Structure of Sleep

Beginning in 1929 with the introduction of the **electro-encephalogram (EEG)**, it was revealed that sleep consists of patterns of changing brain waves that present in cycles of about 90 minutes throughout the night. Within these cycles, different stages of sleep are identified by the frequency and amplitude of the brain waves. When comparing the EEG readings of waking and sleep stages, researchers and clinicians assess the frequency of the brain waves, measured in hertz (Hz), and the size, or amplitude, of the brain waves, measured in microvolts, which differ for various stages of wakefulness and sleep.

Sleep Stages and Architecture

The stages of sleep fall into two categories: **rapid eye movement sleep** or **REM**, in which most dreaming occurs, and **nonrapid eye movement sleep**, called **NREM** or non-REM, which displays progressively deeper stages identified as NREM1, NREM2, and NREM3. Infants and children have higher proportions of REM sleep than adults.

Transition from wakefulness begins with light sleep, known as stage 1 (NREM1), and deepens to stage 2 sleep (NREM2). In early cycles of the night, slow brain waves with low frequency and high amplitude characteristic of stage 3 or deep sleep (NREM3) are common. As morning approaches, the proportion of time in deep sleep drops, whereas the proportion in REM sleep—characterized by higher frequency and lower amplitude brain waves—increases. During REM sleep, there is diminished muscle tone, preventing the sleeper from acting out dream experiences. The map of a typical adult night's sleep showing the REM and NREM stages in 90-minute cycles through the night is called a **hypnogram** (Figure 54-1).

Current sleep medicine research explores the roles of REM and NREM sleep stages in contributing to specific functions, including emotional regulation, cognition, learning, and memory consolidation (American Academy of Sleep Medicine [AASM], 2009; Haack & Mullington, 2005; Poe et al., 2010; Stickgold, 2005; Walker & Stickgold, 2004).

Sleep Drives

Two processes interact to determine the drive for sleep: **sleep-wake homeostasis** and the **circadian biological clock**. The **homeostatic drive** increases with accumulated time awake. The circadian biological clock organizes a physiological cycle of body temperature and hormone release regulating the variability of sleepiness and wakefulness throughout the night and day. These two drives are not simply additive because with an increase in accumulated **sleep debt**, the circadian drive has been shown to exert greater impact on sleepiness (Figure 54-2).

The **suprachiasmatic nucleus (SCN)**, a group of cells in the hypothalamus that respond to light and dark, controls the circadian biological clock. Signals generated by

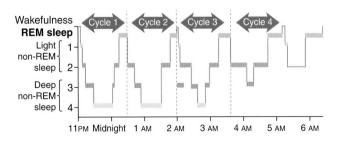

FIGURE 54-1 Sleep cycles across the night "hypnogram." *REM*, rapid eye movement.

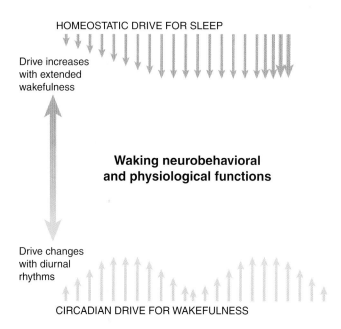

FIGURE 54-2 Sleep and wakefulness are regulated by two processes.

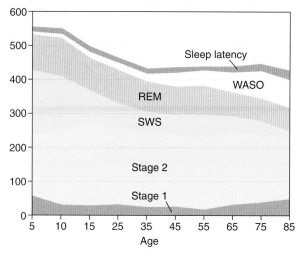

WASO: Wake after sleep onset (more with age)
REM: Rapid eye movement sleep (slightly less with age)
SWS: Non-REM, deep stages 3 and 4 combined (less with age)

FIGURE 54-3 Sleep: less and lighter with aging. (Source: Reprinted with permission from Ohayon, N. M., Carskadon, M. A., Guilleminault, C., & Vitiello, M. V. [2004]. Meta-analysis of quantitative sleep parameters from childhood to old age in healthy individuals: Developing normative sleep values across the human lifespan. *SLEEP, 27,* 1255–1273.)

light reaching the optic nerve through the eyes travel to the SCN, carrying the message to the internal clock for wakefulness. With exposure to morning light, the SCN orchestrates signals to other parts of the brain, raising body temperature and regulating certain hormone levels. Light delays the release of the hormone **melatonin**, which rises in the evening and stays elevated through the night, promoting sleep (Brendel, Florman, Roberts, & Solet, 2001; Edlund, 2003).

Sleep and the Life Cycle

Sleep changes through the life cycle, becoming shorter and lighter with aging (Figure 54-3). The period it takes to fall asleep, known as **sleep latency**, changes little over the life course, but the amount of time in restorative deep sleep drops off and the time spent **awake after sleep onset (WASO)** increases. The proportion of individuals with sleep-wake impairments also increases substantially with age (Hale, 2005; Ohayon, 2002; Ohayon & Vecchierini, 2005). As the baby boomers age, disordered sleep will require substantial attention and consumption of health care resources (Leland, Marcione, Schepens, Kelkar, & Fogelberg, 2014).

Sleep and Modern Life

Epidemiology

The average sleep time for Americans has dropped over the past five decades from 8.5 to 7 hours at the same time as obesity and diabetes rates have risen (Ayas, 2010; Flier & Elmquist, 2004; Hale, 2005; Patel & Hu, 2008; Quan,

Parthasarathy, & Budhiraja, 2010; Watanabe, Kikuchi, Katsutoshi, & Takahashi, 2010; Watson, Buchwald, Vitiello, Noonan, & Goldberg, 2010). Furthermore, Centers for Disease Control and Prevention (CDC) overlay maps show an alarming congruence; states, especially in the Deep South, with populations having the most limited sleep also have the highest rates of obesity and diabetes (Figure 54-4) (see CDC Website). Not only does inadequate sleep increase appetite, lower satiation, and alter glucose metabolism, but as part of a dangerous cycle, obesity also increases the risk for disordered sleep. Insufficient sleep is common even among children. Parents may not be aware of child sleep requirements and or may not enforce consistent sleep schedules (Owens & Mindell, 2005). Many believe that insufficient sleep is in part responsible for the alarming rise in childhood obesity.

Individual Health Impacts

The range of negative health impacts from insufficient or disrupted sleep includes elevated stress hormones, impaired glucose tolerance, diabetes (Zizi et al., 2011), obesity (Flier & Elmquist, 2004), cardiovascular disease, and stroke (Ayas, White, Al-Delaimy, et al., 2003; Ayas, White, Manson, et al., 2003). In addition, insufficient or disrupted

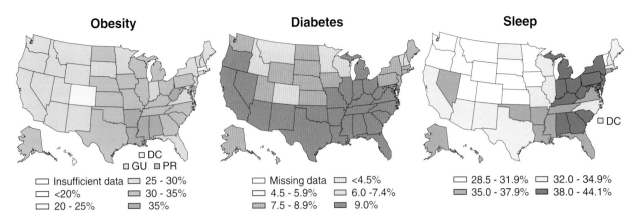

FIGURE 54-4 Intersecting epidemics. (Sources: Data from the following sources: Obesity: Centers for Disease Control and Prevention. [2016]. *Overweight and obesity: U.S. obesity trends.* Retrieved from https://www.cdc.gov/obesity/data/prevalence-maps.html; Diabetes: Centers for Disease Control and Prevention, Division of Diabetes Translation. [2015]. *Maps of trends in diagnosed diabetes.* Retrieved from https://www.cdc.gov/diabetes/statistics/slides/maps_diabetes_trends.pdf; Insufficient sleep: Centers for Disease Control and Prevention, National Center for Chronic Disease Prevention and Health Promotion. [2014]. *Sleep and sleep disorders: Data and statistics.* Retrieved from http://www.cdc.gov/sleep/data_statistics.htm.)

sleep may be associated with **hyperalgesia** (Chhangani et al., 2009; Hamilton, Catley, & Karlson, 2007; Kristiansen et al., 2011; Roehrs, Hyde, Blaisdell, Greenwald, & Roth, 2006), lowered mood, irritability, aggressiveness, and psychosocial difficulties (AASM, 2009; Owens, Belon, & Moss, 2010). Decreased memory consolidation (Poe et al., 2010; Stickgold, 2005; Walker & Stickgold, 2004), impairments in concentration, impaired task completion, and decreased occupational performance have also been documented (Banks, Van Dongen, Mailsen, & Dinges, 2010; Cohen et al., 2010; Durmer & Dinges, 2005; Ohayon & Vecchierini, 2005). Industrial, truck, and auto accidents are also associated with insufficient sleep (Classen et al., 2011; Connor et al., 2002; Drake et al., 2010; Pizza et al., 2010; Smith & Phillips, 2011; Tregear, Reston, Schoelles, & Phillips, 2009) (Figure 54-5).

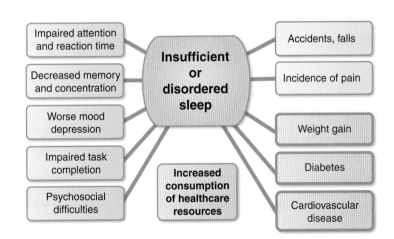

FIGURE 54-5 Insufficient or disordered sleep. (Copyright Jo Solet, MS, EdM, PhD, OTR/L; Data from Ancoli-Israel, S., & Cooke, J. R. [2005]. Prevalence and comorbidity of insomnia and effect on functioning in elderly populations. *Journal of the American Geriatrics Society, 54,* S264–S271; Choi, S. W., Peek-Asa, C., Sprince, N. L., Rautiainen, R. H., Flamme, G. A., Whitten, P. S., & Zwerling, C. [2006]. Sleep quantity and quality as a predictor of injuries in a rural population. *American Journal of Emergency Medicine, 24,* 189–196; and Spiegel, K., Knutson, K., Leproult, R., Tasali, E., & Van Cauter, E. [2005]. Sleep loss: A novel risk factor for insulin resistance and Type 2 diabetes. *Journal of Applied Physiology, 99,* 2008–2019.; Chien, K. L., Chen, P. C., Hsu, H. C., Su, T. C., Sung, F. C., Chen, M. F., & Lee, Y. T. [2010]. Habitual sleep duration and insomnia and the risk of cardiovascular events and all-cause death: Report from a community-based cohort. *SLEEP, 33,* 177–184.)

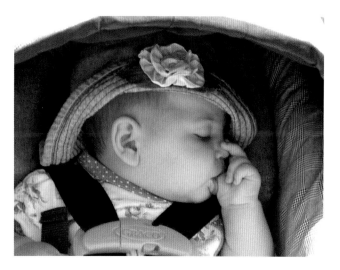

FIGURE 54-6 Infants have a faster sleep homeostasis and a greater percentage of REM sleep than older children. (Courtesy of Jo Solet, MS, EdM, PhD, OTR/L.)

Sleep Requirements through the Life Cycle

Whereas newborns sleep as much as 16 hours a day, by 6 months, babies typically sleep 12 hours during the night, plus two naps during the day (Figure 54-6). Well-rested preschoolers may still take an afternoon nap while sleeping 12 consolidated hours at night. Elementary school children require as much as 10 to 12 hours. Teenagers are understood as a group to experience **delayed sleep phase**—their natural sleep inclinations, based on timing release of the sleep inducing hormone melatonin, are often toward later bedtime and later wake up. This is in conflict with typical school schedules and may leave students who must awaken early feeling underslept and inattentive. Experiments with later high school start times showed improvements in multiple areas, including mood and academic performance as well as positive reactions from teachers (Owens et al., 2010). These findings are now driving policy initiatives supported by the American Academy of Pediatrics to delay junior and high school start times. School-based occupational therapists are in the position to bring awareness of sleep impacts to parents, teachers, and administrators.

Along with changes during growth and development, there are individual differences in adult sleep requirements and schedule preferences. Ideally, individuals choose occupations that match their natural proclivities. However, it may be that many of us have become accustomed to a level of functioning that results from less than optimal sleep. In sleep restriction vigilance studies, subjects actually show limited insight into their deepening performance decrements over a 2-week period (Van Dongen et al., 2003) (Figure 54-7). Although 7.5 hours is frequently cited as adequate for healthy adults, recent sleep extension studies with college athletes showed performance enhancements at 10 hours of time in bed (TIB) (Mah, Mah, Kezerian, & Dement, 2011).

Although elderly people may sleep less, in part due to higher levels of medical disorders and pain, or because they lack a consolidated night sleep period, napping on and off during the day, there is no evidence to support the common belief that elderly people actually require less sleep.

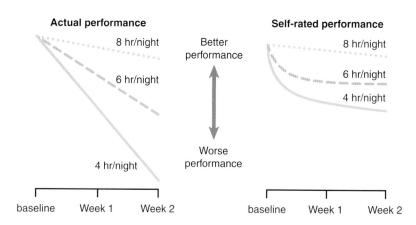

FIGURE 54-7 Restricting sleep impairs vigilance without parallel insight into increased deficits. (Source: Reprinted with permission from Van Dongen, H. P., Maislin, G., Mullington, J. M., & Dinges, D. F. [2003]. The cumulative cost of additional wakefulness: Dose-response effects on neurobehavioral functions and sleep physiology from chronic sleep restriction and total sleep deprivation. *SLEEP, 26,* 117–126. As redrawn by Orfeu Buxton.)

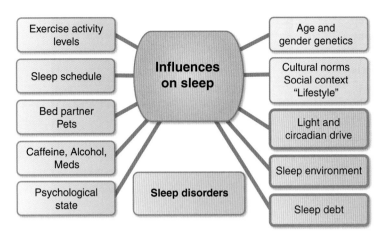

FIGURE 54-8 Influences on sleep: Many of these influences are open to modification as a part of occupational therapy collaborative treatment. (Courtesy of Jo Solet, MS, EdM, PhD, OTR/L.)

Influences on Sleep

As part of the clinical reasoning process and treatment planning, the occupational therapist is aware of multiple influences on sleep (Figure 54-8), which fall into five realms of concern: (1) common medical conditions and psychiatric disorders, (2) health habits and behaviors, (3) stress and occupational balance, (4) sleep environments, and (5) sleep disorders. The next sections of the chapter review each of these realms of concern with reference to these influences.

Sleep and Common Medical Conditions and Psychiatric Disorders

The majority of conditions and disorders treated by occupational therapists (see Appendix I) may either impact client sleep, be exacerbated by insufficient or disordered sleep, or both (Stroe et al., 2010; Zee & Turek, 2006). The examples shown in Box 54-1 include possible mechanisms through which sleep may mediate functional disability.

BOX 54-1 MECHANISMS THROUGH WHICH SLEEP MAY MEDIATE FUNCTIONAL DISABILITY IN COMMON CONDITIONS AND DISORDERS

Acute or Chronic Pain
- Arthritis
- Burns
- Low back pain

Central Nervous System Disease or Injury
- Alzheimer disease, dementias
- Parkinson disease
- Head injury
- Stroke/cerebrovascular disease
- Spinal cord injury
- Multiple sclerosis

Reward System, Appetite Satiation, or Metabolic Dysregulation
- Substance abuse
- Eating disorders
- Obesity
- Diabetes
- Cardiovascular disease

Respiratory Compromise, Disordered Breathing
- Chronic obstructive pulmonary disease
- Asthma
- Allergies

Perceived Lack of Safety, Insufficient Environmental Resources
- Posttraumatic stress disorder
- Anxiety disorders
- Poverty
- Homelessness

Failure of Self-Care, Isolation
- Major mental illness
- Developmental delays
- Autism

Compiled from Bondoc and Siebert (2008); Braley and Chervin (2010); Brown et al. (2011); Burton, Rahman, Kadota, Lloyd, and Vollmer-Conna (2010); Buxton and Marcelli (2010); Chandola, Ferrie, Perski, Akbaraly, and Marmor (2010); Coelho, Georgsson, Narayansingh, Swartz, and Murray (2010); Copinschi (2005); Epstein and Brown (2010); Fogelberg, Hoffman, Dikmen, Temkin, and Bell (2012); Fogelberg, Hughes, Vitiello, Hoffman, and Amtmann (2016); Fogelberg, Leland, Blanchard, Rich, and Clark (2017); Irwin et al. (2008); Johnson and Johnson (2010); Jozwiak et al. (2017); Luyster, Chasens, Wasko, and Dunbar-Jacob (2011); McCall et al. (2009); Ownby et al. (2010); Parcell, Ponsford, Redman, and Rajaratnam (2008); Redline (2009); Sixel-Döring, Schweitzer, Mollenhauer, and Trenkwalder (2011); Spiegel, Knutson, Leproult, Tasali, and Van Cauter (2005); Spiegel, Tasali, Penev, and Van Cauter (2004); Watson (2010); as well as comprehensive sleep textbook Kryger, Roth, and Dement (2011).

Additional common medical conditions with sleep disrupting symptoms include **adenotonsillar hypertrophy** (breathing difficulties, especially in childhood), ulcers and gastroesophageal reflux disease, pain, **benign prostatic hypertrophy (nocturia)**, and **atopic dermatitis** (itching). Pregnancy, especially the last trimester (discomfort, difficulty breathing, nocturia), postpartum (infant care), and menopause (autonomic instability, hot flashes) may compromise sleep for some women. Although it is beyond the scope of this chapter to fully describe sleep issues associated with each of these disorders, the occupational therapist becomes familiar with this information for the specific diagnostic categories that present in his or her clinical practice, using chapter references and other resources. The "Practice Dilemma" box describes a client with a sleep disorder.

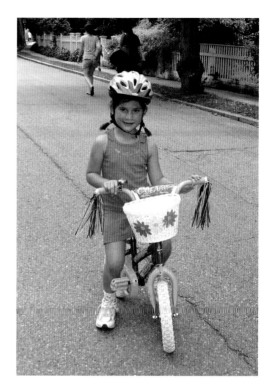

FIGURE 54-9 Exercise enhances sleep. (Courtesy of Jo Solet, MS, EdM, PhD, OTR/L.)

⚓ PRACTICE DILEMMA

Celia is an occupational therapist called for a bedside activities of daily living (ADL) evaluation of Elvira, a 40-year-old naturalized citizen, following colostomy reversal surgery. Communicating with the help of a Spanish interpreter, Elvira complains that her pain is still "so so bad," that she is having "fears and visions" about her surgical experiences and that "her legs are kicking and waking her up at night." Yet, in terms of ADL, Celia finds Elvira only requires minimal assistance.

Questions

1. How should Celia prioritize the multiple concerns which Elvira has raised?
2. Are there possible interactions between Elvira's pain report and her other complaints?
3. Which members of the clinical team should be called for consultation?
4. How might cultural competency help Celia and other team members address Elvira's complaints?

Health Habits and Behaviors

Exercise for both adults and children is sleep enhancing (Buxton, Lee, L'Hermite-Baleriaux, Turek, & Van Cauter, 2003; Passos et al., 2010; Youngstedt & Buxton, 2003; Figure 54-9). Ideally, it is undertaken several hours before sleep. Following evening exercise, at least 2 hours are thought to be required for body temperature cooldown into sleep; a tepid shower may speed the process.

Caffeine—as coffee, colas, or energy drinks—is very commonly used at "wake up" and to fight fatigue and sleepiness. Caffeine can be an asset when used judiciously. Individuals develop tolerance for caffeine, needing more and more to provide the same effect. Especially when used to fight the midafternoon energy decline, caffeine may delay night sleep onset and reduce deep sleep (Roehrs & Roth, 2008). Depending on the planned sleep schedule, it is often recommended that the last caffeine be no later than early afternoon. Caffeine withdrawal can produce headache, fatigue, and drowsiness.

Although tobacco has multiple well-known negative health impacts, it remains among the chosen substances individuals use to manage mood and energy. Smokers are more likely to report problems falling asleep and staying asleep and may experience decreased REM sleep as compared with nonsmokers. Increased arousals from sleep may be reported with smoking cessation efforts (Roehrs & Roth, 2011a).

Alcohol is used by some to help bring on sleep. In healthy adults, alcohol has an initial sedative effect, but later during the night, following completed metabolism of alcohol, a rebound effect may actually interfere with sleep. In addition to effects on sleep initiation and sleep maintenance, alcohol also can also affect the proportion of the various sleep stages, including suppressing REM sleep. There is some evidence that alcohol may behave differently in insomniacs. Many questions remain, including whether insomniacs develop tolerance to alcohol's sedative effects and then increase intake (Roehrs & Roth, 2011b). A new category of beverage is one that combines caffeine and alcohol. These drinks are thought to be dangerous because caffeine can produce a perception of wakefulness and mask insight into deficits caused by alcohol.

Numerous drugs, recreational, over-the-counter, and prescription medications, including marijuana, herbs, and "nutraceuticals," can impact sleep (Albert, Roth, Toscani, Vitiello, &

Zee, 2017; Schweitzer, 2011). Chart review and careful history taking may identify these substances; information can be brought to the attention of the treating physician for review, including analysis of drug interactions and polypharmacy, the latter especially common in the elderly (Frazier, 2005).

Stress and Occupational Balance

The ideal sleep-wake pattern dedicates sufficient time for uninterrupted sleep, is congruent with natural circadian clock rhythms, and is regular and consistent. Yet, compelling opportunities and requirements for night activity, as well as situational stressors, at times override sleep needs. For some, these reflect lifestyle choices and leisure pursuits, with the option for easy reversal to increased TIB. For others, it is a challenge to complete work, school, family caregiving, and home responsibilities within a schedule that leaves adequate time for self-care and sleep (Berkman, Buxton, Ertel, & Okechukwu, 2010; Bibbs, 2011; Luckhaupt, Tak, & Calvert, 2010). For example, an increasing number of mothers of young children have joined the workforce and may struggle to maintain occupational balance (Anaby, Backman, & Jarus, 2010). Technologies bring work into the home setting, even well after normal work hours, demanding immediate attention. Occupations such as nursing, medicine, and air traffic controller must be accomplished around the clock, requiring night shift work (Edlund, 2003; Levine, Adusumilli, & Landrigan, 2010; Nurok, Czeisler, & Lehmann, 2010). Daytime sleep must then be undertaken against natural circadian rhythms. Travel to other time zones can disrupt natural sleep patterns, requiring alertness and high functioning during natural circadian sleep periods. This experience is colloquially known as jet lag (Youngstedt & Buxton, 2003). Finally, situations of grief, loss, and trauma, common in client populations that OT practitioners encounter, have ripple effects that can damage sleep.

The "Ethical Dilemma" box illustrates some of the difficulties clients and occupational therapists can encounter while addressing sleep and occupational performance. The reader is urged to develop initial responses to the questions posed here and then to return to them after completing the chapter for discussion with colleagues.

⚖ ETHICAL DILEMMA

Stanley is an occupational therapist working in an outpatient facility. During evaluation of Mr. Chevy, a 58-year-old overweight truck driver with high blood pressure (partially controlled by medication), he notices the client falling asleep midmorning.

Upon questioning, Mr. Chevy admits he sometimes "feels himself falling asleep" even while driving, especially on long hauls at night. In answering some basic screening questions about his sleep schedule, sleep experience, and sleep environment, he mentions that his wife gets angry with him on nights when he sleeps at home because his snoring wakes her up repeatedly at night.

Mr. Chevy has been referred to occupational by orthopedics for "energy conservation training and back school" to improve his driving comfort and lifting safety. He is afraid that any mention of sleep problems in his record could cause him to lose his job. He has just 2 years left before planned retirement. Mr. Chevy threatens to leave treatment entirely if Stanley will not agree to keep sleep problems off his record.

Questions

1. What should Stanley do in this situation?
2. What additional information should Stanley seek to help with his decision?
3. How might Stanley help educate Mr. Chevy about risks to himself and others?
4. Should Stanley reach out to Mrs. Chevy for help in supporting diagnosis or treatment?
5. Should Stanley make a referral for further assessment?

Social Context

Eliciting the client's social context as part of the occupational profile and initial assessment can be particularly relevant with regard to sleep behaviors and occupational balance. For example, presleep stimulating computer use and video games and all-night texting are documented peer-driven sleep hazards for many young people (American College of Chest Physicians, 2010; Weaver, Gradisar, Dohnt, Lovato, & Douglas, 2010). Developing and maintaining balance in an environment where this is far from the norm, such as in a college dormitory, can be difficult.

A social context of emotional isolation experienced as loneliness has been identified as an independent risk factor for sleep problems (Hawkley, Cacioppo, & Preacher, 2011; Hawkley, Preacher, & Cacioppo, 2010; McHugh & Lawlor, 2011). In addition, individuals who have little contact with others, due to advanced age or disability, may have insufficient daily life structure. They may spend much of their TIB, napping on and off. Providing for daily activities and companionship, which are common goals of OT intervention, may help to consolidate and improve sleep.

Naps and Safe Management of Fatigue

Naps have historically been part of occupational balance in some cultures, especially in the heat of midday. Like exercise, planned napping can be integrated into daily routines to enhance health and well-being. Even brief naps can have restorative effects. However, misplaced or extended napping can interfere with daily activities, social integration, and night sleep (Leland et al., 2016). There are times when the OT practitioner may recommend napping to manage fatigue and to improve safety and alertness, especially in anticipation of night performance requirements, such as driving, infant care, or medical shift work.

Short naps of 20 to 30 minutes, or longer naps of a full sleep cycle, 90 minutes, are more likely to allow for awakening without significant sleep inertia (Mednick & Ehrman, 2006). The sleep stage content of the nap is thought to affect the resulting enhancements, with REM-containing naps shown to decrease negative emotional bias and amplify recognition of positive emotions (Gujar, McDonald, Nishida, & Walker, 2010). When naps are required even after adequate TIB, it can be a signal that further assessment is required. Chronic illnesses such as multiple sclerosis (MS) may increase fatigue levels for extended periods (Stout & Finlayson, 2011); under these circumstances, it may be useful to schedule naps and rest periods into the daily routine. In cases of excessive daytime sleepiness, safety must be given the highest priority, including arrangements for alternative transportation rather than driving and extra attention given to fall and accident prevention.

Sleep Environments

Along with healthy sleep habits, an optimal sleep environment is a component of **sleep hygiene**. The ideal sleep environment is *quiet*, *dark*, *cool*, *comfortable*, *clean*, and *safe*. As part of a home visit or review of a long-term care facility, the occupational therapist helps to adapt and organize the sleep environment (Figure 54-10).

Numerous studies document the disruptive effects of noise on sleep (Basner, Müller, & Elmenhorst, 2011; Buxton et al., 2012; Hume, 2011; Solet, Buxton, Ellenbogen, Wang,

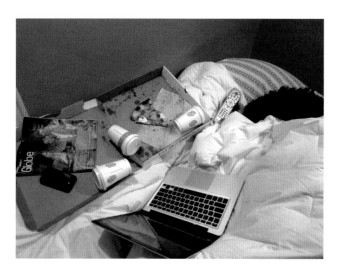

FIGURE 54-10 **Inappropriate environment for sleep. (Courtesy of Jo Solet, MS, EdM, PhD, OTR/L.)**

& Carballiera, 2010). Ensuring quiet includes blocking disturbances from within the room, home, or building. This may include simple solutions such as closing doors and soliciting family and partner (or roommate) commitments to limit noisy activities after an agreed on hour. Sometimes, external noise sources from the streetscape, such as truck deliveries and cycling air-handling equipment, disrupt sleep. Soothing sound and white noise machines or earplugs may be successful in blocking these disturbances. Be sure smoke alarms, phone signals, and other emergency alerts can penetrate.

Some communities have noise ordinances that limit decibel levels, especially during night hours. Night noise, from airplane overflights and truck traffic, for example, may be quite prevalent in some communities. Many American cities have homeless populations, limited shelter beds, and people sleeping on the streets. Availability of a safe, quiet place for sleep is an occupational justice issue. According to Blakeney and Marshall (2009), occupational justice rests on two important principles: that "occupational participation is a determinant of health" and the "principle of empowerment through occupation" (p. 47). Sleep qualifies on both counts (see Chapter 45).

Ironically, some of the most difficult sleep environments are health care facilities, including critical care units (Busch-Vishniac et al., 2005; Dogan, Ertekin, & Dogan, 2005; Friese, Diaz-Arrastia, McBride, Frankel, & Gentilello, 2003; Solet & Barach, 2012; Weinhouse & Schwab, 2006). Complaints of "noise around room" are among the most common in hospital quality-of-care surveys. In most states, since 2006, construction codes for new hospitals require single-bed patient rooms, preventing disturbance through roommates. Research demonstrating the sleep disruptive character of common hospital sounds has informed the most recent edition of *Design and Construction Guidelines for Healthcare Facilities*, which now includes acoustic guidelines for hospital rooms (Facility Guidelines Institute, 2010; Solet et al., 2010). Patient sleep disruption by hospital night staff led to the development of the Somerville Protocol, an evidence-based night routine solution that can be implemented by staff in health care settings to preserve patient sleep (Bartick, Thai, Schmidt, Altaye, & Solet, 2010).

Because light is naturally alerting, providing darkness in the sleep environment is also an important protector of sleep (Edlund, 2003). As the negative impacts of night lighting on sleep are being documented, community efforts to limit LED streetlights have become vigorous (Solet, 2016). Light sources within the room such as bright digital clocks should be dimmed or removed. The bedroom can be conditioned for sleep and sex, not meals, technology, and TV. Ideally, space allows the TV and computer to be placed elsewhere; screens including cellphones should be shut down well before sleep. This can be part of a consistent "wind-down period" with a relaxing presleep ritual, such as a bath and reading, or "story time" for children.

Night shift workers, who are at special risk because they sleep during daylight against natural circadian rhythms, are found to sleep more efficiently when true darkness is provided. Eye masks or "blackout" window shades may be useful in the effort to limit ambient light intrusion.

Body temperature drops as part of the sleep cycle. A cool bedroom is thus most conducive to sleep. Most people report the mid to high 60s as quite comfortable. Conflicts between bed partners over room temperature are legendary. For this and other reasons, partners sometimes do not sleep well next to each other. Mismatched sleep schedules or even specific disorders in one partner (e.g., excessive movement during sleep, use of equipment to normalize breathing) may disturb the sleep of the other. Splitting into individual beds in the same room may be sufficient to preserve sleep; separate rooms, if available, may serve to protect sleep and ultimately preserve relationships. "Visits" can be planned.

A significant percentage of Americans responding to the U.S. census listed pets as family members. Pets are common bed partners. However, pets may have natural sleep cycles that are different from their owners', for example, becoming most active as the sun rises. Many people report that sleeping with their pets is a great comfort. This decision should be made in consideration of the degree of pet induced sleep disruption and the individual's health status. A separate comfortable pet bed should be an option (Figure 54-11).

A clean environment is especially important to those with allergies, who may experience breathing difficulties during sleep due to accumulated allergens, such as pet hair.

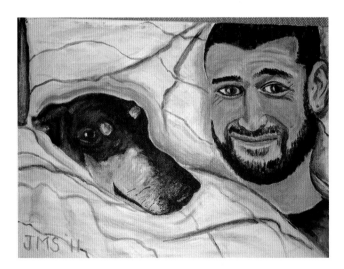

FIGURE 54-11 **Sleeping with a pet may be comforting yet at times may disrupt sleep. (Courtesy of Jo Solet, MS, EdM, PhD, OTR/L.)**

HEPA air cleaning machines may be helpful. A clean environment is also safer, with clothes and other items off the floor. Any cords, equipment, or furniture that blocks the exit or the path to the bathroom should be relocated as part of fall prevention. Availability of a full set of fresh bedclothes should be assured, and a weekly room cleaning schedule put in place.

Sleep Disorders

Patients may describe significant distress related to impairment in occupational and social functioning and yet have little insight that disordered sleep is driving their difficulties. Although making a diagnosis of a sleep disorder is outside the professional expertise of occupational therapists, it is important to be aware of the International Classification of Sleep Disorders (ICSD-2) (available for download), to have access to criteria and standards as resources, and to recognize sleep disorders that are commonly diagnosed. The newest edition of the *Diagnostic and Statistical Manual of Mental Disorders* (*DSM-5*), published in 2013, offers a revised categorization of sleep disorders.

Sleep disorders can be understood through descriptions of the ways in which sleep is disturbed: inability to fall asleep, multiple awakenings, inability to fall back asleep, nonrestorative sleep, inadequate breathing during sleep (may be described as snoring and or gasping for breath), disruptive movements during sleep, nonsleep activities intruding into sleep, and mistimed or uncontrolled sleep. Although shortened sleep conveys health risks and decreases longevity, when sleep is disrupted and discontinuous, this impact is even greater.

Insomnias

The **insomnias** are defined by repeated problems of sleep initiation, duration, consolidation, or quality that occur despite adequate time and opportunity for sleep and result in some form of daytime impairment (Haynes, 2009; Passos et al., 2010; Roth, Roehrs, & Pies, 2007; Vitiello, Rybarczk, Von Korff, & Stepanski, 2009). Using stringent criteria of sleep disturbance every night for 2 weeks or more, a consistent prevalence ranging between 9% and 17.7% of the adult population has been documented as affected (Ohayon, 2002). This translates into 30 to 40 million Americans. Historically, the insomnias have been organized into multiple subtypes with variable patterns at different phases of the life course: pediatric, pregnancy, menopause, and geriatric. Insomnia can be primary or **secondary insomnia** that is comorbid, at times related to pain, depression, posttraumatic stress disorder, and other medical conditions that should be identified and addressed in treatment planning.

Treatments may include use of the relaxation response such as meditation, progressive muscle relaxation, or

biofeedback; cognitive-behavioral therapy (especially addressing sleep-related anxieties and conditioning the bed for sleep only); improved sleep habits and environments; limits on caffeine and alcohol; and sometimes prescription medications.

Obstructive Sleep Apnea

Obstructive sleep apnea (OSA) is caused by partial or complete blockage of airway passages during sleep. Diagnosis typically follows from laboratory sleep testing, frequently after the individual's roommate or sleep partner has reported hearing "loud snoring" or "gasping for breath" during the night. The index of OSA severity, called the **apnea/hypopnea index** or **AHI**, typically increases in untreated individuals with age and relates to the number of repeated awakenings per hour driven by decreased **oxygen saturation**. Awakenings may occur dozens or even hundreds of times a night; individuals may have no awareness, perhaps only reporting excessive daytime sleepiness. Morning headache is a common complaint (Vaughn & D'Cruz, 2011). Certain jaw, overbite, tongue and soft tissue proportions, and large neck girth as well as excessive weight are recognized as anatomical risk factors. OSA can be a serious disorder, depriving the brain of oxygen, leading to **hypertension**, metabolic changes, weight gain, diabetes, and cardiovascular disease (O'Connor et al., 2009; Peppard, 2009; Redline, 2009). Increased risks for dementia documented with OSA may be due to retention of toxic metabolites, normally drained through increased interstitial space during adequate sleep (Xie et al., 2013). Excessive sleepiness also places these individuals, like others with serious sleep disorders, at increased risk for auto and industrial accidents (Tregear et al., 2009).

Treatments for OSA include use of a **continuous positive airway pressure (CPAP)** system that pushes air through the nose (Tomfohr, Ancoli-Israel, Loredo, & Dimsdale, 2011), sleep positioning to side-lying, dental devices, corrective surgery (Verse & Hörmann, 2011), and weight loss to decrease obstructive tissue. CPAP "machines" now include technology to monitor their use. Some individuals find the masks inconvenient or uncomfortable or feel the devices negatively impact intimate relationships. The consequences of untreated chronic OSA can be severe; support for seeking a comfortable CPAP mask fit and reinforcing treatment adherence through continuous monitoring are valuable therapeutic interventions (Cooke et al., 2009).

See instructional video http://healthysleep.med.harvard.edu/sleep-apnea.

Restless Legs Syndrome and Periodic Limb Movement Disorder

Restless legs syndrome (RLS) is a sleep disorder in which there is an urge to move the legs in order to stop unpleasant leg sensations that may be described as "crawling" or "tingling." During sleep, involuntary leg movements can lead to awakenings and may occur repeatedly without being remembered (Bayard, Avonda, & Wadzinski, 2008; Kushida, 2007). Risk factors include peripheral neuropathy, chronic kidney disease, iron deficiency, Parkinson disease, and side effects of certain medications; there is also higher prevalence among clients with a history of stroke (Coelho et al., 2010) and fibromyalgia (Viola-Saltzman, Watson, Bogart, Goldberg, & Buchwald, 2010). Genetic factors are implicated because certain families as well as populations, especially northern Europeans, show higher incidence. Some individuals experience movements without the sensations; upper extremities can also be involved. This is called **periodic limb movement disorder (PLMD)**. Along with treatment of predisposing conditions, exercise, stretching, massage, and warm baths may provide some relief. In some cases, medications may be prescribed.

Parasomnias

Parasomnias are nonsleep behaviors that intrude during sleep. Sleepwalking and sleep-eating episodes can occur during deep sleep through partial awakening (Howell, Schenck, & Crow, 2009). Typically, individuals have no memory of these behaviors, which are reported to them by others or are discovered through evidence found in the morning. Sleepwalking is more common in children, who often outgrow the disorder. Organizing secure environments and alerting systems for parents or partners are practical safety measures.

Healthy REM sleep involves muscle paralysis (**atonia**). In **REM sleep behavior disorder (RBD)**, this paralysis fails and the individual moves, as if acting out a dream. Bed partners can be at risk of injury from these uncontrolled actions and may be the initiators of the search for diagnosis. Research demonstrates RBD may be a precursor to dementia or Parkinson disease (Sixel-Döring et al., 2011). When it does occur, RBD in Parkinson disease is associated with a more impaired cognitive profile and more severe and widespread neurodegeneration (Jozwiak et al., 2017).

Other parasomnias include **night terrors**, **rhythmic movement disorders in children**, **bruxism** (tooth grinding), and **confusional arousals** in adults. Secondary insomnia can result from an effort to block frightening parasomnia experiences by avoiding sleep.

Narcolepsy

Narcolepsy is characterized by an excessive uncontrollable daytime sleepiness even after adequate sleep at night. According to the National Institutes of Health, it is estimated to be as common as Parkinson disease or MS but is underdiagnosed. Experiences that affect some, but not all, narcoleptics include **cataplexy**: a sudden loss of muscle function ranging from weakness to full collapse, which may have an emotional trigger; inability to talk or move while falling asleep or waking up; and vivid, sometimes frightening, images in transition to sleep, called **hypnagogic hallucinations**. In narcolepsy, the architecture of sleep is disturbed with REM rather than NREM occurring at sleep onset and REM experiences actually intruding into waking periods. The main treatments are lifestyle adaptations to maintain safety, central nervous system stimulants, and antidepressant or other medications that suppress REM sleep.

Additional Resources for Sleep Disorders

Readers are also encouraged to visit http://healthysleep .med.harvard.edu/healthy/getting/treatment/an-overview -of-sleep-disorders. This is a section of online resources provided by the Division of Sleep Medicine at Harvard Medical School in collaboration with the WGBH (public television) Educational Foundation.

The National Institutes of Health also offers valuable online sleep disorder information: http://www.nhlbi.nih .gov/health/public/sleep.

National Sleep Foundation: http://www.sleepfoundation .org/articles/sleep-disorders?

Also see the comprehensive text: Kryger, M. H., Roth, T., & Dement, W. C. (Eds.). (2011). *Principles and practice of sleep medicine* (5th ed.). St. Louis, MO: Elsevier Saunders.

Sleep Screening and Referral

Because the majority of medical and psychiatric disorders treated by occupational therapists may affect or be affected by sleep, and because sleep disorders are so common, brief sleep screening as part of initial OT assessment is valuable (Zee & Turek, 2006). The attuned occupational therapist will be alert to a history or current report of excessive daytime sleepiness and will probe for the degree to which sleep is experienced as nonrestorative and the extent to which daytime activities may be impaired. Some clients will report functional problems without recognizing any link to their sleep difficulties. Others, despite complaints of excessive sleepiness, may have little insight even into multiple night arousals, for example, due to OSA or RLS. Bed partners or family members of clients may be resources for supplying additional details and documentation, especially women (Umberson, 1992). As always, to protect privacy, clients' permission must be sought before these discussions.

Sleep History and Self-reports

Standardized client self-report questionnaires, such as the Epworth Sleepiness Scale, supplement the occupational profile and may be useful for screening and for tracking effectiveness of certain treatments (Box 54-2) (Johns, 1991). Many clinical settings make available preferred tools for sleep screening that have been validated for the specific treated population, such as school-age children (Owens, Spirito, & McGuinn, 2000).

When clients complain of *excessive daytime sleepiness*, a **sleep diary** or a wrist-worn sleep-monitoring device, showing sleep timing and perceived refreshment, can be useful in collaborating to gain a picture defining sleep patterns (Figure 54-12). **Sleep inertia** is the normal period at awakening in which full alertness is not yet achieved. Diary rating of sleep should be completed after the individual is fully awake and through this transition period.

When diary or device results confirm insufficient TIB or an erratic schedule, a critical OT sleep education and

---

BOX 54-2   EPWORTH SLEEPINESS SCALE

The Epworth Sleepiness Scale is used to determine the level of daytime sleepiness. A score of 10 or more is considered sleepy.

Use the following scale to choose the most appropriate number for each situation:

0 = would *never* doze or sleep
1 = *slight* chance of dozing or sleeping
2 = *moderate* chance of dozing or sleeping
3 = *high* chance of dozing or sleeping

Situations: Chance of Dozing or Sleeping

1. Sitting and reading   _____
2. Watching TV   _____
3. Sitting inactive in a public place   _____
4. Being a passenger in a motor vehicle for an hour or more   _____
5. Lying down in the afternoon   _____
6. Sitting and talking to someone   _____
7. Sitting quietly after lunch (no alcohol)   _____
8. Stopped for a few minutes in traffic while driving   _____

Total (add the scores up)   _____

Johns, M. W. (1991). A new method for measuring daytime sleepiness: The Epworth Sleepiness Scale. *SLEEP, 14,* 540–545.

SLEEP HEALTHCENTERS®
...better sleep. better health.

SLEEP DIARY

NAME: ______________________

WEEK OF: ______________________

Day	Duration of Naps (minutes)	Bedtime	Time to Fall Asleep (minutes)	Number of Awakenings	Duration of Awakenings (minutes)	Final Waketime	Out of Bed Time	Time Spent Asleep (hours)	Medications Taken	Next Day Alertness 1-10 (10=most alert)
Monday										
Tuesday										
Wednesday										
Thursday										
Friday										
Saturday										
Sunday										

- Please begin to complete the sleep diary on a daily basis. It will provide a subjective tracking of your sleep schedule for you and your sleep clinician to use as you work together to improve your sleep.
- Do not look at the clock to complete this form. You should complete this diary each morning with respect to your previous night of sleep. Do not complete it during the night or keep it in your bedroom.
- Use it only as a guideline and spend no more than 30 seconds filling it out in the morning.

BSM-DIRY-0002_1 Reviewed 3/05/10

FIGURE 54-12 Sleep diary. (Source: Reprinted with permission from Sleep HealthCenters, LLC: http://www.sleephealth.com.)

treatment goal is to evoke a cognitive shift: away from perceiving limited sleep as "no problem," "heroic," or "efficient," toward perceiving it as "a drain on well-being and performance," "an unwise health risk," or "a factor complicating recovery." Individuals suffering from certain medical, psychiatric, or sleep disorders can be doubly challenged and health risks raised further by poor sleep habits. This cognitive shift initiates readiness for a program to include sleep as a priority. The occupational therapist helps clients develop strategies to incorporate energy conservation and fatigue management techniques to cope with the extra demands associated with these conditions.

Recent research suggests that sleep symptoms are common but are not routinely screened for in primary care settings (Haponik et al., 1996; Senthilvel, Auckley, & Dasarathy, 2011; Sorscher, 2008). Although efforts are underway to enhance medical attention to sleep, an OT encounter could include the first sleep screening a client receives. Referral for follow-up, potentially including a home or laboratory sleep study, may be made to neurology, pulmonology, psychiatry, occupational health, or directly to sleep medicine, depending on comorbid diagnosis, potential severity, and available resources.

As part of the referral process and in follow-up team meetings, the occupational therapist takes the opportunity to make colleagues aware of his or her tools for addressing sleep problems and documents sleep interventions in care notes.

Sleep Evaluation

The technology used for sleep evaluation is evolving toward more complete home testing. **Actigraphy** is a wristband mounted accelerometer system that records periods of motion during sleep and indicates sleep latency, arousals, and time of awakening (Sadeh, 2011; Sánchez-Ortuño, Edinger, Means, & Almirall, 2010). Actigraphy systems for personal use can now be run through downloadable apps for smartphones. Consumer/home sleep tracking devices paired with smartphone apps can provide a more accurate picture of sleep than diary recording alone.

Polysomnography is comprehensive testing that includes three simultaneously recorded parts: the EEG, which traces brain wave activity through scalp electrodes, recording differing frequencies identified as alpha, beta, delta, and theta rhythms; **electrooculograms**, which measure eye movements through electrodes placed on the skin around the eyes; and **electromyograms**, which measure motor activity through electrodes placed on the skin over muscles. As part of sleep evaluation, sensors may be used to track breathing and oxygen saturation in the blood. Video recordings are used for monitoring client positioning and movements during sleep, especially as coordinated with other readouts. Sleep stages (REM and NREM1, NREM2, and NREM3) have specific "fingerprints" based on brain activity and coordinated muscle and eye movements. Certain sleep disorders are more likely to occur during specific stages. Furthermore, alterations in architecture of sleep, as shown in the hypnogram, can be produced by environmental or medical conditions. Standardized scoring criteria are applied to analyze these recordings to identify stages, arousals, and anomalies supporting diagnoses (Chervin, 2010).

Summary: Sleep and Occupational Therapy Interventions

Occupational therapy interventions to improve sleep and manage fatigue are based in client education, self-care and health habits, occupational balance, and optimal environments (Case Study 54-1). As part of the continuum of care provided by occupational therapists, sleep-enhancing interventions may be adapted for primary prevention and health promotion, such as work-based and school wellness programs (Beebe, Ris, Kramer, Long, & Amin, 2010; Gangwisch et al., 2010; Gangwisch, Malaspina, Boden-Albala, & Heymsfield, 2005; Quan et al., 2010); may address sleep problems related to aging, injury, illness, or disability; and may contribute to treatments directed specifically at sleep disorders. School and work wellness programs focus on life cycle sleep requirements and schedules, health habits and behaviors that influence sleep, and adequate sleep environments.

Occupational therapy treatments for common medical conditions and psychiatric disorders, many of which carry comorbid sleep difficulties, may be directed toward pain, anxiety, depression, limited mobility, poor self-care,

---

CASE STUDY 54-1   ALBERTA

Alberta is a 15-year-old private high school student who complains of "being so tired." Although she showed early academic ability, the high school "scene" has posed increasing problems. A large girl at 5 ft 9 in, 170 lb, her athletic activities are restricted due to asthma, which she has suffered since early childhood. She recently had an experience of social network bullying, which left her isolated from and unable to trust her female classmates. Her strong interest in math and science has allowed her to forge some friendships with boys in the class. Her mother has described her as "depressed." Alberta has been referred to a group private OT practice by her long-time pediatrician for help with "fatigue, fitness, and fitting in."

1. What information should Alberta's OT seek from the pediatrician?

2. Describe components of a first OT meeting with Alberta?

   What could be helpful in establishing rapport?

   What screening and assessments might shed light on her fatigue?

3. Could bullying and isolation affect adolescent sleep?

4. Through what mechanisms might sleep affect fitness, mood?

5. Suggest possible components for an OT treatment program to improve adolescent self-care and sleep.

Case Discussion

1. The OT should ask for a developmental and medical history, information related to specific asthma symptoms and triggers, treatments, medications and their side effects, and restrictions.

   Any available information about mood and childhood sleep should be examined. Has the doctor discussed the referral with Alberta and has she agreed on specific goals? What kind of parental support can be anticipated?

2. The first meeting is critical for establishing rapport. Initial questions can include:

   "What do you hope to get out of our time together? How will we know that we are heading in the right direction? What will be different?

   Please describe your typical day. Are some times of day better/easier than others?

   When you are feeling your best, what are you doing?

respiratory compromise, substance abuse, insufficient resources, and/or social isolation. Broad components of treatment for these clients, which may also improve comorbid sleep difficulties, include (but are not limited to) cognitive behavioral therapy, relaxation response, graded exercise, activities to increase social integration, and resources for safety (Solet, 2014). Improvement in any of these complaint areas can also be expected to improve sleep; the effects are reciprocal (Zee & Turek, 2006).

Treatment components directed specifically at sleep either as a primary problem or a comorbidity include reinforcing consistent sleep schedules, sufficient TIB, conditioning bed for sleep only, and sleep environment modifications: quiet, dark, cool, safe, and clean. Sleep interventions also target related health habits including use of caffeine, alcohol, tobacco, or other substances; exercise; and support for treatment adherence such as use of CPAP equipment and weight loss programs (Barnes, Goldsworthy, Cary, & Hill, 2009).

Although the primary focus of this chapter is sleep, occupational balance encompasses both patterns and cycles of activity, including periods of **rest**. Yoga, meditation, and other spiritual or relaxation practices, especially when undertaken consistently, may not only improve sleep by lowering autonomic arousal and bringing mindful attention to the present but also have important independent adaptive and restorative qualities (Benson & Proctor, 2010; Solet, 2014). In *The Power of Rest*, Dr. Matthew Edlund (2010) offers an accessible, comprehensive review of the benefits of rest including through music and companionship.

Conclusion

Sleep medicine is a new frontier, an opportunity to enhance health, safety, well-being, performance, and even longevity. As occupational therapists, our unique perspective on daily living, together with the relationships we enjoy with our clients and colleagues, puts us in a unique position to contribute to this dynamic area of science and health care.

As part of your professional commitment, improve sleep awareness, evaluation, and treatment and sleep well!

Resources for More Information about Sleep and Rest

Websites

Centers for Disease Control and Prevention: http://www.cdc.gov/sleep/
Center for Health Design: http://www.healthdesign.org/chd/research/validating-acoustic-guidelines-healthcare-facilities

Harvard Medical School, Division of Sleep Medicine: http://healthysleep.med.harvard.edu/portal/; Section on Sleep Disorders: http://healthysleep.med.harvard.edu/healthy/getting/treatment/an-overview-of-sleep-disorders
International Network for Occupational Therapists Interested in Sleep: http://www.sleepOT.org (new resource to empower OT practitioners, students, and researchers to consider, identify, and address sleep and sleep problems)
National Institute of Alcohol Abuse and Alcoholism: http://www.niaaa.nih.gov/
National Sleep Foundation Sleep in America Polls: http://www.sleepfoundation.org/category/article-type/sleep-america-polls
National Sleep Foundation: http://www.sleepfoundation.org/articles/sleep-disorders?
YMCA: http://www.ymca.net/healthy-family-home/sleep-well.html

Additional Resources

American Academy of Sleep Medicine: http://www.aasmnet.org
Journal of Clinical Sleep Medicine: http://www.aasmnet.org/JCSM
Sleep Centers: http://www.sleepcenters.org
SLEEP: http://www.journalsleep.org

Acknowledgments

I would like to thank the patients who have been my teachers for the more than 40 years I have been an occupational therapist as well as Jenny Lee Olsen, former director of Library Services at Cambridge Health Alliance, for help in the literature search, the chapter peer reviewers for their careful attention and thoughtful comments, and the editors for offering me the opportunity to contribute this chapter on sleep, an important emerging area of practice.

REFERENCES

Albert, S. M., Roth, T., Toscani, M., Vitiello, M. V., & Zee, P. (2017). Sleep health and appropriate use of OTC sleep aids in older adults. *The Gerontologist, 57*, 163–170.

American Academy of Sleep Medicine. (2009). *Naps with rapid eye movement sleep increase receptiveness to positive emotion.* Retrieved from http://www.aasmnet.org/articles.aspx?id=1317

American College of Chest Physicians. (2010, November). *Electronic media taking its toll on teens.* Paper presented at the 76th CHEST Annual Meeting of American College of Chest Physicians, Vancouver, Canada. Retrieved from http://www.chestnet.org/accp/article/electronic-media-taking-its-toll-teens

American Occupational Therapy Association. (2008). Occupational therapy practice framework: Domain and process, 2nd edition. *American Journal of Occupational Therapy, 62*, 625–683.

Anaby, D. R., Backman, C. L., & Jarus, T. (2010). Measuring occupational balance: Theoretical exploration of two approaches to occupational balance. *Canadian Journal of Occupational Therapy, 77*, 280–288.

Ancoli-Israel, S., & Cooke, J. R. (2005). Prevalence and comorbidity of insomnia and effect on functioning in elderly populations. *Journal of the American Geriatrics Society, 53*, S264–S271.

Ayas, N. T. (2010). If you weigh too much, maybe you should try sleeping more. *SLEEP, 33*, 143–144.

Ayas, N. T., White, D. P., Al-Delaimy, W. K., Manson, J. E., Stampfer, M. J., Speizer, F. E., & Hu, F. B. (2003). A prospective study of self-reported sleep duration and incipient diabetes in women. *Diabetes Care, 26*, 380–384.

Ayas, N. T., White, D. P., Manson, J. E., Stampfer, M. J., Speizer, F. E., Malhotra, A., & Hu, F. B. (2003). A prospective study of sleep duration and coronary heart disease in women. *Archives of Internal Medicine, 163*, 205–209.

Banks, S., Van Dongen, H. P., Mailsen, G., & Dinges, D. F. (2010). Neurobehavioral dynamics following chronic sleep restriction: Dose-response effects of one night for recovery. *SLEEP, 33*, 1013–1026.

Barnes, M., Goldsworthy, U. R., Cary, B. A., & Hill, C. J. (2009). A diet and exercise program to improve clinical outcomes on patients with obstructive sleep apnea—A feasibility study. *Journal of Clinical Sleep Medicine, 5*, 409–421.

Bartick, M. C., Thai, X., Schmidt, T., Altaye, A., & Solet, J. M. (2010). Decrease in as needed sedative use by limiting nighttime sleep disruptions from hospital staff. *Journal of Hospital Medicine, 5*, E20–E24.

Basner, M., Fomberstein, K. M., Razavi, F. M., Banks, S., William, J. H., Rosa, R. R., & Dinges, D. F. (2007). American time use survey: Sleep time and its relationship to waking activities. *SLEEP, 30*, 1085–1095.

Basner, M., Müller, U., & Elmenhorst, E. M. (2011). Single and combined effects of air, road, and rail traffic noise on sleep and recuperation. *SLEEP, 34*, 11–23.

Bayard, M., Avonda, T., & Wadzinski, J. (2008). Restless legs syndrome. *American Family Physician, 78*, 235–240.

Beebe, D. W., Ris, D. M., Kramer, M. E., Long, E., & Amin, R. (2010). The association between sleep disordered breathing, academic grades, and cognitive and behavioral functioning among overweight subjects during middle to late childhood. *SLEEP, 33*, 1447–1457.

Benson, H., & Proctor, W. (2010). *Relaxation revolution: Enhancing your personal health through the science and genetics of mind body healing.* New York, NY: Scribner.

Berkman, L. F., Buxton, O., Ertel, K., & Okechukwu, C. (2010). Managers' practices related to work-family balance predict employee cardiovascular risk and sleep duration in extended care settings. *Journal of Occupational Health Psychology, 15*, 316–329.

Bibbs, M. (2011). A wake up call to sleepy workers. *Sleep Diagnosis and Therapy, 6*, 14.

Blakeney, A., & Marshall, A. (2009). Water quality, health, and human occupations. *American Journal of Occupational Therapy, 63*, 46–57.

Bondoc, S., & Siebert, C. (2008). *The role of occupational therapy in chronic disease management.* Bethesda, MD: American Occupational Therapy Association.

Braley, T. J., & Chervin, R. D. (2010). Fatigue in multiple sclerosis: Mechanisms, evaluation, and treatment. *SLEEP, 33*, 1061–1067.

Brendel, D. H., Florman, J., Roberts, S., & Solet, J. M. (2001). "In sleep I almost never grope": Blindness, neuropsychiatric deficits, and a chaotic upbringing. *Harvard Review of Psychiatry, 9*, 178–188.

Brown, C. A., Berry, R., Tan, M. C., Khoshia, A., Turlapati, L., & Swedlove, F. (2011). A critique of the evidence-base for non-pharmacological sleep interventions for persons with dementia. *Dementia, 12*, 174–201.

Burton, A. R., Rahman, K., Kadota, Y., Lloyd, A., & Vollmer-Conna, U. (2010). Reduced heart rate variability predicts poor sleep quality in a case-control study of chronic fatigue syndrome. *Experimental Brain Research, 204*, 71–78.

Busch-Vishniac, I. J., West, J. E., Barnhill, C., Hunter, T., Orellana, D., & Chivukula, R. (2005). Noise levels in Johns Hopkins Hospital. *The Journal of the Acoustical Society of America, 118*, 3629–3645.

Buxton, O. M., Ellenbogen, J. M., Wang, W., Carballeira, A., O'Connor, S., Cooper, D., . . . Solet, J. M. (2012). Sleep disruption due to hospital noises: A prospective evaluation. *Annals of Internal Medicine, 157*, 170–179.

Buxton, O. M., Lee, C. W., L'Hermite-Baleriaux, M., Turek, F. W., & Van Cauter, E. (2003). Exercise elicits phase shifts and acute alterations of melatonin that vary with circadian phase. *American Journal of Physiology. Regulatory, Integrative and Comparative Physiology, 284*, R714–R724.

Buxton, O. M., & Marcelli, E. (2010). Short and long sleep are positively associated with obesity, diabetes, hypertension, and cardiovascular disease among adults in the United States. *Social Science and Medicine, 71*, 1027–1036.

Chandola, T., Ferrie, J. E., Perski, A., Akbaraly, T., & Marmor, M. G. (2010). The effect of short sleep duration on coronary heart disease risk is greatest among those with sleep disturbance: A prospective study from Whitehall II cohort. *SLEEP, 33*, 739–744.

Chervin, R. D. (2010). Use of clinical tools and tests in sleep medicine. In M. H. Kryger, T. Roth, & W. C. Dement (Eds.), *Principles and practice of sleep medicine* (5th ed., pp. 666–679). St. Louis, MO: Elsevier Saunders.

Chhangani, B. S., Roehrs, T. A., Harris, E. J., Hyde, M., Drake, C., Hudgel, D. W., & Roth, T. (2009). Pain sensitivity in sleepy pain-free normals. *SLEEP, 32*, 1011–1017.

Chien, K. L., Chen, P. C., Hsu, H. C., Su, T. C., Sung, F. C., Chen, M. F., & Lee, Y. T. (2010). Habitual sleep duration and insomnia and the risk of cardiovascular events and all-cause death: Report from a community-based cohort. *SLEEP, 33*, 177–184.

Choi, S. W., Peek-Asa, C., Sprince, N. L., Rautiainen, R. H., Flamme, G. A., Whitten, P. S., & Zwerling, C. (2006). Sleep quantity and quality as a predictor of injuries in a rural population. *American Journal of Emergency Medicine, 24*, 189–196.

Classen, S., Levy, C., Meyer, D. L., Bewernitz, M., Lanford, D. N., & Mann, W. C. (2011). Simulated driving performance of combat veterans with mild traumatic brain injury and posttraumatic stress disorder: A pilot study. *American Journal of Occupational Therapy, 65*, 419–427.

Coelho, F. M., Georgsson, H., Narayansingh, M., Swartz, R. H., & Murray, B. J. (2010). Higher prevalence of periodic limb movements of sleep in patients with history of stroke. *Journal of Clinical Sleep Medicine, 6*, 428–430.

Cohen, D. A., Wang, W., Wyatt, J. K., Kronauer, R. E., Dijk, D. J., Czeisler, C. A., & Klerman, E. B. (2010). Uncovering residual effects of chronic sleep loss on human performance. *Science Translational Medicine, 2*, 14ra3.

Connor, J., Norton, R., Ameratunga, S., Robinson, E., Civil, I., Dunn, R., . . . Jackson, R. (2002). Driver sleepiness and risk of serious injury to car occupants: Population-based case control study. *BMJ, 324*, 1125.

Cooke, J. R., Ayalon, L., Palmer, B. W., Loredo, J. S., Corey-Bloom, J., Natarajan, L., . . . Ancoli-Israel, S. (2009). Sustained use of CPAP slows deterioration of cognition, sleep, and mood in patients with Alzheimer's disease and obstructive sleep apnea: A preliminary study. *Journal of Clinical Sleep Medicine, 5*, 305–309.

Copinschi, G. (2005). Metabolic and endocrine effects of sleep deprivation. *Essentials of Psychopharmacology, 6*, 341–347.

Dogan, O., Ertekin, S., & Dogan, S. (2005). Sleep quality in hospitalized patients. *Journal of Clinical Nursing, 14*, 107–113.

Dorrian, J., Sweeney, M., & Dawson, D. (2011). Modeling fatigue-related truck accidents: Prior sleep duration, recency and continuity. *Sleep and Biological Rhythms, 9*, 3–11.

Drake, C., Roehrs, T., Breslau, N., Johnson, E., Jefferson, C., Scofield, H., & Roth, T. (2010). The 10-year risk of verified motor vehicle crashes in relation to physiologic sleepiness. *SLEEP, 33*, 745–752.

Dunton, W. R. (1917). History of occupational therapy. *The Modern Hospital, 8*, 380–382.

Durmer, J. S., & Dinges, D. F. (2005). Neurocognitive consequences of sleep deprivation. *Seminars in Neurology, 25*, 117–129.

Edlund, M. (2003). *The body clock advantage: Finding your best time to succeed in love, work, play, and exercise.* Avon, MA: Adams Media.

Edlund, M. (2010). *The power of rest: Why sleep alone is not enough. A 30-day plan to reset your body.* New York, NY: HarperOne.

Epstein, J. E., & Brown, R. (2010). Sleep disorders in spinal cord injury. In V. W. Lin (Ed.), *Spinal cord medicine: Principles and practice* (2nd ed., pp. 230–240). New York, NY: Demos.

Facility Guidelines Institute. (2010). *Guidelines for design and construction of health care facilities—2010 edition.* Chicago, IL: American Hospital Association Services.

Flier, J. S., & Elmquist, J. K. (2004). A good night's sleep: Future antidote to the obesity epidemic? *Annals of Internal Medicine, 141,* 885–886.

Fogelberg, D. J., Hoffman, J. M., Dikmen, S., Temkin, N. R., & Bell, K. R. (2012). Association of sleep and co-occurring psychological conditions at 1 year after traumatic head injury. *Archives of Physical Medicine Rehabilitation, 93,* 1313–1318.

Fogelberg, D. J., Hughes, A. B., Vitiello, M. V., Hoffman, J. M., & Amtmann, D. (2016). Comparison of sleep problems in individuals with spinal cord injury and multiple sclerosis. *Journal of Clinical Sleep Medicine, 12,* 695–701.

Fogelberg, D. J., Leland, N. E., Blanchard, J., Rich, T. J., & Clark, F. A. (2017). Qualitative experience of sleep in individuals with spinal cord injury. *OTJR: Occupation, Participation and Health, 37,* 89–97.

Frazier, S. C. (2005). Health outcomes and polypharmacy in elderly individuals: An integrated literature review. *Journal of Gerontological Nursing, 31,* 4–11.

Friese, R. S., Diaz-Arrastia, R., McBride, D., Frankel, H., & Gentilello, L. M. (2007). Quantity and quality of sleep in the surgical intensive care unit: Are our patients sleeping? *The Journal of Trauma, 63,* 1210–1214.

Gangwisch, J. E., Babiss, L. A., Malaspina, D., Turner, B., Zammit, G. K., & Posner, K. (2010). Earlier parental set bedtimes as a protective factor against depression and suicidal ideation. *SLEEP, 33,* 97–106.

Gangwisch, J. E., Malaspina, D., Boden-Albala, B., & Heymsfield, S. B. (2005). Inadequate sleep as a risk factor for obesity: Analyses of the NHANES I. *SLEEP, 28,* 1289–1296.

Gujar, N., McDonald, S. A., Nishida, M., & Walker, M. P. (2010). A role for REM sleep in recalibrating the sensitivity of the human brain to specific emotions. *Cerebral Cortex, 21,* 115–123.

Haack, G., & Mullington, J. M. (2005). Sustained sleep restriction reduces emotional and physical well-being. *Pain, 119,* 56–64.

Hale, L. (2005). Who has time to sleep? *Journal of Public Health, 27,* 205–211.

Hale, L., & Do, D. P. (2007). Racial differences in self-reports of sleep duration in a population-based study. *SLEEP, 30,* 1096–1103.

Hamilton, N. A., Catley, D., & Karlson, C. (2007). Sleep and affective response to stress and pain. *Health Psychology, 26,* 288–295.

Haponik, E. F., Frye, A. W., Richards, B., Wymer, A., Hinds, A., Pearce, K., . . . Konen, J. (1996). Sleep history is neglected diagnostic information. Challenges for primary care physicians. *Journal of General Internal Medicine, 11,* 759–761.

Hawkley, L. C., Cacioppo, J. T., & Preacher, K. J. (2011). As we said, loneliness (not living alone) explains individual differences in sleep quality: Reply. *Health Psychology, 30,* 136.

Hawkley, L. C., Preacher, K. J., & Cacioppo, J. T. (2010). Loneliness impairs daytime functioning but not sleep duration. *Health Psychology, 29,* 124–129.

Haynes, P. L. (2009). Is CBT-I effective for pain? *Journal of Clinical Sleep Medicine, 5,* 363–364.

Hobson, J. A. (2011). *Dream life: An experimental memoir.* London, United Kingdom: MIT Press.

Howell, M. J., Schenck, C. H., & Crow, S. J. (2009). A review of nighttime eating disorders. *Sleep Medicine Reviews, 13,* 23–34.

Hume, K. I. (2011). Noise pollution: A ubiquitous unrecognized disruptor of sleep? *SLEEP, 34,* 7–8.

Irwin, M. R., Wang, M., Ribeiro, D., Cho, H. J., Olmstead, R., Breen, E. C., . . . Cole, S. (2008). Sleep loss activates cellular inflammatory signaling. *Biological Psychiatry, 64,* 538–554.

Johns, M. W. (1991). A new method for measuring daytime sleepiness: The Epworth Sleepiness Scale. *SLEEP, 14,* 540–545.

Johnson, K. G., & Johnson, C. D. (2010). Frequency of sleep apnea in stroke and TIA patients: A meta-analysis. *Journal of Clinical Sleep Medicine, 6,* 131–137.

Jozwiak, N., Postuma, R. B., Montplaisir, J., Latreille, V., Panisset, M., Chouinard, S., . . . Gagnon, J. F. (2017). REM sleep behavior disorder and cognitive impairment in Parkinson's disease. *SLEEP, 40,* zsx101. doi:10.1093/sleep/zsx101

Kim, H., & Young, T. (2005). Subjective daytime sleepiness: Dimensions and correlates in the general population. *SLEEP, 28,* 625–634.

Kristiansen, J., Perrson, R., Björk, J., Albin, M., Jakobsson, K., Ostergren, P. O., & Ardö, J. (2011). Work stress, worries, and pain intersect synergistically with modeled traffic noise on cross-sectional associations with self-reported sleep problems. *International Archives of Occupational and Environmental Health, 84,* 211–224.

Kryger, M. H., Roth, T., & Dement, W. C. (Eds.). (2011). *Principles and practice of sleep medicine* (5th ed.). St. Louis, MO: Elsevier Saunders.

Kushida, C. A. (2007). Clinical presentation, diagnosis, and quality of life issues in restless legs syndrome. *American Journal of Medicine, 120,* S4–S12.

Leland, N. E., Fogelberg, D., Sleight, A., Mallinson, T., Vigen, C., Blanchard, J., . . . Clark, F. (2016). Napping and nighttime sleep: Findings from an occupation-based intervention. *American Journal of Occupational Therapy, 70,* 7004270010p1–7004270010p7.

Leland, N. E., Marcione, N., Schepens, S. L., Kelkar, K., & Fogelberg, D. (2014). What is occupational therapy's role in addressing sleep problems among older adults? *OTJR: Occupation, Participation and Health, 4,* 141–149.

Levine, A. C., Adusumilli, J., & Landrigan, C. P. (2010). Effects of reducing or eliminating resident work shifts over 16 hours: A systematic review. *SLEEP, 32,* 1043–1053.

Luckhaupt, S. E., Tak, S., & Calvert, G. M., (2010). The prevalence of short sleep by industry and occupation in the National Health Interview Survey. *SLEEP, 33,* 149–159.

Luyster, F. S., Chasens, E. R., Wasko, M. C., & Dunbar-Jacob, J. (2011). Sleep quality and functional disability in patients with rheumatoid arthritis. *Journal of Clinical Sleep Medicine, 7,* 49–55.

Mah, C. D., Mah, K. E., Kezerian, E. J., & Dement, W. C. (2011). The effects of sleep extension on the athletic performance of collegiate basketball players. *SLEEP, 34,* 943–950.

McCall, W. V., Kimball, J., Boggs, N., Lasater, B., D'Agostino, R. B., & Rosenquist, P. B. (2009). Prevalence and prediction of primary sleep disorders in a clinical trial of depressed patients with insomnia. *Journal of Clinical Sleep Medicine, 5,* 454–458.

McHugh, J., & Lawlor, B. (2011). Commentary: Living alone does not account for the association between loneliness and sleep in older adults: Response to Hawkley, Preacher, and Cacioppo, 2010. *Health Psychology, 30,* 135.

Mednick, S. C., & Ehrman, M. (2006). *Take a nap! Change your life.* New York, NY: Workman.

Nurok, M., Czeisler, C. A., & Lehmann, L. S. (2010). Sleep deprivation, elective surgical procedures, and informed consent. *The New England Journal of Medicine, 36,* 2577–2579.

O'Connor, G. T., Caffo, B., Newman, A. B., Quan, S. F., Rapoport, D. M., Redline, S., . . . Shahar, E. (2009). Prospective study of sleep-disordered breathing and hypertension: The Sleep Heart Health Study. *American Journal of Respiratory Critical Care Medicine, 179,* 1159–1164.

Ohayon, M. M. (2002). Epidemiology of insomnia: What we know and what we still need to learn. *Sleep Medicine Reviews, 6,* 97–111.

Ohayon, M. M., Carskadon, M. A., Guilleminault, C., & Vitiello, M. V. (2004). Meta-analysis of quantitative sleep parameters from childhood to old age in healthy individuals: Developing normative sleep values across the human lifespan. *SLEEP, 27,* 1255–1273.

Ohayon, M. M., & Vecchierini, M. F. (2005). Normative sleep data, cognitive function and daily living activities in older adults in the community. *SLEEP, 28,* 981–989.

Owens, J. A., Belon, K., & Moss, P. (2010). Impact of delaying school start time on adolescent sleep, mood, and behavior. *Archives of Pediatrics and Adolescent Medicine, 164,* 608–614.

Owens, J. A., & Mindell, J. A. (2005). *Take charge of your child's sleep: The all-in-one resource for solving sleep problems in kids and teens.* New York, NY: Marlowe & Company.

Owens, J. A., Spirito, A., & McGuinn, M. (2000). The Children's Sleep Habits Questionnaire (CSHQ): Psychometric properties of a survey instrument for school-aged children. *SLEEP, 23,* 1043–1051.

Owens, J. A., Spirito, A., McGuinn, M., & Nobile, C. (2000). Sleep habits and sleep disturbance in elementary school-aged children. *Journal of Developmental and Behavioral Pediatrics, 21,* 27–36.

Ownby, R. L., Saeed, M., Wohlgemuth, W., Capasso, R., Acevedo, A., Peruyera, G., & Sevush, S. (2010). Caregiver reports of sleep problems in non-Hispanic white, Hispanic, and African American patients with Alzheimer dementia. *Journal of Clinical Sleep Medicine, 6,* 281–289.

Parcell, D. L., Ponsford, J. L., Redman, J. R., & Rajaratnam, S. M. (2008). Poor sleep quality and changes in objectively recorded sleep after traumatic brain injury: A preliminary study *Archives of Physical Medicine and Rehabilitation, 89,* 843–850.

Passos, G. S., Poyares, D., Santana, M. G., Garbuio, S., Tufik, S., & Mello, M. T. (2010). Effect of acute physical exercise on patients with chronic primary insomnia. *Journal of Clinical Sleep Medicine, 6,* 270–275.

Patel, S. R., Ayas, N. T., Malhotra, M. R., White, D. P., Schernhammer, E. S., Speizer, F. E., . . . Hu, F. B. (2004). A prospective study of sleep duration and mortality risk in women. *SLEEP, 27,* 440–444.

Patel, S. R., & Hu, F. B. (2008). Short sleep duration and weight gain: A systematic review. *Obesity, 16,* 643–653.

Peppard, P. E. (2009). Is obstructive sleep apnea a risk factor for hypertension?—Differences between the Wisconsin sleep cohort and the Sleep heart health study. *Journal of Clinical Sleep Medicine, 5,* 404–405.

Pizza, F., Contardi, S., Antognini, A. B., Zagoraiou, M., Borrotti, M., Mostacci, B., . . . Cirignotta, F. (2010). Sleep quality and motor vehicle crashes in adolescents. *Journal of Clinical Sleep Medicine, 6,* 41–45.

Poe, G. R., Walsh, C. M., & Bjorness, T. E. (2010). Both duration and timing of sleep are important to memory consolidation. *SLEEP, 33,* 1277–1280.

Quan, S. F., Parthasarathy, S., & Budhiraja, R. (2010). Healthy sleep education—a salve for obesity? *Journal of Clinical Sleep Medicine, 6,* 18–19.

Redline, S. (2009). Does sleep disordered breathing increase hypertension risk? A practical perspective on interpreting the evidence. *Journal of Clinical Sleep Medicine, 5,* 406–408.

Roehrs, T., Hyde, M., Blaisdell, B., Greenwald, M., & Roth, T. (2006). Sleep loss and REM sleep loss are hyperalgesic. *SLEEP, 29,* 145–151.

Roehrs, T., & Roth, T. (2008). Caffeine: Sleep and daytime sleepiness. *Sleep Medicine Reviews, 12,* 153–162.

Roehrs, T., & Roth, T. (2011a). Medication and substance abuse. In M. H. Kryger, T. Roth, W. C. Dement (Eds.), *Principles and practice of sleep medicine* (5th ed., pp. 1512–1523). St. Louis, MO: Elsevier Saunders.

Roehrs, T., & Roth, T. (2011b). *Sleep, sleepiness, and alcohol use.* Retrieved from http://pubs.niaaa.nih.gov/publications/arh25-2/101-109.htm

Roth, T., Roehrs, T., & Pies, R. (2007). Insomnia: Pathophysiology and implications for treatment. *Sleep Medicine Reviews, 11,* 71–79.

Sadeh, A. (2011). The role and validity of actigraphy in sleep medicine: An update. *Sleep Medicine Reviews, 15,* 259–267.

Sánchez-Ortuño, M. M., Edinger, J. D., Means, M. K., & Almirall, D. (2010). Home is where the sleep is: An ecological approach to test the validity of actigraphy for the assessment of insomnia. *Journal of Clinical Sleep Medicine, 6,* 21–29.

Schweitzer, P. (2011). Drugs that disturb sleep and wakefulness. In M. H. Kryger, T. Roth, W. C. Dement (Eds.), *Principles and practice of sleep medicine* (5th ed., pp. 542–562). St. Louis, MO: Elsevier Saunders.

Senthilvel, E., Auckley, D., & Dasarathy, J. (2011). Evaluation of sleep disorders in the primary care setting: History taking compared to questionnaires. *Journal of Clinical Sleep Medicine, 7,* 41–48.

Shepard, J. W., Buyesse, D. J., Chesson, A. L., Dement, W. C., Goldberg, R., Guilleinault, C., . . . White, D. P. (2005). History of the development of sleep medicine in the United States. *Journal of Clinical Sleep Medicine, 1,* 61–81.

Sixel-Döring, F., Schweitzer, M., Mollenhauer, B., & Trenkwalder, C. (2011). Intraindividual variability of REM sleep behavior disorder in Parkinson's disease: A comparative assessment using a new REM Sleep Behavior Disorder Severity Scale (RBDSS) for clinical routine. *Journal of Clinical Sleep Medicine, 7,* 75–80.

Slagle, E. C. (1934). The occupational therapy programme in the State of New York. *Journal of Mental Science, 80,* 639–649.

Smith, B., & Phillips, B. A. (2011). Truckers drive their own assessment for obstructive sleep apnea: A collaborative approach to online self-assessment for obstructive sleep apnea. *Journal of Clinical Sleep Medicine, 7,* 241–245.

Solet, J. M. (2014). Optimizing personal and social adaptation. In M. V. Radomski & C. A. Trombly Latham (Eds.), *Occupational therapy for physical dysfunction* (7th ed., pp. 925–954). Philadelphia, PA: Lippincott Williams & Wilkins.

Solet, J. M. (2016). Translating sleep science into policy. *Sleep Health, 2,* 264–265. doi:10.1016/j.sleh.2016.09.005

Solet, J. M., & Barach, P. (2012). Managing alarm fatigue in cardiac care. *Progress in Pediatric Cardiology, 33,* 85–90.

Solet, J. M., Buxton, O. M., Ellenbogen, J. M., Wang, W., & Carballiera, A. (2010). *Validating acoustic guidelines for healthcare facilities. Evidence-based design meets evidence-based medicine: The sound sleep study.* Concord, CA: The Center for Health Design. Retrieved from http://www.healthdesign.org/chd/research/validating-acoustic-guidelines-healthcare-facilities

Sorscher, A. J. (2008). How is your sleep: A neglected topic for health care screening. *Journal of the American Board of Family Medicine, 21,* 141–148.

Spiegel, K., Knutson, K., Leproult, R., Tasali, E., & Van Cauter, E. (2005). Sleep loss: A novel risk factor for insulin resistance and Type 2 diabetes. *Journal of Applied Physiology, 99,* 2008–2019.

Spiegel, K., Tasali, E., Penev, P., & Van Cauter, E. (2004). Brief communication: Sleep curtailment in healthy young men is associated with decreased leptin levels, elevated ghrelin levels, and increased hunger and appetite. *Annals of Internal Medicine, 141,* 846–850.

Stickgold, R. (2005). Sleep-dependent memory consolidation. *Nature, 437,* 1272–1285.

Stout, K., & Finlayson, M. (2011). Fatigue management in chronic illness: The role of occupational therapy. *OT Practice, 16*(1), 16–19.

Stroe, A. F., Roth, T., Jefferson, C., Hudgel, D. W., Roehrs, T., Moss, K., & Drake, C. L. (2010). Comparative levels of excessive daytime sleepiness in common medical disorders. *Sleep Medicine, 11,* 890–896.

Tomfohr, L. M., Ancoli-Israel, S., Loredo, J. S., & Dimsdale, J. E. (2011). Effects of continuous positive airway pressure on fatigue and sleepiness in patients with obstructive sleep apnea: Data from a randomized controlled trial. *SLEEP, 34,* 121–126.

Tregear, S., Reston, J., Schoelles, K., & Phillips, B. (2009). Obstructive sleep apnea and risk of motor vehicle crash: A systematic review and meta-analysis. *Journal of Clinical Sleep Medicine, 5,* 573–581.

Umberson, D. (1992). Gender, marital status and the social control of health behaviors. *Social Science & Medicine, 34,* 907–917.

Van Dongen, H. P., Maislin, G., Mullington, J. M., & Dinges, D. (2003). The cumulative cost of additional wakefulness: Dose-response effects on neurobehavioral functions and sleep physiology from chronic sleep restriction and total sleep deprivation. *SLEEP, 26,* 117–126.

Vaughn, B. V., & D'Cruz, O. (2011). Cardinal manifestations of sleep disorders. In M. H. Kryger, T. Roth, & W. C. Dement (Eds.), *Principles and practice of sleep medicine* (5th ed., pp. 647–657). St. Louis, MO: Elsevier Saunders.

Verse, T., & Hörmann, K. (2011). The surgical treatment of sleep-related upper airway obstruction. *Deutsches Ärzteblatt International, 108,* 216–221.

Viola-Saltzman, M., Watson, N. F., Bogart, A., Goldberg, J., & Buchwald, D. (2010). High prevalence of restless legs syndrome among patients with fibromyalgia: A controlled cross-sectional study. *Journal of Clinical Sleep Medicine, 6,* 423–427.

Vitiello, M. V., Rybarczk, B., Von Korff, M., & Stepanski, E. J. (2009). Cognitive behavioral therapy for insomnia improves sleep and decreases pain in older adults with co-morbid insomnia and osteoarthritis. *Journal of Clinical Sleep Medicine, 5,* 355–362.

Walker, M. P., & Stickgold, R. (2004). Sleep-dependent learning and memory consolidation. *Neuron, 44,* 121–133.

Watanabe, M., Kikuchi, H., Katsutoshi, T., & Takahashi, M. (2010). Association of short sleep duration with weight gain and obesity at 1 year follow-up: A large-scale prospective study. *SLEEP, 33,* 161–167.

Watson, N. F. (2010). Stroke and sleep specialists: An opportunity to intervene? *Journal of Clinical Sleep Medicine, 6,* 138–139.

Watson, N. F., Buchwald, D., Vitiello, M. V., Noonan, C., & Goldberg, J. (2010). A twin study of sleep duration and body mass index. *Journal of Clinical Sleep Medicine, 6,* 11–17.

Weaver, E., Gradisar, M., Dohnt, H., Lovato, N., & Douglas, P. (2010). The effect of presleep video-game playing in adolescent sleep. *Journal of Clinical Sleep Medicine, 6,* 184–185.

Weinhouse, G. L., & Schwab, R. J. (2006). Sleep in the critically ill patient. *SLEEP, 29,* 707–716.

Xie, C., Kang, H., Xu, Q., Chen, M. J., Liao, Y., Thiyagarajan, M., . . . Nedergaard, M. (2013). Sleep drives metabolite clearance from the adult brain. *Science, 342,* 373–377.

Youngstedt, S. D., & Buxton, O. M. (2003). Jet lag and athletic performance. *American Journal of Medicine and Sports, 5,* 219–226.

Zee, P. C., & Turek, F. W. (2006). Sleep and health: Everywhere and in both directions. *Archives of Internal Medicine, 166,* 1686–1688.

Zizi, F., Jean-Louis, G., Brown, C. D., Ogedegbe, G., Boutin-Foster, C., & McFarlane, S. I. (2011). Sleep duration and risk of diabetes mellitus: Epidemiologic evidence and pathophysiologic insights. *Current Diabetes Reports, 10,* 43–47.

the **Point®** *For additional resources on the subjects discussed in this chapter, visit* **http://thePoint.lww.com /Willard-Spackman13e**. *See* **Appendix I, Resources and Evidence for Common Conditions Addressed in OT** *for more information on sleep and common medical conditions and psychiatric disorders.*

Social Participation

Mary Alunkal Khetani, Wendy J. Coster

LEARNING OBJECTIVES

After reading this chapter, you will be able to:

1. Describe how social participation is defined in comparison to performance and quality of life.
2. Evaluate the strengths and limitations of available assessments to develop participation profiles of clients seeking occupational therapy services.
   a. Describe ways that you might appraise a client's participation using available measures.
   b. Describe ways that you can incorporate information about environmental supports and barriers in your appraisal of a client's participation.
3. Describe ways of intervening to promote participation at the individual, group, or organizational level.

Introduction

More than one billion people or 15% of the world's population live with disability (World Health Organization [WHO] & World Bank, 2011), and approximately 53 million Americans live with a disability (Frontera et al., 2017). Estimates of global disability from the *World Report on Disability* are striking, especially when you consider the likelihood that this is an underestimate of the prevalence of disability because the estimates were based on the presence or absence of a select group of impairments.

Current models of disability reflect a broader understanding of the construct. Disability is not conceptualized as a stable characteristic of a person but rather as a state in which the individual experiences functional limitations (e.g., grasping utensils) (Lollar & Andresen, 2011). According to the *International Classification of Functioning, Disability and Health* (ICF) and the *ICF Version for Children and Youth* (ICF-CY), functional limitations may, in turn, lead to difficulties participating in society on an equal basis with others (WHO, 2001, 2007).

CENTENNIAL NOTES

Consistent Conceptualization of Client Participation in Occupation

Between 2001 and 2007, the WHO released the ICF and ICF-CY frameworks, which drew international attention to participation as a key rehabilitation outcome (WHO, 2001, 2007). In an editorial speaking to these documents and the profession's role in them, Baum (2003) noted, "The profession of occupational therapy was founded on the principles of occupation and participation, and now, these principles have become central concepts in the definition of health" (p. 46). She went on to credit Adolph Meyer, from the 1920s; Mary Reilly, from the 1960s; Tristam Englehart, from the 1970s; and Gary Kielhofner, from the 1990s, as key figures whose work contributed to increasing the focus on participation. The AOTA and American Occupational Therapy Foundation (AOTF) are also credited for staging scholarship on participation, such as Mary Law's Distinguished Scholar Lecture on participation in 2002. Occupational therapists, with their expertise and commitment to advancing knowledge regarding participation in occupation, are suited to contribute to the ongoing evolution of the ICF and ICF-CY frameworks (Hemmingsson & Jonsson, 2005).

There is a need for greater conceptual clarity in our own practice framework to support clear and consistent measurement of participation as a "patient-important"

outcome. In our profession, social participation has been simultaneously viewed as a separate area of occupation and as an outcome of engagement in all areas of occupation. Current work is providing greater consistency in how the concept is described in our profession. This conceptual clarity should translate to greater consistency in how we gather information about client participation to create the occupational profile for intervention planning, implementation, and outcomes monitoring.

We (Mary A. Khetani and Wendy J. Coster) have been fortunate to be among a number of OT researchers and practitioners who have developed conceptually grounded participation assessments. These assessments have been used to build stronger evidence of disparities in participation across multiple diagnoses, ages, and contexts. More recently, these assessments have helped to elucidate the important role of the environment in shaping opportunities for meaningful participation in occupations. This knowledge, in turn, has increased the need for interventions that focus on minimizing disparities in participation. In particular, a shift toward environmentally focused interventions targeting individuals and organizations holds promise. This multipronged approach to intervention research parallels our profession's shift to preparing entry-level practitioners to improve participation outcomes with individual clients and within broader systems of care.

This contemporary definition of disability emphasizes the importance of understanding individuals' experiences of disability when they attempt to participate in meaningful occupation (Cutchin, 2004).

Information about participation is of particular importance for occupational therapists because a major focus of our profession is on promoting participation in everyday occupations that give meaning and purpose to people's lives (American Occupational Therapy Association [AOTA], 2014). To practice at our best, it is imperative to understand the concept of social participation. This knowledge can help us to determine how to partner with our clients to minimize their disablement experience(s) when attempting to participate in occupations that they need and want to do.

As a student en route to a career in occupational therapy (OT), this chapter is intended to provide you with an introduction to contemporary thinking about social participation—how it is currently understood, assessed, and promoted. It is a primer for shaping your clinical lens toward supporting client participation in occupation.

Defining Social Participation

The Distinction between Performance and Social Participation

A client's social participation is related to, but different from, his or her competence performing discrete tasks of everyday life (e.g., putting on shoes, eating with a utensil, following directions in a small group activity, asking permission before using someone else's property). Clients with different task-related competencies can actively participate and derive equal value from the same occupations (Imms, Adair, Keen, Ullenhag, Rosenbaum, & Granlund, 2015). Thus, a client with a spinal cord injury may still show enjoyment when participating in team sports like his or her peers, although he or she may move about the court using a wheelchair. Similarly, a client with a sensory

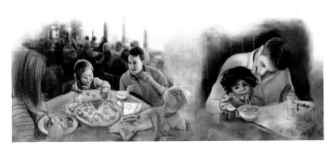

FIGURE 55-1 Clients with different task-related competencies can actively participate and derive equal value from the same occupations. (Used with permission from artist Christina Sidorowych.)

processing disorder may still participate like his or her siblings in the family ritual of dining out at a local restaurant, although the client may request a modified meal, use technology to interact with family members while waiting for the meal to arrive, and use adaptive utensils that were brought from home to eat his or her meal. In these examples, the clients each perform functional tasks in different ways to meet an expected standard (e.g., using regular or adapted utensils to eat food, a typical standard when dining out at a restaurant). However, regardless of their differences when performing these tasks, both clients have satisfying experiences when taking part in the occupation. They demonstrate their presence and interest in the occupation, and they each derive personal or social connection to the occupation (Figure 55-1).

The Distinction between Social Participation and Quality of Life

A second important distinction is between the concepts of social participation and quality of life. The WHO provides definitions of both concepts but does not clearly describe their relationship. Whereas participation is defined as a person's "involvement in life situations," quality of life is defined as a person's overall well-being, including "perceptions of their position in life in the context of the culture and value system where they live and in relation to their goals, expectations, standards, and concerns" (Quality of Life Assessment by World Health Organization Quality of Life [WHOQOL] Group, as cited in WHO, 1998, p. 27). These definitions suggest an objective quality to participation and a subjective aspect of quality of life.

However, this standard way of distinguishing the concepts of *social participation* and *quality of life* may be inadequate for guiding our work as occupational therapists. From an OT perspective, information about whether individuals are participating in the activities that matter to them determines whether or not there is a participation

problem (Hemmingsson & Jonsson, 2005; Ueda & Okawa, 2003). Therefore, we need to gather information about the objective component of social participation, such as how often the client participates (i.e., their attendance) and their level of involvement in the activity (Imms et al., 2015). However, what we observe a person doing may be different from what that person experiences when taking part in the activity, so we need to also evaluate the subjective component of a client's social participation. The subjective component of social participation may describe whether the person is doing what he or she wants to do and in a way that is satisfying to him or her. This way of thinking about social participation as having both objective and subjective qualities reflects the perspectives of parents of children with disabilities (Bedell, Khetani, Cousins, Coster, & Law, 2011; Khetani, Cohn, Orsmond, Law, & Coster, 2013) and adults with disabilities (Hammel et al., 2008). In contrast, quality of life measures were developed without input from people with disabilities (Hays, Hahn, & Marshall, 2002).

Put together, we can think about participation and quality of life as closely related domains (Whiteneck, 2006). A client's social participation can be considered as an indicator of their overall quality of life as described in the Occupational Therapy Practice Framework (AOTA, 2014) and by McDougall, Wright, Schmidt, Miller, and Lowry (2011).

The Relationship between Participation and Social Participation

Current thinking about *participation* and *social participation* is that they are interchangeable terms. This definition of social participation is congruent with the Occupational Therapy Practice Framework (AOTA, 2014) that defines social participation broadly as "the interweaving of occupations to support desired engagement in community and family activities as well as those involving peers and friends" and can occur in person or remotely using technology such as telephone, computer, or video interaction (p. S21) (Figure 55-2). This broad definition of participation is also congruent with the ICF and ICF-CY definition of participation as "involvement in life situations" (WHO, 2001, 2007) without specific reference made to social participation as a separate concept.

Although the concepts of *participation* and *social participation* are considered interchangeable, there has been much dialogue about how to define the key features of the participation concept to consistently guide assessment and intervention. For children, McConachie, Colver, Forsyth, Jarvis, and Parkinson (2006) classified "life situations" as sets of activities that were pursued because they were

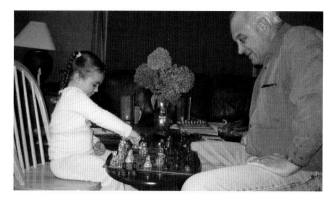

FIGURE 55-2 For children, life situations are organized sets and sequences of activities that typically involve the presence and engagement of others. These life situations may be directed toward development of skills and capacities as well as enjoyment.

essential for survival, supporting the child's development, discretionary, or educationally enriching. For young children as well as older children and youth, life situations have been defined as organized sets and sequences of activities that typically involve the presence and engagement of others, are setting-specific, and are directed toward a personally or socially meaningful goal such as sustenance and physical health, development of skills and capacities, and enjoyment and emotional well-being (Coster & Khetani, 2008; Khetani et al., 2013). Similarly, for adults, participation is intrinsically social and entails engagement in productivity, social, and community situations (Chang & Coster, 2014) (Figure 55-3).

Although each of these definitions is targeted for a different age group (infants and young children, children and youth, adults and older adults), the definitions share common features. Across these definitions, there are two

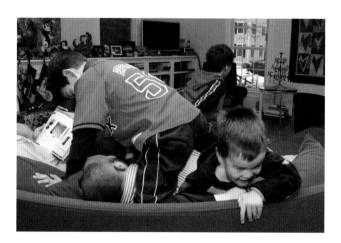

FIGURE 55-3 Social participation and participation are considered interchangeable terms.

common underlying assumptions: (1) Any life situation can be social, and (2) we can classify areas of social participation according to where the situations take place rather than whether they include a social element.

Thinking about social participation in this way will help us to consistently organize our thinking about social participation when working with clients across the life course. We can assume all important life situations for a client, can have a social element, and we can proceed to appraising a host of features, including specific features of the activity setting that influence the client's social participation. For example, we might consider the availability and adequacy of resources to play basketball in a driveway at home, which may be different from resources needed to feel safe and supported to play basketball at the local playground after school (Heinemann, 2010).

This approach places high demand on contextual thinking because client desires and expectations may differ from others of the same age as well as across activities and settings (Khetani et al., 2013) and over time (Tamis-Monda et al., 2007). Even for adults, defining participation by degree of fit to a predefined social role may not be accurate if, for example, they have redefined caregiving to accommodate living with a mobility impairment (Jackson, 1998a, 1998b). As an example, Gloria Dickerson (see Chapter 13) describes how her lived experience as an adult with mental illness shaped her role as an educator:

> Dr. Spaniol mentored me and gave me a valued role facilitating recovery groups and co-facilitating statewide workshops . . . I now have a newly found identity of educator. This was a dream of mine when as a little girl. I played school with my childhood friends. These experiences allowed me a glimpse into the land of being accepted and well respected. And now, I am forever changed, and giving up is simply harder because of them. Their use of the universal concept that difficulties are caused by barriers took me out of the land of a defective human being failing to function and placed me squarely back in the land of human beings striving to overcome environmental obstacles without judgments about my intellect, character, or motivation. I was on an equal playing field with all others.

In the remainder of this chapter, we choose to use the term *participation* only. We discuss ways to evaluate and intervene to achieve participation outcomes with reference to a broad range of activities that an individual client might engage in with others across the life course.

Evaluating Participation

As occupational therapists, one of our first tasks when working with clients is to gather information about their experiences engaging in everyday activities. This occupational profile that we create focuses on the client's current and desired participation (AOTA, 2014).

Because participation is a *multidimensional* and *context-dependent* concept, we need to approach this task recognizing that there is more than one way to ascertain whether or not our clients are participating in the activities they need and want to do (i.e., multidimensional) and how our clients' participation may differ depending on what they are doing and where the activity takes place (i.e., context-dependent). Hence, the task of gathering useful information about how our diverse clients participate across a full range of relevant activities and settings is complex at best.

Because participation is influenced by the environment in which activities take place, there is also need to appraise whether changes to the environment may directly improve participation. There are many features of environments that can facilitate or hinder a client's participation, including products and technology, the natural environment and human-made changes to the environment, support and relationships, attitudes, services, systems, and policies (Khetani, Bedell, Coster, Cousins, & Law, 2012; WHO, 2001, 2007). Thus, understanding the client's participation requires consideration of the environments the client encounters in the course of his or her daily life.

There is no single measure of participation that is suitable for use with all of our potential clients across age groups, functional profiles, and activity contexts. In addition, measures can be more or less useful depending on whether we are using an assessment as it was intended to be used (e.g., for individualized service planning, program evaluation, intervention or population-based studies) (Bedell & Coster, 2008). In the next section, we describe the work that has been done to develop assessments of participation for individuals across the life course, with a focus on those approaches that can be used to guide our assessment of participation to support individualized service planning.

Common Features of Participation Assessments

Evaluation approaches described in this section support the use of a top–down and client-centered approach to addressing our clients' occupational needs. When using a top–down approach, we first focus on obtaining the client's occupational profile by identifying what the client does, wants to do, needs to do, or is expected to do. We then focus on determining the major factors, both personal and contextual, that are limiting the client's ability to do what he or she needs or wants to do as well as the capacities and strengths that he or she has available. Finally, we identify services to address the identified impairments, functional limitations, and contextual factors restricting their participation in a particular activity context. Assessments described in this section provide a

way to systematically obtain information that is relevant to developing clients' occupational profiles. This information can help practitioners to more sharply focus our services toward those subsets of activities that clients most want or need to participate in but where they are experiencing restriction(s).

We can gather information about what our clients want or need to participate in by asking them directly using an interview or survey format. This assessment process is one important way that we build therapeutic alliance. Understanding the results of the participation assessment enables us to partner effectively with clients to make decisions about services (see Chapter 35).

Assessments themselves may vary in their client centeredness. The extent to which the assessments have been developed with consumer input about what to include in the measure is an important indicator of whose voice is represented in the information we use to guide decision-making efforts with clients (Brown & Gordon, 2004; Coster, 2006). Consumers whose perspectives have been gathered on the topic of participation include adults with disabilities (Hammel et al., 2008), parents of children with and without disabilities (Bedell, Cohn, & Dumas, 2005; Bedell et al., 2011; Dunst, Hamby, Trivette, Raab, & Bruder, 2002; Khetani et al., 2013; Lawlor, 2003; Mactavish & Schleien, 1998), and children and youth with disabilities themselves (Heah, Case, McGuire, & Law, 2007; Kramer & Hammel, 2011; Majnemer et al., 2010; Shikako-Thomas et al., 2009).

Overview of Selected Participation Measures

For this chapter, we build on what has been covered in other chapters and review a set of measures that explicitly address participation in a broad range of activities and that have some psychometric evidence to support their use in practice (McConachie et al., 2006; Morris, Kurinczuk, & Fitzpatrick, 2005). Most of these measures were developed since the ICF and ICF-CY were published and so offer ideas for how to think about and measure participation for individuals with disabilities across the life course.

The measures reviewed in this chapter vary in terms of their comprehensiveness, how they are administered, how long they take to complete, the target population they are designed for, and the extent to which they include assessment of environmental impact on client participation. In this section, we describe assessments of participation that have been developed for young children, children and youth, and adults and older adults.

Table 55-1 provides a brief overview of what information each assessment can help you gather as you begin the assessment process with your clients. For each measure selected for review, we have indicated (1) whether its

TABLE 55-1 Overview of Select Participation Measures for Young Children, Children and Youth, Adults and Older Adults

Assessment	Area(s) of Participation Addressed			Dimensions Addressed		Environmental Impact Addressed
	Home	School or Work	Community	Objective Assessment	Subjective Assessment	
Participation Measures for Young Children						
Preschooler Activity Card Sort (PACS)	✓		✓	Frequency, Extent	Importance, Satisfaction	✓
Routines-Based Interview (RBI)	✓	✓	✓	Engagement, Independence, Interaction	Satisfaction	✓
Asset-Based Context Matrix (ABC Matrix)	✓	✓	✓	Capabilities, Interactions	Interests	✓
Assessment of Preschool Children's Participation (APCP)	✓	✓	✓	Diversity, Intensity, Where, With whom	Enjoyment, Preferences	
Children's Engagement in Daily Life (CEDL)	✓		✓	Frequency	Enjoyment	
Children's Participation Questionnaire (CPQ)	✓	✓	✓	Diversity, Intensity	Enjoyment, Satisfaction	
Young Children's Participation and Environment Measure (YC-PEM)	✓	✓	✓	Frequency, Involvement	Desire for change	✓
Participation Measures for Children and Youth						
Pediatric Activity Card Sort (PACS)	✓	✓	✓	Frequency	Preference	
Children's Assessment of Participation and Enjoyment (CAPE) and Preferences for Activities (PAC)	✓	✓	✓	Diversity, Intensity, Where, With whom	Enjoyment, Preferences	
School Function Assessment (SFA)		✓	✓	Involvement		✓
Child and Adolescent Scale of Participation (CASP)	✓	✓	✓	Degree of restriction		✓
Assessment of LIFE-Habits for Children (LIFE-H)	✓	✓	✓	Accomplishment	Satisfaction	✓
Participation and Environment Measure for Children and Youth (PEM-CY)	✓	✓	✓	Frequency, Involvement	Desire for change	✓
Meaningful Activity Participation Assessment (MAPA)	✓		✓	Frequency	Meaning	
Engagement in Meaningful Activities Scale (EMAS)	✓		✓	Frequency	Meaning	
Activity Card Sort (ACS)	✓		✓	% Maintained		
Craig Handicap Assessment and Reporting Technique (CHART)		✓	✓	Time spent, No. of social contacts		✓
Participation Objective, Participation Subjective	✓		✓	How often	Importance	
Community Integration Questionnaire (CIQ)	✓	✓	✓	How often, With whom, Assistance		
The Participation Measure for Post-Acute Care (PM-PAC)			✓	Frequency, Extent of limitation	Satisfaction	

content addresses home, school, work, and/or community participation; (2) whether it gathers objective or subjective data, or both; and (3) whether it includes an assessment of environment.

Many participation assessments are now endorsed as common data elements in intervention studies involving individuals with disabilities (e.g., National Institutes of Health Common Data Elements Initiative [National Institutes of Health, 2017]). Many details of the assessments, including their culturally adapted versions, are also summarized and routinely updated for immediate access by practitioners (e.g., Rehabilitation Measures Database [Shirley Ryan AbilityLab, 2010]).

Selected Participation Measures for Young Children

Young children's participation is one of the four primary service outcomes addressed by OT practitioners working in early intervention (Guralnick, 2005) and is considered to be an important indicator of preschool inclusion. All of the available instruments rely on parent report but vary in their content and mode of administration (paper vs. electronic). Young children are typically in close contact with and guided by their parents or caregivers to participate in home and community-based activities. Therefore, parent-report measures are commonly used to make inferences about the young child's participation. We review seven measures of young children's participation (Figure 55-4).

Preschooler Activity Card Sort

The Preschooler Activity Card Sort (Berg & LaVesser, 2006) is a semistructured interview for use with parents of children 3 to 6 years of age that is available in English and Spanish (Stoffel & Berg, 2008). The primary purpose of this tool is intervention planning. In its current edition, the Preschooler Activity Card Sort contains

85 photographs of children engaged in one of seven types of activities: self-care, community mobility, leisure (both high physical demand and low physical demand), social interaction, domestic chores, and education. Parents are asked to view each of the 85 photographs and respond to the question "Does your child participate in this activity?" using one of the following response options: (1) yes, child participates; (2) yes, child participates but requires adult assistance beyond that typically required of preschoolers; (3) yes, with environmental assistance (e.g., can ride a bike on some surfaces—hard, smooth surfaces but not grass); (4) no (does not participate in the activity), for child reasons (e.g., due to pain, balance, vision); (5) no, for adult reasons (e.g., financial, fear, feels child is too young); or (6) no, for environmental reasons (e.g., community resources unavailable, neighborhood safety). Parents are then asked to identify five activities that they would like to be the focus of intervention and rate the relative importance of each activity, the frequency that the activity is performed, the extent of participation (from 0 = *currently not participating at all* to 10 = *fully participating*), and satisfaction with participation.

Routines-Based Interview

The Routines-Based Interview (RBI) (McWilliam, Casey, & Sims, 2009) is a semistructured interview designed to obtain a rich picture of each routine within a young child's day. The interviewer goes through a typical day for a family, and for each routine (i.e., time of day or activity) that the parent identifies, the interviewer proceeds to ask the following questions: (1) What is everyone else doing? (2) What is the child doing? (3) What is the child's engagement like? (4) What is the child's independence like? (5) What are the child's social relationships like? and (6) How satisfactory is this time of day (from 1 *not at all* to 5 *very satisfied*)? The interviewer then recaps family concerns and asks the parent or caregiver to prioritize their concerns by importance. The RBI can be used with the Scale for Assessment of Family Enjoyment within Routines

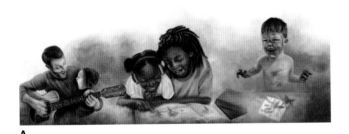
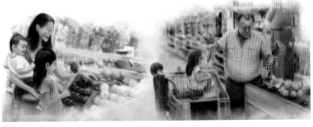

A   **B**

FIGURE 55-4 Young children are typically in close contact with and guided by their parents or caregivers to participate in **(A)** home-based and **(B)** community-based activities. Therefore, parent-report measures are commonly used to make inferences about the young child's participation. (Used with permission from artist Christina Sidorowych.)

(SAFER) (Scott & McWilliam, 2000) and the Scale for the Assessment of Teachers' Impressions of Routines and Engagement (SATIRE) (Clingenpeel & McWilliam, 2003) to obtain an estimate of the teacher's perceptions of the child's functioning in classroom routines. The RBI can be used to obtain a narrative description of the child's performance (independence) and participation (engagement) in activities over the course of a 90-minute interview (McWilliam, 2009).

Asset-Based Context Matrix

The Asset-Based Context Matrix (ABCM) (Wilson, Mott, & Batman, 2004) combines semistructured interview and observation to help practitioners identify the child's interests and abilities (i.e., assets) so that contextually based goals can be developed. The information is gathered in an informal manner rather than by formal administration of a scale. Parents are asked to describe a typical day and the everyday, weekly, and special activities and events in which the child and family participate. The ABCM focuses on activities and events in family life, community life, and early childhood programming, and the parent reports on the following for each activity setting: the child's interests, the child's assets/capabilities, the child's functional/meaningful interactions with others, the amount of opportunity that the child has to participate in the activity or event, and the child's participation.

Assessment of Preschool Children's Participation

The Assessment of Preschool Children's Participation (APCP) scale (Law, King, Petrenchik, Kertoy, & Anaby, 2012) has been modeled after the Children's Assessment of Participation and Enjoyment (CAPE) and the Preferences for Activities of Children (PAC) (King et al., 2004) and is designed for use with children ages 2 to 5 years and 11 months. The APCP assesses young children's participation in voluntary, day-to-day activities outside of preschool. The APCP is a parent-report, paper-pencil survey that contains 45 drawings of activities across the areas of play (9 items); skill development (15 items); active physical recreation (10 items); and social activities (11 items). Parents identify activities that their child has participated in during the past 4 months (yes/no) and, if yes, how often they did them (7-point scale). Diversity and intensity scores can be generated for each activity area.

Children's Participation Questionnaire

The Children's Participation Questionnaire (CPQ) (Rosenberg, Jarus, & Bart, 2010) is a parent-report questionnaire for use with children with and without disabilities who are 4 to 6 years old. The CPQ contains 40 items that address six areas of participation: activities of daily living (5 items), instrumental activities of daily living

(5 items), play (5 items), leisure (10 items), social participation (9 items), and education (11 items). For each activity, the parent is asked to report on the child's intensity (how often the child participates, from 0 = *never* to 5 = *every day*), the child's independence level (need for assistance, from 1 = *needs much assistance* to 6 = *fully independent*), the child's enjoyment (from 1 = *does not take pleasure* to 6 = *takes much pleasure*), and the parent's level of satisfaction with the child's performance (from 1 = *not at all satisfied* to 6 = *very satisfied*). Total summary scores and summary scores for each of the six participation areas can be computed for diversity (number of activities the child participates in), intensity (mean frequency), enjoyment (mean enjoyment), and satisfaction (mean satisfaction).

Young Children's Participation and Environment Measure

The Young Children's Participation and Environment Measure (YC-PEM) (Khetani, 2015; Khetani, Graham, Davies, Law, & Simeonsson, 2015) is a parent-report questionnaire designed to assess the child's current and desired participation as well as the perceived impact of the child's environment on participation in specific settings. This measure can be used with families of children ages 0 to 5 years old. The YC-PEM allows parents to rate their child's frequency of participation (0 = *never* to 7 = *once or more each day*), the extent of involvement (0 = *not very involved* to 5 = *very involved*), and their desire for change (*yes/no*) relating to sets of activities that typically occur in home, daycare/preschool, and community environments. If parents desire change related to their child's participation in a given activity, they can specify ways that they want the child's participation to change (e.g., participate in a broader variety of activities). Parents are also asked to identify aspects of each environment in terms of the perceived impact on the child's participation. Parents evaluate the impact of a broad range of environmental features and resources, including the demands of activities, on participation in occupation. A clinimetric approach (Coster et al., 2012) makes it possible to create composite or summary scores by administering a portion of the measure (e.g., home section) or by pulling items together to address a specific area of participation (e.g., participation in work-related activities that occur in the home, school, and community).

Child Engagement in Daily Life

The Child Engagement in Daily Life measure (CEDL) (Chiarello et al., 2014) is a parent-completed measure that was designed for use with young children with and without cerebral palsy who are 18 months to 5 years old. The CEDL contains 18 items that address participation in family and recreational activities (11 items) and self-care (7 items). For each activity in the Family and Recreational Activities section, the parent is asked to report on the child's frequency of participation (how often the child participates, from 1 = *never* to 5 = *very often*) and the child's enjoyment of participation (from 1 = *not at all* to 5 = *a great deal*). For each activity in the Self-Care section, the parent is asked to report on the child's degree of participation in his or her daily self-care activities (from 1 = *no, unable* to 5 = *yes, initiates and performs consistently*). Summary scores for each area of participation can be computed separately to provide raw and scaled scores of frequency of participation in family and recreational activities (sum frequency), enjoyment of participation in family and recreational activities (average enjoyment), and participation in self-care (sum participation).

Selected Participation Measures for Children and Youth

We review six participation measures that were designed for school-age children.

Pediatric Activity Card Sort

The Pediatric Activity Card Sort (PACS) (Mandich, Polatajko, Miller, & Baum, 2004) is an adaptation of the Activity Card Sort (ACS) (Baum & Edwards, 2008) that was developed for adults. The PACS uses Q-sort methodology and involves the use of pictures of children engaging in various activities to elicit the child's perspective of their level of occupational participation. The PACS includes 83 sorting cards that depict 75 activities addressing personal care, school/productivity, hobbies/social activities, and sports as well as eight blank cards for additional activities that the child might report on during the course of the interview. The child is instructed to place the card in a "yes" or "no" pile based on whether he or she had participated in the activity within the last 4 months and, if he or she participates, is asked how often he or she participates (daily, weekly, monthly, yearly). Scoring involves recording the five activities that are most important for the child to do and the activities that the child would like to do the most. The PACS can be administered to the parent or child and takes 20 to 25 minutes to complete with children who are between 5 and 14 years old.

Children's Assessment of Participation and Enjoyment

The CAPE (King et al., 2004) is a 55-item measure designed to obtain a participation profile specific to leisure and recreation activities that take place outside of the school setting (e.g., hobbies, crafts, games, organized sports, clubs, groups, arts, and entertainment). The CAPE contains activity drawings on cards and visual response forms to help enable children to complete this assessment via self-report or interview. The CAPE assesses five dimensions of participation in reference to a 4-month time frame: (1) diversity of activities (whether child participates), (2) intensity or how often the child participates, (3) with whom the child participates, (4) where the child participates, and (5) extent of enjoyment in activities. The CAPE can be completed separately from the PAC by either the child or his or her parent and takes 30 to 45 minutes to complete.

School Function Assessment

The School Function Assessment (SFA) (Coster, Deeney, Haltiwanger, & Haley, 1998) begins with a section on participation in the elementary school setting. The SFA participation scale examines six different school settings: (1) classroom (regular or specialized), (2) playground or recess, (3) transportation, (4) bathroom or toileting, (5) transitions, and (6) mealtime or snack time, with one item for each section. The SFA participation section consists of six items. Each item pertains to one of the six settings previously described and includes examples of tasks and activities that are typically part of that setting. Items are rated on a 6-point scale that reflects the extent to which the child participates in the tasks and activities compared to peers (from 1 = *extremely limited* to 6 = *child fully participates in all tasks and activities within each setting*). The SFA participation subscale can be completed by the child's teacher in about 5 to 10 minutes when used separately from the larger measure and has reported evidence of test–retest reliability and internal consistency. The SFA addresses the environment in separate scales that assess the use of adult assistance and/or adaptations (modifications of equipment, environment, activity, program) to complete school tasks.

Child and Adolescent Scale of Participation

The Child and Adolescent Scale of Participation (CASP) (Bedell, 2009) was developed as part of the Child and Family Follow-up Survey (CFFS) to monitor outcomes and needs of children with acquired brain injuries and subsequently has been used separately from the CFFS to assess children with other diagnoses (Bedell, 2004, 2009; Bedell & Dumas, 2004). The CASP includes four subsections that address the extent to which children ages 5 years and older participate in broad types of home, school, and community activities compared to same-aged peers. All items are rated on a 4-point scale (from 1 = *unable* to 4 = *age expected*). The CASP includes open-ended questions that ask about effective strategies and supports and barriers that affect participation. The CASP alone takes about 10 minutes to complete and has reported evidence of test–retest reliability, internal consistency, and construct and discriminant validity (Bedell, 2004, 2009; Bedell & Dumas, 2004; Golos & Bedell, 2016). The 18-item Child and Adolescent Scale of Environment (CASE) is a separate but compatible measure that can be used with the CASP to obtain information about environmental barriers to participation (from 1 = *no problem* to 3 = *big problem*).

Assessment of Life Habits in Children

The Assessment of Life Habits (LIFE-H) (Noreau, Fougeyrollas, Post, & Asano, 2005; Noreau et al., 2007) was initially designed for adults but has been adapted for use as a parent-report survey for families of children ages 5 years and older. Its purpose is to identify disruptions in the accomplishment of 11 types of life habits that are described as "regular activities or social roles valued by the person or his or her sociocultural context according to his or her characteristics . . ." (Noreau et al., 2005). There are six categories of life habits that fall into the daily activities domain (communication, personal care, housing, mobility, nutrition, fitness) and five life habits that fall into the social roles domain (recreation, responsibility, education, community life, interpersonal relationships). The LIFE-H has a long form (197 items) that takes 1 to 2 hours to complete and a short form (64 items) that is estimated to take 30 to 45 minutes to complete. The LIFE-H assesses (1) level of accomplishment (according to level of difficulty and type of assistance) and (2) level of satisfaction. Level of accomplishment and satisfaction scores can be computed for items, life habit categories, and global scores.

Participation and Environment Measure for Children and Youth

The Participation and Environment Measure for Children and Youth (PEM-CY) (Coster, Law, & Bedell, 2010) is a caregiver-report instrument that combines assessment of participation and environment in a single measure. The PEM-CY contains 25 participation items reflecting broad types of activities that are typically done at home, at school, or in the community. Each participation item is rated in three ways: (1) frequency (from 0 = *never* to 7 = *daily*), (2) involvement (from 1 = *minimally* to 5 = *very involved*), and (3) desire for change (parents are asked if they want their child's participation to change [yes/no], and if yes, the parent is asked to indicate all of the ways in which change is desired [e.g., more or less frequency, more or less involvement, and/or more variety]). For each setting, parents are asked about whether features of the environment help or hinder their child's participation and whether there are available or adequate resources to support their child's participation. When administered online, the PEM-CY takes 20 to 30 minutes to complete and is a reliable and valid measure for children and youth ages 5 to 17 years (Coster et al., 2011).

Selected Participation Measures for Adults and Older Adults

We describe six adult participation measures, some of which have been reviewed in greater detail in other chapters in this text.

Meaningful Activity Participation Assessment

The Meaningful Activity Participation Assessment (MAPA) is a survey checklist that was developed in the context of the USC Well Elderly 2 study and is designed to capture the meaningfulness of activities for older adults. The MAPA contains 28 activities ranging from using public transportation to physical exercise to musical activities to computer use. The respondent is asked to indicate how frequently he or she participates in each activity (from 0 = *not at all* to 7 = *every day*). The client is also asked to rate the meaningfulness of each activity or "how much it matters or is personally fulfilling to you" (from 0 = *not at all meaningful* to 4 = *extremely meaningful*). The total score reflects the individual's overall level of meaningful activity participation by taking the frequency ratings and multiplying it by the meaning rating for each of the 28 activities. When summed, a total score is obtained such that higher scores indicate higher meaningful activity participation.

Engagement in Meaningful Activity Scale

The Engagement in Meaningful Activity Scale (EMAS) is a 12-item survey initially developed by Goldberg, Brintnell, and Goldberg (2002) and subsequently revised and validated (Eakman, 2011; Eakman, Carlson, & Clark, 2010a, 2010b). The EMAS also addresses meaningful participation, and the respondent is asked to identify the accuracy of each statement to himself or herself (from 1 = *never* to 5 = *always*).

Activity Card Sort

The ACS (Baum & Edwards, 2008) is intended to help practitioners document the client's participation in instrumental, leisure, and social activities. The ACS uses Q-sort methodology, which is a rank-order procedure in which the client sorts a series of photographs into categories based on the question being posed by the person administering the assessment. There are 89 photographs that fall into one of the following domains: 20 instrumental activities, 35 low-physical-demand leisure activities, 17 high-physical-demand leisure activities, and 17 social activities. There are three versions of the ACS. The first version is for healthy older adults and involves clients sorting 80 photographs into the following five categories: never done, not doing as an older adult, do now, do less, and given up. The second version is intended for use with clients receiving services in a hospital, rehabilitation, or skilled nursing facility and uses the same 80 photographs that are sorted into two groups—done prior to illness or not done. The third version is intended for use with clients to record changes in activity patterns, and the client sorts photographs into the following categories: not done in the last 5 years, gave up due to illness, beginning to do again, and do now. The score for each version of the ACS reflects the percentage of activities that the client maintains or retains.

Craig Handicap Assessment and Reporting Technique

The Craig Handicap Assessment and Reporting Technique (CHART) (Whiteneck, Charlifue, Gerhart, Overholser, & Richardson, 1992) was originally developed as a self-report instrument for persons with spinal cord injury, but it has since been used with other groups of individuals with physical disabilities. Content development was guided by the International Classification of Impairments, Disabilities, and Handicaps (ICIDH). There are 27 questions grouped into subscales addressing physical independence, mobility, occupation, social integration, and economic self-sufficiency. Questions focus on objective indicators such as time spent on a given activity or number of social contacts.

Participation Objective, Participation Subjective

The Participation Objective, Participation Subjective (POPS) (Brown, 2006; Brown et al., 2004) is a self-report survey that can be completed in about 10 to 20 minutes. It consists of 26 items that are situations of participation (e.g., going out, doing housework). Two types of questions are asked for each item: an objective question (e.g., "How often do you do this activity in a typical month?") and a subjective question (e.g., "How important is this activity?" "Are you satisfied with your level of participation?"). The items are grouped into five categories that reflect several chapters of the ICF: domestic life; major life activities; transportation; interpersonal interactions and relationships; and community, recreational, and civic life. Although it was developed in the context of traumatic brain injury, its content is broadly relevant to other adult populations.

Community Integration Questionnaire

The Community Integration Questionnaire (CIQ) (Corrigan & Deming, 1995; Sander et al., 2007; Willer, Rosenthal, Kreutzer, Gordon, & Rempel, 1993) is a brief semistructured phone interview that was developed for assessment of individuals after traumatic brain injury. The CIQ contains 15 items relevant to home integration, school integration, and productive activities. The respondent is asked how often the activity is performed and whether he or she performs the activity alone, with another person, or if it is performed by someone else. Subscores and a total community integration score can be computed based on frequency of performing activities or roles and whether or not activities are done jointly with others.

Participation Measure for Post-Acute Care

The Participation Measure for Post-Acute Care (PM-PAC) (Gandek, Sinclair, Jette, & Ware, 2007) contains 51 items that assess a person's degree of perceived participation restriction in nine areas. Most of the PM-PAC items ask respondents to rate the extent to which they are currently limited in a life situation, from 1 = *not at all limited* to 5 = *extremely limited*. Items measure frequency of participation (1 = *every day* to 5 = *never*) and satisfaction (1 = *very satisfied* to 5 = *very dissatisfied*).

In summary, the measures reviewed in this section offer different approaches to gathering information about your client's participation. When selecting the best measure for your information-gathering needs, it is important to first identify your assessment purpose and then identify those measures that best match that need by considering the following: (1) the characteristics of your target population (e.g., a 3-year-old child with developmental delay, in which case only a subset of measures that have been validated on young children would be appropriate); (2) the type of information you are interested in gathering (e.g., areas where a child is least satisfied with his or her participation in community activities, which would require gathering information about the subjective qualities of participation in a comprehensive set of activities within a specific setting); (3) whether it is important for you to obtain estimates of change in your client's participation, in which case you would want to identify measures that have some reported evidence of responsiveness to change or that have the potential to detect clinically meaningful change, as is the case with measures that ask about participation in discrete activities versus broader areas of activities; and (4) how much time you have to gather this information in the context of your daily practice (Bedell & Coster, 2008).

Interventions to Promote Social Participation

The measures described in this chapter have helped to develop a robust knowledge base about participation that can begin to inform the implementation of evidence-based practice (see Chapter 31). As a result, there is growing evidence of disparities in participation across multiple contexts (Bedell et al., 2013; Benjamin, Lucas-Thompson, Little, Davies, & Khetani, 2017; Khetani et al. 2014) and determinants of participation outcomes, with an emphasis on the role of the environment in predicting participation outcomes (Albrecht & Khetani, 2017; Anaby et al., 2013; Anaby et al., 2014; Di Marino, Tremblay, Khetani, & Anaby, 2018; Vaughan et al., 2017). There are a growing number of large-scale studies on participation outcomes (King et al., 2013) and longitudinal studies of participation change (Imms & Adair, 2017; Khetani, 2017). This evidence suggests that there is need to build and test interventions to promote participation.

Participation in everyday occupation is the reason for OT (Law, 2002) and the promise of rehabilitation (Baum, 2011). Assuming that individuals have a strong motivation to be engaged in meaningful activities within a social context, participation should always be considered when designing OT intervention. Participation may be incorporated into intervention in one of two ways: (1) participation as an *end goal* of intervention and (2) participation as a *component* of a multifaceted intervention program.

Promoting Participation as End Goal of Intervention

When participation is the end goal, interventions are often designed to empower individuals who are socially isolated due to stigmatization, remove barriers that limit their access to desired social activities, and/or help facilitate changes in their major life roles following the onset of a chronic health condition. There is more than one valid way to develop interventions to promote a client's participation. These interventions may be directed toward the client or the client's environment. Law and colleagues (2011) recently examined child-focused and context-focused intervention approaches for young children with cerebral palsy and found them to be equally effective (Figure 55-5).

Client-Centered Approaches to Promoting Participation as End Goal

Occupational therapists can intervene with individual clients to help them become participating members of a community, such as by linking the individual clients to various services and supports before a crisis occurs and by helping them develop peer networks. As an example, Kramer and colleagues applied a participatory action research approach to develop and pilot test a Teens Making Environment and Activity Modifications (TEAM) intervention to help youth with disabilities identify and advocate for removal of environmental barriers that prevent them from participating in school and community life (Kramer et al., 2013; Kramer, Roemer, Liljenquist, Shin, & Hart, 2014). More recently,

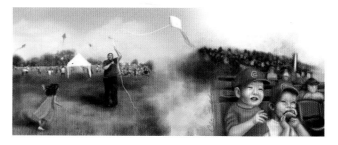

FIGURE 55-5 There is more than one valid way to develop interventions to promote a client's participation. These interventions may be directed toward the client or the client's environment. (Used with permission from artist Christina Sidorowych.)

Anaby and colleagues have developed and evaluated a similar type of intervention approach called Pathways and Resources for Engagement and Participation (PREP) (Anaby, Law, Majnemer, & Feldman, 2016; Anaby, Law, Teplicky, & Turner, 2015). As another example, Schelly, Davies, and Spooner (2011) at the Center for Community Partnerships at Colorado State University are implementing a peer-mentored approach to help students with an autism spectrum disorder (ASD) develop strategies to navigate challenges associated with college life such as time management and study skills, effective communication, forming relationships, and learning to advocate for themselves in the educational setting. As seen by these examples, the methods of intervention depend on the nature of the identified barriers limiting participation. Barriers related to lack of knowledge about available resources may be addressed through client education and guided exploration. On the other hand, barriers due to lack of accessibility may need to be addressed through advocacy with planning, building, and policy groups.

When participation is the client's primary goal, it is important to ensure that the client's own definition of meaningful and satisfying participation guides the design of the intervention. Individuals have different preferences for how they engage with others: Some are "group" people, whereas others may be seeking a closer friendship with a few people; some enjoy and are comfortable with conversation as a main activity, others prefer to engage in the context of doing an activity together. Therefore, it is not enough to simply identify situations that offer opportunities for participation: The nature of the setting and their activities need to fit with individuals' values, interests, and preferences. The opportunity for choice is an important component to facilitating meaningful participation, and clients may need a period of guided exploration to discover the options that offer the best fit.

Recently, there have been efforts to explore the use of technology to provide guided support for client engagement by designing interventions that focus on participation as the end goal. For example, Bedell, Wade, Turkstra, Haarbauer-Krupa, and King (2016) have developed an app-based coaching intervention to support social participation among youth with traumatic brain injury. As another example, Khetani, Lim, and Corden (2017) have examined the user experience of an e-health option to accelerate family engaged care planning toward participation-level outcomes when the child is engaged in early childhood intervention services.

Context-Based Interventions to Promote Participation as End Goal

Use of universal design principles to directly intervene on the environment have been applied by OT practitioners to promote participation (see Chapter 33). For example, ensuring that residences have a single-level entrance and 32-in wide access to a bathroom on the main level are ways to ensure the "visitability" of a home (Maisel, 2006). The ACCESS project through the Center for Community Partnerships at Colorado State University builds on Universal Design for Learning (UDL) principles and strategies to improve the learning experience and persistence of college students with disabilities (Schelly et al., 2011). As yet another example of this environmentally focused approach to intervention, OT researchers have provided guidance on how to consult with museums and other community agencies to increase access to and learning by visitors with and without intellectual and developmental disabilities (Umeda et al., 2017).

Although most of this discussion has focused on planned activities to facilitate participation, spontaneous occurrences may offer unexpected opportunities. Cohn (2001) provides an example in her description of the "waiting room," where parents whose children were attending therapy appointments began to connect with each other to share experiences. This example serves as a reminder of the important role the therapist can play in facilitating participation simply by arranging the environments they work in. For example, one could experiment to see which arrangement of seating seems to facilitate social exchanges among clients in a waiting room area or among adults in a supported living environment. Evidence regarding the impact of color, lighting, organization of space, and available play materials may help maximize the opportunities for spontaneous participation within a particular clinic, school, or community setting.

Another focus of a context-based intervention approach is one that considers the human dimensions of environments, particularly in supported work and living situations such as group homes or assisted living facilities. Staff in these programs may view their primary role to be enabling clients to complete necessary daily tasks such as dressing, grooming, or eating and may not recognize the important role that meaningful social participation can play in supporting health and well-being. Educating staff to facilitate client participation in meaningful occupation may be an important role for the occupational therapist in these settings. For example, studies have shown the positive impact of appropriate training of direct-care staff in group homes to increase the participation of residents with intellectual and developmental disabilities in social interactions and daily activities (Jones et al., 1999).

Interventions to Promote Participation as a Component of a Broader Program

Some interventions address social participation because it is believed to enhance the therapeutic value of the program. This is a key idea underlying various health promotion initiatives such as the Well Elderly Study 2 (Clark et al., 1997; Clark et al., 2011) and programs that apply concepts from this key study, including adult day programs (Horowitz & Chang, 2004) and older adults in senior housing (Matsuka, Giles-Heinz, Flinn, Neighbor, & Bass-Haugen, 2003). This is also the underlying premise of peer support groups, where it is believed that connecting with others who face similar challenges will decrease the sense of social isolation and provide additional emotional support and resources for managing the day-to-day impact of a health condition. Examples include symptom self-management programs for people with multiple sclerosis (Finlayson, Preissner, Cho, & Plow, 2011), stroke (Lee, Fischer, Zera, Robertson, & Hammel, 2017; Wolf, Baum, Lee, & Hammel, 2016), or Parkinson disease (Tickle-Degnen, Ellis, Saint-Hilaire, Thomas, & Wagenaar, 2010). Some intervention programs may have more specific goals to provide positive social experiences as a component of an overall prevention effort. For example, Bazyk and Bazyk (2009) have developed social-skills groups for urban youth. Anti-bullying efforts share this goal of reducing risk by enhancing the overall social climate of the school community, as do programs designed to foster respect for diversity by engaging individuals from different groups in collaborative learning experiences. It is important to realize that simply incorporating social interaction into a group is not sufficient to ensure that meaningful participation that truly facilitates achievement of other group goals will occur. Just as activities need to be carefully selected to support achieving client skill development goals, the process and activities of the group also need to be carefully selected to facilitate meaningful social participation. Relevant considerations include the size and makeup of group, type of leadership and decision-making processes, and member roles and responsibilities.

Conclusions and Future Directions

Participation in everyday occupations is the central focus of OT. Given its importance, we recommend that practitioners try to say current about developments in the following key areas and consider ways of contributing to them while in practice: (1) development and testing of new measures of participation; (2) applying measures of participation to generate occupational profiles; and (3) design and testing of new interventions to promote participation, including technology-based approaches to intervention.

Acknowledgments

We thank University of Illinois at Chicago graduate OT students Andrea Gurga, Briana Rigau, and Jessica Jarvis who have helped with updating descriptions of selected measures, inserting references, and/or providing critical feedback. We also thank Christina Sidorowych, a graduate student in biomedical visualization at University of Illinois at Chicago, whose illustrations of social participation across the life course have enhanced our mode of delivery on this important topic.

 Visit thePoint to watch a video about community participation.

REFERENCES

Albrecht, E., & Khetani, M. A. (2017). Environmental impact on young children's participation in home-based activities. *Developmental Medicine and Child Neurology, 59,* 388–394. doi:10.1111/dmcn.13360

American Occupational Therapy Association. (2014). Occupational therapy practice framework: Domain and process, 3rd edition. *American Journal of Occupational Therapy, 68,* S1–S48. doi:10.5014/ajot.2014.682006

Anaby, D., Law, M. C., Coster, W. J., Bedell, G. M., Khetani, M. A., Avery, L., & Teplicky, R. (2014). The mediating role of the environment in explaining participation of children and youth with and without disabilities across home, school, and community. *Archives of Physical Medicine and Rehabilitation, 95,* 908–917. doi:10.1016/j.apmr.2014.01.005

Anaby, D., Hand, C., Bradley, L., DiRezze, B., Forhan, M., DiGiacomo, A., & Law, M. (2013). The effect of the environment on participation of children and youth with disabilities: a scoping review. *Disability and Rehabilitation, 35,* 1589–1598.

Anaby, D., Law, M., Majnemer, A., & Feldman, D. (2016). Improving the participation of youth with physical disabilities: The effectiveness of the Pathways and Resources for Engagement and Participation (PREP) intervention. *Developmental Medicine and Child Neurology, 58,* 41–41. doi:10.1111/dmcn.56_13224

Anaby, D., Law, M., Teplicky, R., & Turner, L. (2015). Focusing on the environment to improve youth participation: Experiences and perspectives of occupational therapists. *International Journal of Environmental Research in Public Health, 12*(10), 13388–13398.

Baum, C. (2003). Participation: Its relationship to occupation and health. *OTJR: Occupation, Participation and Health, 23*(2), 46–47.

Baum, C. M. (2011). Fulfilling the promise: Supporting participation in daily life. *Archives of Physical Medicine and Rehabilitation, 92,* 169–175.

Baum, C., & Edwards, D. (2008). *Activity Card Sort* (2nd ed.). Bethesda, MD: American Occupational Therapy Association.

Bazyk, S., & Bazyk, J. (2009). Meaning of occupation-based groups for low-income urban youths attending after-school care. *American Journal of Occupational Therapy, 63,* 69–80.

Bedell, G. M. (2004). Developing a follow-up survey focused on participation of children and youth with acquired brain injuries after discharge from inpatient rehabilitation. *Neuro Rehabilitation, 19,* 191–205.

Bedell, G. M. (2009). Further validation of the Child and Adolescent Scale of Participation (CASP). *Developmental Neurorehabilitation, 12,* 342–351.

Bedell, G. M., Cohn, E., & Dumas, H. (2005). Exploring parents' use of strategies to promote social participation of school-age children with acquired brain injuries. ; Clark et al. *American Journal of Occupational Therapy, 59,* 273–284.

Bedell, G. M., & Coster, W. (2008). Measuring participation of school-aged children with traumatic brain injuries: Considerations and approaches. *The Journal of Head Trauma Rehabilitation, 23,* 220–229.

Bedell, G. M., Coster, W. J., Law, M., Liljenquist, K., Kao, Y. C., Teplicky, R., . . . Khetani, M. A. (2013). Community participation, supports, and barriers of school-age children with and without disabilities. *Archives of Physical Medicine and Rehabilitation, 94,* 315–323.

Bedell, G. M., & Dumas, H. M. (2004). Social participation of children and youth with acquired brain injuries discharged from inpatient rehabilitation: A follow-up study. *Brain Injury, 18,* 65–82.

Bedell, G. M., Khetani, M. A., Cousins, M. A., Coster, W. J., & Law, M. C. (2011). Parent perspectives to inform development of measures of children's participation and environment. *Archives of Physical Medicine and Rehabilitation, 92,* 765–773.

Bedell, G. M., Wade, S. L., Turkstra, L. S., Haarbauer-Krupa, J., & King, J. A. (2016). Informing design of an app-based coaching intervention to promote social participation of teenagers with traumatic brain injury. *Developmental Neurorehabilitation,* 1–10.

Benjamin, T. E., Lucas-Thompson, R. G., Little, L. M., Davies, P. L., & Khetani, M. A. (2017). Participation in early childhood educational environments for young children with and without developmental disabilities. *Physical & Occupational Therapy in Pediatrics, 37,* 87–107.

Berg, C., & LaVesser, P. (2006). The Preschool Activity Card Sort. *OTJR: Occupation, Participation and Health, 26,* 143–151.

Brown, M. (2006). *Participation Objective, Participation Subjective. The center for outcome measurement in brain injury.* Retrieved from http://www.tbims.org/combi/pops

Brown, M., Dijkers, M., Gordon, W., Ashman, T., Charatz, H., & Cheng, Z. (2004). Participation objective, participation subjective: A measure of participation combining outsider and insider perspectives. *The Journal of Head Trauma Rehabilitation, 19,* 459–481.

Brown, M., & Gordon, W. (2004). Empowerment in measurement: "muscle," "voice," and subjective quality of life as a gold standard. *Archives of Physical Medicine and Rehabilitation, 85,* S13–S20.

Chang, F. H., & Coster, W. J. (2014). Conceptualizing the construct of participation in adults with disabilities. *Archives of Physical Medicine and Rehabilitation, 95,* 1791–1798. doi:10.1016/j.apmr.2014.05.008

Chiarello, L. A., Palisano, R. J., McCoy, S. W., Bartlett, D. J., Wood, A., Chang, H., . . . Avery, L. (2014). Child engagement in daily life: A measure of participation for young children with cerebral palsy. *Disability and Rehabilitation, 36,* 1804–1816. doi:10.3109/09638288.2014.88241

Clark, F. A., Azen, S. P., Zemke, R., Jackson, J. M., Carlson, M. E., Hay, J., . . . Lipson, L. (1997). Occupational therapy for independent-living older adults: A randomized controlled trial. *JAMA, 278,* 1321–1326.

Clark, F. A., Jackson, J. M., Carlson, M. E., Chou, C. P., Cherry, B. J., Jordan-Marsh, M., . . . Azen, S. P. (2011). Effectiveness of a lifestyle intervention in promoting the well-being of independently living older people: Results of the Well Elderly 2 Randomised Controlled Trial. *Journal of Epidemiology and Community Health, 66,* 782–790. doi:10.1136/jech.2009.099754

Clingenpeel, B. T., & McWilliam, R. A. (2003). *Scale for the Assessment of Teachers' Impressions of Routines and Engagement (SATIRE).* Nashville, TN: Vanderbilt University Medical Center: Center for Child Development.

Cohn, E. S. (2001). From waiting to relating: Parents' experiences in the waiting room of an occupational therapy clinic. *American Journal of Occupational Therapy, 55,* 167–174.

Corrigan, J. D., & Deming, R. (1995). Psychometric characteristics of the Community Integration Questionnaire: Replication and extension. *The Journal of Head Trauma Rehabilitation, 10,* 41–53.

Coster, W. J. (2006). Guest editorial. The road forward to better measures for practice and research. *OTJR: Occupation, Participation and Health, 26,* 131.

Coster, W. J., Bedell, G. M., Law, M., Khetani, M., Teplicky, R., Liljenquist, K., . . . Kao, Y. (2011). Psychometric evaluation of the Participation and Environment Measure for Children and Youth. *Developmental Medicine and Child Neurology, 53,* 1030–1037.

Coster, W. J., Deeney, T., Haltiwanger, J., & Haley, S. M. (1998). *School function assessment.* San Antonio, TX: PsychCorp.

Coster, W. J., & Khetani, M. (2008). Measuring participation of children with disabilities: Issues and challenges. *Disability and Rehabilitation, 30,* 639–648.

Coster, W. J., Law, M., & Bedell, G. M. (2010). *Participation and Environment Measure for Children and Youth (PEM-CY).* Boston, MA: Boston University.

Coster, W. J., Law, M., Bedell, G. M., Khetani, M., Cousins, M., & Teplicky, R. (2012). Development of the participation and environment measure for children and youth: Conceptual basis. *Disability and Rehabilitation, 34,* 238–246.

Cutchin, M. (2004). Using Deweyan philosophy to rename and reframe adaptation-to-environment. *American Journal of Occupational Therapy, 58,* 303–312.

Di Marino, E., Tremblay, S., Khetani, M. A., & Anaby, D. (2018). The effect of child, family and environmental factors on the participation of young children with disabilities. *Disability and Health Journal, 11,* 36–42. doi:10.1016/j.dhjo.2017.05.005

Dunst, C., Hamby, D., Trivette, C., Raab, M., & Bruder, M. (2002). Young children's participation in everyday family and community activity. *Psychological Reports, 91,* 875–897.

Eakman, A. (2011). Convergent validity of the engagement in meaningful activities survey in a college sample. *OTJR: Occupation, Participation and Health, 31,* 23–32. doi:10.3928/15394492-20100122-02

Eakman, A., Carlson, M., & Clark, F. (2010a). Factor structure, reliability, and convergent validity of the engagement in meaningful activities survey for older adults. *OTJR: Occupation, Participation and Health, 30,* 111–121.

Eakman, A. M., Carlson, M., & Clark, F. (2010b). The Meaningful Activity Participation Assessment: A measure of engagement in personally valued activities. *International Journal of Aging & Human Development, 70,* 339–357.

Finlayson, M., Preissner, K., Cho, C., & Plow, M. (2011). Randomized trial of a teleconference-delivered fatigue management program for people with multiple sclerosis. *Multiple Sclerosis, 17,* 1130–1140.

Frontera, W. R., Bean, J. F., Damiano, D., Ehrlich-Jones, L., Fried-Oken, M., Jette, A., . . . Thompson, A. (2017). Rehabilitation research at the National Institutes of Health: Moving the field forward. *American Journal of Occupational Therapy, 71.* doi:10.5014/ajot.2017.713003

Gandek, B., Sinclair, S. J., Jette, A. M., & Ware, J. E., Jr. (2007). Development and initial psychometric evaluation of the participation measure for post-acute care (PM-PAC). *American Journal of Physical Medicine & Rehabilitation, 86,* 57–71. doi:10.1097/01.phm.0000233200.43822.21

Goldberg, B., Brintnell, E., & Goldberg, J. (2002). The relationship between engagement in meaningful activities and quality of life in persons disabled by mental illness. *Occupational Therapy in Mental Health, 18,* 17–44.

Golos, A., & Bedell, G. (2016). Psychometric properties of the Child and Adolescent Scale of Participation (CASP) across a 3-year period for children and youth with traumatic brain injury. *NeuroRehabilitation, 38,* 311–319. doi:10.3233/NRE-161322

Guralnick, M. J. (2005). Early intervention for children with intellectual disabilities: Current knowledge and future prospects. *Journal of Applied Research in Intellectual Disabilities, 18,* 313–324. doi:10.1111/j.1468-3148.2005.00270.x

Hammel, J., Magasi, S., Heinemann, A., Whiteneck, G., Bogner, J., & Rodriguez, E. (2008). What does participation mean? An insider perspective from people with disabilities. *Disability and Rehabilitation, 30,* 1445–1460.

Hays, R., Hahn, H., & Marshall, G. (2002). Use of the SF-36 and other health-related quality of life measures to assess persons with disabilities. *Archives of Physical Medicine and Rehabilitation, 83,* S4–S9.

Heah, T., Case, T., McGuire, B., & Law, M. (2007). Successful participation: The lived experience among children with disabilities. *Canadian Journal of Occupational Therapy, 74,* 38–47.

Heinemann, A. W. (2010). Measurement of participation in rehabilitation research. *Archives of Physical Medicine and Rehabilitation, 92,* 1729–1730.

Hemmingsson, H., & Jonsson, H. (2005). An occupational perspective on the concept of participation in the International Classification of Functioning, Disability and Health—Some critical remarks. *American Journal of Occupational Therapy, 59,* 569–576.

Horowitz, B. P., & Chang, P. F. J. (2004). Promoting well-being and engagement in life through occupational therapy lifestyle redesign: A pilot study with adult day programs. *Topics in Geriatric Rehabilitation, 20,* 46–58.

Imms, C., & Adair, B. (2017). Participation trajectories: Impact of school transitions on children and adolescents with cerebral palsy. *Developmental Medicine and Child Neurology, 59,* 174–182.

Imms, C., Adair, B., Keen, D., Ullenhag, A., Rosenbaum, P., & Granlund, M. (2015). 'Participation': A systematic review of language, definitions, and constructs used in intervention research with children with disabilities. *Developmental Medicine and Child Neurology, 58,* 29–38.

Jackson, J. (1998a). Contemporary criticisms of role theory . . . part 1. *Journal of Occupational Science, 5,* 49–55.

Jackson, J. (1998b). Is there a place for role theory in occupational science? . . . part 2. *Journal of Occupational Science, 5,* 56–65.

Jones, E., Perry, J., Lowe, K., Felce, D., Toogood, S., Dunstan, F., . . . Pagler, J. (1999). Opportunity and the promotion of activity among adults with severe intellectual disability living in community residences: The impact of training staff in active support. *Journal of Intellectual Disability Research, 43,* 164–178.

Khetani, M. A. (2015). Validation of environmental content in the Young Children's Participation and Environment Measure. *Archives of Physical Medicine and Rehabilitation, 96,* 317–322.

Khetani, M. A. (2017). Capturing change: Participation trajectories in cerebral palsy during life transitions. *Developmental Medicine and Child Neurology, 59*(2), 118–119.

Khetani, M. A., Bedell, G., Coster, W., Cousins, M., & Law, M. (2012). Physical, social and attitudinal environment. In A. Majnemer (Ed.), *Measures for children with developmental disabilities: An ICF-CY approach* (pp. 440–454). London, United Kingdom: MacKeith Press.

Khetani, M. A., Cohn, E., Orsmond, G., Law, M., & Coster, W. (2013). Parent perspectives of participation in home and community life when receiving Part C early intervention services. *Topics in Early Childhood Special Education. 32*(4), 234–245. doi:10.1177 /0271121411418004

Khetani, M. A., Graham, J. E., Davies, P. L., Law, M. C., & Simeonsson, R. J. (2015). Psychometric properties of the Young Children's Participation and Environment Measure (YC-PEM). *Archives of Physical Medicine and Rehabilitation, 96*, 307–316.

Khetani, M. A., Lim, H., & Corden, M. (2017). Caregiver input to optimize the design of a pediatric care planning guide for rehabilitation: Descriptive study. *JMIR Rehabilitation and Assistive Technologies, 4*, e10. doi:10.2196/rehab.7566

Khetani, M. A., Marley, J., Baker, M., Albrecht, E., Bedell, G., Coster, W., . . . Law, M. (2014). Validity of the Participation and Environment Measure for Children and Youth (PEM-CY) for Health Impact Assessment (HIA) in sustainable development projects. *Disability and Health Journal, 7*, 226–235.

King, G., Imms, C., Palisano, R., Majnemer, A., Chiarello, L., Orlin, M., . . . Avery, L. (2013). Geographical patterns in the recreation and leisure participation of children and youth with cerebral palsy: A CAPE international collaborative network study. *Developmental Neurorehabilitation, 16*, 196–206.

King, G. A., Law, M., King, S., Hurley, P., Rosenbaum, P., Hanna, S., . . . Young, N. (2004). *Children's Assessment of Participation & Enjoyment (CAPE) and Preferences for Activities of Children (PAC)*. San Antonio, TX: PsychCorp.

Kramer, J., Barth, Y., Curtis, K., Livingston, K., O'Neil, M., Smith, Z., . . . Wolfe, A. (2013). Involving youth with disabilities in the development and evaluation of a new advocacy training: Project TEAM. *Disability and Rehabilitation, 35*, 614–622.

Kramer, J., & Hammel, J. (2011). "I do lots of things": Children with cerebral palsy perceptions of competence for everyday activities. *International Journal of Disability, Development, and Education, 58*, 121–136.

Kramer, J. M., Roemer, K., Liljenquist, K., Shin, J., & Hart, S. (2014). Formative evaluation of project TEAM (Teens Making Environment and Activity Modifications). *Intellectual and Developmental Disabilities, 52*, 258–272.

Law, M. (2002). Participation in the occupations of everyday life. *American Journal of Occupational Therapy, 56*, 640–649.

Law, M., Darrah, J., Pollock, N., Wilson, B., Russell, D., Walter, S., . . . Galuppi, B. (2011). Focus on function: A cluster, randomized controlled trial comparing child- versus context-focused intervention for young children with cerebral palsy. *Developmental Medicine and Child Neurology, 53*, 621–629.

Law, M., King, G., Petrenchik, T., Kertoy, M., & Anaby, D. (2012). The assessment of preschool children's participation: Internal consistency and construct validity. *Physical & Occupational Therapy in Pediatrics, 32*, 272–287. doi:10.3109/01942638.2012.662584

Lawlor, M. (2003). The significance of being occupied: The social construction of childhood occupations. *American Journal of Occupational Therapy, 57*, 424–434.

Lee, D., Fischer, H., Zera, S., Robertson, R., & Hammel, J. (2017). Examining a participation-focused stroke self-management intervention in a day rehabilitation setting: A quasi-experimental pilot study. *Topics in Stroke Rehabilitation, 24*, 601–607.

Lollar, D. J., & Andresen, E. M. (Eds.). (2011). Introduction. In *Public health perspectives on disability: Epidemiology to ethics and beyond* (pp. 3–12). New York, NY: Springer.

Mactavish, J., & Schleien, S. (1998). Playing together growing together: Parents' perspectives on the benefits of family recreation in families that include children with a developmental disability. *Therapeutic Recreation Journal, 32*, 207–230.

Maisel, J. L. (2006). Toward inclusive housing and neighborhood design: A look at visitability. *Community Development, 37*, 26–34.

Majnemer, A., Shikako-Thomas, K., Chokron, N., Law, M., Shevell, M., Chlingaryan, G., . . . Rosenbaum, P. (2010). Leisure activity preferences for 6- to 12-year-old children with cerebral palsy. *Developmental Medicine and Child Neurology, 52*, 167–173.

Mandich, A., Polatajko, H., Miller, L., & Baum, C. (2004). *The Pediatric Activity Card Sort (PACS)*. Ontario, Canada: Canadian Association of Occupational Therapists.

Matsuka, K., Giles-Heinz, A., Flinn, N., Neighbor, M., & Bass-Haugen, J. (2003). Outcomes of a pilot occupational therapy wellness program for older adults. *American Journal of Occupational Therapy, 57*, 220–224.

McConachie, H., Colver, A., Forsyth, R., Jarvis, S., & Parkinson, K. (2006). Participation of disabled children: How should it be characterised and measured? *Disability and Rehabilitation, 28*, 1157–1164.

McDougall, J., Wright, V., Schmidt, J., Miller, L., & Lowry, K. (2011). Applying the ICF framework to study changes in quality-of-life for youth with chronic conditions. *Developmental Neurorehabilitation, 14*, 41–53.

McWilliam, R. A. (2009). *Protocol for the routines-based interview*. Chattanooga, TN: Siskin Children's Institute.

McWilliam, R. A., Casey, A. M., & Sims, J. (2009). The routines-based interview: A method for gathering information and assessing needs. *Infants and Young Children, 22*, 224–233.

Morris, C., Kurinczuk, J., & Fitzpatrick, R. (2005). Child or family assessed measures of activity performance and participation for children with cerebral palsy: A structured review. *Child: Care, Health and Development, 31*, 397–407.

National Institutes of Health. (2017). *NINDS common data elements*. Retrieved from https://www.commondataelements.ninds.nih.gov /#page=Default

Noreau, L., Fougeyrollas, P., Post, M., & Asano, M. (2005). Participation after spinal cord injury: The evolution of conceptualization and measurement. *Journal of Neurologic Physical Therapy, 29*, 147–156.

Noreau, L., Lepage, C., Boissiere, L., Picard, R., Fougeyrollas, P., Mathieu, J., . . . Nadeau, L. (2007). Measuring participation in children with disabilities using the Assessment of Life Habits. *Developmental Medicine and Child Neurology, 49*, 666–671.

Rosenberg, L., Jarus, T., & Bart, O. (2010). Development and initial validation of the Children Participation Questionnaire (CPQ). *Disability and Rehabilitation, 32*, 1633–1644. doi:10.3109 /09638281003611086

Sander, A. M., Seel, R. T., Kreutzer, J. S., Hall, K. M., High, W. M., & Rosenthal, M. (2007). Agreement between persons with traumatic brain injury and their relatives regarding psychosocial outcome using the Community Integration Questionnaire. *Archives of Physical Medicine and Rehabilitation, 78*, 353–357.

Schelly, C., Davies, P., & Spooner, C. (2011). Student perceptions of faculty implementation of universal design for learning. *Journal of Postsecondary Education and Disability, 24*, 17–28.

Scott, S., & McWilliam, R. A. (2000). *Scale for Assessment of Family Enjoyment within Routines (SAFER)*. Chapel Hill, NC Frank Porter Graham Child Development Center, University of North Carolina at Chapel Hill.

Shikako-Thomas, K., Lach, L., Majnemer, A., Nimignon, J., Cameron, K., & Shevell, M. (2009). Quality of life from the perspective of adolescents with cerebral palsy: "I just think I'm a normal kid, I just happen to have a disability." *Quality of Life Research, 18*, 825–832.

Shirley Ryan AbilityLab. (2010). *Rehabilitation measures database.* Retrieved from http://www.rehabmeasures.org/default.aspx

Stoffel, A., & Berg, C. (2008). Spanish translation and validation of the Preschool Activity Card Sort. *Physical & Occupational Therapy in Pediatrics, 28,* 171–189.

Tamis-Monda, C. S., Way, N., Hughes, D., Yoshikawa, H., Kalman, R. K., & Niwa, E. Y. (2007). Parents' goals for children: The dynamic coexistence of individualism and collectivism in cultures and individuals. *Social Development, 17,* 183–209.

Tickle-Degnen, L., Ellis, T., Saint-Hilaire, M. H., Thomas, C. A., & Wagenaar, R. (2010). Self-management rehabilitation and health-related quality of life in Parkinson's disease: A randomized controlled trial. *Movement Disorders, 25,* 194–204.

Ueda, S., & Okawa, Y. (2003). The subjective dimension of functioning and disability: What is it and what is it for? *Disability and Rehabilitation, 25,* 596–601.

Umeda, C. J., Fogelberg, D., Jirikowic, T., Pitonyak, J. S., Mroz, T., & Ideishi, R. (2017). Expanding the implementation of the Americans with Disabilities Act for populations with intellectual and developmental disabilities: The role of organization-level occupational therapy consultation. *American Journal of Occupational Therapy, 71,* 7104090010p1–7104090010p6.

Vaughan, M. W., Felson, D. T., LaValley, M. P., Orsmond, G. I., Niu, J., Lewis, C. E., . . . Keysor, J. J. (2017). Perceived community environmental factors and risk of five-year participation restriction among older adults with or at risk of knee osteoarthritis. *Arthritis Care & Research (Hoboken), 69,* 952–958.

Whiteneck, G. (2006). Conceptual models of disability: Past, present, and future. In M. J. Field & A. M. Jette (Eds.), *The future of disability in America* (pp. 50–64). Washington, DC: The National Academies Press.

Whiteneck, G., Charlifue, S., Gerhart, K., Overholser, J., & Richardson, G. (1992). Quantifying handicap: A new measure of long-term rehabilitation outcomes. *Archives of Physical Medicine and Rehabilitation, 73,* 519–526.

Willer, B., Rosenthal, M., Kreutzer, J. S., Gordon, W. A., & Rempel, R. (1993). Assessment of community integration following rehabilitation for traumatic brain injury. *The Journal of Head Trauma Rehabilitation, 8,* 75–87.

Wilson, L., Mott, D. W., & Batman, D. (2004). The Asset-Based Context Matrix: A tool for assessing children's learning opportunities and participation in natural environments. *Topics in Early Childhood Special Education, 24,* 110–120.

Wolf, T., Baum, C. M., Lee, D., & Hammel, J. (2016). The development of the Improving Participation after Stroke Self-Management Program (IPASS): An exploratory randomized clinical study. *Topics in Stroke Rehabilitation, 23,* 284–292.

World Health Organization. (1998). *Quality of life.* Retrieved from http://www.who.int/healthpromotion/about/HPR%20Glossary%201998.pdf

World Health Organization. (2001). *International classification of functioning, disability and health: ICF.* Geneva, Switzerland: Author.

World Health Organization. (2007). *International classification of functioning, disability and health: Version for children and youth.* Geneva, Switzerland: Author.

World Health Organization & World Bank. (2011). *World report on disability.* Retrieved from http://www.who.int/disabilities/world_report/en/index.html

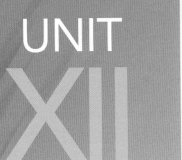

UNIT XII

Theory Guided Interventions: Examples from the Field

"The secret of getting ahead is getting started. The secret of getting started is breaking down complex overwhelming tasks into small manageable tasks, and then starting on the first one."

—Mark Twain

CHAPTER 56

Overview of Theory Guided Intervention

Barbara A. Boyt Schell, Glen Gillen

LEARNING OBJECTIVES

After reading this chapter, you will be able to:

1. Discuss the importance of client subjective experiences in considering therapy approaches.
2. Explore the limitations of deficit-oriented theories in light of the strength-based models.
3. Critically examine both the benefits and limitations of restorative approaches in improving client participation.
4. Examine opportunities for improving participation by attending to client preferences, occupational needs, and the timing and duration of theoretical approaches focused on client impairments.

Introduction

Occupational therapy (OT) is a profession that demands much from its practitioners. Excellence in OT practice presumes that practitioners appreciate the complexity of occupation and are committed to helping those we serve to be able to participate meaningfully in society. As discussed in many previous chapters, in this text, occupation is seen as having curative powers as a therapeutic medium, but it is also seen as an end in itself. For those seeking to use occupation in a way that restores bodily impairments or promote improved bodily function, extensive knowledge of a range of scientifically based information from medical, educational, social, and psychological as well as occupational sciences is required. Occupational therapy researchers and expert practitioners blend knowledge from these fields with OT theories and as a result develop evaluation and intervention methods that are informed by these interdisciplinary perspectives. In this unit, we introduce you to some of the major theoretical perspectives that are commonly used in OT practice and have growing bodies of evidence indicating that they are effective approaches. Topics addressed include motor function, cognition and perception, sensory processing, emotional regulation, and communication/social interaction. Note that each chapter addresses these in the context of occupational performance and participation. Chapters include in-depth summaries of current practice theories and models that guide intervention, examples of standardized assessments used to document change, and available evidence to guide practitioners using these approaches.

Before moving on to these chapters, it is important to gain a sense of perspective about how these theories "fit" within effective OT practice. Important perspectives drawn from philosophy, from disability studies, and from leaders within the profession are provided as guides on how to think about and use the theories discussed in this unit. Although all of these perspectives are addressed in other ways throughout this text, we feel it is especially important to consider in a unit such as this, where attention to the vast array of important information about each aspect of performance can threaten to overshadow the focus on each person and the uniqueness of each person as an occupational being. Therefore, this chapter is designed to help the reader approach the theories and practices covered in this unit in light of the core knowledge of occupation that guides the profession.

The "I" and the "It"

Perhaps the most therapeutic action that OT practitioners can do is to always hold in mind each person's hopes, dreams, and experiences and at the same time understand all the many person and environmental factors that affect that person and his or her occupations. As discussed earlier in Chapter 30, therapists have to use many different perspectives to pull off this therapy tall order. Adding to the complexity, much of the practice of OT occurs within systems of health care and education, which are focused on measurable results (see for instance, Sandhu, Furniss, & Metzler, 2018). These efforts are intended to guide policy makers on how to efficiently parcel out social resources—in other words, to figure out what is worth paying for. Unfortunately, a focus on these results can either intentionally or unintentionally depersonalize the person receiving services.

Renowned leader and scholar Dr. Elizabeth "Betty" Yerxa (2009) provided an effective metaphor for appreciating the dueling perspectives which challenge OT in her discussion entitled "Infinite Distance Between the I and the It" (p. 490). In the abstract of this article, she notes that

traditional science and medical practice in the 21st century often separates the *I* consciousness, the person who experiences daily life, from the *it* of an object that can be probed, tested, and fixed. This separation may also influence the development of occupational science and the practice of occupational therapy to the detriment of the profession.

Attention to theories focused on restoring bodily functions runs the risk of creating therapy situations in which practitioners lose track of their clients as individuals who have unique desires and needs. The caution here is not to avoid using effective theoretical approaches to restore function but to be very mindful that these theories are used in service of the "I." The purpose of working on motor control is not to "fix" someone's arm, but it is to help that person who wants to move his or her arm in order to fix his or her hair. The purpose of understanding theories of cognition is not to focus on someone's problems with memory that are affecting his or her ability to work but to figure out how to help him or her get back to work on a job he or she really cares about. The purpose of understanding how we all vary in our neurological processes is not to classify a child into a particular category. It is to find the best way for that child and his or her family to play, learn, and do all the things that the child and his or her family want to do.

Strength-Based Approaches

Winnie Dunn (2011), another renowned occupational therapist and scholar, raises an additional important set of issues to consider: the need to focus on strengths as the basis for effective intervention. She notes that although professions and programs logically develop out of an attempt to respond to needs, she goes on to say,

There is certainly a place for finding out what is interfering with participation. . . . However, what has happened is that, in doing the detective work to identify needs, professionals have gotten caught up in the empty places and have forgotten to consider what is working! (p. 7)

In many instances, the chapters that follow discuss adaptive approaches, strategy training approaches, and/or environmental modifications as effective interventions that indeed tap into our client's strength to overcome performance deficits. The theories provided in this unit provide a rich wealth of resources to notice what is working for the individuals being served. Dr. Dunn's (2011) advice can be taken as a call to document the "full" places as well as to notice the empty ones. When combined with Dr. Yerxa's (2009) advice to stay focused on the *I*, the opportunities to use these theories to support participations in occupation become even more visible.

Challenging Assumptions about Learning Transfer and Skills

Beyond the need to deal with people as unique individuals and to consider their strengths as the basis for improving performance, there is another perspective to consider.

In many aspects of modern society, there are pervasive assumptions about the presumed sequencing of development and learning. The saying, "You must crawl before you can walk," presumes a developmental sequence to the process. Likewise, in some universities, one must have an algebra course as a prerequisite to a statistics course. Once again, the presumption is that there are foundation skills on which higher level performance is required. Yet, many of us likely know children who went right from sitting to walking, with little "crawling" involved. Likewise, there are many students who have successfully taken college level statistics without a prior college level algebra course. In spite of these examples to the contrary, there appears to be a durable assumption that one must have certain skills or abilities in order to engage in higher level activities. Therefore, it is not surprising that this assumption underlies clinical decisions that focus on the need to remediate impairments and build component skills in preparation for engaging in occupations. Even the American Occupational Therapy Association's (AOTA) "Occupational Therapy Practice Framework: Domain and Process (3rd ed.)" (AOTA, 2014) adopts the term *preparatory* for one category of interventions.

It is important that practitioners not lose focus when helping clients manage their impairments. A recent study of OT practice patterns for stroke survivors clearly demonstrates potential pitfalls when we "can't see the forest through the trees." Smallfield and Karges (2009) investigated the specific type of OT intervention used by occupational therapists during inpatient stroke rehabilitation to determine the frequency of preparatory or prefunctional versus functional activity use. Of concern is that they found that most sessions (65.77%) consisted of activities that were prefunctional in nature compared with 48.26% that focused on activities of daily living. In other words, occupational therapists used prefunctional activities that aim to improve performance skills and body structures more often than occupation-based activities that incorporate meaningful activities into therapy sessions. This is clearly in contrast to our professions current philosophy (AOTA, 2014).

The philosophy of OT includes the premise that meaningful activity is essential to OT intervention because occupation is the power of intervention. If occupational therapists believe in the use of occupation-based activities, it is contradictory for them to use prefunctional activities more often than functional activities with this diagnostic group (Smallfield & Karges, 2009, p. 411).

More recently, Proffitt (2016) surveyed occupational therapists regarding usage and prescription of and clinical reasoning process supporting home programs. Unfortunately, preparatory activities were again most commonly prescribed. In fact, the most common interventions were active range of motion, active assistive range of motion, passive range of motion, and stretching. Proffitt concluded that client goals should guide treatment planning, strategies, and choice of activities to ensure true client-centered care in the provision of a home program.

There are several studies across a wide variety of disciplines that are challenging these assumptions that you must "do this" before you can "do that." In Chapter 7, Humphry and Womack provide a convincing summary of how the demands of the performance context (both physical and social) as well as engaging in the actual occupation itself explain performance variance in daily life. Consideration of sociological and ecological perspectives tempers our understanding of developmental hierarchies by acknowledging the power of actual performance to draw out needed skills. Likewise, educational scholars over the last several decades have challenged the reliance on learning transfer in schools (Detterman & Sternberg, 1996; Lave, 1988; Lave & Wenger, 1991). Mounting evidence suggests that learning transfer is unpredictable and is context and task dependent. Similar findings in the motor control literature strongly suggest that practitioners should be moving away from impairment-based hierarchical approaches to approaches that are best described as task and context specific. These approaches are clearly better aligned with past and current philosophies of our profession. These and other developments have influenced many occupational therapists to critically examine the assumption that improving an impairment will automatically transfer into the improvement of occupational performance and related social participation (Box 56-1).

Blended Approaches and a Focus on Participation

Perhaps the best way for practitioners to use the focused theories designed to manage impairments is to blend them with theories that provide a broader understanding of human learning and motivation as it occurs within the context of occupation. There is promising evidence to suggest that by directly working on the occupational tasks that the client wants or needs to do, occupational participation is enhanced. The focused theories presented in this unit can be used *in the context of assisting the client to perform actual occupations.* That is different than trying to "fix" the person. Rather, it involves harnessing sound-focused therapy techniques to enhance the likelihood of success and at the same time doing the "real thing." Furthermore, working on occupational participation directly and almost automatically ensures opportunities to recognize and build

BOX 56-1   IS RESTORATION THE BEST CHOICE? CONSIDERATIONS FOR PRACTICE

Just because someone has an impairment, it doesn't necessarily follow that OT intervention focused directly on that impairment is the best approach. The following questions are intended to provoke careful reflection about the assumptions underlying the choice to use a restorative approach.

- What is the client interested in being able to do? If the client is focused on a bodily impairment, why does it matter? How does it affect the client's ability to live life?
- Why restore impairments versus choosing to work directly on the occupational areas the client wants to improve?
- Can engaging in relevant occupations serves to remediate an underlying impairment? If we are engaged in housekeeping activities such as making a bed, don't our analysis skills lead us to think that we are simultaneously "working on" balance, strength, motor planning, attention skills, and so forth?
- How much evidence is there to suggest that an intervention aimed at a body function will actually result in improved occupational performance?

- If you choose remediation, how do you know which impairment to focus on to best improve performance?
- How do we know that the impairment is amenable to remediation?
- What strengths do the client have that can be marshaled to improve performance as well as restore bodily function?
- Can the bodily impairment be used to enhance performance (e.g., a woman with spasticity in her arm might be able to use the extra tension to hold a purse)?
- Have you chosen outcome measures that are indicative of improved occupational performance versus just a change in bodily function?
- How might your own cultural lenses, both your personal one and the ones imbedded in your workplace, affect the intervention options you present to your client?
- How open are you to exploring and negotiating differences with your clients over therapy goals and expectations?

on strengths and further serves to reinforce the identity of the client as one who can participate as a valued member of society.

REFERENCES

American Occupational Therapy Association. (2014). Occupational therapy practice framework: Domain and process (3rd ed.). *American Journal of Occupational Therapy, 68*, S1–S48.

Detterman, D. K., & Sternberg, R. J. (1996). *Transfer on trial: Intelligence, cognition, & instruction.* Norwood, NJ: Ablex.

Dunn, W. (2011). *Best practice occupational therapy for children and families in community settings* (2nd ed.). Thorofare, NJ: SLACK.

Lave, J. (1988). *Cognition in practice: Mind, mathematics, and culture in everyday life.* Cambridge, United Kingdom: Cambridge University Press.

Lave, J., & Wenger, E. (1991). *Situated learning: Legitimate peripheral participation.* Cambridge, United Kingdom: Cambridge University Press.

Proffitt, R. (2016). Home exercise programs for adults with neurological injuries: A survey. *American Journal of Occupational Therapy, 70,* 7003290020p1–7003290020p8.

Sandhu, S., Furniss, J., & Metzler, C. (2018). Using the new postacute care quality measures to demonstrate the value of occupational therapy. *American Journal of Occupational Therapy, 72,* 7202090010p1–7202090010p6. doi:10.5014/ajot.2018.722002

Smallfield, S., & Karges, J. (2009). Classification of occupational therapy intervention for inpatient stroke rehabilitation. *American Journal of Occupational Therapy, 63,* 408–413.

Yerxa, E. J. (2009). Infinite distance between the I and the it. *American Journal of Occupational Therapy, 63,* 490–497.

thePoint® *For additional resources on the subjects discussed in this chapter, visit* **http://thePoint.lww.com /Willard-Spackman13e.**

Motor Function and Occupational Performance

Glen Gillen, Dawn M. Nilsen

LEARNING OBJECTIVES

After reading this chapter, you will be able to:

1. Understand how motor function supports occupational performance throughout the life course.
2. Explain how impairments related to motor function limit occupational performance across the life course.
3. Compare and contrast the approaches that are used to guide the occupational therapy process related to improving occupational performance for those with motor impairments.
4. Become familiar with assessments that are used to measure motor function across the life course.
5. Begin to construct evidence-based intervention plans that improve occupational performance for those living with motor impairments.

Introduction: Motor Function and Everyday Living

This morning, you may have rolled over in bed, reached over to your nightstand to turn off the alarm, and transitioned to a seated position on your bed, followed by a transition to a standing posture prior to walking to the bathroom. On your way to the bathroom, you might step into your slippers by shifting your weight from one foot to the other. Your **postural control** system combined with your trunk and limb function worked together to support your functional mobility and activities of daily living (ADL).

Samuel is taking care of his child. As he lifts his child from the crib, he must generate enough force in his upper limbs to move his child, calibrate this force as to not harm his child with too much pressure in his hands, maintain his balance as he lifts his child toward him, and coordinate/plan his movements so that his hand supports his child's head as he lifts. Samuel's parenting role is being supported by various motor functions.

Danielle is going ice-skating for the first time today at the age of 4 years. To be successful, she will need to learn to maintain her center of gravity, use various postural reflexes (e.g., righting and equilibrium responses) to

CENTENNIAL NOTES

Motor Function and Occupational Performance

The first documented case study in our journals that described OT interventions for motor control deficits after stroke was in Volume 1, Issue 1 of the *Archives of Occupational Therapy* in 1922. Occupational therapist Evelyn Lawrence Collins described providing home care on the Lower East Side of Manhattan. She described her case as a woman being bedridden after a "paralytic stroke" and the woman's neighbor describing that "she can't do nothing; she has only got one hand" (p. 36). Collins went on to give a short description of what we now mistakenly call a "contemporary" approach to motor control rehabilitation. She described engaging the affected hand using a bilateral activity as the means to remediate hand function. This activity of creating three small purses had all the makings of what we have now proven from a science perspective; that repetitive and purposeful activity has the powerful potential to remediate motor function.

Our approach to remediating motor control was clear from the birth of our profession; we were remediating motor control in the context of using every day activities. Occupational therapy interventions for this population were described over the years as bilateral crafts, toy making, tool use, working looms, making rugs, use of a metronome during typing training, engaging our lower functioning clients in activity by unweighting the upper limb using a suspension sling, project making, activities that provide graded resistance, remedial games, bilateral activities, etc. (Gillen, 2013).

On the basis of the current evidence summarized in this chapter, the "contemporary" interventions that are effective in improving occupational performance would be described as practicing, doing, active, activity, repetitive, life related, skill building, and relearning, etc. This is what we have been doing as a profession for 100 years. This is to be celebrated.

---

maintain an upright position, learn that she can integrate her upper limbs to maintain her balance, and coordinate her limbs to glide over the ice. In addition, she requires enough strength and endurance to complete the task. Danielle's ability to engage in play is supported by multiple systems and structures related to motor function. To be successful, Danielle must also process and adapt to incoming information from her sensory systems (e.g., vestibular, proprioception, vision) (see Chapter 59 for more details).

Most of the day (and night albeit to a much lesser extent) is spent engaging in occupations that require motor functions to support performance. Occupational therapy (OT) practitioners treat various conditions (see Appendix I) that result in limited motor function and loss of motor control. As you can infer from the examples earlier, any change in motor function has a tremendous impact on our ability to engage in meaningful occupations. The following two cases illustrate these points.

Approaches That Guide Therapy

Various approaches may be used when working with clients with motor deficits. Many times, approaches are combined and/or the therapist may switch from one to another based on the client's response or preference (see Chapter 30).

Biomechanical Approach

The **biomechanical approach** is considered a remediation approach. It is focused at the client factor/impairment level when these said impairments are limiting occupational performance. Examples of impairments that are addressed by this approach include weakness, limitations in joint **range of motion**, edema, pain, low endurance, sensory changes, joint instability, poor coordination, etc. Clients living with cardiopulmonary diseases, various forms of arthritis, burns, cumulative trauma disorders/repetitive strain injuries, tendon tears or lacerations, fractures, etc., may be appropriate for interventions based on the biomechanical approach.

More recently, components of this approach (e.g., **strengthening**) have been applied to those living with acquired brain injuries such as a stroke (Harris & Eng, 2010). Further research is recommended to determine the appropriate candidate (e.g., the Harris and Eng paper included those with mild spasticity) as well as the ability to generalize to improved occupational performance.

This approach is based on several assumptions:

- The underlying impairment is amenable to remediation.
- Engagement in occupation and various other therapeutic activities has the potential to remediate the underlying impairment(s).
- This remediation will result in improved occupational performance.

CASE STUDY 57-1   JACOB: LIMITED OCCUPATIONAL PERFORMANCE DUE TO HEMIPARESIS

Jacob is an 8-year-old boy with a hemiparetic right upper limb secondary to cerebral palsy. See Appendix I for more details on cerebral palsy. Jacob's parents are frustrated because he does have minimal movement in his arm and hand. They report constantly "nagging" Jacob to use his arm when he is outside of a structured therapy session. They also describe that his arm appears "useless" when he is at school or play. Both Jacob and his parents are getting frustrated with therapy. Specifically, his parents would like to see "carryover" from his present therapy. Jacob's occupational therapist informed the parents that there was a local therapeutic camp held during school holidays. Jacob was enrolled in this camp that incorporated an intervention called constraint-induced movement therapy (CI therapy).

The occupational therapist at the camp evaluated Jacob via observing his arm use during unstructured play in addition to two standardized assessments of motor function (the speed and dexterity subtest of the Bruininks-Oseretsky Test and the Jebsen-Taylor Test of Hand Function). Jacob's goals were established as (1) Jacob will use his right hand to drink without cues, (2) Jacob will be able to apply paste to his toothbrush using his right hand, and (3) Jacob will swing a bat using both hands.

The CI therapy intervention consisted of the following components (Gordon, Charles, & Wolf, 2005; Morris, Taub, & Mark, 2006):

- Restraint of Jacob's less involved extremity (left) using a sling.
- Encouraging the involved side to be active via engaging Jacob in unimanual activities with the involved extremity (right) 6 hours a day for 10 days (60 hours).
- Repetitive practice embedded in play and functional activities. Examples of activities include arts and crafts, board games, card games, puzzles, cleaning a table after a meal, etc.
- The technique of shaping was used. Shaping involves approaching a behavioral objective (task) in small steps by successive approximation. As Jacob's performance improved, the task was made more challenging, taking into consideration his abilities. The occupational therapist graded the tasks accordingly to target movements he wanted Jacob to achieve.
- Adherence-enhancing behavioral strategies ("the transfer package") such as a caregiver contract, home diary, home practice, etc.

Following the therapy, Jacob's parents reported that he was using his involved arm more spontaneously and automatically. Jacob was able to meet his goals.

The key to successfully using this approach is linking the underlying impairment to the occupational performance deficit. This linking must occur in both the intervention planning process as well as in goal writing. See Box 57-1 for examples of goal writing for those with motor deficits. See Tables 57-1 to 57-4 for examples of assessments/evaluations and interventions that are commonly used when the biomechanical approach is adopted. See Table 57-2 for examples of evidence that supports interventions used in the biomechanical approach.

Rehabilitative Approach

The **rehabilitative approach** includes the concepts of adaptation, compensation, and environmental modifications (see Chapter 30 for more details). It may be used in conjunction with other approaches or in isolation. This approach places an emphasis on the client's strengths as opposed to their limitations. The ultimate goal is to maximize independence despite the presence of persistent impairments. This approach may be most appropriate for client's who are living with impairments that are permanent, including both static and progressive

impairments. This approach may also be useful when an underlying impairment is potentially amenable to remediation but the client is not motivated to participate in the sometimes long and difficult process of remediation. Contextual factors such as limited therapy visits may also lead therapists to adopt this approach because some may argue that functional independence is achieved quicker.

Clients living with the following diagnoses may be candidates for the rehabilitative approach in isolation or in conjunction with the other approaches discussed: multiple sclerosis, amyotrophic lateral sclerosis, severe stroke, advanced arthritis, advancing Parkinson disease, spinal cord injuries, etc. Readers should note that the rehabilitative approach is used for various impairments beyond motor deficits.

In many cases, the occupational therapist takes on the role of "teacher" when using this approach and must consider the following questions:

1. What is the client's potential to learn?
2. Is the client motivated to learn?
3. What is the client's optimal learning style?

CASE STUDY 57-2   SAMUEL: LIMITED OCCUPATIONAL PERFORMANCE DUE TO A MUSCULOSKELETAL INJURY

Samuel (as discussed in the opening paragraphs) fell while jogging. He landed on his dominant right shoulder and returned home complaining of weakness and excruciating pain. Samuel's orthopedist diagnosed him with a full thickness tear of his rotator cuff. See Appendix I for more details on orthopedic injuries. Surgery was scheduled, and the tear was repaired. Postoperatively, Samuel was referred for occupational therapy. The occupational therapist performed evaluations focused on Samuel's impairments and activity limitations related to areas of occupation. Various standardized measures were used. A Visual Analogue Scale documented that his pain was rated as 8 on a 0–10 scale. His active **range of motion** and strength, as tested by a manual muscle test, were intact with the exception of his right shoulder. These tests were deferred for his injured shoulder because the medical orders allowed only passive motion until the repair site began to heal. **Passive range of motion** of his involved shoulder was limited by pain as expected. Samuel reported and demonstrated difficulty with both basic and instrumental activities of daily living (ADL), stating, "I am very right dominant." The occupational therapist administered the Disabilities of the Arm, Shoulder, and Hand (DASH) Outcome Measure including the work module because Samuel was employed as a grocery store manager. The DASH is a 30-item, self-report questionnaire designed to measure physical function and symptoms in people with any of several musculoskeletal disorders of the upper limb. The DASH provided the occupational therapist with specific information regarding how Samuel's shoulder injury was impacting his daily functioning. Samuel's long-term goals were defined as (1) independent in all basic ADL, (2) independent in child care, and (3) return to work part-time.

The occupational therapist used various interventions that were graded as Samuel's tendons healed over time. The interventions were based on both rehabilitative and biomechanical approaches. These included the following:

- Activities of daily living retraining using one-handed techniques and assistive devices. This was an early focus because Samuel was not allowed to actively move his right shoulder for several weeks. Although he lived with his wife, he did not want to be a burden as she was taking care of their newborn. Therefore, he was highly motivated to be as independent as possible. These techniques were only employed temporarily.
- Physical agent modalities such as ice (**cryotherapy**) for pain control
- Education related to sleep postures
- Progressive mobilization of Samuel's shoulder (passive range of motion, active assisted range of motion, active range of motion, and strengthening)
- Physical agent modalities such as therapeutic heat to increase flexibility prior to therapy
- Engaging Samuel's right arm to support performance of occupations that were graded over time. The occupational therapist began with low-height activities such as reaching into cabinets under the sink, followed by medium-height activities (e.g., applying deodorant), and followed by overhead reach activities such as hanging up clothing and putting groceries away on to high shelves.
- Resumption of bilateral ADL
- Simulated work activities

Using the aforementioned approaches and interventions, Samuel was able to meet his goals and soon after resumed full-time duties at work.

Motor learning principles to promote skill acquisition will be discussed later in this chapter. See Table 57-5 for a summary of assessments/evaluation and interventions used when adopting this approach.

Task-Oriented Approaches

Task-oriented approaches—also described as task-specific training, repetitive task practice, goal-directed training, and functional task practice—are considered the most current approach related to impaired motor function and motor control for those living with brain damage. Timmermans, Spooren, Kingma, and Seelen (2010) describe the components of task-oriented training (Box 57-2). In this

approach, movement emerges as an interaction between many systems in the brain and is organized around a goal and constrained by the environment (Shumway-Cook & Woollacott, 2017). Rensink, Schuurmans, Lindeman, and Hafsteinsdóttir (2009) describe task-oriented training as including a wide range of interventions such as walking training on the ground, bicycling programs, endurance training and circuit training, sit-to-stand exercises, and reaching tasks for improving balance. A major focus of task-oriented training is on arm training using functional tasks, such as grasping objects, and constraint-induced movement therapy (CI therapy) (S. L. Wolf et al., 2006). This approach is task- and client-focused and not therapist-focused (Rensink et al., 2009). See Table 57-6

BOX 57-1 | **KEEPING AN OCCUPATION-BASED PERSPECTIVE WHEN USING THE BIOMECHANICAL APPROACH DURING GOAL WRITING FOR REIMBURSEMENT**

Goal 1 incorrectly focused on the impairment: *Client will demonstrate improved grip strength of 15 lb.*

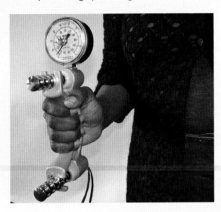

Goal 2 incorrectly focused on impairment: *Client will demonstrate a 20-degree increase in shoulder external rotation.*

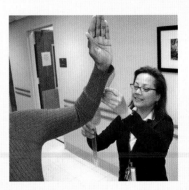

Goal 1 rewritten to reflect the change in performance: *Client will demonstrate improved grip strength of 15 lb in order to independently open a previously unopened jar.* It is assumed that the therapist has documented this client's difficulties with meal preparation in relation to her pattern of weakness. The goal should reflect an improvement in areas of occupation not an isolated change in impairment.

Goal 2 rewritten to reflect the change in performance: *Client will demonstrate a 20-degree increase in shoulder external rotation in order to comb the back of her hair with minimal assistance.* It is assumed that a self-care evaluation has been documented to demonstrate the impact of the loss of range of motion on basic activities of daily living.

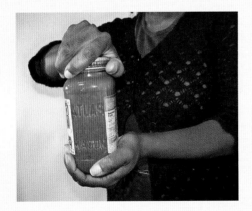

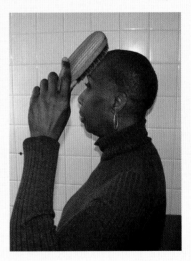

for examples of evidence that supports the use of a task-oriented approach.

Training components of the task-oriented approach have been described (adapted from Timmermans et al., 2010).

1. *Functional movements*: A movement involving task execution that is not directed toward a clear ADL goal.

2. *Clear functional goal*: A goal that is set during everyday life activities and/or hobbies (e.g., washing dishes, grooming activity, dressing oneself, playing golf).

3. *Client-centered patient goal*: Therapy goals that are set through the involvement of the patient himself or herself in the therapy goal decision process. The goals respect patients' values, preferences, and expressed needs and recognize the clients' experience and knowledge.

TABLE 57-1 Assessments/Evaluations and Interventions Commonly Associated with the Biomechanical Approach

Assessments/Evaluations[a]	Sample Interventions
• Standardized objective tests of occupational performance (see Unit XI) • Self-report measures of how impairments limit occupational performance (e.g., DASH, Manual Ability Measure) • Goniometry: active and passive range of motion • Manual muscle tests • Dynamometry (grip and pinch strength testing) • Sensory testing (e.g., Semmes Weinstein Monofilament Examination, 2-point discrimination) • Coordination testing • Provocative tests (tests used to provoke underlying symptoms) • Circumferential or volumetric measures to quantify edema • Pain scales • Examination of skin integrity/wounds • Borg Rating of Perceived Exertion Scale (endurance) • Ergonomic evaluations	• ADL retraining • Work hardening • Active, **active assistive**, passive **range of motion** exercises • High-load brief stretch • Low-load prolonged stretch • Orthoses (static and dynamic) (see Figures 57-1 and 57-2) • Strengthening • Endurance training • Joint protection techniques • Physical agent modalities (see Table 57-3) • Therapeutic exercise (see Table 57-4) • Edema control techniques (e.g., massage and mobilization, positional elevation, wrapping techniques) • Desensitization for hypersensitivity • Sensory retraining • Scar management • Joint mobilization • Tendon gliding • Nerve gliding

[a]See Table 57-11 and Appendix II for more details on standardized assessments for this population.

ADL, activities of daily living; DASH, Disabilities of the Arm, Shoulder, and Hand.

Orthosis type	Associated diagnoses
Wrist cock up 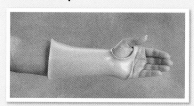	Carpal tunnel syndrome Radial nerve palsy Tenosynovitis/tendinitis Wrist fractures Rheumatoid arthritis Osteoarthritis Reflex sympathetic dystrophy Wrist sprains
Resting orthosis 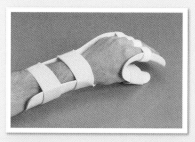	Rheumatoid arthritis Traumatic injuries: crush, contusion Burns Tendon injuries Stroke Spinal cord injury Central nervous system disease and injury Postop Dupuytren's Infections
Thumb spica 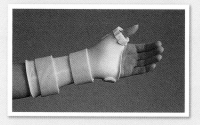	De Quervain's tendinitis Degenerative arthritis/basilar joint arthritis Rheumatoid arthritis Thumb sprains Median nerve injuries

FIGURE 57-1 Common static orthoses associated with diagnostic conditions. (Photos courtesy of the Rehabilitation Division of Smith & Nephew, Germantown, WI.)

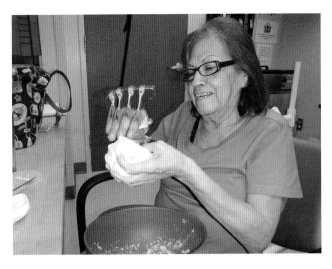

FIGURE 57-2 Using a dynamic orthosis to support engagement in occupation. (Photo courtesy of Lauro A. Munoz, OTR, MOT.)

4. *Overload*: Overload is determined by the total time spent on therapeutic activity, the number of repetitions, the difficulty of the activity in terms of coordination, muscle activity type and resistance load, and the intensity, that is, number of repetitions per time unit.

5. *Real-life object manipulation*: Manipulation that makes use of objects that are handled in normal everyday life activities (e.g., cutlery, hairbrush).

6. *Context-specific environment*: A training environment (supporting surface, objects, people, room, etc.) that equals or mimics the natural environment for a specific task execution in order to include task characteristic sensory/perceptual information, task-specific context characteristics, and cognitive processes involved.

7. *Exercise progression*: Exercises with an increasing difficulty level that is in line with the increasing abilities of the patient in order to keep the demands of the exercises and challenges optimal for motor learning.

8. *Exercise variety*: Various exercises are offered to support motor skill learning of a certain task because of the person experiencing different movement and context characteristics (within task variety) and problem-solving strategies.

9. *Feedback*: Specific information on the patient's motor performance that enhances motor learning and positively influences patient motivation.

10. *Multiple movement planes*: Movement that uses more than one degree of freedom of a joint, therefore occurring around multiple joint axes.

TABLE 57-2   Sample Evidence that Supports Interventions Used when Adopting the Biomechanical Approach

Author/Year	Objective	Conclusion
Egan and Brousseau (2007)	To review the evidence regarding the effectiveness of splinting for carpometacarpal osteoarthritis	Research to date indicates that splinting may help relieve pain in persons with carpometacarpal osteoarthritis.
Page, Massy-Westropp, O'Connor, and Pitt (2012)	To compare the effectiveness of splinting for carpal tunnel syndrome (CTS) with no treatment, placebo, or another non-surgical intervention	Overall, limited evidence that a splint worn at night is more effective than no treatment, but insufficient evidence regarding safety/effectiveness of one type of splint or wearing schedules over others, and of splinting over other nonsurgical interventions.
Harris and Eng (2010)	To evaluate the effects of strengthening on upper limb function after stroke via a meta-analysis	There is evidence that strength training can improve upper limb strength and function without increasing tone or pain in individuals with stroke.
Hurkmans, van der Giesen, Vliet Vlieland, Schoones, and Van den Ende (2009)	To assess the effectiveness and safety of short-term and long-term dynamic exercise therapy programs (aerobic capacity and/or muscle strength training) for people with rheumatoid arthritis (RA)	Based on the evidence, aerobic capacity training combined with muscle strength training is recommended as routine practice in patients with RA.
Saunders and colleagues (2016)	To determine whether fitness training after stroke reduces death, dependence, and disability and to assess the effects of training regarding adverse events, risk factors, physical fitness, mobility, physical function, quality of life, mood, and cognitive function	Cardiorespiratory training and, to a lesser extent, mixed training reduce disability during or after usual stroke care. Sufficient evidence to incorporate cardiorespiratory and mixed training, involving walking, within poststroke rehabilitation programs. Insufficient evidence to support the use of resistance training. The effects of training on death and dependence are unclear. Impact on cognitive function is under investigated.
Werner, Franzblau, and Gell (2005)	To determine whether night splinting of workers identified through active surveillance with symptoms consistent with CTS would improve symptoms and median nerve function as well as impact medical care	The results suggest that a short course of nocturnal splinting may reduce wrist, hand, and/or finger discomfort among active workers with symptoms consistent with CTS.

TABLE 57-3	Physical Agent Modalities	
Modality	**Indications**	**Contraindications/Precautions**
Superficial heat • Hot packs, heating pads • Paraffin wax • Fluidotherapy • Whirlpool	Prior to active exercise, passive stretching, and joint mobilization Before traction and soft tissue mobilization Reduce pain and muscle spasms After acute inflammation to increase tissue healing	Decreased circulation Decreased sensibility Altered cardiorespiratory status Open wounds or recently healed burns (paraffin) Significant areas of edema Over tissue during acute inflammation
Deep heat • Ultrasound and phonophoresis	Soft tissue tightness Subacute and chronic inflammation (e.g., tendinitis) Bone fracture Wound healing	Do not use over or near the eyes, ears, heart, pregnant uterus, testes, known or expected malignant tumor, pacemaker, joint replacements or metal implants, or insensate areas
Therapeutic cold • Cold packs and cold baths • Ice massage	Minimize acute inflammation associated with therapeutic intervention Reduce edema and bleeding Reduce spasticity	Temperature sensation deficits Circulation deficits Altered cardiorespiratory status Cold hypersensitivity such as Raynaud phenomenon
Contrast baths	Promotes tissue healing and may control edema	Cardiovascular problems as fluctuations in pulse and blood pressure may occur Peripheral vascular diseases Loss of sensation Pregnancy Cold hypersensitivity such as Raynaud phenomenon
Electrotherapy • Functional electrical stimulation (neuromuscular electrical stimulation) • Transcutaneous electrical nerve stimulation • Iontophoresis	Modulate pain Decrease inflammation (e.g., bursitis, tendinitis) Reduce edema Improve motor control Improve strength	Do not use over or near the eyes, ears, chest of person with cardiac disease, pregnant uterus, wounds or skin breaks, known or expected malignant tumor, pacemaker, blood vessels susceptible to hemorrhage, thrombosis or embolus, or insensate areas

Adapted from Poole, J. L. (2008). Musculoskeletal factors. In E. B. Crepeau, E. S. Cohn, & B. A. B. Schell (Eds.), *Willard & Spackman's occupational therapy* (11th ed., pp. 658–680). Baltimore, MD: Lippincott Williams & Wilkins.

11. *Patient-customized training load*: A training load that suits the individualized treatment targets (e.g., endurance, coordination, or strength training) as well as the patient's capabilities.

12. *Total skill practice*: The skill is practiced in total, with or without preceding skill component training (e.g., via chaining).

13. *Random practice*: In each practice session, the tasks are randomly ordered.

14. *Distributed practice*: A practice schedule with relatively long rest periods.

15. *Bimanual practice*: Tasks where both arms and hands are involved.

Occupational Therapy Task-Oriented Approach

In the early 1990s, Mathiowetz and Bass-Haugen (1994) argued for a shift away from the traditional neurophysiologic approaches that were being used in occupational therapy. They proposed the Occupational Therapy Task-Oriented Approach that continues to develop (Mathiowetz, 2016; Mathiowetz & Bass-Haugen, 2008). The approach is based on current understandings of motor control, recovery, and development as well as contemporary motor learning principles (Boxes 57-2 and 57-3).

Motor Relearning Program

The Motor Relearning Program (Carr & Shepherd, 1987, 2003) is specific to the rehabilitation of patients following stroke. The program is based on four factors that are thought to be essential for the learning of motor skill and assumed to be essential for the relearning of motor control: (1) elimination of unnecessary muscle activity, (2) feedback, (3) practice, and (4) the interrelationship of postural adjustment and movement. In this program, treatment is directed toward relearning of control rather than to activities incorporating exercise or to facilitation or inhibition techniques. Treatment is directed toward enhancing motor performance, and the emphasis is on the practice of

TABLE 57-4   Therapeutic Exercise Programs

Type	Definition	Resistance	Muscles Grades	Precautions
Passive exercise	Involves passive range of motion and passive stretch, usually done by a practitioner	None Stretch may be held 15–30 seconds	Zero Trace	Inflammation Limited sensation for pain Prolonged immobilization
Isotonic active assistive exercise	Client moves the joint as far as possible, then an outside force such as a practitioner or equipment assists with moving the joint through the rest of the range	None	Trace Poor minus Fair minus	None
Isotonic active exercise	Client moves the joint through available range of motion without any assistance. The muscle shortens and lengthens.	None	Poor Fair	Poor muscles: Move in gravity eliminated plane Fair muscles: Move in against gravity plane
Isometric without resistance	Client contracts the muscle, increasing the tension, and holds the position for 5 seconds. Used when motion of a joint is prohibited.	None	Trace Poor Fair Good	Clients with cardiac conditions and high blood pressure
Isotonic resistive exercise	An isotonic contraction against resistance	Resistance provided by wrist weights, dumbbells, Thera-Band, Theraputty, elastic bands, springs, weights	Fair plus Good	Inflammation Unstable joint Recent or unhealed fracture Use with caution with conditions that are exacerbated by fatigue
Isometric resistive exercise	An isometric contraction against a load	Resistance could be an immovable surface (e.g., pushing the palm against a wall).	Fair plus Good	Clients with cardiac conditions and high blood pressure
Isokinetic exercise	Exercise that uses a machine that controls the speed of contraction within the range of motion	Resistance controlled by machine and is variable in proportion to the change in muscle length throughout the range of motion	Fair plus Good	Inflammation Unstable joint Recent or unhealed fracture Use with caution with conditions that are exacerbated by fatigue

Reprinted from Poole, J. L. (2008). Musculoskeletal factors. In E. B. Crepeau, E. S. Cohn, & B. A. B. Schell (Eds.), *Willard & Spackman's occupational therapy* (11th ed., pp. 658–680). Baltimore, MD: Lippincott Williams & Wilkins.

TABLE 57-5   Assessments/Evaluations and Interventions Commonly Associated with the Rehabilitative Approach as It Relates to Motor Deficits

Assessments/Evaluations[a]	Sample Interventions

• Standardized objective tests of occupational performance (see Unit XI)
 • Self-report measures of occupational performance
 • Ergonomic evaluations
 • Evaluations to determine client's strengths
   – Cognitive evaluations (to evaluate learning potential)
   – Range of motion and strength testing of nonaffected limbs
   – Balance testing
 • Evaluations of environmental and social contexts to determine supports and limitations
	• Energy conservation
	 • Work simplification
	 • Recommending and training with assistive devices to support occupational performance
	 • Recommending and training with durable medical equipment
	 • Recommending and training with assistive technology
	 • Home modifications
	 • Work modifications
	 • Wheeled mobility and seating recommendations
	 • Fabrication of orthoses that support function

[a]See Table 57-11 and Appendix II for more details on standardized assessments for this population.

BOX 57-2 ASSUMPTIONS OF THE OCCUPATIONAL THERAPY TASK-ORIENTED APPROACH BASED ON A SYSTEMS MODEL OF MOTOR BEHAVIOR

- Functional tasks help organize behavior.
- Personal and environmental systems, including the central nervous system, are heterarchically organized.
- Occupational performance emerges from the interaction of persons and their environment.
- Experimentation with various strategies leads to optimal solutions to motor problems.
- Recovery is variable because patient factors and environmental contexts are unique.
- Behavioral changes reflect attempts to compensate and to achieve task performance.

specific tasks, the training of controllable muscle action, and control over the movement components of these tasks. The major assumptions about motor control underlying this approach are listed in Box 57-4. A four-step sequence is followed for skill acquisition (Carr & Shepherd, 1987):

1. Analysis of the task, including observation
2. Practice of missing components, including goal identification, instruction, practice, and feedback with some manual guidance
3. Practice of the task with the addition of reevaluation and encouraging of task flexibility
4. Targets transfer of training

Motor Control and Motor Learning

Motor control is "the ability to regulate or direct the mechanisms essential to movement" (Shumway-Cook & Woollacott, 2017, p. 3), and motor control

TABLE 57-6 Sample Evidence That Supports Interventions Used when Adopting the Task-Oriented Approach

Author/Year	Objective	Conclusion
Almhdawi (2011)	To evaluate the functional and the impairment effects of the Occupational Therapy Task-Oriented Approach on upper limb function via a randomized clinical trial using a crossover design	The results supported the approach as indicated by significant and clinically meaningful changes in the Canadian Occupational Performance Measure, the Motor Activity Log, and the time scale of the Wolf Motor Function Test. The author concluded that the approach is an effective upper extremity (UE) poststroke rehabilitation approach in improving the UE functional abilities.
Arya and colleagues (2012)	To evaluate the effectiveness of the meaningful task-specific training (MTST) on the upper extremity motor recovery during the subacute phase after a stroke	The MTST produced statistically significant and clinically relevant improvements in the upper extremity motor recovery of the patients who had a subacute stroke.
Nilsen and colleagues (2015)	To determine the effectiveness of interventions to improve occupational performance in people with motor impairments after stroke	Evidence suggests that repetitive task practice, constraint-induced or modified constraint-induced movement therapy can improve upper extremity function, balance and mobility, and/or activity and participation. Commonalities among several of the effective interventions include the use of goal-directed, individualized tasks that promote frequent repetitions of task-related or task-specific movements.
Rensink and colleagues (2009)	To examine the effectiveness of task-oriented training after stroke via a systematic review	"Studies of task-related training showed benefits for functional outcome compared with traditional therapies. Active use of task-oriented training with stroke survivors will lead to improvements in functional outcomes and overall health-related quality of life" (p. 737). The authors recommended "creating opportunities to practise meaningful functional tasks outside of regular therapy sessions" (p. 737).
S. L. Wolf and colleagues (2010)	To compare functional improvements between stroke participants randomized to receive constraint-induced movement therapy (CI therapy) within 3–9 mo (early group) to participants randomized on recruitment to receive the identical intervention 15–21 mo after stroke (delayed group)	CI therapy can be delivered to eligible patients 3–9 mo or 15–21 mo after stroke. Both groups achieved approximately the same level of significant arm motor function 24 mo after enrollment.

BOX 57-3   EVALUATION PROCEDURES AND INTERVENTIONS BASED ON THE OCCUPATIONAL THERAPY TASK-ORIENTED APPROACH

Occupational Therapy Task-Oriented Approach Evaluation Framework

There are five main areas to assess using this approach.

1. Role performance (social participation)

Roles: worker, student, volunteer, home maintainer, hobbyist/amateur, participant in organizations, friend, family member, caregiver, religious participant, other

- Identify past roles and whether they can be maintained or need to be changed.
- Determine how future roles will be balanced.

2. Occupational performance tasks (areas of occupation)

- Activities of daily living: bathing, feeding, bowel and bladder management, dressing, functional mobility, and personal hygiene and grooming
- Instrumental activities of daily living: home management, meal preparation and cleanup, care of others and pets, community mobility, shopping, financial management, and safety procedures
- Work and/or education: employment seeking, job performance, volunteer exploration and participation, retirement activities, and formal and informal educational participation
- Play/leisure: exploration and participation
- Rest and sleep: preparation and participation

3. Task selection and analysis

- What client factors, performance skills and patterns, and/or contexts and activity demands limit or enhance occupational performance?

4. Person (client factors; performance skills and patterns)

- Cognitive: orientation, attention span, memory, problem solving, sequencing, calculations, learning, and generalization

- Psychosocial: interests, coping skills, self-concept, interpersonal skills, self-expression, time management, and emotional regulation and self-control
- Sensorimotor: strength, endurance, range of motion, sensory functions and pain, perceptual function, and postural control

5. Environment (context and activity demands)

- Physical: objects, tools, devices, furniture, plants, animals, and built and natural environment
- Socioeconomic: social supports: family, friends, caregivers, social groups, and community and financial resources
- Cultural: customs, beliefs, activity patterns, behavior standards, and societal expectations

Intervention Principles

- Interventions are occupation-based and client-focused.
- Keep clients active during treatment.
- Use natural objects and environments.
- Help patients adjust to role and task performance limitations.
- Create an environment that uses the common challenges of everyday life.
- Practice functional tasks or close simulations to find effective and efficient strategies for performance.
- Provide opportunities for practice outside of therapy time.
- Structure practice of the task to promote motor learning.
- Minimize ineffective and inefficient movement patterns.
- Remediate a client factor (impairment) if it is the critical control parameter.
- Adapt the environment, modify the task, use assistive technology, and/or reduce the effects of gravity.
- For persons with poor control of movement, constrain the degrees of freedom.
- For persons who do not use returned function in their involved extremities, use constraint-induced movement therapy (CI therapy).

theories "describe viewpoints regarding how movement is controlled" (Shumway-Cook & Woollacott, 2017, p. 7). In contrast, **motor learning** is defined as "a set of processes associated with practice or experience leading to relatively permanent changes in the capability for skilled movement" (Schmidt & Lee, 2011, p. 327). Thus, motor learning theories describe the processes involved in motor skill acquisition, retention, and generalization. Motor learning is a key component of many of the earlier described intervention approaches. Over the years, various *motor control* and *motor learning* theories have been proposed, each with its own merit. These theories are summarized in Table 57-7.

See Table 57-8 for a summary of motor learning principles that have evolved from these theories and Table 57-9 for examples of evidence that support the use of motor learning principles in clinical populations.

As our clients are learning or relearning skills, they must first acquire the skill (acquisition phase). This occurs during initial instruction on and practice of a skill or task. This usually occurs in the initial occupational therapy sessions. Following acquisition, the client must retain the skill (retention phase); this refers to *persistence of performance*. This occurs after the initial practice period, and the client is asked to demonstrate how he or she performs the newly

BOX 57-4   ASSUMPTIONS UNDERLYING THE MOTOR RELEARNING APPROACH

- In regaining motor control, learning is required. This learning follows the same principles and factors as those incurred in normal learning. Therefore, practice, receiving feedback, and understanding the goal are essential for treatment.
- Motor control is exercised in both anticipatory and ongoing modes.
- Sensory input is related to motor output and helps to modulate action.
- Control of a specific task can be effectively regained by practice of that specific motor task in various contexts.
- Conscious practice of tasks builds up awareness of the ability to elicit motor control activity.
- Progression of practice is from conscious awareness to practice at a more automatic level in order to ensure that a skill is learned.
- Cognitive function is emphasized. If the client is to learn, then the environment must encourage the learning process.

- When clients can perform a task effectively and efficiently without thinking about it in a variety of contexts, learning has occurred.
- Contemporary theories of motor control emphasize distributed control rather than a top–down or bottom–up approach. Therefore, in the Motor Relearning Program, recovery is directed to relearning control through many systems.
- The client is defined as an active participant in the treatment process. The major goal in rehabilitation is to relearn effective strategies for performing functional activities.
- The role of the therapist is to prevent the use of inefficient strategies by the client.
- The program addresses seven categories of functional daily activities: upper limb function, orofacial function, sitting up over the side of the bed, balanced sitting, standing up and sitting down, balanced standing, and walking.

---

acquired skill. Clients must then be able to transfer their performance (transfer phase). *Transfer of learning* refers to the gain in capability for performance in one task as a result of practice on another task. The individual can use the skill in a new context. Our clients can generalize the strategies learned in the therapy setting and use them in real-life situations (Sabari, 2016; Schmidt & Lee, 2011) (Figure 57-3).

Sabari (2016) summarized the literature about skill acquisition and therapeutic interventions that promote generalization of learning. These concepts can be categorized into three major groups: type of feedback, development of underlying strategies, and practice conditions (Figure 57-4).

An Overview of Motor Development

Motor development is a process during which a person acquires skills and movement patterns. Malina (2004) has described motor development as

a continuous process of modification that involves the interaction of several factors:

1. Neuromuscular maturation;
2. The physical growth and behavioral characteristics of the child;
3. The tempo of physical growth, biological maturation, and behavioral development;
4. The residual effects of prior movement experiences;
5. The new movement experiences. (p. 50)

Although many consider motor development a process specific to children, it is in fact a lifelong process that should be considered from a life course perspective. Typical developmental changes that occur in infancy and childhood are considered positive when milestones are met and new skills are acquired. Maximum performance may be reached in adolescence and adulthood. As the aging process continues, there comes a decline in performance with loss of speed, accuracy, and precision of movement. That being said, "a progression to regression" of skills description of motor development may not be completely accurate. Older adults have the potential to acquire quite intricate new motor skills as well. Think of older adults in your life who have mastered new leisure activities such as knitting, paddle boarding, or ballroom dancing (Figure 57-5).

Although neurodevelopment follows a predictable course, it is important to understand that intrinsic and extrinsic forces produce individual variation, making each child's developmental path unique. Intrinsic influences include genetically determined attributes (e.g., physical characteristics, temperament) as well as the child's overall state of wellness. Extrinsic influences during infancy and childhood originate primarily from the family. Parent and sibling personalities, the nurturing methods used

TABLE 57-7 Summary of Motor Control and Motor Learning Theories

Theory	Key Components of Theory
Motor Control Theories[a] (Shumway-Cook & Woollacott, 2017)	
Reflex Theory	• Stimulus–response view of motor control • Complex patterns of movement are the result of combining individual reflexes.
Hierarchical Theory	• Top–down organizational control of movement with higher levels always exerting full control over lower levels.
Motor Programming Theory	• *Central motor program* contains the "rules" for generating an action. • Program can be activated by sensory input or by central processes.
System Theory	• Describes the body as a *mechanical system* that is subject to both external (e.g., gravity) and internal forces (e.g., inertial forces) • *Self-organization*: movement emerges from an interaction of multiple systems—no need for "higher centers" or "central motor program." • *Nonlinearity*: motor output is not proportional to input—variability expected and needed in the system. • *Control parameters*: a variable that regulates a change in behavior (e.g., velocity may be considered the control parameter that shifts the action of walking to running) • *Attractor states*: preferred patterns of movements that are highly stable • *Attractor wells*: the degree of flexibility to change an attractor state: *shallow well*—unstable pattern that is easy to change; *deep well*—stable pattern that is difficult to change
Ecological Theory	• Motor control evolved so that animals can cope with their environment: *perception–action coupling* • Gibson's theory of affordances—perception of environmental factors that are critical to the task
Motor Learning Theories (Shumway-Cook & Woollacott, 2017)	
Schmidt Schema Theory	• Draws heavily on *motor programming theory* of motor control • Emphasis on open loop control processes and the development of the *generalized motor program* (GMP), which contains the "*rules*" for creating the pattern of muscle activity needed to perform the movement • After a movement is made, there are four elements available for short-term memory storage: (1) initial movement conditions, (2) parameters used in the GMP, (3) outcome of the movement (knowledge of results), and (4) sensory consequences of the movement (knowledge of performance). This information is stored as two schemas: *recall schema* (motor) and *recognition schema* (sensory). • Recall schema is used to select a specific set of responses and the response schema is used to evaluate the responses. • *Learning* occurs as a result of the updating of the two schemas each time a movement is attempted, and it is augmented by the amount of practice and variability of practice.
Ecological Theory	• Draws heavily on *systems* and *ecological theories* of motor control • During practice, there is a search for *optimal strategy* to solve the task problem—search for most salient perceptual cues and optimal motor response. • Learning occurs as a performer searches for the optimal solution; this process strengthens perception–action coupling and is augmented by helping the learner understand the nature of the perceptual/motor workspace, identifying the natural search strategies employed by the learner, and using augmented feedback to aid the search for the optimal solution.
Fitts and Posner Three-Stage Model	• *Cognitive stage*: learner is figuring out what is to be done; determining appropriate strategies to complete the task. Effective strategies are maintained and ineffective ones are discarded. Performance is variable, but improvements are large. High cognitive demands are placed on the learner. The therapist uses instructions, models, feedback, etc., to assist in learning the task at hand. • *Associative stage*: learner has determined the best strategy for the task and is now refining it. Performance is less variable and improvements are slower. Cognitive demands decrease. • *Autonomous stage*: skill is performed automatically requiring little attention.
Bernstien Three-Stage Model	• Draws heavily on the *systems theory* of motor control and solving the *degrees of freedom* problem • *Stage 1*: reduction in the number of degrees of freedom that must be controlled—learner will constrain the degrees of freedom and develop an *effective strategy* for task performance, but the *strategy is not energy efficient or flexible*. • *Stage 2*: release of additional degrees of freedom and muscle synergies are used across multiple joints resulting in *well-coordinated movement* that is more efficient and flexible • *Stage 3*: release of all the degrees of freedom needed for task performance; performer has *learned to exploit external and internal forces* acting on the system to produce the most coordinated and efficient movement pattern.
Gentile Two-Stage Model	• *Initial stage*: learner develops an understanding of the task and generates a movement pattern that enables some degree of success; key element of this stage is learning to discriminating between *regulatory features* (characteristic of environment that determine movement requirements) and *non-regulatory features* in the environment; high cognitive load • *Later stage* (a.k.a. *fixation/diversification*): learner is refining the movement so that it can be performed to meet the demands of any situation, and so that it is performed consistently and efficiently. • *Closed tasks*: environmental conditions are stable and little variability is needed—*fixation*. • *Open tasks*: environmental conditions are changing requiring multiple movement patterns—*diversification*.

[a]No single theory accounts for all of the experimental evidence to date.

TABLE 57-8	Summary of Motor Learning Principles/Considerations

Principles/Considerations	Examples
Classification of tasks to be learned: Learning is contingent on the type of task that is being learned.	
• Discrete tasks: Tasks with a recognizable beginning and end.	Kick a ball, push a button
• Continuous tasks: There is no recognizable beginning and end. Tasks are performed until they are arbitrarily stopped.	Jogging, driving, swimming
• Serial tasks: Comprised a series of movements linked together to make a "whole."	Play an instrument, dressing, light a fireplace
• Closed tasks: Performed in a predictable and stable environment. Movements can be planned in advance.	Oral care, signing a check, bowling
• Open tasks: Performed in a constantly changing environment that may be unpredictable.	Driving in traffic, catching an insect, soccer
• Variable motionless tasks: Involve interacting with a stable and predictable environment, but specific features of the environment are likely to vary between performance trials.	Performance of ADL outside of the usual home environment
• Consistent motion tasks: An individual must deal with environmental conditions that are in motion during activity performance; the motion is consistent and predictable between trials.	Stepping onto an escalator, assembly line work, retrieving luggage from an airport baggage carousel
Practice conditions: The law of practice refers to performance changing linearly with the amount of time spent in practice.	
• Massed practice: Rest time is much less than practice time.	Constraint-induced movement therapy
• Distributed practice: Practice time is equal to or less than rest time.	Practice sessions of a tub transfer are spaced to include rest breaks.
• Blocked practice: Repetitive practice of the same task, uninterrupted by practice of other tasks	Practicing moving from sit to stand multiple times in a row. Practice sequence of tasks "A," "B," and "C": AAAAABBBBBBBCCCCC.
• Random or variable practice: Tasks being practiced are ordered randomly. Attempt multiple tasks or variations of a task before mastering any one of the tasks.	Practice transferring to multiple surfaces (couch, toilet, bench, chair, stool, car) in one occupational therapy session. Practice sequence of tasks "A," "B," and "C": ACBACABCCBACABCACABBACCACB.
• Whole practice: The task is practiced in its entirety and not broken into parts.	Practicing dressing.
• Part practice: The task is broken down into its parts for separate practice.	Don/doff shirt.
Feedback: A key feature of practice is the information the learners receive about their attempts to learn a skill.	
• Inherent (intrinsic) feedback: Feedback normally received while performing a task.	Knowing you made an error as you spill water when trying to pour from a pitcher to a cup
• Augmented feedback: Information about task performance that is supplemental to inherent feedback.	A therapist provides feedback related to task performance: "You need to lock your wheelchair brakes."
• Concurrent feedback: Given during task performance.	While practicing reaching, the therapist says, "Don't hike your shoulder."
• Terminal feedback: Given after task performance.	After practice of reaching, the therapist says, "You didn't open your hand wide enough."
• Immediate feedback: Given immediately after performance.	Right after an attempt at a tub transfer, the therapist says, "That was perfect."
• Delayed feedback: Feedback is delayed by some amount of time.	The occupational therapist says, "You did better this morning but keep checking your brakes."
• Knowledge of results (KR): Feedback given after task performance about the outcome.	The occupational therapist says, "Your shirt is on backwards" or "You dropped the cup."
• Knowledge of performance (KP): Feedback given after task about the nature of performance.	The occupational therapist says, "Next time, dress your right arm first" or "Your elbow was bent."

ADL, activities of daily living.

Data from Schmidt, R. A., & Lee, T. D. (2011). *Motor control and learning: A behavioral emphasis* (5th ed.). Champaign, IL: Human Kinetics; Sabari, J. (2016). Activity-based interventions in stroke rehabilitation. In G. Gillen (Ed.), *Stroke rehabilitation: A function-based approach* (4th ed., pp. 79–95). St. Louis, MO: Elsevier; and Zwicker, J. G., & Harris, S. R. (2009). A reflection on motor learning theory in pediatric occupational therapy practice. *Canadian Journal of Occupational Therapy, 76,* 29–37.

| TABLE 57-9 | Sample Evidence That Supports Motor Learning–Based Interventions |

Author/Year	Objective	Conclusion
Bar-Haim and colleagues (2010)	To evaluate effectiveness of motor learning coaching on retention and transfer of gross motor function in children with cerebral palsy	In higher functioning children with cerebral palsy, the motor learning coaching treatment resulted in significantly greater retention of gross motor function and transfer of mobility performance to unstructured environments than neurodevelopmental treatment.
Nilsen and colleagues (2015)	To determine the effectiveness of interventions to improve occupational performance in people with motor impairments after stroke	Evidence suggests that mental practice, virtual reality, mirror therapy, and action observation can improve upper-extremity function, balance and mobility, and/or activity and participation.
Ste-Marie, Clark, Findlay, and Latimer (2004)	To examine whether introducing high levels of **contextual interference** is useful in handwriting skill acquisition	Overall, the results showed that the random practice schedule leads to enhanced retention and transfer performance of handwriting skill acquisition.
Subramanian, Massie, Malcolm, and Levin (2010)	To determine if the provision of extrinsic feedback results in improved motor learning in the upper limb poststroke	The author's systematic review "found strong evidence supporting the provision of explicit feedback for implicit motor learning in the upper limb of stroke survivors." The results suggest that "stroke survivors are able to use explicit feedback and preserve motor learning abilities despite having underlying upper limb motor control deficits. An important consideration is that the ability to use explicit feedback applies to both the less- and more-affected sides" (p. 121).
Timmermans and colleagues (2010)	To investigate the influence of each task-oriented arm training component on the functional outcome, that is, skill or activity level	There was no correlation between the number of task-oriented training components used in a study and the treatment effect size. "Distributed practice" and "feedback" were associated with the largest postintervention effect sizes. "Random practice" and "use of clear functional goals" were associated with the largest follow-up effect sizes.

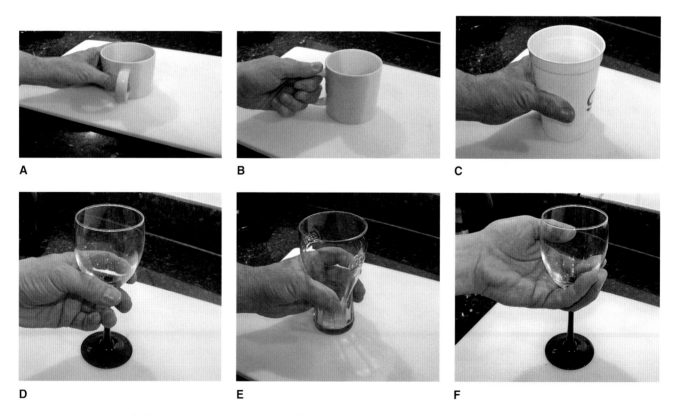

A   B   C

D   E   F

FIGURE 57-3 Variability in practice promotes both generalization and learning.

Feedback/instructions	Strategy	Practice conditions
• Capacity to generate intrinsic feedback • Low extrinsic KR feedback • Ballpark instructions about desired kinematics • Instructions to focus on activity demands	A foundational set of guidelines that guide action in a variety of situations	• Variable • Random • High contextual interference • Match with task category of the functional goal • Naturalistic setting • Self-selected practice challenges

Generalization of learning

FIGURE 57-4 Factors that contribute to generalization of learning. *KR*, knowledge of results. (Reprinted with permission from Sabari, J. [2016]. Activity-based interventions in stroke rehabilitation. In G. Gillen [Ed.], *Stroke rehabilitation a function-based approach* [3rd ed., pp. 80991. St. Louis, MO: Mosby.)

by caregivers, the cultural environment, and the family's socioeconomic status with its effect on resources of time and money all play a role in the development of children. Developmental theory has, itself, developed as clinicians have tried to grapple with which influence is more predominant (Gerber, Wilks, & Erdie-Lalena, 2010, p. 267).

Although there is a typical order of motor development that is commonly discussed and described (Table 57-10), it is important to remember that individuals may achieve their developmental milestones in various orders, may skip a milestone step, may achieve them within different time periods (Figure 57-6), etc.

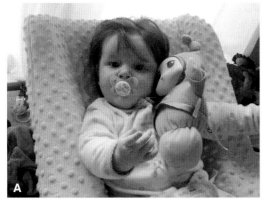
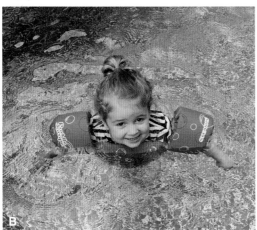
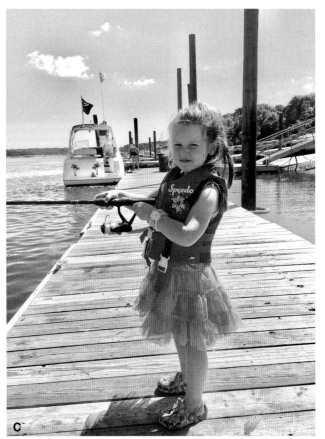

FIGURE 57-5 Development of motor control.

TABLE 57-10 Examples of Developmental Motor Milestones

Age	Gross Motor	Fine Motor
1 mo	Chin up in prone position. Turns head in supine position.	Keeps hands fisted near face.
2 mo	Can hold head up and begins to push up when lying prone. Makes smoother movements with arms and legs.	Hands not fisted 50% of the time. Retains rattle if placed in hand. Holds hands together.
4 mo	Holds head steady, unsupported. Pushes down on legs when feet are on a hard surface. May be able to roll over from prone to supine. Brings hands to mouth. When lying on stomach, pushes up to elbows.	Hands held predominately open. Clutches at clothes. Reaches persistently. Can hold a toy and shake it and swing at dangling toys.
6 mo	Rolls over in both directions (front to back, back to front). Begins to sit without support. When standing, supports weight on legs and might bounce. Rocks back and forth, sometimes crawling backward before moving forward.	Transfers hand to hand. Rakes pellet. Takes a second cube in hand and holds on to first. Reaches with one hand.
9 mo	Stands, holding on. Can get into sitting position. Sits without support. Pulls to stand. Crawls.	Radial-digital grasp of cube. Bangs two cubes together.
1 y	Gets to a sitting position without help. Pulls up to stand, walks holding on to furniture ("cruising"). May take a few steps without holding on. May stand alone.	Scribbles after demonstration. Fine pincer grasp of pellet. Holds crayon. Attempts tower of two cubes.
18 mo	Walks alone. May walk up steps and run. Pulls toys while walking. Can help undress himself or herself.	Drinks from a cup. Eats with a spoon. Makes a four cube tower. Crudely imitates vertical stroke.
2 y	Stands on tiptoes. Kicks a ball. Begins to run. Climbs onto and down from furniture without help. Walks up and down stairs holding on. Throws ball overhand. Makes or copies straight lines and circles.	Makes a single-line "train" of cubes. Imitates circle. Imitates horizontal line.
3 y	Climbs well. Runs easily. Pedals a tricycle. Walks up and down stairs, one foot on each step.	Copies circle. Begins to cut awkwardly with scissors. Strings small beads well. Imitates bridge of cubes.
4 y	Hops and stands on one foot up to 2 s. Catches a bounced ball most of the time. Pours liquid.	Cuts food with supervision and mashes own food. Copies square. Ties single knot. Cuts 5-in circle. Uses tongs to transfer. Writes part of first name.
5 y	Stands on one foot for 10 s or longer. Hops; may be able to skip. Can do a somersault. Can use the toilet on his or her own. Swings and climbs.	Uses a fork and spoon and sometimes a table knife. Copies triangle. Puts paper clip on paper. Can use clothespins to transfer small objects. Cuts with scissors. Writes first name. Builds stairs from model.

Data from Centers for Disease Control and Prevention. (2017). *Learn the signs. Act early.* Retrieved from http://www.cdc.gov/ncbddd/actearly/index .html and Gerber, R. J., Wilks, T., & Erdie-Lalena, C. (2010). Developmental milestones: Motor development. *Pediatrics in Review, 31,* 267–277.

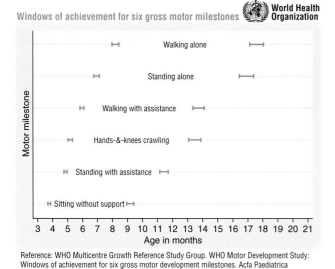

Reference: WHO Multicentre Growth Reference Study Group. WHO Motor Development Study: Windows of achievement for six gross motor development milestones. Acfa Paediatrica Supplement 2006;450:86-95.

FIGURE 57-6 Windows of achievement for six gross motor milestones.

For example, Gerber et al. (2010) note that crawling is not a prerequisite to walking; pulling to stand is the skill infants must develop before they take their first steps.

It is of critical importance that therapists and parents are aware of the warning signs that indicate delays in motor development. Gerber et al. (2010) discuss three key "red flags":

1. Lack of steady head control at 4 months while sitting
2. Inability to sit by 9 months
3. Inability to walk by 18 months

As part of their "Act Early" initiative, the Centers for Disease Control and Prevention (2017) has provided a summary of behaviors that may be indicative of delays in motor development (Table 57-11).

As will be discussed next, there are various standardized tools that occupational therapists can use to monitor motor development.

Evaluation and Assessment of Motor Function

Many tools and procedures are available to document our client's level of motor function. These include developmental assessments, neurological screening methods, self-report measures, assessments of postural control, assessments of limb function, and assessments performed

TABLE 57-11	Delays in Motor Development
Age	**Examples of Signs of Potential Delay in Motor Development**
2 mo	Doesn't bring hands to mouth. Can't hold head up when pushing up when prone.
4 mo	Can't hold head steady. Doesn't bring things to mouth. Doesn't push down with legs when feet are placed on a hard surface. Has trouble moving one or both eyes in all directions.
6 mo	Doesn't try to get objects that are in reach. Has difficulty getting things to mouth. Doesn't roll over in either direction. Seems very stiff with tight muscles (increased tone). Seems very floppy like a rag doll (low tone).
9 mo	Doesn't bear weight on legs with support. Doesn't sit with help. Doesn't transfer toys from one hand to the other.
1 y	Doesn't crawl. Can't stand when supported. Doesn't learn gestures like waving or shaking head. Doesn't point to things. Loses skills he or she once had.
18 mo	Doesn't point to show things to others. Can't walk. Doesn't know what familiar things are for. Doesn't copy others. Loses skills he or she once had.
2 y	Doesn't know what to do with common things like a brush, phone, fork, or spoon. Doesn't copy actions and words. Doesn't walk steadily. Loses skills he or she once had.
3 y	Falls down a lot. Has trouble with stairs. Drools or has very unclear speech. Can't work simple toys (such as peg boards, simple puzzles, turning handle). Loses skills he or she once had.
4 y	Can't jump in place. Has trouble scribbling. Loses skills he or she once had.
5 y	Doesn't draw pictures. Can't brush teeth, wash and dry hands, or get undressed without help. Loses skills he or she once had.

Data from Centers for Disease Control and Prevention. (2017). *Learn the signs. Act early.* Retrieved from http://www.cdc.gov/ncbddd/actearly/index.html.

in natural contexts. The following paragraphs and Table 57-12 gives examples of each.

Developmental Assessments

These tools are used to assess the development and capability of functional skills in children. The assessments in this category consist of screening instruments,

TABLE 57-12	Standardized Assessments of Motor Function

Assessment	Areas of Occupation			Client Factors		
	Activity	Participation	Quality of Life	Body Structures and Functions	Values, Beliefs, and Spirituality	Performance Skills
ABILHAND Questionnaire and ABILHAND-Kids	X					
Action Research Arm Test				X		X
Activities-Specific Balance Confidence (ABC) Scale	X					
Arm Motor Ability Test	X					
Ashworth Scale				X		
Assessment of Motor and Process Skills	X	X				X
Assisting Hand Assessment	X					X
Bayley Scales of Infant Development, Second Edition				X		X
Bennett Hand-Tool Dexterity Test	X					X
Berg Balance Scale (adult and pediatric versions)	X			X		X
Box and Block Test				X		X
Bruininks-Oseretsky Test of Motor Proficiency, Second Edition	X			X		
Chedoke Arm and Hand Activity Inventory	X					
Clinical Observations of Motor and Postural Skills-Second Edition				X		
Complete Minnesota Dexterity Test				X		X
Crawford Small Parts Dexterity Test				X		X
Disabilities of the Arm, Shoulder, and Hand (DASH)	X	X				
Dynamometry				X		
Erhardt Developmental Prehension Assessment	X					X
Evaluation Tool of Children's Handwriting	X					X
FirstSTEp: Screening Test for Evaluating Preschoolers	X			X		
Frenchay Arm Test	X					X
Fugl-Meyer Sensorimotor Assessment				X		
Functional Reach Test and Multi-Directional Functional Reach Test						X
Goniometry				X		
Grooved Pegboard Test				X		
Gross Motor Function Measure	X					
Infant Neurological International Battery (INFANIB)				X		
Jebsen-Taylor Test of Hand Function	X					
Manual Ability Measure	X					
Manual Muscle Testing				X		
Melbourne Assessment of Unilateral Upper Limb Function	X					X
Miller Assessment for Preschoolers	X			X		
Miller Function and Participation Scales	X	X		X		
Minnesota Rate of Manipulation Test				X		
Modified Ashworth Scale				X		
Motor Activity Log (adult and pediatric versions)	X					
Motor Assessment Scale	X			X		X
Motricity Index			X			X
Movement Assessment Battery for Children (Movement ABC)				X		X

TABLE 57-12   ## Standardized Assessments of Motor Function *(continued)*

Assessment	Areas of Occupation			Client Factors		
	Activity	Participation	Quality of Life	Body Structures and Functions	Values, Beliefs, and Spirituality	Performance Skills
National Institutes of Health (NIH) Pain Scales				X		
Nine-Hole Peg Test				X		
O'Connor Dexterity Tests				X		X
Peabody Developmental Motor Scales, Second Edition				X		X
Pediatric Evaluation of Disability Inventory	X	X				
Postural Assessment Scale for Stroke Patients	X					
Purdue Pegboard Test				X		
Quick Neurological Screening Test (QNST)				X		
Reflex Testing				X		
Rivermead Motor Assessment	X			X		
Sensory Organization Test				X		
School Assessment of Motor and Process Skills	X	X				X
School Function Assessment	X	X				
Tardieu Scale				X		
Tinetti Balance and Gait Evaluation	X			X		
Timed Up and Go Test	X					
Trunk Control Test	X					
Upper Extremity Performance Test for the Elderly or *Test d'Evaluation des Membres Supérieurs de Personnes Agées* (TEMPA)	X					
Wolf Motor Function Test	X					X

See Appendix II for more details related to these tools.

criterion-referenced measures, rating scales, and norm-referenced measures, some of which can be completed by a teacher or caregiver or through direct interaction with the child being assessed.

The Pediatric Evaluation of Disability Inventory (PEDI) examines three categories: self-care, mobility, and social function. This test is designed for use with children, ages 6 months to 7 years, who have various disabilities that result in functional problems. The PEDI is standardized on a normative sample; therefore, one can calculate both standard and scaled performance scores. The PEDI provides resources to assess a child on three different measurement scales. The first, Functional Skills, establishes the ability of the child to complete discrete functional skills. The Caregiver Assessment scale determines the amount of assistance that the child is provided with during complex functional skills. And finally, the Modification Skills scale assesses what types of modifications the child requires to complete and support his or her function. The scales can be used concurrently or independently of one another depending on the domain of interest for each individual child (Haley, Coster, Ludlow, Haltiwanger, & Andrellos, 1992).

The Peabody Gross Motor Scale (2nd edition) compares fine and gross motor skills to normally developing children ages 0 to 5 years. There are 170 activities that are assessed regarding reflexes, stationary skills, locomotion, object manipulation, grasping, and visual motor integration. Results from these subtests are used to generate the three composite scores: Gross Motor Quotient, Fine Motor Quotient, and Total Motor Quotient. Scores are presented as percentiles, standard scores, and age equivalents. Norms, based on a nationally representative sample of more than 2,000 children, are stratified by age (Folio & Fewell, 2000).

The Erhardt Developmental Prehension Assessment was designed to measure components of arm and hand development in children of all ages and cognitive levels who have cerebral palsy, multiple disabilities, and developmental delays. It can be used to identify intervention needs, modify programs with ongoing assessment, and provide accountability with retesting. Three hundred forty-one items are divided into three sections: (1) positional-reflexive: involuntary arm–hand patterns; (2) cognitively directed: voluntary movements of approach, grasp, manipulation, and release; and (3) prewriting skills: pencil grasp and drawing (Erhardt, 1994).

TABLE 57-13	Neurological Disorders and Their Stereotypical Coordination Patterns	

Category	Description	Test
Cerebellar Dysfunction		
Intention tremor	• Occurs during voluntary movement, is less apparent or absent during rest, and intensifies at the termination of the movement. • Evident in multiple sclerosis.	• Finger-to-finger test, finger-to-nose test. • May have trouble performing tasks that require accuracy and precision of limb placement (e.g., drinking from a cup or inserting a key in a lock).
Essential familial tremor	• Inherited as an autosomal-dominant trait, visible when client is carrying out a fine precision and accuracy task.	• Have the person reach for an item. Positive if tremors are present during the reach.
Adiadochokinesis	• Inability to perform rapid alternating movements (e.g., pronation/supination, elbow flexion/extension).	• Tests by counting how many cycles of alternating movements in 10-second time frame. Best to test unaffected/less affected side first and then compare performance to affected side.
Dysdiadochokinesia	• Decreased ability to perform rapid alternating movements smoothly.	• Supinate/pronate, flex/extend elbow, grasp/release hand, alternating bilateral tasks. Number of alternations within a time period and the differences between extremities are noted.
Dysmetria	• Inability to control muscle length results in overshooting when pointing to target objects. • Inability to estimate range of motion necessary to reach a target. Two types include hypermetria (overshoot) and hypometria (undershoot).	• Finger-to-finger or finger-to-nose tests.
Dyssynergia	• Movements are broken up into their component parts and appear jerky. Jerky movements are due to lack of synergy between agonist/antagonist. • Can cause problems in articulation and phonation.	• Alternating movement, finger-to-nose, finger-to-finger tests.
Ataxia	• Delayed initiation of movement responses, errors in range and force of movement, errors in rate and regularity of movement. Poor agonist/antagonist coordination, results in jerky, poorly controlled movements, poor postural stability.	• When reaching for object, shortest distance between the client and object is not a straight line.
Ataxic gait	• Unsteady, wide-based gait, tendency to veer or fall toward side of lesion. • Staggering, wide-based gait with reduced or no arm swing, uneven step length and tendency to fall.	• Observation of walking, turning quickly, walking toe to heel along straight line.
Rebound phenomenon of Holmes	• Lack of a check reflex. • Inability to stop a motion quickly to avoid striking something.	• Therapist releases resistance to client's elbow flexion unexpectedly; client's hand hits his or her own chest if unable to check motion.
Hypotonia	• Decreased muscle tone, decreased resistance to passive movement.	• Can observe clinically and perform a quick stretch.
Nystagmus	• Involuntary (oscillating) movement of eyes. Interferes with head control and balance. Can occur as result of vestibular system, brainstem, or cerebellar lesions.	• Can observe by having the person look at a fixed object. Is positive if the eyes make small rapid oscillations (tremor-like movements).
Dysarthria	• Explosive or slurred speech caused by incoordination of the speech mechanism. • Speech may vary in pitch, seem nasal or tremulous.	• Can observe if ability to articulate words due to the oral-motor and/or larynx musculature. This is a motor problem, not due to aphasia.
Posterior Column Dysfunction		
Ataxia	• Wide-based gait results from loss of proprioception, but client can self-correct using vision by watching their feet (compare with cerebellar dysfunction).	• Can observe in any part of the body. Is characterized by "large" tremors.
Romberg sign	• Inability to maintain standing balance with feet together and eyes closed.	• The test is the same as the definition.

TABLE 57-13	**Neurological Disorders and Their Stereotypical Coordination Patterns** *(continued)*	

Category	Description	Test
Basal Ganglia Dysfunction		
Athetoid movements	• Continuous, slow, wormlike, arrhythmic movements that primarily affect the distal portions of the extremities. Occur in the same patterns in the same subject, not present during sleep. Co-occurrence with athetosis = choreoathetosis.	• Therapist should note proximal or distal involvement extremities involved, pattern of motions, and which stimuli increase/decrease abnormal movements. Its occurrence can be documented through observation.
Dystonia	• A form of athetosis that causes twisting movements of the trunk and proximal muscles of the extremities, distorted postures, and torsion spasms. • Persistent posturing of the extremities (e.g., hyperextension or hyperflexion of the wrist and fingers) often with concurrent torsion of the spine and twisting of the trunk. Movements are often continuous and seen in conjunction with spasticity. Subtypes included segmental, generalized, focal, and multifocal.	• Its occurrence can be documented through observation.
Chorea	• Irregular, purposeless, involuntary, coarse, quick, jerky, and dysrhythmic movements of variable distribution. May occur in sleep.	• Its occurrence can be documented through observation.
Ballism	• A rare symptom produced by continuous, abrupt contraction of axial and proximal musculature of the extremity. Causes the limb to fly out suddenly. Occurs on one side (hemiballism) and is caused by lesions of the opposite subthalamic nucleus.	• Its occurrence can be documented through observation.
Resting tremors	• Stop at the initiation of voluntary movement, resume during holding phase of motor task (e.g., pill rolling tremor of Parkinsonism). • Occurs at rest and subsides when voluntary movement is attempted. Seen in Parkinson's disease.	• Have the person reach for an item. Positive if tremors are present before initiation of the reach but stop when the reach begins.
Bradykinesia	• Movement is very slow or even nonexistent, with accompanying rigidity.	• Ask the person to move; on attempting to move, the person's motions are extremely slow, if at all. Tone appears to be high.

Reprinted from Giuffrida, C. G., & Rice, M. S. (2008). Motor skills and occupational performance: Assessments and interventions. In E. B. Crepeau, E. S. Cohn, & B. A. B. Schell (Eds.), *Willard & Spackman's occupational therapy* (11th ed., pp. 658–680). Baltimore, MD: Lippincott Williams & Wilkins.

Neurological Screening Methods

Various procedures are used to document the presence of atypical motor performance and movements. These screening procedures related to motor function are outlined in Table 57-13.

Self-Report Measures

Several measures are available that allow clients to report their level of motor function. The Disabilities of the Arm, Shoulder, and Hand (DASH), as described in Case Study 57-2, is an example of this level of measurement that is typically used by therapists. The Motor Activity Log is also a self-report questionnaire (report by patient or family) related to actual use of the involved

upper extremity outside of structured therapy time. It uses a semistructured interview format. Quality of movement ("How well" scale) and amount of use ("How much" scale) are graded on a 6-point scale. At present, there are 30, 28, and 14 item versions of the tool. Sample items include hold book, use a towel, pick up a glass, write/type, steady myself, and etc. (Uswatte, Taub, Morris, Light, & Thompson, 2006; Uswatte, Taub, Morris, Vignolo, & McCulloch, 2005). The Pediatric Motor Activity Log is a structured interview intended to examine how often and how well a child uses his or her involved upper extremity in his or her natural environment outside the therapeutic setting. The child's primary caregiver is asked standardized questions about the amount of use of the child's involved arm and the quality of the child's movement during the functional activities specified in the instrument (e.g., point to a picture, turn pages in a book) (Uswatte et al., 2012; Wallen, Bundy, Pont, & Ziviani, 2009).

The 36-item Manual Ability Measure (MAM-36) is a Rasch-developed, self-report disability outcome measure. It contains 36 gender-neutral, commonly performed everyday hand tasks. The patient is asked to report the ease or difficulty of performing such items. It uses a 4-point rating scale, with 1 indicating *unable* ("I am unable to do the task all by myself"), 2 indicating *very hard* ("It is very hard for me to do the task and I usually ask others to do it for me unless no one is around"), 3 indicating *a little hard* ("I usually do the task myself, although it takes longer or more effort now than before"), and 4 indicating *easy* ("I can do the task without any problem"). Item examples include zip a jacket, turn a key, and take things/cards out of a wallet. The MAM-36 can be accessed (Chen, Kasven, Karpatkin, & Sylvester, 2007). A lookup table from raw scores to converted 0 to 100 Rasch measures is available (Chen & Bode, 2009).

The ABILHAND questionnaire asks clients to use a 3-point scale (0 = *impossible*, 1 = *difficult*, 2 = *easy*) to rate how difficult it would be to complete 23 bimanual activities (e.g., hammering a nail, wrapping a gift, thread a needle, file nails, cut meat, peel onions, open jar) (Penta, Tesio, Arnould, Zancan, & Thonnard, 2001). The ABILHAND-Kids is comprised of 21 mainly bimanual daily activities. The difficulty experienced by the child to perform the required tasks is scored on a 3-point ordinal scale (Arnould, Penta, Renders, & Thonnard, 2004).

Assessments of Postural Control

Various postural control measures are available based on client status. Examples follow. The Trunk Control Test examines four functional movements: roll from supine to the weak side, roll from supine to the strong side, sitting up from supine, and sitting on the edge of the bed for 30 seconds (feet off the ground). Each task is scored as follows: 0, unable to perform with assistance; 12, able to perform but in an abnormal manner; and 25, able to complete movement normally. The range of scores is 0 to 100 (Collin & Wade, 1990).

The Postural Assessment Scale for Stroke Patients contains 12 4-point items graded from 0 to 3 (Benaim, Pérennou, Villy, Rousseaux, & Pelissier, 1999). Higher scores indicate better performance. Items include sitting without support, standing with and without support, standing on the nonparetic leg, standing on the paretic leg, supine to affected side, supine to unaffected side, supine to sit, sit to supine, sit to stand, stand to sit, and standing and picking up a pencil from the floor.

The Berg Balance Scale (BBS) was developed to measure balance among older people with impairment in balance function by assessing the performance of functional tasks. It is a valid instrument used for evaluation of the effectiveness of interventions and for quantitative

descriptions of function in clinical practice and research. It includes 14 items such as sit to stand, transfers, and retrieving an object from the floor (Berg, Wood-Dauphinee, Williams, & Gayton, 1989).

Assessments of Limb Function

Assessments of limb function are usually composed of items that are best described as simulated ADL or movements that mimic those required to engage in daily activities. The Fugl-Meyer Upper Extremity subscale (FM-UE) (Fugl-Meyer, Jääskö, Leyman, Olsson, & Steglind, 1975) has been used to reliably measure change in the upper extremity in a variety of stroke motor intervention trials (Bushnell et al., 2015). It assesses movement of the upper extremity via the performance of 33 tasks. Performance of each task is rated on a 3-point ordinal scale from 0 (cannot perform) to 2 (performs fully). Velozo and Woodbury (2011) developed a key form recovery map for use with the FM-UE. Recording patient responses to the standardized items on the form allows the therapist to quickly see what items the patient is struggling with. This information can then be used to tailor upper extremity training to the specific needs of the patient. In addition, minimally clinically important differences (MCID) have been established for the FM-UE for stroke survivors across various stages of recovery (Arya, Verma, & Garg, 2011; S. J. Page, Fulk, & Boyne, 2012; Shelton, Volpe, & Reding, 2001).

The Arm Motor Ability Test has been used to determine the effectiveness of interventions and includes 13 unilateral and bilateral tasks. Sample items include tying a shoe, opening a jar, wiping up spilled water, using a light switch, using utensils, and drinking. The therapist times task performance and rates movement quality on a 6-point scale. The test is appropriate for evaluating motor skills in high-level clients with active wrist and finger extension (Kopp et al., 1997).

The Wolf Motor Function Test has been used to document the outcomes related to CI therapy and other interventions and includes various tasks such as basic reaching tasks (e.g., lifting arm from lap to table, extending elbow with and without a weight attached) as well as more functional activities that involve fine motor control (e.g., picking up a pencil, turning a key in a lock). All tasks but one are unilateral and appropriate for both the dominant and nondominant arm. Because many tasks do not require distal control, it is appropriate for people with a more involved upper extremity. The therapist times task performance and qualitatively grades movement (S. L. Wolf et al., 2001).

The Jebsen-Taylor Test of Hand Function includes the performance of seven test activities: writing a short sentence, turning over index cards, picking up small objects and placing them in a container, stacking checkers, simulating eating, moving empty large cans, and moving weighted large cans during timed trials. The original paper is based on data collected from 360 normal subjects and patients, including patients with hemiparesis resulting from a stroke. The mean times and standard deviations for normal subjects (with their dominant and nondominant hand) are published in the paper. The test is standardized and reliable and does not have a practice effect. Therapists must be aware that some of the tasks are simulated activities, and some tasks cannot be considered ADL tasks (Jebsen, Taylor, Trieschmann, Trotter, & Howard, 1969).

The Melbourne Assessment of Unilateral Upper Limb Function measures quality of unilateral upper limb movement in children with neurological conditions aged 5 to 15 years. The assessment is designed to provide general information about levels of ability/disability rather than specific diagnostic information. The tool consists of 16 items that involve reach, grasp, release, and manipulation. A child's performance is recorded on videotape for subsequent scoring. Each test item has an individual scoring system so that various aspects of the movement can be considered such as range of movement, accuracy of reach and placement, fluency of reach and release, and developmental level of grasp. The test items and scoring system aim to be representative of the most important components of upper limb function (Randall, Johnson, & Reddihough, 1999).

The Assisting Hand Assessment (Krumlinde-Sundholm & Eliasson, 2003) examines how effectively a child's hemiplegic hand is actually used in bimanual activities. The spontaneous use is evaluated during a semistructured play session with toys requiring bimanual handling. The items that are scored include general use, arm use, grasp and release, fine motor adjustments, and coordination and pace. All items are scored from 0 (*does not do*) to 4 (*effective use*).

Assessments Performed in Natural Contexts

There are a limited number of tools that measure motor skills in a naturalistic context. The Assessment of Motor and Process Skills (AMPS) and School AMPS are two examples. The therapist evaluates motor and process skills within the context of basic ADL and instrumental ADL. The quality of the person's ADL performance is assessed by rating the effort, efficiency, safety, and independence of 16 ADL motor and 20 ADL process skill items while the person is doing chosen, familiar, and life-relevant ADL tasks. There are more than 100 tasks to choose from, thus promoting a client-centered approach to assessment. Evaluated motor skills include skills related to body position (stabilizes, aligns, positions), obtaining and holding objects (reaches, bends, grips, manipulates, coordinates), moving self and objects (moves, lifts, walks, transports, calibrates, flows), and sustaining performance (endures, paces) (Fisher & Jones, 2014). See Chapter 26 for more details.

The School AMPS is a naturalistic, observation-based assessment that is administered in the natural classroom setting while the student performs schoolwork tasks assigned by the teacher. No disruption of the normal classroom routine occurs during its administration. The School AMPS helps an occupational therapist answer the following questions:

- What is the quality of this student's schoolwork task performance?
- How does the quality of this student's task performance compare with that of his or her same-age peers?
- Which school motor and/or school process skills are most impacting this student's occupational performance in the classroom?
- What intervention strategies will have the most impact on this student's performance in the classroom?
- Was there a change in this student's quality of schoolwork task performance since the last School AMPS evaluation?

The School AMPS examines the transaction between a student, a schoolwork task, and a classroom environment and evaluates the quality of the student's schoolwork task performance, measured at the level of complex activity and participation, not body functions (Fingerhut, Madill, Darrah, Hodge, & Warren, 2002; Fisher, Bryze, & Atchison, 2000; Fisher, Bryze, Hume, & Griswold, 2007).

Examples of Evidence-Based Interventions

Since the last edition of this book, there has been a substantial increase and focus on testing interventions for those with limitations in motor function. When using evidence to guide practice, it is important to reflect on the type of outcome measures used as described previously. One should consider the following questions when interpreting evidence:

1. Is the population that was tested similar to my client?
2. Has the intervention been shown to be effective related to measures of activity and participation (areas of occupation) in addition to impairment measures (measurement of client factors)?

Although interventions have been discussed throughout this chapter (orthoses, strengthening, physical agent modalities, task-oriented training, motor learning techniques such as mental practice, etc.), the following paragraphs provide the reader with further examples of contemporary evidence-based interventions.

Task-Oriented Training Interventions

Constraint-Induced Movement Therapy

The term **learned nonuse** was coined by Taub et al. (1993). The learned nonuse phenomenon originally was identified in animal studies and later was applied to chronic stroke survivors and others. Taub et al. hypothesized that the nonuse or limited use of an affected upper extremity in human beings after a neurologic event results from a phenomenon of learned suppression. CI therapy is an intervention developed to reverse the effects of learned nonuse. This intervention has become the gold standard to improve daily use of neurologically impaired upper extremities in both the adult population (stroke) and children with cerebral palsy who meet the motor inclusion criteria. Refer back to Case Study 57-2

for a description of pediatric applications. Boxes 57-5 and 57-6 provide more details related to how to implement this intervention.

Repetitive Task Practice/ Task-Specific Training

Repetitive Task Practice and Task-Specific Training (Arya et al., 2012; Waddell et al., 2014) are terms used to describe training approaches that include the performance of goal-directed activities that require high-intensity repetition of task-related or task-specific movements. They are frequently used to remediate upper and lower limb dysfunction in persons who have sustained neurological injuries, such as stroke (French et al., 2010).

Bilateral Arm Training/ Bimanual Training

Bilateral arm training has emerged as a promising intervention to improve arm function after stroke. Stoykov, Lewis, and Corcos (2009) summarized that the technique:

- Has been shown to be efficacious not only with stroke survivors who are only mildly impaired but also those with moderate and severe motor impairments

---

BOX 57-5   SUMMARY OF CONSTRAINT-INDUCED MOVEMENT THERAPY

- Use to counteract learned nonuse. Hypothesized causes of learned nonuse include therapeutic interventions implemented during the acute period of neurologic suppression after stroke or other neurologic event, an early focus on adaptations to meet functional goals, negative reinforcement experienced by the patients as they unsuccessfully attempt to use the affected limb, and positive reinforcement experienced by using the less involved hand and/or use of successful adaptations.
- Motor inclusion criteria. Control of the wrist and digits is necessary to engage in this type of intervention. Current and past protocols have used the following inclusion criteria: 20 degrees of extension of the wrist and 10 degrees of extension of each finger; 10 degrees extension of the wrist, 10 degrees abduction of the thumb, and 10 degrees extension of any two other digits; or able to lift a wash rag off a table using any type of prehension and then release it.
- Main therapeutic factor. Massed practice and shaping of the affected limb during repetitive functional activities appears to be the therapeutic change agent.

- Activity choices and therapist's interventions. Select tasks that address the motor deficits of the individual patient; assist the patient to carry out parts of a movement sequence if they are incapable of completing the movement on their own at first, providing explicit verbal feedback and verbal reward for small improvements in task performance, use modeling and prompting of task performance, use tasks that are of interest and motivating to the patient, ignore regression of function, and use tasks that can be quantified related to improvements.
- Outcome measures. The Motor Activity Log (actual use outside of structured therapy or "real-world use"), Arm Motor Ability Test, Wolf Motor Function Test, and the Action Research Arm Test have been used to document outcomes.
- Cortical reorganization. Constraint-induced movement therapy is the first rehabilitation intervention that has been demonstrated to induce changes in the cortical representation of the affected upper limb.

BOX 57-6 CONSTRAINT-INDUCED MOVEMENT THERAPY PROTOCOLS

Traditional Protocol

The EXCITE trial defined the intervention as: "Participants in the intervention group were taught to apply an instrumented protective safety mitt and encouraged to wear it on their less-impaired upper extremity for a goal of 90% of their waking hours over a 2-week period, including 2 weekends, for a total of 14 days. On each weekday, participants received shaping (adaptive task practice) and standard task training of the paretic limb for up to 6 hours per day. The former is based on the principles of behavioral training that can also be described in terms of motor learning derived from adaptive or part-task practice. Standard task practice is less structured (i.e., repetition of tasks is not conducted as individual trials of discrete movements); it involves functional activities performed continuously for a period of 15 to 20 minutes (e.g., eating, writing)" (Wolf et al., 2006).

Modified Protocols

Page, Levine, Leonard, Szaflarski, and Kissela (2008) described the following protocol consisting of 2 components. "The first component consisted of half-hour, one-on-one sessions of more affected arm therapy occurring 3 days per week during a 10-week period. This component included shaping in which operant conditioning was applied in such a way that subjects received positive verbal encouragement to more fully perform selected motor skills with their more affected arm. Shaping was applied with 2 or 3 upper-limb activities (e.g., writing, using a fork) chosen by the subjects with help from their therapist. In the second component of the mCIT intervention, during the same 10-week period, subjects' less affected arms were restrained every weekday for 5 hours identified as a time of frequent arm use, as identified by the subjects with assistance from the therapist. Their arms were restrained using a cotton hemi-sling, while their hands were placed in mesh, polystyrene-filled mitts with Velcro straps around the wrist."

Lin, Wu, Liu, Chen, and Hsu (2009) defined their protocol as "restraint of the less affected limb combined with intensive training of the affected limb for 2 hours daily 5 days per week for 3 weeks and restraint of the less affected hand for 5 hours outside of the rehabilitation training."

Sterr and colleagues (2002) defined their protocol as 14 consecutive days; constraint of unaffected hand for a target of 90% of waking hours, with 3 hours of shaping training with the affected hand per day. To note, they concluded that: "The 3-hour CIMT training schedule significantly improved motor function in chronic hemiparesis, but it was less effective than the 6-hour training schedule."

CIMT, constraint-induced movement therapy; EXCITE, Extremity Constraint-Induced Therapy Evaluation; mCIT, modified constraint-induced movement therapy.
Reprinted with permission from Gillen, G. (Ed.). (2016). Upper extremity function and management. In *Stroke rehabilitation: A function-based approach* (4th ed., pp. 424–485). St. Louis, MO: Elsevier.

- Protocols reported in the literature are diverse and can be categorized as categories: repetitive reaching with and fixed, isolated muscle repetitive training, and whole arm functioning
- May be combined with rhythmic auditory cueing and is coupled with repetitive reaching with hand-fixed activities

Examples of treatment activities include opening and closing two identical drawers, wiping a table with both arms using both arms symmetrically, bilateral reaching and placing objects, etc. Stoykov et al. (2009) compare the effectiveness of bilateral training with unilateral training for individuals with moderate upper limb hemiparesis. They concluded that both bilateral and unilateral training are efficacious for moderately impaired chronic stroke survivors and that bilateral training may be more advantageous for proximal arm function.

Gordon, Schneider, Chinnan, and Charles (2007) developed a bimanual intervention, Hand-Arm Bimanual Intensive Therapy (HABIT), which is specifically aimed at upper extremity impairments in congenital hemiplegia. The authors describe HABIT as

- A form of functional training
- Focusing on intensive practice

- Focused on improving coordination of the two hands using structured task practice embedded in bimanual play and functional activities
- Using principles of motor learning (practice specificity, types of practice, feedback)
- Using principles of neuroplasticity (practice-induced brain changes arising from repetition, increasing movement complexity, motivation, and reward)

The authors conducted a randomized trial to examine the effectiveness of this intervention. Children were engaged in play and functional activities that provided structured bimanual practice 6 hours per day for 10 days. They concluded that for this carefully selected subgroup of children with hemiplegic cerebral palsy, HABIT appears to be efficacious in improving bimanual hand use.

Of note is that Gordon et al. (2011) conducted a randomized trial comparing CI therapy and HABIT that maintains the intensity of practice associated with CI therapy but where children are engaged in functional bimanual tasks. The children received 90 hours of CI therapy or HABIT. They concluded that both CI therapy and bimanual training lead to similar improvements in hand function. They note that a potential benefit of bimanual training is that participants may improve more on self-determined goals.

Use of Cognitive Strategies to Improve Performance

The use of cognitive strategies is emerging as an effective intervention for children with *developmental coordination disorder* (DCD). This term is used to describe children with motor skill impairment who experience problems with the performance of various motor-based tasks, such as catching/throwing a ball, playing on a jungle gym, dressing, feeding, riding a bicycle, and handwriting.

Hyland and Polatajko (2012) describe the Cognitive Orientation to daily Occupational Performance (CO-OP) approach as a multifaceted top–down approach that combines elements from various disciplines such as behavioral and cognitive psychology, health, and human movement science. They further describe it as a verbally based individualized approach that focuses on teaching children to use self-talk and problem-solving strategies to solve their motor-based performance problems. The children choose their own goals, and problem-solving strategies are used to identify and address performance issues.

The CO-OP therapist guides the child in the learning of a global problem solving strategy and the discovery of domain specific cognitive strategies that improve motor performance. The global cognitive strategy is a problem-solving strategy taken from the work of Meichenbaum (1977), which provides a structure within which the child can learn to talk through occupational performance problems. Domain specific strategies (DSS) are used in specific tasks or situations to help achieve specific occupational performance goals (Sangster, Beninger, Polatajko, & Mandich, 2005, p. 70).

Sangster et al. (2005) argue that it is the development of skills in using cognitive strategies that has supported the reported improvement in occupational performance. They state that the CO-OP approach has two hypotheses: (1) that children with DCD do not independently generate effective cognitive strategies to solve performance problems and (2) that cognitive strategy use changes with the CO-OP intervention. Examples of strategies that are employed include verbal guidance, feeling the movement, attention to doing, practice, etc. Indeed, the authors' pilot work has support the use of a cognitively based approach such as CO-OP in assisting children with DCD in developing cognitive strategies when solving occupational performance problems.

Cognitive strategies have also been used to enhance motor skill acquisition poststroke. McEwen, Huijbregts, Ryan, and Polatajko (2009) examined the literature and concluded that

- Research investigating cognitive strategies to improve motor skill acquisition in people with stroke is emerging in the peer-reviewed literature.
- The cognitive strategies studied included three general strategies (those that are applicable in many different situations) and four task-specific strategies: motor imagery (MI) (also known as *mental practice*); Feldenkrais Attention to Movement; goal setting with assigned, high, specific goals and preparatory arousal.
- None of the strategies have been studied exhaustively.
- There is strong evidence that general strategy training combined with MI during practice improves and maintains performance in both trained and untrained ADL compared to traditional functional training in people in the early rehabilitation phase after a stroke.
- There is strong evidence that general strategy training improves performance in untrained ADL compared to traditional occupational therapy in people with apraxia as a result of stroke (see Chapter 58 for more information on apraxia).

Wolf et al. (2016) examined the impact of combining CO-OP with task-specific training on cognition and upper-extremity function in subacute stroke survivors. They found that the group receiving CO-OP had measurable improvements over usual care on all of the included outcome measures related to arm function, cognition, and participation.

Additionally, combining repetitive task practice with cognitive strategies such as mirror therapy (MT) and action observation (AO) have also been shown to be effective at improving upper extremity function in adults poststroke (Nilsen et al., 2015) and children with cerebral palsy (Buccino et al., 2012; Park, Baek, & Park, 2016; Sgandurra et al., 2013).

Postural Control/ Balance Interventions

Adding purpose to daily occupations has been shown to improve standing balance (Hsieh, Nelson, Smith, & Peterson, 1996) in those with hemiplegia. Hsieh et al. (1996) examined three types of standing balance interventions. They hypothesized that the two added-purpose occupations would elicit more exercise repetitions than a rote exercise. They examined a dynamic standing balance exercise that involved bending down, reaching, standing up, and extending the arm. One condition of added purpose involved the use of materials (small balls and target); a second added-purpose condition involved the subjects' imagination of the small balls. The third condition was the rote exercise without added purpose. The subjects did significantly more exercise repetitions in the added-materials condition and in the imagery-based condition than in the rote exercise condition. The authors concluded that this study demonstrates how added purpose can enhance motor performance in persons with hemiplegia. They demonstrated that purpose may be effectively added to an exercise through the use of materials or imagery.

The concept of using reaching activities has also been shown to be effective in retraining seated postural control (Dean & Shepherd, 1997). As technology continued to be more and more common place, games such as the Wii are being used in rehabilitation settings to address multiple impairments including improving balance (Gil-Gómez, Lloréns, Alcañiz, & Colomer, 2011).

Physical Agent Modalities

Electrical stimulation and electromyography (EMG)-triggered electrical stimulation are being used for those with impaired motor function. Electrical stimulation has been used in poststroke upper extremity rehabilitation for many years. Potential uses have included reduction of shoulder subluxation, reduction of pain, improved motor control, and increasing use of the involved extremity. In general, the effects of electrical stimulation have been the most consistent at improving limb impairments such as range of motion and reducing pain. The effects on function and ADL have received less attention and have been inconsistent. Electrical stimulation can be triggered by voluntary movement or nontriggered. The EMG-triggered stimulation detects underlying muscle activity when it reaches a threshold level prior to providing the stimulation. The stroke survivor must voluntarily activate the correct muscles prior to the stimulation facilitating the motor response. This type of stimulation assures that the intervention is not passive in nature. Triggered electrical stimulation may be more effective than nontriggered electrical stimulation in facilitating upper extremity motor recovery following stroke (de Kroon, Ijzerman, Chae, Lankhorst, & Zilvold, 2005). This intervention has been shown to be effective at improving wrist extension, a key movement to be considered a candidate for some task-oriented approaches such as CI therapy. Findings from systematic reviews and meta-analyses have been inconsistent. However, there is enough evidence to continue to integrate these modalities with other task-oriented training activities. Further investigation is warranted (see Figure 57-7A–B).

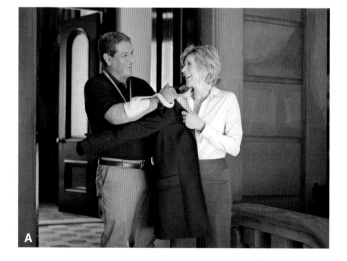
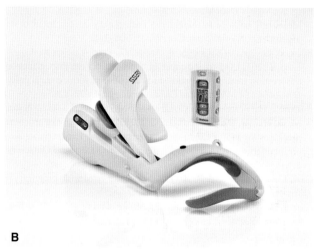

FIGURE 57-7 A neuroprosthesis (H200 Wireless) used to support occupational performance. This device combines a wrist/hand orthosis (to provide stabilization) with integrated surface electrodes to activate muscles of a paralyzed forearm and hand. (Photo courtesy of Bioness, Inc., Valencia, California.)

Conclusion

Motor function and control is a multifaceted concept that relies on multiple body structures and functions, performance skills, etc. Successful rehabilitation is based on the adoption of a clear therapeutic approach or approaches; the interpretation of standardized, valid, and reliable assessments; and the adoption of evidence-based interventions. Remember, the goal of motor-based interventions is to improve overall occupational performance and *not* only reduce motor impairment.

 Visit thePoint to watch a video about motor function.

REFERENCES

Almhdawi, K. (2011). *Effects of occupational therapy task-oriented approach in upper extremity post-stroke rehabilitation* (Unpublished doctoral dissertation). University of Minnesota, Twin Cities.

Arnould, C., Penta, M., Renders, A., & Thonnard, J. L. (2004). ABILHAND-Kids: A measure of manual ability in children with cerebral palsy. *Neurology, 63*, 1045–1052.

Arya, K. N., Verma, R., & Garg, R. K. (2011). Estimating the minimal clinically important difference of an upper extremity recovery measure in subacute stroke patients. *Topics in Stroke Rehabilitation, 18*(Suppl. 1), 599–610.

Arya, K. N., Verma, R., Garg, R. K., Sharma, V. P., Agarwal, M., & Aggarwal, G. G. (2012). Meaningful task-specific training (MTST) for stroke rehabilitation: A randomized controlled trial. *Topics in Stroke Rehabilitation, 19*, 193–211.

Bar-Haim, S., Harries, N., Nammourah, I., Oraibi, S., Malhees, W., Loeppky, J., . . . Lahat, E. (2010). Effectiveness of motor learning coaching in children with cerebral palsy: a randomized controlled trial. *Clinical Rehabilitation, 24*, 1009–1020.

Benaim, C., Pérennou, D. A., Villy, J., Rousseaux, M., & Pelissier, J. Y. (1999). Validation of a standardized assessment of postural control in stroke patients: The Postural Assessment Scale for Stroke Patients (PASS). *Stroke, 30*, 1862–1868.

Berg, K., Wood-Dauphinee, S., Williams, J. I., & Gayton, D. (1989). Measuring balance in the elderly: Preliminary development of an instrument. *Physiotherapy Canada, 41*, 304–311.

Buccino, G., Arisi, D., Gough, P., Aprile, D., Ferri, C., Serotti, L., . . . Fazzi, E. (2012). Improving upper limb motor functions through action observation treatment: A pilot study in children with cerebral palsy. *Developmental Medicine and Child Neurology, 54*, 822–828.

Bushnell, C., Bettger, J. P., Cockroft, K. M., Cramer, S. C., Edelen, M. O., Hanley, D., . . . Yenokyan, G. (2015). Chronic stroke outcome measures for motor function intervention trials: Expert panel recommendations. *Circulation: Cardiovascular Quality and Outcomes, 8*, S163–S169. doi:10.1161/CIRCOUTCOMES.115.002098

Carr, J. H., & Shepherd, R. B. (1987). *A motor relearning program for stroke* (2nd ed.). Rockville, MD: Aspen.

Carr, J. H., & Shepherd, R. B. (2003). *Stroke rehabilitation: Guidelines for exercise and training to optimize motor skill*. New York, NY: Butterworth-Heinemann.

Centers for Disease Control and Prevention. (2017). *Learn the signs. Act early*. Retrieved from http://www.cdc.gov/ncbddd/actearly/index.html

Chen, C. C., & Bode, R. K. (2009, April). *MAM-36: Psychometric properties and differential item functioning in neurologic and orthopedic patients*. Paper presented at the AOTA 88th Annual Conference, Long Beach, CA.

Chen, C. C., Kasven, N., Karpatkin, H. I., & Sylvester, A. (2007). Hand strength and perceived manual ability among patients with multiple sclerosis. *Archives of Physical Medicine and Rehabilitation, 88*, 794–797.

Collin, C., & Wade, D. (1990). Assessing motor impairment after stroke: A pilot reliability study. *Journal of Neurology, Neurosurgery, and Psychiatry, 53*, 576–579.

Collins, E. L. (1922). Occupational therapy for the homebound. *Archives of Occupational Therapy, 1*, 33–40.

Dean, C. M., & Shepherd, R. B. (1997). Task-related training improves performance of seated reaching tasks after stroke. A randomized controlled trial. *Stroke, 28*, 722–728.

de Kroon, J., Ijzerman, M., Chae, J., Lankhorst, G., & Zilvold, G. (2005). Relation between stimulation characteristics and clinical outcome in studies using electrical stimulation to improve motor control of the upper extremity in stroke. *Journal of Rehabilitation Medicine, 37*, 65–74.

Egan, M. Y., & Brousseau, L. (2007). Splinting for osteoarthritis of the carpometacarpal joint: A review of the evidence. *American Journal of Occupational Therapy, 61*, 70–78.

Erhardt, R. (1994). *Developmental hand dysfunction: Theory, assessment, and treatment* (2nd ed.). Austin, TX: Pro-Ed.

Fingerhut, P., Madill, H., Darrah, J., Hodge, M., & Warren, S. (2002). Classroom-based assessment: Validation for the school AMPS. *American Journal of Occupational Therapy, 56*, 210–213.

Fisher, A. G., Bryze, K., & Atchison, B. T. (2000). Naturalistic assessment of functional performance in school settings: Reliability and validity of the School AMPS. *Journal of Outcome Measurement, 4*, 504–522.

Fisher, A. G., Bryze, K., Hume, V., & Griswold, L. A. (2007). *School AMPS: School Version of the Assessment of Motor and Process Skills* (2nd ed.). Fort Collins, CO: Three Star Press.

Fisher, A. G., & Jones, K. B. (2014). *Assessment of Motor and Process Skills: User manual* (8th ed.). Fort Collins, CO: Three Star Press.

Folio, M. R., & Fewell, R. R. (2000). *Peabody Developmental Motor Scales: Examiner's Manual* (2nd ed.). Austin, TX: Pro-ED.

French, B., Thomas, L., Leathley, M., Sutton, C., McAdam, J., Forster, A., . . . Watkins, C. (2010). Does repetitive task training improve functional activity after stroke? A Cochrane systematic review and meta-analysis. *Journal of Rehabilitation Medicine, 42*, 9–14.

Fugl-Meyer, A. R., Jääskö, L., Leyman, I., Olsson, S., & Steglind, S. (1975). The post-stroke hemiplegic patient. 1. A method for evaluation of physical performance. *Scandinavian Journal of Rehabilitation Medicine, 7*, 13–31.

Gerber, R. J., Wilks, T., & Erdie-Lalena, C. (2010). Developmental milestones: Motor development. *Pediatrics in Review, 31*, 267–277.

Gil-Gómez, J. A., Lloréns, R., Alcañiz, M., & Colomer, C. (2011). Effectiveness of a Wii balance board-based system (eBaViR) for balance rehabilitation: A pilot randomized clinical trial in patients with acquired brain injury. *Journal of Neuroengineering and Rehabilitation, 8*, 30.

Gillen, G. (2013). A fork in the road: An occupational hazard? (Eleanor Clarke Slagle Lecture). *American Journal of Occupational Therapy, 67*, 641–652.

Gillen, G. (Ed.). (2016). Upper extremity function and management. In *Stroke rehabilitation: A function-based approach* (4th ed., pp. 658–680). St. Louis, MO: Elsevier.

Giuffrida, C. G., & Rice, M. S. (2008). Motor skills and occupational performance: Assessments and interventions. In E. B. Crepeau, E. S. Cohn, & B. A. B. Schell (Eds.), *Willard & Spackman's occupational therapy* (11th ed. pp. 424–485). Baltimore, MD: Lippincott Williams & Wilkins.

Gordon, A. M., Charles, J., & Wolf, S. L. (2005). Methods of constraint–induced movement therapy for children with hemiplegic cerebral palsy: Development of a child-friendly intervention for improving upper-extremity function. *Archives of Physical Medicine and Rehabilitation, 86,* 837–844.

Gordon, A. M., Hung, Y. C., Brandao, M., Ferre, C. L., Kuo, H. C., Friel, K., . . . Charles, J. R. (2011). Bimanual training and constraint-induced movement therapy in children with hemiplegic cerebral palsy: A randomized trial. *Neurorehabilitation and Neural Repair, 25,* 692–702.

Gordon, A. M., Schneider, J. A., Chinnan, A., & Charles, J. R. (2007). Efficacy of hand-arm bimanual intensive therapy (HABIT) for children with hemiplegic cerebral palsy: A randomized control trial. *Developmental Medicine and Child Neurology, 49,* 830–838.

Haley, S., Coster, W., Ludlow, L., Haltiwanger, J., & Andrellos, J. (1992). *Pediatric Evaluation of Disability Inventory (PEDI).* Boston, MA: Trustees of Boston University.

Harris, J. E., & Eng, J. J. (2010). Strength training improves upper limb function in individuals with stroke. *Stroke, 41,* 136–140.

Hsieh, C. L., Nelson, D. L., Smith, D. A., & Peterson, C. Q. (1996). A comparison of performance in added-purpose occupations and rote exercise for dynamic standing balance in persons with hemiplegia. *American Journal of Occupational Therapy, 50,* 10–16.

Hurkmans, E., van der Giesen, F. J., Vliet Vlieland, T. P., Schoones, J., & Van den Ende, E. C. (2009). Dynamic exercise programs (aerobic capacity and/or muscle strength training) in patients with rheumatoid arthritis. *Cochrane Database of Systematic Reviews,* CD006853. doi:10.1002/14651858.CD006853.pub2

Hyland, M., & Polatajko, H. J. (2012). Enabling children with developmental coordination disorder to self-regulate through the use of dynamic performance analysis: Evidence from the CO-OP approach. *Human Movement Science, 31,* 987–998. doi:10.1016/j.humov.2011.09.003

Jebsen, R. H., Taylor, N., Trieschmann, R. B., Trotter, M. J., & Howard, L. A. (1969). An objective and standardized test of hand function. *Archives of Physical Medicine and Rehabilitation, 50,* 311–319.

Kopp, B., Kunkel, A., Flor, H., Platz, T., Rose, U., Mauritz, K. H., . . . Taub, E. (1997). The Arm Motor Ability Test: Reliability, validity, and sensitivity to change of an instrument for assessing disabilities in activities of daily living. *Archives of Physical Medicine and Rehabilitation, 78,* 615–620.

Krumlinde-Sundholm, L., & Eliasson, A. C. (2003). Development of the Assisting Hand Assessment, a rash-built measure intended for children with unilateral upper limb impairments. *Scandinavian Journal of Occupational Therapy, 10,* 16–26.

Lin, K. C., Wu, C. Y., Liu, J. S., Chen, Y. T., & Hsu, C. J. (2009). Constraint-induced therapy versus dose-matched control intervention to improve motor ability, basic/extended daily functions, and quality of life in stroke. *Neurorehabilitation and Neural Repair, 23,* 160–165.

Malina, R. (2004). Motor development during infancy and early childhood: Overview and suggested directions for research. *International Journal of Sport and Health Science, 2,* 50–66.

Mathiowetz, V. (2016). Task-oriented approach to stroke rehabilitation. In G. Gillen (Ed.), *Stroke rehabilitation a function-based approach* (4th ed., pp. 59–78). St. Louis, MO: Elsevier.

Mathiowetz, V., & Bass-Haugen, J. (1994). Motor behavior research: Implications for therapeutic approaches to central nervous system dysfunction. *American Journal of Occupational Therapy, 48,* 733–745.

Mathiowetz, V., & Bass-Haugen, J. (2008). Assessing abilities and capacities: Motor behavior. In M. V. Radomski & C. A. Trombly-Latham (Eds.), *Occupational therapy for physical dysfunction* (6th ed., pp. 186–211). Baltimore, MD: Lippincott Williams & Wilkins.

McEwen, S. E., Huijbregts, M. P., Ryan, J. D., & Polatajko, H. J. (2009). Cognitive strategy use to enhance motor skill acquisition poststroke: A critical review. *Brain Injury, 23,* 263–277.

Meichenbaum, D. (1977). *Cognitive-behaviour modification: An integrative approach.* New York, NY: Plenum Press.

Morris, D. M., Taub, E., & Mark, V. W. (2006). Constraint-induced movement therapy: Characterizing the intervention protocol. *Europa Medicophysica, 42*(3), 257–268.

Nilsen, D. M., Gillen, G., Geller, D., Hreha, K., Osei, E., & Saleem, G. T. (2015). Effectiveness of interventions to improve occupational performance of people with motor impairments after stroke: An evidence-based review. *American Journal of Occupational Therapy, 69,* 6901180030p1. doi:10.5014/ajot.2015.011965

Page, M. J., Massy-Westropp, N., O'Connor, D., & Pitt, V. (2012). Splinting for carpal tunnel syndrome. *Cochrane Database of Systematic Reviews,* CD010003. doi:10.1002/14651858.CD010003

Page, S. J., Fulk, G. D., & Boyne, P. (2012). Clinically important differences for the upper-extremity Fugl-Meyer scale in people with minimal to moderate impairment due to chronic stroke. *Physical Therapy, 92,* 791–798.

Page, S. J., Levine, P., Leonard, A., Szaflarski, J. P., & Kissela, B. M. (2008). Modified constraint-induced therapy in chronic stroke: Results of a single-blinded randomized controlled trial. *Physical Therapy, 88,* 333–340.

Park, E., Baek, S., & Park, S. (2016). Systematic review of the effects of mirror therapy in children with cerebral palsy. *Journal of Physical Therapy Science, 28,* 3227–3231.

Penta, M., Tesio, L., Arnould, C., Zancan, A., & Thonnard, J. L. (2001). The ABILHAND questionnaire as a measure of manual ability in chronic stroke patients: Rasch-based validation and relationship to upper limb impairment. *Stroke, 32,* 1627–1634.

Poole, J. L. (2008). Musculoskeletal factors. In E. B. Crepeau, E. S. Cohn, & B. A. B. Schell (Eds.), *Willard & Spackman's occupational therapy* (11th ed. pp. 658-680). Baltimore, MD: Lippincott Williams & Wilkins.

Randall, M., Johnson, L., & Reddihough, D. (1999). *The Melbourne Assessment of Unilateral Upper Limb Function: Test administration manual.* Melbourne, Australia: Royal Children's Hospital.

Rensink, M., Schuurmans, M., Lindeman, E., & Hafsteinsdóttir, T. (2009). Task-oriented training in rehabilitation after stroke: Systematic review. *Journal of Advanced Nursing, 65,* 737–754.

Sabari, J. (2016). Activity-based interventions in stroke rehabilitation. In G. Gillen (Ed.), *Stroke rehabilitation: A function-based approach* (4th ed., pp. 79–95). St. Louis, MO: Elsevier.

Sangster, C. A., Beninger, C., Polatajko, H. J., & Mandich, A. (2005). Cognitive strategy generation in children with developmental coordination disorder. *Canadian Journal of Occupational Therapy, 72,* 67–77.

Saunders, D. H, Sanderson, M., Hayes, S., Kilrane, M., Greig, C. A., Brazzelli, M., & Mead, G. E. (2016). Physical fitness training for stroke patients. *Cochrane Database of Systematic Reviews,* CD003316. doi:10.1002/14651858.CD003316.pub6

Schmidt, R. A., & Lee, T. D. (2011). *Motor control and learning: A behavioral emphasis* (5th ed.). Champaign, IL: Human Kinetics.

Sgandurra, G., Ferrari, A., Cossu, G., Guzzetta, A., Fogassi, L., & Cioni, G. (2013). Randomized trial of observation and execution of upper extremity actions versus action alone in children with unilateral cerebral palsy. *Neurorehabilitation and Neural Repair, 27,* 808–815.

Shelton, F., Volpe, B. T., & Reding, M. (2001). Motor impairment as a predictor of functional recovery and guide to rehabilitation treatment after stroke. *Neurorehabilitation and Neural Repair, 15,* 229–237.

Shumway-Cook, A., & Woollacott, M. (2017). *Motor control: Translating research into clinical practice* (5th ed.). Baltimore, MD: Lippincott Williams & Wilkins.

Ste-Marie, D. M., Clark, S. E., Findlay, L. C., & Latimer, A. E. (2004). High levels of contextual interference enhance handwriting skill acquisition. *Journal of Motor Behavior, 36,* 115–126.

Sterr, A., Elbert, T., Berthold, I., Kölbel, S., Rockstroh, B., & Taub, E. (2002). Longer versus shorter daily constraint-induced movement therapy of chronic hemiparesis: an exploratory study. *Archives of Physical Medicine and Rehabilitation, 83,* 1374–1377.

Stoykov, M. E., Lewis, G. N., & Corcos, D. M. (2009). Comparison of bilateral and unilateral training for upper extremity hemiparesis in stroke. *Neurorehabilitation and Neural Repair, 23,* 945–953.

Subramanian, S. K., Massie, C. L., Malcolm, M. P., & Levin, M. F. (2010). Does provision of extrinsic feedback result in improved motor learning in the upper limb poststroke? A systematic review of the evidence. *Neurorehabilitation and Neural Repair, 24,* 113–124.

Taub, E., Miller, N. E., Novack, T. A., Cook, E. W., III, Fleming, W. C., Nepomuceno, C. S., . . . Crago, J. E. (1993). Technique to improve chronic motor deficit after stroke. *Archives of Physical Medicine and Rehabilitation, 74,* 347–354.

Timmermans, A. A. A., Spooren, A. I. F., Kingma, H., & Seelen, H. A. M. (2010). Influence of task-oriented training content on skilled arm-hand performance in stroke: A systematic review. *Neurorehabilitation and Neural Repair, 24,* 858–870.

Uswatte, G., Taub, E., Griffin, M. A., Vogtle, L., Rowe, J., & Barman, J. (2012). The Pediatric Motor Activity Log-revised: Assessing real-world arm use in children with cerebral palsy. *Rehabilitation Psychology, 57,* 149–158.

Uswatte, G., Taub, E., Morris, D., Light, K., & Thompson, P. A. (2006). The Motor Activity Log-28: Assessing daily use of the hemiparetic arm after stroke. *Neurology, 67,* 1189–1194.

Uswatte, G., Taub, E., Morris, D., Vignolo, M., & McCulloch, K. (2005). Reliability and validity of the upper-extremity Motor Activity Log-14 for measuring real-world arm use. *Stroke, 36,* 2493.

Velozo, G. A., & Woodbury, M. L. (2011). Translating measurement findings into rehabilitation practice: An example using Fugl-Meyer Assessment-Upper Extremity with patients following stroke. *Journal of Rehabilitation Research and Development, 48,* 1211–1222. doi:10.1682/JRRD.2010.10.0203

Waddell, K. J., Birkenmeier, R. L., Moore, J. L., Hornby, T. G., & Lang, C. E. (2014). Feasibility of high-repetition, task-specific training for individuals with upper-extremity paresis. *American Journal of Occupational Therapy, 68,* 444–453.

Wallen, M., Bundy, A., Pont, K., & Ziviani, J. (2009). Psychometric properties of the Pediatric Motor Activity Log used for children with cerebral palsy. *Developmental Medicine and Child Neurology, 51,* 200–208.

Werner, R. A., Franzblau, A., & Gell, N. (2005). Randomized controlled trial of nocturnal splinting for active workers with symptoms of carpal tunnel syndrome. *Archives of Physical Medicine and Rehabilitation, 86,* 1–7.

Wolf, S. L., Catlin, P. A., Ellis, M., Archer, A. L., Morgan, B., & Piacentino, A. (2001). Assessing Wolf Motor Function Test as outcome measure for research in patients after stroke. *Stroke, 32,* 1635–1639.

Wolf, S. L., Thompson, P. A., Winstein, C. J., Miller, J. P., Blanton, S. R., Nichols-Larsen, D. S., . . . Sawaki, L. (2010). The EXCITE stroke trial: Comparing early and delayed constraint-induced movement therapy. *Stroke, 41,* 2309–2315.

Wolf, S. L., Winstein, C. J., Miller, J. P., Taub, E., Uswatte, G., Morris, D., . . . Nichols-Larsen, D. (2006). Effect of constraint-induced movement therapy on upper extremity function 3 to 9 months after stroke: The EXCITE randomized clinical trial. *JAMA, 296,* 2095–2104.

Wolf, T. J., Polatajko, H., Baum, C., Rios, J., Cirone, D., Doherty, M., & McEwen, S. (2016). Combined cognitive-strategy and task-specific training affects cognition and upper-extremity function in subacute stroke: An exploratory randomized controlled trial. *American Journal of Occupational Therapy, 70,* 7002290010p10. doi:10.5014/ajot.2016.017293

Zwicker, J. G., & Harris, S. R. (2009). A reflection on motor learning theory in pediatric occupational therapy practice. *Canadian Journal of Occupational Therapy, 76,* 29–37.

the**Point**® *For additional resources on the subjects discussed in this chapter, visit* http://thePoint.lww.com /Willard-Spackman13e. *See* **Appendix I, Resources and Evidence for Common Conditions Addressed in OT** *for more details on developmental coordination disorder, cerebral palsy, orthopedic injuries, and other diagnoses discussed in this chapter. See* **Appendix II, Table of Assessments** *for a comprehensive list of assessments and descriptions respectively.*

CHAPTER 58

Cognition, Perception, and Occupational Performance

Joan Pascale Toglia, Kathleen M. Golisz, Yael Goverover

LEARNING OBJECTIVES

After reading this chapter, you will be able to:

1. Define cognition and describe how cognitive impairments can limit performance of activities and decrease participation in meaningful occupations.
2. Discuss the role of occupational therapy practitioners in cognitive rehabilitation.
3. Describe the key characteristics and process of a comprehensive approach to evaluate cognition and perception.
4. Compare and contrast different models and theories of cognition.
5. Discuss the factors that need to be considered when choosing evaluation and intervention approaches, including the evidence that supports decisions.
6. Define specific cognitive and perceptual skills.
7. Identify appropriate assessment tools for specific cognitive impairments.
8. Discuss the different approaches for therapy to address specific cognitive impairments.

Introduction

"Thinking, remembering, reasoning, and making sense of the world around us are fundamental to carrying out everyday living activities" (Unsworth, 1999, p. 3). **Cognition** involves many interrelated processes, including the ability to perceive, organize, assimilate, and manipulate information to enable the person to process information, learn, and generalize (Salthouse, 2016).

Cognitive impairments can result from developmental or learning problems, brain injury or disease, psychiatric dysfunction, and/or socio-cultural conditions (American Occupational Therapy Association [AOTA], 2013). These impairments can significantly limit an individual's activity and restrict participation in meaningful occupations, potentially compromising his or her safety, health, and well-being. For example, a decreased ability to recognize potential hazards, anticipate consequences of actions and behaviors, follow safety precautions, and respond to emergencies can significantly interfere with independence and compromise health and well-being. Cognitive limitations can also diminish one's sense of competence, self-efficacy, and self-esteem, further compounding difficulties in adapting to the demands of everyday living.

The aim of occupational therapy (OT) intervention for people with cognitive-perceptual impairments is to decrease activity limitations, enhance participation in everyday activities, and help individuals gain the abilities they need to take control over their lives and develop healthy and satisfying ways of living. Although the ultimate goal of intervention with this population is clear and similar to other type of rehabilitation, there are different perspectives and rehabilitation approaches to accomplish the goal.

Overview of Models and Theories of Cognition

Models and theories of cognitive rehabilitation and recovery reflect different perspectives on learning and the ability to generalize information. Each model incorporates several approaches; however, they differ in the areas targeted for change or emphasized in intervention. For example, some models emphasize change in the task or environment (e.g., functional cognitive models), whereas others emphasize change in the person's skills (e.g., remedial). Evaluation and treatment guidelines reflect these different areas of focus. This section describes various models, theories, and intervention approaches to cognition as well as factors that are critical in the application of theory to the selection of intervention approaches and the methods for systematically integrating them.

Cognitive Functional Models: Functional Skill Training and Task or Environmental Adaptations

Cognitive functional models emphasize the ability to successfully perform everyday tasks and routines by building on the person's assets and/or residual skills. Activity limitations and participation restrictions are reduced by changing the task and environment or enhancing specific

CENTENNIAL NOTES

Evolution in Occupational Therapy Practice in Cognitive Rehabilitation

Cognitive rehabilitation first became a standard component of medical care around the time of World War I with the establishment of facilities to treat soldiers recovering from battle injuries, including brain injuries. As more soldiers with brain injuries survived, physicians advocated for a holistic approach, providing both cognitive and physical rehabilitation (Koehler, Wilhelm, & Shoulson, 2011; Parente & Stapleton, 1997). Although treatment was not labeled "cognitive rehabilitation," one might wonder whether some of the symptoms of injuries that were originally classified as "mental" injuries may actually have been descriptions of cognitive impairments.

Cognition has been identified as an area of OT practice since 1940 when the topic first appeared in OT literature (Abreu & Toglia, 1987). In the 1970s and 1980s, occupational therapists focused on perceptual functioning and sensory integration using a remediation approach. Neistadt (1987) was the first researcher in OT to compare both remedial and functional approaches to treating perceptual impairments and advocated for a functional approach. Occupational therapists began to draw on the work of neuropsychologists Diller (1976), Ben-Yishay (1978), and Prigatano (1986) to address cognitive dysfunction in adults with neurological impairments.

The mid to late 1980s saw a surge of interest and publications on cognitive rehabilitation in the *American Journal of Occupational Therapy*. Abreu and Toglia (1987) introduced a cognitive rehabilitation model for OT based on information processing and learning concepts, which included promoting cognitive strategies and self-monitoring skills; the environment; and body alignment, position, and movement patterns. Giles developed the neurofunctional approach in the 1980s and emphasized the value of task-specific training in individuals with chronic cognitive disabilities (Giles & Clark-Wilson, 1988). Allen (1987) developed a functional cognitive approach that identified levels of cognitive function in individuals with mental illness.

Over the past 30 to 40 years, OT practitioners have continued to provide cognitive rehabilitation to clients with various diagnoses across the lifespan and in populations beyond the acute neurological population. An emerging area of interest involves subtle neurological and functional signs that can lead to decline in cognition and a focus on prevention, health promotion, and early intervention (Toglia & Katz, 2018). Systematic reviews and practice guidelines (Brown, 2012; Preissner, 2014; Wheeler & Acord-Vira, 2016; Wolf & Nilsen, 2015) by occupational therapists and other health care professionals (Cicerone et al., 2011) have supported reimbursement for cognitive rehabilitation.

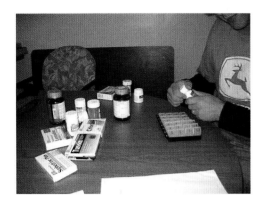

FIGURE 58-1 A pillbox organizer can be an important contextual cue to help those with memory impairments to safely self-administer medications.

task performance rather than remediating or restoring impaired skills (Figure 58-1). Common approaches used within cognitive functional models include the following:

- Adapting the environment
- Matching or prescribing activities appropriate to the person's level (Allen, 1985)
- Using task modifications and compensatory methods
- Providing caregiver education and training (Döpp et al., 2015; Gitlin et al., 2016)
- Using task-specific methods such as errorless learning (i.e., the person is prevented from making incorrect or inappropriate responses during the learning process), vanishing cues, and spaced retrieval (Giles, 2018)
- Employing everyday technologies such as mobile phones, iPads, or computers to support cognitive abilities (Gentry, 2018)

The effectiveness of these methods has been demonstrated in persons with schizophrenia (Kessler, Rhodes, & Giovannetti, 2015; Velligan et al., 2009), brain injury (Clark-Wilson, Giles, & Baxter, 2014), dementia (Bier et al., 2008; de Werd, Boelen, Rikkert, & Kessels, 2013), and autism (Ducharme & Ng, 2012).

It is important to acknowledge that functional methods can require different levels of learning, environmental supports, and awareness. For example, adaptations, task modifications, and/or technologies may be set up, implemented, and monitored by others or practiced repeatedly to encourage automatic learning. On the other hand, individuals can be taught methods to modify or adapt activities themselves. This latter approach requires higher levels of learning and is integrated with strategy approaches that are discussed later in this chapter.

The Cognitive Disability Model

Allen (1985) developed a Cognitive Disability Model (CDM), which provides guidelines for matching and

adapting the individual's functional cognitive capacities with activity demands and contexts. In this model, function is organized into six ordinal levels of global functional cognitive capacities ranging from normal (level 6) to profoundly disabled (level 1). Modes of performance within each level further qualify behavior variations and allow for more sensitive measurement of the person's global functional capacity. To obtain a comprehensive description of the CDM and Allen Cognitive Levels, refer to Allen (1985), McCraith and Earhart (2018), and Levy (2018).

Environmental Skill Building Program

Gitlin et al. (2016) and Gitlin, Winter, Dennis, Hodgson, and Hauck (2010a, 2010b) developed an environmental skill-building program (ESP) for persons with dementia and their caregivers that was influenced by the CDM and includes a system of matching environmental demands with the individual's capabilities. The ESP is a home-based, individually tailored, client-centered program implemented by occupational therapists. It includes collaboration with caregivers to identify concerns and strategies that are practiced within the home environment. Studies have found that ESP reduces the frequency of behavioral symptoms and functional dependence in clients with dementia, caregiver upset, and the need for assistance from others; in addition, it improves caregiver skill, efficacy, and mood (Gitlin et al., 2016; Gitlin, Winter, et al., 2010a, 2010b; Gitlin et al., 2009).

Cognitive Adaptation Training

Cognitive adaptation training is another approach that shares some similarities with the CDM. Cognitive adaptation training is described (Velligan et al., 2015) as an evidence-based strategy to improve functional performance by teaching people ways to modify their environment (e.g., signs, reminders, organizing the home environment). Velligan et al. (2006) collaborated with occupational therapists to create a systematic approach for the use of environmental supports and compensatory strategies for persons with schizophrenia. Velligan et al. found that cognitive adaptation training improved functional behaviors for patients with schizophrenia (Velligan et al., 2009; Velligan et al., 2006; Velligan et al., 2015). Persons with different cognitive behaviors (e.g., decreased initiation vs. disinhibition) were found to benefit from different types of adaptations (Velligan et al., 2009).

Adaptations and environmental supports should address the problems and needs identified by the client and/or family/caregivers as well as be appropriate to the client's cognitive symptoms. Recent studies provided more support for this approach in countries outside the United States (Quee et al., 2014), with shorter implementation time (Kidd et al., 2014) and focused on families (i.e., Family-Directed Cognitive Adaptation; Friedman-Yakoobian, Mueser, Giuliano, Goff, & Seidman, 2016).

Functional Task Training: The Neurofunctional Approach

The neurofunctional approach (NFA) was initially designed for persons with chronic or severe cognitive impairments as a result of traumatic brain injury (TBI) (Clark-Wilson et al., 2014; Giles, 2018). Similar approaches have been applied to persons with a history of cerebrovascular accidents (CVA; Rotenberg-Shpigelman, Erez, Nahaloni, & Maeir, 2012), dementia (Clare et al., 2010), and persons with TBI in acute rehabilitation (Trevena-Peters et al., 2018).

Neurofunctional approach emphasizes the use of task-specific training or rote repetition of specific tasks or routines within natural contexts to develop habits or functional behavioral routines. Repetitive practice reduces the demands on cognitive resources needed for task performance and increases automaticity of performance. Emphasis is on the mastery of functional task performance through the practice of "doing" meaningful activities. Intervention involves systematically breaking down a functional task into essential subcomponents for the person (Clark-Wilson et al., 2014). Behavioral techniques including feedback, reinforcement, and chaining are incorporated into structured practice sessions. Key techniques such as goal setting, task analysis, repetition, practice, cue experimentation, errorless learning, feedback, and reinforcement methods (Giles, 2018) may be used to promote skill acquisition.

Functional task training capitalizes on procedural or implicit memory of "how to" do something rather than verbal memory for facts and events. Electronic cueing devices, including tablets and smart phones, can be used to promote internalization of habits and routines during task-specific training. Functional task training can produce significant changes in performance of activities of daily living (ADL) and work tasks in people with severe or long-term cognitive impairments (Giles, 2018). Evidence to support this approach includes a large randomized controlled trial (RCT) of interdisciplinary acute rehabilitation after TBI (Vanderploeg et al., 2008).

Remedial Models

Remedial models place an emphasis on evaluating and restoring impaired cognitive-perceptual skills. They focus on identifying and targeting the person's underlying deficits or skills rather than manipulating the activity demands or context (Neistadt, 1990; Zoltan, 2007). This approach assumes that repetitive training on impaired tasks stimulates neuroplasticity and allows the brain to reorganize its structural and functional connections (Chiaravalloti, Genova, & DeLuca, 2015).

In traditional cognitive-perceptual remedial approaches, cognitive skills are conceptualized in terms of higher cortical skills, which are divided into a hierarchy of discrete subskills, such as attention, discrimination, memory, sequencing, categorization, concept formation, and problem solving. The lower level skills provide the foundation for more complex skills and behaviors (Toglia, 2011). For example, attention skills are addressed before higher level cognitive skills such as problem solving. Cognitive remedial training has been applied to diverse populations; however, treatment appears to be most successful with individuals who have mild and discrete deficits, particularly in working memory (Klingberg, 2010), and demonstrate strong motivation for improvement.

Improvement in underlying cognitive or perceptual deficits is thought to promote recovery or reorganization of the impaired skill. Information on functional reorganization and adult brain plasticity supports this view.

Targeted and intense training of discrete skills using new technology that automatically adjusts the challenge level based on the person's ability level and response is different than use of repetitive memory drills or general cognitive stimulation activities. Remedial interventions, however, have been criticized because a person can show changes in specific cognitive exercises without changes in everyday function (Cicerone et al., 2011; Goverover, Chiaravalloti, O'Brien, DeLuca, 2018).

Remedial interventions have been found to be more effective when combined with other intervention techniques such as coaching, goal setting, peer support (Dymowski, Ponsford, & Willmott, 2016; Johansson & Tornmalm, 2012), self-monitoring techniques, and strategy training or when used to enhance a rehabilitation program. Although remedial cognitive activities can supplement comprehensive programs that address meaningful activities and motivational or affective components, the isolated use of computer-based tasks is not recommended because of limited evidence of generalization to function (Cicerone et al., 2011).

Cognitive Strategy Models

Cognitive strategy models emphasize the use of cognitive strategies and view such strategies as part of normal cognition. Strategies are described as methods or tactics that are used to increase information processing, learning, and/or performance. Cognitive strategies can be internal and include self-talk, self-cues, self-questions, or use of mental practice, or they can be external and include the use of a checklist. They can also be situational or specific to certain tasks or environments or general and used across a wide variety (Toglia, 2018; Toglia, Rodger, & Polatajko, 2012).

Rather than focusing on discrete cognitive skills, strategy models focus on methods or approaches to enhance learning and performance. Typically, healthy people use multiple strategies simultaneously to cope with cognitively challenging situations. Use of strategies typically requires metacognitive skills such as the ability to anticipate challenges, monitor performance, detect errors, and self-evaluate performance. Models that focus on strategies, therefore, also emphasize metacognitive skills.

Cognitive strategy approaches have been used with both children and adults. Examples of models and approaches that use strategies include the multicontext approach (Foster, Spence, & Toglia, 2018; Toglia, 2018) and the Cognitive Orientation to Occupational Performance (CO-OP) approach (Dawson, McEwen, & Polatajko, 2017; Polatajko, Mandich, & McEwen, 2011). These two models are discussed in detail later in this chapter.

The Dynamic Interactional Model of Cognition

The Dynamic Interactional Model of Cognition integrates information on learning from cognitive and educational psychology with OT practice. The Dynamic Interactional Model explains how cognitive symptoms and occupational performance change depending on the interaction between personal factors as well as activity and environmental demands. Personal characteristics that influence learning and performance include the person's lifestyle, beliefs, self-efficacy, emotional status, and motivation. Self-awareness and processing strategies are identified as key components of cognitive function. The ability to effectively use strategies and monitor performance varies with external factors such as activity demands and the social, cultural, or physical environment as well as personal characteristics. Assessment, therefore, uses dynamic interactive methods to determine how external variables such as activity demands, alterations in the environment, and mediation from others influence a person's strategy use and self-awareness during task performance (Toglia, 2018).

Because dynamic assessment examines *how* performance can be facilitated, it is naturally linked to intervention. During an evaluation, the therapist intervenes to change, guide, or improve the person's performance using guided questioning, suggesting strategies, facilitating error detection, or modifying the activity (Toglia, 2011; Toglia & Cermak, 2009). This information directly relates to intervention planning. For example, if performance cannot

be modified through dynamic procedures, an intervention approach that seeks to change the environment or train caregivers might be more appropriate than an approach that focuses on changing a person's abilities or behaviors. Intervention may address the person's self-awareness and use of strategies, modification of the task or environment, or a combination of all three to optimize the fit between the person's abilities and the task and environment. The Dynamic Interactional Model of Cognition provides a broad view of cognition that accommodates multiple intervention approaches.

The Multicontext Approach

The multicontext approach is based on the Dynamic Interactional Model of Cognition and provides a specific framework for facilitating awareness and strategy use within activities or environments that may need to be adapted so that they are at a "just right" challenge level for the client (i.e., activities that are not only not too difficult but also not too easy). The key features of the multicontext approach include (1) consideration of personal context, (2) structured methods to promote self-monitoring and self-awareness, (3) strategy self-generation and training, and (4) practice across multiple activities and contexts using a transfer continuum. Intervention strategies vary depending on the client and his or her cognitive symptoms. Examples of the wide range of internal and external strategies that can be used in treatment are provided by Toglia (2018). This approach focuses on assisting clients in anticipating challenges and generating strategies themselves (i.e., enhancing the ability to apply and transfer use of strategies across different situations). For example, in the multicontext approach, the person practices application of a targeted strategy such as the use of a checklist, mental rehearsal, or self-cues across purposeful and occupation-based activities that systematically differ in appearance yet remain at a similar level of difficulty. This places gradual demands on the ability to transfer learning because the more two situations or activities are physically similar, the easier it is to transfer strategies learned in one situation to another (Toglia, 1991b). Table 58-1 shows an example of intervention activities presented along the transfer continuum. Activity

TABLE 58-1 The Transfer Continuum

Strategy emphasized in all activities: Use a checklist to gather and keep track of items to:							
Very Similar		Somewhat Similar		Different		Very Different	
Make vegetable salad (6–8 items).	Make fruit salad (6–8 items).	Set a table for dinner (for 6–8).	Pack 6–8 items in a lunchbox.	Pack 6–8 items in a bag for an overnight stay.	Put a list of 6–8 appointments in a calendar.	Use a list to complete 6–8 party invitations.	Use a list to complete 6–8 errands.

The multicontext approach was originally developed for use with adults with traumatic brain injury (Toglia, 2011); however, it has been applied to persons with schizophrenia (Josman, 2011), adults with lupus and MS, as well as with children and adolescents (Cermak & Maeir, 2011; Josman & Rosenblum, 2011).

demands are not graded in difficulty until evidence of spontaneous strategy use along the entire transfer continuum is observed. The use of awareness and metacognitive training techniques to facilitate self-monitoring skills and self-evaluation is deeply embedded throughout intervention. There is now evidence to support this treatment approach as a treatment guideline for persons with acquired brain injury (ABI; Goverover, Johnston, Toglia, & DeLuca, 2007b), TBI (Toglia, Goverover, Johnston, & Dain, 2011; Toglia, Johnston, Goverover, & Dain, 2010), multiple sclerosis (MS; Goverover, Genova, Griswold, Chiaravalloti, & DeLuca, 2014), and, more recently, with Parkinson disease (Foster et al., 2018). The multicontext approach was originally developed for use with adults with TBI (Toglia, 2018); however, it has been applied to persons with schizophrenia (Josman, 2011), adults with lupus and MS, and with children and adolescents (Cermak & Maeir, 2011; Josman & Rosenblum, 2011).

The Cognitive Orientation to Occupational Performance Approach

The CO-OP approach was originally developed in 2001 to enhance skill acquisition in children with developmental coordination disorder (DCD; Polatajko, Mandich, Miller, & Macnab, 2001) and subsequently applied to children with autism (Rodger & Vishram, 2010), cerebral palsy (Mandich, Polatajko, & Zilberbrant, 2008), and pervasive developmental disorder (Phelan, Steinke, & Mandich, 2009), as well as adults with stroke (Henshaw, Polatajko, McEwen, Ryan, & Baum, 2011; Skidmore et al., 2015), chronic stroke (Imms & Nott, 2012; Polatajko, McEwen, Ryan, & Baum, 2012), brain injury (Dawson et al., 2009), elderly adults with mild cognitive impairment (Dawson et al., 2014), and recently with women with chemotherapy-induced cognitive impairment (Wolf et al., 2016) with promising outcomes.

The CO-OP approach emphasizes the use of cognitive strategies in the development and acquisition of motor skills and daily living skills. It draws on dynamic systems theory as well as literature in motor performance, educational or cognitive psychology, and OT. Key components of the CO-OP approach include the following:

- Client-centered goals
- Dynamic performance analysis
- Cognitive strategy use
- Guided discovery
- Principles that include methods for promoting client engagement and learning,
- Parent or significant other involvement
- A structured intervention format (i.e., preparation phase, acquisition phase, and check verification phase)

The CO-OP approach is embedded within a client-centered framework and uses several techniques to ensure that the skills to be acquired are goals that the client wants, needs, or is expected to acquire. Evaluation involves several different tools to establish and assess client goals. In addition, dynamic performance analysis (DPA) is used as a top–down, structured method of observation to identify performance problems or breakdowns within activities that are chosen by the client and performed in context.

The CO-OP approach uses a combination of a global strategy (Goal, Plan, Do, Check) and task-specific strategies to acquire skills that will support the person's daily functioning (Dawson et al., 2017). For example, Rodger and Vishram (2010) describe the use of the CO-OP approach with two children with Asperger syndrome. Goals for one child included getting organized for school in the morning, managing anger in the playground, and managing time to complete homework. The global "goal, plan, do, check" strategy was used as an overall problem-solving framework throughout intervention. Domain-specific strategies such as visual charts, lists, walking away, counting to 10, and punching a bag when feeling angry to manage specific tasks or situations were facilitated using guided discovery and enabling principles. The children created and wrote their own goals and plans, reward charts, and time logs, and were encouraged to discover their own solutions using coaching, modeling, and feedback.

The Cognitive Rehabilitation Model

Averbuch and Katz (2011) describe a comprehensive OT cognitive rehabilitation model for adolescents and adults with neurological disabilities that integrates remedial principles with strategy use and awareness of abilities to broaden the capacity for learning. The model draws on neurophysiological, neurobiological, and neuropsychological theories to provide a framework for cognitive learning. Different approaches may be emphasized at various stages of the injury. Training is directed at initially enhancing remaining abilities and improving functional task performance within the context of client and/or family goals. Cognitive training is structured according to different levels and involves a gradual increase in the amount and complexity of information presented. Intervention involves systematic and structured activities including visual scanning, categorization or classification, sequencing, planning, and thinking operations. At the same time, there is an emphasis on teaching new learning strategies (e.g., systematic visual scanning strategy) to perform skills related to the different areas of cognitive function. Once clients learn to use strategies in various activities within the clinic, strategies are practiced in real-life situations.

The approach uses a combination of paper-and-pencil exercises, tabletop and computer activities, functional activities, compensatory methods, and virtual reality. If the client is incapable of using learning strategies, procedural strategies that focus on training the component parts of a task are used to promote the ability to perform ADL (Averbuch & Katz, 2011; Y. Schwartz & Sagiv, 2018). Strong evidence supports the combination of remedial training with strategy training. For example, Dymowski et al. (2016) combined attention processing training with individualized strategy training in persons with TBI. Peng and Fuchs (2017) showed that training of verbal working memory with a strategy of rehearsal improved verbal working memory and passage listening comprehension compared with training without strategy instruction. Cicerone et al. (2011) recommended a combined approach in cognitive rehabilitation.

Evaluation

Comprehensive cognitive evaluations are used for two primary reasons: First, evaluations provide evidence and information about the presence of impairments and performance competencies. Such information can be used to establish baselines, estimate functional cognitive abilities, plan discharge, and measure intervention effectiveness (e.g., rehabilitation outcomes). Second, evaluations gather information for intervention planning. This section provides detailed information about cognitive evaluation factors that practitioners need to consider when choosing and performing appropriate assessments.

The Cognition Evaluation Process

Occupational therapists approach the evaluation process with the goal of identifying functional cognitive challenges that influence "how an individual uses and integrates thinking and processing skills to accomplish everyday activities in clinical and community living environments" (Giles, Edwards, Morrison, Baum & Wolf, 2017, p. 2).

Using a Cognitive Functional Evaluation Process (Hartman-Maeir, Katz, & Baum, 2009), therapists intentionally select and sequence evaluations that provide information about a client's cognitive capabilities. Initial interviews or questionnaires along with cognitive and functional screenings may be followed by more domain-specific assessments, specific cognitive measures in occupation-based tasks, and an environmental assessment. When combined, the data from the cognitive evaluation process provides the therapist with a comprehensive perspective of the potential interaction of the person-occupation-environment and the influence of cognitive symptoms. Table 58-2 outlines

specific assessment tools for different aspects of client evaluation, including the following:

- Interview—perspective of client and others
- Cognitive screening instruments
- Functional assessments of cognition: performance-based testing
- Cognitive tests for specific domains
- Ratings of everyday cognitive symptoms and behaviors
- Environmental assessments

The role of the occupational therapist in evaluating cognition and perception is to provide clear, comprehensive information on the effect of cognitive-perceptual impairments on ADL, instrumental activities of daily living (IADL), education, work, play and leisure, and social participation. All team members need to consider that other factors, in addition to cognitive impairments, may impact the client's performance; for example, the client's true cognitive abilities may be masked by language impairments, pain, fatigue, low motivation, depression, anxiety, or psychological distress.

Interviews—Perspectives of the Client and Others

Occupational therapists typically begin the evaluation process by gathering information directly from the client and/or family members. A structured interview that considers the client's typical routines and occupations helps the therapist develop an occupational profile of the client's past functioning and goals for the future (AOTA, 2014). The client is usually asked to identify everyday activities that he or she is most concerned about or would like to be able to do with greater ease (see Table 58-2).

Interviews with community-dwelling clients to identify current levels of participation and desired changes may involve the use of participation scales such as the Mayo-Portland Adaptability Inventory (MPAI-4; Malec & Lezak, 2008), the Community Integration Questionnaire (CIQ; Willer, Ottenbacher, & Coad, 1994), or the Participation Objective, Participation Subjective (POPS; Curtin et al., 2011). These scales typically ask the client to rate the frequency and satisfaction of their current participation in various tasks; most of which can be impacted by the presence of cognitive symptoms.

Because people with cognitive impairments often have limited awareness of their impairments and limited understanding of the implications of these impairments (Goverover, Chiaravalloti, & DeLuca, 2005), a close relative or friend should participate in identifying concerns and priorities for intervention. In acute or rehabilitation inpatient settings where clients' daily occupations are often structured and limited in nature, client's relatives may be unaware of the presence of mild cognitive impairments; subtle cognitive symptoms tend to be apparent only in higher level activities such as driving, social participation,

TABLE 58-2 Cognitive Perceptual Assessments

Interview—Perspective of Client and Others	**Occupational Profile** Canadian Occupational Performance Measure (COPM) (Law et al., 2005) Activity Card Sort (ACS) (Baum & Edwards, 2001); pediatric version: Paediatric Activity Card Sort (PACS) (Mandich, Polatajko, Miller, & Baum, 2004) **Awareness Assessments** Assessment of Awareness of Disability (AAD) (Tham, Bernspang, & Fisher, 1999) Awareness Questionnaire (AQ) (Sherer, Bergloff, Boake, High, & Levin, 1998) Patient Competency Rating Scale (PCRS) (Prigatano, 1986) Self-Awareness of Deficits Interview (SADI) (Fleming, Strong, & Ashton, 1996) Self-Regulation Skills Interview (SRSI) (Ownsworth, McFarland, & Young, 2000)
Cognitive Screening Instruments	**Mental Status Exams** Blessed Dementia Rating Scale (BDRS) (Blessed, Tomlinson, & Roth, 1968) Medi-Cog (Anderson, Jue, & Madaras Kelly, 2008) Mini-Mental State Exam (MMSE) (Folstein, Folstein, & McHugh, 1975) Modified Mini-Mental State Examination (3MS) (Teng & Chui, 1987) Montreal Cognitive Assessment (MoCA) (Nasreddine et al., 2005) Saint Louis University Mental Status (SLUMS) (Tariq, Tumosa, Chibnall, Perry, & Morley, 2006) **Comprehensive Cognitive Screenings** Addenbrooke's Cognitive Examination-III (ACE-III) (Noone, 2015) Cognitive Assessment of Minnesota (CAM) (Rustad et al., 1993) Cognistat (Kiernan, Mueller, & Langston, 2011) Dynamic Loewenstein Occupational Therapy Cognitive Assessment (DLOTCA) (Katz, Livni, Bar-Haim Erez, & Averbuch, 2011); pediatric version: Dynamic Occupational Therapy Cognitive Assessment for Children (DOTCA-Ch) (Katz, Parush, & Traub Bar-Ilan, 2005) Lowenstein Occupational Therapy Cognitive Assessment (LOTCA) (Katz, Itzkovich, Averbuch, & Elazar, 1990); geriatric version available: Loewenstein Occupational Therapy Cognitive Assessment-Geriatric (LOTCA-G) (Elazar, Itzkovich, & Katz, 1996); functional version available: Functional Loewenstein Occupational Therapy Cognitive Assessment (FLOTCA) (Y. Schwartz, Averbuch, Katz, & Sagiv, 2016) Safe at Home (Robnett, Hopkins, & Kimball, 2003)
Functional Assessments of Cognition: Performance Based Testing	**Assessments Measuring Competency or Assistance Required** Independent Living Scales (ILS) (Loeb, 1996) Kettle Test (Hartman-Maeir, Harel, & Katz, 2009) Kitchen Task Assessment (KTA) (Baum & Edwards, 1993); pediatric version available: Children's Kitchen Task Assessment (CKTA) (Rocke, Hays, Edwards, & Berg, 2008) Kohlman Evaluation of Living Skills (KELS) 4th edition (Thomson & Robnett, 2016) Performance Assessment of Self-Care Skills, Version 4.0 (Rogers & Holm, 2014) Test of Grocery Shopping Skills (TOGSS) (Hamera & Brown, 2000) Texas Functional Living Scale (TFLS) (Cullum, Weiner, & Saine, 2009) University of California, San Diego Performance-Based Skills Assessment-Brief (UPSA-Brief) (Mausbach, Harvey, Goldman, Jeste, & Patterson, 2007) **Assessments Observing Factors Interfering with Performance** Actual Reality Task (Goverover, O'Brien, Moore, & DeLuca, 2010) ADL-Focused Occupation-Based Neurobehavioral Evaluation (A-ONE; formerly, Árnadóttir OT-ADL Neurobehavioral Evaluation) (Arnadottir, 1990) Allen Cognitive Level Test (ACL) (Allen, Earhart, & Blue, 1992) Assessment of Motor and Process Skills (AMPS) (Fisher, 1993a, 1993b) Cognitive Performance Test (CPT) (Allen et al., 1992) Complex Task Performance Assessment (Wolf, Dahl, Auen, & Doherty, 2017) Do-Eat Assessment for Children (Josman, Goffer, & Rosenblum, 2010) Executive Function Performance Test (EFPT) (Baum, Edwards, Morrison, & Hahn, 2003) Instrumental Activities of Daily Living (IADL) Profile (Bottari, Gosseli, Guillemette, LaMoureux, & Ptito, 2011) Multiple Errands Test–Revised (MET-R) (Morrison et al., 2013) Naturalistic Action Test (NAT) (M. F. Schwartz, Segal, Veramonti, Ferraro, & Buxbaum, 2002) Perceive, Recall, Plan, and Perform (PRPP) (Nott & Ch200, 2012) Routine Task Inventory-Expanded (RTI-E) (Katz, 2006) Weekly Calendar Planning Activity (WCPA) (Toglia, 2015)

TABLE 58-2	**Cognitive Perceptual Assessments** *(continued)*
Cognitive Tests for Specific Domains	**Attention Assessments** Test of Everyday Attention (TEA) (Robertson, Ward, Ridgeway, & Nimmo-Smith, 1994); pediatric version: Test of Everyday Attention for Child (TEA-CH) (Manly, Robertson, Anderson, & Nimmo-Smith, 1998) Trail Making Test (Reitan, 1955) **Spatial Neglect Assessments** The Baking Tray Test (Tham & Tegnér, 1996)[a] The Balloons Test (Edgeworth, Robertson, & McMillan, 1998) Behavioral Inattention Test (BIT) (Wilson, Cockburn, & Baddeley, 1987) Indented Paragraph Test (Caplan, 1987) Kessler Foundation Neglect Assessment Process (KF-NAP) (Chen & Hreha, 2015)[a] Line Cancellation (Albert, 1973) Verbal and Nonverbal Cancellation Tasks (Mesulam, 2000) **Memory Assessments** Contextual Memory Test (CMT) (Toglia, 1993b) Memory for Intentions Test (MIST) (Raskin & Buckheit, 2010) Prospective Memory Screening (PROMS) (Sohlberg & Mateer, 1989b) Rivermead Behavioral Memory Test-Extended version (RBMT-E) (Wilson, Clare, Baddeley, Watson, & Tate, 1998); pediatric version: Rivermead Behavioural Memory Test for Children (RBMT-C) (Aldrich & Wilson, 1991) **Visual Perception Assessments** Brain Injury Visual Assessment Battery for Adults (biVABA) (Warren, 1998) Motor-Free Visual Perception Test (MVPT-3) (Colarusso & Hammill, 2002) Occupational Therapy Adult Perceptual Screening Test (OT-APST) (Cooke, McKenna, & Fleming, 2005) **Executive Function Assessments** Behavioral Assessment of Dysexecutive Syndrome (BADS) (Wilson, Alderman, Burgess, Emslie, & Evans, 1996); pediatric version: Behavioral Assessment of Dysexecutive Syndrome for Children (BADS-C) (Emslie, Wilson, Burden, Nimmo-Smith, & Wilson, 2003) Toglia Category Assessment (TCA) (Toglia, 1994) **Motor Planning Assessments** Assessment of Apraxic Disabilities (van Heugten et al., 2000) Test of Upper Limb Apraxia (TULIA) (Vanbellingen et al., 2010) Test of Ideational Praxis (TIP for children) (May-Benson & Cermak, 2007)
Ratings of Everyday Cognitive Symptoms and Behaviors	Behavior Rating Inventory of Executive Function-Adult Version (BRIEF-A) (Roth, Isquith, & Gioia, 2005); pediatric version: Behavior Rating Inventory of Executive Function, Second Edition (BRIEF-2) (Gioia, Isquith, Guy, & Kenworthy, 2015). Brief Assessment of Prospective Memory (BAPM) (Man, Fleming, Hohaus, & Shum, 2011) Catherine Bergego Scale (CBS) for Unilateral Neglect (Azouvi et al., 2003) Cognitive Failures Questionnaire (CFQ) (Broadbent, Cooper, FitzGerald, & Parkes, 1982; Wilhelm, Witthöft, & Schipolowski, 2010) Moss Attentional Rating Scale (MARS) (Whyte, Hart, Bode, & Malec, 2003) Prospective and Retrospective Memory Questionnaire (PRMQ) (Crawford, Smith, Maylor, Della Sala, & Logie, 2003)
Environmental Assessments	Analysis of Cognitive Environmental Support (ACES) (Ryan et al., 2011) Home Environmental Assessment Protocol (HEAP) (Gitlin et al., 2002) Home Occupational-Environmental Assessment (HOEA) (Baum & Edwards, 1998) Safety Assessment of Function and the Environment for Rehabilitation (SAFER tool) (Chui et al., 2006)

[a]These assessments are functional cognitive assessments of neglect.

shopping, and using public transportation. A clearer picture of the impact of the client's cognitive impairments may emerge when the client is discharged home and resumes these higher level community activities (Toglia & Golisz, 2012).

Interview and rating scales for self-awareness (see Table 58-2) generally evaluate awareness of limitations and strengths, the ability to generalize the impact of limitations on functional tasks, and concerns regarding disability judgment (i.e., intellectual awareness). Typically, the person's self-ratings are compared with those of a relative or clinician (Toglia & Maier, 2018). Alternatively, some scales such as the Self-Awareness of Deficits Interview (Fleming et al., 1996) use a semistructured interview in which the clinician directly rates the person's level of awareness, depending on the response to questions. Both methods of assessing awareness examine intellectual awareness outside the context of an activity.

Although interviews and rating scales are the most common method of assessing awareness, it can also be assessed within the context of an activity by asking the client to estimate his or her performance before (i.e., anticipatory awareness) and immediately after (i.e., emergent awareness) performing a task. Differences between estimated performance and actual performance are then compared. Task estimation including normative comparison is used within the Contextual Memory Test (CMT) (Toglia, 1993b). The Assessment of Awareness of Disability includes self-rating of performance that is compared with Assessment of Motor and Process Skills (AMPS) performance (Anderson, Doble, Merritt, & Kottorp, 2010). A task-specific awareness scale may ask clients to identify challenges prior to task performance (Toglia, Goverover, et al., 2011; Toglia et al., 2010). Changes in awareness that may occur during the experience of an activity can be examined by comparing responses to awareness questions before, during, and immediately after performance.

Cognitive Screening Instruments

Cognitive-screening instruments are standardized assessments that are designed to identify problems that need special or further attention. Mental status exams provide an overall score or diagnostic cutoff score that differentiates normal from suspect or impaired cognitive functioning. In choosing a screening, the published sensitivity (i.e., persons correctly identified as having cognitive impairment) and specificity (i.e., correct identification of persons without cognitive impairment) need to be considered within the population that is being tested.

Typically, mental status exams are 5- to 10-minute assessments that do not require equipment other than paper and pencil, making them convenient to bedside and office testing. In addition, many of these exams are in the public domain or freely available on the Internet. Mental status exams such as the popular Mini-Mental State Examination (MMSE; Folstein et al., 1975) were originally developed for clients with dementia of the Alzheimer type but have been used and validated in other populations (Mackin, Ayalon, Feliciano, & Areán, 2010; Swirsky-Sacchetti et al., 1992; Toglia, Fitzgerald, O'Dell, Mastrogiovanni, & Lin, 2011).

Most mental status exams provide global ratings of the client's orientation, attention, memory, language, and judgment. The Montreal Cognitive Assessment (MoCA; Nasreddine et al., 2005) also includes an executive function component and has been shown to be more predictive of functional status and improvement than the MMSE in acute inpatients with stroke and mild cognitive impairment

(Toglia, Fitzgerald, et al., 2011). Mental status screenings generally identify the types of cognitive impairments that may be present; however, results need to be examined in combination with direct observation of functional performance to provide a complete picture of the client. Results of cognitive standardized assessments do not always translate clearly to functional performance.

Mental status exams have some additional disadvantages because they rely heavily on verbal skills, can be culturally biased, and have substantial false-negative rates (i.e., missing possible cognitive impairments). The deficits of clients with focal lesions, particularly right hemisphere lesions and mild diffuse cognitive disorders, are often missed (Nelson, Fogel, & Faust, 1986). In general, cognitive screening assessments may miss more subtle impairments that are displayed by higher level clients because the breadth and depth of item content are limited. Toglia et al. (2017) found that approximately one-third of people with stroke who do not show impairment on the MoCA at admission to an acute rehabilitation unit exhibited IADL deficits on discharge (see Table 58-2).

Performance-Based Testing of Functional Cognition

Direct observation of functional performance, or performance-based testing, incorporates everyday activities (real or simulated) as another method used to assess functional cognition. Clients with agitation or severely limited attention may be unable to engage in a standardized evaluation process; however, a task analysis system such as the Perceive, Recall, Plan, and Perform (PRPP) system may be used to assess information processing during functional or everyday tasks of clients in this phase of recovery (Nott & Chapparo, 2008; Nott, Chapparo, & Heard, 2009). The PRPP approach requires the occupational therapist to analyze the behavioral steps and typical cognitive processing strategies (i.e., sensory processing [Perceive], memory [Recall], response planning and evaluation [Plan], and performance monitoring [Perform]) used to successfully complete a task. Any functional task may be selected for observation and systematic rating of the efficacy of the information processing strategy demonstrated by the client. This method has been validated in adults with schizophrenia (Aubin, Chapparo, Gélinas, Stip, & Rainville, 2009), dementia (Steultjens, Voigt-Radloff, Leonhart, & Graff, 2012), Parkinson disease (Van Keulen-Rouweler et al., 2017), and brain injury (Nott & Chapparo, 2008).

Some performance-based assessments such as the Kettle Test (Hartman-Maeir, Harel et al., 2009) rate the degree of assistance required for each substep of an IADL task within a functional context. This information can help determine the level of assistance needed for discharge planning. Other performance-based assessments are also designed to identify the cognitive and perceptual impairments that interfere with successful performance on such tasks. For example, in the ADL-Focused Occupation-Based Neurobehavioral Evaluation (A-ONE; formerly, Árnadóttir OT-ADL Neurobehavioral Evaluation) (Árnadóttir, 1990), a client is observed performing a basic ADL (e.g., putting on a shirt) for possible cognitive impairments such as spatial relation difficulties, spatial or body neglect, and the like.

The Executive Function Performance Test (Baum et al., 2003; Goverover et al., 2005) is a functional performance test that analyzes the need for assistance in executive components such as initiation, organization, and safety by observing client performance on IADL such as making a phone call. The Naturalistic Action Test (M. F. Schwartz et al., 2002) scores the accuracy of steps completed and types of error made (e.g., omissions, perseveration, spatial estimation, reversals, substitutions, quality) during the completion of three functional tasks (e.g., making toast and coffee, gift wrapping a present, and packing a child's lunchbox and schoolbag) under standardized conditions. Pediatric assessments such as the DO-Eat (Josman et al., 2010) and the Children's Kitchen Task Assessment (CKTA; Rocke et al., 2008) also consider the impact of executive function components on task performance.

The development of cognitive domain assessments that use real-world objects or tasks has enabled therapists to make clearer links between observed functional task performance and the underlying cognitive impairments. The area of executive functioning is particularly robust with assessments that use function-based tasks. Tests such as the Multiple Errands Test–Revised (Morrison et al., 2013) and WCPA (Toglia, 2015) provide more specific information on a client's performance of tasks requiring executive functioning skills.

It is important to acknowledge that performance-based assessments that simulate performance in a treatment setting may not be predictive of performance in natural contexts in which the person must establish goals, plan, initiate, problem-solve, and manage both subtle and complex environmental cues. Questionnaires or rating scales such as the Behavior Rating Inventory of Executive Function (BRIEF; Roth et al., 2005) and the Brief Assessment of Prospective Memory (BAPM; Man et al., 2011) can be completed by the client, clinician, and/or significant other. Although these assessments do not require actual performance of the functional task, they provide additional insight into how the cognitive symptoms impact everyday occupational performance (see Table 58-2).

Domain-Specific Cognitive Assessments

When the client's performance in either cognitive or occupation-based screenings indicates the potential for cognitive impairments, the occupational therapist may administer more specific standardized cognitive assessments. Comparing the client's performance with normative data can determine whether a cognitive impairment exists and quantify the severity of such impairments. This step in the evaluation process provides a more in-depth understanding of the client's cognitive impairments. Standardized cognitive assessments are typically static in nature, evaluating "here and now" performance and providing a baseline against which changes in condition or ability can be measured over time.

Cognitive impairments may also be assessed more specifically with assessments that simulate functional tasks or use functional objects (see Table 58-2). Many of these assessments have versions specifically designed for children, and several assessments have been validated in individuals with schizophrenia.

Assessments based on the dynamic model of cognition such as the CMT (Toglia, 1993b), the Toglia Category Assessment (TCA; Toglia, 1994), or the Weekly Calendar Planning Activity (WCPA; Toglia, 2015) can provide information about underlying impairments and the ability to change the client's performance with cues and task modifications. Dynamic assessment methods have been applied to a wide range of ages and people with cognitive disabilities. However, research applications and specific tools are limited.

Environmental Assessment of Cognition Supports and Barriers

The environment in which cognitive tasks are performed may either support or hinder a client's occupational performance. Situations that require higher level cognitive-perceptual skills are difficult to create in structured treatment environments. In addition, contextual factors can increase or decrease cognitive demands of performance, so it is important to consider the context in which an activity is performed. For example, Hamera and Brown (2000) developed the Test of Grocery Shopping Skills as a real-world measure of community function for people with chronic schizophrenia. In hospital-based treatment settings, the occupational therapist, however, might not be able to create a close enough approximation of a real-world environment. The contextual influence on performance needs to be considered; if feasible, performance should be observed across real-world contexts.

Occupational therapists may use one of several environmental assessments to specifically analyze the supports and barriers contributed by the environment to the performance of cognitive-based tasks. These assessments do not measure occupational performance or quantify the presence or severity of a cognitive impairment; rather, they provide additional information on how the environment influenced the client's performance. The Analysis of Cognitive Environmental Support (ACES; Ryan et al., 2011) assesses the cognitive supports and barriers of the environment, the client's awareness of the cognitive supports/barriers, who introduced the support/barrier (e.g., client or someone else), and how recent the support/barrier is in relation to the client's cognitive impairment.

Other environmental assessments such as the Safety Assessment of Function and the Environment for Rehabilitation (SAFER; Chui et al., 2006) focus on the client's ability to safely perform functional tasks within the home. Risks within the physical environment are rated in severity, and environmental modifications are suggested. Some environmental assessments were designed for specific cognitively impaired populations, such as the Home Environmental Assessment Protocol (HEAP; Gitlin et al., 2002), which was developed for individuals with dementia.

Choosing the Most Appropriate Type of Assessment

Within a structured cognitive evaluation process, an occupational therapist must first decide what questions need to be answered. The therapist can then select the assessment that will most effectively address such questions. Some factors to consider before choosing an assessment include the following:

1. *The need to screen for the presence of cognitive impairments*—The therapist may use an assessment with normative comparison or cutoff scores with diagnostic-based sensitivity and specificity. The extent to which the person's scores deviates from expected performance identifies the presence and/ or severity of cognitive impairments. In clients with moderate-to-severe impairments, occupational therapists may also use functional assessments such as the A-ONE to confirm the presence of deficits. If possible cognitive deficits are identified, the client may be referred to a neuropsychologist for a more comprehensive cognitive-perceptual assessment.

2. *The need to perform a comprehensive evaluation on a client who is confused, disoriented, and unable to identify common objects*—A client who presents with disorientation and possible agnosia will most likely be unable to follow the instructions of a standardized assessment. The therapist should monitor the client's orientation level and ability to appropriately identify and use common objects within functional tasks. If or when the confusion clears, and the client can follow simple commands, the therapist may engage in more formal evaluation of the client's cognitive-perceptual skills.

3. *The need to understand the effect of cognitive-perceptual impairments on occupational performance (i.e., the activity limitation and participation restrictions from the International Classification of Function [ICF]; World Health Organization, 2001)*—When the existence of impairments has been validated by neuropsychological testing, the occupational therapist's role in evaluation typically focuses on describing the impact of cognitive dysfunction on functional performance or analysis of the influence of different activity demands and contexts on everyday activities.

4. *Concern about cognitive-perceptual deficits in a patient who scores within normal range on cognitive screenings and demonstrates no difficulty when completing self-care or routine activities*—Even when a client appears to be doing well in routine activities, the therapist should consider complex activities or IADL tasks that the patient may need to perform as well as the ability to resume former roles and lifestyle. Testing the patient's ability to perform within unstructured IADL tasks and crowded environments requiring multitasking or executive skills will enable the therapist to identify any subtle impairment that may benefit from outpatient intervention. Participation measures can also identify difficulties in everyday life that may reflect subtle cognitive impairments.

5. *The need for information to guide intervention*—The model of cognitive intervention that the therapist is using often guides the selection of evaluation tools. Dynamic assessments emphasize the processes that are involved in learning and change and may provide information that is needed to plan and guide intervention that focuses on changing skills or behaviors (Toglia, 2011).

6. *The need to establish a baseline as a measurement of change or outcome of intervention*—The therapist needs to take into consideration short- and long-term intervention goals. In documenting outcomes, it is important to take into consideration the three levels of disability described by the ICF: impairment, activity limitation, and participation restriction. Therefore, a cognitive-perceptual evaluation that includes these three components will provide a more comprehensive view of the person's functioning.

Selecting Intervention Approaches

Given the wide ranges of severity, symptoms, ages, populations, and performance challenges that characterize individuals with cognitive-perceptual dysfunction, there is not one model or approach that will fit all clients. Intervention approaches can result in different outcomes, depending on these client characteristics.

In planning intervention, the clinician uses therapeutic reasoning and considers questions such as the following:

- How much change is expected from the person?
- How much learning and generalization are expected?
- How much do the activity demands or context need to be changed or altered to meet the person's capabilities?
- Is the person responsive to cues?
- Is the person aware of his or her difficulties?

For a person who is completely unaware of his or her difficulties, is unresponsive to cues, has severe global deficits, and does not show potential for change within the intervention time frame, a treatment approach that targets changes in strategy use such as the multicontext approach, CO-OP approach, or the cognitive retraining approach might not be appropriate. The CDM or the ESP, which focuses on teaching others to change the environment or activity rather than the person, may result in greater functional outcomes. The NFA, which uses repetitive practice to change performance on a specific task, might also be indicated to increase functional performance.

Alternatively, a person who is highly motivated with focal cognitive deficits who is aware of weaknesses and able to engage in intense and consistent practice may benefit from a remedial approach that targets specific cognitive skills. Another client who shows only partial or incomplete self-awareness, task error patterns that affect performance across situations, and decreased use of strategies might benefit from a cognitive strategy approach.

Considerations of the severity of the cognitive and functional deficits as well as assumptions regarding awareness and learning and the type of change expected within intervention models need to be carefully considered in planning intervention (Toglia, 2018). This process is reflected in the scenarios described in the case example.

Cognitive Impairments: Definitions, Evaluations, and Interventions

This section explains the main constructs involved in cognition, including their definitions, evaluation, and treatment. These constructs are as follows:

- Self-awareness
- Orientation
- Attention
- Spatial neglect
- Visual processing and visual motor
- Motor planning
- Memory
- Executive functions, organization, and problem solving

Although each of these constructs is discussed separately for the purposes of description, it is important to recognize that cognitive problems are interrelated and rarely occur in isolation. Similarly, examples of intervention strategies and task or environmental adaptations for specific cognitive-perceptual domains are discussed; however, in clinical practice, various intervention methods are used in combination with each other and within the context of different models. The context of the person's life needs to be considered in planning and choosing intervention activities (Johnston, Goverover, & Dijkers, 2005). This includes the person's occupations, personality, interests, premorbid level of functioning, culture, values, external supports, and resources. Interventions that address cognitive impairments need to be blended with those that address interpersonal skills; social participation; and everyday activities, routines, and roles (Abreu & Peloquin, 2005).

Self-Awareness

Self-awareness is discussed first because lack of awareness can affect the motivation, effort, and sustained participation that are needed for intervention (Toglia & Maeir, 2018).

Impaired self-awareness includes lack of knowledge about one's own cognitive-perceptual limitations and/or his or her functional implications as well as deficiencies in metacognitive skills (e.g., the ability to anticipate difficulties, recognize errors, and/or monitor performance within the context of an activity) (Toglia & Kirk, 2000). Impaired self-awareness presents obstacles to adjustment, collaborative goal setting, and active participation in intervention (G. Gillen, 2009). Decreased awareness results in poor motivation and compliance, lack of sustained effort, unrealistic expectations, incongruence between goals of the client and family, impaired judgment and safety, inability to adopt the use of compensatory strategies, and increased caregiver burden (Kelleher, Tolea, & Galvin, 2015; Toglia & Maeir, 2018). Studies support the association between awareness and functional outcome across different populations (Engel, Chui, Goverover, & Dawson, 2017; Gould et al., 2015; Goverover, Chiaravalloti, Gaudino-Goering, Moore, & DeLuca, 2009; Robertson & Schmitter-Edgecomb, 2015).

Lack of awareness may be related to psychological or neurological sources. Denial is a psychological defense mechanism that is related to premorbid personality traits and is characterized by overrationalization, hostility, resistance to feedback, and an unwillingness to confront problems (Prigatano, 1999). A person who has a history of denying inadequacies and resisting help from others and a strong desire to be "in control" is more likely to use denial as a coping strategy.

Impaired self-awareness resulting from neurological lesions represents a lack of access to information regarding one's cognitive state and is characterized by

CASE STUDY 58-1   COGNITION AND PERFORMANCE CONTEXTS

Scenario 1

Mr. James is a 24-year-old male with a 10-year history of attention and memory problems related to a head trauma that he sustained at age 14 years. He has difficulty in recalling conversations and events that occurred just hours before. During performance of a task, he easily loses track of the steps and repeats some steps twice while omitting other steps altogether. Mr. James denies any difficulty with his concentration or memory and would like to return to school. He currently lives with his parents who care for him.

Scenario 2

Mr. Cornwall is a 64-year-old male with attention and memory problems related to head trauma that he sustained 3 weeks ago. He has difficulty in recalling conversations and events that occurred just hours before. During performance of a task, he easily loses track of the steps and repeats some steps twice while omitting other steps altogether. Mr. Cornwall is well aware of his difficulties and is depressed by them. For example, he states, "I can't even remember what I ate for breakfast. What good am I? If I have to give up my business, my life is over." Mr. Cornwall was recently widowed and lived alone before his accident.

Questions

The two scenarios describe the same clinical symptoms, but the performance contexts are different.

1. How do the differences in context influence the emphasis in intervention that you would use?
2. What influenced your selection?

Discussion

There are no absolute right or wrong answers to these questions. In scenario 1, Mr. James is 10 years postinjury, so the potential for change in the underlying cognitive skills is assumed to be minimal. A remedial approach that focuses on improving memory and attention skills would not be warranted unless there was some evidence of potential for further improvement. Compensatory strategies such as the use of a memory aids could be considered. However, Mr. James denies any difficulty in memory or attention. This lack of self-awareness will present a major obstacle to independent initiation and the use of compensatory strategies.

Caregiver training, task and environmental adaptation, and the possibility of functional skill training to increase performance of a specified task appear to be the most appropriate areas for intervention. Techniques to increase awareness may be attempted as a prerequisite for using compensatory aids. External memory aids such as memory notebook training may be introduced by using task-specific training methods in combination with maximum prompts and external cues for their use; however, success likely depends on Mr. James's ability to gain awareness and accept his disability.

In scenario 2, Mr. Cornwall is only 3 weeks postinjury so that the potential for change in the underlying skills is presumably present. In addition, Mr. Cornwall is aware of his problems. This would appear to make him a potential candidate for remedial techniques. However, he is also depressed by his difficulties. He might not be able to cope emotionally with an approach that focuses on the underlying client factors.

An approach that will provide opportunities for success and control over his environment could be the initial intervention emphasis. For example, adaptive techniques in which the caregiver or practitioner presents directions one step at a time might make it easier for Mr. Cornwall to follow task instructions. Training in the use of compensatory strategies such as the use of a memory notebook or digital journal to keep track of daily events and conversations and the use of a checklist to assist in keeping track of task steps that have already been completed could enhance task performance. As Mr. Cornwall gains self-confidence and control, remedial tasks that focus on improving attention may be gradually introduced if he is able to tolerate them.

---

surprise, indifference, or perplexity in response to feedback (Prigatano, 1999). In many cases, the neurological and psychological sources of unawareness coexist and cannot be easily differentiated. If denial is the predominant source of unawareness, methods of awareness training might not be effective (Toglia & Maeir, 2018).

Crosson et al. (1989) described a hierarchical pyramid model of awareness that distinguishes between intellectual awareness, emergent awareness, and anticipatory awareness. Clients with *intellectual awareness* verbally describe limitations in functioning, whereas clients with *emergent awareness* recognize a problem only when it is actually happening. Clients with *anticipatory awareness* are able to anticipate that an impairment will likely cause a challenge before performing a given activity (Crosson et al., 1989). The hierarchical nature of this model has not been empirically demonstrated, and there is some indication that the interrelationships among these concepts are complex and nonhierarchical (Abreu et al., 2001).

Toglia and Kirk (2000) proposed a dynamic model of awareness that includes self-knowledge or beliefs about knowledge and abilities that exists prior to an activity (i.e., intellectual awareness) and "online" awareness that includes self-monitoring and self-regulatory processes that are activated within the context of an activity. This view of awareness is nonhierarchical and proposes that levels of awareness vary across different tasks and contexts within the same domain. It implies that awareness needs to be assessed both outside and inside the context of an activity (Toglia & Kirk, 2000). In addition, it suggests that awareness involves both an interplay between neurological mechanisms as well as the task, context, and personal factors such as personality, coping mechanisms, and culture.

Evaluation

A comprehensive evaluation of awareness plays a key role in guiding and selecting methods of intervention. Self-awareness training is a key component of the multicontext approach but not of other approaches such as the NFA. For example, in some cases, potential for changes in awareness may be limited, particularly within the intervention time frame or because of the disease course (e.g., Alzheimer disease). In these situations, intervention methods that do not require awareness, such as functional skill training, errorless learning, and adaptation of the environment, may be most appropriate in facilitating occupational performance. If a lack of understanding of one's own strengths and limitations prevents a person from choosing goals that are realistic and attainable, the therapist should assist the client in focusing on skills or tasks that are needed for the "here and now."

Intervention

Models that focus on helping individuals learn to monitor performance and increase understanding about their own strengths and limitations include the cognitive retraining approach, multicontext approach, and the CO-OP approach. The two latter approaches stress the importance of helping a person discover his or her own errors and generate his or her own solutions. The multicontext approach places a greater emphasis on enhancing awareness of limitations across different activities, whereas the CO-OP approach focuses on discovering performance errors in specific tasks.

Toglia and Kirk (2000) emphasize that directly pointing out errors or telling clients that they have problems is least effective in increasing awareness, as this approach tends to elicit defensive reactions. They recommend a therapeutically supportive context, use of familiar activities at the "just right challenge level," and structured experiences to enhance the emergence of awareness. Goverover et al. (2007a, 2007b) found that, compared with a control group, a structured, occupation-based intervention based on Toglia and Kirk's (2000) self-awareness model significantly improved IADL performances and self-regulation in persons with ABI. Recently, a systematic review by Engel et al. (2017) found support for use of multiple awareness intervention techniques including metacognitive strategy intervention, guided discussion, external feedback, and multimodal feedback within the context of experiential participation and functional task practice to produce positive outcomes at an activity and participation level.

Clearly, awareness interventions are critical to improving function. Following are descriptions of specific techniques that can be used in a wide range of activities to enhance awareness, including self-prediction, specific goal ratings, videotape feedback, self-evaluation, and self-questioning. These techniques are often used in combination with one other, can be blended with strategy training, and may be incorporated into all treatment sessions. The multicontext approach provides additional guidelines for simultaneously addressing awareness and strategy use (Toglia, 2018).

Self-Prediction. Self-prediction is the ability of a person to anticipate difficulties or predict his or her performance on a task. In an OT evaluation, the client might be asked to indicate on a rating scale whether the activity will be easy or hard or to identify the type of challenges or obstacles that he or she might encounter before actual performance of an activity. Immediately following performance, the actual results are compared with the predicted results, and any discrepancies are discussed (Goverover et al., 2007a, 2007b; Toglia, 2011).

Specific Goal Ratings. Daily or weekly self-ratings of clearly defined behaviors or targeted strategies can be used to help a person focus on what he or she can do in the present. Goal attainment scales offer a concrete, individualized focus that can increase self-awareness and realistic goal orientation (Rockwood, Joyce, & Stolee, 1997). Client self-ratings of goal attainment can be compared with the ratings of the therapist or a significant other, and any discrepancies can be discussed. Self-ratings can be charted or graphed over time and tracked to improve awareness (Sohlberg & Turkstra, 2011).

Videotape Feedback. A videotape of a client that illustrates difficulties in performing an activity can be used to enhance awareness. Videotape feedback is concrete, and it allows clients to reexperience their performance and evaluate their difficulties as they are occurring rather than simply discussing them after the fact. Videotape feedback has been used successfully in treating people with stroke and brain injury (Engel et al., 2017; Liu & Chan; 2014; Schmidt, Fleming, Ownsworth, & Lannin, 2015).

Self-Evaluation. With self-evaluation, the practitioner provides a structured system, such as a set of questions, a checklist, or a rating system that the client uses as a guide to evaluate his or her own performance (Goverover et al., 2007a, 2007b; Toglia et al., 1991a, 2011). Examples of self-evaluation questions are "Have I attended to all the necessary information?" and "Did I check over my work?"

Self-Questioning. With self-questioning, questions that are designed to cue the client to monitor his or her behavior are written on an index card or memorized. At specific time intervals during a task, the client is expected to stop and answer the same two or three questions, such as "Am I sure that I am looking all the way to the left?" "Am I paying attention to the details?" and "Am I going too quickly?" (Fertherlin & Kurland, 1989).

Journaling. In journaling practice, the client keeps a journal in which he or she records activity experiences and performance results. The client is encouraged to reflect on and interpret activity experiences, think about what he or she has learned about himself or herself, and summarize strengths and weaknesses (Goverover et al., 2007a, 2007b).

Orientation

Orientation is the ability to understand the self and the relationships between the self and the past and present environment. Orientation relies on the integration of several mental activities that are represented in different areas of the brain. Disorientation is indicative of significant impairments in attention and memory (Lezak, Howieson, & Loring, 2004).

Evaluation

Evaluation of orientation traditionally includes the client's orientation to person, place, and time. Orientation to person involves both the self and others. Orientation to place is demonstrated by the client's ability to understand the type of place he or she is in (e.g., hospital or home), to report the name and location of the place, and to appreciate distance and direction. Orientation to time requires an ability to report the current point in time (e.g., day, month, and year), to show understanding of the continuity and sequence of time (i.e., estimation), and to associate events with time.

Topographical orientation, often considered a component of orientation to place, is the ability to follow a familiar route or a new route once given an opportunity to become familiar with it (e.g., for a person to find his or her way from the therapy area to his or her room or describe and draw the layout of a familiar room or route) (Zoltan, 2007). Difficulties with the visual-spatial and memory aspects of topographical orientation need to be identified during evaluation (Brunsdon, Nickels, & Coltheart, 2007).

Orientation assessments are traditionally covered in mental status examinations (see Table 58-2). However, occupational therapists frequently use nonstandardized measures of orientation, such as interviews with open-ended questions asked in a conversational or informal manner. Most practitioners use cues to determine the severity of the disorientation. If the client is unable to answer the questions independently, the practitioner might offer a multiple-choice array or verbal cues. Cues usually move from general or abstract to more concrete, as determined by the severity of disorientation (e.g., "Today is the beginning of the work week" vs. "Today is the day after Sunday"). The number and type of cues offer a method for

scoring and monitoring progress. Fluctuations in orientation during the day should be noted because clients might experience sundowning, a syndrome in which they become confused in the evening because of fatigue.

Intervention

Interventions to address orientation focus on adaptations of the task or environment. Adaptations that increase the saliency of external cues can be used to help a person feel less confused. For example, an information poster that contains orientation facts and pictures of family members can be placed on a wall or a key location within the room. Or, a family member can create an audio or video recording that reviews orientation information at set times during the day or whenever the person feels confused. Care must be taken to match the amount of information presented at one time with the person's processing abilities.

A calendar posted in an accessible place can help orient a person to time. If the client has poor selective attention, a single piece of paper with the day and date written daily rather than a monthly calendar might be helpful. Electronic devices such as a talking clock or watch can also be preset to automatically announce the day and time on an hourly basis.

To assist the client in finding his or her room, directional arrows can be placed in the hallway, and tape indicating the route can be placed on the floor. Key landmarks can be pointed out and made more prominent with arrows or colored tape, and a sign with the person's picture can be placed on the door of his or her room.

These adaptations are key characteristics of functional cognitive models and can be used directly with clients or as part of caregiver training programs. Task-specific training techniques used within the NFA such as errorless learning or spaced retrieval techniques can also be used to train use of specific external aids such as referring to a daily calendar through structured repetition and practice. Spaced retrieval involves systematically lengthening the period of retention and recall. There is evidence that this technique is more effective than cueing hierarchies in treating people with dementia (Bourgeois et al., 2003).

Attention

Attention encompasses a number of cognitive processes from basic alertness or arousal to higher level attentional processes that overlap with executive function, such as dual tasking or divided attention, multitasking skills, and error monitoring (Hart, Whyte, & Kennedy, 2016). Several aspects of attention, such as the ability to keep track of information within a task, shift or alternate attention between tasks, and selectively attend to relevant information while inhibiting distractions, are now conceptualized under the umbrella of executive function and discussed later in this chapter.

Fundamentally, attention includes the ability to detect and react to changes in the environment. At a basic level, this includes *orienting functions* or *the ability to detect* and react to gross environmental changes (e.g., a telephone ringing, a name being called, or a ball that is thrown). At higher levels of function, measures of reaction time or processing speed are commonly used as indicators of generalized attentional function. The time required to press a button whenever a stimulus appears on the computer screen or the time it takes to press on the brake during driving when an obstacle is detected on the road are examples of measures of processing speed. *Sustained attention* is described as the ability to persist or consistently engage in an activity over time, such as reading for 15 minutes without losing concentration.

Evaluation

Attention is typically assessed within mental status screenings or in conjunction with other cognitive skills such as executive functions. Standardized assessments such as the Test of Everyday Attention (Robertson et al., 1994) evaluate multiple components of attention; however, attention is affected by the task and environmental context and should be observed across different situations.

Clinician-rated observational ratings scales such as the Moss Attentional Rating Scale (MARS) (Whyte, Hart, Bode, & Malec, 2003), which was developed for persons with TBI, can be used to characterize everyday attentional related behavior. Observations of functional performance across different tasks and contexts provide the opportunity to evaluate attentional behaviors such as the ability to stay on task, detect hazards, and notice important details.

Intervention

Interventions for addressing attention include strategy training, adaptations of task or environment, and remedial training.

Strategy Training for Attention. Strategy training for attention deficits during postacute rehabilitation for people with TBI has been recommended as a practice standard based on a review of evidence. Successful interventions included strategy training and self-awareness techniques such as training participants to recognize when they are experiencing information overload, they are off task, and need to take a time-out from a task when concentration begins to fade (Cicerone et al., 2011). Time pressure management strategies have been found to help people cope with situations in which the speed of information presented exceeds processing capacity (Fasotti, Kovacs, Eling, & Brouwer, 2000).

Metacognitive strategy attention training programs for children with brain injury have been reported by several studies (Luton, Reed-Knight, Loiselle, O'Toole, & Blount,

2011; Séguin, Lahaie, Matte-Gagné, & Beauchamp, 2017). For example, Luton et al. (2011) developed an attentional strategy training program that was applied to children ages 6 to 15 years with various neurological deficits. Children were taught strategies such as key phrases or "magic words" to help alert and prepare themselves for focusing. They were also taught to restate task directions in their own words and write down or draw visual cues to remind them what to do. The strategy program was associated with improvement in several aspects of parent-reported attention and children's performance on tasks measuring attention (see "Executive Functions, Organization, and Problem Solving" section).

Adaptations of Task or Environment. Adaptations can minimize attention demands within everyday activities, using techniques such as increasing saliency of items that require attention and reducing or limiting the amount of information presented to the client at one time. An example includes placing colored tape on house keys or on operating buttons of appliances (Toglia, 1993a).

The enhancement of salient cues in the environment can be used to promote desired behaviors, as emphasized in the environmental adaptation component of the NFA. In the task of brushing teeth, for example, unnecessary items should be removed from the sink, and the items that are required for use can be made prominent with contrasting colors. The contrasting colors of the toothbrush, toothpaste, and cup provide a cue to assist the client in attending to the different items. Other examples are described under "Executive Functions, Organization, and Problem Solving" section.

Remedial Training. Computer-based training that focuses on processing speed and/or working memory (see "Executive Functions, Organization, and Problem Solving" section) is most commonly used to treat attentional deficits. The Attention Process Training program is a popular remedial program for children and adults (Zickefoose, Hux, Brown, & Wulf, 2013). Recent evidence suggests that attention, especially in relation to processing speed, may be strongly related to functional abilities in healthy older adults (Ball, Edwards, & Ross, 2007). Processing speed training resulted in improved cognitive abilities in healthy adults after 10 years, less decline in self-reported IADL (Rebok et al., 2014), prolonged driving mobility (Ross et al., 2016), and lowered risk of dementia after a 10-year follow-up compared with untreated controls (Edwards et al., 2017). These results have not yet been replicated in persons with brain injury or other neurological impairments. An evidence-based review recommended that computer-based interventions for attention may be considered as an adjunct to treatment after TBI or stroke but did not recommend computer-based attentional tasks without some involvement and intervention by a therapist (Cicerone et al., 2011). (See the "Executive Functions, Organization, and Problem Solving" section.)

Spatial Neglect

Spatial neglect is a failure to orient to, respond to, or report stimuli that are presented on the side contralateral to the cerebral lesion in clients who do not have primary sensory or motor impairments (Heilman, Watson, & Valenstein, 2003). Because spatial neglect is more common after right hemisphere lesions, the left side of space is typically neglected. The term *neglect* connotes a volitional component to the disorder, but this is a misnomer. The client with spatial neglect is unaware of the incompleteness of his or her perception and responses to the environment. He or she often behaves as though one-half of the world does not exist. For example, following right hemisphere strokes, clients often begin scanning on the right side and miss or fail to explore most of the stimuli on the left.

Asymmetry may be observed in functional activities, drawing tasks, reading, and writing. In severe cases, clients may eat food on one side of their plate, shave one-half of their face, or dress one-half of their body without recognizing the problem. In milder cases, they may misread the first letter of a particular word or fail to attend information while crossing a street, shopping, or driving. Many clients with spatial neglect also exhibit anxiety or flattened affect (Toglia, 1991b).

Spatial neglect has been identified as a major factor impeding functional recovery in clients who have sustained strokes (Di Monaco et al., 2011; Spaccavento, Cellamare, Falcone, Loverre, & Nardulli, 2017; Viken, Samuelsson, Jern, Jood, & Blomstrand, 2012). Individuals with spatial neglect have more difficulty resuming ADL, have longer hospital stays (Chen, Hreha, Kong, & Barrett, 2015; R. Gillen, Tennen, & McKee, 2005), and are at increased risk for falls or accidents (Chen et al., 2015). In addition, neglect has been found to be a predictor of upper arm use during ADL, suggesting that neglect treatment could positively impact motor recovery (Vanbellingen et al., 2017).

Spatial neglect has been described as a heterogeneous disorder that includes different clinical subtypes and behavioral components (Barrett et al., 2006; Rode, Pagliari, Huchon, Rossetti, & Pisella, 2017). Spatial neglect can involve one or more modalities, can vary with the nature of the stimuli (e.g., verbal vs. nonverbal), and can encompass single objects or different spatial frames of space (i.e., extrapersonal or large space, peripersonal or space within reach, and personal or body space). For example, some clients demonstrate neglect symptoms in large spaces, such as a room (extrapersonal neglect) but do not have reduced awareness of their body (personal neglect) or difficulty on paper-and-pencil tasks (peripersonal neglect).

Neglect subtypes have also been proposed that involve internal mental images (representational neglect), decreased movement into or toward the contralesional space (motor neglect), or decreased ability to perceive sensory stimuli in contralesional space (sensory neglect) (Rode et al., 2017).

Evaluation

When evaluating clients with spatial neglect, occupational therapists must first distinguish between hemianopsia and spatial neglect. Visual field cuts (hemianopsia) are hemiretinal, whereas neglect is hemispatial. Clients with visual field cuts typically have awareness of their visual field loss and make compensatory head movements and turns. Spatial neglect may exist with or without hemianopsia, and one syndrome does not cause the other.

Assessment of spatial neglect typically involves cancellation tasks that require detection of target stimuli, distributed on both sides of space (see Table 58-2). Typically, most targets on the contralesional side of space are missed. The complexity of spatial neglect symptoms is not fully captured by traditional tests of neglect. Therefore, do not rely completely on test instruments in identifying spatial neglect.

The tasks used to assess neglect consist primarily of paper-and-pencil types of assessments. These tools suffer from two main limitations. First, some of the most commonly used tests, such as the cancellation task, do not provide information regarding different forms of neglect. The cancellation test provides information of spatial biases in attention in peripersonal space but not on personal neglect. Second, the traditional paper-and-pencil tests may be insensitive to mild forms of neglect. Azouvi, Jacquin-Courtois, and Luauté (2003) found that the Catherine Bergego Scale (CBS), a 10-item behavioral assessment of neglect that involves rating neglect in everyday tasks, was more sensitive than conventional tests. This was supported by Chen et al. (2015), who further developed the observational methods for assessment and scoring of the CBS and modified it as the Kessler Foundation Neglect Assessment Process (KF-NAP; Chen & Hreha, 2015).

Neglect symptoms that are not observed in structured or quiet environments may emerge under busy, real-world environments; therefore, environmental conditions need to be considered in assessment (Barrett et al., 2006). The different behavioral manifestations and subtypes of neglect also need to be considered during observation of performance (Barrett et al., 2006; Rode et al., 2017).

Dynamic assessment of spatial neglect provides information about task conditions that increase or decrease the symptoms of spatial neglect as well as the person's ability to respond to different types of cues or implement and carryover learned strategies to different situations. Toglia and Cermak (2009) describe a dynamic object search task that analyzes the ability to learn and apply a strategy across a series of search tasks in people with spatial neglect.

Intervention

Interventions aimed at spatial neglect include remedial training, strategy training, and adaptations of task or environment.

Remedial Training. A variety of interventions have been used to remediate disorders of spatial neglect, including visual scanning training (VST), prism adaptation (PA), eye patching, and neck vibration (Azouvi et al., 2017; G. Gillen et al., 2015). More recently, use of brain stimulation, mirror therapy (Wang et al., 2015), music (Guilbert, Clément, & Moroni, 2017), virtual reality (Ogourtsova, Souza Silva, Archambault, & Lamontagne, 2017), exergames (Tobler-Ammann et al., 2017), repetitive task specific practice (Grattan et al., 2016), and pharmacological agents have emerged as interventions, but evidence is limited.

Several systematic reviews have found the strongest level of evidence for VST or eye pursuit training in reducing neglect symptoms (Azouvi et al., 2017; Cicerone et al., 2011; G. Gillen et al., 2015). In spatial neglect, clients demonstrate decreased eye movements to the affected side, reflecting diminished attention to one side of the environment (Antonucci et al., 1995). Averbuch and Katz (2011) described systematic training in visual scanning that gradually increases the amount and complexity of information presented but, at the same time, teaches new strategies to improve impaired functioning. Cicerone et al. (2011) concluded that there is Level I evidence to support the use of visuospatial interventions that include practice in visual scanning because it improves compensation for spatial neglect and generalizes to everyday activities. Visual scanning training was therefore recommended as a practice standard for individuals with visual neglect after right hemisphere stroke (Cicerone et al., 2011).

The combination of forced limb activation or movements of the left arm or hand on the left side of space in conjunction with visual scanning also shows positive results, suggesting that a combination of treatment techniques may be more effective than one technique alone (Saevarsson, Halsband, & Kristjánsson, 2011). Nilsen, Gillen, Arbesman, and Lieberman (2015) illustrated the application of evidence on VST and other treatment techniques to OT intervention in a case description of a person with a stroke and spatial neglect.

General alertness training has been described in the treatment of neglect based on the premise that nonlateralized deficits in sustained attention and alertness frequently accompany the asymmetrical attentional deficits observed in neglect (Van Vleet & DeGutis, 2013). Gross motor activities involving vestibular input and whole-body movement in space increase general arousal and alertness and have been used in combination with visual scanning

activities to increase gaze and attention to the affected side (Cappa, Sterzi, Vallar, & Bisiach, 1987). Bilateral activities such as balloon volleyball, with the client hitting the balloon with his or her hands clasped together, are encouraged to incorporate the use of the affected side of the body. Also, the use of neck muscle vibration for 5 minutes before OT has been found to be beneficial for reducing the symptoms of neglect (Kamada, Shimodozono, Hamada, & Kawahira, 2011).

Other intervention techniques that have been recommended for clients with spatial neglect include the use of prisms and visual occlusion techniques. Partial visual occlusion methods attempt to force the person to use the neglected visual field by patching the eye ipsilateral to the lesion, patching the non-neglected half field of eyeglasses (Ianes et al., 2012; Tsang, Sze, & Fong, 2009), or darkening the non-neglected half field of eyeglasses (hemispatial sunglasses; Arai, Ohi, Sasaki, Nobuto, & Tanaka, 1997).

Prism adaptation has been shown to alleviate the symptoms of spatial neglect following stroke. Prisms cause an optical deviation of the visual field to the right so that objects appear to be moved farther to the right than they actually are. A systematic review of the impact of PA on daily life activities found evidence suggesting that PA improves daily functioning, particularly in the area of reading and writing (Champod, Frank, Taylor, & Eskes, 2018). Vaes et al. (2016) found an effect of PA after seven sessions on navigational skills up to 3 months posttreatment. Prism adaptation may affect some aspects of function more than others.

A study comparing VST, limb activation, and PA found that all three techniques were equally effective (Priftis, Passarini, Pilosio, Meneghello, & Pitteri, 2013). Similarly, there is limited evidence that virtual reality is more effective than conventional therapy in improving neglect symptoms (Ogourtsova et al., 2017).

It has been recommended that intervention for spatial neglect be tailored to the types of neglect symptoms that the person exhibits (Spaccavento et al., 2017). Although there is no gold standard for treatment of spatial neglect, it is clear that specific neglect training is effective in helping to reduce neglect symptoms and improve functional recovery in some clients, and individuals who do not respond to intervention have poorer functional outcomes (Matano, Iosa, Guariglia, Pizzamiglio, & Paolucci, 2015).

Strategy Training. Strategies for spatial neglect can be practiced within everyday tasks such as setting a table for several people, dealing a deck of cards to six people, identifying appointments on a wall calendar, reading a newspaper, addressing envelopes of different sizes, and identifying all of the pictures or chairs in the room. Because spatial neglect symptoms vary with the size of space, arrangement of space, and amount and density of information presented, these activity parameters need to be matched with the neglect symptoms and systematically varied and graded in treatment to match the task to the "just right level"; this is particularly emphasized in the multicontext approach. In some cases, intervention should emphasize large space activities; in other situations, activities should focus on tabletop tasks that involve visual detail. In general, activities that are unpredictable or involve stimuli randomly scattered on a table or page are more sensitive to the symptoms of spatial neglect than the activities that are arranged in a predictable, structured, or horizontal array (Ferber & Karnath, 2001). Intervention should include practice in identifying situations in which neglect symptoms are most likely to occur, such as filling multiple bowls with salad, placing cookie dough on a baking sheet, and arranging photographs in a picture album.

Individuals with spatial neglect do not always know when they are attending to the left side; therefore, intervention should assist clients in finding external cues that provide feedback about when they are indeed attending to the left. Before beginning a task, the client can find the edges of a page or table or the periphery of stimuli and mark it with an anchor or spatial point of reference such as colored tape, a colored highlighter, a bright object, or placement of his or her arm on the left border.

Auditory cueing using a beeper or alarm device can be combined with strategy training to remind the person to use a strategy or visual cue. The alarm device can require the client to scan space and attend to the left to turn off the sound (Seron, Deloche, & Coyette, 1989). Alternatively, devices with vibrating or auditory cues can be placed in left pockets, clipped on the left side of a belt, or placed on a wrist to encourage attention to the left side of the body (personal neglect). These are examples of combining compensation with environmental adaptation approaches. Occupational therapy practitioners are encouraged to use clinical reasoning skills to determine when a combination of approaches is beneficial for patients.

Other intervention strategies for spatial neglect include tactile search, use of mental imagery, and general alerting techniques. *Tactile search* includes teaching the client to feel the left side of space with eyes closed or to feel the left edges of objects before visual search. *Mental imagery* teaches imagining and describing familiar scenes or routes and using mental images during movement of limbs or visual scanning (Welfringer, Leifert-Fiebach, Babinsky, & Brandt, 2011). For example, reduction in neglect symptoms and increased performance on functional tasks were reported after a mental imagery program that involved teaching people with neglect to imagine their eyes as sweeping beams of a lighthouse from left to right across the visual field. Clients were cued to use this mental image during functional and therapy training tasks (McCarthy, Beaumont, Thompson, & Pringle, 2002; Niemeier, Cifu, & Kishore, 2001).

In addition to strategies specifically aimed at facilitating attention to the left side, strategies that focus on the general ability to sustain attention, or *general alerting techniques*, have also been found to reduce spatial neglect. For example, Robertson, Tegnér, Tham, Lo, and Nimmo-Smith (1995) taught clients with chronic spatial neglect to mentally tell themselves to "pay attention" and to tap loudly on a table.

It has been observed that response to strategy training depends on whether people with spatial neglect show improvements in their awareness (Tham, Ginsburg, Fisher, & Tegnér, 2001). This observation supports the use of the multicontext approach in the treatment of neglect. It underscores the importance of deeply embedding awareness training techniques, such as those described earlier, into all intervention activities. In addition, intervention activities that are meaningful and functional in nature have more effect on the discovery of disability and developing self-awareness (Tham et al., 2001). The integration of methods to promote awareness and strategy use is illustrated in a case description by Toglia (2011).

Adaptations of Task or Environment. Adaptation of the task or environment to enhance functional performance, even in the presence of neglect, is a key element of the functional cognitive approaches. Collaboration with caregivers and family members to minimize the effects of neglect within everyday environments involves identifying specific activities that are impacted by neglect symptoms and discussing potential solutions. This may include increasing the saliency of items on the left side, such as placing red tape on the client's wheelchair brakes, edges of doorways, and furniture, or placing brightly colored objects such as a napkin or cup on the left side. Techniques may also include rearranging the position or placement of items within a task or environment (Golisz, 1998).

Visual Processing and Visual Motor Impairments

Visual processing and visual motor impairments are associated with difficulties in ADL, mobility, and reduced participation (Beaudoin et al., 2013; G. Gillen, 2009). They are frequently observed after stroke, ABI, Parkinson disease, and other neurological disorders and have also been identified in adults with schizophrenia (P. D. Butler, Silverstein, & Dakin, 2008). Visual perceptual impairments are also a key feature of nonverbal learning disorders and have been hypothesized to contribute to difficulties in interpreting facial expressions and mathematics (Liddell & Rasmussen, 2005).

Visual perception can be viewed on an information-processing continuum involving the reception, organization, and assimilation of visual information.

On one end of the continuum, simple visual-processing tasks such as matching shapes or objects occur quickly and automatically with minimal effort. On the opposite end of the continuum, complex visual tasks that include unfamiliar stimuli or subtle discriminations within visually crowded arrays require slower and effortful processing. In this conceptualization, visual-processing dysfunction is defined as a decrease in the amount that the visual system is able to assimilate at any one time (Toglia, 1989). To understand a client's visual perceptual skills and the effects of impairments on functioning, OT practitioners analyze the activity conditions (complexity, amount, familiarity, and predictability) and context.

Problems in simple visual processing include the following:

- Difficulty in discriminating between objects, pictures of objects, and basic shapes
- Difficulty in detecting gross differences in size, position, direction, angles, and rotations
- Decreased ability to visually locate single visual targets in space or judge gross distance between two objects
- Decreased ability to detect simple part–whole relationships in objects or basic shapes

The person may have difficulty in familiar and routine activities and may easily misinterpret or misidentify objects. Failure to recognize an object is labeled visual agnosia. Toglia (1989) proposes that labels such as visual agnosia are too broad for the purposes of intervention because there are many different underlying reasons for object recognition difficulties. For example, a person might fail to attend to the critical feature of an object or the part of the object that identifies what it is (e.g., prongs of a fork). Attention might be captured by salient but irrelevant aspects of the object (e.g., the utensil's decorative handle). There might be an inability to process the overall shape and the details simultaneously, so the person might miss important details.

Complex visual processing skills are required in visually confusing environments; when there is abstract, unfamiliar, or detailed visual information; or in conditions under which the distinctive visual features are partially obscured (e.g., the object is rotated and partially hidden on a crowded desk). Dysfunction of complex visual perceptual skills may include decreased ability to detect subtle differences in shapes, features, objects, angles, size, location, distance, and position. A client might have difficulty recognizing and interpreting facial expressions or making sense out of ambiguous, incomplete, fragmented, or distorted visual stimuli. The client might misinterpret an object when it is in an unusual position or partially hidden. The person might experience increased difficulty in visually confusing, crowded, or dynamic environments. Everyday tasks such as finding items in a crowded closet, drawer, desk, or supermarket shelf; locating key information on a bill, map, or schedule; and copying or following a diagram might present difficulty. On these tasks, the person might misinterpret information, miss key visual details, or become sidetracked by irrelevant visual stimuli.

Visual motor skills include writing, copying, and drawing tasks (e.g., drawing a map, copying a design), or construction of tasks that involve assembling pieces into a whole (e.g., assembling a coffeepot). Clients may demonstrate difficulty on visual motor tasks for many reasons. For example, a client might have difficulty copying a diagram of a room because of a poor ability to scan, locate, align, position, or rotate items accurately; decreased planning and organization; spatial neglect; or impaired discrimination of size and angle.

The term *constructional apraxia* is used to refer to difficulty with drawing or assembly tasks that cannot be attributed to primary motor or sensory impairment, ideomotor apraxia, or general cognitive impairments (Farah, 2003). Constructional abilities are closely related to ADL performance (Neistadt, 1992; Warren, 1981). Clients may have difficulty dressing (dressing apraxia), orienting clothes correctly on a hanger, or assembling a sandwich or coffeepot. People with left-hemisphere parietal lesions tend to omit individual pieces or details in constructional tasks, whereas those with right-hemisphere lesions demonstrate spatial disorganization of the pieces and lose the overall gestalt (Kramer, Kaplan, Blusewicz, & Preston, 1991). Constructional apraxia is not a unitary syndrome. Impairments in different types of perceptual processing or spatial relations are thought to underlie constructional apraxia in both right- and left-hemisphere lesions (Laeng, 2006).

Evaluation

Evaluation of individuals with visual perceptual impairments involves examining visual foundations skills, visual abilities without a motor response, and visual motor skills. Visual foundation skills include visual acuity; ocular alignment; visual pursuits, or smooth tracking of moving objects; and saccades, or quick eye movements to place an object of interest in view. Visual fields should be evaluated prior to a visual processing evaluation to screen out visual problems that will interfere with the accuracy of perceptual testing (Cate & Richards, 2000).

Several clinical observations during functional tasks can alert occupational therapists to the need for a formal visual assessment, such as compensatory head movements and tilting, squinting, shutting of one eye, or a tendency to lose one's place while reading. The Brain Injury Visual Assessment Battery for Adults (biVABA) (Warren, 1998) is an example of an evaluation that includes screening of visual foundation skills. Any disruptions of foundational skills can affect interpretations of higher level visual processing assessments (Warren, 1993). Hanna, Hepworth, and Rowe (2017) present an updated review of screening methods for post-stroke visual impairment.

Standardized nonmotor assessments of visual perception (see Table 58-2) categorize visual perception into specific skills such as figure-ground, position in space, form constancy, spatial relations, and visual recognition. Persons with visual perceptual impairments may have difficulty performing various types of visual processing tasks for similar reasons (e.g., a tendency to over focus on parts, a tendency to miss visual details, failure to simultaneously attend to the details as well as the whole, and difficulty in keeping track of what was just seen). Therefore, Toglia (1989) recommended an approach that conceptualizes visual processing on a continuum and evaluates both conventional and unconventional objects under a variety of different activity conditions. In a dynamic approach to visual perception, the therapist systematically manipulates activity parameters and analyzes responses to cues to understand why a client is having difficulty accurately discriminating objects or visual stimuli (Toglia, 1989; Toglia & Cermak, 2009). Visual perceptual assessment should examine responses to activities with and without a motor response to examine differences in performance.

Visual motor skills are typically evaluated with contrived tasks such as block designs, puzzles, or copying designs; however, observation of everyday tasks provides the opportunity to analyze visual motor performance. The A-ONE standardized assessment (Árnadóttir, 1990) identifies the effect of visual spatial impairments on self-care tasks such as grooming, feeding, and dressing (G. Gillen, 2009). Informal observations in tasks such as copying a map route, assembling a coffeepot or woodworking project, wrapping a package, packing a lunchbox, or folding clothes can provide additional information on visual motor abilities (Figure 58-2). Symptoms of visual perceptual impairments may include angular deviations; improper position,

location, spacing, or alignment of parts; and spatial distortions. The client's ability to recognize and correct errors in alignment or position should be investigated. For example, some clients do not recognize visual spatial errors even when attention is directed to the problem area, whereas other clients recognize errors but are unable to correct them.

Intervention

Interventions may address visual foundation skills or visual processing skills with or without a motor response. Following are descriptions of interventions for visual foundation skills, strategy training, and adaptations of task or environment.

Visual Foundation Skills. Treatment of impairments in visual foundation skills such as visual acuity and contrast sensitivity, oculomotor skills, and visual fields generally involves adaptations such as large-print reading materials; magnifiers; talking devices; increasing contrast of edges, borders, or backgrounds; and changes in lighting. However, remedial exercises may be recommended for individuals with oculomotor or visual field deficits. For example, range of motion eye exercises to the involved muscle have been advocated for individuals with eye muscle paresis. Occlusion of the intact visual field with eye patching has been used to force use of the impaired visual field (Warren, 1993), and an Internet-based visual scanning application (Jacquin-Courtois, Bays, Salemme, Leff, & Husain, 2013) has been used to increase rapid visual search for individuals with visual field deficits. These treatments involve repetitions of graded activities and are linked directly to the remedial deficit specific approach.

Strategy Training. Strategies that maximize the client's ability to process visual information can include getting a sense of the whole before looking at the parts (Chen, Hartman, Galarza, & DeLuca, 2012); teaching the person to partition space before localizing details; using one's finger to scan, trace visual stimuli, or focus on details; covering or blocking visual stimuli when too much information is presented at once; verbalizing salient visual features or subtle differences; and mentally visualizing a particular item before looking for it (Toglia, 1989, 2011). These strategies can be trained within everyday activities that involve choosing among objects that are similar in shape and size (e.g., matching socks, sorting teaspoons and soup spoons); locating information within supermarket circulars, calendars, maps, or schedules; arranging information within grids or spreadsheets; copying patterns in arts and craft activities; or finding information in crowded drawers, shelves, tables, or bulletin boards.

Intervention involves careful manipulation of activity parameters. Activities that involve familiar items or

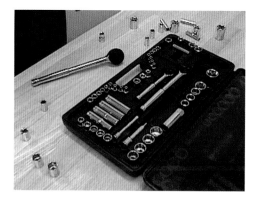

FIGURE 58-2 Organizing the components of a ratchet tool kit requires perception of size and shape as well as organizational skills.

contexts, high contrast (e.g., red socks and white socks), distinctive features, little detail, and solid colors or backgrounds require less attention, effort, and visual analysis than do activities that involve choosing among items that have low contrast (e.g., light beige and white socks), are in unusual positions, are embedded within crowded or distracting visual backgrounds, or are partially obscured. Changes in the familiarity, number of items, and degree of detail can place greater demands on visual processing. In addition, verbal mediation, including repeating a list of step-by-step instructions during a functional activity such as dressing, capitalizes on strengths in verbal abilities and can be effective in facilitating functional performance (Sunderland, Walker, & Walker, 2006). Strategies can be trained within a multicontext paradigm, in which activities are graded within the "just right challenging level" for each client, or within a compensational paradigm in which strategy is trained within a specific task context.

Adaptations of Task or Environment. The key guideline in minimizing the effects of visual perceptual difficulties is to make the distinctive features of objects more salient with color cues. An example is placing colored tape on buttons to operate appliances or using salient color cues on objects to make them easier to locate and discriminate (e.g., bright pink tape on a medication bottle). Cues such as colored marks or tape at spatial landmarks (e.g., tape recorder, wheelchair footrests, or label of a shirt) reduce spatial demands and make it easier to orient and align parts of an item. Visual stimuli such as items on a shelf or sentences on a page that are large and arranged in an organized manner with large spaces between items are easier to perceive. Consistent locations for objects (e.g., in the refrigerator, closet, drawer, or a countertop) increase predictability and provide contextual cues for recognition. Caregivers and family should be instructed to decrease visual distractions in rooms and within tasks by limiting designs and patterns and by using solid colors with high contrast. Patterns, designs, and decorations make it harder to select and recognize critical features of an object. They should also be trained to introduce only a small amount of visual information at one time.

Motor Planning

Motor planning, or **praxis**, is the ability to execute learned and purposeful activities. **Apraxia** is defined as a disorder of skilled movement that cannot be adequately explained by primary motor or sensory impairments, visual spatial problems, language comprehension difficulties, or cognitive problems alone (Heilman & Rothi, 2003). Apraxia has also been described as action disorganization syndrome, characterized by difficulty with tool use and multistep actions (Worthington, 2016).

It has been suggested that apraxia is primarily a disorder of *learned* movement, whereas **developmental dyspraxia** or DCD represents difficulties in the *acquisition* of motor skills in the absence of a physical or neurological disorder in children (Tempest & Roden, 2008). Decreased motor learning, however, has also been observed in adults with apraxia (Poole, 1998). A study comparing adults with apraxia and children with dyspraxia found that both groups made similar types of errors, suggesting similarities in behavioral manifestations (Poole, 2000).

Apraxia occurs most commonly after stroke; however, it can also be seen in persons with dementia, Parkinson disease, and movement disorders such as Huntington's chorea (Vanbellingen & Bohlhalter, 2011). Apraxia may be seen after lesions in either hemisphere, although it is more frequently encountered in clients who have sustained a left-hemisphere lesion. Aphasia is often associated with apraxia because the left hemisphere is also dominant for language (Heilman & Rothi, 2003).

Apraxia can significantly impact ADL, functional outcome, and the ability to engage in meaningful activities (G. Gillen, 2009; Vanbellingen & Bohlhalter, 2011). Wetter, Poole, and Haaland (2005) found that limb apraxia is a better predictor of functional motor skills after left hemisphere damage than aphasia. Further, apraxia can increase caregiver burden (Lindsten-McQueen, Weiner, Wang, Josman, & Connor, 2014). Apraxia can persist over time, and individuals can continue to have significant functional limitations in both the learning of new motor tasks, such as one-handed shoe tying, and in the efficiency and accuracy of actions to verbal command or demonstration (Poole, 2000). Similarly, children with dyspraxia or DCD may present with functional difficulties in writing, riding a bike, self-care tasks, and engaging in sports (Kirby, 2011).

Roy (1978) identifies two major subsystems in apraxia: the conceptual and the production subsystems. Difficulties in motor planning may reflect disorders in one or both subsystems. The production aspect of motor planning, traditionally called *ideomotor apraxia*, involves generating the action plan, sequencing and organizing the appropriate elements, and carrying out the plan (e.g., reaching for a glass of water to take a drink). The greatest difficulty is observed when the client is asked to pretend to use a tool or object or to perform limb gestures. Some improvement may be seen when the client is asked to imitate the motion or perform the motion with the actual object, but the movement is still imprecise. These clients know what they want to do, but actions are carried out in an awkward, inefficient, or clumsy manner. Errors of preservation, sequencing, or omissions may be observed.

The conceptual aspect of motor planning (Roy, 1978) includes knowledge about the functional properties of an object, the object action, and the sequence of action. Conceptual or ideation errors, traditionally called *ideational apraxia*, involve object function, action knowledge, and knowledge of sequence. Clients might be able to accurately identify and match objects, but difficulties in sequencing or choosing appropriate objects or tools may be observed. For example, the client might try to brush his or her hair with a toothbrush. Although object recognition may be intact, the person might be unable to associate the object with its correct action plan. Dressing apraxia and constructional apraxia are additional subtypes of apraxia, previously described in the section on visual processing and visual motor impairments. Traditional labels of apraxia are narrow in scope and do not account for the wide range of skills that underlie motor planning and constructional abilities.

Evaluation

Motor planning and action sequencing involve an integration of multiple skills including visual spatial, executive functions, language, and somatosensory skills as well as knowledge and understanding of object properties and sequences. Occupational therapy practitioners are encouraged to analyze error patterns and the underlying factors contributing to difficulties in performance rather than attempt to classify clients within traditional categories. If aphasia and apraxia coexist, information on the client's language skills should be obtained from a speech-language pathologist or be screened for by testing for "yes" or "no" comprehension and ability to follow one-step commands.

In evaluating apraxia, the clinician typically observes the client's performance of different types of functional movements and tasks, noting the method of evocation (e.g., command, imitation, or object use), quality of movement, type of errors made, and the influence of familiarity and context (Haaland, 1993). Error patterns can be generally categorized into errors of production or errors of ideation. Assessments for apraxia are listed in Table 58-2. An observational method for assessing apraxia in ADL, adapted from the A-ONE, has been validated for people with stroke (van Heugten et al., 2000). May-Benson and Cermak (2007) developed the Test of Ideational Praxis (TIP) to objectively assess conceptual or ideational abilities in children. The CO-OP method has described DPA to identify breakdowns in task performance in children with DCD. In addition, Toglia (2011) described a dynamic assessment approach for adults with aphasia and apraxia that analyzes response to cues across functional tasks with increasing number of steps.

Intervention

Worthington (2016) and Lindsten-McQueen et al. (2014) describe treatment for limb apraxia with adults, and Zwicker, Missiuna, Harris, and Boyd (2012) and Wilson, Ruddock, Smits-Engelsman, Polatajko, and Blank (2013) describe treatment for children. Interventions to overcome motor planning deficits may emphasize either the production aspect or the conceptual aspect of motor planning (Roy, 1985).

Techniques that address the orientation of an object or limb in space or the timing, sequence, and organization of the motor elements aim to enhance the production aspect of motor planning. For example, the practitioner can provide physical contact (i.e., hand-over-hand assistance or light touch) to limit inappropriate or extraneous movements while using guiding methods to facilitate a smooth motor pattern or guide the manipulation of objects within functional tasks. Through repeated practice in different tasks using task-specific methods or errorless learning, the client begins to learn the movement patterns that feel "right," and the practitioner gradually withdraws assistance. G. Gillen (2009) provides detailed suggestions for guiding limbs during functional activities, including guidance of both sides of the body when possible, providing changes in resistance during the activity, and keeping talking to a minimum.

Familiar tasks that are performed in context are easier for people with motor planning disorders because the context provide cues that facilitate the desired action. Interventions can be graded by gradually increasing the number of tools and distractors, increasing the degrees of freedom (G. Gillen, 2009), or introducing activities and environments that have less stability and predictability, such as negotiating around obstacles in a crowded store.

Intervention addressing the conceptual aspect of motor planning focuses on facilitating the client's understanding of how an object is used or how a gesture is performed (Pilgrim & Humphreys, 1994; Smania et al., 2006).

Strategy Training. Clients may be taught to generate or use verbal, visual, and tactile cues to enhance movement. For example, before performing an activity, the client can mentally practice or imagine the task performance (e.g., making tea), or imagine how an object should look in his or her hand before picking it up. Audiotapes or verbal scripts can be used to guide mental practice (Wu, Radel, & Hanna-Pladdy, 2011). Incorrect patterns of movement, such as holding an object in the wrong way, can also be visualized with an emphasis on having the client solve the problem and mentally practice correcting the movement.

Talking to a client through action sequences or use of step-by-step written lists or illustrations can be useful in facilitating functional performance in tasks such as drinking from a cup (J. A. Butler, 1999). The person can be taught to verbally rehearse an action sequence or associate the movement with a rhyme, rhythm, or musical tune with a gradual fading of the verbalization. Self-monitoring strategies can be used to teach a client to monitor unnecessary contraction, incomplete actions, and difficulty in switching direction of movements.

Treatment can also focus on a task analysis of the movements and articulation of goal-directed tasks. The treatment begins with physical manipulation plus verbalization of task elements (e.g., "reach the cup, grab the cup, carry to my lips, drink, stop"), and those cues are systematically withdrawn as performance improved (Pilgrim & Humphreys, 1994).

The use of strategies typically requires metacognitive skills. Models that focus on strategies, therefore, also typically emphasize metacognitive skills (as in the compensatory approach or multicontextual approach). Reviews of apraxia interventions have indicated that strategy training is the most promising intervention for improving everyday function (Geusgens et al., 2006; Lindsten-McQueen et al., 2014; Worthington, 2016). For example, in a randomized study design, changes on nontrained ADL were greater in a group of people with stroke who had received strategy training as compared with those receiving usual OT. This suggests that the strategies are generalized to everyday activities (Geusgens et al., 2006). Similarly, the CO-OP approach, which emphasizes strategy use, has been demonstrated to be effective in improving impairments, activity, and participation in children with DCD (Thornton et al., 2016). Strategy training has been recommended as a practice standard due to the evidence supporting it (Cicerone et al., 2011).

Adaptations of Task or Environment. Simple adaptations to objects that draw attention to the critical features of the object or activity can facilitate action and motor planning (e.g., colored tape on the knife handle or toothbrush handle). Patterns and designs on utensils or clothing might draw attention to the wrong detail and result in an inappropriate motor response.

Tool use should be minimized (Poole, 2000), and adaptive equipment should be selected with caution for clients with apraxia. For example, some adaptations such as a button hook, one-handed shoe tying, or a one arm drive wheelchair might be confusing for clients with apraxia and place greater demands on motor planning abilities. Other adaptations, such as adaptive clothing closures, may simplify the task or motor pattern required to manipulate or hold objects, reduce the number of steps, and facilitate function in the client with apraxia.

Training caregivers to modify instructions so that the activity is broken into one command at a time and to use simple whole commands (e.g., "Get up") can put the activity on an automatic level and effectively enhance motor planning (Zoltan, 2007). Another treatment that is in line with this approach is the multiple-cues treatment method (Maher, Rothi, & Greenwald, 1991), which uses presentation of multiple cues including tools, objects, visual models, and feedback. Errors are corrected using imitation and physical manipulation. As performance improves, cues

are systematically withdrawn. This method of treatment is based on the NFA, which emphasizes mastery of functional task performance through practice rather than on the underlying skills that are needed to perform the task. Intervention involves breaking down a functional task into small subcomponents and provides reinforcement and chaining when needed (Giles, 2018).

Memory

Memory gives individuals the ability to draw on past experiences and learn new information (Dudai, Karni, & Born, 2015). This provides us with a sense of continuity in the environment and frees us from dependency in here-and-now situations. Memory is conceptualized as a multistep process involving encoding (i.e., input of information), storage (i.e., holding information), and retrieval (i.e., getting information, Levy, 2011b). There are different types of memory. *Declarative memory* is an aspect of long-term memory that includes conscious memory for events, knowledge, or facts. *Procedural (nondeclarative) memory* involves the ability to remember how to perform an activity or procedure without conscious awareness. *Prospective memory* involves the ability to remember intentions or activities that will be required in the future (Levy, 2011b).

Evaluation

It is important to distinguish whether everyday memory problems are due to failures to keep track of a conversation or what was just said (e.g., working memory), recall of past events or conversations from the day before (e.g., declarative, event-based memory), or failures in carrying out future activities (e.g., prospective memory). A comprehensive evaluation of memory, whether static or dynamic, must address the different types of memory and methods of retrieval (see Table 58-2). Assessments must consider factors such as the modality in which the information is presented (auditory, verbal, or visual), the type of instructions (general or specific), the amount of stimuli presented, the familiarity and meaningfulness of the information, the presence of contextual cues during recall phases, the type of information to be remembered (factual or skill related), and the length of retention. Dynamic assessment of memory such as Toglia's (1993b) CMT evaluates awareness of memory capabilities and use of strategies.

Intervention

Memory impairments can be closely related to other cognitive impairments, particularly attention and processing speed. Some investigators have suggested that an indirect approach that addresses other cognitive skills such as attention, organization, and processing speed (Chiaravalloti, Christodoulou, Demaree, & DeLuca, 2003; Leavitt, Lengenfelder, Moore, Chiaravalloti, & DeLuca,

2011) rather than memory may be effective. For example, Sohlberg and Mateer (1989a) reported improvement in memory function after attentional training using a remedial approach. Interventions for memory impairments include memory strategy training; external aids and devices; and adaptations as well as techniques of errorless learning, vanishing cues, and spaced retrieval, which were discussed earlier in this chapter. In addition, some researchers found that in order to benefit from memory treatment and use of strategies, one needs to present with good working memory (Sandry, Chiou, DeLuca, & Chiaravalloti, 2016) and executive functions (Goverover, Chiaravallot, & DeLuca, 2013).

Strategy Training.

Training of internal memory strategies is most appropriate for people with mild memory deficits and those in whom other areas of cognition are intact (Cicerone et al., 2011). The client practices one or two targeted memory strategies in various different tasks such as remembering telephone numbers, news headlines, a sequence of errands, items that need to be bought in a store, and instructions to an activity. During practice on different memory tasks, various awareness training techniques are used if the therapist selects the multicontext approach to guide intervention. The client may be trained on a specific strategy to facilitate performance of one specific task, or treatment could emphasize learning several strategies and determining which works best based on the content to be remembered and the task.

Memory strategies may be directed primarily at encoding operations (i.e., getting information in) or the retrieval phase of memory (i.e., getting information out). Recently, some RCTs were conducted to test the efficacy of memory strategies. For example, Chiaravalloti, Moore, Nikelshpur, and DeLuca (2013) and Chiaravalloti, Sandry, Moore, and DeLuca (2016) examined the efficacy of the modified Story Memory Technique (mSMT) to improve learning (i.e., acquisition) and memory in participants with MS and TBI. The mSMT is a behavioral intervention that teaches context and imagery to facilitate learning. The studies found that the mSMT is effective for improving learning and memory in TBI and MS.

Recently, Goverover, Chiaravalloti, Genova, and DeLuca (2017) examined the efficacy of the self-generation learning program (self-GEN trial), which consists of behavioral intervention sessions, teaching self-generation technique while using metacognitive strategies to improve learning and memory abilities in persons with MS. Additionally, the treatment aimed to address generalization of the inatervention to ADL. They found that the study provided evidence that the self-GEN behavioral intervention improves memory, self-regulation, functional status, affective symptomatology, and quality of life in patients with MS.

Memory External Strategies, Aids, and Technology.

Everyday technology such as smartphones, notebooks (digital or paper), voice recorders, tablets, and computers can store information that a person may have difficulty remembering. In addition, preprogrammed text messages and alarms can remind a person to perform an action (prospective memory) (Gentry, 2018). Intervention programs can use a combination of external aids and strategies with awareness training to improve prospective memory (Shum, Fleming, Gill, Gullo, & Strong, 2011). Devices and aids that can support memory function include the following: timers, voice recorders, alarm messages on smart devices, electronic devices such as pillbox organizers, lists, daily planners or notebooks, smart watches, and commercially available applications (i.e., apps) for mobile/smart phones, tablets, and computers (Figure 58-3). Studies have documented the effectiveness of technology and aids to support memory (Bos, Babbage, & Leathem, 2017; Dewar, Kapur, & Kopelman, 2018; Evald, 2017). Intervention is most effective when the client is motivated, involved in identifying the memory problem, and fairly independent in daily function (Cicerone et al., 2011).

Evidence obtained from case studies supports the use of technology and aids in reducing everyday memory failures for people with moderate-to-severe memory impairments (Bos et al., 2017; Cicerone et al., 2011; Goodwin, Lincoln, das Nair, & Bateman, 2017; McDonald et al., 2011). More individuals with and without memory impairments are using technologies that support memory such as online calendars and smart watches, making them more socially acceptable. Recent studies support the use of online calendars that are synced with smart phones in

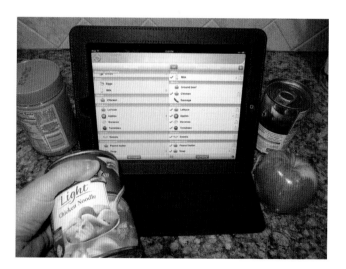

FIGURE 58-3 Use of an iPad app to aid organizing grocery shopping for clients with memory and executive function impairments.

reducing everyday memory failures (Cruz, Petrie, Goudie, Kersel, & Evans, 2016; Evald, 2017). Use of electronic reminder systems has been recommended as a practice guideline in supporting the everyday functioning of people with ABI (Charters, Gillett, & Simpson, 2015).

The successful use of a new device or memory aid may require extensive training and may not fit every client who present with memory problems. In a recent RCT, Dewar et al. (2018) found a significant treatment effect of training within a Memory Aids Service on the goal attainment diary but only at 12 weeks follow-up. Treatment was effective for participants with a nonprogressive condition but not for participants with a progressive condition. Importantly, the client may need to practice initiating and using the device or aid in various situations.

The use of external devices may need to be graded. In the initial stages, the client might be expected to use the aid or device only when it is initiated by another person. Gradually, the client can be trained to initiate the use of the aid independently. Errorless learning, spaced retrieval, and other task-specific training methods that capitalize on procedural memory and are core components of the NFA may be used in training clients with moderate or severe memory impairments to use an external aid.

Researchers have also examined how memory aids and technology can be adapted and developed for other users such as the older adult (Bayen et al., 2013). These technologies are focused on supporting the users' abilities rather than strengthening them. Compensation systems that have been developed for older adults range from simple reminder systems to home robotic support systems (Bayen et al., 2013). The person's needs and lifestyle should be considered when selecting devices or memory aids (McKerracher, Powell, & Oyebode, 2005). Devices that were used previous to the memory impairment may tap into procedural memory and be more easily accepted and used to support memory.

Training to use aids or devices as memory support needs to take place in the context of various everyday activities. Therapy sessions should include role-playing and practice in the use of the aid. For example, memory notebook training protocols have been described in the literature that incorporate the memory system within treatment sessions (Greenaway, Duncan, & Smith, 2013). Greenaway et al. (2013) found the use of a notebook/calendar system with individuals with amnestic mild cognitive impairment significantly improved functional ability and memory self-efficacy up to 8 weeks later, compared to a control group.

The continued development of mobile devices (e.g., smart phones, tablets, smart watches, and apps) and smart home technology offers emerging technology and opportunities to support individuals with memory impairments.

Some of the current trends in the use of technology in rehabilitation include the following:

- Smart home voice-activated "assistants" can be programmed with reminders and instructions to support performance of everyday activities (Boman, Bartfai, Borell, Tham, & Hemmingsson, 2010; Gentry, 2018) as well as enable remote monitoring of the individual by family.
- Reminder apps for smartphones and tablets can send text reminders or alarms to remind individuals to complete tasks.
- Wearable devices, such as smart glasses, watches, or cameras such as SenseCam (Silva, Pinho, Macedo, & Moulin, 2018), allow for continuous recording of everyday life in the real world over an extended period of time.
- Apps for IADL tasks such as grocery shopping can help clients categorize and arrange items in a logical manner (see Figure 58-3). Other apps may help the individual correctly sequence a task through video/photo modeling and/or voice instructions.

Adaptations of Task or Environment. A therapist applying the principles of the CDM can rearrange tasks and environments so that they place fewer demands on memory. For example:

- Cue cards or signs in key places (e.g., a sign on door where it will be seen before leaving: "Take keys and . . . ")
- Labeling the outside of drawers or closets to minimize the need to recall the location of items
- Providing step-by-step directions to reduce memory demands
- Providing checklists to assist in keeping track of task steps (Figure 58-4)

Significant others can be trained to use methods that increase the likelihood that the client will remember

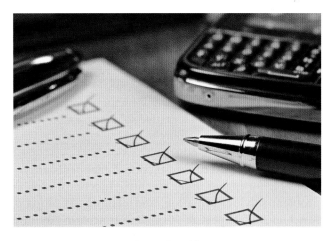

FIGURE 58-4 Providing checklists to assist in keeping track of task steps.

material, such as asking the client to repeat any instructions or important information in his or her own words; encouraging the client to ask questions; and presenting material in small groups, clusters, or categories (Levy, 2011a).

Executive Functions, Organization, and Problem Solving

Executive functions encompass a broad range of skills that allow a person to engage in independent, purposeful, and self-directed behavior. There are three core executive functions: inhibition, working memory, and cognitive flexibility.

Inhibition, or inhibitory control, includes self-control and interference control (selective attention and cognitive inhibition). Examples include resisting distractions when finding specific items in a closet, restraining impulsive responses, and staying within a fixed budget when shopping. In these cases, executive functions demands are increased as the number of items presented simultaneously increase; at times, it is easier to give into temptation than to resist it (Theeuwes, 2010).

Working memory involves holding information in mind and mentally working with it (i.e., working with information no longer perceptually present) (McCabe, Roediger, McDaniel, Balota, & Hambrick, 2010). Examples include keeping track of what has already been done in a multistep cooking task and remembering which medication or pill was just taken. Children who have trouble with their working memory skills may have difficulty remembering their teachers' instructions, recalling the rules to a game, and paying attention. Working memory skills enable remembering details that otherwise require further attention if impairment exist.

Cognitive flexibility (also referred to as set shifting, mental flexibility, and mental set shifting) is closely linked to creativity. Examples include the ability to shift between adding and subtracting when balancing a checkbook, answering the telephone, and going back to typing, or baking a cake while following a written recipe. In addition, limitations in the ability to view information from different perspectives, generate alternative solutions, and respond flexibly can reduce the ability to cope, adapt to everyday demands, and relate to others.

These three executive function components are responsible for higher order executive functions, such as problem solving, initiation, and planning (Collins & Koechlin 2012; Lunt et al., 2012). Impairments in executive functions are associated with prefrontal lesions and may involve all of these components, with one or two areas of impairment especially prominent (Alvarez & Emory, 2006).

Impairments in executive functions can affect mental and physical health; success in school and in life; and cognitive, social, and psychological development (Diamond, 2013; Voelbel et al., 2011). In addition, impaired executive function can affect the ability to benefit from treatment (Goverover et al., 2013; Sandry et al., 2016).

Executive function impairments represent a distinct challenge because they can be masked within familiar ADL or routines but are most apparent when the client is required to function in situations that are less structured, require multitasking, and require managing novel and unexpected situations (Redick et al., 2016).

Evaluation

Most standardized cognitive assessments are structured and do not adequately examine the area of executive functions (Sohlberg & Mateer, 2001) (see Table 58-2). Newer ecologically valid evaluations for executive function have been designed such as the Multiple Errands Test (Morrison et al., 2013), its home version (Burns & Neville, 2017), a virtual version (Cipresso et al., 2014), the Executive Function Performance Test (Baum et al., 2008), and the WCPA (Toglia, 2015).

Intervention

Interventions for impairments in executive functions include remedial deficit specific training, strategy training, and adaptations of task or environment.

Remedial Deficit Specific Training. Recently, several commercial, computer-based, working memory training programs have been developed. A well-known program is CogMed (http://www.cogmed.com/), which is widely used in schools and clinics. This program is based on eight different exercises involving both visuospatial and verbal working memory tasks, in which the difficulty level varies adaptively during training. Other commercially available working memory training programs include Jungle Memory (http://www.junglememory.com/), which is based on three different tasks, and CogniFit (http://www.cognifit.com/), which is based on auditory, visual, and cross-modal working memory tasks. Melby-Lervåg and Hulme (2013) conducted a meta-analysis on the benefit of computerized programs in children with attention-deficit/hyperactivity disorder (ADHD) and concluded that working memory training programs appear to produce short-term, specific training effects that do not generalize. Additionally, Lampit, Hallock, and Valenzuela, (2014) conducted a meta-analysis related to the use of computerized cognitive training in older adults. However, no significant effects were found for executive functions and attention. Thus, more research is needed on the effect of remedial deficit specific executive functions treatment; specifically, data about its transfer and generalization is needed.

Strategy Training. Strategies that maximize executive functioning can be practiced in various unstructured tasks, such as organizing medications according to a schedule, planning an overnight trip and packing a suitcase, obtaining and organizing a list of local business phone numbers, and organizing tools. Strategy training can be learned using the multicontext approach (Toglia, Goverover, et al., 2011; Toglia et al., 2010). Toglia, Goverover, et al. (2011) and Foster et al. (2018) used a case study design to examine the application of the multicontext approach in the treatment of clients with brain injury and Parkinson and executive deficits. They demonstrated that a checklist strategy combined with self-awareness training and practice across multiple tasks improved the occupational performance of clients with executive function impairments.

Training in problem-solving strategies involves teaching the person to break down complex activities into smaller, more manageable steps. Strategies may also aim to help the person maintain the focus of goals and intentions (Skidmore et al., 2015; Skidmore et al., 2014). For example, a goal management training procedure was proposed (Levine et al., 2000; Levine et al., 2007), in which participants had to (1) "stop" and define what they are going to do, (2) "define" the main task, (3) "list" the steps, (4) "learn" the steps and *do* it, and (5) "check" if am I doing what I planned to do. A systematic review concluded that goal management training can be effective when integrated with other approaches such as problem-solving therapy, personal goal setting, external cueing or prompting apply goal management training to the current task, personal homework to increase patients' commitment and training intensity, and ecological and daily life training activities rather than paper-and-pencil, office-type tasks (Krasny-Pacini, Chevignard, & Evans, 2014). Cicerone et al. (2011) recommended such training as a practice guideline for people with stroke or brain injury during post-acute rehabilitation. The steps of the problem-solving process can be reinforced with the use of self-questioning techniques (as discussed earlier in this chapter) (e.g., Casaletto et al., 2016)

Broad checklists and task guidance systems are commonly used to assist clients in initiating, planning, and carrying out an activity systematically (e.g., Levine et al., 2000; Levine et al., 2007). Interventions should incorporate practice in identifying the situations or activities in which the use of a checklist could be helpful, as described in the multicontext approach (Foster et al., 2018; Toglia, Goverover, et al., 2011; Toglia et al., 2010). The client may be given the opportunity to practice the same activity with and without the use of a checklist to enhance awareness. Initially, the goal might be to have a client follow a checklist established by the practitioner, caregiver, or family member. Eventually, the client might be given checklists with missing steps and be asked to review the lists to identify the missing components. Finally, the client might be required to create a checklist

independently. Burke, Zencius, Wesolowski, and Doubleday (1991) describe four cases of individuals with executive dysfunction for whom checklists were successfully used to improve the ability to carry out routine vocational tasks.

Another example of intervention directed at enhancing strategy use is provided by a pilot study that examined the applicability of the CO-OP approach for use with adults with executive dysfunction arising from TBI. The intervention entailed guiding participants to use a metacognitive problem-solving strategy to perform self-identified daily tasks that they needed and wanted to do and with which they were having difficulties (Dawson et al., 2009).

Decreased initiation can interfere with the ability to use and apply a learned strategy. For example, a person with deficits in executive functions might use a strategy effectively when cued but not use the strategy spontaneously because of a failure to initiate its use. Therefore, external cues such as alarm signals or text messages can be used to prompt the client to initiate a task, switch to a different task component, use a strategy within an activity, or mentally review intentions (Evans, Emslie, & Wilson, 1998; Gracey et al., 2017).

Adaptations of Task or Environment. Adaptations that minimize demands on executive functions include training the caregiver or family to reduce the number of items or choices presented to the client at one time, decrease distractions such as clutter or interruptions, and preorganize an activity or activity materials. For example, all the items needed for grooming can be prearranged on the sink in the sequence in which they are used. As an alternative, one task step can be introduced at a time. These adaptations reduce demands on working memory, inhibitory control, and flexibility and limit the need for planning and organization (Sohlberg & Mateer, 2001).

People who have difficulty with initiation, organization, and decision making require structure. Open-ended questions such as "What do you want to eat" should be avoided. Clients who have difficulty in initiation will have a great deal of difficulty in answering open-ended questions. Questions should provide a limited number of choices whenever feasible.

A predictable and structured daily routine enhances the client's ability to initiate tasks and should be established and monitored by the caregiver or family. Audiotape instructions that cue the client to initiate an activity and perform each step at a time in its proper sequence have been reported to be successful within the context of daily routines (S. M. Schwartz, 1995).

Group Interventions

Cognitive rehabilitation principles and strategies can be incorporated within group programs and combined with psychosocial or psychoeducational interventions.

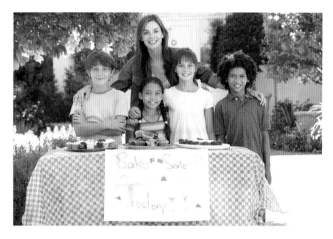

FIGURE 58-5 Planning and carrying out a bake sale is an appropriate group activity for those with executive function impairments.

The group format can be used to target specific cognitive skills, train the use of compensatory task methods, and facilitate the use of cognitive strategies (Revheim & Marcopulos, 2006; Stuss et al., 2007). Group activities can emphasize interpersonal skills within cooperative tasks such as planning a bake sale; publishing a newsletter; and role-playing scenarios involving interviews, conflicts, or on-the-spot problem solving (Figure 58-5). Strategies that include monitoring the tendency to respond impulsively, become stuck in one viewpoint, or wander off task can be practiced within social contexts (Toglia, 2018).

Group programs that center on teaching self-monitoring techniques and strategies for paying attention, remembering, organization, or problem solving can be applied to a wide spectrum of clients such as individuals with MS (Shevil & Finlayson, 2010), mental illness (Revheim & Marcopulos, 2006), lupus (Harrison et al., 2005), and ADHD (Hahn-Markowitz, Manor, & Maeir, 2011). Activities such as remembering names and facts about group members, recalling directions for operating a new electronic device, and creating a checklist for a complex task can provide opportunities to practice different strategies and share experiences within a group context. Group members can be encouraged to reflect on performance and identify strategies that would be useful in their everyday activities.

Group interventions that simultaneously address subtle cognitive difficulties and emotional issues have demonstrated value in improving self-awareness, self-efficacy, coping skills, psychosocial skills, and perceived daily functioning (Harrison et al., 2005; Rilo et al., 2018; Shevil & Finlayson, 2010; Toglia, 2018; Twamley et al., 2015). See Chapter 39 for more information on group process and intervention.

Occupational Therapy Role within the Rehabilitation Team

A strong interdisciplinary approach is needed to address the complex issues that arise from cognitive-perceptual problems. Team goals should be identified as well as specific discipline goals. The family, client, and caregivers, when appropriate, are also members of the team; they should be involved in team discussions and provide input into the overall intervention plan.

Once the targeted behaviors for intervention have been clearly identified, the occupational therapist and OT assistant collaborate to identify various activities that can be used to reinforce the desired behaviors. The work environment in which the therapist practices may determine the depth of the OT practitioner's involvement because of the nature of the practice setting and the client's length of stay.

An interdisciplinary intervention program should emphasize the same major goals during treatment rather than working on separate skills. For example, a speech-language pathologist might address attention problems within the context of language material such as listening to tapes or conversations; a neuropsychologist might use remedial attentional exercises; a physical therapist might reinforce attention through motor tasks; and an OT practitioner might address attentional strategies within the context of self-care, leisure, community, and/or work activities. An integrated approach that assists the person in seeing patterns of behaviors across different activities is strongly advocated rather than a fragmented approach.

Summary

Evidence supports the use of comprehensive cognitive rehabilitation programs that address a combination of cognitive, emotional, functional, and social participation skills in people with brain injury (Cappa et al., 2005; Cicerone et al., 2011; Cicerone, Mott, Azulay, & Friel, 2004; Sarajuuri et al., 2005; Tiersky et al., 2005). The need to blend cognitive interventions with those that address interpersonal and real-world functioning has been emphasized in recent literature; however, the outcome of cognitive rehabilitation is most commonly measured at the impairment level.

As occupational therapists return to more community-focused intervention, it is important to widen the perspective on the influence that cognitive-perceptual impairments have on clients' ability to engage in the occupations they need or want to do within the contexts of their lives. The effect of cognitive rehabilitation on occupational engagement and social participation need to be explored because even subtle cognitive impairments can decrease satisfaction, participation, and quality of life, preventing clients from leading enriching lives (McDowd, Filion, Pohl, Richards, & Stiers, 2003).

The outcome or benefit of cognitive rehabilitation needs to be examined broadly across different populations including effects on changing existing habits, routines, or increasing productive activity patterns; increasing the frequency and quality of social participation; decreasing caregiver assistance, stress, or burden; improving subjective well-being including self-efficacy, self-esteem, satisfaction, and quality of life; and preventing functional decline.

 Visit thePoint to watch a video about cognition and perception.

REFERENCES

Abreu, B. C., & Peloquin, S. M. (2005). The quadraphonic approach: A holistic rehabilitation model for brain injury. In N. Katz (Ed.), *Cognition and occupation across the life span* (2nd ed., pp. 73–112). Bethesda, MD: American Occupational Therapy Association.

Abreu, B. C., Seale, G., Scheibel, R. S., Huddleston, N., Zhang, L., & Ottenbacher, K. J. (2001). Levels of self-awareness after acute brain injury: How patients' and rehabilitation specialists' perceptions compare. *Archives of Physical Medicine and Rehabilitation, 82,* 49–55. doi:10.1053/apmr.2001.9167

Abreu, B. C., & Toglia, J. P. (1987). Cognitive rehabilitation: A model for occupational therapy. *American Journal of Occupational Therapy, 41,* 439–448.

Albert, M. L. (1973). A simple test of visual neglect. *Neurology, 23,* 658–665. doi:10.1212/wnl.23.6.658

Aldrich, F. K., & Wilson, B. (1991). Rivermead Behavioural Memory Test for Children (RBMTC): A preliminary evaluation. *British Journal of Clinical Psychology, 30,* 161–168. doi:10.1111/j.2044-8260.1991.tb00931.x

Allen, C. K. (1985). *Occupational therapy for psychiatric diseases: Measurement and management of cognitive disabilities.* Boston, MA: Little Brown.

Allen, C. K. (1987). Activity: Occupational therapy's treatment method. 1987 Eleanor Clarke Slagle. *American Journal of Occupational Therapy, 41,* 563–575. doi:10.5014/ajot.41.9.563

Allen, C. K., Earhart, C. A., & Blue, T. (1992). *Occupational therapy treatment goals for the physically and cognitively disabled.* Bethesda, MD: AOTA Press.

Alvarez, J., & Emory, E. (2006). Executive function and the frontal lobes: A meta-analytic review. *Neuropsychology Review, 16,* 17–42. doi:10.1007/s11065-006-9002-x

American Occupational Therapy Association. (2013). Management of occupational therapy services for persons with cognitive impairments. *American Journal of Occupational Therapy, 67,* S9–S31. doi:10.5014/ajot.2013.67S9

American Occupational Therapy Association. (2014). Occupational therapy practice framework: Domain and process (3rd ed.). *American Journal of Occupational Therapy, 68*(Suppl. 1), S1–S48. doi:10.5014/ajot.2014.682006

Anderson, R. L., Doble, S. E., Merritt, B. K., & Kottorp, A. (2010). Assessment of Awareness of Disability measures among persons with acquired brain injury. *Canadian Journal of Occupational Therapy, 77,* 22–29. doi:10.2182/cjot.2010.77.1.4

Anderson, K., Jue, S. G., & Madaras-Kelly, K. J. (2008). Identifying patients at risk for medication mismanagement: Using cognitive screens to predict a patient's accuracy in filling a pillbox. *The Consultant Pharmacist, 23,* 459–472.

Antonucci, G., Guariglia, C., Judica, A., Magnotti, L., Paolucci, S., Pizzamiglio, L., & Zoccolotti, P. (1995). Effectiveness of neglect rehabilitation in a randomized group study. *Journal of Clinical and Experimental Neuropsychology, 17,* 383–389. doi:10.1080/01688639508405131

Arai, T., Ohi, H., Sasaki, H., Nobuto, H., & Tanaka, K. (1997). Hemispatial sunglasses: Effect on unilateral spatial neglect. *Archives of Physical Medicine and Rehabilitation, 78,* 230–232. doi:10.1016/s0003-9993(97)90269-0

Árnadóttir, G. (1990). *The brain and behavior: Assessing cortical dysfunction through activities of daily living.* St. Louis, MO: Mosby.

Aubin, G., Chapparo, C., Gélinas, I., Stip, E., & Rainville, C. (2009). Use of the perceive, recall, plan and perform system of task analysis for persons with schizophrenia: A preliminary study. *Australian Occupational Therapy Journal, 56,* 189–199. doi:10.1111/j.1440-1630.2007.00725.x

Averbuch, S., & Katz, N. (2011). Cognitive rehabilitation: A retraining model for clients with neurological disabilities. In N. Katz (Ed.), *Cognition, occupation, and participation across the life span: Neuroscience, neurorehabilitation, and models of intervention in occupational therapy* (3rd ed., pp. 277–298). Bethesda, MD: AOTA Press.

Azouvi, P., Jacquin-Courtois, S., & Luauté, J. (2017). Rehabilitation of unilateral neglect: Evidence based medicine. *Annals of Physical and Rehabilitation Medicine, 60,* 191–197. doi:10.1016/j.rehab.2016.10.006

Azouvi, P., Olivier, S., Montety, G., Samuel, C., Louise-Dreyfus, A., & Luigi, T. (2003). Behavioral assessment of unilateral neglect: Study of the psychometric properties of the Catherine Bergego Scale. *Archives of Physical Medicine and Rehabilitation, 84,* 51–57. doi:10.1053/apmr.2003.50062

Ball, K., Edwards, J. D., & Ross, L. A. (2007). The impact of speed of processing training on cognitive and everyday functions. *The Journals of Gerontology. Series B: Psychological Sciences and Social Sciences, 62,* 19–31. doi:10.1093/geronb/62.special_issue_1.19

Barrett, A. M., Buxbaum, L. J., Coslett, H. B., Edwards, E., Heilman, K. M., Hillis, A. E., . . . Robertson, I. H. (2006). Cognitive rehabilitation interventions for neglect and related disorders: Moving from bench to bedside in stroke patients. *Journal of Cognitive Neuroscience, 18,* 1223–1236. doi:10.1162/jocn.2006.18.7.1223

Baum, C. M., Connor, L. T., Morrison, T., Hahn, M., Dromerick, A. W., & Edwards, D. F. (2008). Reliability, validity, and clinical utility of the Executive Function Performance Test: A measure of executive function in a sample of people with stroke. *American Journal of Occupational Therapy, 62,* 446–455. doi:10.5014/ajot.62.4.446

Baum, C. M., & Edwards, D. F. (1993). Cognitive performance in senile dementia of the Alzheimer's type: The Kitchen Task Assessment. *American Journal of Occupational Therapy, 47,* 431–436. doi:10.5014/ajot.47.5.431

Baum, C. M., & Edwards, D. F. (1998). *Home Occupational Environmental Assessment: An environmental checklist for treatment planning.* Unpublished manuscript, University School of Medicine, St. Louis, MO.

Baum, C. M., & Edwards, D. F. (2001). *ACS: Activity Card Sort.* St. Louis, MO: Washington University School of Medicine.

Baum, C. M., Edwards, D. F., Morrison, T., & Hahn, M. (2003). *Executive Function Performance Test.* St. Louis, MO: Washington University School of Medicine.

Bayen, U. J., Dogangün, A., Grundgeiger, T., Haese, A., Stockmanns, G., & Ziegler, J. (2013). Evaluating the effectiveness of a memory aid system. *Gerontology, 59,* 77–84. doi:10.1159/000339096

Beaudoin, A., Fournier, B., Julie-Caron, L., Moleski, L., Simard, J., Mercier, L., & Desrosiers, J. (2013). Visuoperceptual deficits and participation in older adults after stroke. *Australian Occupational Therapy Journal, 60,* 260–266. doi:10.1111/1440-1630.12046

Ben-Yishay, Y. (1978). *Working approaches to remediation of cognitive deficits in brain damaged persons* (Rehabilitation Monograph No. 59). New York, NY: New York University Medical Center.

Bier, N., Provencher, V., Gagnon, L., Van der Linden, M., Adam, S., & Desrosiers, J. (2008). New learning in dementia: Transfer and spontaneous use of learning in everyday life functioning. Two case studies. *Neuropsychological Rehabilitation, 18*, 204–235. doi:10.1080/09602010701406581

Blessed, G., Tomlinson, B. E., & Roth, M. (1968). The association between quantitative measures of dementia and of senile change in the cerebral gray matter of elderly subjects. *The British Journal of Psychiatry, 114*, 797–811. doi:10.1192/bjp.114.512.797

Boman, I. L., Bartfai, A., Borell, L., Tham, K., & Hemmingsson, H. (2010). Support in everyday activities with a home-based electronic memory aid for persons with memory impairments. *Disability and Rehabilitation, 5*, 339–350. doi:10.3109/17483100903131777

Bos, H. R., Babbage, D. R., & Leathem, J. M. (2017). Efficacy of memory aids after traumatic brain injury: A single case series. *NeuroRehabilitation, 41*, 463–481. doi:10.3233/NRE-151528

Bottari, C., Gosselin, N., Guillemette, M., Lamoureux, J., & Ptito, A. (2011). Independence in managing one's finances after traumatic brain injury. *Brain Injury, 25*, 1306–1317. doi:10.3109/02699052.2011.624570

Bourgeois, M. S., Camp, C., Rose, M., White, B., Malone, M., Carr, J., & Rovine, M. (2003). A comparison of training strategies to enhance use of external aids by persons with dementia. *Journal of Communication Disorders, 36*, 361–378. doi:10.1016/s0021-9924(03)00051-0

Broadbent, D. E., Cooper, P. F., FitzGerald, P., & Parkes, K. R. (1982). The Cognitive Failures Questionnaire (CFQ) and its correlates. *The British Journal of Clinical Psychology, 21*(Pt. 1), 1–16. doi:10.1111/j.2044-8260.1982.tb01421.x

Brown, C. (2012). *Occupational therapy practice guidelines for adults with serious mental illness.* Bethesda, MD: AOTA Press.

Brunsdon, R., Nickels, L., & Coltheart, M. (2007). Topographical disorientation: Towards an integrated framework for assessment. *Neuropsychological Rehabilitation, 17*, 34–52. doi:10.1080/09602010500505021

Burke, W. H., Zencius, A. H., Wesolowski, M. D., & Doubleday, F. (1991). Improving executive function disorders in brain injured clients. *Brain Injury, 5*, 241–252. doi:10.3109/02699059109008095

Burns, S., & Neville, M. (2017). Assessing the impact of real-life cognitive functioning in the home: Development and psychometric study of the Multiple Errands Test–Home. *American Journal of Occupational Therapy, 71*. doi:10.5014/ajot.2017.71S1-PO2138

Butler, J. A. (1999). Evaluation and intervention with apraxia. In C. Unsworth (Ed.), *Cognitive and perceptual dysfunction* (pp. 257–298). Philadelphia, PA: F. A. Davis.

Butler, P. D., Silverstein, S. M., & Dakin, S. C. (2008). Visual perception and its impairment in schizophrenia. *Biological Psychiatry, 64*, 40–47. doi:10.1016/j.biopsych.2008.03.023

Caplan, B. (1987). Assessment of unilateral neglect: A new reading test. *Journal of Clinical and Experimental Neuropsychology, 9*, 359–364. doi:10.1080/01688638708405056

Cappa, S. F., Benke, T., Clarke, S., Rossi, B., Stemmer, B., & van Heugten, C. M. (2005). EFNS guidelines on cognitive rehabilitation: Report of an EFNS task force. *European Journal of Neurology, 12*, 665–680. doi:10.1111/j.1468-1331.2005.01330.x

Cappa, S. F., Sterzi, R., Vallar, G., & Bisiach, E. (1987). Remission of hemineglect and anosognosia during vestibular stimulation. *Neuropsychologia, 25*, 775–782. doi:10.1016/0028-3932(87)90115-1

Casaletto, K. B., Moore, D. J., Woods, S. P., Umlauf, A., Scott, J. C., & Heaton, R. K. (2016). Abbreviated goal management training shows preliminary evidence as a neurorehabilitation tool for HIV-associated neurocognitive disorders among substance users. *The Clinical Neuropsychologist, 30*, 107–130. doi:10.1080/13854046.2015.1129437

Cate, Y., & Richards, L. (2000). Relationship between performance on tests of basic visual functions and visual-perceptual processing in persons after brain injury. *American Journal of Occupational Therapy, 54*, 326–334. doi:10.5014/ajot.54.3.326

Cermak, S. A., & Maeir, A. (2011). Cognitive rehabilitation of children and adults with attention-deficit hyperactivity disorder. In N. Katz (Ed.), *Cognition, occupation, and participation across the life span: Neuroscience, neurorehabilitation, and models of intervention in occupational therapy* (3rd ed., pp. 249–276). Bethesda, MD: AOTA Press.

Champod, A., Frank, R., Taylor, K., & Eskes, G. (2018). The effects of prism adaptation on daily life activities in patients with visuospatial neglect: A systematic review. *Neuropsychological Rehabilitation, 28*, 491–514. doi:10.1080/09602011.2016.1182032

Charters, E., Gillett, L., & Simpson, G. (2015). Efficacy of electronic portable assistive devices for people with acquired brain injury: A systematic review. *Neuropsychological Rehabilitation, 25*, 82–121. doi:10.1080/09602011.2014.942672

Chen, P., Hartman, A. J., Galarza, C. P., & DeLuca, J. (2012). Global processing training to improve visuospatial memory deficits after right-brain stroke. *Archives of Clinical Neuropsychology, 27*, 891–905. doi:10.1093/arclin/acs089

Chen, P., & Hreha, K. (2015). *KF-NAP 2015 manual.* West Orange, NJ: Kessler Foundation.

Chen, P., Hreha, K., Kong, Y., & Barrett, A. (2015). Impact of spatial neglect on stroke rehabilitation: Evidence from the setting of an inpatient rehabilitation facility. *Archives of Physical Medicine and Rehabilitation, 96*, 1458–1466. doi:10.1016/j.apmr.2015.03.019

Chiaravalloti, N., Christodoulou, C., Demaree, H., & DeLuca, J. (2003). Differentiating simple versus complex processing speed: Influence on new learning and memory performance. *Journal of Clinical and Experimental Neuropsychology, 25*, 489–501. doi:10.1076/jcen.25.4.489.13878

Chiaravalloti, N. D., Genova, H. M., & DeLuca, J. (2015). Cognitive rehabilitation in multiple sclerosis: The role of plasticity. *Frontiers in Neurology, 6*, 67. doi:10.3389/fneur.2015.00067

Chiaravalloti, N. D., Moore, N. B., Nikelshpur, O. M., & DeLuca, J. (2013). An RCT to treat learning impairment in multiple sclerosis: The MEMREHAB trial. *Neurology, 81*, 2066–2072. doi:10.1212/01.wnl.0000437295.97946.a8

Chiaravalloti, N. D., Sandry, J., Moore, N. B., & DeLuca, J. (2016). An RCT to treat learning impairment in traumatic brain injury: The TBI-MEM trial. *Neurorehabilitation and Neural Repair, 30*, 539–550. doi:10.1177/1545968315604395

Chui, T., Oliver, R., Ascott, P., Choo, L. C., Davis, T., Gaya, A., . . . Letts, L. (2006). *Safety Assessment of Function and the Environment for Rehabilitation (SAFER)* (Version 3). Ontario, Canada: COTA Health. Retrieved from http://www.cotahealth.ca

Cicerone, K. D., Langenbahn, D. M., Braden, C., Malec, J. F., Kalmar, K., Fraas, M., . . . Ashman, T. (2011). Evidence-based cognitive rehabilitation: Updated review of the literature from 2003 through 2008. *Archives of Physical Medicine and Rehabilitation, 92*, 519–530. doi:10.1016/j.apmr.2010.11.015

Cicerone, K., Mott, T., Azulay, J., & Friel, J. (2004). Community integration and satisfaction with functioning after intensive cognitive rehabilitation for traumatic brain injury. *Archives of Physical Medicine and Rehabilitation, 85*, 943–950. doi:10.1016/j.apmr.2003.07.019

Cipresso, P., Albani, G., Serino, S., Pedroli, E., Pallavicini, F., Mauro, A., & Riva, G. (2014). Virtual Multiple Errands Test (VMET): A virtual reality-based tool to detect early executive functions deficit in Parkinson's disease. *Frontiers in Behavioral Neuroscience, 8*, 405. doi:10.3389/fnbeh.2014.00405

Clare, L., Linden, D. E. J., Woods, R. T., Whitaker, R., Evans, S. J., Parkinson, C. H., . . . Rugg, M. D. (2010). Goal-oriented cognitive rehabilitation for people with early-stage Alzheimer disease: A single-blind randomized controlled trial of clinical efficacy. *The American Journal of Geriatric Psychiatry, 18,* 928–939. doi:10.1097/JGP.0b013e3181d5792a

Clark-Wilson, J., Giles, G. M., & Baxter, D. M. (2014). Revisiting the neurofunctional approach: Conceptualizing the core components for the rehabilitation of everyday living skills. *Brain Injury, 28,* 1646–1656. doi:10.3109/02699052.2014.946449

Colarusso, R. P., & Hammill, D. D. (2002). *Motor-Free Visual Perception Test (MVPT-3).* Austin, TX: PRO-ED.

Collins, A., & Koechlin, E. (2012). Reasoning, learning, and creativity: Frontal lobe function and human decision-making. *PLoS Biology, 10,* e1001293. doi:10.1371/journal.pbio.1001293

Cooke, D. M., McKenna, K., & Fleming, J. (2005). Development of a standardized occupational therapy screening tool for visual perception in adults. *Scandinavian Journal of Occupational Therapy, 12,* 59–71. doi:10.1080/11038120410020683-1

Crawford, J. R., Smith, G. V., Maylor, E. A. M., Della Sala, S., & Logie, R. H. (2003). The Prospective and Retrospective Memory Questionnaire (PMRQ): Normative data and latent structure in a large non-clinical sample. *Memory, 11,* 261–265. doi:10.1080/09658210244000027

Crosson, C., Barco, P. P., Velozo, C., Bolesta, M. M., Cooper, P. V., Werts, D., & Brobeck, T. C. (1989). Awareness and compensation in postacute head injury rehabilitation. *Journal of Clinical and Experimental Neuropsychology, 2,* 355–363. doi:10.1097/00001199-198909000-00008

Cruz, G., Petrie, S., Goudie, N., Kersel, D., & Evans, J. (2016). Text messages reduce memory failures in adults with brain injury: A single-case experimental design. *British Journal of Occupational Therapy, 79,* 598–606. doi:10.1177/0308022616640299

Cullum, C. M., Weiner, M. F., & Saine, K. (2009). *Texas Functional Living Scale.* San Antonio, TX: Pearson.

Curtin, M., Jones, J., Tyson, G. A., Mitsch, V., Alston, M., & McAllister, L. (2011). Outcomes of Participation Objective, Participation Subjective (POPS) measure following traumatic brain injury. *Brain Injury, 25,* 266–273. doi:10.3109/02699052.2010.542793

Dawson, D., Gaya, A., Hunt, A., Levine, B., Lemsky, C., & Polatajko, H. J. (2009). Using the Cognitive Orientation to Occupational Performance (CO-OP) with adults with executive dysfunction following traumatic brain injury. *Canadian Journal of Occupational Therapy, 76,* 115–127. doi:10.1177/000841740907600209

Dawson, D., McEwen, S., & Polatajko, H. (2017). *Cognitive orientation to daily occupational performance in occupational therapy: Using the CO-OP approach to enable participation across the lifespan.* Bethesda, MD: AOTA Press.

Dawson, D., Richardson, J., Troyer, A., Binns, M., Clark, A., Polatajko, H., . . . Bar, Y. (2014). An occupation-based strategy training approach to managing age-related executive changes: A pilot randomized controlled trial. *Clinical Rehabilitation, 28,* 118–127. doi:10.1177/0269215513492541

Dewar, B. K., Kapur, N., & Kopelman, M. (2018). Do memory aids help everyday memory? A controlled trial of a Memory Aids Service. *Neuropsychological Rehabilitation,* 1–19. doi:10.1080/09602011.2016.1189342

de Werd, M. M. E., Boelen, D., Rikkert, M. G. M. O., & Kessels, R. P. C. (2013). Errorless learning of everyday tasks in people with dementia. *Clinical Interventions in Aging, 8,* 1177–1190. doi:10.2147/CIA.S46809

Diamond, A. (2013). Executive functions. *Annual Review of Psychology, 64,* 135–168. doi:10.1146/annurev-psych-113011-143750

Di Monaco, M., Schintu, S., Dotta, M., Barba, S., Tappero, R., & Gindri, P. (2011). Severity of unilateral spatial neglect is an independent predictor of functional outcome after acute inpatient rehabilitation in individuals with right hemispheric stroke. *Archives of Physical Medicine and Rehabilitation, 92,* 1250–1256. doi:10.1016/j.apmr.2011.03.018

Diller, L. (1976). A model for cognitive retraining in rehabilitation. *Clinical Psychology, 29,* 13–15. doi:10.1037/e544562009-010

Döpp, C. M. E., Graff, M. J. L., Teerenstra, S., Olde Rikkert, M. G. M., Nijhuis–van der Sanden, M. W. G., & Vernooij-Dassen, M. J. F. J. (2015). Effectiveness of a training package for implementing a community-based occupational therapy program in dementia: A cluster randomized controlled trial. *Clinical Rehabilitation, 29,* 974–986. doi:10.1177/0269215514564699

Ducharme, J. M., & Ng, O. (2012). Errorless academic compliance training: A school-based application for young students with autism. *Behavior Modification, 36,* 650–669. doi:10.1177/0145445511436006

Dudai, Y., Karni, A., & Born, J. (2015). The consolidation and transformation of memory. *Neuron, 88,* 20–32. doi:10.1016/j.neuron.2015.09.004

Dymowski, A. R., Ponsford, J. L., & Willmott, C. (2016). Cognitive training approaches to remediate attention and executive dysfunction after traumatic brain injury: A single-case series. *Neuropsychological Rehabilitation, 26,* 866–894. doi:10.1080/09602011.2015.1102746

Edgeworth, J. A., Robertson, I. H., & McMillan, T. M. (1998). *The Balloons Test.* Bury St. Edmunds, United Kingdom: Thames Valley Test Company.

Edwards, J. D., Xu, H., Clark, D., Guey, L., Ross, L., & Unverzagt, F. (2017). Speed of processing training results in lower risk of dementia. *Alzheimer's & Dementia (New York, N. Y.), 3,* 603–611. doi:10.1016/j.trci.2017.09.002

Elazar, B., Itzkovich, M., & Katz, N. (1996). *Geriatric version: Lowenstein Occupational Therapy Cognitive Assessment (LOTCA-G) battery.* Pequannock, NJ: Maddak.

Emslie, H., Wilson, F. C., Burden, V., Nimmo-Smith, I., & Wilson, B. A. (2003). *Behavioural Assessment of the Dysexecutive Syndrome for Children (BADS-C).* London, United Kingdom: Harcourt Assessment/The Psychological Corporation.

Engel, L., Chui, A., Goverover, Y., & Dawson, D. (2017). Optimising activity and participation outcomes for people with self-awareness impairments related to acquired brain injury: An interventions systematic review. *Neuropsychological Rehabilitation,* 1–36. doi:10.1080/09602011.2017.1292923

Evald, L. (2017). Prospective memory rehabilitation using smartphones in patients with TBI. *Disability and Rehabilitation.* Advance online publication. doi:10.1080/09638288.2017.1333633

Evans, J. J., Emslie, H., & Wilson, B. A. (1998). External cueing systems in the rehabilitation of executive impairments of action. *Journal of the International Neuropsychological Society, 4,* 399–408.

Farah, M. J. (2003). Disorders of visual-spatial perception and cognition: Visuoperceptual, visuospatial, and visuoconstructive disorders. In K. M. Heilman & E. Valenstein (Eds.), *Clinical neuropsychology* (4th ed., pp. 146–160). New York, NY: Oxford University Press.

Fasotti, L., Kovacs, F., Eling, P., & Brouwer, W. H. (2000). Time pressure management as a compensatory strategy training after closed head injury. *Neuropsychological Rehabilitation, 10,* 47–65. doi:10.1080/096020100389291

Ferber, S., & Karnath, H. (2001). How to assess spatial neglect—line bisection or cancellation tasks? *Journal of Clinical and Experimental Neuropsychology, 23,* 599–607. doi:10.1076/jcen.23.5.599.1243

Fertherlin, J. M., & Kurland, L. (1989). Self-instruction: A compensatory strategy to increase functional independence with brain injured adults. *Occupational Therapy Practice, 1,* 75–78.

Fisher, A. G. (1993a). Functional measures: Part 1. What is function, what should we measure and how should we measure it? *American Journal of Occupational Therapy, 46*, 183–185. doi:10.5014/ajot.46.2.183

Fisher, A. G. (1993b). Functional measures: Part 2. Selecting the right test, minimizing the limitations. *American Journal of Occupational Therapy, 46*, 278–281. doi:10.5014/ajot.46.3.278

Fleming, J. M., Strong, J., & Ashton, R. (1996). Self-awareness of deficits in adults with traumatic brain injury: How best to measure? *Brain Injury, 10*, 1–15. doi:10.1080/026990596124674

Folstein, M. F., Folstein, S. E., & McHugh, P. R. (1975). "Mini-mental state." A practical method for grading the cognitive state of patients for the clinician. *Journal of Psychiatric Research, 12*, 189–198.

Foster, E. R., Spence, D., & Toglia, J. (2018). Feasibility of a cognitive strategy training intervention for people with Parkinson's disease. *Disability and Rehabilitation, 40*, 1127–1134. doi:10.1080/09638288.2017.1288275

Friedman-Yakoobian, M. S., Mueser, K. T., Giuliano, A. J., Goff, D. C., & Seidman, L. J. (2016). Family-directed cognitive adaptation pilot: Teaching cognitive adaptation to families of individuals with schizophrenia. *American Journal of Psychiatric Rehabilitation, 19*, 62–74. doi:10.1080/15487768.2015.1125401

Gentry, T. (2018). Consumer technologies as cognitive aids. In N. Katz (Ed.), *Cognition, occupation, and participation across the life span: Neuroscience, neurorehabilitation, and models of intervention in occupational therapy* (4th ed. pp. 219–230). Bethesda, MD: AOTA Press.

Geusgens, C., van Heugten, C., Donkervoort, M., van den Ende, E., Jolles, J., & van den Heuvel, W. (2006). Transfer of training effects in stroke patients with apraxia: An exploratory study. *Neuropsychological Rehabilitation, 16*, 213–229.

Giles, G. M. (2018). Neurofunctional approach to rehabilitation following brain injury. In N. Katz (Ed.), *Cognition, occupation, and participation across the life span: Neuroscience, neurorehabilitation, and models of intervention in occupational therapy* (4th ed. pp. 419–442). Bethesda, MD: AOTA Press.

Giles, G. M., & Clark-Wilson, J. (1988). The use of behavioral techniques in functional skills training after severe brain injury. *American Journal of Occupational Therapy, 42*, 658–665.

Giles, G. M., Edwards, D. F., Morrison, M. T., Baum, C., & Wolf, T. J. (2017). Screening for functional cognition in postacute care and the Improving Medicare Post-Acute Care Transformation (IMPACT) Act of 2014. *American Journal of Occupational Therapy, 71*, 7105090010p1–7105090010p6. doi:10.5014/ajot.2017.715001

Gillen, G. (2009). *Cognitive and perceptual rehabilitation: Optimizing function.* St. Louis, MO: Mosby.

Gillen, G., Nilsen, D., Attridge, J., Banakos, E., Morgan, M., Winterbottom, L., & York, W. (2015). Effectiveness of interventions to improve occupational performance of people with cognitive impairments after stroke: An evidence-based review. *American Journal of Occupational Therapy, 69*, 6901180040p1–6901180040p9. doi:10.5014/ajot.2015.012138

Gillen, R., Tennen, H., & McKee, T. (2005). Unilateral spatial neglect: Relation to rehabilitation outcomes in patients with right hemisphere stroke. *Archives of Physical Medicine and Rehabilitation, 86*, 763–767. doi:10.1016/j.apmr.2004.10.029

Gioia, G. A., Isquith, P. K., Guy, S. C., & Kenworthy, L. (2015). *Behavior Rating Inventory of Executive Function (BRIEF-2)* (2nd ed.). Lutz, FL: Psychological Assessment Resources.

Gitlin, L. N., Piersol, C. V., Hodgson, N., Marx, K., Roth, D. L., Johnston, D., . . . Lyketsos, C. G. (2016). Reducing neuropsychiatric symptoms in persons with dementia and associated burden in family caregivers using tailored activities: Design and methods of a randomized clinical trial. *Contemporary Clinical Trials, 49*, 92–102. doi:10.1016/j.cct.2016.06.006

Gitlin, L. N., Schinfeld, S., Winter, L., Corcoran, M., Boyce, A. A., & Hauck, W. W. (2002). Evaluating home environments of persons with dementia: Interrater reliability and validity of the Home Environmental Assessment Protocol (HEAP). *Disability and Rehabilitation, 24*, 59–71. doi:10.1080/09638280110066325

Gitlin, L. N., Winter, L., Dennis, M. P., Hodgson, N., & Hauck, W. W. (2010a). A biobehavioral home-based intervention and the well-being of patients with dementia and their caregivers: The COPE randomized trial. *JAMA, 304*, 983–991. doi:10.1001/jama.2010.1253

Gitlin, L. N., Winter, L., Dennis, M. P., Hodgson, N., & Hauck, W. W. (2010b). Targeting and managing behavioral symptoms in individuals with dementia: A randomized trial of a nonpharmacological intervention. *Journal of the American Geriatrics Society, 58*, 1465–1474. doi:10.1111/j.1532-5415.2010.02971.x

Gitlin, L. N., Winter, L., Vause Earland, T., Adel Herge, E., Chernett, N. L., Piersol, C. V., & Burke, J. P. (2009). The tailored activity program to reduce behavioral symptoms in individuals with dementia: Feasibility, acceptability, and replication potential. *The Gerontologist, 49*, 428–439. doi:10.1093/geront/gnp087

Golisz, K. M. (1998). Dynamic assessment and multicontext treatment of unilateral neglect. *Topics in Stroke Rehabilitation, 5*, 11–28. doi:10.1310/c5eu-a605-l7uq-1qxb

Goodwin, R., Lincoln, N., das Nair, R., & Bateman, A. (2017). External memory aids for memory problems in people with multiple sclerosis: A systematic review. *Neuropsychological Rehabilitation, 27*, 1081–1102. doi:10.1080/09602011.2015.1113997

Gould, F., McGuire, L. S., Durand, D., Sabbag, S., Larrauri, C., Patterson, T. L., . . . Harvey, P. D. (2015). Self-assessment in schizophrenia: Accuracy of evaluation of cognition and everyday functioning. *Neuropsychology, 29*, 675–682. doi:10.1037/neu0000175

Goverover, Y., Chiaravalloti, N., & DeLuca, J. (2005). The relationship between self-awareness of neurobehavioral symptoms, cognitive functioning, and emotional symptoms in multiple sclerosis. *Multiple Sclerosis (Houndmills, Basingstoke, England), 11*, 203–212. doi:10.1191/1352458505ms1153oa

Goverover, Y., Chiaravalloti, N., & DeLuca, J. (2013). The influence of executive functions and memory on self-generation benefit in persons with multiple sclerosis. *Journal of Clinical and Experimental Neuropsychology, 35*, 775–783. doi:10.1080/13803395.2013.824553

Goverover, Y., Chiaravalloti, N., Gaudino-Goering, E., Moore, N. B., & DeLuca, J. (2009). The relationship among performance of instrumental activities of daily living, self-report of quality of life, and self-awareness of functional status in individuals with multiple sclerosis. *Rehabilitation Psychology, 54*, 60–68. doi:10.1037/a0014556

Goverover, Y., Chiaravalloti, N., Genova, H., & DeLuca, J. (2017). A randomized controlled trial to treat impaired learning and memory in multiple sclerosis: The self-GEN trial. *Multiple Sclerosis.* Advance Online Publication. doi:10.1177/1352458517709955

Goverover, Y., Chiaravalloti, N., O'Brien, A., & DeLuca, J. (2018). Evidenced based cognitive rehabilitation for persons with multiple sclerosis: An updated review of the literature from 2007 to 2016. *Archives of Physical Medicine and Rehabilitation, 99*, 390–407. doi:10.1016/j.apmr.2017.07.021

Goverover, Y., Genova, H., Griswold, H., Chiaravalloti, N., & DeLuca, J. (2014). Metacognitive knowledge and online awareness in persons with multiple sclerosis. *NeuroRehabilitation, 35*, 315–323. doi:10.3233/NRE-141113

Goverover, Y., Johnston, M. V., Toglia, J., & DeLuca, J. (2007a, February). *Treatment to improve self-awareness and functional independence for persons with TBI: A pilot randomized trial.* Paper presented at the Neuropsychological Society 35th Annual Meeting, Portland, OR.

Goverover, Y., Johnston, M. V., Toglia, J., & DeLuca, J. (2007b). Treatment to improve self-awareness in persons with acquired brain injury. *Brain Injury, 21*, 913–923. doi:10.1080/02699050701553205

Goverover, Y., O'Brien, A., Moore, N., & DeLuca, J. (2010). Actual reality: A new approach to functional assessment in persons with multiple sclerosis. *Archives of Physical Medicine and Rehabilitation, 91,* 252–260. doi:10.1016/j.apmr.2009.09.022

Gracey, F., Fish, J., Greenfield, E., Bateman, A., Malley, D., Hardy, G., . . . Manly, T. (2017). A randomized controlled trial of assisted intention monitoring for the rehabilitation of executive impairments following acquired brain injury. *Neurorehabilitation and Neural Repair, 31,* 323–333. doi:10.1177/1545968316680484

Grattan, E., Lang, C., Birkenmeier, R., Holm, M., Rubinstein, E., Van Swearingen, J., & Skidmore, E. (2016). Examining the feasibility, tolerability, and preliminary efficacy of repetitive task-specific practice for people with unilateral spatial neglect. *American Journal of Occupational Therapy, 70,* 7004290020p1–7004290020p8. doi:10.5014/ajot.2016.019471

Greenaway, M. C., Duncan, N. L., & Smith, G. E. (2013). The memory support system for mild cognitive impairment: Randomized trial of a cognitive rehabilitation intervention. *International Journal of Geriatric Psychiatry, 28,* 402–409. doi:10.1002/gps.3838

Guilbert, A., Clément, S., & Moroni, C. (2017). A rehabilitation program based on music practice for patients with unilateral spatial neglect: A single-case study. *Neurocase, 23*(1), 12–21. doi:10.1080/13554794.2016.1265652

Haaland, K. Y. (1993, March). *Assessment of limb apraxia.* Paper presented at the AOTA Neuroscience Institute Treating Adults with Apraxia, Baltimore, MD.

Hahn-Markowitz, J., Manor, I., & Maeir, A. (2011). Effectiveness of cognitive-functional (cog-fun) intervention with children with attention deficit hyperactivity disorder: A pilot study. *American Journal of Occupational Therapy, 65,* 384–392. doi:10.5014/ajot.2011.000901

Hamera, E., & Brown, C. E. (2000). Developing a context-based performance measure for persons with schizophrenia: The test of grocery shopping skills. *American Journal of Occupational Therapy, 54,* 20–25. doi:10.5014/ajot.54.1.20

Hanna, K., Hepworth, L., & Rowe, F. (2017). Screening methods for post-stroke visual impairment: A systematic review. *Disability and Rehabilitation, 39,* 2531–2543. doi:10.1080/09638288.2016.1231846

Harrison, M. J., Morris, K. A., Horton, R., Toglia, J., Barsky, J., Chait, S., . . . Robbins, L. (2005). Results of an intervention for lupus patients with self-perceived cognitive difficulties. *Neurology, 65,* 1325–1327. doi:10.1212/01.wnl.0000180938.69146.5e

Hart, T., Whyte, J., & Kennedy, D. (2016). *Moss Attention Rating Scale (MARS).* Retrieved from http://mrri.org/moss-attention-rating-scale-mars

Hartman-Maeir, A., Harel, H., & Katz, N. (2009). Kettle Test—a brief measure of cognitive functional performance. Reliability and validity in stroke rehabilitation. *American Journal of Occupational Therapy, 63,* 592–599. doi:10.5014/ajot.63.5.592

Hartman-Maeir, A., Katz, N., & Baum, C. M. (2009). Cognitive Functional Evaluation (CFE) process for individuals with suspected cognitive disabilities. *Occupational Therapy in Health Care, 23,* 1–23. doi:10.1080/07380570802455516

Heilman, K. M., & Rothi, L. J. (2003). Apraxia. In K. M. Heilman & E. Valenstein (Eds.), *Clinical neuropsychology* (4th ed., pp. 215–245). New York, NY: Oxford University Press.

Heilman, K. M., Watson, R. T., & Valenstein, E. (2003). Neglect and related disorders. In K. M. Heilman & E. Valenstein (Eds.), *Clinical neuropsychology* (4th ed., pp. 296–346). New York, NY: Oxford University Press.

Henshaw, E., Polatajko, H., McEwen, S., Ryan, J. D., & Baum, C. M. (2011). Cognitive approach to improving participation after stroke: Two case studies. *American Journal of Occupational Therapy, 65,* 55–63. doi:10.5014/ajot.2011.09010

Ianes, P., Varalta, V., Gandolfi, M., Picelli, A., Corno, M., Di Matteo, A., . . . Smania, N. (2012). Stimulating visual exploration of the neglected space in the early stage of stroke by hemifield eye-patching: A randomized controlled trial in patients with right brain damage. *European Journal of Physical and Rehabilitation Medicine, 48,* 189–196.

Imms, C., & Nott, M. (2012). Single subject experimental design study demonstrated cognitive orientation to daily occupational performance (CO-OP) improved performance of self-selected goals in adults with chronic stroke. *Australian Occupational Therapy Journal, 59,* 467–468. doi:10.1111/1440-1630.12013

Jacquin-Courtois, S., Bays, P. M., Salemme, R., Leff, A. P., & Husain, M. (2013). Rapid compensation of visual search strategy in patients with chronic visual field defects. *Cortex, 49,* 994–1000. doi:10.1016/j.cortex.2012.03.025

Johansson, B., & Tornmalm, M. (2012). Working memory training for patients with acquired brain injury: Effects in daily life. *Scandinavian Journal of Occupational Therapy, 19,* 176–183. doi:10.3109/11038128.2011.603352

Johnston, M. V., Goverover, Y., & Dijkers, M. (2005). Community activities and individuals' satisfaction about them: Quality of life in the first year after traumatic brain injury. *Archives of Physical Medicine and Rehabilitation, 86,* 735–745. doi:10.1016/j.apmr.2004.10.031

Josman, N. (2011). The dynamic interactional model in schizophrenia. In N. Katz (Ed.), *Cognition, occupation, and participation across the life span: Neuroscience, neurorehabilitation, and models of intervention in occupational therapy* (3rd ed., pp. 203–222). Bethesda, MD: AOTA Press.

Josman, N., Goffer, A., & Rosenblum, S. (2010). Development and standardization of a "do-eat" activity of daily living performance test for children. *American Journal of Occupational Therapy, 64,* 47–58. doi:10.5014/ajot.64.1.47

Josman, N., & Rosenblum, S. (2011). A metacognitive model for children with atypical brain development. In N. Katz (Ed.), *Cognition, occupation, and participation across the life span: Neuroscience, neurorehabilitation, and models of intervention in occupational therapy* (3rd ed., pp. 223–248). Bethesda, MD: AOTA Press.

Kamada, K., Shimodozono, M., Hamada, H., & Kawahira, K. (2011). Effects of 5 minutes of neck-muscle vibration immediately before occupational therapy on unilateral spatial neglect. *Disability and Rehabilitation, 33,* 2322–2328. doi:10.3109/09638288.2011.570411

Katz, N. (2006). *Routine Task Inventory—Expanded (RTI-E) manual, prepared and elaborated on the basis of Allen, C. K. (1989 unpublished).* Unpublished manuscript. Retrieved from http://www.allen_cognitive_network.org

Katz, N., Itzkovich, M., Averbuch, S., & Elazar, B. (1990). *Lowenstein Occupational Therapy Cognitive Assessment (LOTCA) manual.* Pequannock, NJ: Maddak.

Katz, N., Livni, L., Bar-Haim Erez, A., & Averbuch, S. (2011). *Dynamic Loewenstein Occupational Therapy Cognitive Assessment (DLOTCA).* Pequannock, NJ: Maddak.

Katz, N., Parush, S., & Traub Bar-Ilan, R. (2005). *Dynamic Occupational Therapy Cognitive Assessment for Children (DOTCA-Ch).* Pequannock, NJ: Maddak.

Kelleher, M., Tolea, M. I., & Galvin, J. E. (2015). Anosognosia increases caregiver burden in mild cognitive impairment. *International Journal of Geriatric Psychiatry, 31,* 799–808. doi:10.1002/gps.4394

Kessler, R. K., Rhodes, E., & Giovannetti, T. (2015). Environmental adaptations improve everyday action in schizophrenia. *Journal of the International Neuropsychological Society, 21,* 319–329. doi:10.1017/S1355617715000260

Kidd, S. A., Herman, Y., Barbic, S., Ganguli, R., George, T. P., Hassan, S., . . . Velligan, D. (2014). Testing a modification of cognitive adaptation training: Streamlining the model for broader implementation. *Schizophrenia Research, 156,* 46–50. doi:10.1016/j.schres.2014.03.026

Kiernan, R. J., Mueller, J., & Langston, J. W. (2011). *Cognistat and Cognistat assessment system manual.* Fairfax, CA: Cognistat.

Kirby, A. (2011). Dyspraxia series: Part one. At sixes and sevens. *The Journal of Family Health Care, 21,* 29–31.

Klingberg, T. (2010). Training and plasticity of working memory. *Trends in Cognitive Sciences, 14,* 317–324. doi:10.1016/j.tics.2010.05.002

Koehler, R., Wilhelm, E. E., & Shoulson, I. (2011). *Cognitive rehabilitation therapy for traumatic brain injury: Evaluating the evidence.* Washington, D.C.: The National Academies Press.

Kramer, J. H., Kaplan, E., Blusewicz, M. J., & Preston, K. A. (1991). Visual hierarchical analysis of block design configural errors. *Journal of Clinical and Experimental Neuropsychology, 13,* 455–465. doi:10.1080/01688639108401063

Krasny-Pacini, A., Chevignard, M., & Evans, J. (2014). Goal management training for rehabilitation of executive functions: A systematic review of effectiveness in patients with acquired brain injury. *Disability and Rehabilitation, 36,* 105–116. doi:10.3109/09638288.2013.777807

Laeng, B. (2006). Constructional apraxia after left or right unilateral stroke. *Neuropsychologia, 44,* 1595–1606. doi:10.1016/j.neuropsychologia.2006.01.023

Lampit, A., Hallock, H., & Valenzuela, M. (2014). Computerized cognitive training in cognitively healthy older adults: A systematic review and meta-analysis of effect modifiers. *PLoS Medicine, 11,* 1–18. doi:10.1371/journal.pmed.1001756

Law, M., Baptiste, S., Carswell, A., McColl, M. A., Polatajko, H., & Pollock, N. (2005). *Canadian occupational performance measure* (3rd ed., Rev. ed.). Ontario, Canada: Canadian Association of Occupational Therapists.

Leavitt, V. M., Lengenfelder, J., Moore, N. B., Chiaravalloti, N. D., & DeLuca, J. (2011). The relative contributions of processing speed and cognitive load to working memory accuracy in multiple sclerosis. *Journal of Clinical and Experimental Neuropsychology, 33,* 580–586. doi:10.1080/13803395.2010.541427

Levine, B., Robertson, I. H., Clare, L., Carter, G., Hong, J., Wilson, B. A., . . . Stuss, D. T. (2000). Rehabilitation of executive functioning: An experimental-clinical validation of goal management training. *Journal of the International Neuropsychological Society, 6,* 299–312. doi:10.1017/s1355617700633052

Levine, B., Stuss, D. T., Winocur, G., Binns, M. A., Fahy, L., Mandic, M., . . . Robertson, I. H. (2007). Cognitive rehabilitation in the elderly: Effects on strategic behavior in relation to goal management. *Journal of the International Neuropsychological Society, 13,* 143–152. doi:10.1017/S1355617707070178

Levy, L. L. (2011a). Cognitive aging. In N. Katz (Ed.), *Cognition, occupation, and participation across the life span: Neuroscience, neurorehabilitation, and models of intervention in occupational therapy* (3rd ed., pp. 93–116). Bethesda, MD: AOTA Press.

Levy, L. L. (2011b). Cognitive information processing. In N. Katz (Ed.), *Cognition, occupation, and participation across the life span: Neuroscience, neurorehabilitation, and models of intervention in occupational therapy* (3rd ed., pp. 117–142). Bethesda, MD: AOTA Press.

Levy, L. L. (2018). Neurocognition and function: Intervention in dementia based on the Cognitive Disabilities Model. In N. Katz (Ed.), *Cognition, occupation, and participation across the life span: Neuroscience, neurorehabilitation, and models of intervention in occupational therapy* (4th ed. pp. 499–522). Bethesda, MD: AOTA Press.

Lezak, M. D., Howieson, D. B., & Loring, D. W. (2004). *Neuropsychological assessment* (4th ed.). New York, NY: Oxford University Press.

Liddell, A., & Rasmussen, C. (2005). Memory profile of children with nonverbal learning disability. *Learning Disabilities Research and Practice, 20,* 137–141. Doi:10.1111/j.1540-5826.2005.00128.x

Lindsten-McQueen, K., Weiner, N. W., Wang, H. Y., Josman, N., & Connor, L. T. (2014). Systematic review of apraxia treatments to improve occupational performance outcomes. *OTJR: Occupation, Participation and Health, 34,* 183–192. doi:10.3928/15394492-20141006-02

Liu, K. P., & Chan, C. C. (2014). Pilot randomized controlled trial of self-regulation in promoting function in acute poststroke patients. *Archives of Physical Medicine and Rehabilitation, 95,* 1262–1267. doi:10.1016/j.apmr.2014.03.018

Loeb, P. A. (1996). *Independent Living Scales (ILS) manual.* San Antonio, TX: The Psychological Corporation.

Lunt, L., Bramham, J., Morris, R. G., Bullock, P. R., Selway, R. P., Xenitidis, K., & David, A. S. (2012). Prefrontal cortex dysfunction and 'jumping to conclusions': Bias or deficit? *Journal of Neuropsychology, 6,* 65–78. doi:10.1111/j.1748-6653.2011.02005.x

Luton, L. M., Reed-Knight, B., Loiselle, K., O'Toole, K., & Blount, R. (2011). A pilot study evaluating an abbreviated version of the cognitive remediation programme for youth with neurocognitive deficits. *Brain Injury, 25,* 409–415. doi:10.3109/02699052.2011.558044

Mackin, R. S., Ayalon, L., Feliciano, L., & Areán, P. A. (2010). The sensitivity and specificity of cognitive screening instruments to detect cognitive impairment in older adults with severe psychiatric illness. *Journal of Geriatric Psychiatry and Neurology, 23,* 94–99. doi:10.1177/0891988709358589

Maher, L., Rothi, L., & Greenwald, M. (1991). Treatment of gesture impairment: A single case. *American Speech and Hearing Association, 33,* 195.

Malec, J. F., & Lezak, M. D. (2008). *Manual for the Mayo-Portland Adaptability Inventory (MPAI-4) for adults, children and adolescents.* Retrieved from http://www.tbims.org/combi/mpai/manual.pdf

Man, D. W., Fleming, J., Hohaus, L., & Shum, D. (2011). Development of the Brief Assessment of Prospective Memory (BAPM) for use with traumatic brain injury populations. *Neuropsychological Rehabilitation, 21,* 884–898. doi:10.1080/09602011.2011.627270

Mandich, A., Polatajko, H. J., Miller, L., & Baum, C. (2004). *The Paediatric Activity Card Sort (PACS).* Ottawa, ON: Canadian Association of Occupational Therapists.

Mandich, A. D., Polatajko, H., & Zilberbrant, A. (2008). A cognitive perspective on intervention. In A. C. Eliasson & P. Burtner (Eds.), *Improving hand function in children with cerebral palsy: Theory, evidence and intervention.* London, United Kingdom: Mac Keith Press.

Manly, T., Robertson, I. H., Anderson, V., & Nimmo-Smith, I. (1998). *Test of Everyday Attention for Children, the (TEA-Ch).* San Antonio, TX: Pearson Clinical.

Matano, A., Iosa, M., Guariglia, C., Pizzamiglio, L., & Paolucci, S. (2015). Does outcome of neuropsychological treatment in patients with unilateral spatial neglect after stroke affect functional outcome? *European Journal of Physical and Rehabilitation Medicine, 51,* 737–743.

Mausbach, B. T., Harvey, P. D., Goldman, S. R., Jeste, D. V., & Patterson, T. L. (2007). Development of a brief scale of everyday functioning in persons with serious mental illness. *Schizophrenia Bulletin, 33,* 1364–1372. doi:10.1093/schbul/sbm014

May-Benson, T. A., & Cermak, S. A. (2007). Development of an assessment for ideational praxis. *American Journal of Occupational Therapy, 61,* 148–153. doi:10.5014/ajot.61.2.148

McCabe, D. P., Roediger, H. L., III, McDaniel, M. A., Balota, D. A., & Hambrick, D. Z. (2010). The relationship between working memory capacity and executive functioning: Evidence for a common executive attention construct. *Neuropsychology, 24,* 222. doi:10.1037/a0017619

McCarthy, M., Beaumont, J. G., Thompson, R., & Pringle, H. (2002). The role of imagery in the rehabilitation of neglect in severely disabled brain-injured adults. *Archives of Clinical Neuropsychology, 17*, 407–422. doi:10.1093/arclin/17.5.407

McCraith, D., & Earhart, C. (2018). Cognitive Disabilities Model: Creating a fit between functional cognitive abilities and activity demands for best ability to function. In N. Katz (Ed.), *Cognition, occupation, and participation across the life span: Neuroscience, neurorehabilitation, and models of intervention in occupational therapy* (4th ed. pp. 469–497). Bethesda, MD: AOTA Press.

McDonald, A., Haslam, C., Yates, P., Gurr, B., Leeder, G., & Sayers, A. (2011). Google calendar: A new memory aid to compensate for prospective memory deficits following acquired brain injury. *Neuropsychological Rehabilitation, 21*, 784–807. doi:10.1080/09602011.2011.598405

McDowd, J. M., Filion, D. L., Pohl, P. S., Richards, L. G., & Stiers, W. (2003). Attentional abilities and functional outcomes following stroke. *The Journals of Gerontology. Series B, Psychological Sciences and Social Sciences, 58*, P45–P53. doi:10.1093/geronb/58.1.p45

McKerracher, G., Powell, T., & Oyebode, J. (2005). A single case experimental design comparing two memory notebook formats for a man with memory problems caused by traumatic brain injury. *Neuropsychological Rehabilitation, 15*, 115–128. doi:10.1080/09602010443000056

Melby-Lervåg, M., & Hulme, C. (2013). Is working memory training effective? A meta-analytic review. *Developmental Psychology, 49*, 270–291. doi:10.1037/a0028228

Mesulam, M. M. (2000). Attentional networks, confusional states and neglect syndromes. In M. Mesulam (Ed.), *Principles of behavioral neurology* (2nd ed., pp. 174–256). New York, NY: Oxford University Press.

Morrison, M. T., Giles, G. M., Ryan, J. D., Baum, C. M., Dromerick, A. W., Polatajko, H. J., & Edwards, D. F. (2013). Multiple Errands Test–Revised (MET-R): A performance-based measure of executive function in people with mild cerebrovascular accident. *American Journal of Occupational Therapy, 67*, 460–468. doi:10.5014/ajot.2013.007880

Nasreddine, Z. S., Phillips, N. A., Bédirian, V., Charbonneau, S., Whitehead, V., Collin, I., . . . Chertkow, H. (2005). The Montreal Cognitive Assessment, MoCA: A brief screening tool for mild cognitive impairment. *Journal of the American Geriatrics Society, 53*, 695–699. doi:10.1111/j.1532-5415.2005.53221.x

Neistadt, M. E. (1987). Occupational therapy for adults with perceptual deficits. *American Journal of Occupational Therapy, 42*, 434–440.

Neistadt, M. E. (1990). A critical analysis of occupational therapy approaches for perceptual deficits in adults with brain injury. *American Journal of Occupational Therapy, 44*, 299–304. doi:10.5014/ajot.44.4.299

Neistadt, M. E. (1992). Occupational therapy treatments for constructional deficits. *American Journal of Occupational Therapy, 46*, 141–148. doi:10.5014/ajot.46.2.141

Nelson, A., Fogel, B. S., & Faust, D. (1986). Bedside cognitive screening instruments. A critical assessment. *The Journal of Nervous and Mental Disease, 174*, 73–83. doi:10.1097/00005053-198602000-00002

Niemeier, J. P., Cifu, D. X., & Kishore, R. (2001). The lighthouse strategy: Improving the functional status of patients with unilateral neglect after stroke and brain injury using a visual imagery intervention. *Topics in Stroke Rehabilitation, 8*(2), 10–18. doi:10.1310/7UKK-HJ0F-GDWF-HHM8

Nilsen, D., Gillen, G., Arbesman, M., & Lieberman, D. (2015). Occupational therapy interventions for adults with stroke. *American Journal of Occupational Therapy, 69*, 6905395010p1. doi:10.5014/ajot.2015.695002

Noone, P. (2015). Addenbrooke's Cognitive Examination-III. *Occupational Medicine (Oxford, England), 65*, 418–420. doi:10.1093/occmed/kqv041

Nott, M. T., & Chapparo, C. (2008). Measuring information processing in a client with extreme agitation following traumatic brain injury using the perceive, recall, plan and perform system of task analysis. *Australian Occupational Therapy Journal, 55*, 188–198. doi:10.1111/j.1440-1630.2007.00685.x

Nott, M. T., Chapparo, C., & Heard, R. (2009). Reliability of the perceive, recall, plan and perform system of task analysis: A criterion-referenced assessment. *Australian Occupational Therapy Journal, 56*, 307–314. doi:10.1111/j.1440-1630.2008.00763.x

Ogourtsova, T., Souza Silva, W., Archambault, P. S., & Lamontagne, A. (2017). Virtual reality treatment and assessments for post-stroke unilateral spatial neglect: A systematic literature review. *Neuropsychological Rehabilitation, 27*, 409–454. doi:10.1080/09602011.2015.1113187

Ownsworth, T. L., McFarland, K., & Young, R. M. (2000). Development and standardization of the Self-Regulation Skills Interview (SRSI): A new clinical assessment tool for acquired brain injury. *The Clinical Neuropsychologist, 14*, 76–92. doi:10.1076/1385-4046(200002)14:1;1-8;FT076

Parente, R., & Stapleton, M. (1997). History and systems of cognitive rehabilitation. *NeuroRehabilitation, 8*, 3–11. doi:10.3233/NRE-1997-8102

Peng, P., & Fuchs, D. (2017). A randomized control trial of working memory training with and without strategy instruction. *Journal of Learning Disabilities, 50*, 62–80. doi:10.1177/0022219415594609

Phelan, S., Steinke, L., & Mandich, A. (2009). Exploring a cognitive intervention for children with pervasive developmental disorder. *Canadian Journal of Occupational Therapy, 76*, 23–28. doi:10.1177/000841740907600107

Pilgrim, E., & Humphreys, G. W. (1994). Rehabilitation of a case of ideomotor apraxia. In M. J. Riddoch & G. W. Humphreys (Eds.), *Cognitive neuropsychology and cognitive rehabilitation* (pp. 271–315). East Sussex, United Kingdom: Lawrence Erlbaum Associates.

Polatajko, H. J., Mandich, A., & McEwen, S. E. (2011). Cognitive orientation to daily occupational performance (CO-OP): A cognitive-based intervention for children and adults. In N. Katz (Ed.), *Cognition, occupation, and participation across the life span: Neuroscience, neurorehabilitation, and models of intervention in occupational therapy* (3rd ed., pp. 299–322). Bethesda, MD: AOTA Press.

Polatajko, H. J., Mandich, A. D., Miller, L. T., & Macnab, J. J. (2001). Cognitive orientation to daily occupational performance (CO-OP): Part II—the evidence. *Physical & Occupational Therapy in Pediatrics, 20*, 83–106.

Polatajko, H. J., McEwen, S. E., Ryan, J. D., & Baum, C. M. (2012). Pilot randomized controlled trial investigating cognitive strategy use to improve goal performance after stroke. *American Journal of Occupational Therapy, 66*, 104–109. doi:10.5014/ajot.2012.001784

Poole, J. L. (1998). Effect of apraxia on the ability to learn one-handed shoe tying. *Occupational Therapy Journal of Research, 18*, 99–104. doi:10.1177/153944929801800303

Poole, J. L. (2000). A comparison of limb praxis abilities of persons with developmental dyspraxia and adult onset apraxia. *Occupational Therapy Journal of Research, 20*, 106–120. doi:10.1177/153944920002000202

Preissner, K. (2014). *Occupational therapy practice guidelines for adults with neurodegenerative diseases.* Bethesda, MD: AOTA Press.

Priftis, K., Passarini, L., Pilosio, C., Meneghello, F., & Pitteri, M. (2013). Visual scanning training, limb activation treatment, and prism adaptation for rehabilitating left neglect: Who is the winner? *Frontiers in Human Neuroscience, 7*, 360. doi:10.3389/fnhum.2013.00360

Prigatano, G. P. (1986). *Neuropsychological rehabilitation after brain injury*. Baltimore, MD: Johns Hopkins University Press.

Prigatano, G. P. (1999). *Principles of neuropsychological rehabilitation*. New York, NY: Oxford University Press.

Quee, P. J., Stiekema, A. P. M., Wigman, J. T. W., Schneider, H., van der Meer, L., Maples, N. J., . . . Bruggeman, R. (2014). Improving functional outcomes for schizophrenia patients in the Netherlands using cognitive adaptation training as a nursing intervention—a pilot study. *Schizophrenia Research, 158*, 120–125. doi:10.1016/j.schres.2014.06.020

Raskin, S., & Buckheit, C. (2010). *Memory for Intentions Test (MIST)*. Lutz, FL: Psychological Assessment Resources.

Rebok, G., Ball, K., Guey, L., Jones, R., Kim, H., King, J., . . . Willis, S. (2014). Ten-year effects of the advanced cognitive training for independent and vital elderly cognitive training trial on cognition and everyday functioning in older adults. *Journal of the American Geriatrics Society, 62*, 16–24. doi:10.1111/jgs.12607

Redick, T., Shipstead, Z., Meier, M., Montroy, J., Hicks, K., Unsworth, N., . . . Engle, R. (2016). Cognitive predictors of a common multitasking ability: Contributions from working memory, attention control, and fluid intelligence. *Journal of Experimental Psychology. 145*, 1473. doi:10.1037/xge0000219

Reitan, R. M. (1955). The relation of the trail making test to organic brain damage. *Journal of Consulting Psychology, 19*, 393–394. doi:10.1037/h0044509

Revheim, N., & Marcopulos, B. A. (2006). Group treatment approaches to address cognitive deficits. *Psychiatric Rehabilitation Journal, 30*, 38–45. doi:10.2975/30.2006.38.45

Rilo, O., Peña, J., Ojeda, N., Rodríguez-Antigüedad, A., Mendibe-Bilbao, M., Gómez-Gastiasoro, A., . . . Ibarretxe-Bilbao, N. (2018). Integrative group-based cognitive rehabilitation efficacy in multiple sclerosis: A randomized clinical trial. *Disability and Rehabilitation, 40*, 208–216. doi:10.1080/09638288.2016.1250168

Robertson, I. H., Tegnér, R., Tham, K., Lo, A., & Nimmo-Smith, I. (1995). Sustained attention training for unilateral neglect: Theoretical and rehabilitation implications. *Journal of Clinical and Experimental Neuropsychology, 17*, 416–430. doi:10.1080/01688639508405133

Robertson, I. H., Ward, T., Ridgeway, V., & Nimmo-Smith, I. (1994). *The Test of Everyday Attention (TEA)*. Bury St. Edmunds, United Kingdom: Thames Valley Test Company.

Robertson, K., & Schmitter-Edgecombe, M. (2015). Self-awareness and traumatic brain injury outcome. *Brain Injury, 29*, 848–858. doi:10.3109/02699052.2015.1005135

Robnett, R. H., Hopkins, V., Kimball, J. G. (2003). The safe at home: A quick home safety assessment. *Physical Occupational Therapy in Geriatrics, 20*, 77–101. doi:10.1300/j148v20n03_06

Rocke, K., Hays, P., Edwards, D., & Berg, C. (2008). Development of a performance assessment of executive function: The Children's Kitchen Task Assessment. *American Journal of Occupational Therapy, 62*, 528–537. doi:10.5014/ajot.62.5.528

Rockwood, K., Joyce, B., & Stolee, P. (1997). Use of goal attainment scaling in measuring clinically important change in cognitive rehabilitation patients. *Journal of Clinical Epidemiology, 50*, 581–588. doi:10.1016/s0895-4356(97)00014-0

Rode, G., Pagliari, C., Huchon, L., Rossetti, Y., & Pisella, L. (2017). Semiology of neglect: An update. *Annals of Physical and Rehabilitation Medicine, 60*, 177–185. doi:10.1016/j.rehab.2016.03.003

Rodger, S., & Vishram, A. (2010). Mastering social and organization goals: Strategy use by two children with Asperger syndrome during cognitive orientation to daily occupational performance. *Physical & Occupational Therapy in Pediatrics, 30*, 264–276. doi:10.3109/01942638.2010.500893

Rogers, J. C., & Holm, M. B. (2014). *Performance Assessment of Self-Care Skills* (Version 4.0). Pittsburgh, PA: University of Pittsburgh.

Ross, L., Edwards, J., O'Connor, M., Ball, K., Wadley, V., & Vance, D. (2016). The transfer of cognitive speed of processing training to older adults' driving mobility across 5 years. *The Journals of Gerontology Series B: Psychological Sciences and Social Sciences, 71*(1), 87–97. doi:10.1093/geronb/gbv022

Rotenberg-Shpigelman, S., Erez, A. B. H., Nahaloni, I., & Maeir, A. (2012). Neurofunctional treatment targeting participation among chronic stroke survivors: A pilot randomised controlled study. *Neuropsychological Rehabilitation, 22*, 532–549. doi:10.1080/09602011.2012.665610

Roth, R. M., Isquith, P. K., & Gioia, G. A. (2005). *Behavior Rating Inventory of Executive Function—Adult version (BRIEF-A)*. Lutz, FL: Psychological Assessment Resources.

Roy, E. A. (1978). Apraxia: A new look at an old syndrome. *Journal of Human Movement Studies, 4*, 191–210.

Roy, E. A. (1985). *Neuropsychological studies of apraxia and related disorders*. Amsterdam, Netherlands: Elsevier Science.

Rustad, R. A., DeGroot, T. L., Jungkunz, M. L., Freeberg, K. S., Borowick, L. G., & Wanttie, A. M. (1993). *The cognitive assessment of minnesota*. Tucson, AZ: Therapy Skill Builders.

Ryan, J. D., Polatajko, H. J., McEwen, S., Peressotti, M., Young, A., Rummel, K., . . . Baum, C. M. (2011). Analysis of Cognitive Environmental Support (ACES): Preliminary testing. *Neuropsychological Rehabilitation, 21*, 401–427. doi:10.1080/09602011.2011.572692

Saevarsson, S., Halsband, U., & Kristjánsson, Á. (2011). Designing rehabilitation programs for neglect: Could 1+1 be more than 2? *Applied Neuropsychology, 18*, 95–106. doi:10.1080/09084282.2010.547774

Salthouse, T. A. (2016). *Theoretical perspectives on cognitive aging*. Hillsdale, NJ: Lawrence Erlbaum Associates.

Sandry, J., Chiou, K. S., DeLuca, J., & Chiaravalloti, N. D. (2016). Individual differences in working memory capacity predicts responsiveness to memory rehabilitation after traumatic brain injury. *Archives of Physical Medicine and Rehabilitation, 97*, 1026–1029.e1. doi:10.1016/j.apmr.2015.10.109

Sarajuuri, J. M., Kaipio, M. L., Koskinen, S. K., Neimela, M. R., Servo, A. R., & Vilkki, J. (2005). Outcome of a comprehensive neurorehabilitation program for persons with traumatic brain injury. *Archives of Physical Medicine and Rehabilitation, 86*, 2296–2302. doi:10.1016/j.apmr.2005.06.018

Schmidt, J., Fleming, J., Ownsworth, T., & Lannin, N. A. (2015). Maintenance of treatment effects of an occupation-based intervention with video feedback for adults with TBI. *NeuroRehabilitation, 36*, 175–186. doi:10.3233/NRE-151205

Schwartz, M. F., Segal, M., Veramonti, T., Ferraro, M., & Buxbaum, L. J. (2002). The Naturalistic Action Test: A standardised assessment for everyday action impairment. *Neuropsychological Rehabilitation, 12*, 311–339. doi:10.1080/09602010244000084

Schwartz, S. M. (1995). Adults with traumatic brain injury: Three case studies of cognitive rehabilitation in the home setting. *American Journal of Occupational Therapy, 49*, 655–668. doi:10.5014/ajot.49.7.655

Schwartz, Y., Averbuch, S., Katz, N., & Sagiv, A. (2016). Validity of the Functional Loewenstein Occupational Therapy Cognitive Assessment (FLOTCA). *American Journal of Occupational Therapy, 70*, 7001290010p1–7001290010p7. doi:10.5014/ajot.2016.016451

Schwartz, Y., & Sagiv, A. (2018). Cognitive rehabilitation: A retraining model for clients with neurological disabilities. In N. Katz (Ed.), *Cognition, occupation, and participation across the life span: Neuroscience, neurorehabilitation, and models of intervention in occupational therapy* (4th ed. pp. 405–418). Bethesda, MD: AOTA Press.

Séguin, M., Lahaie, A., Matte-Gagné, C., & Beauchamp, M. (2017). Ready! Set? Let's train! Feasibility of an intensive attention training program and its beneficial effect after childhood traumatic brain injury. *Annals of Physical and Rehabilitation Medicine*, doi:10.1016/j.rehab.2017.05.001

Seron, X., Deloche, G., & Coyette, F. (1989). A retrospective analysis of a single case of neglect therapy: A point of theory. In X. Seron & G. Deloche (Eds.), *Cognitive approaches in neuropsychological rehabilitation*. Hillsdale, NJ: Lawrence Erlbaum Associates.

Sherer, M., Bergloff, P., Boake, C., High, W., Jr., & Levin, E. (1998). The Awareness Questionnaire: Factor structure and internal consistency. *Brain Injury*, *12*, 63–68. doi:10.1080/026990598122863

Shevil, E., & Finlayson, M. (2010). Pilot study of a cognitive intervention program for persons with multiple sclerosis. *Health Education Research*, *25*, 41–53. doi:10.1093/her/cyp037

Shum, D., Fleming, J., Gill, H., Gullo, M. J., & Strong, J. (2011). A randomized controlled trial of prospective memory rehabilitation in adults with traumatic brain injury. *Journal of Rehabilitation Medicine*, *43*, 216–223. doi:10.2340/16501977-0647

Silva, A. R., Pinho, M. S., Macedo, L., & Moulin, C. J. A. (2018). A critical review of the effects of wearable cameras on memory. *Neuropsychological Rehabilitation*, *28*, 117–141. doi:10.1080/09602011.2015.1128450

Skidmore, E. R., Dawson, D. R., Butters, M. A., Grattan, E. S., Juengst, S. B., Whyte, E. M., . . . Becker, J. T. (2015). Strategy training shows promise for addressing disability in the first 6 months after stroke. *Neurorehabilitation and Neural Repair*, *29*, 668–676. doi:10.1177/1545968314562113

Skidmore, E. R., Dawson, D. R., Whyte, E. M., Butters, M. A., Dew, M. A., Grattan, E. S., . . . Holm, M. B. (2014). Developing complex interventions: Lessons learned from a pilot study examining strategy training in acute stroke rehabilitation. *Clinical Rehabilitation*, *28*, 378–387. doi:10.1177/0269215513502799

Smania, N., Aglioti, S. M., Girardi, F., Tinazzi, M., Fiaschi, A., Cosentino, A., & Corato, E. (2006). Rehabilitation of limb apraxia improves daily life activities in patients with stroke. *Neurology*, *67*, 2050–2052. doi:10.1212/01.wnl.0000247279.63483.1f

Sohlberg, M. M., & Mateer, C. A. (1989a). *Attention Process Training*. San Antonio, TX: The Psychological Corporation.

Sohlberg, M. M., & Mateer, C. A. (1989b). *Introduction to cognitive rehabilitation: Theory and practice*. New York, NY: Guilford Press.

Sohlberg, M. M., & Mateer, C. A. (2001). *Cognitive rehabilitation: An integrative neuropsychological approach*. New York, NY: Guilford Press.

Sohlberg, M. M., & Turkstra, L. S. (2011). *Optimizing cognitive rehabilitation: Effective instructional methods*. New York, NY: Guilford Press.

Spaccavento, S., Cellamare, F., Falcone, R., Loverre, A., & Nardulli, R. (2017). Effect of subtypes of neglect on functional outcome in stroke patients. *Annals of Physical and Rehabilitation Medicine*, *60*, 376–381. doi:10.1016/j.rehab.2017.07.245

Steultjens, E. M., Voigt-Radloff, S., Leonhart, R., & Graff, M. J. (2012). Reliability of the Perceive, Recall, Plan, and Perform (PRPP) assessment in community-dwelling dementia patients: Test consistency and inter-rater agreement. *International Psychogeriatrics*, *24*, 659–665. doi:10.1017/S1041610211002249

Stuss, D. T., Robertson, I. H., Craik, F. I., Levine, B., Alexander, M. P., Black, S., . . . Winocur, G. (2007). Cognitive rehabilitation in the elderly: A randomized trial to evaluate a new protocol. *Journal of the International Neuropsychological Society*, *13*, 120–131. doi:10.1017/S1355617707070154

Sunderland, A., Walker, C. M., & Walker, M. F. (2006). Action errors and dressing disability after stroke: An ecological approach to neuropsychological assessment and intervention. *Neuropsychological Rehabilitation*, *16*, 666–683. doi:10.1080/09602010500204385

Swirsky-Sacchetti, T., Field, H. L., Mitchell, D. R., Seward, J., Lublin, F. D., Knobler, R. L., & Gonzalez, C. F. (1992). The sensitivity of the Mini-Mental State Exam in the white matter dementia of multiple sclerosis. *Journal of Clinical Psychology*, *48*, 779–786. doi:10.1002/1097-4679(199211)48:6<779::AID-JCLP2270480612>3.0.CO;2-B

Tariq, S. H., Tumosa, N., Chibnall, J. T., Perry, M. H., III, & Morley, J. E. (2006). Comparison of the Saint Louis University Mental Status Examination and the Mini-Mental State Examination for detecting dementia and mild neurocognitive disorder—a pilot study. *American Journal of Geriatric Psychology*, *14*, 900–910. doi:10.1097/01.JGP.0000221510.33817.86

Tempest, S., & Roden, P. (2008). Exploring evidence-based practice by occupational therapists when working with people with apraxia. *British Journal of Occupational Therapy*, *71*, 33–37. doi:10.1177/030802260807100106

Teng, E., & Chui, H. (1987). The Modified Mini-Mental State (3MS) examination. *The Journal of Clinical Psychiatry*, *48*, 314–318.

Tham, K., Bernspang, B., & Fisher, A. G. (1999). Development of the Assessment of Awareness of Disability. *Scandinavian Journal of Occupational Therapy*, *6*, 101–190. doi:10.1080/110381299443663

Tham, K., Ginsburg, E., Fisher, A., & Tegnér, R. (2001). Training to improve awareness of disabilities in clients with unilateral neglect. *American Journal of Occupational Therapy*, *55*, 46–54. doi:10.5014/ajot.55.1.46

Tham, K., & Tegnér, R. (1996). The baking tray task: A test of spatial neglect. *Neuropsychological Rehabilitation*, *6*, 19–25. doi:10.1080/713755496

Theeuwes, J. (2010). Top-down and bottom-up control of visual selection. *Acta Psychologica*, *135*, 77–99. doi:10.1016/j.actpsy.2010.02.006

Thomson, L. K., & Robnett, R. (2016). *The Kohlman Evaluation of Living Skills (KELS)* (4th ed.). Bethesda, MD: AOTA Press.

Thornton, A., Licari, M., Reid, S., Armstrong, J., Fallows, R., & Elliott, C. (2016). Cognitive orientation to (daily) occupational performance intervention leads to improvements in impairments, activity and participation in children with developmental coordination disorder. *Disability and Rehabilitation*, *38*, 979–986. doi:10.3109/09638288.2015.1070298

Tiersky, L. A., Anselmi, V., Johnston, M. V., Kurtyka, J., Roosen, E., Schwartz, T., & DeLuca, J. (2005). A trial of neuropsychologic rehabilitation in mild-spectrum traumatic brain injury. *Archives of Physical Medicine and Rehabilitation*, *86*, 1565–1574. doi:10.1016/j.apmr.2005.03.013

Tobler-Ammann, B. C., Surer, E., de Bruin, E. D., Rabuffetti, M., Borghese, N. A., Mainetti, R., . . . Knols, R. H. (2017). Exergames encouraging exploration of hemineglected space in stroke patients with visuospatial neglect: A feasibility study. *JMIR Serious Games*, *5*, e17. doi:10.2196/games.7923

Toglia, J. P. (1989). Visual perception of objects: An approach to assessment and intervention. *American Journal of Occupational Therapy*, *43*, 587–595. doi:10.5014/ajot.43.9.587

Toglia, J. P. (1991a). Generalization of treatment: A multicontextual approach to cognitive perceptual impairment in the brain injured adult. *American Journal of Occupational Therapy*, *45*, 505–516. doi:10.5014/ajot.45.6.505

Toglia, J. P. (1991b). Unilateral visual inattention: Multidimensional components. *Occupational Therapy Practice*, *3*, 18–34.

Toglia, J. P. (1993a). Attention and memory. In C. B. Royeen (Ed.), *AOTA self-study series: Cognitive rehabilitation* (pp. 4–72). Bethesda, MD: AOTA Press.

Toglia, J. P. (1993b). *The Contextual Memory Test*. Tucson, AZ: Therapy Skill Builders.

Toglia, J. P. (1994). *Toglia Category Assessment (TCA)*. Pequannock, NJ: Maddak.

Toglia, J. P. (2011). A dynamic interactional model of cognition in cognitive rehabilitation. In N. Katz (Ed.), *Cognition, occupation, and participation across the life span: Neuroscience, neurorehabilitation, and models of intervention in occupational therapy* (3rd ed., pp. 161–202). Bethesda, MD: AOTA Press.

Toglia, J. P. (2015). *Weekly Calendar Planning Activity.* Bethesda, MD: AOTA

Toglia, J. P. (2018). Dynamic interactional model and the multicontext approach. In N. Katz (Ed.), *Cognition, occupation, and participation across the life span: Neuroscience, neurorehabilitation, and models of intervention in occupational therapy.* (4th ed. pp. 355–385). Bethesda, MD: AOTA Press.

Toglia, J., Askin, G., Gerber, L. M., Taub, M. C., Mastrogiovanni, A. R., & O'Dell, M. W. (2017). Association between 2 measures of cognitive instrumental activities of daily living and their relationship to the Montreal Cognitive Assessment in persons with stroke. *Archives of Physical Medicine and Rehabilitation, 98,* 2280–2287. doi:10.1016/j.apmr.2017.04.007

Toglia, J. P., & Cermak, S. (2009). Dynamic assessment and prediction of learning potential in clients with unilateral neglect. *American Journal of Occupational Therapy, 64,* 569–579. doi:10.5014/ajot.63.5.569

Toglia, J. P., Fitzgerald, K. A., O'Dell, M. W., Mastrogiovanni, A. R., & Lin, C. D. (2011). The Mini-Mental State Examination and Montreal Cognitive Assessment in persons with mild subacute stroke: Relationship to functional outcome. *Archives of Physical Medicine and Rehabilitation, 92,* 792–798. doi:10.1016/j.apmr.2010.12.034

Toglia, J. P., & Golisz, K. M. (2012). Therapy for activities of daily living: Theoretical and practical perspectives. In N. D. Zasler, D. I. Katz, & R. D. Zafonte (Eds.), *Brain injury medicine* (2nd ed., pp. 1162–1177). New York, NY: Demos Medical.

Toglia, J. P., Goverover, Y., Johnston, M. V., & Dain, B. (2011). Application of the multicontextual approach in promoting learning and transfer of strategy use in an individual with TBI and executive dysfunction. *OTJR: Occupation, Participation and Health, 31,* S53–S60. doi:10.3928/15394492-20101108-09

Toglia, J. P., Johnston, M. V., Goverover, Y., & Dain, B. (2010). A multicontext approach to promoting transfer of strategy use and self regulation after brain injury: An exploratory study. *Brain Injury, 24,* 664–677. doi:10.3109/02699051003610474

Toglia, J., & Katz, N. (2018). *Cognition, occupation, and participation across the lifespan* (4th ed.). Bethesda, MD: American Occupational Therapy Association.

Toglia, J. P., & Kirk, U. (2000). Understanding awareness deficits following brain injury. *NeuroRehabilitation, 15,* 57–70.

Toglia, J. P., & Maeir, A. (2018). Self-awareness and metacognition: Impact on occupational performance and outcome across the lifespan. In N. Katz (Ed.), *Cognition, occupation, and participation across the life span: Neuroscience, neurorehabilitation, and models of intervention in occupational therapy* (4th ed. pp. 143–163). Bethesda, MD: AOTA Press.

Toglia, J., Rodger, S. A., & Polatajko, H. J. (2012). Anatomy of cognitive strategies: A therapist's primer for enabling occupational performance. *Canadian Journal of Occupational Therapy, 79,* 225–236. doi:10.2182/cjot.2012.79.4.4

Trevena-Peters, J., McKay, A., Spitz, G., Suda, R., Renison, B., & Ponsford, J. (2018). Efficacy of activities of daily living retraining during posttraumatic amnesia: A randomized controlled trial. *Archives of Physical Medicine and Rehabilitation, 99,* 329–337. doi:10.1016/j.apmr.2017.08.486

Tsang, M. H. M., Sze, K. H., & Fong, K. N. K. (2009). Occupational therapy treatment with right half-field eye patching for patients with subacute stroke and unilateral neglect: A randomized controlled trial. *Disability and Rehabilitation, 31,* 630–637. doi:10.1080/09638280802240621

Twamley, E. W., Thomas, K. R., Gregory, A. M., Jak, A. J., Bondi, M. W., Delis, D. C., & Lohr, J. B. (2015). CogSMART compensatory cognitive training for traumatic brain injury: Effects over 1 year. *The Journal of Head Trauma Rehabilitation, 30,* 391–401. doi:10.1097/HTR.0000000000000076

Unsworth, C. (Ed.). (1999). Introduction to cognitive and perceptual dysfunction: Theoretical approaches to therapy. In *Cognitive and perceptual dysfunction: A clinical reasoning approach to evaluation and intervention* (pp. 1–41). Philadelphia, PA: F. A. Davis.

Vaes, N., Nys, G., Lafosse, C., Dereymaeker, L., Oostra, K., Hemelsoet, D., & Vingerhoets, G. (2016). Rehabilitation of visuospatial neglect by prism adaptation: Effects of a mild treatment regime. A randomised controlled trial. *Neuropsychological Rehabilitation.* Advance online publication. doi:10.1080/09602011.2016.1208617

Vanbellingen, T., & Bohlhalter, S. (2011). Apraxia in neurorehabilitation: Classification, assessment and treatment. *NeuroRehabilitation, 28,* 91–98. doi:10.3233/NRE-2011-0637

Vanbellingen, T., Kersten, B., Hemelrijk, B. V., Van de Winckel, A., Bertschi, M., Müri, R., . . . Bohlhalter, S. (2010). Comprehensive assessment of gesture production: A new Test of Upper Limb Apraxia (TULIA). *European Journal of Neurology, 17,* 59–66. doi:10.1111/j.1468-1331.2009.02741.x

Vanbellingen, T., Ottiger, B., Maaijwee, N., Pflugshaupt, T., Bohlhalter, S., Müri, R., . . . Nyffeler, T. (2017). Spatial neglect predicts upper limb use in the activities of daily living. *Cerebrovascular Diseases (Basel, Switzerland), 44,* 122–127. doi:10.1159/000477500

Vanderploeg, R. D., Schwab, K., Walker, W. C., Fraser, J. A., Sigford, B. J., Date, E. S., . . . Warden, D. L. (2008). Rehabilitation of traumatic brain injury in active duty military personnel and veterans: Defense and veterans brain injury center randomized controlled trial of two rehabilitation approaches. *Archives of Physical Medicine and Rehabilitation, 89,* 2227–2238. doi:10.1016/j.apmr.2008.06.015

van Heugten, C. M., Dekker, J., Deelman, B. G., van Dijk, A. J., Stehmann-Saris, J. C., & Kinebanian, A. (2000). Measuring disabilities in stroke patients with apraxia: A validation study of an observational method. *Neuropsychological Rehabilitation, 10,* 401–414. doi:10.1080/096020100411989

Van Keulen-Rouweler, B. J., Sturkenboom, I. H. W. M., Kottorp, A., Graff, M. J. L., Nijhuis-Van der Sanden, M. W. G. M., & Steultjens, E. M. J. (2017). The Perceive, Recall, Plan and Perform (PRPP) system for persons with Parkinson's disease: A psychometric study. *Scandinavian Journal of Occupational Therapy, 24,* 65–73. doi:10.1080/11038128.2016.1233291

Van Vleet, T., & DeGutis, J. (2013). Cross-training in hemispatial neglect: Auditory sustained attention training ameliorates visual attention deficits. *Cortex, 49,* 679–690. doi:10.1016/j.cortex.2012.03.020

Velligan, D. I., Diamond, P., Mueller, J., Li, X., Maples, N., Wang, M., & Miller, A. L. (2009). The short-term impact of generic versus individualized environmental supports on functional outcomes and target behaviors in schizophrenia. *Psychiatry Research, 168,* 94–101. doi:10.1016/j.psychres.2008.03.016

Velligan, D. I., Mueller, J., Wang, M., Dicocco, M., Diamond, P. M., Maples, N. J., & Davis, B. (2006). Use of environmental supports among patients with schizophrenia. *Psychiatric Services, 57,* 219–224. doi:10.1176/appi.ps.57.2.219

Velligan, D. I., Roberts, D., Mintz, J., Maples, N., Li, X., Medellin, E., & Brown, M. (2015). A randomized pilot study of MOtiVation and Enhancement (MOVE) training for negative symptoms in schizophrenia. *Schizophrenia Research, 165,* 175–180. doi:10.1016/j.schres.2015.04.008

Viken, J. I., Samuelsson, H., Jern, C., Jood, K., & Blomstrand, C. (2012). The prediction of functional dependency by lateralized and non-lateralized neglect in a large prospective stroke sample. *European Journal of Neurology, 19,* 128–134. doi:10.1111/j.1468-1331.2011.03449.x

Voelbel, G. T., Goverover, Y., Gaudino, E. A., Moore, N. B., Chiaravalloti, N., & DeLuca, J. (2011). The relationship between neurocognitive behavior of executive functions and the EFPT in individuals with multiple sclerosis. *OTJR: Occupation, Participation and Health, 31*, S30–S37. doi:10.3928/15394492 -20101108-06

Wang, W., Zhang, X., Ji, X., Ye, Q., Chen, W., Ni, J., . . . Shan, C. (2015). Mirror neuron therapy for hemispatial neglect patients. *Scientific Reports, 5*, 8664. doi:10.1038/srep08664

Warren, M. (1981). Relationship of constructional apraxia and body scheme disorders to dressing performance in CVA. *American Journal of Occupational Therapy, 35*, 431–442. doi:10.5014/ajot.35.7.431

Warren, M. (1993). Visuospatial skills: Assessment and intervention strategies. In C. B. Royeen (Ed.), *AOTA self-study series: Cognitive rehabilitation* (pp. 6–76). Bethesda, MD: AOTA Press.

Warren, M. (1998). *The brain injury visual assessment battery for adults.* Lenexa, KS: visABILITIES Rehab Services.

Welfringer, A., Leifert-Fiebach, G., Babinsky, R., & Brandt, T. (2011). Visuomotor imagery as a new tool in the rehabilitation of neglect: A randomised controlled study of feasibility and efficacy. *Disability and Rehabilitation, 33*, 2033–2043. doi:10.3109/09638288.2011 .556208

Wetter, S., Poole, J. L., & Haaland, K. Y. (2005). Functional implications of ipsilesional motor deficits after unilateral stroke. *Archives of Physical Medicine and Rehabilitation, 86*, 776–781. doi:10.1016 /j.apmr.2004.08.009

Wheeler, S., & Acord-Vira, A. (2016). *Occupational therapy practice guidelines for adults with traumatic brain injury.* Bethesda, MD: AOTA Press.

Whyte, J., Hart, T., Bode, R., & Malec, J. (2003). The Moss Attention Rating Scale for traumatic brain injury: Initial psychometric assessment. *Archives of Physical Medicine and Rehabilitation, 84*, 268–276. doi:10.1053/apmr.2003.50108

Wilhelm, O., Witthöft, M., & Schipolowski, S. (2010). Self-reported cognitive failures: Competing measurement models and self-report correlates. *Journal of Individual Differences, 31*, 1–14. doi:10.1027/1614-0001/a000001

Willer, B., Ottenbacher, K. J., & Coad, M. L. (1994). The Community Integration Questionnaire. A comparative examination. *American Journal of Physical Medicine & Rehabilitation, 73*, 103–111. doi:10.1097/00002060-199404000-00006

Wilson, B. A., Alderman, N., Burgess, P., Emslie, H., & Evans, J. (1996). *Behavioural Assessment of the Dysexecutive Syndrome.* Bury St. Edmunds, United Kingdom: Thames Valley Test Company.

Wilson, B. A., Clare, L., Baddeley, A., Watson, P., & Tate, R. (1998). *The Rivermead Behavioral Memory Test–Extended version (RBMT-E).* Bury St. Edmunds, United Kingdom: Thames Valley Test Company.

Wilson, B. A., Cockburn, J., & Baddeley, A. (1987). *Behavioral Inattention Test (BIT).* Bury St. Edmunds, United Kingdom: Thames Valley Test Company.

Wolf, T. J., Dahl, A., Auen, C., & Doherty, M. (2017). The reliability and validity of the Complex Task Performance Assessment: A performance-based assessment of executive function. *Neuropsychological Rehabilitation, 27*, 707–721. doi:10.1080/09602011.2015.1037771

Wolf, T. J., Doherty, M., Kallogjeri, D., Coalson, R. S., Nicklaus, J., Ma, C. X., . . . Piccirillo, J. (2016). The feasibility of using metacognitive strategy training to improve cognitive performance and neural connectivity in women with chemotherapy-induced cognitive impairment. *Oncology (Switzerland), 91*, 143–152. doi:10.1159/000447744

Wolf, T. J., & Nilsen, D. M. (2015). *Occupational therapy practice guidelines for adults with stroke.* Bethesda, MD: AOTA Press.

World Health Organization. (2001). *ICIDH-2: International classification of functioning, disability and health.* Geneva, Switzerland: Author.

Worthington, A. (2016). Treatments and technologies in the rehabilitation of apraxia and action disorganisation syndrome: A review. *NeuroRehabilitation, 39*, 163–174. doi:10.3233/NRE-161348

Wu, A. J., Radel, J., & Hanna-Pladdy, B. (2011). Improved function after combined physical and mental practice after stroke: A case of hemiparesis and apraxia. *American Journal of Occupational Therapy, 65*, 161–168. doi:10.5014/ajot.2011.000786

Zickefoose, S., Hux, K., Brown, J., & Wulf, K. (2013). Let the games begin: A preliminary study using Attention Process Training-3 and Lumosity™ brain games to remediate attention deficits following traumatic brain injury. *Brain Injury, 27*, 707–716. doi:10.3109 /02699052.2013.775484

Zoltan, B. (2007). *Vision, perception, and cognition: A manual for the evaluation and treatment of the adult with acquired brain injury* (4th ed.). Thorofare, NJ: SLACK.

Zwicker, J., Missiuna, C., Harris, S., & Boyd, L. (2012). Developmental coordination disorder: A review and update. *European Journal of Paediatric Neurology, 16*, 573–581. doi:10.1016/j.ejpn.2012.05.005

the**Point**® *For additional resources on the subjects discussed in this chapter, visit* http://thePoint.lww.com /Willard-Spackman13e.

CHAPTER 59

Sensory Processing in Everyday Life

Evan E. Dean, Lauren M. Little, Anna Wallisch, Winnie Dunn

LEARNING OBJECTIVES

After reading this chapter, you will be able to:

1. Examine the history that has led to occupational therapy becoming a leader in applying sensory processing ideas to daily life.
2. Explain the core concepts of sensory processing using Dunn's Sensory Processing Framework.
3. Using the Ecology of Human Performance (EHP) as a conceptual basis, apply sensory processing concepts to the daily life routines and adaptations of the general population.
4. Assess the current evidence about sensory processing concepts and its application to people's everyday lives.
5. Assess the current evidence related to intervention and explain how adjusting routines and contexts can support sensory processing patterns.
6. Design ways to discuss sensory processing intervention options with families, individuals, and other colleagues.

Introduction

Individuals experience the world through their senses. The ways in which we structure our days, coordinate routines, and engage in social activities are all influenced by how we prefer sensory experiences. **Sensory processing** is a key factor that occupational therapists assess to understand the participation of clients they serve. When occupational therapists are able to understand how an individual's sensory processing patterns influence participation, they are able to design intervention approaches to meet the individual's needs.

There have been decades of research about sensory processing in the occupational therapy (OT) literature, and ideas continue to develop. This chapter discusses the history of sensory processing theory as it has evolved from Dr. Jean Ayres's original ideas. It explains Dunn's Sensory Processing Framework and outlines how different behaviors fit within each sensory processing pattern (i.e., registration, seeking, sensitivity, and avoidance). Additionally, it examines current evidence about how sensory processing influences everyday activities among a variety of populations. Using the

CENTENNIAL NOTES

Sensory Processing Has Emerged as a Critical Construct in Understanding Daily Life

Sensory processing is one content area that has arisen from OT scholars. Since the 1960s, when Dr. Jean Ayres first considered an alternate way to derive meaning from her skilled observations (Ayres, 1968, 1971, 1972), many OT researchers and practitioners have thought deeply about this topic and have shared their ideas with individuals, families, and other professionals from other disciplines. Sensory processing has become one of the defining aspects of OT's unique contribution to science and practice. Just as more mature disciplines have shared

their knowledge to help build the OT profession, OT practitioners share what they have learned about sensory processing with others (Dunn, Little, Dean, Robertson, & Evans, 2016). Today, many disciplines rely on the contributions of sensory processing knowledge to support interdisciplinary intervention approaches. This area of expertise has elevated the standing of the OT profession.

The truth that sensory processing has existed all along was hiding behind the ingrained perceptions of who we are that we did not notice their impact on everyday choices. It took the daily life perspective of OT to bring this important area of knowledge into the light for application to many situations (Dunn, 1997, 2007).

Ecological Model of Human Performance (Dean, Wallisch, & Dunn, in press; Dunn, Brown, & McGuigan, 1994), sensory processing concepts are applied to different intervention approaches (e.g., Establish/Restore, Alter, Adapt/Modify, Prevent). This chapter also identifies how specific methods of assessing sensory processing, including observation, interview, and self-report, may be combined with direct measures of participation. Lastly, it synthesizes evidence related to sensory processing and sensory integration (SI) intervention research.

History of Sensory Processing in Occupational Therapy

From the 1950s to 1970s, Dr. Jean Ayres was unsettled about some of the children she encountered in her work as an occupational therapist. Dr. Ayres dared to ask questions that others had not considered; in doing so, she opened the floodgates of what is possible to know about sensory processing and its impact on everyday life. It is important to remember the context of Dr. Ayres's work. During this time period, children with disabilities were segregated in care centers or special schools outside of public education. Prior to the passage of the Education of All Handicapped Children Act of 1975, some children were not allowed in school at all. Dr. Ayres noticed certain children who had characteristics that did not receive attention because the focus at the time was on serving children with more frank disorders such as cerebral palsy and intellectual disabilities. As a further reflection of the time, people started using the term "minimal brain dysfunction" to describe these children's conditions.

As Dr. Ayres worked, she observed details about how children with less noticeable conditions and subtle differences responded to sensory stimuli in their play and other routines. Based on her work with these children, she identified the possible relationship between children's responses to sensory events and subsequent behaviors. Being one of the few occupational therapists with a background in research, Dr. Ayres began to examine what she observed in practice. She designed a standardized test to document and measure her observations about sensory processing, the Southern California Sensory Integration Tests (SCSIT; Ayres, 1980). Dr. Ayres used the data from the SCSIT to create a model of SI that linked the findings to her background in neuroscience. Basically, the model incorporated sensory input, integration of sensory inputs, and behavioral outputs into a cohesive set of ideas. She hypothesized that when sensory input works differently than expected, the integration and outputs are affected as well; in this way, she linked sensory input to behavioral output. These ideas were revolutionary for the time. They had great appeal and spread quickly, especially within the OT community.

After the passage of Education of All Handicapped Children Act of 1975 in the United States (which later became the Individuals with Disabilities Education Act [IDEA], 1990), there were many more possibilities for serving all children. Dr. Ayres's ideas about the impact of sensory processing on children's behavior became tools for therapists and teachers working with school-aged children in public education. Implementation of Dr. Ayres's ideas and the passage of Education of All Handicapped Children Act of 1975 occurred at a time when all children were given the opportunity to obtain services, which would have been impossible to consider before this point. Although Education of All Handicapped Children Act of

1975 explicitly stated that children were to be served in the "least restrictive environment," "clinical" settings continued to exist within public schools. In creating these separate spaces for children and removing them from natural environments, the approach to serving children reflected a medical model (i.e., fix what is wrong with the child).

Over time, therapists began to recognize opportunities for applying OT knowledge in a more integrated way in school routines and settings. For example, tools from traditional "sensory integration" clinical settings started to be used in preschools (e.g., scooter boards). Therapists began to embrace their role as *related service* professionals at school, which compelled them to examine how they contributed to educational outcomes. This cultural shift in service delivery, specifically how to deliver OT using sensory processing theory, reflected how ideas evolve when contexts and environmental opportunities change.

The professional culture also changed over the next two decades. There were strong calls for professionals to test their ideas systematically and create convincing methods of applying such ideas (i.e., evidence-based practices). Occupational therapists started going to graduate school to learn about research. People designed systematic ways to evaluate children; standardized tests became more available, and therapists used them more often in practice. Over time, data accumulated from studies, leading the way for both practical application and research. (These research trends are reviewed in a later section of this chapter.)

The history of OT and the cultural shifts that impact service delivery affect our ability to understand the evolution of ideas and subsequent application of such ideas. A significant benchmark in the development of the OT profession is Dr. Ayres's explication of the impact of sensory processing on behavior and therapists' ability to interpret behavior. Many researchers have followed her to provide further research about this topic, and their contributions build on the strong scaffolding Dr. Ayres created. Today, work in sensory processing looks very different from Dr. Ayres's original ideas and work. We draw from her innovative thinking for her time; however, because contexts change and scientific methods and approaches evolve, new ways to study sensory processing and apply its concepts in practice have been developed.

Application of Sensory Processing to the General Population

It is important to note that this chapter places sensory processing concepts and research within the context of the general population or all people. Occupational therapy practitioners recognize that all sensory processing occurs on a continuum, and individuals have distinct sensory preferences and aversions. **Sensory processing** can be defined as how an individual detects sensory information from the environment and regulates behavioral responses associated with such sensory information (Dunn, 2014). To describe how people process sensory information and behave in accordance, researchers and clinicians have used various terms. Terminology can become confusing because individuals from different fields (e.g., OT vs. neuroscience) often use different words to describe similar behaviors (Baranek, Little, Parham, Ausderau, & Sabatos-DeVito, 2014; Cascio, Woynaroski, Baranek, & Wallace, 2016; Schaaf & Lane, 2015). Although there is a significant body of research concerning children with autism spectrum disorder (ASD) and other childhood conditions because children in these groups have different ways of responding to sensory events in everyday life, sensory processing is actually about everyone. The terms "sensory processing differences" and "sensory features" are used to describe all people's sensory experiences. Certainly, research shows that some groups (e.g., children with ASD and attention-deficit/hyperactivity disorder [ADHD]) demonstrate distinct sensory processing preferences and aversions; however, such differences should not be considered as dysfunction, abnormalities, or deficits. In the book *Saving Normal: An Insider's Look at What Caused the Epidemic of Mental Illness and How to Cure It*, Frances (2013) argues against pathologizing people's experiences by stating the following:

> This brings us to the question of the moment—can we use statistics in some simple and precise way to define mental normality? Can the bell curve provide a scientific guide in deciding who is mentally normal and who is not? Conceptually, the answer is "why not," but practically the answer is "hell no". . . . There are just too many statistical, contextual, and value judgments that perplex a simple statistical solution. (p. 7)

Just as other person characteristics (e.g., cognition, emotion) occur on a bell curve, sensory processing characteristics present on a bell curve: Most people display responses to sensory stimuli in a similar range, but there will always be people who demonstrate responses outside of that range who can still participate successfully in their daily lives. Consider yourself or any other individual. You may be in the top 5% on height but still appear in the middle of the bell curve because you have brown eyes, which are more common. In sensory processing, you might be in the "just like others" range for seeking and respond "much more than others" in sensitivity. Perhaps your motor coordination is in the bottom 20% compared with others. This places your characteristics all over the bell curve, so you cannot be classified as "normal" or "not normal" as a person. Individuals can adapt to their situations no matter where their characteristics might be on the bell curve, so difference cannot be used to identify dysfunction. Frances (2013) continues,

> We must reconcile to there not being any simple standard to decide the question of how many of us are abnormal. The normal curve tells us a great deal about the distribution of everything from quarks to koalas, but it doesn't dictate to us where normal ends and abnormal begins. . . . Human difference was never meant to be reducible to an exhaustive list of diagnoses . . . it takes all types to make a successful tribe and a full palette of emotions to make a fully lived life. We shouldn't medicalize difference and attempt to treat it away. . . . (p. 8)

Again, sensory processing is a characteristic that applies to everyone; it is not associated with abnormality. Although some people use the term "sensory processing disorder," it is not an official term in diagnostic manuals such as the *Diagnostic and Statistical Manual of Mental Disorders*, 5th edition (*DSM-5*) (American Psychiatric Association, 2013). The American Academy of Pediatrics (Zimmer et al., 2012) issued a statement on *sensory processing disorder* for pediatricians, which suggests that the term should not be used. Rather, the American Academy of Pediatrics emphasizes that services should focus on daily life, which supports OT's core tenets.

Due to the diligent work of many occupational therapists and other researchers, sensory processing concepts have permeated people's work and lives. Many people recognize that sensory processing differences, just as other human differences, are reflective of how people prefer to live. Words such as "sensory seeker" and "sensory avoider" have become everyday language to describe an individual's responses to sensory events. People's sensory preferences influence the ways in which they prefer to contribute to work and relationships. For example, Seekers create new ideas, Avoiders create structure, and Bystanders are easy-going in challenging situations. In summary, a core assumption in this chapter is that everyone has particular sensory processing patterns that affect their lives. Occupational therapy practitioners can contribute by helping individuals gain insight into their own patterns so they can mindfully plan how to create a satisfying life.

Dunn's Sensory Processing Framework

This section describes a commonly used model of sensory processing, Dunn's Sensory Processing Framework (Dunn, 2014); explains the terminology and concepts used in this model; and provides examples of behaviors within each sensory processing pattern. Additionally, it describes the ways in which researchers in OT have organized sensory processing knowledge by grouping individuals according to their particular sensory patterns.

In a recent scoping review of how sensory factors impact children's everyday lives and occupations (Dunn et al., 2016), evidence showed that the most commonly used model to investigate sensory features is Dunn's Sensory Processing Framework. In 1997, Dunn proposed a model of sensory processing describing the interaction of individual sensory detection thresholds (i.e., how quickly one detects a sensation) and self-regulation strategies (i.e., one's behavioral responses to the sensation) (Dunn, 1997). Since then, the model has been updated and is now referred to as Dunn's Sensory Processing Framework (Dunn, 2014). In this model, detection thresholds range from high (i.e., slow to notice or perceive a sensation) to low (i.e., quick to notice or perceive a sensation). Self-regulation ranges from passive to active. These two continua interact to create four sensory processing patterns (Figure 59-1):

1. **Registration**: high threshold and passive self-regulation
2. **Seeking**: high threshold and active self-regulation
3. **Sensitivity**: low threshold and passive self-regulation
4. **Avoiding**: low threshold and active self-regulation

Sensory processing patterns occur across systems (e.g., tactile, auditory, olfactory) and reflect behaviors affected by neurological thresholds and self-regulation strategies. Individuals can exhibit specific behaviors that align with each sensory processing pattern, referred to as bystanders, seekers, avoiders, and sensors. *Bystanders* are individuals who have difficulty with registration and may take longer to notice sensory information or need sensory events to be more intense to notice. Examples of behaviors that bystanders may show include lack of response to one's name or not noticing when someone new enters a room.

Sensory seekers are individuals who crave intense sensory experiences. Sensory seeking behaviors include active involvement in activities or actions that provide intense sensory input (e.g., a lot of movement), preferring environments that are colorful or bright, and needing busy or loud environments.

Individuals who detect sensory stimuli very quickly and exhibit active behavior responses in an attempt to disengage from such stimuli are referred to as *avoiders*. Avoidance behaviors include covering one's ears to block noise, not attending an event or place that is known to be loud or bright, and not being willing to try a novel food.

Individuals who detect sensory information quickly but do not use active strategies to disengage are referred to as *sensors*. Sensors may prefer specific brands of foods or clothing and may have distinct preferences about what restaurants or stores are acceptable (Figures 59-2 and 59-3).

Sensory Processing Classifications

As you read descriptions of behaviors that fall within each sensory processing pattern, you may wonder about the senses themselves. You may think, "I am a seeker with

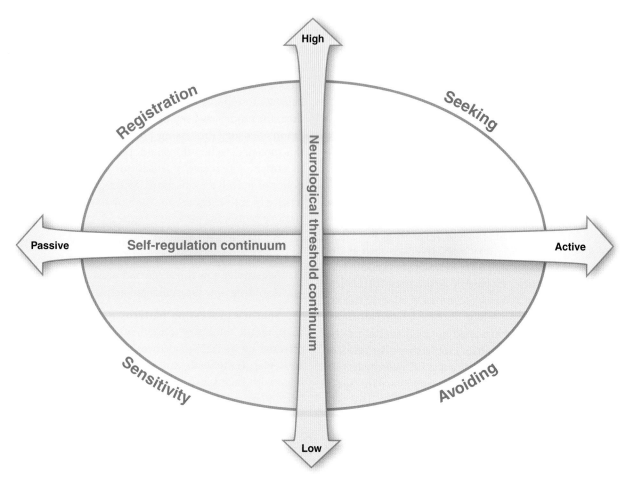

FIGURE 59-1 Dunn's Sensory Processing Framework.

movement, but I am very sensitive to smells." Occupational therapy researchers have been interested in this topic and have therefore studied the heterogeneity or different combinations of sensory features among individuals with typical development as well as those with conditions. Evidence shows that individuals can show unique combinations of sensory patterns based on activity contexts and task demands (Baranek et al., 2014; Little, Ausderau, Sideris, & Baranek, 2015). That is, individuals' behavior is affected by a combination of the sensory aspects of contexts, task factors, and their own sensory preferences. For example, a bright, loud sporting stadium may expose a person's

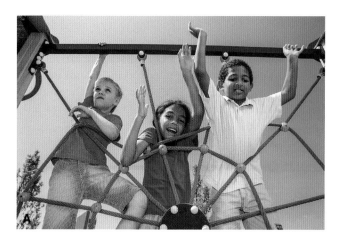
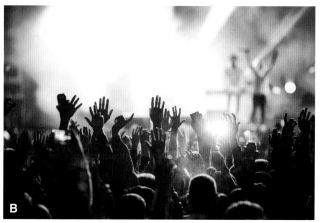

FIGURE 59-2 Sensory seekers are individuals who crave intense sensory experiences.

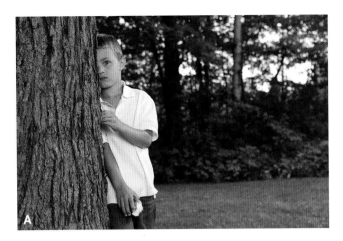 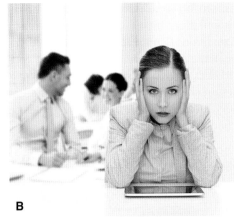

FIGURE 59-3 Avoiders seek less sensory input.

sensitivity, but a dark movie theater may not activate such sensitivity. Additionally, a child may show aversion to playing with play dough due to the sticky texture; however, the same child may play at a water table without hesitation.

When an individual shows different sensory responses across different tasks and environments, therapists may need to use a variety of strategies to increase adaptation. One study, using the Sensory Profile (Dunn, 1999), showed that parents and teachers rated children's sensory processing differently (N. B. Brown & Dunn, 2010). This suggests that children may show varying sensory-related behaviors based on contextual characteristics. For example, children may be more avoidant at school or engage in more sensory seeking due to the noise in the environment and number of other children. First-hand accounts from individuals with ASD (Grandin, 1986) suggest that busy, multisensory, and social environments may become overstimulating. Such overstimulation results in some individuals becoming withdrawn or unable to select the most relevant sensory stimuli.

Researchers have tried to understand how certain groups of people show differing sensory patterns across different situations. In an attempt to group or cluster people, researchers have investigated how to characterize people based on their sensory responses. Based on previous research, Miller and colleagues (Miller, Anzalone, Lane, Cermak, & Osten, 2007) suggested a nosology of sensory processing characteristics that grouped people together in the following categories: sensory modulation disorder ("respond faster, with more intensity, or for a longer duration," p. 136), sensory-based motor disorder ("crave an unusual amount or type of sensory input," p. 137), and sensory discrimination disorder ("difficulty interpreting qualities of sensory stimuli," p. 138). Each group of people was hypothesized to show distinct sensory features, based on different combinations of sensory patterns and motor characteristics.

Subsequent research has focused on how sensory patterns can be grouped to characterize people into "sensory subtypes." Many of these studies have focused on children with ASD because they have high rates of sensory features. A few studies have identified four groups that characterize children with ASD. Lane and colleagues (Lane, Molloy, & Bishop, 2014) used the Short Sensory Profile (McIntosh, Miller, Shyu, & Dunn, 1999) to examine sensory subtypes of children with ASD and found four subtypes: (1) sensory adaptive, (2) taste smell sensitive, (3) postural inattentive, and (4) generalized sensory difference. Another group of researchers used the Sensory Experiences Questionnaire (Baranek, 2009) and also found four sensory subtypes of children with ASD: (1) mild, (2) sensitive-distressed, (3) attenuated-preoccupied, and (4) extreme-mixed (Ausderau et al., 2014). These studies suggest that four subtypes describe the combinations of sensory responses among children with ASD. Subtypes were characterized by overall intensity of sensory features and the different presentation of sensory responses. Specifically:

- The mild group was similar to the sensory adaptive group; these children with ASD showed very few sensory processing differences.
- Children in the sensitive-distressed group were somewhat similar to the taste-smell sensitive subtype and showed high rates of sensory sensitivities, particularly in taste and olfactory processing.
- Children in the attenuated-preoccupied group were similar to the postural inattentive group, showing high rates of sensory seeking and registration.
- The extreme-mixed group was similar to the generalized sensory difference group; these children showed high rates of sensory processing differences across all sensory processing patterns.

The abovementioned studies showed that children with ASD may be grouped according to their sensory responses. However, all individuals have sensory preferences and aversions; sensory processing patterns occur across the general population, including among children with and without conditions (Dunn, Tomchek, Little, & Dean, 2016). Therefore, Little and colleagues (Little, Dean, Tomchek, & Dunn, 2017) examined sensory subtypes among a general population of children with and without conditions using the Sensory Profile-2 (Dunn, 2014). Five groups characterized all children and included the following:

1. Balanced: characterized by evenly distributed and low frequency of sensory behaviors
2. Interested: increased sensory seeking behaviors with other sensory patterns in the expected range
3. Intense: high frequencies of all sensory patterns; that is, they concurrently show high avoidance, sensitivities, registration, and seeking.
4. Mellow until . . . : increased scores in avoidance and registration (i.e., misses more cues). Children in this profile may not notice sensory stimuli (low registration) as quickly as other children. However, when a stimulus becomes salient enough for the child to notice, the stimuli may quickly become aversive (avoiding).
5. Vigilant: increased sensitivity and avoidance. This group of children likely avoids sensory experiences and shows aversion to different types of sensory stimuli.

The Balanced Sensory Profile showed overall low sensory processing scores, whereas the Intense Sensory Profile showed high sensory scores. The Vigilant Sensory Profile showed increased sensitivity and avoidance to sensory stimuli with low seeking and registration scores. The Mellow Until . . . Sensory Profile showed a high frequency of registration (i.e., misses more sensory cues) and avoidance, whereas the Interested Sensory Profile was characterized by high rates of sensory seeking with low scores on other sensory patterns. All five subtypes included children with and without conditions, such as ASD, ADHD, learning disabilities, and typical development. The findings suggest that sensory subtypes reflect the variability in all children, not just those with conditions. Future research may continue to investigate how the variability in sensory responses across individuals in the general population as well as those with ASD may be used to characterize groups.

⚖ ETHICAL DILEMMA

The Situation

A mother named Rachel reached out to you about her son Jeffery. Jeffery is a 5-year-old boy diagnosed with ASD who is getting ready to transition to kindergarten. Although Rachel reports many concerns, her primary concern is getting Jeffery's "sensory issues" under control prior to starting kindergarten. She further explains that Jeffery used to see an outpatient occupational therapist who said Jeffery may have sensory processing disorder (SPD). Due to a recent move, Rachel reports they never received the diagnosis. Rachel has indicated communication with Jeffery's school is especially difficult, and she fears the new classroom environment may need to make certain accommodations for Jeffery's "sensory issues." Without an SPD diagnosis, she worries the school will not accommodate Jeffery. Rachel requests help with receiving the SPD diagnosis to ease Jeffery's transition into a new classroom.

The Dilemma

As a new occupational therapist with this family, you want to support them and build rapport; however, you find yourself in a dilemma. That is, a dilemma between the controversial evidence on SPD and supporting Rachel's request for an SPD diagnosis.

The Take Home Message

From listening to your concerns, it seems the SPD diagnosis is important for environmental accommodations within Jeffery's new school. I too think it's important for Jeffery to receive the accommodations he needs to participate in the classroom. Although some occupational therapists discuss SPD, this diagnosis is currently controversial. Specifically, a recent policy statement from the American Academy of Pediatrics recommends not using the SPD diagnosis. This is because it is difficult to distinguish if this is an actual disorder of our sensory systems or if it is characteristic of other diagnoses (Zimmer et al., 2012). With Jeffery's ASD diagnosis, the school should accommodate his sensory preferences, especially if this is written into his Individualized Education Plan (IEP). If not, I would be happy to work with you on adding OT consultation to his IEP so we can make adjustments that honor his sensory patterns and support his learning.

Also, from a strengths-based perspective, I like to think of Jeffery's "sensory issues" as sensory preferences. Specifically, we all have preferences on which environments are too loud, too bright, or just right. When we find environments with sensory features that match our preferences, we are able to participate and feel more comfortable. However, when environments do not match our preferences, we can develop strategies to help us. For example, some individuals with certain sensory patterns may be very detail oriented; however, this may mean certain environments are very distracting. For instance, sitting at the front of a classroom may help to avoid visual distractions, whereas sitting at the back of the classroom may create too many distractions. From this perspective, we think about a child's preferences and finding sensory features within environments that support participation.

The Ecology of Human Performance: A Framework to Understand Sensory Processing

As explained above, a person's response to sensory stimuli is a result of the person's sensory preferences as well as the demands of the context and task. Given this relationship, the Ecology of Human Performance (EHP) provides a guiding framework for understanding aspects of sensory processing and identifying an appropriate intervention focus (Dean et al., in press; Dunn et al., 1994). Four primary factors guide EHP: person, task, context, and performance. Five therapeutic intervention approaches (i.e., Establish/Restore, Adapt/Modify, Alter, Prevent, and Create) address the dynamic relationship among the four constructs. (These factors and intervention approaches are examined in more detail below.)

Similarly, the underlying assumptions of Dunn's Sensory Processing Framework also focus on the importance of matching an individual's characteristics with contextual factors and task demands to increase participation and performance in meaningful activities. The theoretical underpinnings of EHP provide a structure for considering one's sensory processing patterns in light of the demands of everyday life. The following section outlines the four primary factors of EHP, which guide an understanding of evidence related to how sensory features impact everyday life. Ecology of Human Performance is covered in more depth in Chapter 43, although the model is briefly described here because the chapter uses EHP to structure the discussions of research related to sensory processing.

Ecology of Human Performance Factors

According to EHP, *person factors* include the combination of sensorimotor and psychosocial abilities as well as a person's interests, values, and experiences (Dean et al., in press; Dunn et al., 2003). Applied to sensory processing, person factors may also include sensory preferences and patterns (i.e., sensors, avoiders, seekers, or bystanders).

Each *task* or activity requires specific behaviors and performance ranges to reach the end goal and therefore places different demands on a person for successful engagement. In the context of sensory processing, each task involves different sensory features (e.g., kneading pizza dough compared to washing dishes) and may either match or not match a person's preferences.

The *performance* construct refers to how an individual engages in tasks. Each person has a performance range based on the interaction of person and context factors (Dunn et al., 2003). Specifically, individuals may perform best in contexts with certain sensory features.

Lastly, **context**, or the environment, is key to the EHP framework and refers to the physical, social, temporal, and cultural environments surrounding a person (Dunn et al., 2003). Each context has inherent sensory features (e.g., sounds in an auditorium). By understanding contextual features, one may better understand how sensory preferences (i.e., person factors) fit best within certain contexts and tasks.

A key assumption of EHP is that the four factors dynamically interact with one another. Particularly, it is not possible from an EHP perspective to truly understand person factors or a person's performance range without understanding the context for performance (Dunn et al., 1994). Contexts may facilitate performance of tasks or serve as a barrier to performance in any given task. For instance, someone who lives far from the ocean who is interested in surfing may not have the same opportunities to learn surfing as someone living on a coast who is also interested in surfing; therefore, the context creates a barrier to surfing for one individual (i.e., the person living far from the ocean) while facilitating performance for another (i.e., individual living on the coast). One's sensory preferences and patterns are an important feature of person factors; consequently, certain sensory patterns may make certain activities or contexts more appealing, whereas other sensory patterns might make people feel more apprehensive.

Ecology of Human Performance Intervention Approaches

As explicated above, sensory processing patterns impact many areas of occupation and shape the ways in which individuals experience the world. As sensory processing patterns impact people's participation, researchers have tried to understand how to best design intervention approaches that incorporate knowledge of or directly address sensory features. This section places sensory processing concepts within the EHP framework, showing how the five intervention approaches of EHP address the dynamic interactions among the four factors (i.e., person, task, performance, context). Table 59-1 provides examples of how each intervention approach can be used with Dunn's Sensory Processing Framework.

Establish/Restore: Learn Something New Every Day

The Establish/Restore approach to intervention focuses on improving person factors by establishing new skills or restoring a person's performance in a task. For instance, the weather during the summer time (i.e., physical context) is

| TABLE 59-1 | Strategies that Exemplify Ecology of Human Performance Interventions by Sensory Processing Pattern | | | |

| | Sensory Processing Pattern | | | |
Intervention Approach	Seeker	Avoider	Sensor	Bystander
Establish/Restore (Learn something new every day.)	Teach individual to recognize what his or her body needs and acceptable ways to get the input.	Teach individual to recognize situations in which he or she might get overloaded and develop strategies to manage input.	Develop strategies to manage input so individual can successfully participate in desired settings.	Develop strategies to create awareness of missed sensory input (e.g., to help you remember to take your bag to work, put car keys in the bag so you can't drive off without the bag).
Adapt/Modify (Make it easier to do.)	Insert ways to move during a computer work task.	Wear ear plugs when in noisy environment.	Use a mixer instead of hands to mix dough.	Gather all ingredients on a tray before starting to follow a recipe.
Alter (Find a better place.)	Choose concert venues that encourage standing, with clear exit and enter points.	Allow students to work in a library when the classroom is noisy.	Divide classroom into small groups to limit input.	Find a grocery store with clear overhead signs and aisle markers.
Prevent (Think ahead.)	Provide magazines and fidget toys in a waiting room.	Make quiet rooms available at a noisy building.	Arrive at class or appointment early to avoid crowds.	Make numerous navigation signs that are easy to see in a building.
Create (Make it work for everyone.)	Serve on the community park board to construct playgrounds that meet diverse sensory needs.	Work with the museum to create "get away" spaces within exhibits.	Consult with designers to find the most "accessible" fabrics for a convention center seating.	Collaborate with the shopping mall to design signage that is easy to see.

more conducive to swimming (i.e., task); however, at the beginning of the summer, the individual may need to focus on restoring swimming skills (i.e., person) and potentially establishing new skills (e.g., back stroke, free style).

Adapt/Modify: Make It Easier to Do

The Adapt/Modify approach focuses on both the context and task demands to best facilitate performance (Dean et al., in press; Dunn et al., 1994). With sensory processing, a therapist can facilitate an individual's performance by adjusting the task features to match his or her sensory preferences or by making the context of the task best match the person's sensory preferences. For example, the sound of a lawn mower may be too loud for sensors and avoiders. To make the task a better match for their sensory preferences, they may wear noise canceling head phones or use a battery-operated lawn mower; both adaptations result in less noise.

Alter: Find a Better Place

The Alter method of intervention focuses on changing contextual factors to support a person's current strengths and abilities as a way to facilitate task performance (Dunn, 2007). This approach aligns with sensory processing in that many people select the places where they engage in activities based on their sensory preferences. For instance, when attending a class, an individual may select a seat based on his or her social context (i.e., friends) or based on our sensory preferences. A seat in the front row provides

fewer visual distractions for a sensor, whereas a seat in the middle may match the preferences of a seeker.

Prevent: Think Ahead

The Prevent intervention method addresses all factors (i.e., person, task, context, performance) to identify and address potential barriers to performance, thus preventing negative events from occurring. When applied to sensory processing, parents may think ahead and address potential contexts that may not be best suited for them or their children. For instance, a music concert may provide a context where seekers may thrive, but it may also provide a context too overwhelming for an avoider or a sensor. Therefore, one may think ahead and prevent the contextual features from impacting engagement in attending a music concert by bringing ear plugs, carefully selecting a seating location, and establishing an exit plan ahead of time.

Create: Make It Work for Everyone

The Create intervention approach focuses on creating strategies to support the performance of a community or population (Dean et al., in press). Similar to the Prevent approach, the Create approach may focus on all four factors to develop an intervention strategy (Dunn et al., 2003). In fact, many Create intervention approaches begin as Alter approaches but result in a solution that benefits the population as a whole (Dean et al., in press). For instance, by having grocery stores of varying sizes, with varying foods and options within a community, people may find a store that

CASE STUDY 59-1   ALTERING THE WORKPLACE TO SUPPORT PARTICIPATION

This case is an example of how altering a workplace environment based on sensory processing patterns can support a person with employment. Jonel is now 20 years old and working as a dish washer at a restaurant. This work required standing for long periods of time and involved little interaction with other people. The restaurant owner considered Jonel a valuable employee who showed up on time and was fun to work with. However, recently, the owner has voiced concerns about Jonel's productivity.

The owner reported that Jonel frequently walked away from his dishwashing station and visited with other workers in the dining room. Jonel's coworkers also expressed that Jonel was sometimes rude when they offered help. Jonel also expressed he was unhappy with his job. Jonel liked working in the restaurant, and the owner wanted to find a way for Jonel to increase his productivity so he could keep his job. His father, who also served as Jonel's legal guardian, contacted vocational rehabilitation to find out how they could support Jonel. Jonel and his father completed an application to gain access to vocational rehabilitation supports.

An occupational therapist who contracted with a vocational rehabilitation agency came to the restaurant to assess Jonel's strengths and preferences related to work. The occupational therapist administered the Adolescent/Adult Sensory Profile (AASP; C. Brown & Dunn, 2002), talked with Jonel and his boss, and observed Jonel at work. The occupational therapist noticed that Jonel stayed on task at his dishwashing station for about 5 minutes before he walked around to either go to the restroom or visit with other employees. The occupational therapist also noticed that when the kitchen was busy and noisy (which is where the dishwashing station was located), Jonel would become irritable and sometimes respond rudely when another employee or the owner asked him a question or directed him back to his task.

The AASP indicated that Jonel scored in the "more than others" range on the "high threshold" quadrants (seeking and registration). Based on this result, along with observations and information from the restaurant owner, the occupational therapist concluded that Jonel was most successful when doing tasks that allowed him to move around frequently and minimized auditory cues (e.g., verbal instructions). She hypothesized that altering Jonel's workplace tasks based on his sensory preferences may make him more successful at work.

The occupational therapist talked with Jonel and the owner about assigning new work tasks for Jonel for a trial period. During the trial period, Jonel's job included seating customers, wiping down tables, and taking dishes to the kitchen. Jonel enjoyed the fast pace of the restaurant. He recognized when he needed to clear a table because he could see that the customers had left, and their plates were still on the table. Additionally, Jonel had brief social interactions with customers, which he and the customers enjoyed.

In this example, the context of the restaurant provided many options for productive work so that Jonel could remain a loyal employee there. The occupational therapist recognized the sensory characteristics of the restaurant context and, with strong activity analysis skills, found the combination of tasks that would match Jonel's sensory patterns throughout his shift. The restaurant did not have to make adjustments to their routines or environment to accommodate Jonel; partnering with the OT, they found a situation that already existed and matched Jonel with these work tasks. From an EHP perspective, this would be an "Alter" intervention, finding a better match without changing the person's characteristics or the context.

best matches their preferences. Specifically, the contextual factors of a small grocery store with more limited options may provide the best match for a sensor or avoider (e.g., less noisy, easier to navigate, less visually stimulating). A larger store, with many options and taste testings may provide a better match for a seeker or bystander (e.g., noisier, more people to talk to, stimulating for tastes and smells).

Measurement

The first step to successful intervention is to administer an appropriate, validated measure to help understand the sensory processing patterns of an individual and how they affect participation in daily life. A variety of assessment tools measure sensory processing through direct observation of behavior or questionnaires completed by family members, caregivers, teachers, and/or self-report.

Measures are designed to reflect differing theoretical foundations (e.g., sensory processing or SI), and therefore, utility and supporting evidence varies by measure. Additionally, the theoretical foundations guide whether a measure is developed with a top–down (i.e., measuring and focusing on the person as a whole or participation-focused) versus a bottom–up approach (i.e., focusing on details first or skill-focused) framework. Because measures guide intervention development, it is important for occupational therapists to understand the theoretical assumptions of a measure as well as the specific type of information gathered. Although sensory processing assessments provide information about sensory features in everyday life contexts, it is helpful for occupational therapists to use additional measures that directly assess participation; participation-based assessments can help practitioners further understand how sensory patterns impact participation and how to develop intervention approaches to best suit the needs of an individual. Table 59-2

TABLE 59-2 **Assessment Measures Related to Sensory Processing, Sensory Integration, and Participation**

Measure	Category	Population	Type	Description	Approach
Measures of Sensory Processing and Sensory Integration					
Sensory Profile-2 (Dunn, 2014) Short Sensory Profile-2 (Dunn, 2014) Adolescent/Adult Sensory Profile (C. Brown & Dunn, 2002)	SP	Across the life course	Questionnaire	Caregiver questionnaire designed to measure sensory preferences in four quadrants: Low Registration, Sensory Seeking, Sensory Sensitivity, and Sensory Avoiding. A short form and adolescent/adult self-report form are also available.	Top–down
Sensory Experiences Questionnaire Version 3.0 (Baranek, 2009)	SP	2–12 yr	Questionnaire	Caregiver-report questionnaire designed to measure behaviors associated with everyday sensory experiences. Measures the frequency of behaviors associated with four sensory response patterns: hyporesponsiveness, hyperresponsiveness, sensory seeking, enhanced perception	Top–down
Sensory Processing Measure (Parham & Ecker, 2007) Sensory Processing Measure-Preschool (SPM-P) (Miller Kuhaneck, Ecker, Parham, Henry, & Glennon, 2010; Parham & Ecker, 2007)	SI	5–12 yr; 2–5 yr	Questionnaire	Parent or teacher questionnaire for assessing SP challenges at school and at home. Detects problem behaviors in sensory processing, praxis, and social participation. The SPM-P provides information on social participation; praxis; and the visual, auditory, tactile, proprioceptive, and vestibular sensory systems.	Bottom–up
The Sensory Perception Quotient (Tavassoli, Hoekstra, & Baron-Cohen, 2014)	SP	Adults	Questionnaire	Self-report questionnaire that assesses sensory perception in adults. Assesses basic hypersensitivity and hyposensitivity across five modalities (touch, hearing, vision, smell, taste). A short form is also available.	Top–down
The Sensory Processing Scales Sensory Over-Responsivity Scales (Schoen, Miller, & Green, 2008)	SI	3–55 yr	Performance-based and Questionnaire	Includes a trained examiner performance-based assessment and a caregiver-report questionnaire. Measures sensory overresponsivity in seven sensory domains (tactile, auditory, visual, proprioceptive, olfactory, gustatory, vestibular)	Bottom–up
Comprehensive Observations of Proprioception (Blanche, Bodison, Chang, & Reinoso, 2012)	SI	2–8 yr	Performance-based	A criterion-based observational and play-based measure assessing two components of proprioception (behavior and sensory-motor abilities) as well as muscle tone and hypermobility	Bottom–up
Observations Based on SI Theory (Blanche, 2002)	SI	3–15 yr	Performance-based	Nonstandardized observational measure that provides guidelines for semistructured play to assess SI skills and behaviors	Bottom–up
Sensory Integration Praxis Tests (Ayres, 1989)	SI	4–8 yr	Performance-based	A performance-based and standardized assessment with 17 subtests designed to measure dysfunctional SI behavior. The subtests include visual, tactile, kinesthetic, and motor tasks.	Bottom–up
Sensory Processing Assessment (Baranek, 1999)	SP	9–6 yr	Performance-based	A play-based observational assessment that measures sensory avoidance and hyporesponsiveness (i.e., approach-avoidance patterns, orienting responses, and habituation to repeated stimuli)	Top–down
Tactile Defensiveness and Discrimination Test-Revised (Baranek, 2010)	SP	3–12 yr	Performance-based	Observational measure with five structured play-based subtests that assesses tactile processing (i.e., hyperresponsiveness and discrimination)	Top–down
The Test of Sensory Functions in Infants (DeGangi & Greenspan, 1989)	SI	4–18 mo	Performance-based	Criterion-referenced measure to assess infants' deficits in SI in the following five subdomains: deep pressure, visual-tactile integration, adaptive motor functioning, ocular-motor control, and vestibular stimulation	Bottom–up
DeGangi-Berk Test of Sensory Integration (Berk & DeGangi, 1983)	SI	3–5 yr	Performance-based	A test requiring children to perform specific tasks that focus on measuring sensory deficits in postural control, bilateral motor integration, and reflex integration.	Bottom–up

| TABLE 59-2 | Assessment Measures Related to Sensory Processing, Sensory Integration, and Participation *(continued)* |

Measure	Category	Population	Type	Description	Approach
Measures of Participation					
Activity Card Sort (Baum & Edwards, 2001)		18–65+ yr	Questionnaire	Individuals sort activity cards (i.e., instrumental, social, and leisure). Examines individual's engagement in the activity and if he or she discontinues an activity	Top–down
Paediatric Activity Card Sort (Mandich, Polatajko, Miller, & Baum, 2004)		5–14 yr	Questionnaire	Children sort activity cards in four domains: personal care, school, hobbies/social, and sports. Examines a child's engagement in the activity and if he or she discontinues an activity	Top–down
Assessment of Preschool Activity Participation (King, Law, Petrenchik, & Kertoy, 2006)		2–5 yr	Questionnaire	Caregiver-report scale that characterizes children's engagement in activities in four categories: play, skill development, active physical recreation, and social activities	Top–down
Child and Adolescent Scale of Participation (Bedell, 2009)		3–22 yr	Questionnaire	Caregiver-report scale that measures child participation in home, school, and community activities in four subdomains: home participation, community participation, school participation, and home and community living participation	Top–down
Participation and Environment Measure for Children and Youth (Coster, Law, Bedell, & Teplicky, 2010)		5–17 yr	Questionnaire	Parent-report measure for participation at home, school, and the community, including environmental features	Top–down
The Young Children's Participation and Environment Measure (Khetani, Coster, Law, & Bedell, 2013)		0–5 yr	Questionnaire	Parent report measure of participation at home, preschool/day care, and the community	Top–down

SP, sensory processing; SI, sensory integration.

presents various measures related to sensory processing, SI, and participation. It is not intended to be an exhaustive list of measures of participation; rather, it provides examples that may be helpful for occupational therapists to administer in conjunction with an assessment of sensory features.

Evidence on Sensory Processing and Everyday Life

As described above, senses can enhance an individual's enjoyment of a place or activity, but sensory experiences can also make daily life challenging. For example, a person may love to cook at home because the smells of their family recipes remind them of childhood, and the repetitive movement of chopping or mixing is relaxing. However, creating the same recipe when multiple children are running around the kitchen may not be so pleasant. The addition of extra noise, touching, and a crowded work environment changes the experience of cooking the same recipe. This section describes the research on how sensory

processing contributes to daily life, with an emphasis on how sensory aspects of the person, task, and context interaction relate to performance.

School and Learning

For all children, success in school is in part dependent on how well the child can attend to instruction and self-regulate behavior to match classroom expectations, the demands of specific learning activities, and teachers' teaching styles. Research has investigated how sensory processing impacts learning and school performance among typically developing children as well as those with conditions. In preschoolers, how quickly children identify and focus on changing stimuli is related to reading and spelling performance (Boets, Wouters, van Wieringen, De Smedt, & Ghesquiére, 2008). Children with a learning disability may struggle to integrate auditory and visual input, which can impact their learning (Boliek, Keintz, Norrix, & Obrzut, 2010). Additionally, children with dyslexia may have more difficulty filtering noise when people are speaking, indicating that a quiet classroom may support learning for these students (Geiger et al., 2008). One study (Jirikowic, Olson, & Kartin, 2008) reported that children with fetal

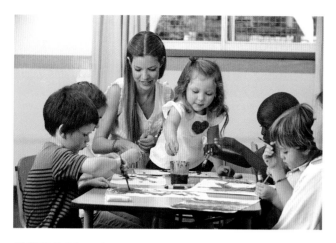

FIGURE 59-4 Sensory processing demands of schools can be different from those at home, indicating the importance of considering sensory processing patterns in the specific context in which the therapist is working with a child.

alcohol spectrum disorder (FASD) have differences in sensory processing that affect academic and behavioral performance. Children with ASD may also need more support to be successful in some learning environments. For instance, Ashburner, Ziviani, and Rodger (2008) reported that academic performance for students with ASD may be affected by a mismatch between the classroom context (e.g., background noise in the classroom) and the students' sensory processing preferences (e.g., toleration of auditory or touch stimuli). This mismatch can lead to difficulties with attention, hyperactivity, and oppositional behaviors.

As shown in Figure 59-4, it is important to note that the sensory processing demands of schools can be different from those at home, indicating the importance of considering sensory processing patterns in the specific context in which the therapist is working with the child (N. B. Brown & Dunn, 2010). See Chapter 51 for details related to the role of OT in educational settings.

Adaptive Behavior

Evidence shows that individuals' adaptive behavior (i.e., how they function in social communication and daily living skills) is impacted by their sensory processing patterns. Among individuals with ASD, the overall degree of sensory features (e.g., how loud, bright, or crowded a room is or how much movement is required in a task; Rogers, Hepburn, & Wehner, 2003) as well as specific sensory response patterns (Ashburner et al., 2008) may be related to adaptive behavior difficulties. Specifically, sensory seeking and registration patterns have been found

to contribute to such difficulties among individuals with ASD (Adams et al., 2011; Baker, Lane, Angley, & Young, 2008; Reynolds, Bendixen, Lawrence, & Lane, 2011). Studies have found similar findings among individuals with FASD and ADHD (Mattard-Labrecque, Ben Amor, & Couture, 2013).

With regard to self-care, a few studies (Stein, Polido, & Cermak, 2013; Stein, Polido, Mailloux, Coleman, & Cermak, 2011) reported that children with ASD struggle with dental care due to the sensory challenges associated with the task; the authors proposed modifications to reduce the sensory input in dental care environments.

Overall, the relationship between adaptive behavior and sensory features is complex. There are many behavioral domains associated with adaptive behavior (e.g., social communication, self-care, community skills), all of which may be differentially impacted by a person's sensory processing characteristics as well as task and contextual demands. In OT, more investigations are needed to unravel the complexities of how specific sensory features support and interfere with adaptive behavior.

Activity Participation

When individuals have certain sensory patterns, they are likely to choose activities that match their sensory preferences and aversions. Overall, studies suggest that sensory avoidance and sensitivities negatively impact the amount of activity participation among individuals with ASD (Hochhauser & Engel-Yeger, 2010; Jasmin et al., 2009; Lane, Young, Baker, & Angley, 2010; Marquenie, Rodger, Mangohig, & Cronin, 2011) and ADHD (Engel-Yeger, Hardal-Nasser, & Gal, 2011). Parents have reported that home activities are more manageable for children with ASD due to the unpredictability of sensory features in community contexts (Bagby, Dickie, & Baranek, 2012). Findings are mixed with regard to the roles that cognition and attention play in how sensory features impact activity participation. Some findings suggest that difficulties are more related to cognition and attention (Zingerevich, 2009), whereas other findings suggest that sensory processing contributes to difficulties in activity participation regardless of cognition (Little et al., 2015).

Although most research has focused on sensory barriers to participation, there are likely sensory features that support children's activity participation. Little et al. (2015) found that enhanced perception (i.e., sensory hyperacuity and attention to details) was associated with increased activity participation among individuals with ASD, and children with increased sensory seeking scores participated in more adult/child play time in the home. Additionally, Dean, Little, Tomchek, and

CASE STUDY 59-2   ADAPTING CLASSROOM EXPECTATIONS TO SUPPORT PARTICIPATION

This case is an example of how adapting a classroom environment based on sensory processing patterns can support classroom participation.

Jonel is a 7-year-old boy who attends a first-grade classroom. He loves his teacher and says that he "has lots of friends" in the class. He says his favorite subject is "recess," but he also likes math but "not too much"—meaning he doesn't like to do math for too long at one time. Jonel also says that he gets frustrated because he gets in trouble a lot but can't seem to "do what I'm supposed to."

Jonel's teacher contacted the school's occupational therapist because she felt that his classroom behavior was preventing him from reaching academic potential. The teacher explained that Jonel was a "sweet kid" but would disrupt the class (especially during quiet, seated work) by walking or running around the classroom, talking to the teacher at her desk, or fidgeting at his desk. Jonel frequently did not complete assignments and would often claim he did not hear the teacher's instructions about completing the assignment. The teacher had tried providing rewards and punishments for completing assignments and staying in his seat, but these interventions frustrated Jonel because he could not seem to meet the teacher's expectation to get the reward or avoid the punishment.

At home, Jonel's mother claimed that she did not have trouble with Jonel being disruptive and stated he spent most of his time riding his bike outside or playing with his four brothers. She did note, however, that Jonel had difficulty following directions, but she didn't think he was being defiant. She stated, "I just don't think he hears me all of the time."

The occupational therapist administered the Sensory Profile School Companion 2 (SPSC2; Dunn, 2014) and observed Jonel in the classroom and on the playground. The occupational therapist noticed that Jonel could sit still for about 5 minutes but then would start shaking his leg. When he came to school in the morning, he was friendly with his classmates, but as the day went on, he would get up from his seat and poke or kick classmates as he walked around the classroom. On the playground, Jonel would play soccer or tag the entire recess and cooperated with classmates.

The SPSC2 indicated that Jonel scored in the "more than others" range on the "high threshold" quadrants (seeking and registration). Based on this result, along with classroom and playground observations and information from his teacher, the occupational therapist concluded that Jonel was most successful when doing tasks that allowed him to move around frequently and minimized auditory cues (e.g., verbal instructions). She hypothesized that adapting classroom expectations would support Jonel's academic performance.

The occupational therapist worked with Jonel's teacher to develop teaching strategies to provide more opportunities for movement and also limit verbal instructions. The teacher said that she would find "errands" for Jonel to run before long periods of sitting time and also experiment with dynamic seating options, such as ball seats for more sensory input. Finally, the teacher said she would ask the class to write down their homework assignments before they finished the lesson and ensure that Jonel wrote down the assignments.

Jonel loved the ball seat, and his teacher noted that Jonel stayed in his seat longer when using it. He still got fidgety and needed to walk around but usually only once an hour rather than every 10 minutes. The teacher designated Jonel as the "assignment collector" which allowed him to walk around the classroom and collect the assignments. On days when Jonel needed extra movement, the class would time him to see how fast he could do the job. When Jonel wrote down his homework assignments, he increased his assignment completion from "almost never" to "about half the time." The teacher resolved to talk with his family about organizational strategies that would enable Jonel to complete his homework more often.

In this example, the classroom environment was not a good match for Jonel's sensory preferences. Jonel did not demonstrate the same behaviors at home because his sensory seeking needs were being met by having more time to play outside and play with his four brothers. Through observation and consultation with the teacher, the occupational therapist identified classroom modifications that would better match Jonel's sensory input needs. From an EHP perspective, this "Adapt" intervention supported Jonel's academic participation by modifying the classroom to meet Jonel's sensory preferences.

Dunn (2018) studied children in the general population and found that the Avoiding and Seeking patterns can affect resiliency and the Avoiding pattern also affects adaptability. The authors concluded that people who notice sensory responses quickly and actively respond to the stimuli (e.g., try to get away or reduce the input) may need more support to overcome obstacles or adjust to changes in routine. Higher frequencies of seeking behaviors, on the other hand, may make children more resilient.

Sensory processing is also related to how individuals participate in social situations. Children with avoidance and sensory sensitivities get more enjoyment out of socializing with family or a few close friends than a larger group of peers (Cosbey, Johnston, & Dunn, 2010). Also, typically developing children and children with ASD who demonstrate higher frequency of sensory processing behaviors also demonstrate more needs for support with social interactions (Hilton, Graver, & LaVesser, 2007; Matsushima & Kato, 2013). Individuals' sensory characteristics contribute to and detract from activity participation. When OT practitioners understand the interface between people's sensory characteristics and the features of the context or task, they can best support activity participation.

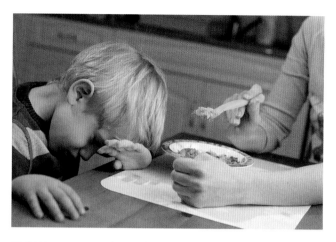

FIGURE 59-5 When children show sensory sensitivities and avoidances, eating and mealtime can become challenging.

Eating and Mealtime

Eating is an important daily activity that involves many sensory features; in fact, the sensory features of food are what can make eating enjoyable for many people. The sights, smells, and tastes of our favorite foods can make eating a central aspect of many social and family activities. When children show sensory sensitivities and avoidances, however, eating and mealtime can become challenging.

Overall, children with ADHD, ASD, and gastrointestinal (GI) conditions tend to show increased taste and smell sensitivities (Davis et al., 2013; Ghanizadeh, 2013; Zobel-Lachiusa, Andrianopoulos, Mailloux, & Cermak, 2015). Children with ASD who show sensory sensitivities also demonstrate more challenges with mealtime, including the number of foods eaten, amount and variety of foods eaten, ability to sit at the table with others, and ability to stay seated at mealtime (Nadon, Feldman, Dunn, & Gisel, 2011).

Among individuals with typical development, sensory processing is related to how people approach novel foods. Research suggests that when trying new food, children are more attracted to foods that are visually similar to familiar foods, whereas adults are more likely to use touch to decide whether they will try a new food (Dovey et al., 2012). Children with taste and smell sensitivities may also be more likely to reject fruits and vegetables than other children (Coulthard & Blissett, 2009). Knowing these issues related to sensory processing and mealtime, occupational therapists can work with families to create mealtime routines that match the sensory processing patterns of all people in the family (Figure 59-5).

Play

Play is a central occupation for children, and children's sensory processing patterns can inform practitioners about the types of play activities that are likely to be more

enjoyable for different children. When typically developing children show more sensory processing differences, they engage in less mature and less socially based play than peers (Cosbey et al., 2010). Additionally, typically developing children with increased sensitivities are less likely to change their body positions during play (Mische Lawson & Dunn, 2008).

The play opportunities of children are likely influenced by their parents' sensory preferences. One study showed that child and parent sensory avoiding and sensitivity scores are significantly related, which contributes to parents offering nonseeking play activities (Welters-Davis & Mische Lawson, 2011). For children with ASD, researchers have shown relationships between sensory processing and social play; specifically, the overall sensory processing scores relate to how children create play opportunities with others (Kuhaneck & Britner, 2013).

When addressing play with children and their families, it is important for occupational therapists to understand the sensory preferences of the child and the sensory experiences that particular activities afford. For example, a child who has a low threshold for movement may not enjoy playing soccer but may enjoy the predictability of swinging on a swing set. When the preference of the child matches the sensory characteristics of the activity, the child is more likely to be successful. See Chapter 53 for more information on OT and play.

Sleep

A child's sleep routines can have a significant impact on a family's quality of life. The relationship between sensory processing and sleep has not been studied extensively; however, research is beginning to focus on these issues, specifically among children with conditions. Children with

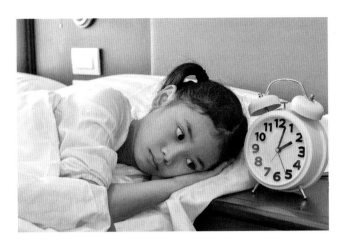

FIGURE 59-6 A child's sleep routines can have a significant impact on a family's quality of life.

FASD, who are more sensitive to sensory input, may not sleep as long and may take longer to go to sleep (Wengel, Hanlon-Dearman, & Fjeldsted, 2011). Similarly, children who seek more sensory input tend to stay awake longer and sleep less. Children with ASD who show increased sensory sensitivities have also been shown to have sleep difficulties (Mazurek & Petroski, 2015; Reynolds, Lane, & Thacker, 2012). Researchers suggest that, when children arouse to more stimuli, it is harder to fall asleep again because they detect more sensory events. They also hypothesize that these sensory and sleep patterns could be associated with anxiety.

When OT practitioners work with individuals on sleep and bedtime routines, it is important to consider the sensory characteristics of the person as well as how the sensory features of the environment may be impacting overall sleep (Figure 59-6). See Chapter 54 for more information related to OT and sleep.

Evidence Related to Intervention

Interventions designed to address sensory processing vary by what aspect of occupational performance they emphasize and therefore differently align with EHP intervention approaches. Similar to sensory measures, sensory-focused interventions use differing theoretical bases (e.g., sensory processing vs. SI) as well as the conceptualization of the mechanism of change (i.e., the process or specific way in which participation increases). This section discusses the evidence related to a number of interventions, including environmental modifications, parent-led interventions, SI, and sensory-based interventions, and explains how each intervention fits within an EHP intervention

approach (i.e., Establish/Restore, Alter, Adapt/Modify, Prevent, Create). (Refer to Table 59-1 for examples of how specific strategies match each sensory pattern and EHP intervention approach.)

🧘 PRACTICE DILEMMA

The Situation

A parent named Keith is interested in understanding more about what he can do to support his daughter, Veronica, with sensory-related activities. He reports he completed many Internet searches and learned occupational therapists are often certified in these activities. He wants to learn more about how these interventions will help Veronica's sensory challenges. He hands you a list of interventions, including auditory integration training and the Wilbarger brushing protocol.

The Dilemma

Parents taking responsibility to research information is especially important; however, you know the evidence for these methods is lacking. Although you want to continue to support Keith, you also have a responsibility to report accurate evidence on the interventions he found during his search.

The Take Home Message

First, we can explore Veronica's sensory preferences, as this may help us target activities that are the most supportive to Veronica's needs. We all have sensory preferences; and over time, we learn strategies to help us when activities do not match our preferences. By understanding Veronica's sensory processing patterns, we can develop strategies to support her.

The Internet research you completed is very important, and I am encouraged that you took the time to learn and understand Veronica this way. I would like to share with you the evidence on the two methods you read about. Studies show different findings with these two methods, and certain studies were stronger than others as well. This makes it especially confusing to sift through the evidence. The idea behind Auditory Integration Training is that by listening to specialized auditory input, this will fix Veronica's central nervous system. However, to date, studies are showing no benefits to Auditory Integration Training for child behavior (Case-Smith, Weaver, & Fristad, 2015). The Wilbarger Protocol is very similar; however, instead of auditory input, you use a small brush to apply pressure to different joints of the body to change the sensory systems of Veronica (Wilbarger & Wilbarger, 1991). However, like Auditory Integration Training, there is little to no evidence indicating the Wilbarger Brushing Protocol will help child behavior.

There are many other strategies we can use to support Veronica. Her sensory preferences are part of how she understands the world; her discerning auditory system can be distracting in noisy places, but this might also mean she hears details in songs that you and I would miss. Her touch sensitivity makes it hard to get dressed, but we can find the right fabrics and textures for her wardrobe so she can fully participate without her clothing bothering her. So we can take advantage of understanding her preferences by planning activities that match her needs and by thinking ahead about activities that might be more challenging.

Environmental Modifications

Most public environments were created for people who fit within the majority of others on the bell curve, which can create challenges for people who process sensory input differently. Environmental modifications can be used to address specific elements of contexts that elicit aversive responses from individuals. Such modifications can be made to match children's sensory preferences. For example, classrooms are bright and loud for many children with sensory differences, and a few studies have investigated the effects of modifying the classroom environment. One study found positive effects on student engagement when classroom lighting and sound were altered for children with ASD (Kinnealey et al., 2012). Specifically, the students in this study expressed that the halogen lighting and sound-absorbing walls helped them focus and feel more comfortable in the classroom. Another study (Bagatell, Mirigliani, Patterson, Reyes, & Test, 2010) found that young children with ASD benefited from using therapy balls in the classroom, particularly if they had frequent seeking behaviors. The therapy balls were not helpful, however, for children with poor postural stability, as they were less engaged.

Visual schedules have been shown to be a very effective environmental modification intervention among children with ASD, likely due to strengths in visual processing (Case-Smith & Arbesman, 2008). Research shows that when using visual schedules, children show decreased problem behavior and increased engagement; the visual schedules seem to offer the children control because they have pictures to sequentially depict activities (for a review, see Lequia, Machalicek, & Rispoli, 2012).

Research findings about environmental modifications show that OT practitioners should consider the individual sensory preferences of each child when designing these types of interventions. Children with differing levels of sensory seeking, registration, sensitivities, and avoidance may respond differently to varying types of modifications. For example, a bright light or strong scent may be activating for some children with registration difficulties;

however, if a child shows sensory avoidance, the bright light or strong scent may lead to more problem behaviors.

In the context of EHP intervention approaches, environmental modifications may be considered to be an Alter intervention. When we alter the sensory elements of contexts, individuals may be better able to participate. For example, dimming florescent lighting and soundproofing walls may help students with sensory sensitivities focus in the classroom.

Although we think about changing the environment to meet the needs of specific individuals with sensory processing challenges and distinct preferences, such environmental modifications may also result in a Create intervention. Interventions that use the Create approach are designed to support optimal performance for all persons and populations. There are few examples in the literature of using the create strategy to support sensory processing, but environmental modifications are being increasingly used to create environments acceptable for various people. For example, therapy balls provide seating for individuals who seek movement; however, some research suggests that therapy balls may help other children maintain focus in a classroom (Fedewa & Erwin, 2011; Schilling, Washington, Billingsley, & Deitz, 2003). Other examples include businesses that understand the potential of matching customers' sensory preferences with sensory friendly environments. Some movie theaters offer "sensory-friendly" times in which the sound is down and the lights are up, which are appealing to a wide variety of people. Some museums offer tactile, visual, and movement opportunities to interact with displays.

Occupational therapists can use their knowledge of sensory processing to play key roles in supporting businesses to create sensory-friendly environments for all people.

Parent-Led Interventions

Parent-led interventions directly involve a child's caregiver and/or other family members. There are a few parent-led intervention approaches that incorporate the therapists' sensory processing knowledge. Although the specific theoretical bases for these interventions vary, the approaches target a wide variety of child skills and often incorporate, or are specific to, parent involvement and/or training. Currently, best practice for young children with sensory differences and conditions such as ASD dictates that caregivers are central to intervention approaches; that is, parents and other family members must be involved in a child's OT for it to be effective. Strategies for involving families in intervention are gaining traction with practitioners and families because there is positive empirical evidence of the effectiveness of these methods on child behavior and parent satisfaction (Little, Pope, Wallisch, Dunn, 2018).

Examples of comprehensive parent-led interventions include Occupational Performance Coaching (OPC), Adapted Responsive Teaching, Early Start Denver Model, and targeted parent education models.

Occupational Performance Coaching

Occupational Performance Coaching directly engages caregivers in identifying their own goals for their children and working with a therapist to understand how to embed sensory-based, communication, and play strategies into everyday activities. In OPC, therapists work with caregivers to gain a deeper understanding of the caregivers' own knowledge and the impact of their strategies on their children's behavior (Rush & Shelden, 2011). The role of the therapist is to support caregivers to generate their own solutions to challenges in everyday life. Therapists ask reflective questions and make reflective comments so that caregivers have opportunities to evaluate their own strategies and daily routines. Differences in sensory preferences among family members often play a role in family life, and parents must understand their children's particular sensory patterns to best provide them with learning opportunities that match their needs.

A number of studies suggest that OPC is an effective intervention method. Among families of children with ASD, a 12-week OPC intervention resulted in positive effects related to parent self-efficacy and child participation (Dunn, Cox, Foster, Mische-Lawson, & Tanquary, 2012). At the end of intervention, families of children with ASD reached goals such as going to the grocery store and having their child engage in a bath time routine. One study implemented OPC via telehealth and found a significant increase in parent self-efficacy and child participation (Little et al., 2018). A recent study using a shorter timeline (4 weeks) for three parents of children with ASD aged 3 to 5 years showed improvements in child behavior (Bulkeley, Bundy, Roberts, & Einfeld, 2016).

The American Academy of Pediatrics identified coaching as a best practice method in early intervention (Baio, 2014) and is a recommended practice from the Division of Early Childhood (DEC, 2014; see http://www.dec-sped.org/dec-recommended-practices for more information). Through coaching, parents become empowered to support their child's everyday routines. Occupational therapists are in a unique position to use the principles of coaching in combination with their knowledge of how children's sensory processing influences participation in everyday routines and activities. More information on coaching can be found at http://www.coachinginearlychildhood.org/.

Adapted Responsive Teaching and Early Start Denver Model

Other parent-led intervention approaches include *Adapted Responsive Teaching* (Baranek et al., 2015) and the *Early*

Start Denver Model (Rogers et al., 2012). In these models, professionals teach parents specific strategies so the parents can then use those strategies in everyday routines with their children. Although similar to coaching practices, these structured interventions include a specific set of strategies that parents should use. In coaching, on the other hand, the strategies evolve through a reflective conversation with each family and are unique to the family's particular circumstances.

Adapted Responsive Teaching, which is a modified version of Responsive Teaching (Mahoney & Perales, 2003), is a model that emphasizes parent responsiveness and sensitivity. This model teaches parents about specific strategies that are aimed at meeting children's needs in a sensitive way and structuring specific activities to meet children's sensory preferences. For example, if a child is fearful of new and unfamiliar experiences due to low threshold responses (i.e., avoiding or sensitivity), a therapist using Adapted Responsive Teaching would provide a specific strategy for parents to implement that would accommodate the child's sensory preferences. Adapted Responsive Teaching for toddlers at risk for ASD has been shown to be effective in increasing children's language and adaptive behavior (Baranek et al., 2015).

The Early Start Denver Model is an intensive program of parent training that promotes positive exchanges between parents and children with ASD, using real-life materials and activities. The focus is on enhancing parent responsivity and sensitivity, and the model incorporates knowledge related to how children respond to sensory information in the specific strategies that therapists teach to parents. Research suggests that among children with ASD, the Early Start Denver Model is effective in increasing children's IQ, social communication, and adaptive behavior (Dawson et al., 2010; Rogers et al., 2012). Additionally, children who have received intensive therapy via the Early Start Denver Model have shown difference in brain responses to social situations compared with children who did not receive this intensive therapy (Dawson et al., 2012).

Targeted Parent Education Models

Another intervention that has shown promise is structured parent education that incorporates sensory processing knowledge. After participating in a 6-week intervention, parents showed a significant increase in self-confidence about their children's particular characteristics as well as a significant decrease in anxiety (Farmer & Reupert, 2013). Other studies have found that the parents were empowered when they understood how to implement sensory strategies at home and take control over their child's therapy (Dunstan & Griffiths, 2008). Gibbs and Toth-Cohen (2011) used structured parent education and sensory diets for four families of children with ASD and found a decrease in self-stimulatory behaviors and an increase in fine-motor skills.

In the context of EHP intervention approaches, parent-led models may be considered as an Adapt/Modify intervention and/or a Prevent intervention. When parents adapt and modify task features to match children's sensory preferences, children may be able to better participate in occupations. For example, if a child needs to attend a siblings' school concert in a crowded and noisy auditorium, an occupational therapist can coach a family to think through strategies to make the event tolerable for the child. On the other hand, when parents engage in parent-led interventions with occupational therapists, they can better understand how to set up environments and tasks for their children in a way that will mitigate negative responses before they occur. For example, a parent may know that a child with taste and smell sensitivity will not eat dinner with the family if ketchup is on anyone's plate. The parent would then simply not use ketchup; by removing something from the task or environment, the parent is preventing a negative reaction to mealtime.

Sensory Integration

Sensory integration or sensory integration therapy (SIT) is a clinic-based, play-focused intervention that uses sensory-enhanced interactions to elicit child adaptive responses (Case-Smith et al., 2015). Sensory integration uses controlled sensory stimulation and provides children with structured opportunities in activities with specific sensory input. Therapists set up activities that provide the "just right" challenge, and the sensory-focused activities are designed to elicit adaptive behavioral responses from children. Such behavioral responses are hypothesized to reflect organization of neural activity that will subsequently generalize to everyday behavior. In other words, gross motor activities activate somatosensory, vestibular, and proprioceptive systems and are believed to help the child integrate environmental sensory information. The hypothesis of SI is that the "integration" that occurs in the clinic will translate to the child's organization of communication and adaptive behavior across everyday contexts.

Research on SI is mixed, and studies that compare SI with other treatment approaches vary in their findings. As compared with Applied Behavior Analysis (ABA), SI showed similar results in reducing challenging behavior among children with ASD (Devlin, Healy, Leader, & Hughes, 2011). When compared with sensorimotor activities, SI resulted in similar play behaviors among children with ASD (Dunbar, Carr-Hertel, Lieberman, Perez, & Ricks, 2012). Additionally, when compared with group therapy that used social skill and communication training,

individuals in SI showed similar improvements in cognition, social communication, and motor skills (Iwanaga et al., 2014). Lastly, children with ASD who received SI showed similar positive goal attainment results compared with children who received fine motor interventions (Pfeiffer, Koenig, Kinnealey, Sheppard, & Henderson, 2011). A few studies suggest that SI may be efficacious compared with usual treatment (Miller, Coll, & Schoen, 2007; Schaaf et al., 2014); however, it should be noted that children in SI received many more hours of therapy than children who received therapy in typical community settings.

The American Academy of Pediatrics suggests that although SI therapy is a widely used intervention, the available evidence does not support its efficacy (Zimmer et al., 2012). Occupational therapists who use SI must consider the child behavior that the therapy is intended to impact. If sensory factors are impacting a child's play or self-care skills, the therapist may use an occupation-based intervention to directly address such play or self-care skills. In order to provide best practice and serve families in an efficient, efficacious manner, occupational therapists must explain how and why therapies work.

In terms of EHP intervention approaches, SI is an Establish/Restore approach. The underlying assumption of SI is to target changes in the person's central nervous system and investigate outcomes related to the child's ability to respond differently to demands. The Establish/Restore intervention is the only approach that aims to directly improve a person's skills. The focus of these interventions is on changing the child's ability to integrate sensory information as opposed to focusing on the environment to meet the needs of the child or changing the task to match a child's preferences.

Sensory-Based Interventions

Sensory-based interventions use "adult-directed sensory modalities that are applied to the child to improve behaviors associated with modulation disorders" (Case-Smith et al., 2015, p. 3). In sensory-based interventions, children are passive recipients of sensory stimulation. Aligned with the theoretical conceptualizations of SI, sensory-based interventions are grounded in the belief that after passive receipt of sensory input, a child's nervous system is organized and ready to adaptively interpret sensory information for functional activities. Some sensory-based approaches can be used in children's natural contexts, whereas others require special equipment. Table 59-3 provides an overview of sensory-based interventions.

 Visit thePoint to watch a video about sensory interventions.

TABLE 59-3 Selected Sensory-Based Interventions

Intervention	Definition	Scientific Reasoning Concerning Mechanism of Change	Evidence	Ecology of Human Performance Intervention Approach
Weighted vest/ Weighted blankets (Olson & Moulton, 2004)	Individual wears a garment that typically has 10% of the child's body weight distributed around the vest.	Deep pressure provides stimulation that is calming and organizing to the child's central nervous system. This calming effect then decreases undesirable behaviors and supports the ability to engage.	Overall, research does not support the use of weighted vests to directly impact child behavior (Davis et al., 2013; Hodgetts, Magill-Evans, & Misiaszek, 2011a, 2011b; Reichow, Barton, Sewell, Good, & Wolery, 2010). Some studies, however, suggest that some individuals may like the feeling of weighted vests/blankets, and parents and teachers may find them helpful (Hodgetts et al., 2011b; Leew, Stein, & Gibbard, 2010).	*Modify/Adapt: Make it easier to do.* Because some individuals have reported that they prefer the input of weighted vests and blankets, this adaptation may provide a calming effect to allow people to better engage in activities while wearing the vest or blanket.
Sound Therapies (e.g., Therapeutic Listening, Auditory Integration Training)	The application of passive, specialized auditory input through specialized sounds and headphones worn while child sits passively for 15–120 min	The specialized sounds will organize a child's central nervous system. The child, then, is ready for learning, participation, and engagement.	Overall, studies show no effects of listening programs on child behavior (Case-Smith & Arbesman, 2008; Tomchek & Koenig, 2016), and it is not recommended as an evidence-based practice.	*Establish/Restore: Learn something new everyday.* Because sound therapies are hypothesized to result in organized nervous system activity, this approach would be considered as one that aims to enhance person factors.
Brushing (e.g., the Wilbarger Brushing Protocol) (Wilbarger & Wilbarger, 1991)	A small surgical brush applies pressure to a child's arms, hands, backs, legs, and feet. The Wilbarger Protocol, which is the specialized version of this method, uses brushing in combination with joint compressions to children's shoulders, elbows, wrists, hips, knees, ankles, fingers, and feet.	This treatment applies systematic input to the child's central nervous system, after which the child demonstrates organized behavior that shows he or she is ready to engage in learning and functional activities.	Researchers have found no effects on children's stereotypical behaviors (Davis, Durand, & Chan, 2011; Moore, Cividini-Motta, Clark, & Ahearn, 2015), and it is not recommended as an evidence-based practice.	*Establish/Restore: Learn something new everyday.* Brushing is hypothesized to be effective through the enhanced organization of a person's central nervous system; therefore, it targets a person factor.

REFERENCES

Adams, J. B., Audhya, T., McDonough-Means, S., Rubin, R. A., Quig, D., Geis, E., . . . Lee, W. (2011). Nutritional and metabolic status of children with autism vs. neurotypical children, and the association with autism severity. *Nutrition & Metabolism, 8*(1), 34.

American Psychiatric Association. (2013). *Diagnostic and statistical manual of mental disorders* (5th ed.). Arlington, VA: Author.

Ashburner, J., Ziviani, J., & Rodger, S. (2008). Sensory processing and classroom emotional, behavioral, and educational outcomes in children with autism spectrum disorder. *American Journal of Occupational Therapy, 62*, 564–573.

Ausderau, K. K., Furlong, M., Sideris, J., Bulluck, J., Little, L. M., Watson, L. R., . . . Baranek, G. T. (2014). Sensory subtypes in children with autism spectrum disorder: Latent profile transition analysis using a national survey of sensory features. *Journal of Child Psychology and Psychiatry, and Allied Disciplines, 55*(8), 935–944.

Ayres, A. J. (1968). Sensory integrative processes and neuropsychological learning disability. *Learning Disorders, 3*, 41–58.

Ayres, A. J. (1971). Characteristics of types of sensory integrative dysfunction. *American Journal of Occupational Therapy, 25*, 329–334.

Ayres, A. J. (1972). *Sensory integration and learning disorders.* Los Angeles, CA: Western Psychological Services.

Ayres, A. J. (1980). *Southern California Sensory Integration Tests manual.* Los Angeles, CA: Western Psychological Services.

Ayres, A. J. (1989). *Sensory Integration and Praxis Tests (SIPT).* Los Angeles, CA: Western Psychological Services.

Bagatell, N., Mirigliani, G., Patterson, C., Reyes, Y., & Test, L. (2010). Effectiveness of therapy ball chairs on classroom participation in children with autism spectrum disorders. *American Journal of Occupational Therapy, 64*, 895–903.

Bagby, M. S., Dickie, V. A., & Baranek, G. T. (2012). How sensory experiences of children with and without autism affect family occupations. *American Journal of Occupational Therapy, 66*, 78–86.

Baio, J. (2014). Prevalence of autism spectrum disorder among children aged 8 years—Autism and developmental disabilities monitoring network, 11 sites, United States, 2010. *Surveillance Summaries, 63*, 1–21.

Baker, A. E., Lane, A., Angley, M. T., & Young, R. L. (2008). The relationship between sensory processing patterns and behavioural responsiveness in autistic disorder: A pilot study. *Journal of Autism and Developmental Disorders, 38*, 867–875.

Baranek, G. T. (1999). *Sensory Processing Assessment for young children (SPA)*. Unpublished manuscript, University of North Carolina at Chapel Hill, North Carolina.

Baranek, G. T. (2009). *Sensory Experiences Questionnaire Version 3.0.* Unpublished manuscript, University of North Carolina at Chapel Hill, North Carolina.

Baranek, G. T. (2010). *Tactile Defensiveness and Discrimination Test-Revised (TDDT-R)*. Unpublished manuscript, University of North Carolina at Chapel Hill, North Carolina.

Baranek, G. T., Little, L. M., Parham, L., Ausderau, K. K., & Sabatos-DeVito, M. G. (2014). Sensory features in autism spectrum disorders. In F. R. Volkmar, S. J. Rogers, R. Paul, & K. Pelphrey (Eds.), *Handbook of autism and pervasive developmental disorders* (4th ed., Vol. 1, pp. 378–408). Hoboken, NJ: Wiley.

Baranek, G. T., Watson, L. R., Turner-Brown, L., Field, S. H., Crais, E. R., Wakeford, L., . . . Reznick, J. S. (2015). Preliminary efficacy of adapted responsive teaching for infants at risk of autism spectrum disorder in a community sample. *Autism Research and Treatment, 2015*, 386951.

Baum, C. M., & Edwards, D. (2001). *ACS: Activity Card Sort*. St. Louis, MO: Washington University School of Medicine.

Bedell, G. (2009). Further validation of the Child and Adolescent Scale of Participation (CASP). *Developmental Neurorehabilitation, 12*, 342–351.

Berk, R. A., & DeGangi, G. A. (1983). *DeGangi-Berk Test of Sensory Integration: Manual*. Los Angeles, CA: Western Psychological Services.

Blanche, E. I. (2002). *Observations based on sensory integration theory.* Los Angeles, CA: Pediatric Therapy Network, Western Psychological Services.

Blanche, E. I., Bodison, S., Chang, M. C., & Reinoso, G. (2012). Development of the Comprehensive Observations of Proprioception (COP): Validity, reliability, and factor analysis. *American Journal of Occupational Therapy, 66*, 691–698.

Boets, B., Wouters, J., van Wieringen, A., De Smedt, B., & Ghesquiére, P. (2008). Modelling relations between sensory processing, speech perception, orthographic and phonological ability, and literacy achievement. *Brain and Language, 106*, 29–40.

Boliek, C., Keintz, C., Norrix, L., & Obrzut, J. (2010). Auditory-visual perception of speech in children with learning disabilities: The McGurk effect. *Canadian Journal of Speech-Language Pathology and Audiology, 34*, 124–131.

Brown, C., & Dunn, W. (2002). *Adolescent/Adult Sensory Profile: User's manual*. Tucson, AZ: Therapy Skill Builders.

Brown, N. B., & Dunn, W. (2010). Relationship between context and sensory processing in children with autism. *American Journal of Occupational Therapy, 64*, 474–483.

Bulkeley, K., Bundy, A., Roberts, J., & Einfeld, S. (2016). Family-centered management of sensory challenges of children with autism: Single-case experimental design. *American Journal of Occupational Therapy, 70*, 7005220040p1–7005220040p8.

Cascio, C. J., Woynaroski, T., Baranek, G. T., & Wallace, M. T. (2016). Toward an interdisciplinary approach to understanding sensory function in autism spectrum disorder. *Autism Research, 9*, 920–925.

Case-Smith, J., & Arbesman, M. (2008). Evidence-based review of interventions for autism used in or of relevance to occupational therapy. *American Journal of Occupational Therapy, 62*, 416–429.

Case-Smith, J., Weaver, L. L., & Fristad, M. A. (2015). A systematic review of sensory processing interventions for children with autism spectrum disorders. *Autism, 19*, 133–148.

Cosbey, J., Johnston, S. S., & Dunn, M. L. (2010). Sensory processing disorders and social participation. *American Journal of Occupational Therapy, 64*, 462–473.

Coster, W., Law, M., Bedell, G., & Teplicky, R. (2010). *Participation and Environment Measure for Children and Youth (PEM-CY)*. Boston, MA: Trustees of Boston University.

Coulthard, H., & Blissett, J. (2009). Fruit and vegetable consumption in children and their mothers. Moderating effects of child sensory sensitivity. *Appetite, 52*, 410–415.

Davis, T. N., Dacus, S., Strickland, E., Copeland, D., Chan, J. M., Blenden, K., . . . Christian, K. (2013). The effects of a weighted vest on aggressive and self-injurious behavior in a child with autism. *Developmental Neurorehabilitation, 16*, 210–215.

Davis, T. N., Durand, S., & Chan, J. M. (2011). The effects of a brushing procedure on stereotypical behavior. *Research in Autism Spectrum Disorders, 5*, 1053–1058.

Davis, A. M., Bruce, A. S., Khasawneh, R., Schulz, T., Fox, C., & Dunn, W. (2013). Sensory processing issues in young children presenting to an outpatient feeding clinic. *Journal of Pediatric Gastroenterology and Nutrition, 56*, 156–160.

Dawson, G., Jones, E. J., Merkle, K., Venema, K., Lowy, R., Faja, S., . . . Webb, S. J. (2012). Early behavioral intervention is associated with normalized brain activity in young children with autism. *Journal of the American Academy of Child and Adolescent Psychiatry, 51*, 1150–1159.

Dawson, G., Rogers, S., Munson, J., Smith, M., Winter, J., Greenson, J., . . . Varley, J. (2010). Randomized, controlled trial of an intervention for toddlers with autism: the Early Start Denver Model. *Pediatrics, 125*, e17–e23.

Dean, E. E., Little, L., Tomchek, S., & Dunn, W. (2018). Sensory processing in the general population: Adaptability, resiliency, and challenging behavior. *American Journal of Occupational Therapy, 72*, 7201195060p1–7201195060p8. doi:10.5014/ajot.2018.019919

Dean, E. E., Wallisch, A., & Dunn, W. (in press). Adaptation as a transaction with the environment: Perspectives from an ecological model of OT. In L. C. Grajo & A. Boisselle (Eds.), *Occupation and adaptation: Multidimensional perspectives*. Thorofare, NJ: SLACK.

DeGangi, G. A., & Greenspan, S. I. (1989). *Test of Sensory Functions in Infants (TSFI)*. Philadelphia, PA: Western Psychological Services.

Devlin, S., Healy, O., Leader, G., & Hughes, B. M. (2011). Comparison of behavioral intervention and sensory-integration therapy in the treatment of challenging behavior. *Journal of Autism and Developmental Disorders, 41*, 1303–1320.

Division for Early Childhood. (2014). *DEC recommended practices in early intervention/early childhood special education 2014*. Retrieved from http://www.dec-sped.org/dec-recommendedpractices

Dovey, T. M., Aldridge, V. K., Dignan, W., Staples, P. A., Gibson, E. L., & Halford, J. C. (2012). Developmental differences in sensory decision making involved in deciding to try a novel fruit. *British Journal of Health Psychology, 17*, 258–272.

Dunbar, S. B., Carr-Hertel, J., Lieberman, H. A., Perez, B., & Ricks, K. (2012). A pilot study comparison of sensory integration treatment and integrated preschool activities for children with autism. *Internet Journal of Allied Health Sciences and Practice, 10*, 6.

Dunn, W. (1997). The impact of sensory processing abilities on the daily lives of young children and their families: A conceptual model. *Infants and Young Children, 9*, 23–35.

Dunn, W. (1999). *The Sensory Profile manual*. San Antonio, TX: The Psychological Corporation.

Dunn, W. (2007). Ecology of human performance model. In S. Dunbar (Ed.), *Occupational therapy models for intervention with children and families* (pp. 127–156). Thorofare, NJ: SLACK.

Dunn, W. (2014). *Sensory Profile-2*. San Antonio, TX: Pearson.

Dunn, W., Brown, C., & McGuigan, A. (1994). The ecology of human performance: A framework for considering the effect of context. *American Journal of Occupational Therapy, 48*, 595–607.

Dunn, W., Brown, C., Youngstrom, M. J., Kramer, P., Hinojosa, J., & Royeen, C. (2003). Ecological model of occupation. In P. Kramer, J. Hinojosa, & C. B. Royeen (Eds.), *Perspectives in human occupation: Participation in life* (pp. 222–263). Philadelphia, PA: Lippincott Williams & Wilkins.

Dunn, W., Cox, J., Foster, L., Mische-Lawson, L., & Tanquary, J. (2012). Impact of a contextual intervention on child participation and parent competence among children with autism spectrum disorders: A pretest-posttest repeated-measures design. *American Journal of Occupational Therapy, 66*, 520–528.

Dunn, W., Tomchek, S., Little, L., & Dean, E. (2016). Prevalence of sensory characteristics in the general population: A person-centered approach. *American Journal of Occupational Therapy, 70*, 7011500001p1. doi:10.5014/ajot.2016.70S1-RP202A.

Dunn, W., Little, L., Dean, E., Robertson, S., & Evans, B. (2016). The state of the science on sensory factors and their impact on daily life for children: A scoping review. *OTJR: Occupation, Participation and Health, 36*(Suppl.), 3S–26S.

Dunstan, E., & Griffiths, S. (2008). Sensory strategies: Practical support to empower families. *New Zealand Journal of Occupational Therapy, 55*, 5.

Education of All Handicapped Children Act of 1975, Pub. L. No. 94-142, 89 Stat. 773, *codified as amended at* title 20 U.S.C. §1401 (1975).

Engel-Yeger, B., Hardal-Nasser, R., & Gal, E. (2011). Sensory processing dysfunctions as expressed among children with different severities of intellectual developmental disabilities. *Research in Developmental Disabilities, 32*, 1770–1775.

Farmer, J., & Reupert, A. (2013). Understanding autism and understanding my child with autism: An evaluation of a group parent education program in rural Australia. *The Australian Journal of Rural Health, 21*, 20–27.

Fedewa, A. L., & Erwin, H. E. (2011). Stability balls and students with attention and hyperactivity concerns: Implications for on-task and in-seat behavior. *American Journal of Occupational Therapy, 65*, 393–399.

Frances, A. (2013). *Saving normal: An insider's look at what caused the epidemic of mental illness and how to cure it.* New York, NY: William Morrow.

Geiger, G., Cattaneo, C., Galli, R., Pozzoli, U., Lorusso, M. L., Facoetti, A., & Molteni, M. (2008). Wide and diffuse perceptual modes characterize dyslexics in vision and audition. *Perception, 37*, 1745–1764.

Ghanizadeh, A. (2013). Parents reported oral sensory sensitivity processing and food preference in ADHD. *Journal of Psychiatric and Mental Health Nursing, 20*, 426–432.

Gibbs, V., & Toth-Cohen, S. (2011). Family-centered occupational therapy and telerehabilitation for children with autism spectrum disorders. *Occupational Therapy in Health Care, 25*, 298–314.

Grandin, T. (1986). *Emergence: Labeled autistic.* Novato, CA: Arena Press.

Hilton, C., Graver, K., & LaVesser, P. (2007). Relationship between social competence and sensory processing in children with high functioning autism spectrum disorders. *Research in Autism Spectrum Disorders, 1*, 164–173.

Hochhauser, M., & Engel-Yeger, B. (2010). Sensory processing abilities and their relation to participation in leisure activities among children with high-functioning autism spectrum disorder (HFASD). *Research in Autism Spectrum Disorders, 4*, 746–754.

Hodgetts, S., Magill-Evans, J., & Misiaszek, J. (2011a). Effects of weighted vests on classroom behavior for children with autism and cognitive impairments. *Research in Autism Spectrum Disorders, 5*, 495–505.

Hodgetts, S., Magill-Evans, J., & Misiaszek, J. E. (2011b). Weighted vests, stereotyped behaviors and arousal in children with autism. *Journal of Autism and Developmental Disorders, 41*, 805–814.

Individuals with Disabilities Education Act, Pub. L. No. 101-476, 104 Stat. 1142, *codified as amended at* title 20 U.S.C. §1400 (1990).

Iwanaga, R., Honda, S., Nakane, H., Tanaka, K., Toeda, H., & Tanaka, G. (2014). Pilot study: Efficacy of sensory integration therapy for Japanese children with high-functioning autism spectrum disorder. *Occupational Therapy International, 21*, 4–11.

Jasmin, E., Couture, M., McKinley, P., Reid, G., Fombonne, E., & Gisel, E. (2009). Sensori-motor and daily living skills of preschool children with autism spectrum disorders. *Journal of Autism and Developmental Disorders, 39*, 231–241.

Jirikowic, T., Olson, H. C., & Kartin, D. (2008). Sensory processing, school performance, and adaptive behavior of young school-age children with fetal alcohol spectrum disorders. *Physical & Occupational Therapy in Pediatrics, 28*, 117–136.

Khetani, M., Coster, W., Law, M., & Bedell, G. (2013). *Young children's Participation and Environment Measure (YC-PEM).* Fort Collins, CO: Colorado State University.

King, G., Law, M., Petrenchik, T., & Kertoy, M. (2006). *Assessment of Preschool Children's Participation (APCP).* Hamilton, Ontario, Canada: CanChild Centre for Childhood Disability Research, McMaster University.

Kinnealey, M., Pfeiffer, B., Miller, J., Roan, C., Shoener, R., & Ellner, M. L. (2012). Effect of classroom modification on attention and engagement of students with autism or dyspraxia. *American Journal of Occupational Therapy, 66*, 511–519.

Kuhaneck, H. M., & Britner, P. A. (2013). A preliminary investigation of the relationship between sensory processing and social play in autism spectrum disorder. *OTJR: Occupation, Participation and Health, 33*, 159–167.

Lane, A. E., Molloy, C. A., & Bishop, S. L. (2014). Classification of children with autism spectrum disorder by sensory subtype: A case for sensory-based phenotypes. *Autism Research, 7*, 322–333.

Lane, A. E., Young, R. L., Baker, A. E., & Angley, M. T. (2010). Sensory processing subtypes in autism: Association with adaptive behavior. *Journal of Autism and Developmental Disorders, 40*, 112–122.

Leew, S. V., Stein, N. G., & Gibbard, W. B. (2010). Weighted vests' effect on social attention for toddlers with autism spectrum disorders. *Canadian Journal of Occupational Therapy, 77*, 113–124.

Lequia, J., Machalicek, W., & Rispoli, M. J. (2012). Effects of activity schedules on challenging behavior exhibited in children with autism spectrum disorders: A systematic review. *Research in Autism Spectrum Disorders, 6*, 480–492.

Little, L. M., Ausderau, K., Sideris, J., & Baranek, G. T. (2015). Activity participation and sensory features among children with autism spectrum disorders. *Journal of Autism and Developmental Disorders, 45*, 2981–2990.

Little, L. M., Dean, E., Tomchek, S. D., & Dunn, W. (2017). Classifying sensory profiles of children in the general population. *Child: Care, Health and Development, 43*, 81–88.

Little, L. M., Pope, E., Wallisch, A., & Dunn, W. (2018). Occupation-based coaching by means of telehealth for families of young children with autism spectrum disorder. *American Journal of Occupational Therapy, 72*, 7202205020.

Mahoney, G., & Perales, F. (2003). Using relationship-focused intervention to enhance the social—emotional functioning of young children with autism spectrum disorders. *Topics in Early Childhood Special Education, 23*, 74–86.

Mandich, A., Polatajko, H., Miller, L., & Baum, C. (2004). *Paediatric Activity Card Sort (PACS).* Ontario, Canada: Canadian Association of Occupational Therapists.

Marquenie, K., Rodger, S., Mangohig, K., & Cronin, A. (2011). Dinnertime and bedtime routines and rituals in families with a young child with an autism spectrum disorder. *Australian Occupational Therapy Journal, 58*, 145–154.

Matsushima, K., & Kato, T. (2013). Social interaction and atypical sensory processing in children with autism spectrum disorders. *Hong Kong Journal of Occupational Therapy, 23*, 89–96.

Mattard-Labrecque, C., Ben Amor, L., & Couture, M. M. (2013). Children with autism and attention difficulties: A pilot study of the association between sensory, motor, and adaptive behaviors. *Journal of the Canadian Academy of Child and Adolescent Psychiatry, 22,* 139–146.

Mazurek, M. O., & Petroski, G. F. (2015). Sleep problems in children with autism spectrum disorder: Examining the contributions of sensory over-responsivity and anxiety. *Sleep Medicine, 16,* 270–279.

McIntosh, D. N., Miller, L. J., Shyu, V., & Dunn, W. (1999). Overview of the Short Sensory Profile (SSP). In W. Dunn (Ed.), *The Sensory Profile: Examiner's manual* (pp. 59–73). San Antonio, TX: The Psychological Corporation.

Miller, L. J., Anzalone, M. E., Lane, S. J., Cermak, S. A., & Osten, E. T. (2007). Concept evolution in sensory integration: A proposed nosology for diagnosis. *American Journal of Occupational Therapy, 61,* 135–140.

Miller, L. J., Coll, J. R., & Schoen, S. A. (2007). A randomized controlled pilot study of the effectiveness of occupational therapy for children with sensory modulation disorder. *American Journal of Occupational Therapy, 61,* 228–238.

Miller Kuhaneck, H., Ecker, C., Parham, L., Henry, D., & Glennon, T. (2010). *Sensory Processing Measure-Preschool (SPM-P): Manual.* Los Angeles, CA: Western Psychological Services.

Mische Lawson, L., & Dunn, W. (2008). Children's sensory processing patterns and play preferences. *Annual in Therapeutic Recreation, 16,* 1–14.

Moore, K. M., Cividini-Motta, C., Clark, K. M., & Ahearn, W. H. (2015). Sensory integration as a treatment for automatically maintained stereotypy. *Behavioral Interventions, 30,* 95–111.

Nadon, G., Feldman, D. E., Dunn, W., & Gisel, E. (2011). Association of sensory processing and eating problems in children with autism spectrum disorders. *Autism Research and Treatment, 2011,* 541926.

Olson, L. J., & Moulton, H. J. (2004). Use of weighted vests in pediatric occupational therapy practice. *Physical & Therapy in Pediatrics, 24,* 45–60.

Parham, L. D., & Ecker, C. (2007). *Sensory Processing Measure (SPM).* Los Angeles, CA: Western Psychological Services.

Pfeiffer, B. A., Koenig, K., Kinnealey, M., Sheppard, M., & Henderson, L. (2011). Effectiveness of sensory integration interventions in children with autism spectrum disorders: A pilot study. *American Journal of Occupational Therapy, 65,* 76–85.

Reichow, B., Barton, E. E., Sewell, J. N., Good, L., & Wolery, M. (2010). Effects of weighted vests on the engagement of children with developmental delays and autism. *Focus on Autism and Other Developmental Disabilities, 25,* 3–11.

Reynolds, S., Bendixen, R. M., Lawrence, T., & Lane, S. J. (2011). A pilot study examining activity participation, sensory responsiveness, and competence in children with high functioning autism spectrum disorder. *Journal of Autism and Developmental Disorders, 41,* 1496–1506.

Reynolds, S., Lane, S. J., & Thacker, L. (2012). Sensory processing, physiological stress, and sleep behaviors in children with and without autism spectrum disorders. *OTJR: Occupation, Participation and Health, 32,* 246–257.

Rogers, S. J., Estes, A., Lord, C., Vismara, L., Winter, J., Fitzpatrick, A., . . . Dawson, G. (2012). Effects of a brief Early Start Denver Model (ESDM)–based parent intervention on toddlers at risk for autism spectrum disorders: A randomized controlled trial. *Journal of the American Academy of Child and Adolescent Psychiatry, 51,* 1052–1065.

Rogers, S. J., Hepburn, S., & Wehner, E. (2003). Parent reports of sensory symptoms in toddlers with autism and those with other developmental disorders. *Journal of Autism and Developmental Disorders, 33,* 631–642.

Rush, D. D., & Shelden, M. L. L. (2011). *The early childhood coaching Handbook.* Baltimore, MD: Brookes.

Schaaf, R. C., Benevides, T., Mailloux, Z., Faller, P., Hunt, J., van Hooydonk, E., . . . Kelly, D. (2014). An intervention for sensory difficulties in children with autism: A randomized trial. *Journal of Autism and Developmental Disorders, 44,* 1493–1506.

Schaaf, R. C., & Lane, A. E. (2015). Toward a best-practice protocol for assessment of sensory features in ASD. *Journal of Autism and Developmental Disorders, 45,* 1380–1395.

Schilling, D. L., Washington, K., Billingsley, F. F., & Deitz, J. (2003). Classroom seating for children with attention deficit hyperactivity disorder: Therapy balls versus chairs. *American Journal of Occupational Therapy, 57,* 534–541.

Schoen, S. A., Miller, L. J., & Green, K. E. (2008). Pilot study of the Sensory Over-Responsibility Scales: Assessment and inventory. *American Journal of Occupational Therapy, 62,* 393–406.

Stein, L. I., Polido, J. C., & Cermak, S. A. (2013). Oral care and sensory over-responsivity in children with autism spectrum disorders. *Pediatric Dentistry, 35,* 230–235.

Stein, L. I., Polido, J. C., Mailloux, Z., Coleman, G. G., & Cermak, S. A. (2011). Oral care and sensory sensitivities in children with autism spectrum disorders. *Special Care in Dentistry, 31,* 102–110.

Tavassoli, T., Hoekstra, R. A., & Baron-Cohen, S. (2014). The Sensory Perception Quotient (SPQ): Development and validation of a new sensory questionnaire for adults with and without autism. *Molecular Autism, 5,* 29.

Tomchek, S. D., & Koenig, K. P. (2016). *Occupational therapy practice guidelines for individuals with autism spectrum disorder.* Bethesda, MD: AOTA Press.

Welters-Davis, M., & Mische Lawson, L. (2011). The relationship between sensory processing and parent–child play preferences. *Journal of Occupational Therapy, Schools, and Early Intervention, 4,* 108–120.

Wengel, T., Hanlon-Dearman, A. C., & Fjeldsted, B. (2011). Sleep and sensory characteristics in young children with fetal alcohol spectrum disorder. *Journal of Developmental and Behavioral Pediatrics, 32,* 384–392. doi:10.1097/DBP.0b013e3182199694

Wilbarger, P., & Wilbarger, J. L. (1991). *Sensory defensiveness in children aged 2–12: An intervention guide for parents and other caretakers.* Framingham, MA: Therapro.

Zimmer, M., Desch, L., Rosen, L. D., Bailey, M. L., Becker, D., Culbert, T. P., . . . Liptak, G. S. (2012). Sensory integration therapies for children with developmental and behavioral disorders. *Pediatrics, 129*(6), 1186–1189.

Zingerevich, C. (2009). The contribution of executive functions to participation in school activities of children with high functioning autism spectrum disorder. *Research in Autism Spectrum Disorders, 3,* 429–437.

Zobel-Lachiusa, J., Andrianopoulos, M. V., Mailloux, Z., & Cermak, S. A. (2015). Sensory differences and mealtime behavior in children with autism. *American Journal of Occupational Therapy, 69,* 6905185050p1–6905185050p8.

thePoint *For additional resources on the subjects discussed in this chapter, visit* **http://thePoint.lww.com /Willard-Spackman13e.** *See* **Appendix I, Resources and Evidence for Common Conditions Addressed in OT** *for more information about ASD and ADHD.*

CHAPTER 60

Emotion Regulation

Marjorie E. Scaffa

LEARNING OBJECTIVES

After reading this chapter, you will be able to:

1. Describe the neurophysiological and developmental aspects of emotion regulation.
2. Discuss the relationship between emotion regulation and trauma.
3. Understand how emotion regulation supports or limits occupational performance.
4. Identify assessments that are used to measure emotion regulation.
5. Develop intervention plans that address the needs of persons with emotion dysregulation and improve occupational performance.
6. Discuss a strength-based approach to emotion regulation.

Introduction

Emotions are an essential component of being human. It is impossible to be alive and not experience emotions. According to Mahoney (2005), "emotional processes are among the most powerful and primitive of human self-organizing processes" (p. 747). Although the term **emotion** is difficult to define, there is consensus that emotions are evaluative mental states that occur in the present moment and consist of neurobiological arousal, perceptual-cognitive processes, subjective experience, and affective expression (Izard, 2010). Emotions arise when a situation appears that has relevance to one's goals. Situations that are likely to enhance goal attainment elicit pleasurable emotions, whereas situations that are likely to inhibit goal attainment elicit negative or unpleasant feelings. Emotions provide us with qualitative information on which to make decisions that result in adaptive responses in our everyday lives. Emotions serve various functions including "motivating and focusing individual endeavors, social interactions, and the development of adaptive and maladaptive behavior" (Izard, 2010, p. 368).

Some emotions are ubiquitous and experienced by all human beings, for example, love, anger, grief/sadness, fear, joy, and disgust. Other emotions are often melds of these primary emotions. For example, surprise could be conceived of as a melding or combination of joy and fear, whereas contempt is a melding of anger and disgust. Emotions vary in intensity. For example, hostility, frustration, and rage are varying intensities of anger,

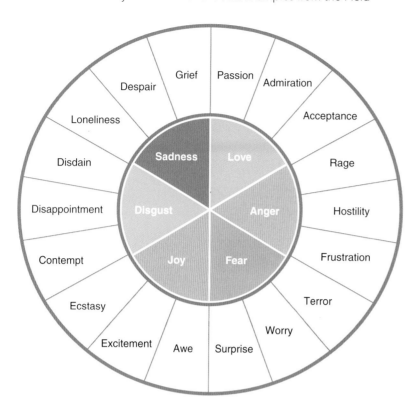

FIGURE 60-1 **Emotions wheel.**

whereas anticipation, happiness, and ecstasy are varying intensities of joy (Nussbaum, 2001). One way to illustrate the variety and intensities of emotion is through an emotions wheel (Figure 60-1).

Emotions can affect health directly and indirectly, and that impact can be either positive or negative. Emotions can influence health directly through their impact on the immune, endocrine, cardiovascular, and nervous systems. Emotions affect health indirectly through adherence to medical regimens and participation in healthy or unhealthy behaviors (Kiecolt-Glaser, McGuire, Robles, & Glaser, 2002).

An Overview of Emotion Regulation

Emotions are rarely obligatory or automatic and are therefore subject to self-regulation and response modulation. Eisenberg and Spinrad (2004) define *emotion-related self-regulation* as

> the process of initiating, avoiding, inhibiting, maintaining, or modulating the occurrence, form, intensity, or duration of internal feeling states, emotion-related physiological, attentional processes, motivational states, and/or the behavioral concomitants of emotion in the service of accomplishing affect-related biological or social adaptation or achieving individual goals. (p. 338)

More simply, *emotion regulation processes* are those behaviors, skills, and strategies that monitor, evaluate,

modulate, modify, inhibit, or enhance emotional experiences in the pursuit of one's goals. **Emotion dysregulation** refers to actions or behaviors related to emotional experience that interfere with goal-directed pursuits, interpersonal relationships, or healthy adaptation (Schore, 2003).

Individuals who are referred for occupational therapy (OT) services with diagnoses of traumatic brain injury, cerebrovascular accident (CVA), autism spectrum disorders, dementia, diabetes, cancer, chronic obstructive pulmonary disease (COPD), heart disease, progressive neurological disorders, attention deficit disorder, eating disorders, addictions of all types, depression, bipolar disorder, posttraumatic stress disorder, and other psychiatric diagnoses often present with emotion dysregulation problems that interfere with their occupational performance and participation.

Emotion regulation may be intrinsic or extrinsic. *Intrinsic* refers to factors within the person that contribute to emotion regulation, for example, temperament, cognitive processes, and neurological and physiological functions. *Extrinsic* refers to social and contextual influences that affect emotion regulation, for example, interactions with caregivers, sibling and peer relationships, and cultural context (Fox & Calkins, 2003). Although typically focused on reducing negative or painful emotions, emotion regulation can also involve heightening positive emotions (Eisenberg & Spinrad, 2004).

The modal model of emotion consists of five components: the situation, attention to the situation, appraisal of the situation, the emotional and behavioral response to the situation based on the appraisal, and feedback on the effects of the response. Emotions can be regulated before (antecedent focused), during, and after (response focused) they occur. Although these regulatory mechanisms are described separately, they are often employed in combination. Antecedent-focused emotion regulation involves selecting and modifying situations that typically give rise to emotional response tendencies. Situation selection involves taking actions that increase or decrease the likelihood that one will end up in a situation that evokes desirable or undesirable emotional reactions. Situation modifying involves consciously altering external environmental conditions to reduce or enhance the likelihood of evoking specific emotions (Gross & Thompson, 2007).

Regulating emotions in the midst of experiencing them may take the form of attentional deployment or cognitive change. *Attentional deployment* refers to "how individuals direct their attention within a given situation to influence their emotions" and includes distraction, or focusing attention away from the situation, and concentration, or focusing on the emotional aspects of the situation in order to gain control over them (Gross & Thompson, 2007, p. 13). *Cognitive change*, sometimes referred to as cognitive reappraisal, involves changing one's evaluation of a situation, its consequences, or one's ability to manage the consequences in order to alter its emotional significance or modify its impact.

Response-focused emotion regulation, also called response modulation, involves modifying the physiological effects, the experiential aspects, and/or the behavioral expression of emotion. Emotional responses are not adaptive or maladaptive in and of themselves but rather are adaptive or maladaptive depending on the context. For example, crying may be adaptive in one situation and maladaptive in another. Cultural values also determine emotional response modulation and the interpretation of what is socially appropriate, desirable, and adaptive (Gross & Thompson, 2007).

Neurophysiological Aspects of Emotion Regulation

Emotion regulation occurs along a continuum from fully automatic and subconscious to conscious and voluntary. Deliberate and effortful attempts to manage emotional reactions are referred to as *intentional emotion regulation*, whereas unintentional and effortless responses are referred to as *incidental emotion regulation*. The neural mechanisms of intentional emotion regulation have been studied fairly extensively, whereas there is much less research on incidental emotion regulation (Berkman & Lieberman, 2009).

Research has demonstrated that the areas of the brain most involved in emotion regulation are the sensory thalamus, amygdala, the hippocampus, and several areas of the prefrontal cortex (PFC) (Davidson, Fox, & Kalin, 2007). The amygdala is the primary brain structure involved in

the generation of normal and pathological emotional behavior and is responsible for directing attention to salient stimuli and determining if further processing is needed. The PFC is often considered the locus of cognitive control, but it also has a role in affective processing. The PFC develops and stores goals and the means to their achievement. Therefore, the PFC appraises the situation to determine if it is a facilitator or threat to one's goals. In stressful situations, threat stimuli are registered in the sensory thalamus and are almost instantaneously relayed to the amygdala, which is the emotional center responsible for fight-or-flight responses. From there, the message travels to the hippocampus and PFC. The hippocampus applies context to the threat situation and regulates the amygdala, whereas the cortex incorporates memory (Davidson et al., 2007).

Research on populations with focal brain damage has yielded the following insights regarding emotional processing and emotion regulation:

- Lesions in the lateral frontal lobes are linked to blunted emotional responses or the absence of expected emotions.
- Right orbital frontal lobe damage is associated with increased anger and depression and inability to maximize positive emotion.
- Lesions in the caudate produce inappropriate laughing or crying.
- Regulation of aversive emotions may not require awareness or memory as evidenced by damage to the temporal lobes (Beer & Lombardo, 2007).

Trauma exposure compromises neurological function particularly in the hippocampus, which is responsible for learning and memory, and in the frontal-limbic systems, which are responsible for emotion regulation (Karl et al., 2006). There is evidence to suggest that at least half of psychiatric disorders are characterized by emotion dysregulation, possibly as a result of dysfunction of the prefrontal-amygdala pathway (Drevets, 2000; Mennin, Heimberg, Turk, & Fresco, 2005; Ochsner & Gross, 2007; Suveg & Zeman, 2004). As a result, OT practitioners should be particularly alert to the presence of emotion dysregulation in children, adolescents, adults, and older adults who have experienced trauma.

Developmental Aspects of Emotion Regulation

The biological foundations for emotion regulation develop prenatally. For example, stress during pregnancy has been associated with "problematic outcomes such as hyperactivity, deficits in attention, and maladaptive social behavior, all of which are characterized by deficits in self-regulation and emotion regulation in particular" (Calkins & Hill, 2007, p. 238). The ability to self-regulate emotional states begins to develop in infancy. Research on infant temperament has demonstrated biologically based tendencies toward the experience and expression of particular emotions. *Temperament* refers to the speed and intensity of emotional reactivity and the ability to modify or self-regulate the intensity and duration of the emotional experience. Babies and toddlers self-regulate using strategies such as gaze aversion, self-sucking, and seeking proximity to their caregiver (Cole, Martin, & Dennis, 2004).

Young children learn to self-regulate through their relationships with their primary caregivers (Figure 60-2). Mothers influence their child's emotional states by interpreting the infant's emotional signals, modulating the baby's level of physiological arousal, and reinforcing the child's efforts at self-regulation. For example, when an infant cries, the caregiver often tries to calm and soothe the child through gentle, rhythmic rocking. Cole et al. (2004) postulate that the "quality of these emotional exchanges . . . is an important precursor of the developing child's ability to regulate his or her own emotions" (p. 324).

Toddlers and preschoolers learn to incorporate these caregiver-directed strategies into their behavioral repertoires for self-regulation of emotion. Children at this age typically demonstrate a decrease in self-soothing strategies and an increase in more complex emotion regulation approaches using objects and interpersonal interactions (Cole et al., 2004). These emotion regulation skills can then be applied across various situations in both deliberate and automatic ways. Failure to develop these early emotion self-regulatory skills may constrain the development of more complex emotional skills later and can lead to poor school adjustment and a low level of social competence (Calkins & Hill, 2007).

For older children, "learning to tolerate distress, correctly label uncomfortable situations, and develop

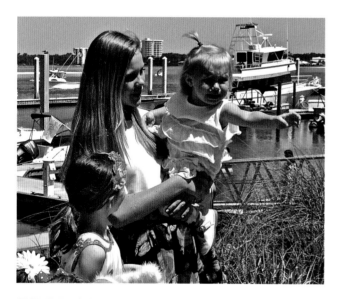

FIGURE 60-2 Learning emotion regulation through relationships with caregivers.

appropriate ways to respond to emotions is central to healthy development" (Scheinholz, 2011, p. 347). This is accomplished through the development of effortful control. **Effortful control** refers to a volitional ability to shift attention, inhibit the tendency to enact a dominant response, and/or activate an alternative response as needed (Rothbart & Bates, 1998). Other factors that impact the development of adaptive emotion regulation are the maturation of language skills that enable the labeling and expression of emotions, observation of the expression of emotions by others in various contexts, and cultural values and mores (Gross & Thompson, 2007). Neurophysiological processes continue to mature during adolescence, enabling teenagers to develop self and other awareness, empathy, impulse control, mastery over the environment, and self-regulation of emotion.

Among healthy adults, emotional experience and emotion regulation are well maintained into late adulthood and typically do not deteriorate with aging. However, the frequency of use of different modes of regulation may change. In middle adulthood, suppression of emotion may be used more frequently to succeed in higher education and work, whereas in older adulthood, there appears to be more of a tendency to use cognitive reappraisal to lessen unpleasant emotional experiences and heighten positive emotional states (Gross & Thompson, 2007). Older adults perceive daily stressors as less threatening and therefore report less negativity as a result when compared to their younger counterparts (Birditt, Fingerman, & Almeida, 2005).

Relationship between Emotion Regulation and Trauma

Many children and adults have been impacted by trauma. The effects of exposure to trauma are dependent, in part, on the developmental stage of the individual when the trauma occurs. Trauma early in life has a negative effect on a child's ability to establish and maintain healthy interpersonal attachments and his or her capacity for emotional self-regulation (Hughes, 2004). This results in poorly moderated affect and impulse control; distrust of others and problems with intimacy; and the lack of a stable, predictable sense of self (van der Kolk, 2003).

Children and adolescents exposed to trauma, in the form of neglect and child abuse in all its forms, as well as witnessing domestic violence, war, and violent crime, have difficulty identifying and describing internal arousal states, labeling and expressing emotions, and making their needs and wants known. Childhood trauma increases the risk of major depressive disorder later in life often with earlier onset and longer duration. The presence of a competent, emotionally supportive caregiver can mitigate these effects. There appear to be three critical factors in a caregiver's response to his or her child's trauma experience that

BOX 60-1 EXTERNALIZING AND INTERNALIZING BEHAVIORS

Acting Out—Externalizing Behaviors
- Anger
- Violence toward others
- Truancy
- Criminal acts

Acting In—Internalizing Behaviors
- Denial, repression
- Substance abuse (self-medicating)
- Eating disorders
- Self-injury
- Dissociation

facilitate adaptive emotional functioning. These are believing and validating the child's experience, accepting and understanding the child's affect, and managing the caregiver's own emotional reactions (Cook et al., 2005).

Even mentally healthy, competent adults demonstrate significant declines in cognitive and emotional functioning when traumatized. Adults with posttraumatic stress disorder experience persistent arousal (e.g., sleep difficulties, concentration problems, irritability, and exaggerated startle responses) and continue to reexperience the traumatic event after it is over through flashbacks, nightmares, and intrusive thoughts, which produce emotional distress. In their attempts to regulate these distressing emotions, persons exposed to trauma may exhibit externalizing and/or internalizing behaviors. These are listed in Box 60-1. Internalizing behaviors are often associated with fearful emotions, whereas externalizing behaviors are typically the result of irritable and angry emotions.

Impact of Emotional Dysregulation on Occupational Performance

Poorly regulated emotions can impair occupational functioning and are therefore important considerations in OT evaluation and intervention. In the second edition of the "Occupational Therapy Practice Framework" (American Occupational Therapy Association [AOTA], 2008), **emotional regulation skills** are defined as "actions or

behaviors a client uses to identify, manage, and express feelings while engaging in activities or interacting with others" (p. 640). In the framework (AOTA, 2008), examples of emotional regulation skills included are the following:

- Responding to the feelings of others
- Controlling anger
- Coping with stressful events
- Expressing emotions appropriately
- Recovering from hurt or disappointment
- Tolerating frustration and persisting in the performance of tasks

There is no specific definition of emotional regulation in the third edition of the Framework (AOTA, 2014).

Gratz and Roemer (2004) suggest emotion regulation skills also include the ability to:

- Accept unpleasant, negative emotional experiences as an inevitable aspect of living
- Redirect and focus one's attention in the presence of intense emotion
- Soothe oneself in response to emotion-related physiological arousal
- Inhibit inappropriate behaviors related to intense emotional experiences
- Initiate, organize, and persist in goal-directed activity regardless of mood state

Under healthy conditions, these skills are acquired as part of the normal developmental process. However, some children demonstrate impairment in self-regulation as a result of emotional hyperreactivity and a poorly organized stress response system. This reflects an excessive reaction of the autonomic nervous system to relatively low levels of stress that results in intense reactions to emotional stimuli and a slow return to baseline or homeostasis. Linehan (1993a) believes that emotion dysregulation results when a child with high emotional vulnerability is exposed to an invalidating, neglectful, or abusive environment. These children demonstrate affective instability, impulsiveness, irritability, and distractibility all of which interfere with school performance, play, and family and peer relationships. Box 60-2 presents a day in the life of Henry, a child with emotional dysregulation.

In adults, affective instability and the accompanying behavior patterns interfere with the development and maintenance of healthy habits and routines and the ability to perform occupational roles effectively. Persons with emotion regulation deficits typically have occupational performance problems in work, instrumental activities of daily living, leisure, and social participation (Figure 60-3) (Scheinholz, 2011).

The manner in which people regulate their emotions affects their social participation, interactions, and relationships. In one study of college students, emotion regulation

BOX 60-2	**THE DYNAMICS OF DYSREGULATION: A DAY IN THE LIFE OF A CHILD WITH EMOTION DYSREGULATION**

Henry is a 7-year-old child who struggles with emotion regulation. Although he has not been formally diagnosed, his parents and teachers agree that many things in life are more difficult for Henry than for his siblings and his peers.

Morning mayhem: *Activities of daily living (ADL)*	Henry has little trouble awakening in the morning, although he is somewhat grouchy. The first thing Henry must do as part of his morning routine is discreetly throw away his "pull-up," being careful not to let any of his siblings see, even though he knows that they know. At 7 years old, Henry is not fully potty trained and bedwetting continues to be a problem despite all of his parent's efforts. Henry feels embarrassed every morning because his 2-year-old brother wears regular underwear to sleep. "What is wrong with me?" He worries and he wonders.
Bad luck on the bus: *Work*	Henry's dad is responsible for making sure that he gets to the bus stop on time. His father makes sure that the morning routine is kept structured to reduce anxiety for Henry and assist with the family's busy morning routine. But today, when Henry climbs on to the bus and attempts to sit down in his assigned seat, a new child is sitting where he is supposed to sit. The bus driver asks Henry to please be seated so that she can continue. Henry's eyes well up with tears because he doesn't know how to explain that someone is sitting in his seat. One of the older boys on the bus sees Henry crying and says tauntingly, "Cry baby!"
Suffering through school: *Education*	At school, Henry's teacher is working with the children on writing paragraphs from a prompt. The class has formed paragraphs together for weeks, and today, the teacher will give the students a prompt and ask the students to write a paragraph on their own. The teacher notes that Henry participates verbally when the class works together but notices that it takes Henry longer to copy the class paragraph from the board to his paper. Today, the teacher notes that as the other children are attempting to write their paragraph, Henry is off-task, playing in his desk. She quietly asks him to please get started, and he appears to be compliant. But when she collects the paragraphs, Henry has only written three sentences, whereas the other children have produced more than double the amount of sentences.
Cafeteria crisis: *Social participation*	Henry has several close friends; most of them are people he has known for a long time because they attended the same preschool as he did. One of the boys is in Henry's class. Henry usually sits next to his friend at the lunch table. But today, his friend is absent from school. Henry sits at the same table but eats his lunch in solitude because he is too shy to talk to any of the other children.
"It's not fair." *Play and leisure*	Henry has three siblings. He usually makes good choices when it comes to following the rules of games. But he gets overly angry when other people do not follow the rules. Often, he storms out in the middle of games with both siblings and peers if he thinks something is "unfair." His peers have difficulty with this pattern of behavior, which often results in them not wanting to include Henry in play.
Homework hostility: *Work*	One of Henry's parents' most difficult tasks is helping Henry complete his homework. They report that Henry has a difficult time focusing, often becomes distracted, and must have a quiet environment with no disruptions to complete even simple assignments. In a busy household, this is seldom possible. Henry also often cries if he cannot quickly figure out new material, and he is sensitive about even gentle corrections from his parents.
Medication complication: **"I can't sleep."** *Rest and sleep*	Recently, the pediatrician has recommended medication for Henry to help alleviate some of his noted anxiety and to improve his level of concentration. Henry's mother feels uncertain but decides to agree with her husband and try the medication. At times, the medication seems to be helping. But at night, Henry cannot sleep. This side effect bothers his parents, and they feel that this sleep disruption may erase any benefit of the medication.

ability was positively correlated with four of eight social interaction quality indicators. These were "self-reports and peer nominations of interpersonal sensitivity, reciprocal friendship nominations, and the proportion of positive versus negative peer nominations" (Lopes, Salovey, Coté, & Beers, 2005, p. 115). In addition, poor emotional regulation can produce both internalizing and externalizing behaviors, which have a negative impact on social functioning (Eisenberg, Fabes, Guthrie, & Reiser, 2000). Box 60-3 presents a day in the life of Rebecca, an adult with emotional dysregulation.

Evaluation and Assessment of Emotion Regulation

Despite the importance of emotion regulation to overall health and well-being, there are few validated assessments to measure emotional regulation skills and none are specific to OT. The social history interview and occupation-based interview assessment tools are useful

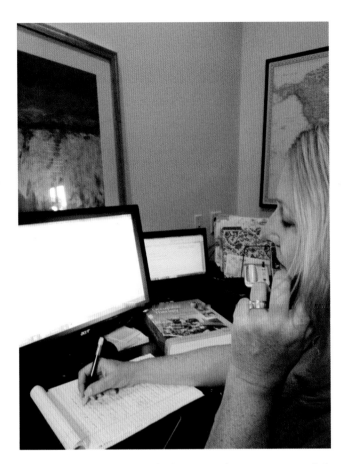

FIGURE 60-3 **The workplace can be very stressful and challenge one's ability to self-regulate emotions.**

in identifying occupational performance issues related to emotion dysregulation. However, naturalistic observation of emotion regulation skills in various contexts may be the most informative.

One assessment developed for adults, the Difficulties in Emotion Regulation Scale (DERS), has demonstrated "high internal consistency, good test-retest reliability, and adequate construct and predictive validity" (Gratz & Roemer, 2004, p. 41). The DERS was validated on a community sample of adolescents (Neumann, van Lier, Gratz, & Koot, 2010).

The DERS was designed to measure the following dimensions of emotion regulation:

- Awareness and acceptance of emotions
- Ability to persist in goal-directed behavior when experiencing negative emotions
- Access to emotion regulation strategies that are perceived to be efficacious

The DERS consists of 36 items that make up the following six subscales with higher scores indicating deficits in emotion regulation:

1. Acceptance of emotional responses
2. Engagement in goal-directed behavior
3. Impulse control
4. Emotional awareness
5. Access to emotion regulation strategies
6. Emotional clarity

One assessment, although not directly measuring emotion regulation, that may be useful to measure affective states is the Positive and Negative Affect Schedule (PANAS). The PANAS is a 20-item assessment that measures positive and negative affective dispositions. High negative affect scores indicate the presence of subjective distress and unpleasant engagement, whereas low negative affect scores represent the absence of these feeling states. High positive affect scores indicate enthusiasm and pleasurable engagement with the environment, whereas low positive affect scores represent a lack of pleasurable engagement and lethargy. Using a large sample of the general adult population, the PANAS demonstrated adequate to good reliability and validity (Crawford & Henry, 2004).

Another assessment that might provide an insight on emotional regulation is the Mayer-Salovey-Caruso Emotional Intelligence Test, Version 2.0 (MSCEIT V2.0). This tool is designed as a performance-based assessment of the ability to reason using emotional information, including the capacity to access, perceive, and understand emotions; to use emotional knowledge; and to regulate emotions. It can be administered individually or in groups and presents the client with eight tasks that require emotional problem solving. The test has norms based on data from over 5,000 participants in various countries and has demonstrated acceptable reliability and validity (Mayer, Salovey, Caruso, & Sitarenios, 2003).

Interventions to Enhance Emotion Regulation

There are few psychological interventions designed specifically for emotion regulation published in the literature, and only one, dialectical behavior therapy (DBT), has an extensive evidence base. Dialectical behavior therapy is described briefly, and its applicability to OT is discussed. Three other approaches, emotional intelligence interventions, social and emotional learning (SEL), and sensory-based approaches, are also described.

Dialectical Behavior Therapy

Dialectical behavior therapy is based on cognitive behavioral principles. Cognitive behavioral intervention approaches are based on evidence that suggests that cognitive processes influence emotional states. These cognitive processes occur when people use situational cues, judgment, and memory to identify the source of their physiological

BOX 60-3	**THE DYNAMICS OF DYSREGULATION: A DAY IN THE LIFE OF AN ADULT WITH EMOTION DYSREGULATION**

Rebecca is a 36-year-old adult who struggles with emotion regulation. Rebecca is married and has one child. She works as a legal secretary in a large law practice. Rebecca is the adult child of an abusive mother who abandoned the family when she was 14 years old. Rebecca was expected to take over the often overwhelming role of helping to raise her siblings after her mother left.

Mad already and it's only morning: *Rest and sleep*	The alarm goes off every day at 5:30 a.m., and every day, Rebecca hits the snooze button because she dreads getting out of bed. Today, she doesn't have the opportunity to hit the snooze button; she has forgotten to set her alarm the night before. Instead, she awakens to her husband who says, "Rebecca, the alarm didn't go off, hurry up, get up, we've overslept." As is frequently the case, her misdirected anger causes her to snap at both her husband and her daughter repeatedly before leaving for work. Her husband, fed up with this treatment, looks at her and says, "It's only morning, and you are already mad. I'm starting to wonder if you wake up this way?"
Breakfast on the run; life on the run: *Activities of daily living (ADL)*	Even though Rebecca considers herself an organized person, she often rushes through tasks because she has so many responsibilities. Most of her life, she has been expected to complete more than the reasonable amount of activities. She has come to believe that if she doesn't get it all done, she will not be valued. She also has difficulty saying "no" when people ask her for help. She feels that her self-worth is dependent on task completion. Throughout her life, her ADL and personal care have taken a backseat to other people's needs. This morning is no different. In her hurry, after oversleeping, Rebecca skips breakfast and hurries out the door, forgetting also the lunch in the refrigerator her husband had packed for her.
"Never mind, I will do it myself." *The world of work*	At work, the firm has hired an additional legal secretary because of expansion. Rebecca feels threatened by the new legal secretary because she is younger and performs many tasks more quickly than Rebecca. Rebecca knows that she should ask the new secretary to share some of her workload, and today, she decides to ask for help because she is running late. After greeting the new coworker, she asks if she can complete the morning summaries for her while Rebecca moves on to the next item. Morning summaries are an area that the new secretary has not done before, and so she agrees to do the work but says she will need to ask a few questions. Before her new colleague can ask the first question, Rebecca snatches the papers from her hand and says, "Never mind, I will just do it myself." Her coworker comments later to their mutual supervisor that, "Rebecca seems a bit passive–aggressive to me." She follows with details of their earlier interaction.
Stop the stress: *Health promotion and maintenance*	Rebecca's job is busy and stressful. A trip to her doctor earlier that month confirmed that Rebecca has extremely high blood pressure, placing her at risk for various illnesses. He had insisted that she begin taking blood pressure medication but also told her that she must find other ways to reduce her stress and anxiety.
Finding friends, no time for play: *Social participation/play and leisure*	Rebecca has difficulty trusting other people and therefore feels that she has little peer support. She had even been to counseling during adulthood to try to cope with the rejection, loneliness, fear of abandonment, and depression that she has experienced since her mother left. Because she had to help raise her siblings and even now takes on more than a reasonable share of responsibility at home and work, Rebecca has little opportunity to pursue hobbies. Also, she has few opportunities for social participation.
Taking care of everything and everyone: *Instrumental activities of daily living (IADL) overload*	Rebecca is still taking care of her siblings in addition to her responsibilities to her spouse and child. As a result, she manages several households and supplements her siblings financially as well. This causes marital stress because Rebecca is unable to say no to her siblings, and her spouse and child suffer as a result. When her spouse and/or child express their concerns or displeasure, Rebecca either retreats into isolation or becomes angry and verbally abusive toward them.
"I can't rest, I can't relax, and I can't SLEEP!" Turning off the emotionally dysregulated brain: *Rest and sleep*	Most nights, Rebecca lays in her bed, and she cannot stop thinking about how many things that she didn't finish that day, worried about how she will finish the next day's responsibilities, and feels that she cannot quiet her brain or her emotions. Rebecca sometimes uses alcohol to "quiet her mind." Her husband worries because this is a pattern that seems to be happening more frequently.

arousal, to recognize other people's emotions, and to interpret and respond effectively to emotionally charged situations (Nussbaum, 2001).

Developed by Linehan (1993a, 1993b), DBT was originally designed as an outpatient psychotherapy protocol to treat persons with borderline personality disorder but has been adapted for use with a variety of populations. The DBT philosophy is based on the following principles and assumptions, which are critical to the effectiveness of the approach:

- The client wants to change and is trying but may not always appear so.
- The client's emotional responses and behaviors are best understood in the context of personal history and present circumstances.
- The client is not to blame for their current situation but is responsible for making changes in his or her life.
- Blaming and labeling the client as manipulative, deceptive, etc. will not enhance the therapeutic intervention.
- A client does not fail at DBT, it is the intervention that is not working and needs to be modified (Linehan, 1993a).

Dialectical behavior therapy combines individual psychotherapy with group-based skills training. Although occupational therapists are not qualified to provide psychotherapy, we are adequately prepared to implement aspects of the skills training component.

Skills taught include mindfulness, interpersonal effectiveness, emotion modulation, and distress tolerance (Linehan, 1993b). Mindfulness training facilitates the awareness of emotional states without judgment and thereby decreases the arousal associated with negative mood states. Mindfulness also encourages living in the moment, observing, interpreting, and experiencing emotions in productive ways to satisfy one's own needs and to meet the demands of the environment. Interpersonal effectiveness training facilitates the development of effective communication skills, social skills, and interpersonal problem solving. Participants learn how to meet their needs in interpersonal encounters without damaging their relationships with their significant others.

Emotion modulation training is designed to help clients understand their emotions, reduce emotional suffering, and increase emotional resilience. Skills taught include identifying emotions, expressing emotions appropriately, and responding to the feelings of others. Distress tolerance training facilitates the ability to cope with stressful events, self-soothe, and persist in tasks despite frustration. This requires the capacity to accept the current reality, experience negative emotions without judgment, and thoughtfully determine a course of action.

Miller, Wyman, Huppert, Glassman, and Rathus (2000) have pioneered the use of DBT with adolescents.

An early study evaluated the use of DBT with 27 adolescents with suicidal ideation. Suicidal adolescents typically demonstrate four characteristic problems: (1) emotional instability, (2) impulsivity, (3) confusion about self, and (4) difficulties with interpersonal relationships. The study intervention consisted of skill modules on mindfulness, distress tolerance, emotion regulation, and interpersonal effectiveness. Based on the *Life Problems Inventory* (Rathus & Miller, 1995), statistically significant improvements were noted in all four problem areas (Miller et al., 2000).

Miller and Smith (2008) described the application of DBT for teens who demonstrate nonsuicidal self-injurious (NSSI) behavior. From a DBT perspective, NSSI behavior is "considered to be a maladaptive solution to overwhelming and intensely painful negative emotions" (Miller & Smith, 2008, p. 180) and a manifestation of emotion dysregulation. They concluded that DBT is a promising intervention for this population, but more research is needed. Dialectical behavior therapy has also been used effectively with adolescents with eating disorders (Safer, Lock, & Couturier, 2007; Salbach-Andrae, Bohnekamp, Pfeiffer, Lehmkuhl, & Miller, 2008) and adults with substance dependence (Dimeff, Rizvi, Brown, & Linehan, 2000; Wagner, Miller, Greene, & Winiarski, 2004).

Anger management programs are typically based on cognitive behavioral principles. Tang (2001), an occupational therapist, designed an anger management intervention for persons with mental disorders that, like DBT, included skills training sessions. This anger management intervention consisted of ten 90-minute group meetings in which participants learned and practiced anger management and relaxation strategies. Homework was assigned, which included readings, journaling, and recording situations that evoked anger in a hassle log. Over a period of 2 years, 64 clients participated in cohorts of 7 to 10 persons per group. A quasi-experimental pretest and posttest study demonstrated declines in the participants' overall experience of angry feelings, anger intensity, and anger duration. Significant reductions in maladaptive cognition and maladaptive behaviors were also noted (Tang, 2001).

The effectiveness of DBT for improving emotion regulation has been validated through research for a variety of populations. Occupational therapists who wish to infuse their practice with DBT principles and strategies should participate in continuing education in order to gain knowledge and skills regarding the science and practice of DBT.

Emotional Intelligence Interventions

The concept of emotional intelligence, first introduced into the popular media by Goleman (1995), has received a great deal of attention over the past decade. The Four-Branch Model of Emotional Intelligence posits that a person's emotional quotient (EQ) consists of four skill sets: perceiving emotions in self and others, understanding emotional information, incorporating emotions into one's thought processes, and managing or regulating one's emotions (Salovey, Mayer, & Caruso, 2002). Emotion management or regulation in this model consists of the ability to:

- Be open to both pleasant and unpleasant emotional experiences
- Monitor and reflect on emotional states
- Access, reduce, or prolong an emotional response
- Manage one's own emotions
- Respond to the emotions of others (Salovey et al., 2002)

Other aspects of emotional intelligence are presented in Box 60-4.

Although there are many studies that have linked emotional intelligence to overall health and well-being, academic and occupational success, quality of life, and resilience, little attention has been paid thus far to the development of interventions that enhance EQ. One experimental study consisting of 37 participants (19 in the intervention group and 18 in the control group) evaluated the effectiveness of a psychoeducational approach based on the Four-Branch Model of Emotional Intelligence. The intervention consisted of four weekly sessions of 2.5 hours each. The sessions consisted of mini-lectures, role-play, group discussions, readings, and homework. Results indicated positive changes in trait emotional intelligence, emotion identification, and emotion management for the intervention group but not for the control group, and the changes were sustained at the 6-month follow-up (Nelis, Quoidbach, Mikolajczak, & Hansenne, 2009). More intervention studies are clearly needed.

BOX 60-4 ASPECTS OF EMOTIONAL INTELLIGENCE

- Knowledge that an individual possesses regarding how and when emotions can be regulated
- Knowledge of strategies for emotion regulation and when to deploy them
- Ability to implement emotion regulation strategies
- Ability to identify and describe one's emotional experience
- Ability to express one's feelings in words or some other symbolic expression

Social and Emotional Learning

Social and emotional learning is a strategy to teach children, adolescents, and adults the skills needed for self-management and the establishment of healthy relationships. These skills include, but are not limited to, identifying and managing one's emotions, initiating and maintaining interpersonal relationships, handling challenges effectively, and making responsible decisions. The overall goal of SEL is to reduce risk factors and enhance resiliency factors for positive adjustment. The five core competencies in SEL are the following: self-awareness, self-management, social awareness, relationship skills, and responsible decision making (Collaborative for Academic, Social, and Emotional Learning [CASEL], 2011).

A large-scale meta-analysis indicated that SEL programs are effective for racially and ethnically diverse students at the elementary, middle, and high school levels and can be implemented successfully in both school and after-school settings. The outcomes identified by this study included higher achievement test scores and improved social-emotional skills, prosocial behavior, and attitudes toward self, others, and school for students who participated in SEL. In addition, a reduction in conduct problems and emotional distress were noted (Durlak, Weissberg, Dymnicki, Taylor, & Schellinger, 2011).

The most effective SEL programs incorporated four best practices. These programs were sequenced (S), active (A), focused (F), and explicit (E). This has become known as the SAFE approach to SEL. The interaction of these practices produces greater results than any single factor alone. *Sequenced* means breaking down complex skills into smaller steps and mastering them sequentially within a developmental perspective. *Active learning* involves incorporating opportunities to experiment and practice the skills being taught in various contexts, for example, through role-play and behavioral rehearsal. *Focused* means that sufficient time and attention are allotted for the development of specific skills, and *explicit* refers to the importance of specific, rather than general, learning objectives (Durlak et al., 2011).

Sensory-Based Approaches

Sensory-based approaches to intervention are based on the biological aspects of emotion regulation and are neuroregulatory in nature. The underlying concept, although not well researched, is by managing and/or controlling physiological responses, it is possible to regulate emotional states.

Sensory integration as a therapeutic approach is designed to help children develop the ability to self-regulate. Self-regulation involves various processes such as sensory modulation and emotion regulation are just some. Sensory integration theory posits that some developmental problems in children are due in part to hyposensitivity or hypersensitivity to sensory stimuli. This undersensitivity or oversensitivity results in emotional hypoarousal or hyperarousal, respectively. Hypoarousal may manifest as flat affect, detachment, withdrawal, depression, and passive–aggressive behavior. Hyperarousal may appear in the form of emotional tantrums, hypervigilance, anxiety, fear, and overreaction to perceived threats (Champagne, 2011). Sensory modulation is the ability to comfort, calm, or alert oneself and to regulate responses to sensory stimuli in order to engage in goal-directed behavior. Self-soothing is an important skill to reduce sensory and emotional arousal when it becomes uncomfortable and distressing. Sensory-based interventions include therapeutic sensorimotor groups, sensory activities, sensory diet, and environmental enhancements such as multisensory rooms (Champagne, Koomar, & Olson, 2010).

Champagne (2006) describes the use of multisensory rooms as an intervention that addresses the emotion regulation needs of adults with psychiatric disorders. Multisensory rooms are designed to reduce a client's exposure to chaotic, sensory overload and thereby elicit a relaxation response. This is typically accomplished through the use of muted, soft paint colors; a variety of comfortable seating options; soothing music; and visually appealing imagery. For more information about sensory integration evaluation and intervention, see Chapter 59.

Use of the arts in OT also improves sensory processing. Art making is a sensory activity that is naturally self-soothing. Because emotion regulation is a mind-body phenomenon, embodied multisensory experiences, such as the arts and mindfulness practices, may prove useful in therapy. One study of adults with a variety of mental health challenges, using a multiple case study design, demonstrated the efficacy of an art-based self-soothing kit. An arts-based self-soothing kit was defined as "a container, such as a box, bag, or a bin, that contains multi-sensory and multi-modal materials that a person uses to engage in meaningful creative and contemplative activities" (Sokmen & Watters, 2016, p. 350). Each participant created their own personalized self-soothing kit. The items chosen to be included in order of frequency were music, gratitude journaling, scented candles, audio meditations, painting, jewelry-making supplies, doodling/coloring, modeling materials, and gardening. During the first 4 weeks, use of the kits varied from every other day to multiple times a day. The length of these self-directed sessions ranged from 15 minutes to 3 hours. The results indicated that making and regularly using the kits fostered self-awareness, interrupted intrusive thoughts and flashbacks, decreased impulsive negative coping behaviors, and improved emotion regulation. An unexpected finding was that the participants used their self-soothing kits as a means of improving social connections and facilitating social participation (Sokmen & Watters, 2016).

Future Directions

Most research in emotion regulation focuses on decreasing and/or managing negative emotions and behaviors. An alternative approach is to focus on enhancing positive emotions, strengths, and resilience. The health benefits of positive emotion are being documented in the literature. For example, greater optimism predicted better health outcomes among persons with heart disease (Scheier et al., 1999). The mechanisms through which positive emotion impacts health are not yet clear but are likely to involve endocrine and immune system functions (Kiecolt-Glaser et al., 2002).

Fredrickson's (2001) Broaden and Build Model provides a framework for enhancing positive emotions and resilience. She asserts that negative, distressing emotions narrow an individual's attention and focus to the problem or source of dissatisfaction, whereas positive emotion broadens the field of attention. The broader field of attention facilitates creative problem solving that builds personal resources and resilience (Fredrickson, 2001). As a result, *broadening* a person's range of attention, cognition, and action and *building* his or her physical, intellectual, emotional, and social resources can enhance resilience and improves physical and mental health. Positive affect, especially curiosity, also encourages exploration and mastery (Peterson & Seligman, 2004).

The ability to access positive emotion is an important aspect of coping. Coping can be described as "conscious, volitional efforts to regulate emotion, cognition, behavior, physiology, and the environment in response to stressful events or circumstances" (Compas, Connor, Saltzman, Thomsen, & Wadsworth, 2001, p. 89). Eliciting positive emotions reduces stressful reactions and returns the body to a more balanced state. For example, prompting positive emotions such as gratitude and joy in response to stressful situations resulted in reduced heart rate, blood pressure, and vasoconstriction (Fredrickson & Levenson, 1998).

Conclusion

Effective OT interventions focus on helping clients participate in meaningful occupations. For some individuals, emotional dysregulation impairs occupational performance and limits participation. In addition, adults with emotion regulation difficulties report more physical and cognitive fatigue, less overall satisfaction with life, and less satisfaction with performance of daily activities (Hebert, 2017).

CENTENNIAL NOTES

Training of Teachers for Occupational Therapy for the Rehabilitation of Disabled Soldiers and Sailors

One of the first references regarding the impact of OT on the management and regulation of emotions was in a document entitled *Training of Teachers for Occupational Therapy for the Rehabilitation of Disabled Soldiers and Sailors* published in 1918 by the United States Federal Board for Vocational Education in response to a Senate Resolution 189 (Figure 60-4):

> In addition to reading from selected medical authorities, the student must prepare a list of processes from agricultural or commercial or industrial pursuits which may be suitable for relaxing, stimulating, coordinating, or concentrating the mind, and which may be used to restore self-confidence, overcome depression, indifference and excitability.

This was an acknowledgment that occupational performance and participation have emotional impacts as well as cognitive and physical effects.

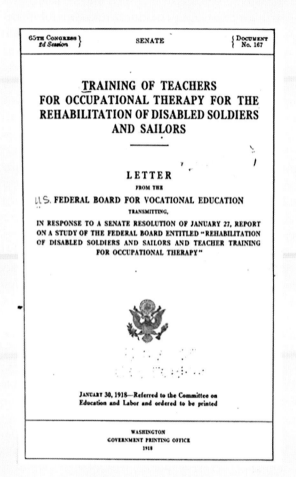

FIGURE 60-4 *Training of Teachers for Occupational Therapy for the Rehabilitation of Disabled Soldiers and Sailors* contains an early reference to the management and regulation of emotions.

It is for this reason that occupational therapists must attend to and attempt to enhance the emotional regulation and emotional intelligence of their clients. However, emotion regulation skills cannot be considered in isolation. They must be addressed in the context of the client's desired and meaningful occupations; his or her habits, roles, and routines; and his or her values and beliefs. In addition, emotion regulation is a complex phenomenon that requires attention to be paid to the physiological, cognitive, affective, behavioral, and motivational aspects of the client. Our unique role as OT practitioners is to help clients manage emotions within the context of occupational performance and identify the appropriate contextual supports that are needed to enhance emotion regulation and thereby facilitate occupational participation.

Although research in this area is limited, there are indications of the effectiveness of various approaches including sensory-based interventions, DBT, emotional intelligence interventions, social-emotional learning, and strengths-based approaches. Occupational therapy practitioners and researchers are in a unique position to develop and evaluate occupation-based assessment tools and interventions related to emotion regulation and emotional intelligence.

CASE STUDY 60-1   MARIA: STRUGGLING WITH THE EMOTION DYSREGULATION ASSOCIATED WITH BIPOLAR DISORDER

I first met Maria when she began participating in a program at the local high school for teenage mothers who were without a high school diploma. At the time, I was teaching and facilitating a grant-based program that provided adult basic education, high school completion, English language literacy services, and parenting classes. Maria was 15 years old at the time, and she had a 6-month-old daughter named Rosie. Maria had limited English language skills and very little family support.

Maria could attend classes 3 days per week for 4 hours each day, and childcare was provided for her daughter. What I remember the most about Maria was that despite her circumstances, she always tried to make everyone else happy. Generally, she would entertain her peers by telling funny jokes (translated by peers and sometimes made even funnier with the attempts at translation). Maria had days of flourishing, with the support of peers, demonstrating the positive effects of social and emotional learning. But sometimes, she would have days where neither her peers nor the teachers recognized her because of her sullen and withdrawn affect and apparent unwillingness to participate.

I also remember that sometimes, Maria and Rosie just wouldn't show up for a week or even several weeks at a time. Because Maria lived near enough to the facility where the classes were taught, she would walk to the classes, bringing her daughter in a stroller. When Maria didn't attend, one of my co-teachers immediately assumed and often verbalized that she felt that Maria's missing class was the result of "laziness, irresponsibility, and lack of motivation." Whereas I and another teacher, although we didn't realize it at the time, consistently chose to focus on what Maria was doing well when she did attend classes. We also factored into our consideration the environmental, social-emotional, and language barriers that were the more likely reasons for her absences.

When Maria had progressed academically, she signed up to take the general Education Development (GED) test. I remember all of us waiting anxiously for her exam results. Unfortunately, Maria did not pass the test on her initial attempt. After that, Maria's attendance to the classes began to wane. When she did attend, she would often express tearful regret about many of the life choices that she had made, was sometimes deeply upset, and especially self-deprecating about her failed attempt at the GED exam. Although the staff made frequent home visits and phone calls to encourage Maria to continue through the classes, she eventually displayed anger about "being bothered" and soon stopped attending classes completely.

Changes in my life led to a change in my career, and today, I am an occupational therapist practicing in a variety of settings. Now nearly a decade later, last week, as I sat to provide a group intervention at a hospital-based inpatient psychiatric unit where I sometimes work, I noticed a young girl sitting in the corner.

I knew that she looked familiar, and although we made eye contact and although I invited her to join the group, I couldn't place her. But as I left, I turned back and asked her name, explaining that she looked familiar to me. And before she even had time to answer, I knew who she was. I knew it was Maria.

I sat and talked with her. In our conversation, she told me that she was at the hospital because she had attempted suicide. She disclosed to me that she had been diagnosed with bipolar disorder not long after she left our program. She also let me know that her daughter was doing well, but she tearfully expressed that " . . . life just doesn't seem to ever get any easier for me."

The *Comprehensive Occupational Therapy Evaluation* (COTE) and *Coping Inventory* were administered. The COTE indicated strengths in reality orientation, cooperation, sociability, following directions, and interest in accomplishments. Deficits identified included problem solving, decision making, and organization. Maria becomes easily overwhelmed with complex tasks and has a low frustration tolerance. Her COTE score indicated moderate impairment in general behaviors and task behaviors; however, she was functional in the category of interpersonal behaviors. Many of the identified problems are directly related to her diagnosis of bipolar disorder. The *Coping Inventory* indicated that Maria has a rigid coping style and a limited repertoire of strategies to reach a goal or solve a problem. She tends to be passive, making little or no effort to initiate or sustain action in response to stressful situations. In addition, Maria demonstrates little resilience in response to disappointment or setbacks. Her adaptive coping behaviors include her ability to talk to others about personal needs, her desire and effectiveness in being liked and accepted by others, and her socially appropriate behavior in various situations.

Intervention goals included increasing Maria's frustration tolerance, improving her ability to problem-solve, expanding her repertoire of coping skills, and enhancing her ability to manage her medications. Maria participated in two individual and five OT group sessions. However, her length of stay was only 5 days for medication stabilization, and as a result, many of her OT goals were not realized.

1. Describe the elements of emotional regulation that are demonstrated in this case.
2. What principles and assumptions of the DBT philosophy apply to this case?
3. Discuss which emotional regulation intervention or approach would be most successful for Maria. Provide a rationale for your choice.
4. Describe the OT theoretical approach(es) that most closely support(s) your emotional regulation intervention.
5. What discharge recommendations would you make for this client?

Source: Case Study courtesy of Courtney Sasse.

REFERENCES

American Occupational Therapy Association. (2008). Occupational therapy practice framework: Domain and process, 2nd edition. *American Journal of Occupational Therapy, 62*, 625–683.

American Occupational Therapy Association. (2014). Occupational therapy practice framework: Domain and process, 3rd edition. *American Journal of Occupational Therapy, 68*, S1–S48.

Beer, J. S., & Lombardo, M. V. (2007). Insights into emotion regulation from neuropsychology. In J. J. Gross (Ed.), *Handbook of emotion regulation* (pp. 69–86). New York, NY: Guilford Press.

Berkman, E. T., & Lieberman, M. D. (2009). Using neuroscience to broaden emotion regulation: Theoretical and methodological considerations. *Social and Personality Psychology Compass, 3*, 475–493. doi:10.1111/j.1751-9004.2009.00186.x

Birditt, K. S., Fingerman, K. L., & Almeida, D. M. (2005). Age differences in exposure and reactions to interpersonal tensions: A daily diary study. *Psychology and Aging, 20*, 330–340.

Calkins, S. D., & Hill, A. (2007). Caregiver influences on emerging emotion regulation: Biological and environmental transactions in early development. In J. J. Gross (Ed.), *Handbook of emotion regulation* (pp. 229–248). New York, NY: Guilford Press.

Champagne, T. (2006). Creating sensory rooms: Environmental enhancements for acute inpatient mental health settings. *Mental Health Special Interest Section Quarterly, 29*(4), 1–4.

Champagne, T. (2011). *Sensory modulation & environment: Essential elements of occupation* (3rd ed.). San Antonio, TX: Pearson.

Champagne, T., Koomar, J., & Olson, L. (2010). Sensory processing evaluation and intervention in mental health. *OT Practice, 15*(5), CE1–CE7.

Cole, P. M., Martin, S. E., & Dennis, R. A. (2004). Emotion regulation as a scientific construct: Methodological challenges and directions for child development research. *Child Development, 75*, 317–333.

Collaborative for Academic, Social, and Emotional Learning. (2011). *What is social and emotional learning?* Retrieved from https://casel.org/what-is-sel/

Compas, B. E., Connor, J. K., Saltzman, H., Thomsen, A. H., & Wadsworth, M. E. (2001). Coping with stress during childhood and adolescence: Problems, progress, and potential in theory and research. *Psychological Bulletin, 127*, 87–127.

Cook, A., Spinazzola, J., Ford, J., Lanktree, C., Blaustein, M., Cloitre, M., . . . van der Kolk, B. (2005). Complex trauma in children and adolescents. *Psychiatric Annals, 35*, 390–398.

Crawford, J. R., & Henry, J. D. (2004). The Positive and Negative Affect Schedule (PANAS): Construct validity, measurement properties and normative data in a large non-clinical sample. *British Journal of Clinical Psychology, 43*, 245–265.

Davidson, R. J., Fox, A., & Kalin, N. H. (2007). Neural bases of emotion regulation in nonhuman primates and humans. In J. J. Gross (Ed.), *Handbook of emotion regulation* (pp. 47–68). New York, NY: Guilford Press.

Dimeff, L., Rizvi, S. L., Brown, M., & Linehan, M. M. (2000). Dialectical behavior therapy for substance abuse: A pilot application to methamphetamine-dependent women with borderline personality disorder. *Cognitive and Behavioral Practice, 7*, 457–468.

Drevets, W. C. (2000). Neuroimaging studies of mood disorders. *Biological Psychiatry, 48*, 813–829.

Durlak, J. A., Weissberg, R. P., Dymnicki, A. B., Taylor, R. D., & Schellinger, K. B. (2011). The impact of enhancing students' social and emotional learning: A meta-analysis of school-based universal interventions. *Child Development, 82*, 405–432.

Eisenberg, N., Fabes, R. A., Guthrie, I. K., & Reiser, M. (2000). Dispositional emotionality and regulation: Their role in predicting quality of social functioning. *Journal of Personality and Social Psychology, 78*, 136–157.

Eisenberg, N., & Spinrad, T. L. (2004). Emotion-related regulation: Sharpening the definition. *Child Development, 75*, 334–339.

Fox, N. A., & Calkins, S. D. (2003). The development of self-control of emotion: Intrinsic and extrinsic influences. *Motivation and Emotion, 27*, 7–26.

Fredrickson, B. L. (2001). The role of positive emotions in positive psychology. The broaden-and-build theory of positive emotions. *American Psychologist, 56*, 218–226.

Fredrickson, B. L., & Levenson, R. W. (1998). Positive emotions speed recovery from the cardiovascular sequelae of negative emotions. *Cognition & Emotion, 12*, 191–220.

Goleman, D. (1995). *Emotional intelligence: Why it can matter more than IQ.* New York, NY: Bantam Books.

Gratz, K. L., & Roemer, L. (2004). Multidimensional assessment of emotion regulation and dysregulation: Development, factor structure, and initial validation of the Difficulties in Emotion Regulation Scale. *Journal of Psychopathology and Behavioral Assessment, 26*, 41–54.

Gross, J. J., & Thompson, R. A. (2007). Emotion regulation: Conceptual foundations. In J. J. Gross (Ed.), *Handbook of emotion regulation* (pp. 3–24). New York, NY: Guilford Press.

Hebert, K. (2017). The relationship between emotion regulation and quality of life in healthy adults: Implications for occupational therapy. *American Journal of Occupational Therapy, 71*, 7111505138p1. doi:10.5014/ajot.2017.71S1-PO5107

Hughes, D. (2004). An attachment-based treatment of maltreated children and young people. *Attachment & Human Development, 6*, 263–278.

Izard, C. E. (2010). The many meanings/aspects of emotion: Definitions, functions, activation, and regulation. *Emotion Review, 2*, 363–370.

Karl, A., Schaefer, M., Malta, L. S., Dörfel, D., Rohleder, N., & Werner, A. (2006). A meta-analysis of structural brain abnormalities in PTSD. *Neuroscience and Biobehavioral Reviews, 30*, 1004–1031.

Kiecolt-Glaser, J. K., McGuire, L., Robles, T., & Glaser, R. (2002). Emotions, morbidity, and mortality: New perspectives from psychoneuroimmunology. *Annual Reviews of Psychology, 53*, 83–107.

Linehan, M. M. (1993a). *Cognitive-behavioral treatment of borderline personality disorder.* New York, NY: Guilford Press.

Linehan, M. M. (1993b). *Skills training manual for treating borderline personality disorder.* New York, NY: Guilford Press.

Lopes, P. N., Salovey, P., Coté, S., & Beers, M. (2005). Emotion regulation abilities and the quality of social interaction. *Emotion, 5*, 113–118.

Mahoney, M. J. (2005). Constructivism and positive psychology. In C. R. Snyder & S. J. Lopez (Eds.), *Handbook of positive psychology* (pp. 745–750). New York, NY: Oxford University Press.

Mayer, J., Salovey, P., Caruso, D., & Sitarenios, G. (2003). Measuring emotional intelligence with the MSCEIT V2.0. *Emotion, 3*, 97–105.

Mennin, D. S., Heimberg, R. G., Turk, C. L., & Fresco, D. M. (2005). Preliminary evidence for an emotion dysregulation model of generalized anxiety disorder. *Behaviour Research and Therapy, 43*, 1281–1310.

Miller, A. L., & Smith, H. L. (2008). Adolescent non-suicidal self-injurious behavior: The latest epidemic to assess and treat. *Applied and Preventative Psychology, 12*, 178–188.

Miller, A. L., Wyman, S. E., Huppert, J. D., Glassman, S. L., & Rathus, J. H. (2000). Analysis of behavioral skills utilized by suicidal adolescents receiving dialectical behavior therapy. *Cognitive and Behavioral Practice, 7*, 183–187.

Nelis, D., Quoidbach, J., Mikolajczak, M., & Hansenne, M. (2009). Increasing emotional intelligence: (How) is it possible? *Personality and Individual Differences, 47*, 36–41.

Neumann, A., van Lier, P. A., Gratz, K. L., & Koot, H. M. (2010). Multidimensional assessment of emotion regulation difficulties in adolescents using the Difficulties in Emotion Regulation Scale. *Assessment, 17,* 138–149.

Nussbaum, M. C. (2001). *Upheavals of thought: The intelligence of emotions.* Cambridge, United Kingdom: Cambridge University Press.

Ochsner, K. N., & Gross, J. J. (2007). The neural architecture of emotion regulation. In J. J. Gross (Ed.), *Handbook of emotion regulation* (pp. 87–109). New York, NY: Guilford Press.

Peterson, C., & Seligman, M. E. P. (2004). *Character strengths and virtues: A handbook and classification.* New York, NY: Oxford University Press.

Rathus, J. H., & Miller, A. L. (1995). *Life problems inventory.* Unpublished manuscript, Montefiore Medical Center, Albert Einstein College of Medicine, Bronx, NY.

Rothbart, M. K., & Bates, J. E. (1998). Temperament. In W. Damon & N. Eisenberg (Eds.), *Handbook of Child Psychology: Vol. 3. Social, emotional, and personality development* (5th ed., pp. 105–176). New York, NY: Wiley.

Safer, D. L., Lock, J., & Couturier, J. L. (2007). Dialectical behavior therapy modified for adolescent binge eating disorder: A case report. *Cognitive and Behavioral Practice, 14,* 157–167.

Salbach-Andrae, H., Bohnekamp, I., Pfeiffer, E., Lehmkuhl, U., & Miller, A. L. (2008). Dialectical behavior therapy of anorexia and bulimia nervosa among adolescents: A case series. *Cognitive and Behavioral Practice, 15,* 415–425.

Salovey, P., Mayer, J. D., & Caruso, D. (2002). The positive psychology of emotional intelligence. In C. R. Snyder & S. J. Lopez (Eds.), *Handbook of positive psychology* (2nd ed., pp. 159–171). New York, NY: Oxford University Press.

Scheier, M. F., Matthews, K. A., Owens, J. F., Schulz, R., Bridges, M. W., Magovern, G. J., & Carver, C. S. (1999). Optimism and rehospitalization after coronary artery bypass graft surgery. *Archives of Internal Medicine, 159,* 829–835.

Scheinholz, M. (2011). Emotion regulation. In C. Brown & V. C. Stoffel (Eds.), *Occupational therapy in mental health: A vision for participation.* Philadelphia, PA: F. A. Davis.

Schore, A. (2003). *Affect dysregulation and disorders of the self.* New York, NY: Norton.

Sokmen, Y. C., & Watters, A. (2016). Emotion regulation with mindful arts activities using a personalized self-soothing kit. *Occupational Therapy in Mental Health, 32,* 345–369. doi:10.1080/016421 2X.2016.1165642

Suveg, C., & Zeman, J. (2004). Emotion regulation in children with anxiety disorders. *Journal of Clinical Child and Adolescent Psychology, 33,* 750–759.

Tang, M. (2001). Clinical outcome and client satisfaction of an anger management group program. *Canadian Journal of Occupational Therapy, 68,* 228–236.

United States Federal Board for Vocational Education. (1918). *Training of teachers for occupational therapy for the rehabilitation of disabled soldiers and sailors.* Washington, DC: U.S. Government Printing Office.

van der Kolk, B. A. (2003). The neurobiology of childhood trauma and abuse. *Child and Adolescent Psychiatric Clinics of North America, 12,* 293–317.

Wagner, E. E., Miller, A. L., Greene, L. I., & Winiarski, M. G. (2004). Dialectical behavior therapy for substance abusers adapted for persons living with HIV/AIDS with substance use diagnoses and borderline personality disorder. *Cognitive and Behavioral Practice, 11,* 202–212.

the **Point®** *For additional resources on the subjects discussed in this chapter, visit* http://thePoint.lww.com /Willard-Spackman13e.

Social Interaction and Occupational Performance

Lou Ann Griswold, C. Douglas Simmons

LEARNING OBJECTIVES

After reading this chapter, you will be able to:

1. Understand the importance of addressing social interaction skills as critical for engagement in all areas of occupation.
2. Compare assessment approaches evaluating social interaction.
3. Consider factors that influence the quality of social interaction.
4. Consider different intervention approaches to support social interaction skills.
5. Discuss how to support the quality of social interaction during a person's occupational engagement.

Introduction to Social Interaction and Occupational Performance

People are social beings, and many occupations in which people engage involve social interaction with others. Although social participation is considered an occupation within the Occupational Therapy Practice Framework (OTPF) (American Occupational Therapy Association [AOTA], 2014), other areas of occupation such as work, leisure, play, education, and instrumental activities of daily living are often social. Children interact with one another as they play together, do school projects, and share information about their day with their families. Teens spend a large amount of their time interacting with their peers inside and outside of school as they participate in music groups, theater, team sports, and other youth activities. Adults interact with others at work, at home, and in the community. Depending on the circumstances, personal activities of daily living and rest and sleep might also involve social interaction with others. It appears, therefore, that social participation supports one's engagement in the many occupations and is not necessarily a distinct or separate occupation.

Regardless of the context, interacting with others requires decision making, collaborating, sharing information, gathering information, and conversing socially—each different intended purposes of social interaction. All social exchanges require similar skills to support interaction (see social interaction skills discussed in Chapter 26). People initiate interaction or respond to another person's greeting to begin an interaction. They communicate using words (i.e., speech, augmentative device, or sign language) and gestures. They ask questions, respond to a social partner, and take turns to support the interaction. A person also responds to messages sent by a social partner, empathizing, clarifying, and encouraging the other person to sustain the interaction. Specific expectations and demands for skills may vary with the context of the social exchange, yet all of these skills are required for social interaction.

Because most occupations require social interaction, having difficulty interacting with others potentially influences all areas of occupation, significantly limiting full occupational engagement. In fact, difficulty with social interaction skills may be *the* limiting factor for full participation in work, leisure, or instrumental activities of daily living. Furthermore, a lack of social interaction skills may have long-lasting negative consequences, particularly for children (Elliott, Sheridan, & Gresham, 1989). Hartup (1992) emphasized the importance of social skills claiming, "the single best childhood predictor of adult adaptation is not school grades, and not classroom behavior, but rather, the adequacy with which the child gets along with other children" (p. 1). More details on the inclusion of social interaction skills in occupational therapy (OT) theory are available on thePoint.

Assessment of Social Interaction

Assessments of social interaction have been primarily developed by psychologists and have taken two forms: report by the person or others and observation. According to Sheridan, Hungelmann, and Maughan (1999), report by self or others indicates a person's *social competence*, reflecting judgment of the person's behavior. Commonly used assessments based on report include the Social Skills Rating System (SSRS) (Gresham & Elliott, 1990), the Behavior Assessment System for Children (BASC) (Reynolds & Kamphaus, 1992), and the Matson Evaluation of Social Skills for Individuals with Severe Retardation (MESSIER) (Matson, 1995). Sheridan et al. (1999) argued that evaluation based on the perspective of another person is limited to that individual's perspective of the person's social interaction within a specific context. For example, when a parent or teacher completes a questionnaire on a child's social interaction, their reports are based on specific settings and situations, such as interacting during activities that occur at home, school, or on a playground and also social partners with whom the child interacts in a given environment (McCabe & Marshall, 2006; McConnell & Odom, 1999; Wight & Chapparro, 2008). Additionally, the persons completing the report may not have a clear understanding of the terms used in the rating scale (McCabe & Marshall, 2006) and may in fact be rating other constructs including psychopathology, self-esteem, adaptive behavior, and academic performance (for children) or work skills (for adults) (Matson & Wilkins, 2009).

Although rating scales of social competence completed by others may be limited to a given context, they indicate the result of a person's quality of social interaction and how the person's social interaction skills interfere with work, education, leisure, and play. Such information may contribute to an occupational profile (the first phase of evaluation in AOTA's OTPF) and may guide the occupational therapist to select an appropriate assessment tool for further evaluation. Assessments based on report by the person or others are easy to administer, convenient for the therapist, and require minimal training to give and interpret, and as

CENTENNIAL NOTES

The History of Social Interaction in Occupational Therapy

The first discussion of promoting social interaction was provided by Dunton, in 1937, when he described using quilt-making for persons with mental illness. Schwartzberg, Howe, and McDermott (1983) further reported other occupational therapists in the profession's early history promoting social interaction for persons with psychiatric disorders by using activity groups. Mosey (1973) provided guidance to occupational therapists in using activity groups to facilitate social interaction among group members.

As the profession began looking at effectiveness of group intervention, evaluating social interaction focused on observation, limited to specific behaviors, for example "talking," "looking at other person," and "laughing" as documented by Nelson, Peterson, Smith, Boughton, and Whalen (1988). Doble, Bonnell, and Magill-Evans (1991) acknowledged that occupational therapists lacked an assessment tool for social interaction to guide intervention and measure change. As a result, Doble and Magill-Evans (1992) developed an OT model of social interaction, which was expanded on and included in Fisher and Kielhofner's (1995) taxonomies of occupational performance skills. Doble and Magill-Evans' model provided the foundation for what is now the Evaluation of Social Interaction Skills (Fisher & Griswold, 2009, 2018).

result, Matson and Wilkins (2009) claimed they will continue to be used. However, it is important for occupational therapists to know the type and extent of information gained from any assessment. Although assessment tools of social interaction based on report by the person or others provide information on one's social competence, they do not identify specific problems in social interaction to guide intervention planning to support improvement in social interaction skills (Elliott et al., 1989).

Observation is the second form of evaluation of social interaction and provides information on behaviors during a social exchange that can guide intervention. Occupational therapists frequently include observation of a person in their evaluation process. Assessments based on observation may be contrived or "set up" to elicit certain behaviors or may be conducted in a natural context. Assessments based on role-play reflect contrived situations based on social situations that are believed to be important to people. Because the role-play situations are predetermined, they allow for a standardized observation. Assessments using role-play are common in mental health settings. An example of such an assessment was developed by Tsang and Pearson (2000) to evaluate social skills, to prepare persons with mental illness for work. Their evaluation included two work-related role-play situations: a job interview and requesting time off from work. Tsang and Pearson's assessment also included a self-report. Bellack, Brown, and Thomas-Lohrman (2006) believed that assessments based on role-play provide information on a person's "behavioral capacity" rather than "real life performance" (p. 350).

Doble and Magill-Evans (1992) and later many others (Case-Smith, 2005; Coster 2008; Gillen, 2013; Law, 2002; Royeen, Grajo, & Luebben, 2014; Wight & Chapparo, 2008) advocated for evaluating a person's performance, including social interaction, in the natural context to gather information to guide intervention to support participation in the contexts that are relevant for clients. Assessment that occurs in a natural context during occupational engagement logically leads to intervention that is occupation-based, using occupation as a means (Fisher, 2009; Law, 2002). More details on evaluating social interaction in a natural context are available on thePoint.

Occupational Therapy Assessment of Social Interaction

Two assessment tools have been developed by occupational therapists to evaluate social interaction skills: the Assessment of Communication and Interaction Skills (ACIS) (Forsyth, Salamy, Simon, & Kielhofner, 1998) and the Evaluation of Social Interaction (ESI) (Fisher & Griswold, 2009, 2018). For both of these assessments, therapists rate the social interaction skills using a 4-point criterion-referenced scale indicating the person's level of competence.

When the ACIS is administered, the person evaluated is observed during more than one situation. Options for situations include interacting during (1) one-on-one conversations with another person to discuss a topic, (2) parallel tasks in which people work individually on tasks but near others, (3) cooperative groups in which several people interact to complete a task or play a game, and (4) open interactions without a preplanned agenda or limited number of persons (e.g., a break room or party) (Forsyth et al., 1998). Using the ACIS, the person can be observed during either naturalistic situations or in simulated situations in which the occupational therapist might become the social partner. The ACIS evaluates 20 skills in categories of (1) physicality, (2) information exchange, and (3) relations (Forsyth et al., 1998).

The psychometric properties of the ACIS were determined primarily with persons with psychiatric diagnoses (81 of the 117 subjects) (Forsyth, Lai, & Kielhofner, 1999, p. 72). Subsequent studies using the ACIS have also included that same client population (Bonsaksen, Myraunet, Celo, Granå, & Ellingham, 2011; Haglund & Thorell, 2004; Hsu, Pan, & Chen, 2008).

Occupational therapists using the ESI only observe the person during social interactions in natural contexts with typical social partners (Fisher & Griswold, 2018). The person and occupational therapist determine what social interactions the occupational therapist will observe by discussing social interactions that are relevant to the person's daily life. The ESI evaluates 27 skills related to (1) initiating and terminating social interaction, (2) producing social interaction, (3) physically supporting social interaction, (4) shaping content of social interaction, (5) maintaining flow of social interaction, (6) verbally supporting social interaction, and (7) adapting social interaction (Fisher & Griswold, 2018).

The ESI has been used with persons of all ages without a diagnosis and with those with various diagnostic conditions, including children with autism, learning disabilities, and anxiety disorders (Griswold & Townsend, 2012); adults with traumatic brain injury (TBI) (Simmons & Griswold, 2010); adults with psychiatric disorders or neurological disorders (Søndergaard & Fisher, 2012); and adults with intellectual disabilities (Fisher, Griswold, Munkholm, & Kottorp, 2017).

Intervention to Enhance Social Interaction Skills

Research on Intervention Strategies

Intervention strategies to support social interaction skills found in the literature differ based on the age and diagnostic condition (Deckers, Muris, Roelofs, & Arntz, 2016).

CASE STUDY 61-1   BETHANY

Evaluating Quality of Social Interaction

Background: Referral and Occupational Therapy Interview

Bethany is 31 years old and a survivor of two traumatic brain injuries (TBIs) (see Appendix I for more details on TBI). She currently lives in an apartment associated with an independent living organization and attends a community-based program for adults with acquired brain injury (ABI). It was in this setting that Bethany sought the services of OT. The occupational therapist, Steve, met with Bethany, at which point he gathered information about Bethany as a person and learned about her goals (Figure 61-1).

Bethany told Steve about herself and her two accidents that resulted in two TBIs. Bethany identified herself as an artist since childhood. She loved painting and had been studying fine arts in college in a large urban area, with plans to become a studio artist and continue living in the city with her friends. On her way to class, she was crossing a busy intersection and was struck by a car and a driver who was texting and not aware of people in the crosswalk. Bethany was thrown 20 ft down the road and sustained a TBI as well as orthopedic injuries. After 10 weeks of rehabilitation, Bethany was discharged to her parents' home where she lived for 1 year and then moved back to the city to pursue an art degree. Bethany reported that she continued to have minimal issues with balance and after a night of clubbing decided to return to her apartment alone. She was on the second flight of stairs up to her third floor apartment when she had a dizzy spell and fell down a flight and a half of stairs, sustaining a second head injury. She was again discharged to her parents' home postrehabilitation. After living with her parents for about a year and a half, she moved into her apartment associated with an independent living organization in the city where her parents live.

At the time of her discharge from rehabilitation services, Bethany had no identified options for employment and had few friends with whom she had contact. She had difficulty speaking and was given an augmentative and alternative communication (AAC) device, which she did not use regularly. She felt isolated. When she learned about a community-based program for adults with ABI, she eagerly attended in hopes of meeting people and finding meaningful activities. In the program, Bethany began exploring new art media and had joined a cake decorating group, both of which she enjoyed. However, she stated that while she enjoyed the activities, she really missed having a strong social network. She recognized that her brain injuries had resulted in difficulty interacting with others.

Bethany's desires were to establish social networks and to use her art talents in some way to supplement her income. Steve and Bethany discussed that improved social interaction skills would be essential in supporting both of Bethany's goals. Bethany stated that when she was engaged in an activity with another program member, she usually did not interact a great deal and they usually worked side by side, not working together or talking. She knew this type of experience was important for her to practice using her AAC in a productive manner and to become more social again, but she did not know how to begin working in this direction.

Steve suggested using the Evaluation of Social Interaction (ESI) to evaluate Bethany's social interaction skills to identify specific problems and plan intervention to address those identified. Bethany agreed, and together they identified two possible social exchanges that naturally occurred in the community program that Bethany reported were relevant and challenging for her. Bethany agreed to have Steve observe her as she (1) created a bulletin board with another program member and (2) decorated a cake with a different program member.

Evaluation Results

Steve followed the steps of implementing a standardized performance analysis using the ESI (refer to Chapter 26 for details of performance analysis and the definition of the 27 ESI items). Steve quietly observed Bethany as she engaged in the two tasks that involved social interaction. He took notes on Bethany's quality of social interaction and scored her performance using the standardized ESI scoring criteria. Bethany's score form for the cake decorating task is shown in Figure 61-2.

Steve entered Bethany's raw ESI scores into his copy of the ESI computer-scoring software to generate a linear measure of the quality of social interaction. Bethany's quality of social interaction measure is reported on the computer-generated ESI graphic report (Figure 61-3).

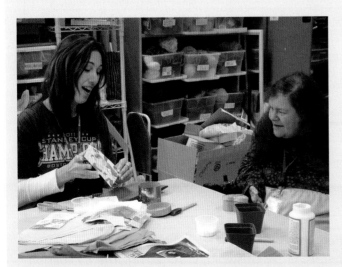

FIGURE 61-1 **Bethany practicing social skills in an occupational therapy group.**

(continues)

CASE STUDY 61-1   BETHANY *(continued)*

EVALUATION OF SOCIAL INTERACTION SCORE FORM (Page 1)

Name: Bethany

Occupational therapist: Steve

Gender: ____ Male   X Female

Date of evaluation: _____

Date of birth: _____   Age: 31

Major diagnosis: Traumatic brain injury

Secondary diagnosis: _____

Observation number: ____1 X 2 ____3 ____4

Intended purpose of social interaction:
____ Gathering information (GI)
____ Sharing information (SI)
____ Problem solving/Decision making (PD)
X Collaborating/Producing (CP)
____ Acquiring goods and services (AG)
____ Conversing socially/Small talk (CS)

Social interaction code: CP-1

Detailed task description: Decorating a cake
_____

Time of day:
____ Morning X Afternoon ____ Evening

Familiarity of the physical environment:
X Familiar
____ Somewhat familiar
____ Unfamiliar

Degree of expected structure:
____ High structure
X Relaxed structure
____ "Free" structure

Noise level:
____ Quiet
X Moderate noise
____ Extreme noise

Number of social partners: 1

Primary social partner: KL

Familiarity of primary the social partner:
X Familiar
____ Somewhat familiar
____ Unknown

Status of pri[mary]
____ Expe[...]
____ Rec[...]
X Frien[...]
____ Fam[...]
____ Othe[...]

Age of prima[ry]
____ Chil[d]
____ Adol[escent]
X Adul[t]
____ Olde[r]

Social part[ner]
____ App[...]
____ Que[...]
____ Mini[...]
X Mod[...]
____ Mar[...]

Overall com[...]
____ Gen[...]
____ Que[...]
____ Unc[...]
X Very[...]

Person's ov[...]
____ App[...]
____ Que[...]
____ Mini[...]
____ Mod[...]
X Mar[...]

EVALUATION OF SOCIAL INTERACTION SCORE FORM (Page 2)

ITEM RAW SCORES

Initiating and Terminating Social Interaction

1. Approaches/Starts   4 3 2 ①
   Did not respond to partner's greeting
2. Concludes/Disengages   4 3 ② 1
   Ended somewhat abruptly

Producing Social Interaction

3. Produces Speech   4 3 2 ①
   Produced very little intelligible speech
4. Gesticulates   4 3 ② 1
   Minimal gestures to support interaction
5. Speaks Fluently   4 3 2 ①
   Very little intelligible speech

Physically Supporting Social Interaction

6. Turns Toward   4 3 ② 1
   Did not turn face toward partner
7. Looks   4 3 ② 1
   Looked at partner out of corner of eye
8. Places Self   4 3 ② 1
   Placed self far away from partner
9. Touches   ④ 3 2 1
10. Regulates   ④ 3 2 1

Shaping Content of Social Interaction

11. Questions   4 3 2 ①
    Did not ask partner questions
12. Replies   4 3 ② 1
    Did not reply to questions and comments
13. Discloses   ④ 3 2 1
14. Expresses Emotion   4 3 2 ①
    Did not express emotion matching partner's messages
15. Disagrees   4 3 2 ①
    Did not respond to partner's suggestions
16. Thanks   4 3 ② 1
    Did not thank partner for frosting tip

Maintaining Flow of Social Interaction

17. Transitions   ④ 3 2 1
18. Times Response   4 3 2 ①
    Long delay to respond and no response
19. Times Duration   4 3 2 ①
    Spoke briefly -- partner needed clarification
20. Takes Turns   4 3 2 ①
    Did not take social turn

Verbally Supporting Social Interaction

21. Matches Language   4 3 2 ①
    Said very little and used simple language
22. Clarifies   4 3 2 ①
    Did not clarify when partner questioned
23. Acknowledges/Encourages   4 3 2 ①
    Did not encourage partner to engage
24. Empathizes   4 3 2 ①
    No support when partner was frustrated

Adapting Social Interaction

25. Heeds   4 3 2 ①
    Did not heed intended purpose: collaborate
26. Accommodates   4 3 2 ①
    Did not prevent problems from occurring
27. Benefits   4 3 2 ①
    Social interaction problems persisted

Additional comments: _____

FIGURE 61-2 Bethany's Evaluation of Social Interaction (ESI) score form for her social interaction supporting decorating a cake with another person. (Fisher, A. G., & Griswold, L. A. [2018]. *The Evaluation of Social Interaction* [4th ed.]. Fort Collins, CO: Three Star Press. Reprinted with permission.)

CASE STUDY 61-1   BETHANY (continued)

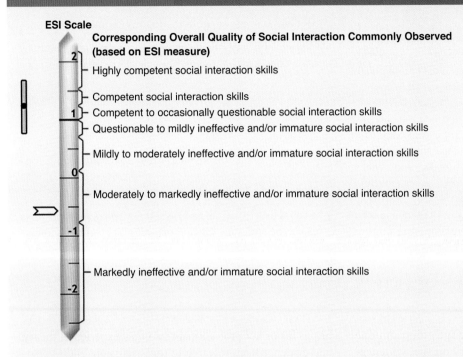

FIGURE 61-3 The Evaluation of Social Interaction (ESI) scale illustrating Bethany's ESI measure, indicated by the arrow to the left. (Fisher, A. G., & Griswold, L. A. [2018]. *The Evaluation of Social Interaction* [4th ed.]. Fort Collins, CO: Three Star Press. Reprinted with permission.)

Bethany's ESI measures can be interpreted from a criterion-based interpretation and norm-based perspective. The arrow to the left of the scale indicates the location of Bethany's ESI measure along the scale at −0.52 logit. At this level, well below the criterion-referenced cutoff point of competent performance (at 1.0 logit, indicated by a heavy black line on the ESI scale), persons commonly have *moderately to markedly ineffective social interaction skills*. When making a norm-referenced interpretation, Steve compared the location of Bethany's ESI measure to the bar to the left of the scale that indicates the range (±2 *SD*) of quality of social interaction of typical adults between the ages of 22 and 59 years. The black dot in the middle of the bar indicates the mean quality of social interaction for typical adults.

Steve began his documentation with a global baseline statement reflecting Bethany's overall quality of social interaction:

When Bethany was engaged in two social interactions, one with a program member to create a bulletin board for the program's hallway and another interaction with a different member to decorate a cake, the quality of her social interaction was moderately to markedly ineffective for both tasks. Bethany chose not to use her augmentative communication device and she did not collaborate with her social partners during either task.

Steve identified clusters of interrelated social interaction skills and wrote the following summary statements to document Bethany's social interaction and support her baseline statement (refer to Chapter 26 for details on clustering interrelated skills). Because Bethany's observed social interaction skills were similar in both social exchanges, creating a bulletin board and decorating a cake, Steve described them together.

- **Produces Speech, Speaks Fluently, and Matches Language:** Bethany spoke very little (two to three words per social exchange), and when she did, her speech was almost always unintelligible, with frequent pauses between words.

- **Times Response, Times Duration, Takes Turns, and Clarifies:** Bethany did not respond to most of her social partners' questions or comments, and when she did, she gave one-word responses, resulting in her partners asking for clarification, to which Bethany did not respond.

- **Expresses Emotion and Empathizes:** Bethany demonstrated little emotion throughout the two social exchanges and did not empathize with her partners' feelings when they were jovial or frustrated when they could not understand what Bethany was saying.

- **Questions, Acknowledges/Encourages, and Heeds:** Bethany did not ask her social partners any questions during either task and did not acknowledge or encourage her social partners to continue the social interaction. The result was that she did not collaborate with her partners when they were to work together to make the bulletin board and decorate the cake.

Steve shared the results of his observations with Bethany so that they could use the information to refine Bethany's goal of improving her interaction with others. Steve's documentation clearly identified skills that Bethany might work on as a means to reaching her overarching goal.

(continues)

CASE STUDY 61-1   BETHANY (continued)

Because Bethany had difficulty with several social interaction skills, Steve and Bethany had to determine which of these to address first. Steve knew that they had two approaches to use: (1) reflect on the skills that seemed to most interfere with Bethany's overall quality of social interaction or (2) address the skills that are relatively easier. The ESI manual (Fisher & Griswold, 2018) includes a hierarchy of the relative difficulty of all ESI skills, based on Rasch analysis of all evaluations for the ESI standardization sample. Working collaboratively, Steve and Bethany used a combination of these two approaches and decided to focus first on skills of *Clarifies, Questions, and Replies*. Steve reasoned that whereas *Replies* was a relatively more difficult skill on the ESI skill hierarchy, Bethany's lack of responding to her social partners had a very large impact on her overall quality of social interaction. Steve also reasoned that if Bethany improved her ability to reply to her social partner even somewhat, her overall social interaction would be enhanced.

Bethany and Steve wrote the following goals:

1. In a collaborative task (e.g., cooking, art project), Bethany will consistently answer her social partner's questions using five or more words.
2. In a collaborative task (e.g., cooking, art project), Bethany will clarify what she had said when prompted by her social partner, responding with five or more words.
3. In a collaborative task (e.g., cooking, art project), Bethany will ask her social partner at least two questions to seek his or her perspective on the task and/or how to proceed.

The measurable goals allow Bethany to know what she is working toward and provide her with objective benchmarks against which to measure progress. Most importantly, Bethany set her own goals with Steve, using the results from her observed performance.

Research typically has focused on one age group and one diagnosis at a time. See "Commentary on the Evidence" box for further details.

Intervention Planning

After setting goals, together, the occupational therapist and person plan intervention. The occupational therapist brings his or her professional reasoning, experience, theory, and evidence from research to the discussion, and the person contributes suggestions related to activities, strategies, and locations in which intervention might occur naturally. Having evaluation results based on observation in a natural context enables the occupational therapist and person to logically plan well-targeted intervention to promote social interaction during occupations that are relevant and meaningful.

" COMMENTARY ON THE EVIDENCE

Odom et al. (1999) organized intervention approaches described throughout the literature to promote social competence in young children with disabilities into four strategies: (1) adapting the environment, which included structuring play activities to promote social interaction, arranging and limiting materials, and matching socially competent peers with children with difficulty with social interaction; (2) teaching social skills to small groups of children and providing opportunity for them to practice the skills in play activities; (3) teaching peers who have good social skills how to support their peers who are having difficulty with social skills; and (4) combining the three other strategies. When Odom et al. (1999) compared the four approaches in a study with 92 preschool-age children with disabilities, they found that having one's peers support social interaction is most effective for improving proxy-reported competence of social interaction. They further found the improved social competence to be maintained 1 year later.

Intervention studies with adult populations have focused on the social interaction needs for people with mental illness, primarily schizophrenia (Shimada, Nishi, Yoshida, Tanaka,

& Kobayashi, 2016). A dominant frame of reference used in these studies is social learning theory, originally described by Bandura (Kurtz & Mueser, 2008). Specific strategies include goal setting, role modeling, practice, and reinforcement. Kurtz and Mueser (2008) conducted a meta-analysis of 23 randomized controlled studies with a total of 1,599 persons with schizophrenia. Although the studies targeted social interaction, Kurtz and Mueser found that only eight of these studies focused on social interaction skills during intervention. Kurtz and Mueser reported that in spite of a lack of focus on social interaction skills, analysis of the studies revealed a strong effect size for self-reported improvements in social interaction.

Simmons and Griswold (2010) used the ESI to evaluate the quality of social interaction for a group of 10 survivors of traumatic brain injury. The ESI provided a pretest measure of quality of social interaction, served as a guide for an 8-week OT intervention program, and was used as a posttest to measure intervention effectiveness. The difference between pre- and post-ESI measures was significant for the group of study participants. Their study demonstrated the utility of the ESI in guiding intervention and measuring change.

Intervention Guided by Theory

Occupational therapists use theory in their professional reasoning to guide the planning of intervention. The Occupational Therapy Intervention Process Model (OTIPM; Fisher, 1998, 2009) guides the evaluation and intervention process in a true top-down model by first understanding the client as a person, the client's performance context, and occupations that are meaningful for the client, followed by observing the client perform meaningful tasks and conducting performance analyses. As discussed in detail in Chapter 26, performance analyses involve determining what specific goal-directed actions are effective and ineffective. This process was illustrated earlier with Bethany. The problems identified in the performance analysis provide the basis for goals and the focus of intervention.

Based on OTIPM, after conducting a performance analysis in which the occupational therapist determines which actions (e.g., social interaction skills) most limit the person's social interaction, the occupational therapist considers the cause of the problem (Fisher, 2009). Considering cause after implementing a performance analysis is the hallmark of true top–down reasoning. Using a top–down reasoning process also keeps the occupational therapist focused on occupations that are important to the client, reflecting client-centered and occupation-based practice (Fisher, 2009; see Chapter 26).

Conceptual Model of Social Interaction and Factors That Impact Quality of Social Interaction.
Fisher and Griswold (2015) proposed a conceptual model of social interaction and identified factors believed to influence a person's quality of social interaction (Figure 61-4). Factors that support or hinder a person's quality of social interaction include societal

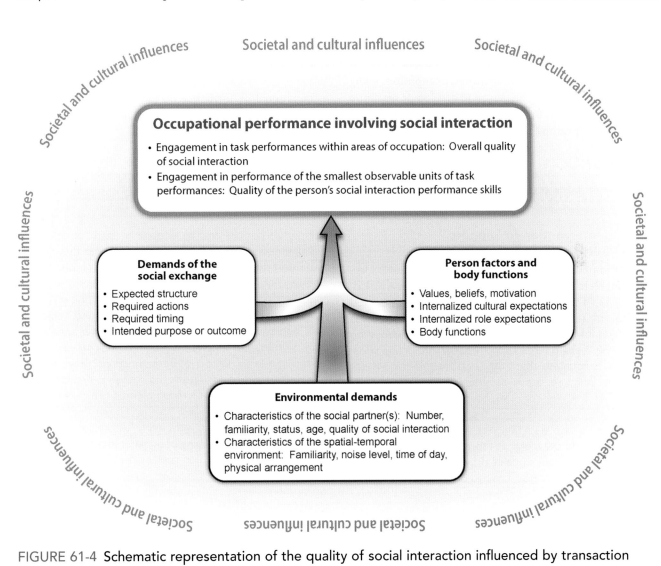

FIGURE 61-4 Schematic representation of the quality of social interaction influenced by transaction among societal and cultural influences, demands of the social exchange, environmental demands, and person factors and body functions. (Adapted from Fisher, A. G., & Griswold, L. A. [2018]. *The Evaluation of Social Interaction* [4th ed.]. Fort Collins, CO: Three Star Press. Reprinted with permission.)

and cultural influences, demands of the social exchange, environmental demands, and influences of person factors and body functions. Because each of the identified factors can impact a person's quality of social interaction, they can also contribute to the "cause" of the person's problems with social interaction. The many factors that influence the quality of one's social interaction can also provide the occupational therapist with options to consider when planning interventions to promote or support a person's quality of social interaction. Refer on thePoint for a detailed discussion of the conceptual model of social interaction by Fisher and Griswold.

Models for Intervention. Once the occupational therapist and the person have considered factors that limited the person's quality of social interaction, they need to select an intervention approach to address the identified concerns and work toward the person's goals. According to OTIPM (Fisher, 2009), there are four models for intervention: **adaptive occupation**, using adapted methods such as adaptive equipment or assistive technology or modifications of the environment or task demands to support performance; **acquisitional occupation**, using occupations to promote the person to develop or reacquire skills; **restorative occupation**, using occupations to facilitate restoring person factors and/or body functions; and

occupation-based education programs, providing education to large groups of people related to common problems and strategies to address problems. The occupational therapist uses the identified cause(s) of the problems to determine the most appropriate intervention model. The case study illustrates Steve's reasoning process in planning intervention for Bethany.

Effectiveness of Intervention

After intervention, it is essential that the occupational therapist reevaluate the person to determine if occupational therapy was effective. Again, using observation in natural context provides information that is relevant to the person's daily needs. A reevaluation might indicate that the person had made significant changes and no longer needs OT. Reevaluation might also reveal new areas of concern, in which case the occupational therapist and person would use the same top–down reasoning process to consider the cause of newly identified problems of social interaction in occupational performance, to identify appropriate intervention models and strategies, and to enhance quality of social interaction.

CASE STUDY 61-2   BETHANY

Planning Intervention to Support Social Interaction

Steve considered how demands of the social exchange contributed to Bethany's quality of social interaction. Specifically, he thought that the challenge of the intended purpose of collaborating with another person was challenging for Bethany. Steve was aware that collaborating with another person requires many social interaction skills. Steve also recognized that both social exchanges did not offer much structure. Steve considered the environmental demands of the two social exchanges. Bethany had two different social partners from the community program, both of whom also had difficulty with social interaction. Steve wondered how much of the partners' lack of social skill influenced Bethany's quality of social interaction. Steve was aware that both interactions had occurred in the natural environments of the hallway (for the bulletin board task) and the kitchen, where other members were passing through or also engaged in a task. Steve considered the influence of the noise from other people on Bethany's quality of social interaction. Steve then considered person factors and body functions. Bethany was motivated to engage

with other people and to engage in both of the tasks. Discussion with Bethany about how well she thought she had interacted with her partners led Steve to reason that Bethany had internalized the expectations, as she reported that she knew her partners had asked questions and made comments, but she had chosen not to respond because it was "too hard." When Bethany did speak, her speech was slow, slurred, and not well articulated, making her speech unintelligible—all factors of body functions. Steve recalled that Bethany reported that she did not use her AAC because she thought it had not been programmed to include phrases that she commonly needed, so she did not find it helpful. Steve realized that there were many factors contributing to Bethany's ineffective quality of social interaction. Although limitation in body function was evident, Steve knew that Bethany was not likely to improve her ability to articulate her words more clearly, at least not very quickly.

As Steve and Bethany discussed the causes of Bethany's difficulty in social interaction, they began considering ways to address many of these factors. Steve considered the first three intervention models from Occupational Therapy Intervention Process Model. Together, they determined that restoring

CASE STUDY 61-2   BETHANY *(continued)*

body function around oral motor control was not going to be fruitful because Bethany had already received a great deal of speech therapy with little to no improvement. They decided that using the AAC would enable other people to better understand Bethany, provided the right phrases and words were programmed into the device. Steve agreed to program Bethany's AAC with phrases that Bethany thought she would need. For example, including the question, "Do you know what I mean?" would help Bethany ensure that her social partners where understanding her and allow her to clarify as needed. Bethany suggested that adding the question, "What do you think?" would promote her to encourage her partners in interactions that were collaborative. Steve knew that Bethany and he had just selected the *adaptive occupation* model of intervention.

Bethany was eager to reacquire skills around social interaction using her AAC, the *acquisitional occupation* model for intervention. However, Bethany stated that she needed assistance to identify when she might use her augmentative device to engage in interaction more successfully. Steve and Bethany discussed the use of a subtle cuing system in which Steve could prompt Bethany to ask questions or respond to her social partner. They practiced the cuing system briefly and then tried it later that day when Bethany engaged in casual conversation with other program members during lunch. Steve explained that he could support Bethany as she acquired skills through practice in the natural opportunities while she attended the community program.

Bethany and Steve concluded that a combination of using two models for intervention would provide the basis to enhance Bethany's social interaction skills: adaptive occupation, using her AAC; and acquisitional occupation, to acquire social interaction skills.

The natural context of the community-based program included many opportunities for Bethany to practice the skills she wanted to acquire. Bethany realized that Steve would not be with her throughout the day and suggested that a few of the other staff also be shown the subtle cues to prompt her as needed. Steve knew that many of the program members wanted to work on social interaction to support their desired occupational participation. Therefore, Steve decided to offer an in-service training session to all staff using another model of intervention—*occupation-based education program* (Fisher, 2009). During the training session, Steve shared the conceptual model for social interaction and led the staff in a discussion of natural strategies for the program to better support social interaction by adapting the environment. The staff and Steve discussed promoting more face-to-face opportunities for members to socially interact

with one another, monitoring noise in areas in which social interactions frequently occurred, and pairing members so that they were better suited to support one another's social interaction. Steve suggested strategies to provide more structure to the activities with clear social interaction demands. For example, when cooking together, members might be organized into small groups of three persons with each person having a defined role for interacting, such as one person reading directions and the other two sharing the actual cooking task. Last, Steve introduced a simple universal system of cuing to prompt members on skills that many wanted to acquire. The in-service training session resulted in support of natural opportunities to acquire and practice social interaction skills throughout the day for all program members.

Determining Effectiveness of Occupational Therapy Intervention

After 8 weeks of working on improving her social interaction skills in the program, Bethany believed that she was meeting her goals. She requested that Steve see how she was doing by observing her again. Bethany and Steve again determined two social exchanges for Steve to observe and score using the ESI. For this evaluation, Bethany taught another member how to use a digital camera that the program had recently purchased and then how to enhance the pictures using a computer. Steve observed the two interactions, scored them, and entered Bethany's scores into the ESI computer software program. The results revealed that Bethany's overall quality of social interaction was now at 0.6 logits. Criterion-referenced interpretation indicated that her overall quality of social interaction was *mildly to moderately ineffective*, a significant improvement from the first evaluation. Steve verified the change by comparing Bethany's ESI measures for both evaluations, finding that the difference in the two measures was greater than the sum of the mean standard error of measurement for each assessment, according to the ESI manual (Fisher & Griswold, 2018). The ESI progress report, obtained from the computer-scoring software, includes the ESI scale indicating Bethany's ESI measure for the first and second assessment, marked with a number 1 and 2 for each respective assessment (Figure 61-5). Using a standardized assessment such as the ESI enabled Steve to confirm that Bethany had indeed made significant progress in the quality of her social interaction skill. The ESI scale in the ESI progress report provided an understandable visual aid. Bethany was eager to further improve her social interaction skills and set new goals based on the last evaluation results.

(continues)

CASE STUDY 61-2   BETHANY (continued)

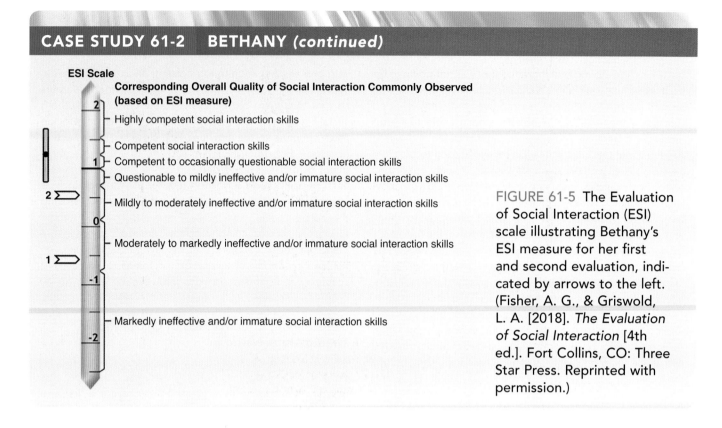

FIGURE 61-5 The Evaluation of Social Interaction (ESI) scale illustrating Bethany's ESI measure for her first and second evaluation, indicated by arrows to the left. (Fisher, A. G., & Griswold, L. A. [2018]. *The Evaluation of Social Interaction* [4th ed.]. Fort Collins, CO: Three Star Press. Reprinted with permission.)

Conclusion

The case study illustrated how the occupational therapist listened to his client as she expressed a desire to interact with others. As Doble et al. (1991) reported, occupational therapists working in all areas of practice reported that their clients had a need to improve their social interaction. In the case study, Steve determined that Bethany had difficulty with social interaction skills and evaluated her social interaction using a standardized assessment. He then used the assessment results to guide intervention. Furthermore, Steve worked with Bethany to select various intervention models and specific strategies based on a conceptual model. Most importantly, Steve provided intervention in natural context to support Bethany's occupational participation.

REFERENCES

American Occupational Therapy Association. (2014). Occupational therapy practice framework: Domain and process, 3rd edition. *American Journal of Occupational Therapy, 68*, S1–S48. doi:10.5014/ajot.2014.682006

Bellack, A. S., Brown, C. H., & Thomas-Lohrman, S. (2006). Psychometric characteristics of role-play assessments of social skill in schizophrenia. *Behavior Therapy, 37*, 339–352.

Bonsaksen, T., Myraunet, I., Celo, C., Granå, K. E., & Ellingham, B. (2011). Experiences of occupational therapists and occupational therapy students in using the Assessment of Communication and Interaction Skills in mental health settings in Norway. *British Journal of Occupational Therapy, 74*, 332–338.

Case-Smith, J. (2005). Contextual evaluation to support participation. In P. Kramer, J. Hinojosa, & P. Crist (Eds.), *Evaluation: Obtaining and interpreting data* (2nd ed., pp. 101–124). Bethesda, MD: American Occupational Therapy Association.

Coster, W. J. (2008). 2008 Eleanor Clarke Slagle Lecture. Embracing ambiguity: facing the challenge of measurement. *American Journal of Occupational Therapy, 62*, 743–752.

Deckers, A., Muris, P., Roelofs, J., & Arntz, A. (2016). A group-administered social skills training for 8- to 12-year-old, high-functioning children with autism spectrum disorders: An evaluation of its effectiveness in a naturalistic outpatient treatment setting. *Journal of Autism and Developmental Disorders, 46*, 3493–3504.

Doble, S. E., Bonnell, J. E., & Magill-Evans, J. (1991). Evaluation of social skills: A survey of current practice. *Canadian Journal of Occupational Therapy, 58*, 241–249.

Doble, S. E., & Magill-Evans, J. (1992). A model of social interaction to guide occupational therapy practice. *Canadian Journal of Occupational Therapy, 59*, 141–150.

Dunton, W. R., Jr. (1937). Quilt making as a socializing measure. *Occupational Therapy and Rehabilitation, 16*, 275–278.

Elliott, S. N., Sheridan, S. M., & Gresham, F. M. (1989). Assessing and treating social skill deficits: A case study for the scientist-practitioner. *Journal of School Psychology, 27*, 197–222.

Fisher, A. G. (1998). Uniting practice and theory in an occupational framework. 1998 Eleanor Clarke Slagle Lecture. *American Journal of Occupational Therapy, 52*, 509–521.

Fisher, A. G. (2009). *Occupational therapy intervention process model: A model for planning and implementing top-down, client-centered, and occupation-based occupational therapy interventions.* Fort Collins, CO: Three Star Press.

Fisher, A. G., & Griswold, L. A. (2009). *Evaluation of Social Interaction.* Fort Collins, CO: Three Star Press.

Fisher, A. G., & Griswold, L. A. (2018). *The Evaluation of Social Interaction* (4th ed.). Fort Collins, CO: Three Star Press.

Fisher, A. G., Griswold, L. A., Munkholm, M., & Kottorp, A. (2017). Evaluating domains of everyday functioning in people with developmental disabilities. *Scandinavian Journal of Occupational Therapy,* *24*, 1–9. doi:10.3109/11038128.2016.1160147

Fisher, A. G., & Kielhofner, G. (1995). Skill in occupational performance. In G. Kielhofner (Ed.), *A model of human occupational: Theory and application* (2nd ed., pp. 113–137). Baltimore, MD: Lippincott Williams & Wilkins.

Forsyth, K., Lai, J., & Kielhofner, G. (1999). The Assessment of Communication and Interaction Skills (ACIS): Measurement properties. *British Journal of Occupational Therapy, 62,* 69–74.

Forsyth, K., Salamy, M., Simon, S., & Kielhofner, G. (1998). *The Assessment of Communication and Interaction Skills (ACIS).* Chicago, IL: Model of Human Occupation Clearinghouse, University of Illinois.

Gillen, G. (2013). A fork in the road: An occupational hazard? *American Journal of Occupational Therapy, 67,* 641–652. doi:10.5014/ajot.2013.676002

Gresham, F. M., & Elliott, S. N. (1990). *Social Skills Rating System.* Circle Pines, MN: American Guidance Service.

Griswold, L. A., & Townsend, S. (2012). Assessing the sensitivity of the evaluation of social interaction: Comparing social skills for children with and without disabilities. *American Journal of Occupational Therapy, 66,* 709–717.

Haglund, L., & Thorell, L. (2004). Clinical perspective on the Swedish version of the Assessment of Communication and Interaction Skills: Stability of assessments. *Scandinavian Journal of Caring Sciences, 18,* 417–423.

Hartup, W. W. (1992). *Having friends, making friends, and keeping friends: Relationships as educational contexts. ERIC Digest (ED345854).* Champaign, IL: ERIC Clearinghouse on Elementary and Early Childhood Education.

Hsu, W., Pan, A., & Chen, T. (2008). A psychometric study of the Chinese version of the Assessment of Communication and Interaction Skills. *Occupational Therapy in Health Care, 22,* 177–185.

Kurtz, M. M., & Mueser, K. T. (2008). A meta-analysis of controlled research on social skills training for schizophrenia. *Journal of Consulting and Clinical Psychology, 76,* 491–504.

Law, M. (2002). Participation in the occupations of everyday life. *American Journal of Occupational Therapy, 56,* 640–649.

Matson, J. L. (1995). *The Matson Evaluation of Social Skills for Individuals with Severe Retardation (MESSIER).* Baton Rouge, LA: Scientific Publishers.

Matson, J. L., & Wilkins, J. (2009). Psychometric testing methods for children's social skills. *Research in Developmental Disabilities, 30,* 249–274.

McCabe, P. C., & Marshall, D. J. (2006). Measuring the social competence of preschool children with specific language impairment: Correspondence among informant ratings and behavioral observations. *Topics in Early Childhood Special Education, 26,* 234–246.

McConnell, S. R., & Odom, S. L. (1999). A multimeasure performance-based assessment of social competence in young children with disabilities. *Topics in Early Childhood Special Education, 19,* 67–74.

Mosey, A. C. (1973). *Activities therapy.* New York, NY: Raven Press.

Nelson, D. L., Peterson, C., Smith, D. A., Boughton, J. A., & Whalen, G. M. (1988). Effects of project versus parallel groups on social interaction and affective responses in senior citizens. *American Journal of Occupational Therapy, 42,* 23–29.

Odom, S., McConnell, S. R., McEvoy, M. A., Peterson, C., Ostrosky, M., Chandler, L. K., . . . Favazza, P. C. (1999). Relative effects of interventions supporting the social competence of young children with disabilities. *Topics in Early Childhood Education, 19,* 75–91.

Reynolds, C. R., & Kamphaus, R. W. (1992). *Behavior assessment system for children.* Circle Pines, MN: American Guidance Service.

Royeen, C. B., Grajo, L. C., & Luebben, A. J. (2014). Nonstandardized assessments. In P. Kramer, J. Hinojosa, & P. Crist (Eds.), *Evaluation in occupational therapy: Obtaining and interpreting data* (4th ed., pp. 121–141). Bethesda, MD: American Occupational Therapy Association.

Schwartzberg, S. L., Howe, M. C., & McDermott, A. (1983). A comparison of three treatment group formats for facilitating social interaction. *Occupational Therapy in Mental Health, 2,* 1–16. doi:10.1300/J004v02n04_01

Sheridan, S. M., Hungelmann, A., & Maughan, D. P. (1999). A contextualized framework for social skills assessment, intervention, and generalization. *School Psychology Review, 28,* 84–103.

Shimada, T., Nishi, A., Yoshida, T., Tanaka, S., & Kobayashi, M. (2016). Development of an individualized occupational therapy programme and its effects on the neurocognition, symptoms and social functioning of patients with schizophrenia. *Occupational Therapy International, 23,* 425–435.

Simmons, C. D., & Griswold, L. A. (2010). Using the evaluation of social interaction in a community-based program for persons with traumatic brain injury. *Scandinavian Journal of Occupational Therapy, 17,* 49–56.

Søndergaard, M., & Fisher, A. G. (2012). Sensitivity of the evaluation of social interaction measures among people with and without neurologic or psychiatric disorders. *American Journal of Occupational Therapy, 66,* 356–362.

Tsang, H., & Pearson, V. (2000). Reliability and validity of a simple measure for assessing the social skills of people with schizophrenia necessary for seeking and securing a job. *Canadian Journal of Occupational Therapy, 67,* 250–259.

Wight, M., & Chapparo, C. (2008). Social competence and learning difficulties: Teacher perceptions. *Australian Occupational Therapy Journal, 55,* 256–265.

the**Point**® *For additional resources on the subjects discussed in this chapter, visit* **http://thePoint.lww.com/Willard-Spackman13e.**

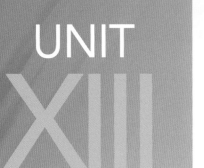

UNIT
XIII

The Practice Context: Therapists in Action

"In theory there is no difference between theory and practice.
In practice there is."

—Yogi Berra

Continuum of Care

Pamela S. Roberts, Mary E. Evenson

LEARNING OBJECTIVES

After reading this chapter, you will be able to:

1. Describe occupational therapy's typical roles in acute care, inpatient, outpatient, and community-based settings as illustrated in vignettes.
2. Value the importance of client-centered care through the collaborative goal-setting process to guide the professional reasoning process and influence the intervention plan throughout the continuum of care.
3. Recognize how client factors and contexts featured in the vignettes influence discharge recommendations and disposition through the continuum.
4. Be aware of key health care system regulations within the United States that affect a client's eligibility for services and length of stay in various settings along the continuum.
5. Acknowledge the opportunities for emerging practice areas to meet the needs of populations with varying access to health care.

This chapter describes an overview of the **continuum of care** that is part of the U.S. health care system. Case vignettes are featured as examples to illustrate how different services can meet an individual client's needs and goals, depending on the level of care and the client's personal factors and occupational performance. A table at the end of the chapter provides an organizing structure to help understand dimensions of the different levels of the continuum at a glance (Table 62-1). This chapter is a preface to the following chapters in this unit that more comprehensively address selected populations and occupational therapy's (OT) role to support optimal function and participation.

Introduction

Occupational therapy practitioners work in facilities that provide a range of services to address the occupational performance needs and concerns of children and adults across the life course (Roberts & Evenson, 2009). The reasons why individuals seek OT evaluation and interventions are often a result of a diagnosis/condition that requires medical, surgical, psychiatric, or rehabilitative intervention. As a consequence, individuals experience

CENTENNIAL NOTES

Health Care Policy and the Continuum of Care

From its earliest days, OT has been embedded in systems which have focused on patients' journeys from acute care hospitals to postacute care and the community. For instance, the care of injured soldiers in World War I (WWI) prompted this comment in a report from the U.S. Federal Board of Education to the U.S. senate:

> Between the time when the disabled soldier or sailor enters the hospital and his final placement in industry, commerce, agriculture, or less frequently in the special workshop or home, there lies a long period of education and adaptation. (Upham, 1918, p. 11)

In Britain in the post–World War II (WWII) years, one debate was whether to develop specialized orthopedic centers for wounded soldiers which mirrored the "custom in civilian practice to discharge a patient when fit for 'light work' and still maintain some supervision of his further recovery as an out-patient" (Malkin & Parker, as cited in Wilcock, 2002, p. 195). Occupational therapy services were discussed for each phases of care.

In the course of the 20th century, inpatient admissions grew in the United States with concomitant increased health care costs. In the 1970s, federal funding policies changed from paying billed charges to *prospective payment systems* in which rates were predetermined based on diagnostic-related categories (Tax Equity and Fiscal Responsibility Act [TEFRA], 1983). In the 1990s, costs increased in other sectors as patients were moved out of acute care into different parts of the continuum. This in turn prompted managed care pricing approaches to cover inpatient rehabilitation, skilled nursing, home care, outpatient services. Thus, each venue had its own patient assessment instrument, case-mix adjusters, documentation system, and payment rules. Occupational therapy services can be seen fitting within each of these shifts.

In the 2000s, U.S. governmental policies started to shift again by focusing on managing patient care starting from community-based services and then to acute care, recovery, and postacute care. The intent is to use dollars for a more seamless and cost-efficient continuum of care. Future health care initiatives will continue to explore value and determine solutions that will include redesigning the continuum of care to address and meet the value, quality, cost, and care. Occupational therapy will continue to both be influenced by and influence these systems.

---

difficulty performing daily life habits and activities and participating in social roles within their homes and communities (World Health Organization [WHO], 2001).

As part of the OT process, practitioners collaborate with clients and their caregivers to identify goals that will influence the intervention plan and subsequent delivery of services to support the individual's optimal functioning, recovery, and desired outcomes (see Chapters 27, 28, and 37). In addition to the client's goals, the evaluation process ideally encompasses a biopsychosocial perspective, addressing safety, client factors, occupational performance, social support, and environmental contexts. In doing so, analysis of client functioning for areas of occupation, activities of daily living (ADL), instrumental activities of daily living (IADL), education, work, play and leisure, rest and sleep, and social participation is assessed throughout the various settings within the continuum of care (American Occupational Therapy Association [AOTA], 2014) (see Unit XI).

Types of Facilities

Hospitals are the largest employer of OT practitioners with more than 114,600 occupational therapists in the United States (Bureau of Labor Statistics, 2015). Various levels of care may be available at an individual hospital, including **acute care**, **long-term acute care**, **inpatient rehabilitation**, and **outpatient rehabilitation**. Schools and **long-term care/skilled nursing facilities** also provide a substantial percentage of job opportunities within the field (AOTA, 2015). Administratively, facilities may be for-profit, not-for-profit, or governmental. Hospital-based health care is a labor-intensive industry operating on a 24-hour-per-day, 7-day-per-week basis, facing complex issues related to finances, workforce, and information technology (American Hospital Association, 2017a, 2017b). Additionally, employment for occupational therapists is projected to increase by 27% from 2014 to 2024 (Bureau of Labor Statistics, 2015).

Once a client's condition is medically stable or in the case that inpatient medical services are not needed or indicated, OT practitioners also work in freestanding outpatient/ambulatory care services, **community agencies**, **private practices**, and home-based services, such as **early intervention** and **home health care**. Community-based settings often afford practitioners the opportunity to work in the client's natural environment, such as home or school, and to focus on authentic occupation, in comparison to the focus on medical stabilization as the priority for inpatient settings.

TABLE 62-1	**Practice Settings**				
Setting	Requirements for Admission to Setting	Typical Setting	Typical Services	Type of Occupational Therapy	Role of Occupational Therapy Service	Legislation and Funding/Payment
Acute medical/ surgical care	• Need for medical or surgical diagnosis or intervention • Admitted from emergency room, direct admission, or transfer from another facility	• Private hospital • Community hospital • Academic hospital • Veteran's Administration hospital • Specialty hospital	• Trauma services • ICU • Monitored unit • Medical services • Surgical services • Consultations by allied health care providers	• Direct • Consultation	• Occupational therapy role for trauma services and ICU may be direct or consultation including positioning, range of motion, splinting/casting, early mobilization, and ADL. • Occupational therapy role for monitored, medical, and surgical services may be direct or consultation including safety assessment, assessment of client's abilities, roles, habits, and routines; and functional skills such as eating/dysphagia, grooming, dressing, bathing, and toileting • Recommendations for continued services at next level of care • Discharge planning	• Prospective payment system • Private insurance or self-pay • Managed care (PPO or HMO) • Indemnity • Workers' compensation • Medicare • Medicaid • Unfunded
Inpatient rehabilitation	• Transfer from a hospital, nursing home, or home • 60% of clients must have a diagnosis within Centers for Medicare & Medicaid Services (CMS) 13 diagnostic groups.[a] • Must be able to tolerate intensive therapy for a minimum of 3 h of therapy for 5 out of 7 d • Must require active and ongoing intervention of multiple therapies, one of which must be physical therapy or occupational therapy • Must actively participate in and benefit from an intensive therapy program • Patient is stable at time of admission. • Requires supervision by a rehabilitation physician, with face-to-face visits at least three times per week	• Freestanding rehabilitation center • Unit within hospital • Veteran's Administration rehabilitation unit	• Rehabilitation physician • Rehabilitation nursing • Physical therapy • Occupational therapy • Speech-language pathology • Recreational therapy • Neuropsychology or psychology • Social services • Respiratory therapy • Dietary • Pharmacy • Other services by consultation	• Direct	• Comprehensive evaluation • Participation in functional outcomes such as the Inpatient Rehabilitation Facility-Patient Assessment Instrument (IRF-PAI) • Self-care skills • Functional mobility • Functional communication • Social cognition • IADL • Community reintegration • Discharge planning • Recommendations for continued services (e.g., driving evaluation) at the next level of care	• Prospective payment system • Private insurance or self-pay • Managed care (PPO or HMO) • Indemnity • Workers' compensation • Medicare • Medicaid • Unfunded

Level of care	Characteristics	Setting	Personnel	Type of service	Treatment focus	Reimbursement
(continued from previous page)					• Therapy treatments must begin within 36 h of admission. • Therapy to be provided in 1:1 treatment sessions; group therapies are to be used as an adjunct. • Must include progress toward rehabilitation goals, problems, or barriers to discharge and any changes in rehabilitation goals or treatment plan • Interdisciplinary weekly team conferences directed by the rehabilitation physician	
Skilled nursing/transitional care	• Require 24-h care for either a short or extended period of time • Bridge the gap with another level of care • Admitted from acute care hospital • Skilled intervention such as intravenous medication, wound care, and so forth • Disability with new functional deficit	• Unit in a hospital • Freestanding nursing home	• Physician • Nursing • Social services • Activity therapy • Physical therapy • Occupational therapy • Speech-language pathology • Other services by consultation	• Direct • Consultation	• Short-term care is more intensive with specified frequency. • Long term care is by consultation. • Self-care skills such as eating/dysphagia, grooming, upper and lower body dressing, bathing, and toileting • Mobility skills during ADL such as bed, chair, and wheelchair transfers; toilet and tub/shower transfers; and locomotion activities • IADL and community skills such as car transfers, homemaking activities, public dining, care of pets, and so forth	• Prospective payment system • Private insurance or self-pay • Managed care (PPO or HMO) • Indemnity • Workers' compensation • Medicare • Medicaid • Unfunded
Outpatient rehabilitation	• Medical/surgical diagnosis with functional limitation that interferes with abilities to participate in activities and roles • Admitted from a variety of places, including institutional care or home	• Part of a freestanding rehabilitation center • Within a hospital • Within the Veteran's Administration hospital • Satellite clinic (affiliated with a health care institution) • Independent, privately owned clinic	• Physician referral • Self-referral for self-pay services	• Direct	• Self-care skills such as eating/dysphagia, grooming, upper and lower body dressing, bathing, and toileting • Mobility skills during ADL such as bed, chair, and wheelchair transfers; toilet and tub/shower transfers; and locomotion activities • IADL skills • Social participation such as student, worker, and caregiver roles	• Prospective payment system • Private insurance or self-pay • Managed care (PPO or HMO) • Indemnity • Workers' compensation • Medicare • Medicaid • Unfunded

(continues)

TABLE 62-1   Practice Settings (continued)

Setting	Requirements for Admission to Setting	Typical Setting	Typical Services	Type of Occupational Therapy	Role of Occupational Therapy Service	Legislation and Funding/Payment
Inpatient psychiatry	• Require 24-h care for either a short or extended period of time • Need for psychiatric diagnosis or intervention • Admitted from the emergency room • Direct admit • Transfer from another facility • Person requires 24-h monitoring for safety • May be court ordered as in the case of forensic cases in which clients require secured (locked) units due to safety risk to self or others	• Freestanding hospital • Private hospital • Unit within hospital • State hospital • Veteran's Administration hospital	• Psychiatry • Psychology • Nursing • Mental health workers • Social services • Occupational therapy • Recreational therapy • Art therapy • Expressive or music therapy • Behavior management • Other services by consultation	• Direct • Consultation	• Assessment of client's abilities, roles, habits, and routines • Safety assessment • Recommendations for continued services at next level of care • Discharge planning • Individual and/or group treatment • Functional skills such as self-care, home, and community function • Reinforce behavioral or therapeutic plan	• Private insurance • Self-pay • Medicare • Medicaid • SSI • Unfunded
Partial hospitalization	• Require episodic focused psychiatric intervention • Transition from inpatient or as an alternative to acute psychiatric hospitalization • Structured program	• Freestanding hospital • Private hospital • Unit within hospital • State hospital • Veteran's Administration hospital	• Psychiatry • Psychology • Nursing • Mental health workers • Social services • Occupational therapy • Recreational therapy	• Direct • Consultation	• Assessment of client's abilities, roles, habits, and routines • Continuity of care for self-management goals with emphasis on productive living for home, community, and work • Individual and/or group treatment • Recommendations for continued services at next level of care	• Private insurance • Self-pay • Medicare • Medicaid • SSI • Unfunded
Long-term care (physical and mental health)	• Require 24-h care for an indefinite period of time • When functional recovery may not be possible • Lack of resources to be safe at home • Transfer from a hospital, nursing home, or home • Bridge gap between inpatient setting and home versus determine need for permanent placement	• Freestanding hospital • Private hospital • State hospital • Veteran's Administration hospital • Freestanding nursing home • Private nursing home • Custodial care such as eating/dysphagia, grooming, and bathing	• Physician/psychiatrists • Nursing • Mental health workers • Therapy consultation as indicated for safety, assessment, self-care skills and routines, positioning, functional mobility during ADL, adaptations, and caregiver training	• Direct • Consultation	• Individual assessment and interventions as indicated • Consultant to program for ADL, environmental adaptations, and behavior management	• Medicare Part B • Medicaid • Private insurance or self-pay supplement

	Eligibility	Settings	Providers	Service Delivery	Services	Funding
Hospice	• Eligible for Medicare Part A • Physician and hospice medical director certify terminal illness, and the patient has 6 mo or less to live if illness runs normal course. • Sign statement choosing hospice care instead of other Medicare-covered benefits to treatment of terminal illness • Care from Medicare-approved hospice program	• Short-term inpatient care • Short-term respite care • Home	• Physician • Nursing • Counselors • Social services • Occupational therapy • Physical therapy • Speech-language pathology • Hospice aides • Homemakers • Volunteers • Dietitian • Grief and loss counseling	• Direct • Consultation	• Assessment (living skills, work, leisure) • Home visits, environmental changes • Provision of aids and adaptations • Training in the use of equipment • Work simplification • Energy conservation, time management • Group activities • Group therapy (touch, role-play psychodrama) • Education in coping with change (patient and family) • Relaxation and stress management • Therapeutic activities (arts, crafts, poetry, music) • Reminiscence therapy	• Medicare
Early intervention	• Developmental delay in one or more area of development or has diagnosis likely to result in developmental delay • Identified disability or condition or be at risk for developing a disability • Demonstrate atypical behaviors • Circumstances that place child and/or parent that places the child at risk for developmental delay • Each state has its own specific eligibility criteria.	• Home • Hospital • Clinic • Child care	• Physician • Occupational therapy • Focus on family-centered model for service delivery	• Direct • Consultation	• Services to promote development • Promotion of parent–child interaction, ADL especially feeding, and play skills • Sensorimotor development • Gross motor skills • Fine motor skills • Self–help skills • Social-emotional development	• Individuals with Disabilities Education Act (IDEA) • Private insurance • Medicaid
Preschool	• Children who are 3 years and older (until enter elementary school) • Fit one of the categories under IDEA	• Public school setting • Childcare • Preschool setting	• Occupational therapy • Preschool teacher	• Direct • Consultation	• Carrying out or suggesting activities that promote the child's overall development and ability to fully participate in preschool activities • Sensorimotor development • Gross motor skills • Fine motor skills • Social-emotional development	• IDEA • Private insurance • Medicaid

(continues)

TABLE 62-1 **Practice Settings** (continued)

Setting	Requirements for Admission to Setting	Typical Setting	Typical Services	Type of Occupational Therapy	Role of Occupational Therapy Service	Legislation and Funding/Payment
School	• Identified disability that fits one of the categories under IDEA • All eligibility and service decision is made by a student's individual educational program.	• Public school • Private school	• Occupational therapy • School teacher	• Direct • Consultation • Supportive service	• Supports student's education program and ability to fully participate in school activities including recess • Organizing the student's daily schedule and materials • Negotiating cafeteria • At the point of planning for transition out of the school system, focus broadens to include independent living and community participation.	• IDEA • Private insurance • Medicaid • No Child Left Behind legislation
Private practice	• Children of all ages • Decreased performance in daily tasks or desired activities	• Private clinic	• Occupational therapy	• Direct • Consultation	• Addressing the child's needs that may not be met at school • Focus on body functions such as sensory processing, motor planning, and visual perception that provide foundation skills needed in school, ADL, and play	• Private insurance • Medicaid • Federal grants • Private pay
Adult day services (social, medical, dementia)	• Provide social/medical programming to increase the quality of life and health status of participants • Social: day programs to provide social/recreational activities, meals, and some health supports • Medical: provides rehabilitation and medical services to provide sufficient supports to forestall nursing home placement • Dementia: programs designed to focus on providing programming with cognitive supports that improve the quality of life	• Freestanding • Associated with other community programs or health agencies such as senior centers, mental health centers, rehabilitation centers, nursing homes, or hospitals	• Personnel from adult day services • Occupational therapy • Physical therapy • Speech-language pathology	• Direct • Consultation	• Assistance with modifying and adapting activity programming for social, medical, and dementia programs • Assessment of ADL, IADL, safety, cognition, and so forth • Educational services to staff and family members regarding ADL, IADL, safety, fall prevention, and so forth	• Federal, state, county, city, or town budgets • Funded through churches or other charitable organizations • Medicaid • Long-term care policies • Scholarships • Sliding fees

Setting	Description	Location	Personnel	Mode	Examples of services	Payment
Assisted living	• Residential care for elders who can no longer live independently but do not require medical services of a nursing home • Provides supportive care that enhances autonomy and choice • Provides supervision and support for ADL, IADL, safety, and so forth caused by dementia, neurological impairment, or other medical problems • Provides activity programming to foster social engagement and participation	• Assisted living facilities	• Personnel from assisted living • Occupational therapy • Physical therapy • Speech-language pathology	• Direct • Consultation	• Consultation to ensure that program engages residents in occupations of their choice and assist facility personnel to modify the physical/social environment to promote safety and independence • Direct services including evaluation and intervention to increase independence in ADL and IADL, prevent falls, and enhance participation in social activities • Education or direct service regarding issues related to aging, occupation, and health promotion	• Private pay • Medicare and Medicaid for people with dementia • Long-term insurance
Community mental health programs	• Provide ongoing support and structure to people who have mental health diagnoses to live in the community by promoting daily routine and sense of belonging to the program community and community at large • Participants may come and go based on program interests.	• Freestanding • Community health facility	• Personnel from community mental health programs • Occupational therapy • Social services • Recreational therapists • Art therapists • Dance movement therapists	• Direct • Consultation	• Establish or restore performance skills or work, self-care, and leisure including coping strategies, interpersonal skills, time management, and decision making • Strategies to support participants' behavior and ability to cope with challenges in social environments and adapt tasks for participant success	• State money • Medicaid
Group homes	• Adults with chronic mental or medical illness, cognitive dysfunction, or developmental disabilities who require 24-h residential care • Foster development of social networks	• Residential facilities designed to create support, structure, and stability in a homelike setting	• Personnel from group home • Occupational therapy	• Direct • Consultation	• Behavioral management techniques • Development of social and recreational programs in the home • Facilitate independence in ADL and IADL by establishing performance patterns or modifying environment or activity demands • Evaluation to identify skills and develop behavioral plans and involvement in social, recreational, and work-related injuries	• State money • Medicaid

(continues)

TABLE 62-1   Practice Settings *(continued)*

Setting	Requirements for Admission to Setting	Typical Setting	Typical Services	Type of Occupational Therapy	Role of Occupational Therapy Service	Legislation and Funding/Payment
Sheltered workshops and vocational training	• Provide support to workers as they perform work tasks such as parts assembly, packing, sorting, and so forth; workers paid at percent of work output based on their performance in relation to typical work performance • Provide social opportunities for workers during the day and after work hours • Goal setting and supports for transition to supported or independent employment in the community	• Freestanding facility	• Personnel from sheltered workshops and vocational training • Occupational therapy	• Direct • Consultation	• Evaluate workers' performance skills to match the activity demands of various possible jobs • Consultants to others to modify the work environment or activity demands for more efficient performance • Establish performance patterns and new performance skills • Maintain performance skills that workers have acquired	• Revenue from contracting company for which being done • State funding • Grants from nonprofit agencies
Supported employment	• Provide supported employment for people with severe chronic mental illness, mental retardation, learning disabilities, traumatic brain injury, and other severe disabilities who desire to work but have disabilities sufficient to preclude employment in traditional settings without ongoing support to perform job	• Work environments in the community	• Personnel from supported employment • Occupational therapy	• Direct • Consultation	• Consultation with worksites to ensure integration of the employee and to provide education regarding adaptation to worksite environment and activity demands • Direct services in the role of job coach to assist the employee to adapt to the worksite and to function effectively by learning job skills and interacting appropriately with other employees at worksite • Involved in matching prospective worker to potential worksites	• Vocational rehabilitation through state funding • Vocational rehabilitation through private funding

Work-related programs	• Serve people with acquired disability who require rehabilitation to return to workforce either on job or new one	• Freestanding • Part of other facilities such as hospital, rehabilitation center, or community program	• Employment specialists • Occupational therapy • Physical therapy • Certified vocational evaluation	• Direct • Consultation	• Provide rehabilitation services to enable the client to return to work • Evaluation of work tolerance • Development of work-related skills primarily using purposeful activities such as work simulation and preparatory methods such as work conditioning, work hardening, and exercise programs • Modification of job demands when necessary and possible to better match the current skills	• Vocational rehabilitation • Workers' compensation • Income from litigation • Private insurance

[a]These include (1) stroke; (2) spinal cord injury; (3) congenital deformity; (4) amputation; (5) major multiple trauma; (6) fracture of femur; (7) brain injury; (8) neurological disorders; (9) burns; (10) active polyarticular rheumatoid arthritis, psoriatic arthritis, and seronegative arthropathies; (11) systematic vasculitides with joint inflammation; (12) severe or advanced osteoarthritis; and (13) knee or hip replacement if one of the following conditions are met: (1) Patient underwent bilateral knee or bilateral hip joint replacement surgery immediately preceding the IRF admission, (2) patient is extremely obese with a body mass index of at least 50 at the time of admission to the IRF, and (3) patient is age 85 years or older at the time of the admission to the IRF.

ICU, intensive care unit; ADL, activities of daily living; PPO, preferred provider organization; HMO, health maintenance organization; IADL, instrumental activities of daily living; SSI, supplemental security income.

Data from Centers for Medicare & Medicaid Services. (2017a). *Medicare benefit policy manual: Chapter 1—inpatient hospital services cover under Part A.* Retrieved from http://www.cms.hhs/gov/manuals /downloads/bp102c13.pdf; Centers for Medicare & Medicaid Services. (2017b). *Medical hospice benefits.* Retrieved from http://www.medicare.gov/Publications/Pubs/pdf/02154.pdf; and Centers for Medicare & Medicaid Services. (2018). *MDS 3.0 RAI manual.* Retrieved from https://www.cms.gov/Medicare/Quality-Initiatives-Patient-Assessment-Instruments/NursinghomeQualityInits/MDS30RAIManual.html.

Dependent on the client's needs, an individual may receive OT services in different types of settings within the **continuum of care**, spanning **emergency**/acute care, inpatient and outpatient rehabilitation, skilled nursing and/or extended care, **partial hospital** or **day programs**, community-based services, home care, and/or **hospice**. Balancing clients' needs, resources, personal factors, and occupational performance in consideration of their future goals also involves review and use of the best available evidence. This complex decision-making process requires practitioners to use their professional reasoning to make appropriate and meaningful recommendations to support and facilitate a client's progression through the continuum of care (see Chapter 34). Individual personal factors and levels of occupational performance, along with the contexts and environments in which one participates, greatly influence the options for discharge both between the levels of care and toward a final discharge disposition, ultimately enabling the client to be in a residential or home context. In a recent health policy study, OT was found to be the only spending category where additional spending has statistically significant association with lower readmission rates for heart failure, pneumonia, and acute myocardial infarction. The study noted that OT places a unique and immediate focus on patients' functional and social needs which are important indicators to address. It was noted that this spending category (OT) affects both the clinical and social determinants of health and that investment in OT in the acute care setting has the potential to improve quality of care without significantly increasing overall hospital spending (Rogers, Bai, Lavin, & Anderson, 2016). In another study involving OT in the community, it was found that a structured Community Aging in Place, Advancing Better Living for Elders (CAPABLE) program was associated with improved physical functioning including improving from four to two difficulties with ADL could enable the person to continue living at home instead of having to move to assisted living or institution (Szanton, Leff, Wolff, Roberts, & Gitlin, 2016). These client dimensions of care intersect with legislative and funding/payment parameters to determine a client's eligibility for the frequency and duration of receiving OT services (see Table 62-1).

Continuum of Care Vignettes

The following vignettes illustrate examples of typical levels of the continuum of care as relevant to an individual's occupational profile, performance, needs, and goals.

Physical Disabilities: Adult with Cerebral Vascular Accident

Jack is a mid–70-year-old male who had a sudden onset of right-sided weakness as well as aphasia at 10 p.m. Jack's wife immediately drove him to the local hospital, which had a certified stroke center. Within an hour of the onset of symptoms, he was assessed by the triage nurse and emergency room physician who consulted the neurologist on call. Jack was taken to imaging for a computed tomography (CT) scan, which showed no evidence of hemorrhage and a left middle cerebral artery infarct. The neurologist determined that Jack was a candidate for tissue plasminogen activator (tPA). Tissue plasminogen activator, if provided within an established time frame, can significantly reduce the effects of stroke and permanent disability. Jack was transferred to the neurointensive care unit where he was continuously monitored.

Occupational therapy was consulted in the neurointensive care unit. The occupational therapist performed an evaluation using an occupational profile to learn of Jack's active lifestyle prior to admission to the hospital. Jack lived with his wife in a one-story home with five steps to enter. Jack is a retired lawyer. He is active with guest lecturing at a local law school and in volunteering at the animal shelter in his community. Jack loves to cook for his wife, two children, and four grandchildren. Additionally, Jack enjoyed driving, going to the theater, and dining at restaurants at least two times per week. Jack's goals are to be able to return to his previous active lifestyle, especially being able to cook for his family.

Jack's past medical history is significant for coronary artery disease, osteoarthritis, and borderline renal insufficiency. The OT assessment revealed right hemiparesis and expressive aphasia, resulting in activity limitations in daily activities requiring maximum assistance for eating, grooming, dressing, bathing, toileting, and mobility. Jack is dependent on others to perform IADL. Occupational therapy started in the intensive care unit and continued on the acute stroke floor, with the focus on improving Jack's participation in daily activities and functional mobility. It was determined that Jack met admission criteria for inpatient rehabilitation (see Table 62-1) based on the diagnosis of stroke and functional limitations. Jack required intervention from multiple therapies, including physical therapy (PT), OT, and speech-language pathology (SLP). During his acute care hospitalization, Jack was actively participating in therapies (PT, OT, and SLP). After 4 days in the acute hospital, Jack was admitted to the inpatient rehabilitation unit with the focus on restoration of function for eventual return to home with his wife.

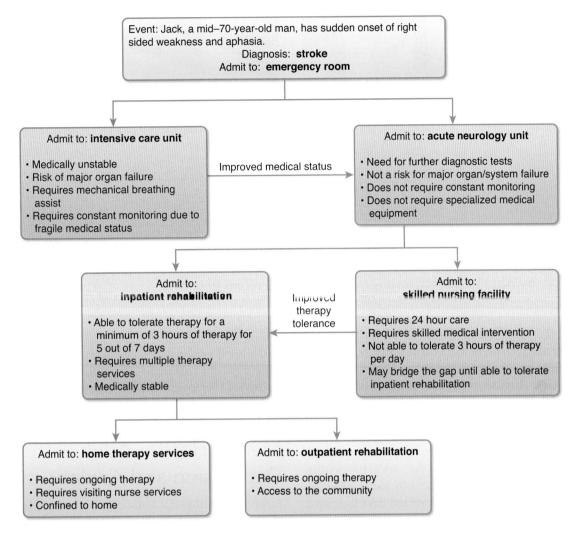

Event: Jack, a mid–70-year-old man, has sudden onset of right sided weakness and aphasia.
Diagnosis: **stroke**
Admit to: **emergency room**

Admit to: **intensive care unit**

• Medically unstable
• Risk of major organ failure
• Requires mechanical breathing assist
• Requires constant monitoring due to fragile medical status

Improved medical status

Admit to: **acute neurology unit**

• Need for further diagnostic tests
• Not a risk for major organ/system failure
• Does not require constant monitoring
• Does not require specialized medical equipment

Admit to: **inpatient rehabilitation**

• Able to tolerate therapy for a minimum of 3 hours of therapy for 5 out of 7 days
• Requires multiple therapy services
• Medically stable

Improved therapy tolerance

Admit to: **skilled nursing facility**

• Requires 24 hour care
• Requires skilled medical intervention
• Not able to tolerate 3 hours of therapy per day
• May bridge the gap until able to tolerate inpatient rehabilitation

Admit to: **home therapy services**

• Requires ongoing therapy
• Requires visiting nurse services
• Confined to home

Admit to: **outpatient rehabilitation**

• Requires ongoing therapy
• Access to the community

FIGURE 62-1 Example of transitioning through the continuum of care.

The OT practitioner performed an evaluation, including the Functional Independence Measure (FIM™) (Hamilton, Granger, Sherwin, Zielezny, & Tashman, 1987) and the Canadian Occupational Performance Measure (COPM) (Law et al., 2014), which revealed that Jack's goals were to be independent in self-care, cooking, and, eventually, to return to his community activities. Within the first week, the interprofessional team had a team conference that included Jack and his wife, discussing Jack's functional status, barriers, and goals. This collaboration provided the foundation for the interprofessional treatment plan with focus on Jack's goals to increase his independence for self-care, functional mobility, and IADL. Jack demonstrated significant improvement throughout his inpatient stay and was able to perform his daily activities with minimal assistance and cook simple meals with moderate assistance. He was able to eat a regular diet; however, he required assistance with cutting his food.

Discharge planning included an evaluation of the home environment, ordering of durable medical equipment, and provision of referrals for community resources and support groups. After discharge, Jack plans to continue his therapy at home with home health services until he is no longer homebound, when he will then plan to transition to outpatient rehabilitation to support his goals of increased independence for home and community reintegration, including eventual return to driving. See Figures 62-1 and 62-2.

Physical Disability: Adult with Total Hip Replacement

Marion is an early 90-year-old Asian female who has severe osteoarthritis. Prior to the hospitalization, Marion was having increasing pain in her right hip, which was

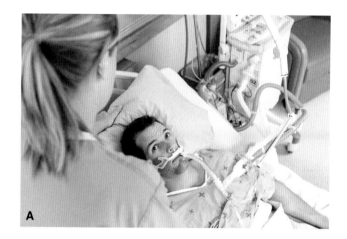

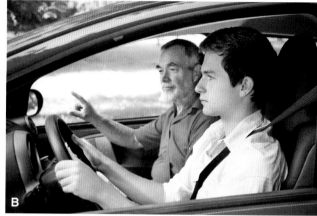

FIGURE 62-2 Occupational therapy practitioners work with clients throughout the continuum. **A.** In severe cases, we may first start to interact as part of early mobilization intensive care unit teams. **B.** Our role may continue all the way through community reentry including return to driving.

limiting her ability to perform her daily activities including walking. She had an elective right total hip arthroplasty. The orthopedic surgeon ordered postsurgery precautions with toe-touch weight bearing on the right lower extremity. Marion's past medical history was significant for hypertension and congestive heart failure, which were controlled with medications. Prior to admission, Marion lived alone in an assisted living community. She was active within this community, participating in the daily social activities. Marion has three sons who are grown and have their own families and do not live locally.

One day after surgery, the acute care occupational therapist was consulted. The occupational profile revealed that Marion's goal was to eventually return to her assisted living residential community. Upon evaluation, Marion required maximum assistance for functional mobility using a walker and for lower body activities of daily living. Marion also had pain and intermittent confusion since surgery, which limited her ability to participate in therapy. It was determined that Marion would continue her rehabilitation at the local skilled nursing facility because she required skilled intervention but did not require an intensive therapy program of 3 hours daily.

The OT practitioner performed the facility's initial evaluation including the Minimum Data Set (Centers for Medicare & Medicaid Services, 2018) and the COPM (Law et al., 2014). The COPM revealed Marion's desire to be independent in self-care and to return to her assisted living community. Intervention at the skilled nursing facility focused on self-care and functional mobility retraining. Within 20 days, Marion was independent in self-care except for minimal assistance for seated bathing in the shower and functional mobility using a front-wheeled walker. The OT practitioner provided caregiver training

to the hired personal care attendant, ordered appropriate equipment for bathroom adaptations, and arranged for continued therapy in Marion's assisted living community to support her optimal recovery.

Mental Health: Adult with Depression and Anxiety

Sarah is a multiracial female in her early 30s who has experienced a history of minor depression and anxiety beginning when she was in college. Initially, her symptoms were most noticeable at the end of the semester, stemming from the pressures of final examinations and erratic study habits, resulting in irregular sleep patterns. Typically, Sarah managed her symptoms through social drinking of alcohol and partying with friends, sometimes binge drinking. On a few occasions, Sarah sought out behavioral health counseling services offered by the university when she faced trouble focusing her attention or feeling panicky. With her parents living abroad, Sarah has relied heavily on classmates and coworkers for her social support. After college graduation, she met her husband-to-be at an after-work social gathering featuring alcoholic drinks and dancing.

Soon after, they were married and immediately started to try to build a family. However, after 2 years of having difficulty getting pregnant, Sarah sought infertility treatments while struggling with feelings of failure and emotional insecurity about the lack of control. Increasing stress and distractions about her infertility treatments started to affect Sarah's job performance. Ultimately, she was laid off when her company was downsizing personnel, and she found herself increasingly distressed, ruminating on her feelings of failure, both personally and professionally. Although she subsequently became pregnant several times, she experienced multiple miscarriages. Consequently, Sarah's emotional condition escalated and she was hospitalized to treat major depression. This hospitalization was precipitated by Sarah experiencing many of the following symptoms nearly every day for at least 2 weeks: feeling sad or empty most of the day (depressed mood), significant loss of interest or pleasure in activities that used to be enjoyable, significant weight gain, fatigue, poor concentration and slowing down of thoughts, sleeping too much, and feelings of worthlessness and guilt that are related to thoughts about death or suicide. After a few days in the hospital and a new medication regimen, Sarah was discharged to home. She felt isolated and alone, whereas her husband was at work and started to drink alcohol during the day, with her husband often finding her still in her pajamas and intoxicated when he got home from work. Her alcohol abuse further compromised her ability to cope with her feelings of depression and anxiety, impacting her ability to consistently perform basic self-care and home management daily activities. Frustrated with Sarah's debilitating symptoms, her marital relationship became significantly strained and her husband moved out of their apartment, asking for a separation and possibly a divorce.

Struggling to manage her symptoms, this change in her marital relationship triggered Sarah's contemplation of suicide. Consequently, Sarah sought voluntary readmission to an inpatient psychiatric hospital unit to treat her **dual diagnosis** of major depression and alcohol abuse. This hospitalization addressed adjustment of her medications, along with Sarah's participation in an OT evaluation and group interventions focusing on the use of **cognitive behavioral therapy** coping strategies (Ellis, 1992) (see Chapters 28 and 38). Sarah's goals are to be able to more effectively cope with and manage her symptoms; to regain her ability to productively engage in basic self-care, home management, and exploration of job search opportunities; and to work on her marital relationship. After a week, Sarah was discharged from the hospital and referred to a partial hospital program to participate in a structured program to support her continued work toward meeting her goals.

Partial hospital programs extend care and serve as a transition from inpatient hospitalization. This level of care enables occupational therapists to support clients' goals for instrumental activities of daily living, work, and social participation. Sarah was a candidate to participate in this type of program based on her motivation to gain coping skills to manage her symptoms and to reengage in her daily routine, including explorations of marital reconciliation and potential to work. Initially, Sarah participated in the program for 5 days each week for a month, then tapered to

3 days a week. She took initiative to explore community resources to build a support network and to begin to volunteer in order to transition into a workplace context, taking steps toward her longer term goal of paid employment. Identifying vocational skills necessary to reenter the workforce became a focus of Sarah's rehabilitation program and volunteer experience. This skill set capitalized on her work experience and included practicing communication skills to foster effective peer and supervisory relationships, sustaining concentration and using problem-solving skills, and regaining confidence and self-reliance for beginning a job search.

Pediatrics: Child with Traumatic Brain Injury, Orthopedic Fracture, and Amputation

Joshua is a sixth-grade African American male who experienced a traumatic brain injury along with multiple fractures and a severe crush injury as a result of being hit by a truck when riding his bike home after a soccer game. Unconscious at the scene of the accident, emergency medical personnel transported Joshua to the nearest Children's Hospital Emergency Services via medic flight. Joshua underwent extensive orthopedic surgery to stabilize his left humeral fracture with an open reduction internal fixation (ORIF) and to amputate his right lower extremity below the knee due to the severe nature of his ankle and foot crush injury. Following surgery, Joshua was treated in the hospital's pediatric intensive care unit (PICU) to closely monitor his status while in a comatose state for 5 days. In the PICU, occupational therapist performed an initial evaluation and found that Joshua responded to localized stimuli before he eventually emerged from the coma. At first signs of consciousness, Joshua was sluggish and complained of feeling tired. He was disoriented, not knowing where he was or what had happened—common symptoms of posttraumatic amnesia.

After a week, Joshua became emotionally agitated, trying to get out of the hospital bed and repeatedly yelling, "It hurts . . . I want to go home!" After a few days, Joshua's confusion and agitation started to subside, and he began to more cooperatively participate in all of his nursing care and therapy sessions. This medical stabilization enabled transfer from the PICU to the hospital's pediatric unit and, eventually, to the inpatient rehabilitation unit. Once in rehabilitation, the OT practitioner worked closely with his mother and the nursing staff to engage Joshua in participating in his basic self-care such as eating, brushing his teeth, and dressing his upper and lower body. Nursing, OT, and PT provided collaborative interventions to assist Joshua with his functional mobility in getting in and out of bed, building up his sitting tolerance, and toileting and bathing with adaptive equipment and assistance. Joshua tended to be impulsive and impatient with the extra time and effort required for getting from one place to another, requiring step-by-step verbal cueing and moderate physical assistance to support his safety. Joshua used a wheelchair and practiced standing pivot functional transfers using his left leg for weight bearing. Therapy involved teaching Joshua and his mother important safety precautions to prevent falls and to adhere to his orthopedic precautions. Another aspect of care that was addressed during inpatient rehabilitation was coordination with Joshua's school. The interprofessional team obtained Joshua's school records, and they were able to address skills necessary for eventual return to school. These skills included improving attention and concentration as well as other executive functioning activities. After 2 weeks in inpatient rehabilitation, Joshua was discharged to home, having progressed to needing only minimal assistance from his mother or nursing staff for his basic self-care and functional transfers. The left distal humerus ORIF was still healing, and he was using a wheelchair for functional mobility until his right lower extremity prosthetic training progressed.

Initially, Joshua received home care OT and PT to ensure a safe transition to home. However, once the left upper extremity ORIF was fully healed, Joshua started outpatient OT and PT 3 days a week with his mother driving him to the hospital. Joshua's goals focused on "being able to do what I did before," requiring the support of the health care team and his mother to help him accept that he will need to find some new ways to do things after his accident. Because his accident was in the summer, Joshua will be returning to his middle school. Joshua's mother is very concerned about him going back to school and being frustrated with the challenges that he will face, especially ambulating with his new prosthesis and crutches while using a backpack. Although the neuropsychological testing in the hospital revealed Joshua's performance to be at the low end of normal for his age, it is unknown to what extent his cognitive deficits as a result of his traumatic brain injury might pose to his academic performance in returning to school. Therefore, Joshua's outpatient rehabilitation program focused on transition to school-based OT (see Chapter 51). The school-based therapists (PT, OT, SLP, and neuropsychology) collaborated with the outpatient rehabilitation therapists to determine the skills and adaptations that would be necessary in order to have a smooth transition back to school in the fall. The individualized learning plan (IEP) identifies aspects of continued care in the school system for participation in adaptive physical education and other identified strategies for taking notes and test taking since Joshua's brain injury. Coping and adaptation to disability within the educational setting is another transitional aspect that will need to be addressed through individual therapy and/or participation in a support group.

Emerging Practice

Emerging practice is commonly viewed as expanding service delivery models and contexts, often beyond traditional medical and health services. An important guiding rationale for emerging practice has been identified as "the successful promotion of participation in occupations among individuals, groups, or communities through the development of occupational therapy services to underserved or unserved clients" (Holmes & Scaffa, 2009, p. 196). However, a common barrier for emerging practice is the lack of third-party reimbursement for populations of all ages, including, but not limited to, children and adults with chronic disabilities, those who are homeless, and at-risk elderly. Opportunities for emerging OT practice are evolving in day programs, transitional housing and employment programs, and specialized services such as low vision and ergonomics.

Some specific examples of OT's contributions in emerging areas of practice involve consultation (see Chapter 73), program development, health promotion education, and grant-funded demonstration projects. Once young adults reach the age of 21 or 22 years, most are no longer eligible for school-based special education services. For this population, parents and guardians are responsible to assume a full-time caregiving role. **Group homes** provide residential options for young adults with disabilities to transition from living with parents/guardians into the community. **Centers for independent living** provide consumer services and resources to promote independent living skills. Occupational therapists can influence the quality of life for this population by offering consultation services to group homes or centers for independent living. Such services may address making recommendations for activity adaptations and environmental modifications and training clients in self-advocacy and support staff in approaches to provide quality care.

For adults with chronic conditions such as HIV/AIDS, fibromyalgia, arthritis, chronic fatigue syndrome, multiple sclerosis, and so forth, performance of desired occupations is often experienced in conjunction with pain and/or fatigue. For these populations, occupational therapists have collaborated and partnered with professional organizations that provide consumer services, resources, and support. Development of educational self-management programs that outline strategies to control and cope with symptoms and to simplify daily activities have been enhanced by OT's unique perspective. Fall prevention programs have been developed targeting at-risk elderly populations with interventions to promote wellness through active lifestyles and healthy habits for exercise as well as to assess home safety risks and to offer assistance with home modifications. The following vignette describes an example of occupational therapy—emerging practice in the area of low vision.

Older Adults: Community-Based Adult with Low Vision

Mr. Gonzales is a Spanish-speaking male in his late 70s who immigrated to the United States from Mexico more than 40 years ago with his wife and brother. When his wife died, he relocated to a subsidized housing development for elderly individuals where he has been living for the past 10 years. Mr. Gonzales has a history of diabetes mellitus with associated visual impairment as a result of glaucoma. He does not seek regular medical care and has not had a recent ophthalmological examination. He is aware that some of his neighbors have taken advantage of free vision screenings that are offered through a grant-funded mobile van service. Mr. Gonzales has told some of his neighbors that his glasses do not work as well as they used to, and his neighbors have encouraged him to go to the mobile van for a vision screening the next time that it comes to the housing development.

Mr. Gonzales voluntarily participated in a low-vision screening that was administered by an occupational therapist with specialty certification in low-vision rehabilitation. Besides recommending and referring him to an ophthalmologist, the therapist suggested that she could also visit his apartment and help to adapt the environment for safety and improved vision. Mr. Gonzales agreed, and the therapist conducted a home safety assessment to identify risks and to recommend environmental adaptations, such as installing an overhead light in both his kitchen and bathroom.

Conclusion

Today's health care environment is ever changing and complex (Porter, 2010; Porter & Teisberg, 2006). Occupational therapy practice focuses on the client based on where they are receiving services within the service delivery continuum, other factors that may affect the client's transition and ultimate outcome are the severity of the disability as well as the client's social and financial support systems. Quality care requires interprofessional teamwork, which can be informal and/or formal. Occupational therapists have the opportunity to advocate for the client by identifying necessary transitions and resources at the next level within the continuum of care. This goal can be accomplished by collaborating with and exchanging information between providers to ensure that the client's needs and preferences for care are understood and provided. It is important for practitioners to keep in mind the client's priorities as related to satisfaction and participation in life roles. Whether transitioning from acute care or long-term care, the role of OT is to support our clients' successful reintegration into the home and community environments.

REFERENCES

American Hospital Association. (2017a). *AHA fast facts on U.S. hospitals*. Retrieved from http://www.aha.org/research/rc/stat-studies/fast-facts.shtml

American Hospital Association. (2017b). *AHA hospital statistics, 2017 edition*. Retrieved from https://ams.aha.org/eweb/DynamicPage.aspx?WebCode=ProdDetailAdd&ivd_prc_prd_key=886dfb06-826f-4258-b843-77ae9416b895

American Occupational Therapy Association. (2014). Occupational therapy practice framework: Domain and process, 3rd edition. *American Journal of Occupational Therapy, 68*, S1–S48. doi:10.5014/ajot.2014.682006

American Occupational Therapy Association. (2015). *Occupational therapy compensation and workforce study*. Retrieved from http://www.aota.org/Education-Careers/Advance-Career/Salary-Workforce-Survey.aspx

Bureau of Labor Statistics. (2015). *Occupational outlook handbook*. Washington, DC: Author. Retrieved from https://www.bls.gov/ooh/healthcare/occupational-therapists.htm

Centers for Medicare & Medicaid Services. (2017a). *Medicare benefit policy manual: Chapter 1—inpatient hospital services cover under Part A*. Retrieved from http://www.cms.hhs.gov/manuals/downloads/bp102c13.pdf

Centers for Medicare & Medicaid Services. (2017b). *Medicare hospice benefits*. Retrieved from http://www.medicare.gov/Publications/Pubs/pdf/02154.pdf

Centers for Medicare & Medicaid Services. (2018). *MDS 3.0 RAI manual*. Retrieved from https://www.cms.gov/Medicare/Quality-Initiatives-Patient-Assessment-Instruments/NursinghomeQualityInits/MDS30RAIManual.html

Ellis, A. (1992). Group rational-emotive and cognitive-behavioral therapy. *International Journal of Group Psychotherapy, 42*, 63–80.

Hamilton, B. B., Granger, C. V., Sherwin, F. S., Zielezny, M., & Tashman, J. S. (1987). A uniform national data system for medical rehabilitation. In M. J. Fuhrer (Ed.), *Rehabilitation outcomes: Analysis and measurement* (pp. 137–147). Baltimore, MD: Paul H. Brookes.

Holmes, W. M., & Scaffa, M. E. (2009). The nature of emerging practice in occupational therapy: A pilot study. *Occupational Therapy in Health Care, 23*, 189–206.

Law, M., Baptiste, S., Carswell, A., McColl, M., Polatajko, H., & Pollock, N. (2014). *Canadian Occupational Performance Measure* (5th ed.). Ottawa, Canada: Canadian Association of Occupational Therapists.

Porter, M. E. (2010). What is value in health care? *The New England Journal of Medicine, 363*, 2477–2481.

Porter, M. E., & Teisberg, E. O. (2006). *Redefining health care*. Boston, MA: Harvard Business School.

Roberts, P., & Evenson, M. E. (2009). Occupational therapy resource summaries: Practice settings. In E. B. Crepeau, E. S. Cohn, & B. A. B. Schell (Eds.), *Willard & Spackman's occupational therapy* (11th ed., pp. 1070–1083). Philadelphia, PA: Lippincott Williams & Wilkins.

Rogers, A. T., Bai, G., Lavin, R. A., & Anderson, G. F. (2016). Higher hospital spending on occupational therapy is associated with lower readmission rates. *Medical Care Research and Review, 74*, 668–686. doi:10.1177/1077558716666981

Szanton, S. L., Leff, B., Wolff, J. L., Roberts, L., & Gitlin, L. N. (2016). Home-based care program reduces disability and promotes aging in place. *Health Affairs, 35,* 1558–1563.

Tax Equity and Fiscal Responsibility Act, Pub. L. No. 97-248, 96 Stat. 324 (1983).

Upham, E. G. (1918). *Training of teachers for occupational therapy for the rehabilitation of disabled soldiers and sailor.* Washington, DC: Federal Board for Vocational Education.

Wilcock, A. (2002). *Occupation for health: V.2: A journey from prescription to self health.* London, United Kingdom: British Association and College of Occupational Therapists.

World Health Organization. (2001). *International classification of functioning, disability, and health (ICF).* Geneva, Switzerland: Author.

the**Point**® *For additional resources on the subjects discussed in this chapter, visit* **http://thePoint.lww.com /Willard-Spackman13e.** *See* **Appendix I, Resources and Evidence for Common Conditions Addressed in OT** *for more information on stroke, orthopedic conditions (joint replacements), mood disorders, traumatic brain injury and amputations, and visual impairments.*

CHAPTER 63

Providing Occupational Therapy for Individuals with Autism

Panagiotis (Panos) A. Rekoutis

LEARNING OBJECTIVES

After reading this chapter, you will be able to:

1. Differentiate the needs of different individuals with autism spectrum disorder (ASD) across different stages in their lives.
2. Outline the scope of occupational therapy practice as it relates to individuals with ASD and their families with different needs of support from childhood through adulthood.
3. Describe the role of occupational therapy evaluation and intervention as part of multidisciplinary team approaches in the field of autism.
4. Explain the daily challenges that individuals with ASD face and how those can shape different life trajectories.

Introduction

> By the time Katie was 18 months, the more manifest sign was no sounds were coming in. We were supposed to have a three-session evaluation with this notable speech therapist. Right before we went over to see her, I got a book on autism. It was like a slow death for me reading that book. Because of all the signs: the crying, the lining up of all the toys, the speech delays with her; the non-relatedness when you called her name. There was no babbling. The only thing Katie would relate to was music, and she would light up with music and maybe "Ring around the Rosy." Very few things would interest her. The worst was when you would call her name, and she would be completely unresponsive (Rekoutis, 2013, p. 144).

According to the Centers for Disease Control and Prevention (CDC, 2017b) and the Autism and Developmental Disabilities Monitoring (ADDM) Network (Christensen et al., 2016), the most recent epidemiological data show that parents and families of 1 in 68 children in the United States find themselves in the same position as Katie's mother: At some point during their child's first 3 years of life, they hear from a diagnostician (whether it is a developmental pediatrician or a neuropsychologist) that their child presents with an autism spectrum disorder (ASD). This rate of occurrence translates into more than 1% of the general population being identified (CDC, 2017a), or more than 3.5 million Americans (Buescher, Cidav, Knapp, & Mandell, 2014). The *Diagnostic and Statistical Manual of Mental Disorders* (5th ed.) (*DSM-5*) (American Psychiatric Association [APA],

TABLE 63-1	Selected Diagnostic Criteria for Autism Spectrum Disorder	
Severity	**Deficits in Social Communication and Interaction**	**Restricted, Repetitive Patterns**
Level 1 (requiring support)	• Decreased interest to interact with others • Challenges with initiating and responding to typical back-and-forth conversations (e.g., difficulty making friends)	• Challenges with demonstrating flexibility in different contexts • Daily performance is affected by difficulties with executive function skills.
Level 2 (requiring substantial support)	• Observable challenges with both verbal and nonverbal communication • Limited ability to engage in communicative exchanges (i.e., poor eye contact, use of short sentences, tendency to only talk about personal special interests)	• Inflexible adherence to routines and insistence on sameness paired with restricted/repetitive behaviors that disrupt daily function • Becoming distressed or having obvious challenges when needing to shift focus between different actions or activities
Level 3 (requiring very substantial support)	• Very limited verbal and nonverbal communication (possibly nonverbal or having few intelligible words) • Social interaction is limited to responding to direct social approaches initiated by others.	• High frequency of repetitive behaviors/motor movements • Ritualized patterns or use of objects • Change or unpredictable events can cause extreme distress and coping difficulties.

Adapted from American Psychiatric Association. (2013). *Diagnostic and statistical manual of mental disorders* (5th ed.). Arlington, VA: Author.

2013) describes the disorder as a confluence of challenges in verbal and nonverbal communication and restricted and repetitive behaviors. Such challenges appear very early in life and are present with different severity among individuals with ASD. The current classification system identifies three distinct severity levels. Each level reflects the need for varying levels and types of supports across the life course of an individual with autism, as seen in Table 63-1.

The role and contributions of occupational therapy (OT) practice for individuals with autism will be presented through the lens of two case studies that exemplify the opposite ends of the autism spectrum. Jonathan's journey is that of an individual requiring a "very substantial level of support" (Level 3), whereas Brandon is a person with autism without intellectual impairment who is classified as Level 1, requiring only some support (APA, 2013). Their struggles and victories from early childhood through late adolescence and adulthood will shed a guiding light on the challenging, but highly rewarding and fascinating, practice of OT in the field of autism.

Providing Occupational Therapy for Individuals with Autism in Early Childhood

Working with the Families

Toddlers and preschool children with autism can demonstrate deficits across all domains of daily performance. Before discussing these challenges in more detailed terms,

it is imperative to consider the children's parents and caregivers at this particular junction. Receiving the diagnosis of autism is an earth-shattering moment in any parent's life (Rekoutis, 2013). Parents may feel relief because for the first time they have a framework that can begin to explain some of their child's challenges. At the same time, parents are required to come to terms with the reality of a "disease" that cannot be cured. They have to reframe their life dreams about their child, and even more so, they need to start paving the path toward acceptance. As they start recruiting their support team, they have to advocate for and navigate through uncharted waters regarding different treatments and approaches, mandates, financial reimbursement, and scheduling. Whether they are ready or not, skillful or not, they need to become—almost overnight—effective and efficient team managers, planners, facilitators, communicators, and decision makers about things they probably have very little prior exposure to, or knowledge of, when it comes to dealing with autism. (In Chapter 11, Laura Horowitz describes this as learning that she needed to "drive the bus.") In that regard, parents of children with autism tend to identify the following as critical qualities of the therapists who interact with their children: respectfulness, consistency, openness, and willingness to collaborate, together with professional knowledge (Grindle, Kovshoff, Hastings, & Remington, 2009; MacKean, Thurston, & Scott, 2005; Rekoutis, 2013). At the very least, parents expect therapists to be "direct, yet gentle and sensitive; and optimistic, yet realistic" (Rekoutis, 2013, p. 270).

Working with the Children

Challenges with communication, social interaction, and cognitive difficulties are at the forefront of issues for children with autism. These are accompanied by preoccupation

CENTENNIAL NOTES

The Changing Views of Autism

Societal and medical/health care beliefs about autism have changed dramatically in the past 75 years. Today, we are light years away from Dr. Kanner's description of "infantile autism" (Kanner, 1943/1985) and the subsequent witch hunt of "refrigerator" parents (Bettelheim, 1967). Autism is now considered a neurodevelopmental disorder that can be triggered by genetic and environmental factors (CDC, 2017b). However, this understanding is fairly recent, and the effort to better determine autism's etiology is ongoing. The shift to identify autism as a developmental disorder instead of a psychiatric condition began in the *Diagnostic and Statistical Manual of Mental Disorders* (3rd ed.) (*DSM-III*) (APA, 1980), although public awareness and understanding remained limited (Grinker, 2007). As a clinician, it was not until the early 2000s that I was finally allowed—through the change in fourth edition of the *DSM* (*DSM-IV-R*) criteria (APA, 2000)—to alert parents of younger children under the age of 3 years about some of their children's significant traits and steer them toward seeking an early diagnosis. In the past 15 years, our understanding of the multifaceted challenges of the disorder has expanded exponentially. Consequently, these advances and developments have helped delineate and signify the important contributions of OT professionals (particularly in the area of sensory processing difficulties) in helping people with autism progress through each stage of their lives.

Beyond the domain of sensory approaches, OT practice in the field of autism addresses a wider range of needs that include social skills and communication, leisure participation and utilization of preferred interests, executive functioning skills, activities of daily living and work skills, parent self-efficacy, and coping (Koenig & Hough Williams, 2017; Kuhaneck & Watling, 2015).

The role of OT continues to be increasingly acknowledged as an integral part of the intensive and comprehensive intervention programming that is recommended for individuals with autism (Bilaver, Cushing, & Cutler, 2016; Christon, Arnold, & Myers 2015; Shattuck, Wagner, Narendorf, Sterzing, & Hensley, 2011; Turcotte, Mathew, Shea, Brusilovskiy, & Nonnemacher, 2016). As a result, qualified occupational therapists are being sought after across many clinical and educational settings. Accordingly, interest in OT research in autism has become a focused topic, and opportunities for associated funded projects are expanding in frequency and scope (American Occupational Therapy Association [AOTA], 2017; Case-Smith, Weaver, & Fristad, 2015; Schaaf, Schoen, et al., 2015; Tomlin & Swinth, 2015). As occupational therapists, we possess a unique lens for understanding the needs of individuals with autism and their families. Our strength-based perspective in developing and implementing interventions places us firmly in the forefront of the service provision system for individuals with ASD and will guide us for the decades to come (Box 63-1).

---

with specific interests, lack of flexibility, ritualistic types of behavior, and insistence on sameness. Children's ability to explore and understand the world around them is hampered by sensory processing deficits (Ben-Sasson, Soto, Martínez-Pedraza, & Carter, 2013; Schaaf, Benevides, Leiby, & Sendecki, 2015; Wigham, Rodgers, South, McConachie, & Freeston, 2015). More specifically, young children with ASD may demonstrate difficulties with how they process different types of tactile (Cascio, Lorenzi, & Baranek, 2016; Puts, Wodka, Tommerdahl, Mostofsky, & Edden, 2014; Tavassoli et al., 2016), visual (Sabatos-DeVito, Schipul, Bulluck, Belger, & Baranek, 2016), auditory (Brandwein et al., 2015; Chang et al., 2012), and proprioceptive and vestibular input (Ament et al., 2015; Hazen, Stornelli, O'Rourke, Koesterer, & McDougle, 2014). They may demonstrate very distinct sensory patterns or combinations of sensory behaviors depending on the environments they find themselves in or the demands that are placed on them. Children may demonstrate sensory over-responsivity (SOR) to sensory input (Baranek, Boyd Poe, David, & Watson, 2007) that is associated with increased

sensitivity (defensiveness), described as "a tendency to react negatively or with alarm to sensory input that is generally considered harmless or nonirritating" (Wilbarger & Wilbarger, 1991, p. 3). Surrounding environments and conditions are perceived as dangerous, and children can be fearful and anxiety ridden (Ben-Sasson et al., 2013). Some children appear as underresponsive (SUR). Often, those children appear to have challenges related to muscle tone and their responses to sensory input are usually slower, or "sluggish." For example, they may demonstrate decreased awareness of temperature or pain (Ausderau et al., 2014). Finally, children with autism may also be described as "sensory seeking" when they present with prolonged and repetitive engagement in sensory experiences that serve no function (e.g., twirling objects, observing lights, looking from the corner of their eyes). See Chapter 59 for more information on sensory processing.

Further deficits include motor coordination and motor planning delays (Green et al., 2009; Jasmin et al., 2009; Liu, 2012) that often result in challenges with the development of self-care skills, play skills, and

BOX 63-1   THERAPIST NARRATIVE—INSIGHTS TO A CLINICIAN'S APPROACH

Across the years, many different elements shape and change one's approach to treatment. The unwavering constants in my work with individuals with autism spectrum disorder (ASD) and their families have been the following three aspects: work with the family and not just the child, know what you do and why you do it, and be part of a village. The common thread and most essential part is effective communication. What may take therapists one step closer is to be direct, yet gentle and sensitive, and optimistic, yet realistic (Rekoutis, 2013).

Challenges in the ability to communicate are the defining criterion for ASDs. Combined with the complexity of other symptoms and a plethora of different therapists involved in the intervention process, the impact on family life can be very stressful, and the need for effective communication can be overwhelming. That aspect constantly ebbs and flows among parents and their children, parents and the therapists, among members of the therapeutic team, and between different agents of the multilayered health care and educational systems. Across all ages, symptoms, and severity, we are working in tandem with the families. Parents value communicative exchanges by their outcome. If deemed successful or effective, they lead to broader shared experiences and promote extended exchanges. On the contrary, when deemed as less effective or not helpful, the underlying message is discarded, the experience devalued, and future exchanges can be met with skepticism and disbelief.

As an occupational therapist, I see myself as uniquely educated and equipped to aid individuals with ASD in making useful sense of their bodies and their environment on their way to living a meaningful and happy life. Children lost within their own bodies, or uncomfortable and threatened by their surroundings, do not know how to regulate, or modulate, or achieve homeostasis for long periods of time. The goal (early on) is to help open up a window to teach skills and strategies so that they can then better negotiate their environment and increase their function. A powerful tool in that direction is finding their hidden interests and turning them into motivating strengths. As a therapist, you need to be good enough, creative enough, quick on your feet enough, and imaginative and resourceful enough to go with the child's flow and embed learning in what the child wants to do. In that regard, occupational therapists can be the ones to help them start connecting their brain to the rest of their body and begin to make sense of the world around them. That leads to being less anxious and better able to maintain socially acceptable behaviors.

Our daily interactions with individuals with ASD do not happen in isolation. More often than not, occupational therapists are parts of distinct teams (in home care, school and clinical settings, vocational and assisted living facilities). They need to be able to navigate the dynamics of those teams, clearly explain their role, and help set appropriate expectations. When successfully doing so, they can become effective advocates for the individuals they work with and their families.

meaningful engagement in age-appropriate occupations (Liu & Breslin, 2013; Lloyd, MacDonald, & Lord, 2013; Tomchek, Little, & Dunn, 2015). For these young children and their families, such issues often translate into frequent behavior and emotional overreactions and meltdowns, problems with eating, and problems with sleeping that can place significant strains on the entire family's life and routines.

Based on the child's age and needs, services can be variable in nature and intensity. Home-based and private practice/clinic instruction programs are usually organized with a primary focus on facilitating skill development across domains. Center-based programs can provide the same focus in addition to exposing children to social participation and integration opportunities (Koegel, Matos-Freden, Lang, & Koegel, 2012; Stahmer & Ingersoll, 2004). Occupational therapists find themselves working hand in hand with speech-language pathologists, special education teachers, mainstream teachers and daycare teachers, psychologists, behavior therapists, and, to a lesser degree, physical therapists and social workers. Depending on the nature of the program and the composition of the team, interventions that occupational therapists may directly or indirectly utilize can include the following: Picture Exchange Communication System (PECS™) or Prompts for Restructuring Oral Muscular Phonetic Targets (PROMPT©) systems to improve communication; classroom protocols such as Treatment and Education of Autistic and Related Communication Handicapped Children (TEACCH); play-based relationship-based therapy (Developmental Individual-difference Relationship-based model [DIR®] Floortime) (Brunner & Seung, 2009); applied behavior analysis (ABA); sensory integration approaches; sensorimotor activities and developmental interventions; strengths-based approaches (Braun, Dunn, & Tomchek, 2017; Dunst, Trivette, & Hamby, 2012; Steiner, 2011; Tomchek & Koenig, 2016), and parent-mediated interventions (PACT) (Tanner, Hand, O'Toole, & Lane, 2015). See Box 63-2 for examples of commonly used interventions, and see Chapter 59 for more information on sensory-based approaches.

BOX 63-2   EXAMPLES OF COMMONLY USED INTERVENTIONS

- Strength-based approaches: The practitioner focuses on identifying and building on the students' abilities versus focusing on their limitations or disabilities.
- Picture Exchange Communication System (PECS™): allows people with little or no communication abilities to communicate using pictures. People using PECS™ are taught to approach another person and give them a picture of a desired item in exchange for that item. By doing so, the person is able to initiate communication. A child or adult with autism can use PECS™ to communicate a request, a thought, or anything that can reasonably be displayed or symbolized on a picture card.
- Prompts for Restructuring Oral Muscular Phonetic Targets (PROMPT©): The technique is a tactile-kinesthetic approach that uses touch cues to a patient's articulators (jaw, tongue, lips) to manually guide them through a targeted word, phrase, or sentence. The technique develops motor control and the development of proper oral muscular movements while eliminating unnecessary muscle movements.
- Developmental Individual-difference Relationship-based model (DIR®) Floortime: a specific technique to both follow the child's natural emotional interests and at the same time challenge the child toward greater and greater mastery of the social, emotional, and intellectual capacities. With young children, these playful interactions may occur on the floor but go on to include conversations and interactions in other places.
- Applied behavior analysis (ABA): the process of systematically applying interventions based on the principles of learning theory to improve socially significant behaviors to a meaningful degree

Providing Occupational Therapy for Individuals with Autism during School Years

By the time children with autism reach elementary school age, the primary intervention setting is school, although children often continue to receive services in a clinical setting or at home (Bilaver et al., 2016) to either complement the school program or to add further layers of necessary intensity. Based on the child's needs, classroom placements can range from inclusion in classrooms with typically developing peers to much more restricted special education settings with highly increased ratios between adults/instructors and students (1:1 or 2:1). Occupational therapists who function within these environments may continue to focus their efforts to help students develop age-appropriate skills in academics, social participation, and play/leisure-related occupations. For students without intellectual impairment, therapy often focuses on strengthening executive functioning skills (Zingerevich & Patricia, 2009). During the middle school years, students who continue to require support engage in OT interventions that address independence across the range of self-care skills, activities of daily living, aspects of self-efficacy, and wellness (Rekoutis & Dimitropoulou, 2018; Tomchek, Koenig, Arbesman, & Lieberman, 2017). Those interventions expand at some point to include prevocational and vocational training (Dunn, Diener, Wright, Wright, & Narumanchi, 2015).

Providing Occupational Therapy for Individuals with Autism in Late Adolescence and Early Adulthood

Recent studies estimate that up to 50,000 teens with autism become adults—thereby losing school-based autism services—each year (Shattuck et al., 2011). For older students in more inclusive settings, occupational therapists may assist with their transition toward college by supporting them in exploring studies and college programs of interest, creating a study path, and helping with the application process. At the same time, both the students and their families may need support while preparing for life away from home. Furthermore, students may need guidance and scaffolding in the area of work skills, including such tasks as learning how to perform job searches, creating resumes, and preparing for job interviews (Seaman & Cannella-Malone, 2016). The latest labor force statistics indicate that 8 out of 10 people with a disability are not part of the active labor force across the Unites States. Among individuals with disabilities who are included in the labor force, only 17.9% were employed in 2016 according to the United States Bureau of Labor Statistics (2017) compared to 65.3% for those without a disability. The chances of employment are even worse for individuals with autism compared to other persons with disabilities and become even more dismal for people with ASD who also have an

CASE STUDY 63-1   JONATHAN (JOHNNIE)

Initial Evaluation and Findings

Johnnie was diagnosed at the age of 18 months with ASD. He received his diagnosis from an early intervention state-funded agency. Using today's diagnostic criteria, he would have been classified as Level 3, "requiring very substantial support." At the time of the evaluation, Johnnie presented as a nonverbal toddler, showing no interest in his surrounding, with a tendency to produce only repetitive sounds and movements when excited. Johnnie would start crying and become emotionally overwhelmed when his parents attempted to take away some of the objects he enjoyed holding in his hands. He also demonstrated fearful reactions to different sounds and noises, types of foods, and textures. He was particularly fearful of large spaces and encounters with groups of people. At the time of his initial evaluation, Johnnie had just started walking independently and demonstrated significant low tone in both large and small muscles. Based on the team's diagnosis and recommendations, he received home-based special education instruction, speech-language pathology, and physical therapy at the time but no OT.

Progress through the Years

The Preschool Years

At age 3 years, 6 months: Johnnie demonstrated minimal progress in communication skills. He was still nonverbal and demonstrated minimal eye contact with peers or adults. Overall sensory processing was severely dysfunctional, and Johnnie presented with fleeting joint attention and poor frustration tolerance. Repetitive behaviors and obsessive-compulsive behaviors were frequent and intensified when he was frustrated. His parents were frustrated with the lack of progress and enrolled Johnnie at a private special education school that provided an intense applied behavior analysis (ABA) program paired with speech-language therapy and OT.

At age 4 years, 2 months: By the end of his first school year, Johnnie was starting to verbalize more and was actively communicating his desire during games by saying "go," using "more" to initiate or continue with a motor task (i.e., swinging or jumping on the trampoline), or using "ball" when he wanted a ball thrown at him. Johnnie would almost always stand up at the sight of the occupational therapist stepping into his classroom and would verbalize "jump—jump." His oral motor skills also improved, as Johnnie was now able to blow bubbles and different types of whistles independently on request. Johnnie's overall tactile sensitivity had decreased, and he could tolerate handling a variety of textures (play dough, finger paint, and lotion). However, he still was not demonstrating any self-driven interest to engage with these materials. Johnnie required physical prompting and/or verbal cues to redirect him during tasks that were repetitive in nature (i.e., climb to reach for an

object and bring it to a specified area in the room). In that first year of school, Johnnie also made improvements in his gross motor skills and overall strength, which seemed to help increase his overall alertness and endurance. However, he still had significant issues with sensory processing and tactile defensiveness. Haircutting was an impossible task for his parents who either had to hold him down or tried to snip his hair while he was asleep. The same applied to nail clipping. For his second year at school, these goals were identified as high priority and became the focus of his OT sessions. An incremental and simplified process of desensitization was initiated, paired with a simple token rewards system was put in place aiming to help Johnnie accommodate to the different steps involved in a haircut (allowing his hair to be combed, tolerate wearing a bib, allowing his hair to be wet, becoming used to the presence of scissors around him). Several of those components were carried over in the classroom during direct instruction time with his ABA teacher (Figure 63-1).

At age 5 years, 3 months: At the end of the second school year, Johnnie had demonstrated measurable improvement across all areas and programs. Although more words were becoming part of his everyday speech, his communicative interactions were still quite limited to sentences of two to three words. His verbalizations were almost exclusively about satisfying basic needs. Johnnie had also started using Picture Exchange Communication System (PECS) and visual schedules successfully. Sensory processing difficulties continued to persist despite gains. For example, although Johnnie had successfully participated in a Therapeutic Listening© auditory integration protocol, he was still immensely scared of the noise during birthday parties. However, he had successfully overcome difficulties that had to do with waking up in the middle of the night from the sound of sirens and not being

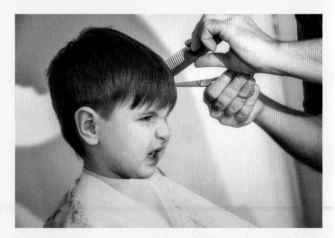

FIGURE 63-1 Johnnie had significant issues with sensory processing and tactile defensiveness. Haircutting became an impossible task.

CASE STUDY 63-1   JONATHAN (JOHNNIE) *(continued)*

TABLE 63-2   Johnnie's Occupational Therapy Evaluation Scores during His First Year at School

Subtest	Beginning of School Year (age equivalent in months)	End of School Year (age equivalent in months)
Stationary	28	35
Locomotion	22	29
Object manipulation	32	32
Grasping	11	28
Visual-motor integration	30	30

TABLE 63-3   Johnnie's Occupational Therapy Evaluation Bruininks-Oseretsky Test of Motor Proficiency, Second Edition Scores

	11-years 3-months	12-years 3-months	Progress Made
Fine motor precision	4:0–4:1	5:0–5:1	+12 months
Fine motor integration	4:10–4:11	5:6–5:7	+8 months
Manual dexterity	5:2–5:3	5:6–5:7	+4 months
Upper-limb coordination	7:3–7:5	7:6–7:8	+3 months
Bilateral coordination	7:3–7:5	8:9–8:11	+18 months
Balance	5:2–5:3	5:4–5:6	+2 months
Running speed and agility	4:2–4:3	4:2–4:3	No change
Strength	4:8–4:9	5:6–5:7	+10 months

able to go back to sleep. While going through the first cycle with the protocol, Johnnie also stopped being annoyed by the ringing of the phone at home. His mother, actually, asked to have him start back on the protocol after about 4 weeks since they had found that Johnnie would participate nicely during dinner at the table when he was listening to the modified music. In the weeks that ensued, Johnnie started becoming more restless again during dinner time. However, by the end of the second cycle, those gains became solidified.

Beyond these gains, Johnnie's engagement in tabletop activities and fine motor tasks led to small improvements that were measurable enough to be identified in his Peabody Developmental Motor Scales, Second Edition (PDMS-2) scoring between the beginning and end of the school year as demonstrated in the Table 63-2.

The School Years

Johnnie's progress through the years across all domains and occupations continued at a slow pace. Each victory and milestone was a big cause of celebration for his family and his team. New skills would come in after targeting them for a number of years and after a lot of plateaus. Often, we would make one step forward, followed by a regression of shorts. Johnnie did not sleep in his own bed until he was 9 years old. Until that point, he was sharing the same bed with his mother and father at home. It took him 5 years before he could tolerate having a haircut with a barber at a hair salon. The day he came back with his first haircut, we threw a big party for him at the school. By that time, he had learned to enjoy parties and other school gatherings. A little time later, he tolerated having an orthodontic retainer placed in his mouth by the dentist with no overreactions. Talking to his mother, at the time, she mentioned that getting to that point really made all the efforts we had put in through the years worthwhile

and worth waiting for. Johnnie spent several years learning how to write his name but was quite proficient with learning to type. Once introduced to computers and electronic tablets, he demonstrated an affinity of scanning the keyboard for the correct letters in order to find his favorite video clips on the Internet. He enjoyed typing up e-mails and telling his mother how his day was going at school. Within this, functional format typing instruction became one of his preferred school tasks. His overall motor skills, motor planning, and coordination continued to be delayed despite concerted efforts to help him in those domains. Table 63-3 demonstrates his performance and overall change in scores when tested with the Bruininks-Oseretsky Test of Motor Proficiency, Second Edition (BOT-2). In all this time, all the areas of needs were addressed collectively by all the team members through sharing of expertise, cross-training, and daily collaboration (Figure 63-2).

Jonathan's verbal skills also improved through the years. Johnnie grew apparently tired of being called "Johnnie" because around the time of his ninth birthday, he announced that his name was Jonathan. The entire school staff never called him Johnnie after that day. At age 10 years, Jonathan was the master of ceremonies (emcee) during a school event announcing the different skits in front of a crowd of more than 100 people. He was wearing a blazer and stood behind a microphone, reading his script and smiling. All of us, who experienced his journey up to that point, were crying tears of joy. Jonathan also revealed an affinity for pranks. His favorite task during his school day was to practice his navigational skills and follow multi-step directions in delivering mail and

(continues)

CASE STUDY 63-1   JONATHAN (JOHNNIE) *(continued)*

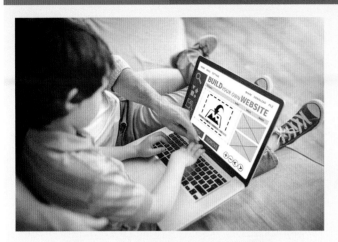

FIGURE 63-2 Johnnie developed an affinity for computers and electronic tablets. Computer skills became one of his strengths and resulted in improved school performance.

different forms to staff. It was his opportunity to come and place plastic bugs at our work stations or give us a handshake and jolt us with a little contraption between his fingers. Our surprised expressions would always crack him up.

By the time Jonathan was 11 years, he had already started participating in different types of prevocational activities that aimed at further developing his organizational skills and also focused on professional behaviors. He learned very quickly how to distribute mail to different staff members. He was also able to file worksheets in alphabetical order. During one of our sessions, he was asked to look at a picture of a kitchen at a fast-food restaurant. I asked him to pretend that he was working there and tell me what he would cook. He quickly replied, "Hamburgers." I then showed him a picture of the same kitchen with a big fire on top of the grill. When I asked him what he would do if there was a big fire, his response was "I will cook a Big Burger." On another occasion, when

I asked him what he would do if there was a fire at the restaurant that he was eating as a customer, he responded that he would leave and go to a different restaurant.

During his school day, Jonathan continued to participate in training programs that targeted aspects of safety awareness in different contexts (home, school, community) whether it was on an individual basis or part of his classroom group curriculum. Occupational therapists, speech-language pathologists, and classroom teachers all contributed in their respective roles. Social skills from an early stage involved learning how to go through a meal at a restaurant, tolerating and eventually enjoying trips to entertainment venues (the zoo, movie theaters, and amusement parks). Jonathan's OT sessions involved meal planning and meal preparation, as he started getting older. In the area of health and wellness, Jonathan—while at his school—learned how to use a gym membership and practiced arriving, checking in, changing into his gym outfit in the locker rooms, using the treadmills there, changing back to his clothes, and returning to school. Beyond the memberships, we were able to develop a collaboration between the school and that particular neighborhood gym, where Jonathan and other students would go and clean up the equipment during low "foot-traffic periods," as part of their vocational training with the occupational therapist being the most knowledgeable team member to act as the liaison.

Latest Update

Jonathan is preparing to graduate his school having surpassed the age of 18 year. His transition team is working toward expanding one of Jonathan's internships into a part-time paid position. Jonathan will continue living with his family for the foreseeable future. A couple of years ago, his parents worked in tandem with a group of other families to create a small residential community for young adults with autism in a suburban area. Their plans fell through because the group could not convince community boards across a handful of different municipalities about the benefits of having such a community in their area.

CASE STUDY 63-2   BRANDON

Initial Evaluation and Findings

Brandon was initially evaluated by a multidisciplinary team at the age of 2 years. The diagnostic center—where he was evaluated—included a developmental pediatrician, psychologist, speech-language pathologist, and an occupational therapist. His parents were concerned about his delay in meeting several milestones, his limited use of language and diminished eye contact. In addition, his parents felt that Brandon was not interested in other people and was shying away from interactions with his parents and

infant brother. During parental interviewing, his mother mentioned characteristically that Brandon "was there, but was practically absent" while the family celebrated his second birthday.

Brandon was seen separately by each clinician but demonstrated consistent behaviors across testing administrations. He had had observable difficulty following verbal directions and tended to simply repeat everything he heard, while requiring visual and gestural prompts to perform simple tasks. At times, he showed signs of

CASE STUDY 63-2   BRANDON (continued)

hyperresponsiveness to sound, covering his ears and/or would sing to himself, in an attempt to disengage from the process. Brandon was particularly drawn to visual stimulation, evidenced by his enjoyment and prolonged looking at spinning and shiny objects. Furthermore, he demonstrated difficulty transitioning from preferred activities (such as playing with train toys) to adult-directed tasks. As a result, he was not able to complete the corresponding standardized expressive and receptive language assessment as well as an intelligence scale. During his evaluation, Brandon appeared very distracted while inside a large sensory gym. He had marked difficulty with visual-vestibular processing, showing signs of gravitational insecurity (a fear of having his feet off the ground), and fear of imposed movement. He further appeared to lack depth perception, necessary for safe navigation around his environment, very frequently tripping over objects. Brandon avoided touching certain textures and walked primarily on his toes, presenting signs of tactile defensiveness. In addition, his mother reported that Brandon almost always resisted having his teeth brushed and frequently refused to try new foods. Brandon presented with low to average muscle tone, normal to slightly increased range of motion (joint laxity), and poor strength and stability throughout his body. Righting, equilibrium, and protective reactions were slow to emerge, causing him to seek out stationary, familiar activities and to resist imposed and novel movements in all planes of motion. Brandon was observed drooling when physical demands were placed on him, demonstrating difficulty with motor planning and dissociation of major muscle groups. Brandon demonstrated similar difficulties with fine motor tasks and age-appropriate self-care tasks, such as taking off his socks and shoes on his own. As was the case with the other assessments, it was not possible to engage Brandon in all the necessary tasks as part of his PDMS-2, and thus, he was not able to receive scores for any of the five subtests.

Brandon received the diagnosis of pervasive developmental disorder not otherwise specified (PDD-NOS). The recommendation to his parent was that he received an intensive early intervention program that included 1-to-1 special education instruction, relationship-based home intervention, speech-therapy, physical therapy, and OT. His early programming amounted to almost 30 hours of weekly intervention time that took place at a private clinic and at home. Brandon's parents were able to fund his program by combining compensation through private pay, their health insurance plans, and early intervention services funded by IDEA part C.

Occupational therapy services were provided in a sensory clinic with additional home consultations to help adapt his environment and teach parents strategies to promote self-care skills. Specific interventions were put in place to address sensory processing difficulties, gross, fine, and visual motor, cognitive, and self-care skill deficits.

Progress Through the Years
The Preschool Years

At Age 3 years 11 months: Brandon had demonstrated impressive gains in expressive language and was able to form short sentences. Repetitive answers and stereotypical speech were still frequent, but considerably reduced since the onset of services. At this point, Brandon had been enrolled in a small preschool class with typically developing peers and a "shadow" teacher in a part-time program. Brandon continued to have a very hard time regulating his behavior and was becoming distracted and disengaged when his environment was too stimulating or expectations were overwhelming. Brandon's ability to process auditory information remained a relative weakness, but following multiple-step verbal directions had improved. The focus of intervention was to further improve response times and ability to remain focused on the task at hand. Walking on tiptoes has diminished with the use of the Wilbarger Brushing protocol. Through direct intervention following the sequential oral sensory (SOS) approach to feeding, his food repertoire and willingness to try new foods in different environments improved tenfold. New foods were added in practically every food category. Brandon's mother attributed a lot of the gains in the trusting bond that he had developed with his therapist. At the same time, defensiveness and avoidance behaviors with toothbrushing, blowing horns, blowing bubbles, and blowing candles were successfully addressed and resolved through gradual exposure and pairing with tangible rewards. Although Brandon demonstrated improvements in tolerating vestibular input and improved balancing and protective reactions, his sensory system was still becoming overwhelmed by the vestibular input that he received. Although still not using a mature running pattern, Brandon could walk up and down stairs alternating feet without the need to hold onto a hand rail. He was also jumping forward, jumping down from a height, and jumping over obstacles by taking off and landing with both feet. Overall gross motor coordination performance, however, was still well below age level expectancy. Brandon continued to be disinterested in catching and throwing ball games. At that point in time, Brandon was much more efficient with fine motor skills and dressing skills. Brandon, nevertheless, was showing a keen interest in all the suspended equipment available to him during his OT sessions. He enjoyed participating in imaginary journeys to faraway places, where he had to overcome ominous creatures and obstacles to reach his destination, while navigating the different parts of elaborate obstacle courses. With the passing of time, he started adding comments and parts to the narrative and enjoyed building his own obstacle courses.

(continues)

CASE STUDY 63-2 BRANDON (*continued*)

TABLE 63-4 Brandon's Occupational Therapy Evaluation Scores at Age 5 Years 3 Months

Brandon's PDMS-2 Scores at 41 Months and 63 Months				
Subtest	Age Equivalent Months 41 Months	Age Equivalent Months 63 Months	Percentile Rank (%) at 63 Months	Progress Made
Stationary	43	58	37	15 months
Locomotion	39	57	37	18 months
Object manipulation	37	41	9	4 months
Grasping	40	40	5	No change
Visual-motor integration	51	62	50	11 months

Beery-Buktenica Developmental Test of Visual-Motor Integration (6th edition) (VMI)			
	VMI	Visual	Motor
Percentile Rank	50%	63%	12%
Age Equivalence	5 years 2 months	5 years 6 months	4 years 6 months

PDMS-2, Peabody Developmental Motor Scales, Second Edition.

At age 5 years 3 months: Brandon continued to make impressive gains across all domains of communication, social interactions, and sensory processing. However, he started demonstrating anxiety-related issues and was placed on medication. Some of his improvements and overall functioning in gross and fine motor skills are presented in the Table 63-4. The team and his parents made the decision—at that point—to prolong his preschool stay for another year, although he would typically be eligible for kindergarten. Throughout this time, Brandon enjoyed participating in OT sessions and continued to excitedly engage in "jungle gym" type of obstacle courses. He was able to show a creative side in organizing his environment and was demonstrating a bubbly personality. His interest in the jungle gym "stories" translated in more elaborate drawings and became a spark-plug for his early forays with letter formation and writing using the vocabulary from his "journeys" (Figure 63-3).

The School Years

At Age 7 years 3 months: After Brandon remained in preschool for a second year, he was then placed at a kindergarten classroom with typically developing peers and a shadow teacher. However, at the end of that year, and because of his increasing anxiety, the decision was made to place him at a school for high functioning students with autism. At that point, Brandon started receiving OT sessions at home instead of the sensory gym environment. Sessions focused on age-appropriate leisure skills, such as learning how to ride his bike and play different types of interactive video games (Wii Sports). Brandon's relationship with his therapist evolved to that of him having an older brother after working together for almost 6 years. Brandon would confide about his problems at school, and we would try to look for solutions together. At the same time, his improvements in communication and social skills did land him in "hot water." For example, Brandon texted one of his home tutors, pretending to be his mother and attempted to cancel his session. More seriously, he managed to also use his parents' credit card information to order a series of religious books (religion becoming one of his special interests at the time). Facilitating his interest in matters of religion allowed Brandon to gain increased social opportunities with other children attending rites and ceremonies. It helped further increase his ability to attend long events with sustained attention and better body control. Brandon was very motivated and decided to participate in the chorus of his church.

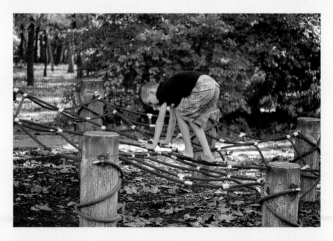

FIGURE 63-3 Brandon enjoyed participating in OT sessions and continued to excitedly engage in "jungle gym" types of obstacle courses.

CASE STUDY 63-2   BRANDON *(continued)*

At age 8 years 11 months: Brandon demonstrated a resolute ability and motivation to overcome difficulties and excelled with his learning at his school. Parent and teacher reports indicated that he was well organized and able to follow classroom instruction. At the same time, Brandon could manage frustration very effectively and would easily follow the "voice of reason." Brandon developed a keen sense of humor, which, combined with strong verbal skills, made him a very affable young boy with strong and well-argued opinions, who was a pleasure to interact with. In his OT sessions, Brandon was working on developing organizational strategies and strengthening his executive functioning to guide him in following specific steps toward completing the task at hand. Progressively, these strategies would translate into habits and routines associated with how he prepares, works through and completes academic projects, and performs during school testing procedures. Furthermore, he continued to explore new movement and exercise strategies that helped him remain regulated. Brandon excelled in learning how to jump rope and used an app to practice yoga and meditation.

A couple of months before his ninth birthday, Brandon managed to wonder off outside his weekend home in a wooded area and got lost for a few hours. Police and rescue parties were notified. He was found about half a mile from his home because he decided to stay in place and wait until somebody would call him for dinner. During one of our sessions—while addressing safety awareness—I asked him what he would do if he woke up at night and smelled fire. He responded that he would run out of the house. When I asked him, if he would alert anybody else in case they were still asleep, he responded, "No, because my life is too precious to lose." Empathy was still a skill that required further development, apparently. In late spring of that school year, we decided to discharge Brandon. He was getting ready to go to sleep away camp in the summer, and he felt that he was ready after 7 years of working together.

About 6 months later, I received an e-mail from his mother. She shared with me what another girl at Brandon's class wrote in an essay at school (sent to Brandon's mother by the girl's mother):

> My friends named Brandon and J. made school a fun place to be because they taught me how to do new things I never did. Some things my friends taught me were how to play box ball, how to jump rope while the rope is spinning, how to use the spinny thing, how to do forward rolls and how to play the fire drill game.

Latest Update

Brandon decided to cut down on commuting time between school and home and has been living in the residential part of his school for the past 2 years. This is the third consecutive year that he has campaigned successfully to be the class president. His latest aspirations include studying political science in college.

intellectual impairment (Taylor & Seltzer, 2011). For many adults with autism, the only available option is sheltered workshops or day activity centers. In addition to addressing work for adolescents with ASD, OT services can address continuing needs for independent daily living, functional limitations with self-care skills, community mobility, work-related practices, and leisure activities.

Conclusion

Occupational therapy practice can play a vital and dynamic role in supporting individuals with autism and their families. Occupational therapy interventions can be very beneficial regardless of level of severity or age. As part of a multidisciplinary team approach, occupational therapists assume distinct parts in both the assessment and intervention process. The two case studies illustrate the strong bonds that therapists can develop with both the individuals with autism and their families.

Recommended Readings

Case-Smith, J., Weaver, L. L., & Fristad, M. A. (2015). A systematic review of sensory processing interventions for children with autism spectrum disorders. *Autism, 19,* 133–148. doi:10.1177/1362361313517762

Dunst, C. J., Trivette, C. M., & Hamby, D. W. (2012). Meta-analysis of studies incorporating the interests of young children with autism spectrum disorders into early intervention practices. *Autism Research and Treatment, 2012,* 462531. doi:10.1155/2012/462531

Grinker, R. P. (2007). *Unstrange minds: Remapping the world of autism.* New York, NY: Basic Books.

Kuhaneck, H. M., & Watling, R. (2015). Occupational therapy: Meeting the needs of families of people with autism spectrum disorder. *American Journal of Occupational Therapy, 69,* 6905170010p1–6905170010p5. doi:10.5014/ajot.2015.019562

Rekoutis, P. A. (2013). *Parents of children with autism: Their perceptions and experiences with occupational therapy.* Saarbrucken, Germany: LAP Lambert Academic Publishing AG & Co. KG.

Tomchek, S., & Koenig, K. P. (2016). *Occupational therapy practice guidelines for individuals with autism spectrum disorder.* Bethesda, MD: AOTA Press.

REFERENCES

Ament, K., Mejia, A., Buhlman, R., Erklin, S., Caffo, B., Mostofsky, S., & Wodka, E. (2015). Evidence for specificity of motor impairments in catching and balance in children with autism. *Journal of Autism and Developmental Disorders, 45,* 742–751.

American Occupational Therapy Association. (2017). Research opportunities in the area of people with autism spectrum disorder. *American Journal of Occupational Therapy, 71,* 7102400010p1–7102400010p2.

American Psychiatric Association. (1980). *Diagnostic and statistical manual of mental disorders* (3rd ed.). Washington, DC: Author.

American Psychiatric Association. (2000). *Diagnostic and statistical manual of mental disorders* (4th ed., Rev. ed.). Washington, DC: Author.

American Psychiatric Association. (2013). *Diagnostic and statistical manual of mental disorders* (5th ed.). Arlington, VA: Author.

Ausderau, K. K., Furlong, M., Sideris, J., Bulluck, J., Little, L. M., Watson, L. R., . . . Baranek, G. T. (2014). Sensory subtypes in children with autism spectrum disorder: Latent profile transition analysis using a national survey of sensory features. *Journal of Child Psychology and Psychiatry, and Allied Disciplines, 55,* 935–944.

Baranek, G. T., Boyd, B. A., Poe, M. D., David, F. J., & Watson, L. R. (2007). Hyperresponsive sensory patterns in young children with autism, developmental delay, and typical development. *American Journal on Mental Retardation, 112,* 233–245.

Ben-Sasson, A., Soto, T. W., Martínez-Pedraza, F., & Carter, A. S. (2013). Early sensory over-responsivity in toddlers with autism spectrum disorders as a predictor of family impairment and parenting stress. *Journal of Child Psychology and Psychiatry, and Allied Disciplines, 54,* 846–853.

Bettelheim, B. (1967). *The empty fortress; infantile autism and the birth of self.* New York, NY: Free Press.

Bilaver, L., Cushing, L., & Cutler, A. (2016). Prevalence and correlates of educational intervention utilization among children with autism spectrum disorder. *Journal of Autism and Developmental Disorders, 46,* 561. doi:10.1007/s10803-015-2598-z

Brandwein, A., Foxe, J., Butler, J., Frey, H., Bates, J., Shulman, L., & Molholm, S. (2015). Neurophysiological indices of atypical auditory processing and multisensory integration are associated with symptom severity in autism. *Journal of Autism and Developmental Disorders, 45,* 230–244. doi:10.1007/s10803-014-2212-9

Braun, M. J., Dunn, W., & Tomchek, S. D. (2017). A pilot study on professional documentation: Do we write from a strengths perspective? *American Journal of Speech-Language Pathology, 26,* 972–981.

Brunner, D. L., & Seung, H. (2009). Evaluation of the efficacy of communication-based treatments for autism spectrum disorders: A literature review. *Communication Disorders Quarterly, 31,* 15–41. doi:10.1177/ 1525740108324097

Buescher, A. V., Cidav, Z., Knapp, M., & Mandell, D. S. (2014). Costs of autism spectrum disorders in the United Kingdom and the United States. *JAMA Pediatrics, 168,* 721–728. doi:10.1001/ jamapediatrics.2014.210

Cascio, C., Lorenzi, J., & Baranek, G. (2016). Self-reported pleasantness ratings and examiner-coded defensiveness in response to touch in children with ASD: Effects of stimulus material and bodily location. *Journal of Autism and Developmental Disorders, 46,* 1528–1537. doi:10.1007/s10803-013-1961-1

Case-Smith, J., Weaver, L. L., & Fristad, M. A. (2015). A systematic review of sensory processing interventions for children with autism spectrum disorders. *Autism, 19,* 133–148. doi:10.1177/1362361313517762

Centers for Disease Control and Prevention. (2017a). *Autism spectrum disorder: Data and statistics.* Retrieved from https://www.cdc.gov /ncbddd/autism/data.html

Centers for Disease Control and Prevention. (2017b). *Facts about ASD.* Retrieved from https://www.cdc.gov/ncbddd/autism/facts.html

Chang, M. C., Parham, L. D., Blanche, E. I., Schell, A., Chou, C.-P., Dawson, M., & Clark, F. (2012). Autonomic and behavioral responses of children with autism to auditory stimuli. *American Journal of Occupational Therapy, 66,* 567–576.

Christensen, D. L., Baio, J., Braun, K. V., Bilder, D., Charles, J., Constantino, J. N., . . . Yeargin-Allsopp, M. (2016). Prevalence and characteristics of autism spectrum disorder among children aged 8 years—Autism and Developmental Disabilities Monitoring Network, 11 sites, United States, 2012. *Morbidity and Mortality Weekly Report, 65,* 1–23. doi:10.15585/mmwr.ss6503a1

Christon, L. M., Arnold, C. C., & Myers, B. J. (2015). Professionals' reported provision and recommendation of psychosocial interventions for youth with autism spectrum disorder. *Behavior Therapy, 46,* 68–82. doi:10.1016/j.beth.2014.02.002

Dunn, L., Diener, M., Wright, C., Wright, S., & Narumanchi, A. (2015). Vocational exploration in an extracurricular technology program for youth with autism. *Work, 52,* 457–468. doi:10.3233/WOR-152160

Dunst, C. J., Trivette, C. M., & Hamby, D. W. (2012). Meta-analysis of studies incorporating the interests of young children with autism spectrum disorders into early intervention practices. *Autism Research and Treatment, 2012,* 462531. doi:10.1155/2012/462531

Green, D., Charman, T., Pickles, A., Chandler, S., Loucas, T., Simonoff, E., & Baird, G. (2009). Impairments in movement skills of children with autistic spectrum disorders. *Developmental Medicine and Child Neurology, 51,* 311–316.

Grindle, C. F., Kovshoff, H., Hastings, R. P., & Remington, B. (2009). Parent's experiences of home-based applied behavior analysis programs for young children with autism. *Journal of Autism and Developmental Disorders, 39,* 42–56.

Grinker, R. P. (2007). *Unstrange minds: Remapping the world of autism.* New York, NY: Basic Books.

Hazen, E. P., Stornelli, J. L., O'Rourke, J. A., Koesterer, K., & McDougle, C. J. (2014). Sensory symptoms in autism spectrum disorders. *Harvard Review of Psychiatry, 22,* 112–124.

Jasmin, E., Couture, M., McKinley, P., Reid, G., Fombonne, E., & Gisel, E. (2009). Sensori-motor and daily living skills of preschool children with autism spectrum disorders. *Journal of Autism and Developmental Disorders, 39,* 231–241.

Kanner, L. (1985). Autistic disturbances of affective contact. In A. M. Donnellan (Ed.), *Classical readings in autism* (pp. 11–50). New York, NY: Teachers College Press. (Original work published 1943)

Koegel, L., Matos-Freden, R., Lang, R., & Koegel, R. (2012). Interventions for children with autism spectrum disorders in inclusive school settings. *Cognitive and Behavioral Practice, 19,* 401–412. doi:10.1016/j.cbpra.2010.11.003

Koenig, K. P., & Hough Williams, L. (2017). Characterization and utilization of preferred interests: A survey of adults on the autism spectrum. *Occupational Therapy in Mental Health, 33,* 129–140. doi:10 .1080/0164212X.2016.1248877

Kuhaneck, H. M., & Watling, R. (2015). Occupational therapy: Meeting the needs of families of people with autism spectrum disorder. *American Journal of Occupational Therapy, 69,* 6905170010p1– 6905170010p5. doi:10.5014/ajot.2015.019562

Liu, T. (2012). Motor milestone development in young children with autism spectrum disorders: An exploratory study. *Educational Psychology in Practice, 28,* 315–326.

Liu, T., & Breslin, C. M. (2013). Fine and gross motor performance of the MABC-2 by children with autism spectrum disorder and typically developing children. *Research in Autism Spectrum Disorders, 7,* 1244–1249.

Lloyd, M., MacDonald, M., & Lord, C. (2013). Motor skills of toddlers with autism spectrum disorder. *Autism, 17,* 133–146.

MacKean, G. L., Thurston, W. E., & Scott, C. M. (2005). Bridging the divide between families and health professionals' perspectives on family-centered care. *Health Expectations, 8,* 74–85.

Puts, N. A., Wodka, E. L., Tommerdahl, M., Mostofsky, S. H., & Edden, R. A. (2014). Impaired tactile processing in children with autism spectrum disorder. *Journal of Neurophysiology, 111,* 1803–1811. doi:10.1152/jn.00890.2013

Rekoutis, P. A. (2013). *Parents of children with autism: Their perceptions and experiences with occupational therapy.* Saarbrucken, Germany: LAP Lambert Academic Publishing AG & Co. KG.

Rekoutis, P. A., & Dimitropoulou, K. A. (2018, April). *Individual movement-based protocols to reduce stereotypies and increase academic participation in school-age children with ASD.* Poster session presented at the 2018 AOTA Annual Conference & Expo, Salt Lake City, UT.

Sabatos-DeVito, M., Schipul, S., Bulluck, J., Belger, A., & Baranek, G. (2016). Eye tracking reveals impaired attentional disengagement associated with sensory response patterns in children with autism. *Journal of Autism and Developmental Disorders, 46,* 1319–1333. doi:10.1007/s10803-015-2681-5

Schaaf, R., Benevides, T., Leiby, B., & Sendecki, J. (2015). Autonomic dysregulation during sensory stimulation in children with autism spectrum disorder. *Journal of Autism and Developmental Disorders, 45,* 461–472. doi:10.1007/s10803-013-1924-6

Schaaf, R. C., Schoen, S. A., May-Benson, T. A., Parham, L. D., Lane, S. J., Roley, S. S., & Mailloux, Z. (2015). State of the science: A road map for research in sensory integration. *American Journal of Occupational Therapy, 69,* 6906360010p1–6906360010p7.

Seaman, R., & Cannella-Malone, H. (2016). Vocational skills interventions for adults with autism spectrum disorder: A review of the literature. *Journal of Developmental and Physical Disabilities, 28,* 479–494. doi:10.1007/s10882-016-9479-z

Shattuck, P., Wagner, M., Narendorf, S., Sterzing, P., & Hensley, M. (2011). Post-high school service use among young adults with an autism spectrum disorder. *Archives of Pediatrics and Adolescent Medicine, 165,* 141–146.

Stahmer, A. C., & Ingersoll, B. (2004). Inclusive programming for toddlers with autism spectrum disorders: Outcomes from the children's toddler school. *Journal of Positive Behavior Interventions, 6,* 67–82.

Steiner, A. M. (2011). A strength-based approach to parent education for children with autism. *Journal of Positive Behavior Interventions, 13,* 178–190.

Tanner, K., Hand, B. N., O'Toole, G., & Lane, A. E. (2015). Effectiveness of interventions to improve social participation, play, leisure, and restricted and repetitive behaviors in people with autism spectrum disorder: A systematic review. *American Journal of Occupational Therapy, 69,* 6905180010.

Tavassoli, T., Bellesheim, K., Tommerdahl, M., Holden, J. M., Kolevzon, A., & Buxbaum, J. D. (2016). Altered tactile processing in children with autism spectrum disorder. *Autism Research, 9,* 616. doi:10.1002/aur.1563

Taylor, J. J., & Seltzer, M. (2011). Employment and post-secondary educational activities for young adults with autism spectrum disorders during the transition to adulthood. *Journal of Autism and Developmental Disorders, 41,* 566–574.

Tomchek, S., & Koenig, K. P. (2016). *Occupational therapy practice guidelines for individuals with autism spectrum disorder.* Bethesda, MD: AOTA Press.

Tomchek, S., Koenig, K. P., Arbesman, M., & Lieberman, D. (2017). Evidence connection—Occupational therapy interventions for adolescents with autism spectrum disorder. *American Journal of Occupational Therapy, 71,* 7101395010.

Tomchek, S. D., Little, L. M., & Dunn, W. (2015). Sensory pattern contributions to developmental performance in children with autism spectrum disorder. *American Journal of Occupational Therapy, 69,* 6905185040p1.

Tomlin, G. S., & Swinth, Y. (2015). Contribution of qualitative research to evidence in practice for people with autism spectrum disorder. *American Journal of Occupational Therapy, 69,* 6905360010p1–6905360010p4. doi:10.5014/ajot.2015.017988

Turcotte, P., Mathew, M., Shea, L., Brusilovskiy, E., & Nonnemacher, S. (2016). Service needs across the lifespan for individuals with autism. *Journal of Autism and Developmental Disorders, 46,* 2480. doi:10.1007/s10803-016-2787-4

United States Bureau of Labor Statistics. (2017). *Persons with a disability: Labor force characteristics summary.* Retrieved from https://www.bls.gov/news.release/disabl.nr0.htm

Wigham, S., Rodgers, J., South, M., McConachie, H., & Freeston, M. (2015). The interplay between sensory processing abnormalities, intolerance of uncertainty, anxiety and restricted and repetitive behaviours in autism spectrum disorder. *Journal of Autism and Developmental Disorders, 45,* 943–952. doi:10.1007/s10803-014-2248-x

Wilbarger, P., & Wilbarger, J. (1991). *Sensory defensiveness in children aged 2–12: An intervention guide for parents and other caretakers.* Santa Barbara, CA: Avanti Educational Programs.

Zingerevich, C., & Patricia, D., L. (2009). The contribution of executive functions to participation in school activities of children with high functioning autism spectrum disorder. *Research in Autism Spectrum Disorders, 3,* 429–437.

thePoint®   *For additional resources on the subjects discussed in this chapter, visit* **http://thePoint.lww.com/Willard-Spackman13e**. See Appendix I, **Resources and Evidence for Common Conditions Addressed in OT** *for more information about ASD.*

Providing Occupational Therapy for Individuals with Traumatic Brain Injury

Intensive Care to Community Reentry

Steven D. Wheeler

LEARNING OBJECTIVES

After reading this chapter, you will be able to:

1. Identify the role of occupational therapy throughout the full spectrum of traumatic brain injury (TBI) recovery.
2. Appreciate the manner in which impairments, activity limitations, personal factors, and environmental barriers interact to impact successful and satisfying occupational performance following TBI.
3. Understand the importance of therapeutic relationship building and occupation-based practice in facilitating optimal community reentry following TBI.

Introduction

Few conditions challenge the diverse knowledge base and skill set of occupational therapy (OT) practitioners like traumatic brain injury (TBI). Traumatic brain injury is a complex condition characterized by varying degrees of cognitive, physical, psychological, behavioral, and emotional impairment. Although successful "community reentry" represents the ultimate goal of the TBI recovery process, for most individuals, the road from intensive care to community reentry is a long and arduous one. One's presentation after TBI depends on the extent and location of damage to the brain mixed with that person's cultural background, personality, and life experiences. As a result, no two individuals presenting to the OT practitioner are exactly alike, necessitating a true client-centered approach to assessment and treatment (see Box 64-1 and Chapter 37).

Persons with TBI can receive medical care and/or rehabilitation in a variety of settings. Senelick and Dougherty (2001) summarize the possibilities for care and rehabilitation following TBI to include the following:

1. Intensive care unit (ICU)/acute care
2. Acute rehabilitation (inpatient)
3. Outpatient rehabilitation
4. Skilled long-term care
5. Skilled residential care
6. Transitional living/work

CENTENNIAL NOTES

Considering the Illness Experience of Individuals with Traumatic Brain Injury

Although humans have undoubtedly sustained brain injuries over the centuries, attention to traumatic brain injury (TBI) emerged in the United States in relation to military traumas because of war. The U.S. military sources indicate that "it wasn't until World War I that medical professionals began seeing head injuries as an area of focus" when researchers recognized that "intellectual abilities made a difference in how they could fight, perform their duties and contribute to the unit" (French as quoted by Smith, 2016). French goes on to note that "Many forms of [definitive] care we use today, such as occupational therapy, evacuation trains, art therapy, canine therapy and sign painting were used to help patients overcome different medical issues in the past."

Early editions of *Willard & Spackman's Occupational Therapy* discussed "lesions" of the brain. In the first edition of the text, authors of one chapter noted that there tended to be an "overemphasis on the mental or physical treatment, the one at the expense of the other, when a well-balanced, coordinated approach to the patient would be better" (Fay & March, 1947, p. 132). It wasn't until the personal narrative of Mary Feldhaus Weber and her 16-year journey following severe TBI (included in the ninth edition of *Willard & Spackman's Occupational Therapy*) that a chapter appeared which prompted discussion of the condition in light of its impact on occupation and the important role of OT in a context similar to our modern day perspective. Although more current rehabilitation efforts focus on conducting standardized, rigorous research to support the effectiveness of interventions, Mary's story, and others like it, highlight the individualized nature of TBI and depict why OT is so critical to the rehabilitation process. As occupational therapists strive for best practice and optimal outcomes, it is crucial that the use of the latest evidence related to any particular method or procedure is implemented in a manner that considers "the illness experience and the influences of illness, cultural systems, socioeconomic systems, and non-human environments on occupation" (Neistadt & Crepeau, 1998, p. 31).

Note: Mary Feldhaus Weber's story and artwork appeared in four editions of *Willard & Spackman's Occupational Therapy* (9th through 12th) and can now be found online on thePoint. Figures 64-1 and 64-2 show two of Mary's many paintings presented in her narrative.

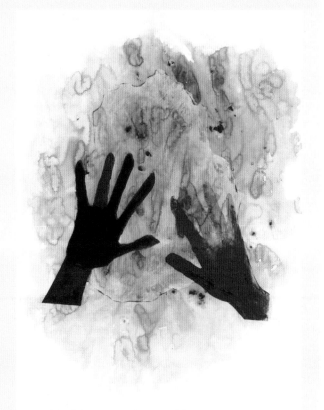

FIGURE 64-1 Mary Feldhaus Weber's painting "Blue Seizure" from her *Willard & Spackman* narrative.

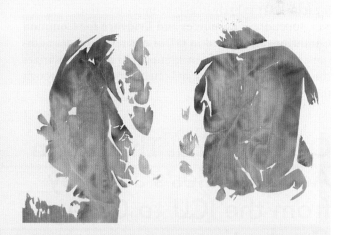

FIGURE 64-2 Mary Feldhaus Weber's painting "Healing Brain" from her *Willard & Spackman* narrative.

BOX 64-1	THERAPIST NARRATIVE: THE IMPORTANCE OF THERAPEUTIC RELATIONSHIP BUILDING IN TBI REHABILITATION

Although the phrase "risk-taking behaviors" is sometimes associated with actions and behaviors contributing to traumatic brain injury (TBI), taking risks is a necessary aspect of successful life functioning. Many of our greatest accomplishments and "self-esteem builders" come as a result of performing a task that carried with it the possibility of failure or rejection—asking someone out on a date, interviewing for a job, or even applying to college and pursuing occupational therapy studies. Those with a high self-esteem are better suited to taking such risks; failures are disappointments that fuel future attempts. If a decision doesn't work out, a high self-esteem can give you the strength and confidence necessary to pursue other avenues to reach your life goals.

Unsuccessful efforts to return to "normal" after TBI can be damaging to one's self-esteem and, subsequently, one's willingness to take chances and risk failure. This can pose a considerable challenge to occupational therapy practitioners responsible for encouraging clients to try new tasks necessary for the attainment of meaningful goals. Working within a client's comfort zone (i.e., doing activities that they're already competent at) can make a session manageable but may not be moving toward those meaningful occupations identified by the client and family in the early stages of therapy. Additionally,

always keeping things "safe" also prevents the client from learning about their deficits, an important component in the development of self-awareness. The inability to recognize one's deficits interferes with the motivation to change behavior or adapt to one's environment (Fleming, Strong, & Ashton, 1998). Impaired self-awareness negatively impacts social participation and the ability to establish a productive daily routine (Trudel, Tryon, & Purdum, 1998).

The development of an unconditional, therapeutic relationship is central to building a climate of trust. Clients who believe that their therapist will remain supportive regardless of whether they succeed or fail at an activity are more likely to take those risks necessary to experience meaningful accomplishments and enhance self-esteem. Unfortunately, rapport building with many clients takes time and may even require the therapist to "prove" his or her commitment to the relationship by staying supportive with the client during periods of acting out, defiance, and other acts. Therapists who discharge or transfer clients to other therapists because of difficult behavior or "noncompliance" may be missing an opportunity to establish the therapeutic relationship needed to encourage clients risk taking and the attainment of major life accomplishments.

There are many factors that influence the continuum of care following TBI. These are summarized in Figure 64-3 and discussed in Box 64-2. Regardless of the path following injury, OT is likely to play an important role.

Appendix I, **Resources and Evidence for Common Conditions Addressed in OT** of this text provides additional background information on TBI and summarizes common OT assessments and interventions used through the continuum of care.

Occupational Therapy in Action: Miles's Journey from the ICU to College Graduation

The case of Miles characterizes the complexity of TBI rehabilitation and the important impact of OT throughout the recovery spectrum. His experience following severe TBI also demonstrates the barriers to full community participation from the standpoint of both the individual and society.

Background Information

At the age of 22 years, Miles sustained a severe TBI in a motor vehicle accident while performing his job as a laborer with a local homebuilder. At the time of the injury, Miles was living with his mother, girlfriend, and infant daughter. He was a high school graduate who enjoyed sports, computers, and social events. Miles's injury was classified as severe. He remained in a coma for approximately 3 months, with computed tomography (CT) scan showing extensive brainstem damage and multiple contusions throughout his brain. Occupational therapy at this stage focuses on both managing impairments resulting from the injury and preventing secondary impairments that can occur over periods of unconsciousness. Sensory stimulation programs may be implemented at this stage. The evidence supports a team-coordinated multimodal approach with close observation of the client designed to improve alertness and arousal (Padilla & Domina, 2016). This approach typically involves stimulation of the visual, auditory, olfactory, gustatory, cutaneous, and/or kinesthetic system tailored to both client tolerance and premorbid preferences. Additionally, interventions such as passive range of motion (PROM), splinting, casting, and positioning are among the "preparatory" methods used to either

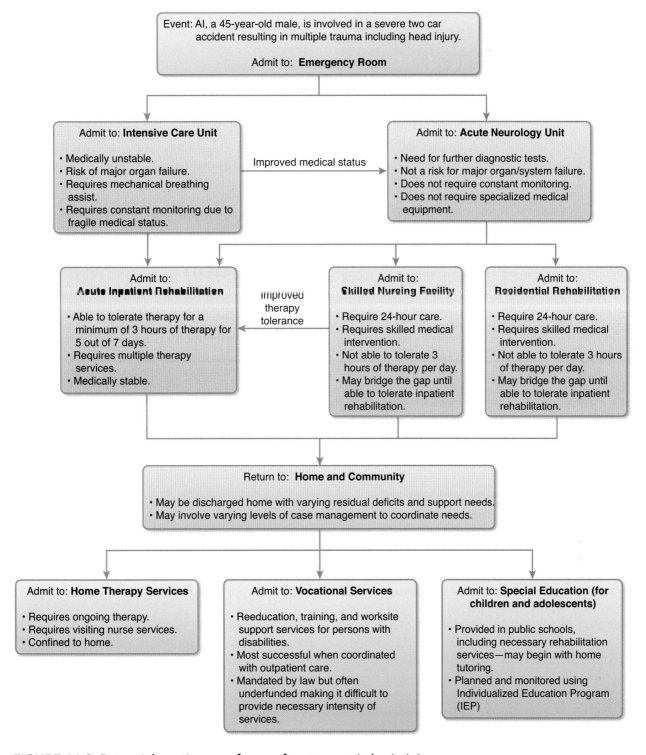

FIGURE 64-3 Potential continuum of care after traumatic brain injury.

restore motor function or prevent secondary complications such as joint and muscle contractures during coma (McNeny, 2015).

Miles had numerous medical complications during his acute care admission, including a lower extremity deep vein thrombosis (DVT), pneumonia, atelectasis, bradycardia, and questionable seizure activity. When his medical status stabilized, he was transferred to a skilled nursing facility where he continued the coma recovery program as described earlier. He remained in this setting until he emerged from coma and became progressively more alert. At that point, he was transferred to a rehabilitation

BOX 64-2	MARKETPLACE REALITIES AFFECTING THE TBI CONTINUUM OF CARE

The need to shift from the medical model of traumatic brain injury (TBI) rehabilitation to a more client-centered philosophy as an individual becomes medically stable is commonly cited in the literature (Lash, 2009). Unfortunately, the realities of the U.S. marketplace present considerable challenges to providing such care for many in need (Katz, Zasler, & Zafonte, 2007). Health insurance coverage for rehabilitation becomes incrementally more difficult across the continuum of care outlined in Figure 64-3—from inpatient to outpatient to residential and community services. For many, funding shifts from private to public sources such as Medicaid or Medicare for longer term care. The adequacy of public funding varies between states as some have developed Medicaid waivers to provide long-term home and community services that would otherwise be covered in institutional settings such as a nursing home (Katz et al., 2007). Understanding the complexities of reimbursement and sources of alternative funding is a challenging but essential element for clinicians, especially those providing services at the community level.

hospital for intensive interdisciplinary rehabilitation—approximately 6 months after the date of his injury. Occupational therapy at this stage employs remedial and compensatory approaches to address sensorimotor and self-care skill deficits, functional cognitive, and environmental modifications, along with caregiver education and training (Mortera, 2015). Depending on the client's level of agitation, structured, basic self-care tasks can be initiated along with structured simple activities requiring physical movements and/or cognitive skills. New learning at this stage is generally limited due to posttraumatic amnesia, agitation, overstimulation, and confusion (Wheeler & Acord-Vira, 2016). After 5 weeks of intensive, inpatient interdisciplinary rehabilitation, Miles's progress was considered to have reached a plateau and he was subsequently transferred back to the skilled nursing facility. At that time, he was assessed at a level V (confused, inappropriate) on the Rancho Los Amigos Levels of Cognitive Functioning Scale (Hagen, 1998). He continued to require assistance with all basic activities of daily living (ADL), had a percutaneous endoscopic gastrostomy (PEG) tube in place, was on a pureed diet with moderately thickened liquids,

and was nonambulatory, dependent on others for wheelchair mobility. His verbal expression was described as "profoundly impaired," and he communicated via a communication board.

Referral

Approximately 2 months into his second admission to the skilled nursing facility, Miles was referred to a TBI postacute, residential rehabilitation program. As part of the community reentry rehabilitation team, I had the opportunity to complete a comprehensive assessment with Miles followed by an intensive rehabilitation program.

Evaluation

Initial Impressions

Given the severity of Miles's injury, I was very aware of the challenges that were to lie ahead for both of us. Schutz and Schutz (2010) noted that for injuries where coma is less than 1 day, most survivors regain independence and perform adequately in a competitive job. However, when coma is counted in months, as was the case for Miles, even the most intense therapy may not restore full functioning in any area (Schutz & Schutz, 2010). While reviewing Miles's medical record, I was able to gain an appreciation of recent positive changes in his level of alertness, initiation, and desire to participate in intensive rehabilitation.

Community-Based Occupational Therapy Assessment—Considerations

Helping people to be productive and satisfied in their least restrictive environment is central to OT regardless of treatment setting or medical diagnosis. McColl, Davies, Carlson, Johnston, and Minnes (2001) categorized meaningful aspects of community integration to include the following:

1. Activities to fill one's time
2. Independence in one's living situation
3. Relationships with other people

Additionally, I've found the constructs of the International Classification of Functioning, Disability, and Health (ICF) (World Health Organization [WHO], 2001) to be particularly helpful in organizing my approach to both assessment and treatment. Both perspectives consider the interaction between person and environment and its impact on participation in meaningful occupations.

Assessment Priority No. 1—Therapeutic Relationship Building

If I were to name one thing that was essential to a positive outcome when working with persons with severe brain injury, it would be the establishment of a strong therapeutic relationship. That process begins with the very first interaction with the client. Standardized interview tools such as the Occupational Performance History Interview II (Kielhofner et al., 2004) and the Canadian Occupational Performance Measure (COPM) (Law et al., 2005) are excellent strategies for collecting important information and establishing client-centered goals. However, care should be taken to ensure that the interview isn't so structured that it hinders rapport building (refer back to Box 64-1). Additionally, for persons with a low frustration tolerance, moderate-to-severe cognitive deficits, and/or difficulty managing environmental stimulation, adaptations to the interview duration, wording of questions, and interview setting may be required in order to collect meaningful data. When initial rapport is established, the therapist is in a better position to encourage participation in home and community assessment tasks likely to be both challenging and frustrating for the client.

Assessment Results

Selected assessment strategies were implemented to complete Miles's occupational profile, a summary of his "history and experiences, patterns of daily living, interests, values, and needs" (American Occupational Therapy Association [AOTA], 2014, p. S13). Miles's initial assessment was completed over a period of approximately 1 week, a time frame that is longer than in many settings but necessary for community-based rehabilitation given the need to observe performance in both home and community settings. The assessments used with Miles are outlined in Table 64-1.

During our initial interview, Miles presented as extremely motivated and eager to participate in assessment tasks. After collecting some background information, Miles was asked to identify long-term goals and areas of life that were most important to him. They included the following:

1. Getting reunited with his girlfriend and infant daughter who had relocated to her parents' home more than 1,000 miles away
2. Being able to move more effectively and walk—"getting out of this wheelchair"
3. Being able to complete morning dressing, grooming, self-feeding, and toileting tasks without assistance from others—"taking care of myself and having some privacy"
4. Being able to communicate more effectively—"talking better without drooling so much"
5. Going back to school—wanted to attend college prior to injury
6. Being able to play sports—expressed a particular interest in basketball and running

Having Miles identify these areas was important. Clients who generate their own goals have been found to be more likely to want to work on them and feel that the goals are important (Doig, Fleming, Kuipers, & Cornwell, 2010). Given the gap between Miles's current and desired level of functioning, his full commitment to the program is especially essential.

Further impairment testing was carried out to determine which impairments limited occupational performance. Sensorimotor testing revealed severe ataxia affecting his ability to coordinate movements throughout the muscles of his extremities and trunk. Balance as evaluated through functional transfers from wheelchair to bed and toilet was poor. Generalized weakness and decreased endurance was also noted. Grip strength, evaluated using a dynamometer, was 20 lb on the dominant right side and 34 lb on the left. Range of motion was within normal limits, with the exception of right shoulder abduction and flexion, which were both limited to approximately 30° actively and 90° passively. It was noted in his medical record that Miles had sustained a severe fracture to his right forearm in his accident, resulting in prolonged immobilization of his right arm. Miles did not report discomfort with movement of his right upper extremity and no exercise restrictions were noted. Sensation was grossly intact.

In addition to the assessments listed in Table 64-1, Miles and I also completed a community living skills assessment (Angle & Buxton, 1991) that, as was hypothesized, demonstrated moderate-to-severe difficulty with all home and community tasks except money management and telephone use, which were mildly impaired. Although it appeared that physical impairments were the primary contributor to these functional difficulties, cognitive issues such as impulsivity and reduced awareness of deficits were also evident during observations. Such "executive cognitive functions" are commonly associated with damage to the brain's frontal lobes. These executive functions significantly influence other higher order cognitive skills such as decision making, goal setting, self-evaluation, and, ultimately, successful performance of the majority of life roles. Short-term memory impairments were also evident but appeared influenced by time of day and nature of the content to be remembered. Vision was tested prior to his admission and was determined to be consistent with pre-injury acuity. Miles demonstrated functional vision during reading, computer keyboard access, and other evaluation activities.

| TABLE 64-1 | **Community-Based Assessment Data Collection to Complete an Occupational Profile** |

Assessment Method	Rationale	Interpretation
Initial interview	Rapport building, establish client goals and meaningful occupations, screen cognitive impairments and orientation	Positive transition from skilled nursing; patient concerned about girlfriend and daughter relocating and not available to visit. Therapeutic relationship initiated with OT practitioners.
Functional Independence Measure (FIM) (Keith, Granger, Hamilton, & Sherwin, 1987) Functional Assessment Measure (FAM) (Hall, 1997)	FIM—assesses dysfunction in the performance of basic activities of daily living; physical deficit based FAM—addresses major functional areas less emphasized in the FIM to include cognitive, behavioral, communication, and community functioning	Moderate (client provides 50%–74% assistance) to maximum (client provides 25%–49% assistance) assist required for all aspects of basic self-care and functional transfers to bed and chair from wheelchair. Total assistance was required for transfer into a standard bathtub.
Community Integration Questionnaire (CIQ) (Willer, Ottenbacher, & Coad, 1994)	Brain injury–specific measure to address actual participation in categories related to community integration 1. Integration into a homelike setting 2. Social integration 3. Integration into productive activities	A total CIQ score can range from 0 to 29, with higher scores indicating greater community integration. Miles's score reflects virtually no current participation in activities inside or outside home.
Satisfaction with Life Scale (SWLS) (Diener, Emmons, Larsen, & Griffin, 1985)	Measure of general life satisfaction, a factor of subjective well-being; quick administration, well established validity and reliability	Scores on the SWLS range from 5 (very dissatisfied) to 35 (highly satisfied). Miles's score of 24 represented "mild satisfaction."
Neurobehavioral Functioning Inventory (Kreutzer, Seel, & Marwitz, 1999)	Completing patient form in concert with family caregiver form allows assessment of awareness of deficits, an important aspect of executive cognitive functioning and an area considered important to rehabilitation program compliance	*Miles Caregiver* Depression 45 51 Somatic complaints 45 74 Memory 46 51 Communication 58 54 Aggression 39 44 Motor impairments 51 60 Comparison of patient and caregiver raw scores suggests possibility of deficit of self-awareness based on Miles reporting less severity of symptoms in all areas except communication.

Treatment Planning: Mapping Out Strategies to Turn Assessment Findings into Performance Outcomes

Assessment findings revealed a large performance discrepancy between Miles's current functioning and his stated goals. Overcoming the factors contributing to reduced community participation following TBI is generally much more challenging for OT practitioners than identifying them. My treatment plan with Miles was heavily influenced by the following:

1. The client-centered philosophy and the person–environment models of OT (see Chapters 37 and 43)
2. The ICF
3. The "Whatever It Takes" approach (Willer & Corrigan, 1994)

Whatever It Takes is a practical approach to fostering community integration after TBI that considers both environmental barriers and needed natural supports that may be necessary for long-term community functioning. The approach is based on the following principles:

- No two individuals with acquired brain injury are alike.
- Skills are more likely to generalize when taught in the environment where they can be used.
- Environments are easier to change than people.
- Community integration should be holistic.
- Life is a place-and-train venture (i.e., placing an individual in an environment of his or her choice and providing the necessary supports and coaching/training to facilitate success).
- Natural supports last longer than professionals.
- Interventions must not do more harm than good.
- The service system prevents many barriers to community integration.
- Needs of individuals last a lifetime, so should their resources

To me, this model represents the "ideal" scenario for a community reentry OT plan because it integrates the client-centered, occupational-based focus of OT with what we've learned about the course of brain injury recovery. Unfortunately, the ability to fully implement the approach in most health care settings and systems is difficult, but clinicians should do all that is possible within the settings that they work. Working in Miles's favor was the fact that his health insurance (Workers Compensation) and case manager appeared supportive of intensive, long-term rehabilitation. More intensive rehabilitation following TBI has been linked to earlier functional gains (Turner-Stokes, Disler, Nair, & Wade, 2005). However, the chronic, complex, and evolving nature of TBI makes it very difficult to determine the optimal and most cost-effective amount of intervention for any particular individual (Wheeler & Acord-Vira, 2016).

Given the gap between Miles's current functional level and desired goals, regular communication with him

regarding his progress was essential so that he could see how small incremental goals were related to his long-term goals. Success experiences are essential to building self-esteem and self-confidence as well as fueling motivation. Encouragement and support from outside his treatment program would be negatively affected by the fact that his girlfriend and child relocated with her parents after his accident and were more than 1,000 miles away. Additionally, although his mother expressed a strong interest in helping Miles recover, both she and Miles acknowledged a turbulent and unstable family history that included little contact with his father. Miles's community-based rehabilitation program included a multidisciplinary treatment team that included, in addition to myself and a certified occupational therapy assistant (COTA), a psychologist, speech-language pathologist, physical therapist, nurse, and social worker. Key target areas of the interdisciplinary treatment program are described in Table 64-2.

Implementing the Treatment Plan

Miles's treatment program tested the strength of our therapeutic relationship right from the onset. His severe ataxia contributed to poor motor coordination and frequent frustration during our sessions. Despite his high drive to participate in tasks with me and the COTA, functional gains were slow, accompanied by growing self-awareness of the fact that getting physically stronger was not going to resolve his severe ataxic movements. Miles was less interested in compensatory strategies than being the person he was prior to his injury, and that contributed to resistance when it came to trying adaptive equipment and compensatory techniques.

Occupational therapy treatment sessions used both home and community settings. In the home, ADL

TABLE 64-2 **Selected Target Areas of the Interdisciplinary Treatment Program**

Occupational Therapy	Speech Therapy	Psychology	Physical Therapy
Basic ADL performance/functional transfers	Speech clarity	Counseling for adjustment to disability	Functional ambulation using walker
Handwriting skills to facilitate day planner/memory notebook use prevocational	Swallowing/oral-motor skills	Memory training and compensation	Strengthening exercises with home exercise program
Meal preparation/home management	Memory—recall of sentences and paragraphs	Family counseling	Balance training
Leisure and social community outings	Augmentative communication	Attention training	Transfers and bed/mat mobility
Prevocational preparation including computer access	Respiratory exercises	Comprehensive neuropsychological assessment	Family/caregiver training related to ambulation and exercises

ADL, activities of daily living.

training and home management activities were in an actual bedroom, bathroom, kitchen, living room, and office area. Whenever possible, we practiced actual tasks at normal times in Miles's typical daily routine—dressing, grooming, transfers, meal preparation, using the computer, handwriting in his memory notebook, planning and participating in community outings, doing household chores, and doing leisure activities. Repetition during activities was used to strengthen muscles and improve performance in conjunction with daily upper extremity strengthening exercises. Although often considered an adjunct to occupation, Miles's upper extremity strengthening program was additionally important as exercising was meaningful occupation for him preinjury.

With repeated struggles, Miles gradually appeared more accepting of adaptive equipment to improve his independence in activities that were particularly important to him. For example, weighted feeding utensils with built-up handles, dishes with higher lips, and cups with a top were effective at improving motor function to improve his ability to feed himself and drink more efficiently without excessive spillage. Building up handles on writing and grooming utensils also improved quality of performance, although to a lesser degree. We attempted to use weighted wrist cuffs to improve movement efficiency during computer keyboard use. However, Miles insisted on a one-handed typing technique that involved stabilizing his wrist using the opposite hand (Figure 64-4).

Miles had his first session in the community approximately 3 weeks into his program—a trip to a department store to purchase a music CD. From that point on, sessions in the community were a regular aspect of his program, occurring approximately two to three times a week. Community outings included visits to restaurants, visiting his mother at her home, and attending sporting events, including a wheelchair basketball game. During outings, OT focused on evaluating skills such as money management, functional mobility, planning, initiative, problem solving, and decision making in relation to his degree of independence for each task.

Although functional gains were positive, the rate of progress was inconsistent. Success was complicated by medical factors such as frequent medication changes attempting to manage upper extremity tremors and severe esophageal reflux, which negatively impacted self-feeding and nutritional intake. His status 3 months after the onset of his postacute, residential program and 8 months from the date of his injury is summarized in

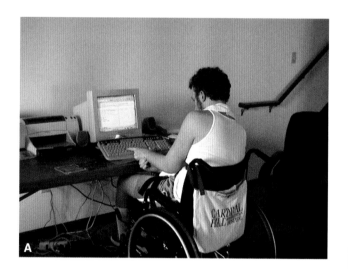

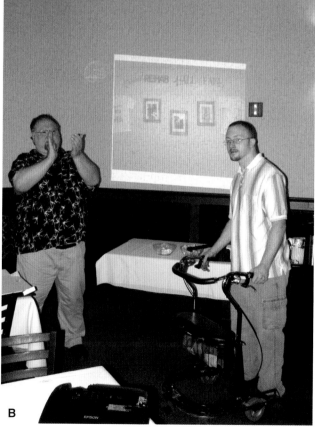

FIGURE 64-4 Miles's educational program progressed from **(A)** basic computer keyboard access to **(B)** speaking to other survivors of brain injury.

TABLE 64-3 Selected Test Scores from 90-Day Evaluation

Evaluation	Baseline	90-Day Reassessment	Interpretation
Community Integration Questionnaire	Home integration, 0 Social integration, 2 Productive activity, 0	Home integration, 3 Social integration, 5 Productive activity, 0	Significant progress in home management and initiation and participation in social activities
FIM/FAM	Feeding, 2 Upper body dressing, 3 Lower body dressing, 2 Grooming, 2 Bathing, 2 Transfers (wheelchair to bed), 2 Transfers (wheelchair to bathtub), 1 Home management, 1	Feeding, 4 Upper body dressing, 5 Lower body dressing, 4 Grooming, 4 Bathing, 4 Transfers, (wheelchair to bed), 4 Transfers, (wheelchair to bathtub), 4 Home management, 2–3	Notable functional gains in ADL independence. Assistance required for tasks requiring balance and fine motor coordination due to continued ataxia. Improved meal planning and money management
SWLS	24	12	Despite progress, significant reduction in self-reported life satisfaction

FIM, Functional Independence Measure; FAM, Functional Assessment Measure; ADL, activities of daily living; SWLS, Satisfaction with Life Scale.

Table 64-3. Despite his functional gains, Miles reported less satisfaction with life, frustration with his current situation, more frequent periods of agitation, and depressed mood. Additionally, he demonstrated increased self-awareness based on statements regarding the severity of his deficits and similarities between his and staff responses on the Neurobehavioral Functioning Inventory (Kreutzer et al., 1999).

Revising the Treatment Plan: Expanding Occupations

With it becoming increasingly clear that Miles would have lifelong physical impairments, especially ataxia, aspects of Miles's program were modified to expand his occupations by putting greater emphasis on productivity and leisure goals. Up to this point in his treatment program, the occupations occupying Miles's typical day were almost entirely centered on self-care. The effort required for basic ADL and home management left little time and energy for other activities. That, combined with an increasing level of awareness of impairments, appeared to be negatively affecting life satisfaction. Although basic self-care and home management are necessary elements of successful community reentry, aspects of leisure and productivity, so central to Miles preinjury daily routine, were very limited and impacted his psychological well-being. It was hoped that by balancing self-care and home management goals with more productive activity and leisure, Miles would develop a greater sense of accomplishment and gain a more positive outlook in life in the face of residual disability.

The plan to increase Miles's productive occupations included two primary objectives, identified by Miles as being of primary importance:

1. Taking college courses to eventually obtain a degree
2. Taking greater responsibility of his finances to demonstrate capacity to become his own legal guardian

Additionally, OT continued working on self-care skills, home management, and community participation to help Miles and the clinical team make decisions on his least restrictive living environment after his discharge from the residential treatment program.

In addition to beginning college studies, planning was also initiated to look at options for community living. During family sessions, it became increasingly clear that Miles would not be residing with his parents, and his girlfriend had expressed an intention to break off their relationship. The therapeutic relationships established with many clinical team members served as a critical source of support during this period of social isolation and an uncertain future. Although supportive of Miles during his struggles, adherence to professional boundaries by the OT team and all staff was essential at all times. Purtilo, Haddad, and Doherty (2012) describe strategies to express genuine care for clients while maintaining some distance. Given Miles's emotional vulnerability, it would be understandable for him to misinterpret the nature of his relationships with health care providers (social friendships, intimacy, etc.). Strategies that the treatment team used to maintain professional boundaries included the following:

- Having Miles participate in team meetings where issues about his progress were discussed
- Dividing outings and activities between team members

Phase 1 (90 days)	Phase 2 (approx. 180 days)	Phase 3 (approx. 180 days)
College course selection	One course fully completed through distance education format—progression to two courses in semester 3	Transition to off campus accessible apartment
College application		Home management and ADL training in new living environment
Investigating online learning options	Continued development of study skills, prioritizing time for study for heavier course load, contacting instructor with questions	Beginning on campus coursework with rehab staff in class to assist with note taking
Computer word processing / e-mail and Internet use		
Functional mobility—in collaboration with physical therapy	Investigated possibility of voice dictation to increase efficiency (problems due to ataxia) in collaboration with speech therapy—unsuccessful due to poor voice quality	Final determination of degree major (psychology)
Functional communication skills—in collaboration with speech therapy		Gradual phasing out of use of treatment program staff with greater use of university disability resources
Functional cognition—memory skills and executive functions—in collaboration with speech therapy and psychology	Attending on-campus events—to experience leisure interest and expand social contacts as well as determine accessibility issues	Leading group session on brain injury and cognition for residential program
Continued home management and basic ADL sessions as part of regular routine	Training in use of public transportation for disabled	Discharge from rehabilitation therapies with residential treatment program with regular follow-up by OT and speech therapy. Continued outpatient physical therapy.
	Exploration of on or off campus living options/accessibility evaluations	
	Participating in group therapy in residential program	

FIGURE 64-5 Stages of Miles's school/independent living progression with occupational therapy (OT) focus areas. *ADL*, activities of daily living.

- Limiting visits/interactions to work hours
- Working with Miles to expand his relationships beyond the rehabilitation setting
- Selectively sharing with Miles's personal incidents from everyday life

The stages of Miles's education, independent living, and leisure goals are detailed in Figure 64-5. Each phase is characterized by significant clinical progress and incorporation of meaningful occupations into his daily routine. Each was also characterized by significant struggle and testing of the therapist–client relationship. On occasion, Miles would appear to sabotage his progress, acting out or refusing to participate in tasks that had been weeks, and sometimes months, in planning. The roles of OT changed throughout the phases, moving from predominantly direct skills teaching to advocate, working with landlords, builders, and professors to help Miles face environmental barriers in terms of accessibility and prejudice.

It took 8 years for Miles to receive his Bachelor of Arts degree in Psychology (Figure 64-6). At the time of graduation, he was living in the community with homemaker support and had successfully gained legal authority

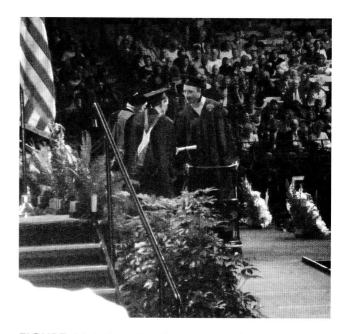

FIGURE 64-6 An intensive, occupation-based rehabilitation program helped Miles accomplish his goal of college graduation.

to manage his own finances. His outcomes defy the expected for persons with severe TBI. But despite these unlikely accomplishments, he also faces an uncertain future. Without secured employment, an absence of leisure activities, few friends, and residual motor impairments, it is likely that Miles will continue to require various rehabilitative and social services as future challenges present.

 Visit thePoint to watch a video about interventions for acquired brain injury.

REFERENCES

American Occupational Therapy Association. (2014). Occupational therapy practice framework: Domain and process, 3rd edition. *American Journal of Occupational Therapy, 68*, S1–S48. doi:10.5014/ajot.2014.682006

Angle, D., & Buxton, J. (1991). *Community living skills workbook for the head injured adult.* New York, NY: Aspen.

Diener, E., Emmons, R. A., Larsen, R. J., & Griffin, S. (1985). The Satisfaction with Life Scale. *Journal of Personality Assessment, 49,* 71–75.

Doig, E., Fleming, J., Kuipers, P., & Cornwell, P. (2010). Clinical utility of the combined use of the Canadian Occupational Performance Measure and Goal Attainment Scaling. *American Journal of Occupational Therapy, 64*, 904–914.

Fay, E. V., & March, I. (1947). Occupational therapy in general and special hospitals. In H. S. Willard & C. S. Spackman (Eds.), *Occupational therapy* (pp. 118–140). Philadelphia, PA: J. B. Lippincott.

Fleming, J., Strong, J., & Ashton, R. (1998). Cluster analysis of self-awareness levels in adults with traumatic brain injury and relationship to outcome. *The Journal of Head Trauma Rehabilitation, 13*, 39–51.

Hagen, C. (1998). Levels of cognitive functioning. In *Rehabilitation of the head injured adult: Comprehensive physical management* (3rd ed.). Dowey, CA: Professional Staff Association of the Rancho Los Amigos Hospital.

Hall, K. (1997). The Functional Assessment Measure (FAM). *Journal of Rehabilitation Outcomes Measures, 1*, 63–65.

Katz, D., Zasler, N., & Zafonte, R. (2007). Clinical continuum of care and natural history. In N. Zasler, D. Katz, & R. Zafonte (Eds.), *Perspectives on rehabilitation care and research* (pp. 1–13). New York, NY: Demos.

Keith, R., Granger, C., Hamilton, B., & Sherwin, F. (1987). The Functional Independence Measure: A new tool for rehabilitation. *Advances in Clinical Rehabilitation, 1*, 6–18.

Kielhofner, G., Mallinson, T., Crawford, C., Nowak, M., Rigby, M., Henry, A., & Walens, D. (2004). *Occupational Performance History Interview—II (version 2.1).* Chicago, IL: MOHO Clearinghouse.

Kreutzer, J., Seel, R., & Marwitz, J. (1999). *Neurobehavioral Functioning Inventory.* San Antonio, TX: The Psychological Corporation.

Lash, M. (2009). *The essential brain injury guide* (4th ed.). Vienna, VA: Brain Injury Association of America.

Law, M., Baptiste, S., Carswell, A., McColl, M., Polatajko, H., & Pollock, N. (2005). *Canadian Occupational Performance Measure.* Ontario, Canada: Canadian Association of Occupational Therapists.

McColl, M., Davies, D., Carlson, P., Johnston, J., & Minnes, P. (2001). The Community Integration Measure: Development and preliminary validation. *Archives of Physical Medicine and Rehabilitation, 82*, 429–434.

McNeny, R. (2015). Rehabilitation of the patient with a disorder of consciousness. In K. Golisz & M. V. Radomski (Eds.), *Traumatic brain injury (TBI): Interventions to support occupational performance* (pp. 139–173). Bethesda, MD: American Occupational Therapy Association.

Mortera, M. (2015). The acute, inpatient, and subacute rehabilitation phases of recovery. In K. Golisz & M. V. Radomski (Eds.), *Traumatic brain injury (TBI): Interventions to support occupational performance* (pp. 175–229). Bethesda, MD: American Occupational Therapy Association.

Neistadt, M., & Crepeau, E. (1998). *Willard & Spackman's occupational therapy* (9th ed.). Philadelphia, PA: Lippincott.

Padilla, R., & Domina, A. (2016). Effectiveness of sensory stimulation to improve arousal and alertness of people in a coma or persistent vegetative state after traumatic brain injury: A systematic review. *American Journal of Occupational Therapy, 70*, 7003180030p1–7003180030p8. doi:10.5014/ajot.2016.021022

Purtilo, R., Haddad, A., & Doherty, R. (2012). *Health professional and patient interaction* (8th ed.). St. Louis, MO: Elsevier.

Schutz, L., & Schutz, M. (2010). *Head injury recovery in real life.* San Diego, CA: Plural.

Senelick, R., & Dougherty, K. (2001). *Living with brain injury.* Birmingham, AL: HealthSouth Press.

Smith, M. D. (2016). *History of military medical advancements in brain injury treatment.* Retrieved from https://health.mil/News/Articles/2016/12/19/History-of-military-medical-advancements-in-brain-injury-treatment

Trudel, T., Tryon, W., & Purdum, C. (1998). Awareness of disability and long-term outcome after traumatic brain injury. *Rehabilitation Psychology, 43*, 267–281.

Turner-Stokes, L., Disler, P., Nair, A., & Wade, D. (2005). Multidisciplinary rehabilitation for acquired brain injury in adults of working age. *Cochrane Database of Systematic Reviews*, (3), CD004170. doi:1002/14651858.CD004170.pub2

Wheeler, S., & Acord-Vira, A. (2016). *Occupational therapy practice guidelines for adults with traumatic brain injury.* Bethesda, MD: American Occupational Therapy Association.

Willer, B., & Corrigan, J. (1994). Whatever it takes: A model for community-based services. *Brain Injury, 8*, 647–659.

Willer, B., Ottenbacher, K., & Coad, M. (1994). The Community Integration Questionnaire. A comparative examination. *American Journal of Physical Medicine & Rehabilitation, 73*, 103–111.

World Health Organization. (2001). *International classification of functioning, disability, and health.* Geneva, Switzerland: Author.

thePoint® *For additional resources on the subjects discussed in this chapter, visit* **http://thePoint.lww.com/Willard-Spackman13e.**

Providing Occupational Therapy Services for Persons with Major Mental Disorders

Promoting Recovery and Wellness

Margaret Swarbrick

LEARNING OBJECTIVES

After reading this chapter, you will be able to:

1. Outline concepts of recovery, wellness, and peer support as they apply to persons with major mental disorders.
2. Describe emerging roles for occupational therapists in mental health and the different settings in which they deliver services to persons with major mental disorders.
3. Compare occupational therapy approaches for persons with major mental disorders.
4. Identify community support services for persons with major mental disorders that facilitate recovery, wellness, and self-determination.

Introduction

Mental disorders are common in the United States. Mental disorders involve changes in thinking, mood, and/or behavior. Mental disorders take many different forms, with some rooted in deep levels of anxiety, extreme changes in mood, or reduced ability to focus. Others involve unwanted, intrusive thoughts, and some may result in hallucinations or false beliefs about basic aspects of reality. Reaching a threshold for a formal diagnosis is related to how much a person's ability to function is impacted. Mental disorders can occur once, reoccur intermittently, or be more long term (chronic) in nature. Mental disorders frequently co-occur with each other and with substance use disorders. Because of this, and because of variation in symptoms even within one type of disorder, individual situations and symptoms are extremely varied (Box 65-1).

In 2015, there were an estimated 43.4 million adults aged 18 years or older in the United States with any mental illness within the past year. This number represented 17.9% of all U.S. adults (Figure 65-1). Any **mental illness** is defined as follows:

- A mental, behavioral, or emotional disorder (excluding developmental and substance use disorders);
- Diagnosable currently or within the past year; and,
- Of sufficient duration to meet diagnostic criteria specified within the *Diagnostic and Statistical Manual of Mental Disorders* (currently in its fifth edition [*DSM-5*]; American Psychiatric Association [APA], 2013).

BOX 65-1 THERAPIST NARRATIVE

While studying to become an occupational therapy (OT) practitioner in the mid-1980s, I learned that the profession had a rich history of promoting mental health in all areas of practice through the use of meaningful and enjoyable occupations (Meyer, 1922). I had no doubt that I would take my first job in mental health practice, as I was committed to help individuals develop and maintain positive mental health and recover from mental health challenges in order to live full and productive lives. I was so very fortunate to start my career as an OT practitioner in a long-term state-run inpatient facility. I had the opportunity to deliver *person-centered* wellness programs many years ago, before the term was in vogue. I worked on the *acute units*—even though, in those days, the length of stay was quite long (ranging from about 3 to 4 months to many years). This often puzzled me because I was so inspired and motivated by the resilience of the people I served, and so many of them seemed like they did not require such a restrictive setting. I was a member of an interprofessional team. I ran time management and health skills management groups and organized functional activities for people who were unable to leave the unit. I used the whole person OT lens to support people in this setting. I wanted to strengthen my skills, so I continued my education to become a registered occupational therapist. Eventually, I was able to learn to design and offer formal whole person wellness programs in this setting (Swarbrick, 1997). I made a commitment to grow professionally by regularly networking with many fellow occupational therapists. This was possible by participating in the local OT association activities and attending the American Occupational Therapy Association (AOTA) conference every year. My desire to develop science-driven, evidence-based approaches for people in the community where they live, learn, and can grow was bolstered as I pursued advanced education. People I served experienced many challenges; yet, despite how much they were impacted, I continued to be inspired by the strength they had that enabled them to endure the challenges of an institutional setting. I started creating and running OT groups in short-term inpatient settings (Gutman & Swarbrick, 1998).

I eventually discovered an exciting nontraditional position in a community-based peer support program (Swarbrick & Duffy, 2000). I have had a great opportunity to use OT knowledge, skills, and techniques to help the peer support agency develop and expand recovery-oriented services, peer-led programs fostering self-sufficiency, and services addressing the eight dimensions of wellness (Swarbrick, 2012). My optimism was confirmed when I noticed fellow employees who were once "clients" who attended wellness groups at the state-run inpatient facility years earlier.

This agency collaborates with OT academic programs to provide fieldwork opportunities for many students who gain a very rich experience. Local OT researchers regularly work with the vast network of people in recovery to craft and engage in research related to recovery, wellness, and OT practice. This research, and related studies by researchers in other disciplines, provides the evidence base for the efficacy of certain interventions, which then need to be disseminated, implemented, and evaluated in the real world. I have appreciated being able to work collaboratively on these efforts. I continue to be involved with a local state OT advocacy group to educate local certified community behavioral health clinic (CCBHC) on the value of OT.

The AOTA has identified *mental health* as a key practice area in the twenty-first century. The World Health Organization has identified mental illness as a growing cause of disability worldwide. It is essential for OT to continue to place emphasis on mental health treatment and prevention services for children, youth, people who are aging, and individuals diagnosed with a severe and persistent mental illness.

From a global perspective, results of a systematic review and meta-analysis indicated that approximately 1 in 5 persons experienced a common mental disorder within a 12-month period across 155 general population surveys undertaken in 59 countries. The aggregate lifetime prevalence of common mental disorder was estimated at 29.2% from 85 surveys undertaken across 39 countries (Steel et al., 2014).

Using this definition, "any mental illness" can range in impact from no or mild impairment to significantly disabling impairment. These estimates of any mental illness do not include substance use disorders, such as drug- or alcohol-related disorders. People with major mental disorders represent a subset of people in the "any mental illness" category who experience "a significant functional impairment that substantially interferes with or limits one or more major activities" (APA, 2013). Major mental disorders impact the individuals diagnosed, their family, and their supporters as well as the communities where they live, work, learn, and contribute to the well-being of others. Individuals with a major mental disorder experience various symptoms that make it very challenging to continue or resume valued life roles, such as living independently, working, or going to school. The symptoms of the illness impact major life activities, including basic daily living skills (e.g., eating, bathing, dressing); instrumental living skills (e.g., maintaining a household, managing money, getting around the community, taking prescribed medication); and functioning in social, family, and vocational/educational contexts.

Major mental illnesses co-occur at a significant rate with other medical conditions. Individuals with serious

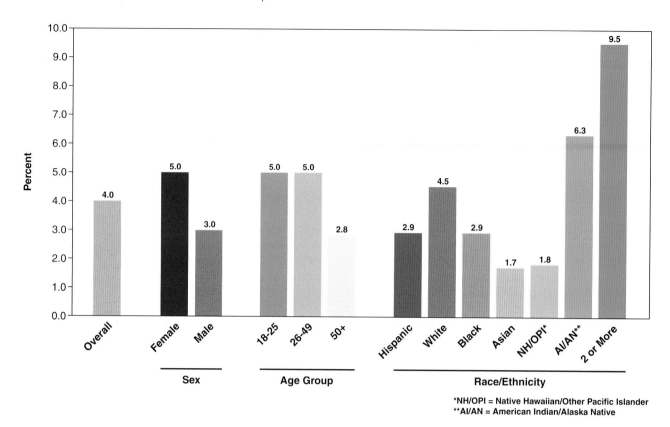

FIGURE 65-1 Prevalence of major mental disorders among U.S. adults. (Source: Substance Abuse and Mental Health Services, 2015.)

major mental illnesses have shorter life courses and worse overall health than nondisabled individuals possibly due to increased vulnerability as a result of poverty; inadequate access to health care; and significantly higher rates of smoking, obesity, and substance abuse than the overall population (Center for Mental Health Services, 2010). Since 2006, published data have documented that these individuals live on average 25 years less than the general population (Druss, Zhao, Von Esenwein, Morrato, & Marcus, 2011). This disturbing disparity can be addressed through effective supports and treatment delivered by interprofessional teams, including occupational therapists, in order to increase life course and quality of life for people served by the public mental health system. Recovery- and wellness-focused social supports in the community have been developed as well as newer less toxic medications that are as effective for some people at lessening troubling symptoms while causing fewer side effects. These new approaches that are helping people with major mental disorders are based on the belief that people can and do recover from major mental disorder (Box 65-2).

Occupational therapy practice is based on a person-centered (or client-centered), holistic approach that fits well with wellness and recovery. Occupational therapists have a strong skill set to bring to serving persons with major mental disorders. Because occupational therapists

have educational grounding in psychology, therapeutic use of self, task analysis, neuroscience, and the teaching of self-care and life skills, they can be effective members of interprofessional teams. Occupational therapists can be found in a wide array of settings and programs for

BOX 65-2 RECOVERY

Recovery has been defined as a process of change through which individuals improve their health and wellness, live a self-directed life, and strive to reach their full potential (Substance Abuse and Mental Health Services Administration [SAMHSA], 2011, para. 3). *Wellness* is defined as a conscious, deliberate process that requires a person to become aware of and make choices for a more satisfying lifestyle. A wellness lifestyle includes a balance of health habits, including adequate sleep and rest, good nutrition, productivity, exercise, participation in meaningful activity, and connections with supportive relationships (Swarbrick, 1997). Wellness views a person holistically, more than simply mental and emotional well-being, and includes physical, intellectual, social, environmental, occupational, financial and spiritual dimensions (Swarbrick, 2012).

BOX 65-3 ADDED VALUE OF OCCUPATIONAL THERAPISTS ON INTERPROFESSIONAL BEHAVIORAL HEALTH CARE TEAMS

- Occupational therapy is a deeply person-centered approach, and OT practitioners are trained to assess cognitive and functional impairments.
- Occupational therapy practitioners help determine the likelihood that an individual will engage in services, effectively participate in treatment, and change his or her behaviors as necessary to sustain recovery.
- Occupational therapy practitioners use performance-based testing, which yields clinical insight and impact from everyday activities that have high potential to engage clients in a relatively brief amount of time.
- Cognitive functioning testing helps a team to more appropriately engage individuals in planning the treatment and recovery support that is right for them

- (i.e., self-care, household management, childcare, and workplace tasks).
- Occupational therapy practitioners assess each client's ability to perform tasks to determine how or whether the client initiates a real-world task, avoids and/or corrects errors, sequences and executes task steps, and demonstrates intrapersonal skill and good time management.
- Occupational therapy practitioners can help calibrate interventions (group or individual treatment based on sensory needs and cognitive capacity), develop health promotion plans, and support chronic disease management (i.e., habits and routines related to medication physical activity, occupational engagement, and sleep).

---

people with major mental disorders such as acute or longer term inpatient units, partial hospitalization programs, intensive outpatient programs, and even with homeless shelters (Gutman, Raphael-Greenfield, & Simon, 2016). Occupational therapists are forging into new terrain working on integrated primary care teams and in certified community behavioral health clinics (CCBHCs). Occupational therapists may be employed in any of these programs in various capacities, from direct service provider to consultant, program coordinator, or director. Occupational therapists can serve as case managers and often facilitate groups that address social skills, work and education, health management, and activities of daily living. In all capacities, occupational therapists contribute their unique expertise to increase the individual's occupational participation and quality of life. Box 65-3 outlines OT value working with interprofessional behavioral health care teams.

Long-Term and Acute Inpatient Facilities

Persons with serious mental disorders often begin to display symptoms in early adulthood. This can lead to the need for intensive services, which may include an acute inpatient hospitalization if the individual is acutely psychotic, depressed, suicidal, manic, or displaying other behaviors that might pose a threat to self or others. Some individuals seek voluntary admission for evaluation and treatment that will enable them to stabilize and resume their lives in a safe environment. In community hospitals, inpatient services are short term (a few days to a few weeks) but are longer in state-run facilities or forensic hospitals for people

often involuntarily committed. While in the hospital, the focus is brief intervention to stabilize symptoms and provide a comprehensive evaluation and diagnosis. At times, hospitalization is needed to start or change medications and monitor significant side effects. An interprofessional team of health care professionals, including physicians, nurses, social workers, and occupational therapists, works together to facilitate recovery. Occupational therapy practitioners working in the inpatient and day hospitals focus on instrumental activities of daily living (IADL), including health management, community navigation, home management, budgeting and money management, meal preparation, and grocery shopping.

Occupational therapists are valued members of inpatient treatment teams, providing individual functional assessment, individual occupation-focused treatment, therapeutic group facilitation, and participation in discharge planning (Lloyd & Williams, 2010). Starting with a comprehensive functional evaluation, they provide practical and functional interventions to help clients establish or reestablish healthy habits of daily living while on the unit and plan for community reintegration after discharge. Interventions may be offered in both group and individual format, and topics include wellness self-care skills to manage illness and prevent relapse; relaxation through leisure; time management; and exploration of leisure activities such as arts and crafts, fitness, and sports. Occupational therapists working in these settings can help facilitate the recovery process, assisting individuals in identifying strengths and challenges, developing treatment/intervention goals, and providing skill building and resources development interventions in group and individual format.

Occupational therapists are also involved in the design, development, and therapeutic application of

CENTENNIAL NOTES

Use of Drama, Puppets, and Marionettes in Occupational Therapy

Lori T. Andersen

In the 1920s and 1930s, occupational therapists started using drama, puppetry, and marionettes as a clinical modality with patients of all age ranges from young children to adults including soldiers serving in the military who had mental health issues, emotional issues, and/or physical problems (Figure 65-2) (Campbell, 1970; Eibeschutz, 1960; Phillips, 1996). The use of drama allowed the patient to dramatize conflicts and express obscure problems (Edgerton, 1947, p. 40–59). This engaging activity could be modified for use with individuals or groups and during the 1920 to 1930s time frame was used with patients in psychiatric facilities. Often in these settings, a full range of activities associated with puppets and marionettes culminated in a theatrical performance. Tasks could be divided up among residents, assigned according to the patient's capability and interests, and graded according to their needs. Tasks could range from singular and simple to multiple and more complex including creation of puppets and marionettes, construction of sets and stage props, writing plays and music, and acting with or handling of puppets or marionettes. The goals were to gain insight, enhance self-concept, promote competence, and improve socialization and social skills.

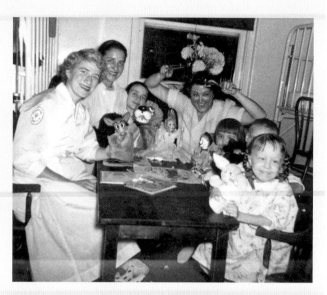

FIGURE 65-2 Occupational therapists using puppets and marionettes with a group of children at Washington University.

"sensory rooms" in these settings. These sensorimotor or multisensory rooms have been developed as environmental enhancements in response to evidence that many people with serious mental disorders experience sensory challenges, especially during times of crisis. The individuals may benefit from interventions designed to calm or stimulate their sensory systems and help them avoid seclusion and restraint (Champagne, 2006; Champagne & Stromberg, 2004). In one study, the rate of seclusion/restraint in the unit was reduced by 54% during the year of sensory room implementation (Champagne, 2006). Multisensory rooms can include calming elements such as weighted blankets for deep pressure, rocking chairs, calming music, and relaxing oils such as lavender or vanilla. Stimulating elements can include exercise equipment, peppermint or citrus oils, art materials, and energetic music.

Partial Hospitalization Programs

Partial hospitalization programs are designed for people who need a more intensive level of support than can be provided by outpatient visits. Persons at this level may be functioning adequately in one or more of their occupational roles but need more support or therapy than traditional outpatient treatment. Partial hospitalization programs are intended to divert the person from expensive and restrictive inpatient settings or serve as an intermediary step toward community living after treatment in an intensive setting. The goal is to reduce acute symptoms and provide crisis intervention. Services include a comprehensive evaluation of client needs and a coordinated array of active treatment components, delivered in a manner that is least disruptive to and/or simulates daily functioning. Services are delivered in the least restrictive environment, rely on client strengths, and use existing family and community supports. Occupational therapy practitioners in these settings focus on comprehensive and accurate assessment of function; preparation for community reintegration; and teaching of coping, stress management, and community living skills. Occupational therapists can assess functional cognition, which is the way an individual utilizes and integrates his or her thinking and processing skills to accomplish everyday activities. The OT practitioner can advise adjustments to the care plan if individuals' cognitive deficits reduce their capacity to understand their diagnosis, effectively participate in care planning, take medication, attend routine appointments, or successfully engage in interventions (especially the modalities rooted in cognitive behavioral therapy).

Community Settings

Community-based settings support individuals who reside outside of an inpatient or forensic facility, and may serve people who live independently, with their families, in structured or supervised residential programs, or on the streets (Swarbrick, 2016). Any of the emerging and evidence-based approaches described in the previous section may be used with people served in these settings.

Certified Community Behavioral Health Clinics

Certified community behavioral health clinics are a new innovation in the field of behavioral health care. Certified community behavioral health clinics are required to provide coordinated integrated care that is person-centered and recovery-oriented and to integrate physical and behavioral health care (SAMHSA, 2015). Licensed occupational therapists are included among the professions that states might require under CCBHC funding guidelines in order to best meet service and quality requirements of the program (SAMHSA, 2015). Because occupational therapists are trained to understand mental health diagnoses, assess functional challenges, and help individuals do what they need and want to do each day, their work complements the work of other staff on the team. Occupational therapists have the expertise to ensure that interprofessional teams identify and address commonly overlooked barriers to wellness and recovery, such as cognitive impairments, sensory needs, and difficulties with activities of daily living and social interactions. Each of these performance areas impacts goals related to housing, education, employment, and other valued occupational roles. As part of a CCBHC team, occupational therapists can contribute to the assessment and treatment by the following:

- Identifying individual strengths, goals, skills, and other factors important for wellness and recovery planning
- Performing psychosocial evaluations, including housing, vocational, and educational status as well as social support networks and community participation
- Assessing basic competency through cognitive impairment screening
- Assessing the need for other supports including family/caregiver support, targeted management, and psychiatric rehabilitation
- Helping persons served develop day-to-day independent living skills and improving their functional capacity

- Teaching compensatory strategies that mitigate the impact of the illness and how to reduce symptoms through engagement in healthy roles and routines
- Promoting health and wellness through the use of everyday activities

Occupational therapists working in a CCBHC can use a wellness- and recovery-oriented approach because it is congruent with the profession's person-centered, occupation-based practice, engages people served in their health management, and promotes independence in living a balanced and satisfying life.

Supported Employment

Supported employment is an approach to vocational rehabilitation that helps people with mental disorders to attain and succeed in competitive jobs. The Individual Placement and Support (IPS) model of supported employment has a strong evidence base that reinforces its value in vocational rehabilitation for people with major mental disorders. The program has a clear procedural manual, fidelity scale, and defined training procedures (Swanson & Becker, 2013) with the results of over 15 randomized control trials showing that about two-thirds of clients enrolled in IPS who supported employment achieved competitive employment within 12 to 18 months (Luciano et al., 2014). Recent research is examining the effectiveness of compensatory cognitive enhancement strategies to enhance employment success (McGuirk et al., 2015), which presents an ideal role for OT practitioners within the IPS model. IPS supported employment is a team-based model often integrated with one or more interprofessional teams (e.g., case management, assertive community treatment, intensive case management, supportive housing). In the area of employment supports, occupational therapists can use their knowledge and skills in the areas of task analysis, grading of tasks, and modifying work environments to help clients achieve success, provide direct services as job coaches, and assist with all phases of vocational services: assessing, planning, developing, acquiring, mastering, retaining, and changing jobs.

Supported Education

Supported education is an emerging best practice to help individuals with major mental disorders succeed in higher education. Educational advancement boosts earning power, preventing people from being stuck in low-wage jobs and poverty. Supported education funding often emphasizes employment-related educational goals rather than just general educational achievement. Educational goals include completing a high school equivalency diploma, obtaining a technical training certificate, taking adult education courses at a community college, or attaining a college degree (Mowbray et al., 2005).

Early supported education models included a classroom model where people with major mental disorders attended closed classes on campus (Arbesman & Logsdon, 2011), but supported education services increasingly involve providing individualized supports for clients taking classes in normalized settings while accessing available supports and accommodations through disability services provided by the educational institution.

Occupational therapists assist prospective students to identify educational skills and interests, enter the educational setting, and access needed resources such as financial aid and tutoring (Schindler & Kientz, 2013; Schindler & Sauerwald, 2013). Occupational therapists can be effective in helping students overcome barriers to school attendance, including self-esteem issues, challenges in social relationships, and managing personal and family issues. Occupational therapists have many relevant areas of expertise, such as strategies for stress and symptom management and improving memory, retention, concentration, and problem solving. Occupational therapists can play an important role in helping people with major mental disorders achieve college success, avoid unemployment, secure economic self-sufficiency, and improve their quality of life.

First Episode Programs

Specialized programs aim to promote recovery and independence among young people experiencing early psychosis or other psychiatric symptoms, with a goal of preventing or reducing long-term disability. Most of these programs, known as **first episode programs**, emphasize individualized plans of care that are developed and implemented with an interprofessional behavioral health care team. Team members often include occupational therapists, psychiatrists, family supporters or therapists, social workers, supported education and employment specialists, peer supporters, and psychologists. Because OT is the only profession that looks at the person–environment–occupation interaction (Waite, 2014), the occupational therapist fills a unique and valuable role in this setting, primarily across the three domains of assessment, intervention, and advocacy (Lloyd, Waghorn, Williams, Harris, & Capra, 2008). Effective assessment by an occupational therapist provides information on the occupational role functioning of a young person. Intervention services provide consultative and direct treatment to assist the young person in engaging in developmentally and culturally appropriate occupational roles. Advocacy involves educating members of the multidisciplinary mental health team about the role and potential outcomes of OT. Depending on each young person's needs and goals, the occupational therapist may provide skill-based assessments, occupational-based interventions, and/or caregiver education. Research on employment and educational outcomes in early intervention programs for early psychosis support the value of these programs (Bond, Drake, & Luciano, 2015; Poon, Siu, & Ming, 2010; Rinaldi, Perkins, McNeil, Hickman, & Singh, 2015). Psychoeducational group interventions for individuals with psychosis and their families also have been beneficial (Calvo et al., 2015).

Peer-Support Services

A growing body of research demonstrates the benefits of peer-led services in behavioral health (Bellamy, Schmutte, & Davidson, 2017). Peer-led or **peer-support services** are a part of the continuum of services available in the community based on the concept of peer support, a belief that people who have faced, endured, or overcome adversity can offer useful support, hope, and encouragement to others in similar situations. The peer-led support service model has been evolving throughout the world and in the United States is considered an essential ingredient in many people's mental health recovery. Occupational therapists link clients to peer resources and also provide consultation and mentoring for the development and growth of peer programs. Peer-led services are based on the premise that people in recovery helping others pursue their recovery foster hope and optimism—people connect most easily with people who have similar experiences (Bellamy et al., 2017; Swarbrick, 2017). Peer-led support services may be offered before, during, and after treatment to facilitate long-term recovery in the community. Peer-led support can be offered in inpatient and community settings. Peers may provide assistance by promoting community integration, developing coping and problem-solving strategies for illness self-management, drawing on their lived experiences, and offering empathy to promote hope, insights, and skills (Bellamy et al., 2017; Swarbrick, 2017). Peer support specialists help clients engage in treatment or access community supports to help reestablish a satisfying life. Many opportunities exist for OT practitioners to collaborate with and promote peer-led support services and peer support specialists. Practitioners who work in all aspects of behavioral health care, including public inpatient state facilities, Veterans Administration services, and community-based settings, have the requisite knowledge and skills to collaborate with peers to develop, implement, and/or evaluate peer-led services regardless of the service setting or model used.

Peer-led support services and working alongside peer support specialists can be an excellent nontraditional student field worksite. For many years, Collaborative Support Programs of New Jersey (Swarbrick & Ellis, 2009) has been a fieldwork site for OT programs and has allowed students to be collaborative research partners. Occupational therapists working at universities collaborate on person-centered projects. For many years, local researchers have engaged the community wellness centers to cocreate research projects through the collaborative efforts of OT researchers, OT students, and center members. Examples of research projects include identifying sensory preferences of members (Gardner, Swarbrick, Kearns, et al., 2017), determining how physical limitations affect occupational functioning (Gardner, Swarbrick, Ackerman, et al., 2017), and studying sleep habits and routines (Gardner, Swarbrick, Dennis, et al., 2017).

Emerging and Evidence-Based Models

Models developed by occupational therapists are increasingly recognized as effective based on research evidence demonstrating positive outcomes.

Action Over Inertia (Krupa et al., 2010), an occupational time use intervention, is a standardized tool to target occupational balance and engagement for people with major mental disorders. *Action Over Inertia* was found to have clinical utility based on feedback from both treatment participants and the occupational therapists involved in the delivery of the treatment. Developed in Canada, this approach has been implemented and researched in Canada, Austria, and Germany. *Action Over Inertia* encourages occupational balance and participation with individuals with major mental disorders living in the community by supporting individuals in overcoming the barriers preventing them from deriving meaning and enjoyment from the wide range of activities that make up their daily life (Edgelow & Krupa, 2011; Krupa, Fossey, Anthony, Brown, & Pitts, 2009). *Action Over Inertia* uses a collaborative approach based on OT techniques. The program lasts for 10 weeks, meeting in hourly sessions to explore the various dimensions of activity engagement. These include balance, physical activity, structure and routine, the experience of meaning and purpose, satisfaction with activities, social interaction through activities, and access to community environments. The program conveys a message of optimism—that a fulfilling life and engagement in meaningful activities and social interaction are possible in spite of the challenges of living with a major mental disorder.

Let's Get Organized is a program designed to help individuals with co-occurring mental and substance use disorders improve their organization and time management skills. The aim of the program is to improve participants' ability to perform life's daily tasks, such as being on time to work. Success at daily tasks leads to success in valued life roles, such as maintaining employment, which, in turn, supports continued sobriety. The results of a small pilot study demonstrated improvements in participants' knowledge and behaviors related to time management, skills

that are critical to successful reentry into the community (White, 2007).

To address the weight gain that commonly occurs when taking psychiatric medication, Catana Brown and collaborators created and revised a weight-loss program now called *Nutrition and Exercise for Weight Loss and Recovery* (NEW-R; Brown et al., 2015). The NEW-R curriculum provides both a leader manual and a participant manual to guide each session over the 2 months of the program, using a 90-minute session format of didactic teaching of nutritional and other health content, followed by active learning in which participants practice skills and make plans to apply the information in their own lives. This format allows the program to be highly individualized to each participant's needs, strengths, interests, and personal situation. The written curriculum is supplemented by free videos for the exercise segments of the program. Designed by occupational therapists, the videos feature OT students and people in recovery dancing, doing yoga, building upper and lower body strength, and performing other exercises. The NEW-R can be taught in mental health or social service agencies, peer-run programs, community health clinics, or in a private space in the community.

The *Housing Transition Program* (Gutman et al., 2016) was designed to support homeless adults with major mental disorders and substance use challenges. This 3-week intervention was offered at a homeless shelter using instructional videos, graphics, and opportunities for hands-on practice of functional skills in a simulated apartment setting. Participants in a pilot study indicated that the program was engaging and helped them better understand the housing transition process.

The following case examples (Case Studies 65-1 and 65-2) illustrate needs of people served and examples of roles for occupational therapists.

Conclusion

Major mental disorders continue to impact people in society at increasing rates. It is inevitable that occupational therapists will encounter individuals with major mental disorders regardless of their chosen practice setting. Because OT is a profession that focuses on occupational engagement and the links to health and well-being, occupational therapists are becoming more valued in new practice arenas working with peer-led programs and peer support specialists; on first episode/early intervention teams; and as members of CCBHCs promoting occupation, wellness, and community integration. Occupational therapists have an important role as a member of interprofessional team collaborating with people served to help increase their involvement in meaningful occupation, providing functional skills assessment, planning and

CASE STUDY 65-1 JOSEPH

Ruth Ramsey

Joseph is a 55-year-old man who has received services from the public mental health system for over 30 years. He has been hospitalized many times and received numerous mental health diagnoses. He was first diagnosed with schizophrenia at age 21 years but is currently diagnosed with bipolar disorder and co-occurring alcohol dependence. Joseph is the second of seven siblings. At age 9 years, he experienced a very stressful traumatic incident (sexual abuse by a relative). He recently was enrolled in a certified community behavioral health clinic (CCBHC) where Julie, an occupational therapist, is a member of the interprofessional team. Julie met with Joseph to complete an Occupational Profile and Activity Engagement measure (Krupa et al., 2010), reviewing his strengths, needs, and goals, and to develop a strengths-based wellness plan.

Joseph recently was diagnosed with fibromyalgia and reports intense pain and bouts of sleeplessness. He reported that he seems to feel better physically, emotionally, and socially when he follows a regular sleep-and-wake schedule. However, he has significant difficulty adhering to a regular routine and was unable to pinpoint and describe the many factors that contribute to this. Joseph is currently prescribed bimonthly medications that make him feel tired, and he believes they have caused his significant weight gain. He is very concerned about his weight. He has been smoking for more than 30 years and is planning to quit smoking sometime soon. He states that he realizes he needs to take medication to maintain stability, although he has major concerns regarding side effects (short- and long-term), especially how the medication slows him down and contributes to weight gain.

Joseph is a high school graduate. He hopes to find volunteer or paid work opportunities to use his talents and skills so he can improve his sense of purpose and meaning. He periodically walks a neighbor's dogs, which he finds quite rewarding. He feels very disheartened because family and professionals often discourage him from working, which they believe would be too stressful for him. He believes that he is capable of getting and keeping a job. He is interested in learning new information, particularly in the areas of the environment, and recently was able to purchase a computer. He likes to share what he learns. Joseph reports that he frequently feels lonely. He is currently living on a very limited budget and receives a housing subsidy to offset the costs for living in a studio apartment. He has the ability to manage money effectively. Joseph takes pride in his appearance and apartment. He has determined a budget so he can do his laundry and purchase good food and household supplies. He wants a part-time job so he can eat out once in a while, purchase new clothing, and eventually plan to save for the future. He reported that walking the dogs provides purpose and a reason to get up in the morning, which helps him prioritize going to bed early on a consistent basis so he can wake up in time to walk the dogs. Julie, the occupational therapist working on the CCBHC team, will help Joseph with the following wellness goals that he identified to help him develop an increased sense of purpose and self-sufficiency.

1. Maintain a daily healthy routine: Wake up and go to sleep at set times and create a daily routine for balance and emotional equilibrium.
2. Secure a part-time job at least three to four times a week (3 to 5 hours per day).
3. Increase physical activity to prevent further weight gain and risk for sedentary lifestyle.

CASE STUDY 65-2 ADAM

Ruth Ramsey

Adam, age 19 years, likes to paint and draw, is gifted musically, and plays guitar and drums. He had a normal childhood and did well in school. In his first year of college, he began to have difficulties, which included inability to attend classes and complete assignments, lack of attention to personal self-care, disturbed sleeping, trouble concentrating, hearing voices, and social withdrawal. He started drinking and smoking marijuana heavily. He was found singing loudly in the halls of his dorm several times at 3 a.m. A friend called his parents, who came to the school and suggested Adam be seen by a physician. By this time, he was sleep-deprived

and became angry and agitated when his parents told him their intention to have him hospitalized as a "danger to self." The police were called, and Adam was escorted to the emergency department of a local community hospital, where he was involuntarily committed. He was able to reestablish normal sleeping and eating patterns while in the hospital and, together with his team, make plans for future treatment.

The psychiatrist diagnosed Adam as having schizophrenia and referred him to a first episode program. Team members included an occupational therapist, psychiatrist, peer support specialist, a supported education and employment specialist, and family support specialist. The family support specialist met with Adam's family to help them understand the implications

CASE STUDY 65-2   ADAM *(continued)*

of his new diagnosis and how they could support him in his recovery. Adam meets with a psychiatrist to evaluate his response to medications and confer with the staff about his progress. The occupational therapist, Rita, met with Adam for an initial OT evaluation to help him identify personally meaningful treatment goals. Adam reported that he decided he would return to live with his parent who converted their garage into a studio apartment for him. He feels this will allow him space to practice his music and art. He reported he will be able to fix himself a sandwich in his mini kitchen.

Rita met with Adam to develop a daily grooming schedule and agreed to review it with him daily before morning meeting. They also made plans to meet individually twice weekly so he could learn some mindfulness approaches. Adam appeared very motivated to go back to school. He adjusted well to the antipsychotic medication with few side effects and started sleeping better. He said that the mindfulness meditation helped him learn to relax, focus, and ignore the voices he

was hearing. Rita and Adam discussed his plans to create a structured routine that would include a balance of sleep, physical activity, and participation in meaningful activity, and Adam planned to live with his parents while he continued his recovery. He continued to meet with his psychiatrist to ensure that the medications were helping to control his symptoms. The supported education and employment specialist helped Adam find a part-time job at a local art supply store and register for one class at a local community college. The peer support specialist provided Adam information about a young adult wellness program for individuals experiencing mental health challenges. Over time, Rita, the occupational therapist, helped Adam with time management and activity engagement, whereas the peer support specialist helped him become more comfortable and empowered to socialize with other young people, use the computers at the college computer lab, attend outings, and take additional classes on topics such as computer graphics and tai chi.

implementing wellness-focused interventions. Time use interventions and activity engagement tools are examples of strategies that can enhance mental health and recovery outcomes. Occupational therapists can play an important role educating and mentoring peer support specialists, frontline direct providers, and professional staff as well as assuming a lead role participating in program development and leadership. Occupational therapists can make meaningful contributions to improving the lives of people with major mental disorders especially in the areas of managing comorbid conditions and promoting wellness.

REFERENCES

American Psychiatric Association. (2013). *Diagnostic and statistical manual of mental disorders.* 5th ed. Arlington, VA: Author.

Arbesman, M., & Logsdon, D. (2011). Occupational therapy interventions for employment and education for adults with serious mental illness: A systematic review. *American Journal of Occupational Therapy, 65,* 238–246.

Bellamy, B., Schmutte, T., & Davidson, L. (2017). An update on the growing evidence base for peer support. *Mental Health and Social Inclusion, 21,* 161–167.

Bond, G. R., Drake, R. E., & Luciano, A. (2015). Employment and educational outcomes in early intervention programmes for early psychosis: A systematic review. *Epidemiologia e Psichiatria Sociale, 24,* 446–457. doi:10.1017/S2045796014000419

Brown, C., Read, H., Stanton, M., Zeeb, M., Jonikas, J., & Cook, J. (2015). A pilot study of the nutrition and exercise for weight loss and recovery (NEW-R): A weight loss program for individuals with serious mental illness. *Psychiatric Rehabilitation Journal, 38,* 371–373.

Calvo, A., Moreno, M., Ruiz-Sancho, A., Rapado-Castro, M., Moreno, C., Sanchez-Gutierrez, T., . . . Mayoral, M. (2015). Psychoeducational group intervention for adolescents with psychosis and their families: A two-year follow-up. *Journal of the American Academy of Child and Adolescent Psychiatry, 54,* 984–990. doi:10.1016/j.jaac.2015.09.018

Campbell, C. M. (1970). The use of puppetry in occupational therapy. *British Journal of Occupational Therapy, 33,* 9–11.

Center for Mental Health Services. (2010). *The 10 by 10 campaign: A national action plan to improve life expectancy by 10 years in 10 years for people with mental illnesses. A report of the 2007 National Wellness Summit* (HHS Publication No. [SMA] 10-4476). Rockville, MD: Center for Mental Health Services, Substance Abuse and Mental Health Administration.

Champagne, T. (2006). *Sensory modulation and environment: Essential elements for occupation. General handbook and references* (2nd ed.). Southampton, MA: Champagne Conferences and Consultation.

Champagne, T., & Stromberg, N. (2004). Sensory approaches in inpatient mental disorders settings: Innovative alternatives to seclusion and restraint. *Journal of Psychosocial Nursing, 42,* 35–44.

Druss, B. G., Zhao, L., Von Esenwein, S., Morrato, E. H., & Marcus, S. C. (2011). Understanding excess mortality in persons with mental illness: 17-year follow up of a nationally representative US survey. *Medical Care, 49,* 599–604. Retrieved from http://journals.lww.com/lww-medicalcare/Fulltext/2011/06000/Understanding_Excess_Mortality_in_Persons_With.11.aspx

Edgelow, M., & Krupa, T. (2011). Randomized controlled pilot study of an occupational time-use intervention for people with serious mental illness. *American Journal of Occupational Therapy, 65,* 267–276.

Edgerton, W. M. (1947). Activities in occupational therapy. In H. S. Willard & C. S. Spackman (Eds.), *Principles of occupational therapy* (pp. 40–59). Philadelphia: PA: J. B. Lippincott.

Eibeschutz, I. (1960). Puppetry in hospital. *British Journal of Occupational Therapy, 23,* 27–29.

Gardner, J., Swarbrick, M., Ackerman, A., Church, T., Rios, V., Valente, L., & Rutledge, J. (2017). Effects of physical limitations on daily activities among adults with mental health disorders: opportunities for nursing and occupational therapy interventions. *Journal of Psychosocial Nursing Mental Health Services, 55*(10), 45-51.

Gardner, J., Swarbrick, M., Dennis, S., Franklin, M., Pricken, M., & Rodriguez, K. (2017). *Sleep habits and routines of individuals diagnosed with mental and/or substance use disorders.* Unpublished manuscript.

Gardner, J., Swarbrick, M., Kearns, D., Suero, L., Moscoe, E., Harder, P., . . . Rutledge, J. (2017, March). *Sensory preferences of community wellness center members*. Poster session presented at American Occupational Therapy Association Annual Conference, Philadelphia, PA.

Gutman, S. A., Raphael-Greenfield, E. I., & Simon, P. M. (2016). Feasibility and acceptability of a pilot housing transition program for homeless adults with mental illness and substance use. *Occupational Therapy in Health Care, 30*, 124–138.

Gutman, S. A., & Swarbrick, P. (1998). The multiple linkages between childhood sexual abuse, adult alcoholism, and traumatic brain injury in women. *Occupational Therapy in Mental Health, 14*, 33–65. doi:10.1300/J004v14n03_03

Krupa, T., Edgelow, M., Chen, S., Mieras, C., Perry, A., Radloff-Gabriel, D., . . . Bransfield, M. (2010). *Action over inertia: Addressing the activity-health needs of individuals with serious mental illness*. Ontario, Canada: Canadian Association of Occupational Therapists.

Krupa, T., Fossey, E., Anthony, W. A., Brown, C., & Pitts, D. B. (2009). Doing daily life: How occupational therapy can inform psychiatric rehabilitation practice. *Psychiatric Rehabilitation Journal, 32*, 155–161.

Lloyd, C., Waghorn, G., Williams, P., Harris, M., & Capra, C. (2008). Early psychosis: Treatment issues and the role of occupational therapy. *British Journal of Occupational Therapy, 71*, 297–304. doi:10.1177/030802260807100708

Lloyd, C., & Williams, P. L. (2010). Occupational therapy in the modern acute mental health setting: A review of current practice. *International Journal of Therapy and Rehabilitation, 17*, 483–493.

Luciano, A., Drake, R. E., Bond, G. R., Becker, D. R., Carpenter-Song, E., Lord, S., & Swanson, S. J. (2014). Evidence-based supported employment for people with severe mental illness: Past, current, and future research. *Journal of Vocational Rehabilitation, 40*, 1–13.

McGuirk, S., Mueser, K., Xie, H., Welsh, J., Kaiser, J., Drake, R., . . . McHugo, G. (2015). Cognitive enhancement treatment for people with a mental illness who do not respond to supported employment: A randomized control trial. *American Journal of Psychiatry, 172*, 852–861.

Meyer, A. (1922). The philosophy of occupational therapy. Reprinted from the *Archives of Occupational Therapy. The British Journal of Psychiatry, 68*, 421–423. doi:10.1192/bjp.68.283.421

Mowbray, C. T., Collins, M. E., Bellamy, C. D., Megivern, D. A., Bybee, D., & Szilvagyi, S. (2005). Supported education for adults with mental disorders: An innovation for social and psychological rehabilitation practice. *Social Work, 50*, 7–20.

Phillips, M. E. (1996). The use of drama and puppetry in occupational therapy during the 1920s and 1930s. *American Journal of Occupational Therapy, 50*, 229–233.

Poon, M. Y. C., Siu, A. M. H., & Ming, S. Y. (2010). Outcome analysis of occupational therapy programme for persons with early psychosis. *Work, 37*, 65–70. doi:10.3233/WOR-2010-1057

Rinaldi, M., Perkins, R., McNeil, K., Hickman, N., & Singh, S. P. (2015). The individual placement and support approach to vocational rehabilitation for young people with first episode psychosis in the UK. *Journal of Mental Health, 19*, 483–491. doi:10.3109/09638230903531100

Schindler, V., & Kientz, M. (2013). Supports and barriers to higher education and employment for individuals diagnosed with mental illness. *The Journal of Vocational Rehabilitation, 39*, 39–41. doi:10.3233/JVR-130640

Schindler, V., & Sauerwald, C. (2013). Outcomes of a 4-year program with higher education and employment goals for individuals diagnosed with mental illness. *Work, 4*, 325–336. doi:10.3233/WOR-121548

Steel, Z., Marnane, C., Iranpour, C., Chey, T., Jackson, J. W., Patel, V., & Silove, D. (2014). The global prevalence of common mental disorders: a systematic review and meta-analysis 1980-2013. *International Journal of Epidemiology, 43*, 476–493.

Substance Abuse and Mental Health Services Administration. (2011). *SAMHSA news release: SAMHSA announces a working definition of "recovery" from mental disorders and substance use disorders*. Retrieved from http://www.samhsa.gov/newsroom/advisories/1112223420.aspx

Substance Abuse and Mental Health Services Administration. (2015). *Criteria for the demonstration program to improve community mental health centers and to establish certified community behavioral health clinics*. Retrieved from https://www.samhsa.gov/sites/default/files/programs_campaigns/ccbhc-criteria.pdf

Swanson, S. J., & Becker, D. R. (2013). *Individual placement and support (IPS) supported employment: A practical guide*. Lebanon, NH: Dartmouth Psychiatric Research Center.

Swarbrick, M. (1997). A wellness model for clients. *Mental Health Special Interest Section Newsletter, 20*, 1–4.

Swarbrick, M. (2012). A wellness approach to mental health recovery. In A. Rudnick (Ed.), *Recovery of people with mental illness: Philosophical and related perspectives* (pp. 30–38). Oxford, United Kingdom: Oxford University Press.

Swarbrick, M. (2016). Support models to enhance community transitions. *SIS Quarterly Practice Connections, 1*(2), 14–16.

Swarbrick, M. (2017). Peer-led treatment. In A. Wenzel (Ed.), *The SAGE encyclopedia of abnormal and clinical psychology* (pp. 2511–2512). Thousand Oaks, CA: Sage. doi:10.4135/9781483365817.n1008

Swarbrick, M., & Duffy, M. (2000). A consumer run self-help program model. *Mental Health Special Interest Section Quarterly, 23*(1), 1–4.

Swarbrick, M., & Ellis, J. (2009). Peer-operated self-help centers. *Occupational Therapy in Mental Health, 25*, 239–251. doi:10.1080/01642120903083960

Waite, A., (2014). On the brink: Occupational therapy helps address early psychosis. *OT Practice, 19*(11), 297–304.

White, S. M. (2007). Let's get organized: An intervention for persons with co-occurring disorders. *Psychiatric Services, 58*, 713. doi:10.1176/appi.ps.58.5.713

the**Point**® *For additional resources on the subjects discussed in this chapter, visit* **http://thePoint.lww.com /Willard-Spackman13e.**

A Woodworker's Hand Injury

Restoring a Life

Karen Roe Garren

LEARNING OBJECTIVES

After reading this chapter, you will be able to:

1. Describe the primary elements found in an evaluation for a person with a hand injury.
2. Identify objective measures that might be used to evaluate a complex injury.
3. Describe client-centered goal setting.
4. Understand the use of functional activities to restore specific anatomical function and client-desired function.
5. Describe the use of physical agent modalities to enhance healing and restoration of function.

THERAPIST NARRATIVE

Over years of practice, I have learned to incorporate methods such as physical agent modalities, manual therapy techniques, and wound care into hand therapy. However, occupational therapy (OT) methods and philosophy have always been the foundation of my therapeutic approach. Helping clients to achieve occupational goals requires more than tissue healing and joint mobility. I have learned that recovery is a fabric woven from psychological, spiritual, and physical pain. Hand therapy is about restoring meaning in client's lives as well as restoring tissue function.

Case Description: Don

It was a shock to hear that the father-in-law of a woman who worked in our building had cut his hand badly in a table saw. When he actually walked into the clinic, it was one of those moments when I could feel my heart sink. Don is a 58-year-old fine woodworker who built spectacular and complex crown moldings and built-ins in very upscale homes. He had indeed put his left hand through a table saw at work 10 days earlier. I had just gotten a call from the hand surgeon upstairs telling me that he was sending Don down to be seen immediately for splinting and to start therapy. This doctor had not done the surgery; Don had been rushed to a hospital near where he worked some distance away and was operated on there

CENTENNIAL NOTES

Occupational Therapists and Hand Therapy

World War II was the catalyst that created the specialty of hand surgery. Dr. Sterling Bunnell, author of the 1944 book, *Surgery of the Hand*, was recruited to educate U.S. Army surgeons and organize hand centers in nine Army hospitals (Omer, 2000; Yakobina, Yakobina, Harrison-Weaver, 2008). In 1955, Bunnell wrote, "Contrary to the degeneration of disuse there is revivification of tissues on voluntary use and the will to do. It is in this respect that occupational therapy is superior to passive physical therapy."

In 1955, in a paper for the U.S. Army on hand surgery, Bunnell said, "In rehabilitation of the injured hand, occupational therapy played an extremely important role.

The patient was assigned a job on the basis of his needs, not just to keep him working. The occupational therapist knew the results desired and devoted her efforts to restoration of the special function which had been lost" (Bunnell, 1955).

In 1964, L. Irene Hollis, OTR, was recruited by Dr. Erle Peacock to help establish the first hand rehabilitation center at the University of North Carolina in Chapel Hill. Hollis, the 1979 Eleanor Clarke Slagle lecturer, authored the first chapter on hand rehabilitation in the fifth edition of *Willard and Spackman's Occupational Therapy*, published in 1978. The work of Hollis and other occupational therapists at the center, including Florence "Bunny" Bearden and Gloria Devore, helped to solidify the role of OT in hand therapy and eventually led to the establishment of the American Society of Hand Therapists (ASHT) in 1977 (Bell-Krotoski, 1989).

---

by a plastic surgeon. The operative report was not available, but from what the doctor was able to ascertain, Don had lacerated his hand through his proximal palm and severed both flexor tendons to his long and ring fingers, amputated his small finger at the metacarpal phalangeal (MP) joint, and lacerated the nerves to all his fingers. The doctor was not sure about the involvement to Don's thumb and index fingers. Don had arrived in his office bandaged and protected only by a wrist support with the fingers free to move at the proximal interphalangeal (PIP) joints. This was not good. I brought Don in immediately and told him not to move anything. He said that the doctor had just told him that, but the only thing that he had been told at discharge from the hospital was to follow up in a week. He thought wiggling his fingers was good because they were not immobilized.

There are critical elements to consider in dealing with a patient who has recently undergone reconstructive surgery of tendons and nerves. The first and foremost concern is to protect the repair. I knew enough history from the brief discussion with the referring surgeon to know that I needed to get Don into a protective splint as quickly as possible to reduce the tension on the tendon and nerve repairs and to stop any active motion of the repaired tendons (Duran & Houser, 1975; Taras, Martyak, & Steelman, 2011). I also needed to assess the wound to determine the integument (skin) condition and, because no operative report was available, to visually assess the exact anatomical level of injury. During this process, I was monitoring his reactions to the situation. It can be an extremely emotional time, and patients often have not even looked at their wounds. I keep ammonia capsules and facial tissues readily available. Don seemed to be coping by focusing on the process and asking questions. At the same time, I needed

to reassure Don that his zeal to get his fingers moving had probably not ruptured the repairs because he assured me that he could wiggle them. I do not deceive patients, but informing Don of all of the possible ramifications at that point would only have distressed him, and I needed him to be focused on where we were going and what he was going to need to do. Once Don's hand was bandaged in a dry dressing and he was safely tucked into a dorsal blocking splint that positioned his wrist in 30 degrees of flexion, his MPs in 70 degrees of flexion, and his PIPs and distal interphalangeal (DIP) joints in as much extension as he could actively produce (the ideal is full extension, but he was already contracted, and applying any force could compromise the repairs), I could safely continue his evaluation.

Note: Those with occupational performance limitations secondary to hand and/or upper extremity injuries, potentially interact with occupational therapists and certified occupational therapy assistants (COTAs) in a variety of settings (Box 66-1).

Don's Evaluation and Goal Setting

The evaluation consisted of the following:

Subjective examination and background
- Age, hand dominance
- Date and mechanism of injury
- Functional capability/work status
- Activities of daily living (ADL) status/help status
- Chief complaints: pain, loss of function, sensory changes, and/or sleep problems
- Rehabilitation expectations/goals

BOX 66-1   PROVISION OF OCCUPATIONAL THERAPY: CLIENTS WITH PERFORMANCE CHALLENGES SECONDARY TO HAND AND UPPER EXTREMITY INJURIES

In many instances, these clients are treated by occupational therapists specializing in this practice area and who carry the additional credential of "certified hand therapist." The majority of these injuries are treated in outpatient hospital settings or private practices. However, the setting and progression through the settings is determined by the type and severity of injury, insurance coverage, and client preference (see Figure 66-1 for two examples).

A variety of sources of funding/reimbursement are available for these services. Examples include the following:

- Medicare Part A. Covers outpatient services. Clients may be seen two to three times per week for up to 3 months.

- Medicaid. Covers 20 visits per year. After this, an authorization request may be sent to the referring physician to continue intervention.
- Private insurance. Coverage varies greatly based on plan. If the plan covers the service, clients are usually seen two to three times per week for up to 3 months as needed.
- Private pay.
- Workmen's compensation. A case file must be opened, and authorization for services varies greatly based on insurance. For example, a client may be authorized for 6 to 12 visits. After this, further authorization is required.

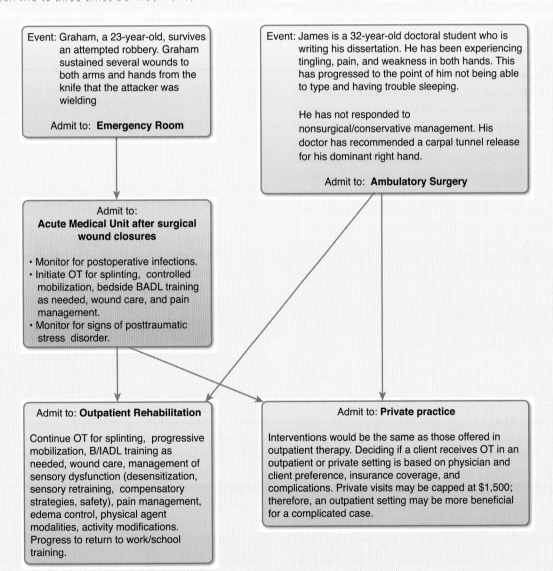

FIGURE 66-1 Two examples of progression through treatment settings. *BADL*, basic activities of daily living; *IADL*, instrumental activities of daily living; *OT*, occupational therapy.

- Medical management and review of medical/surgical records, including available radiographic summaries
- Awareness of pathology/precautions/contraindications/physician orders
- Past relevant medical history

Don was 58 years old at the time of the accident, right-handed, and married. He worked full-time as a woodworker and loved his job. He wanted to return to his occupation as soon as it was possible to do so; he needed to be able to lift and carry wood supplies, hold and manipulate tools and hardware, and stabilize wood with his left hand. Secondary to being immobilized in the splint, Don was unable to use his left hand for any self-care; however, over the previous week, he had become sufficiently proficient with his right hand alone to manage to dress, feed, bathe, and even drive himself. His wife managed the meals and household tasks. Initially, his chief complaints were loss of function, inability to move his hand, and numbness in all of his fingers. Don could not describe exactly how the accident had happened except that he was cutting wood on the table saw and it caught, pulling his hand down on the blade. This is a familiar story. The blade spins at an incredible speed, and when things go wrong, it is too fast to actually see or react. A table saw blade does not cut like a knife but consists of teeth that are a series of angled chisels that are an eighth of an inch wide or more. It leaves a fairly wide slot when it cuts wood. The same happened to Don's hand. The blade had amputated his small finger and continued across his proximal palm in zone 3. When the tendons and nerves were cut, the result was that several millimeters of tissue were missing as well as skin and thenar and hypothenar muscle. It follows that when the ends of the tendons and nerves were sutured together, the result was shortening of the muscles, tendons, and nerves, creating additional tension on the repair.

Objective examination
- Integument
- Range of motion (ROM)
- Sensation
- Edema

To evaluate Don's hand, I needed to keep in mind the protocol that I would use to guide his physical recovery. There are multiple protocols to choose from, with extensive research supporting advantages and disadvantages. Most surgeons have a preferred pathway or protocol, and the therapist must be aware of these differences in preference. Pettengill (2005) has written a historical perspective on the research of tendon rehabilitation, with a comparison of the most recent early active motion protocols. My input is usually taken into consideration; however, it is the doctor who decides which protocol he or she wants to follow. The doctor who made this referral does not like to use any of the early active motion protocols because he thinks that

research has shown that there is a greater risk of rupture. In Don's case, it was not an option because his was not a clean and simple wound, we were not starting therapy 3 days after surgery, and we had no knowledge of what suturing technique had been used to repair the tendons. In fact, we were beginning at the 10th day, which is when research has demonstrated that the tendon tissue actually softens and is at the highest risk of rupture. The doctor was concerned about the amount of trauma and the significant amount of scarring and wanted to minimize adhesions (bands of scar tissue that binds together two anatomic surfaces that are normally separated), so I used the modified Duran protocol (Duran & Houser, 1975) to begin early passive flexion with restricted active extension of the fingers but held any active motion until the sixth week. With his wrist and MPs splinted in flexion and his interphalangeal (IP) joints in extension, I taught Don to passively flex his fingers into his palm and actively extend his fingers as far as the splint would allow. This allowed a few millimeters of tendon excursion with minimal resistance on the repair and has been shown by research to reduce tendon adhesions. On visual inspection, his hand was moderately swollen, indicative of inflammation, and he was not able to fully flex his fingers to his palm. Don had multiple system trauma involving not only the tendons but also nerves, muscle, palmar fascia, and skin. I tested his sensation with the Semmes-Weinstein monofilament test (Bell-Krotoski, 2002) because I was not sure whether all the digital nerve branches were severed. The test revealed loss of protective sensation or complete numbness in the median and ulnar nerves to his index, long, and ring fingers.

Setting goals for Don's therapy ultimately centered on what Don wanted to accomplish. The doctor always pushes for a perfect physical outcome, and usually, the patient is in agreement; however, returning the patient to his or her previous job is not automatically a goal. I often do not set a return-to-work goal in the initial evaluation when there is a traumatic injury because it can be too early to determine what the patient wants and what the potential might be in terms of ability, time, and opportunity. Woodworking was Don's passion, not just his job. He had built something for each of his grandchildren, and he was anxious to build a rocking horse for his new grandchild.

For the next 5 weeks, the goals for Don were to understand the pathology, precautions, and home exercise program to increase his passive finger flexion; facilitate wound healing; and remodel scar to ensure necessary restoration of strength to the tendon tissues while safely allowing mobility through the adjacent tissues (Pettengill, 2011). The splint would not come off until the sixth week after surgery, so there could be no functional use of his hand. Don was diligent in his exercises and quickly recovered full passive finger flexion. He reported that he was keeping his hand elevated as much as possible to help decrease the swelling. The sutures were removed at 21 days with full skin closure. It was not until 4 weeks after his surgery that we finally got a copy of his original operative report revealing that there had been repair to his palmar arch, flexor pollicis longus to his thumb, and flexor digitorum superficialis (FDS) and flexor digitorum profundus (FDP) to his index finger, which had been only partially lacerated. The additional information helped me to anticipate what limitations there might be when the splint came off. Potential limitations included difficulty or inability to actively flex his thumb IP joint and index PIP and DIP joints due to scar adhesions or rupture from lack of protection in the first week postop.

Interventions and Ongoing Evaluation

Don's treatment initially consisted of manual ROM; dressing changes; and, when the sutures were removed, moist heat, low-intensity ultrasound, and manual scar massage to increase the soft tissue extensibility and remodel the scar. His treatment was a team effort with Erin (the other therapist in the clinic), Don, and me. This partnership required mutual attentiveness, the act of listening, and engaging in conversation in order for Don's feelings, needs, and desires to become part of the common understanding between Don, Erin, and myself (Crepeau, 1991; Crepeau & Garren, 2011; Rosendahl & Ross, 1982; Tickle-Degnen, 2008).

Six weeks after surgery was the next major hurdle for Don. The splint came off, and he was allowed to start moving his fingers (Table 66-1). It was hard to prepare Don for the disappointment that he felt when his fingers did not actively flex into a fist. His hope was beyond realistic expectation, but Don just wanted to move forward and do whatever it took to be able to use his hand again. He still had no sensation in his fingers.

TABLE 66-1 | **Active Range of Motion (in Degrees) at 6 Weeks Postsurgery**

6 Weeks Postsurgery	MP (0–90)	PIP (0–100)	DIP (0–80)
Index	0–60	−30–60	−10–30
Long	0–55	−30–45	−10–10
Ring	0–30	−35–45	−5–5
Thumb	−10–35		0–25
Wrist: 25–60			

MP, metacarpal phalangeal joint; PIP, proximal interphalangeal joint; DIP, distal interphalangeal joint.

His goals were to increase the active range of motion (AROM) of his fingers and wrist to pull up his pants, button his pants, hold a washcloth to bathe, and eventually hold tools to return to work. This required heat modalities; low-intensity 3-MHz ultrasound (Michlovitz, 2005); and manual therapy to facilitate healing, increase soft tissue mobility, and remodel scar. We used occupational coaching (Clark, Ennevor, & Richardson, 1996) to teach Don the skills and strategies he needed for attaining the mutually agreed-on goals. Occupational coaching involves several techniques aimed at moving Don toward a positive view of engagement in occupations. Examples of techniques include giving encouragement, making positive remarks, and teaching about occupation's role in recovery. We created a therapeutic alliance in which we worked in the presence of one another. Erin and I served as supportive function while guiding Don in an occupation-based intervention (Tickle-Degnen, 2008). As Don presented with a loss of protective sensation as measured by the Semmes-Weinstein monofilament test, we taught Don sensory loss precautions so that he would not accidentally burn or cut himself. His home program was expanded to include paraffin (to improve soft tissue extensibility) and a mini-vibrator (for scar remodeling and desensitization); however, he discovered that his hot tub water jets worked perfectly. Exercise and functional activities were initiated to increase his active motion and encourage grasp and pinch for pulling on clothes, holding utensils, and washing himself. He began desensitization for the scar and nerve hypersensitivity in his palm with particle immersion (submerging and moving the hand in rice and progressively more textured particles) and vibration (Pettengill, 2011).

For the next 6 weeks, Don used the dexerciser (a handheld wire maze that requires wrist and/or finger motion to move a washer along the wire), Chinese balls (2 to 2 ¾ in diameter smooth metal or enamel balls that are rotated around each other in the palm), pegboards, paper wadding, page turning, manipulating buttons, and pinching out beads in putty to regain active motion of his fingers. Experience guided the choice of these activities to promote tendon excursion through the very dense scar tissue in his palm and to train Don to begin to use his hand for light resistive functional activities. With this guided experience of how much pinch and grip force was safe, Don confidently began to try to use his hand safely at home for daily tasks. At 10 weeks, the tendons had healed sufficiently to add resistance using the hand gripper to pick up checkers (a strengthening device that uses graded rubber band resistance that when gripped separates two parallel bars held together by the rubber bands and when opened wide enough can fit and hold checkers, which can then be released into a container) and the BTE (work simulator/exercise machine) to increase the force against the scar adhesions that limited tendon excursion (Table 66-2).

| TABLE 66-2 | Active Range of Motion (in Degrees) at 10 Weeks Postsurgery |

10 Weeks Postsurgery	MP (0–90)	PIP (0–100)	DIP (0–80)
Index	0–80	−20–100	−10–65
Long	0–80	−35–92	−15–45
Ring	0–30	−35–70	0–25
Thumb	−10–50		−20–75
Wrist: 55–70			

MP, metacarpal phalangeal joint; PIP, proximal interphalangeal joint; DIP, distal interphalangeal joint.

Sensation had begun to return in his distal palm, but his fingers remained numb.

His thumb, index, and long fingers progressed to full active flexion, but his ring finger had only 90 degrees of total motion. The loss of his small finger and severe limitation in active flexion of his ring finger due to adhesion of the FDP in his palm resulted in the syndrome of quadriga described by Verdan (1960), causing incomplete terminal flexion of his long and index fingers during grip. Quadriga is a phenomenon that results when one FDP tendon is tethered by proximal adhesions. This in turn will limit the remaining FDP tendons from proximal excursion and result in the inability to completely flex the fingers into a fist. It will also result in significant weakness in grip strength.

Don could not functionally grip a steering wheel or hold tools for work simulation. He was able to pinch and grip sufficiently to pull on clothes and bathe; however, buttoning and holding screws, boards, or nails were impaired by the sensory deficit.

Don's Second Surgery

At 12 weeks, the hand surgeon who had referred Don decided to take him back to surgery for a tenolysis (i.e., freeing the tendons from adhesions) or possible tendon repair depending on what he found when he opened Don's hand, so we discharged him to a home exercise program until he returned from surgery.

Surgery revealed that the ulnar digital nerve to Don's ring finger was ruptured with a 2-cm defect between the proximal and distal ends. The proximal end of the digital nerve that had previously gone to his amputated small finger was in the immediate vicinity, so the surgeon connected that to the distal end of the ring finger ulnar digital nerve. On evaluation of the flexor tendons to the ring finger, it was discovered that both not only were extremely scarred down but also were attached only by pseudotendons (repaired tendons that fail to regenerate tendon tissue in the repair

site but contain a section of scar tissue that lacks the tensile strength of tendon tissue). After tenolysis of both tendons, it was decided to leave the FDS alone and excise the pseudotendon to the FDP. A primary repair to the FDP was successfully performed with minimal loss of tendon excursion.

Don's Referral Back to Occupational Therapy

Don was referred to therapy 1 week after surgery for evaluation and initiation of treatment. His original splint was modified to free his index finger and thumb, and his dressings were changed. Don was familiar with the Duran protocol and started passively ranging his long and ring fingers immediately. He required only one follow-up visit after the evaluation to achieve full passive range of motion (PROM) and was discharged to a home program until he came out of the splint to begin AROM. The biggest difference in the course of rehabilitation this time was that Don returned to work in a supervisory capacity as soon as the sutures were removed.

The doctor again decided to hold all active motion until the sixth week after surgery. Even though Don was ready this time for his finger not to move immediately, by the end of the first week of therapy, he was extremely frustrated and disappointed by the lack of progress. By the third week of therapy (9 weeks postoperative), Don was finally beginning to find it easier to do his self-care. Lack of sensation in the fingertips continued to be a problem, but Don was beginning to compensate. As patients progress through the healing process and therapy, they become more cognizant of their own physical and emotional capacity to return to previous occupations or accomplish their goals. Our goal at this juncture was to help Don begin to identify the problems that interfered with reentering or performing his occupation and to begin to plan possible solutions with him. Clark and colleagues (1996) identified this process as evoking insights in occupational storymaking. We chose many of the same activities to gain grip and pinch; however, we geared them as much as possible toward work using the nut and bolt board, pegs to simulate nails, and grasping of various-sized objects. Don had already learned how to use his hand safely for self-care tasks after the first surgery and expressed his desire to concentrate specifically on tasks that would restore function related to work.

At the 10th week, a dynamic PIP extension splint was added to reduce the flexion contracture in his ring finger and to mobilize the tendon distally through the scar adhesions by applying a low-load long duration force to manipulate the scar tissue (Pettengill, 2005). Don worked relentlessly at home, gripping putty in an attempt to force

TABLE 66-3	Active Range of Motion (in Degrees) at 12 Weeks After Second Surgery		
12 Weeks (Second Surgery)	MP (0–90)	PIP (0–100)	DIP (0–80)
Ring	WNL	−25–90	0–50

MP, metacarpal phalangeal joint; PIP, proximal interphalangeal joint; DIP, distal interphalangeal joint; WNL, within normal limits.

the tendon through the thick scar, but there was still no appreciable difference in flexion, and Don was devastated. At 12 weeks, the repair site had developed enough tendon tissue growth through the anastomosis to almost eliminate the possibility of rupture. On the basis of our experience, we decided to use iontophoresis with dexamethasone to reduce the inflammation and adhesions around the healing tendon. Within 1 week, Don had increased his ring finger flexion and was able to flex to his central palm (Table 66-3).

Don's therapeutic activities expanded to gripping tools and swinging a hammer into a pillow for controlled grip

even though he was not left-handed. He began to notice a significant decrease in hypersensitivity in his palm and reported that he was picking up small pieces of wood at work with some success. At 15 weeks, he returned to full duty but was in a position to modify his activities when needed, lifting Sheetrock with his wrist instead of his fingers. At 18 weeks, he was discharged with L42/R130 lb of grip, L19/R27 lb of lateral pinch, and L12/R20 lb of three-point pinch; he was able to do his job and was working at home on his grandchild's rocking horse.

Epilogue

It has been many years since Don left therapy, but he stopped by to drop off a *Fine Homebuilding* magazine in which there were pictures of him building complicated wainscot on a curved stairwell. Most notable in the pictures which Don proudly showed was his left hand holding a measuring triangle, holding a caulking gun, and supporting molding securely against the wall (Figures 66-2, 66-3, and 66-4).

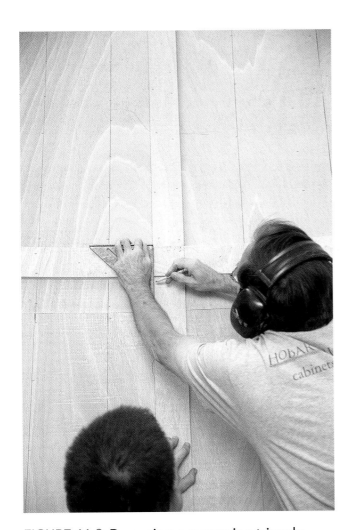

FIGURE 66-2 Don using a measuring triangle.

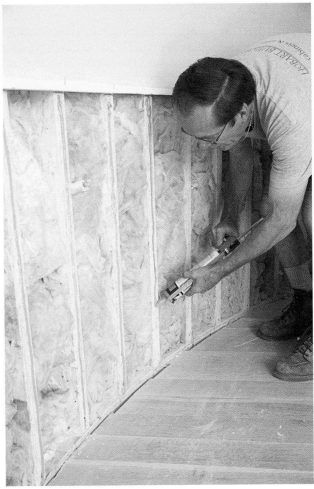

FIGURE 66-3 Don using a caulking gun.

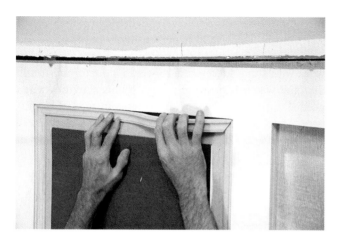

FIGURE 66-4 **Don supporting molding against a wall.**

▶ Visit thePoint to watch a video about orthopedic assessment and intervention.

REFERENCES

Bell-Krotoski, J. A. (1989). Hands research and success. *Journal of Hand Therapy, 2,* 5–11.

Bell-Krotoski, J. A. (2002). Sensibility testing with the Semmes-Weinstein Monofilaments. In E. Mackin, A. Callahan, T. Skirven, L. Schneider, & A. Osterman (Eds.), *Rehabilitation of the hand and upper extremity* (5th ed., pp. 194–213). St. Louis, MO: Mosby.

Bunnell, S. (1955). *Hand surgery.* Washington, DC: Medical Department, United States Army.

Clark, F., Ennevor, B. L., & Richardson, P. L. (1996). A grounded theory of techniques for occupational storytelling and occupational storymaking. In R. Zemke & F. Clark (Eds.), *Occupational science: The evolving discipline* (pp. 373–392). Philadelphia, PA: F. A. Davis.

Crepeau, E. B. (1991). Achieving intersubjective understanding: Examples from an occupational therapy treatment session. *American Journal of Occupational Therapy, 45,* 1016–1025.

Crepeau, E. B., & Garren, K. R. (2011). I looked to her as a guide: The therapeutic relationship in hand therapy. *Disability and Rehabilitation, 33,* 872–881.

Duran, R., & Houser, R. (1975). Controlled passive motion following flexor tendon repair in zones 2 and 3. In *AAOS symposium on tendon surgery in the hand* (pp. 105–114). St. Louis, MO: Mosby.

Michlovitz, S. L. (2005). Is there a role for ultrasound and electrical stimulation following injury to tendon and nerve? *Journal of Hand Therapy, 18,* 292–296.

Omer, G. E., Jr. (2000). Development of hand surgery: Education of hand surgeons. *Journal of Hand Surgery, 25,* 616–628.

Pettengill, K. (2005). The evolution of early mobilization of the repaired flexor tendon. *Journal of Hand Therapy, 18,* 157–168.

Pettengill, K. (2011). Therapist's management of the complex injury. In T. M. Skirven, A. Osterman, J. Fedorczyk, & P. C. Amadio (Eds.), *Rehabilitation of the hand and upper extremity* (6th ed., pp. 1238–1251). St. Louis, MO: Mosby.

Rosendahl, P. P., & Ross, V. (1982). Does your behaviour affect your patient's response? *Journal of Gerontological Nursing, 8,* 572–575.

Taras, J. S., Martyak, G. G., & Steelman, P. J. (2011). Primary care of flexor tendon injuries. In T. M. Skirven, A. Osterman, J. Fedorczyk, & P. C. Amadio (Eds.), *Rehabilitation of the hand and upper extremity* (6th ed., pp. 445–456). St. Louis, MO: Mosby.

Tickle-Degnen, L. (2008). Therapeutic rapport. In M. V. Radomski & C. A. Trombly Latham (Eds.), *Occupational therapy for physical dysfunction* (6th ed., pp. 402–420). Philadelphia, PA: Lippincott Williams & Wilkins.

Verdan, C. (1960). Syndrome of the quadriga. *The Surgical Clinics of North America, 40,* 425–426.

Yakobina, S. C., Yakobina, S. R., & Harrison-Weaver, S. (2008). War, what is it good for? Historical contribution of the military and war to occupational therapy and hand therapy. *Journal of Hand Therapy, 21,* 106–113.

the**Point**® *For additional resources on the subjects discussed in this chapter, visit* **http://thePoint.lww.com /Willard-Spackman13e**.

Providing Occupational Therapy for Older Adults with Changing Needs

Bette R. Bonder, Glenn David Goodman

LEARNING OBJECTIVES

After reading this chapter, you will be able to:

1. Discuss normal age-related changes that affect occupational performance.
2. Describe health conditions and trajectories in later life as these affect occupational performance.
3. Describe environmental factors that influence the experience of growing older.
4. Discuss unique considerations in evaluating and intervening to support successful aging and minimize dysfunction in later life.
5. Describe characteristics of health care systems that serve older adults.
6. Describe social factors that support or impede successful aging.
7. Discuss unique considerations in providing occupational therapy services to older adults throughout late life development.
8. Analyze common ethical issues in providing occupational therapy services for older adults.

Introduction: Understanding the Life Course in Later Life

Older adults constitute the fastest growing segment of the population in the United States and in much of the world. In 2010, persons older than age 65 years constituted roughly 13% of the U.S. population; by 2030, it is expected that they will be more than 19% (Vincent & Velkoff, 2010). Those over 65 years are living longer than ever in the past; life expectancy for men is more than 76 years, and for women, more than 81 years. In addition, the older population, like the U.S. population as a whole, is becoming more racially and ethnically diverse (National Center for Health Statistics, 2016), with implications for continued issues related to health disparities. This rapid increase in older adults has significant implications for every aspect of life—workforce, education, economic development, and, of course, health care.

Although opinions vary about the precise consequences of an aging population for health care, there is no question that preventing health problems is both possible and desirable from an individual and a societal perspective. Researchers have increasingly focused on strategies for ensuring **successful aging**, maintaining positive quality of life as normal

CENTENNIAL NOTES

Aging: 1917 versus 2017

In 1917, life expectancy was roughly 54 years for white men, 46 years for African-American men, 66 years for white women, and 45 years for African-American women (Roser, 2017). Although this reflects, in part, significant early mortality from infectious disease and injury (e.g., the virulent flu epidemic of 1917 to 1918 [National Archives, n.d.]), living past age 65 years was much less common in 1917 than it is in 2017 when the fastest growing population group in the United States is individuals over age 90 years (U.S. Census Bureau, 2016). The oldest living adult in 2017 is 117 years old, and in the United States, a woman living in South Carolina is 113 years old (Lewis, 2017). Thus, in 1917, there was not much call for emphasis on care of older adults, whereas in 2017, it is one of the largest practice areas in health care.

The concept of "successful aging" emerged in the 1960s, altering considerations about health care for older adults from strictly medical intervention to a focus on quality of life (Bearon, 1996). Individuals of all ages note that well-being is the most important consideration in later life (Kelly & Lazarus, 2015). A Harvard University study found that relationships and how happy individuals are in those relationships is one of the most powerful influences on health of older adults (Harvard Second Generation Study, 2017). Research on centenarians suggests that engaged lifestyles are predictive of better functional capacity in the oldest old (Martin et al., 2011). The landmark Well Elderly Treatment Program, developed by occupational therapists and occupational scientists, provided evidence about the effectiveness of occupational therapy (OT) not only in rehabilitation of elders but also in promotion of continued engagement in life activities through lifestyle redesign (Jackson, Carlson, Mandel, Zemke, & Clark, 1998). Such research has increased recognition of OT as a vital service in the care and health promotion of older adults.

---

age-related physical and cognitive changes occur (Wahl, Deeg, & Litwin, 2016). Rowe and Kahn (1998) theorized that successful aging is based on three factors: avoiding disease and disability, maintaining mental and physical function, and maintaining active engagement with life. There is general agreement that this model captures essential components of well-being in later life, although the framework has been refined and elaborated by numerous other researchers (Nimrod & Ben-Shem, 2015).

There are many actions that individuals of all ages can take to avoid disease and disability; however, to some extent, this is not within personal control. Likewise, it is possible to take several positive steps to maintain mental and physical function, although again, these do not guarantee that function will not decline. In fact, some degree of functional decline is a fact of life in later life (National Institutes of Health [NIH], 2013). The third factor, maintaining active engagement with life, is within individual control and is the central emphasis of OT (American Occupational Therapy Association [AOTA], 2014).

Occupational Therapy in Action: Mrs. Ramirez's Path through Later Life

In general, there has been a reduction in disabling health conditions in late life (NIH, 2013). A common experience of aging is a gradual decline in aspects of body function and performance skills. Vision almost universally deteriorates;

a condition known as *presbyopia* is readily accommodated using reading glasses. Hearing often worsens. Muscle mass decreases. These and other body function changes can affect motor and sensory-perceptual skills. Decline is often gradual for long periods of time, punctuated by acute health problems that can accelerate functional loss. A bout of pneumonia may severely reduce cardiovascular

THERAPIST NARRATIVE

One of my early experiences in working with older adults came when I was a research assistant on a study focused on the causes of falls. The study was undertaken in a low-income residential facility in an urban inner city. Participants were asked to rate how happy they were. The researchers expected a low level of happiness because the participants were so economically disadvantaged. It was a surprise to learn that these individuals indicated they were very happy with their current lives, largely because they had the freedom to do what interested them, typically after many years earning a living at needed but unfulfilling work. As I have interacted with older adults, it has become increasingly evident to me that once basic needs for shelter and food are met, it is what one does and not what one has that makes for happiness in later life. Occupational therapists are central to promoting the ability of these individuals to do what matters most to them.

—Bette R. Bonder

endurance, a situation compounded by the fact that elders also take longer to recover and may never return to their pre-illness baseline (Bray & Bonder, 2018).

Superimposed on this gradual decline with occasional acute episodes is the development of chronic health conditions such as arthritis, osteoporosis, and dementia, which have profound consequences for function and quality of life. Issues requiring special attention in later life include the following:

- Health conditions may have more benign (some cancers) or severe (pneumonia, influenza) consequences in late life.
- Decrements in sensory systems, cardiovascular and musculoskeletal function, and cognition are universal, although variable in degree.
- Multiple, sometimes conflicting, health conditions can complicate treatment choices (e.g., osteoporosis and arthritis).
- Social, economic, and environmental factors profoundly influence aging.

Background Information

Mrs. Estelle Ramirez is a 78-year-old widow when she first receives OT services. She lives alone in a third floor walk-up apartment in Brooklyn, New York—the apartment in which she raised her three daughters, now aged 56, 53, and 51 years. It is also where she and her husband lived together after the girls left home for college. Mrs. Ramirez and her husband moved to New York from Puerto Rico when Mr. Ramirez took a job in a factory 50 years ago. Mrs. Ramirez began working as an accountant when her girls were in high school. She retired at age 66 years to take care of her husband and then in the late stages of Alzheimer's disease (AD). He died 4 years later.

Mrs. Ramirez believes herself to be in good health. She is of normal weight, and although she has joint pain that she characterizes as *artritis* (arthritis), it does not interfere very much with her function. She wears glasses, now trifocals, but sees reasonably well with them. She has noted lately that she has some difficulty seeing at night and as a result has chosen not to drive after sunset. She never drove much, preferring as do many New Yorkers to use public transportation but does not feel safe doing so after dark. These two factors have limited her evening activities, which causes her some distress. She has also begun to complain to her daughters about her memory. They note that she tends to repeat herself when speaking with them and that she sometimes forgets appointments.

Puerto Rican culture has a strong emphasis on *familismo*, a belief in the importance of strong family ties. In Mrs. Ramirez's case, this is reflected in the conversations that her daughters have had about whether Mrs. Ramirez should be living by herself, and there is growing tension regarding possible alternate arrangements. One daughter is

adamant that Mrs. Ramirez should stay in her own home with the three girls providing supportive care; one believes her mother should come live with her, and one strongly favors moving her to an assisted living facility.

Since her husband's death, Mrs. Ramirez volunteers at the local elementary school reading to the children. She sees her daughters frequently. She takes great pleasure in spending time with her nine grandchildren and her first great-grandchild who was born last year; she particularly likes cooking traditional Puerto Rican meals and telling them about their heritage. She spends time at the local Hispanic Senior Center. She misses her husband and regrets that she had to stop working earlier than she would have liked, but she is reasonably satisfied with her current life and enjoys her apartment and neighbors.

First Encounter

Mrs. Ramirez was present when the consulting occupational therapist at the senior center made a presentation about home safety and provided a checklist for the participants so that they could assess their environments. As the therapist knows, falls are common among older populations and can have dire consequences (Kramarow, Chen, Hedegaard, & Warner, 2015), including significant disability or death. Mrs. Ramirez was very interested in the presentation, but funding is typically available for this service only for individuals with an identified disability (Beattie & Peterson, 2007).

Reimbursement Issues and Ethical Dilemmas in Working with Older Adults

The funding difficulty that Mrs. Ramirez has encountered is not an unusual one for older adults. Although in the United States, individuals older than age 65 years benefit from being eligible for Medicare, a nearly universal form of health insurance for elders, Medicare has numerous—and frequently changing—limitations and regulations (Richman, 2018). Medical services associated with preventive care (e.g., vaccinations, mammography, diabetes care) are covered, but preventive OT services are not. This is particularly unfortunate because there is strong research evidence that early intervention focused on lifestyle issues can maintain health and reduce costs (Clark et al., 2012; Lood, Häggblom-Kronlöf, & Dahlin-Ivanoff, 2015).

Even when some OT services are covered, numerous regulations limit the specific types of services covered. This creates one of the many ethical dilemmas that confront occupational therapists working with elders. How can one ensure that vital services are made available in a reimbursement environment that regulates the goals that will be covered while also limiting providers' ability to impose charges for services not covered? Creativity in selecting activities that address multiple goals can be an essential component of an effective intervention plan.

The involvement of family can also create ethical challenges for therapists. It is not unusual for family members to have divergent views regarding the best interests of the older adult. It is important for the occupational therapist to recognize that the elder is his or her client and to remain focused on what is best for that individual even in the face of sometimes intense lobbying by family. Mrs. Ramirez's family is supportive, but it is evident early on that they have different views about what is best for her.

Wellness and Prevention

Evaluation

As described previously, funding for wellness and prevention can be challenging. Most often, occupational therapists provide such services by consulting with organizations rather than caring for individual clients (Bass, 2018). The process by which this occurs mirrors individual evaluation and intervention but requires focus on the needs and interests of groups of individuals as well as epidemiological data that suggest what kinds of problems are most common and what health indicators can identify need and measure progress (Morrow & Johnson, 2014). Poor diet, physical inactivity, and smoking cause significant disability and premature morbidity around the world (Scarborough et al., 2011). Such information would be useful in framing goals of senior center activities, educational programs, and health screenings. Furthermore, data demonstrate that cognitive decline and falls are among the most common and, particularly in the case of falls, preventable health problems in later life.

Interventions to Support Successful Aging

In wellness and prevention services for older adults, the occupational therapist's most typical role is to assist in understanding the needs of clients and in designing programs that will be delivered by activity therapists, aides, and, often, volunteers (Bass, 2018). Based on the information gleaned from the participants and a review of literature about common health problems, the therapist generates a list of program goals and explores best practice about effective programming to address those goals. In the case of the Hispanic Senior Center that Mrs. Ramirez attends, one of the activities that participants most enjoy is the lunch, which includes typical Puerto Rican foods. They also enjoy listening to Hispanic music on the radio and watching Spanish-language soap operas.

Thus, the therapist suggests that senior center programming focus on culturally relevant activities that encourage physical activity through meaningful and enjoyable activities such as dancing while listening to the music they enjoy, gardening, and nature hikes; maintain supportive social interaction and cognitive wellness through interactive, challenging activities such as a book club, lectures with discussion, creative writing, journaling, or scrapbooking and discussion of the soap opera that they enjoy; encourage positive health promotion behaviors through nutrition and cooking demonstrations and discussions, safety awareness activities, and group discussion; and provide opportunities for altruistic activities such as visits to a local preschool to read to children, food drives, and care for program participants who become ill.

The occupational therapist attends team meetings during which the activity therapist, part-time nurse, nutritionist, and consulting physician discuss the needs of the center's participants. Along with occupation-based programming, a series of wellness events is designed and implemented. These include blood pressure, vision and hearing screening, quarterly visits by a dentist, and an invitation to a physical therapist to plan an appropriate exercise program for participants. These activities are relevant to Mrs. Ramirez's situation because she has not had regular screenings for common health problems and has become increasingly sedentary.

Naturally Occurring Retirement Communities

Mrs. Ramirez's apartment building is now populated almost exclusively by individuals older than age 65 years. This occurred gradually over time because children of residents became adults and moved away, whereas Mrs. Ramirez and her age cohorts remained in place. The building now constitutes a naturally occurring retirement community (NORC) (Ivery, 2014; Naturally Occurring Retirement Communities Programs, 2012). The emergence of NORCs reflects the wish of many older adults to age in place; that is, to remain in their lifelong homes as they grow older. There are many advantages to doing so, including the familiarity of the surroundings, social support from long-time neighbors, and access to family and to health care professionals who know their histories and needs.

Recognizing the opportunity offered by NORCs to support successful aging, government and social agencies have begun to provide various wellness and health promotion services in these facilities. In 2008, the Administration on Aging (AoA, 2011) established a funding initiative designed to

• Enhance the ability of older adults living in a residential community to continue living independently;

- Increase healthy aging behaviors through exercise, recreation, socialization, education, and culturally appropriate activities; and
- Identify needs of at-risk residents, facilitate access to existing community/government resources, and create gap-filling supportive services.

This initiative and its goals offer significant opportunities for occupational therapists to serve community-residing, well older adults. In particular, offering evidence-based services such as lifestyle redesign (Clark et al., 2012) can promote the goals of the AoA NORC program. Based on Mrs. Ramirez's current status, transportation services would be of particular value, as would evening activities in her apartment building to reduce her sense of loss as a result of her nighttime transportation difficulties.

Primary Care

Occupational therapists' involvement with traditional primary care for older adults has evolved over the past few decades. Their role emphasizes assessment and management of function related to activities of daily living (ADL) that patients identify as important in their lives (Donnelly, Brenchley, Crawford, & Letts, 2014). Interventions might emphasize pain management, community mobility, environmental redesign, and other strategies for supporting and maximizing occupational engagement.

Inpatient Care

Several months after her first encounter with the occupational therapist, Mrs. Ramirez misses a week at the senior center. Concerned staff calls her home and, when they cannot reach her, her oldest daughter. They discover to their dismay that she recently fell on the steps leading to her apartment and sustained a fracture of the femur.

Evaluation

Mrs. Ramirez is hospitalized, and surgery to stabilize the fracture is performed. A metal plate with several screws is inserted, although the surgeon is somewhat concerned about the outcome, given the osteoporotic condition of her bones. The occupational therapist is involved immediately, both to help minimize any hospital-induced cognitive loss and to help Mrs. Ramirez prepare for the rehabilitation that will follow her surgery.

The occupational therapist spends some time talking with Mrs. Ramirez to get to know about her interests and her life before the accident. The AOTA Practice Framework (AOTA, 2014) encourages the completion of an occupational profile as a starting point for evaluation. The therapist is pleased when two of Mrs. Ramirez's daughters stop by to visit while she is

in the room so that she can meet them and get a sense of the kind of support Mrs. Ramirez may have on her eventual return home. The therapist also administers the Mini-Cog (Borson, Scanlan, Brush, Vitaliano, & Dokmak, 2000), a quick screening instrument for cognitive impairment, and the Functional Independence Measure (FIM) (Heinemann, Linacre, Wright, Hamilton, & Granger, 1994) to evaluate Mrs. Ramirez's current physical capacity. She finds that Mrs. Ramirez has some memory loss but does not meet the standard for dementia. In addition, Mrs. Ramirez is now struggling with basic self-care such as dressing, getting herself to and from the bed to a chair or wheelchair, and moving from the wheelchair to the toilet safely.

Interventions to Minimize Dysfunction

Mrs. Ramirez will be transferred very soon to a skilled nursing facility where she can receive rehabilitation services. The therapist and Mrs. Ramirez agree that the focus of intervention will be on planning for a smooth discharge to the rehabilitation setting. For the brief time that they are together, they work on safe transfers from bed to chair and from wheelchair to toilet. They also focus on dressing in part because Mrs. Ramirez expresses unhappiness that she looks so disheveled.

The therapist makes a point of dropping in to Mrs. Ramirez's room several times a day, and she encourages some of the hospital volunteers to do likewise. The daughters have expressed concern that Mrs. Ramirez seems more confused than usual. For an older adult who already has memory problems, hospital stays can lead to rapid deterioration (Ehlenbach, Larson, Curtis, & Hough, 2015). Thus, the treatment plan includes strategies to provide stimulation and orientation to time and place: providing Mrs. Ramirez a newspaper each day; discussing current events; talking about events happening in her own day ("What did you have for breakfast?" or "Have you had company today?"); and conversing about the events in the Spanish-language soap opera that Mrs. Ramirez likes to watch.

Skilled Nursing

Three days after her surgery, Mrs. Ramirez is transferred to a skilled nursing facility. She expresses relief at being out of the hospital but great concern about whether she will be able to go home. She is adamant that this is what she wants and expresses this wish to every staff member she meets as well as to her daughters.

Evaluation

Skilled nursing facilities are among the most highly regulated health care institutions with both federal and state guidelines about the nature of services, expectations for improvement, requirements about length of stay, and outcome reporting (Centers for Medicare & Medicaid Services, 2007; DeJong, 2016). Mrs. Ramirez will receive care from a comprehensive team as long as she shows improvement. If her condition stabilizes before she can safely go home, other arrangements will need to be made. Mrs. Ramirez is highly motivated to regain function. The occupational therapist is involved early based on evidence that intensive OT is associated with shorter stay and better functional outcomes (Cimarolli & Jung, 2016).

Medicare guidelines are quite specific about the services to be provided. The occupational therapist is aware that his evaluation and interventions must focus on Mrs. Ramirez's ADL and instrumental activities of daily living (IADL). He reviews the report from the occupational therapist at the inpatient facility and participates with others on the team in completing the Minimum Data Set (MDS) (Centers for Medicare & Medicaid Services, 2012). In addition, he repeats the FIM and interviews Mrs. Ramirez about her goals. He requests her permission to involve her family in the intervention process, to which Mrs. Ramirez readily agrees.

Intervention

Mrs. Ramirez wants to regain independence in self-care and to resume her usual activities. She and the therapist begin to practice fundamental skills like dressing, bathing, toileting, and grooming. One goal of their sessions is to identify ways to minimize the difficulties of some of these activities, using, where appropriate, modified clothing (especially for lower extremity dressing), assistive devices (reachers, bath seat), and task modification to reduce energy expenditure.

During these treatment sessions, the therapist inquires about Mrs. Ramirez's typical patterns at home and about the environment to which she wants to return. The therapist talks with the physical therapist about the challenges of a third floor apartment, and both agree this may be quite difficult for Mrs. Ramirez. They suggest to the social worker that she explore the possibility of moving Mrs. Ramirez to a first-floor apartment in the same building, realizing that this may not be acceptable to Mrs. Ramirez or feasible in New York's tight housing market.

It becomes apparent to the therapist that Mrs. Ramirez's cognitive difficulties are interfering with her ability to master the changes in her typical occupational patterns required by her new physical status. The therapist requests an evaluation by the psychologist who indicates that Mrs. Ramirez has mild cognitive impairment (MCI) (Parikh, Troyer, Maione, & Murphy, 2016). Unlike AD and other frank dementias, MCI is characterized by forgetfulness and poor short-term memory. Well-learned functions tend to remain intact so that individuals with MCI can

manage their daily activities in their accustomed environments. Function becomes much more challenging when the individual is in a new setting or when physical changes require new patterns for ADL and IADL. Mrs. Ramirez's hip fracture and subsequent stay in inpatient care and now in a skilled nursing facility has increased her confusion. The occupational therapist finds that her retention from session to session is poor so begins to focus on low-tech memory aids (lists, labeling, mnemonic strategies) that will help her.

Transition to Home Care

Reimbursement rules from Medicare limit the amount of time that an individual can remain in skilled nursing. Very early in Mrs. Ramirez's stay, the social worker and the treatment team begin conversations with her and, with her permission, her daughters regarding a plan for her discharge. Although only one daughter supports her wish, Mrs. Ramirez remains determined to return to her home. Ultimately, one of the daughters agrees to stay with her for several weeks to help her readjust to the apartment. However, all three of them and the treatment team are concerned about her ability to manage the stairs.

A week before her scheduled departure, the social worker contacts a home health agency. Given Mrs. Ramirez's continued physical limitations and the fact that she has had inpatient care, she is eligible for home health services paid for by Medicare. All agree that these services will be very helpful, and the social worker arranges for the intake nurse from the home health agency to visit Mrs. Ramirez on her first full day at home.

Home Care

As is true for rehabilitation, Medicare coverage of home health care is based on very specific rules guiding the kinds of services that can be provided (Centers for Medicare & Medicaid Services, 2014a). Occupational therapy is a covered service, as is supportive care provided by a home health aide (although supportive care must be in concert with rehabilitation). A challenge for OT is that the guidelines specify that services must focus on ADL and IADL, not on other activities that focus on quality of life. This may create an ethical dilemma for the therapist who believes that she has an obligation to provide comprehensive services to meet client needs. One strategy for addressing this dilemma is to provide intervention that can generalize to multiple activities. So, for instance, efforts to improve Mrs. Ramirez's balance might incorporate a few minutes salsa dancing rather than more straightforward balance exercises, and practice using the phone to report emergencies might also include a call to the senior center to reestablish contact.

Evaluation

Home health reimbursement guidelines require that there should be an initial intake assessment, typically completed by a nurse. The Outcomes and Assessment Information Set (OASIS) (Centers for Medicare & Medicaid Services, 2014b) must be administered, and the intake worker then determines what other services should be provided. These may include OT, physical therapy (PT), speech-language therapy, home aide services (but only in conjunction with therapeutic services), and nursing care. In Mrs. Ramirez's case, it is evident that OT is important to a positive outcome.

Occupational therapy evaluation in the client's own environment is often the most meaningful in terms of occupational performance. Familiarity with the environment and the psychological comfort of being at home can enhance a client's function. For Mrs. Ramirez, whose cognitive status has affected her performance greatly, this is particularly true. On her first visit, the occupational therapist asks Mrs. Ramirez to demonstrate her daily routine: getting out of bed, toileting, grooming, bathing, and dressing. Mrs. Ramirez is able to dress independently, sitting in a chair as she was shown during her rehabilitation. However, she struggles with bathing and is unsafe getting on and off the toilet. The therapist completes a home safety evaluation (Horowitz, Nochajski, & Schweitzer, 2013), looking for unstable area rugs, inadequate lighting, and clutter.

In addition to ADL, Mrs. Ramirez will need to be able to manage some IADL for herself. Her daughters are willing to stop by to help with laundry, grocery shopping, and light cleaning, but Mrs. Ramirez will need to fix some meals for herself and read and respond to mail, including bills. The therapist asks her to demonstrate these activities.

Intervention

If Mrs. Ramirez is to be able to manage in her home, there is much to do. The therapist orders appropriate durable medical equipment (bath seat, grab bars, raised toilet seat) to assist with safety and function. She and Mrs. Ramirez reorganize the kitchen so that frequently used items are within easy reach (Figure 67-1). With Mrs. Ramirez's approval, the therapist works with the daughters to remove safety hazards from the home. They continue to work on self-care skills, bathing in particular, that are giving Mrs. Ramirez difficulty.

As a way to address leisure and social activities, the therapist structures conversation while they work on self-care so that Mrs. Ramirez can identify what she would like to be able to do and can problem-solve about how to make those activities possible. She is eager to return to the Hispanic Senior Center as soon as possible, and the therapist helps her make the phone call that will arrange transportation. The therapist incorporates elements of these tasks to promote problem solving and endurance in support of ADL and IADL.

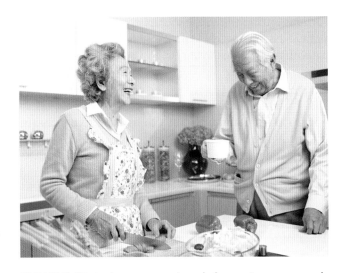

FIGURE 67-1 An occupational therapist may work with a client to organize a kitchen for ease of use.

Throughout their time together, the therapist notes that Mrs. Ramirez's increasing cognitive deficits create problems for her independent function. They work on organizing her space to help her find commonly used items, to lay out her grooming supplies in the bathroom, to label cabinets, and to use lists to help her remember important procedures and events; but the lists are frequently mislaid or forgotten, and the therapist is increasingly concerned about Mrs. Ramirez's safety. Mrs. Ramirez continues to be unsteady on her feet and seems unable to remember the precautions that the therapist showed her regarding standing carefully from a seated position, using her cane effectively to move around the apartment, and using the grab bars that have been installed in the bathroom.

Assisted Living

Although Mrs. Ramirez is very motivated to live on her own, ultimately, the challenges of her environment are simply too much. There are two daunting difficulties. One is the three steep flights of stairs leading to the apartment. Although Mrs. Ramirez is increasingly functional at home, leaving and returning are painful and exhausting. Using the stairs does not fall strictly within the goals for home health services (which are intended for individuals who are homebound, not to assist such individuals with return to their community activities), the therapist feels comfortable having Mrs. Ramirez practice as a way to regain strength and endurance. However, her progress is painfully slow. Mrs. Ramirez feels increasingly isolated and depressed.

The second dilemma is Mrs. Ramirez's failing memory, which causes concern for the therapist and for Mrs. Ramirez's daughters. The therapist arranges a visit from the social worker to discuss the options. The daughters are not in agreement, and there are several very intense sessions during which the therapist, with Mrs. Ramirez's permission, reviews her skills and abilities. Ultimately, they agree that an assisted living facility is the best solution.

Evaluation

For OT, Mrs. Ramirez's move to assisted living means coming full circle in terms of services. Occupational therapists typically serve as consultants to such facilities, advising on programming, environmental considerations, and staff training. Residents of assisted living facilities may be referred for outpatient OT as needed, but assisted living is not designed to provide such services within the facility. Their purpose is to provide a supportive environment where meals, housekeeping, and activities are provided and health care can be accessed easily. Thus, Mrs. Ramirez will not be formally evaluated by an occupational therapist at the assisted living facility.

Intervention

There is evidence that function-focused interventions are very helpful in assisted living facilities (Egan, Dubouloz, Leonard, Paquet, & Carter, 2014). The occupational therapist encourages an array of activities that support wellness (physical activity, socialization at mealtime to encourage adequate nutrition) and quality of life (culturally appropriate, creative, spiritual, altruistic, and other meaningful and enjoyable occupations). In addition, the occupational therapist works with staff to assist in creating strategies for monitoring Mrs. Ramirez's well-being and for interacting with and supporting the family. Effective intervention and monitoring in assisted living can provide support for residents and families to prolong high quality and meaningful life.

Summary

Occupational therapy practitioners have a well-defined and critical role in the care of older adults. Our roles and methods change based on the evolving needs of these clients. However, as shown in Table 67-1, our OT goals remain the same:

1. Prevent functional decline.
2. Maximize our client's performance in areas of occupation.
3. Decrease participation restrictions and maximize quality of life.

| TABLE 67-1 | Typical Areas of Emphasis in Prevention, Inpatient Care, Skilled Nursing, Home Health, and Assisted Living |

Prevention	Inpatient Care	Skilled Nursing	Home Health	Assisted Living
Consult on design of programs to support meaningful activity.	Evaluate ADL in preparation for discharge/transition planning.	Evaluate ADL/IADL.	Evaluate ADL/IADL.	Design wellness programs.
Consult on design of physical activities.	Provide stimulation to prevent cognitive loss.	As feasible, explore meaningful occupations.	As feasible, explore meaningful occupations.	Design leisure programs with an emphasis on function and meaning.
Train staff.	As appropriate, discuss needs with family/other informal caregivers.	Provide interventions to increase functional ability in ADL/IADL, increase physical capacity.	Provide interventions to increase functional ability in ADL/IADL.	Consider development of day care programming.
Advise on physical design of facilities.	Low vision services	Provide assistive devices as appropriate and provide training in their use.	Provide interventions to promote wellness.	Train staff.
			Complete safety assessment.	Advise on physical design of facilities.
			Support environmental modifications to enhance safety and function.	
			Provide assistive devices as appropriate and provide training in their use.	
			Low vision services	
			Fall prevention	

ADL, activities of daily living; IADL, instrumental activities of daily living.

Visit thePoint to watch a video about interventions for older adults.

REFERENCES

Administration on Aging. (2011). *Naturally occurring retirement communities.* Retrieved from http://www.aoa.gov/AoARoot /AoA_Programs/HCLTC/NORC/index.aspx

American Occupational Therapy Association. (2014). Occupational therapy practice framework: Domain and process, 3rd edition. *American Journal of Occupational Therapy, 68,* S1–S48. doi:10.5014 /ajot.2014.682006

Bass, J. D. (2018). Health and wellness. In B. R. Bonder & V. Dal Bello-Haas (Eds.), *Functional performance in older adults* (4th ed., pp. 421–436). Philadelphia, PA: F. A. Davis.

Bearon, L. D. (1996). Successful aging: What does the "good life" look like? *The Forum for Family and Consumer Issues, 1.* Retrieved from https://ncsu.edu/ffci/publications/1996/v1-n3-1996-summer /successful-aging.php

Beattie, B. L., & Peterson, F. W. (2007). *Exploring practice in home safety for fall prevention: The creative practices in home safety assessment and modification study.* Washington, DC: National Council on Aging.

Borson, S., Scanlan, J., Brush, M., Vitaliano, P., & Dokmak, A. (2000). The mini-cog: A cognitive "vital signs" measure for dementia screening in multi-lingual elderly. *International Journal of Geriatric Psychiatry, 15,* 1021–1027.

Bray, P., & Bonder, B. (2018). Considerations for medical care of older adults. In B. R. Bonder & V. Dal Bello-Haas (Eds.), *Functional performance in older adults* (4th ed., pp. 263–276). Philadelphia, PA: F. A. Davis.

Centers for Medicare & Medicaid Services. (2007). *Medicare coverage of skilled nursing facility care.* Retrieved from http://www.medicare .gov/Pubs/pdf/10153.pdf

Centers for Medicare & Medicaid Services. (2012). *Nursing home quality initiative.* Retrieved from https://www.cms.gov /Medicare/Quality-Initiatives-Patient-Assessment-Instruments /NursingHomeQualityInits/index.html

Centers for Medicare & Medicaid Services. (2014a). *Medicare benefit policy manual.* Retrieved from http://www.cms.gov /Regulations-and-Guidance/Guidance/Manuals/Internet-Only -Manuals-IOMs-Items/CMS012673.html and http://www.cms .gov/Regulations-and-Guidance/Guidance/Manuals/downloads /bp102c07.pdf

Centers for Medicare & Medicaid Services. (2014b). *OASIS users manual.* Retrieved from http://cms.hhs.gov/Medicare/Quality-Initiatives -Patient-Assessment-Instruments/HomeHealthQualityInits /HHQIOASISUserManual.html

Cimarolli, V. R., & Jung, S. (2016). Intensity of occupational therapy utilization in nursing home residents: The role of sensory impairments. *Journal of the American Medical Directors Association, 17,* 939–942. doi:10.1016/j.jamda.2016.06.023

Clark, F., Jackson, J., Carlson, M., Chou, C., Cherry, B. J., Jordan-Marsh, M., . . . Azen, S. (2012). Effectiveness of a lifestyle intervention in promoting the well-being of independently living older people: Results of the Well Elderly 2 Randomised Controlled Trial. *Journal of Epidemiology and Community Health, 66,* 782–790. doi:10.1136/jech.2009.099754

DeJong, G. (2016). Coming to terms with the IMPACT Act of 2014. *American Journal of Occupational Therapy, 70,* 7003090010p1–7003090010p6. doi:10.5014/ajot.2016.703003

Donnelly, C. A., Brenchley, C., Crawford, C., & Letts, L. (2014). The emerging role of occupational therapy in primary care. *Canadian Journal of Occupational Therapy, 81,* 51–61.

Egan, M. Y., Dubouloz, C., Leonard, C., Paquet, N., & Carter, M. (2014). Engagement in personally valued occupations following stroke and a move to assisted living. *Physical & Occupational Therapy in Geriatrics, 32,* 25–41.

Ehlenbach, W. J., Larson, E. B., Curtis, J. R., & Hough, C. L. (2015). Physical function and disability after acute care and critical illness hospitalizations in a prospective cohort of older adults. *Journal of the American Geriatrics Society, 63,* 2061–2069.

Harvard Second Generation Study. (2017). *Welcome to the Harvard study of adult development.* Retrieved from http://www.adult developmentstudy.org/

Heinemann, A. W., Linacre, J. M., Wright, B. D., Hamilton, B. B., & Granger, C. (1994). Prediction of rehabilitation outcomes with disability measures. *Archives of Physical Medicine and Rehabilitation, 75,* 133–143.

Horowitz, B. P., Nochajski, S. M., & Schweitzer, J. A. (2013). Occupational therapy community practice and home assessments: use of the home safety self-assessment tool (HSSAT) to support aging in place. *Occupational Therapy in Health Care, 27,* 216–227.

Ivery, J. M. (2014). The NORC supportive services model: The role of social capital in community aging initiatives. *Journal of Community Practice, 22,* 451–471.

Jackson, J., Carlson, M., Mandel, D., Zemke, R., & Clark, F. (1998). Occupation in lifestyle redesign: The well elderly study occupational therapy program. *American Journal of Occupational Therapy, 52,* 326–336.

Kelly, G. A., & Lazarus, J. (2015). Perceptions of successful aging: Intergenerational voices value well-being. *International Journal of Aging & Human Development, 80,* 233–247.

Kramarow, E., Chen, L., Hedegaard, H., & Warner, M. (2015). Deaths from unintentional injury among adults aged 65 and over: United States, 2000–2013. *NCHS Data Brief, 199.* Retrieved from https:// www.cdc.gov/nchs/data/databriefs/db199.pdf

Lewis, S. (2017, April 17). There's a new world's oldest woman. *CNN.* Retrieved from http://www.cnn.com/2017/04/17/health/worlds-oldest -woman-trnd/index.html

Lood, Q., Häggblom-Kronlöf, G., & Dahlin-Ivanoff, S. (2015). Health promotion programme design and efficacy in relation to ageing persons with culturally and linguistically diverse backgrounds: a systematic literature review and meta-analysis. *BMC Health Services Research, 15,* 560.

Martin, P., MacDonald, M., Margrett, J., Siegler, I., Poon, L. W., Jazwinski, S. M., . . . Arnold, J. (2011). Correlates of functional capacity among centenarians. *Journal of Applied Gerontology, 32,* 324–346.

Morrow, C. B., & Johnson, J. A. (2014). Public health administration and practice framework. In L. Shi & J. A. Johnson (Eds.), *Novick & Morrow's public health administration: Principles for population-based management* (3rd ed., pp. 53–78). New York, NY: Jones & Bartlett Learning.

National Archives. (n.d.). *The deadly virus.* Retrieved from https:// www.archives.gov/exhibits/influenza-epidemic/

National Center for Health Statistics. (2016). *Health, United States, 2015: With special feature on racial and ethnic health disparities.* Retrieved from https://www.cdc.gov/nchs/data/hus/hus15.pdf#014

National Institutes of Health. (2013). *Disability in older adults.* Retrieved from https://report.nih.gov/nihfactsheets/ViewFactSheet .aspx?csid=37

Naturally Occurring Retirement Communities Programs. (2012). *NORC blueprint: A guide to community action.* Retrieved from http://www.norcblueprint.org/

Nimrod, G., & Ben-Shem, I. (2015). Successful aging as a lifelong process. *Educational Gerontology, 41,* 814–824.

Parikh, P. K., Troyer, A. K., Maione, A. M., & Murphy, K. J. (2016). The impact of memory change on daily life in normal aging and mild cognitive impairment. *The Gerontologist*, 56, 877–885.

Richman, N. Z. (2018). Public policy and advocacy in North America. In B. R. Bonder & V. Dal Bello-Haas (Eds.), *Functional performance in older adults* (4th ed., pp. 33–44). Philadelphia, PA: F. A. Davis.

Roser, M. (2017). *Life expectancy*. Retrieved from https://ourworldindata.org/life-expectancy/

Rowe, J. W., & Kahn, R. L. (1998). *Successful aging*. New York, NY: Dell.

Scarborough, P., Bhatnagar, P., Wickramasinghe, K. K., Allender, S., Foster, C., & Rayner, M. (2011). The economic burden of ill health due to diet, physical inactivity, smoking, alcohol and obesity in the UK: An update to 2006–07 NHS costs. *Journal of Public Health*, 33, 527–535. doi:10.1093/pubmed/fdr033

U.S. Census Bureau. (2016). *Quick facts: United States*. Retrieved from https://www.census.gov/quickfacts/fact/table/US/RHI325216#viewtop

Vincent, G. K., & Velkoff, V. A. (2010). *The next four decades. The older population of the United States. 2010 to 2050: Population estimates and projections*. Retrieved from https://www.census.gov/prod/2010pubs/p25-1138.pdf

Wahl, H., Deeg, D., & Litwin, H. (2016). Successful ageing as a persistent priority in ageing research. *European Journal of Ageing*, 13, 1–3. doi:10.1007/s10433-016-0364-5

the Point® *For additional resources on the subjects discussed in this chapter, visit* http://thePoint.lww.com/Willard-Spackman13e.

Providing Occupational Therapy for Disaster Survivors

Theresa M. Smith, Nicole M. Picone

LEARNING OBJECTIVES

After reading this chapter, you will be able to:

1. Describe the impact of disasters on mental health including factors that may predispose a person to posttraumatic stress disorder.
2. Discuss the role of occupational therapy practitioners in addressing the needs of individuals, families, and communities in the different stages of disasters.
3. Describe how occupational therapy practitioners might address the needs of special populations during disasters.
4. Identify potential training needs of occupational therapy practitioners in order to more effectively participate in disaster work.

Introduction

I (Theresa Smith) first became interested in effects of disasters after being evacuated before Hurricane Katrina struck New Orleans on August 29, 2005. At that time, I was working as a faculty member at Louisiana State University Health Science Center (LSUHSC), New Orleans. After the storm, the heavily damaged parts of New Orleans were not accessible for months. I was not allowed to visit my property until October. Some residents were never able to move back into their homes including myself. In July 2009, the Corps of Engineers paid me for my home taken under eminent domain in January 2006.

After Hurricane Ike hit the Gulf Coast of Texas in September 2008, I was again displaced from my home. In writing this chapter, we have drawn on our own personal experiences; the occupational therapy (OT) and other literature on disaster preparation, response, and recovery; and from personal communication with other occupational therapists involved in disaster work. Our intent is to help illuminate the complexity and need for occupation-based interventions after disasters.

Impact of Disasters

It is estimated that between 13% and 30% of the U.S. population have been exposed to one or more disasters in their lifetime (Briere & Elliott, 2000). The term **disaster** refers to dangerous, accidental, or uncontrollable situations

CASE STUDY 68-1   NICOLE'S CASE STUDY

My (Nicole Picone) high school peers and I were briefly labeled "the 9/11 Generation," but I didn't question the impact of collective trauma on community health until I traveled to Nicaragua, South Africa, Israel, and the West Bank as an undergraduate. There, I learned how political and social conflict could affect how citizens talked about the right to access health care. People with the fewest material resources also seemed more savvy in tapping local networks to meet their needs compared to my American friends. In some ways, I felt like the illusion of "security" and our culture of convenience made us more vulnerable in emergencies. While completing the master's program at the Boston School of Occupational Therapy at Tufts University, I studied abroad at Oxford Brookes University in England, when the 2013 Boston Marathon bombing occurred. I read the disturbing media reports alongside international students and wondered, what could I do to define the OT role in disaster response?

When I began my doctoral studies in the fall of 2014, I aimed to add to the knowledge base of disaster preparedness and response for OT practitioners. To start, I read about pilot educational programs for physicians and nurses, federal recommendations following Hurricanes Katrina and Sandy, and took a class to learn how the Federal Emergency Management Agency's (FEMA) use of the

Incident Command System could be adapted for health care settings. Over the next 2 years, I attended trainings hosted by state and federal partners through Boston's DelValle Institute for Emergency Preparedness. There, we completed tabletop exercises and observed barriers in communication as "live" chemical spills, storms, and pandemics unfolded. Hospital administrators and public health and law enforcement officers welcomed a new face at the table. I also registered with the Massachusetts registration system, "MA Responds," to identify my credentials as a medical professional willing to train and deploy for mass events.

I used these experiences and concepts from the 2006 AOTA position paper on disaster preparedness to design free workshops for OT practitioners to introduce them to key emergency management concepts. We reviewed the FEMA's Family Emergency Communication Plan, contents of an emergency kit, and alert notification systems. Participants contemplated ways to tailor their services to their specific population. For example, should school-based practitioners contribute input on "grab and go" kits, and should home health agencies assess the level of support required during emergencies? There is enormous potential for OT practitioners to identify and address areas of need. So start where you're most familiar: at home and work.

CASE STUDY 68-2   SHANNON MANGUM'S CASE STUDY

Shannon Mangum, MPS, LOTR, has been involved in disaster work for over 12 years. She specializes in mental health practice and teaches in the Occupational Therapy Department at LSUHSC in New Orleans. Shannon's disaster work after Katrina began during the recovery period. She organized students, and they gutted people's homes to prepare the houses for rebuilding. More recently (S. Mangum, personal communication, June 7, 2017), she reports the LSUHSC faculty dedicated a day of service for two classes of students. The classes divided themselves among four projects: (1) gutting three houses flooded in Baton Rouge from August 2016 flood waters; (2) working at shelters with kids and families assisting with food preparation and distribution, organizing children's activities, distributing basic items, and visiting with individuals; (3) volunteering at the animal shelters in the surrounding area, helping with walking, bathing, cleaning out kennels/stalls; and (4) collecting items such as school uniforms, baby items, and basic cleaning supplies to distribute directly to some of the home owners. Many of the students then voluntarily returned on their own time with faculty to continue with their efforts they had started on the day of service. Many of the students who helped with the gutting had either gutted their own homes or had gotten

assistance after Katrina, and they were highly motivated as well as skilled in the whole process (Figure 68-1).

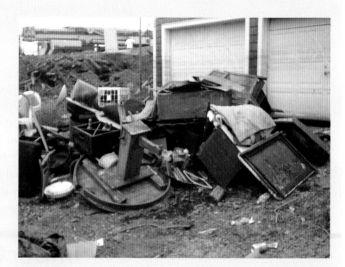

FIGURE 68-1 **Contents of the first floor of Theresa Smith's townhouse gutted by LSUHSC students in 2005.**

or events that cause significant environmental destruction, loss of life, and disruption of social structure and normal daily life routines. Disasters overwhelm the local capacity to respond and necessitate requests for external assistance (Centre for Research on the Epidemiology of Disasters, 2009). Due to growing number of natural and technological disasters and continued terrorist threats, it can be expected that the number of individuals affected by disasters will rise. This increase is due to significant population density in flood plains and along vulnerable coasts and earthquake fault lines, an increase in climate-related disasters as evidenced by the average number of Atlantic hurricanes doubling in the last century (Holland & Webster, 2007), technological failures such as the Gulf Oil Spill and the subsequent use of dispersant to clean it up (Hollis, 2010), and international terrorist attacks resulting in thousands of fatalities (LaFranchi, 2010).

Disasters are not delineated as a singular event but rather conceptualized as progressing through a sequence of stages (American Occupational Therapy Association [AOTA], 2011). The five stages of preimpact period, impact period, immediate postimpact period, recovery period, and reconstruction period require different responses. Disasters can result in great personal loss, fragmented social support, and community destruction (Lowe, Chan, & Rhodes, 2010). Personal loss can include not only injury to oneself but also the injury or death of a loved one, property damage, and/or financial loss. Social support can be affected due to widespread evacuations, and lack of social connections has been determined to be a risk factor for the development of posttraumatic stress disorder (PTSD) (Hobfoll et al., 2007). The destruction of a community leads to loss of community support and the social structure where "individuals routinely, and habitually, enact and shape identity through doing within everyday social interactions" (Huot & Rudman, 2010, p. 72) (Figure 68-2).

Following disasters, most survivors experience acute stress reactions including emotional, physical, cognitive, and interpersonal effects (AOTA, 2011). Emotional reactions such as grief, fear, guilt, numbness, and despair (Rao, 2006) are usually more severe and last longer than physical effects (Carroll, Morbey, Balogh, & Araoz, 2009). Long-term physical disabilities can result (Parente et al., 2017) including the most frequent disabilities of spinal cord injury, traumatic brain injury, fracture, limb amputation, peripheral nerve injury, and crush injury (Khan, Amatya, Gosney, Rathore, & Burkle, 2015). In addition, disaster survivors have reported cognitive effects such as confusion and inability to concentrate and interpersonal problems secondary to avoidance of social interaction (AOTA, 2011). Health problems or injuries were evident in approximately one-third of the Katrina evacuees in Houston shelters (Brodie, Weltzien, Altman, Blendon, & Benson, 2006). Recent research has shown that the psychosocial and health effects of disasters can sometimes last for years (Te Brake et al., 2009).

Postdisaster distress is nearly universal and important to address among disaster survivors (North, 2010). Psychosocial responses vary depending on the disaster, affected population and setting, so no one mental health model can adequately address all postdisaster scenarios. The range of people's reactions posttrauma will vary from a transient stress reaction needing support and provision of resources to those reactions that need psychological assessment and intensive intervention (Hobfoll et al., 2007). Some survivors may develop psychiatric disorders including PTSD, depression, prolonged grief, or substance abuse (Rao, 2006). Rao (2006) lists the following predisposing and posttraumatic factors that may contribute to the development of these disorders.

Predisposing factors

- Childhood sexual abuse
- Previous unresolved losses and traumas
- Substance use
- Previous psychiatric history
- Minority or disadvantage status (economic, social)
- Multiple life stressors

Posttraumatic factors

- Severe and acute psychological reactions after the event
- Lack of social and family supports
- Extensive personal loss
- Adverse reactions from others (blame or rejection)
- Survivor's guilt

Other factors that may predispose a person to a postdisaster psychiatric disorder include sustaining injuries (Norris, Sherrieb, & Galea, 2010), viewing upsetting events, the death of family or friend, displacement (Fullilove, 1996), property loss, and a perceived decrease in social support (Hobfoll et al., 2007; Lowe et al., 2010). Survivors with postdisaster psychiatric disorders require

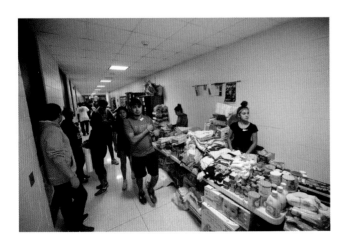

FIGURE 68-2 **Creating shelters during the immediate postimpact stage of Hurricane Harvey.**

rapid mental health interventions and long-term continuation of services (North, 2010).

Not all effects from disasters are detrimental. **Posttraumatic growth** can occur when survivors find something positive in a tragedy and try to make sense of it (Kessler, Galea, Jones, & Parker, 2006). Personal growth may manifest as increased emotional closeness to loved ones, faith in the ability to reconstruct life, spirituality, meaning or purpose in life, and/or recognition of inner strength. Posttraumatic growth can be facilitated as an individual reflects through journaling or talking with friends and establishes a support system or creates a positive vision of life (Cancer.Net, 2011).

Addressing the Needs of Individuals and Families

During disaster work, practitioners can focus on supporting people's health and participation through engagement in occupation. Many areas of occupation are essential in managing the ensuing disorder of a disaster. Disaster survivors commonly face disrupted habits, routines, and roles, and participation in occupation can help restore these (AOTA, 2011, 2017).

Occupational therapy practitioners can contribute at every stage of a disaster and on an individual, family, or community level. In the predisaster stage, they can assist by addressing emergency plans with individuals and providing consultation for community agencies. An emergency plan should be considered a living document to be revised in detail and practiced regularly in the home and workplace. The FEMA's "Family Emergency Communication Plan" (FEMA, 2015) lists extensive considerations for shelter-in-place and evacuation planning. In areas more susceptible to natural disasters, practitioners can assist with planning culturally sensitive shelter accommodations that provide equal access for all persons including those with disabilities. Postdisaster, practitioners can provide mental health services to mitigate acute stress reactions and facilitate adaptation to changed contexts. Some of the distress experienced in later stages of a disaster can be prevented or mitigated by being organized during the preparation and impact stages. Box 68-1 contains information on how to prepare individuals and families for the different disaster stages.

A majority of states have also passed laws regarding disaster planning for pets partly to ensure evacuation is not delayed. All individuals can access guidelines for creating a Pet Emergency Plan (https://www.ready.gov/animals) and can consult the local veterinarian or animal shelter (Ready, n.d.).

BOX 68-1	INDIVIDUAL AND FAMILY NEEDS AT DIFFERENT STAGES OF DISASTER

Preparation Stage for Individuals and Family	
Personal	• A plastic container for all important documents: legal (birth certificate, marriage certificate, passport, social security card), medical (history, medications, allergies, insurance cards), monthly bills (e.g., utilities, mortgage) with phone numbers, insurance policies (e.g., homeowners, renters, flood), pictures of your property • Licensing information (e.g., license, continuing education certificates) • Chargers and batteries for durable medical equipment (e.g., motorized wheelchair) • Glasses and contact lenses • Hand sanitizer and antibacterial wipes • Cash, debit/credit cards, and traveler's checks • Written list of phone numbers and e-mail addresses for household members • Consult providers to plan for replacing medical supplies used daily, refrigerated medication, or maintaining life-support devices (e.g., dialysis machines) • Create emergency plan with your local pharmacy for access to refills and to maintain 2-week supply of prescription medications • Hard of hearing: Ensure access to relay services to landline phones, computers, or cell phones. • If dependent on electricity for life-support devices: Notify local fire department, electric company, and equipment suppliers (some states have a "priority reconnection service" list).
Home	• Portable chargers and external battery packs for cell phone, rechargeable flashlight, candles, and waterproof matches, radio (battery-operated, solar-powered, or hand crank) • At least 5-day supply of nonperishable foods (e.g., canned food, fruits, vegetables, cereal, granola bars, nuts) and a manual can opener; bottled water (1 gallon per person/per day) and water purification tablets; extra tanks of oxygen, insulin, catheters, or medical supplies; basic tools (to shut off natural gas or water valves); comfort items (to promote self-regulation)
Cars	• Keep your gas tank at least half full; have a phone charger for the car, flashlight, first aid kit; cash • Paper maps of local area (to take alternate routes for evacuation)

BOX 68-1 INDIVIDUAL AND FAMILY NEEDS AT DIFFERENT STAGES OF DISASTER (continued)

Impact Stage for Individuals and Family: Evacuation and Shelter in Place

	Evacuation	Shelter in Place
Personal	• Everything from the preparation stage plus clothing for a week • Pay monthly bills ahead if possible. • Pets: Follow your Pet Emergency Plan, or call your local animal shelter for instructions.	• Assess immediate danger.
Home	• Arrange temporary housing.	• Clear outdoor spaces. • Close storm shutters if present. • Fill bathtubs with water. • Prepare closets or tubs with bedding.
Car(s)	• Use radio to follow instructions on accessing evacuation routes and the appropriate shelter. • Do not take shortcuts (routes may be blocked).	• Park in the garage or a covered parking lot on at least the second level.

Immediate Postimpact Stage for Individuals and Family

Personal	• Stay away from oversensationalized news reports. • When safe to return, determine if protective clothing (face masks, rubber boots, and gloves) are needed. • Buy items outside the impact area.
Home	• If necessary, continue in temporary housing and call insurance companies. • Make sure your smoke and carbon monoxide detectors are working. • Assess damages, take pictures, and do not remove any damaged items until an insurance representative has arrived. • Determine through local news if the tap water is safe to drink before using. • If electricity has been off more than several hours, cook frozen food and discard refrigerated food. • Update your status, or search for loved ones, on the American Red Cross "Safe and Well" Website: https://safeandwell.communityos.org/cms/index.php.
Cars	• Assess for damages and call insurance company as needed.

Recovery and Reconstruction Stage for Individuals and Family

Personal	• Return to routines (Te Brake et al., 2009). • Use stress management techniques (e.g., exercise, meditate, pray, relax). • Ensure sleep quality through environmental and behavioral changes. • Participate in valued leisure activities (AOTA, 2011). • Ventilation (e.g., talk about your experiences) (Rao, 2006) • Restore social connections (Lowe et al., 2010). • Reconnect with community.
Home	• If the area has been declared a disaster area, register with FEMA. • Remove items like wet wallboard and carpeting to prevent further damage. • Save all receipts for any replacement items. • Organize insurance claims, and keep copies of all documents. • Consider new modifications or home arrangements, as you rebuild. • If interested in volunteering for your community, listen to instructions from local authorities. Help your neighbors, if appropriate, but do not "self-deploy" and place a greater burden on first responders. You can also contact your local Red Cross agency or faith-based organization.

FEMA, Federal Emergency Management Agency.

Addressing the Needs of Communities

Disasters impact whole communities, resulting in potential community-wide economic, environmental, governmental, social, and cultural disruptions that can themselves contribute to psychological distress (Norris et al., 2010). Practitioners can also contribute at the community level during different disaster stages, but if they expect to work at this level, they should be involved in the community disaster response agencies prior to a disaster occurring (AOTA, 2011; Stone, 2006; Taylor, Jacobs, & Marsh, 2011).

Preparation Stage for Communities

It's important to learn fundamental principles of disaster planning, which includes shelter-in-place and evacuation procedures. FEMA (2011) has modeled the "Whole Community Approach" to emergency planning, promoting collaborations between private and nonprofit agencies, academia, government officials, and individual residents. All OT practitioners can identify ways to contribute to emergency planning efforts, particularly to meet the significant need in community-based contexts. As with recent trends in telehealth, there is an interest in adapting technology to deliver disaster preparedness education to populations who are traditionally isolated (e.g., older adults in rural communities).

In the preparation stage, Taylor et al. (2011) recommend that practitioners assist in planning evacuations and in advising communities on shelter accommodations for vulnerable individuals. Some practitioners have taken active roles to educate the public on this subject. Michael Steinhauer, OTR/L, MPH, FAOTA, brings to emergency planning both public health and emergency management experiences, having served two counties as the county public health officer by overseeing natural and public health disasters, and chief county planner in Madison, Wisconsin. He emphasizes three avenues of interprofessional collaboration (M. Steinhauer, personal communication, June 25, 2017):

- Public health (local, county, state): All local public health departments are mandated to have an emergency preparedness unit. Practitioners should make contact and identify ways to attend volunteer events or take leadership roles to revise emergency plans.
- Emergency management (local, county, state): All towns and counties have a local emergency manager. Depending on the state, practitioners can volunteer in different capacities (American Red Cross, community emergency response teams [CERT], or a volunteer-management system where specific credentials are recognized).

- Human services: Federal recommendations emphasize collaboration with health care practitioners and community-based organizations, including mental and behavioral health agencies. There is great potential for practitioners to address the overwhelming gap in disaster planning, response, and recovery for populations that require special considerations.

Throughout the impact stage, it's critical to ensure access to verified methods of communication. In the community, practitioners should be familiar with specific alert notification systems to receive official instructions from local authorities. In the workplace, it's important to understand the chain of command, operational procedures, and how to signal a supervisor when necessary.

Organizations like the American Red Cross provide free informational smartphone apps to facilitate collaboration during disaster responses. Practitioners can learn about smartphone apps that operate without cellular service or Internet connection. One app worth noting: In Case of Emergency (ICE) can store contacts related to medical information (physicians, insurance, medications, allergies, and special instructions). If the phone screen and password are locked, there is a feature that grants access to first responders seeking critical information.

Addressing the Needs of Special Populations

Traditionally, the terms *at-risk*, *vulnerable*, or *special needs* populations have been used in the literature. FEMA's guidance to emergency managers now includes references to "access and functional needs," reflecting a recent shift to reconceptualize the services required for shelter planning and evacuation. The term *inclusive planning* typically refers to the act of including such persons in disaster planning and emergency management. Special populations traditionally include, but are not limited to, children, older adults, those with chronic medical needs, racial and ethnic minorities, undocumented immigrants, and non-English speakers as well as those with low literacy rates and lower socioeconomic status (Lemyre, Gibson, Zlepnig, Meyer-Macleod, & Boutette, 2009). Practitioners have skills that can address the needs of special populations before, during, and after disasters.

First Responders

To participate in disaster planning and response, it's critical to become familiar with the key players and organizations involved in disaster management (AOTA, 2011). The term *first responders* can refer to a range of positions in public safety, law enforcement, public health, and health care. Depending on the scale of the emergency, local, county, state, or federal levels are activated. To effectively collaborate, practitioners should consider ways to register or become affiliated with organizations like the Medical Reserve Corps, the Red Cross, CERT, or local public health branches (AOTA, 2011). Practitioners can establish greater credibility by learning to articulate their role within a common organizational structure. Every responder in the country should be familiar with FEMA's Incident Command System (ICS), which promotes an integrated response between all personnel on site. Practitioners can locate free introductory courses by registering for a FEMA Student Identification Number on FEMA's Website (https://training.fema.gov).

The response to the 2013 Boston Marathon bombing demonstrated the value of integrating preparedness training among public safety, law enforcement, public health, and health care workers (Krisberg, 2013). Efficient information sharing and medical surge capacities ensured the survival of every injured person who arrived at a hospital (Massachusetts Emergency Management Agency et al., 2014), where OT practitioners supported the long-term rehabilitation of survivors. Two survivors, Patrick Downes and Jessica Kensky, would later present as keynote speakers at AOTA's 2016 Annual Conference. The lack of a disaster mental health coordination plan after the bombings resulted in several need areas, including support for non-public personnel and health care providers (Massachusetts Emergency Management Agency et al., 2014). This gap in service highlights the ongoing need for practitioners in community-based and mental health settings to be more proactive with registering in appropriate systems (i.e., Medical Reserve Corps, mental health response teams) and listing specific credentials.

First responders work long, difficult hours under poor conditions and are often required to perform tasks that can potentially result in injury or even death. In addition, they can be exposed to horrifying images of people with significant injuries, observe grieving family members, and view body parts or corpses (Evans, Patt, Giosan, Spielman, & Difede, 2009). Occupational therapy practitioners working in disaster situations must be mindful of the need to prevent compassion fatigue for other disaster responders and for themselves. Compassion fatigue can occur when the helper (volunteer or professional) becomes preoccupied with the suffering and distress experienced by the recipients of care which results in spiritual exhaustion accompanied by acute emotional pain (Pfifferling & Gilley, 2000). Prevention requires personal self-care including good nutrition, adequate sleep, enjoyable physical activity, spending time with family and friends, prayer, and meditation.

Some first responders are at risk for developing more severe psychological problems. Approximately 12% of the utility workers cutting and restoring power at the World Trade Center had substantial symptoms of PTSD (Evans et al., 2009). Because each disaster site is unique, the psychological needs of first responders at different disasters will vary. As Precin (2006) said of providing counseling to firefighters after 9/11, "There were no manuals or books written on how to do firehouse counseling in the wake of a devastating disaster of this magnitude" (p. 47).

Children

Children in disaster zones are subject to the same tragedy observations and frightening media coverage as adults (Figure 68-3). In the chaos immediately after a disaster, they may be separated from family members, and if lacking identification, they may be displaced from a stable environment for years (Nadkarni & Leonard, 2007). It is estimated that at least 20,000 of the 160,000 children displaced by Hurricane Katrina have developed serious emotional or behavioral problems (Donnelly, 2010). These problems have been attributed to children not possessing the coping mechanisms adults do. Researchers have suggested means to combat the fear and anxiety children experience from disasters. Therapeutic play can be initiated in shelters during the impact stage of a disaster or postimpact stage of a disaster (Nadkarni & Leonard, 2007). One play activity for which it is easy to transport supplies and that allows children to express their emotions is drawing. Goenjian and colleagues (as cited in Hobfoll et al., 2007) found that teaching children emotional regulation skills and enhanced problem-solving skills help them address adversities in a disaster's wake. Children also need to return to a normal routine as soon as possible and that means returning to school even if in a temporary setting (Rao, 2006).

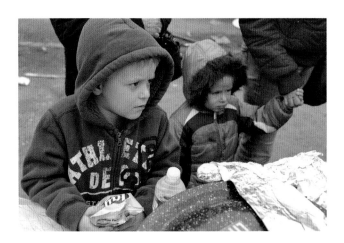

FIGURE 68-3 **Children getting basic needs met after Super Storm Sandy.**

Persons with Disabilities

Persons with disabilities and activity limitations are at particular risk during emergency and disaster situations. Reduced abilities to see, speak, hear, walk, understand, learn, remember, and manipulate significantly affect a person's ability to respond in disaster situations. In addition, activity limitations may decrease a person's adaptability during disasters and predispose them to emotional trauma. After a disaster, lack of food and water, extremes of temperature, stress, interruptions in medication regimens, lack of access to medical care, and exposure to contaminants can contribute to the exacerbation of a chronic illness that was previously well managed (Aldrich & Benson, 2008). Due to the near limitless variety of potential activity limitations, there is no "one size fits all" when it comes to addressing the needs of people with disabilities before, during, and after disasters. The breakdown of infrastructure during and after disaster disadvantages persons with disabilities disproportionally, limiting their ability to access transportation, shelter, health care, and communication services (Priestley & Hemingway, 2006). Occupational therapy practitioners can participate in the design of shelters for persons with disabilities, training of shelter managers and staff, planning of accessible services after a disaster, and educating individuals and families on strategies for sheltering in place.

Limited English Proficient Persons and Refugees

In the past decade, there has been an increased focus on addressing the gaps in disaster planning for limited English proficient persons. This population includes immigrant families, students, and refugees living in the United States. Few county and city agencies have adequate resources to provide rapid translations of emergency instructions. Practitioners can assist in raising awareness and developing community partnerships for populations that are isolated from mainstream American organizations.

In August 2016, an OT graduate student spent 2 weeks at "The Jungle," a refugee camp in Calais, France, as a volunteer with a U.S. nonprofit. She worked with children, teenagers, and adult refugees from Afghanistan, Syria, Iraq, Sudan, Eritrea, and Ethiopia: "In our circus workshops we aimed to provide inclusive space for those from different cultures to solve problems and depend on each other in a crucial survival setting. Supporting the need for adults to develop language skills, facilitators taught English through teaching circus skills, by linking words to an action with the toss of a ball or the spin of a hoop. I saw roles emerge in these workshops: participants who had learned a basic juggling sequence would demonstrate to others. In times of nothing is where we humans are forced to re-examine the ways in which we live with one another. This is where

learning occurs, this is where we give up what we've relied on and learn to adapt quickly" (S. Arrigo, personal communication, June 1, 2017).

The Role of Occupational Therapy Organizations

On an international and national level, OT practitioners have contributed to emergency preparedness and disaster response (AOTA, 2011; Hasselkus, 2001; McColl, 2002; World Federation of Occupational Therapists [WFOT], 2016a). The WFOT has a manual on disaster response and recently posted an online module for disaster management training (WFOT, 2016b). The AOTA has facilitated online communication from members affected by disasters in the past such as Hurricane Katrina.

Occupational therapy practitioners and OT students (AOTA, 2011; Persh, 2003; Pizzi, 2015; Precin, 2003; Smith, Dreyfus, & Hersch, 2011; Smith & Scaffa, 2014; Taylor et al., 2011) are also victims and survivors of disasters. Universities in disaster areas experience crisis, and their faculty, students, and infrastructures are forced to operate in survival mode (Morris, 2008). Whole communities and supporting institutions in disaster zones are unable to function, remain closed for extended periods of time, or never reopen. In these times, entities outside the impact zone must be prepared to respond.

A Professional Responsibility

Practitioners have a professional responsibility to participate in disaster work. By promoting access to occupation to ensure health and quality of life for individuals and populations affected by disasters, they can uphold the commitment of the profession to promote occupational justice (AOTA, 2011).

Training for Disaster Work

Education and training for OT practitioners in evidence-based, trauma-informed care is critical. **Trauma-informed care** refers to assessment and intervention that includes "a basic understanding of how trauma affects the life of an individual seeking services . . . so that these services and programs can be more supportive and avoid re-traumatization" (Substance Abuse and Mental Health Services Administration, n.d., p. 1). It is a strengths-based approach that represents a paradigm shift from focusing on dysfunction and diagnosis to focusing on what happened to the person, recognizing that the individual's reaction may be a normal response to an abnormal situation.

CENTENNIAL NOTES

Disaster Response

Historically in the United States, OT practitioners were not considered able to assist in disaster response in a professional capacity due to their lack of training in caring for injuries or wounds, taking vital signs, administering injections or medicine, or caring for people in a state of mental distress (McDaniel, 1960). Rosenfeld (1982) did recognize the ability of practitioners in disaster rehabilitation efforts, stating they could assist disaster victims "remake their world" (p. 229). For years, the Army has deployed practitioners on mental health teams (Oakley, Caswell, & Parks, 2008). In the 1990s, the number of journal articles on disaster work increased with a focus on safety for vulnerable populations (Valluzzi, 1995) and issues relating to veterans (Gerardi, 1996, 1999, Rice & Gerardi, 1999). But in the weeks and months after 9/11, practitioners did provide wound care, scar management, splinting, psychosocial care, and job restoration (Precin, 2003). In 2005, practitioners came out in numbers to work with evacuees from Hurricane Katrina in the Houston Reliant Center. Occupational therapy students in New Orleans worked for many months gutting houses damaged or destroyed by Hurricane Katrina. Through responding to the very different disasters, practitioners gained confidence in the services they had to offer over and above survivors' physical needs and an undeniable press to provide their services. As the need for disaster response has grown and a better understanding of survivors' needs grew, so has the number and type of resources OT practitioners can utilize. In 2006, AOTA published its first position paper on OT and disaster relief (Scaffa, Gerardi, Herzberg, & McColl, 2006), and a second position paper was written in 2011 (AOTA, 2011). Most recently, AOTA (2017) published a societal statement on disaster response consistent with the WFOT's most recent position statement (WFOT, 2016a). In 2014, a chapter devoted to disaster response in *Willard & Spackman's Occupational Therapy* 12th edition was published (Smith & Scaffa, 2014), and in 2015, an entire text on the occupational perspective on disaster was published (Rushford & Thomas, 2015). As stated earlier, the WFOT has a manual on disaster response and an online module for disaster management training (WFOT, 2016b). Although we now have more resources, there has not been any slowing in global warming effects, terrorists' acts, or forced migrations of large populations including vulnerable populations. This means that we must prepare and stand at ready to mobilize.

Trauma-informed care has become the standard of care in mental health and is compatible with several OT theories and models or models used in OT, including the Model of Human Occupation, Occupational Adaptation, and the Canadian Model of Occupational Performance and Engagement. The Model of Human Occupation was found to be useful in evaluation of and intervention for older adults with a history of trauma in Israel "because of its emphasis on the ongoing possibility of people to maintain, reinforce, shape, and change their own capacities, beliefs, dispositions, and life stories through occupation" (Ziv & Roitman, 2008, p. 91). It was also used to examine changes in students' roles after Hurricane Ike (Smith et al., 2011). The theory of Occupational Adaptation is helpful in understanding and facilitating mature adaptive response behaviors, which, in turn, allow "individuals to meet the demands of the environment, cope with the problems of everyday living, and fulfill age-specific roles" (Johnson, 2006, p. 75), The Canadian Model of Occupational Performance is valuable because it is a client-centered approach that incorporates spirituality (Law et al., 1997). More recently, Pizzi (2015) used the Recovery Model for students coping with the aftermath of Hurricane Sandy. See Unit IX for more information on theory and practice.

Prior to a disaster, practitioners should become involved with organizations like the American Red Cross, CERT, mental health crisis services, critical incident stress management teams, and employee assistance programs to increase the probability of being called on to serve during a disaster (AOTA, 2011). To ensure our participation in disaster work, it is incumbent on practitioners to educate the agency they have joined as to the scope and value of OT services (Taylor et al., 2011).

REFERENCES

Aldrich, N., & Benson, W. F. (2008). Disaster preparedness and the chronic disease needs of vulnerable older adults. *Preventing Chronic Disease: Public Health Research, Practice and Policy, 5*, A27. Retrieved from http://www.cdc.gov/pcd/issues/2008/jan/07_0135.htm

American Occupational Therapy Association. (2011). The role of occupational therapy in disaster preparedness, response, and recovery. *American Journal of Occupational Therapy, 65*, S11–S25. Retrieved from http://www.aota.org/Practitioners/Official /Concept/39464.aspx?FT=.pdf

American Occupational Therapy Association. (2017). AOTA's societal statement on disaster response and risk reduction. *American Journal of Occupational Therapy, 71*, 7112410060p1–7112410060p3. doi:10.5014/ajot.2017.716S11

Briere, J., & Elliott, D. (2000). Prevalence, characteristics, and long-term sequelae of natural disaster exposure in the general population. *Journal of Traumatic Stress, 13*, 661–679.

Brodie, M., Weltzien, E., Altman, D., Blendon, R., & Benson, J. (2006). Experiences of Hurricane Katrina evacuees in Houston shelters: Implications for future planning. *American Journal of Public Health, 96*, 1402–1408.

Cancer.Net. (2011). *Post-traumatic growth and cancer*. Retrieved from http://www.cancer.net/patient/All+About+Cancer/Cancer.Net +Feature+Articles/After+Treatment+and+Survivorship/Post -Traumatic+Growth+and+Cancer

Carroll, B., Morbey, H., Balogh, R., & Araoz, G. (2009). Flooded homes, broken bonds, the meaning of home, psychological processes and their impact on psychological health in a disaster. *Health & Place, 15*, 540–547. doi:10.1016/j.healthplace.2008.08.009

Centre for Research on the Epidemiology of Disasters. (2009). *What's new*. Retrieved from http://www.cred.be/

Donnelly, B. (2010). *Katrina five years after: Hurricane left a legacy of health concerns*. Retrieved from http://www.foxnews.com/health/2010/08/27 /katrina-years-hurricane-left-legacy-health-concerns.html

Evans, S., Patt, I., Giosan, C., Spielman, L., & Difede, J. (2009). Disability and posttraumatic stress disorder in disaster relief workers responding to September 11, 2001 World Trade Center disaster. *Journal of Clinical Psychology, 65*, 684–694. doi:10.1002/jclp.20575

Federal Emergency Management Agency. (2011). *A whole community approach to emergency management: Principles, themes, and pathways for action*. Retrieved from https://www.fema.gov/media-library -data/20130726-1813-25045-0649/whole_community_dec2011__2_.pdf

Federal Emergency Management Agency. (2015). *Create your family emergency communication plan*. Retrieved from https://www.fema .gov/media-library-data/1440449346150-1ff18127345615d8b7e1ef fb4752b668/Family_Comm_Plan_508_20150820.pdf

Fullilove, M. T. (1996). Psychiatric implications of displacement: Contributions from the psychology of place. *American Journal of Psychiatry, 153*, 1516–1523.

Gerardi, S. M. (1996). The management of battle-fatigued soldiers: An occupational therapy model. *Military Medicine, 161*, 483–488.

Gerardi, S. M. (1999). Part I. Work hardening for warriors: Occupational therapy for combat stress casualties. *Work, 13*, 185–195.

Hasselkus, B. R. (2001). From the desk of the editor—Unspeakable occupations. *American Journal of Occupational Therapy, 5*, 606–607.

Hobfoll, S. E., Watson, P., Bell, C. C., Bryant, R. A., Brymer, M. J., Friedman, M. J., . . . Ursano, R. J. (2007). Five essential elements of immediate and mid-term mass trauma intervention: Empirical evidence. *Psychiatry, 70*, 283–315.

Holland, G., & Webster, P. (2007). Heightened tropical cyclone activity in the North Atlantic: Natural variability or climate trend? *Philosophical Transactions, 365*, 2695–2716.

Hollis, P. (2010). *Gulf oil spill disaster latest example in list of technological blunders*. Retrieved from http://southeastfarmpress.com /gulf-oil-spill-disaster-latest-example-list-technological-blunders

Huot, S., & Rudman, D. L. (2010). The performances and places of identity: Conceptualizing intersections of occupation, identity and place in the process of migration. *Journal of Occupational Science, 17*, 68–77.

Johnson, J. A. (2006). Describing the phenomenon of homelessness through the theory of occupational adaptation. *Occupational Therapy in Health Care, 20*, 63–80.

Kessler, R. C., Galea, S., Jones, R. T., & Parker, H. A. (2006). Mental illness and suicidality after Hurricane Katrina. *Bulletin of the World Health Organization, 84*, 930–939.

Khan, F., Amatya, B., Gosney, J., Rathore, F. A., & Burkle, F. M., Jr., (2015). Medical rehabilitation in natural disasters: A review. *Archives of Physical Medicine and Rehabilitation, 96*, 1709–1727.

Krisberg, K. (2013). Public health workers at center of Boston bombing response: Preparedness pays off during crisis. *The Nation's Health, 43*(5), 1–14.

LaFranchi, H. (2010). *Last year, 10,999 terrorist attacks worldwide—A decline from 2008*. Retrieved from http://www.csmonitor .com/USA/Foreign-Policy/2010/0805/Last-year-10-999-terrorist -attacks-worldwide-a-decline-from-2008

Law, M. L., Cooper, B. A., Strong, S., Stewart, D., Rigby, P., & Letts, L. (1997). Theoretical contexts for the practice of occupational therapy.

In C. Christiansen & C. Baum (Eds.), *Occupational therapy: Enabling function and well-being* (2nd ed., pp. 73–103). Thorofare, NJ: SLACK.

Lemyre, L., Gibson, S., Zlepnig, J., Meyer-Macleod, R., & Boutette, P. (2009). Emergency preparedness for higher risk populations: Psychosocial considerations. *Radiation Protection Dosimetry, 134*, 207–214. doi:10.1093/rpd/ncp084

Lowe, S. R., Chan, C. S., & Rhodes, J. E. (2010). Pre-hurricane perceived social support protects against psychological distress: A longitudinal analysis of low-income mothers. *Journal of Consulting and Clinical Psychology, 78*, 551–560. doi:10.1037/a0018317

Massachusetts Emergency Management Agency, Massachusetts Department of Public Health, City of Boston, City of Cambridge, Town of Watertown, Massachusetts Bay Transportation Authority Transit Police Department, Massachusetts National Guard, Massachusetts State Police. (2014). *After action report for the response to the 2013 Boston marathon bombings*. Retrieved from http://www.mass.gov/eopss/docs/mema/after-action-report-for-the -response-to-the-2013-boston-marathon-bombings.pdf

McColl, M. (2002). Occupation in stressful times. *American Journal of Occupational Therapy, 56*, 350–353.

McDaniel, M. L. (1960). The role of the occupational therapist in natural disaster situations. *American Journal of Occupational Therapy, 14*, 195–198.

Morris, A. S. (2008). Making it through a traumatic life experience: Applications for teaching, research, and personal adjustment. *Training and Education in Professional Psychology, 2*, 89–95. doi:10.1037/1931-3918.2.2.89

Nadkarni, M., & Leonard, R. B. (2007). Immediate psychological support for children after a disaster: A concept. *The Internet Journal of Rescue and Disaster Medicine, 6*, 127–131.

Norris, F. H., Sherrieb, K., & Galea, S. (2010). Prevalence and consequences of disaster-related illness and injury from Hurricane Ike. *Rehabilitation Psychology, 55*, 221–230.

North, C. S. (2010). A tale of two studies of two disasters: Comparing psychosocial responses to disaster among Oklahoma city bombing survivors and Hurricane Katrina evacuees. *Rehabilitation Psychology, 55*, 241–246. doi:10.1037/a0020119

Oakley, F., Caswell, S., & Parks, R. (2008). Occupational therapists' role on U.S. army and U.S. Public Health Service Commissioned Corps disaster mental health response teams. *American Journal of Occupational Therapy, 62*, 361–364. doi:10.5014/ajot.62.3.361

Parente, M., Tofani, M., De Santis, R., Esposito, G., Santilli, V., & Galeoto, G. (2017). The role of the occupational therapist in disaster areas: Systematic review. *Occupational Therapy International, 2017*, 6474761. doi:10.1155/2017/6474761

Persh, J. (2003). Coping with tragedy: A fieldwork student's experience with FEMA crisis counseling. In P. Precin (Ed.), *Surviving 9/11. Impact and experiences of occupational therapy practitioners* (pp. 129–151). New York, NY: Haworth Press.

Pfifferling, J. H., & Gilley, K. (2000). Overcoming compassion fatigue. *Family Practice Management, 7*(4), 39–44.

Pizzi, M. A. (2015). Hurricane Sandy, disaster preparedness, and the recovery model. *American Journal of Occupational Therapy, 69*, 6904250010p1–6904250010p10. doi:10.5014/ajot.2015.015990

Precin, P. (2003). Introduction: Surviving 9/11: Impact and experiences of occupational therapy practitioners. *Occupational Therapy in Mental Health, 19*, 1–4.

Precin, P. (2006). *Healing 9/11: Creative programming by occupational therapists*. New York, NY: Haworth Press.

Priestley, M., & Hemingway, L. (2006). Disability and disaster recovery: A tale of two cities? *Journal of Social Work in Disability & Rehabilitation, 5*(3–4), 23–42.

Rao, K. (2006). Psychosocial support in disaster-affected communities. *International Review of Psychiatry, 18*, 501–505. doi:10.1080/09540260601038472

Ready. (n.d.). *Pets and animals*. Retrieved from https://www.ready.gov/animals

Rice, V. J., & Gerardi, S. M. (1999). Part II. Work hardening for warriors: Training military occupational therapy professionals in the management of combat stress casualties. *Work, 13*, 197–209.

Rosenfeld, M. S. (1982). A model for activity intervention in disaster-stricken communities. *American Journal of Occupational Therapy, 36*, 229–235.

Rushford, N., & Thomas, K. (2015). *Disaster and development: An occupational perspective*. London, United Kingdom: Elsevier Health Sciences.

Scaffa, M. E., Gerardi, S., Herzberg, G., & McColl, M. A. (2006). The role of occupational therapy in disaster preparedness, response, and recovery. *American Journal of Occupational Therapy, 60*, 642–649.

Smith, T. M., Drefus, A., & Hersch, G. (2011). Habits, routines, and roles of graduate students: effects of Hurricane Ike. *Occupational Therapy in Health Care, 25*, 283–297.

Smith, T. M., & Scaffa, M. (2014). Providing occupational therapy for disaster survivors. In B. Schell, G. Gillen, & M. Scaffa (Eds.), *Willard & Spackman's occupational therapy* (12th ed., pp. 962–971). Baltimore, MD: Lippincott Williams & Wilkins.

Stone, G. V. M. (2006). Occupational therapy in times of disaster. *American Journal of Occupational Therapy, 60*, 7–8.

Substance Abuse and Mental Health Services Administration. (n.d.). *Trauma-informed care and trauma services*. Retrieved from http://www.samhsa.gov/nctic/trauma.asp

Taylor, E., Jacobs, R., & Marsh, E. D. (2011). First year post-Katrina: Changes in occupational performance and emotional responses. *Occupational Therapy in Mental Health, 27*, 3–25. doi:10.1080/0164212X.2011.543454

Te Brake, H., Dückers, M., De Vries, M., Van Duin, D., Rooze, M., & Spreeuwenberg, C. (2009). Early psychosocial interventions after disasters, terrorism, and other shocking events: Guideline development. *Nursing & Health Sciences, 11*, 336–343. doi:10.1111/j.1442-2018.2009.00491.x

Valluzzi, J. I. (1995). Safety issues in community-based settings for children who are medically fragile: Program planning for natural disasters. *Infants and Young Children, 7*, 62–76.

World Federation of Occupational Therapists. (2016a). *Disaster preparedness and response (DP&R)*. Retrieved from http://www.wfot.org/Practice/DisasterPreparednessandResponseDPR.aspx

World Federation of Occupational Therapists. (2016b). *Responding internationally to disasters*. Retrieved from http://www.wfot.org/Portals/0/PDF/2016/Dos%20and%20Donts%20in%20Disasters%20April%202016.pdf

Ziv, N., & Roitman, D. M. (2008). Addressing the needs of elderly clients whose lives have been compounded by traumatic histories. *Occupational Therapy in Health Care, 22*, 83–93.

the**Point**® *For additional resources on the subjects discussed in this chapter, visit* **http://thePoint.lww.com/Willard-Spackman13e.**

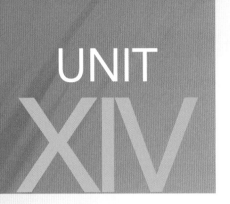

UNIT XIV

Professional Development

"The capacity to learn is a gift;
the ability to learn is a skill;
the willingness to learn is a choice."

—Brian Herbert
Dune: House Harkonnen

CHAPTER 69

Fieldwork, Practice Education, and Professional Entry

Mary E. Evenson, Debra J. Hanson

LEARNING OBJECTIVES

After reading this chapter, you will be able to:

1. Comprehend how fieldwork or practice education is integral to the educational curriculum and one's own professional development.
2. Identify the requirements, types, and levels of experiential learning, fieldwork, and practice education in United States and international academic occupational therapy programs.
3. Compare traditional and innovative types of fieldwork settings and supervision models.
4. Analyze the roles and responsibilities of those stakeholders who are involved in the fieldwork education process.
5. Analyze the process and types of competencies that are used to evaluate student fieldwork performance.
6. Explore the dynamic nature of the personal and professional transitions that are inherent in the role shifts from that of being a student to assuming the role of a professional.
7. Explain individual responsibilities for meeting professional credentialing requirements for certification and licensure/registration.
8. Compare the entry-level competencies for both occupational therapists and occupational therapy assistants.

Introduction

This chapter addresses the purpose and goals of fieldwork or practice education, along with various models associated with that form of education. Roles and responsibilities of students and educators are identified. Shifts in the learning context and expectations related to the transition from student to professional are discussed including special considerations for students with disabilities. Lastly, factors associated with professional entry into employment are described.

Fieldwork or **practice placements** are structured learning experiences that are formally administered by academic programs in partnership with facilities that offer training experiences. Whereas hospitals serve as traditional fieldwork settings, increasing numbers of placements are occurring in skilled nursing and long-term care facilities, community health, schools, private practice, and home-based settings (Rodger et al., 2008). Fieldwork or practice education provides students with opportunities to apply theoretical and scientific knowledge to address the occupational performance needs of individuals and/or groups in authentic practice contexts (American Occupational Therapy Association [AOTA], International Fieldwork Ad Hoc Committee for the Commission on Education, 2009). The consensus within the occupational therapy (OT) profession is that the fieldwork experience plays an integral role in professional development. Through progressively more challenging fieldwork requirements, designed as a part of each academic program's curriculum, students gain exposure to a "variety of clients across the lifespan and to a variety of settings" (Accreditation Council for Occupational Therapy Education [ACOTE], 2012).

Participating in fieldwork and practice education affords students the opportunity to develop collaborative supervisory relationships that evolve and shift as competency grows, along with professional development of coping skills and strategies. Both students and supervisors experience the rewards of effective communication to nurture the teaching-learning process within the dynamic context of real-life practice. Optimally, supervisors use teaching techniques such as grading and scaffolding to support students in taking an active role in providing client services. Doing so requires flexibility because the supervisor delegates selected responsibilities to the student, whereas the student builds confidence in taking risks that are inherent in new learning and skill development. These formative fieldwork experiences significantly influence each student's future career choices.

Labor projections for the growth of the profession, coinciding with changes in governmental and health care regulations have spurred increased enrollments in academic programs (Evenson, Roberts, Kaldenberg, Barnes, & Ozelie, 2015; Hamilton et al., 2015). It is anticipated that the profession will expand to meet growing global health needs through the creation of population-based approaches (World Federation of Occupational Therapists [WFOT], 2016, p. 6). Frameworks such as the World Health Organization's (WHO) community-based rehabilitation (CBR) guidelines serve as valuable resources to support occupational therapists' roles and involvement to address clients' health, education, livelihood and economic status, social, and empowerment needs (WHO, 2010). As a result, education accreditation is evolving to include a broader range of teaching methods to supplement students' participation in traditional fieldwork or practice placements. In response to competition for clinical site placements and patient safety needs in the United States, the AOTA Board of Directors has proposed the use of simulation, standardized patient encounters, faculty-led practice

experiences, and consumer education as alternative experiential learning to some of the hours in mentored practice settings (AOTA, 2017a; Bethea, Castillo, & Harvison, 2014). Occupational therapy educators are embracing innovations in practice education (Hamilton et al., 2015). For example, your academic program may designate a certain number of hours or require that specific conditions be met for learning experiences such as simulation, faculty-led or student-run clinics, faculty-led site visits, consumer education, and role-emerging or project-based placements.

Purpose and Goals of Fieldwork

The purpose of fieldwork education is to provide students with opportunities to apply the knowledge, skills, and attitudes learned in the classroom by putting them into practice in the fieldwork setting (AOTA, 2016; Costa, 2015). Fieldwork experiences are intended to provide students with opportunities to carry out professional responsibilities under supervision of professionals who also act as role models (ACOTE, 2012). Working in the context of real-life practice enables students to develop a multitude of skills. The two main categories of skill development that are inherent in participating in fieldwork are (1) the core skills and techniques that are relevant to OT service delivery for a given setting and (2) the personal skills that evolve and transform one's level of professional behavior (Missiuna, Polatajko, & Ernest-Conibear, 1992). For example, fieldwork interactions with clients and team members from other disciplines provide significant learning opportunities in the development of one's therapeutic use of self (Taylor, Lee, Kielhofner, & Ketkar, 2009) and in gaining awareness of the impact of cultural diversity on service provision (Murden et al., 2008).

Fieldwork also provides a venue for enculturation into the field. The interplay among the student as a person, the profession, and the environment supports the development of a professional identity along with a set of basic professional competencies (Alsop & Donald, 1996). This component of education functions as the gateway into the profession because it enables students to establish the fundamental skills of the profession that will support them in transitioning from the role of student into employment as a practitioner. The ultimate goal of fieldwork is to prepare students who possess the necessary competencies to be able to enter the workforce as a generalist practitioner. Beyond establishing basic skills in service provision, fieldwork also enables students to engage in advocacy, leadership, and managerial/administrative learning activities that require critical thinking, communication, collaboration, and ethical reasoning.

CENTENNIAL NOTES

Subject Areas in Clinical/Fieldwork Section of the Minimum (Accreditation) Standards and Essentials

Reflective of health care changes and the expansion of the profession, focus area designations for Level II fieldwork were constantly changing in the United States from 1923 to 1973 (AOTA, 1924, 1950; Lewis, 2005; Written History Committee of the American Occupational Therapy Association, 1983).

Note that fieldwork expectations as reflected in the 1973 accreditation standards are very similar to those of

today, with the exception of time documented in hours rather than months.

The future requirements for amount of time and areas of focus for fieldwork training are under evaluation in the United States. The AOTA (2017a) has proposed a residency model that would likely reduce the total number of hours required. Implementation of a residency will require changes in state licensure regulations which may prove to be a challenge across 50 states.

Focus Areas for Clinical Training	1923	1931	1938	1949	1965	1973
No specifics on clinical training areas just total time	3 mo	3 mo	3 mo			6 mo
Mental hospitals		2 mo	2 mo			
Tuberculosis sanatoriums		1 mo	1 mo	4–8 wk.		
General hospitals		1 mo	1 mo			
Children's hospitals or services		1 mo	1 mo	4–8 wk.		
Orthopedic hospitals or services		1 mo	1 mo			
Psychiatric conditions				12 wk		
Physical disabilities				8 wk	3 mo	
General medicine and surgery				4–8 wk		
Psychosocial dysfunction					3 mo	
Total Time Required	**3 mo**	**9 mo**	**9 mo**	**36 wk**	**6 mo**	**6 mo**

Experiential Learning: United States

The ACOTE (2012) outlines the general fieldwork requirements for doctoral-level degree and master's-level degree OT students and for OT assistant students. The requirements are divided into two classifications: Level I and Level II fieldwork. Additionally, entry-level doctoral students must complete a doctoral experiential component as a capstone experience. In this section, we first summarize the kinds of experiential learning approaches, followed by a discussion of each level of fieldwork.

Types of Experiential Learning Approaches

Simulation and Standardized Patient Encounters. Simulation may refer to a person, device, or set of conditions that attempts to authentically present education and evaluation problems, requiring learners to respond as they would under natural conditions. Simulation activities are provided on a continuum from *low to high fidelity* (Maran & Glavin, 2003). *Low-fidelity*

activities are not interactive in nature but do provide opportunity for students to practice discrete tasks or discuss potential responses to a hypothetical situation. Practicing one-handed dressing techniques or role-playing how to respond to a given practice scenario are examples of low fidelity simulation (Herge et al., 2013). *High-fidelity* simulation involves integration of knowledge, skills, and concepts and immersing the participant in a situation that mimics an actual circumstance. This might involve the use of equipment or mannequins that enable students to respond as though they were with a real patient or computer software that generates a realistic situation. Alternatively, live actors, known as *simulated* or *standardized patients* might be hired and trained to play the part of a patient in a standardized way for educational purposes (Giles, Carson, Breland, Coker-Bolt, & Bowman, 2014). Other simulation possibilities involve use of computerized technology to simulate various practice conditions. See Table 69-1 for a description of categories of simulation.

Faculty-Led Experiences, Student-Run Clinics and Interprofessional Education. Innovative health professions education methods are being explored

TABLE 69-1   Categories of Simulation

Term	Definition of Term	Example
Low-fidelity simulation (Herge et al., 2013; Maran & Glavin, 2003)	Provides opportunity for students to practice discrete tasks/discuss potential responses to situation	Practicing one-handed dressing; role-play simulation
High-fidelity simulation (Herge et al., 2013; Maran & Glavin, 2003)	Immersion in a situation that mimics an actual circumstance	The use of equipment, mannequins, a real patient, or computer software that generates a realistic situation
Standardized patient simulation (Giles et al., 2014)	Live actors hired and trained to play the part of a patient in a standardized way for educational purposes	Actor plays the role of a patient who recently acquired a CVA
Human patient simulation (Rosen, 2008)	Computerized full-body low-, medium-, or high-fidelity mannequin capable of providing real-time physiological and pharmacological responses to various health conditions and interventions	Mannequin with ability to project someone's voice, elicit a blood pressure reading, and produce a pulse
Computerized software simulation (Bradley, 2006)	Use of computer-based programs to practice decision making and skills	Advanced cardiac life support, trauma management training
Virtual immersive-reality simulation (Bradley, 2006)	Allows learning by projecting or immersing the person into the computerized environment or setting.	The person's movement becomes the actual motion of the game, such as the Wii sports program

CVA, cerebrovascular accident.

for promoting interprofessional collaboration and community service (Institute of Medicine [IOM], 2015). Core competencies for all health professions have been identified as strategies to promote client-centered care that is accessible and cost effective while taking into account the work life of health providers to prevent burnout and dissatisfaction (Bodenheimer & Sinsky, 2014; Interprofessional Education Collaborative [IPEC], 2016). Client-centered care places the client's interests, goals, and preferences at the center of interprofessional practice, giving attention to ethical, quality services that respectfully acknowledge shared values and uphold privacy and dignity. Understanding the roles and responsibilities of other providers and colleagues is essential to working together to assess and address the health needs of individuals and populations. Teamwork and communication skills are foundational to promoting meaningful, effective, and efficient health care.

Faculty-led, student-assisted programs and clinics can provide a venue to role-model teamwork while also providing community-based services to underserved populations. Similarly, student-led clinics are providing opportunities to address a specific community need and may also involve interprofessional learning experiences (Copley et al., 2007). These learning experiences may occur on campus, or within the community context. Examples include occupational therapists' role in assessing clients' functional capacities in relation to daily habits and routines to facilitate coordination services, such as primary care with families, physicians, and nurses (Donnelly, Brenchley, Crawford, & Letts, 2013), or school-based programming with school staff and teachers for refugee students (Copley, Turpin, Gordon, & McLaren, 2011). The diversification of practice education has, in some cases, been responsive to addressing community needs

(Copley et al., 2007; Fortune & McKinstry, 2012). Future research is needed as evidence to demonstrate the relationship between occupation-based interventions and targeted health outcomes (Leland, Fogelberg, Halle, & Mroz, 2017). Faculty are positioned to address this need by mentoring and actively engaging students in studying and publishing outcomes related to community-based, interprofessional services, along with dissemination of successes and failures (IOM, 2015, p. 77).

Consumer Education. Increasingly, occupational therapists, along with other health professionals, are involved with consumer instruction and education as another population-based approach for individuals and groups with chronic diseases. Such self-management interventions are often disease-specific, such as arthritis, diabetes, heart disease, breast cancer, etc., and based on behavior change theories (Richardson et al., 2014). Education typically addresses coping strategies and activity adaptations for common symptoms such as pain and fatigue (Boogard, Gater, Mori, Trincao, & Smith-Turchyn, 2016). Evidence reveals improved occupational outcomes for adults with chronic diseases who received community-based OT interventions (Hand, Law, & McColl, 2011).

Level I Experience

Level I fieldwork offers students practical experiences that are integrated throughout the academic program. The ACOTE standards describe **Level I fieldwork** as "experiences designed to enrich didactic course work through directed observation and participation in selected aspects of the occupational therapy process" (ACOTE, 2012, p. S61). For both OT and OT assistant students, the goal of

Level I fieldwork is to introduce students to the experience, "to apply knowledge to practice, and to develop understanding of the needs of clients" (ACOTE, 2012, p. S61).

Through Level I experiences, students are exposed to the values and traditions of OT practice and have the opportunity to examine their reactions to clients, systems of service delivery, related personnel, and potential role(s) within the profession. Because the academic Level I performance expectations and specific purposes of the Level I fieldwork experience vary in each OT curriculum, the timing, length, requirements, and specific focus of the experience are determined by each academic program on an individual basis (AOTA, Commission on Education, 1999). For example, schedule options may include full or half days throughout an academic term, a 1-week placement, or otherwise prearranged visits to fieldwork sites. Schedule flexibility can occur based on a community-identified need with various learning activities involving more than one visit that may evolve during a semester or at multiple points across a curriculum in a programmatic approach. Level I fieldwork or a project-based practice placement in a community-based setting may be organized as a service learning experience (Hansen et al., 2007). Simulation, standardized patients/clients, faculty-led site visits, faculty practice, and consumer instruction may also be considered Level I experiences according to the academic program's curricular design.

A study of contexts and perceptions of Level I fieldwork in practice revealed that the number of placements in emerging practice is growing and that students generally rated their Level I fieldwork experiences as positive (Johnson, Koenig, Piersol, Santalucia, & Wachter-Schutz, 2006). In examining the types of learning opportunities that are afforded to Level I students, observation and communication skills were the most commonly practiced skills across all types of settings (Johnson et al., 2006). The learning experiences available to students varied by practice setting. For example, in physical disabilities settings 72% had opportunity to practice activities of daily living (ADL), whereas 47% practiced ADL in pediatric settings (Haynes, 2011). Practice of additional clinical skills during Level I fieldwork most frequently included fine and gross motor activities in pediatrics (94%), range of motion in physical disabilities (82%), interviewing in emerging practice settings (77%), and behavioral management in mental health settings (73%) (Johnson et al., 2006, p. 281). Overall, Level I fieldwork students can maximize their learning experiences by proactively seeking opportunities to practice skills and to experience occupation-based practice.

Level II Fieldwork Experience

The goal of **Level II fieldwork** for the OT and OT assistant student is "to develop competent, entry-level generalist" practitioners (ACOTE, 2012, p. S62). Accreditation standards state that "Level II fieldwork must be integral to the program's curriculum design and must include an in-depth experience in delivering OT services to clients, focusing on the application of purposeful and meaningful occupation" (ACOTE, 2012, p. S62). Although 24 weeks of full-time Level II is required, it may be completed on a part-time basis as long as it is at least 50% of a full-time position at the placement site (ACOTE, 2012). The goal of students participating in administration and management of OT services and research is differentiated for OT Level II fieldwork when applicable. Additional learning outcomes for OT Level II fieldwork are to "promote clinical reasoning and reflective practice; to transmit the values, beliefs, that enable ethical practice; and to develop professionalism and competence as career responsibilities" (ACOTE, 2012, pp. S62–S63). For OT assistant students, the purpose of Level II fieldwork is to "promote clinical reasoning, appropriate to the occupational therapy assistant role" as well as to achieve professionalism and competence (ACOTE, 2012, pp. S62–S63). For more information about duration of placements, settings, and supervisor qualifications, see Table 69-2.

Doctoral Experiential Component

In the United States, entry-level doctoral degree programs must include a doctoral experiential component that is completed after finishing Level II fieldwork (ACOTE, 2012, pp. S63–S65). Students participate in a semester-long, full-time capstone experience, working under a mentor, for an in-depth experience that includes one or more of the following areas: clinical practice, research, program and policy development, education, administration, leadership, advocacy, or theory development (ACOTE, 2012). Each academic program structures and designs the doctoral capstone to

TABLE 69-2 Educational Requirements for Level II Fieldwork

	Occupational Therapy (ACOTE, 2012)	Occupational Therapy Assistant (ACOTE, 2012)	WFOT (2016)
Duration	24 wk full time	16 wk full time	1,000 h, some placements—8 wk
Settings	Minimum of one setting if reflective of more than one practice setting; maximum of four settings	Minimum of one setting if reflective of more than one practice setting; maximum of four settings	Different levels of health care: acute care, rehab, disability, community, and wellness
Supervisor qualifications	Occupational therapist with 1 y of experience	Occupational therapist or OT assistant with 1 y of experience	No requirement for on-site supervisor

ACOTE, Accreditation Council for Occupational Therapy Education; WFOT, World Federation of Occupational Therapists.

align with the curriculum. Determination of faculty, student, and site mentor roles and responsibilities, as well as individualized learning objectives, are agreed on and documented in a memorandum of understanding (ACOTE, 2012). For example, some students may participate in faculty-led research, whereas others may be leading a pilot implementation of community-based educational services in a role-emerging setting (Evenson & Connor, 2015).

Initially working under direct supervision, students test firsthand the theories and facts learned in academic study and have a chance to refine skills through interaction with clients across the life course, with clients' families, and with team members while working in various service delivery settings and systems. As students' abilities grow, supervision may become less direct as appropriate for the setting and the severity of the client's condition. A developmental model of supervision can be applied as an approach for planning, intervening, and evaluating the students' readiness for learning and participation throughout the trajectory of a fieldwork placement. Within a developmental framework, the learner and supervisor relationship progresses through four different phases: directive, coaching, supportive, and delegation (Barnes & Evenson, 2000). Throughout the placement, the fieldwork educator is responsible to assess the level of student competency for engaging in direct care and retains legal obligations for service provision in the fieldwork setting. In all, supervision of students must meet existing local, state/provincial, and/or federal/national safety and health requirements for relevant policies, laws, and regulations for OT practice.

PRACTICE DILEMMA

You are participating in an outpatient fieldwork placement finishing up your fourth week. Your skills and confidence are growing, and your supervisor has assigned you primary responsibilities for several individuals on your shared caseload. You are treating a woman who sustained a wrist fracture as a result of a fall (unknown etiology). You have established a friendly and open rapport in working with this client over the past couple of weeks. However, the client comes into the clinic for her intervention session noticeably distressed. It is apparent that she has been crying with red, puffy eyes, and she is acting withdrawn, not making eye contact, and limiting her normal conversation with you to short answers. You notice that she has a bandage on her arm with a cut/wound that appears to need stitches. The client's cell phone continues to ring/buzz throughout the session. Finally, she tells you that is her boyfriend calling and that she is afraid to talk with him because they had a fight before her coming into the clinic. The client breaks down crying as she explains to you that she does not feel safe to go back home. Other clients in the clinic are noticing that there is a problem. What do you do?

Practice Placements: International Perspectives

Educational Standards

Internationally, the WFOT *Minimum Standards for the Education of Occupational Therapists, Revised 2016* require that students complete 1,000 practice placement hours in different health care settings. Within these settings, practice education must provide students with the opportunity to implement an OT process "involving human interaction" with clients (individual, family, group or community to business, institution, agency, or government) delivering interventions that focus on the person, the occupation, and the environment (WFOT, 2016, p. 49). Targeted learning outcomes for graduates of WFOT-approved educational programs are to demonstrate knowledge, skills, and attitudes in the following competencies: the person-occupation-environment and its relationship to health, therapeutic and professional relationships, OT processes, professional reasoning and behavior, the context of professional practice, and the application of evidence to promote best practice (WFOT, 2016, p. 29). The Minimum Standards for Education are aligned with the WHO and United Nations Educational, Scientific and Cultural Organization (UNESCO) with the goal of advancing "human rights in global society" (WFOT, 2016, p. 3). Position statements on a variety of topics serve as resources for educators, practitioners, and students, including environmental sustainability, human displacement, universal design, vocational rehabilitation, and diversity and culture (WFOT, 2016, p. 19).

Placements

For students who are interested in international placements, the WFOT Website lists "Country Profiles" with contact details for national OT associations. It is recommended that students and academic programs allow at least 18 months for advance planning, working through the resources of the WFOT member country association in order to understand the supervision requirements of the country of interest as well as to assess individual student qualifications (AOTA, International Fieldwork Ad Hoc Committee for the Commission on Education, 2009; WFOT, n.d.) (Box 69-1). As an alternative, nonfieldwork experiences abroad may be more readily accessible with wider choices and greater flexibility for scheduling when organized through volunteer organizations, charitable mission trips, faculty initiatives, or university global center institutes. With any type of intercultural learning experience, it is important to explicitly acknowledge and address differences between health care providers and recipients of services, including belief systems, political systems, social structures, health status, educational level, and wealth (Whiteford & McAllister, 2007). Internationally, health

BOX 69-1	REQUIREMENTS AND QUALIFICATIONS FOR FOREIGN FIELDWORK OR PRACTICE PLACEMENTS

- Language fluency
- Support on local dialects and customs
- Knowledge of health care regulations and practices
- Personal safety
- Insurance
- Criminal records/police checks
- Travel advisories
- Conflict areas

- Housing
- Finances
- Contract between academic program and training facility
- Presence of qualified supervisors
- Duration of placement (meets curricular/accreditation standards)

educators have identified a number of factors that are influencing fieldwork education (see Box 69-1).

Models of Fieldwork or Practice Education: Placement Settings and Supervision

Traditionally, fieldwork or practice education has taken place in the context of a hospital or primary health care setting in which students may spend 6 weeks to 3 months at one facility with a single supervisor. However, a number of factors such as increasing demand for OT services, personnel shortages, and increasing needs for student placements are influencing the profession to develop and expand innovative fieldwork opportunities (Box 69-2). Fieldwork or practice education is now taking place in settings such as community-based day treatment programs, senior centers, assisted living facilities, sheltered workshops, homeless shelters, after-school programs, home health care, rural settings, and international placements (AOTA, Commission on Education and Fieldwork Issues Committee, 2000; AOTA, Education Department, 1999; Johnson et al., 2006; Thomas, Penman, & Williamson, 2005). For a summary of various fieldwork models and their benefits and challenges, see Table 69-3.

Roles and Responsibilities of Students and Educators

Students are eligible to begin fieldwork experiences upon completion of the prerequisite academic coursework or concurrently aligned with specific course(s) within the curriculum. Academic fieldwork coordinators

BOX 69-2	COMMENTARY: INTERNATIONAL TRENDS IN HEALTH CLINICAL EDUCATION

A multitude of factors are influencing fieldwork and practice placements and expectations of students and educators. Increasingly, university educators are facing challenges in providing sufficient placements for students with a trend of rising enrollments (Rodger et al., 2008). Health care environments are experiencing significant issues with staffing and decreased funding that are contributing to increased workloads. Work demands involving care provision to individuals with more acute health conditions and growing documentation demands create time constraints. At the organizational level, these issues are resulting in training facilities that have diminishing resources to effectively support students. These workplace demands, along with new educational requirements/standards, have shaped increased expectations of students, especially in the areas of initiative, judgment, and taking responsibility for independent learning (Vogel, Grice, Hill, & Moody, 2004). Preparing students to be competent practitioners in an increasingly complex and culturally diverse global health environment requires evidence-based care, reflective professional reasoning skills, population-based and preventive services, interprofessional collaboration, and a commitment to lifelong learning (Rodger et al., 2008).

TABLE 69-3   Fieldwork Models

Fieldwork Model and Definition	Benefits/Opportunities	Challenges/Drawbacks
Same-Site Model of Fieldwork (Diambra, Cole-Zakrzewski, & Booher, 2004; Evenson, Barnes, & Cohn, 2002) *Level I and Level II fieldwork in the same site employing developmental learning approach*	• Gain familiarity with site • Increase comfort, decrease anxiety • Early learning experience builds foundational skills and confidence for Level II Fieldwork	• Decreased exposure to alternative practice settings in the profession • Negative Level I can increase anxiety
Project-Focused/Role-Emerging Models (Clarke, Martin, de Visser, & Sadlo, 2015; Dancza et al., 2013; Hanson & Nielsen, 2016) *Designed to promote OT services in settings where the occupational therapist role has not yet been established; focuses on occupational needs, with emphasis on skills in direct practice and program development; often in community settings*	• Increased self-confidence, flexibility, perseverance, and problem solving • Project management skills • Develop skills for consultancy role • Strengthened professional identity • Opportunity to integrate theory into practice and program planning	• Coordination of on-site supervision with occupational therapist supervision • Students experience wide variety of emotions • Time challenges • Lack of occupational therapist role modeling • Purpose of placement may be obscured if on-site staff have alternative expectations • Additional support needed from academic program
Collaborative/Peer-Assisted Learning Models (Flood, Haslam, & Hocking, 2010; Hanson & Deluliis, 2015; Hong Meng Tai, Canny, Haines, & Molloy, 2016; Price & Whiteside, 2016) *Students at a similar level of education work together collaboratively to acquire knowledge and skills; usually with one supervisor*	• Positive interdependence • Face-to-face interaction skills • Cooperative, group problem solving • Supports both collaborative and autonomous learning • Equips students to be peer educators • More supportive of adult learning principles and development of teamwork skills commonly applied in OT education • Social support for students	• Interpersonal difficulties or incompatibility between students • Individualization of student grading and maintenance of student confidentiality • Requires established structure and practices along with advance orientation for all parties to support optimal outcome • Supervisor workload • Client safety in high acuity medical settings • Clinician buy-in due to unfamiliarity with the model and expectations of medical hierarchy
International Fieldwork Placement (Shields, Quilty, Dharamsi, & Drynan, 2016; Sim & Mackenzie, 2016; Simonelis, Njelesani, Novak, Kuzma, & Cameron, 2011) *Fieldwork placements which allow students to share knowledge of their field abroad while acquiring new clinical and cultural skills*	• Development of personal and professional maturity • Appreciation for differing health care systems • Cultural appreciation and sensitivity • Broader view of opportunities to make a difference • Learning to be creative with limited resources • Understanding of global issues • Participation in collaborative learning	• Flexibility is required to minimize disappointment • Cultural shock • Language barriers • Need to develop new coping strategies • Risk of harassment or financial harm • Need to develop strategies to sustain work upon departure
Intraprofessional OT–OT Assistant Education (Costa, Molinsky, & Sauerwald, 2012; Jung, Salvatori, & Martin, 2008) *OT and OT assistant students share practice activities to explore roles and promote understanding.*	• Develops relationship of trust, mutual respect • Facilitates understanding of roles • Enhanced communication skills • Development of competence and confidence in skills and abilities	• Care given to site selection and preceptor preparation • Coordinating schedule between occupational therapist and OT assistant programs • Additional tutorial once per week with resources binder
Interprofessional Clinical Experience (Ford et al., 2013; Precin, 2007; Sheppard et al., 2015) *Trainees collaborate with two or more professions in provision of client intervention.*	• Increased respect for the benefits of teamwork • Increased understanding of own role and the role of other professions • Development of skills for collaborative interprofessional communication • Increased quality of client care	• Students may underestimate skills and knowledge until they orient the next cohort • Coordination of placement schedules across disciplines may be challenging • Inconsistency in discipline participation
Multiple Mentoring Model (Copley & Nelson, 2012; Nelson, Copley, & Salama, 2010; O'Connor, Cahill, & McKay, 2012) *Multiple mentors share in the supervision of one or more students.*	• Mentors learn from one another. • Increased access of students to multiple mentors and practice areas • Increased independence and development of a range of skills	• Preplanned structure and organization needed to support student learning • Consistency among mentors in grading or expectations

ACOTE, Accreditation Council for Occupational Therapy Education.

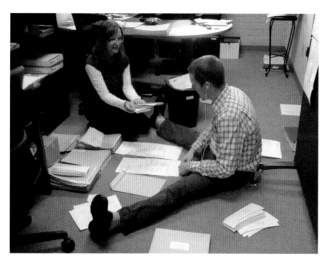

FIGURE 69-1 A fieldwork coordinator and her assistant sort through required paperwork.

or designated faculty are responsible for administrative arrangements to support student participation in fieldwork experiences, commensurate with the goals of the curriculum and accreditation standards as well as with the policies of affiliated practice settings and health care systems (Figure 69-1). Clearly defined objectives and guidelines can help to organize student efforts toward achieving

professional competence. Working toward mastery of the entry-level skills required for high-quality client care is a mutual undertaking between fieldwork educators in academic and professional practice and students. Fieldwork or practice educators assume primary responsibility for the process of evaluating student progress and modifying the learning experience within the environment, in consultation with the academic fieldwork coordinator, as appropriate. Professional confidence, which is "an understanding of and a belief in the role, scope of practice, and significance of the profession" (Holland, Middleton, & Uys, 2012a, p. 222) is also nurtured during the Level II fieldwork experience. See Table 69-4 to gain insight into how each person contributes to and participates in the overall fieldwork process.

Fieldwork Educator Guidelines

The role for the people who are responsible for providing student supervision is formally titled **fieldwork educator**, although the terms *clinical educator, fieldwork supervisor, student supervisor* (AOTA, Commission on Education and Fieldwork Issues Committee, 2000), or *practice educator* (Turpin, Fitzgerald, & Rodger, 2011) are also commonly and interchangeably used. Although the minimum requirement is 1 year of experience to supervise Level II students in the United States, fieldwork educators should

TABLE 69-4 Roles and Responsibilities in Fieldwork

Roles	Responsibilities
Academic fieldwork coordinator (AFWC)	• Serves as a liaison and collaborator with faculty and fieldwork educators to ensure integration of curricular goals with fieldwork (ACOTE, 2012) • Selects training sites and assigns students • Oversees administrative requirements, such as contracts and student health records • Available for consultation to fieldwork educators and students
Site coordinator of fieldwork	• Addresses administrative details of the fieldwork placement on behalf of the facility, serving as the fieldwork sites formal representative and liaison to the academic institution • Serves as a resource/support to the fieldwork educator
Fieldwork/practice educator	• As a credentialed occupational therapist or OT assistant, meets requisite eligibility for supervisory role as applicable (ACOTE, 2012; Committee on University Fieldwork Education, Association of Canadian Occupational Therapy University Programs [CUFE-ACOTUP], 2011) • Engages in administrative collaboration with site coordinator of fieldwork (if applicable) and AFWC to determine and schedule assignments • Provides day-to-day student supervision • Completes evaluation of student performance as designated • Structures learning and create a positive learning environment
Site educator	• Represents a professional discipline at the site, not a credentialed occupational therapist or OT assistant • Provides direct day-to-day supervision when a role-emerging model is used or during a Level I fieldwork
Student	• Fulfills all duties identified by the fieldwork educators and academic fieldwork coordinators within the designated time lines • Complies with the professional standards identified by the fieldwork facility, the education program, and the Occupational Therapy Code of Ethics (AOTA, 2015)

ACOTE, Accreditation Council for Occupational Therapy Education.

be competent practitioners who meet governmental practices acts and regulations and serve as good role models or mentors for future practitioners. Supervising students can be beneficial in keeping up to date with research evidence and professional theoretical frameworks to guide occupation-based interventions. Additionally, serving in the role as a fieldwork educator enables practitioners to hone their teaching skills in fostering the professional development of future colleagues.

Beyond training students, supervision is fundamentally viewed as underlying to the quality of service provision and development of the workforce (College of Occupational Therapists [COT], 2015). National initiatives are providing training to support the professional development of fieldwork educators in response to identified needs (Gaitskell & Morley, 2008). In the United States, AOTA has implemented a Fieldwork Education Certificate Program with the curriculum centered on the Self-Assessment Tool for Fieldwork Educator Competency (AOTA, Commission on Education, 2009) that addresses five areas: professional practice, education, supervision, evaluation, and administration. Regional workshops are instructed by a team of a practice and an academic educator. Online training programs have been developed in Canada and Australia. The Preceptor Education Certification Program for Health Professionals and Students consists of seven modules to guide learning (Bossers et al., n.d.). Developed in Australia, an online training package is freely available to support the use of the Student Placement Evaluation Form–Revised (SPEF-R), including resources addressing the use of the tool, various assessment processes, and approaches for providing feedback (Turpin et al., 2011). Each of these training programs serve as tools to assist the fieldwork educators who strive to develop and provide the best opportunity for the implementation of theoretical concepts offered as part of the academic educational program while creating an environment that facilitates learning, inquiry, self-direction, and reflection on one's practice.

Evaluation of Student Performance

Both formal and informal mechanisms for providing feedback and evaluation of performance, judgment, and attitude are built into the fieldwork experience. These evaluations have two distinct purposes, which are referred to as **formative** and **summative** processes. The formative process occurs throughout the fieldwork experience so that students and their fieldwork educators can compare perceptions, assess which learning activities are important and which are less so, review objectives, plan new learning opportunities, and make necessary modifications in behaviors and expectations. The summative process serves

to document the level of skills attained. This cumulative review requires documentation of performance at the midpoint of the placement and upon completion of the fieldwork experience.

In the United States, a Level I Fieldwork Competency Evaluation for OT and OT assistant students has been designed to assess performance skills that build a foundation for Level II fieldwork (AOTA, 2017c). The Level I Evaluation addresses skill assessment in the areas of fundamentals of practice, foundations of OT, professional behaviors, screening and evaluation, and intervention. For Level II, the Fieldwork Performance Evaluation for the Occupational Therapy Student (FWPE/OTS) (AOTA, 2002b) and the Fieldwork Performance Evaluation for the Occupational Therapy Assistant Student (FWPE/OTAS) (AOTA, 2002a) are companion instruments, adopted by AOTA's Commission on Education in 2002 (Atler, 2003). A validation study is underway to examine revised versions of the FWPE "to evaluate evidence of internal structure, response processes, and fairness in testing" (AOTA, 2017b, p. 4). Apart from a numeric rating system, the forms provide space and opportunity for supervisors to add or qualify their scoring with written descriptions and comments (Atler, 2003). The intent of the fieldwork evaluation is not to differentiate between students but to measure one's achievement of specific entry-level competencies. A profession usually defines its boundaries by setting up criteria for entry. In OT, the fieldwork experience is an essential component of the entry criteria. Successful completion of Level II fieldwork is a requirement for certification as a credentialed occupational therapist or credentialed OT assistant (National Board for Certification in Occupational Therapy [NBCOT], n.d.). Future employers want assurance that students satisfy the entry-level requirements. The FWPE data may be synthesized to provide the foundation for employment references.

Internationally, there is a trend toward the use of standardized approaches for the evaluation of student fieldwork performance. However, students are advised to verify the tool being used by their individual academic program. The Competency Based Fieldwork Evaluation for Occupational Therapists (CBFE-OT) (Bossers, Miller, Polatajko, & Hartley, 2007), widely used across English Canada and the United Kingdom, is designed for use in any level of fieldwork and within any placement area. This instrument is used in conjunction with a learning contract associated with each competency. In Australia, SPEF-R has been revised and included as part of an online package of resources (Allison & Turpin, 2004; Turpin et al., 2011). A unique aspect of the SPEF-R tool is the option to select domains that relate to the streams of either direct service provision or project management/consultancy. Additionally, a comment bank has been developed to support selection of comments that are consistent with the rating scale

TABLE 69-5 Fieldwork Evaluation in the United States, Australia, Canada, and the United Kingdom

	FWPE/OTS (United States)	FWPE/OTAS (United States)	SPEF-R (Australia)	CBFE-OT (Canada, United Kingdom)
Fieldwork evaluations and authors	AOTA (2002b)	AOTA (2002a)	Turpin et al. (2011)	Bossers et al. (2007)
Purpose	To measure entry-level competence of the OT student	To measure entry-level competence of the OT assistant student	To assess student performance for professional practice and behavior	To evaluate a student's performance and learning
Content: areas of competency	• Fundamentals of practice • Basic tenets • Evaluation/screening • Intervention • Management of OT services • Communication • Professional behavior	• Fundamentals of practice • Basic tenets • Evaluation/screening • Intervention • Communication • Professional behavior	• Professional behavior • Self-management skills • Coworker communication • Communication skills • Documentation • Information gathering • Service provision • Service evaluation	• Practice knowledge • Clinical reasoning • Facilitating change with a practice process • Professional interactions • Communication • Professional development • Performance management
Number of items	42	25	Variable; stream selected by practice educator; items vary for • Direct client contact, including case management • Project management/ consultancy	Variable; learning objectives are written by each fieldwork site as relevant to the setting.
Rating scale	4 points	4 points	5 points	3 points
Evaluation	Midterm, final	Midterm, final	Midterm (halfway), final	Midterm, final

FWPE/OTS, Fieldwork Performance Evaluation for the Occupational Therapy Student; FWPE/OTAS, Fieldwork Performance Evaluation for the Occupational Therapy Assistant Student; SPEF-R, Student Practice Evaluation Form–Revised; CBFE-OT, Competency Based Fieldwork Evaluation for Occupational Therapists.

(Rodger, Turpin, et al., 2014). Studies have been conducted to investigate the validity and reliability of the SPEF-R (Rodger et al., 2016; Rodger, Coleman, et al., 2014). It is noteworthy that each of these fieldwork evaluation tools is intended to be used across and within all practice settings. Furthermore, similar content and competency areas are evident among these tools, as noted in Table 69-5.

Student Evaluation of the Fieldwork Experience

Students also have the opportunity to provide their fieldwork or practice educators and the placement facility with feedback. The AOTA Student Evaluation of Fieldwork Experience Task Force (2016) recommends the Student Evaluation of Fieldwork Experiences (SEFWE) form. This form allows students to provide feedback about orientation, caseload, and OT process; theory, frames of reference, and models of practice; fieldwork assignments; supervisor interactions; aspects of the environment, such as team relationships; and how the entire learning experience related to the academic curriculum and to one's own professional development. In Canada and Australia, similar forms are used for students to provide feedback to placement sites. Overall, documentation of students' feedback regarding their participation in fieldwork experiences provides valuable program evaluation information to both the training site and the academic program.

Transition from Classroom to Fieldwork

The shift from the academic setting to the fieldwork setting is an obvious, yet often underestimated, life change. As a student, this entails making the environmental transition from the classroom to the fieldwork setting while simultaneously emerging from the role of student into the role of OT practitioner (Figure 69-2). As with any transition, leaving academia triggers a process of change from one structure, role, or sense of self to another. The struggle to assimilate into a new environment and to develop a new

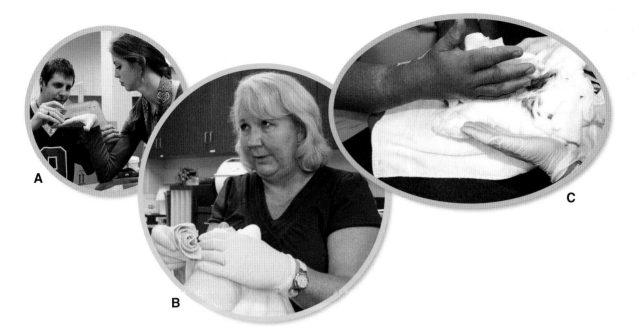

FIGURE 69-2 Moving from classroom to fieldwork: a lot to think about. Practicing techniques in the classroom can be very different than doing them with a client, as shown in these examples related to assessing wrist range of motion. **A.** The students are practicing how to measure wrist motion. **B.** The occupational therapist is unwrapping a man's hand during his first therapy session after hand surgery. This requires her to remove his dressings and manage any postoperative bleeding from his wound. **C.** The occupational therapist is observing how well he can move his wrist. She may eventually measure his wrist mobility using a similar technique as the students did during lab. Note how in the classroom, students can worry less about the client's fear and pain and focus on the technique. In practice, the therapist has to carefully monitor the client's response and postsurgical precautions while observing universal precautions and functional range of motion. (Photos courtesy of Krisi Probert and Barbara Schell.)

role can jolt students into disequilibrium, and some students have trouble adjusting to the new role. As is true of all life changes, this disequilibrium can be an opportunity for growth, especially in the context of a supportive supervisory relationship.

This time of transition results in changes in assumptions about one's self and the world, requiring a corresponding change in behaviors, relationships, learning styles, and self-perceptions. In fieldwork settings, students may begin to reassess suppositions about OT; the theories learned in school; and their views of themselves as a practitioners, learners, and individuals. Because individuals differ in their ability to adapt to change and because each student is placed in a different fieldwork setting, these transitions have different effects on each student.

The nature of the fieldwork environment is fundamentally different from that of the academic environment. Knowing and acknowledging some of the distinctions between the two settings can ease the transition and provide support and insight to accept the challenges of fieldwork experiences (Table 69-6). Within the fieldwork environment, the learning focus shifts to the application

or implementation of therapy techniques in an applied interpersonal context. Techniques that were introduced in a simulated context now must be mastered and applied with attention to the client's emotional needs.

Abstract questions that are appropriate in the academic environment shift to pragmatic questions to reduce the possibility of error in one's thinking. For example, rather than thinking about a client's function in the kitchen from an abstract perspective, one has to think about the client's function in the context of a specific kitchen in a certain small apartment and attend to the client's concerns about his or her roles, activities, family, and home environment. Recognizing that actions have an influence on the client's life, supervisor tolerance for ambiguity or uncertainty declines during fieldwork.

In the academic setting, students are accountable primarily to self and peers, and performance is evaluated on a summative basis through tests, assignments, and grades. Students can choose whether to disclose grades to family or peers, and performance may have little effect on others. In the fieldwork placement, a student's performance is evaluated on a formative basis and may be observed by

TABLE 69-6	Distinctions between Academic and Fieldwork Settings	
Characteristic	Academic Setting	Fieldwork Setting
Purpose	Dissemination of knowledge, development of creative thought, student growth	Provide high-quality client care
Faculty/supervisor accountability	To student, to university/college	To client and significant others, to fieldwork center and team, to student
Student accountability	To self	To clients and significant others, to supervisor and team, to fieldwork center
Pace	Depends on curriculum; adaptable to student and faculty needs	Depends on clients' needs; less adaptable; shaped by facility procedures
Student/educator ratio	Many students to one faculty member	One student to one supervisor, small group of students to one supervisor, one or two students to two supervisors
Source of feedback	Summative at midterm or end of term; provided by faculty	Provided by clients and significant others, supervisor, and other staff; formative
Degree of faculty/supervisor control of educational experience	Able to plan, controlled	Limited control; various diagnoses and length of client stay, pace of setting, and size of caseload varies from setting to setting.
Primary learning tool	Books, journal articles, lectures, audiovisual aids, case studies, simulations, technology, Internet	Situation of practice; clients, families, significant others, and staff; may be face to face or electronic (e.g., webcams, e-mail, telehealth)
Conceptual learning	Abstract, theoretical	Pragmatic, applied in interpersonal context
Learning process	Teacher directed	Client, self, peer, supervisor-directed
Tolerance for ambiguity	High	Low
Lifestyle	Flexible, able to plan time around class schedule	Structured, flexible time limited to evenings and weekends or days off
Contexts	University or college classroom, online learning	Hospitals, schools, nursing homes, day care centers, day treatment programs, community-based agencies, clients' homes

the entire health care team, especially at team meetings. Performance is no longer the private matter that it was at school but is publicly observed because it has direct and critical consequences for clients. Colleagues, clients, and their families may offer meaningful feedback. Although all these opportunities may create disequilibrium or tension, they also constitute new ways to learn about one's self and the profession. The broad and diverse experience within fieldwork settings presents challenges to redefine one's sense of self and evolving professional identity. Staying open to learning can counter negative feelings related to criticism, judgment, failure, and self-doubt. This personal and professional growth can be supported through the use of mindful, self-care protocols to mitigate stress and burnout. Resources and strategies about mindful awareness and self-care may enable students to access adaptive coping skills to orchestrate their student role with personal life (Zeman & Harvison, 2017).

Fieldwork takes place in a situation over which fieldwork educators have little control. The organizational factors of the health care setting, combined with client care factors, such as the nature and complexity of the client's problem, the length of stay, and fluctuation in the client load, make planning difficult, especially in acute care settings (Britton, Rosenwax, & McNamara, 2015). In settings that provide extended care for clients, however, the fieldwork educators are able to plan ahead because the client population is more constant and the fieldwork educator knows which clients will be available during student placements.

Fieldwork/professional practice educators' primary responsibility is client care; they have an ethical imperative to ensure the welfare of clients. This appropriate professional ethic may constrain activities that are desirable from the standpoint of education. However, the supervisory relationship allows fieldwork educators to adapt to the constraints of the setting. This unique relationship is

BOX 69-3 STUDENT CHARACTERISTICS DESIRED BY FIELDWORK EDUCATORS

- Having theoretical knowledge in and enthusiasm for the profession
- Knowing how to assess information when there is a gap
- Willingness to problem-solve and take responsibility for learning
- Willingness to receive feedback/constructive criticism
- Being on time, dressed appropriately and prepared

- Demonstrating effective communication skills with broad audiences
- Managing stress effectively
- Good time management skills
- Exploring new approaches or projects
- Engaging in creative problem solving

(Chipchase, et al., 2012, p. 6)

a positive aspect of the fieldwork environment because fieldwork educators can adapt the fieldwork experiences to meet the learner's needs.

Examination of supervisor perceptions of what makes up a quality fieldwork experience includes the need for students to be well prepared for the caseload and to demonstrate professional work behaviors (Jensen & Daniel, 2010; Rodger, Fitzgerald, Davila, Millar, & Allison, 2011). A Delphi study of 49 fieldwork educators revealed adaptability and teamwork as essential professional behaviors as well as being open to constructive criticism (Campbell et al., 2015). Characteristics desired by fieldwork educators across health care professions included student willingness to take responsibility for their own learning and willingness to engage in learning activities (Chipchase et al., 2012). See the full list of characteristics desired in Box 69-3 (Chipchase et al., 2012, p. 6). Awareness of these attributes and characteristics, in addition to positive coping strategies, can aid students in preparing for and participating in their fieldwork.

Both internal and external factors impact the development of professional confidence in OT students during fieldwork (Holland, Middleton, & Uys, 2012b). External factors include positive role modeling by an occupational therapist; opportunities for practice; positive grades during fieldwork; a supportive, encouraging supervisor; the support of peers; positive feedback from patients, family members, and supervisors; increased competence; and the overall reputation of the profession within the facility as well as the reputation of the facility for providing quality care. Internal determinants of confidence included students' ownership and personal responsibility for their professional confidence, use of a variety of coping mechanisms to address stress and anxiety, and ability to adapt to language and cultural differences.

A student experiencing difficulty during fieldwork should communicate directly with his or her fieldwork supervisor and contact the academic program as a resource. See Box 69-4 for a listing of behaviors that may

BOX 69-4 BEHAVIORS THAT PUT STUDENTS AT RISK

Affective Behaviors

- Making excuses or blaming others
- Being defensive, not receptive to feedback
- Allowing fear/anxiety to interfere with new learning and risk taking
- Making insensitive/unfiltered comments to others
- Difficulty upholding professional demeanor, appearing sleepy/sluggish, disinterested, distracted
- Becoming avoidant/passive or overwhelmed/shut down

Performance and Judgment Behaviors

- Arriving late in the morning to client sessions or to meetings

- Being disorganized or unprepared, such as misplacing schedule, documentation, etc.
- Failing to change behavior/performance after repeated feedback and redirection from supervisor
- Inconsistently maintaining your level of performance, "backsliding," regressing
- Violating facility policies, such as dress code, cell phone usage/texting
- Lacking ability to "think on your feet"
- Demonstrating poor safety awareness and adherence to precautions
- Breeching confidentiality by posting client or facility-related information to social networking Websites

put students at risk for not succeeding in fieldwork placements. Often, an action plan can be developed with specific strategies to address any identified challenges. The Fieldwork Experience Assessment Tool (FEAT) can be a useful method to help clarify which key components of fieldwork might be posing the greatest challenges, whether related to the student, the fieldwork educator, and/or the learning environment (AOTA, The Fieldwork Research Team, 2001).

Considerations for Students with Disabilities

Although occupational therapists are skilled in adaptation, the context of fieldwork education in the practice environment presents legal, administrative, and emotional issues that impact supervision, especially for students with disabilities (Tee & Cowen, 2012). The demands of fieldwork are different from the classroom portion of academic programs and may push a student with disabilities past his or her ability to effectively compensate (Grosemans, Coertjens, & Kyndt, 2017).

In the United States, Section 504 of the Rehabilitation Act of 1973 and Titles II and III of the Americans with Disabilities Act of 1990 (ADA) as well as the amendment in 2008 provides for equal access to educational opportunities for students with a physical or mental disability. Students with a documented disability may request "reasonable accommodations" to help them meet the academic and technical standards of their educational program, including the fieldwork component of the program. Accommodations must be provided by the institution as long as the accommodations or aids do not result in fundamental alteration of the program or cause undue burden to the institution. Students may find that the physical or behavioral requirements of the fieldwork setting differ from academic requirements and that difficulties that might have been manageable during the academic program become significant during fieldwork education. For example, the academic class schedule typically allows for breaks during the day and across the week, whereas placements are generally full-time, which may require a schedule accommodation for part-time accommodations. There may be challenges for students with complex or multiple disabilities in determining, from the fieldwork site perspective, whether a proposed accommodation is reasonable, and from the academic program perspective, whether an accommodation fundamentally alters program requirements (Katsiyannis, Zhang, Landmark, & Reber, 2009).

Prior to the start of the placement, students are advised to review with an OT faculty member (usually the academic fieldwork coordinator) the technical standards of the academic program to determine institutional expectations and the need to request accommodations prior to fieldwork placement (Dupler, Allen, Maheady, Fleming, & Allen, 2012). Students who decide to disclose their disability will find that campus resources, such as student support services and disability services will help them to determine what accommodations might be needed for fieldwork and to complete the paperwork associated with an accommodation request (Meeks & Jain, 2016). Academic fieldwork coordinators are often knowledgeable about specific site requirements and can advise on performance expectations to students determine what accommodations might be helpful (Taguchi Meyer, 2014). In contrast, a student who chooses not to self-identify disability status to the fieldwork site is not entitled to accommodations as provided by the law and risks the possibility of failing fieldwork if unable to meet the performance expectations without accommodations (Griffiths, Worth, Scullard, & Gilbert, 2010).

There are both benefits and drawbacks to advance disclosure for students who have a disability. A survey of students and OT practice educators with experience supervising students with disabilities revealed that most educators were able to implement reasonable accommodations for students with disabilities once they disclosed and the majority felt that the placement environment had the facilities to support students with disabilities to demonstrate competency (Nolan, Gleeson, Treanor, & Madigan, 2015). Practice educators did express concerns about being able to give extra time to students with disabilities. The most common concern reported by practitioners occurred when the disability was not disclosed until the clear emergence of a health issue interfered with the student's ability to meet the placement requirements. In these situations, they were uncertain how to maintain safety for their clients while also supporting student performance. The main reason offered by students surveyed for not disclosing was fear of being treated differently or judged as less capable. On the other hand, factors encouraging disclosure were knowing that supports were available, reduced fear, discrimination or stigma, and supportive staff. It is hoped that the awareness of the experiences of these educators and students will help to motivate students with disabilities to be courageous and proactive in their communication to plan and prepare for participation in fieldwork.

Disclosure of disability status is a personal choice, and students are not required to disclose their disability diagnoses to a faculty member or fieldwork educator, only their request for accommodation, based on a recognized disability status (Sharby & Roush, 2009). Students who are aware of their disability have an opportunity to be self-advocates and disclose their status in advance of fieldwork to enable collaboration between themselves, the academic program and fieldwork coordinator, other health professionals, and the prospective fieldwork site(s) (Brown, James, & Mackenzie, 2006). The decision to disclose can promote an open dialogue in exploring strategies and barriers and types of support available from the university, placement site, family and friends, and personal health care providers (Brown et al., 2006; Griffiths et al., 2010). Recommendations in advance of placements are to obtain a job description and to clarify the essential performance requirements. When possible, it can be useful for the student to also visit the fieldwork facility to plan ahead for accommodations and to explore what modifications may be necessary and those which are deemed reasonable by the training facility (Tee & Cowen, 2012). In addition to these preparatory steps, key strategies identified by individuals with disabilities include setting personal goals, learning from prior experiences, identifying coping actions, and maintaining a positive attitude (Brown et al., 2006). Regardless of the degree of advance planning, it is also possible that the student may not realize all accommodation needs until fully immersed in the training setting, and therefore, communication between the student and fieldwork educator should be ongoing throughout the placement (Andrews et al., 2013).

A qualitative study of practitioners with disabilities revealed advantages to being a therapist with a disability experience. Occupational therapists reported a broader understanding of the realities of disabled and other marginalized people and heightened attention to therapeutic use of self to enhance connection with their clients (Chacala, McCormack, Collins, & Beagan, 2014). Resonating with these findings, a pilot study of health professional students with disabilities discovered that each individual reported a "unique experience" and the use of individual strategies were used to overcome individual barriers (Brown et al., 2006, p. 36). Overall, students identified the value of support during placements as an important component contributing to a positive educational experience (Brown et al., 2006; Nolan et al., 2015). Students who seek assistance in building confidence to take initiative in identifying and negotiating strategies and accommodations can plan for positive placement experiences and develop self-advocacy skills that will be needed in the future.

Transition from Fieldwork to Employment

For all students, the overarching purpose of the fieldwork and placement experience is to gain mastery of OT professional reasoning and techniques to develop entry-level competence. Effective oral and written communication of ideas and objectives that are relevant to the roles and duties of an occupational therapist or OT assistant, including professional interaction with clients and staff, is expected of all students. Students are responsible for demonstrating sensitivity to and respect for client confidentiality, establishing and sustaining therapeutic relationships, and working collaboratively with others. Another expectation, more internal to the students' development of positive professional identity, includes taking responsibility for maintaining, assessing, and improving self-competence. Students are responsible for articulating their understanding of theoretical information and identifying their abilities to implement evaluation or intervention techniques. Moreover, the ability to benefit from supervision as a resource for self-directed learning is *crucial* to professional development, establishing valuable habits that will support and sustain growth as a new practitioner.

Fieldwork has long been associated with employment, with students gaining important insights into practice demands, their preferences, and directions for the future (Rodger et al., 2007). Christie, Joyce, and Moeller (1985) highlighted that value by documenting the fieldwork experience as having the greatest influence on the development of a therapist's preference for a specific area of practice. Of the 131 therapists who were surveyed, 55% indicated that practice preferences were either formed or changed during the fieldwork experience, and another 24% noted that fieldwork experience expanded their interests to other areas of practice. A more recent study confirmed the critical influence of fieldwork on preferred future practice areas. Findings from a study of 152 entry-level OT students indicate the most influential factors for future practice area preference are fieldwork experiences with clinical supervisors, fieldwork experiences with peers, social factors, college course, and future work experiences (Chiang et al., 2013). Thus, the fieldwork experience can be rich and rewarding, and as such, it is likely to have a tremendous bearing on one's career choices.

Recruitment of students into paid employment positions has been identified as a benefit to organizations offering fieldwork placements (Hanson, 2011; Rodger et al., 2007). However, in order to be eligible for employment, students must first apply for and successfully meet requirements for national certification and state licensure or registration, as applicable to laws and regulations for health care practitioners. Initial certification often involves successfully passing a national examination once all degree requirements are completed and verified by the university or college. New graduates must take responsibility to investigate and adhere to professional credentialing requirements and procedures. Once certification and licensure/registration, as applicable, have been granted, new graduates are ready to search for and accept a job position.

Studies report that new graduates may experience a range of feelings and stages of adjustment in regard to professional confidence and competence as they enter the workforce. Novice therapists describe professional confidence as a phenomenological experience, rooted in knowing and believing in yourself, your professional skills and knowledge, and your role (Holland, Middleton, & Uys, 2013). Hodgetts et al. (2007) identify that 6 months to 2 years of practice is often required for practitioners to feel competent. An online survey of new graduate occupational therapists in Australia and Aotearoa/New Zealand found that new graduates felt competent in "managing inwards" such as interpersonal and technical skills for assessment and intervention but less confident in tasks requiring interactions with other professionals and using evidence/resources (Gray et al., 2012).

Tryssenaar and Perkins (2001) describe four stages associated with the first year of practice: "Transition, Euphoria and Angst, Reality of Practice, and Adaptation" (p. 19). Seah, Mackenzie, and Gamble (2011) found similar themes in their study of graduate students transitioning to the practitioner role. They noted the excitement of challenging work and the need to normalize the challenges by gaining emotional and practical support from a community of practice, including OT colleagues, other professionals on site, and networking with peers.

Viewing the entry to employment as a time of predictable stress and rapid professional development can aid new graduates in seeking jobs that provide support and supervision to ease this transition (Robertson & Griffiths, 2009). For example, the United Kingdom has implemented a 1-year preceptorship, whereby newly qualified National Health Service (NHS) practitioners are paired with senior colleagues who serve as day-to-day role models and resources (Morley, Rugg, & Drew, 2007). Evaluation of this model revealed that new graduates were experiencing increased demands for autonomy and valued access to informal, accessible support from coworkers and opportunity to observe more experienced practitioners (Morley, 2009). In Australia, an Occupational Therapy Clinical Learning Framework (OTCLF) was developed and refined to support new graduates in their clinical learning and professional development (Fitzgerald, Moores, Coleman, & Fleming, 2015). Overall, these studies illustrate the importance of acknowledging that a transition period is normal for new practitioners entering employment.

This recognition is apparent in a survey of what attributes employers seek when hiring therapists, with less or modified expectations for new graduates (Adam, Gibson, Strong, & Lyle, 2011; Mulholland & Derdall, 2004). Beside background experience, employers sought job candidates who possess attributes in teamwork, communication, interpersonal skills, and specific practice competencies.

These findings can offer important insights to new graduates who are marketing themselves to prospective employers along with a realistic understanding of expectations for entry-level competencies.

Entry-Level Competencies and Credentialing Requirements: OT Practitioner and OT Assistant

The outcome of successful classroom and fieldwork preparation is considered the achievement of **entry-level competence**. The occupational therapist and the OT assistant have different entry-level competencies when each begins practice. In the United States, the occupational therapist receives a postbaccalaureate degree, which may either be a master's or entry-level doctorate degree, and the OT assistant typically receives an associate's degree. By July 1, 2027, ACOTE has mandated that OT programs will only be the entry-level doctoral degree and that OT assistant programs will move to the baccalaureate degree (ACOTE, 2017). The Accreditation Council is engaging stakeholders to gather evidence to inform the transition toward single points of entry for the respective degrees.

Although there are differences in the depth of learning, both practitioners receive education in the liberal arts; take prerequisites in the biological, physical, social, and behavioral sciences; and learn about the basic tenets of OT (ACOTE, 2012). The occupational therapist comprehends and knows how to apply the various theoretical perspectives of OT and understands the evaluation process, which emphasizes the interpretation of assessments in terms of the underlying factors contributing to occupational performance needs and concerns as well as how the environment presents barriers to and supports for participation in daily life. The OT assistant may assist with the screening and assessment process through data collection depending on institutional regulations and policies.

The occupational therapist uses the interpretation of the assessment data to formulate an intervention plan—in collaboration with the client and the OT assistant—designed to improve occupational performance and daily life participation. Both practitioners may implement the intervention plan, but the occupational therapist is ultimately responsible for the entire OT process. The occupational therapist is trained in service management within various types of service delivery models. The OT assistant supports the occupational therapist in service management and understands the influence of these service delivery models, such as educational, medical, or community. Both practitioners read the professional literature, but the occupational therapist is able to determine how to use and apply research evidence for specific clients or populations. There is an emphasis in the education of both practitioners on advocacy, lifelong learning, professional ethics, values, and responsibilities. Upon successful completion of the academic degree, new graduates need to take initiative to investigate the requirements and apply for professional credentialing for certification and licensure/registration according to the geographic jurisdiction of the country and state/province.

See Chapter 72 for more information about the roles responsibilities of occupational therapists and OT assistants.

Conclusion

Participating in fieldwork or practice placements, successfully completing this component of an academic program, and entering employment are influential rites of passage in becoming an OT practitioner. Historically and in contemporary practice, fieldwork functions as a critical link between the academic world of theory, the scientific world of research, and the world of practice, now and in the future (Costa, 2015; Santalucia & Johnson, 2015). Quality fieldwork involves an investment of all parties to promote successful experiences (Kirke, Layton, & Sim, 2007; Rodger et al., 2011). The depth of the experience depends greatly on the degree to which students and fieldwork educators share the responsibility for teaching and learning. Today's rapidly changing health and human service delivery systems are providing new opportunities for OT practice and fieldwork education. Globally, the profession is giving attention to innovative approaches to improving the quality of fieldwork while taking into consideration each country's health, economic, educational, and social status (McAllister, Paterson, Higgs, & Bithell, 2010). To be successful in these dynamic and complex situations, practitioners must be able to make judgments based on thoughtful inquiry, analysis, and reflection on practice working effectively with interprofessional colleagues, groups, and communities in order to support their clients in improving their participation in daily and social activities and overall quality of life.

Acknowledgments

A special "thank you" to Dr. Jodie Copley, The University of Queensland, Australia, for her collaboration with Australian colleagues to contribute to the research evidence updates for this chapter. Additionally, we would like to acknowledge everyone involved in the fieldwork and practice education process: academic faculty and educators, students, and our dedicated fieldwork and practice

education educators, along with their interprofessional colleagues.

REFERENCES

Accreditation Council for Occupational Therapy Education. (2012). Accreditation standards for a doctoral-degree level educational program for the occupational therapist; accreditation standards for a master's-degree level educational program for the occupational therapist; accreditation standards for an educational program for the occupational therapy assistant. *American Journal of Occupational Therapy, 66*, S6–S74.

Accreditation Council for Occupational Therapy Education. (2017). *ACOTE 2027 mandate and FAQs.* Retrieved from https://www.aota.org /Education-Careers/Accreditation/acote-doctoral-mandate-2027.aspx

Adam, K., Gibson, E., Strong, J., & Lyle, A. (2011). Knowledge, skills and professional behaviours needed for occupational therapists and physiotherapists new to work-related practice. *Work, 38*, 309–318. doi:10.3233/WOR-2011-1134

Allison, H., & Turpin, M. (2004). Development of the Student Placement Evaluation Form: A tool for assessing student fieldwork performance. *Australian Occupational Therapy Journal, 51*, 125–132.

Alsop, A., & Donald, M. (1996). Taking stock and taking chances: Creating new opportunities for fieldwork education. *British Journal of Occupational Therapy, 59*, 498–502.

American Occupational Therapy Association. (1924). Minimum standards for courses of training in occupational therapy. *Archives of Occupational Therapy, 3*(4), 295–298.

American Occupational Therapy Association. (1950). Essentials of an acceptable school of occupational therapy. *American Journal of Occupational Therapy, 4*, 125–128.

American Occupational Therapy Association. (2002a). *Fieldwork Performance Evaluation for the Occupational Therapy Assistant Student.* Bethesda, MD: Author.

American Occupational Therapy Association. (2002b). *Fieldwork Performance Evaluation for the Occupational Therapy Student.* Bethesda, MD: Author.

American Occupational Therapy Association. (2015). Occupational therapy code of ethics. *American Journal of Occupational Therapy, 69*, 6913410030p1–6913410030p8. doi:10.5014/ajot.2015.696S03

American Occupational Therapy Association. (2016). Occupational therapy fieldwork education: Value and purpose. *American Journal of Occupational Therapy, 70*, 7012410060p1–7012410060p2. doi:10.5014 /ajot.2016.706S06

American Occupational Therapy Association. (2017a). *Fieldwork (experiential learning) Ad Hoc Committee report and recommendations to the AOTA Board of Directors.* Retrieved from https://www .aota.org/~/media/Corporate/Files/EducationCareers/Educators /Fieldwork/AOTA-Fieldwork/Residency-for-OTs-considered-by -AOTA-ad-hoc-committee-report.pdf

American Occupational Therapy Association. (2017b). Fieldwork performance evaluation validation study. *OT Practice, 22*(14), 4.

American Occupational Therapy Association. (2017c). *Level I fieldwork competency evaluation for OT and OTA students.* Retrieved from https://www.aota.org/~/media/Corporate/Files/EducationCareers /Educators/Fieldwork/LevelI/Level-I-Fieldwork-Competency -Evaluation-for-ot-and-ota-students.pdf

American Occupational Therapy Association, Commission on Education. (1999). *Guidelines for an occupational therapy fieldwork experience: Level I.* Bethesda, MD: Author.

American Occupational Therapy Association, Commission on Education. (2009). *The AOTA Self-Assessment Tool for Fieldwork Educator Competency.* Bethesda, MD: Author. Retrieved from http://www.aota .org/Educate/EdRes/Fieldwork/Supervisor/Forms/38251.aspx?FT.pdf

American Occupational Therapy Association, Commission on Education and Fieldwork Issues Committee. (2000). *Guidelines for an occupational therapy fieldwork experience: Level II*. Bethesda, MD: Author.

American Occupational Therapy Association, Education Department. (1999). *Innovative fieldwork annotated bibliography*. Bethesda, MD: Author. Retrieved from http://www.aota.org/Educate/EdRes/Fieldwork/38240.aspx

American Occupational Therapy Association, International Fieldwork Ad Hoc Committee for the Commission on Education. (2009). *Recommended international fieldwork timelines for academic OT/OTA programs and fieldwork sites*. Retrieved from http://www.aota.org/Educate/EdRes/International/International-Fieldwork-Timelines.aspx?FT=.pdf

American Occupational Therapy Association, Student Evaluation of Fieldwork Experience Task Force. (2016). *Student evaluation of fieldwork experience*. Bethesda, MD: Author. Retrieved from https://www.aota.org/Education-Careers/Fieldwork/StuSuprvsn.aspx

American Occupational Therapy Association, The Fieldwork Research Team. (2001). *Fieldwork Experience Assessment Tool (FEAT)*. Bethesda, MD: Author. Retrieved from http://www.aota.org/Students/Current/Fieldwork/FEAT.aspx?FT=.pdf

Americans with Disabilities Act Amendments of 2008, Pub. L. No. 110-325, § 122 Stat. 3553 (2008).

Andrews, E., Kuemmel, A., Williams, J., Pilarski, C., Dunn, M., & Lund, E. (2013). Providing culturally competent supervision to trainees with disabilities in rehabilitation settings. *Rehabilitation Psychology*, 58, 233–244. doi:10.1037/a0033338

Atler, K. (2003). *Using the Fieldwork Performance Evaluation forms: The complete guide*. Bethesda, MD: American Occupational Therapy Association.

Barnes, M. A., & Evenson, M. E. (2000). Supervision and mentoring. In S. C. Merrill & P. A. Crist (Eds.), *Meeting the fieldwork challenge: A self-paced clinical course* (pp. 9–12). Bethesda, MD: American Occupational Therapy Association.

Bethea, D. P., Castillo, D. C., & Harvison, N. (2014). Use of simulation in occupational therapy education: Way of the future? *American Journal of Occupational Therapy*, 68, S32–S39. doi:10.5014/ajot.2014.012716

Bodenheimer, T., & Sinsky, C. (2014). From triple to quadruple aim: Care of the patient requires care of the provider. *Annals of Family Medicine*, 12, 573–576. doi:10.1370/afm.1713

Boogard, L., Gater, L., Mori, M., Trincao, A., & Smith-Turchyn, J. (2016). Efficacy of self-management programs in managing side effects of breast cancer: A systematic review and meta-analysis of randomized control trials. *Rehabilitation Oncology*, 34, 14–26. doi:10.1097/01.REO.0000475835.78984.41

Bossers, A., Bezzina, M. B., Hobson, S., Kinsella, A., MacPhail, A., Schurrs, S., & Jenkins, K. (n.d.). *Preceptor education program (PEP) for health professionals and students*. Ontario, Canada: University of Western Ontario. Retrieved from http://www.preceptor.ca

Bossers, A., Miller, L. T., Polatajko, H. J., & Hartley, M. (2007). *Competency Based Fieldwork Evaluation for Occupational Therapists*. Albany, NY: Delmar Thomson Learning.

Bradley, P. (2006). The history of simulation in medical education and possible future directions. *Medical Education*, 40, 254–262. doi:10.1111/j.1365-2929.2006.02394.x

Britton, L., Rosenwax, L., & McNamara, B. (2015). Occupational therapy practice in acute physical hospital settings. *Australian Occupational Therapy Journal*, 62, 370–377. doi:10.1111/1440-1630.12227

Brown, K., James, C., & Mackenzie, L. (2006). The practice placement education experience: An Australian pilot study exploring the perspectives of health professional students with a disability. *British Journal of Occupational Therapy*, 69, 31–37.

Campbell, M., Corpus, K., Wussow, T., Plummer, T., Gibbs, D., & Hix, S. (2015). Fieldwork educators' perspectives: Professional behavior attributes of level II fieldwork students. *The Open Journal of Occupational Therapy*, 3, 7. doi:10.15453/2168-6408.1146

Chacala, A., McCormack, C., Collins, B., & Beagan, B. (2014). "My view that disability is okay sometimes clashes": Experiences of two disabled occupational therapists. *Scandinavian Journal of Occupational Therapy*, 21, 107–115. doi:10.3109/11038128.2013.861016

Chiang, J. A., Liu, C. H., Chen, Y., Wang, S. H., Lin, W. S., Su, F. Y., . . . Wang, C. A. (2013). A survey of how occupational therapy fieldwork influences future professional preference. *Hong Kong Journal of Occupational Therapy*, 23, 62–68. doi:10.1016/j.hkjot.2013.09.003

Chipchase, L., Buttrum, P., Dunwoodie, R., Hill, A., Mandrusiak, A., & Moran, M. (2012). Characteristics of student preparedness for clinical learning: Clinical educator perspectives using the Delphi approach. *BMC Medical Education*, 12, 112. Retrieved from http://www.biomedcentral.com/1472-6920/12/112

Christie, B. A., Joyce, P. C., & Moeller, P. L. (1985). Fieldwork experience 1: Impact on practice preference. *American Journal of Occupational Therapy*, 39, 671–674.

Clarke, C., Martin, M., de Visser, R., & Sadlo, G. (2015). Sustaining professional identity in practice following role-emerging placements: Opportunities and challenges for occupational therapists. *British Journal of Occupational Therapy*, 78, 42–50.

College of Occupational Therapists. (2015). *Supervision: Guidance for occupational therapists and their managers*. London, United Kingdom: Royal College of Occupational Therapists Limited. Retrieved from https://www.rcot.co.uk/sites/default/files/supervision.pdf

Committee on University Fieldwork Education, Association of Canadian Occupational Therapy University Programs. (2011). *Canadian guidelines for fieldwork education in occupational therapy (CGFEOT): Guiding principles, responsibilities and continuous quality improvement process*. Retrieved from http://www.caot.ca/pdfs/Exam/June7.pdf

Copley, J., Allison, H. D., Hill, A. E., Moran, M. C., Tait, J., & Day, T. (2007). Making interprofessional education real: A university clinic model. *Australian Health Review*, 31, 351–357.

Copley, J., & Nelson, A. (2012). Practice educator perspectives of multiple mentoring in diverse clinical settings. *British Journal of Occupational Therapy*, 75, 456–462.

Copley, J., Turpin, M., Gordon, S., & McLaren, C. (2011). Development and evaluation of an occupational therapy program for refugee high school students. *Australian Occupational Therapy Journal*, 58, 310–316. doi:10.1111/j.1440-1630.2011.00933.x

Costa, D. (Ed.). (2015). *The essential guide to occupational therapy fieldwork education: Resources for today's educators and practitioners* (2nd ed.). Bethesda, MD: American Occupational Therapy Association.

Costa, D., Molinsky, R., & Sauerwald, C. (2012). Collaborative intraprofessional education with occupational therapy and occupational therapy assistant students. *OT Practice*, 17(21), CE1–CE7.

Dancza, K., Warren, A., Copley, J., Rodger, S., Moran, M., McKay, E., & Taylor, A. (2013). Learning experiences on role-emerging placements: An exploration from the students' perspective. *Australian Occupational Therapy Journal*, 60, 427–435. doi:10.1111/1440-1630.12079

Diambra, C., Cole-Zakrzewski, K., & Booher, J. (2004). A comparison of internship stage models: Evidence from intern experiences. *Journal of Experiential Education*, 27, 191–212. doi:10.1177/105382590402700206

Donnelly, C., Brenchley, C., Crawford, C., & Letts, L. (2013). The integration of occupational therapy into primary care: A multiple case study design. *BMC Family Practice*, 14, 60. Retrieved from http://www.biomedcentral.com/1471-2296/14/60

Dupler, A. E., Allen, C., Maheady, D. C., Fleming, S. E., & Allen, M. (2012). Leveling the playing field for nursing students with disabilities: Implications of the amendments to the Americans with Disabilities Act. *Journal of Nursing Education, 51*, 140–144.

Evenson, M. E., Barnes, M. A., & Cohn, E. S. (2002). Brief report: Perceptions of level I and level II fieldwork in the same site. *American Journal of Occupational Therapy, 56*, 103–106.

Evenson, M. E., & Connor, L. T. (2015). Perspectives on the doctoral experiential component. *OT Practice, 20*(8), 17–19.

Evenson, M. E., Roberts, M., Kaldenberg, J., Barnes, M. A., & Ozelie, R. (2015). A national survey of fieldwork educators: Implications for OT education. *American Journal of Occupational Therapy, 69*, 6912350020p1–6912350020p5.

Fitzgerald, C., Moores, A., Coleman, A., & Fleming, J. (2015). Supporting new graduate professional development: A clinical learning framework. *Australian Occupational Therapy Journal, 62*, 13–20. doi:10.1111/1440-1630.12165

Flood, B., Haslam, L., & Hocking, C. (2010). Implementing a collaborative model of student supervision in New Zealand: Enhancing therapist and student experiences. *New Zealand Journal of Occupational Therapy, 57*, 22–26.

Ford, C., Foley, K., Ritchie, C., Sheppard, K., Sawyer, P., & Swanson, M. (2013). Creation of an interprofessional clinical experience for healthcare professions trainees in a nursing home setting. *Medical Teacher, 35*, 544–548. doi:10.3109/0142159x.2013.787138

Fortune, T., & McKinstry, C. (2012). Project-based fieldwork: Perspectives of graduate entry students and project sponsors. *Australian Occupational Therapy Journal, 59*, 265–275. doi:10.1111/j.1440-1630.2012.01026.x

Gaitskell, S., & Morley, M. (2008). Supervision in occupational therapy: How are we doing? *British Journal of Occupational Therapy, 71*, 119–121.

Giles, A., Carson, N., Breland, H., Coker-Bolt, P., & Bowman, P. (2014). Conference proceedings—use of simulated patients and reflective video analysis to assess occupational therapy students' preparedness for fieldwork. *American Journal of Occupational Therapy, 68*, S57–S66. doi:10.5014/ajot.2014.685S03

Gray, M., Clark, M., Penman, M., Smith, J., Bell, J., Thomas, Y., & Trevan-Hawke, J. (2012). New graduate occupational therapists feelings of preparedness for practice in Australia and Aotearoa/New Zealand. *Australian Occupational Therapy Journal, 59*, 445–455. doi:10.1111/j.1440-1630.2012.01029.x

Griffiths, L., Worth, P., Scullard, Z., & Gilbert, D. (2010). Supporting disabled students in practice: A tripartite approach. *Nurse Education in Practice, 10*, 132–137. doi:10.1016/j.nepr.2009.05.001

Grosemans, I., Coertjens, L., & Kyndt, E. (2017). Exploring learning and fit in the transition from higher education to the labour market: A systematic review. *Educational Research Review, 21*, 67–84. doi:10.1016/j.edurev.2017.03.001

Hamilton, A., Copley, J., Thomas, Y., Edwards, A., Broadbridge, J., Bonassi, M., . . . Newton, J. (2015). Responding to the growing demand for practice education: Are we building sustainable solutions? *Australian Occupational Therapy Journal, 62*, 265–270. doi:10.1111/1440-1630.12181

Hand, C., Law, M., & McColl, M. A. (2011). Occupational therapy interventions for chronic diseases: A scoping review. *American Journal of Occupational Therapy, 65*, 428–436.

Hansen, A. W., Munoz, J., Crist, P. A., Gupta, J., Ideishi, R. I., Primeau, L. A., & Tupe, D. (2007). Service learning: Meaningful, community-centered professional skill development for occupational therapy students. *Occupational Therapy in Health Care, 21*, 25–48. doi:10.1300/J003v21n01_03

Hanson, D. J. (2011). The perspectives of fieldwork educators regarding Level II fieldwork students. *Occupational Therapy in Health Care, 25*, 164–177. doi:10.3109/07380577.2011:561420

Hanson, D. J., & DeIulis, E. D. (2015). The collaborative model of fieldwork education: A blueprint for group supervision of students. *Occupational Therapy in Health Care, 29*, 223–239. doi:10.3109/07380577,2015.1011297

Hanson, D., & Nielsen, S. K. (2016). Introduction to role-emerging fieldwork. In D. Costa (Ed.), *The essential guide to fieldwork education* (2nd ed.). Bethesda, MD: American Occupational Therapy Association.

Haynes, C. J. (2011). Active participation in Fieldwork Level I: Fieldwork educator and student perceptions. *Occupational Therapy in Health Care, 25*, 257–269. doi:10.3109/07380577.2011.595477

Herge, A., Lorch, A., DeAngelis, T., Vause-Earland, T., Mollo, K., & Zapletal, A. (2013). The standardized patient encounter: A dynamic educational approach to enhance students' clinical healthcare skills. *Journal of Allied Health, 42*, 229–235.

Hodgetts, S., Hollis, V., Triska, O., Dennis, S., Madill, H., & Taylor, E. (2007). Occupational therapy students' and graduates' satisfaction with professional education and preparedness for practice. *Canadian Journal of Occupational Therapy, 74*, 148–160.

Holland, K., Middleton, L., & Uys, L. (2012a). Professional confidence: A concept analysis. *Scandinavian Journal of Occupational Therapy, 19*, 214–224. doi:10.3109/11038128.2011.583939

Holland, K., Middleton, L., & Uys, L. (2012b). The sources of professional confidence in occupational therapy students. *South African Journal of Occupational Therapy, 42*, 19–25.

Holland, K., Middleton, L., & Uys, L. (2013). Professional confidence: Conceptions held by novice occupational therapists in South Africa. *Occupational Therapy International, 20*, 105–113.

Hong Meng Tai, J., Canny, B. J., Haines, T. P., & Molloy, E. K. (2016). Implementing peer learning in clinical education: A framework to address challenges in the "real world." *Teaching and Learning in Medicine, 29*, 162–172. doi:10.1080/10401334.2016.1247000

Institute of Medicine. (2015). *Building health workforce capacity through community-based health professional education: Workshop summary.* Washington, DC: National Academies Press. Retrieved from https://www.nap.edu/catalog/18973/building-health-workforce-capacity-through-community-based-health-professional-education

Interprofessional Education Collaborative. (2016). *Core competencies for interprofessional collaborative practice: 2016 Update.* Washington, DC: Interprofessional Education Collaborative.

Jensen, L. R., & Daniel, C (2010). A descriptive study on Level II fieldwork supervision in hospital settings. *Occupational Therapy in Health Care, 24*, 335–347. doi:10.3109/07380577.2010.502211

Johnson, C. R., Koenig, K. P., Piersol, C. V., Santalucia, S. E., & Wachter-Schutz, W. (2006). Level I fieldwork today: A study of contexts and perceptions. *American Journal of Occupational Therapy, 60*, 275–287.

Jung, B., Salvatori, P., & Martin, A. (2008). Intraprofessional fieldwork education: Occupational therapy and occupational therapy assistant students learning together. *Canadian Journal of Occupational Therapy, 75*, 42–50.

Katsiyannis, A., Zhang, D., Landmark, L., & Reber, A. (2009). Postsecondary education for individuals with disabilities: Legal and practice considerations. *Journal of Disability Policy Studies, 20*, 35–45. doi:10.1177/1044207308324896

Kirke, P., Layton, N., & Sim, J. (2007). Informing fieldwork design: Key elements to quality fieldwork education for undergraduate occupational therapy students. *Australian Occupational Therapy Journal, 54*, S13–S22.

Leland, N. E., Fogelberg, D. J., Halle, A. D., & Mroz, T. (2017). Occupational therapy and management of multiple chronic conditions in the context of health care reform. *American Journal of Occupational Therapy, 71*, 7101090010p1–7101090010p6. doi:10.5014/ajot.2017.711001

Lewis, L. M. (2005). Fieldwork requirements of the past, present and future. *American Occupational Therapy Association: Education Special Interest Quarterly, 15*(3), 1–4.

Maran, N., & Glavin, R. (2003). Low- to high-fidelity simulation—A continuum of medical education? *Medical Education, 37,* 22–28.

McAllister, L., Paterson, M., Higgs, J., & Bithell, C. (2010). *Innovations in allied health fieldwork education: A critical appraisal.* Rotterdam, The Netherlands: Sense.

Meeks, L. M., & Jain, N. R. (Eds.). (2016). *The guide to assisting students with disabilities: Equal access in health science and professional education.* New York, NY: Springer.

Missiuna, C. A., Polatajko, H. I., & Ernest-Conibear, M. (1992). Skill acquisition during fieldwork placements in occupational therapy. *Canadian Journal of Occupational Therapy, 59,* 28–39.

Morley, M. (2009). Contextual factors that have an impact on the transition experience of newly qualified occupational therapists. *British Journal of Occupational Therapy, 72,* 507–514.

Morley, M., Rugg, S., & Drew, J. (2007). Before preceptorship: New occupational therapists' expectations of practice and experience of supervision. *British Journal of Occupational Therapy, 70,* 243–253.

Mulholland, S., & Derdall, M. (2004). Exploring what employers seek when hiring occupational therapists. *Canadian Journal of Occupational Therapy, 71,* 223–229.

Murden, R., Norman, A., Ross, J., Sturdivant, E., Kedia, M., & Shah, S. (2008). Occupational therapy students' perceptions of their cultural awareness and competency. *Occupational Therapy International, 15,* 191–203. doi:10.1002/oti.253

National Board for Certification in Occupational Therapy. (n.d.). *Online certification examination handbook.* Gaithersburg, MD: Author. Retrieved from http://www.nbcot.org/pdf/eligibility_01.pdf

Nelson, A., Copley, J., & Salama, R. (2010). Occupational therapy students' perceptions of the multiple mentoring model of clinical supervision. *Focus on Health Professional Education, 11,* 14–27.

Nolan, C., Gleeson, C., Treanor, D., & Madigan, S. (2015). Higher education students registered with disability services and practice educators: Issues and concerns for professional placements. *International Journal of Inclusive Education, 19,* 487–502. doi:10.1080/13603116.2014.943306

O'Connor, A., Cahill, M., & McKay, E. (2012). Revisiting 1:1 and 2:1 clinical placement models: Student and clinical educator perspectives. *Australian Occupational Therapy Journal, 59,* 276–283. doi:10.1111/j.1440-1630.2012.01025.x

Precin, P. (2007). An aggregate fieldwork model: Interdisciplinary training/intervention component. *Occupational Therapy in Health Care, 21,* 123–131.

Price, D., & Whiteside, M. (2016). Implementing the 2:1 student placement model in occupational therapy: Strategies for practice. *Australian Occupational Therapy Journal, 63,* 123–129. doi:10.1111/1440-1630.12257

Richardson, J., Loyola-Sanchez, A., Sinclair, S., Harris, J., Letts, L., MacIntyre, N. J., . . . Martin Ginis, K. (2014). Self-management interventions for chronic disease: A systematic scoping review. *Clinical Rehabilitation, 28,* 1067–1077. doi:10.1177/0269215514532478

Robertson, L., & Griffiths, S. (2009). Graduates' reflections on their preparation for practice. *British Journal of Occupational Therapy, 72,* 125–132.

Rodger, S., Chien, C. W., Turpin, M., Copley, J., Coleman, A., Brown, T., & Caine, A. M. (2016). Establishing the validity and reliability of the Student Practice Evaluation Form-Revised (SPEF-R) in occupational therapy practice education: A Rasch analysis. *Evaluation and the Health Professions, 39,* 33–48.

Rodger, S., Coleman, A., Caine, A., Chien, C., Copley, J., Turpin, M., & Brown, T. (2014). Examining the inter-rater and test-retest reliability of the Student Practice Evaluation Form-Revised (SPEF-R) for occupational therapy students. *Australian Occupational Therapy Journal, 61,* 353–363. doi:10.1111/1440-1630

Rodger, S., Fitzgerald, C., Davila, W., Millar, F., & Allison, H. (2011). What makes a quality occupational therapy practice placement? Students' and practice educators' perspectives. *Australian Occupational Therapy Journal, 58,* 195–202. doi:10.1111/j.1440-1630.2010.00903.x

Rodger, S., Thomas, Y., Dickson, D., McBryde, C., Broadbridge, J., Hawkins, R., & Edwards, A. (2007). Putting students to work: Valuing fieldwork placements as a mechanism for recruitment and shaping the future occupational therapy workforce. *Australian Occupational Therapy Journal, 54,* S94–S97. doi:10.1111/j.1440-1630.2007.00691.x

Rodger, S., Turpin, M., Copley, J., Coleman, A., Chien, C., Caine, A., & Brown, T. (2014). Student Practice Evaluation Form–Revised edition online comment bank: Development and reliability analysis. *Australian Occupational Therapy Journal, 61,* 241–248. doi:10.1111/1440-1630

Rodger, S., Webb, G., Devitt, L., Gilbert, J., Wrightson, P., & McMeeken, J. (2008). Clinical education and practice placements in the allied health professions: An international perspective. *Journal of Allied Health, 37,* 53–62.

Rosen, K. R. (2008). The history of medical simulation. *Journal of Critical Care, 23,* 157–166. doi:10.1016/j.jcrc.2007.12.004

Santalucia, S., & Johnson, C. (2015). Transformative learning: Facilitating growth and change through fieldwork. In D. Costa (Ed), *The essential guide to occupational therapy fieldwork education: Resources for educators and practitioners* (2nd ed., pp. 15–24). Bethesda, MD: American Occupational Therapy Association.

Seah, C., Mackenzie, L., & Gamble, J. (2011). Transition of graduates of the master of occupational therapy to practice. *Australian Occupational Therapy Journal, 58,* 103–110. doi:10.1111/j.1440-1630.2010.00899.x

Sharby, N., & Roush, S. E. (2009). Analytical decision-making model for addressing the needs of allied health students with disabilities. *Journal of Allied Health, 38,* 54–62.

Sheppard, K. D., Ford, C. R., Sawyer, P., Foley, K. T., Harada, C. N., Brown, C. J., & Ritchie, C. S. (2015). The interprofessional clinical experience: Interprofessional education in the nursing home. *Journal of Interprofessional Care, 29,* 170–172.

Shields, M., Quilty, J., Dharamsi, S., & Drynan, D. (2016). International fieldwork placements in low-income countries: Exploring community perspectives. *Australian Occupational Therapy Journal, 63,* 321–328. doi:10.1111/1440-1630.12291

Sim, I., & Mackenzie, L. (2016). Graduate perspectives of fieldwork placements in developing countries: Contributions to occupational therapy practice. *Australian Occupational Therapy Journal, 63,* 244–256. doi:10.1111/1440.1630.12282

Simonelis, J., Njelesani, J., Novak, L., Kuzma, C., & Cameron, D. (2011). International fieldwork placements and occupational therapy: Lived experiences of the major stakeholders. *Australian Occupational Therapy Journal, 58,* 370–377. doi:10.1111/j.1440-1630.2011.00942.x

Taguchi Meyer, J. T. (2014). Ensuring a diverse workforce: Fieldwork success for occupational therapy students with disabilities [Fieldwork issues]. *OT Practice, 19*(20), 18–19.

Taylor, R. R., Lee, S. W., Kielhofner, G., & Ketkar, M. (2009). Therapeutic use of self: A nationwide survey of practitioners' attitudes and experiences. *American Journal of Occupational Therapy, 63,* 198–207.

Tee, S., & Cowen, M. (2012). Supporting students with disabilities—Promoting understanding amongst mentors in practice. *Nurse Education in Practice, 12,* 6–10. doi:10.1016/j.nepr.2011.03.020

Thomas, Y., Penman, M., & Williamson, P. (2005). Australian and New Zealand fieldwork: Charting the territory for future practice. *Australian Occupational Therapy Journal, 52,* 78–81.

Tryssenaar, J., & Perkins, J. (2001). From student to therapist: Exploring the first year of practice. *American Journal of Occupational Therapy, 55,* 19–27.

Turpin, M., Fitzgerald, C., & Rodger, S. (2011). Development of the Student Practice Evaluation Form revised edition package. *Australian Occupational Therapy Journal, 58,* 67–73.

Vogel, K. A., Grice, K. O., Hill, S., & Moody, J. (2004). Supervisor and student expectations of level II fieldwork. *Occupational Therapy in Health Care, 18*, 5–19. doi:10.1300/J003v18n01_02

Whiteford, G. E., & McAllister, L. (2007). Politics and complexity in intercultural fieldwork: The Vietnam experience. *Australian Occupational Therapy Journal, 54*, S74–S83.

World Federation of Occupational Therapists. (2016). *Minimum standards for the education of occupational therapists, revised 2016.* Retrieved from http://www.wfot.org/

World Federation of Occupational Therapists. (n.d.). *FAQ—Education.* Retrieved from http://www.wfot.org/FAQs/Education

World Health Organization. (2010). *Community-based rehabilitation guidelines.* Retrieved from http://www.who.int/disabilities/cbr/guidelines/en/

Written History Committee of the American Occupational Therapy Association. (1983). *Written History Symposium, 1984.* Rockville, MD: American Occupational Therapy Association.

Zeman, E., & Harvison, N. (2017). *Burnout, stress and compassion fatigue in occupational therapy practice and education: A call for mindful, self-care protocols* [Commentary]. Washington, DC: National Academy of Medicine. Retrieved from https://nam.edu/Burnout-Stress-and-Compassion-Fatigue-in-Occupational-Therapy-Practice-and-Education-A-Call-for-Mindful-Self-Care-Protocols/

the Point® *For additional resources on the subjects discussed in this chapter, visit* **http://thePoint.lww.com/Willard-Spackman13e.**

CHAPTER 70

Competence and Professional Development

Winifred Schultz-Krohn

LEARNING OBJECTIVES

After reading this chapter, you will be able to:

1. Discuss the professional expectation of and individual accountability for pursuing continuing competence and professional development.
2. Differentiate the terms *competency* and *continuing competence* and explain the variables influencing each concept.
3. Examine the basic differences in competency expectations for occupational therapists and occupational therapy assistants.
4. Explain how to engage in continuing competence on an ongoing basis through self-assessment, individualized professional development, and clear outcomes.
5. Identify available resources and the steps in the process of creating a professional development plan including beneficial learning activities for plan implementation.
6. Assess the role of certification, licensure, and advanced and specialty certifications for practice.
7. Compare and contrast the merits of practice competence and practice excellence.

Introduction

Occupational therapy (OT) practitioners are expected to deliver competent services. The delivery of these services is guided by an ethical foundation as described by the American Occupational Therapy Association (AOTA) 2015 Code of Ethics (AOTA, 2015b) and the World Federation of Occupational Therapy (WFOT) Code of Ethics (WFOT, 2016). Included in these documents is a clear recognition that the profession of OT and the provision of these services are dynamic, being responsive to society needs and proactive in promoting participation and inclusion in occupational pursuits. The dynamic nature of OT services requires the practitioner to consider the complexities of clients' occupational needs, various models of service delivery, reimbursement issues, along with laws and regulations governing services. Given the dynamic nature of the profession, there is a need for all OT practitioners to engage in continuing competence and professional development to meet the changing needs of clients and societies (AOTA, 2015d). The WFOT supports the development of

CENTENNIAL NOTES

The Importance of "Refresher" Work

Lori T. Andersen

I am convinced, however, that alike for the best interests of the work itself, and of the patients to whom you are devoting your lives, and also for your own professional advancement, it should be your constant effort to improve your skill, to refresh your hearts, and to renew your faith in the value of curative occupations and related activities by every legitimate means in your power. Only in that way can our very human tendency to be satisfied, after a time, with our past acquirements and a routine performance of our duties, be overcome; our work and ourselves grow in value.

THOMAS KIDNER (1929, p. 403)

Shortly after the forming of the National Society for the Promotion of Occupational Therapy (NSPOT), as discussions began to determine minimum standards for training courses in OT, founders Eleanor Clarke Slagle and Thomas B. Kidner recognized the importance of continuing training during one's career. Kidner supported the idea

that refresher courses were needed to prevent "staleness" and to keep one apprised of new discoveries and methods in the field. Unfortunately, financial limitations prevented AOTA's dream of developing short, intensive summer courses to meet this objective; however, the official publication of the AOTA starting in 1925, *Occupational Therapy and Rehabilitation*, provided informative articles on OT as "refreshment." In 1924, Eleanor Clarke Slagle, in her position of Director of Occupational Therapy for the New York State Department of Mental Hygiene, started an Annual Institute of the Chief Occupational Therapists of the New York State Hospitals for the purpose of sharing information, working together to solve common problems, and providing refreshment and renewed inspiration to occupational therapists. Additionally, in the 1920s, the movers and shakers of the New York State Association of Occupational Therapists arranged monthly lectures and demonstrations as refresher work. Nearly 100 years later, Slagle and Kidner would surely be pleased with the numerous AOTA programs to support "refresher" work and continuing competence, especially the 2017 Annual AOTA Conference and Centennial Celebration in Philadelphia with its record-setting 14,000 attendees.

competency standards within all member countries (WFOT, 2012). In this chapter, the examples are drawn primarily from the United States; however, the concepts are likely to be applicable to other countries and cultures.

This chapter describes the process of moving from initial (entry-level) competencies to advanced skills through continuing competence and professional development. This process is self-directed and requires the practitioner to systematically examine current skills and abilities while anticipating future service demands. The process is applicable to all OT practitioners regardless of the entry-level education.

Continuing Competence

The terms *continuing competence* and *competency* are not interchangeable. A **competency** refers to a specified skill or ability (AOTA, 2002) and **continuing competence** "is a process involving the examination of current competence and the development of capacity for the future" (AOTA, 2015d). The AOTA Standards for Continuing Competence identify a need for every OT practitioner to not only maintain the skills needed to competently practice but also develop skills needed for future demands. This process of

engaging in continuing competence requires "knowledge, performance skills, interpersonal abilities, critical reasoning, and ethical reasoning" (AOTA, 2015d). The OT practitioner seeks to provide service that is more effective by expanding knowledge base, improving skills, and further developing reasoning abilities and, in through this process, moves from an entry-level practitioner to one with more advanced skills (Unsworth, 2001).

Entry-Level Competencies

The Accreditation Council for Occupational Therapy Education (ACOTE) Standards, adopted in 2011, identifies the entry-level expectations for OT practitioners at the associate, master's, and doctoral degree levels of educational preparation in the United States (ACOTE, 2012). These entry-level competencies identify the performance expectations at each level of educational preparation. The **entry-level competencies** are directed toward delivery of OT services as a generalist and specify that an entry-level OT practitioner is one who has less than 1 year of experience (Table 70-1).

| TABLE 70-1 | Differences in Occupational Therapists and Occupational Therapy Assistant Standards of Practice—United States |

Occupational Therapy Process	Occupational Therapist Master's or Doctoral Degree	Occupational Therapy Assistant
Education, Examination, and Licensure Requirements		
1. Graduated from an occupational therapist program accredited by ACOTE	x	x
2. Successfully completed a period of supervised fieldwork	Master's: 24 weeks Doctoral: 24 weeks + 16 weeks experiential	16 weeks
3. Passed nationally recognized entry-level examination for occupational therapist	x	x
4. Fulfills state requirements for licensure, certification, or registration	x	x
Professional Standing and Responsibility		
1. Delivers OT services that reflect the philosophical base of OT and are consistent with the established principles and concepts of theory and practice	x	x
2. Knowledgeable about and delivers OT services in accordance with AOTA standards, policies, and guidelines and state, federal, and other regulatory and payer requirements relevant to practice and service delivery	x	x
3. Maintains current licensure, registration, credentialing, or certification as required by law or regulation	x	x
4. Abides by the Occupational Therapy Code of Ethics (AOTA, 2015b)	x	x
5. Abides by the Standards for Continuing Competence (AOTA, 2015d) by establishing, maintaining, and updating professional performance, knowledge, and skills	x	x
6. Responsible for all aspects of OT service delivery and is accountable for the safety and effectiveness of the OT service delivery process	x	
7. Responsible for providing safe and effective OT services under the supervision of and in partnership with the occupational therapist and in accordance with laws or regulations and AOTA documents		x
8. Maintains current knowledge of legislative, political, social, cultural, societal, and reimbursement issues that affect clients and the practice of OT	x	x
9. Knowledgeable about evidence-based research and applies it ethically and appropriately to provide OT services consistent with best practice approaches	x	x—service implementation
10. Respects the client's sociocultural background and provides client-centered and family-centered OT services	x	x
Screening, Evaluation, and Reevaluation		
1. Responsible for all aspects of the screening, evaluation, and reevaluation process	x	
2. Accepts and responds to referrals in compliance with state laws or other regulatory requirements	x	
3. In collaboration with the client, evaluates the client's ability to participate in daily life activities by considering the client's capacities, the activities, and the environments in which these activities occur	x	
4. Initiates and directs the screening, evaluation, and reevaluation process and analyzes and interprets the data	x	Contributes as delegated by occupational therapist
5. Uses current assessments and follows defined protocols when standardized assessments are used	x	x as delegated by occupational therapist
6. Completes and documents OT evaluation results	x	Contributes as delegated by occupational therapist

TABLE 70-1 **Differences in Occupational Therapists and Occupational Therapy Assistant Standards of Practice—United States** *(continued)*

Occupational Therapy Process	Occupational Therapist Master's or Doctoral Degree	Occupational Therapy Assistant
Screening, Evaluation, and Reevaluation		
7. Communicates screening, evaluation, and reevaluation results within the boundaries of client confidentiality to the appropriate person, group, or organization	x	
8. Recommends additional consultations or refers clients to appropriate resources when the needs of the client can best be served by the expertise of other professionals or services	x	
9. Educates current and potential referral sources about the scope of OT services and the process of initiating OT services	x	x as delegated by occupational therapist
Intervention		
1. Has overall responsibility for the development, documentation, and implementation of the OT intervention based on the evaluation, client goals, current best evidence, and clinical reasoning	x	
2. Ensures that the intervention plan is documented within the time frames, formats, and standards	x	Contributes as delegated by occupational therapist
3. Collaborates with the client to develop and implement the intervention plan based on the client's needs and priorities, safety issues, and relative benefits and risks	x	x
4. Coordinates the development and implementation of the OT intervention with the intervention provided by other professionals when appropriate	x	x
5. Selects, implements, and makes modifications to therapeutic activities and interventions	x	x as delegated by occupational therapist
6. Modifies the intervention plan throughout the intervention process and documents the changes in the client's needs, goals, and performance	x	Contributes as delegated by occupational therapist
7. Documents the OT services provided within the time frames, formats, and standards	x	x
Outcomes		
1. Selects, measures, documents, and interprets expected or achieved outcomes that are related to the client's ability to engage in occupations	x	
2. Documents changes in the client's performance and capacities and for transitioning the client to other types or intensities of service or discontinuing services when the client has achieved identified goals, reached maximum benefit, or does not desire to continue services	x	Contributes as delegated by occupational therapist
3. Prepares and implements a transition or discontinuation plan based on the client's needs, goals, performance, and appropriate follow-up resources	x	Contributes as delegated by occupational therapist
4. Facilitates the transition or discharge process in collaboration with the client, family members, significant others, team, other professionals, and community resources when appropriate	x	x
5. Evaluates the safety and effectiveness of the OT processes and intervention within the practice setting	x	Contributes as delegated by occupational therapist

ACOTE, Accreditation Council for Occupational Therapy Education.

Adapted from American Occupational Therapy Association. (2015e). Standards of practice for occupational therapy. *American Journal of Occupational Therapy, 69*, 6913410057p1–6913410057p6. doi:10.5014/ajot.2015.696S06; and American Occupational Therapy Association. (2014a). Guidelines for supervision, roles, and responsibilities during the delivery of occupational therapy services. *American Journal of Occupational Therapy, 68*, S16–S22. doi:10.5014/ajot.2014.686S03.

The ACOTE Standards and Interpretive Guide differentiates entry-level competencies for OT practitioners by the level of educational preparation (AOTA, 2012). The entry-level competencies of the OT assistant are different from the expectations of the occupational therapist educated at either the master's or doctoral degree level. These are the entry-level skills to practice as an OT generalist at the designated practitioner level (OT assistant or occupational therapist; occupational therapist being further differentiated at the master's and doctoral degree levels). There are also specific areas where the entry-level skills are somewhat similar across the educational degrees. Foundational skills in the biological, social, and behavioral sciences are expected for all practitioners, as are the basic tenets of the profession. The depth and application of this knowledge differ across the educational levels. There are specific differences in the entry-level competencies expected from the OT assistant compared to the occupational therapist in the area of OT theoretical perspectives. Further, the entry-level competencies of the occupational therapist prepared at the doctoral degree level differ from those professionals prepared at the master's degree level in the area of theoretical perspectives of the profession. The differentiation of entry-level competencies is described throughout the document for entry-level OT practice as a generalist. The minimum standards of practice for OT delineate the occupational therapist and OTA roles and provide a starting point as the individual enters the field of practice. (AOTA, 2015e; see Chapter 72 for more information on these roles). So how does the OT practitioner advance his or her skills and how would an OT practitioner, at all levels of educational preparation, engage in continuing competence and professional development?

Continuing Professional Development

Advancing practice skills is not a matter of longevity in a specific job or position but a process of engaging in self-directed professional development (AOTA, 2017b). Occupational therapy practice is constantly changing in response to new practice evidence, advancements in technology, health policy modifications, institutional changes, and emerging areas of practice that create new employment options. In addition, practitioners may seek new employment opportunities necessitating new knowledge to meet job expectations, practice setting, or both. Clients, employers, third-party reimbursement resources, licensure boards, accreditation agencies, and society in general expect occupational therapists and OT assistants to proactively anticipate and meet changes in practice by

maintaining and upgrading their skills and abilities to deliver effective OT services.

Meeting these expectations can be challenging for several reasons (Moyers, 2009, p. 241):

- The skills and abilities of all practitioners fade with lack of practice, feedback, or administrative/systems support.
- The rapid expansion of information makes it challenging to systematically focus on learning and upgrade practice knowledge and skills.
- Significant sophistication is required to translate new knowledge into practice that meets the client-centered and culturally appropriate services.
- The pressure from complex health care and social systems creates barriers to practice enhancements.
- Rapid shifts in health policy and third-party reimbursement processes modify intervention delivery and outcome expectations.

The AOTA provides a guide with a five-step process to support OT practitioners as they engage in continuing professional development (AOTA, 2017b).

Step 1: Reflect

First, the practitioner reflects on current service delivery demands with anticipated advancements or changes in practice. This first step is not only an externally driven process but also includes intrinsic motivation and personal goals.

Step 2: Assess Practice

The next step in the process is assessing professional development in terms of the AOTA Standards for Continuing Competence (AOTA, 2015d). These standards identify the components to address during this step and include the practitioner's *knowledge* related to current and anticipated future demands. For example, an OT assistant and an occupational therapist are practicing in a school system. The school system is considering the use of new technology to enhance student learning. Both levels of practitioners would need to become familiar with the basic skills needed to use the technology to support student access. *Critical reasoning skills*, another standard for continuing competence, would need to be assessed as the practitioner considers how new evidence can be incorporated into current practice and what decisions need to be made to upgrade practice. *Interpersonal skills* are critical in the process of assessing practice and require the practitioner to consider the relationships and communications with others. For example, a hospital is providing a new oncology service to support clients in their homes. An occupational therapist who had developed relationships within the hospital could advocate for OT services to be included to support clients. **Performance skills** are the standards that address the OT practitioner's therapeutic use of self, client-centered occupations and activities, consultation, and education as part of service delivery (AOTA, 2014b, 2015d). An example is seen with the arena of telehealth and access to service. An OT practitioner, working in early intervention in a rural area, plans to provide services using telehealth. The practitioner would need to acquire the performance skills to competently deliver OT services using this model (Fitzgerald, Moores, Coleman, & Fleming, 2015; Moyers & Metzler, 2014). The final standard is that of *ethical practice* and refers to the application of ethical principles and adherence to the Occupational Therapy Code of Ethics (AOTA, 2015b). In examining one's practice, these standards are used and combined with feedback obtained from performance reviews, self-assessment tools, and consumer ratings.

Step 3: Develop the Continuing Professional Development Plan

Developing the plan is the third step in the process and includes setting measureable goals with strategies to meet these goals. This includes reflecting on learning styles and abilities (Fitzgerald et al., 2015; Haywood, Pain, Ryan, & Adams, 2012). These goals should provide incremental steps to be successfully implemented along with a completion date.

Step 4: Implement the Plan

The fourth step includes selecting opportunities that will best fit the goals. For example, an OT practitioner plans to pursue the AOTA Specialty Certification in Feeding, Eating and Swallowing (SCFES) to meet a personal goal and better serve clients in a skilled nursing facility. To meet this goal, the practitioner selects a variety of strategies such as online educational courses, in-person workshops with the opportunity to practice new techniques, and engaging in a mentorship relationship with another practitioner who holds a current SCFES.

Step 5: Document Effectiveness of the Continuing Professional Development Plan

The final step considers the completion of the plan in terms of client outcomes, external expectations, and personal satisfaction. The benefits of using a systematic plan can be seen in the trajectory of professional growth (Haywood et al., 2012; Roessger, 2015). If the plan has brought about improved client outcomes, greater job satisfaction in performance, and better service delivery, the plan would be considered a success. Often, a plan produces a pattern of strengths and weaknesses. As the OT practitioner evaluates

the effectiveness of the plan, the practitioner may need to return to the first step of engaging in reflection and consider why the client outcomes improved but personal job satisfaction did not substantially change. This may be the impetus to initiate a new plan.

What Does It Mean to Be Competent?

The term *competent* refers to the knowledge, skills, and ability to practice as an occupational therapist or OT assistant. This does not only refer to entry-level competence but also refer to practitioners as they shift areas of practice. For example, an occupational therapist practicing in an acute care hospital setting accepts a new position in a skilled nursing facility. A majority of the clients in this setting have unique sensory needs due to vision and hearing loss. The occupational therapist has the foundational skills to practice but needs to expand knowledge and practice skills to competently work with clients who have vision and hearing compromises (Wittich, Jarry, Barstow, & Thomas, 2017). **Competency** is the *actual performance* of competence; an example of competency would be safely parking a car during the on-the-road driving test. The driver demonstrates competent parking skills with this action (competency). **Competence** is the result of combining one's knowledge base, current practice skills, and abilities along with client outcomes and comparing your competence with a specific criterion such as using evidence-based practice on a consistent basis. Substantiating competence implies internal self-determination coupled with external validation regarding one's effectiveness in performing certain skills or behaviors. Although practice guidelines are available for specific arenas of services, this poses a problem for emerging practice areas (Knightbridge, 2014). For emerging practice areas, the OT practitioner will have far fewer external benchmarks to use as a comparison between current performance and desired performance skills. This will require a greater degree of reflection on professional behaviors and further development of professional reasoning skills (Unsworth & Baker, 2016).

Ensuring competence and practicing competently is a dynamic and evolving process requiring lifelong learning. Determining the currency of one's competence requires self-evaluation of existing abilities according to criteria such as completing a self-development tool, a periodic peer review, a knowledge examination, a refresher course offered by the employer, or even recalibrating oneself against published standardized procedures published for an assessment tool or meeting continuing education (CE) requirements for licensing or certification. Also, one may seek out professional development opportunities to identify and enhance a skill set to ensure implementation of contemporary approaches during practice. Common approaches include pursuing post-professional education or workshops, reading scholarly publications and/or evidence-based practice briefs, securing additional certifications, participating in local special interest practitioner groups, or attending focused in-service or conference presentations. Participation in these activities provides several benefits such as validation of current practice skills, acquisition of advanced knowledge and practice skills, and opportunities for further inquiry in the selected topic.

American Occupational Therapy Association and the Choosing Wisely Campaign

As of 2017, AOTA joined the Choosing Wisely Campaign initiated by the American Board of Internal Medicine (ABIM) in 2012 (Gillen, Leiberman, Stutzbach, & Arbesman, 2017). The impetus for this campaign was to foster meaningful conversations between practitioners and clients in the selection and implementation of services. Overuse of medical procedures has substantially increased health care spending and generated concern (Morgan, Dhruva, Wright, & Korenstein, 2016). A systematic review of medical literature found overuse of medications, advanced technological treatments and tests, and that clinicians were slow to discontinue use of these options when evidence identified approaches that were more effective. The AOTA joined this campaign as a member-driven organization to improve communication among OT practitioners, clients, consumers, and other service providers. The purpose of joining this effort is specifically to improve communication to implement the most effective OT service, not as a guide for reimbursement (Gillen et al., 2017).

Costs of Ineffective Practice

Competent service delivery is a core professional value to effectively serve clients (AOTA, 2015e). The consequences of providing ineffective OT service harm not only the client/consumer but also the profession. All stakeholders, including the clients, their family, employers, payers, and social service agencies, expect at least minimally effective practice, and for the most part, the use of best practices grounded in evidence that suggests the intervention selected will lead to desired outcomes. This requires the OT practitioner to systematically monitor advances in practice and upgrade skills to provide effective service. Examples can be seen when new evidence reports an effective method of functional retraining for individuals who sustained a stroke, or an investigation identifies better outcomes using an intervention for individuals who have autism compared to current interventions. Professional ethics and accountability requires the practitioner to be aware of such innovations and engage in continuing competence and professional development on an ongoing basis. Not knowing about new evidence or seeking relevant training for practice approaches supported by evidence represents unethical and neglectful practice and may lead to charges of malpractice. Waiting for external funding from employers or others to be educated is not sufficient. An ethical, responsible OT practitioner needs to proactively advocate for and complete continuing competence activities to ensure the provision of best practice in the delivery of OT services. Self-funding is a clear option to enhance one's professional responsibility to prevent neglect or harm, which includes delivering the most effective intervention available.

Evidence-Based Practice

Evidence-based practice has been adopted by the profession of OT for several decades and was a clear directive for OT practitioners in Dr. Holm's 2000 Eleanor Clarke Slagle address (Holm, 2000). The foundation of evidence-based practice combines clinical expertise, client input with the best current evidence to direct decisions regarding client services (Holm, 2000; Sackett, Rosenberg, Gray, Haynes, & Richardson, 1996). This requires all OT practitioners to carefully and consistently examine available evidence with an understanding of current and future client needs. With the expansion of available information, this can appear to be a daunting task, but a systematic approach can offer guidance in examining available evidence. The process may begin with a review and discussion of a specific publication related to the area of practice and expands into a journal club where articles are selected and reviewed periodically (Davis, 2014). The AOTA Website provides evidence-based practice resources to support OT practitioners (AOTA, 2017a). Further examination of the topic may result in the OT practitioner(s) generating a critically appraised topic (CAT) that can be shared with other OT practitioners to advance the professional use of evidence. The AOTA provides a CAT Website with topics aligned with client occupational needs, practice settings, and intervention approaches. These can serve as an avenue to enhance the continuing competence of the OT practitioner and affords an opportunity to share expertise with other practitioners. Refer to Chapter 35 for an in-depth discussion of evidence-based practice.

Professional Development and Resources in the United States

The continuing competency journey begins with becoming familiar with external guides and resources. These resources and guides are often developed by organizations and agencies committed to ensuring a work force well equipped to provide quality OT services. Professional organizations, certification agencies, institutional accreditation programs, and state regulatory groups each play a unique and pivotal role in defining and applying standards related to competence and continuing competence. For OT in the United States, the primary ones are AOTA, state professional organizations supporting OT, National Board for Certification in Occupational Therapy (NBCOT), governmental programs, state regulatory agencies, and institutional accreditation bodies. Each of these previous mentioned groups has a unique mission and purpose, and as a result, a healthy tension exists that supports quality service delivery, promotes the profession, honors all the stakeholders, and protects professional domains of concerns. The focus of these groups varies as can be seen in Table 70-2.

TABLE 70-2 Organizations and Focus Related to Continuing Professional Development in Occupational Therapy

Name	American Occupational Therapy Association (AOTA; state professional associations)	National Board for Certification in Occupational Therapy (NBCOT)	State Regulatory Agencies	Institutional Accreditation Bodies
Website	AOTA http://www.aota.org (state associations parallel)	NBCOT http://www.nbcot.org	Check each state's government site.	Example: The Joint Commission
Purpose	Support the profession by setting standards to assure high-quality services; represent the interests and concerns of OT practitioners, students, and educational programs to the public and to policy groups; improve consumer access to health care services; and promote the professional development of members.	Initial certification of OT practitioners; develop, administer, and continually review a certification process based on current and valid standards that provide reliable indicators of competence for the practice of OT.	Oversee implementation of laws or statutes enacted by legislators who are elected public officials; regulations specifically describe how the intent of the laws will be carried out.	Quality assurance; indicate service provider's commitment to continually improve services, encourage feedback, and serve the community.
Oversight responsibilities	Profession, member driven	Certificants (initial) and those who voluntarily recertify after initial certification	State government regulators who are appointed public officials of various departments or boards in state government to enact state law	Nonprofit agencies offering accreditation to institutions
Responsible to	Profession, members of the association	Consumers of practice or intervention	Citizens of the state	Consumers of services
Occupational therapist input	Occupational therapist and OTA members elect key leaders and representatives who make decisions. Appointed or elected volunteer committees make recommendations to decision makers.	OTR® and COTA® representatives along with public representatives appointed by the governing board	Government-appointed board members oversee regulations (writing and ensuring implementation). Occupational therapists can be appointed to a board.	Experts invited by agency to set standards and accredit institutions. Standards developed independently but seek input from related professions
Professional development	Provides standards and guidelines for practice, self-assessment tools, profession-focused continuing education, and advanced board and specialty certification processes	Certification renewal requires acquisition of professional development unit, self-assessment tools, and verification documents	Requirements for continuing education established by each state	Standards related to continuing competency promote institutional supports.
Value	Supports occupational therapist and OTA members by promoting the profession, educating the public, and advancing the profession	Public, regulatory groups, and employers by providing certification examination, verification of credentials, disciplinary actions, and oversight of ongoing general professional certification	Public health and welfare	Public health and welfare, including third parties who provide service reimbursement

COTA®, certified occupational therapy assistant; OTA, occupational therapy assistant; OTR®, certified (registered) occupational therapist

The promotion of the profession comes from each of these organizations being well established to oversee and promote valuable change in practice in response to challenges and opportunities. Engaging in continuing competency is complex and multifactorial endeavor. Thus, it benefits practitioners to have several resources to guide and/or support professional development in OT.

The AOTA is committed to ensuring quality service delivery and has several resources that are useful: "AOTA Standards for Continuing Competence" (AOTA, 2015d) and the "AOTA Standards of Practice for Occupational Therapy" (AOTA, 2015e). Together, these outline core performance expectations that oversee all practice. The *Standards for Continuing Competence* describes the process as multidimensional including the following standards to support the individual practitioner's roles and responsibilities:

- *Knowledge* about multiple roles and responsibilities
- *Critical reasoning* is used to make sound decisions.
- *Interpersonal skills* for professional relationships and communication
- *Performance skill* demonstrates the expertise, proficiencies, and abilities to competently provide OT services.
- *Ethical practice* responding responsibly to issues and dilemmas in the changing context

In addition, AOTA publishes various practice guidelines and related documents that are specific to practice with specific populations, conditions, and/or contexts. The AOTA (2003) *Professional Development Tool* provides a process for self-assessing professional development interests and needs and then presents a guide for planning. The AOTA also provides a Continuing Education Recording Form (https://www.aota.org/~/media/Corporate/Files/EducationCareers/CE/CE-Recording-Form.pdf) that fosters the application of new knowledge to practice. The recording form is more than a simple log of attendance. This form prompts the OT practitioner to consider the application of the new knowledge to practice with a prompt to return to the form to reflect on the changes in practice upon using this form (Schultz-Krohn, James, & Nonaillada, 2017). This AOTA CE Recording Form can be used in conjunction with a larger professional development plan as the form includes sections for the OT practitioner to decide on next steps and future pursuits.

An OT practitioner may want to pursue advanced certification such as the AOTA Board and Specialty Certifications. These certifications are focused on continuing competence and quality service delivery in advanced or specialty practice areas that exceed the profession's core expectations. For these, the competencies outlined serve as a guide for self-assessment as well as documenting evidence of advanced or specialty practice competency. In addition to a demonstration of current performance skills, the AOTA Board and Specialty Certification portfolio constructed by the applicant includes a plan for future development to engage in continuing competence and professional development on an ongoing basis.

State professional associations provide similar activities as AOTA but are designed to serve specific state interests, particularly as desired by the state government agencies or programs. The goal of state professional associations is to represent and advocate for practice opportunities and challenges at the state level, whereas many require some form of continuing competence engagement. State associations also closely monitor and even provide suggestions regarding the state regulations on continuing competency. The AOTA provides a list of licensure requirements for occupational therapist (AOTA, 2017c) and OT assistant (AOTA, 2017c) in each state.

Some form of *government-based state regulation of practice* is present in all 50 states plus the District of Columbia, Puerto Rico, and Guam for OT practitioners in some capacity. The major purpose of regulation is to protect consumers in a state or jurisdiction from unqualified or unscrupulous practitioners (AOTA, 2017c). State laws and regulations significantly affect the practice of OT. Over 90% of the states have a continuing competency or education requirements for renewal of a license (AOTA, 2015c). These requirements may be in terms of submitting evidence of CE units (CEUs) or professional development units (PDUs) (Box 70-1).

The NBCOT (http://www.nbcot.org) is known for its role in conducting the initial certification examination for occupational therapists and OT assistants, which, when successfully passed, allows the applicant use of the occupational therapist, registered (OTR) or certified OT assistant (COTA©) credential. The "NBCOT also serves the public interest by developing, administering, and continually reviewing a certification process that reflects current standards of competent practice in occupational therapy" (NBCOT 2012a; NBCOT 2012b). The professional development requirement for NBCOT recertification is to be able to demonstrate continuing competency of the certificants to the public, be it consumers, employers, agencies, etc. To retain use of the OTR or COTA© professional certification designations, one must apply for certification renewal every 3 years and be able to present documentation regarding continuing competency activities. One of the goals regarding recertification is to engage certificants of all levels of experience in self-reflective assessment of one's current levels of proficiency or efficacy leading to ongoing, role-related engagement in continuing competency activities. Certification renewal requires assembling documentation of continuing competence activities called PDUs. In addition, NBCOT provides self-assessment tools to self-identify professional developmental needs in the highest frequency practice areas for the OTR and COTA. Case Study 70-1 provides an illustration of creating and implementing a professional development plan for an occupational therapist.

BOX 70-1   WHAT IS A CONTINUING EDUCATION UNIT?

The award of a continuing education units (CEU) is often dependent on the number of hours of instruction, where 10 hours of formal instruction equals 1 CEU. Courses can be approved for CEUs through the International Association for Continuing Education and Training (IACET), but CEUs can also be obtained by completing post-professional academic coursework offered by an accredited institution. Professional development units (PDUs) can include a wider variety of activities such as engagement in journal clubs, involvement in a mentee/mentor relationship with specific objectives, or by attending post-professional workshops or seminars. The AOTA provides a voluntary, approved CE provider screening and designating process called the AOTA Approved Provider Program (APP) that aligns with the professional association's mission. Generally, 1 CEU equals 10 PDUs. The decision to select the CEU or PDU activity is based on several variables including professional goals, client needs, emerging practice demands, and workplace expectations, along with the costs of engaging in these continuing competence activities. Engaging in self-assessment and then searching for literature in rigorous journals is a frequent method of professional development by OT practitioners (Coffelt & Gabriel, 2017). The use of journal clubs and literature search to support professional development may be accepted for state licensure purposes (AOTA, 2015c); however, the types and amount of qualified professional development activities vary among states.

CASE STUDY 70-1   AN ENTRY-LEVEL PRACTITIONER INITIATES A PROFESSIONAL DEVELOPMENT PLAN

Andrea, a new graduate has just accepted a position in a school district. The current OT services consist of a full-time occupational therapist (Carol) and a ¾ position OT assistant (Sarah). Andrea is replacing an occupational therapist who recently resigned to pursue another job opportunity. Andrea completed one of her 3-month fieldwork placements at a public school and has reviewed the laws and regulations related to school-based practice. The other occupational therapist, Carol, has been at the school district for 4 years and Sarah, the OT assistant, has been at the school for 7 years.

Both Carol and Sarah are active in the state OT association and participate in a journal club with other OT school-based practitioners. Additionally, Carol recently contacted a local university with an OT program to provide Level I fieldwork (FWE) experiences at the school. Andrea knows that with less than 1 year of experience, she would not be able to supervise a Level II FWE OT student but is interested in participating in the Level I FWE program. Andrea examines her knowledge base regarding expectations and support she could offer in the Level I FWE program. As a newly hired employee of the school district, she had to complete several training modules regarding the federal law Individuals with Disabilities Education Act (IDEA). She also needed to complete training modules addressing the Family Educational Rights and Privacy Act (FERPA), Every Student Succeeds Act, and the Americans with Disabilities Act (ADA). Andrea asks Carol if she could help with the Level I FWE program by providing a brief orientation to the students regarding the laws guiding school-based OT practice. Carol and Andrea collaborate on the development of the program including the orientation of the Level I FWE students and the selection of teachers and classrooms where student could complete the Level I FWE requirements. Andrea's initial step of self-assessment and consideration of how she could become involved in the Level I FWE program represents the basic start of a professional development plan.

Andrea was excited to participate in the Level I FWE program with Carol. The collaborative interactions provided the support for Andrea to begin the process of developing a systematic professional development plan. She discussed her short- and long-range goals with Carol and Sarah during the next OT staff meeting. Andrea had a goal of obtaining her Fieldwork Educator Certificate from AOTA. This required completing the program outlined by AOTA. Sarah suggested reaching out to the school-based OT journal club to see if other members were interested in pursuing this program. Sarah, the OT assistant at the school, was pursuing her Specialty Certification in School Systems–Assistant (SCSS-A) and was in a small journal club. She was specifically examining information related to foster social interaction skills for children with mental health issues such as anxiety and autism. Another occupational therapist in the journal club was working on the requirements to obtain his SCSS. He and Sarah had exchanged various articles to address social participation within the school system. This collaborative process had supported both in meeting the knowledge requirements for the SCSS/SCSS-A, and both were able to incorporate evidence into practice to meet these specific needs.

Following the staff meeting, Andrea developed a plan with clear goals to work toward obtaining her Fieldwork Educators Certificate from AOTA and orienting students in the Level I FWE program. She discussed that an additional goal would be to expand the Level II FWE program that Carol started by connecting with other universities and potentially adding OT assistant level fieldwork at the school within 2 years. She knew that a substantial number of OT practitioners provide

(continues)

CASE STUDY 70-1 AN ENTRY-LEVEL PRACTITIONER INITIATES A PROFESSIONAL DEVELOPMENT PLAN *(continued)*

school-based OT and many school systems faced difficulties in recruiting and retaining OT practitioners. Her professional interests seemed well aligned with supporting students to understand the role of the OT practitioner in schools. Andrea used the suggestions provided by Carol and Sarah to identify the steps to take to reach these goals using the journal club, contact with the local OT program, and connecting with her previous professors to ask for guidance.

Andrea engaged in the process of professional development by creating a plan with systematic steps and clear outcomes. She developed a method to meet her goals that included several activities not only attending conferences but also engaging in additional professional development activities. She collaborated with other practitioners and sought their support and guidance as she moved toward her goal.

Factors Motivating Continuing Competence

The process of engaging in continuing competence is dynamic with multiple factors influencing decisions (Moyers, 2009). The new OT practitioner may have specific goals to accomplish within the first few years of practice. The transition from student to OT practitioner requires both time and systematic planning to gain the skills needed to be proficient in the practice area (Fitzgerald et al., 2015; Wallingford, Knecht-Sabres, Lee, & St. Amand, 2016). This process requires the OT practitioner to consider the knowledge necessary to provide service within the specific setting, the critical reasoning needed to select the best intervention for clients, and the skills to ethically implement these services (AOTA, 2015d, 2015e). Additionally, interactions with others involved with the client require a clear understanding of the role of OT. Consider the many factors evident in Case Study 70-1 in which Andrea as a new OT practitioner is seeking guidance and support from coworkers, whereas Carol is initiating a fieldwork program and Sarah is pursuing her Specialty Certification in School Systems–Assistant (SCSS-A) as a means to recognize her expertise and guide her further development as a school-based OT assistant. Factors motivating continuing competence can be viewed along a continuum from self-determined to primarily external factors. Practitioners often have specific professional interests, and with experience, they learn what their particular therapy talents are. These internal motivations may also be influenced by their desire to provide more expert care for specific groups of clients. In addition to these more personal motivations, external requirements from employers, regulators, and accreditation agencies provide external pressure to gain skills. All of these factors may influence practitioner's choices to engage in continuing competence programs, obtain advanced certification or credentials, seek additional knowledge to support evidence-based practice, or add new skills in preparation for new job responsibilities.

Regardless of the motivating factors, engagement in thoughtful, continuous professional development processes is essential for all OT practitioners (AOTA 2015d; Coffelt & Gabriel, 2017). A practitioner must also critically evaluate who determines competence when implementing a continuous, goal-directed competency development plan that is not only individually relevant but also judiciously and ethically reflects external practice demands.

Who Determines Whether Someone Is Competent?

Competent practice is the expectation and responsibility of every OT practitioner (AOTA 2015e; Coffelt & Gabriel, 2017; Fitzgerald et al., 2015). In addition, the profession and public use credentials as indicators that the OT practitioner has met minimal standards to provide safe, quality practice. The most common approaches to determining competency are entry-level education expectations, testing, credentialing, and requiring position-related CE (Coffelt & Gabriel, 2017; Fitzgerald et al., 2015; Moyers, 2009; Wallingford et al., 2016). Graduation from an accredited educational program, meeting licensure requirements from state or government agencies, and/or professional certification is presumed to protect the public from incompetent practitioners. Entry-level OT practitioners and those practitioners with several years of experience both report consistent expectation when asked about the import entry-level competence (Wallingford et al., 2016).

State regulatory authorities and NBCOT protect the public by providing practice credentials to qualified individuals: This is referred to as **credentialing**. In the United States, initial credentialing is met by graduating from an academic program accredited by ACOTE, completing the required fieldwork experience and then successfully passing the NBCOT examination. State credentialing involves licensure to practice and may require additional documentation from the applicant. Both state regulatory boards and the NBCOT grant credentials to practitioners who meet the required standards, and they also remove credentials from individuals if the practitioner is either not able or unwilling to act according to established standards. This information is of particular interest to current or future employers. On finding significant misconduct or malpractice, practice credentials can be removed, reprimanded, or censored. Most states have licensure portals that readily identify the current state-credentialed practitioners.

Planning and Engaging in Continuing Professional Development

Continuing professional development (CPD) refers to the process of engaging in "lifelong learning aimed at maintaining practice competence, ensuring client safety and quality outcomes, enhancing or expanding professional practice, and reaching career goals" (AOTA, 2017b). This process is self-directed and requires a reflective process to establish goals and a plan to meet the goals. The OT practitioner considers not only current skills but also skills needed to meet future client needs, anticipated roles, and educational activities suited to meet these goals (Dik, Sargent, & Steger, 2008; Haywood et al., 2012; McMahon, Forde, & Dickson, 2015). All professional development planning is based on continuous self-reflection and critical analysis regarding one's current practice competence and one's career aspirations coupled with sustained environmental scanning of practice standards and expectations.

Evaluating the quality of professional development opportunities is essential in order to develop a productive CPD plan (AOTA, 2017b). The process is more than just acquiring specific skills or enhancing competence-related knowledge. The OT practitioner seeks to also improve critical and ethical reasoning processes and requisite interactional skills. Use of audio or video recording of the OT practitioner's intervention session can be used for both experiential self-learning and during a mentor/mentee session. Consent should always be obtained when recording a session with a client. Numerous approaches and tools are available to implement a CPD plan. Literature reviews including critically appraised papers and CATs, journal clubs, and mentee/mentor relationship in addition to attending CE courses are only a few examples of professional development activities that can be used to reach a CPD goal. **Competence is continually enhancing "best practice" to achieve the highest potential or outcome for the client that is possible according to evidence and applied knowledge in the practice area.**

The outcomes of CPD are only as good as the quality of learning activities and the successful integration of the knowledge and skills into more competent practice (Coffelt & Gabriel, 2017). Selecting activities that best support the achievement of CPD goals is an important part of the CPD process. For example, gaining information about billing and documentation may be achieved through literature review, but learning a new intervention approach often requires guided practice and support from a mentor. Because competence is usually not achieved on the first attempt, repeated practice including systematic reflection on and comparing results to benchmark outcomes is expected. The following questions guide individual reflection on the results of competency-based learning:

- What are my outcomes in relation to predicted ones?
- How can I improve effective, efficient competency use?
- When does the approach work best or worst?
- What are cues that I can use to move forward?
- When is use beneficial?
- When should I withhold using this approach when cues suggest difficulty or failure in achieving desired results?

Regardless of the educational program attended, learning will not be translated into practice competencies without practice to test and refine skills to guide future application (Coffelt & Gabriel, 2017; O'Brien et al., 2007). Evidence found in systematic reviews indicates that workshops that mix interactive components with didactic information are better integrated into intervention processes than educational meetings that only have didactic components. Experiential learning activities such as case history reviews and simulated practice adapted to self-study can all be effective. Problem-based learning can be implemented through the use of study groups, conference calls, and networking through electronic systems. Assistance from a more expert practitioner can include mentoring and structured observation of your practice in which newly acquired skills are used (O'Brien et al., 2007). The key in self-directed learning is to consider integrating any continuing competency into practice coupled with continuous feedback and reflection regarding practice results.

Specialty and Advanced Certification

Specialization refers to becoming proficient in a particular practice area, diagnostic procedure or evaluation tool, or intervention approach (Moyers, 2009). The growing use of the words **advanced practice** and *advanced practitioner* raises the issue of what is meant by the term *advanced*. Advanced practitioners possess a higher level of practice expertise resulting from engagement in theory-informed, evidence-based practice. In addition, expertise is developed and improved with proactively planned CPD with sustained focus on reflections, skill enhancement, applied ethics, and strategically planning a career. An example is seen in the area of providing OT services for those with compromised vision and hearing (Wittich et al., 2017).

The AOTA provides both *board certifications* of advance practice (for occupational therapists only) and *specialty certifications* (for occupational therapists and OT assistants). The AOTA defines advanced practice as knowledge and skills regarding both the breadth and depth of a major practice area such as mental health, pediatrics, gerontology, and physical rehabilitation. In contrast, specialty certification reflects expertise in a more precise or definitive intervention skill area such as community mobility, school-based practice, or low vision, each of which is a subcomponent of a larger practice area. Additionally, post-professional credentialing is available from other groups invested in being able to document and attest to specific practitioner competencies (see Table 70-3).

TABLE 70-3 Entry-Level (Initial) and Post–Entry-Level (Specialty) Certifications for Practice in the United States

Credentials[a]		Granting Organization	
Entry-Level Credentialing and Certification Renewal			
OTR®	Occupational therapist, registered (professional level)	NBCOT	http://www.nbcot.org/
COTA®	Certified OT assistant (technical level)	NBCOT	http://www.nbcot.org/
AOTA Board Certification (Advanced Practice for Occupational Therapists Only)			
BCG	Board Certification in Gerontology	AOTA-BASC	https://www.aota.org/Education-Careers/Advance-Career/Board-Specialty-Certifications/Gerontology.aspx
BCMH	Board Certification in Mental Health	AOTA-BASC	https://www.aota.org/Education-Careers/Advance-Career/Board-Specialty-Certifications/MentalHealth.aspx
BCP	Board Certification in Pediatrics	AOTA-BASC	https://www.aota.org/Education-Careers/Advance-Career/Board-Specialty-Certifications/Pediatrics.aspx
BCPR	Board Certification in Physical Rehabilitation	AOTA-BASC	https://www.aota.org/Education-Careers/Advance-Career/Board-Specialty-Certifications/Physical-Rehabilitation.aspx
AOTA Specialty Certifications (Specific Advanced Practice for Occupational Therapists and Occupational Therapy Assistants)			
SCDCM or SCDCM-A	Specialty Certification in Driving and Community Mobility	AOTA-BASC	https://www.aota.org/Education-Careers/Advance-Career/Board-Specialty-Certifications/Driving-Community-Mobility.aspx
SCEM or SCEM-A	Specialty Certification in Environmental Modification	AOTA-BASC	https://www.aota.org/Education-Careers/Advance-Career/Board-Specialty-Certifications/EnvironmentalModification.aspx
SCFES or SCFES-A	Specialty Certification in Feeding, Eating, and Swallowing	AOTA-BASC	https://www.aota.org/Education-Careers/Advance-Career/Board-Specialty-Certifications/Feeding.aspx
SCLV or SCLV-A	Specialty Certification in Low Vision	AOTA-BASC	https://www.aota.org/Education-Careers/Advance-Career/Board-Specialty-Certifications/Low-vision.aspx
SCSS or SCSS-A	Specialty Certification in School Systems	AOTA-BASC	https://www.aota.org/Education-Careers/Advance-Career/Board-Specialty-Certifications/School-system.aspx
Other Specialty Certifications (Professional Level Varies)			
ATP	Assistive Technology Practitioner	RESNA	http://resna.org/
CCM	Certified Case Managers	CCMC	http://www.ccmcertification.org/
CDRS	Certified Driver Rehabilitation Specialist	ADED	http://www.driver-ed.org/
CHT	Certified Hand Therapist	HTCC	http://www.htcc.org/
CLVT	Certification in Low Vision Therapy	ACVREP	http://www.acvrep.org/
CPE	Certified Professional Ergonomist	BCPE	http://www.bcpe.org/
CVE	Certified Vocational Evaluation Specialist	CRCC	http://www.crccertification.com/
PC or CC	Professional Coach Certification	ICF	(PC) http://www.coachfederation.org/
MPC, CMC, or MMC	Masteries Practitioner Coach, Certified Masteries Coach, or Master Masteries Coach	IAC	(CC) https://certifiedcoach.org/about/
SMS	Seating and Mobility Specialist	RESNA	http://resna.org/certification/

[a]Note that credentialing starts with graduation from Accreditation Council for Occupational Therapy Education (ACOTE)-accredited educational program. AOTA-BASC, American Occupational Therapy Association: Board and Specialty Certification; ACVREP, Academy for Certification of Vision Rehabilitation & Education Professionals; ADED, Association for Driver Rehabilitation Specialists; BCPE, Board of Certification in Professional Ergonomics; CCMC, Commission for Case Manager Certification; CRCC, Commission on Rehabilitation Counselor Certification; HTCC, Hand Therapy Certification Commission; IAC, International Association of Coaching; ICF, International Coach Federation; NBCOT, National Board for Certification in Occupational Therapy; RESNA, Rehabilitation Engineering and Assistive Technology Society of North America.

Changing Areas of Practice, Pursuing Emerging Areas, or Reentering the Field

Sometimes during one's career, the opportunity presents itself to take one's professional work in a new direction such as with changing practice focus, seeking a new emerging practice area, or reentering after a leave of absence from practicing. All these require professional development considerations. Changing practice areas requires careful analysis of specific theories and skills relevant to the new or emerging practice area, with attention to both prospective clients and the practice context. Further work is often necessary when practitioners have opted to leave practice and then return.

For a variety of reasons, an OT practitioner may choose to leave the field for a period of time and then return. In these cases, guidelines have been established to support the practitioner who has left OT practice for over 24 months and decides to return to provide OT services (AOTA, 2015a). These Guidelines for Reentry into the Field of Occupational Therapy identify basic expectations to return practice as an OT practitioner, but all state licensure and regulatory requirements must be met in addition to workplace requirements.

Reentering occupational therapists and OT assistants are defined as individuals who have practiced in the field for a minimum of 1 year, who have not engaged in the practice of OT for a minimum of 18 months, and who wish to return to the profession in the capacity of delivering OT services to clients (AOTA, 2015a). Regardless of the reason for change, practitioners have the ethical accountability to ensure high standards of practice competency and skills. The AOTA's (2015a) "Guidelines for Reentry into the Field of Occupational Therapy" contains procedural recommendations to follow for returning to practice after an extended absence. These strategies could be adapted to entering new areas of unfamiliar practice.

Professional Sustainability: Mapping and Documenting

Sustainability is the capacity to persist. For OT practitioners, engagement in CPD is sustainability. Responsible, long-term maintenance of knowledge and skills enables the OT practitioner to remain productive and effective over time. Professional development stems from a commitment not only to personal competence but also to maintaining ethical practice and upholding the social justice of providing the best practice possible coupled with the economic value associated with this promise and obligation. Sustaining professional competence reflects continuous, dynamic engagement in one's professional development.

Beneficial tools and resources to sustain professional development processes specific to OT are the following:

> The AOTA:
> *Professional Development Tool* (AOTA, 2003)
> *Board and Specialty Portfolio Process for Certification* (AOTA, 2018a)
> *Fieldwork Educators Certificate* (AOTA 2018b)
> The NBCOT:
> *COTA Self-Assessment Tool* (NBCOT, 2012a)
> *OTR Self-Assessment Tool* (NBCOT, 2012b)

Integrating information from the professional development self-assessment process becomes the basis on which to develop an individualized, professional development plan. Effective development plans answer the following questions:

- Where are the gaps between my current competence and what is expected or possible?
- What new learning will fill these gaps in my practice competence to ensure best practice?
- What evidence can I accumulate to demonstrate my acquired competencies?

Reflection on the first two questions provides a personalized map or plan for professional development. The last one calls for the development of a **reflective portfolio** to collect ongoing activities and evidence of competence.

A reflective portfolio is a dynamic, flexible, self-directed tool designed to document CPD through thoughtful engagement with artifacts created and accumulated in pursuit to achieve professional goals and desired roles (Schultz-Krohn et al., 2017). The CPD is a cyclical process initiated by reflection. The OT practitioner reflects on current practice skills by identifying triggers within the environment and the ability to respond to those triggers. Triggers can be external factors such as changes to reimbursement, changes in practice area, or derived from internal personal goals. The OT practitioner then completes an analysis of practice that may include consumer ratings, peer reviews, or assessing skills through use of the continuing competence document (AOTA, 2015d). A CPD plan is then developed including specific goals with the methods to achieve the stated goal. The next phase of the process is the implementation of the CDP plan. The final step is documenting the effectiveness of the plan which then returns to the OT practitioner to the first step of reflection to determine new goals to be addressed. This circular process provides an ongoing and advancing systematic approach to engage in CPD.

Conclusion

Rapid changes in health care, knowledge, and technology require constant reevaluation and modification of the role and functions of every OT practitioner. Our clients, their families, our employers, the profession, and the public expect occupational therapists and OT assistants to provide the highest quality services possible. Engaging in CPD is an essential responsibility for every OT practitioner to ensure continuing competence and competency. Professional development results from continuous, reflective self-assessment accounting for client outcomes, job responsibilities, and context as well as future trends in practice (AOTA, 2017b; Schultz-Krohn et al., 2017). Professional development is individualized, goal-directed learning that not only responds to but also advocates and initiates change in practice delivery, sustains practice competence, and enhances the profession.

The universal standard is to deliver best practices with encouragement to strive for practice excellence. Self-responsibility for engaging in continuous professional development is primary. Seeking support and guidance to engage in CPD and assistance in selecting the best suited activities to meet CPD goals is beneficial for all OT practitioners.

REFERENCES

Accreditation Council for Occupational Therapy Education. (2012). *2011 Accreditation Council for Occupational Therapy Education (ACOTE) standards and interpretative guide: January 2012 interpretative guide version*. Retrieved from https://www.aota.org/~/media/Corporate/Files/EducationCareers/Accredit/Standards/2011-Standards-and-Interpretive-Guide.pdf

American Occupational Therapy Association. (2002). *Fieldwork performance evaluation for the occupational therapy student*. Bethesda, MD: Author.

American Occupational Therapy Association. (2003). *Professional development tool*. Bethesda, MD: Author. Retrieved from https://www1.aota.org/pdt/index.asp

American Occupational Therapy Association. (2012). 2011 Accreditation Council for Occupational Therapy Education (ACOTE) standards. *American Journal of Occupational Therapy, 66*, S6–S74.

American Occupational Therapy Association. (2014a). Guidelines for supervision, roles, and responsibilities during the delivery of occupational therapy services. *American Journal of Occupational Therapy, 68*, S16–S22. doi:10.5014/ajot.2014.686S03

American Occupational Therapy Association. (2014b). Occupational therapy practice framework: Domain and process (3rd ed.). *American Journal of Occupational Therapy, 68*, S1–S48. doi:10.5014/ajot.2014.682006

American Occupational Therapy Association. (2015a). Guidelines for reentry into the field of occupational therapy. *American Journal of Occupational Therapy, 69*, 6913410015p1–6913410015p3. doi:10.5014/ajot.2015.696S15

American Occupational Therapy Association. (2015b). Occupational therapy code of ethics. (2015). *American Journal of Occupational Therapy, 69*, 6913410030p1–6913410030p8. doi:10.5014/ajot.2015.696S03

American Occupational Therapy Association. (2015c). *Occupational therapy profession—Continuing competence requirements*. Retrieved from https://www.aota.org/~/media/Corporate/Files/Advocacy/Licensure/StateRegs/ContComp/Continuing-Competence-Chart-2016.pdf

American Occupational Therapy Association. (2015d). Standards for continuing competence. *American Journal of Occupational Therapy, 69*, 6913410055p1–6913410055p3. doi:10.5014/ajot.2015.696S16

American Occupational Therapy Association. (2015e). Standards of practice for occupational therapy. *American Journal of Occupational Therapy, 69*, 6913410057p1–6913410057p6. doi:10.5014/ajot.2015.696S06

American Occupational Therapy Association. (2017a). *AOTA's evidence-based practice resources*. Retrieved from https://www.aota.org/~/media/Corporate/Files/Practice/Researcher/EBP-Resources.pdf

American Occupational Therapy Association. (2017b). Continuing professional development in occupational therapy. *American Journal of Occupational Therapy, 71*, 7112410017p1–7112410017p5. doi:10.5014/ajot.2017.716S13

American Occupational Therapy Association. (2017c). *Licensure*. Retrieved from https://www.aota.org/~/media/Corporate/Files/Secure/Advocacy/Licensure/StateRegs/Qualifications/OT-qualifications-licensure-requirements-by-state.pdf

American Occupational Therapy Association. (2018a). *Board and specialty certifications*. Retrieved from https://www.aota.org/Education-Careers/Advance-Career/Board-Specialty-Certifications.aspx

American Occupational Therapy Association. (2018b). *Fieldwork educators certificate workshop*. Retrieved from https://www.aota.org/Education-Careers/Fieldwork/Workshop.aspx

Coffelt, K. J., & Gabriel, L. S. (2017). Continuing competence trends of occupational therapy practitioners. *The Open Journal of Occupational Therapy, 5*(1), 4. doi:10.15453/2168-6408.1268

Davis, S. (2014). Evidence-based practice and the new practitioner. *OT Practice, 19*(22), 17–18.

Dik, B. J., Sargent, A. M., & Steger, M. F. (2008). Career development strivings: Assessing goals and motivation in career decision-making and planning. *Journal of Career Development, 35*, 23–41. doi:10.1177/0894845308317934

Fitzgerald, C., Moores, A., Coleman, A., & Fleming, J. (2015). Supporting new graduate professional development: A clinical learning framework. *Australian Occupational Therapy Journal, 62*, 13–20. doi:10.1111/1440-1630.12165

Gillen, G., Lieberman, D., Stutzbach, M., & Arbesman, M. (2017). Five interventions/assessments our clients should question: AOTA joins Choosing Wisely. *OT Practice, 22*(15), 19–20.

Haywood, H., Pain, H., Ryan, S., & Adams, J. (2012). Engagement with continuing professional development: Development of a service model. *Journal of Allied Health, 41*, 83–89.

Holm, M. B. (2000). The 2000 Eleanor Clarke Slagle lecture. Our mandate for the new millennium: Evidence-based practice. *American Journal of Occupational Therapy, 54*, 575–585.

Kidner, T. B. (1929). The importance of "refresher" work for individual and professional advancement. *Psychiatric Quarterly, 3*(3), 398–403.

Knightbridge, L. (2014). Experiential learning on an alternative practice education placement: Student reflections on entry-level competency, personal growth, and future practice. *British Journal of Occupational Therapy, 77*, 438–446. doi:10.4276/030802214X14098207540956

McMahon, M., Forde, C., & Dickson, B. (2015). Reshaping teacher education through the professional continuum. *Educational Review, 67*, 158–178. doi:10.1080/00131911.2013.846298

Morgan, D. J., Dhruva, S. S., Wright, S. M., & Korenstein, D. (2016). 2016 Update on medical overuse: A systematic review. *JAMA International Medicine, 176*, 1687–1692. doi:10.1001/jamainternmed.2016.5381

Moyers, P. (2009). Occupational therapy practitioners: Competence and professional development. In E. B. Crepeau, E. S. Cohn, & B. A. B. Schell (Eds.), *Willard & Spackman's occupational therapy* (11th ed., pp. 240–251). Philadelphia, PA: Lippincott Williams & Wilkins.

Moyers, P. A., & Metzler, C. A. (2014). Interprofessional collaborative practice in care coordination. *American Journal of Occupational Therapy, 68*, 500–505. doi:ajot.2014.685002

National Board for Certification in Occupational Therapy. (2012a). *COTA self-assessment tool manual*. Retrieved from http://www.nbcot.org/pdf/cota-Self-Assessment-Manual.pdf?phpMyAdmin=3710605fd34365e380b9ab41a5078545

National Board for Certification in Occupational Therapy. (2012b). *OTR self-assessment tool manual*. Retrieved from http://www.nbcot.org/pdf/OTR-Self-Assessment-Manual.pdf?phpMyAdmin=3710605fd34365e380b9ab41a5078545

O'Brien, M. A., Rogers, S., Jamtvedt, G., Oxman, A. D., Odgaard-Jensen, J., Kristofferson, D. T., . . . Harvey, E. (2007). Educational outreach visits: Effects on professional practice and health care outcomes. *Cochrane Database Systematic Reviews,* (4), CD000409. doi:10.1002/14651858.CD000409.pub2

Roessger, K. M. (2015). But does it work? Reflective activities, learning outcomes and instrumental learning in continuing professional development. *Journal of Education and Work, 28*, 83–105. doi:10.1080/13639080.2013.805186

Sackett, D. L., Rosenberg, W. M., Gray, J. A.M., Haynes, R. B., & Richardson, W. S. (1996). Evidence-based medicine: What it is and what it isn't. *British Medical Journal, 312*, 71–72.

Schultz-Krohn, W., James, A., & Nonaillada, J. (2017). Continuing professional development—How if fits with practice. *OT Practice, 22*(5), 22–24.

Unsworth, C. A. (2001). The clinical reasoning of novice and expert occupational therapists. *Scandinavian Journal of Occupational Therapy, 8*, 163–173.

Unsworth, C., & Baker, A. (2016). A systematic review of professional reasoning literature in occupational therapy. *British Journal of Occupational Therapy, 79*, 5–16. doi:10.1177/0308022615599994

Wallingford, M., Knecht-Sabres, L. J., Lee, M. M., & St.Amand, L. E. (2016). OT practitioners' and OT students' perceptions of entry-level competency for occupational therapy practice. *The Open Journal of Occupational Therapy, 4*(4), 10. doi:10.15453/2168-6408.1243

Wittich, W., Jarry, J., Barstow, E., & Thomas, A. (2017). Vision and hearing impairment and occupational therapy education: Needs and current practice. *British Journal of Occupational Therapy, 80*, 384–391.

World Federation of Occupational Therapists. (2012). *The World Federation of Occupational Therapists (WFOT) Position Statement on Competency and Maintaining Competency* (CM2012). Retrieved from http://www.wfot.org/ResourceCentre.aspx

World Federation of Occupational Therapists. (2016). *The World Federation of Occupational Therapists (WFOT) Code of Ethic (Revised CM2016)*. Retrieved from http://www.wfot.org/ResourceCentre.aspx

the**Point**® *For additional resources on the subjects discussed in this chapter, visit* **http://thePoint.lww.com /Willard-Spackman13e.**

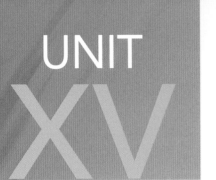

UNIT XV

Occupational Therapy Management

"When it comes to health care delivery,
the issue goes past the logic that we must manage care
to this question:
Shall we inspire it?"

—Suzanne M. Peloquin

From Peloquin, S.M. (1996).
The issue is: Now that we have managed care,
shall we inspire it?
American Journal of Occupational Therapy, 50, p. 459.

CHAPTER 71

Management of Occupational Therapy Services

Brent Braveman

LEARNING OBJECTIVES

After reading this chapter, you will be able to:

1. Analyze and explain the relationship and differences between administrators, managers, supervisors, and leaders in the oversight of work activities in organizations.
2. Identify and explain examples of the common roles, functions, and responsibilities of managers.
3. Identify and explain the areas of knowledge and skills necessary for a manager to demonstrate competency.

Management Can Mean Many Things

Becoming an occupational therapy (OT) or interdisciplinary manager is just one of the many professional roles that an OT practitioner may assume over his or her career. Being a "manager" can mean many different things depending on the setting in which you practice, the scope of duties included in your job description, and the related roles and functions assumed by others in that setting. There is a wealth of information to guide management practice, including theory, research and other types of evidence, formal education, continuing education and training, publications, and other scholarly forms. Investigators and practitioners in a variety of disciplines such as organizational development, business psychology, business administration, and human resource management have contributed to this knowledge base over the past decades. Consequently, many resources to guide managers in their jobs are readily available on the Internet, in bookstores, and through educational courses offered at colleges and universities or at continuing education events, such as professional conferences. Resources are also available from the American Occupational Therapy Association (AOTA).

Similar to clinical practice within OT, demonstrating effective practice as an OT manager is dependent on familiarity with the relevant theories and the ability to apply these theories based on the most current evidence. Just as there are multiple clinical practice models that OT practitioners draw on depending on the area of practice and the needs of the

TABLE 71-1	**Administration, Management, Supervision, and Leadership Defined**
Administration	The process of guiding an organization through the authoritative control of others and overseen by the governing body of the organization
Management	The process of guiding a work unit by planning for future work obligations, organizing employees into functional units, directing employees in the process of completing daily work tasks, and controlling work processes and systems to ensure adequate quality of work output
Supervision	The control and direction of the work of one or more employees in a manner that promotes improved performance and a higher quality outcome
Leadership	The process of creating structural change where the values, vision, and ethics of individuals are integrated into the culture of a community as a means of achieving sustainable change

client, there are multiple theories and skill sets on which a manager draws to guide effective managerial practice. Becoming an effective OT manager is a complicated and time-intensive process. Therefore, this chapter focuses on introducing the reader to the scope of what an OT manager *is* and what an OT manager *does*. Chapter 72 provides a complementary discussion that focuses on supervision and the roles and functions that OT supervisors perform.

In order to truly understand and appreciate the variety of roles and functions that an OT manager can serve, it is critical to recognize that most managers function in ways often described as supervisors and leaders. Table 71-1 provides definitions of **administration**, **management**, **supervision**, and **leadership**.

An administrator may be defined as a member of a *governing body*, such as a board of directors of an organization; the top officials, such as the president or chief executive officer of an organization; or that official's leadership team. Together, administrators perform the key function of being responsible for the overall welfare and direction of the organization, including oversight of financial affairs, establishing the major policies that guide operations, and planning for the health and future of the organization. Administrators typically supervise others but usually are only indirectly responsible for the oversight of the day-to-day work of the organization. They frequently delegate authority for much of the day-to-day coordination of organizational functioning to managers.

Managers are responsible for oversight of work units (such as an OT department or a program for head injury survivors) and of their contributions to the organization's mission. Managers put the policies and directives of administration into action in measurable and visible ways. The specific responsibilities of a manager have been traditionally categorized according to four major functions, which are (1) **planning**, (2) **organizing**, (3) **directing**, and (4) **controlling**. Staffing is a management function that is sometimes grouped with organizing (e.g., organizing and staffing). These four functions are briefly defined

in Table 71-1 and further discussed in the next sections of this chapter.

Supervisors are responsible for direct oversight of employees who perform the work of the organization. Although managers are typically given the ability to decide who becomes part of their work unit through the ability to hire and fire, there are many supervisory roles in organizations that do not perform this or many other functions of the manager. Understanding the important concept of **requisite managerial authority** can help us to further clarify how an OT manager is different from an organizational administrator or from an OT supervisor. Elliot Jaques (1998) defined minimum requisite managerial authority as

> the level of control and discretion that a manager must have to be fairly held responsible for the outcomes of work groups. (p. 69)

For example, requisite managerial authority includes the authority to hire and fire employees and to determine within reason how rewards are distributed. However, in OT, it is not uncommon for a therapist to accept a formally named position within an organization in which he or she has supervisory responsibilities but does not have requisite managerial authority. An example of such a position would be that of a *senior therapist*—an individual who might have specialized or advanced skills and who might provide clinical supervision to other therapists but who does not have the full range of managerial responsibilities.

Administrators, managers, and supervisors may often be viewed as *leaders* by virtue of their formally named positions in an organization, although there are typically many informal leaders in organizations as well. One conceptualization of the relationship between management and leadership is that the role of a manager is to maintain stability in the organization, whereas a leader guides change. Effective leadership is a topic that has been the focus of much research, and several leadership theories have been investigated in depth. A brief description of five of the most commonly cited theories of leadership are presented in Table 71-2.

TABLE 71-2 Common Theories of Leadership

Theories of Leadership	Primary Focus
Supervisory Theories	
Path–Goal	Leaders increase personal payoffs for subordinates for goal attainment and make the path to these payoffs easier to travel by reducing obstacles, thereby improving performance.
Transactional	Leaders promise rewards and benefits to subordinates for meeting work goals, and leaders and subordinates agree through transactions on what will lead to reward and how to avoid punishment.
Strategic Theories	
Charismatic	Stresses the personal identification of followers with the leader who formulates an inspirational vision and impression that the leader's mission is extraordinary
Transformational	Leaders achieve change by expressing the value associated with outcomes and by articulating a vision of the future, resulting in commitment, effort, and improved performance on the part of subordinates.
Situational	Leaders should adopt a leadership style that best fits the developmental level of their subordinates' competence and commitment.

🧘 PRACTICE DILEMMA

Finding Solid Ground as an Occupational Therapy Manager

Six years after accepting a position as the director of the department of rehabilitation services at a large, internationally renowned cancer research and treatment center, Brent is just beginning to feel that he is standing on solid ground. Thirty years earlier in his career, Brent accepted his first management position as the director of OT at a small acute care hospital. In that first job, Brent treated patients half the time and supervised just four OT practitioners. Today, he works full days as a manager and leads a department of over 130 OT and physical therapy practitioners and support staff.

Reflecting on his experiences, Brent realizes that despite the many changes that have occurred in health care over 30 years and the differences in size and scope, his current job holds many of the same challenges as his first. In both experiences, he had to (1) manage the expectations, satisfaction, and performance of employees as well as the expectations of patients and those of his boss; (2) navigate complex organizations while promoting the distinct value of OT; (3) promote the development of clinical competencies and the professional development of the therapy practitioners; and (4) develop a variety of skills including human resources, program development and evaluation, continuous quality improvement, financial planning and budgeting and others.

Questions

As you read this chapter, consider Brent's situation and ask yourself the following questions:
1. What challenges face OT managers no matter how big or small the department they lead?
2. What types of managerial knowledge and skills do all OT managers need to develop?
3. What would be examples of the traditionally identified management functions of planning, organizing, directing, and controlling that most managers perform?
4. What questions can any OT manager ask to guide him or her toward useful management theory and evidence to make his practice as a manager more effective?

Administrators, managers, and supervisors all perform various tasks related to the four functions of management described in Table 71-3, but the scope of these tasks varies for the different levels of leadership. Table 71-4 provides a comparison of sample functions of administrators, managers, and supervisors organized according to the traditional four functions of management.

TABLE 71-3 The Four Traditional Functions of Management

Planning	The process of deciding what to do by setting performance goals and identifying the specific objectives and activities that need to be carried out to accomplish these objectives
Organizing	Designing workable units, determining lines of authority and communication, and developing and managing patterns of coordination
Controlling	Providing guidance and leadership so that the work that is performed is congruent with goals
Directing	Establishing performance standards, measuring, evaluating, and correcting performance

TABLE 71-4 **Comparisons of Sample Functions of Administrators, Managers, and Supervisors**

Management Function	Organizational Administration	Occupational Therapy Managers	Occupational Therapy Supervisors
Planning	• Establishment of organizational mission and vision • Creation of an organizational culture • Strategic planning • Financial forecasting • Establishing organization policies and procedures	• Interpreting the organizational mission and vision for the staff • Aligning the departmental mission and vision with the organizational mission and vision • Establishing departmental objectives • Creating and implementing the departmental budget • Establishing departmental policies and procedures	• Integration of the mission and vision of the organization and department in the daily work of the department and staff • Oversight of work tasks related to achievement of departmental objectives • Ensuring that work is completed effectively and efficiently
Organizing and staffing	• Oversight of the organizational chart and determination of primary organizational structure • Establishing systems for staff functions such as human resources and marketing[a]	• Recruiting, hiring, orienting, and training staff • Appraising performance, determining rewards, and overseeing disciplinary actions	• Providing management with feedback related to the appropriateness of staffing levels • Provide daily supervision, coaching, and feedback to line staff
Directing	• Development of parameters for staff training, education, and development • Mentoring and coaching middle managers	• Mentoring and coaching supervisors • Implementing staff training, education, and development programs	
Controlling	• Establishing systems to measure organizational performance and achievement of key organizational goals • Setting expectations for performance for management	• Oversight and implementation of departmental continuous quality improvement and quality control systems • Establishing performance expectations and measures for department functions and outputs	• Ensuring compliance with policies and procedures • Measuring and recording quality indicators • Alerting management to systems problems

[a]Staff functions relate to the overall maintenance and management of an organization (e.g., human resources, housekeeping, or marketing). Line functions relate to carrying out the primary work of the organization (e.g., OT, physical therapy, or social work in medically oriented organizations).

The Four Functions of Management

Planning

Planning is the first of four critical functions that managers perform in an organization. Planning is the process of establishing short- and long-term goals, measurable objectives, and action plans that are both congruent with the mission of the organization and consistent with the vision that current organizational leaders have established. An organization's mission is typically established by its founders and remains relatively stable. It is often expressed in the form of a mission statement that sets forth the organization's purpose, products, and services. **Mission statements** succinctly describe (1) why an organization exists or the function the organization performs in society or in a community, (2) who the organization serves or who its customers are, and (3) an indication of how an organization goes about achieving its purpose.

A **vision statement**, by contrast, expresses an aspirational message about what a department or organization would like to become as it seeks to fulfill its mission. Vision statements are inherently future-oriented and therefore are helpful management tools in long-term planning. Both missions and visions are often communicated in *statements*, but the process itself of developing a mission statement or vision statement can be of tremendous value to an organization.

One example of a mission statement and vision statement are those developed by the University of Texas MD Anderson Cancer Center in Houston, Texas. The mission of the University of Texas MD Anderson Cancer Center is to "eliminate cancer in Texas, the nation, and the world through outstanding programs that integrate patient care, research and prevention, and through education for undergraduate and graduate students, trainees, professionals, employees and the public" (MD Anderson Cancer Center, 2017, para. 1). The vision statement for MD Anderson reads, "We shall be the premier cancer center in the world, based on the excellence of our people, our research-driven patient care and our science. We are Making Cancer History" (MD Anderson Cancer Center, 2017, para. 2).

It is common to distinguish between strategic planning or long-range planning and the shorter term day-to-day planning that most managers complete. **Strategic planning** is "a deliberative, disciplined effort to produce fundamental decisions and actions that shape and guide what an organization (or other entity) is, what it does, and why" (Bryson, Edwards, & Van Slyke, 2017, p. 317). Strategic plans are often developed with 3- to 5-year time frames in mind, although hopefully the top leadership of an organization (e.g., administration) is thinking much further into the future. The *goals* included in the strategic plan are a reflection of the scope of the desired outcomes such that they can be broad and encompass the full breadth of organizational activities or they can be more focused on critical segments of an organization. *Objectives* are the measurable steps that are taken to reach each goal. The discreet objectives for each goal are commonly based on a 1-year period that corresponds with an organization's financial cycle, or *fiscal year*. Fiscal years may correspond with a calendar year or may be reflective of some other time cycle such as an academic calendar. It is common for organizations to have fiscal years that begin on July 1st and end on June 30th.

Operating in an environment in which change occurs frequently, such as the health care arena, may make long-term planning more difficult than in industries or environments that are more stable. When an organization experiences significant change, the processes of mission review and visioning previously discussed become even more important (Braveman, 2016c). The scholarship on change management has focused on four principal aspects: (1) theoretical models and frameworks that reveal and guide organization members' and researchers' thinking about organization change, (2) approaches and tools for creating and managing change, (3) factors that are important to successful change management, and (4) outcomes and consequences of the process of change management (Inalhan, 2009; Kuipers et al., 2014). It is strongly recommended that new managers become familiar with theories of change and strategies for promoting successful change. For example, Kurt Lewin (1997) proposed a prominent and relatively simple approach to understanding change still commonly employed today that includes three stages (Figure 71-1). These three stages are (1) unfreezing or recognizing the need to change, (2) changing, and (3) refreezing or standardizing new procedures or ways of behaving. Managers can apply this theory by identifying different strategies to use with employees during each of the three stages to facilitate the change process. Two other theories that are often used to understand change include the following:

- Prochaska and DiClemente's transtheoretical stages of change model, which conceptualizes change in five stages: (1) precontemplation, (2) contemplation, (3) preparation,

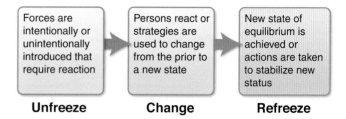

Unfreeze   **Change**   **Refreeze**

FIGURE 71-1 Lewin's three-stage model of change.

(4) action, and (5) maintenance (Franche, Corbière, Lee, Breslin, & Hepburn, 2007; Prochaska, 2013)
- Social cognitive theory, which focuses on change in individuals who can learn by direct experiences, human dialogue and interaction, and observation (Cervone & Pervin, 2008; University of Twente, 2017)

Although the transtheoretical stages of change model and social cognitive theory have most often been applied to change as it relates to health behaviors, they can also be useful in understanding how humans interpret and respond to change in the workplace.

In addition to establishing goals and objectives, planning includes determining the needs for the human resources, materials, supplies, facilities, and equipment required to meet goals and objectives. Financial planning and budgeting and the writing of policies and procedures that guide the use of materials, supplies, facilities, and equipment are also commonly considered components of planning.

Organizing and Staffing

Typically, an organization's administration will determine the overall structure of the organization, including how line authority will be organized and how employees may be grouped into departments. Organizational structures can vary in complexity. An organizational chart helps to facilitate understanding of an organization's structure. Liebler and McConnell (2017) explain that an organizational chart is a management tool that visually depicts the following aspects of an organization:

- Major functions, usually by department
- Relationships of functions or departments
- Channels of supervision
- Lines of authority and of communication
- Positions by job title within departments or units

When one examines an organizational chart, one must keep in mind that it is a static picture of how the organization is structured at one point in time. It might not reflect recent changes, vacancies, or informal relationships because written charts typically indicate only formal lines of command. Earlier, it was noted that there are many

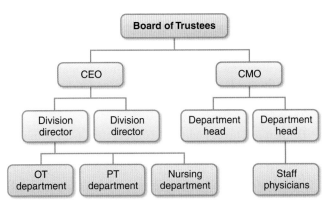

FIGURE 71-2 A sample dual-pyramid form of organizing. *CEO*, chief executive officer; *CMO*, chief medical officer; *PT*, physical therapy.

informal leaders in organizations, and these sources of knowledge, power, and influence are not communicated in an organizational chart. The organizational charts of many large organizations support the notion that systems are often quite organic in how they grow and are restructured over time.

Although few large organizations fit the perfect theoretical profile of any formal organizational form or structure, there are a few basic structures commonly found in health care and service organizations and systems that are useful for a new manager or practitioner to understand. These structures include the dual-pyramid form of organizing, product line or service line organizations, and hybrid or matrix organizations.

The term *dual-pyramid* has been used to describe the common structure found in many medical model settings, such as acute and general hospitals. The pyramid structure is also commonly found in community-based organizations, although the second pyramid representing medical staff might be absent in these cases. A pyramid is typically used to represent an organization of personnel with upper management at the top and line staff at the bottom (Figure 71-2).

In the dual-pyramid form of organizing, the traditional relationship between medical staff and administration

results in the structure shown in Figure 71-2, in which two supervisory pyramids are arranged side by side. One pyramid represents the structure of the professional staff that is organized in departments, including administration (with the chief executive officer at the top of the pyramid); health professionals such as occupational therapists, physical therapists, and social workers; and all support services such as engineering, housekeeping, and human resource personnel. A second pyramid mimics that structure but represents the organization of the medical staff with the chief medical officer at the top of the pyramid, department heads as middle management, and staff physicians as line employees (Braveman, 2016c). Although the medical staff, professional staff, and support staff all ultimately report to a board of trustees or board of directors, there are two distinct chains of command that result in the authority and accountability systems being separated. So, for example, physicians, nurses, occupational therapists, and physical therapists all work together as part of an interdisciplinary team. However, the physicians on a particular service (e.g., cardiovascular) report to a department head (also a physician) who reports to the chief medical officer, who in return reports to the chief executive officer. The other members of the team report to a supervisor and/or a department director who in turn may report to a vice president who reports to the same chief executive officer as the chief medical officer.

A second common form of organizational structure is the *product line*, or *service line*, structure. In a product line structure, personnel are organized according to the service or product that they provide rather than according to the specific function that they complete or their departments. A board of directors maintains ultimate authority, and the chief executive officer and chief medical officer often still maintain parallel but distinct responsibilities and authority. An example of the organizational chart for a product line form is provided in Figure 71-3. Additional ways of structuring organizations may combine elements of the dual-pyramid and product line structures and may function in a more *matrixed* manner with many interconnections between departments, dual reporting structures

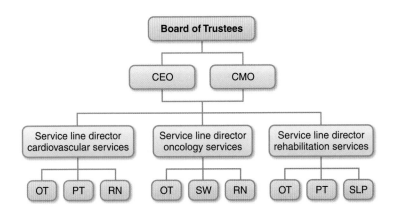

FIGURE 71-3 A sample product line management form of organizing. *CEO*, chief executive officer; *CMO*, chief medical officer; *OT*, occupational therapist; *PT*, physical therapist; *RN*, registered nurse; *SLP*, speech-language pathologist; *SW*, social worker.

where some employees report to more than one manager, and heavy use of internal consultants.

Each of the methods of organization has advantages and disadvantages, and understanding how structure influences the function of an organization can help one to capitalize on the system's benefits and compensate for its limitations. For example, health care organizations that have a dual-pyramid structure rely on departments structured by discipline or professional education and training to provide for strong supervision of staff and their clinical performance. Thus, communication within a professional discipline is facilitated, and the discipline-specific daily work of a unit may be completed more efficiently. Because a department manager or supervisor representing each discipline has direct access to staff and to the data related to routine processes and interventions, performance improvement and outcome measurement using these data may also be easier in a dual-pyramid organization. Nonetheless, in this form of organizing, communication across disciplines (e.g., from OT to nursing) might be more complicated, which can pose potential hazards for developing and managing new programs. Problem-solving and process improvement in existing programming can be cumbersome when staff members feel that it is necessary to communicate up through the chains of command. The advantages and disadvantages of the dual pyramid and the product line forms of organizing are summarized in Table 71-5.

Once decisions have been made about how an organization or a department is to be structured, administrators and managers ideally work together to develop plans for staffing and human resources management. Functions related to recruitment and staffing, such as advertising job vacancies or the development of policies and procedures related to employment, may be performed by a human resources department. Occupational therapy managers are frequently involved in a number of other staffing-related activities. The following is a list of some of these activities:

- Human resources planning: collaborating with administrators and supervisors at all levels of the organization to forecast the short- and long-term personnel needs of the organization based on the organizational mission, leadership vision, and strategic plans
- Recruitment: seeking out and attracting adequate numbers of qualified personnel to meet ongoing organizational needs, including contingencies, such as resignations and leaves of absence for medical or personal reasons
- Hiring: selecting the appropriate personnel for vacant positions and activities related to the hiring process, such as benefits counseling and overseeing background and reference checks
- Orientation: introducing the new employee to organizational policies, benefits, procedures, values, personnel, and environments
- Training and development: meeting the short- and long-term educational and professional development needs of employees at all levels of the organization
- Separation: terminating the employment of personnel due to resignation or inadequate job performance or that which may come about as the result of a decrease in organizational resources

TABLE 71-5 Advantages and Disadvantages of Common Forms of Organizing

	Pyramid	Product Line
Communication	• Communication within a discipline is facilitated.	• Communication between disciplines becomes harder.
Planning	• Planning for activities such as professional development and clinical supervision is facilitated, but program planning becomes harder.	• Program planning and planning for interdisciplinary activities such as program evaluation is facilitated, but planning functions within disciplines becomes harder.
Budgeting	• Tracking and planning for finances related to single-discipline costs are facilitated, but tracking and planning for interdisciplinary activities (e.g., cost per unit of care) are harder.	• Tracking and planning for finances related to programmatic costs are facilitated (e.g., cost per unit of care), but tracking and planning for discipline-specific activities are harder.
Staffing	• Some needs such as providing coverage for leaves or vacancies may be easier, but the need to communicate with other managers increases. Recruitment activities are facilitated.	• Staffing activities influenced by other disciplines such as scheduling programmatic elements may be facilitated, but coverage for leaves or vacancies becomes more difficult. Recruitment of staff may be more difficult, or you might need to rely on managers from other disciplines for assistance.
Process improvement, program evaluation, and outcomes	• Improving discipline-specific processes is easier as is measuring single-discipline outcomes and indicators of program evaluation, but interdisciplinary programs require extra effort.	• Improving interdisciplinary or program processes is easier, as is measuring program outcomes and indicators of program evaluation, but discipline-specific elements require extra effort.
Professional development	• Development of discipline-specific skills related to assessment and intervention may be facilitated by the ease of access to disciplinary specialists.	• Development of interdisciplinary skills related to the needs of a population or program development or implementation may be facilitated.

Maintaining a viable workforce by retaining a qualified and competent staff is perhaps one of the most important functions of the manager for an organization. Retention of staff can also be very difficult in professions such as OT and physical therapy where much of the workforce is young and mobile, and the demand for staff far outnumbers the supply. Maintaining staff satisfaction and retention of staff are two areas where the OT manager can benefit from considerable research and evidence (Ashby, Ryan, Gray, & James, 2013; Scanlan, Meredith, & Poulsen, 2013). Similar to the topics of leadership and change, an in-depth discussion of theories related to staff retention and satisfaction are beyond the scope of this chapter, and managers would benefit from a thorough review of contemporary literature. A few examples of theories that have evolved regarding employee satisfaction and retention are the following:

- Self-determination theory, which explores the relationship of intrinsic and extrinsic motivators to work motivation (Adams, Little, & Ryan, 2017)
- Need theories such as Maslow's hierarchy of needs and McClelland's need theory that focus on identifying physiological and psychological needs of employees with the rationale that satisfying these needs will lead to employee satisfaction (Champoux, 2017)
- Expectancy theory, which holds that people are motivated to behave in ways that produce expected and desired combinations of outcomes (Baumann & Bonner, 2017)

Directing

Directing is the management function that involves giving guidance, instruction, and leadership to subordinates so that work that is performed is goal oriented and contributes to meeting organizational or departmental requirements. More specifically, a manager could assign and manage the workload, develop and implement policies and procedures to guide others in uniform completion of their work, provide mentoring and coaching for improved future performance, and appraise performance by providing feedback to employees about current performance.

Managing the workload is a complicated and multistep process that involves projecting the amount of work to be done, determining which resources are necessary to complete the work, and managing these resources to make certain that the appropriate person with the right skills and right equipment and space is available when needed. The workload is typically projected on a yearly basis as part of planning a departmental budget, but it may also be done on a week-to-week, day-to-day, or even hourly basis. Effective workload management requires flexibility, creativity, a commitment to planning, and advanced problem-solving skills.

Writing policies and procedures to guide staff in their daily tasks in a standardized manner, as well as their use of

materials, supplies, facilities, and equipment in ways that are compliant with accreditation and other standards, is a specific aspect of directing that is typically the responsibility of a department manager. Policies are statements of values that are congruent with the organizational or departmental mission and justify the boundaries that govern the services provided. They set parameters for making decisions about day-to-day operations. Procedures outline the specific tasks that should be completed or that provide specific direction about how a policy should be implemented. A manager should not only be able to cite a policy or procedure but also be able to give the underlying logic for the policy's existence.

Most organizations follow a prescribed standard format that guides managers in deciding what to include in a department's policy and procedure manual. If a policy and procedures format is not provided, the organization may purchase existing customizable resources on the Internet. It is typical for managers to network with others, both locally and nationally, and most managers will freely share nonproprietary information such as a policy and procedure. The basic components of a policy and procedure protocol are presented in Box 71-1.

Managers also serve as mentors, coaches, and appraisers of overall work performance; resources to develop the skills and knowledge necessary for these functions should be sought out both from within the profession of OT and

BOX 71-1 BASIC COMPONENTS OF A POLICY AND PROCEDURE

Organizations often have policy manuals either in print or stored on-line. Manuals consist of many policies and related procedure statements, each of which typically includes the component listed below.

- Policy statement(s): brief statements of the guiding principles to be communicated
- Purpose statement(s): brief statements that outline the reasons for inclusion of the policies or procedures
- Applicability: lists the employee groups to which the policy and procedure applies (e.g., all OT department staff members)
- Procedures: statements outlining the specific actions to be taken by the identified employee groups and criteria for determining adherence to the policy
- Responsibility: identifying the individuals who are responsible for oversight of the policy and procedure (e.g., all OT team leaders)
- Review period: lists the date of the last review and update of the policy and procedures (typically, policies and procedures are reviewed on an annual basis)

CENTENNIAL NOTES

Management in Occupational Therapy

From the earliest days, management and administration were integral to OT practice. The first educational standards included expectations that students would receive lectures in "hospital ethics and management" (AOTA, 1924, p. 297). Perhaps one of the first in a yearly series of OT management meetings was convened in 1924 (Figure 71-4) by Eleanor Clarke Slagle ("Occupational Therapy Institute Is Arranged," 1924). The first edition of *Willard & Spackman's Occupational Therapy* published in 1947 included a chapter by Mary Merritt entitled, "Factors in the Organization of Occupational Therapy." Chapter topics included period of hospitalization and rate of turnover, space requirements, supplies, personnel requirements, remuneration, working schedules, personal attitudes, records, reports, and bookkeeping. One area of debate at the time was the sale of patient-generated products and the use of those funds for department activities as well as the disposal of finished products.

More than 60 years after Slagle's "institutes," Celestine Hamant convened the first organizational meeting of what would become the AOTA Administration & Management Special Interest Section (AMSIS). The AMSIS was officially formed in May of 1984. Marylou Hymen and Barbara Schell cochaired the formation committee while Ruth Ann Watkins was elected as the first chairperson (Watkins, 1985). The first AMSIS Quarterly was published in 1985. A scan of the first AMSIS Quarterly indicates that although much has changed since 1985, managers at that time were concerned with many of the issues that consume managerial attention today including personnel management, productivity, time management, marketing, efficacy, and competition for the health care dollar (Watkins, 1985). The AOTA publications in the 1970s, 1980s, and 1990s reveal topics including continuous quality improvement, policy issues such as the role of managers in implementing the Americans with Disabilities Act, leadership and job satisfaction, management of change, management and marketing, ethical dilemmas, and getting started in private practice (Baum, 1986; Bell, 1993; Bowman, 1991; Chilton, 1989; Hightower-Vandamm, 1980). As we move forward into the second 100 years of OT, it seems likely that many of the same topics will continue to consume much of the OT manager's attention.

The dairy company will remain on the property, as tenants, for several months during which they will erect the new plant.

OCCUPATIONAL THERAPY INSTITUTE IS ARRANGED

A four-day institute of the chief occupational therapists in New York state hospitals has been arranged by Mrs. Eleanor C. Slagle, who is the director of occupational therapy in the New York state system.

The opening session will be held in the office of the State Hospital Commission in New York city on April 21, at 10 a. m. and a program for the following three days, including April 24, will take up all matters in reference to the work which is planned for the rehabilitation of mental patients throughout the state.

Commissioner Harriet May Mills will welcome the delegates from the hospitals in the opening address and throughout the session papers dealing with all phases of the work will be presented by Dr. C. Floyd Haviland, and other state officials.

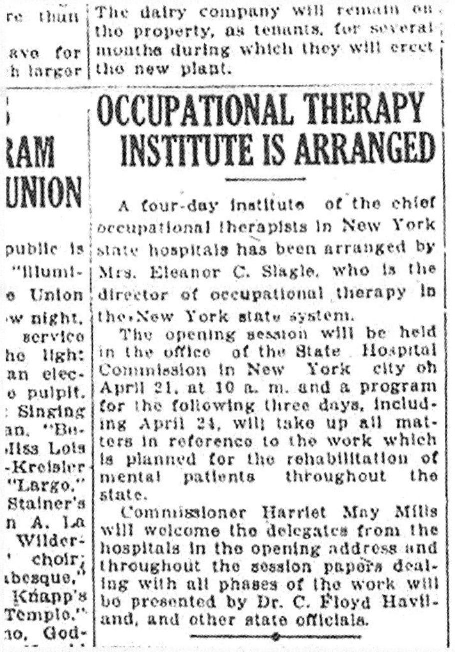

FIGURE 71-4 News article about the first Occupational Therapy Institute arranged by Eleanor Clarke Slagle in *The Binghamton Press*, April 19, 1924.

from outside of it. The AOTA has a number of resources related to supervisory tasks specific to OT assistants or to OT aides (http://www.aota.org). For more generic information on models of supervision, theories of motivating others, developing effective performance appraisal systems, or providing effective mentoring or coaching, managers should look outside the OT literature. For example, associations such as the American Management Association (http://www.amanet.org) or the National Association for Employee Recognition (http://www.recognition.org/) provide resources about how one may become an effective supervisor.

Controlling

Controlling is a management function that relates to the processes of establishing specific work performance standards and the measurement, evaluation, and correction of performance. A key responsibility of managers is to promote the delivery of appropriate intervention through the use of quality control (QC) mechanisms and performance improvement (PI), which is sometimes also called continuous quality improvement (CQI). The QC and PI are related functions, but each serves a different purpose and relies on

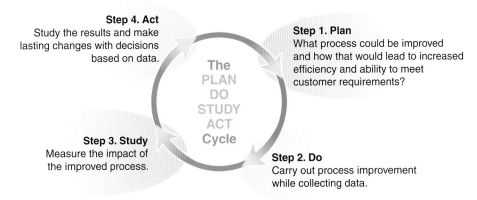

Step 4. Act
Study the results and make lasting changes with decisions based on data.

The PLAN DO STUDY ACT Cycle

Step 1. Plan
What process could be improved and how that would lead to increased efficiency and ability to meet customer requirements?

Step 3. Study
Measure the impact of the improved process.

Step 2. Do
Carry out process improvement while collecting data.

FIGURE 71-5 The Plan, Do, Study, Act (PDSA) Cycle.

different philosophies, strategies, tools, and techniques. The focus of QC is to intervene when the quality or quantity of work output falls below predetermined measures (indicators). The focus of PI is to improve customer satisfaction by constantly striving to meet customer expectations through enhancing critical processes. A critical process is defined as any process that is performed to produce the work of an organization. Examples of OT critical processes include responding to referrals for service, administering assessments, fabricating adaptive equipment, and making postdischarge referrals. PI projects may be complex and time intensive because they rely on decision making based on data and therefore require an organized and structured approach to gathering and analyzing data. Explaining PI in depth is beyond the scope of this chapter, but Figure 71-5 provides a brief overview of commonly identified steps to choose a critical process and implementing steps that improve its performance. The Plan, Do, Study, Act (PDSA) Cycle may be invoked under other names or acronyms, but the steps of the PI process remain constant (Figure 71-6).

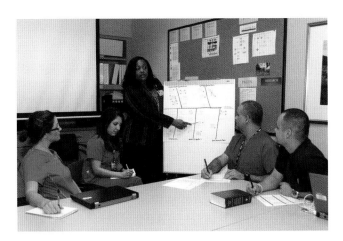

FIGURE 71-6 Staff members complete a cause-and-effect diagram to identify potential root causes of a problem as part of a formal performance improvement project.

The most common tools and techniques and their uses are presented in Table 71-6.

Financial Management

An important function of most managers is the planning and controlling of a department budget. Budgets are typically planned for a calendar year or a fiscal year (e.g., many organizations operate on a fiscal year that runs from July 1 to June 30). The process of planning and managing a budget requires that a manager have a comprehensive understanding of the goals and objectives of the larger organization so that he or she can establish priorities for funding that support this mission over time.

Occupational therapy practitioners who want to become managers or directors of an OT department or to own and operate their own businesses are encouraged to learn financial planning and management and to become well versed in the use of information management technologies, such as spreadsheets or other financial management tools. Braveman (2016b) notes that effective financial planning and management requires a working knowledge of the following:

- Health care systems, including city, county, state, and national systems
- Payment and reimbursement structures, such as Medicare, Medicaid, Workers' Compensation, private insurance, and grants or foundation support
- Human resources systems and costs, including salary and benefit administration, training and educational costs and systems, and recruitment and retention structures
- Equipment and materials purchasing and management, including medical supplies such as splinting or assistive and adaptive equipment, office supplies, and other supportive supplies
- Facilities management, maintenance, and improvement protocols, including cleaning and maintenance of physical plant structures

| TABLE 71-6 | Common Process Improvement Concepts, Tools, and Techniques |

Core Concepts	Use/Importance/Summary
• The Plan, Do, Study, Act (PDSA) Cycle	• The overarching framework for guiding and ordering process improvement activities
• Critical processes	• The important processes that are repeated again and again to complete the organization's or department's work
• Operational definitions	• A quantifiable description of what to measure and the steps to follow to measure it consistently
• Customers and customer requirements	• Identifying internal and external customers or individuals who receive the output of your work and their valid requirements
• Quality indicators	• Quantitative measures of compliance to valid customer requirements
• Variation	• The spread of process output over time; discriminating between natural "common cause" variation that is inherent in a process and the uncommon "special cause" variation that you want to eliminate from a process or emulate if positive
Strategies	
• Ground rules for meetings	• Explicit agreements about how a team will work together and behave as team members
• Roles for effective meetings	• Assigning roles such as the leader, scribe, facilitator, and timekeeper can lead to more effective meetings
• Consensus	• A method for reaching agreement whereby all members agree to fully support a decision even if it is not how they would act if they were acting alone
Tools	
• Process flowcharts	• A visual representation of the steps in a process used to highlight redundancies, rework, or bottlenecks
• Control charts	• A chart with statistically determined upper and lower control limits used to determine whether a process has changed and to highlight variation
• Cause-and-effect diagrams	• A tool to assist in determining possible root causes to a problem
• Proposed options matrix	• A tool for comparing possible options for action against a set of predetermined criteria
Techniques	
• Data stratification	• Methods for categorizing collection of data; it is important to decide how to stratify data before you collect it.
• Designing an effective data collection tool	• Tools to gather facts on how a process works or its effectiveness that allows for accurate collection of data in the simplest manner
• Balancing tasks and people	• Attending to both the needs of team members and the work to be completed to maintain team motivation
• Icebreakers	• Short activities to help team members learn about each other or to become more comfortable interacting with each other
• Brainstorming	• A method for creatively generating lists of possible causes of problems, solutions, or processes to improve
• Multivoting	• A decision-making method to narrow a larger number of options to a number that can be reasonably discussed individually

Budgets may also include revenue and expenses, although it is not uncommon for a community-based organization manager to have oversight of only expenses with no control over direct sources of revenue. Typically, the revenues and expenses associated with each department in an organization are given some sort of marker or code in the organization's accounting system that indicates how the subset of revenues and expenses relate to that department. These subsets of revenues and expenses are commonly referred to as *cost centers*. They may represent the budget of a single department or of several related services. Common examples of revenues and expenses are shown in Table 71-7 and are further explained in the following section.

Forecasting revenue requires that the manager be able to accurately predict the volume of work that a department

will deliver and how that work will happen. In some settings, almost all OT intervention is provided to consumers on a one-to-one basis, whereas in some settings, intervention is provided in groups, and elsewhere, there can be a combination.

Regulations regarding group treatment or treating more than one patient at a time has changed over time, and managers must remain current in their understanding of regulations regarding billing and coding of services. By accurately predicting the total volume of work for a year, managers are able to predict the total gross revenue by multiplying the number of work units (e.g., a 15-minute unit of therapy) by the charge for each unit of service. It is important to note that in the current managed care environment, few payers reimburse at the full

Pressures to Increase Revenue and Service

Shammi is a new manager in a community hospital in a small town. The hospital provides acute care services and has a small rehabilitation unit that focuses on orthopedic patients and some patients who have had strokes. Staffing including recruitment and retention is an ongoing challenge because there are no academic programs near her community. Few therapists are willing to make the commute from the nearest large city even though her facility pays an excellent salary and a sign-on bonus.

Because of the problems she has in recruiting staff, it is difficult to provide patients on the rehabilitation unit the 3 hours of skilled therapy that is required by payers. Shammi realizes that if patients do not receive the required therapy, the hospital may receive denials for payment, but if she shifts staff to the rehabilitation unit, other patients on acute care units will not receive adequate attention. The prior manager directed staff to run a therapy group and to send all patients on the unit to the group even if they were not always appropriate for the focus of the group. Shammi discontinued this practice and directed staff members to only include patients in the group if the focus of the group was directly related to their plan of care. This has increased the pressure on her staff, and now, this practice is being questioned by the case manager on the rehabilitation unit and her boss. For a moment, Shammi considered reversing her decision but instead decided that charging patients for therapy that was not appropriate violated the AOTA Code of Ethics and the ethical practices laid out in her state practice act. Despite pressure, Shammi expressed her concern about ethical practice to her boss and set up a meeting with her human resources representative to brainstorm new recruitment strategies.

TABLE 71-7	Examples of Revenues and Expenses

Revenues	Expenses
Individual 15 minutes: ADL treatment	Variable expense—salary
Individual 15 minutes: cognitive remediation	Variable expense—wages
Individual 15 minutes: community reintegration	Variable expense—office supplies
Individual 15 minutes: neuromuscular facilitation	Variable expense—splinting supplies
Group 15 minutes: home management	Fixed expense—phone
Group 15 minutes: communication skills	Fixed expense—rent
Group 15 minutes: community reintegration	Fixed expense—utilities

ADL, activities of daily living.

rate that is billed, and the net revenue, or the amount of revenue after all discounts to insurers and nonreimbursed charges are accounted for, is typically much less than gross revenue.

Expenses typically include costs associated with personnel, supplies, facilities management, and equipment. As part of the process of forecasting the expense budget, managers determine the number of full-time equivalent (FTE) employees that will be required to handle the projected work volume. Generally, an FTE represents an employee who will be paid 2,080 hours in a year (i.e., 40 hours × 52 weeks). Setting productivity standards (e.g., the amount of work a practitioner is expected to perform in a given period such as a day or week) and helping staff to meet such standards is a common challenge faced by OT managers. Personnel expenses can include salary expenses for professional staff who are exempt from the labor laws that require an organization to pay extra for overtime effort and wages for support staff who are nonexempt. Occupational therapists are often categorized as exempt, and OT assistants and OT aides are often categorized as nonexempt.

Nonpersonnel expenses such as supplies, equipment, food, phone, continuing education, or travel allowances must also be projected. In private businesses, expenses for utilities and rent must also be considered. These expenses are categorized as either fixed or variable expenses. Fixed expenses are costs that are not directly influenced by changes in client volume, such as expenses budgeted for employee continuing education, heating costs, or monthly rent if space is leased. Variable expenses are those that are directly influenced by changes in client volume. For example, you may use more of some types of office supplies, food used for meal preparation activities, or splinting or medical supplies if patient volumes rise and less if they are lower. Although there might not always be a direct correlation, over time, one will be able to estimate how an increase or decrease in volume might affect expenses.

To effectively plan and control a budget, managers must learn many useful concepts and strategies. Some organizations may provide training or orientation for new managers, but, most often, it is assumed that a new manager understands the basic information needed to develop and oversee a budget. People who are assuming their first management position would benefit from additional education or training in financial management and from networking with experienced managers. The AOTA provides networking opportunities such as the professional networking site *OT Connection* and resources for managers through its Administration & Management Special Interest Section (AMSIS). More information on AMSIS, *OT Connection*, and other resources can be found at http://www.aota.org. Occupational therapy associations in other countries should be consulted for resources relevant to OT management in systems outside the United States.

Technology and Management

The technological advances in medicine, information management, communication, and related areas that have occurred over the last few decades are astounding. Managers must evaluate and integrate a wide range of technology into their departments, ranging from computer software programs to clinical equipment, such as driving simulators or environmental controls. Choosing and successfully integrating a new technology requires that managers synthesize information, including costs of initial purchase, maintenance, space, and training requirements and the rate at which the specific technology is advancing so that an estimate can be made of when the current technology may become outdated.

One major area of technology used by managers is that employed in information management, which includes the use of computers for documentation, billing, and financial management as well as data collection and analysis for outcomes management. Table 71-8 lists common types of data and information that must be collected and managed and their possible uses. Becoming skilled at the use of common software programs such as managing a spreadsheet to organize and analyze the large amount of data available to most managers has become a common expectation of most managers.

Marketing

Occupational therapy managers are often responsible for assessing the needs of the target populations served by their department or organization; determining programmatic strategies for meeting these needs; designing, implementing, and evaluating the interventions to meet identified needs; and promoting the intervention to consumers, payers, physicians, and others. These processes, collectively, are called *marketing*. Traditionally, the following four steps are identified in the marketing process:

- *Organizational assessment*: examination of the factors within an organization that will influence the development and promotion of a new product or service
- *Environmental assessment*: examination of the data and other forms of evidence, including the needs of the target population that will guide the development and promotion of a new product or service
- *Market analysis*: use of the information gained during organizational and environmental assessments to validate perceptions of the wants and needs of the target populations that will receive a new product or service
- *Marketing communications*: packaging and promoting a product so the target populations and other key stakeholders in the new product or service have a clear understanding of what the product or service is and how it may be accessed

In larger organizations, other professionals, such as members of a marketing department, often perform portions of the marketing process such as collecting

| TABLE 71-8 | Common Types of Data, Sources, and Possible Uses |

Types of Data	Sources	Uses
Demographics (age, sex, educational level, etc.)	• Admissions records • Public data sets	• Program planning • Program evaluation
Revenue (payer source, rates, discounts)	• Accounting • Budget reports	• Budgeting • Program planning
Expense (accounts payable)	• Financial reports • Purchasing records	• Budgeting • Program planning and evaluation
Payroll (salary, benefits, leave usage)	• Accounting • Budget reports	• Staffing plans • Recruitment and retention
Productivity (visits, staff activity)	• Automated charge systems • Department billing records or productivity tracking sheets	• Staffing plans • Performance appraisal • Recruitment
Personnel (licensure, competencies, professional development, performance)	• Human resources • Departmental personnel files • Professional association data sets	• Accreditation visits • Staffing plan development • Professional development plans
Clinical (diagnosis, intervention, outcomes)	• Medical records • Outcome databases	• Process improvement • Program evaluation
Legal (contracts, leases)	• Legal or grants and contracts department	• Facility planning

BOX 71-2 SAMPLE AREAS FOR ASSESSMENT OF COMPETENCY FOR MANAGERS

- Planning
  - Use of goal setting
  - Financial management skills
  - Understanding the changing health care environment
- Organizing and staffing
  - Understanding team structure and flexible work design
  - Designing and leading effective teams
  - Applying coordination techniques
- Directing
- Interpersonal competencies
  - Communication skills
  - Communicating with the boss

- Communicating with peers and others
- Communicating with employees
- Being politically astute
- Managing conflict
- Managing diversity
- Role model competencies
  - Demonstrating professionalism in conduct and demeanor
  - Enhancing technical competence
- Controlling
  - Empowering employees
  - Applying continuous quality improvement efforts

demographic and other data about potential consumers or may be called on to collaborate with a manager to perform these functions. However, OT managers who are also business owners or who work in community-based, nonprofit organizations might need to learn the marketing process in greater depth. These managers benefit from establishing effective networks with other managers and becoming active in professional organizations, such as their state and national OT associations and business-oriented groups such as the local chamber of commerce.

Who Should Be a Manager?

Over the last two decades, numerous professions have addressed managerial competencies with increasing urgency and concern, emphasizing the need to determine the initial competence of health professionals, to assess specific job competencies as professionals are hired and begin to work, and to promote the professionals' continuing development of competence (Braveman, 2016a). The assessment of initial competency and facilitation of continuing development of staff competency is a function of the OT manager.

Before assuming a role as an OT manager, one should assess one's own level of preparedness to perform the tasks associated with the role. Although the assessment of competencies for managers has not received the same attention by certifying or regulatory bodies such as accrediting agencies, competency development and assessment have been addressed, and some empirical investigations of managerial competencies have been conducted by a number of professions (Braveman, 2016a).

Some competencies might be considered "universal" for managers. One method of identifying managerial competence is to compare their performance against the "yardstick" of previously described traditional managerial functions (e.g., planning, organizing and staffing, directing, controlling). As a guide for this process, each of the management functions is listed subsequently with sample areas for assessment of competency provided for each. (See Box 71-2 for additional areas for development of competencies.)

Other managerial competencies will depend on the nature of the manager's job. Not all managers perform the same tasks and functions, so it is important that before accepting a management position, one understands what will be expected of one and have done a thorough assessment of readiness by identifying strengths and areas in which help might be needed.

Conclusion

This chapter has provided an overview of the numerous tasks, functions, and responsibilities that an OT manager may perform. Readers are encouraged to appreciate the variety and complexities of a manager's responsibilities and the need for a beginning manager to get appropriate training and education. Managers work closely with the administrators and supervisors in large organizations, but small business owners and entrepreneurs also function independently as managers. Fortunately, many resources are available that are specific to OT managers, and more resources may be found in other fields, including business, psychology, and organizational development, that are useful guides for a manager performing his or her job.

> ## COMMENTARY ON THE EVIDENCE
>
> ### The State of Evidence Related to Management

Decades of evidence on management theory, effective managerial strategies, and practices have been produced by multiple disciplines and fields such as business, organizational development, organizational psychology, social work, and nursing. The topics that have been investigated are quite diverse; examples include effective leadership strategies, performance appraisal processes, factors affecting recruitment and retention, effective recognition and reward structures, change management, and performance improvement.

A variety of forms of evidence, including the results of empirical studies, program descriptions, and descriptions of managerial interventions, are published widely in a range of professional journals, Websites, and books. Although the body of evidence specifically related to management in health care organizations might be more limited, it is growing, and OT managers who wish to use an *evidence-based* approach to management will benefit from research and science conducted by other disciplines such as those mentioned.

Particularly in the last decade, there has been a movement toward discussions of *evidence-based management* as the role of evidence in guiding decision making has become more prevalent in health care and other industries. However, caution has been advised to address the worry that application of evidence can become too rote and prescriptive. For example, Arndt and Bigelow (2009) cautioned,

Managers should use all available information and data when planning and implementing decisions, and evidence from research should play a role in that. At the same time, in a turbulent and uncertain environment, creativity and risk taking also will be important, and unanticipated outcomes may result from, among other factors, limits on human cognition, unknowable differences in initial conditions in organizations, and adaptive responses to change as it is implemented. (p. 206)

Current trends in management research include efficient and effective use of technology including the electronic health record, change management, and managing access to care (Hoff, Sutcliffe, & Young, 2016). There continues to be a growing body of experimental management research such as a randomized controlled trial to examine whether an intervention designed to increase self-efficacy for transformational leadership results in more transformational leadership self-efficacy and a higher level of transformational leadership (Richter et al., 2016).

Although OT managers can certainly make valuable judgments by generalizing from evidence produced in other disciplines, the profession would benefit from research specifically related to OT. Questions for investigation might include the following:

- How will health care reform and other societal influences affect the profession?
- How might OT managers influence the delivery of culturally relevant services as we become more globally connected?
- What are the most effective strategies for retaining OT practitioners within the profession across the life course to prevent attrition from the discipline?

REFERENCES

Adams, N., Little, T. D., & Ryan, R. M. (2017). Self-determination theory. In M. L. Wehmeyer, K. Shogren, T. D. Little, & S. J. Lopez (Eds.), *Development of self-determination through the life-course* (pp. 47–54). Dordrecht, The Netherlands: Springer.

American Occupational Therapy Association. (1924). Minimum standards for courses of training in occupational therapy. *Archives of Occupational Therapy, 3*(4), 295–298.

Arndt, M., & Bigelow, B. (2009). Evidence-based management in health care organizations: A cautionary note. *Health Care Management Review, 34*, 206–213.

Ashby, S. E., Ryan, S., Gray, M., & James, C. (2013). Factors that influence the professional resilience of occupational therapists in mental health practice. *Australian Occupational Therapy Journal, 60*, 110–119.

Baum, C. M. (1986). The manager's challenge in a changing marketplace. *Administration & Management Special Interest Section Newsletter, 2*(2), 3.

Baumann, M. R., & Bonner, B. L. (2017). An expectancy theory approach to group coordination: Expertise, task features, and member behavior. *Journal of Behavioral Decision Making, 30*, 407–419.

Bell, E. (1993). Continuous quality improvement can be fun. *Administration & Management Special Interest Section Newsletter, 9*(1), 5–6.

Bowman, O. J. (1991). Managers to play an important role in implementing the Americans with Disabilities Act. *Administration & Management Special Interest Section Newsletter, 7*(3), 1–2.

Braveman, B. (Ed.). (2016a). Assessing and promoting clinical and managerial competency. In *Leading and managing occupational therapy services: An evidence-based approach* (pp. 297–326). Philadelphia, PA: F. A. Davis.

Braveman, B. (Ed.). (2016b). Roles and functions of managers: Planning, organizing, controlling and directing. In *Leading and managing occupational therapy services: An evidence-based approach* (pp. 159–184). Philadelphia, PA: F. A. Davis.

Braveman, B. (Ed.). (2016c). Understanding and working within organizations. In *Leading and managing occupational therapy services: An evidence-based approach* (pp. 93–125). Philadelphia, PA: F. A. Davis.

Bryson, J. M., Edwards, L. H., & Van Slyke, D. M. (2017). Getting strategic about strategic planning research. *Public Management Review, 20*(3), 317–339. Retrieved from http://www.tandfonline.com/doi/abs/10.1080/14719037.2017.1285111

Cervone, D., & Pervin, L. A. (2008). *Personality theory and research* (10th ed.). Hoboken, NJ: Wiley.

Champoux, J. E. (2017). *Organizational behavior: Integrating individuals, groups, and organizations* (5th ed.). Abingdon, United Kingdom: Routledge.

Chilton, H. (1989). Today's occupational therapy managers as managers of change. *Administration & Management Special Interest Section Newsletter, 5*(3), 3–4.

Franche, R., Corbière, M., Lee, H., Breslin, F. C., & Hepburn, C. G. (2007). The Readiness for Return-to-Work (RRTW) scale: Development and validation of a self-report staging scale in lose-time claimants with musculoskeletal disorders. *Journal of Occupational Rehabilitation, 17,* 450–472.

Hightower-Vandamm, M. D. (1980). Nationally speaking: Presidential address: Management, marketing, and the real hard facts. *American Journal of Occupational Therapy, 34,* 833–843.

Hoff, T., Sutcliffe, K. M., & Young, G. J. (2016). *The healthcare professional workforce: New directions in theory and practice.* Oxford, United Kingdom: Oxford University Press.

Inalhan, G. (2009). Attachments: The unrecognised link between employees and their workplace (in change management projects). *Journal of Corporate Real Estate, 11*(1), 17–37.

Jaques, E. (1998). *Requisite organization.* Arlington, VA: Cason Hall.

Kuipers, B. S., Higgs, M., Kickert, W., Tummers, L., Grandia, J., & Van der Voet, J. (2014). The management of change in public organizations: A literature review. *Public Administration, 92,* 1–20.

Lewin, K. (1997). *Resolving social conflict and field theory in social sciences.* Washington, DC: American Psychological Association.

Liebler, J. G., & McConnell, C. R. (2017). *Management principles for health professionals* (7th ed.). Boston, MA: Jones & Bartlett.

MD Anderson Cancer Center. (2017). *About MD Anderson.* Retrieved from https://www.mdanderson.org/about-md-anderson.html

Occupational Therapy Institute Is Arranged. (1924, April 19). *The Binghamton Press,* p. 3. Retrieved from http://www.fultonhistory.com/Fulton.html

Prochaska, J. O. (2013). Transtheoretical model of behavior change. In *Encyclopedia of behavioral medicine* (pp. 1997–2000). New York, NY: Springer.

Richter, A., von Thiele Schwarz, U., Lornudd, C., Lundmark, R., Mosson, R., & Hasson, H. (2016). iLead—A transformational leadership intervention to train healthcare managers' implementation leadership. *Implementation Science, 11,* 108.

Scanlan, J. N., Meredith, P., & Poulsen, A. A. (2013). Enhancing retention of occupational therapists working in mental health: Relationships between wellbeing at work and turnover intention. *Australian Occupational Therapy Journal, 60,* 395–403.

University of Twente. (2017). *Social cognitive theory.* Retrieved from https://www.utwente.nl/en/bms/communication-theories/sorted-by-cluster/Health%20Communication/Social_cognitive_theory/

Watkins, R. A. (1985). *Report from the chairperson. Administration & Management Special Interest Section Newsletter.* Rockville, MD: American Occupational Therapy Association.

thePoint® *For additional resources on the subjects discussed in this chapter, visit* http://thePoint.lww.com/Willard-Spackman13e.

CHAPTER 72

Supervision

Mary Jane Youngstrom, Patricia A. Gentile

LEARNING OBJECTIVES

After reading this chapter, you will be able to:

1. Explain the roles and functions of supervision.
2. Differentiate types of supervision.
3. Examine supervisory processes and implementation.
4. Compare and contrast approaches to managing performance.
5. Apply American Occupational Therapy Association (AOTA) guidelines for appropriate supervision of occupational therapy personnel in the United States.

Introduction

Supervision is a distinct professional activity that is an integral part of occupational therapy (OT) service provision. The supervisory process is consciously used in our profession to ensure that our clients receive safe, effective, and evidence-based OT services. Although the ability to supervise skillfully is developed throughout one's practice career, the entry-level practitioner must be knowledgeable about the supervisory process and have a beginning understanding of how to give and receive supervision in a manner that is consistent with the profession's values and expectations. This chapter provides you with an overview of what supervision is and introduces you to basic information you will need to develop positive and effective supervisory relationships. Supervisory expectations in general are explained, along with supervisory standards specific to practice in the United States.

Supervision Embedded in Practice

The supervision process is an everyday feature of each practitioner's work experience. It is a process that supports effective job performance as well as personal growth. Read the case study about Marta, an OT practitioner, and Kim, an OT assistant, which describes their career experiences with supervision (Case Study 72-1).

CASE STUDY 72-1 MARTA AND KIM: SUPERVISION EMBEDDED IN PRACTICE

Marta began her career as an occupational therapist in a pediatric hospital. She worked with two other therapists and was supervised by Sarah, the senior occupational therapist in the setting. Although she met regularly with Sarah, Marta also sought and received feedback and guidance from the other occupational therapist, who was particularly experienced in working with children with head injuries. Marta used input from both therapists to expand her knowledge and develop her professional reasoning skills. Six months after taking the job, Marta was given the responsibility of supervising volunteers who provided service in a playtime program for hospitalized children. She was responsible for orienting and training the volunteers. Periodically, she would observe their interactions with the children and was always available for questions. During her first year of practice, Marta was regularly involved in supervising both Level I OT practitioner and OT assistant students. She found these experiences to be rewarding. At the end of her second year of work, she was assigned her first Level II clinical fieldwork student, whom she supervised on a daily basis. As the department's caseload expanded, an OT assistant, Kim, was hired, and Marta supervised Kim as they collaboratively worked to provide OT services to referred patients. Marta oriented Kim to the hospital and the department's policies and procedures. Initially, Marta closely observed Kim's treatments and/or cotreated with her. Kim came to the hospital with 3 years of experience with children, but her prior work had been in a school setting, so she was not as familiar with OT interventions involving acute medical conditions. Several months after Kim joined the department, she was given the responsibility

for supervising the volunteers in the playtime program. She consulted with the recreational therapist, Terry, who worked on a different unit in the hospital, about strategies for expanding the play activities and improving volunteer participation.

In the case scenario, supervision was a regular feature of Marta's and Kim's daily work experience. Supervision provided feedback, direction, and support for Marta and Kim as they learned to carry out their responsibilities effectively and supported them in their personal professional development to gain additional competencies. Each practitioner had a designated formal supervisor, but both Marta and Kim received informal peer supervision from other therapists. The close-knit nature of the work group and everyone's interest in providing the best possible care allowed this type of supervision to occur naturally. Adding supervisory responsibilities to their jobs expanded both Marta's and Kim's job roles and offered opportunities for personal growth.

As the case study illustrates, practitioners are involved in giving as well as receiving supervision. In the United States, supervisory skills are an expected entry-level competency for occupational therapists who are responsible for supervising OT assistants (AOTA, 2014). Entry-level OT assistants may be responsible for supervising OT aides and later may move into supervisory roles with other OT assistants. All practitioners should know how to effectively provide supervision and benefit from it. Before exploring how to best provide supervision, let us first look at what supervision is and how it fits into the overall management structure of a work setting.

Formal Supervision

Definition and Focus

Dictionaries trace the roots of the term *supervise* to the Latin roots *super-*, "over," + *videre-*, "to see" (Stevenson, 2010). Supervision is a process that involves "overseeing" or "watching" the work of another. The employer gives a supervisor formal authority to watch the work of others and ensure that the work meets the organization's goals and objectives. To effectively oversee the work of others, supervisors need to be familiar with the work of the positions they supervise. Individuals assuming supervisor positions who do not have advanced knowledge or experience in the job positions they will supervise are expected to familiarize themselves with the job

tasks and responsibilities. This background allows them to provide the support and direction that supervisees need to solve work problems, to learn and grow in their jobs, and to better meet the organization's objectives (Figure 72-1).

It is important to consider where a supervisor fits in the management structure of an organization. Braveman (2016) offers insight into the relationship of the two by defining *supervision* as "the control and direction of the work of one or more employees in a manner that promotes improved performance and a higher quality outcome" (p. 187). Although supervisors may participate in all functions of management (planning, organizing, directing, and controlling), they typically spend the majority of their time focused on the directing and controlling functions by overseeing employee progress and productivity in their daily work (Braveman, 2016, p. 187). (See Chapter 71 for a

CENTENNIAL NOTES

Supervision in Occupational Therapy

Supervision has always been an important part of OT practice. Looking back over the last 100 years, one can see the evolution of supervision in response to changes within the profession and the health care system at large.

One of the first references to supervision in OT can be traced back to 1918 when the U.S. Army included the need for a "head aide" to oversee the early reconstruction aides. At that time, occupational therapists worked under a medical model, which was to persist for many years. This model placed physicians as supervisors. Physician influence can be seen in the 1931 article "Necessity of Medical Supervision in Occupational Therapy" (Coulter & McNary, 1931). This medical model was reinforced by the fact that early on occupational therapists primarily worked in large hospital settings. As a result, structure and focus of supervision in these settings mirrored the framework within these institutions.

With the expansion of OT outside of the hospital and the creation of the OT assistant, the profession moved out from under the umbrella of the medical profession and needed to reexamine its supervisory model. American Occupational Therapy Association (AOTA) responded in the 1970s by authoring several papers and practice standards on the roles and functions of supervision, eventually publishing the first "Guide for Supervision of Occupational Therapy Personnel" in 1981. These guidelines identified the occupational therapist as ultimately responsible for services but emphasized the collaborative nature of the supervisory relationship. They also elaborated on a framework based on the type of practitioner and years of experience. Over time, guideline revisions reflected changes in both education and practice. Currently known as the "AOTA Guidelines for Supervision, Roles, and Responsibilities during the Delivery of Occupational Therapy Services" (AOTA, 2014), they now offer a less prescriptive, competency-based model that is useful across practice settings. Core principles that remain constant are the ultimate responsibility of the professional level occupational therapist for all aspects of the therapy process along with the recognition and importance of mutual collaboration among all levels of OT personnel in the process. As we move ahead, the profession needs to continue to examine effective supervisory models to address the challenges facing new practice opportunities and settings.

discussion of management functions.) When we consider the supervisor's placement within the management hierarchy, this becomes easier to understand (Figure 72-2). Supervisors are placed closest to the staff level of the organization and typically do not supervise others who are in management positions. Supervisors are generally considered to be the first line of management. Although they have some management responsibilities, they are not considered to be managers.

The emphasis primarily on the directing and controlling functions of management rather than the planning and organizing functions does not diminish the importance of the supervisor's role. Formal supervisors because of their placement within the organization, serve as a bridge between the staff and higher levels of management. In this position, the supervisor must support, interpret, and implement management decisions as well as relay staff concerns to higher management, which can influence planning and organizing functions. How well the supervisor can convey management concerns to staff and staff concerns to management can make or break the organization's effectiveness and ability to adapt to change.

Up to this point, we have been emphasizing the supervisor's responsibility to the organization—to oversee work to ensure the organization's success. Supervision takes on an added dimension and responsibility when people who are members of a profession (e.g., OT, nursing, psychology) take on responsibilities to supervise other members of their profession in a work setting. Providing professional supervision that is consistent with the profession's values and standards and supports the professional

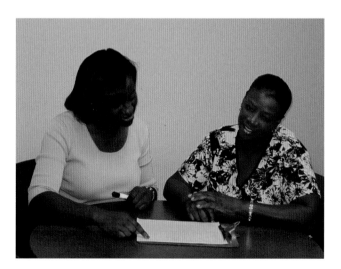

FIGURE 72-1 Discussing weekend coverage plans and how they will be implemented is a common supervisory task in hospital-based OT.

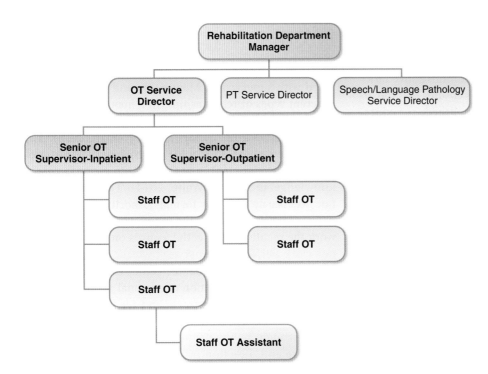

FIGURE 72-2 In this organization, the senior occupational therapists are supervisors, and the OT service director is a manager. *PT*, physical therapist.

growth and development of the professionals who are being supervised is integrated with the supervisor's responsibility to meet the organization's needs. For example, the supervisor must not assign tasks and responsibilities that are outside of the supervisee's professional scope of practice. The supervisor must be cognizant of the profession's standards and guidelines regarding frequency of supervision and requirements for training and competency. Overall, the supervisor must manage and supervise work in a manner that respects the profession's scope and that supports the supervisee's development of continuing competence.

The supervisor who is providing professional supervision must continually ask two related but different questions, which will guide the supervisor's observations, analysis, decisions, and actions:

1. Is the supervisee successfully accomplishing the work?
2. Is the supervisee demonstrating continued professional growth and development?

Supporting the supervisees' efforts to maintain and develop continuing competence does not conflict with supporting the supervisee to successfully accomplish the work. As individuals develop new skills and abilities, clients receive better care and organizations benefit from workers' improved expertise. The supervisor should be concurrently providing feedback on performance and assessing the supervisee's learning and professional development needs.

Functions of Supervision in a Professional Practice Setting

The supervisor's role in a professional practice setting encompasses three broad functions that are carried out under the broader management functions of directing and controlling. These functions are administrative, educational, and supportive functions (Kadushin, 1992). Table 72-1 lists examples of supervisory tasks for each function.

TABLE 72-1 **Examples of Supervisory Tasks within Different Supervisory Functions**

Administrative Function	Educational Function	Supportive Function
• Plan and assign workload • Make schedules • Set priorities for department's work activities • Check performance against work standards • Interpret policies and procedures • Delegate work • Provide written and verbal reports to managers	• Orient new staff • Identify training needs • Develop and provide training programs • Identify and provide educational resources • Assess performance and provide feedback • Discipline	• Hold group meetings to allow for expression of concerns • Meet individually with supervisee on a quarterly basis to check on progress toward work goals • Provide informal and formal support for performance

Administrative functions are directed toward managing the day-to-day work performance and process. Checking that all clients were seen and assigning clients to specific supervisees are examples of administrative tasks. Carrying out administrative functions ensures that the organization's day-to-day work is accomplished. The educational function is focused on the worker and is concerned with teaching and training, providing feedback about performance, and disciplining, if necessary. Educational functions assist the supervisee to be effective in meeting job demands and also can help to promote the supervisee's own professional growth and development. The supportive function is directed toward relationships—both individual and group relationships within the workplace. This function focuses on developing harmonious relationships that will maintain a positive work environment in which people can be productive and successful.

Informal Supervision: Peer Supervision

Supervision is typically understood as a formalized process that occurs in a work setting in which a person's work is supervised by a formally designated supervisor. In a health care professional practice environment where all staff members are committed to providing the best quality of service, informal peer supervision may also occur. Peer supervision is oversight that is provided by another professional who has no formal authority to provide supervision. The peer supervisor provides feedback and shares knowledge with the intent of influencing the peer professional's practices to improve client outcomes.

Peer supervision is a natural extension of each professional's responsibility to ensure that clients receive the highest quality of care. It may or may not be solicited by the "supervisee" practitioner. In Case Study 72-1, Marta did seek input from her peers as a way of continuing to learn and grow as a professional, but not all practitioners seek input from others. When a peer therapist provides peer supervision and feedback that is not requested, the intent is to improve client outcomes by offering information that could help other practitioners to improve their services.

In a professional and collegial work environment, peer supervision often occurs spontaneously and is seen as a benefit of working with others. Exchange and feedback among practitioners frequently occur as colleagues explore how to solve clinical problems and seek the best solutions for their clients. Such exchanges can be energizing for both parties. Engaging in peer supervision can be perceived as a method of mutual accountability and commitment to the profession's obligation to provide the best quality of services to clients.

Mentoring

Being mentored by another professional is often confused with supervision. Mentorship and supervision are different types of relationships. In a mentor relationship, the mentor's primary concern is the personal and professional growth of the mentee (Braveman, 2016). The goal of the mentor is to "guide, counsel and support professional development in regards to the mentee's career, knowledge and skill" (Waite, 2014). The mentor does not necessarily have any formal authority to oversee the mentee's work. Although the mentor is interested in the work the mentee is doing, the focus is on the mentee and not work performance per se. Instead, discussions between the mentor and mentee center on career options and decisions, identification of personal and professional growth needs and resources, and feedback about the mentee's behaviors and choices. A mentor relationship may be sought by the mentee who is feeling the need of guidance and direction in professional growth and development. Mentoring relationships have been found to improve staff satisfaction and increase productivity, and many organizations have implemented formal mentoring programs (Newstrom, 2013). Generally, the mentor is a more experienced professional and is seen as a trusted adviser.

Mentor–mentee relationships may also occur spontaneously between two professionals. In these instances, the mentee usually is attracted to the mentor's knowledge, skills, and accomplishments, and the mentor is attracted to the mentee's talent and potential as well as the opportunity to contribute to another professional's development.

True mentoring relationships are acknowledged by both parties and require formal commitment of time and effort. Mentor and mentee discuss and agree on learning needs and goals for the relationship as well as the structure for the mentoring process.

Mentee–mentor relationship may develop within a supervisory relationship. When this happens, both parties need to be clear about the different purposes and responsibilities of the two types of relationships. It is possible that what the mentor might counsel would not be what the supervisor would counsel. For example, a person who is functioning in the role of a mentor might recognize that a mentee would benefit from staying in one clinical setting for several months to allow for solidification of learning. However, this same person, functioning as a supervisor, recognizes that staffing limitations require that the supervisee must be rotated to a new clinical setting each month. Holding both roles simultaneously can lead to role conflicts, highlighting the need to be very clear about the different responsibilities of each role. Table 72-2 offers a comparison of supervision, mentorship, and peer supervision.

TABLE 72-2	Comparison of Supervision, Mentorship, and Peer Supervision		
	Supervision	**Mentorship**	**Peer Supervision**
Authority	Provided by the work organization	No formal authority	No formal authority; supported by professional responsibility
Nature of relationship and how it is established	Formal—established by the workplace	Personal, voluntary	Informal, spontaneous
Purpose	To support growth and development that will benefit the organization	To foster personal and professional growth and development that will benefit the mentee	To support growth and development that will ensure best outcomes for clients
How established	Assigned	Sought by the mentee and mutually agreed on	Offered by a peer or may be solicited by a practitioner
Accountability for performance	Organizational	Personal	Professional
Whose needs are met—outcomes expected	Needs of organization—work meets organizational objectives and needs	Needs of mentee—mentee achieves personal and professional growth	Needs of mentee and clients—clients receive best services

Mentoring should not be confused with role modeling. A role model is usually watched and admired by a practitioner, but the role model does not have a reciprocating active interest in the person's development and might not even be aware that he or she is serving as a role model (Urish, 2004).

The Supervisory Process

The overseeing of work is an *ongoing* process: It occurs repeatedly across time and is embedded in the everyday work experience. A supervisor, both formally and informally, observes and checks on the work of supervisees by talking to them about their work as well as observing them on a regular basis. A supervisor who observes the work of supervisees only occasionally and meets with them during an annual performance review is not providing appropriate supervision. Supervisors should be regularly present in the workplace and have regular contact with their supervisees.

Supervision is an *orderly* process. A good supervisor establishes a process in which the supervisee understands when regular contacts and meetings will occur. The supervisor is clear about performance expectations and consistent in providing feedback. The supervisory process, although orderly and expected, is also *dynamic*. It changes as people grow and work demands shift. Upon initial hiring, the supervisor might observe an employee daily and meet weekly. However, after several weeks, the employee might practice more independently without daily observation.

Finally, the supervision is an *interactive* process. It is based on an exchange or communication between the supervisor and the supervisee. The exchange that occurs between the OT supervisor and supervisee is central to the development and maintenance of professional competence. For example, the AOTA (2014) document "Guidelines for Supervision, Roles, and Responsibilities during the Delivery of Occupational Therapy Services" describes supervision as "a cooperative process in which two or more people participate in a joint effort to establish, maintain, and/or elevate a level of competence and performance" (p. S16).

Observe, in this description, that AOTA authors see supervision as a two-way street. Supervision is viewed as a cooperative process in which both parties have professional responsibility. This cooperative approach to supervision stems from the profession's ethical responsibility to demonstrate concern for the safety and well-being of their clients (e.g., see Principle 1: Beneficence; AOTA, 2015a) and the profession's responsibility to abide by standards directed to developing and maintaining competent practice (AOTA, 2015b, 2015c).

The AOTA (2014) "Guidelines for Supervision, Roles, and Responsibilities during the Delivery of Occupational Therapy Services" describes the supervisory process as having two purposes that relate to these responsibilities: (1) to ensure safe and effective delivery of OT services and (2) to foster professional competence and development (p. S16). These objectives reflect the organizational duties of the supervisor as well as professional practice obligations. All practitioners have a common interest in providing the best possible care to their clients, and all practitioners are obligated to demonstrate continuing competence. The supervisory process is the tool that occupational therapists and OT assistants use to reach these goals.

Developing a Supervisory Relationship

The supervisory relationship is central to the supervisory process. An effective supervisory relationship is built on trust and integrity. To develop trust and integrity, the supervisor must be approachable and open to the supervisee's questions and concerns; the supervisee, likewise, must be open and willing to share his or her observations, perceptions, and ideas. Both must value and respect the input of the other. The supervisor must be responsive and follow through with actions that indicate that the supervisee's concerns were considered; the supervisee will feel valued and confident in his or her personal abilities, and commitment to the organization will increase. The supervisor must be clear about expectations and provide regular objective feedback about performance; the supervisee will understand what is expected and feel more comfortable in the job. The supervisor must be consistent in his or her interactions; the supervisee will develop a level of trust in how he or she will be treated. When the supervisor is approachable and responsive, the supervisory relationship can thrive. Box 72-1 provides some additional examples of supervisory behaviors that build trust and integrity.

BOX 72-1 IMPORTANT BEHAVIORS IN SUPERVISION

Key Positive Supervisory Behaviors
- Praises others
- Accepts criticism and suggestion without judging
- Tells the truth
- Is supportive of supervisee—goes to bat for supervisees
- Gives credit for accomplishments
- Abides by the same rules as expects others to abide by
- Gives clear and frequent feedback
- Is dependable
- Is loyal to organization—makes decisions that are in best interest of organization
- Is respectful of differences

Key Positive Supervisee Behaviors
- Accepts feedback
- Seeks feedback
- Provides information
- Asks for clarification
- Attempts to integrate feedback to improve performance
- Shares ideas and concerns in a direct but not critical manner
- Sensitive to feelings and needs of supervisor

Supervisor's Role in Building the Relationship

Both supervisee and supervisor bring their own values, beliefs, and attitudes about supervision to the relationship. Each brings past experiences with other supervisors and authority figures, which may have been positive or negative. It is the supervisor's responsibility to set the tone for the relationship in a job setting and to take actions that will support an ongoing positive relationship. The following four steps will help to ensure that a positive supervisory relationship is initiated and developed:

1. Learn about the supervisee. Remember that you are responsible for guiding the learning of this new employee. To do this effectively, you need to understand what your new supervisee knows and how he or she learns best. You should be particularly interested in the person's knowledge and skills match with those that are needed for this job. Interviewing the new employee about past experiences and asking for current strengths and learning needs sends the message that you are interested in building on what the person knows and you value the person's experiences. You might wish to develop a skills checklist that the employee can fill out to supplement the interview process. Although the supervisor never stops learning about the supervisee's abilities, gathering this information formally during orientation to use as you begin to design training and learning experiences is very helpful. Identifying the employee's learning styles and preferences can facilitate the learning process on the new job and avoid wasted time and effort for both parties.

2. Be clear about job expectations. During the initial orientation and training, the supervisor needs to clearly outline the performance expectations for the job. The job requirements and expectations should have been broadly discussed during the job interview and hiring process. Now is a good time to revisit this discussion and provide more specifics. Reviewing the job description is an objective method for beginning this discussion. Expectations about productivity and quality of work should be made clear to the employee. Be honest and open about consequences for various behaviors—rewards as well as punishments. In addition, organizational cultural expectations such as attitudes and behaviors employees are expected to exhibit in interdisciplinary, peer, and client/family interactions should be addressed. These expectations are often not included in a job description but are central to acceptable performance. Discuss your expectations regarding the supervisee's responsibility to learn and grow.

3. Develop and implement a supervisory plan. As noted earlier, the supervisory process is a collaborative one.

During the orientation, discuss how you view the supervisory process and work together to develop a supervisory plan. Discuss topics such as frequency of supervisory contact (e.g., daily, three times per week, weekly), types of contact (e.g., informal, spontaneous, formal scheduled meeting), methods of contact (e.g., face-to-face, e-mail, phone, text, written), and preferred supervisory methods (e.g., observation, cotreatment, dialogue, documentation review). Be clear about the obligations and expectations you have of the supervisee; for example, explain that you expect the supervisee to initiate contact with you if more frequent feedback or supervision is needed.

4. Document supervision that is provided. Document when you meet with your supervisee and what was discussed. Maintain a supervisory log to keep a record of incidents, observations, and meetings. This log allows you to track and note changes in performance. The log record provides concrete examples that can be used to provide feedback and during performance review meetings. Regulatory laws in some states in the United States require that supervisory logs be kept to document the supervisory process that occurs between an occupational therapist and an OT assistant to maintain current licensure.

Supervisee's Role in Building the Relationship

Supervision occurs as an ongoing process of involving the exchange of information about the job and feedback about performance. The feedback process is a two-way street, with both the supervisor and supervisee playing important roles. Positive feedback and constructive criticism should be provided on a regular basis by the supervisor as described in the next section. However, the supervisee also has a responsibility to regularly seek feedback as a way to validate work performance and identify areas for further professional development. In order to be effective, this is a reciprocal process. The supervisor needs to be skilled in delivering feedback, and the supervisee needs to be skilled in seeking and responding to feedback.

How does a supervisee respond effectively to feedback? First and most importantly, the supervisee needs to view the supervisory relationship positively and be open to receiving feedback. Feedback provided by a supervisor provides honest information about how work is to be done and behaviors and performance are perceived. This information can be used to develop new skills, refine current skills, and monitor personal growth and development. Sometimes, hearing how others see you can be difficult to accept. Avoid responding defensively by explaining your behavior or by discounting the feedback as uninformed. Neither strategy will promote the supervisory relationship nor lead to professional growth. If aspects of the information received are unclear because the feedback may not have been behaviorally specific enough, the supervisee should ask for clarification and/or concrete examples of the performance in question. If the feedback is based on incomplete information, the supervisee should provide more information in a calm and matter-of-fact manner. Exchanges that occur during supervisory sessions can help to clarify performance for both the supervisee as well as the supervisor and contribute to the collaborative supervisory relationship. Some general guidelines for receiving feedback are outlined in Box 72-2.

After feedback has been received, the supervisee needs to reflect on how he or she may respond to it. Consideration should be given as to how this new information can be integrated into your daily work performance and how this new information can influence your professional development.

Perhaps, your supervisor pointed out how your ability to communicate succinctly in team meetings has improved. Based on this feedback, you decide you would like to offer to more frequently attend team meetings when others cannot. Perhaps, your supervisor has observed that your skill in wheelchair assessment and positioning are weaker than required by your role. Based on this feedback, you decide to look for a continuing education opportunity in this skill area. Feedback can sensitize you to behaviors, attitudes, and skills that validate your abilities and can also help to provide direction for new learning and growth.

BOX 72-2 GUIDELINES FOR RECEIVING FEEDBACK

- Listen openly. Assume feedback is being shared with positive intentions.
- Make sure you understand what is being said. Paraphrase what you have heard to check for accuracy.
- Ask for clarification or examples if feedback is unclear.
- Pause and think before you respond. If you want some time to consider feedback, ask for it.
- Acknowledge mistakes.
- Avoid interrupting or becoming defensive. Provide justification only if asked.
- Seek a solution to problems presented. Ask for examples of how you could perform better.
- Thank the person for providing you with the feedback.
- Make appropriate changes.
- Initiate a follow-up discussion to assure that needed changes have occurred as expected.

Performance Evaluation: A Supervisory Responsibility

All supervisory actions are directed toward managing the supervisee's work performance. The purpose of performance management is to encourage the supervisee to meet or exceed the established job performance standards and behave safely and appropriately at work (Newstrom, 2013, p. 265). Supervisors use a variety of methods in managing performance (e.g., incentives, job structure), but providing ongoing evaluation of performance by providing both formal and informal feedback is a central supervisory responsibility and skill.

Providing Feedback

Effective feedback is the supervisor's primary tool in influencing the employee's job performance. The supervisor is responsible for letting employees know if they are meeting job performance standards or not. When positive supervisory relationships have been established, feedback occurs naturally and informally throughout the work week. The supervisor comments on what he or she observes and uses the feedback to point out when performance needs to be changed as well as to verify and praise effective performance. Effective feedback needs to be descriptive rather than evaluative.

> Evaluative: The splint you fabricated does not fit well.
> Descriptive: The splint you fabricated has rough edges that may cause skin breakdown.

Effective feedback also needs to be specific rather than general.

> General: Your time management skills are poor.
> Specific: Your treatment notes are not filed in the medical record within 24 hours of completion in accordance with the department policy.

It is important to provide feedback that is descriptive and specific. This will keep the focus on the effectiveness of the supervisee's work behaviors and not on his or her personal characteristics or personality. This distinction is critical to the supervisee's being able to "hear" and respond to the feedback. Other suggestions for giving feedback are listed in Box 72-3.

Remember that the purpose of supervision is to support effective work performance. When supervisors evaluate employees, they are evaluating what employees do—how they behave, how they act, and how effectively they are accomplishing the work. The focus of feedback in supervision—both informal and formal—should be on the

task, not the person. The purpose is to relay information about performance to the performer so that actions can be taken to maintain or improve performance.

BOX 72-3 GUIDELINES FOR GIVING FEEDBACK

- Provide timely feedback—give feedback as close to when the behavior was observed as is possible.
- Provide balanced feedback—point out what is working as well as what needs to be changed.
- Provide feedback on behaviors that can be changed.
- Use "I" statements.
- Avoid the use of generalizations such as "always," "never," and "all."
- Ask the supervisee if he or she understood what you said; ask the supervisee to restate it in his or her own words.
- Ask for feedback about your feedback—how did you do?

Performance Evaluation and Appraisal

Newstrom (2013, p. 311) points out four basic reasons for appraising an employee's performance:

1. To encourage good behavior or to correct and discourage below-standard performance
2. To satisfy employee's curiosity to know how they are doing
3. To provide an opportunity for developing employee skills
4. To provide a firm foundation for later judgments that concern an employee's career such as promotions, pay raises, and transfers

A supervisor should be regularly evaluating the supervisee's performance and providing feedback. However, at least once or twice a year, the supervisor should meet with the employer and provide a formal and systematic evaluation of how the person is performing, using a structured performance appraisal format. Most organizations have formal performance appraisal systems and appraisal forms. Appraisal methods and formats may vary and could include written narratives, behaviorally anchored rating scales, management by objectives, or 360-degree feedback. In a formal performance appraisal, the employee's performance is compared to established standards.

As a supervisor, you might be asked to develop job standards for OT personnel. Professional organizations such as the AOTA can help you to identify standards.

For example, AOTA's "Standards of Practice" (AOTA, 2015c) and the "Guidelines for Supervision, Roles, and Responsibilities during the Delivery of Occupational Therapy Services" (AOTA, 2014) are important resources for supervisors practicing in the United States. The World Federation of Occupational Therapists (WFOT) (http://www.wfot.org) provides a listing of member OT professional organizations throughout the world, each of which are likely to have resources relevant to practice within that region. Refer to Chapter 5 for more information on professional organizations in OT. Equally important are worksite job descriptions. Standards will vary by workplace, but all standards should include *what* performance or behaviors are expected, *how* performance will be *measured*, and *when* performance is to occur. An example of a standard that includes all of these criteria is "Evaluations are completed and distributed within 24 hours of initial contact with the client." Standards for each job title should be clearly outlined in the employee's job description.

In preparing a formal performance appraisal, the supervisor needs to complete three steps:

1. Gather information about the employee's performance. Review your supervisory logs, noting key incidents that you recorded. Record additional information that might have been overlooked. Review other employee records, such as attendance, training and educational records, and competency check off completions. Review the previous year's performance appraisal. Talk to other members of the team both within and outside of your department to understand how the employee's performance is viewed by others. Ask the employee to perform a self-appraisal of his or her work, identifying accomplishments, strengths, and weaknesses. You can ask the employee to give this to you before the performance appraisal or have the employee bring it to the performance appraisal meeting.
2. Compare current performance to standards. Note areas of strength and areas in which improvement may be needed.
3. Reflect on and synthesize information. Consider the needs of the department as well as the professional growth needs of the supervisee. Provide feedback about the effectiveness, efficiency, and safety of performance. Note how the employee has contributed to the department's achievements. Document your comments, including both positive feedback and constructive criticism. Avoid allowing an employee's positive or negative qualities in one area to influence your assessment in other areas. Be objective and balanced and focus feedback on task performance. Numerous Websites and management literature offer information on how to perform effective performance evaluations and can alert you to additional factors to be aware of.

When the performance appraisal is completed, it is time to meet with the employee. The purpose of this meeting is to provide an opportunity for the supervisor and supervisee to discuss the employee's job performance and to collaborate on ways to improve it. Unfortunately, performance appraisal meetings are often viewed as anxiety-provoking events that focus on what the employee has done wrong. The common emphasis on the supervisor's rating of the employee tends to detract from a collaborative educational process during which supervisee and supervisor share perspectives and work together to identify barriers to improved performance. The supervisor can use several approaches to correct this problem:

1. Demystify the process. Make sure the employee is familiar with the evaluation process ahead of time. If a standard form is used, make sure the employee has seen it and understands any terminology or rating scales that are used. Make sure the employee is aware of the job expectations and standards. Involve the employee in the appraisal process by using a self-assessment.
2. Plan ahead. Notify the employee ahead of time as to when the meeting will be and allow the employee time to prepare.
3. Establish a comfortable climate for the exchange. Meet in private. Avoid interruptions. Allow adequate time for discussion. Put the employee at ease in the beginning and explain that you view this time as an opportunity for mutual sharing on how to improve job performance for the benefit of the employee and the organization.

During the performance appraisal interview, be prepared to collaborate with the employee and exchange ideas. Share accomplishments and review what has not been accomplished. If performance ratings are provided, be sure to provide reasons for your ratings that are based on actual job performance. If the employee is surprised by any of your ratings or comments, you probably have not provided enough regular feedback during the year. Take note and work to correct that. The appraisal interview offers another opportunity to realign expectations about job performance and to target goals for the future.

Handling Work Performance Problems

Although there are numerous types of performance problems in professional practice settings, the most common ones are behavior or conduct problems in which a rule is broken, performance that falls below the expected standards, and interpersonal issues that interfere with department morale and effectiveness. Each type of problem is handled differently, but in all situations, the actions that are taken are directed toward helping the employee to improve performance and meet job expectations.

Behavior or Conduct Problems

Behavior or conduct problems are handled by disciplining. Behavior or conduct problems may include absenteeism, chronic late arrival, intoxication, insubordination, sexual harassment, negligence in following procedures, and falsification of records. These are all serious infractions and should not be allowed to persist. Although individual facilities may adopt their own specific procedures for disciplining a variety of infractions. In unionized environments, the disciplinary process is highly prescribed. Regardless of setting, disciplining is generally handled in a progressive manner. In a progressive discipline approach, the employee is counseled repeatedly if performance does not improve, and the penalties for noncompliance with the rules become increasingly harsh (Figure 72-3). In rare cases, conduct problems may be grounds for immediate dismissal as delineated in organizational policies.

In the first stage of progressive disciplining, the performance problem is discussed with the employee, clear expectations for acceptable performance are outlined, and consequences of not improving are described. In the second stage, the process is repeated, and this time, a written record of the exchange is documented. Both the supervisor and the employee signs it, and it is placed in the employee's personnel file. If the behavior persists, in the third stage, the employee is suspended for a period of time and is told that when he or she returns to work, the behavior must be corrected or the employee will be terminated. The last stage occurs if the employee returns to work and another infraction occurs, at which time the employee is terminated.

A useful analogy for administering any discipline is the "red-hot stove" rule. The analogy likens the process

of administering discipline to that of touching a red-hot stove and points out the four essential characteristics of a good disciplinary policy and practice. Discipline should be administered in the following manner:

- With advance warning. When you see a red-hot stove, you know that if you touch it, you will be burned. An employee should know what will happen if he or she breaks a rule or policy.
- Immediately. When you touch a red-hot stove, you will be burned right away. Administration of discipline should be done as soon after the occurrence of the behavior as possible.
- Impartially. No matter who touches a red-hot stove, the person will be burned. Supervisors should not play favorites in administering discipline. Everyone should receive the same penalty for the same infraction.
- Consistently. Every time you touch a red-hot stove, you get burned. Discipline should be administered the same way with each occurrence.

Performance Problems

Problems of substandard performance may occur in professional practice. When dealing with these types of problems, the supervisor needs to adopt an approach of collaborating with the supervisee and enlisting his or her help in resolving the problem. Typical steps in dealing with this type of problem after the performance problem is identified include the following:

1. Meet with supervisee and point out the performance problem. Review the standard and describe the expected performance.
2. Collaborate with the supervisee to determine reasons for the problem.
3. Work together to develop and implement an action plan with time frames to improve performance.
4. Monitor performance.
5. Repeat the process if needed.
6. Inform employee of consequences if the standard is achieved and if the standard is not achieved.

Interpersonal Work Issues

Interpersonal work issues vary in scope and complexity and are common in all work groups. In a professional practice environment in which teamwork is central to the department's effectiveness and to the achievement of positive client outcomes, problems among workers should not be ignored. Interpersonal issues can arise among practitioners in the OT department or among team members from different disciplines. These types of work problems often stem from miscommunication and/or differences in communication styles or personalities. Lack of clarity about job roles or about expectations can also lead to interpersonal problems.

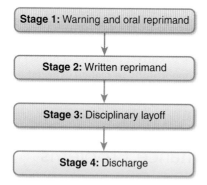

FIGURE 72-3 Using a standard sequence for dealing with performance problems is required in many formal organizations and is considered good practice in most settings.

Just because two people are different or disagree does not mean that they cannot work effectively together. The supervisor's role in resolving these types of performance issues should focus not on personalities, individuals, or differences but on the job tasks and mutual goals that need to be accomplished. The first approach to take when an employee complains to you about another employee is to listen carefully and encourage the person with the complaint to talk directly to the other individual. You should help the person to clarify his or her concerns and frame them in terms of how the other person's actions are affecting the person's ability to get his or her own job done. This approach often works and begins the process of opening communication.

When this approach does not work, you might need to take further action by talking to each of the parties involved. You might want to do this individually at first and then together, or you might want to approach the problem by talking to the parties at the same time. In either case, you will want to interview both to understand all of the facts and frame the issues or problems in terms of specific behavior and job performance expectations that are being affected. As the supervisor, you also must be clear about your expectations for job performance actions and attitudes and remind both of them about the department's expectations. During this discussion, each party should become more aware of his or her own behaviors as well as the behaviors of the other and how the interaction of their choices is affecting their work. Your goal in this exchange is for both parties to work out a solution that does not compromise the work of either and allows the work of the department to continue more effectively.

Supervision of Occupational Therapy Personnel

Effective supervision of OT personnel is necessary to ensure safe and effective delivery of services. As was mentioned at the beginning of this chapter, supervision is embedded within the OT process. However, OT practitioners work in a broad range of work environments (medical, educational, and community-based settings). To guide practitioners in developing effective supervisory practices in these different situations, professional organizations may develop supervisory guidelines that can be applied in all settings. These guidelines describe how the profession views the supervisory process, who needs to be supervised, the methods and frequency of supervision, and supervisory responsibilities of different OT personnel.

Occupational Therapists

The AOTA describes occupational therapists as "autonomous practitioners who are able to deliver services independently" (AOTA, 2014, p. S16). Likewise, the WFOT endorses the autonomy of the profession (WFOT, 2007) and describes the minimum qualifications for OT practitioners (WFOT, 2008). Entry-level occupational therapists are qualified to practice without supervision. The therapist's preparation to deliver services independently is based on education and training, which in the United States includes a minimum of 6 months of supervised fieldwork experience and successful completion of the initial certification exam. Entry-level occupational therapists are trained as generalists and are qualified to enter general practice settings as autonomous therapists. Although entry-level therapists do not require supervision, "occupational therapists are encouraged to seek peer supervision and mentoring for ongoing development of best practice approaches and to promote professional growth" (AOTA, 2014, p. S16). This statement underscores each therapist's professional responsibility to maintain the competencies that are needed to provide safe and effective services. The therapist who enters a work setting where professional supervision is not provided should carefully compare his or her current competencies with the demands of the work setting. When this comparison reveals that current knowledge and skills may need further support or development, the therapist should seek supervision or mentoring to ensure competent practice and professional growth. Although this is not required, many entry-level therapists seek first-time jobs in which supervision will be available. These positions allow them more time to solidify clinical skills and develop confidence. Therapists beyond entry level should continue to assess their need for professional supervision if it is not provided in their work setting. Career changes, such as switching practice settings (from school to nursing home) or types of clients treated (children with autism to adults with spinal cord injuries), may challenge the therapist's current competency and alert the therapist to the need to seek supervision or mentoring (AOTA, 2015b; Youngstrom, 1998).

In many OT practice settings, there may be no formal supervision by another OT practitioner. In these situations, OT practitioners often seek informal peer supervision from OT practitioners in similar settings. They ask for feedback from each other and share case information, often problem solving together to plan effective interventions. The advent of social networking and Web-based resources has expanded the informal consultation resources available to practitioners. This is a positive and proactive approach that helps to ensure effective professional practice and personal competence. See Chapter 70 for an extended discussion of competence and professional development.

Occupational Therapy Assistants

Although OT assistants are used in as many as 22 other countries throughout the world (WFOT, 2016), supervisory guidelines are most fully developed in the United States. Our discussion of OT assistant supervision is based on current practice in the United States. Occupational therapists working with OT assistants in other countries will want to contact the professional association in those countries to determine if supervision requirements are different.

In the United States, OT assistants who deliver OT services must be supervised by an occupational therapist (AOTA, 2014, 2015c). Occupational therapy assistants are trained and educated in basic OT approaches and techniques, and their role is one of assisting the professional level therapist with the delivery of services. The occupational therapist is responsible for all aspects of service delivery and works in partnership and collaboration with the OT assistant to provide appropriate services to clients. Entry-level occupational therapists are expected to be able to supervise OT assistants and to be knowledgeable about the collaborative supervisory relationship that the profession values (Accreditation Council for Occupational Therapy Education [ACOTE], 2011). Entry-level OT assistants are expected to be knowledgeable of the supervisory partnership and to seek supervision appropriately. Occupational therapy assistants, by virtue of their training and education, are often well qualified to take on related work roles (e.g., assistive technologists, activity program directors). When they do assume these roles, they are not providing OT services and consequently do not need to be supervised by an occupational therapist.

Fieldwork Students

Level II fieldwork students at the therapist and assistant level both must be supervised by OT practitioners. In the United States, OT students must be supervised by an occupational therapist who has at least 1 year of experience after being initially certified by the National Board for Certification in Occupational Therapy (ACOTE, 2011). Occupational therapy assistant students may be supervised by either an occupational therapist or an OT assistant, both of whom also must have at least 1 year of experience after initial certification (ACOTE, 2011). If an OT assistant is providing the Level II supervision for the OT assistant student, it is understood that the supervising assistant is supervised by an occupational therapist. According to ACOTE, personnel who are qualified to supervise Level I OT or OT assistant students include all credentialed OT personnel as well as individuals from other disciplines such as psychology, social work, and teaching (ACOTE, 2011).

To benefit from Level II fieldwork supervision, the OT student needs to seek and respond to feedback that is given. The supervisory relationship that is established during fieldwork is similar to a professional supervisory relationship. Chapter 69 discusses the nature of supervision in the fieldwork setting.

Other Personnel

Other types of personnel who may assist with the provision of OT services or the management of services delivery, such as administrative assistants, OT aides, or volunteers, may be supervised by either occupational therapists or OT assistants. Table 72-3 provides an overview of whom various personnel may supervise.

Types of Supervision: Overseeing Various Aspects of Work

Work is a complex activity. The responsibility for supervising various aspects of work is sometimes assigned to

TABLE 72-3   Patterns of Supervision: Who Can Supervise Whom?

Type of Supervisor	OTA	OT Aide	Volunteer	OT Fieldwork Student Level I	OT Fieldwork Student Level II	OTA Fieldwork Student Level I	OTA Fieldwork Student Level II	Occupational Therapist
Entry-level occupational therapist	X	X	X	X	X			
Occupational therapist with more than 1 year of experience	X	X	X	X	X	X	X	X
Entry-level OTA		X	X					
OTA with more than 1 year of experience	X	X	X	X		X	X	

OTA, occupational therapy assistant.

different people. It is not uncommon for an OT practitioner to receive supervision from more than one person for different aspects of their work performance. Discussion of three distinct aspects of work performance and the type of supervision used to oversee that performance will help you to see how supervision in some settings may require a multifaceted approach.

Administrative Supervision

Administrative supervision is focused on monitoring performance and making sure that the supervisee's work performance and professional development meet the objectives and standards of the employing organization. Administrative supervisors focus on the administrative aspects of job performance, such as attendance, schedules, benefit usage, and checking for appropriate completion of assigned job tasks. This type of supervision correlates closely with the administrative function of supervision discussed earlier.

Administrative supervision can be provided by an occupational therapist or an OT assistant to other occupational therapists and OT assistants or to members of other disciplines. Likewise, members of other disciplines can administratively supervise OT practitioners and OT assistants. This type of supervision commonly occurs in public school settings in which school principals or special education administrators are the designated supervisors for the OT staffs. As the supervisor, the principal or special education administrator would be supervising the administrative aspects of the OT's work. Similarly, in rehabilitation settings, an occupational therapist may function in a management role, and thus provide administrative supervision to members of other disciplines such as physical therapy or speech-language pathology.

Clinical or Professional Practice Supervision

Supervision that is aimed at providing support, training, and evaluation of a supervisee's professional performance and development is called **professional practice supervision** or **clinical supervision**. The term *clinical supervision* was the most commonly used term in the past to describe this type of supervision. However, as more OT practitioners have moved into work settings outside the clinical medical model (e.g., school settings, community centers), the term *clinical supervision* seems less appropriate than the broader term *professional practice supervision*. In professional practice supervision, the supervisor's responsibilities extend beyond the purely administrative aspects of job performance and are additionally aimed at assisting and supporting the supervisee's development of professional discipline-specific skills, such as interviewing skills, appropriate use of selected therapeutic techniques, and professional reasoning.

Professional practice supervision can appropriately be provided only by a member of the supervisee's discipline. Consequently, it would not be appropriate for a physical therapist to provide professional practice supervision or clinical supervision to an occupational therapist. Likewise, an occupational therapist cannot be expected to provide professional practice or clinical supervision for a physical therapist. Professional practice supervision is the type of supervision that is provided by fieldwork educators during Level II fieldwork experiences. (Fieldwork educators also provide administrative supervision to students.) An occupational therapist may provide professional practice supervision to other occupational therapists and OT assistants, and an OT assistant may provide professional practice supervision to other OT assistants. This type of supervision correlates closely with the educational and supportive supervisory functions.

Functional Supervision

A third type of supervision that is seen in some OT practice environments is **functional supervision** (AOTA, 1993, p. 1088). In this type of supervision, a specific aspect of work or a "function" of professional practice is delegated to a specified individual to provide training and oversight in that aspect of work. The supervisor who is providing only functional supervision generally has advanced knowledge, skill, and competence in the area being supervised. For example, an OT supervisor of a new employee might request that another OT who is experienced in wheelchair assessment and positioning provide functional supervision to the new employee in this area. When providing functional supervision, the supervisor is not responsible for the entire supervisory process but rather supervises the person's performance and development of specific skills or competency in only the selected job function area.

Methods of Supervision

A professional practice supervisor needs to consider what supervisory methods will be most effective in developing and monitoring performance. Supervisees have different learning styles. Worksites have varying caseload demands, administrative requirements for supervision, and time available to provide supervision. Supervisory methods need to be selected to meet the supervisee's needs and the demands of the worksite.

The supervisor is responsible for initially orienting and training the supervisee and then supporting the supervisee's professional growth and development. From the organization's perspective, it is important that information provided while training the supervisee be delivered in a

BOX 72-4   EXAMPLES OF LEARNING METHODS

- Provide written protocols or instructions.
- Have the learner report back on what he or she learned from reading.
- Provide articles or books to read or use as reference.
- Demonstrate and have the learner return the demonstration.
- Provide a verbal explanation or lecture that covers the content.
- Provide videotapes with questions about content to answer at end.

- Have the learner participate in small group discussion to problem-solve clinical situations.
- Discuss cases or problems presented, either one on one or in small groups.
- Role-play situations.
- Provide repeated practice opportunities to apply new knowledge and skills.
- Observe others carrying out tasks; ask the learner to describe what he or she observed.
- Model desired performance and behaviors.

manner to promote safe and effective outcomes and positive client experiences (Laverdure, Smith, DuPrey, Lynn, & Swope, 2017). To achieve this, consideration should be given to the type of teaching methods that will be most effective in learning new information and developing work skills. Varying the methods used and selecting the

ones that will mesh with the learner's skill and comfort level can be most effective. Involve the supervisee in the process by asking what learning approaches he or she prefers. Box 72-4 lists examples of various learning methods.

To monitor and evaluate performance, the supervisor can use direct and indirect approaches.

❝ COMMENTARY ON THE EVIDENCE

Supervision in Occupational Therapy

The majority of research in supervision has been conducted by business and management researchers. Within the health care professions, nurses, social workers, and counseling psychologists have been the primary contributors to the research on clinical supervision. In OT, direct empirical evidence to support effective supervisory practice is lacking. The research that is available in OT is often related to management issues and/or is descriptive in focus. For example, OT managers, concerned with employee satisfaction and retention, have shown that factors such as feedback and recognition of accomplishments, realistic workloads, and autonomy and opportunities for professional growth and skill development all influence job satisfaction (Barnes, 1998; Smith, 2000). Although these studies did not directly look at supervision, the factors that were identified are all factors that a supervisor can affect, so effective supervision should attend to these factors.

Two studies have provided some insight into current supervisory practices. Johnson, Koenig, Piersol, Santalucia, and Wachter-Schutz (2006) reported that more fieldwork educators who supervise Level I fieldwork students are not occupational therapists (OT practitioners) than in the past. In April 2006, the National Board for Certification in Occupational Therapy reported the results of a 2005 online survey of OT and OT assistant certification exam candidates that included data on who the practitioner's primary supervisor was and the number of hours of direct supervision

received per week (Bent & Conway, 2006). Thirty-eight percent of occupational therapists and 23% of OT assistants were supervised by members of other disciplines. Thirty-one percent of occupational therapists and 18% of OT assistants received zero hours of direct supervision per week. Descriptive statistics such as these prompt us to ask other questions: How does being supervised by someone who is not an OT practitioner affect practitioners' professional growth and commitment to occupation-based practice? Does frequency of direct supervision affect the quality of services delivered and the rate of professional growth?

Research about supervision practices with OT fieldwork students is somewhat more prevalent. Some researchers have explored the supervisory experiences of fieldwork educators (Richard, 2008) to identify supervision issues. Others have studied the effectiveness of different models of supervision: use of non-OT supervisors for Level I fieldwork experiences (Heine & Bennett, 2003) and use of an aggregate fieldwork model (Precin, 2009).

Both descriptive and empirical studies of supervision in OT are needed. How do supervisory practices vary by setting? What is the most efficient and effective way to establish service competency with an OT assistant? What supervisory approaches are most effective in supporting professional growth and development with supervisees? These are only a few of the many questions that need to be answered to provide supervisors with the evidence they need to supervise effectively.

Direct or Line-of-Sight Supervision

In direct or line-of-sight methods of supervision, the supervisor is present when the employee is performing the job and actually observes performance. When we think of supervision methods, this approach is generally the first one that comes to mind. Direct observation gives first-hand information to the supervisor, but this approach is time-consuming, and it is not always practical to use as the only method of supervision.

Indirect Supervision

Indirect methods allow the supervisor to ascertain how the job was performed by gathering this information after performance occurs. Indirect methods include communicating with the supervisee (via phone, e-mail, or written correspondence) after performance, looking at written records (attendance records, documentation), or receiving reports from others (clients, parents, other staff, or team members) about the supervisee's performance. Listening to what others say provides information about the employee's performance and provides feedback about how others perceive the performance. Supervising performance in a clinical setting by reading the supervisee's documentation is a frequently used indirect method in OT practice. Reading documentation tells the supervisor what happened when clients were seen and provides insight into the supervisee's clinical reasoning and documentation skills. However, using only the indirect method of supervision without also periodically observing performance would not give the supervisor a well-rounded picture of the employee's performance in areas such as interpersonal skill, technique application, adaptability in spontaneous clinical situations, and problem solving. Both indirect and direct methods need to be used to develop an accurate and complete picture of employee performance.

Telesupervision

With the advances in and widespread access to technology, increased attention has been given to the use of telesupervision in the health professions, including OT (Brandoff & Lombardi, 2012). **Telesupervision** refers to clinical supervision provided with communication technology and includes the use of video conferencing, telephone, e-mails, chats, podcasts, or the use of social networks (Brandoff & Lombardi, 2012; Kind, Patel, Lie, & Chretien, 2014). At this time, telesupervision has primarily been used in rural or remote areas, or when having to supervise staff working in multiple sites (Dudding & Justice, 2004; Martin, Kumar, Lizarondo, & VanErp, 2015).

The format of telesupervision varies and depends on the particular setting, available technology, supervisee's needs, and supervisor availability (Miller, Miller, Burton, Sprang, & Adams, 2003). For instance, an OT supervisor may lead a chat session with a group of supervisees to review documentation requirements, whereas another OT supervisor may observe a supervisee via videoconference to assess his or her ability to perform a seating assessment.

Factors that have been identified as contributing to effective use of telesupervision include previous face-to-face contact, access to high-quality technical systems, continuity, careful participant selection, and well-planned supervisory sessions (Martin, Kumar, & Lizarondo, 2017; Martin, Lizarondo, & Kumar, 2017). Occupational therapy supervisors planning to use telesupervision should consider these factors when developing these programs. Supervisors will also need to be aware of and comply with any applicable governmental regulations or institutional policies related to employee and patient privacy when using telesupervision (e.g., the need to obtain consent for videotaping and the use of encrypted transmitted data).

Frequency of Supervision

One of the first decisions a supervisor must make when developing a supervision plan is to determine how frequently to have contact with the supervisee to teach, train, monitor, and evaluate performance. The members of the profession have considered this question in relation to how frequency of supervision should be determined in supervising OT assistants (AOTA, 2014, p. S2). The factors that are outlined next can be considered in all supervisory situations. In determining frequency of supervisory contact, the supervisor should consider the following:

1. His or her own supervisory skills. Supervisors who are new and just developing their skills might require more frequent contact with the supervisee because they are less efficient in observing and analyzing performance. They might need more time to recognize possible performance issues and to provide supervisory interventions. The supervisor who has had more experience and/or who has previously supervised in a similar setting might be clearer about performance expectations and able to anticipate problems and provide guidance and direction sooner.

2. The skills of the supervisee. New employees who come to a job with background and experience in a similar job probably bring the needed skills to the new job. Generally, these employees will require less initial training and often move very quickly to a point at which they need less frequent supervision. The supervisor, however, must individually evaluate each employee because experience does not always guarantee effective performance. The employee's speed and style of learning will also affect the frequency of supervision needed.

3. The nature of the work. Work that is more varied and complex might require more frequent supervisory contact to allow the supervisor to observe performance at different times under various conditions and levels of complexity. The new practitioner working in a rehabilitation hospital whose caseload consists only of patients who had stroke might require less frequent supervision than the new practitioner who is working in an acute care setting seeing clients with orthopedic, neurological, and acute medical conditions.

4. The expectations and requirements of the work setting. In various work settings, standards and expectations may have developed, based on experience in that setting, that require certain levels of supervision. Although an experienced supervisor might think that weekly contact is sufficient, a worksite might require daily contact.

5. The expectations and requirements of external regulatory or legislative agencies. Federal or state laws and regulations and accrediting agencies may specify certain methods of oversight and contact that must occur between the occupational therapist and the OT assistant.

Frequency of supervision is generally viewed as occurring on a continuum. At the high end of the continuum, the supervisor is continually in sight of the supervisee who is working. At the low end of the continuum, the supervisor contacts the supervisee only as needed. The supervisor needs to be flexible in dealing with the wide variety of practice setting and supervisory demands that exist within the profession and consider these demands carefully when determining supervision frequency.

There are, however, two firm directives regarding need for supervision based on professional documents:

1. Entry-level OT practitioners do not *require* supervision. They are, however, "encouraged to seek peer supervision and mentoring for ongoing development of best practice approaches and to promote professional growth" (AOTA, 2014, p. S16; WFOT, 2007).

2. OT assistants must *always* receive some level of regular supervision from an occupational therapist when they are providing OT services in the United States (AOTA, 2014).

The Occupational Therapist/Occupational Therapy Assistant Supervisory Relationship

In the United States, where the role of the OT assistant has been developed over a longer period of time, the supervisory relationship between the OT practitioner and OT assistant is characterized as a partnership. The discussion that follows describing the OT practitioner–OT assistant supervisory relationship is based on this partnership perspective.

Both levels of practitioners in the United States are trained and educated within the profession but at different levels. The occupational therapist is educated at the professional knowledge and skill level and receives an entry-level graduate degree. The OT assistant is currently educated at the technical level and receives an associate of arts degree. Each level of practitioner has complementary but distinct roles. The occupational therapist is responsible for overall service provision and can carry out all facets of service provision (i.e., evaluation, intervention planning, intervention implementation and review, and outcomes assessment). The OT assistant's primary role is in the implementation phase of service provision. They may contribute to other aspects of service provision, such as performing selected assessments for which they have demonstrated service competence, or recommending intervention changes, but only under the supervision of the occupational therapist.

The "Guidelines for Supervision, Roles, and Responsibilities during the Delivery of Occupational Therapy Services" (AOTA, 2014) outline the roles and responsibilities of each level of practitioner during the delivery of services. For the partnership to be successful, each practitioner must have a clear understanding of each other's role and respect and value the contribution that each practitioner makes. When the occupational therapists and OT assistants work as a team, they are able to use and build on each other's skills and expand the number and kinds of services that can be provided to clients. When an occupational therapist partners with an OT assistant, the professional level therapist is often able to see more clients and to use the assistant's personal expertise in specific practice areas or techniques to improve client care. See the "Practice Dilemma" box for a discussion of dilemmas that can occur when supervising an OT assistant.

Changing Practice Patterns: Taylor Supervises an Occupational Therapy Assistant

Taylor recently started a new job as an occupational therapist at a large long-term care facility in her community. She works with a team of two other occupational therapist and two OT assistants. She is responsible for supervising Diane, one of the OT assistants. Diane has been working at this facility for 5 years and considers herself very experienced in dealing with this population. When Taylor started the job, she met with Diane to discuss their supervisory relationship and to determine how they would conduct their partnership. Taylor spent time observing and working with Diane and found Diane to be very helpful in orienting her to the facility and familiarizing her with the patients and the typical OT interventions that were being used.

Taylor has now worked at the facility for more than 6 months and is more familiar with the clients and their individual needs. She is interested in developing intervention plans that are more individualized and that use intervention activities that relate to each patient's own needs and personal lifestyle choices, whether they will return home or remain in the nursing home's long-term care wing. Interventions in the past have been focused primarily on self-care issues, and Taylor, although not wanting to ignore these occupations, would like to emphasize more instrumental activities of daily living and leisure occupations in which patients will want to engage if they return home or that might allow them to increase their sense of self-efficacy and control if they remain in long-term care. She has communicated this goal to Diane, and when they develop intervention plans, individualized goals are developed in these areas. However, as she follows up with Diane and observes interventions and monitors patient progress, Taylor has noted that Diane is not choosing to address these goals and continues to use the routine types of tasks and activities that she was previously using.

Questions

1. How would you define the supervisory issues and problems in this situation?
2. As a supervisor in this scenario, what are Taylor's responsibilities?
3. As a supervisee in this scenario, what are Diane's responsibilities?
4. What do you think might be some of the reasons for Diane's behavior?
5. How would you suggest that Taylor approach Diane and address this problem?
6. What do you think might be some supervisory interventions that Taylor could take that would help to improve this situation?

Service Competency

The purpose of the supervisory process is to ensure that safe and effective services are delivered and that professional competence is fostered. The occupational therapist who carries the responsibility for overall service delivery must ensure that OT assistants she supervises performing effectively. To ensure that services provided by both levels of practitioners are safe and effective, the occupational therapist establishes service competency with the OT assistant.

Service competency is the process of teaching, training, and evaluating in which the occupational therapist determines that the OT assistant performs tasks in the same way that the occupational therapist would and achieves the same outcomes (AOTA, 1999).

When the occupational therapist and OT assistant initially start working together, the occupational therapist will establish service competency for overall job performance. In the early stages of the work relationship, the therapist will need to determine what knowledge and skills the OT assistant has. The establishment of service competency is integrated into the normal supervisory process as the supervisor orients and trains the new employee and begins comparing the employee's performance to the established professional and worksite standards and expectations. The occupational therapist should identify the primary job tasks and skills that are needed for the OT assistant's job. These tasks will vary by site and service setting. The therapist will observe and train the assistant and note whether the he or she can perform the identified skills and tasks and whether intervention outcomes are similar to those normally achieved by the occupational therapist. Examples of job tasks or skills for which service competency may be established include reading the medical record, being able to record appropriate and pertinent information, and being able to appropriately grade an activity to increase its cognitive difficulty.

The concept of service competency is based on the assumption that the supervising therapist is competent in the skills for which competency is being established. Both levels of practitioners are responsible for being aware of each other's competent behaviors and providing feedback to inform each other of possible problem areas.

It is important that the supervisor establish an acceptable standard of performance or level of agreement for skills and tasks on which service competency is being established. For example, when observing client dressing performance, the OT assistant will rate the client's level of independence at the same level as the occupational therapist 95% of the time. The comparison of outcomes between practitioners is an approach that helps to ensure that services clients receive are of comparable quality. It supports the validity of delegating to the OT assistant and ensures consistency of services. The methods the therapist can use while establishing service competency could include observation, cotreatment, return demonstration of techniques or skills, review of documentation, testing for knowledge and its application, and discussion of cases to ascertain clinical reasoning and judgment.

After initial service competency is established, the therapist supervisor will need to periodically recheck service competency to ensure that it is maintained. The occupational therapist may also select new tasks and skills in which to establish service competency with the OT assistant. For example, the occupational therapist might decide to train the assistant in how to carry out and score a particular structured assessment tool. After service competency has been established, the therapist can delegate the administration of this assessment to the assistant and be assured that the results of the assistant's giving the test will be comparable to the results that would be obtained if the occupational therapist administered the test. Service competency does not mean that the OT assistant will perform the task in exactly the same manner as the OT assistant would—only that the outcomes will be similar. Note that in all cases, the occupational therapist is responsible for interpreting the assessment results as part of the overall evaluation process.

Frequency and Type of Occupational Therapy Assistant Supervision

The decisions about frequency of supervision for the OT assistant will vary with practice setting and should be decided based on the five factors previously discussed: skills of the supervisor, skills of the supervisee, nature of the work, expectations and requirements of the work setting, and expectations and requirements of external regulatory or legislative agencies. The OT assistant's level of service competency and skill will influence the frequency of supervision needed. If service competency has already been established, the need for supervision might be less frequent. When service competency is being established in a new area or skill, the supervisor will need to change the frequency of supervision until competency is established.

Work factors that can affect frequency of supervision needed by an OT assistant include increased complexity of client's needs and diagnoses, rapidity of client change, more involved or complex types of interventions, and increased number and diversity of clients in the assistant's caseload. When the client population is complex and/or rapidly changing, frequent reevaluation and adjustment in types of interventions and implementation plans are needed, which require the clinical reasoning and evaluation skills of the OT practitioner. Frequency of supervision needs should be

regularly reassessed as workplace demands, client needs, and supervisee skills change.

Because the supervisory process with the OT assistant is collaborative and both practitioners are responsible for providing safe and effective services, the occupational therapist and OT assistant should discuss the decision about the frequency of supervision. Supervision frequency and methods should be mutually decided on.

Although frequency of supervision can vary, OT assistants who are providing OT services will always need some level of regular supervision. Supervision of the OT assistant on an irregular, spontaneous, or as-needed basis is not appropriate. It does not demonstrate that the OT is providing the ongoing oversight required to ensure safe and effective services nor does it validate that high-quality OT is being provided. Many external regulatory and legislative agencies now specify the frequency and type of supervisory contact that must take place between the occupational therapist and OT assistant. The Centers for Medicare & Medicaid Services (CMS) states that the OT assistant providing services to Medicare patients under an occupational therapist working in a physician's office must have direct or on-site (in the building but not in the line of sight) supervision on the day of treatment (CMS, 2012). In February 2006, CMS also clarified that occupational therapists are required to write a progress report every 10 treatment days or once every 30-day interval and requires that the they perform or actively participate in treatments at this frequency level if the treatments have been delegated to an OT assistant (Thomas, 2006). This requirement necessitates that the therapists have regular contact with the client and with the OT assistant who is providing services. Many state regulatory agencies outline specific supervision requirements in their laws for OT assistant supervision, and CMS requires that the supervisor provided complies with these regulations. Occupational therapy practitioners should contact their regulatory boards for information about specific supervisory requirements.

Effective Occupational Therapy Assistant Supervisory Relationships

The occupational therapist–OT assistant relationship should be collaborative in nature. The OT supervisor has the obligation and responsibility to supervise the OT assistant, and the OT assistant has the obligation and responsibility to seek supervision. In writing about their own collaborative relationship, Barbara Hanft and Barbara Banks (1999) identified six qualities that support the development of collaborative supervisory relationships:

- *Sensitivity*, for perceiving and responding to one another's professional and personal needs

BOX 72-5 SUMMARY OF STEPS TO TAKE IN SUPERVISING AN OCCUPATIONAL THERAPY ASSISTANT

1. Orient OT assistant to worksite.
2. Share job and professional expectations.
3. Identify OT assistant's skill level.
4. Identify OT assistant's learning needs and methods of learning—ASK!
5. Establish service competency.
6. Collaborate with OT assistant to establish ongoing supervisory plan:
   Select methods.
   Select frequency.
7. Document ongoing supervision.

- *Dependability*, for keeping commitments and responding to unexpected situations
- *Attentiveness*, for actively listening to one another
- *Respectfulness*, for appreciating one another's distinct knowledge, experiences and judgment
- *Collaborativeness*, for working toward a common goal and representing OT services together as a unit
- *Reflection*, for an ability to use self-observation to review situations objectively from different perspectives (p. 31)

In a collaborative relationship, both parties understand their unique roles and responsibilities and respect their differences and similarities (Sands, 1998).

The occupational therapists needs to actively involve the OT assistant in the supervisory process and needs to tailor the experience to meet individual needs of the OT assistant and the worksite. Box 72-5 presents a summary of the primary steps that should be taken in supervising an OT assistant.

⚖ ETHICAL DILEMMA

Joel Supervises an Employee with Depression

Joel is a supervising occupational therapist in a large metropolitan acute care hospital. He oversees a group of three occupational therapists and one OT assistant. Recently, one of his supervisees, Naomi, met with him and told him that she has been diagnosed with clinical depression. Joel is not surprised. He had noted that Naomi's work performance had changed, and he was even beginning to become concerned about the quality of Naomi's patient care decisions and her ability to handle the normally fast-paced caseload. Naomi has asked for Joel's help and support by decreasing her caseload so that she may continue to work in an effective manner.

Questions

1. Who are the different players in this scenario to whom Joel has an obligation or duty?
2. As a supervisor, what are Joel's obligations to each player?
3. How are the different needs of the players conflicting?

Supervising Occupational Therapy Aides

Occupational therapy aides are individuals with no formalized education in the provision of OT services who are hired to provide supportive services to OT practitioners. Aides are trained on the job to meet the specific needs of the individual department. Aides do not provide skilled OT services, and the types of activities they can perform with clients are clearly prescribed for therapists in the United States in the "Guidelines for Supervision, Roles, and Responsibilities during the Delivery of Occupational Therapy Services" (AOTA, 2014). Aides can perform two types of tasks within the department: They can carry out (1) non–client-related tasks such as clerical work, clinic maintenance tasks, and preparation of work areas and equipment and (2) selected client-related tasks that are routine and supervised by an occupational therapist or an OT assistant (AOTA, 2014). For a task to be considered routine, it must meet the following four criteria:

1. The outcome anticipated for the delegated task is predictable.
2. The situation of the client and the environment is stable and will not require that judgments, interpretations, or adaptations be made by the aide.
3. The client has demonstrated some previous performance ability in executing the task.
4. The task routine and process have been clearly established (AOTA, 2014).

These criteria are based on the understanding that aides do not have the knowledge and skill to evaluate or make changes in an intervention activity but can be helpful in providing oversight or practice of selected activities when change and judgment are not anticipated.

Before a selected task can be delegated to an aide, the practitioner must be assured that the aide can carry out the task safely and effectively. They must instruct the aide and assess his or her competency in performing the delegated task. The aide also must be aware of all precautions and signs or symptoms that a particular client might demonstrate that would indicate that the aide needs to seek assistance (AOTA, 2014). Each of these requirements is intended to ensure that the aide's interaction with the client will be safe and effective. Practitioners can appropriately use aides to oversee clients who are practicing certain skills after the process has been set up (e.g., one-handed shoe tying and activity routines). Aides can also provide another pair of hands during physical activities when additional help is needed to engage the client in an activity as when providing assistance to transfer a patient. Aides can be supervised by either an occupational therapist or an OT assistant. However, when the OT assistant supervises the aide, the occupational therapist maintains overall responsibility for the process through the occupational therapist's supervision of the OT assistant.

Frequency of supervision will vary with tasks assigned and the aide's skill. Client-related tasks may require closer supervision because of the importance of patient safety and intervention effectiveness. The supervisory plan and process need to be documented to demonstrate accountability.

Supervising Non-occupational Therapy Personnel

The same basic guidelines and process for effective supervision should be followed in supervising non-OT personnel. The OT practitioner who assumes a supervisory or management role may supervise personnel from other disciplines who provide direct services to clients (e.g., physical therapists, psychologists, recreational therapists) as well as personnel who provide support services for the department (e.g., administrative assistants, reimbursement specialists, information technology specialists). The type of supervision the OT practitioner will provide to personnel from other disciplines will be administrative. Occupational therapy practitioners cannot provide professional practice supervision or clinical supervision because OT practitioners are not trained in the other individuals' professions. Astute supervisors will ensure that their supervisees from other disciplines seek and have access to professional practice supervision or mentoring and will consult with members of the supervisee's discipline to assist them in evaluating the supervisee's professional practice performance.

Conclusion

Supervision is a person-oriented process—much like OT. The OT supervisor must continually balance the needs of the organization with the needs of supervisees to provide safe and effective services to clients. Awareness of the basic functions of supervision and an understanding of the supervisory process make up the first step in preparing practitioners for the supervisory role.

REFERENCES

Accreditation Council for Occupational Education. (2011). Accreditation Council for Occupational Therapy Education (ACOTE®) standards. *American Journal of Occupational Therapy*, 66, S6–S74. doi:10.5014/ajot.2012.66S6

American Occupational Therapy Association. (1981). Official document: Guide for supervision of occupational therapy personnel. *American Journal of Occupational Therapy*, 35, 815–816.

American Occupational Therapy Association. (1993). Occupational therapy roles. *American Journal of Occupational Therapy*, 47, 1087–1099.

American Occupational Therapy Association. (1999). Guide for the supervision of occupational therapy personnel in the delivery of occupational therapy services. *American Journal of Occupational Therapy*, 53, 592–594.

American Occupational Therapy Association. (2014). Guidelines for supervision, roles, and responsibilities during the delivery of occupational therapy services. *American Journal of Occupational Therapy*, 64, S1–S22. doi:10.5014/ajot.2014.686S03

American Occupational Therapy Association. (2015a). Occupational therapy code of ethics (2015). *American Journal of Occupational Therapy*, 69, 6913410030p1–6913410030p8. doi:10.5014/ajot.2015.696S03

American Occupational Therapy Association. (2015b). Standards for continuing competence. *American Journal of Occupational Therapy*, 69, 6913410055p1–6913410055p3. doi:10.5014/ajot.2015.696S16

American Occupational Therapy Association. (2015c). Standards of practice for occupational therapy. *American Journal of Occupational Therapy*, 69, 6913410057p1–6913410057p6. doi:10.5014/ajot.2015.696S06

Barnes, D. S. (1998). Job satisfaction and the rehabilitation professional. *Administration & Management Special Interest Section Quarterly*, 14(4), 1–2.

Bent, M. A., & Conway, S. (2006). *Results of a national study profiling the 2005 certification candidate population*. Retrieved from http://www.nbcot.org

Brandoff, R., & Lombardi, R. (2012). Miles apart: Two art therapists' experience of distance supervision. *Art Therapy*, 29(2), 93–96.

Braveman, B. (2016). *Leading and managing occupational therapy services: An evidence-based approach* (2nd ed.). Philadelphia, PA: F. A. Davis.

Centers for Medicare & Medicaid Services. (2012). *Part B billing scenarios for PTs and OTs*. Retrieved from https://www.cms.gov/Medicare/Billing/TherapyServices/Downloads/11_Part_B_Billing_Scenarios_for_PTs_and_OTs.pdf

Coulter, J. S., & McNary, H. (1931). Necessity of medical supervision in occupational therapy. *Occupational Therapy and Rehabilitation*, 10, 19–24.

Dudding, C. C., & Justice, L. M. (2004). An e-supervision model: Videoconferencing as a clinical training tool. *Communication Disorder Quarterly*, 25(3), 145–151.

Hanft, B., & Banks, B. (1999). Competent supervision: A collaborative process. *OT Practice*, 4(5), 32–34.

Heine, D., & Bennett, N. (2003). Student perceptions of level I fieldwork supervision. *Occupational Therapy in Health Care*, 17, 89–97.

Johnson, C. R., Koenig, K. P., Piersol, C. V., Santalucia, S. E., & Wachter-Schutz, W. (2006). Level I fieldwork today: A study of contexts and perceptions. *American Journal of Occupational Therapy*, 60, 275–287.

Kadushin, A. (1992). *Supervision in social work* (3rd ed.). New York, NY: Columbia University Press.

Kind, T., Patel, P. D., Lie, D. L., & Chretien, K. C. (2014). Twelve tips for using social media as a medical educator. *Medical Teacher, 36*(4), 165–169.

Laverdure, P., Smith, L. C., DuPrey, J., Lynn, J., & Swope, K. (2017). Beyond the badge: Supporting the orientation and training of new employees across practice settings. *OT Practice, 22*(17), 8–13.

Martin, P., Kumar, S., & Lizarondo, L. (2017). Effective use of technology in clinical supervision. *Internet Interventions, 8,* 35–39. doi:10.1016/j.invent.2017.03.001

Martin, P., Kumar, S., Lizarondo, L., & VanErp, A. (2015). Enablers of and barriers to high quality clinical supervision among occupational therapists across Queensland in Australia: Findings from a qualitative study. *BMC Health Services Research, 15,* 413. doi:10.1186/s12913-015-1085-8

Martin, P., Lizarondo, L., & Kumar, S. (2017). A systematic review of the factors that influence the quality and effectiveness of telesupervision for health professionals. *Journal of Telemedicine and Telecare.* Advance online publication. doi:10.1177/1357633X17698868

Miller, T. W., Miller, J. M., Burton, D., Sprang, R., & Adams, J. (2003). Telehealth: A model for clinical supervision in allied health. *The Internet Journal of Allied Health Sciences and Practice, 1*(2), 6. Retrieved from http://nsuworks.nova.edu/ijahsp/vol1/iss2/6/

Newstrom, J. W. (2013). *Supervision: Managing for results* (10th ed.). Boston, MA: McGraw-Hill.

Precin, P. (2009). An aggregate fieldwork model: Cooperative learning, research, and clinical project publication components. *Occupational Therapy in Mental Health, 25,* 62–82.

Richard, L. F. (2008). Exploring connections between theory and practice: Stories from fieldwork supervisors. *Occupational Therapy in Mental Health, 24,* 154–175.

Sands, M. (1998). Practitioner's perspective of the occupational therapist and occupational therapy assistant partnership. In M. E. Neistadt & E. B. Crepeau (Eds.), *Willard & Spackman's occupational therapy* (9th ed., pp. 83–89). Philadelphia, PA: Lippincott.

Smith, V. (2000). Survey of occupational therapy job satisfaction in today's health care environment. *Administration & Management Special Interest Section Quarterly, 16*(4), 1–2.

Stevenson, A. (Ed.). (2010). *The new Oxford American dictionary* (3rd ed.). New York, NY: Oxford University Press.

Thomas, J. (2006). Interpreting Medicare's documentation requirements. *OT Practice, 11*(7), 8.

Urish, C. (2004). Ongoing competence through mentoring. *OT Practice, 9*(3), 10.

Waite, A. (2014). Guiding forces: Finding and benefiting from occupational therapy mentors. *OT Practice, 19*(17), 7–10.

World Federation of Occupational Therapists. (2007). *Professional OT autonomy—Revised 2007.* Retrieved from http://www.wfot /ResourceCentre/positionstatements.aspx

World Federation of Occupational Therapists. (2008). *Occupational therapy entry-level qualifications* (CM2008). Retrieved from http://www.wfot.org/ResourceCentre/positionstatements.aspx

World Federation of Occupational Therapists. (2016). *OT human resources project 2016—Numerical.* Retrieved from http://www.wfot .org/ResourceCentre/humanresourceproject.aspx

Youngstrom, M. J. (1998). Evolving competence in the practitioner role. *American Journal of Occupational Therapy, 52,* 716–720.

thePoint® *For additional resources on the subjects discussed in this chapter, visit* **http://thePoint.lww.com /Willard-Spackman13e.**

CHAPTER 73

Consulting as an Occupational Therapy Practitioner

Linda S. Fazio

LEARNING OBJECTIVES

After reading this chapter, you will be able to:

1. Analyze the skills and knowledge necessary to be successful as a consultant.
2. Appraise the content areas where occupational therapy practitioners may choose to build a career path toward consulting.
3. Distinguish between the process and the content in a consulting relationship.
4. Articulate the elements of the consulting process to include marketing, establishing consulting relationships, developing the contract for engagement, and completing the work.
5. Analyze the challenges and ethical considerations associated with the role of consultant.
6. Explore the opportunities for occupational therapy consultants to make a difference in their communities and in the world.

Introduction

This chapter discusses consultation as a role for the occupational therapist and the occupational therapy (OT) assistant. Occupational therapy practitioners have always advised and consulted with clients and patients as a primary core of their work as helping professionals. This chapter introduces the role of consulting as an extension of the helping relationship and of our work with clients and patients.

Clients and practitioners often operate within a network of complex systems. These systems impact everyday functions and thus the effectiveness of interventions. Providing supportive consultation within our own existing organizations as well as to external organizations becomes important to maximize services and support client participation.

An Overview of Consultation

Just What Is Consultation?

As we have indicated, consultation has its roots in a desire to help, and it is a collaborative process that may take place at many levels. The desire to help translates to clients, families, other professionals, organizations, and communities. Framing consultation in this way may suggest that it is a process of giving advice; something we often engage in with friends and family. It is important to remember, though, that as consultants, we are contracted to help our client reach a desired outcome, and further, we are accountable for doing so. *Accountability* distinguishes what we do as consultants from the general giving of advice. In its most general use, **consultation** describes any action one might take with a system expressing a need for assistance in moving forward (Block, 2011, p. 2). According to Block (2011), a **consultant** is a person in a position to have some influence over an individual, a group, or an organization but has no direct power to make changes or implement a program (p. 2). In this regard, a consultant may be contrasted with a manager who has direct responsibility over the actions of his or her organization's functioning in matters of change and program implementation (Braveman, 2016). Consultants typically work with managers.

In most cases, the recipients of the consultant's expertise are called clients; although in the world of management and marketing, they may be referred to as customers (Anastasi, 2014; Block, 2011). Sometimes, the client is a single individual, other times an organization, or several organizations. The client is the person or persons whom the consultant wants to influence. Schein (2016) describes consulting as the process of establishing a relationship with the client that is collaborative, personal, and empathetic rather than prescriptive (p. xiii). The consultant utilizes his or her knowledge and expertise to help the client achieve his or her goals and the goals of the organization.

What Is the Consulting Process?

The consulting process has a structure that ensures the successful completion of the work, the project. This process can be summarized through the following phases:

1. Entry into the consulting environment and establishing the agreement
2. Discovery and dialogue with the client and those who are involved in the project
3. Analysis, goal setting, and the decision to take action in one or more ways
4. Full engagement and implementation of the plan
5. Extension of the work, establishing new or altered goals, or completion of the agreement/contract (Block, 2011, pp. 6–8; Lowe, 2016, pp. 1–13).

In order to successfully complete the aforementioned phases of the work, you (as the consultant) have goals for yourself that include the following (Block, 2011, pp. 19–21):

1. Establish a collaborative relationship.
2. Help to solve problems so they stay solved.
3. Ensure attention is given to both the technical/content problem and the relationship.

Perhaps viewed from a somewhat different perspective, the purpose and process of consultation to organizations and communities is similar to our OT clinical process. When consulting to organizations and communities, we help evaluate and remediate problems, we assist in goal setting and attainment, we recommend and assist in monitoring a plan, or plans; along the way, we may offer modifications and adaptations, and we provide our specific expertise and strategies

CENTENNIAL NOTES

Committee for Installations and Advice

Lori T. Andersen

The Constitution of the National Society for the Promotion of Occupational Therapy adopted at the inaugural meeting in 1917 established a Committee for Installations and Advice specifying, "It shall be the duty of the Committee on Installations and Advice to keep in touch with the changing conditions of institutions, to formulate methods by which Occupational Therapy may be introduced, and to confer with and advise any person or body desirous of investigating Occupational Therapy" (NSPOT, 1917, pp. 9–10). Eleanor Clarke Slagle was named chairperson of this committee, consulting with numerous organizations, nationally and internationally, on developing OT programs. Additionally, she was appointed as a consultant to the Department of Reconstruction in the Public Health Service in 1920 (Slagle, 1917, 1919, 1920).

The role of occupational therapists as consultants to private organizations, industry, and government agencies has, through the years, become more formalized and has helped influence the development and direction of the profession. The Foto Group, led by past President of American Occupational Therapy Association (AOTA) Mary Foto (AOTA president 1995 to 1998), exemplifies a group of occupational therapists working in consultant roles with government, educational, private, and other organizations (Foto, 1998; The Foto Group, 2018).

(Anastasi, 2014; Block, 2011). Certainly, we alter the lives of individuals along the way, but our intent is to assist the larger organization, and often, our work extends to the needs of the community. For OT practitioners, this kind of consulting most often occurs within the organizations (hospitals, educational institutions, etc.) where they have gained experience and expertise related to practice, education, administration, or research. The previous *Centennial Vision* of the AOTA (2006) identified trending populations where occupational therapists were providing direction and gaining expertise to meet client and community needs. The populations include children and youth; mental health; rehabilitation, disability, and participation; health and wellness; productive aging; and work and industry. All of these groups function within systems which may require occupation-centered consultation in order to improve opportunities for effective and meaningful occupational participation by the target population. Change occurs at many levels.

As you develop your professional career, you will likely follow a trajectory of interest and opportunity to develop your expertise in one or more of the systems: practice, education, administration, and/or research. And, within these systems, you may choose to engage in program development (something new), program remediation (fixing something), and/or program maintenance (improving what's already there). These often represent a continuum of work. For example, in the realm of practice, you might consult to help a division develop a documentation system or improve the one they have. At another level, you may be helping a department or division become more occupation-centered, guiding them in the choice of theories, frames, and approaches. Perhaps you may help them develop new user or training manuals or other documents to improve practice. In Case Study 73-1, the therapist's knowledge and experience comes together to develop needed programming in a new context.

As you read through R.D.'s experience, you will recognize how his expertise, knowledge, and interests have evolved to prepare him for his consulting goals. You may also anticipate that he has a realistic assessment of the needs and attributes of his proposed clients. As you develop your career, you will select your advanced experience, education, and general knowledge building to prepare, and as you do so, you develop your potential as a consultant and perhaps your professional obligation to practice this role. We become subject matter experts; however, the journey from subject matter expert to valuable and trusted consultant is sometimes long and disappointing. Managing that process is as important as knowing the content you wish to share. According to Anastasi (2014), subject matter expertise for which you are hired and paid account roughly for only about 75% of what is required to deliver successful consulting professional services. The remaining skills are those that will help you successfully manage your relationship with your client(s) (p. 19).

Preparing Ourselves for Effective Consultation

Understanding Working within Systems

Our selected venues for consultation are very complex, layered, integrated systems that the consultant needs to understand. Even our designations of the larger potential systems available to us for consulting: practice, education, administration, and research are themselves so complex and interrelated, that the astute consultant must be familiar with all of them and the multisystems each of these

---

CASE STUDY 73-1　DEVELOPMENT OF A THERAPY PROGRAM FOR RETURNING VETERANS ON ISSUES OF INTIMACY AND SEXUAL FUNCTIONING

R.D. was an enlisted officer in the U.S. Army who had completed his Level II internships with the Army and who practiced 8 years as an officer/occupational therapist. He is newly retired and is planning to enter civilian practice. Over the course of his practice career, he has treated many returning combat veterans as well as active military and knows a good deal about their physical and emotional needs. He is particularly interested in sexuality and adaptations for sexual functioning. He has obtained additional certification with the Association of Sex Educators, Counselors, and Therapists (ASECT), taking continuing education courses and extensive self-study. He is thinking of opening a private practice in the community and/or

consulting to rehabilitation facilities regarding expanding their ability to meet the sexual needs of their patients. Consider some questions you might want to ask.

1. In many ways, opening a private practice and developing a consulting business involve similar skills. What might R.D. need to know? Does he need a consultant himself? How would you advise him?
2. What might be questions R.D. will have when making the transition into civilian practice? Is there information he will need? Should he begin by working in a rehabilitation facility before he ventures out on his own?

BOX 73-1　RESOURCES FOR SYSTEMS THINKING

A good deal has been written about systems, and it is wise for the reader to refresh his or her knowledge of the literature. *General systems theory* is the term used to describe the scientific efforts to identify the structural, behavioral, and developmental features of living organisms and how they influence each other (Boulding, 1956; von Bertalanffy, 1968). The use of systems thinking is a way to help us understand things that interact, to help us anticipate and prepare for possible outcomes.

Several OT authors have discussed how systems thinking relates to their work. Gray, Kennedy, and Zemke (1997) offer a good discussion of ways in which dynamic systems theory may be applied to the understanding of occupation. Fazio (2017) discusses systems thinking as a way to approach and

understand the complexity presented by community-centered program development and practice. She emphasizes how the population of interest is shaped by the environment of multiple communities and, in turn, how these communities may be altered and shaped by populations and by programming. Putting what he describes as *whole-system* process to work, Block (2011) identifies the complex process of bringing about change in a community by bringing large groups of people together, crossing boundaries to assess a situation, define a future, and talk about action toward change. Recognizing and understanding the interactive layers of community, the systems you will encounter as a consultant, regardless of the kind of work you do, create a map for you to follow that will serve you well as you help your client toward change.

---

functions within and between (Box 73-1). Consulting typically starts with investigation of the immediate environment of the client; however, it rarely ends there. The client's environment may consist of many involved agencies and organizations and, ultimately, may interact with various governmental agencies at local, state, national, and international levels. Sometimes, the client may not be fully aware how all of these interrelated systems assist or constrain the goals of his or her organization. In some cases, the environment may be fraught with ambiguity in the form of misinformation and resulting misaligned expectations. In order to assist your client, it will be your task to adapt to this environment, to come to understand its complexity, and to work effectively within it.

Understanding and Managing Change

All of consulting is about *change*, sometimes chosen and sometimes imposed. Regardless of the area where you choose to consult, you can anticipate that some or all of your client's goals will be about trying to stay afloat in a competitive marketplace. This, likely, will require all of your existing skills plus those that are specific to understanding and managing the change process (Block, 2011; Heifetz, Linsky, & Grashow, 2009). If you want to help your organization, your community, and your society thrive in the world today, you must anticipate working with the change process.

In general, there are four issues or themes common to all change efforts (Armenakis & Bedeian, 1999; Suddaby & Foster, 2016):

1. *Content issues* that focus on the substance of organizational change (i.e., more cost-effective rehabilitation service delivery)

2. *Contextual issues* that focus on the conditions existing in an organization's external and internal environments (i.e., service documentation, existing intake and discharge processes, medicare policies, etc.)

3. *Process issues* that address the actions undertaken during the enactment of an intended change (i.e., implementing changes in procedures and policies regarding documentation and service provided, etc.)

4. *Criterion issues* which deal with outcomes commonly assessed in organizational change efforts (i.e., quality of care as measured by patient responses to care, recovery rates; dollars expended and recovered) (Armenakis & Bedeian, 1999)

Levels of organizational change include individuals, groups, and larger systems. At the individual level, such actions as employee selection and sometimes replacement and displacement may be included as well as training, coaching, and counseling. Handling resistance and helping individuals cope with change is also relevant. At the group level, agendas may include team building and intergroup relations. Changes at the larger systems level will include managing the previous concerns plus the management of policy and procedures of the larger institutional influences that may be local, state, national, and international.

Organizational change management (OCM) is a structured approach in an organization for ensuring that changes are smoothly and successfully implemented and that the lasting benefits of change are achieved (Gilley, McMillen, & Gilley, 2009). *Organizational change models*, as with most other models, link theory with practice. They help us to understand what happens during the change process, why it happens, the predictability, and/or randomness of the actions and reactions (Burke, 2018, pp. 24–26). There have been numerous conceptual models for content (what to change) and process (how to change) as well as practice frameworks to explain phases of planned change such as Lewin's Three Step Model of Change (Lewin, as cited in Burke, 2018, pp. 177–179). Lewin's classic work in the 1940s and 1950s focused on changing food habits related to war needs and was described through three steps: (1) unfreezing (behaviors/thoughts), (2) changing (generally cognitive restructuring), and (3) freezing at a new level (of behavior and thinking) (or refreezing). There have been numerous other models to describe the change process, but Lewin's work is remembered as groundbreaking.

Some authors suggest that organizational change in such times of economic and political chaos is problematic at best (Pascale, Milleman, & Gioja, 2000). This coupled with the complexity and unpredictability of human behavior will ensure that the field of change management will continuously produce more frameworks to study and more models to try (Burke, 2018).

As someone who wants to consult, you likely desire to mobilize greater progress on the issues that are important to you, and in doing so, you want to strengthen your practice of leadership and you want to help others strengthen their capacity for change (Block, 2011; McKnight & Block, 2010). To do this, you will train, coach, and facilitate.

Consultation is most often about change, and change is never easy. As there are models to help us understand the dynamics of organizational change, there are models to assist us in understanding human response to the change process and how to assess whether or not members of an organization are ready for change and, further, how to help them manage inevitable change and continue to do their best work. The Transtheoretical Model of Health Behavior Change (also referred to as the *Stages of Change Model*) is one of these models (Prochaska, Norcross, & DiClemente, 1994). Although this model was designed to help practitioners understand how people made changes to negative health behavior or not, it is helpful in designing coaching programs to move employees from resistance to acceptance when institutional change is in process. This model includes six stages of the change process: precontemplation, contemplation, preparation, action, maintenance, and relapse/recycling (see Chapter 47 for a discussion of this model in the context of health promotion). There are processes associated with each of the change levels where the actions of a therapist (or therapist as consultant) may be instrumental in helping one to move forward through the stages. Particularly relevant to consulting are the stages of precontemplation, contemplation, preparation, and action. Such actions by management as offering information and answering questions early in the change process as well as involving employees in preparations for change, along with offering choice making, can help alleviate resistance and distress.

Much of our work will involve organizational change that will ultimately impact employees, participants, and shareholders among others. Attention to change management early on will help the consultant to help the client(s) anticipate and deal with change before resistance can occur. We can understand the change process and identify where people are relative to change, but that may not be enough to help us when change is inevitable as it often is in our consulting work: best to be proactive with both employees and management. Often, one of the biggest challenges for the consultant is how to manage the inevitable negotiation, resistance, and stress in response to change within an organization. As OT practitioners, we are far better prepared academically and have more therapeutic "tools" at our disposal to help people through emotionally distressing times than most other consultants.

Motivational interviewing is one of these "tools." Miller and Rollnick (2013) describe motivational interviewing as a communication style that has proven to be very useful when helping people deal with ambivalence as they struggle with change (pp. 4–5). As individuals, we often wish to change something in our lives, most often a behavior that we would like to alter or one we'd like to add. Either of these circumstances produces reluctance and ambivalence. As occupational therapists, we find motivational interviewing helpful with our clients who may need to adopt a new health promoting behavior or deal with a medication regimen that is imposed by illness and to help them identify and deal with the ambivalence they feel when making difficult health choices. Motivational interviewing has now moved beyond its initial therapeutic applications (see Chapter 48) to businesses and other organizations in an effort to help their managers and supervisors recognize ambivalence regarding change and to deal with it effectively while moving their companies forward. Forced or imposed change is one of the most difficult situations an employee may face. Even seemingly positive change opportunities offered by an employer such as a promotion may include many benefits but often carries more challenging tasks and expectations, more demands on time, and, often, work circumstances such as supervision of colleagues all of which can produce ambivalence (e.g., stay in my comfort zone or step out of it). It is in this vein that motivational interviewing is a useful communication approach for the consultant (Case Study 73-2).

The process of motivational interviewing follows the same structure regardless of the source of ambivalence. The dialogue is altered specific to the content the client/employee expresses. In addition to the earlier Miller and Rollnick (2013) reference on motivational interviewing and for examples of motivational interviewing dialogue between client and therapist, see Rosengren (2017).

CASE STUDY 73-2	HELPING FACULTY DEAL WITH THE AMBIVALENCE ASSOCIATED WITH NEW PROGRAM DEVELOPMENT

The author has consulted to several OT academic programs as they prepare to move from master's entry-level to doctoral entry-level. Often, this process is driven by administration and a few selected faculty. In many instances, there are existing faculty who hold master's degrees and have a long and productive history with the department and the college. Others may be preparing to obtain doctoral degrees but feel uncertain about their career path. If any of the faculty is restricted from the discussions and/or their opinions not validated, harmful factions may develop that can begin to involve students and much needed off-site support such as fieldwork supervisors. Bringing groups of faculty together early in the planning process, continuing on a regular basis to provide information regarding the accreditation requirements for faculty in entry-level doctoral programs, and sharing what the administration hopes to achieve with new academic programming set a precedent for transparency and support. During these meetings, the consultant uses group process/active listening and motivational interviewing to first identify where faculty demonstrate resistance. Smaller groups are then used to help faculty and staff resolve any ambivalence they may have with the assumption of new roles and responsibilities that new programming will likely require. The administrative expectations of teaching new content, initiating grant submissions and conducting research programs, and conducting on-line instruction as well as initiating and/or continuing their own doctoral education can create uncomfortable ambivalence about moving forward with an academic career particularly when the faculty member may be a caregiver of a young family. Motivational interviewing is a useful tool in that it helps individuals identify their options, determine where they are ambivalent regarding these options, and reach a solution and direction without coercion. Ultimately, the climate of the department is improved, and the process of program development can progress with fewer problems.

Foundation Skills for the Consultant

As you likely already know, there is a general business career path called *management consulting*. Most of the consultants in this career are experts in business/management/leadership and/or technology and consult to their specific expertise. Peter Block (2011) has had a long career as an author and management consultant. He describes his work as being about empowerment, stewardship, chosen accountability, and the reconciliation of community. In his continuing career, he has come to the realization that "[we] must begin to organize consulting from its' original model of providing information and solutions to one that focuses on discovering the strengths, positive examples, and "gifts" of the client organization" (Block, 2011, pp. 10–11). Differing from earlier approaches to the consulting relationship seen in management consulting, today's consultant must develop a capacity for authentic behavior, deeper relatedness, and partnership in his or her consulting roles (Block, 2011; Wickham & Wilcock, 2016). It would seem that the core beliefs of OT are now being touted as the way for consultants to make positive change in the world.

In this same vein, Edgar Schein (2016) describes what he refers to as *humble consulting*. Also a leader in organization and management, he evolved a consulting model called *Process Consultation* in 1969 which was then and still may be considered an innovative approach which involved the client in the process of figuring out what is wrong and what can be done about it. *Humble consulting*, according to Schein, "will be the new leadership skill" (p. 25). He goes on to suggest that consultants, as well, must be open, authentic, and innovative in the relationship with clients. Occupational therapy practitioners are well prepared to assume this kind of consulting relationship and as they gain information and expertise in their subject matter should have no difficulty in helping their clients meet the challenges of the evolving health and wellness industry.

Helping, Coaching, and Consultation

The prerequisite practice underlying any work with people, including consulting, is that of being mindful. Jon Kabat-Zinn (2003) offers an operational working definition of *mindfulness* as "the awareness that emerges through paying attention on purpose, in the present moment, and nonjudgmentally to the unfolding of experience moment by moment" (p. 144). Most certainly, the initial and ongoing interviews so important to the consulting process are greatly improved with active and effective listening that is companion to mindfulness (Fazio, 2017, pp. 47–48).

Listening is an art, and it is at the core of the helping relationship and the consulting relationship (Green & Howe, 2012; Maister, Green, & Galford, 2001). Active listening transforms what we might describe as simple listening to a true therapeutic skill, and it is critical to the quality of the consultant–client relationship (Figure 73-1).

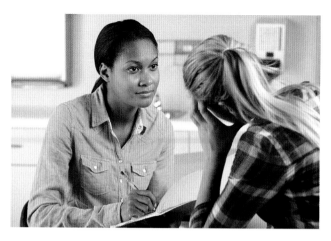

FIGURE 73-1 Active listening is a therapeutic skill that is critical to the act of coaching.

Mindfulness, active listening, and a genuine desire to help come together in what may be described as the act of coaching. Elements of coaching such as empowering and supporting can be useful in forming and maintaining the consulting relationship with our client(s).

As mentioned previously, occupational therapists and occupational therapy assistants are quite comfortable in the helping skills that are coming somewhat late to the world of the management consultant. We know how to actively listen to people and how to communicate, and we have worked to develop our therapeutic self. See Chapter 37 for Renée Taylor's detailed discussion of the intentional relationship that is yet another way to frame the skills and knowledge that come together to inform our work as therapists and as consultants.

We have the foundation skills to effectively communicate with people, and it's critical to remember these are important and not to be abandoned because we think our consulting process is different than our therapy process. Although we will layer other skills on top of these, our core caring and helping skills are our strengths (Box 73-2).

BOX 73-2	WILL YOU BE A GOOD CONSULTANT?

As you're learning more about what it means to be a consultant, consider these basic questions:

- Are you a good manager of time and tasks?
- Are you a good communicator?
- Can you negotiate?
- Are you assertive?
- Do you know your strengths? Your limitations?
- Do you know your biases?

The Professional Parameters for Consulting

Getting Started

Occupational therapy consultants must first have a firm foundation in the theories and skills that support entry-level practice. An awareness of our professional history is also useful in that what we think is new likely happened before, and there's always something to learn from a remix of content and context. Beyond this, most consultants have some years of clinical practice, and many have achieved advanced education and practice in one or more areas of interest. Advanced doctoral education is common for those who consult in education and in research. Consulting in community programming and nonprofit development is being done by all levels of practitioner generally with an entrepreneur's ability to explore and learn as you go.

Alongside your foundation knowledge and skills, you have established a professional arena where you are comfortable with your expertise. How do you get started consulting? First, there are some questions to answer: Am I thinking about this because someone asked for my help in my own organization?

The facility where I am working has asked me to develop an outpatient program at a sister facility or a new clinic at my own facility.

Maybe, it doesn't sound like it, but this is consulting. This is a common beginning, and similar experiences are often bulleted on our resumes when we begin to consult more widely or open our own freestanding consulting business. There are certainly differences when we are *consulting* as part of our present employment, but when we outline the structure of the consultation process, you'll see that the nature of the consulting relationship when it is a support function inside an organization may be similar in many ways to what we would experience in external consultation.

I've developed significant knowledge and experience and I'm ready to share it outside my own organization.

This one may get at our motivation for consulting a little more directly. I would assume that you wouldn't consult outside of your expertise. Review your targeted resume, does it show this expertise? Have you published? Presented at conferences? Maybe your expertise is in helping an organization develop an effective fieldwork/internship/residence model. Have you functioned as an internship supervisor? As an academic fieldwork coordinator? Have you developed an innovative program that assists the student, the academic institution, and the facility? Perhaps the profession? See Case Study 73-3.

For many of us, consulting opportunities came to us through our professional networks. Presenting posters or

CASE STUDY 73-3   A CAREER PATH LEADING TO EXPERT CONSULTATION IN CLINICAL INTERNSHIP DESIGN

J.A. is an occupational therapist with 9 years of practice experience in adult rehabilitation. Seven of those years, she also supervised Level I and Level II OT and OT assistant fieldwork students. Two years ago, she completed her occupational therapy post-professional doctorate with specialty in fieldwork supervision. She is now a clinical faculty member in an OT academic program, and she is the academic fieldwork coordinator (AFC). She has always been an active member of AOTA and her state association, and she has frequently presented posters on fieldwork supervision and fieldwork programming topics at national and state meetings.

1. Is J.A. ready to market herself to other academic programs and/or facilities offering fieldwork to OT and OT assistant students?
2. Do you think there may be gaps in her experience? If so, what might they be and how can she better prepare as a consultant?

workshops at state, national, and perhaps international conferences may have offered our first consulting invitations outside of our internal employment. The author served much of her professional career in volunteer-appointed and elected positions for AOTA and state agencies and associations. In these roles, she gained significant expertise and knowledge but also expanded her professional networks. Some consultants choose to actively market their services, often through social media, particularly those who develop consulting businesses. When people need consultants, they tend to contact each other for recommendations so the more you work, the more work you'll have. In the world of marketing, there is nothing more powerful than a personal recommendation (Lowe, 2016; Weiss, 2009).

Documents to Initiate and Support the Consulting Relationship

Developing a Proposal for Your Work

In our first scenario earlier, being asked to consult within your own facility, it might seem like we can skip the preliminary steps but not so; we need to establish parameters. At this juncture, you know that someone trusts that you have the knowledge and expertise to complete a task within a specified time frame for a specific amount of money; maybe you don't know for how much money that can sometimes be difficult but will need to be resolved. You also know that when you do a good job, they will likely recommend you for other consulting.

The strongest points for marketing yourself are what Fazio (2017) describes as *personal selling*. You represent yourself as a professional with skills and expertise, and most of all, you have unfailing integrity. You do what you promise, and you don't promise what you can't do.

You have the basic information that you need so this is likely the point where you sit down with your client(s) for the first time and you have the *engagement kick-off* meeting. This is where you identify and begin to manage inherent expectations for the outcome and your ability to bring it about. You have likely already gleaned information from your first contact person and perhaps others in the organization. There are always inherent expectations and preconceptions for what needs to be done, and what you can and will offer. This meeting brings these expectations to the surface so that they can be managed before the work is detailed in a more formal document that will follow.

Following the first meeting with your potential client(s), it is usually advisable to draft a *proposal* of work that can be done and that you are recommending. This can also occur if you've had an inquiry received by telephone or e-mail or even a brief in-person encounter, perhaps at a conference. The proposal isn't a finished document and will likely be altered by both your client and by you but rather is a summation that will precede further written agreements. You may wish to ask for a meeting, or a conference call, after your client(s) have read the proposal. This meeting will be a continuation of your proposal process.

Weiss (2009) warns that the proposal is never intended to be confused with a contract; rather, it serves to place the earlier brief discussion in context with the other elements of the proposal (accountabilities, terms, etc.) (p. 147). In some cases, the proposal may take the form of a **letter of intent (LOI)** or a **memorandum of understanding (MOU)**. Neither of these is a contract; however, they may be used in lieu of a proposal. In most cases, there is a good deal of verbal exchange during this process. Whether or not you end the agreement process with a thorough statement of work followed by a formal and legal contract is usually the decision of your client, however, with your approval.

If you are taking on a project for your present employer (as we described previously), you are a consultant, and you should have a document that describes the scope of the work, the proposed outcome, and the pay (or release time). Depending on your circumstances, this may be more of a social contract with a present employer designed not so much for enforcement but for clear communication.

Developing the Statement of Work

Together with the people who are hiring you, your client or clients, you now create a detailed **statement of work (SOW)** (Lowe, 2016). This document follows the proposal that some consultants wish to have signed by the client(s). Others choose not to have a signature but rather rely on the several discussions that have resulted in a proposal that all parties verbally agree on and is now the basis for the more formal SOW. Some authors refer to the culmination of the proposal in a document referred to as a *conceptual agreement* (Biswas & Twitchell, 2002, p. 36; Weiss, 2009, p. 138). In this more informal written agreement, you and your potential client(s) agree on these basic issues (Weiss, 2009, pp. 138–139):

- What are the objectives to be achieved through this project?
- How will progress be measured? How will success be measured?
- What is the value or impact of the project to the organization?

Your client's most critical expectations are written into your SOW and your contract if such is used. Your final SOW or contract details the *scope* of your engagement, the necessary *effort* required for you and your client(s) to achieve it, and the expected *time* for that effort to be exerted. Sometimes referred to as the *triple constraints*, these three elements combine together to create the overall quality of the service being provided (Anastasi, 2014, pp. 105–106). This interdependence means that if any one ingredient shifts during the course of the work, the others must also shift proportionally to compensate and ensure that the level of quality is retained.

Figure 73-2 illustrates the relationship between scope, effort, and time as they influence the quality of the consulting work/product. It is in the elements of the triple constraints that client expectations may become misaligned if the written agreements lack specificity. If false expectations surface, the consultant must address them immediately even for something as seemingly simple as the client expecting you to deliver a document on Tuesday, and you plan to send it on Thursday. Lowe (2016) suggests that a significant function of a detailed SOW is to clear assumptions. Something as simple as who provides the word processing can become a major barrier, as can who covers travel expenses.

Anastasi (2014) also describes the nature of the SOW, and most importantly, he sees it as the first version of *done*. By that, he means that this agreement not only initiates the work together but most significantly

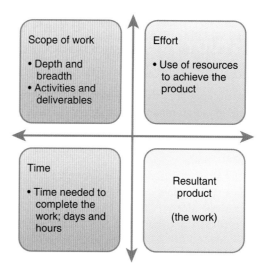

FIGURE 73-2 Combined constraints and quality of the consulting work.

also makes clear how everyone will know the project is finished (Box 73-3).

Anastasi (2014) suggests that, in its' simplest form, the first written agreement generated should include the following:

- A detailed description of the engagement (the *scope* of an engagement)
- The effort it is expected to take to achieve the scope
- The price to be charged

In a very large project that may include several phases over the course of a year or years to complete, a *pilot* may be conducted to assist both the consultant and the client. This is particularly true if you are developing something

BOX 73-3 WHEN IS IT DONE?

Early on, the author consulted via verbal agreements and very quickly realized that there was always "one more thing to do." There had been no hard and fast agreement on what *done* looked like! Knowing what *done* looks like requires that everyone (consultant and client[s]) understands the mutually agreed criteria that will determine the engagements successful conclusion. If your client is more than one person or agency, you likely have many two-way communications, and with each of these misunderstandings can be generated about just when the project is completed/done. In some cases, you may actually have several different clients within the same consulting situation. In academic settings, you may be reporting to the chair of the department, the dean of the division, and sometimes the president of the university, all with their own agendas and "to do lists." Whenever possible, reduce the lines of communication and/or generate separate SOWs.

(i.e., a program, curriculum, course, or a product). If you choose to do a pilot, an SOW is developed for it that is separate from the SOW for the completed, full project. The purpose of the pilot is to validate or define assumptions, risks, estimates, and schedules/timelines.

Neither the SOW nor the conceptual agreements are legal documents that are enforceable in a court of law. Therefore, the next step is the formal, legal contract; however, in some cases, no legal contract is generated, and the work proceeds following agreement and signatures on the detailed SOW. This is acceptable, particularly if you have worked together without problems before. Ultimately, you hope that your client will engage you for repeat business because they were delighted with your first work together. Subsequent engagements are almost always calmer and more effective environments to work in. If you mutually agree to continue to work together without a legal contract and as your work together commences, it is possible that new tasks will emerge either recognized by you or your client. If this is the case, a new SOW will need to be generated and signed by both parties.

If you choose to use a formal contract, this final legal agreement provides a clear vision of the plan to complete the project and to ensure that the vision to complete the engagement aligns perfectly with the previous discussions and the earlier proposed plan.

Legal Contracts

Anastasi (2014) cautions the consultant that an explicit and detailed contract is critical because it is the most effective way to manage expectations for all concerned (p. 126). When the contract is being drafted, using a simple formula to be sure you've included everything is recommended. Identifying *who*, *what*, *when*, and *how* is important (Anastasi, 2014; Biswas & Twitchell, 2002; Nelson & Economy, 2008). Anastasi suggests that there are actually three *how's* to consider: *how well* (refers to the expectations for quality of the draft [or] finished document), *how will it be delivered* (in a meeting?), and *how much* (the price/cost to be paid for the deliverable product) (pp. 124–125).

Block (2011) describes the formal contract as simply an explicit agreement of what the consultant and client expect from each other and how they are going to work together (p. 52). He goes on to suggest that contracts with external consultants who are not well known by the client are more often formal because they are trusted less, especially when it comes to money (Block, 2011, p. 52).

Following the Statement of Work

The author's consulting experience has been primarily in community and academic program design, support, and development. This work is generally initiated with a SOW and often a formal contract. Sometimes a proposal is developed early on particularly when there is more than one client, which is often the case, and substantial negotiations are required. The actual work most often begins with a series of interviews with all persons involved who will continue to carry out the work and sustain the project following the consultant's exit. These interviews are critical, and you may wish to review the characteristics of conducting good interviews (Fazio, 2017, pp. 123–124; Rasiel, 1999, pp. 77–92). Alongside are interviews with stakeholders. In an academic setting, these may be facilities offering fieldwork and potential employers. These interviews are part of the need and asset assessment and are important to any consultant who is developing or helping to improve an OT practice, an educational program, a research program, or an administrative structure or network. For the external consultant, these interviews help you to understand the *engagement environment* where you will do your work (Anastasi, 2014, pp. 23–39). Each setting and work environment is different, and to help them achieve their goals, it is important to understand how they function. Who does what? Who has control? How they deal with change? A detailed description of this kind of need and asset assessment is provided by Fazio (2017, pp. 135–147). Beginning with a series of interviews is not as common in management consulting where it's more likely work is initiated with only one or two representatives from the company/organization as the client. Because sustainability is so important to social entrepreneurship and community-based not-for-profit consulting, all of the stakeholders are identified and involved early on, and there is likely more transparency than there might be in for-profit business environments. If you feel that early interviews will be helpful to your process, always come to agreement regarding the details with your client(s). They will be needed to assist you with identification of whom to interview and to help you gain access.

In community and academic program development, as well as in the other areas where OT practitioners consult, there are a number of actions and resulting documents to generate in a sequential order, and the timeline for these is an important part of the SOW. Your client likely is not aware of these time commitments, and it must be made clear. These may be accreditation applications, grant and funding applications, certification and credentialing for organizations and for people, and public relations actions and documents as well as formal and informal communications within and between involved organizations. All communications (paper and electronic) are retained and tracked. In all of the author's consulting, an externally imposed timeline has been critical to the process, and it is generally in regard to the above actions and accompanying applications and documents. The generation of all of these processes and documents relies on the cooperation of your client(s) (the organization or organizations and their administrators and employees) which further validates the importance of your early need and asset assessment process where you are meeting people and, in the process of doing so, demonstrating your integrity and your skills as well as your commitment to their goals that you share.

Clients change their minds and may often have unrealistic expectations of the time and funds required to achieve their desired goals. These are their goals, not yours, but most clients rely on you to help refine them and make them measurable and achievable. Any change that may occur to goals and therefore *done* along the way requires change management at a contract level. Any change to *done* will also create a new and differing version of the contract (i.e., done 1.0, done 1.1, etc.). If these new versions require approval by one or more people, then you will want to keep a written history of their status and note when they are actually approved.

When you have developed your expertise in one or more of the suggested consultation practice settings (practice, education, administration, research), you will recognize the nature of the *content* work you will need to do in response to a consultative request; therefore, it is not discussed at length here.

Challenges to Consider in Bringing All Consultation Projects to Completion

Controlling Chaos

Chaos isn't a given in consulting arrangements but can often occur and derail a project. Most consultants would say that you begin with good communication with your client. This will include meetings, e-mails, and phone calls to maintain an open and two-way communication at all times (Block, 2011; Lowe, 2016). Controlling chaos begins with your first conversation, what Block (2011) refers to as the discovery period of the developing consultation relationship. Discovery, for you, will include the following (Block, 2011, pp. 41–42):

- Negotiating client wants
- Coping with mixed motivation that may be demonstrated by a client
- Bringing client concerns about exposure and loss of control to the surface
- Understanding how many clients you actually have and putting them all in your contract

The client has responsibilities as well in this discovery process. Typically, a client commits to providing the following during your work together (Anastasi, 2014; Block, 2011; Robinson, Robinson, Phillips, Phillips, & Handshaw, 2015):

- To provide feedback on anything pertinent to achieving outcomes in a timely and specific manner
- To provide a safe and professional work environment as necessary

- To provide access to the necessary employees, administrators, sometimes also stakeholders and others such as advisory board members
- To agree to and sign off documents and specifications in a timely manner
- To provide people and materials necessary to assist in making decisions or completing products
- To provide the agreed on resources so that work can proceed according to the timeline
- To pay for your services in accordance with the terms of the contract

Chaos and problems in your consulting relationship often can be a direct result of your inability to manage the project. Projects and their progress and outcomes are an extension of the way you, the consultant, work. If you tend not to respond to deadlines or manage your own life very well, then you may not be ready to help larger groups attain their goals (Hattori, 2015; Rasiel & Friga, 2002). This is something to consider carefully as you review your skills and attributes in preparation to consult.

Managing Expectations, Assumptions, and Difficult Conversations

Management consultants talk about honesty and integrity as foundation skills for the consultant and the need to have difficult conversations early on as well as managing the expectations of your client(s) (Anastasi, 2014; Beck, 2013; Block, 2011; Lowe, 2016). It is important to remember that you, the consultant, have assumptions, expectations, and perhaps biases. Know what they are and try to work through them to stay focused on the client and his or her needs. One of the most difficult conversations you may have either early on or midway through the process is to correct a misalignment in expectations for what the finished product will include. This isn't easy because likely, either you or your client or both of you will have to accept a different, perhaps less optimal, outcome than what you are currently expecting. This is less likely if you have a well-developed SOW and contract; however, there are often extenuating circumstances beyond anyone's control. Anastasi (2014) suggests that "a consultants true worth is measured by the speed at which issues are brought to the customer's attention regardless of who is at fault, or the difficulty of the conversation" (p. 134). Remember that your client is taking risks. It is your task, as the consultant, to mitigate these risks. In our work, that element of risk often extends beyond the immediate client. As a consultant in educational program design and implementation, the potential risk can extend from the level of the department or school to the college and to the university and may ultimately risk the integrity of the profession and the multiple contributors and consumers of each. You can see how consulting in any of our OT and occupation-centered arenas can have similar potential for risk. To handle difficult concerns and misalignment of goals, go to your clinical (listening) skills—empathy, understanding, and resolution. With patients or consulting clients, this is the best way to approach and guide difficult conversations toward a successful outcome.

Establishing Costs and Fees

For most of our early consulting projects, our consulting costs are composed of our fee, travel, and our communications. As you continue to consult, you will be far better able to anticipate a fairly accurate budget, although there may still be some unanticipated surprises. With experience, you'll come to a point where you know well what a project is worth and how much time and work it will require, particularly if you specialize in an area and consult with different organizations. Certainly, not all organizations you choose to consult with have similar monies in their budgets, particularly for consultants. If you consult with nonprofit organizations, you likely know this well, although the designation of nonprofit isn't necessarily synonymous with poor funding (McKenna, 2010; Meehan & Jonker, 2017a).

Some would suggest that the first "difficult conversation" you may have is the negotiation of your fee (Lowe, 2016; Meehan & Jonker, 2017b). Of course, your fee is first specified in the SOW when you define the deliverables of the project and establish the estimated timeline to completion of the project (when it is *done*). How and when you will be paid is included as well. Many consultants prefer to be paid in phases, receiving payment in advance of the completion of the phase. This reduces risk for all parties involved (Anastasi, 2014; Lowe, 2016).

Consulting fees are subjective, and consultants are usually not forthcoming when it comes to disclosing their fees. You can ask around, particularly of those who have hired consultants who do what you are proposing, and you may be able to get a range for hourly or project task fees. It is seldom that consultants work for hourly fees but rather charge completion fees for phases of the project, or for small projects one fee. Some do work for a daily fee for a small project or a phase of a larger project (such as conducting training sessions for staff). There are resources to help you set your fees (Meehan & Jonker, 2017b; Nelson & Economy, 2008); however, tapping into your professional network may be a better resource.

Consultants and those in the helping professions, most particularly, sometimes find it difficult to put a price on their "helping." These charitable tendencies don't work as a consultant, and if your consultancy is your business, they really don't work. Working pro bono is most likely to occur with a pilot, or not charging for a needs assessment or other preliminary work, paying project-necessary travel out of your own pocket, and/or not charging for changes in the project. If changes occur in the process, meet with your client and reach a solution. If you're responsible for the change (i.e., you missed a deadline, such as an application or certification) and the timeline is pushed forward, then you should absorb the cost of the delay. Your SOW should specify how you will deal with changes and when the client might be assessed an additional fee. Occasionally, things happen that can't be avoided, and neither you nor the client is responsible. On one occasion, a project the author was working on was severely delayed because of a hurricane and resultant flooding.

It is common that there is not sufficient information when the SOW is drafted to accurately estimate the cost/budget (your fee and project costs). However, it is often an assumption of the client that the estimated fee is the actual fee, and it prompts a breach in communications if you must come in later with a fee adjustment (and this is seldom lower than your SOW estimate). Thus, it is better to be specific that the fee/cost quotes may change once the needs assessment and analysis of the project details are complete and assumptions are validated. Do this verbally as well as point it out in your written agreement. Your client has a budget for this project but may not have any idea what it will actually cost.

Lowe (2016) suggests that the estimate of fees and costs of the project can be managed better if they are presented and managed in phases. When the first phase is done (i.e., needs and assets assessment), the project is reestimated, and if needed, an adjustment is made to your fee and/or the cost budget you've developed for the project, the cost budget your client has approved.

One other area where confusion may occur is in the management of actual materials you may produce as part of your work. Other than publicly available materials, no other documentation, preexisting or created specifically for the client, should exchange hands. If you are providing materials as part of the agreed on contract, then you will specify how that material will be used. If the information/documents/handbooks/manuals are deemed your own intellectual property in the contract, they are protected from plagiarism, inappropriate use, or that your clients could sell or publish the information as their own.

Consulting with a Board or Large Group of Participants: Managing Meetings for Action

When possible, it is more efficient for the consultant to report to one person who will then share findings with other board or organization members and stakeholders rather than hold meetings with large groups. The author's experience consulting in academic settings as well as in community settings has suggested that larger report meetings where everyone involved has the opportunity to hear what is happening directly from the consultant as well as provide feedback maintains a much better engagement environment, helping to avoid resistance, frustration, and false assumption about outcomes. Meetings of this nature function like a large focus group or town hall and require more skill in managing them than a simple report meeting. Preparing carefully and conducting a meeting, whether large or small, is a critical skill that all consultants must master (Robinson et al., 2015). In addition, developing comfort in public speaking and developing presentations contributes greatly to a good meeting (Adler, Elmhorst, & Lucas, 2013).

Wide participation and transparency about the work of the organization and the consultant require direction by an administrator who is comfortable with such a structure. This is not always the case, and the consultant needs to be aware of the administrator's style and work with it. The SOW will specify the kind of reporting the consultant will recommend and will help to avoid any confusion.

Ethical Responsibilities of the Consultant: Building Credibility and Trust

Consultants have an obligation to provide services that meet the standards for the profession. The work of occupational therapists enacts a unique form of justice centered on capabilities and opportunities for individuals and for groups to engage in occupations (AOTA, 2015; World Federation of Occupational Therapists [WFOT], 2016). Throughout this chapter, we've discussed numerous situations where the consultant's ethical responsibilities may be challenged and/or compromised. Consultants are more likely to work alone as they engage in the consulting process and, inevitably may not fully appreciate the complexity involved in working within so many systems. The role of consultant that some describe as expert advisor can create situations where the pressure to provide services creates an environment fraught with potential ethical problems and dilemmas (Purtillo, 2005). As the consultant, you are generally considered the expert. As the *expert*, your clients are relying on your ability to guide them to realistic and achievable expectations while delivering on your commitment to their success. *Guide* is an important word here. As a consultant, you may be an expert, but you

seldom have all the answers; however, you can likely find the answers through your clients and their participants and your own colleagues and resources. The challenges of the consulting relationship and your need to help may test your integrity; best to hold fast and admit you don't know something, but that you can find out. Regardless of the practice area, OT practitioners always demonstrate personal integrity, reliability, open-mindedness, and loyalty in all aspects of their professional roles (WFOT, 2016). As the consultant builds a relationship with the client, he or she becomes a *trusted (accountable) advisor* and, as such, assumes responsibility for at least half of the engagement relationship (Maister et al., 2001, pp. 85–90). Building credibility and trust is never ending; each communication and transaction is carefully crafted and articulated, the best that you can offer (Robinson et al., 2015; Verlander, 2012). It is critical that all practitioners, consultants, and private practitioners, in particular, understand ethical principles and related standards so that they are prepared to resolve ethical dilemmas that may occur (See Chapter 36 for an in-depth discussion of ethics as they may apply to the OT practitioner).

⚖ ETHICAL **DILEMMA**

Consulting on Grant Development and Applications

T.R. is an academic instructor who also directs two training grants and one research grant for the department of occupational therapy and the university where she is employed. She is a credentialed occupational therapist, and although she has limited practice experience with patients, beyond her Level II fieldwork, she has utilized patients in numerous research studies so is familiar with the conditions occupational therapists treat. T.R. also serves on a prestigious National Institute of Mental Health (NIMH) committee and has experience reviewing grant applications. She has been asked to assist faculty in another academic institution (one of who is a colleague) to become more proficient in federal grant applications. T.R. would be paid a salary as a consultant and/or a visiting instructor to do this. There are several possible ethical dilemmas here, but maybe not? Consider these questions:

1. Just what are the potential ethical dilemmas in this scenario?
2. Which principles of the Occupational Therapy Code of Ethics and Ethics Standards (AOTA, 2015) are relevant to consider?
3. What additional information might you need to better evaluate whether or not there are actual ethical concerns?
4. How should T.R. proceed moving forward?

Consulting as a Business

A number of authors have written about consulting as a business (Block, 2011; Lowe, 2016; Weiss, 2009). And, for the most part, the actual work of consulting doesn't vary from what has been described in this chapter. The differences are in the process of starting a business and likely won't be greatly different than what you would need to know and do to start your own practice. Weiss (2009) points out that in starting a business, any business, you must first establish your goals and expectations and determine whether or not you're willing to do what's necessary to meet them (pp. 2–21). With any new venture, such as this, a trusted mentor is a prerequisite, not just about the business but about the personal investment that is necessary to make it successful. As with any freestanding business, you'll need a physical space, you'll likely need financial and legal assistance, and you'll need a good business plan and marketing strategy. You'll also need good self-management strategies and be willing to prioritize your time to support the business, at least until you hire additional people.

The Consultant as Social Entrepreneur

In recent years, the term *social entrepreneur* has become a popular way to define those entrepreneurs who have the public good as their agenda. Scofield (2011) refers to this as "righting the unrightable wrong and finding your mission possible" (p. 1). He goes on to say that it's likely that many of these social entrepreneurs will come from the health care sector where they have been exposed to frequent inequities in the distribution of opportunity for health promoting environments. Block (2011) has identified both health care and education as two sectors of society where the call for change and reform has been blatant for years (pp. xiv–xv). The OT practitioner fits this description, and many are being prepared for this entrepreneurial work in their basic education as they develop the skills and knowledge for program design and development, particularly those who are engaged in OT doctoral education (Fazio, 2017). It makes sense that as these students enter the practice environment, they will gravitate toward social entrepreneurship and/or engage in the consulting role to bring about positive change wherever they choose to work.

Conclusion

Providing consultation in a chosen area of expertise offers the opportunity for OT practitioners to extend their ability to make a difference in the world. As consultants, these practitioners have become proficient in a content area and use their substantial helping and relationship-building skills and knowledge to influence the process that brings the content forward. Content areas may include one or more of the following: practice, education, administration/supervision, and research. We have borrowed the structure of the consulting model from the disciplines of business and leadership/management consulting, but it is through our own foundational knowledge and skill building in the attributes of the "helping relationship" that we bring our own professional uniqueness to the consulting relationship.

REFERENCES

Adler, R., Elmhorst, J., & Lucas, K. (2013). *Communicating at work: Strategies for success in business and the professions* (11th ed.). New York, NY: McGraw-Hill.

American Occupational Therapy Association. (2006). *Centennial vision*. Bethesda, MD: Author.

American Occupational Therapy Association. (2015). Occupational therapy code of ethics (2015). *American Journal of Occupational Therapy*, 69, 6913410030p1–6913410030p8. doi:10.5014/ajot.2015.696S03

Anastasi, S. (2014). *The seven principles of professional services*. Chicago, IL: PS Principles.

Armenakis, A., & Bedeian, A. (1999). Organizational change: A review of theory and research in the 1990's. *Journal of Management*, 25, 293.

Beck, H. P. (2013). *Management consulting essentials*. Klampenborg, Denmark: TBK Consult.

Biswas, S., & Twitchell, D. (2002). *Management consulting: A complete guide to the industry*. New York, NY: Wiley.

Block, P. (2011). *Flawless consulting: A guide to getting your expertise used* (3rd ed.). San Francisco, CA: Jossey-Bass.

Boulding, K. E. (1956). General systems theory: The skeleton of science. *Management Science*, 2, 197–208.

Braveman, B. (2016). *Leading & managing occupational therapy services: An evidence-based approach* (2nd ed.). Philadelphia, PA: F. A. Davis.

Burke, W. (2018). *Organization change: Theory and practice* (5th ed.). Thousand Oaks, CA: Sage.

Fazio, L. S. (2017). *Developing occupation-centered programs with the community* (3rd ed.). Thorofare, NJ: SLACK.

Foto, M. (1998). Competence and the occupational therapy entrepreneur. *American Journal of Occupational Therapy*, 52, 765–769. doi:10.5014/ajot.52.9.765

Gilley, A., McMillen, H., & Gilley, J. (2009). Organizational change and characteristics of leadership effectiveness. *Journal of Leadership and Organizational Studies*, 16, 38–47.

Gray, J. M., Kennedy, B. L., & Zemke, R. (1997). Application of dynamic systems theory to occupation. In R. Zemke & J. F. Clark (Eds.), *Occupational science: The evolving discipline* (pp. 309–324). Philadelphia, PA: F. A. Davis.

Green, C. H., & Howe, A. P. (2012). *The trusted advisor fieldbook: A comprehensive toolkit for leading with trust*. Hoboken, NJ: Wiley.

Hattori, S. (2015). *The McKinsey edge: Success principles from the world's most powerful consulting firm*. New York, NY: McGraw-Hill.

Heifetz, R., Linsky, R. A., & Grashow, A. (2009). *The practice of adaptive leadership: Tools and tactics for changing your organization and the world*. Boston, MA: Harvard Business Press.

Kabat-Zinn, J. (2003). Mindfulness-based interventions in context: Past, present, and future. *Clinical Psychology: Science and Practice*, 10, 144–156.

Lowe, R. (2016). *How to manage a consulting project*. San Bernardino, CA: The Writing King.

Maister, D., Green, C., & Galford, R. (2001). *The trusted advisor.* New York, NY: Simon & Schuster.

McKenna, C. D. (2010). *The world's newest profession: Management consulting in the twentieth century.* New York, NY: Cambridge University Press.

McKnight, J., & Block, P. (2010). *The abundant community: Awakening the power of families and neighborhoods.* San Francisco, CA: Berrett-Koehler.

Meehan, W. F., & Jonker, K. (2017a). *Engine of impact: Essentials of strategic leadership in the nonprofit sector.* Palo Alto, CA: Stanford Business Books.

Meehan, W. F., & Jonker, K. (2017b). *The four questions to ask when serving on a nonprofit board.* Palo Alto, CA: Stanford Business Books.

Miller, W., & Rollnick, S. (2013). *Motivational interviewing: Helping people change* (3rd ed.). New York, NY: Guilford Press.

National Society for the Promotion of Occupational Therapy. (1917). *Constitution of the National Society for the Promotion of Occupational Therapy.* Baltimore, MD: Sheppard Hospital Press.

Nelson, B., & Economy, P. (2008). *Consulting for dummies* (2nd ed.). Hoboken, NJ: Wiley.

Pascale, R., Milleman, M., & Gioja, L. (2000). *Surfing the edge of chaos: The laws of nature and the new laws of business.* New York, NY: Random House.

Prochaska, J., Norcross, J., & DiClemente, C. (1994). *Changing for good: A revolutionary six-stage program for overcoming bad habits and moving your life positively forward.* New York, NY: HarperCollins.

Purtillo, R. (2005). *Ethical dimensions in the health professions* (4th ed.). Philadelphia, PA: Elsevier Saunders.

Rasiel, E. (1999). *The McKinsey way.* New York, NY: McGraw-Hill.

Rasiel, E., & Friga, P. (2002). *The McKinsey mind: Understanding and implementing the problem-solving tools and management techniques of the world's top strategic consulting firm.* New York, NY: McGraw-Hill.

Robinson, D. G., Robinson, J. C., Phillips, J. J., Phillips, P. P., & Handshaw, D. (2015). *Performance consulting: A strategic process to improve, measure, and sustain organizational results.* Oakland, CA: Berrett-Koehler.

Rosengren, D. B. (2017). *Building motivational interviewing skills: A practitioner workbook* (2nd ed.). New York, NY: Guilford Press.

Schein, E. (2016). *Humble consulting: How to provide real help faster.* Oakland, CA: Berrett-Koehler.

Scofield, R. (2011). *The social entrepreneur's handbook: How to start, build, and run a business that improves the world.* New York, NY: McGraw-Hill.

Slagle, E. C. (1917). Report of the Committee on Installations and Advice. In *Proceedings of the First Annual Meeting of the National Society for the Promotion of Occupational Therapy* (p. 28). Towson, MD: Spring Grove State Hospital and Sheppard and Enoch Pratt Hospital.

Slagle, E. C. (1919). Report of the Committee on Installations and Advice. In *Proceedings of the Third Annual Meeting of the National Society for the Promotion of Occupational Therapy* (pp. 26–28). Towson, MD: Spring Grove State Hospital and Sheppard and Enoch Pratt Hospital.

Slagle, E. C. (1920). Report of the Committee on Installations and Advice. In *Proceedings of the Fourth Annual Meeting of the National Society for the Promotion of Occupational Therapy* (p. 22). Towson, MD: Spring Grove State Hospital and Sheppard and Enoch Pratt Hospital.

Suddaby, R., & Foster, W. (2016). History and organizational change. *Journal of Management, 43,* 19–38.

The Foto Group. (2018). *The Foto Group.* Retrieved from http://www.thefotogroup.com/default.aspx

Verlander, E. G. (2012). *The practice of professional consulting: The journey of the trusted consultant.* San Francisco, CA: Wiley.

von Bertalanffy, L. (1968). *General systems theory: Foundations, development, and applications.* New York, NY: Braziller.

Weiss, A. (2009). *Getting started in consulting* (3rd ed.). Hoboken, NJ: Wiley.

Wickham, L., & Wilcock, J. (2016). *Management consulting: Delivering an effective project* (5th ed.). London, United Kingdom: Pearson.

World Federation of Occupational Therapists. (2016). *World Federation of Occupational Therapists code of ethics.* Retrieved from http://www.wfot.org/ResourceCentre/tabid/132/did/780/Default.aspx

the**Point**® *For additional resources on the subjects discussed in this chapter, visit* **http://thePoint.lww.com/Willard-Spackman13e.**

CHAPTER 74

Payment for Services in the United States

Helene Lohman, Angela Lampe, Angela Patterson

LEARNING OBJECTIVES

After reading this chapter, you will be able to:

1. Describe the impact of policy related to payment of occupational therapy (OT) services in the U.S.
2. Explain the key types of payment accessed by clients in OT practice.
3. Comprehend payment terminology for Medicare reimbursement.
4. Distinguish between skilled and unskilled services.
5. Discuss emerging payment systems in the U.S.
6. Explain the status of the uninsured and underinsured in the U.S. and what practitioners can do to advocate for reimbursement of OT services.
7. Discuss how practitioners can be advocates for clients related to payment issues impacting practice.

Introduction: Overview of Payment

With nearly 18% of the American gross domestic product, approximately $3.2 trillion dollars, spent on health care (Centers for Disease Control and Prevention [CDC], 2017), payment for health care is of high importance to many stakeholders, including occupational therapy (OT) practitioners. Payment structures and systems change frequently. All practitioners must be knowledgeable about payment sources, have a professional responsibility to understand how payment systems influence practice, and advocate for payment of needed services. Some practitioners may depend on the facility's billing department or the therapy manager to keep them abreast of payment policies and procedures, but regardless they should stay informed (Sieck, Lohman, Stupica, Minthorne-Brown, & Stoffer, 2017). Other practitioners, who handle their own billing for services, must be intimately aware of the regulations affecting payment.

A Historical Look at How Policy Has Influenced Payment

Legislation, the economy, and technology have all influenced the profession of OT. The success of any profession depends on how well it responds to and adapts to such changes. Since the inception of OT in 1917, numerous forces have influenced its trajectory. The major events that have influenced OT payment and practice beginning with the growth of private insurance in the 1940s are summarized in a table on thePoint. Prior to the growth of private insurance, OT services were paid for from the hospital charges and in other settings services were paid out of pocket or provided free of charge (V. Gessert, personal communication, February 15, 2017).

Types of Payment

This section briefly describes varied methods of payment for OT services. The status of how Americans are insured is presented in Figure 74-1 to guide this discussion. Figure 74-2 presents national spending figures of where the nation's health care dollars are spent.

Private Employer-Based Insurance

Nearly half of insurance in the U.S. is employer-based or purchased privately. Health insurers, such as Blue Cross/Blue Shield, Aetna, MetLife, and Prudential, offer a range of for-profit and not-for-profit options for consumers. Most health insurance plans include varying levels of inpatient coverage; however, not all plans include outpatient coverage, and those that do can vary greatly. See Box 74-1 for a list of common abbreviations used in the insurance industry.

The original employer-based insurance was based on a fee-for-service model in which the insured paid 20% of costs. In 1974, federal regulation, the Employee Retirement Income Security Act encouraged larger employers to develop self-funded plans. In self-funded plans, the employer takes fiscal responsibility for the cost of the enrollee's medical claims (Kaiser Family Foundation [KFF], 2015a).

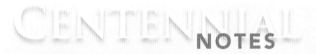

NOTES

Occupational Therapy and the Junior League

Lori T. Andersen

In the early years of the OT profession, federal legislation required that the U.S. government cover the costs of OT services in military and veterans hospitals. State legislatures and other agencies, such as New York City Department of Public Charities, and private agencies provided funding for OT services (Johnson, 1917; Phillips, 1928). In 1917, the Women's Auxiliary Board of the Presbyterian Hospital of Chicago paid Susan E. Tracy to consult on starting an OT department and continued to fund the program as it grew (Brainerd, 1932). In New England, several hospital-based OT programs were funded by auxiliaries (Adams, 1922).

In 1916, the Junior League of the City of New York started occupational work for patients in city hospital. Over the next 10 years, their work extended to Bellevue, St. Luke's, Ruptured and Crippled, and Presbyterian Hospitals. In addition to providing equipment, supplies, and volunteer help, this charitable organization funded salaries for two therapists in 1923 and an additional therapist in 1929 (Howard, 1939).

The Junior League expanded to other cities providing support including the following:

- Funding to establish OT departments in the three university hospitals in Indianapolis (MacDonald, 1930)
- Funding to start the Occupational Therapy Workshop in St. Louis to help with the war relief effort in 1917 (State Historical Society of Missouri, n.d.)
- Equipping and funding an OT department at Columbia Hospital in Milwaukee (Phillips, 1928)
- Starting an OT program in Detroit for those injured in the World War I (Gordon & Reische, 1982)

The Junior League earned funds to support the OT programs through sale of patient-made products, sales at gift shops, sales at secondhand stores, and annual entertainment events. Additionally, these Junior Leagues, as well as other hospital organizations supporting OT programs, solicited donations of money, equipment, and supplies (MacDonald, 1930).

Throughout the 1920s and 1930s, Eleanor Clarke Slagle, in her role as secretary-treasurer of American Occupational Therapy Association (AOTA), provided many Junior Leagues with information on how to develop OT programs. These included Junior Leagues in Albany, New York; Dayton, Ohio; Englewood, New Jersey; and Winnipeg, Canada (Slagle, 1930). In many cases, the Junior League support of OT programs has continued through the years.

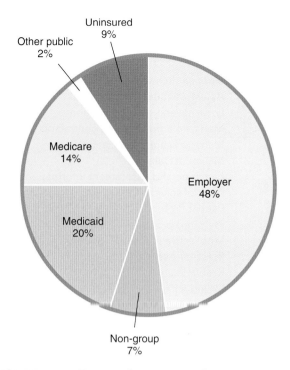

FIGURE 74-1 Types of payment. (Source: Kaiser Family Foundation. [2016b]. *Health insurance of the total population.* Retrieved from https://www.kff.org/other/state-indicator/total-population/?dataView=0&currentTimeframe=0&sortModel=%7B%22colId%22:%22Location%22,%22sort%22:%22asc%22%7D.)

Self-funded health plans currently cover 61% of workers in the U.S. (KFF, 2016a). Forty-eight percent of employer-based insurance (in 2016) is a type of managed care plan called preferred provider organization (PPO) (KFF, 2016a). These PPOs involve a group of providers that the insured can access. The second most common plan type is a **high-deductible health plan** (HDHP) with a health savings account (HSA) (29% in 2016) (KFF, 2016a). As the name implies, the insured pays a high deductible (typically a dollar amount paid by the insured before insurance benefits apply) for coverage and contributes to medical costs through a tax-free savings account. With most employer-based plans, the employee pays a percentage of the charge or coinsurance (typically a percentage of total charges to be paid by the insuree) and a deductible out-of-pocket amount per year. More information about managed care and HDHP/HSAs is discussed later in this chapter.

Managed Care

Managed care, and specifically PPOs, have dominated the employer-based health care market for several years (KFF, 2016a). The many definitions of managed care emphasize controlling and reducing health care costs. Managed care "integrates the functions of financing, insurance, delivery, and payment within one organization" (Shi & Singh, 2004, p. 326). Most managed care organizations (MCOs) include primary and preventive care services (Shi & Singh, 2004). Health maintenance organizations (HMOs), PPOs, and point of service (POS) plans are examples of managed care

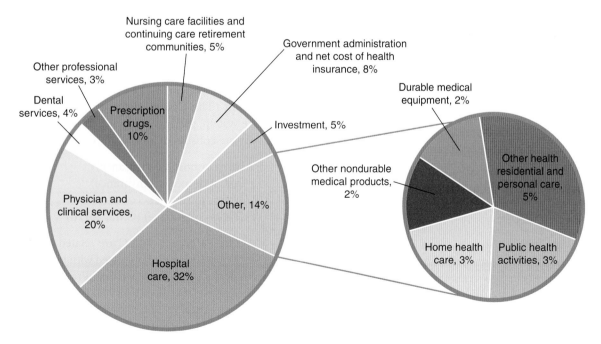

FIGURE 74-2 The nation's health dollar, 2014. (From Centers for Medicare & Medicaid Services. [2014b]. *The nation's health dollar ($3.0 trillion), calendar year 2014, where it went.* Retrieved from https://www.cms.gov/Research-Statistics-Data-and-Systems/Statistics-Trends-and-Reports/NationalHealthExpendData/Downloads/PieChartSourcesExpenditures2014.pdf/).

BOX 74-1   FREQUENTLY USED ABBREVIATIONS

CDHP	Consumer-directed health plan	IRF-PAI	Inpatient Rehabilitation Facility-Patient Assessment Instrument
CHAMPVA	Military insurance plan		
CHIP	Children's Health Insurance Program	LCD	Local coverage determination
CMS	Centers for Medicare & Medicaid Services	MAC	Medicare administrative contractor
COBRA	Consolidated Omnibus Budget Reconciliation Act of 1985	MCO	Managed care organization
		MDS	Minimum Data Set
CPT	Current Procedural Terminology	OASIS	Outcome and Assessment Information Set
DME	Durable medical equipment	POS	Point of service
DRG	Diagnostic-related group	PPACA	Patient Protection and Affordable Care Act
EPSDT	Early and Periodic Screening, Diagnosis, and Treatment	PPO	Preferred provider organization
		PPS	Prospective payment system
HSA	Health savings account	RAI	Resident Assessment Instrument
HCPCS	Healthcare Common Procedure Coding System	RUG	Resource utilization group
		SNF	Skilled nursing facility
HDHP	High-deductible health plan	TRICARE	Military insurance plan
HHA	Home health agency	VA	Department of Veteran's Affairs
HMO	Health maintenance organization	VD-HCBS	Veteran-Directed Home and Community Based Services
IDEA	Individuals with Disabilities Education Act		
IRF	Inpatient rehabilitation facility	VHA	Veterans Health Administration

CHAMPVA, Civilian Health and Medical Program of the Department of Veterans Affairs.

options. As discussed, PPO plans, which allow participants to choose from a limited number of health care providers, have proven to be the most popular plan type because of increased consumer choice (KFF, 2016a).

To receive payment, OT practitioners need to understand how specific managed care plans work and recognize managed care plans often include strategies to reduce cost. For example, some plans require preauthorization or precertification before beginning intervention and may require authorization for the number of treatments and treatment continuation. Managed care has not been without controversy; issues have occurred from both consumers and health care providers (Lohman, 2003). As new systems evolve, it is possible managed care will have a decreased role in the private health care market place.

Government Payment in the United States

Although we do not have universal health care in the U.S. as in other major industrial countries (e.g., Canada, the United Kingdom), government funding accounts for a large percentage of the U.S. health care dollar. The following sections outline key government payers including Medicare, a federal program; Medicaid; the *Children's Health Insurance Program (CHIP)*; **Individuals with Disabilities Education Act (IDEA)**; a combined federal/state programs; and Workers' Compensation, which is a state-administered program.

Medicare

Medicare is a federal health insurance system overseen by the Centers for Medicare & Medicaid Services (CMS, 2017d). It is the largest purchaser of health care and the biggest government health insurance program in the U.S. (Medicare Payment Advisory Commission [MedPAC], 2016a). Medicare covers "people who are 65 or older, people under 65 with certain disabilities, and people of any age with end-stage renal disease (ESRD)" (CMS, 2017d, p. 15). Medicare is financed by payroll taxes, insurance premiums, and general revenue funding from the federal government (The Commonwealth Fund, 2014). In the Medicare system, patients are called "beneficiaries."

Medicare consists of four main parts:

- A (inpatient or hospital insurance)
- B (outpatient or medical insurance)
- C (Medicare Advantage)
- D (prescription coverage) (CMS, 2017d)

Medicare Parts A, B, and C are related to reimbursement for OT practice and is discussed with information that is current at the time of this writing. Practitioners should be knowledgeable of skilled (Box 74-2) as compared to unskilled services (Box 74-3) and guidelines for determining OT coverage in all Medicare practice settings (Box 74-4).

Medicare Part A.   All Medicare beneficiaries are covered under Part A, which incorporates inpatient hospitalization and *critical access hospitals*, skilled nursing facilities (SNFs),

CENTENNIAL NOTES

Occupational Therapy and Medicare

Metzler (2017) reflected on the role of OT when Medicare was developed out of the Social Security Acts in 1965. When Medicare was introduced, OT was almost a 50-year-old established profession; however, Medicare greatly expanded OT services and practice settings. Prior to Medicare, the health system was less integrated than today with separate "siloed" acute care hospitals (Metzler, 2017). The inception of Medicare included Part A for hospital insurance and Part B for optional medical insurance typically covering nonacute care settings. In 1965, OT practitioners practiced in a medical model and were not well reimbursed outside of the institutional hospital setting. After the introduction of Medicare, OT began to have a greater presence for the health care treatment of individuals over the age of 65 years. In the 1970s, Medicare expanded services to individuals under the age of 65 years with long-term disabilities and end-stage renal disease, which increased the number of clients that OT practitioners could treat and subsequently receive reimbursement. At this time of expansion, AOTA made state licensure of OT practitioners important because Medicare wanted consumer protection for clients served through home health. State licensure allowed for growth of the OT profession in the overall health care system (Metzler, 2017). As Medicare continued to grow, so did the OT profession. In the 1980s, OT practitioners began to utilize Part B, outpatient, Medicare benefits. Private practitioners were allowed the right to a Medicare provider number allowing direct reimbursement for OT services covered under Part B. Expansion continued with Medicare reimbursing services for hospice care and additional growth in long-term care and outpatient. The advocacy and forward thinking of OT leaders benefited the profession in the 1990s. The Balanced Budget Act established caps for reimbursement of outpatient services. Occupational therapists were part of a therapy cap separate from other rehabilitation professionals, meaning that OT practitioners received $1,500 per person for OT services, whereas physical therapy (PT) and speech-language pathology (SLP) services were lumped together for the same amount. The caps associated with Medicare Part B have changed numerous times with the legislative Medicare changes. Currently, in 2018, outpatient therapy services are covered if the services provided are reasonable and medically necessary for the recovery of function but may be subject to review beyond a certain amount.

Today, the health care environment is very different than when Medicare was established. Life expectancy has increased by over 15% and the complexity of the aging population's health care needs is escalating (Blumenthal, Davis, & Guterman, 2015). The demands on OT services are complex which will require continued vigilance to adapt as Medicare continues to change. Moving the AOTA headquarters to Bethesda, Maryland, in 1995 to be near the federal offices (Metzler, 2017) and developing policy and payment resources for therapists on the AOTA Website (http://www.aota.org) reflects how the association is attentive to the profession's needs.

Medicare has not been free of controversy, and OT professionals must be knowledgeable and trained in Medicare regulations not only for reimbursement but also for advocacy of the profession for continued growth and distinction (Sieck, Lohman, Stupica, Minthorne-Brown, & Stoffer, 2017). Medicare not only provides coverage for clients with Medicare Part A, Medicare Part B, and Medicare Part C but also has become the framework for which reimbursement is provided through private insurance. Without Medicare, OT would not be the profession it is today.

BOX 74-2 SKILLED THERAPY SERVICES FOR PAYMENT WITH MEDICARE

Skilled therapy services must be reasonable and necessary for the treatment of the patient's illness or injury. Coverage does not turn on the presence or absence of an individual's potential for improvement, but rather on his or her need for skilled care. Skilled care may be necessary to improve a patient's current condition, to maintain the patient's current condition, or to prevent or slow further deterioration of the patient's condition. This means that the therapy services must be:

- Inherently complex, which means that they can be performed safely and/or effectively only by, or under the general supervision of, a skilled therapist
- Consistent with the nature and severity of the illness or injury and the patient's particular medical needs, which include services that are reasonable in amount, frequency, and duration
- Considered specific, safe, and effective treatment for the patient's condition under accepted standards of medical practice

From Centers for Medicare & Medicaid Services. (2017a). Home health prospective payment system. Retrieved from https://www.cms.gov/Outreach-and-Education/Medicare-Learning-Network-MLN/MLNProducts/Downloads/Home-Health-PPS-Fact-Sheet-ICN006816.pdf

BOX 74-3 UNSKILLED THERAPY SERVICES AND REASONS FOR NONPAYMENT WITH MEDICARE

- Services not reasonable and necessary for treatment
- Services inappropriate to the setting or condition (CMS, 2017f) (e.g., mental health intervention in a skilled nursing facility)
- Services performed by an unqualified person (CMS, 2017f) (e.g., by certified nursing assistant [CNA])
- Services that do not require the skills of a therapist or carried out by an unskilled person (CMS, 2017f) (e.g., caregiver doing repetitive range of motion program)
- Services that are for fitness, diversion, motivation, or for a transitory condition (CMS, 2017f) (e.g., endurance training with an older adult)

- Services not under a therapy plan of care that supports the diagnosis being treated (CMS, 2017f)
- Services that do not document minutes when required by setting. Therapists should be aware of what counts as minutes (e.g., documentation cannot be included in timed codes) (CMS, 2017f, p. 184).
- Services that are too long for the condition and do not benefit the patient (CMS, 2017f)
- Services with unclear vague documentation about the skilled need for therapy
- Documentation does not include objective evaluations (CMS, 2012b), therapy provided, and patient response (CMS, 2017f).

home health agencies (HHAs), inpatient rehabilitation facilities (IRFs), and hospice care. Medicare beneficiaries pay deductibles and may purchase coinsurance plans to supplement coverage in these practice settings. The payment method for Part A is a **prospective payment system (PPS)** related to the different practice settings. (Refer to Table 74-1 for an overview of Medicare Part A payment in different settings.)

Medicare Part A Coverage in Acute Care Hospitals. Acute care hospitals receive payment for all services under a prospective, predetermined, payment rate based on **diagnostic-related groups** (DRGs). A DRG is a statistical system of classifying possible diagnoses of patients into groups for the purposes of inpatient hospital stay payment. All services (e.g., treatments provided, such as OT) and treatment

supplies (e.g., medication and equipment) are included in the DRG rate. Hospitals are responsible for determining which services and supplies are provided and the length of stay for each patient. Recent research found higher utilization (spending) of OT services lowered hospital readmission rates for persons with heart failure, pneumonia, and myocardial infarction (Rogers, Bai, Lavin, & Anderson, 2016).

Medicare Part A Coverage in Skilled Nursing Facilities. The PPS system in SNFs involves a mandated assessment structure, the Resident Assessment Instrument (RAI). The Minimum Data Set 3.0 (MDS 3.0) is the screening form used as part of this structure. The MDS 3.0 considers the resident's status, includes quality measures (Thomas, 2010), and determines clinical care and payment.

BOX 74-4 GUIDELINES FOR DETERMINING OCCUPATIONAL THERAPY COVERAGE

- Treatment must be provided under a plan of care certified by a physician or non-physician practitioner. Physician order recommended, not required, and plan of care created before beginning of treatment (CMS, 2017f).
- Treatment must be completed by a qualified occupational therapist (OT) or occupational therapy assistant (OTA) under the supervision of a qualified OT. The OT provides correct level of supervision for the OTA based on state and local law with a minimum of general supervision (CMS, 2017f).
- Treatment must be of reasonable duration, and necessary intervention must be at the level of complexity requiring the "skilled" intervention of an OT. Treatment must be appropriate for the patient's condition and must result

in improvement of the patient's condition within a reasonable time frame.
- Medicare typically does not cover long-term supportive care.
- Documentation should be legible, signed, and include a national provider number.
- Documentation follows Medicare guidelines for type of documentation (e.g., evaluation includes medical history, rehabilitation potential, start of care date, prior therapy, treatment plan, and functional G-codes [Part B]).
- OT must follow Medicare policies and should refer to CMS Benefit Policy Manual 100-02 Chapter 15, Section 220-230 for specific payment and documentation requirements.

TABLE 74-1	An Overview of Medicare Part A Payment in Different Settings

Facility Type	Basis of Payment
Inpatient prospective payment system (IPPS hospital) acute hospital	Diagnostic-related group (DRG)
Inpatient rehabilitation facility	Case mix group based on patient assessment instrument
Critical access hospitals	Rehabilitation services are paid at cost
Inpatient psychological hospitals	DRG
Part A skilled nursing facility	Resource utilization groups based on Minimum Data Set
Home health	Case mix based on the Outcome and Assessment Information Set

The MDS contains "extensive information on the resident's nursing needs, activities of daily living (ADL) impairments, cognitive status, behavioral problems, and medical diagnoses" (CMS, 2010, p. 2) as well as "preferences and lifestyle wishes" (Thomas, 2010, p. 386). Sections of the RAI help establish the classification categories for residents and ultimately the allocation of therapy time the resident receives skilled rehabilitation services.

A resident qualifies for admittance to a SNF under Medicare Part A if he or she meets the following qualifications: has remaining days of Medicare Part A coverage,

is being admitted following a 3-day hospital stay, admission to the SNF occurs within 30 days of hospitalization, and a physician has ordered the SNF stay. Residents must have a "skilled" need to be admitted to an SNF for either nursing care and/or rehabilitation services (CMS, 2016b). The MDS 3.0 is completed on each qualified resident and divides residents into one of six resource utilization groups (RUGs) ranging from ultrahigh to low and rehabilitation plus extensive services. Each RUG has a set total amount of weekly therapy minutes and which skilled services (PT, OT, or speech-language pathology [SLP]) a resident can receive. In addition, RUGs establish the number of days for rehabilitation services. For example, a resident who qualifies to be in the "very high" RUG category receives 500 minutes of skilled services 5 days per week (CMS, 2016c). Specific regulations exist for payment of minutes accrued as individual, group, and concurrent minutes. Because of the need for coordination of these minutes across multiple providers, OT practitioners working in SNFs need to be efficient and have good communication with other disciplines (Case Study 74-1) (Brayford et al., 2002).

Medicare Part A Coverage in Inpatient Rehabilitation Facilities. Patients are admitted to intensive rehabilitation facilities (IRFs) when they require complex nursing, medical care, and rehabilitation from an interprofessional team (CMS, 2012c). Payment in IRFs is through a PPS and includes an evaluation tool called the Inpatient Rehabilitation Facility-Patient Assessment Instrument (IRF-PAI). Medicare beneficiaries receiving services in an IRF are classified in several ways including by impairment

CASE STUDY 74-1 FIELDWORK STUDENT IN SKILLED NURSING FACILITY

Kelly is an OT student on Level II fieldwork at a skilled nursing facility (SNF). She has been treating an 82-year-old Medicare beneficiary, Kay, under the supervision of her fieldwork educator Ben. Kay has been a patient at the SNF for 10 days due to a stroke. Kay has made good progress during OT sessions but continues to require minimal assistance with bathing and toileting. Kay uses a raised toilet seat for toileting and an extended tub bench for bathing. Kay is reaching the end of her allotted days in the SNF. The interprofessional team meets to discuss Kay's progress and discharge planning. Kelly reports that Kay is having difficulty with toileting and bathing and will require durable medical equipment (DME) upon discharge. PT reports similar findings with mobility and transfers and recommend that Kay stay at the SNF for 1 additional week and discharge with a hemi walker. The speech-language pathologist states that Kay has met all speech-language pathology (SLP) goals, and she will be discharged from SLP. Kay's family agrees Kay should stay 1 more week and wants

the recommended DME for discharge, only if covered by insurance. Kelly informs Ben that she has 1 week to order the DME and mentions that it is positive that insurance will cover the DME for toileting and bathing. Ben corrects the student's misperception and responds that Kay's insurance coverage is Medicare and that Medicare does not cover bathroom DME. Ben advises Kelly that she needs to inform the family that Medicare does not cover the raised toilet seat and extended tub bench. Ben educates Kelly that Medicare will reimburse the cost of the hemi walker because it is utilized for safe mobility and PT obtained a prescription for the device. The next day, Kelly discusses with Kay and her family the DME Medicare will cover. Kay states, "Well I guess I will not be able to go home." Kelly states she is happy to work with Kay and her family to find an alternative to purchasing the bathroom DME out of pocket. By discharge, Kelly found a used DME supplier in the local community that had a raised toiled seat and extended tub bench for a cost that Kay's family was able to afford.

group code, rehabilitation impairment category, case mix group, and presence of comorbidities (CMS, 2017b).

There are specific regulations for inpatient rehabilitation that guide patient care and are required for reimbursement. Regulations necessitate 60% of patients in an IRF have 1 of 13 diagnoses (CMS, 2017b) including but not limited to stroke, spinal cord injury, brain injury, amputation, major multiple trauma, and burns. Patients with knee or hip replacement must be 85 years or older to be admitted to an IRF under the 60% rule (CMS, 2012c). Additionally, therapy provided in an IRF setting must equate to a minimum of 3 hours of skilled services 5 days per week.

Medicare Part A Coverage in Home Health Agencies. Home health agencies provide a variety of services in the patient's home including skilled nursing care, PT, OT, SLP, medical social work, and aide services. Medicare beneficiaries utilizing HHAs must meet eligibility criteria for coverage including being *homebound*, which is defined as a situation where leaving home would be difficult for the beneficiary due to transportation needs, ambulatory devices, and/or requiring assistance from others. In most cases, beneficiaries should only leave home for unique or infrequent events (CMS, 2017a). Other eligibility requirements for HHA include the patient's need for skilled services (nursing and/or therapy), having a plan of care created by the physician, and a visit with a physician or allowed nonphysician practitioner in an established timeframe.

Prior to the provision of OT services paid through Medicare in an HHA, another health care professional (nursing, PT, or SLP) must first skill-qualify a beneficiary, which means "according to law, to receive services under the Medicare home health care benefit, a Medicare beneficiary must [initially] be in need of nursing, physical therapy, or speech therapy" (Metzler, 2000, para. 1). Once a beneficiary is qualified for home health coverage, OT can be initiated for medically necessary services. Occupational therapy can continue to follow the patient even after other rehabilitation services have ended, as OT services alone allow for continued home health eligibility (AOTA, 2013; CMS, 2017i).

Home health agencies use a screening tool called the Outcome and Assessment Information Set (OASIS) which is completed by nursing and used to evaluate the beneficiary's status and monitor outcomes for quality of care. Occupational therapists consult with nursing regarding the primary diagnosis for which home health care is needed and the patient's functional status. HHA agencies are paid prospectively an established amount based on calculations every 60 days on a case mix classification system (MedPAC, 2015). This case mix classification system utilizes data from the OASIS, including therapy information (CMS, 2017i), to determine payment. In a home health setting, therapists

follow specific guidelines for timing of assessment (e.g., initial assessment must be completed within 48 hours of referral or the beneficiary's return to home) and reassessment, utilization of objective measurements, and the provision of skilled services. To receive payment, Medicare stipulates that occupational therapists, not OT assistants, must perform the ordered service visit, assessments, and documentation of evaluation and therapy (CMS, 2017e). The reimbursement rate made to HHA under the PPS includes all services provided (e.g., therapy) and medical supplies. The DME is not included in HHA PPS.

At the time of this writing, changes are in discussion for Medicare Part A. For example, SNF payment for each RUG category is based on the total lump cost for resident care rather than on a fee-for-service model, as is currently done with Medicare Part B (CMS, 2017f). However, Medicare is proposing changes with therapy payments in SNFs based on the necessity of therapy (AOTA, 2017g). Eliminating the current minute-based requirements for treatment is among the proposed changes (Halstead, 2017). Furthermore, CMS is proposing changing the HHA payment structure to a 30-day payment with payment more focused on medical complexity (CMS, 2018). Another proposed change for HHA is eliminating the therapy thresholds. Currently, thresholds involve a gradual increase of payment for therapy after day 6 up to day 20 (AOTA, 2018a). Eventually, Medicare may take away the different payment structures that are discussed in this chapter for each of Medicare Part A settings and develop a payment system for all practice settings based on patient acuity (Deloitte, 2017).

Medicare Part B. Some consumers purchase optional Medicare Part B coverage, which includes diagnostic tests; outpatient surgery; outpatient OT, PT, and SLP; HHA services; blood tests; SNF services; some preventive tests; and some DME (CMS, 2017d). In many Medicare Part A settings, people can also be reimbursed under Medicare Part B guidelines at a less intensive level for therapy (e.g., HHA, SNF) (CMS, 2017a). Medicare Part B beneficiaries pay a set fee per month, and 20% of costs after a yearly deductible to cover utilized services. The highest utilization of rehabilitation services under Part B occurs with PT (71%) followed by OT (20%) and SLP (9%) (MedPAC, 2016b). OT services provided to beneficiaries under Part B are generally less intense than Part A services.

Figure 74-3 illustrates the distribution of outpatient (Part B) spending by setting (MedPAC, 2016b).

Durable Medical Equipment. To qualify for reimbursement under Medicare Part B, DME must be prescribed by a physician to be used for a medical reason by the beneficiary in the home environment (Medicare.gov, n.d.). Examples of covered DME include commodes, walkers, wheelchairs, hospital beds, and patient lifts. Items like bathtub grab bars and

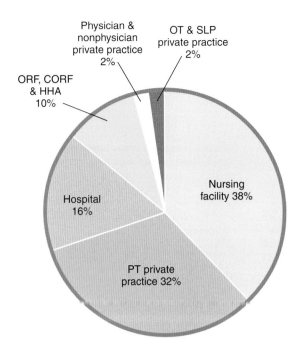

FIGURE 74-3 **Distribution of outpatient therapy spending by setting, 2014 (MedPAC, 2016b). CORF, comprehensive outpatient rehabilitation Facility; HHA, home health agency; ORF, outpatient rehabilitation facility; PT, physical therapy; SLP, speech-language pathology.**

raised toilet seats are not reimbursed under Medicare Part B coverage.

G-Codes. Starting with the Middle Class Tax Relief and Jobs Creation Act of 2012 (Pub. L. 112-96), OTs, PTs, and SLPs have been documenting functional limitation reports, which include G-codes for Medicare Part B beneficiaries (CMS, 2014a). Under the Physician Quality Reporting System, there are a total of 42 G-codes organized into 14 specialty categories (CMS, 2012d). Therapists must select the most appropriate G-code based on the patient's primary functional limitation from all available therapy disciplines (OT, SLP, and PT) along with the appropriate severity/complexity modifier. With G-codes, therapists consider present status, projected goal status, and discharge status (CMS, 2017f). The CMS has established a specific timeline for completing G-code reporting in therapy practice (AOTA, 2017d, 2017h; CMS, 2017f). Reimbursement will not occur if G-codes are not documented or if the patient's functional limitations are not consistent with the long-term goals established in the therapy plan of care (CMS, 2017f). Data collected from G-codes provides information about function, services rendered, and outcomes and may lead to a new payment system for Medicare Part B linking payment to "efficient and effective" therapy services based on function and conditions (CMS, 2012a, p. 1–483). Thus, G-codes will go away with new payment system.

Current Procedural Terminology and Medicare Physician Fee Schedule. Currently, payment for Medicare Part B is completed using the Medicare Physician Fee Schedule (MPFS), which is established by the American Medical Association (AMA) and lists the fees used by physicians and other providers for a variety of health care services and products. All health care services with Medicare Part B are categorized and documented using the Healthcare Common Procedure Coding System (HCPCS) or Current Procedural Terminology (CPT) codes (CMS, 2015a). The CPT codes describe specific services provided by health care personnel, were developed by the AMA, and are updated annually. Each CPT code listed on the MPFS has a detailed payment amount. In 2017, major changes occurred with the CPT codes for OT evaluation and reevaluation. New service-based evaluation codes were added based on the patient's level of complexity (AMA, 2016, 2017; AOTA, 2016). Language from the Occupational Therapy Practice Framework: Domain and Process, third edition, (AOTA, 2014b, 2016) informed these coding changes.

Choosing the right code involves critically assessing the beneficiaries' profile and history, occupational performance, and the degree of clinical decision making involved with intervention. The CPT language clearly describes the difference between the code levels (AOTA, 2016). When documenting the plan of care, it is suggested OT practitioners include an occupational profile, history, standardized or nonstandardized assessments, and analysis of occupational performance (AMA, 2017; AOTA, 2016). (Refer to Table 74-2 for an explanation of payment terminology for Medicare Part B.)

Therapy Cap. The therapy cap was an annual payment maximum or "limit" established in 1997 for Medicare Part B outpatient therapy coverage (Medicare.gov, n.d.). Under the therapy cap, outpatient claims by any given client that exceeded the limit required application for extension of services. This application, called an exception to the therapy limits (Medicare.gov, n.d.), involved the addition of a modifier (KX) to the outpatient claim. The modifier attested that services billed and provided were medically necessary. A CMS-"targeted" medical review by Medicare contractors occurred when OT service charges reached a second larger amount or "threshold" (CMS, 2016d, 2018; MedPAC, 2016b). Therapy caps were repealed in 2018 when Congress voted to end the caps. However, the usage of the KX modifier and the targeted medical review continue (AOTA, 2018b; American Physical Therapy Association, 2018).

Providing thorough documentation supporting OT services is always important for payment and essential for CMS review. Medicare beneficiaries may have supplemental insurance called a **Medigap policy** or pay out of pocket for services not fully covered by Medicare (CMS, 2015b).

TABLE 74-2 Payment Terminology for Medicare Part B

Type	Definition	Application
MPFS: Medicare Physician Fee Schedule	Fee schedule used for Medicare billing in outpatient settings. Each unit of payment is for each individual outpatient service as identified by the Healthcare Common Procedure Coding System codes (MedPAC, 2016b, p. 2)	Used by therapists and other qualified health care providers to bill Medicare Part B
CPT codes: Level I Healthcare Current Procedural Terminology	"Identifies medical services and procedures" (CMS, 2013, para. 2)	Typically, therapists apply timed and untimed codes. Timed codes are based on an *8-min rule* for 15 minute units of service (CMS, 2016a) and untimed or service codes are billed once daily (CMS, 2016a)
HCPCS codes: Level II Healthcare Common Procedure Coding System	"Identifies products, supplies, and services not included in the CPT-4 codes such as durable medical equipment, prosthetics, and orthotics and supplies" (CMS, 2013, para. 4)	Used for payment of "**durable medical equipment**, prosthetics, orthotics, and supplies (DMEPOS)" (CMS, 2015a)
RVU: Relative Value Unit	Payment rate for CPT codes "based on a relative weight . . . which account for the relative costliness of the inputs used to provide the service: the clinician's work, practice expense and professional liability insurance" (MedPAC, 2016b, p. 2).	Therapists should bill appropriately for services provided.
CCI: Correct Coding Initiative	"National correct coding methodologies and to control improper coding leading to inappropriate payment in Part B claims" (CMS, 2017g, para. 2)	Used to review claims for improper bundling of pairs of CPT codes. There are specific requirements for billing certain codes together (Robinson, 2007).
MPPR: Multiple Procedure Payment Reduction	Method of avoiding duplication of services when "more than one unit or procedure is provided to the same patient on the same day" (Medicare Learning Network, 2013)	Therapists should be aware that full payment is made for the unit or procedure with the highest practice expense (PE) payment. Beyond that, 50% of the PE is paid daily for second and additional codes for the same Medicare beneficiary and same provider (AOTA, 2017f)
ICD-10 codes: *International Statistical Classifications of Diseases* codes	"Standard diagnostic tool for epidemiology, health management and clinical purposes" (World Health Organization, 2016). These codes are found on billing claims forms.	Therapists select the most appropriate codes to explain the primary medical condition and primary and secondary therapy diagnoses. With the ICD-10 version, there are more codes and more detail.

Medicare Part C. Medicare Advantage, or Medicare Part C, is the private part of Medicare that beneficiaries can elect to use instead of the traditional program. Medicare Part C plans are typically overseen by managed care commercial payers, such as HMOs or PPOs, and may provide expanded services (e.g., vision, dental, hearing). Each Medicare Part C plan administers Medicare Part A and Part B benefits, including therapy. However, each Part C plan is different with its own requirements for patient out-of-pocket expenses and authorization for therapy services.

Keeping Up with Medicare-Related Payment Changes. Medicare regulations related to therapy are continuously updated, and OT practitioners must keep current with the changes. The CMS Website (https://www.cms.gov/) is a good source for current information on Medicare. Practitioners should access the CMS Internet-only manuals and specifically the Benefit Policy Manual

100-02 Chapter 15, Section 220-230 (CMS, 2017f). The AOTA Website is another good source of information practitioners can utilize to stay abreast of health care changes impacting payment.

Practitioners must also be aware of regional Medicare Administrative Contractors (MACs) who oversee regional Medicare coverage and payment. Each regional MAC may have its own interpretation for therapy coverage (AOTA, 2015b, 2017e). Among other duties, MACs process claims and handle audits and appeals (CMS, 2017j). Personnel in MACs can be valuable resources with payment questions. Practitioners should pay close attention to policies related to payment established by the MACs, called local coverage determinations (LCDs) (AOTA, 2015b, 2017e). It is suggested that practitioners download the LCDs specific to therapy coverage from their regional MACs (AOTA, 2017i). Box 74-5 overviews an example of a significant change related to Medicare clients who have chronic conditions as a result of *Jimmo v. Sebelius* court case.

BOX 74-5 | *JIMMO V. SEBELIUS COURT CASE*

An example of a significant change for coverage considerations resulted from the settlement of the *Jimmo v. Sebelius* case. The Jimmo case clarified that Medicare coverage is based on skilled services of both nursing and therapy and not on the "improvement standard" (AOTA, 2014a). The Jimmo settlement reinstated the "maintenance coverage standard" for therapy (CMS, 2017c). Thus, qualified therapists need to consider whether there is a skilled need for their expertise and utilize critical judgment for intervention, even if the patient has a chronic condition, or therapy services are solely for maintenance. For instance, this change would apply to a patient with the chronic condition of multiple sclerosis who requires the "skilled" expertise of the occupational therapist to help him adapt to doing ADLs safely even if he will not improve in function.

Medicaid

Medicaid, or Title XIX of the Social Security Act, was enacted in 1965 to help persons of low income status including older adults, children, parents of dependent children, parents of other nonelderly adults, pregnant women, and people with disabilities who meet the eligibility requirements KFF, 2015a; Medicaid.gov (n.d.b). Medicaid is the largest government program for low-income Americans. Nearly 50% of Medicaid recipients are children, and they make up 40% of all children in the U.S. (KFF, 2017c). Yet, older adults and disabled persons covered through Medicaid account for two-thirds of Medicaid spending because of extensive use of acute and long-term care services (KFF, 2017c). Medicaid pays for long-term care services in the home/community and nursing homes.

Medicaid is jointly financed by federal and state governments and regulated differently in each state (KFF, 2015b, 2017c). It is a *means tested* program as people qualify if their assets and income levels are below standards set by the program (Shi & Singh, 2004). States can choose to expand their baseline Medicaid coverage and income eligibility requirements beyond the federal minimal requirements. Medicaid programs vary as each state provides different services and different systems for delivery. Quite often, programs are administered with a managed care approach (KFF, 2016c). Each state has a plan that documents how the program is administered, eligibility requirements, as well as required and optional health services. Occupational therapy is one of the optional services; therefore, in some states, OT might not be a covered benefit. However, even in states where OT is included as an optional benefit, states have minimized the benefit by limiting the number of therapy visits or by cutting fee schedule rates for services (C. Willmarth, personal communication, December, 11, 2017).

Medicaid and Related Programs Covering Children. Medicaid covers 60% of children with disabilities in the U.S. (KFF, 2017c). However, the CHIP provides health coverage for families that are low income but earn too much to meet Medicaid qualifications (HealthCare.gov, n.d.). The CHIP is financed through federal and state governments; however, states administer their own programs Medicaid.gov (n.d.a). The Early and Periodic Screening, Diagnosis, and Treatment (EPSDT) benefit covers a large amount of screening and diagnostic services for children up to the age of 21 years, such as medical, vision, hearing, and dental screenings (KFF, 2017b, Thomas, 2010). With Medicaid, OT services are covered for children, including EPSDT benefits.

The Patient Protection and Affordable Care Act

The Patient Protection and Affordable Care Act (PPACA) was signed into law in 2010. Factors behind the development of PPACA were the large numbers of uninsured and underinsured, the rising contribution of health care to the gross national product, and the inefficiencies in the health care market (ObamaCareFacts.com, n.d.). The PPACA was a primary piece of legislation reforming the U.S. health care system and intended to address many problems of the health care system. The PPACA contains over 2,000 pages of provisions expanding access to affordable and quality health care. The PPACA has many important provisions impacting payment for OT including, for example, expanded coverage of preventive health services, enhanced support for Medicaid and CHIP programs, linking payment to outcomes for Medicare, and creating healthier communities through prevention of chronic disease and access to preventive services (PPACA, 2010).

The PPACA impacts the quality, accessibility, and affordability of health care by extending insurance to over 30 million uninsured Americans through expanded Medicaid coverage and requiring most Americans to have health insurance coverage (Affordable Health California, 2017). Insurance "exchanges" or marketplaces were created for the purchase of private health insurance by individuals, families, and small businesses. The exchanges allow consumers to compare different health insurance plans. The PPACA requires an individual and dependents of the individual to have minimum essential health insurance or pay a monthly penalty.

Other provisions impacting payment for OT services under the PPACA include the following:

1. Requiring insurers to cover mental health, substance abuse, rehabilitation, habilitative, and chronic disease management services
2. Improving coverage through eliminating lifetime and annual limits and extending dependent coverage
3. Prohibiting insurance companies to deny coverage or raise rates for preexisting conditions, guaranteeing renewability of coverage, and prohibiting discrimination in health care (PPACA, 2010)

The PPACA is the largest effort to date to improve quality of care and contain health care costs in the U.S. At the time of this writing, the PPACA may be altered or even repealed based on court decisions, the composition of the Congress, or the residing president. It is the authors' beliefs that regardless of what happens to the PPACA, large-scale efforts to improve the quality of care and reduce costs will continue to influence practice.

Veteran's Administration

The Department of Veterans Affairs (VA) is the single largest employer of OT practitioners in the U.S. (VA Careers, 2012). Veterans receiving free or reduced health care must have actively served in a branch of the military and be enrolled in the VA's comprehensive Medical Benefits Package. The Veterans Health Administration (VHA) manages the Medical Benefits Package (Benefits.gov, n.d.). Occupational therapy practitioners work for the VA in all practice settings. They also treat uniformed military and veterans in private health care facilities. Interventions and DME are covered under various forms of VA insurance plans such as TRICARE for Life, TRICARE, CHAMPVA for Life, or Veteran-Directed Home and Community Based Services (VD-HCBS) (Paying for Senior Care, 2017). Active uniformed service members and their families are covered under TRICARE as well as others with a military connection (TRICARE, 2016). Prior to 2018, TRICARE covered services for occupational therapists but not OTA (AOTA, 2017c). The National Defense Authorization Act signed into law for fiscal year 2018 designated OTA as providers under TRICARE, allowing them to submit reimbursement for their services (AOTA, 2017b).

Workers' Compensation

Workers' Compensation programs are state programs that address multiple needs of people who are ill/injured because of work. Occupational therapy practitioners may provide services with the primary goal of returning the

ill/injured person to work. Programs financially support medical and rehabilitation services, partial payment of lost wages, and short- and long-term disability. Programs also reimburse partial as well as permanent disability. Payment for permanent disability may be provided if the condition is expected to last greater than 1 year or result in death (Social Security Administration, 2017). Programs include services such as vocational rehabilitation, medical rehabilitation, job placement for someone with a permanent disability, and social services. Many of these programs are instituted with a managed care approach. Each state has a governing body that determines the administration and funding; therefore, Workers' Compensation programs vary from state to state.

Consolidated Omnibus Budget Reconciliation Act of 1985

The *Consolidated Omnibus Budget Reconciliation Act of 1985 (COBRA)* gives workers and their families who lose health benefits the right to temporary group health benefits. Several circumstances may result in the loss of health benefits. Qualification for COBRA includes voluntary or involuntary loss of employment, reduction in hours worked, transition between jobs, death, divorce, and other life events (United States Department of Labor, n.d.). Occupational therapy practitioners may provide services to persons covered by COBRA insurance.

⚖ PRACTICE DILEMMA

Katie: An Occupational Therapist Working with a Pediatric Client over the Years in Different Settings with Different Payment Issues

Katie has followed John, a 10-year-old child with Down syndrome, for OT since he was born. Katie found that over the course of treating John, she has had to learn about obtaining payment for OT based on insurance coverage and practice setting. Katie first saw John when in the neonatal intensive care unit (NICU) when she worked at the inpatient acute care hospital. The NICU nurse mentioned to Katie that John could benefit from OT intervention and Katie should communicate this with his physician. The physician was reluctant to order OT to evaluate and treat in the NICU. Therefore, Katie advocated with the physician sharing the benefits of OT for John's medical and developmental needs and received an order to evaluate and treat. John's OT treatment in the NICU was covered by a managed care organization. Six years later, Katie saw John again, this time, through the school district where she worked part-time when she was not at the hospital. New to school-based practice, Katie had to learn to change her focus and become familiar with reimbursement in an educationally based model versus a medical model. John's insurance was now Medicaid. Because Katie was unfamiliar with the state Medicaid program and how it related to payment for John's OT in the school system, she decided to seek out education about Medicaid. When John was 8 years old, he fell and broke his wrist and sustained a complex fracture. Katie was able to follow John in the hospital's outpatient OT clinic; John's outpatient OT was reimbursed by Medicaid. A managed care approach was used by the state Medicaid program to guide and monitor therapy. John's intervention goals were based on regaining the functional use of his upper extremity. John was authorized to receive a set number of therapy visits from Medicaid, which Katie felt were not adequate to meet John's therapy goals.

Questions

1. Katie's initial practice dilemma with John was the need to advocate for OT services with the physician. Discuss why it was essential that Katie receive a physician's order to see John and the physician's support for OT treatment.
2. Katie's second practice dilemma was her identified need to learn more about the state Medicaid system and payment for John's school-based treatment. Discuss how you would learn more about Medicaid in your state and how it relates to school-based practice and practice in other settings.
3. Katie's third practice dilemma was figuring out how to gain additional Medicaid therapy coverage beyond school-based treatments to reimburse John's outpatient OT. Discuss how you would go about requesting additional OT visits.

Emerging Payment Systems

Two trends to reduce the cost of care have emerged in the health care marketplace: consumer-driven health care and value-based care.

Consumer-Driven Health Care and a Movement toward Community Partnerships

Consumer-driven health care is an economically driven approach involving lowering health care expenditures while simultaneously providing consumer control over health plans. Thus, decision making about health care moves to the consumer instead of to the insurer, and consumers with these plans become engaged in researching health care options and costs (Vanetine & Masters, 2017). An example of consumer-driven health care is a HDHP, which is often accompanied by an HSA. The HDHPs and HSAs, also known as consumer-directed health plans (CDHPs), allow people to save and apply pretax dollars to health-related payments. Pretax dollars can be used to pay for deductibles, coinsurance, copayments, and health insurance premiums, which are traditionally paid for with after-tax dollars. The consumer can choose areas for health care intervention that are not always covered by traditional insurance. Consumer-driven plans are growing and are predicted to continue to grow, with recent data indicating 39% of persons younger than 65 years old with private health insurance are enrolled in an HDHP, 15.2% are enrolled in a CDHP, and 24% are enrolled in an HDHP without an HSA (CDC, 2016). Because these plans provide an incentive not to spend health care dollars, practitioners need to educate consumers about the value of therapy services.

Value-Based Care

There are many unknowns in health care today; however, the shift from paying for quantity of care (volume based) to paying for the value of care (value based) will likely continue. Increasing cost of health care coupled with subpar outcomes, the aging population, and health care reform all support a continued focus on expanding value-based care payment models (Bristol & Joshi, 2014).

One feature of **value-based care** includes health care institution's public reporting of data related to the quality of care. Transparency in reporting of the quality of care allows third-party payers to determine the value of care. Consumers also have access to quality data through Websites such as CMS's Hospital Compare (http://www.hospitalcompare.hhs.gov). Therefore, value-based care is patient-centered care and includes several different models of care.

Accountable care organizations are a type of value-based care and include networks of physicians, hospitals, and other health care providers who coordinate and deliver care for their patient members. After review of over 90 different payment reform programs, Schneider, Hussey, and Schnyer (2011) categorized them into 11 categories shown in Box 74-6.

Occupational therapy practitioners should be knowledgeable about the aim of value-based payment models and utilize patient-centered and evidenced-based care to reduce cost and improve the quality and safety of patient care regardless of practice setting. Such knowledge is supportive of the strategic goals and objectives of the profession as developed by AOTA. The fourth strategic

---

BOX 74-6 **PAYMENT REFORM: ANALYSIS OF MODELS AND PERFORMANCE MEASUREMENT IMPLICATIONS**

- *Model 1: Global Payment.* A single per-member per-month payment made for all services delivered to a patient with payment adjustments based on measured performance and patient risk
- *Model 2: Accountable Care Organizations Shared Savings Program.* Groups of providers (known as accountable care organizations [ACOs]) voluntarily assume responsibility for the care of a population of patients and share payer savings if they meet quality and cost performance benchmarks.
- *Model 3: Medical Home.* A physician practice or other provider is eligible to receive additional payments if medical home criteria are met. Payment may include calculations based on quality and cost performance using a P4P-like mechanism.
- *Model 4: Bundled Payment.* A single "bundled" payment, which may include multiple providers in multiple care settings, is made for services delivered during an episode of care related to a medical condition or procedure.
- *Model 5: Hospital–Physician Gainsharing.* Hospitals are permitted to provide payments to physicians that represent a share of savings resulting from collaborative

efforts between the hospital and physicians to improve quality and efficiency.
- *Model 6: Payment for Coordination.* Payments are made to providers furnishing care coordination services that integrate care between providers.
- *Model 7: Hospital P4P.* Hospitals receive differential payments for meeting or missing performance benchmarks.
- *Model 8: Payment Adjustment for Readmissions.* Payments to hospitals are adjusted based on the rate of potentially avoidable readmissions.
- *Model 9: Payment Adjustment for Hospital-Acquired Conditions.* Hospitals with high rates of hospital-acquired conditions are subject to a payment penalty, or treatment of hospital-acquired conditions or serious reportable events is not reimbursed.
- *Model 10: Physician P4P.* Physicians receive differential payments for meeting or missing performance benchmarks.
- *Model 11: Payment for Shared Decision Making.* Payment is made for the provision of shared decision making services.

P4P, pay for performance.

Source: Schneider, E. C., Hussey, P. S., & Schnyer, C. (2011). Payment reform: Analysis of models and performance measurement implications. *Rand Health Quarterly, 1*(1), 3.

---

goal identified by AOTA is to "advance quality and recognition of occupational therapy practice [and] foster widespread adoption of evidence-based approaches in occupational therapy that reduce cost, increase access, and improve outcomes across the continuum of care" (AOTA, 2017a, Goal #4). Additionally, such knowledge is supportive of AOTA's centennial vision journey which calls for practitioners to promote the distinct value of OT: "to improve health and quality of life through facilitating participation and engagement in occupations, the meaningful, necessary, and familiar activities of everyday life. Occupational therapy is client-centered, achieves positive outcomes, and is cost-effective" (AOTA, 2015a, para. 5).

Telehealth

Occupational therapists utilize **telehealth** technologies for the provision of OT evaluation, intervention, supervision, and education. Reimbursement for telehealth is not widespread among the various types of reimbursement mentioned in this chapter (Cason, 2014). Medicare does not cover OT services provided through telehealth.

Occupational therapy telehealth reimbursement under Medicaid varies by state. Refer to the state regulatory board within the state you practice to determine Medicaid coverage as well as private insurance reimbursement. The VHA covers telehealth including OT (Cason, 2014).

The Uninsured, Underinsured, and Pro Bono Therapy Intervention

Health insurance is important to people in the U.S.; however, there are people who are either uninsured or underinsured. Without insurance, severe consequences can happen, especially if a preventable condition could have been treated (KFF, 2016d). Public concern about the large number of Americans lacking insurance (44 million in 2013) was behind much of the discussion leading to the PPACA. Due to the PPACA, gains have been made resulting in less uninsured people (28 million uninsured in 2016) (KFF, 2017a). The question remains who are the uninsured 28 million people and why are they still uninsured? The uninsured are lower income, more likely to be people of color, have one employed worker in a family, or are undocumented immigrants (KFF, 2017a). Approximately 45% of uninsured citizens claim the high cost of insurance premiums prohibited purchase of health insurance (KFF, 2017a), and they must consider the costs of paying for health care against other life necessities (KFF, 2016d). As discussed with the PPACA, there was lack of Medicaid expansion in some states. This lack of expansion left certain citizens caught between not qualifying for Medicaid and unable to afford insurance in the marketplaces (or places where uninsured can purchase insurance). This is because the original intent of the PPACA was to expand Medicaid coverage in all states. Not understanding the insurance system is another reason for people being uninsured.

Even with insurance, approximately 31 million U.S. citizens are underinsured. Underinsured adults may have insurance, but coverage is limited often because their deductibles are too high in relationship to their income. Underinsurance can lead to increased medical debt and not seeking out health services (The Commonwealth Fund, 2014), including OT.

The uninsured or underinsured individual can elect to privately pay for OT services, but often, they must pay the full cost of service versus the negotiated rates of insured individuals (KFF, 2016d). As alternatives, the therapy practitioner can look for community-based grants or provide pro bono services. Providing pro bono services is supported by the OT profession as stated in the Occupational Therapy Code of Ethics: Practitioners should "address barriers in access to occupational therapy services by offering or referring clients to financial aid, charity care, or pro bono services within the parameters of organizational policies" (AOTA, 2015c, p. 5). Refer to Chapter 45, which addresses occupational justice.

When Payment Gets Denied

Therapy documentation is reviewed by third-party payers for payment with private and public insurance and services can be denied. Within the Medicare system, MACs and other private contractors are responsible for reviewing therapy records. As discussed, MACs establish guidelines, LCDs, which describe criteria for coverage. Medicare denials can be for many reasons. A common reason is for technical errors, such as incomplete billing codes, not having legible documentation or a missing physician signature on a Medicare Plan of Care. Other reasons are for not following the Medicare regulations, such as the therapy service provided is not reasonable or necessary or a skilled level of therapy is not provided (refer to Boxes 74-2 and 74-3, the guidelines for therapy coverage for skilled and unskilled services in Medicare). Beyond Medicare, knowledge about how OT services are covered in any insurance plan can prevent denials. Appealing a denial for therapy that is perceived as justifiable is one way to advocate for our clients. With Medicare, there is a specific time line to determine "redeterminations" (Morse, 2005). Suggested information provided for an appeal should be a detailed and objective explanation of the patient's status that supports the need for therapy. It is valuable to include physicians, nurses, and other disciplinary notes that discuss the patient's functional status (Costiera, 2014), and needs and benefits from receiving therapy may help the appeals process.

Advocacy for Payment

Every time practitioners experience problems with payment for services, they should critically consider how best to obtain and advocate for reimbursement. Advocacy for payment can occur in many ways. For example, effective communication with case managers or other key people in an insurance system may be all it takes to obtain payment. Providing evidence of the efficacy and value of the intervention is often helpful. Following through with the processes in place, such as an appeals system, can result in payment for services. Accessing resources beyond the traditional system to get funds through charitable and/or community organizations may be an option. Beyond advocating for your client in a clinical situation, practitioners can advocate for improved payment in the health care system when patient-centered care and quality is compromised.

Conclusion

Dealing with payment issues is a regular part of therapy practice. Practitioners may work with a variety of payment systems. On the surface, knowledge about payment systems might seem overwhelming because the financial system for health care and social services in the U.S. is very complex. Yet, it is every practitioner's professional duty to learn about these systems to provide needed OT services and to advocate for payment or changes with policies/systems when considered necessary (AOTA, 2015c). Payment systems change, and these changes often occur because of new or amended legislation. Keeping current with policy and legislation that affect payment for one's area of practice is essential for successful practice.

REFERENCES

Adams, J. D. (1922). The training of the occupational aide. *Archives of Occupational Therapy, 1*(3), 187–192.

Affordable Health California. (2017). *Affordable care act history*. Retrieved from http://affordablehealthca.com/history-affordable-care-act/

American Medical Association. (2016). *Occupational therapy evaluations as described in CPT Code Manual*. Retrieved from https://www.aota.org/~/media/Corporate/Files/Advocacy/Federal/coding/Descriptors-of-New-CPT-Occupational-Therapy-Evaluation-Codes.pdf/

American Medical Association. (2017). 2017 *CPT® for occupational therapy*. Retrieved from https://www.aota.org/~/media/corporate/files/secure/advocacy/federal/coding/2017%20selected%20occupational%20therapy%20cpt%20codes.pdf

American Occupational Therapy Association. (2013). *Fact sheet: Occupational therapy's role in home health*. Retrieved from https://www.aota.org/About-Occupational-Therapy/Professionals/PA/Facts/Home-Health.aspx

American Occupational Therapy Association. (2014a). *Jimmo v. Sebelius: The so called Medicare "improvement standard" deemed illegal, skilled maintenance care now covered*. Retrieved from https://www.aota.org/Advocacy-Policy/Federal-Reg-Affairs/News/2013/Improvement-standard.aspx

American Occupational Therapy Association. (2014b). Occupational therapy practice framework: Domain and process (3rd ed.). *American Journal of Occupational Therapy, 68*, S1–S48. doi:10.5014/ajot.2014.682006

American Occupational Therapy Association. (2015a). *Articulating the distinct value of occupational therapy*. Retrieved from https://www.aota.org/Publications-News/AOTANews/2015/distinct-value-of-occupational-therapy.aspx

American Occupational Therapy Association. (2015b). *Get to know your Medicare Administrative Contractor (MAC)*. Retrieved from https://www.aota.org/Advocacy-Policy/Federal-Reg-Affairs/Medicare/medicare-administrative-contractor.aspx

American Occupational Therapy Association. (2015c). Occupational Therapy Code of Ethics (2015). *American Journal of Occupational Therapy, 69*, 1–8. doi:10.5014/ajot.2015.696S03

American Occupational Therapy Association. (2016). *New occupational therapy evaluation coding overview*. Retrieved from https://www.aota.org/~/media/Corporate/Files/Advocacy/Federal/Evaluation-Codes-Overview-2016.pdf

American Occupational Therapy Association. (2017a). *AOTA 2018-2020 strategic plan*. Retrieved from https://www.aota.org/~/media/Corporate/Files/AboutAOTA/Governance/AOTA-Strategic-Goals-and-Objectives-2018-2020.pdf

American Occupational Therapy Association. (2017b). *Bill to designate OTAs as Tricare providers signed into law*. Retrieved from https://www.aota.org/Advocacy-Policy/Congressional-Affairs/Legislative-Issues-Update/2017/Bill-To-Designate-OTAs-as-Tricare-Providers-Signed-into-Law.aspx

American Occupational Therapy Association. (2017c). *Does Tricare cover services provided by occupational therapy assistants?* Retrieved from https://www.aota.org/Advocacy-Policy/Federal-Reg-Affairs/News/2017/Does-TRICARE-Cover-Services-Provided-by-Occupational-Therapy-Assistants.aspx

American Occupational Therapy Association. (2017d). *G-code functional data reporting*. Retrieved from https://www.aota.org/Advocacy-Policy/Federal-Reg-Affairs/News/2013/Functional-Data-CY2013.aspx

American Occupational Therapy Association. (2017e). *Medicare: Local coverage determinations (LCDs)*. Retrieved from https://www.aota.org/Advocacy-Policy/Federal-Reg-Affairs/Medicare.aspx

American Occupational Therapy Association. (2017f). *Medicare outpatient therapy cap: Implementation fact sheet*. Retrieved from https://www.aota.org/Advocacy-Policy/Federal-Reg-Affairs/Medicare/therapy-cap/fact-sheet.aspx

American Occupational Therapy Association. (2017g). *Medicare proposing changes to SNF therapy payments in future: What can you do to promote OT?* Retrieved from https://www.aota.org/Advocacy-Policy/Federal-Reg-Affairs/News/2017/Medicare-Proposing-Changes-to-SNF-Therapy-Payments-in-Future-What-Can-You-Do-to-Promote-OT.aspx

American Occupational Therapy Association. (2017h). *Resources for G code functional data reporting*. Retrieved from https://www.aota.org/Advocacy-Policy/Federal-Reg-Affairs/Coding/G-Code.aspx/

American Occupational Therapy Association. (2017i). *Take proactive steps to better payment*. Retrieved from https://www.aota.org/Advocacy-Policy/Federal-Reg-Affairs/Medicare/get-better-payment.aspx

American Occupational Therapy Association. (2018a). *Home health changes for therapy*. Retrieved from https://www.aota.org/Advocacy-Policy/Congressional-Affairs/Legislative-Issues-Update/2018/Home-Health-Changes-For-Therapy.aspx

American Occupational Therapy Association. (2018b). *Victory in sight: Permanent repeal of therapy cap in house budget bill being voted on today*. Retrieved from https://www.aota.org/Advocacy-Policy/Congressional-Affairs/Legislative-Issues-Update/2018/Victory-in-Sight-Permanent-Repeal-Therapy-Cap-House-Budget-Bill-Vote.aspx

American Physical Therapy Association. (2018). *A permanent fix to the therapy cap: Improved access for Medicare patients comes with pending APTA-opposed cut to PTA payment*. Retrieved from http://www.apta.org/PTinMotion/News/2018/02/09/TherapyCapRepeal/

Benefits.gov. (n.d.). *Basic medical benefits package for veterans*. Retrieved from https://www.benefits.gov/benefits/benefit-details/303

Blumenthal, D., Davis, K., & Guterman, S. (2015). Medicare at 50—Origins and evolution. *The New England Journal of Medicine, 372*, 479–486.

Brainerd, W. (1932). The evolution of an occupational therapy department in a general hospital. *Occupational Therapy and Rehabilitation, 11*, 33–40.

Brayford, S., Muscatine, J., Dunbar, C., Frank, A., Nguyen, P., & Fisher, G. S. (2002). A pilot study of delivery of occupational therapy in long term care settings under the Medicare prospective payment system. *Occupational Therapy in Health Care, 15*, 67–76.

Bristol, S., & Joshi, M. S. (2014). Transforming the healthcare system for improved quality. In M. S. Joshi, E. R. Ransom, D. B. Nash, & S. B. Ranson (Eds.), *The healthcare quality book: Vision, strategy, and tools* (3rd ed., pp. 541–559). Chicago, IL: Health Administration Press.

Cason, J. (2014). Telehealth: A rapidly developing service delivery model for occupational therapy. *International Journal of Telerehabilitation, 6*, 29–35. doi:10.5195/ijt.2014.6148

Centers for Disease Control and Prevention. (2016). *Health insurance coverage: Early release of estimates form the National Health Interview Survey, January-September 2016*. Retrieved from https://www.cdc.gov/nchs/data/nhis/earlyrelease/insur201702.pdf

Centers for Disease Control and Prevention. (2017). *Health insurance coverage: Early release of estimates form the National Health Interview Survey, January-September 2016*. Retrieved from https://www.cdc.gov/nchs/data/nhis/earlyrelease/insur201702.pdf

Centers for Medicare & Medicaid Services. (2010). *Chapter 6: Medicare skilled nursing facility prospective payment system (SNF PPS)*. Retrieved from https://www.ahcancal.org/facility_operations/Documents/UpdatedFilesRAI3.0/MDS%203.0%20Chapter%206%20V1.02%20July%202010.pdf

Centers for Medicare & Medicaid Services. (2012a). *Medicare program, revisions to payment policies under the physician fee schedule: G. Therapy services. Federal Register, 77, 1–483.* Retrieved from https://www.gpo.gov/fdsys/pkg/FR-2012-11-16/pdf/2012-26900.pdf

Centers for Medicare & Medicaid Services. (2012b). *Physical, occupational, and speech therapy services,* 1-483. Retrieved from https://www.cms.gov/Research-Statistics-Data-and-Systems/Monitoring-Programs/Medical-Review/Downloads/TherapyCapSlidesv10_09052012.pdf

Centers for Medicare & Medicaid Services. (2012c). *The Inpatient Rehabilitation Facility-Patient Assessment Instrument (IRF-PAI) training manual.* Retrieved from https://www.cms.gov/Medicare/Medicare-Fee-for-Service-Payment/InpatientRehabFacPPS/Downloads/IRFPAI-manual-2012.pdf

Centers for Medicare & Medicaid Services. (2012d). *Therapy functional reporting G-codes—Short descriptors.* Retrieved from https://www.aota.org/~/media/Corporate/Files/Advocacy/Reimb/Coding/G%20Codes/G%20Codes%20Descriptors.pdf

Centers for Medicare & Medicaid Services. (2013). *HCPCS coding questions.* Retrieved https://www.cms.gov/Medicare/Coding/MedHCPCSGenInfo/HCPCS_Coding_Questions.html

Centers for Medicare & Medicaid Services. (2014a). *Functional reporting.* Retrieved from https://www.cms.gov/Medicare/Billing/TherapyServices/Functional-Reporting.html

Centers for Medicare & Medicaid Services. (2014b). *The nation's health dollar ($3.0 trillion), calendar year 2014, where it went.* Retrieved from https://www.cms.gov/Research-Statistics-Data-and-Systems/Statistics-Trends-and-Reports/NationalHealthExpendData/Downloads/PieChartSourcesExpenditures2014.pdf/

Centers for Medicare & Medicaid Services. (2015a). *Healthcare Common Procedure Coding System (HCPCS) level II coding procedures.* Retrieved from https://www.cms.gov/Medicare/Coding/MedHCPCSGenInfo/Downloads/HCPCSLevelIICodingProcedures7-2011.pdf

Centers for Medicare & Medicaid Services. (2015b). *Medigap (Medicare supplement insurance policies).* Retrieved from https://www.cms.gov/Outreach-and-Education/Training/CMSNationalTrainingProgram/Downloads/2015-Medigap-Workbook.pdf

Centers for Medicare & Medicaid Services. (2016a). *CMS manual system, Pub 100-04 Medicare claims processing: Transmittal 3670.* Retrieved from https://www.cms.gov/Regulations-and-Guidance/Guidance/Transmittals/Downloads/R3670CP.pdf

Centers for Medicare & Medicaid Services. (2016b). *Medicare benefit policy manual. Chapter 8—Coverage of extended care (SNF) services under hospital insurance.* Retrieved from https://www.cms.gov/Regulations-and-Guidance/Guidance/Manuals/downloads/bp102c08.pdf

Centers for Medicare & Medicaid Services. (2016c). *Medicare skilled nursing facility (SNF) transparency data.* Retrieved from https://www.cms.gov/Regulations-and-Guidance/Guidance/Manuals/downloads/bp102c08.pdf

Centers for Medicare & Medicaid Services. (2016d). *Therapy cap: Manual medical review of therapy claims above the $3,700 threshold.* Retrieved from https://www.cms.gov/Research-Statistics-Data-and-Systems/Monitoring-Programs/Medicare-FFS-Compliance-Programs/Medical-Review/TherapyCap.html

Centers for Medicare & Medicaid Services. (2017a). *Home health prospective payment system.* Retrieved from https://www.cms.gov/Outreach-and-Education/Medicare-Learning-Network-MLN/MLNProducts/Downloads/Home-Health-PPS-Fact-Sheet-ICN006816.pdf

Centers for Medicare & Medicaid Services. (2017b). *Inpatient rehabilitation facility prospective payment system.* Retrieved from https://www.cms.gov/Outreach-and-Education/Medicare-Learning-Network-MLN/MLNProducts/Downloads/Inpatient-Rehabilitation-Facility-Prospective-Payment-System-Text-Only.pdf

Centers for Medicare & Medicaid Services. (2017c). *Jimmo settlement: Important message about the Jimmo settlement.* Retrieved from https://www.cms.gov/Center/Special-Topic/Jimmo-Center.html

Centers for Medicare & Medicaid Services. (2017d). *Medicare & you 2017.* Retrieved from https://www.medicare.gov/pubs/pdf/10050-Medicare-and-You.pdf

Centers for Medicare & Medicaid Services. (2017e). *Medicare benefit policy manual. Chapter 7—Home health services.* Retrieved from https://www.cms.gov/Regulations-and-Guidance/Guidance/Manuals/downloads/bp102c07.pdf

Centers for Medicare & Medicaid Services. (2017f). *Medicare benefit policy manual. Chapter 15—Covered medical and other health services: Part B.* Retrieved from http://www.cms.gov/manuals/Downloads/bp102c15.pdf

Centers for Medicare & Medicaid Services. (2017g). *National correct coding initiative edits.* Retrieved from https://www.cms.gov/Medicare/Coding/NationalCorrectCodInitEd/index.html

Centers for Medicare & Medicaid Services. (2017h). *New a history.*

Centers for Medicare & Medicaid Services. (2017i). *Outcome and assessment information set OASIS-C2 guidance manual.* Retrieved from https://www.cms.gov/Medicare/Quality-Initiatives-Patient-Assessment-Instruments/HomeHealthQualityInits/Downloads/OASIS-C2-Guidance-Manual-6-17-16.pdf

Centers for Medicare & Medicaid Services. (2017j). *What is a MAC?* Retrieved from https://www.cms.gov/Medicare/Medicare-Contracting/Medicare-Administrative-Contractors/What-is-a-MAC.html

Centers for Medicare & Medicaid Services. (2018). *Home health agency (HHA) center.* Retrieved from https://www.cms.gov/Center/Provider-Type/Home-Health-Agency-HHA-Center.html

Costiera, R. (2014). *Appealing a denial for skilled therapy services.* Retrieved from http://www.healthpro-heritage.com/blog/bid/189200/Appealing-a-Denial-for-Skilled-Therapy-Services

Deloitte. (2017). *Medicare changes in post-acute care payment: Shaking up the way acute care hospitals approach post-acute care.* Retrieved from https://www2.deloitte.com/us/en/pages/life-sciences-and-health-care/articles/post-acute-care-payment-changes.html

Gordon, J., & Reische, D. (1982). *The volunteer powerhouse.* New York, NY: Routledge.

Halstead, N. (2017). *CMS simultaneously releases proposed rule to update SNF PPS for FY 2018 & advanced notice of proposed rulemaking (ANPRM) to replace RUG-IV case-mix methodology as early as FY 2019.* Retrieved from https://www.healthindustrywashingtonwatch.com/2017/05/articles/regulatory-developments/medicare-medicaid-services-regulations/cms-releases-proposed-fy-2018-snf-pps-and-case-mix-anprm/

HealthCare.gov. (n.d.). *The Children's Health Insurance Program (CHIP).* Retrieved from https://www.healthcare.gov/medicaid-chip/childrens-health-insurance-program/

Howard, F. M. (1939). Growth of the Occupational Therapy Committee of the Junior League of the City of New York. *Occupational Therapy and Rehabilitation, 18,* 395–398.

Johnson, S. C. (1917). Occupational therapy in New York City institutions. *The Modern Hospital, 8,* 414–415.

Kaiser Family Foundation. (2015a). *2015 Employer health benefits survey: Section ten: Plan funding.* Retrieved from https://www.kff.org/report-section/ehbs-2015-section-ten-plan-funding/

Kaiser Family Foundation. (2015b). *Medicaid at 50.* Retrieved from https://www.kff.org/medicaid/report/medicaid-at-50/

Kaiser Family Foundation. (2016a). *2016 Employer health benefits survey.* Retrieved from https://www.kff.org/report-section/ehbs-2016-summary-of-findings/

Kaiser Family Foundation. (2016b). *Health insurance of the total population.* Retrieved from https://www.kff.org/other/state-indicator/total-population/?dataView=0&currentTimeframe=0&sortModel=%7B%22colId%22:%22Location%22,%22sort%22:%22asc%22%7D

Kaiser Family Foundation. (2016c). *Medicaid financing: The basics*. Retrieved from https://www.kff.org/medicaid/issue-brief/medicaid-financing-the-basics/

Kaiser Family Foundation. (2016d). *The uninsured: A primer-key facts about health insurance and the uninsured in the wake of national health reform*. Retrieved from https://www.kff.org/uninsured/report/the-uninsured-a-primer-key-facts-about-health-insurance-and-the-uninsured-in-the-wake-of-national-health-reform/

Kaiser Family Foundation. (2017a). *Key facts about the uninsured population*. Retrieved from https://www.kff.org/uninsured/fact-sheet/key-facts-about-the-uninsured-population/

Kaiser Family Foundation. (2017b). *Key issues in children's health coverage*. Retrieved from http://www.kff.org/medicaid/issue-brief/key-issues-in-childrens-health-coverage/

Kaiser Family Foundation. (2017c). *Medicaid pocket primer*. Retrieved from https://www.kff.org/medicaid/fact-sheet/medicaid-pocket-primer/

Lohman, H. (2003). Critical analysis of a public policy: An occupational therapist's experience with the patient bill of rights. *American Journal of Occupational Therapy, 57*, 468–472.

MacDonald, J. H. (1930). Curative occupational therapy as conducted by the Junior League of Indianapolis in the Indiana University Hospitals. *Occupational Therapy and Rehabilitation, 9*, 39–44.

Medicaid.gov. (n.d.a). *CHIP state program information*. Retrieved from https://www.medicaid.gov/chip/state-program-information/index.html

Medicaid.gov. (n.d.b). *Medicaid*. Retrieved from https://www.medicaid.gov/medicaid/index.html

Medicare.gov. (n.d.). *Durable medical equipment (DME) coverage*. Retrieved from https://www.medicare.gov/coverage/durable-medical-equipment-coverage.html

Medicare Learning Network. (2013). *Multiple Procedure Payment Reduction (MPPR) for selected therapy services*. Retrieved from https://www.cms.gov/Outreach-and-Education/Medicare-Learning-Network-MLN/MLNMattersArticles/downloads/MM7050.pdf

Medicare Payment Advisory Commission. (2015). *Home health services payment system*. Retrieved from http://www.medpac.gov/docs/default-source/payment-basics/home-health-care-services-payment-system-15.pdf

Medicare Payment Advisory Commission. (2016a). *Health care spending and the Medicare program*. Retrieved from http://www.medpac.gov/docs/default-source/data-book/june-2016-data-book-health-care-spending-and-the-medicare-program.pdf

Medicare Payment Advisory Commission. (2016b). *Outpatient therapy services payment system*. Retrieved from http://www.medpac.gov/docs/default-source/payment-basics/medpac_payment_basics_16_opt_final.pdf

Metzler, C. (2000). *Advocate for OT in home health*. Retrieved from http://www.aota.org/Pubs/OTP/1997-2007/Columns/CapitalBriefing/2000/cb-060500.aspx

Metzler, C. (2017). *Reflecting on 50 years of occupational therapy in the Medicare Program*. Retrieved from http://www.otcentennial.org/article/reflecting-on-50-years-of-occupational-therapy-in-the-medicare-program

Morse, J. (2005). Government affairs. Seeking to simplify Medicare claim appeals. *PT: Magazine of Physical Therapy, 13*(10), 20–24.

ObamaCareFacts.com. (n.d.). *ObamaCare: Everything you need to know about the ACA*. Retrieved from https://obamacarefacts.com/obamacare-everything-you-need-to-know-about-the-aca/

Patient Protection and Affordable Care Act, 42 U.S.C. § 18001 (2010). Retrieved from https://www.gpo.gov/fdsys/pkg/PLAW-111publ148/pdf/PLAW-111publ148.pdf

Paying for Senior Care. (2017). *Veterans financial assistance for durable medical equipment*. Retrieved from https://www.payingforseniorcare.com/durable-medical-equipment/help-for-veterans.html

Phillips, R. F. (1928). The Junior League's occupational therapy work for children in Milwaukee: Organization and financing. *Occupational Therapy and Rehabilitation, 7*, 261–266.

Robinson, M. (2007). Medicare 101: Understanding the basics. *OT Practice, 12*(2), CE1–CE7.

Rogers, A. T., Bai, G., Lavin, R. A., & Anderson, G. F. (2016). Higher hospital spending on occupational therapy is associated with lower readmission rates. *Medical Care Research and Review, 74*, 1–19. doi:10.1177/1077558716666981

Schneider, E. C., Hussey, P. S., & Schnyer, C. (2011). Payment reform: Analysis of models and performance measurement implications. *Rand Health Quarterly, 1*(1), 3.

Shi, L., & Singh, D. A. (2004). *Delivering health care in America: A systems approach* (3rd ed.). Boston, MA: Jones & Bartlett Learning.

Sieck, R., Lohman, H., Stupica, K., Minthorne-Brown, L., & Stoffer, K. (2017). Awareness of Medicare regulation changes: Occupational therapists' perceptions and implications for practice, *Physical & Occupational Therapy in Geriatrics, 35*, 67–80.

Slagle, E. C. (1930). Report of the secretary-treasurer. *Occupational Therapy and Rehabilitation, 9*, 379–393.

Social Security Administration. (2017). *Disability benefits* (Publication No. 05-10029. ICN 456000). Retrieved from https://www.ssa.gov/pubs/EN-05-10029.pdf

State Historical Society of Missouri. (n.d.). *The Junior League of St. Louis, records, 1914-2000*. Retrieved from http://shs.umsystem.edu/stlouis/manuscripts/s0628.pdf

Stevens, R. A. (1996). Health care in the early 1960s. *Health Care Financing Review, 18*(2), 11–22. Retrieved from https://www.ssa.gov/history/pdf/HealthCareEarly1960s.pdf

The Commonwealth Fund. (2014). *The problem of underinsurance and how rising deductibles will make it worse: Findings from the Commonwealth Fund Biennial Health Insurance Survey, 2014*. Retrieved from http://www.commonwealthfund.org/publications/issue-briefs/2015/may/problem-of-underinsurance

Thomas, J. V. (2010). Reimbursement. In K. Jacobs & G. L. McCormack (Eds.), *The occupational therapy manager* (5th ed., pp. 385–405). Bethesda, MD: American Occupational Therapy Association.

TRICARE. (2016). *Eligibility*. Retrieved from https://tricare.mil/Plans/Eligibility

United States Department of Labor. (n.d.). *Health plans & benefits: Continuation of health coverage—COBRA*. Retrieved from https://www.dol.gov/general/topic/health-plans/cobra

VA Careers. (2012). *Become a VA occupational therapist*. Retrieved from https://www.vacareers.va.gov/assets/common/print/OT_Brochure.pdf

Vanetine, S. T., & Masters, G. M. (2017). *Healthcare forecast 2017: Top trends driving board strategic priorities*. Retrieved from https://nrchealth.com/resource/healthcare-forecast-2017-top-trends-driving-board-strategic-priorities/

World Health Organization. (2016). *International classification of diseases*. Retrieved from http://www.who.int/classifications/icd/en/

Available on thePoint (http://thePoint.lww.com/ Willard-Spackman13e)

Appendix I: Resources and Evidence for Common Conditions Addressed in OT

Edited by Ellen S. Cohn

Contributors: Katherine Appelbe, Megan Bailey, Gregory Blocki, Emily Briggs, Ashley Chung, Madeleine Emerson, Nikoletta Evangelatos, Libby Gross, Colleen Hogan, Grace Kelso, Ereann Kilpatrick, Jade LaRochelle, Kristen Layo, Elana Lerner, Estie Martin, Morgan McGoey, Richard McGuire, Emily Moran, Nicole Murgas, Rachel Newman, Jack Norcross, Natalie Petrone, Annie Poole, Casey Primeau, Alicia Quach, Jeanette Stitik, Nicole Strausser, Sarah Tuberty, Taryn Wells

Appendix I is a quick reference for students and practitioners who need summary information about a particular condition or diagnosis. In this appendix, each condition is described, incidence and prevalence data are provided, and causes and etiologies are discussed, followed by a description of the typical course of the disease, symptomatology, and related conditions.

Following the overview of the condition, precautions are noted in addition to interdisciplinary interventions. Occupational therapy (OT) evaluations are listed and, depending on the condition, may include activities of daily living assessments, assessment of client factors and performance skills, and/or occupation-focused assessments. Potential OT interventions are then discussed followed by a summary of OT and evidence. Finally, caregiver concerns and a list of resources (organizations, books, Websites) are provided.

Appendix II: Table of Assessments: Listed Alphabetically by Title

Cheryl Lynne Trautman Boop

Appendix II summarizes many of the assessments mentioned in the 13th edition. For each assessment, the following information is included: the assessment name and author, the publisher and/or contact information, the ages for which it is intended, the stated purpose, and the areas assessed.

Appendix III: First-Person Narratives

Appendix III includes three additional narratives that appeared in previous editions of *Willard & Spackman's Occupational Therapy*:

● "An Excerpt from *The Book of Sorrow, Book of Dreams: A First-Person Narrative*" by Mary Feldhaus-Weber and Sally A. Schreiber-Cohn
● "He's Not Broken—He's Alex: Three Perspectives" by Alexander McIntosh, Laurie S. McIntosh, and Lou McIntosh
● "The Privilege of Giving Care" by Donald M. Murray

GLOSSARY

The following definitions are drawn from the chapters in this book and are intended as a resource for understanding. Chapter numbers appear in parentheses at the end of each definition so that readers can refer to the cited chapters for concepts and definitions listed here. The Glossary also includes definitions from the American Occupational Therapy Association (AOTA) "Occupational Therapy Practice Framework, 3rd Edition." These definitions are indicated by the abbreviations OTPF-III. Likewise, there are definitions from the World Health Organization (indicated by WHO) and the WHO International Classification of Functioning, Disability and Health (indicated by the abbreviation ICF). Readers should cite the appropriate authors or original citations when referring to these constructs.

Accessible design Also referred to as barrier-free design, adds accessibility to otherwise inaccessible buildings, products, and services to enable persons with disabilities to function independently (33).

Accommodation Method for enabling individuals to access or perform work through technology and adjustments or modifications to a job or work environment (52).

Accountable care organization An organization of health care providers that agrees to be accountable for the quality, cost, and overall care of Medicare beneficiaries who are enrolled in the traditional fee-for-service program who are assigned to it (74).

Acquisitional occupation Using occupations to promote the person to develop or reacquire skills (61).

Actigraphy The use of recordings of body motion to display activity patterns across many consecutive days and nights (54).

Active assistive range of motion (AAROM) Arc of motion through which the joint passes when moved by muscles acting on the joint in conjunction with external assistance (57).

Active range of motion (AROM) Arc of motion through which a client can move a joint (without assistance) using the adjacent muscles (57).

Activities of daily living (ADL) Activities that are oriented toward taking care of one's own body such as bathing/showering, bowel and bladder management, dressing, feeding, functional mobility, personal device care, personal hygiene and grooming, sexual activity, and toilet hygiene (50).

Activity The execution of a task or series of actions (ICF, 25, 49).

Activity analysis An analytical analysis intended for purposes of determining the typically required demands of a task within a given culture; addresses the required body functions, personal factors, and environmental characteristics needed to successfully perform the task. It is used in occupational therapy to design therapeutic activities and identify ways to modify activities for improved performance (25, 26).

Activity choices Activities that are engaged in during play and leisure (53).

Activity interests/preferences Affective responses to play and leisure activities, perceptions and awareness of self and environments in relation to play and leisure activities, and motivation to participate in specific play and leisure activities (53).

Activity limitations Difficulties an individual may have in executing activities (ICF, 21, 49).

Acute care Short-term medical treatment, usually in a hospital, for individuals having an acute illness of injury, recovering from surgery, or requiring medical stabilization due to safety concerns (62).

Adaptation A change in response approach generated when encountering a challenge. It also refers to therapeutic intervention in which task demands are changed to be consistent with the individual's ability level; may involve modification by reducing demands, use of assistive devices, or changes in the physical or social environment (30, 44, 52).

Adaptation gestalt Relative balance of sensorimotor, cognitive, and psychosocial functioning that the individual creates internally in order to carry out an adaptive response (44).

Adaptation rate The rate at which afferent sensory receptors discharge into their afferent axons (59).

Adaptive capacity Apparent capability of the individual to perceive the need for change and draw from a repertoire of adaptive responses that will enable him or her to experience mastery over the environment (44).

Adaptive occupation Using adapted methods such as adaptive equipment or assistive technology or modifications of the environment or task demands to support performance (61).

Adaptive response (adaptiveness) A successful environmental interaction in which the individual meets the demands of the task demand; requires adequate sensory integration (44, 59).

Adenotonsillar hypertrophy Adenoid and tonsillar enlargement that may cause airway obstruction (54).

Administration The process of guiding an organization through the authoritative control of others completed by the governing body of the organization (71).

Administrative controls Changes in the nature of work such as scheduling, worker rotation, or the assignment of work tasks (52).

Administrative supervision Aspect of supervision directed toward managing the day-to-day work performance and process; includes tasks such as scheduling, monitoring performance, and delegating (72).

Advanced practice (practitioner) Practice or practitioners who possess a higher level of expertise in professional practice (70).

Advocacy (advocating, advocating mode) The act or process of supporting a cause or proposal such as public policy or resource allocation within political, economic, and social systems and institutions to directly affect people's lives. In occupational therapy, it often refers to actions to advance a profession and to assure that the client rights and resources are secured (5, 33, 37).

Affect Description of general observable emotional expression (37).

Affordances Qualities or properties of objects or the environment that elicit action possibilities (59).

Ageism Stereotypic and often negative bias against older adults; a form of discrimination based on age (20).

Aging in place Designing dwelling units such that residents, if they so choose, can occupy their home from childhood to old age unless illness or impairment come into play (22).

Agnosia Inability to recognize incoming sensory information in spite of intact sensory capacities (58).

Alternative plausible explanations Scientific explanations for the findings beyond the conclusions drawn from the study and its researchers (35).

Americans with Disabilities Act Federal law preventing discrimination against persons with disabilities (2).

Anthropometry Field of science that studies and defines the physical measures of a person's size (e.g., overall height and weight, length of leg, elbow, height in sitting and standing, size of head) and functional capacities (e.g., range of motion, strength, and aerobic capacity) (52).

Apnea A cessation of breathing (54).

Apnea/hypopnea index (AHI) An index of obstructive sleep apnea severity (54).

Apraxia Inability to perform motor activities, although sensory motor function is intact and the individual understands the requirements of the task (58).

Areas of occupation Various kinds of life activities in which people engage, including the following categories: ADL, IADL, rest and sleep, education, work, play, leisure, and social participation (49).

Arena Describes the places in which activities occur, such as a library, school, or hospital (25).

Arousal Level of alertness and responsiveness to stimuli (59).

Arts and Crafts Movement A movement originating in England that championed design and manual craftsmanship as a form of cultural resistance to the mechanization and impersonal production of industrialism (2, 45).

Assessment Specific method, instrument, tool, or strategy that is used as part of the evaluation process (28, 50, 51).

Assets Resources and attributes that might be used to achieve desired intervention outcomes (31).

Assistive technology(ies) Devices, adaptive equipment, or products that are designed to enable persons with disabilities to engage in daily occupations within their home, school, workplace, and communities (33).

Assumptions Thoughts, ideas, beliefs, values, and habits that are taken for granted as true or correct; often form the foundation for a viewpoint or action; may include ideas that cannot be demonstrated to be true or false (3, 41).

Ataxia An inability to coordinate voluntary muscular movements that is symptomatic of some central nervous system disorders and injuries and not due to muscle weakness (50).

At-homeness The taken-for-granted situation of feeling completely comfortable and intimately familiar with the world in which one lives his or her everyday life (22).

Atonia Muscle paralysis (54).

Atopic dermatitis An inflammatory, chronically relapsing, noncontagious, and pruritic skin disorder (54).

Attention The cognitive ability to focus on a task, issue, or object (58).

Attrition In the context of research, it refers to loss of participants from a sample during the course of data collection (35).

Avoiding A sensory pattern characterized by low thresholds and an active self-regulation approach; avoiders want less input (59).

Axiology The theory of values (3).

Background question A type of question used to obtain general knowledge about a disorder or condition (35).

Beliefs Cognitive content held as true (OTPF-III, 3, 24).

Benign prostatic hypertrophy Benign enlargement of the prostate (54).

Bias In quantitative research designs, refers to systematic (as compared to a random) distortion of the results (35).

Biofeedback The process of becoming aware of various physiological functions using instruments that provide information on the activity of those same systems, with a goal of being able to manipulate them at will (54).

Biological needs Requirements for survival, such as air, water, food, and shelter (5).

Biomechanical approach Therapeutic intervention focused on improving body movement and strength; typically identified with remediation or improvements in strength, range of motion, or endurance (52, 57).

Biomechanics (biomechanical) The study of mechanical laws and their application to living organisms, especially the human body and its locomotor system (52).

Biomedical model Model based on scientific knowledge that attributes health and illness to physiological, biological, and scientifically explainable changes in one's body (19).

Bipolar disorder A mental illness characterized by severe mood swings, episodes of depression, and at least one episode of mania (65).

Birth cohorts Groups of people who were born about the same time and for which the sum effects of the times and the people around them affect the trajectory for their lives (7).

Blinding Research term use for when a subject and/or researcher is not aware of the status of the subject in the study (35).

Body functions Physiological processes of the body (ICF, 23).

Body routines Sets of coordinated, habitual bodily actions sustaining a specific task or aim, for example, driving, cooking, or lawn mowing; see also *Body-subject* and *Time-space routines* (22).

Body structures Anatomical parts of the body such as bones and organs (ICF, 23).

Body-subject The prereflective but intelligent awareness of the body manifested through habitual action and typically in sync with the environment in which the action unfolds; plays a major role in the habitual, routine aspects of the lifeworld; see also *Body routines* and *Time-space routines* (22).

Boundary crossing Ways in which people who come from different lived worlds and have different life experiences find commonalities and areas of mutual interest, bridge differences, negotiate multiple and diverse perspectives, develop understandings, and respect multiple and, at times, divergent perspectives (17).

Brain-computer interface (BCI) A developing digital and electronic technology that allows objects and images to be manipulated via sensory devices registering brain waves or eye and facial movements (22).

Broad theory Overarching model that helps to explain a large set of findings or observations (41).

Bruxism Grinding of the teeth (during sleep); typically includes the clenching of the jaw (54).

Capacities Refers to a person's potential for occupation and includes aspects of human anatomy (e.g., bipedal locomotion, opposable thumbs, binocular vision), cognitive functions (e.g., consciousness, attention), and the abilities developed through maturational processes (e.g., strength, coordination, language, problem solving). Capacities are age and gender specific; may not yet be developed; and are shaped by a person's genetic heritage, aptitudes, traits, context, and occupational history (8).

Case-control studies A retrospective study in which subjects with the outcome of interest (cases) are selected and matched to subjects without the outcome of interest (controls). The presence of risk factors or predictors is determined through self-report or chart review, and the relationship between these retrospective predictors and the outcome of interest is determined (35).

Case management A collaborative process that assesses, plans, implements, coordinates, monitors, and evaluates options and services to meet an individual's health needs through communication and available resources to promote quality cost-effective outcomes (52).

Case series A study that tracks several patients over the course of a disease. The results are not aggregated, and detailed information on the diagnosis, treatment, and outcomes is provided for each individual patient (a case study tracks a single patient in a like manner) (35).

Cataplexy An abnormal sudden paralysis of some or all skeletal muscles brought on by strong emotions such as accompany laughter and anger (54).

Centers for independent living A nonresidential, private, nonprofit agency providing an array of independent living services that are consumer controlled, community based, cross disability, and designed and operated within a local community by individuals with disabilities. Core services include information and referral, independent living skills training, individual and systems advocacy, and peer counseling (62).

Certified Community Behavioral Health Clinics (CCBHCs) Clinics that are required to provide coordinated integrated care that is person centered and recovery oriented and to integrate physical and behavioral health care (65).

Chaining A stepwise process for teaching a multistep task (48).

Change talk Statements made by the client revealing consideration of, motivation for, or commitment to change (48).

Circadian biological clock See *Suprachiasmic nucleus (SCN).*

Class Ranking of people into a hierarchy within a culture, arising from interdependent economic relationships such as "middle class," "upper class," or "lower class" (20).

Classical test theory (CTT) Also called classical reliability theory; centers around the notion that each observation or test score has a single true score and yields a single reliability coefficient and that the observed or test score has two components: the true score and the measurement error score (29).

Classroom model A supported education model where students attend closed classes on campus (65).

Client-centered care (client-centered practice) An approach to service that incorporates respect for and partnership with clients as active participants in the therapy process. This approach emphasizes clients' knowledge and experience, strengths, capacity for choice, and overall autonomy (19, 37, 57).

Client characteristics Features of a client's interpersonal behavior that are important to observe and understand during therapy (37).

Clinical reasoning Process used by practitioners to plan, direct, perform, and reflect on client care. See *Professional reasoning* for a term that is considered to be broader (34).

Clinical supervision Supervision that is aimed at providing support, training, and evaluation of a supervisee's professional performance and development (72).

Code of ethics A set of conventional principles and expectations based on values and the standards of conduct to which practitioners of a profession are expected to conform; a public statement of principles used to promote and maintain high standards of conduct within the profession (5).

Cognition Mental processes including attention, memory, motivation, emotional control, motor control, sensory processing, and thinking; ability to think and reason to solve problems (58).

Cognitive behavioral therapy (CBT) A psychotherapeutic approach that combines cognitive and behavioral therapy techniques, aiming to solve problems concerning dysfunctional emotions, behaviors, and cognitions through a goal-oriented, systematic procedure (62).

Cognitive flexibility Mental ability to switch between thinking about two different concepts and to think about multiple concepts simultaneously (58).

Cognitive work hardening Uses graded work tasks to simulate a person's actual work tasks and/or the cognitive demands of the person's job to develop the cognitive skills required for job performance (52).

Cohort studies A study in which subjects who represent a particular population are measured on suspected risk factors/predictors of outcome(s) of interest and are followed over time to determine (a) the incidence/natural history of the outcome and (b) the relationship between the predictors and the outcome(s) (35).

Collaboration The complex interpretative acts in which the practitioner must understand the meanings of interventions, the meanings of illness or disability in a person and family's life, and the feelings that accompany these experiences (17).

Collaborative supervision (in fieldwork) Involves one or more supervisors working with multiple students with all participants viewed as more equal partners in the learning process (69).

Collectivist societies Those that put more value on the family structure than the individual. Interdependence is valued, and decisions are made by the group or family who consider what is good for the entire group before focusing on the individual (19).

Communication style Interpersonal characteristic that describes a person's ability and approach to communication. In therapy, it can refer to therapist or client's style (37).

Community(ies) Collective(s) of people who share common values and demonstrate mutual concern for the development and well-being of the group; may share interests, interactions, and sense of identity (31, 33).

Community agencies Provide services for all ages of individuals, often funded by local communities or states or private payment. For children, services may include early intervention, school based, and/or private practice. For adults, services are often supplemental for individuals who are living at home with the need for socialization and supervision, medical services, and/or dementia supports. Such services may be available in freestanding agencies but may be associated with other community programs or health agencies such as senior centers, assisted living facilities, mental health centers, rehabilitation centers, nursing homes, or hospitals (62).

Community development Community consultation, deliberation, and action to promote individual, family, and community-wide responsibility for self-sustaining development, health, and well-being (33).

Community level Social networks, norms, trends, and standards that facilitate or constrain desired occupational performance and/or participation and impact health (31).

Community participation Participation refers to active participation of individuals who both benefit and contribute to the community through their actions, ideas, knowledge, or skills. And so, community participation is about relating to others, to be in some sort of relationship with them (33).

Compassion fatigue Painful emotional reaction that occurs when the helper (volunteer or professional) becomes preoccupied with the suffering and distress being experienced by the recipients of care, resulting in deep physical, emotional, and spiritual exhaustion; sometimes referred to as secondary traumatic stress reaction (68).

Compelling occupations Occupational pursuits that evoke a deep, intense sense of engagement and meaningfulness (9).

Competency A specified skill or ability. Refers to possession of a required skill (70).

Complementarity The quality or state of being complementary, meaning both parties together make a whole (17).

Concealed random allocation In randomized controlled trials (RCTs), it refers to the a priori development of a randomization sequence so as to prevent investigators and subjects from knowing beforehand to which group a subject will be assigned (35).

Conditioning Designing situations that increase or decrease the likelihood of a behavior being performed (48).

Confidence interval Based on sample scores or outcomes, it is the likely range within which the population scores or outcomes would occur (35).

Confusional arousals Parasomnia sleep disorder that causes the affected person to act in a nonresponsive and confused manner (54).

Conservatorship A legal relationship, like guardianship, but is limited to managing the protected individual's financial affairs and property (50).

Constraint-induced movement therapy (CI or CI therapy) A form of rehabilitation therapy that improves limb function after central nervous system damage and is aimed at increasing the use of the affected upper limb (57).

Construct validity Establishes whether the assessment measures a construct and the theoretical components underlying the construct. A construct is an abstract idea that cannot be observed directly (29).

Consultant Person in a position to have some influences over an individual, a group, or an organization but has no direct power to make changes or implement a program (73).

Consultation A collaborative process completed with clients, families, other professionals, organizations, or communities to identify and solve problems with participation in occupations (73).

Consumer-driven health care An economically driven approach involving lowering health care expenditures while simultaneously providing consumer control over health plans. A high-deductible health plan accompanied by a health savings account is an example of a consumer-driven health care approach (74).

Content validity The extent to which an empirical measurement reflects a specific domain of content (29).

Context Factors that transact with the performance of occupations including personal, physical, cultural, social, spiritual, temporal, and virtual environments (1, 25, 33, 59).

Context-focused therapy Occupational therapy in which the environment and environmentally situated occupations are modified as the mode of intervention (9).

Contextual influences Interrelated conditions within and surrounding people that influence their occupational performance and experience (OTPF-III, 33).

Contextual interference A learning phenomenon where interference during practice is beneficial to skill learning (57).

Contextualism A view in which the person and situation are seen as integrated and cannot be understood separately (7).

Continuing competence A process involving the examination of current competence and the development of capacity for the future (70).

Continuing professional development (CPD) The process of engaging in lifelong learning aimed at maintaining practice competence, ensuring client safety and quality outcomes, enhancing or expanding professional practice, and reaching career goals (70).

Continuous positive airway pressure (CPAP) A treatment for obstructive sleep apnea in which a continuous stream of air under pressure is delivered through a mask worn over the nose, or nose and mouth, to keep the sleeper's airway open (54).

Continuous reinforcement Reinforcement for every instance of the behavior (48).

Continuum of care Term used to summarize the range of health care, educational, residential, employment, and social settings, which may be necessary to meet a client's needs over time (62).

Contraindication A therapeutic procedure that should be avoided because it could potentially harm a client because of the client's condition or medications (40).

Control group (control arm) Group in experimental research that receives the placebo or other comparison treatment against which the intervention is being tested (35).

Controlling Management function that relates to the processes of establishing specific work performance standards and the measurement, evaluation, and correction of performance (71).

Convergence Coming together, joining; applied to neural processes, occurs when input from multiple sources synapse together in one region (59).

Convergent validity Level of agreement between two tests that are being used to measure the same construct (29).

Co-occupation An occupation that implicitly involves two or more individuals (25).

Coping Conscious, volitional efforts to regulate emotion, cognition, behavior, physiology, and the environment in response to stressful events or circumstances (60).

Core values (organizational) Values that provide purpose and guide an organization's decisions and future direction (5).

Covariate A variable that is possibly predictive of the outcome (35).

Credentialing Process of obtaining or demonstrating accepted forms of proof of professional knowledge and skills (70).

Credentials Abbreviations after a person's name that designate that person's educational level and/or professional designation (40).

Criterion-referenced tests Assessments that measure activity mastery and often incorporate activity analyses. The degree of structure that is imposed on testing is usually more flexible than those for norm-referenced testing, allowing therapists to tailor tests appropriately (50).

Criterion validity Implies that the outcome of one assessment can be used as a substitute test for the established gold standard criterion test. Criterion validity can be tested as concurrent validity or predictive validity (29).

Cross-sectional studies A study in which subjects who represent a particular population are measured simultaneously for suspected risk factors/predictors and outcome(s) of interest to determine the prevalence of the outcome and the relationship between the predictors and the outcome(s) (35).

Cryotherapy The use of therapeutic low temperatures such as ice packs to relieve symptoms (57).

Cultural competence The ability to effectively interact with those who differ from oneself (19).

Cultural congruence The degree to which health professionals think and act in ways that "fit" with a person or group's beliefs and cultural style (19).

Cultural emergent A model that suggests that the symbolic aspects of culture and cultural identity emerge in interaction and are displayed primarily through talk and through action (19).

Culturally responsive care An approach that communicates a state of being open to the process of building mutuality with a client and to accepting that the cultural-specific knowledge one has about a group may or may not apply to the client they were currently treating (19).

Culture The sum total of a way of living, including values, beliefs, standards, linguistic expression, patterns of thinking, behavioral norms, and styles of communication that influence the behavior(s) of a group of people [and] is transmitted from generation to generation (19).

Day programs A subset of an outpatient rehabilitation facility in which a patient spends a major part of the day in an outpatient rehabilitation facility (62).

Deinstitutionalization The process of releasing institutionalized individuals from an institution such as a state hospital (2).

Delayed sleep phase syndrome A daily sleep/wake rhythm in which the onset of sleep and the time of awakening are later than desired (54).

Descriptive research A type of research whose purpose is to provide information about a population, for example, the prevalence of a disorder or specific characteristics of a disorder (35).

Diagnosis The process of assessing the presence and degree of disorders and their effect on a client's current status (35).

Diagnostic-related group (DRG) Classification system for Medicare Part A payments based on groups of diagnoses and procedures (74).

Differential reinforcement A technique that teaches individuals to discriminate between desired and undesired behavior and can be used to increase or decrease behavior (48).

Directing Management function that involves giving guidance, instruction, and leadership to subordinates so that work that is performed is goal oriented and contributes to meeting organizational or departmental requirements (71).

Disability Disability is an umbrella term, covering impairments, activity limitations, and participation restrictions. An impairment is a problem in body function or structure, an activity limitation is a difficulty encountered by an individual in executing a task or action, whereas a participation restriction is a problem experienced by an individual in involvement in life situations. Disability is thus not just a health problem. It is a complex phenomenon, reflecting the interaction between features of a person's body and features of the society in which he or she lives (WHO, 21).

Disability Rights Movement (DRM) A worldwide, member-driven sociopolitical movement dedicated to the acquisition of full and equal opportunities for people with disabilities to enjoy full social participation without discrimination in housing, transportation, leisure, education, and civic participation (21).

Disaster A dangerous accidental or uncontrollable situation or event that causes significant environmental destruction, loss of life, and disruption of social structure and normal daily life routines (68).

Discontinuation (discharge) summary Documentation written at the termination of services to summarize the course of a client's intervention (40).

Discrete theory Hypothesis assumed for the sake of argument or investigation (41).

Discretionary time Time not devoted to productive occupations (53).

Discriminant validity Level of disagreement (poor or zero correlation) when two tests measure a trait, behavior, or characteristic.

Discrimination Denial of equal treatment to people because of their membership in some group that occurs at many levels including individual, institutional or organizational, or structural (19).

Distributive occupations Elements that produce occupation distributed among multiple individuals working within a particular system (42).

Divergence Moving apart or separating; applied to neural processes, occurs when fibers from one source split, connecting to many other regions (59).

Diversity Having distinct forms and qualities (19).

Domotics The science of using digital applications to integrate home services with technology in order to improve residents' comfort, communication, safety, and health; see also *Smart house* (22).

Dual diagnosis A comorbid condition of a person who has been diagnosed with substance abuse and a concurrent mental health issue, such as a mood disorder, anxiety, or other mental illness (62).

Durable medical equipment Hardware, tools, and devices used by individuals to manage disease or disability or which provides therapeutic benefits (74).

Dyspraxia (developmental) A developmental condition in which the ability to plan unfamiliar motor tasks is impaired (59).

Early intervention (early intervening) services Multidisciplinary academic and support services provided to children who have developmental delays or special needs, generally from birth until the child turns three, or five, dependent on individual state laws/regulations. State law also determines context for service delivery, provided either in a child's home or in an early intervention program facility (51, 62).

Effectiveness The effect of an intervention in the real world (e.g., clinical settings) under nonideal conditions (35).

Effectiveness evidence Evidence obtained from effectiveness studies (35).

Effect size The strength of an association between variables or the strength of the difference between the outcomes of different conditions (35).

Efficacy The effect of an intervention under ideal conditions (35).

Efficacy expectations A person's belief about how successful or unsuccessful he or she will be at performing a skill or occupation (48).

Effortful control A volitional ability to shift attention, inhibit the tendency to enact a dominant response, and/or activate an alternative response as needed (60).

Eleanor Clarke Slagle Lectureship An AOTA academic honor established as a memorial to Eleanor Clarke Slagle, a pioneer in the profession of occupational therapy (2).

Electroencephalogram (EEG) A recording of brain waves obtained by attaching flat metal discs (electrodes) to the scalp (54).

Electromyogram Technology that measures motor activity through electrodes placed on the skin over muscles (54).

Electronic aids to independent living (EADL) Provide the user with control over appliances and other electronic devices within the environment; a wide variety of switches interface with EADL to allow individuals with a variety of skills and impairments to use them (50).

Electronic health record Computerized medical record created in an organization that delivers care (40).

Electrooculogram Technology that measures eye movements through electrodes placed on the skin around the eyes (54).

Embodied Used to reflect a view that the mind and body are not separate but rather one entity. In relation to occupational therapy, refers to the wholistic nature of therapeutic actions as experienced by the therapist and the client (34).

Embodied action A view of action in which thoughts, sociality, and emotions are considered part of the lived body as opposed to the dualistic view of the mind as planning actions and the body carrying out actions (7).

Emergency A situation that poses an immediate risk to health, life, property, or environment (62).

Emergent performance The process whereby a person puts together actions to engage in a way that is functional drawing on intrinsic capacities and an understanding of the dynamics of the situation as performance unfolds (7).

Emmanuelism A community-based health care approach started in the early nineteenth century that incorporated the use of volunteer providers, education, and arts and crafts as part of its regimen for treating chronic illnesses, including tuberculosis and alcoholism (2).

Emotion An evaluative mental state that occurs in the present moment and consists of neurobiological arousal, perceptual-cognitive processes, subjective experience, and affective expression (60).

Emotional regulation skills Actions or behaviors a client uses to identify, manage, and express feelings while engaging in activities or interacting with others (60).

Emotion dysregulation Actions or behaviors related to emotional experience that interfere with goal-directed pursuits, interpersonal relationships, or healthy adaptation (60).

Empathy Awareness of and insight into the feelings, emotions, and behavior of another person and their meaning and significance; not the same as sympathy, which is usually nonobjective and noncritical (36, 37).

Empowerment Process of becoming stronger and more confident, especially in controlling one's life and claiming one's rights (45).

Engineering controls Equipment and workplace designs or changes that reduce the human efforts needed (52).

Entry-level competence Denotes successful completion of academic program requirements, classroom, and fieldwork, resulting in eligibility to apply for professional credentials required for employment (69, 70).

Environment(s) Particular physical, social, cultural, economic, and political features within a person's everyday life that affect the motivation, organization, and performance (33, 42, 43).

Environmental control units Devices that enable individuals with mobility impairments to have control over their environment, including lights, appliances, television, air/heat units, window blinds, and more (50).

Environmental embodiment The various ways, both sensorially and movement wise, that the lived body engages and coordinates with the world at hand, especially its environmental aspects (22).

Environmental modifications Internal and external physical adaptations to environments that are necessary to maximize independence and to ensure health and safety (30).

Epidemiology (epidemiological) The study of the distribution and determinants of disease, injury, or dysfunction in human populations (52).

Epistemology The theory of knowledge (3).

Epworth Sleepiness Scale A self-report scale intended to measure daytime sleepiness (54).

Ergonomics The scientific discipline concerned with the understanding of interactions among humans and other elements of a system, and the profession that applies theory, principles, data, and methods to design in order to optimize human well-being and overall system performance (52).

Essential functions The basic job duties that all employees must be able to perform with or without reasonable accommodation (52).

Ethical problem Problem in which there are competing possible responses and which requires a morally defensible course of action (36).

Ethnicity A social grouping of people who share cultural or national similarities. The most common characteristics of an ethnic group include kinship, family rituals, food preferences, special clothing, and particular celebrations (19).

Ethnocentrism Tendency of people to put their own group (*ethnos*) at the center; to see things through the narrow lens of their own culture and use the standards of that culture to judge others (19).

Evaluation Process of gathering and interpreting qualitative and/or quantitative data to understand client needs and desires, describe function, predict future function, plan intervention, or measure outcome of occupational therapy intervention; the process of obtaining and interpreting data necessary for intervention. This includes planning for and documenting the evaluation process and results (OTPF-III, 27, 28, 40, 50, 51).

Evidence Knowledge gained through systematic appraisal of experience and of scientific studies (27).

Evidence-based practice Professional practice that integrates the results of scientific research into the clinical decision-making process (35, 39).

Executive functions Encompass a broad range of skills that allow a person to engage in independent, purposeful, and self-directed behavior. There are three core executive functions: inhibition, working memory, and cognitive flexibility (58).

Existential anxiety Fear and anxiety of one's own disablement when confronted by people with disabilities (21).

Existentialism A philosophy (often associated with Kierkegaard) that focuses on the essence of a human that is realized through self-determination (3).

Experimental research Compares two or more conditions in order to determine cause and effect relationships (35).

Exploratory research Research that examines a specific phenomenon and its relationship to other factors (35).

External validity Refers to whether generalizations be made to the general population (29).

Extinction (in behavioral theory) The process of reducing the frequency of a behavior by withholding reinforcement (48).

Extinction burst In behavioral theory, term is used for the phenomenon in which the behavior being extinguished gets worse before it gets better (48).

Face validity Indicates that a measure's items are viewed as plausible (29).

Facilitation A neural process that promotes the conduction of impulses or a response to them. Facilitation is the opposite of inhibition (59).

Factor analysis Statistical process used to identify one or more underlying dimensions of a construct (29).

Fading Systematic reduction of support (scaffold) to clients so that task demands increase; used when clients improve their skills (48).

Family The basic unit in society traditionally consisting of two parents rearing their children; also any of various social units differing from but regarded as equivalent to the traditional family (17).

Family-centered care An experience that happens when practitioners effectively and compassionately listen to the concerns, address the needs, and support the hopes of people and their families (17).

Family routines Observable and repetitive patterns involving two or more family members and occur with predictable regularity in family life (18).

Feedback Information arising from the response itself (i.e., production feedback) or from changes that occur in the environment as a result of the response (outcome feedback) (59).

Feed forward Neural information sent from the motor cortex to the cerebellum in parallel with the motor command sent to the alpha motor neurons; a "preview" of the intended motor action. It permits the cerebellum to exert its role as comparator of expected movement with actual movement (59).

Fee-for-service Retrospective reimbursement for medical services based on "reasonable and necessary" criteria (74).

Fiber diameter Neuronal diameter; fiber diameter plays a role in determining how fast a neural signal is transmitted; bigger fibers transmit information more quickly because there is less resistance to the flow of ions (59).

Fieldwork (practice placements) Structured learning experiences that are formally administered by academic programs in partnership with facilities that offer supervised training experiences (69).

Fieldwork educator Person responsible for providing student supervision; interchangeable terms include clinical educator, fieldwork supervisor, student supervisor, or practice educator (69).

First episode programs Specialized programs that aim to promote recovery and independence among young people experiencing early psychosis or other psychiatric symptoms, with a goal of preventing or reducing long-term disability (65).

Folk healer A person who is recognized within the culture who uses traditional magico-religious practices and rituals to help heal the sick (19).

Folk practices Traditional home remedies used by certain family, ethnic, and cultural groups to counteract illness and support wellness (19).

Foreground questions A type of question used to obtain current knowledge related to best practice treatment of a disorder/condition (35).

Form (of an occupation) The observable features of an occupation such as the sequence of actions in doing an occupation (9).

Formative Evaluation or feedback designed to support continued learning and development (69).

Framing (of play/leisure) Cues that separate play or leisure from "real life"; generally the cues tell others how a player or leisure participant wishes to be viewed by others (53).

Fraud (in relation to therapy billing) The act of intentionally being deceptive in relation to the provision of services; can include fabricating documentation for services that were not really rendered, billing for more services than were provided in a visit, or accepting bribes or kickbacks for referrals (40).

Free appropriate public education (FAPE) Special education and related services provided at public expense that meets the standards of the state education agency (SEA) (51, 74).

Freestanding model A supported education model that provides support at the organization which sponsors program (65).

Function (of an occupation) Is what an occupation achieves, such as volunteering for a local service might achieve integration into the community (9).

Functional assessment Observation of behavior in a natural context or one that closely simulates the natural context in order to understand how environmental factors affect performance or specific behaviors (48).

Functional capacity evaluation An individual's functional abilities and/or limitations in the context of safe, productive work tasks (52).

Functional group A group designed to promote adaptation and health through group action and engagement in occupation (38).

Functional job descriptions Reports that identify essential job functions and critical demands; employers can use them in hiring, making return to work decisions, and determining necessary accommodation (52).

Functionally illiterate Reading below the fifth-grade level (32).

Functional supervision Supervision over a specific aspect of work or job function (72).

Generalizability (in research) The applicability of a study result to the population (35).

Generalizability theory A measurement theory that recognizes multiple different sources of error and attempts to quantify the sources from those various errors (29).

Generalize The ability to apply what has been learned in therapy to a variety of new situations and environments (58).

Grading Systematically increasing the demands of an activity or occupation to stimulate improved function or reducing the demands to respond to client difficulties in performance (30).

Group An aggregate of people who share a common purpose that can only be achieved through collaboration (38).

Group-centered action Member actions that are interdependent (38).

Group cohesiveness The degree of understanding, acceptance, and feelings of closeness group members have toward each other and the value they place on the group (38).

Group goal A future state toward which a majority of group members' efforts are directed (38).

Group home Small, residential facility located within a community, designed to serve children or adults with chronic disabilities. These homes usually have six or fewer occupants and are staffed 24 hours a day by trained caregivers (62).

Group norms The value system of the group; what members believe are appropriate ways of thinking, feeling, and behaving (38).

Group process The interrelationships and interactions among members, leaders, and within the group as a whole (38).

Group protocol (in therapy) An intervention plan for a specific client population (38).

Guardianship A legal association in which a protected individual's personal affairs are managed by one or more people or an agency. Conservatorship is a legal relationship, like guardianship, but is limited to managing the protected individual's financial affairs and property (50).

Habits Acquired tendencies to respond and perform in certain consistent ways in familiar environments or situation; specific, automatic behaviors performed repeatedly, relatively automatically, and with little variation (18, 42).

Habituation Internalized readiness to exhibit consistent patterns of behavior guided by habits and roles and fitted to the characteristics of routine temporal, physical, and social environment. It also refers to a decrease in neural response as a result of continued presentation of a stimulus and to the personal responses in which there is a decreased behavioral response to a repeated stimulus (42, 59).

Health The complete state of physical, mental, and social well-being and not just the absence of disease or infirmity (WHO, 47).

Health disparity Gap in the quality of health and health care across racial and ethnic groups; population-specific difference in the presence of disease, health outcomes, or access to health care (20).

Health literacy The degree to which individuals have the capacity to obtain, process, and understand basic health information and services needed to make appropriate health decisions (32).

Health promotion The movement toward optimal health and high-level wellness; the use of discipline-specific techniques to assist people in achieving their health-related goals (47, 52).

Health savings account Savings account used for medical bills that is not subject to income tax (synonym: *Health reimbursement accounts*) (74).

High-deductible health plan (HDHP) A health insurance plan with lower premiums and higher deductibles than a traditional health plan. Being covered by HDHP is also a requirement for having a health savings account (74).

High-touch societies Those whose members may seek out touch as a means of communication and are comfortable with casual touch (19).

Historically controlled study The control group of the experimental trial is a group of patients observed sometime in the past or for whom data are available only through records (35).

Home health care Provision of predominantly medically related services to patients in a home setting rather than in a medical facility (62).

Homeostatic sleep drive The drive to sleep that accumulates during prolonged wakefulness and lessens during sleep. Sleep homeostasis is one of the primary modulators of sleep in humans (54).

Hospice Palliative care designed to provide medical, emotional, social, and spiritual support to individuals in the final phase of a terminal illness, focusing on comfort and quality of life rather than curative interventions. Aggressive methods of pain control may be used. It is generally provided as home care but can be delivered in free-standing facilities, nursing homes, or within hospitals (62).

Humanism A philosophy of human nature, human interests, welfare, and dignity that upholds humans as having inherent worth and potential (3).

Hyperalgesia An increased sensitivity to pain (54).

Hypertension High blood pressure (54).

Hypnagogic hallucinations Vivid, sometimes frightening images in transition to sleep (54).

Hypnogram A graph that summarizes the pattern of sleep stages across a night, for instance, as recorded in the sleep laboratory (54).

Hypothesis testing Statistical process used to determine the likelihood that assumptions (hypotheses) are true or supported by data (29).

Impairment A problem with part of a person's anatomy or his or her physiological or psychological functioning due to a significant deviation from normal or loss (ICF, 8, 21).

Inception cohort study A cohort study in which all subjects are in the early stages of their disorder when they enter the study (35).

Inclusion State of being able to participate in life activities—often used in relation to removing social and physical obstacles to participation (33).

Incompetence Acting without appropriate knowledge, skill, or ability (40).

Indemnity plans Insurance plans that pay for costs associated with a medical condition or injury; associated with fee-for-service method of payment (74).

Independent Living Movement (ILM) Movement that started in the 1960s with a mission of deinstitutionalization and promoting disability rights based on the fact that disability is a natural part of life and that society has created and maintained barriers for people with disabilities (21).

Indigenous worldview Indigenous worldviews are characterized people's close relationship with the environment; see *Worldview* (9).

Indirect assessment Includes interviews, questionnaires, role-playing, consulting with other professionals, and client self-monitoring (48).

Individual controls The physical, cognitive, and social skills and performance of the workers. Safe, efficient job design is dependent on coordination of all aspects of the system (52).

Individualistic societies Societies that value self-expression, personal choice, autonomy, individual responsibility, and independence (19).

Individualized Education Programs (IEPs) Written plan for the delivery of educationally related services to children ages 3 to 21 years with disabilities, as mandated by IDEA (40).

Individualized Family Service Plans (IFSPs) Written plan for the delivery of services to children with disabilities ages birth through 2 years; prepares children with disabilities to enter the educational system at age 3 years (40).

Individuals with Disabilities Education Act (IDEA) Federal law that mandates that educational services must be provided to a child with a disability from birth to age 21 years (2, 74).

Inevitable interpersonal events Naturally occurring communications, reactions, processes, tasks, or general circumstances of therapy that carry an emotional valence (37).

Inferential statistics Statistics that are used to infer the degree to which a study result from a sample can confidentially be applied to the population (35).

Information and communication technologies (ICT) An umbrella term referring to broadband, wireless, and mobile computing as they combine with the Internet and with social media such as blogging, social networking, gaming, and e-mail (22).

Inhibition A neural process that reduces the likelihood that the postsynaptic neuron will reach threshold (signal level) required for an action potential to occur (59).

Inner drive Motivation and self-direction that come from within a child to develop sensory integration (59).

Inpatient rehabilitation Intensive interdisciplinary services (at least 3 hours a day, 5 to 7 days a week of at least two different types of therapy) performed on a discrete, licensed unit either within a hospital or in a freestanding hospital. Specific admission criteria must be met in order for individuals to be eligible for inpatient rehabilitation (62).

Insomnia Trouble falling asleep, staying asleep, or waking up too early (54).

Institutional review board (IRB) A panel of diverse individuals, including organization staff and at least one community member, who are responsible for reviewing all research proposals and grants to ensure that adequate protections for research participants are in place (36).

Instructing mode One of the six therapist interpersonal modes defined by a therapist's efforts to carefully structure therapy activities and to be explicit with clients about the plan, sequence, and events of therapy (37).

Instrumental activities of daily living (IADL) Activities to support daily life within the home and community that often require more complex interactions than self-care used in ADL. IADL include 12 activity categories: care of others, care of pets, child rearing, communication management, community mobility, financial management, health management and maintenance, home establishment and management, meal preparation and clean up, religious observance, safety and emergency maintenance, and shopping (50).

Integration Intermixing of people or groups previously segregated (51).

Intensive outpatient programs (IOPs) A step down from partial hospitalization programs. Persons at this level may be functioning adequately in one or more of their occupational roles but need more support or therapy than traditional outpatient treatment (65).

Intentional use of self The therapist's ability to deliberately anticipate, formulate, reason, and reflect about the use of modes and other interpersonal skills in light of the client's unique interpersonal characteristics and the inevitable interpersonal events that emerge during the therapy process (37).

Interdisciplinary team Individuals representing different professional disciplines that work together to identify goals and plan intervention collaboratively (39).

Interests What one finds enjoyable and satisfying (42).

Intermittent reinforcement Reinforcement only after certain demonstrations of the behavior (48).

Internal validity Refers to whether or not the assessment measure what it is supposed to measure, that is, a specific trait, behavior, construct, or performance (29).

International Code of Sleep Disorders (ICSD-2) Published by the American Academy of Sleep Medicine. This system classifies sleep disorders into eight major categories (54).

Interpersonal event A naturally occurring communication, reaction, process, task, or general circumstance that occurs during therapy and that has the potential to fortify or weaken the therapeutic relationship, depending on how it is handled (37).

Interpersonal level Relationships among family, friends, peers, and groups that provide support, identity, and role definition and facilitate or constrain occupational performance and/or participation and impact health (31).

Interpersonal reasoning A stepwise process by which a therapist decides what to say, do, or otherwise express in reaction to a client's interpersonal characteristics and behavior (37).

Interpersonal style Defined by the therapist's primary mode or set of modes used during therapy (37).

Interrater reliability With a statistical approach, it is used to detect differences in scoring between two or more raters who measure the same clients on the same attributes (29).

Intervention Process and skilled actions taken by occupational therapy practitioners in collaboration with the client to facilitate engagement in occupations related to health and participation. The intervention process includes the plan, implementation, and review (OTPF-III, 27).

Intrapersonal level Characteristics of individuals within the organization or population that influence behavior and impact occupational performance, participation, and health (31).

Intrarater reliability A statistical approach used to detect differences in scoring obtained by the same rater when measuring the same client on the same attributes (29).

Intrinsic motivation Motivated by the experience itself, not by the promise of external rewards. Self-determined extrinsic motivation: activities chosen by the individual for the long-term gain associated with them or for another's benefit (53).

Job accommodations Accommodations may involve the office, industrial, service, and medical industries and can extend to personal needs (33).

Job analysis Includes a formal methodology that details the interaction between the worker and the equipment of a system (52).

Job description A statement that defines the essential functions of the job and how the job relates to other jobs and to the workplace (52).

Just-right challenge A task that is manageably demanding, neither too difficult nor too easy; promotes central nervous system integration (59).

Leadership The process of creating structural change where the values, vision, and ethics of individuals are integrated into the culture of a community as a means of achieving sustainable change (71).

Learned nonuse A learning phenomenon whereby movement is suppressed initially due to adverse reactions and failure of any activity attempted with the affected limb, which then results in the suppression of behavior (57).

Least restrictive environment (LRE) Environment that provides maximum interaction with nondisabled peers and is consistent with the needs of the child/student (51).

Leisure A transaction characterized by relative intrinsic, or self-determined extrinsic, motivation; relative internal control; and disengagement from reality; and that is framed in such a way as to separate it from "real life" (53).

Letter of intent (LOI) In consulting, refers to a summary of the work that can be done and that the consultant recommending (73).

Level I fieldwork Experiences designed to enrich didactic course work through directed observation and participation in selected aspects of the occupational therapy process (69).

Level II fieldwork An in-depth experience in delivering occupational therapy services to clients, focusing on the application of purposeful and meaningful occupation, as integral to the academic program's curriculum design (69).

Liability A legal term pertaining to personal responsibility (73).

Life balance A satisfying pattern of daily activity that is healthful, meaningful, and sustainable to an individual within the context of his or her current life circumstances (18).

Life coaches Professionals who facilitate positive life changes in their clients using a conversation and question-based process to help clients become more self-aware, assess their values and strengths that lead to self-directed change (18).

Life course A term (and a field of study) used to describe the patterns of people's lives in context. It considers the determinants and consequences of social relationships, historic events, and government policy for how people live their lives (7).

Life imbalance A state in which one's activity configurations limit or compromise participation in valued relationships; are incongruent for establishing or maintaining physiological health and a satisfactory identity; or are mundane, uninteresting, or unchallenging (18).

Life span development A broad phrase from developmental psychology and developmental science that connotes systematic changes within a person from conception to the end of life as they are reflected by changes in behavior. Although change occurs through interacting with the social and physical world, the focus is on the changing functions of the person (7).

Lifeworld The tacit, taken-for-granted context, tenor, and pace of daily life to which normally people give no reflective attention; a major focus of phenomenological investigation (22).

Lived body A phenomenological concept referring to the ways in which our existence as bodily beings contributes to the constitution of human experience and to the human lifeworld; the phenomenologist argues that the lived body is the primary means of being in, experiencing, and encountering the world; see also *Body-subject* (22).

Local independence An indication of whether the items of an assessment independently contribute to the measurement of a particular trait. That is, some items are redundant or not adding anything new to the measuring of a particular trait (29).

Long-term acute care (LTAC) Specialized acute care for medically complex patients who are critically ill with multisystem complications or failures and require long-term hospitalizations, performed on a discrete, licensed unit either within a hospital or in a freestanding hospital (62).

Long-term care (LTC) A combination of medical, nursing, custodial, social, and community services designed to help people who have disabilities or chronic care needs, including dementia, who cannot care for themselves for long periods of time. Services may be provided in the person's home, in the community, in assisted living facilities, or in nursing homes (62).

Low-touch societies Those that tend to avoid touch, especially in public, except in prescribed situations such as the handshake during a greeting. For many, a casual touch between members of the opposite sex may be interpreted as a sexual overture and should be avoided (19).

Lures Use of play, leisure, or other incentives as motivation to participate in therapeutic activities or as rewards for participation in them (54).

Macro level The broadest factors from the external environment that affect policy, funding, services, and sociopolitical influences on the consultation process (73).

Major depressive disorder A mental illness characterized by depressed mood, reduced interest in activities that used to be enjoyed, sleep disturbances, loss of energy, difficulty concentrating, holding a conversation, paying attention, making decisions that used to be made fairly easily, and suicidal thoughts or intentions (65).

Malpractice Misconduct on the part of a professional that results in harm to a client (40).

Managed care Comprehensive health care system that provides a variety of health services and facilities with a focus on controlling costs (74).

Management The process of guiding a work unit by planning for future work obligations, organizing employees into functional units, directing employees in the process of completing daily work tasks, and controlling work processes and systems to assure adequate quality of work output (71).

Marginal functions Tasks that are not essential to the specific job or tasks that could, if necessary, be completed by another worker (52).

Marked Noticeable (26).

Meaning (of an occupation) The significance of an occupation and what is expressed through doing; includes personal, societal, cultural, and historical expressions (9).

Measurement Process of assigning numbers to represent quantities of a trait, attribute, or characteristic or to classify objects (29).

Mechanism-based reasoning Obtaining evidence by extrapolating the results of basic science and applying them to clinical situations (35).

Mechanisms of action An understanding of how specific intervention strategies lead to particular outcomes including how change proceeds and the particular conditions under which an intervention achieves the desired results (41).

Medicaid A governmental insurance program in the United States for older adults, children and parents of dependent children, pregnant women, and people with disabilities who meet the eligibility requirements (74).

Medicare A U.S. national social insurance program that guarantees access to health insurance for Americans ages 65 years and older and younger people with disabilities as well as people with end-stage renal disease (74).

Medigap policy Private health insurance designed to supplement original Medicare; helps pay some of the health care costs ("gaps") that original Medicare does not cover (e.g., copayments, coinsurance, and deductibles) (74).

Melatonin A hormone secreted by the pineal gland in the brain. It helps regulate other hormones and maintains the body's circadian rhythm (54).

Memorandum of understanding (MOU) Memorandum summarizing agreements between parties; see also *Letter of intent* (73).

Memory Ability to register, retain, and recall past experience, knowledge, and sensation (58).

Mental health A state of well-being in which every individual realizes his or her own potential, can cope with the normal stresses of life, can work productively and fruitfully, and is able to make a contribution to his or her community (59).

Mental illness Mental, behavioral, or emotional disorder (excluding developmental and substance use disorders) (65).

Mental status examinations Formal procedure to examine and diagnose mental functioning, including a general description of a person, notation of emotional expression, identification of perceptual disturbances, and exploration of thought processes and thought content (58).

Metacognitive Form of cognitive process in which one thinks about one's own thinking (34).

Methods (methodology) A general approach to practice; the design and approach used to collect data in research (3, 35).

Mezzo level The factors of the environment external to the client receiving consultation services including cultural, physical, temporal, and virtual elements (73).

Micro level The person, interpersonal factors, cultural, and personal contexts of the individual receiving occupational therapy services (73).

Minimal clinically important difference (MCID) The smallest change in an outcome that indicates a clinically important change in a client's condition (35).

Mission The core purpose of an organization, often includes why an organization exists, who the organization serves, and how an organization goes about achieving its purpose (71).

Mission statement A written summary of the core purpose of an organization, often includes why an organization exists, who the organization serves, and how an organization goes about achieving its purpose (71).

Mobile support model A supported education model that meets students with psychiatric disabilities in the community to provide individualized educational support (65).

Mode An aspect of the therapist's therapeutic personality that defines a specific approach to relating with a client (37).

Mode shift A conscious change in one's way of relating to a client when a therapist changes the communication approach from one approach to another (37).

Mood disorder A category of disorders that includes those where the primary symptom is inappropriate, exaggerated, or limited range of feelings or moods; includes depression and bipolar disorders (62).

Moral distress A problem that occurs when practitioners know the right thing to do but cannot achieve it because of external barriers or uncertainty about the outcome (36).

Moral reasoning The process of reflecting on ethical issues; includes reasoning about norms and values, ideas of right and wrong, and how practitioners make decisions in professional work (36).

Moral treatment Term given for a movement characterized by the provision of humane conditions of care for persons with mental illness, influenced by the ideas emanating from the age of enlightenment (2).

Motor control The ability to regulate or direct the mechanisms essential to movement (57).

Motor learning A set of processes associated with practice or experience leading to relatively permanent changes in the capability for skilled movement (57).

Motor planning Ability to carry out a skilled, nonhabitual motor activity; process that bridges ideation and motor execution to enable an adaptive response (58).

Motor skills Occupational performance skills observed as the person interacts with and moves task objects and moves oneself around the task environment (26).

Multiculturalism An ideal in which diverse groups in a society coexist amicably, retaining their individual cultural identities (19).

Multidisciplinary team A group of individuals from different professional disciplines that serves the client; each individual is responsible for identifying and carrying out one's own discipline-related assessment, intervention plan and implementation, and communicating with each other (39).

Multimodal An interpersonal style that describes therapists who have an ability to use all six of the modes flexibly and comfortably and an ability to match those modes to the client and the situation (37).

Muscle tone The continuous and passive partial contraction of the muscles or the muscle's resistance to passive stretch during resting state (59).

Narcolepsy A rare sleep disorder marked by excessive sleepiness or sudden sleep attacks (54).

National Board for Certification in Occupational Therapy (NBCOT) The credentialing body for occupational therapists and occupational therapy assistants practicing in the United States; organization which develops and administers the initial certification examinations for occupational therapists and occupational therapy assistants (5, 36, 70).

National Society for the Promotion of Occupational Therapy The name given to the professional society founded in 1917 that organized workers in the curative occupations, leading to what is now known as the American Occupational Therapy Association (2).

Need for control An interpersonal characteristic describing the role taken within a relationship; ranges from active versus passive (37).

Negative predictive value A statistic indicating the likelihood that people with a negative test result would not have a condition (29).

Negative reinforcement Response or behavior is strengthened by stopping, removing, or avoiding a negative outcome or aversive stimulus (48).

Negligence Failing to do something that ought to be done to prevent harm to a client (40).

Neurasthenia The name given to a nervous condition characterized by fatigue and listlessness that was widely diagnosed during the period from 1880 to 1910. Originally, neurasthenia was treated using "the rest cure," but the rise of the curative occupation movement and its success with these patients helped create legitimacy for this approach to therapy, helping lead to the founding of occupational therapy (2).

Neurologic threshold The smallest change in membrane potential required for the production of an action potential (59).

Neuroplasticity Brain's ability to reorganize itself by forming new neural connections; may be either developmental (occurring throughout life) or reactive (in response to insult or injury). Neuroplasticity entails the activity-dependent shaping of connections at synapses where information is transferred from one nerve cell to another. It is influenced profoundly by sensory input, behavioral output, and practice (59).

New poor Unexpected poverty with inability to meet most basic needs; major factors contributing to growing numbers of new poor are job layoffs, family breakdown, and sudden illness (20).

Night terrors Episodes of fear, flailing, and screaming while asleep; also known as sleep terrors, night terrors often are paired with sleepwalking (54).

Nocturia The need to get up in the night to urinate, thus interrupting sleep (54).

Noncompete clause A statement limiting a person, or company, from competing in a stated business after termination, or resignation, for a specific time, in a particular geographic area, or other specified way (73).

Nonconsecutive cohort study A cohort study in which the sample includes only some of the eligible patients identified during the study recruitment period (35).

Nonrapid eye movement sleep (NREM) The stages of sleep that do not include rapid eye movement patterns. According to current guidelines for sleep stage classification, NREM consists of three different stages: N1, N2, and N3 (54).

Nonstandardized assessments Assessments that do not follow a standard approach or protocol. For instance, they may not involve a consistent set of questions, directions, or conditions for administration, testing, or scoring (29).

Nonverbal cues Communications that do not involve the use of formal language. Some examples of these are facial expressions, movement patterns, body posture, and eye contact (37).

Normative expectations Activities or occupations viewed as standard behavior expected of other people in the same circumstances; may be encouraged by members of the community (7).

Norm-referenced test A type of test, assessment, or evaluation that yields an estimate of the position of the tested individual in a predefined population, with respect to the trait being measured. This estimate is derived from the analysis of test scores and possibly other relevant data from a sample drawn from the population (50).

Objective Not influenced by personal feelings, interpretations, or prejudice; based on facts; unbiased (23).

Observational study Another term for either an associative or descriptive research; called observational studies because the subjects do not receive an experimental intervention but are simply observed (35).

Obstructive sleep apnea (OSA) Apnea caused by partial or complete blockage of airway passages during sleep (54).

Occupation The daily life activities in which people engage (1, 8, 25, 27, 45).

Occupational activities Tasks that are directly related to the individual's preferred occupational role. Such tasks must have personal meaning and occupational relevance; the individual must be the primary actor in the activity (44).

Occupational adaptation Normative internal process that is activated by the individual when approaching and adapting to challenges in life; constructing a positive occupational identity and achieving occupational competence over time in the context of one's environment (42, 44).

Occupational analysis Analysis of an occupation that is relevant to an individual within the actual context of performance. Occupational analysis refers to systematically analyzing what and how a person or groups of people actually do an activity (25, 26, 40).

Occupational apartheid Separation between those who have meaningful, useful occupations and those who are deprived of, isolated from, or otherwise constrained in their daily life occupations (20).

Occupational choice Determination of meaningful activities based on one's values; interests and beliefs; social situation; gender and gender identity; age; and physical, cognitive, and emotional abilities (19).

Occupational competence The degree to which one is able to sustain a pattern of occupational participation that reflects one's occupational identity (42).

Occupational deprivation Lack of access to engagement in an array of self-selected occupations that have meaning to the individual, family, or community (47).

Occupational dysadaptation Performance problems arising from a mismatch between environmental demands and the person's motivation or capacity for response (44).

Occupational engagement One's doing, thinking, and feeling under certain environmental conditions in the midst of or as a planned consequence of therapy (42).

Occupational environment One of the three primary elements in the theory of occupational adaptation. In contrast with other environments, the occupational environment calls for an occupational response from the individual in the context of work, play/leisure, or self-maintenance. The contexts are shaped by unique physical, social, and cultural influences (44).

Occupational form The preexisting structure that elicits, guides, or structures performance of daily life activities (1).

Occupational identity Composite sense of who one is and wishes to become as an occupational being generated from one's history of occupational participation (42).

Occupational justice Concerned with ethical, moral, and civic issues such as equity and fairness for individuals and collectives, specific to engagement in diverse and meaningful occupation that is inclusive of "doing, being, belonging, and becoming" (45).

Occupational knowledge The experiential, observational, and investigatory information acquired by occupational therapy practitioners to understand the form, function, and meaning of engaging in occupations for individuals and society (1).

Occupational orchestration The capacity of individuals to enact their occupations on a daily basis to meet their own needs and the expectations of the many environments in which they are required to function. This may include attention to habits and routines and the interface of these with the needs and expectations of others (25).

Occupational participation Engagement in work, play, or activities of daily living that are part of one's socio-cultural context and that are desired and/or necessary to one's well-being (42).

Occupational patterns Habits, routines, roles, and rituals used in the process of engaging in occupations or activities (18).

Occupational performance Human actions in response to an occupational form (1).

Occupational possibilities Refers to the ways through which accessing and engaging in occupations come to be viewed as ideal and are supported and promoted by broader systems and structures through a specific sociohistorical context (1).

Occupational profile A summary of information that describes the client's occupational history and experiences, patterns of daily living, interests, values, and needs (OTPF-III, 30, 40).

Occupational readiness A term that characterizes interventions that are designed to affect the individual's sensorimotor, cognitive, and/or psychosocial deficits (44).

Occupational rights Ethical, moral, and civic issues such as equity and fairness for both individuals and collectives specific to engagement in diverse and meaningful occupation (45).

Occupational role The personally experienced situation of the individual (25).

Occupational science The study of the things people do; interdisciplinary academic discipline in the social and behavioral sciences dedicated to the study of the form, the function, and the meaning of human occupations (9).

Occupational skill acquisition Increased proficiency in performance and skill related to a meaningful occupation (30).

Occupational transition Major change in the occupational repertoire of a person in which one or several occupations change, disappear, and/or are replaced by others (52).

Occupation as end Occupations that constitute the end product of therapy, that is, the occupations to be learned or relearned (30).

Occupation as means Occupations that act as the therapeutic change agent to remediate impaired abilities or capacities (30).

Occupation-based education programs Providing education to large groups of people related to common problems and strategies to address problems (61).

Occupation-based or occupation-focused practice An approach to intervention that incorporates the real-life interests and activities of the client and typically harness activities naturally occurring in the person's life for therapeutic purposes (9).

Occupation-focused lifestyle interventions An intervention approach that takes account of the unique constellation of circumstances that comprise a person's everyday life (9).

Onsite model A supported education model that provides individualized support sponsored by an educational institution (65).

Ontology An element of philosophy that is concerned with the nature of reality (3).

Operant conditioning Skinner's basic principle that a response followed by some reinforcement is likely to be strengthened (48).

Organizational level (of ecologically based interventions) Rules, regulations, policies, procedures, programs, and resources within agencies and organizations that impact occupational performance and/or participation and impact health (31).

Organizing In management, refers to the overall structure of the organization, including how line authority will be organized and how employees may be grouped into departments and relative expectations of employees and groups (71).

Orientation Awareness of self in relation to time, place, and identification of others (58).

Orientation toward relating Personal characteristic that describes a client's need for interpersonal closeness versus professional distance within the therapeutic relationship (37).

Orthosis (splint) An orthopedic appliance or apparatus used to support, align, prevent, or correct deformities or to improve function of movable parts of the body (57).

Outcome(s) Measurable result(s) or consequence(s) of an intervention or other factors (27, 35).

Outpatient rehabilitation Rehabilitation performed in an outpatient facility that is either attached to an acute care hospital, rehabilitation hospital, or freestanding facility (62).

Oxygen saturation A measure of how much oxygen the blood is carrying (54).

Palliative (palliation) Providing clients with relief from the symptoms, pain, and stress of a serious illness regardless of the diagnosis with a goal of improving quality of life for both the clients and their family (30).

Paradigm A set of broad assumptions and perspectives that unifies a field and defines its purpose and nature. These assumptions and perspectives are believed to underlie a discipline's science and practice at a given time (1, 2).

Parasomnias Nonsleep behaviors that intrude during sleep, such as sleepwalking and sleep eating (54).

Parasympathetic Relating to the division of the autonomic nervous system that acts in opposition to the sympathetic system by slowing the heartbeat, constricting the bronchi of the lungs, stimulating the smooth muscles of the digestive tract, etc. (59).

Partial hospital, partial hospitalization programs (PHPs) Programs that are intended to divert the person from hospitalization or serve as an intermediary step toward community living after an acute inpatient course of treatment. Also, an outpatient program specifically designed for the diagnosis or active treatment of a serious mental disorder when there is a reasonable expectation for improvement or when it is necessary to maintain an individual's functional level and prevent relapse or full hospitalization (62, 65).

Participation Involvement in life situations (e.g., self-care tasks, domestic life, education, employment, social, and civic life). Participation encompasses passive participation (e.g., observing others or listening). Occupational therapists generally include additional elements such as the meaning of participation and people's subjective experience of participating (ICF, 8, 49, 55).

Participation restriction A persons difficulty engaging in a "life situation" (engaging in roles or occupations) (ICF, 21).

Passive range of motion (PROM) Arc of motion through which the joint passes when moved by an outside force (57).

Peer-operated services Part of the continuum of services available in the community for people with psychiatric disabilities and are based on a belief that people who have faced, endured, or overcome adversity can offer useful support, hope, and encouragement to others in similar situations (65).

Peer review When work is reviewed by experts in the field who provide feedback and contribute to the decision of whether or not the work meets specified criteria for dissemination (39).

Peer-support services Services offered before, during, and after treatment to facilitate long-term recovery, promote community integration, develop coping and problem-solving strategies for illness self-management, and offer empathy to promote hope, insights, and skills (65).

Perception(s) The identification, organization, and interpretation of sensation, leading to a mental representation (59).

Performance analysis The evaluation of the quality or effectiveness of the motor, process, and/or social interaction skills based on the observation of a person as he or she is engaged in the performance of a desired or needed daily life task and with the goal of evaluating the person's quality of occupational performance (26).

Performance capacity Ability to do things provided by the status of underlying objective, physical and mental components, and corresponding subjective experience (42).

Performance skills The smallest observable units of occupational performance; goal-directed actions a person carries out one by one when engaged in naturalistic and relevant daily life task performances (26, 70).

Periodic limb movement disorder (PLMD) A sleep disorder characterized by leg movements or jerks that typically occur every 20 to 40 seconds during sleep, causing sleep to be disrupted and leaving the person with excessive daytime sleepiness (54).

Perseveration Unnecessary and prolonged repetition of a word, phase, or movement (58).

Personal causation Sense of capacity and effectiveness (42).

Personal factors Aspects of the human condition such as body structures and body functions (23).

Personal meaning Satisfaction of conscious or unconscious needs and/or attribution of benefits derived from activities (53).

Phenomenology (phenomenological) A philosophical tradition that focuses on describing and interpreting human experience. It is also used to indicate experience of occupation (9, 22).

Philosophy An academic discipline that studies the essence and limits of human beings, reality, knowledge, and action among other fundamental principles pertaining to existence (3).

Physical agent modalities (PAM) Treatment that uses energy in the form of heat, light, sound, cold, electricity, or mechanical devices (57).

Physical environment Natural and built nonhuman surroundings and the objects in them. The natural environment includes geographic terrain, plants, and animals as well as the sensory qualities of the natural surroundings. The built environment includes buildings, furniture, tools, and devices (OTPF-III, 42).

Physiological Pertaining to the functioning of an organ as governed by the interactions between its physical and chemical conditions (52).

Place Any environmental locus that gathers individual or group meanings, intentions, and actions spatially; a fusion of human and natural order and any significance spatial center of a person or group's lived experience; see also *Lifeworld* (22).

Planning In management, refers to process of establishing short- and long-term goals, measurable objectives, and action plans that are both congruent with the mission of the organization and consistent with the vision that current organizational leaders have established (71).

Plan of care A written document that describes the client's occupational therapy goals and how those goals will be achieved; can also be called a care plan, intervention plan, or treatment plan (40).

Play A transaction characterized by relative intrinsic motivation, relative internal control, and suspension of reality, and that is framed in such a way as to separate it from "real life" (53).

Play and leisure experience Subjective experience, personal meaning, and satisfaction with experience related to play and leisure performance (53).

Policies Written statements of direction and responsibility (40).

Political Action Committee A committee in the United States that provides fiscal support to political candidates. In the United States, the Occupational Therapy Political Action Committee (OTPAC) supports candidate with positions important to occupational therapy and its clients (71).

Polysomnography (PSG) The recording of a person's sleep using several physiologic signals such as the brain waves (electroencephalography), eye movements (electrooculography), and muscle activity (electromyography) as well as breathing, the amount of oxygen in the bloodstream, heart rate, etc.; used to evaluate patients in a sleep laboratory for potential sleep disorders (54).

Population health Health outcomes of a group of individuals, including the distribution of such outcomes within the group; an approach to health that aims to improve the health of an entire human population (52).

Populations Groups of people within a community who share common characteristics, for example, homeless persons, veterans, refugees, and people with chronic mental and/or physical disabilities (31).

Positive predictive value Indicates the likelihood that a person with a positive test result would actually have the condition for which the test is used (29).

Positive reinforcement Offering of desirable effects or consequences for a behavior with the intention of increasing the chance of that behavior being repeated in the future (48).

Posttraumatic growth Occurs when survivors find something positive in a tragedy and try to make sense of it. Personal growth may manifest as increased emotional closeness to loved ones, faith in the ability to reconstruct life, spirituality, meaning or purpose in life, and/or recognition of inner strength (68).

Postural control Controlling or regulating the body's position in space to maintain stability and orientation (57).

Postural disorder Deficits characterized by difficulty with proximal stability, low extensor muscle tone, poor prone extension, poor neck flexion against gravity, and, often, poor equilibrium (59).

Pragmatism A philosophic perspective that focuses in experience, science, and logic as the basis for knowledge; associated with the progressive movement (3).

Praxis The ability to conceptualize, plan, and execute skilled tasks. It is goal-directed motor action, supported through the processing of sensation (59).

Precautions Actions to prevent harm to an individual (40).

Precision The accuracy or confidence in the results of a measure or assessment (29).

Predictor variables Variables expected to have an effect on an outcome (35).

Predisposition to giving feedback An interpersonal characteristic that describes a person's ability to provide another with appropriate negative or positive comments about his or her reactions and experiences (37).

Preference for touch An interpersonal characteristic that describes a person's observed or expressed comfort or discomfort with or expressed reaction to any type of physical touch, whether it be a necessary part of treatment or an expression of caring (37).

Prejudice Preconceived ideas and attitudes—usually negative about a particular group of people, often without full examination of the facts (19).

Preparatory interventions Methods and tasks that prepare the client for occupational performance (OTPF-III, 30).

Press The demands of the environment (43).

Preventative strategies Actions people take to avoid negative health consequences (9).

Prevention Measures not only taken to prevent disease but also to arrest its progress and reduce its consequences once established. This also refers to injury prevention and prevention of secondary impairments (30, 67).

Private practices Work of a professional practitioner who is self-employed (62).

Problem solving mode An interpersonal mode defined by a therapist's efforts to facilitate pragmatic thinking and solve dilemmas by outlining choices, posing strategic questions, and providing opportunities for comparative or analytical thinking (37).

Procedures Written statements that describe how policies should be implemented (40).

Process skills Occupational performance skills observed as a person (a) selects, interacts with, and uses task tools and materials; (b) carries out individual actions and steps; and (c) modifies performance when problems are encountered (26).

Professional development Continuous process of acquiring new knowledge and skills that relate to one's profession (5).

Professional identity formation A socialization process that involves both the acquisition of specific knowledge and skills required for professional practice as well as the internalization of attitudes, dispositions, and self-identity that connect the individual to the larger profession (5).

Professionalism The embodiment and demonstration of characteristics that exemplify a profession and its members (39).

Professional organizations Nonprofit organizations seeking to further a profession, the interests of individuals engaged in that profession, and the public interest by building a strong community of students and practitioners that collectively contribute power in numbers (5).

Professional practice supervision Supervision of others in the same profession undertaken with an understanding of the profession's values, standards, and ethics aimed at providing support, training, and evaluation of the supervisee's professional performance (72).

Professional reasoning Process used by practitioners to plan, direct, perform, and reflect on client care; includes processes by supervisors, fieldwork educators, and occupational therapy managers as they conceptualize and manage occupational therapy practice (34).

Prognosis An estimate of the probable course and outcome of a disorder/condition (35).

Programs Systematic efforts to achieve preplanned objectives such as changes in knowledge, attitudes, skills, and behaviors to maintain or improve function and/or health (31).

Progressive era A period during the early twentieth century in the United States characterized by bold ideas, ambitious projects, life-changing inventions, and reforms that created general social optimism and confidence in the future (2).

Progress notes Any note written about a client that explains what the client did in occupational therapy (40).

Project-focused fieldwork A field-based learning experience in which the learner manages a project, such as developing new programs or resources, or evaluating an existing program, involving skill acquisition of conducting a needs assessment/analysis, proposal preparation, and development of reporting structures and time lines (69).

Propositions Formal statements about causes and effects or the nature of relationships among features of the world (41).

Prospective payment system (PPS) A method of reimbursement commonly associated in the United States with Medicare. Payment is made based on a predetermined, fixed amount; derived from the classification system of that service (e.g., diagnosis-related groups for inpatient hospital services) (74).

Proxemics The measureable distance between people as they interact (19).

Psychiatric overlay The circumstance where a client being treated for a primary illness or impairment might also have a coexisting psychiatric diagnosis or other psychosocial issue (37).

Psychosis A thought disorder in which reality testing is grossly impaired. Symptoms can include seeing, hearing, smelling, or tasting things that are not there; paranoia; and delusional thoughts (65).

Psychosocial Referring to the mind's ability to, consciously or unconsciously, adjust and relate the body to its social environment (52).

Public policy level Local, state, and federal policies, laws, and programs that regulate, support, or constrain desired occupational performance and/or participation and impact health (31).

Punishment A negative response to an undesired behavior (48).

Purposeful action Activities that have meaning for individuals and/or groups as a whole (38).

Purposeful activities Specifically selected activities that allow the client to develop skills that enhance occupational engagement (25).

p value The probability that a study effect, or a larger effect, would be found if in actuality there were no true effect or the effect was due to chance (35).

Qualitative studies A research paradigm based on the assumption that there are multiple constructed realities and that the purpose of research is to describe and analyze these realities to facilitate the understanding of the phenomena (35).

Quality of life A measure of well-being and encompasses individuals' perceptions of their position in life in the context of culture and value systems in which they live and in relation to their goals, expectations, standards, and concerns (55).

Quasi-experimental studies An intervention study in which subjects are nonrandomly assigned to the experimental treatment group or the control group (35).

Race A social construction that separates people into groups based on physical characteristics, especially skin color (19).

Racism The assessment of individual worth on the basis of real or imputed group characteristics, most notably skin color (19).

Randomized clinical trials (RCTs) An intervention study in which subjects are randomly assigned to the experimental treatment group or the control group (35).

Range of motion (ROM) Arc of motion through which a joint moves (57).

Rapid eye movement sleep (REM) The stage of sleep characterized by a period of intense brain activity often associated with dreams; named for the rapid eye movements that occur during this time. It is also called paradoxical or dreaming sleep (54).

Reading level Grade level at which one reads; academic level and reading level are often not equivalent (32).

Reasonable accommodation Any change or adjustment to a job or work environment that permits a qualified applicant or employee with a disability to participate in the job application process, to perform the essential functions or a job, or to enjoy benefits and privileges of employment equal to those enjoyed by employees without disabilities (52).

Reasonable and necessary Terms used by payers to determine if services should be covered; based on payer criteria about the likelihood of client change and importance of that change (74).

Receptive fields Region of space in which the presence of a stimulus will alter neural firing (59).

Reconstruction aides Volunteer workers recruited to help care for wounded soldiers in World War I using physical agents and curative occupations. The traditions of this approach to treatment led to the development of physical therapy, occupational therapy, and, eventually, rehabilitation medicine (2).

Recovery (in mental health) A process of change through which individuals with mental disorders and substance abuse disorders improve their health and wellness, live a self-directed life, and strive to reach their full potential (46, 65).

Reductionism A simplification and narrowing of phenomena in which the whole is understood in terms of its parts. In occupational therapy, reductionism refers to focusing intervention on the parts of the person (physical, emotional, or cognitive) or parts of the occupation rather than the whole person and related context (1, 3).

Reevaluation A systematic evaluation conducted to determine change from initial evaluation; typically performed to determine need for changes in course of intervention (27, 28).

Reference standard An existing diagnostic test that can most accurately identify the disease. The results of the assessment being studied are compared to the results of the reference standard (35).

Reflection A form of self-assessment that can be used to improve practice. Developing reflective capacity is a critical element in professional development and competence (36).

Reflective portfolio A dynamic, flexible, self-directed tool designed to document continuing professional development through thoughtful engagement with artifacts created and accumulated in pursuit to achieve professional goals and desired roles (70).

Registration A sensory pattern characterized by high thresholds and a passive self-regulation approach; bystanders do not know what they are missing (59).

Rehabilitation (rehabilitative) approach A therapeutic approach aimed at making people as independent as possible in spite of any residual impairment; includes the concepts of adaptation, compensation, and environmental modifications. This approach places an emphasis on the client's strengths as opposed to their limitations. The ultimate goal is to maximize independence despite the presence of persistent impairments (57).

Reinforcement Something that causes a behavior to be strengthened and performed again (48).

Reinforcement schedule A schedule that indicates which instances of behavior, if any, will be reinforced (48).

Related services (in schools) In a school setting, services that help a child with a disability to benefit from special education, such as those provided by occupational or physical therapy practitioners, school nurse, psychologist, or social worker or special transportation services (40, 51).

Relative mastery A person's phenomenological evaluation of the quality of his or her occupational response. This evaluation has four aspects: efficiency (use of time, energy, resources), effectiveness (the extent to which the desired goal was achieved), satisfaction to self, and satisfaction to society (44).

Relevance The degree to which a research study answers the clinical question and how well its methods fit within the constraints and resources of the practitioner's context of practice (35).

Reliability Consistency and repeatability of the outcome of administration of a test across time, parallel forms of the test, and raters. It also refers to the consistency of the internal structure of the test (29, 35).

Religion An integrated system of beliefs with their attendant practices (24).

Remediation An intervention approach designed to change client variables to establish a skill or ability that has not yet developed or to restore a skill or ability that has been impaired (30).

REM sleep behavior disorder (RBD) A sleep disorder in which one appears to physically act out vivid, often unpleasant dreams with abnormal vocal sounds and movements during REM sleep (54).

Requisite managerial authority The level of control and discretion that a manager must have to be fairly held responsible for the outcomes of work groups (71).

Response The reaction to the stimulus (48).

Response to change and challenge The ability to adapt to things that are new or challenging (37).

Response to human diversity A reaction to another based on how much the other is the same or different. These differences may occur in terms of observable sociodemographic characteristics (e.g., race, ethnicity, gender, age) or other interpretations of outward appearance or perceived worldview (37).

Rest Period of relaxing or ceasing to engage in strenuous or stressful activity (54).

Restless leg syndrome (RLS) A disorder in which there is an urge to move the legs to stop unpleasant sensations (54).

Restorative occupation Using occupations to facilitate restoring person factors and/or body functions (61).

Retrospective payment Payment made based on what was billed; contrasted with prospective payment in which payment is set in advance of intervention (74).

Rhythmic movement disorders in children Neurological disorder characterized by involuntary (however may sometimes be voluntary), repetitive movements of large muscle groups immediately before and during sleep (54).

Rituals Symbolic actions with spiritual, cultural, or social meaning contributing to the client's identity and reinforcing values and beliefs; have a strong affective component and consist of a collection of events (OTPF-III, 18).

Role(s) A set of socially agreed-on behavioral expectations, rights, and responsibilities for a specific position or status in a group or in society. These may be further conceptualized and defined by individuals enacting the role(s) (25, 38, 42).

Role-emerging supervision A form of fieldwork in which placement occurs where there is no occupational therapist on site; generally provides opportunities for students to be more autonomous and independent, promoting increased professional growth (69).

Routines A type of higher order habits that involves sequencing and combining processes, procedures, steps, or occupations and provide a structure for daily life (18).

Same-site model of fieldwork Entails students completing a Level I and Level II fieldwork experience at the same training site (69).

Satisfaction with experience Overall feelings and perceptions related to experiences (53).

Schizophrenia One of several brain diseases whose symptoms may include loss of personality (flat affect), agitation, catatonia, confusion, psychosis, unusual behavior, and withdrawal. The illness usually begins in early adulthood (65).

Screening Obtaining and reviewing data that are relevant to a potential client to determine the need for further evaluation and intervention (28, 40).

Secondary insomnia When insomnia is a result of another medical condition, a side effect of a drug, or another similar cause, it is called secondary insomnia (54).

Seeking A sensory pattern characterized by high thresholds and an active self-regulation approach; seekers want more input (59).

Segregated settings Special schools that are primarily for children with orthopedic and neurological impairments (51).

Self-awareness Includes lack of knowledge about one's own cognitive-perceptual limitations and/or his or her functional implications as well as deficiencies in metacognitive skills (58).

Self-efficacy Confidence in one's ability to take action (47).

Self-initiated action Individual takes initiative verbally or nonverbally (38).

Self-regulation The individual's ability to alter behavior to match environmental demand; in relationship to sensory integration and processing, this involves intake, integration, and processing of sensation and using it as a foundation for appropriate environmental interaction (59).

Sensitivity The predictor test's ability to obtain a positive test when the condition really exists (a true positive) (29).

Sensitivity (sensory) A sensory pattern characterized by low thresholds and a passive self-regulation approach; sensors are particular about their input (59).

Sensitization Progressive increases in response to a stimulus with repeated exposure (59).

Sensory integration Clinic-based, play-focused intervention that uses sensory-enhanced interactions to elicit child adaptive responses (59).

Sensory modulation The ability to regulate and organize reactions to sensory input in a graded and adaptive manner; the balancing of excitatory and inhibitory inputs and adapting to environmental changes (59).

Sensory processing The way a person makes meaning of the sensory input (59).

Sensory registration Detection of sensory information by the central nervous system (59).

Sensory-related affordances The sensory possibilities or qualities of things in the environment and of the environment itself (59).

Serious mental illness (psychiatric disability) (SMI) A diagnosable mental disorder found in persons aged 18 years and older that is so long lasting and severe that it seriously interferes with a person's ability to take part in major life activities (65).

Service competency The specific knowledge, skills, and attitudes to perform at an expected level that matches the requirements of the area of practice or service (73).

Service coordinators In educational settings, the person responsible for managing a student's IFSP or IEP (40).

Service learning Learning experiences, based on a community-identified need, that tend to be aligned with academic course objectives. Learning activities can involve more than one visit and may evolve during a semester or at multiple points across a curriculum in a programmatic approach (69).

Setting Describes those aspects of the context or arena to which the person attends (25).

Shaping A strategy to develop closer and closer approximations of behavior (48, 57).

Sheltered workshops Noncompetitive employment settings intended to provide many of the positive benefits of a work atmosphere for individuals with disabilities (52).

Shift work A general term to describe a job that requires an individual to work other than the standard working hours of midmorning to late afternoon, Monday through Friday. For instance, shift work may involve working from midnight until 7:00 a.m. (54).

Single subject (*n* of 1) studies An intervention study in which a single subject is the total population of the study (35).

Situated activities This concept calls for the study of activities in the real-life contexts and examination of the practices of social institutions where activities occur naturally. To understand situated activities, the practitioner pays special attention to the innovative solutions that unfold as the activities are carried out in that particular context (7).

Skilled nursing facility (SNF) A hospital unit, nursing home, or distinct part of a nursing home that provides skilled nursing care, medical treatments, and rehabilitation services (62).

Skills (skilled) Observable, goal-directed actions that a person uses while performing (42, 74).

Sleep debt An individual's accumulated sleep loss from insufficient sleep, regardless of cause (54).

Sleep diary Self-report system for tracking sleep time and restorative experience (54).

Sleep disordered breathing (SDB) Describes a group of disorders characterized by abnormalities of respiratory pattern (pauses in breathing) or the quantity of ventilation during sleep (54).

Sleep hygiene Habits, environmental factors, and practices that may influence the length and quality of one's sleep (54).

Sleep inertia Period after awakening before full alertness (54).

Sleep latency Period awake in bed before falling asleep (54).

Sleep-wake homeostasis Regulated balance between sleep and waking (54).

Slow wave sleep (SWS) Often referred to as deep sleep, consists of stages 3 and 4 of NREM sleep (54).

Smart house (smart house technology) Dwelling design using computer technologies to incorporate robotics, networked appliances, and other digital devices connecting residents with their home and wider community; the house is "smart" in the sense that it can respond, through digital directives, to the residents' everyday needs in terms of lighting, thermal comfort, security, and so forth; see also *Domotics* (22, 33).

SOAP note A type of progress note written in a standard format of subjective, objective, assessment, and plan so that specific information is easy to find (40).

Social environment Particular social features (i.e., social groups and occupational tasks) of the specific context in which one does something that impacts on what one does and how it is done (42).

Social health Having a standard of living adequate for health and well-being, with equal rights to work, to free choice of employment; to rest, leisure, and holidays; to participate in the cultural life of a community; to the arts and scientific advancement; to take part in national governments; and to education directed to the full development of the human personality (45).

Social inequality Unequal rewards and opportunities that accrue to different individuals and groups, particularly rewards and opportunities that are judged to be unfair, unjust, avoidable, and unnecessary; often linked to unequal distribution of economic assets and power within a society (20).

Social interaction skills Occupational performance skills observed during the ongoing stream of a social exchange (26).

Social justice Ethical distribution and sharing of resources, rights, and responsibilities between people recognizing their equal worth as citizens (45).

Social media Internet-based tools that enable one to communicate quickly and to a very wide audience (39).

Social mobility The degree to which, in a given society, an individual's social status can change throughout the life course or the degree to which that individual's offspring and subsequent generations move up and down the class system (20).

Social participation Involvement in a subset of activities that involve social interactions with others and that support social interdependence; organized patterns of behavior that are characteristic and expected of an individual or a given position within a social system and encompasses the individual's engagement with family, peers and friends, and community members (55).

Social structures Distinctive, stable arrangements of institutions whereby human beings in a society interact and live together (33).

Social supports Support systems that provide assistance and encouragement to individuals with physical or emotional disabilities in order that they may better cope. Informal social support is usually provided by friends, relatives, or peers, whereas formal assistance is provided by churches, groups, etc. (33).

Socioeconomic status (SES) Status- or prestige-based measure of place in the social hierarchy; measurement of SES includes occupational attainment, education, and income (20).

Somatodyspraxia A relatively severe form of sensory integrative–based dyspraxia characterized by difficulty with both easy (feedback dependent) and more difficult (feed forward dependent) motor tasks; thought to be based on poor processing of tactile and likely vestibular and proprioceptive sensations (59).

Spatial neglect A condition in which, after damage to one hemisphere of the brain (usually right) is sustained, a deficit in attention to and awareness of the opposite side (usually left) of space is observed (58).

Spatial summation Involves activating several receptors and summing the excitation from each to produce a response (59).

Special education Educational services that are designed to help a child with a disability learn in a way that is consistent with that child's unique needs (40).

Specificity The predictor test's ability to obtain a negative result when the condition is really absent (a true negative) (29).

Spirituality A deep experience of meaning brought about by engaging in occupations that involve the enacting of personal values and beliefs, reflection, and intention within a supportive contextual environment (24).

Spontaneous action Action occurs in the here and now (38).

Spontaneous recovery Reemergence of a previously extinguished conditioned response after a delay (48).

Stage theory Assumes that there are discontinuous, qualitative shifts that reflect a transition from one stage into the next stage in a predictable manner. The focus is on different organizational or structural change over age-related phases such as infancy, early adulthood, and late adulthood. Classic theorists include Erikson, Kohlberg, and Piaget who provide descriptions of distinctly different psychosocial issues, moral reasoning, and cognition (7).

Standardized assessments Measurement instrument that has been developed in a rigorous, scientific manner for a defined construct and population with a prescribed process of administration and scoring and with demonstrated psychometric properties (29, 50).

Standard setting A professional association's role and methodology for defining levels of achievement (5).

Statement of work (SOW) Formal summary of work to be done by a contractor (such as a consultant), typically signed by both parties (73).

State professional associations Nonprofit organizations in the United States that seek to further a profession, the interests of individuals engaged in that profession, and the public interest by building a strong community of students and practitioners that collectively contribute power in numbers (5).

Stereotyping Preconceived ideas and attitudes, usually negative, about a particular group of people, often without full examination of the facts (19).

Stimulus Something that prompts a behavior (48).

Stimulus discrimination learning A procedure by which an individual can learn to emit a behavior under certain conditions instead of others (48).

Stimulus generalization Occurs when a behavior becomes more probable in the presence of one stimulus as a result of being reinforced in the presence of another similar stimulus (48).

Strategic planning The process of ensuring that an organization's current purpose, aspirations, goals, activities, and strategies connect to plans and support its mission (71).

Strengthening A variety of techniques aimed at increasing the amount of force a muscle can produce (57).

Structuralism Philosophical inquiry focused on understanding the elements that comprise a phenomenon or system (3).

Subjective experience (subjectively experienced) State of mind with which activities are approached and the affective experience of engaging in them (23, 53).

Substrates of occupation The human capacities required for engagement in an occupation (9).

Successful aging Moving through late life in a way that enables participation in valued activities and sustains life satisfaction (67).

Summative Evaluation or feedback desired to summarize current skills or related current skills to set criteria (69).

Sundowning Increased confusion or disorientation that occurs at the end of the day; typically seen in people with Alzheimer disease or other dementias (58).

Supervision The process of guiding individuals or an organization through the authoritative control of others authorized by the governing body of the organization (71, 72).

Supported education An emerging best practice to help individuals with major mental disorders succeed in higher education. Participants receive the education and training they need to achieve their learning and recovery goals and become gainfully employed in the job or career of their choice (65).

Supported employment An evidence-based approach that helps people with mental disorders to attain and succeed in competitive jobs (65).

Suprachiasmic nucleus (SCN) Also referred to as circadian clock, circadian pacemaker, or internal biological clock. The internal circadian pacemaker is a small group of nerve cells located in the hypothalamus that controls the circadian cycles and influences many physiological and behavioral rhythms occurring over a 24-hour period, including the sleep/wake cycle (54).

Suspension of reality In the context of play: being free of unnecessary constraints of reality; the individual determines the degree to which a transaction resembles objective reality (53).

Sympathetic nervous system Part of the autonomic nervous system. The sympathetic nervous system activates what is often termed the "fight-or-flight response." Like other parts of the nervous system, the sympathetic nervous system operates through a series of interconnected neurons (59).

Synaptic activity Transfer of information from one cell to another at a synapse; facilitated if the firing of the presynaptic cell increases the likelihood that the postsynaptic cell with reach threshold and fire an action potential (excitatory synapse) or inhibited if the firing of the presynaptic cell reduces the likelihood of the post-synaptic cell firing (inhibitory synapse) (59).

Synaptic function Entails the transfer of information from one cell (presynaptic neuron) to another (postsynaptic neuron) at the synaptic cleft; commonly referred to as synaptic transmission (59).

Systematic review A literature review pertinent to a specific question that aims at identifying, appraising, and synthesizing all the research evidence relevant to that question (35).

Systems approach Views the properties of the "whole," or system, as arising from interactions and relationships among the parts (52).

Tacit Implicit or based on information or experiences that we cannot easily put into language (41).

Tactile defensiveness A sensory integrative dysfunction in which the tactile sensations cause excessive emotional reactions, hyperactivity, or other behavioral problems (59).

Task analysis An analytical analysis intended for purposes of identifying what environmental, task-related, person-related (i.e., person factors and body functions), and/or societal and cultural factors may have been the reason for a person's diminished quality of occupational performance; most often based on professional reasoning and speculation following the occupational therapist's observation of the person's task performance (26).

Task-oriented approaches Includes a wide range of interventions such as treadmill training, walking training on the ground, bicycling programs, endurance training and circuit training, sit-to-stand exercises, and reaching tasks for improving balance. In addition, use is made of arm training using functional tasks such as grasping objects, CI therapy, and mental imagery. Such training is task and patient focused and not therapist focused (57).

Taxonomies Broad classifications; a way to group things together (4).

Teamwork When more than one health care provider collaborates on the care of the client (39).

Telehealth The application of evaluative, consultative, preventative, and therapeutic services delivered through telecommunication and information technologies (74).

Telesupervision Clinical supervision provided with communication technology and includes the use of videoconferencing, telephone, e-mails, chats, podcasts, or the use of social networks (72).

Temporal Denoting time (9).

Temporal summation Occurs when a stimulus of limited strength is repeated in quick succession, such that the strength of the second stimulus is "added to" the strength of the first stimulus, and so forth, until threshold is reached and the signal is sent forward (59).

Temporarily able-bodied individuals (TABs) The potentially temporary status of able bodied-ness,

because everyone is only one concussion, car accident, or disabling illness away from falling into disability (21).

Therapeutic mode A specific way of relating to a client (37).

Therapeutic reasoning Term used to characterize theory-based reasoning associated with the occupational therapy process; see also *Clinical reasoning* and *Professional reasoning* (34).

Therapeutic relationship Client–therapist interactions (37).

Therapeutic use of self Planned use of practitioner's personality, insights, perceptions, and judgments as part of the therapeutic process (30, 37).

Therapy cap A limit for the payment of therapy services for Medicare Part B of an established monetary amount per year, which began in 1997 and was eliminated in 2018 (74).

Third-party payer Private company or government agency that provides payment for medical expenses (50).

Time-space routines Sets of more or less habitual bodily actions extending through a considerable portion of time, for example, a getting-up routine, a going-to-the-gym routine, or a going-to-church-and-lunch routine; see also *Body-subject* and *Body routines* (22).

Tort law limits The parameters a court can award for a wrongful act or injury. These usually fluctuate based on state law and severity of the type of injury or act (73).

Toxic stress Term used to describe the kinds of experiences, particularly in childhood, that can affect brain architecture and brain chemistry; typically experiences that are bad for an individual during development such as severe abuse (20).

Transactional perspective of occupations Offered as an alternative to individualism that presumes the person is separate from life situations; a transactional way of thinking sees interrelated elements where occupations forms relationships between the person and life situations. This idea is compatible with contextualism (7).

Transactional process Where people, the physical space, time, and objects interconnect to form a functional whole (7).

Transdisciplinary team Individuals representing different professional disciplines whose role-related functions become interchangeable (39).

Transduction With respect to neural activity, the process of changing stimulus energy into a coded action potential that can be propagated and interpreted by the central nervous system (59).

Transitional portfolio A dynamic, flexible, and reflective tool for one to self-direct and document professional development through thoughtful engagement with artifacts created and accumulated during one's career in relationship to professional goals and desired roles (70).

Transitional work Process performed at the client's actual job location and uses the client's job duties to assist in a safe gradual return to work process (52).

Transition planning The education and rehabilitation team prepare the student to leave the school setting and enter into employment and community living (52).

Translational science Theory-driven research focused on developing practical applications that resolve peoples' real-world needs (9).

Trauma-informed care Assessment and intervention services that include attention to the impact of trauma on client lives, designed to minimize trauma and avoid retraumatization (68).

Treatment group (intervention group) In experimental research, it is the group that receives the treatment or intervention being tested (35).

Unidimensionality The determination of whether an assessment measures a single trait (29).

Universal design (UD) Also called "inclusive design" and "life-span design"; design of environments and products to be usable by all people to the greatest extent possible without the need for special arrangements or adaptations; intended to simplify life for everyone by making products, communications, and the built environment more usable by as many people as possible at little or no extra cost (22, 33).

Universal housing Dwellings, housing, and neighborhoods that address the needs of all users, whatever their age or ability (22).

Validation study A second study, using either a subset of data or collecting new data, which is used to confirm the results of a previous study. This term is most often used with prognostic studies (35).

Validity The degree to which a measurement tool measures what it is supposed to measure (accuracy) (35).

Value-based care As a component of a larger strategy to reform health care delivery and payment, the Centers for Medicare & Medicaid rewards providers for quality versus quantity of care, adherence to best practices, and the patient's experience of care (74).

Values Principles, standards, or qualities considered worthwhile by the client who holds them (OTPF-III, 24, 42).

Vestibular-based bilateral integration and sequencing disorder A sensory integrative dysfunction characterized by shortened duration nystagmus, poor integration of the two sides of the body and brain, and difficulty in learning to read or compute (59).

Vision (vision statement) in management An aspirational statement about what a department or organization would like to become as it seeks to fulfill its mission (5, 71).

Visual perceptual (perception) Cognitive process of obtaining and interpreting visual information from the environment; involves the reception, organization, and assimilation of visual information (58).

Vocational rehabilitation A multiprofessional evidence-based approach that is provided in different settings, services, and activities to working age individuals with health-related impairments, limitations, or restrictions with work functioning and whose primary aim is to optimize work participation (52).

Volition Pattern of thoughts and feelings about oneself as an actor in one's world that occurs as one anticipates, chooses, experiences, and interprets what one does (42).

Wake after sleep onset (WASO) The time spent awake from sleep onset to final awakening (54).

Well-being Implies that basic survival needs are met and encompasses ideas such as health, happiness, and prosperity (8).

Wellness The individual's perception of and responsibility for psychological and physical well-being as these contribute to overall satisfaction with one's life situation. It is also the outcome of health promotion (47, 52, 67).

Work Exertion or effort directed to produce or accomplish something (52).

Work conditioning Intervention that emphasizes physical conditioning and addresses issues of strength, endurance, flexibility, motor control, and cardiopulmonary function (52).

Work engagement Performance of work participation occupations in which the activities are a "result of choice, motivation, and meaning within a supportive context and environment" (52).

Workers' compensation State programs that address multiple needs of people who are ill/injured because of work (74).

Work hardening A highly structured, goal-oriented, individualized treatment program designed to maximize the individual's ability to return to work (52).

Working memory Involves holding information in mind and mentally working with it (i.e., working with information no longer perceptually present) (58).

Working poor People who maintain full-time jobs but remain in relative poverty according to government-established poverty standards; may have negative net worth and lack the ability to escape their situations (20).

Work integration program A program designed to coordinate the clinical features of the injured worker into the organizational and ergonomic aspects of the system (52).

Work participation Describes involvement in situations and activities that explore, support, or engage in work (52).

Worldview Cognitive, perceptual, and affective maps developed throughout a lifetime through socialization, which are used to make sense of the social landscape and develop goals (9).

INDEX

Page numbers followed by *f* denote figures, those followed by *t* denote tables, and those followed by *b* denote boxes.